HANDBOOK OF PHYSIOLOGY

SECTION 1: The Nervous System, VOLUME II, PART 1

PUBLICATIONS COMMITTEE

HOWARD E. MORGAN, *Chairman*
ROBERT M. BERNE
LEON E. FARHI

Nancy A. Winchester, Cay Butler,
Catherine B. Carlston, Mary L. Crabill,
Marcia G. Lawson, Susie P. Mann,
Barbara E. Patterson, *Editorial Staff*

Brenda B. Rauner, *Production Manager*

Constantine J. Gillespie, *Indexer*

HANDBOOK OF PHYSIOLOGY

A critical, comprehensive presentation of physiological knowledge and concepts

SECTION 1: # The Nervous System

Formerly SECTION 1: Neurophysiology

VOLUME II.
Motor Control, Part 1

Section Editors: JOHN M. BROOKHART
VERNON B. MOUNTCASTLE

Volume Editor: VERNON B. BROOKS

Executive Editor: STEPHEN R. GEIGER

American Physiological Society, BETHESDA, MARYLAND, 1981

© *Copyright 1959 (Volume I), American Physiological Society*
© *Copyright 1960 (Volume II), American Physiological Society*
© *Copyright 1960 (Volume III), American Physiological Society*

© *Copyright 1981, American Physiological Society*

Library of Congress Catalog Card Number 78–315957

International Standard Book Number 0-683-01105-7

Printed in the United States of America by Waverly Press, Inc., Baltimore, Maryland 21202

Distributed by The Williams & Wilkins Company, Baltimore, Maryland 21202

Preface

Motor Control presents a systematic interdisciplinary view of the control of posture and movement. This volume assesses current understanding of the neural control of motor actions and the directions in which this rapidly expanding field is moving. Each chapter sets the concepts, facts, and methods of current research against the essentials of their background. Much effort has been made by the authors to bridge physiology, anatomy, the behavioral sciences, control theory, and related areas. The relevance of motor control to human performance is kept in view throughout. *Motor Control* is a natural follow-up to the first volume of *The Nervous System, Cellular Biology of Neurons*, which concluded with selected examples of sensorimotor integration.

In the first edition of the *Handbook of Physiology* (*Neurophysiology*, 1959–1960), the search for an understanding of motor actions concentrated on motor control by various parts of the brain. The three volumes of *Neurophysiology* barely approached multidisciplinary coordination let alone integration. Spinal motor mechanisms were considered in separate volumes from central regulatory mechanisms; skilled motor patterns were even further removed in an additional volume dealing with higher functions. The separation of these topics reflects the distances between separate lines of research as practiced twenty years ago. Since that time, questions and methods have come to focus on common problems.

The overall theme of this volume is the current emphasis on how the individual deals with its environment, which dictates the dimensions of motor efforts and hence of their controls. This topic has generated numerous questions. For instance, what are the controlled variables in different circumstances, and how are the contributions of diverse neurons encoded? How is intent translated into action by preset programs and ongoing controls with optimal use of the available information and of the neurons processing it? Enormous strides have been made in the last twenty years to relate structure to function, observations to theory, and "unknowing" neurons to a "purposive" brain and to heuristic performance. It would be too much to expect all these aspects to have fused in so short a time. The promise and the approaches, however, are clear in *Motor Control*. The volume begins with introductory comments by Granit, who traces the history of the quest to define neural mechanisms of motor control.

Topics in this volume are grouped to take the reader on a journey that begins with peripheral conditions and events, moves inward through automatic, unconscious adjustments, proceeds on to voluntary, conscious adjustments, and ends with an analysis of behavioral motor performance. *Motor Control* is divided into sections only for convenience: there are no real boundaries in the continuum of exciting and authoritative accounts. If an anatomical orientation remains in the sequence, it is because many neuroscientists still labor to unravel the functional mysteries of the components of a "computer" that arrived without explanations for either hardware or software.

Important advances have been made in understanding how the peripheral machinery of *bones* and *muscles* is fitted to behavioral use. This is the first area of consideration, and the actions of various kinds of joints and the properties of the muscles that move them are examined. The growing array of synaptic *transmitters* and new modulators is considered next. This account provides important detail for subsequent chapters on central processing, particularly regarding mechanisms that could change central "states" of responsiveness. Use of motor protheses that can assist the nervous system in directing nonfunctional limbs or their artificial replacements is an emerging topic of increasing practicality and completes the first section. Common threads woven through these chapters by Alexander, Partridge and Benton, Krnjević, and Mortimer are the ranges of time and intensity of peripheral actions imposed on parts of the nervous system that drive or are driven by them.

Far-reaching conceptual changes have occurred in ideas on the formerly undoubted hierarchical arrangement of the nervous system. Twenty years ago, low-level reflexes could easily be distinguished from high-level voluntary efforts. Such ease vanished with the unfolding scope of supraspinal controls on inputs and outputs of spinal motor centers, whose processed information is now known to travel both up and down the neuraxis. This is reflected in the section on *reflexes, neural organization, and control systems*. The messages forwarded by muscle spindles and their central control are reconsidered as a functional entity, with reassessments of muscular and neural contributions to posture and movement. The reasoning behind control systems is applied systematically to information that is fed back or fed forward to determine the controlled variables. These chapters by Matthews, Rack, and Houk and Rymer are followed by an analysis by Stein and Lee of the many causes of tremors, which are potentially important for diagnosis and treatment.

New fundamental insights into *spinal integration* have emerged from extensive studies of the functional organization of motoneurons that innervate muscle fibers having different mechanical and biochemical properties. The confirmation that motoneurons can be recruited in the same order for voluntary as for reflex movements has important implications for the whole spectrum of motor management, from delegation of repetitive locomotion to concentration on making intended movements. Two aspects of supraspinal influences stand out: *1*) descending pathways can reach interneurons that link muscles into functional units acting on joints, and *2*) these controls are overlaid on, and therefore can use, the segmental arrangements for governing motoneuron excitability. These subjects are considered in the chapters by Burke, Henneman and Mendell, and Baldissera, Hultborn, and Illert. Their reviews are based on findings obtained with diverse methods, including such new ones as statistical correlation between firing probabilities of motoneurons and muscle fibers, histochemical demonstrations of metabolic capabilities, and unit recording from decerebrate animals walking on a treadmill.

We are gaining assurance from the intense investigations of the roles of *descending control pathways* conducted during the past two decades. The inputs of these pathways have been detailed and correlated with their outputs on both motoneurons and interneurons, as related by Kuypers, Wilson and Peterson, and Asanuma. Behavioral tests of trained animals, single-unit recording, and cortical microstimulation have replaced or amended deductions reached through older methods—for example, performance after lesions in (mostly) acute preparations. Pathways originating in cortex and brain stem have been traced by a plethora of new anatomical techniques and by the effects of lesions in behaviorally trained animals. Comparative phylogenetic studies of the changing role of the corticospinal system, for instance, have pinpointed fine adjustments of the fingers. Vestibulo- and reticulospinal systems have been analyzed with respect to coordination of the head, neck, limb, and trunk, plotting out their excitatory and inhibitory effects. Input-output relations of the pyramidal tract have been examined in relation to afferent and efferent zones of cortical neurons, as established by adequate stimulation of peripheral receptors and by electrical microstimulation of motor cortex. Descending pathways may participate to varying degrees in motor functions, but none ever work in isolation. They reach spinal neurons through fairly direct lines, through less direct ones conveying reprocessed information from cerebellum and basal ganglia, and through the least direct routes that descend from cerebral cortex after having reentered from cerebellum and basal ganglia. The next two sections are structured accordingly.

Important realizations have accumulated about how the *cerebellum and basal ganglia* start, manage, and stop movements properly. How do they reprocess and redirect information? Neither one nor the other subcortical center can be considered as a functional entity without the circuits to which it is linked. Outstanding recognitions have been that the supplementary motor cortex regulates transfer of higher information for subcortical processing, that sensory input reaches cerebellum but not basal ganglia, and that the cerebellum is linked more closely to muscle action than are basal ganglia. There are many new facts but little agreement on the cellular or integrative functions of these centers in learning, programming, or executing movements. Cerebellar afferent systems have been reexamined according to their modes of termination as mossy or climbing fibers and as the new aminergic system, with consideration of their functional roles. Microphysiology of cerebellar cortex and nuclei have been studied increasingly with intracellular recording in excised tissue slices, revealing a role of calcium ions in governing responsiveness in, for example, Purkinje cells and inferior olivary neurons. Overall cerebellar regulatory and triggering functions in posture and movement, both programmed and otherwise, have received much attention. Methods such as unit recording and the effects of reversible and permanent lesions have been studied in behaviorally trained animals. These matters are reviewed by Bloedel and Courville, Llinás, and Brooks and Thach. Striatal and brain stem integrating systems are reviewed by Carpenter and by Kitai, leading from anatomical demonstrations of orderly corticofugal projections to electrophysiological studies of the time frame and of the inhibitory outputs of these systems. The section concludes with a chapter by DeLong and Georgopoulos that gives an overview of motor functions of the basal ganglia and highlights unit recording in behaviorally trained animals, which separates motor functions of the putamen from cognitive ones of the caudate nucleus.

Exciting new perspectives have been gained about how higher control becomes transmuted into motor language in motor cortex; that has been studied most intensively. Integration of inputs from the periphery, cerebellum, basal ganglia, and cerebral cortex has been found to be processed repeatedly, in different ways, in these reentrant circuits and even in individual neurons. Conversely a particular aspect of sensorimotor integration may be embodied in nearly simultaneous activities of many neurons located in different parts of the brain. These revolutionary suggestions of distributed function imply that different parts of the brain are unlikely to serve the production of only one kind of movement. The section on *cerebral control mechanisms* consists of four chapters, beginning with a review by Porter of the internal organization of motor cortex. This lays a base for future circuit solving by emphasizing laminar and radial arrangements. The motor cortex, reviewed by Evarts, has been the main focus for many new integrative approaches. Study of neurons that have been identified antidromically and/or orthodromically in behaviorally trained animals has yielded functional quantitative relations, such as to application of muscular force or to other motor characteristics. Processed information from muscle receptors has been detected in precentral discharge. Uses of this are examined in terms of α-γ-coactivation with possible cerebellar participation. The roles of newly discovered multiple representations of the body in sensory and motor cortices have been investigated in relation to task-related input processing. The dynamic properties of precentral neurons have led to consideration of their participation in centrally programmed movements. Secondary motor areas are reviewed by Wiesendanger, and the prefrontal cortex is treated by Fuster. Anatomical and physiological evidence has shown that these cortical areas lack tight relationships with the spinal motor apparatus. The supplementary motor cortex is a way station to motor cortex from prefrontal cortex, which is furthest removed from motor linkage. Dorsolateral prefrontal cortex, however, emerges as essential for orderly execution, perhaps through basal ganglia and cerebellum.

It is becoming clear how automatic and voluntary controls can cooperate through the study of *rhythmical movements and their voluntary engagement*. Central pattern generators for locomotion have been discovered in many vertebrates, and Grillner reviews their properties in detail and examines how they can be accessed by peripheral feedback and voluntary control. Mastication and voluntary biting are considered by Luschei and Goldberg in relation to neural mechanisms of mandibular control. *Visuomotor control* is another topic that illustrates the relation between involuntary and voluntary control. It is introduced in a chapter by Robinson on the control of eye movements and in one by Bizzi on eye-head coordination. Robinson systematically presents theory and findings on saccadic, pursuit, and vergence systems, and Bizzi compares the physiology for coordinated tracking and anticipatory and "triggered" movements. Both chapters consider long-lasting changes brought about by learning or lesions. Bizzi relates the monkey's performance after deafferentation to learning and to the structure of motor programs.

New vistas have been opened by studies of *behavioral motor performance* in conjuction with physiological experiments. Studies of human manual control have generated models of behavior that are reviewed by Poulton, who combines development of theories with practical advice about evaluation and avoidance of systematic errors. Another approach to behavioral analysis is based on information processing, the limits of which are explored by Keele with detailed comparisons of human and animal motor behavior under controlled conditions. Motor commands and perception are considered by McCloskey from the point of view of corollary discharges. He examines trunk, limb, and eye-head coordination, stressing experiments with muscle vibration. *Motor Control* concludes with a conceptual analysis by Arbib of perceptual structures and distributed motor control. Arbib emphasizes visuomotor coordination and the structure of motor programs and concludes by relating concepts of physiology and computer science. The volume thus ends appropriately with a development begun by von Neumann's milestone Theory of Automata, which stemmed from the now classic assertion by McCulloch and Pitts that the brain is a computing machine made of neurons.

It has been a pleasurable adventure to fashion and edit *Motor Control*. All authors have been very helpful, particularly in cooperating with mutual and external peer reviews. I wish to thank the Section Editors, Vernon B. Mountcastle and John M. Brookhart, who encouraged me in the planning of this volume and advised me throughout two years of intensive work.

VERNON B. BROOKS
Volume Editor

Contents

Part 1

1. Comments on history of motor control
   RAGNAR GRANIT 1

Bones, Muscles, and Transmitters

2. Mechanics of skeleton and tendons
   R. MCNEILL ALEXANDER 17
3. Muscle, the motor
   L. D. PARTRIDGE
   L. A. BENTON 43
4. Transmitters in motor systems
   K. KRNJEVIĆ 107
5. Motor prostheses
   J. THOMAS MORTIMER 155

Reflexes, Neural Organization, and Control Systems

6. Muscle spindles: their messages and their fusimotor supply
   PETER B. C. MATTHEWS 189
7. Limitations of somatosensory feedback in control of posture and movement
   PETER M. H. RACK 229
8. Neural control of muscle length and tension
   JAMES C. HOUK
   W. ZEV RYMER 257
9. Tremor and clonus
   RICHARD B. STEIN
   ROBERT G. LEE 325
10. Motor units: anatomy, physiology, and functional organization
    R. E. BURKE 345
11. Functional organization of motoneuron pool and its inputs
    ELWOOD HENNEMAN
    LORNE M. MENDELL 423

12. Integration in spinal neuronal systems
    FAUSTO BALDISSERA
    HANS HULTBORN
    MICHAEL ILLERT 509

Descending Control Pathways

13. Anatomy of the descending pathways
    H. G. J. M. KUYPERS 597
14. Vestibulospinal and reticulospinal systems
    VICTOR J. WILSON
    BARRY W. PETERSON 667
15. The pyramidal tract
    HIROSHI ASANUMA 703

Index xi

Part 2

Cerebellum and Basal Ganglia

16. Cerebellar afferent systems
    JAMES R. BLOEDEL
    JACQUES COURVILLE 735
17. Electrophysiology of the cerebellar networks
    RODOLFO LLINÁS 831
18. Cerebellar control of posture and movement
    VERNON B. BROOKS
    W. THOMAS THACH 877
19. Anatomy of the corpus striatum and brain stem integrating systems
    MALCOLM B. CARPENTER 947
20. Electrophysiology of the corpus striatum and brain stem integrating systems
    S. T. KITAI 997

21. Motor functions of the basal ganglia
   MAHLON DELONG
   APOSTOLOS P. GEORGOPOULOS 1017

Cerebral Control Mechanisms

22. Internal organization of the motor cortex for input-output arrangements
   R. PORTER 1063
23. Role of motor cortex in voluntary movements in primates
   EDWARD V. EVARTS 1083
24. Organization of secondary motor areas of cerebral cortex
   MARIO WIESENDANGER 1121
25. Prefrontal cortex in motor control
   JOAQUIN M. FUSTER 1149

Rhythmical Movements and Their Voluntary Engagement

26. Control of locomotion in bipeds, tetrapods, and fish
   STEN GRILLNER 1179

27. Neural mechanisms of mandibular control: mastication and voluntary biting
   ERICH S. LUSCHEI
   LOUIS J. GOLDBERG 1237

Visuomotor Control

28. Control of eye movements
   DAVID A. ROBINSON 1275
29. Eye-head coordination
   EMILIO BIZZI 1321

Behavioral Motor Performance

30. Human manual control
   E. C. POULTON 1337
31. Behavioral analysis of movement
   STEVEN W. KEELE 1391
32. Corollary discharges: motor commands and perception
   D. I. MCCLOSKEY 1415
33. Perceptual structures and distributed motor control
   MICHAEL A. ARBIB 1449

Index xi

CHAPTER 1

Comments on history of motor control

RAGNAR GRANIT | *Nobel Institute for Neurophysiology, Karolinska Institutet, Stockholm, Sweden*

CHAPTER CONTENTS

Early Attempts at Quantifying Control Functions
Reflex Origin of Basic Ideas on Motor Control
Early Influence of Electronics: Microelectrodes
Intracellular Approach
Back to Muscular End Organs
Impact of Cybernetics on Motor Physiology
Feedback Problems in Motor Control
Advent of Stereotaxis: Subcortical Motor Centers
Stretch Reflex in Motor Control
Comments on Cortical Localization
Reorientation in Concepts and Interests

INASMUCH AS THIS CHAPTER is devoted to the history of research on motor control, it is centered on the period from the 1920s onwards. This was my own time of acquiring the knowledge necessary for offering a bird's-eye view of what to me seemed exciting and important. In some cases a glance is thrown backwards to indicate how a particular line of advance started. A very limited number of special papers are mentioned, as the theme is far too expansive for detailed references. Moreover, the subject presents a changing pattern of problems, hypotheses, and techniques, all of which for a time have yielded a rich crop of papers. Most of these have not pretended to do more than to illuminate one particular aspect that at the moment seemed highly relevant. It is assumed that such papers generally have served both current needs for clarity and have kept up an interest in the field. Some of the more decisive contributions are pointed out in the text. My original intention had been to go far back searching for the roots of a history of motor control. This lost much of its attraction, however, when so much of the old experimental work was found to have been carried out with techniques that were insufficient for dealing with the issues at stake.

As a concept "control" implies a considerable degree of precision and not merely the discovery of an active site capable of eliciting a movement. For example, this side of the turn of the century the Einthoven string galvanometer made electromyography an enticing proposition. The interference pictures that were obtained led to disputes over the frequencies of the basic rhythms of the oscillations observed. There were Piper rhythms and Dusser de Barenne-Buytendijk vibrations, and the interpretations of the recorded frequencies varied, as was well reviewed by Fulton (53). This controversy lasted until 1929 when Denny-Brown (32) showed that it actually was possible to record from single motor units with the string galvanometer. At that time single-fiber records had already been provided by Adrian and Zotterman (6) using frog muscular afferents and amplification, and in that same year Adrian and Bronk (5) invented the needle electrode and applied it to investigations on the reflex discharge of motoneurons. Before those results on naturally active cat motoneurons were published, the three most important contributions of electromyography were that it *1*) showed up inhibitions, *2*) facilitated precise timing, and *3*) confirmed the notion that motor innervation is based on rhythmic activity. Paul Hoffmann (82) had described the silent period (his Hemmungsreflex), and in 1923 von Kries (103) had declared rhythmic innervation of skeletal muscles a certainty.

While amplification came to the rescue of electromyographers, a less fortunate end, oblivion, was in store for the papers maintaining that tonus was a function of the autonomous nervous system. A good orientation is given by de Boer (14) who defended this theory in a paper with 178 references beginning with Brondgeest (20) in 1860 whose evidence really was in favor of the still prevailing concept that tonus is a postural reflex while autonomic control of muscular activity is exerted on the blood vessels. In 1866 Vulpian (176) had stated that muscular tone is a reflex act, and Sherrington never faltered in his adherence to the same view.

These two approaches to control problems were contemporary with Sherrington's (163) farsighted use of the reflex to analyze the nature of synaptic interaction. In the end Sherrington also added electromyography to his tools of analysis, but essentially his results were obtained with myography. Isotonic and isometric muscular contractions were old concepts developed by Adolf Fick (44) in 1882. The torsion-wire, isometric myograph, which in the end rendered

Sherrington's results on spinal mechanisms of control to be quantitative, was his own invention.

EARLY ATTEMPTS AT QUANTIFYING
CONTROL FUNCTIONS

As a scientific term, "motor control" implies knowledge of what is being controlled, how the process is organized, and what purpose it serves. Given this definition, the physiology of motor control is a very late arrival to the laboratories of the world. In a general way it was understood from the beginning of physiology that we are capable of anticipatorily adjusting our commands to the motoneurons in proportion to the requirements of expected performance, e.g., Müller's (132) textbook of 1840. However, no experimental approach to brain control was possible before the discovery of the motor area by electrical stimulation of the cortex in 1870 by Fritsch and Hitzig (52).

The neurologists were, of course, constantly reminded in their clinics of the importance of the influence of spinal and supraspinal structures on movement. They saw, for example, the symptoms of tabes, Parkinson's disease, and Friedreich's ataxia and felt the need for explanations. These tended to be in terms of localization. Hughlings Jackson's epilepsy (171) and his idea on its origin in a cortical focus is a well-known example; Broca's area for speech another (see ref. 17 for historical notes). Reflex action provided one important framework for theorizing, and a constant issue was always whether an observed symptom was mainly "centrifugal" or "centripetal." Operative techniques had long been available in the laboratory. In his textbook of 1859, Schiff (159) pointed out that acute afferent root section caused locomotor ataxia. Nathan and Sears (134) have reviewed the old literature on root section.

In the historical development of experimentation within the motor field, it is curious to note that the earliest quantitative approach was addressed to the "muscle sense." This undoubtedly was motivated by a belief in its role for the regulation of motor activity, the centripetal factor of the day. Another major source of inspiration is likely to have been the brilliant success of sensory psychophysics in vision, acoustics, and the skin senses. And so, for a time, the muscle sense became more important than the muscles' motor function. An exception is Duchenne (35) who in 1867 combined the simple expedients of skillful palpation and stimulation of different muscles with his precise anatomical knowledge. He made remarkably accurate observations on the sequence of participation of different muscles in voluntary movements of normal subjects and patients.

In 1826, Bell (11, 12) had described the muscular sense as one of exertion. This notion has remained with us as the "Kraftempfindung" (sensation of force or resistance) that later, in 1914–1926, was studied in such detail by von Frey (48–51). The second major component of the common muscle sense was called "sensation of movement" by Goldscheider (58) who had studied it in an important series of papers (1887–1898). To describe this sensation Bastian (10) coined the term "kinaesthetic sense." This he did at a meeting of the Neurological Society of London whose selected theme of discussion was the muscular sense. Brief comments to Bastian's introduction of the subject were made by the leading neurologists of the day. The mere existence of such a discussion is evidence for the lively interest in the centripetal aspects of the regulation of movement and posture. Alongside pathological anatomy the only avenue of advance was really the psychophysical and this, in those days, meant threshold studies.

These two components of the muscle sense—of movement and of force—became established in physiological textbooks such as those of Tigerstedt and Schäfer. Under the influx of new information, since held to be more important for medical students, the muscle sense has now lost this position and unjustly fallen into oblivion.

Goldscheider was in agreement with Duchenne and thought that the capacity for perceiving passive movement (Kinaesthesis) is the basis of all other experiences of sensory origin from the muscles. Of his large experimental material, paper no. 6 in the *Gesammelte Abhandlungen* contains most of the relevant information on thresholds for movement. These thresholds were greatly elevated after faradization of the joint, but were not influenced by applying his narrow sponge electrode elsewhere on the tip of the index finger whose flexor action was studied. Although Goldscheider ascribed the kinesthetic sense to endings in the joints, he allowed for a contribution from the muscular end organs, because faradization did not completely obliterate the sensation of movement. On the basis of a limited number of experiments, he was prepared to admit that the thresholds for active movement were a little lower than those for passive ones. For this conclusion there is today convincing evidence, for example, Lashley (106); Paillard and Brouchon (136); and Skavenski (165). The percepts of direction and resistance Goldscheider held to be complex ones.

The sense of force or resistance Goldscheider also accepted as genuine and referable to a peripheral cause. Nevertheless, it remained for von Frey to produce the precise threshold measurements, which proved it to be extremely sensitive. His method consisted of applying weights to hoops inserted at different points along a plaster of paris cast surrounding the forearm. The perceived torsional forces (Drehmomente) were identical for all locations. Because changes of the order of 1% could be distinguished, this meant that muscular tensions differing by the same amount were discernible. In the end, von Frey also studied the kinesthetic sense in surgically resected joints (50) and in the finger (51) after cutting the cutaneous nerve. His final conclusion was that the sense organs in the ligaments (Pacini bodies and Golgi-Mazzoni endings) were the decisive ones.

Renqvist (151), in von Frey's laboratory, later studied the absolute threshold of force in the fingers of three subjects. After having anesthetized the finger with an injection of 5-ml Novocain (with suprarenin), it was insensitive both to the application of weights of 20-25 g on its surface and to small, slow, unloaded movements, but with active movements force or resistance was felt for a load of about 10 g. In the light of present knowledge this finding suggests spindle coactivation in the active movements (see the section BACK TO MUSCULAR END ORGANS, p. 6). Later Renqvist (150) used Hill's (80) inertia ergometer to study voluntary flexion and extension at the elbow joint. His subjects perceived equal force when the physical forces were equal: the variables being mass and acceleration (whose product defines force). All this early work, largely neglected today, still seems to me unsurpassed in care and precision. [For later contributions, see ref. 66 and the useful review by Howard and Templeton (87).] In the face of this evidence, it seems to me unjustified to deny that there are perceptions originating from the muscular nerve endings. They are perhaps normally of little perceptual interest. The central projections from muscle afferents are small compared with those of eyes, ears, and skin. For this reason, they require a concentration of attention mobilized in properly designed experiments [cf. Skavenski (165) for a discussion of eye muscles].

At the present time, we are well informed about the properties of sensory endings in muscles, joints, and skin, and we are less willing to assign individual roles to specific endings in suprathreshold motor activities than we were at the turn of the century. It seems more likely that the peripheral information used for both automatic and conscious control has the character of a composite message, whose evaluation takes place against a stored program. But the psychophysics of the last century was much concerned with definitions of end organs, and the clinicians wanted tests for a reliable identification of a peripheral disturbance that was reflected in deficient motor control. The "centrifugal" aspect was known in principle and was emphasized, for instance, when Duchenne (35) pointed out that locomotor ataxia could exist despite normal performance of all the testable senses tested by methods available at the time.

REFLEX ORIGIN OF BASIC IDEAS
ON MOTOR CONTROL

Some may hold that the reflex as an automatic response to a stimulus is too narrow a concept to deserve being taken up under the heading of motor control. It did provide, however, the first insight into the nature of a controlling mechanism and does satisfy the three criteria set up above: *1)* one knows what neurons are being controlled; *2)* no other mechanism of motor control is equally well analyzed; and *3)* something at least is understood about the purposiveness in the reflex responses. As to automatism, the final aim even in motor learning is to practice complex actions until they become automatic.

Reflexes were well-established processes by the middle of the last century. An excellent historical account is available in Liddell's *Discovery of Reflexes* (109). This work ends with the contributions of Sherrington that have also been reviewed in two monographs, Granit (64) and Swazey (170), and in the *Selected Writings of Sir Charles Sherrington* thoughtfully compiled by Denny-Brown (164).

At an early date observations on decapitated frogs introduced the idea that the reflex mechanism resides in the spinal cord. In the textbooks of Schiff (159) and of Foster (47) this was generally accepted, as was the idea of supraspinal control. Foster stated that "in the ordinary actions of life the spinal cord is to a large extent a mere instrument of the cerebral hemispheres." Inhibition was a recognized process of unknown nature. At Strasbourg Goltz (60) had noted inhibitions of micturition and other spinal reflexes. The effect of stimulus summation was known and studied in measurements of the reflex latent period, which Foster called a "busy time" for the spinal cord. Even the intriguing concept of "release" from a tonic inhibition had been derived in 1863 from experimental work by Setchenov (161) working in Ludwig's laboratory (see ref. 64 for description). But what actually took place in the spinal cord segments was still a complete mystery.

In 1880 William James (94) had formulated his "law of forward conduction" implying that central nervous structures differ from peripheral nerves by conducting in one direction only. This was reformulated by Ramón y Cajal in terms of axons and dendrites, which were actually identified. At about that time the great era of histology rose to prominence, as is well described by Liddell (109). From this decennium onwards, such structural knowledge gradually became available as was needed for developing precise ideas on neural activity including motor control.

It is impossible to review the large field of histology in the present context. Only a few relevant dates from Liddell's *Discovery of Reflexes* are mentioned for general orientation. The Golgi silver chromate stain was introduced in 1875. Cajal used it on embryological material and he developed the reduced silver method in the eighties. The contact or neuron theory was formulated in 1891 by Waldeyer, based largely on the evidence provided by Cajal. In 1897 before the actual contact points had been described as "end feet" by Held, Sherrington had decided in favor of the evidence for the neuron theory and had introduced the term "synapse" (synapsis) in his contribution to a new edition of Foster's textbook. The first volume of Cajal's chef d'oeuvre, *Histologie du Système Nerveux* (147), appeared in Spanish in 1899.

Several reflexes were known before Sherrington entered the field and added some more. But the new attitude he brought to their study implied thinking of reflex excitation and inhibition in terms of synaptic action at individual neurons or at neuron pools of definite muscles. Sherrington, the well-trained microscopist, always drew a substantial part of his inspiration from histology, in particular from that of Cajal. "Nowhere in physiology does the cell-theory reveal its presence more frequently in the very framework of the argument than at the present time in the study of nervous reaction." These are the opening words—still valid today—of his Silliman Lectures of 1904, which in 1906 became the well-known classic *Integrative Action of the Nervous System* (163). Sherrington spent a lifetime on the verification of these ideas. Fulton's bibliography of Sherrington's writings was updated by Cohen (27). The best final summary is found in the book by Sherrington, himself, and his co-workers, *Reflex Activity of the Spinal Cord* (28).

The controlled element now became Sherrington's "final common path" (the α-motoneuron of today), which is a cell in the ventral horn of the spinal cord innervating a number of muscle fibers. This complex ultimately became known as the motor unit. The controlled motoneuron responded differentially to afferent stimulation from different receptive fields. Sometimes these were localized in the skin and in other cases defined by afferents of known muscular provenance. The stimuli either excited or inhibited the motoneuron; the two opposite effects often being reciprocally connected with respect to flexor and extensor motoneurons. Summation became the functional equivalent of histological convergence on the motoneuron. Excitation (E) and inhibition (I) were regarded as independent, synaptic activities of opposite nature capable of an interaction on the motoneuron that most likely was algebraically additive. They were shown to produce measurable states of E or I, more longlasting than nerve impulses, whether subliminal or supraliminal, as the case might be.

To the clashing of convergent E or I on the motoneuron the isometric myograph delivers only the algebraic sum. For this reason, the properties of the inhibitory process had to be studied against a state of excitation such as the one prevailing in the decerebrate preparation. In the end it proved possible also to show that inhibition could exist by itself without demonstrable excitation. This was an important conclusion, because postexcitatory depressions of excitability had suggested inhibitory processes different from the one ascribed to independent I-synapses. Sherrington's central inhibition was conceived as a genuine process comparable to the inhibitory action of Biedermann's (13) specific nerve fibers to invertebrate muscles or the classic vagal inhibition on the heart that Gaskell (55) in 1887 had found accompanied by a slow, positive change of potential at the sinus region.

Sherrington, familiar with the work on the muscle sense [see, e.g., his contribution to Schäfer's (162) textbook], and in need of definite knowledge about muscular end organs for progress in the understanding of postural reflexes and decerebrate rigidity, proved by afferent root section and degeneration experiments that the muscle spindles and golgi tendon organs were real sensory endings. His anatomical descriptions of the spindles agreed with the slightly earlier one of Ruffini (157, 158) who had shown that these organs, second only to the eye and the ear, are the most intricately innervated sensory endings in the body. Sectioning of the afferent input was shown to abolish decerebrate rigidity. The functional counterpart to all this work was Sherrington's original observation on the reflex "lengthening" and "shortening" reactions that culminated in the experiments with Liddell (110) on the stretch reflex, equally interesting today as at the time of its discovery (84).

EARLY INFLUENCE OF ELECTRONICS:
MICROELECTRODES

The inspiring work of Adrian (3, 4) brought in the single-fiber preparation and converged with that of Sherrington on the motoneuron or final common path, thereby motivating their joint Nobel Prize in 1932. With the advent of amplification the era of unitary analysis opened up fascinating prospects for neurophysiology. The cathode-ray oscillograph became incorporated in physiology by the work of Erlanger and Gasser (41) in the twenties (summarized in 1937). Their results introduced the conduction velocity of a nerve fiber as a function of its diameter. This was an essential contribution to motor control, because it made possible precise timing of conducted information and established definite constraints on the interpretation of input-output time relations. In addition, when Lorente de Nó (116, 117) in 1938 had measured synaptic transmission time, all the ingredients were on hand for circuit analysis of a kind that now is part of our routine in the study of control problems.

Although neurophysiologists in the thirties still built their own electrical equipment, soon the electronic specialists entered their laboratories and devised more intricate amplifiers, sweep circuits, and many other kinds of timing and recording devices, which in the end also became available commercially. Renshaw (152) and Lloyd (113) took up for study the monosynaptic reflex. Paul Hoffmann (83) had come to the very likely conclusion that the tendon jerks were monosynaptic ones carried by the largest afferents directly to the motoneuron. This could now be verified and Lloyd (114) showed them to be set up by end organs sensitive to stretch, exciting their own motoneurons, and inhibiting the antagonists in reciprocal action.

By restricting stimulation to the largest monosynaptic fibers it became possible to measure the time course of a "purified" excitatory state: a conditioning shock mobilized a certain percentage of a pool of motoneurons, excited the others subliminally; a subsequent test shock raised a number of the subliminally excited ones above the firing threshold along a curve obtained by varying the interval between conditioning and test shock. In both Renshaw's and Lloyd's versions of monosynaptic testing, the size of the efferent volley in the ventral root illustrated the time course of motoneuronal excitability by the variable number of activated motoneurons. This method has been widely used in the studies of control of the final executive cell (the α-motoneuron) on humans at an early date as the Hoffmann reflex by Magladery and McDougal (120).

For work on functionally isolated motoneurons another index was necessary. The work I did with Ström (71) introduced the "probability of firing" indicator for studies on both E and I, and this approach was later standardized by Lloyd and McIntyre (115).

Already by the end of the 1930s the fiber-splitting techniques had yielded so much new information on the discharge of sense organs and motoneurons that unitary studies of the rest of the central nervous system became an irresistible temptation, at least to us young neurophysiologists then in our most active years. The obvious answer to this challenge was the microelectrode technique that, steadily perfected in the next 10 to 15 years, began to dominate neurophysiology. Today, this still remains a powerful, analytical instrument, the only one alongside of chemical techniques which is capable of bridging the gap to modern histology. For notes on the early history of microrecording, see Granit (62). Technical improvements by Graham and Gerard (61) and by Ling and Gerard (112) made it possible to penetrate the membrane of muscle fibers in order to record their resting potential. In 1950 Nastuk and Hodgkin (133) carried the microelectrode technique one step further and succeeded in recording also the muscle fiber's intracellular action potential.

INTRACELLULAR APPROACH

The intracellular electrode was successfully applied to motoneurons by Woodbury and Patton (179) and at much the same time by Eccles and his colleagues (see refs. 36, 38 for his summaries). With his basic knowledge of reflexology acquired in Sherrington's laboratory, Eccles realized what could and should be done with the monosynaptic reflex from muscular afferents. His group soon delivered the final, intracellular evidence for the conclusion that excitation and inhibition are two opposite shifts of membrane potential—as adumbrated by his predecessors—and they interpreted these effects in terms of the ionic theory of Hodgkin and Huxley (81).

Another intracellular approach was that of Bernhard Katz and his co-workers [see Katz (98) for summary] on the motor end plates and their miniature potentials in relation to acetylcholine. When Hanson, H. E. Huxley, and A. F. Huxley (see ref. 90 for summary) initiated their experiments on the mechanism of muscular contraction, the whole chain of events, from synaptic effects on the membrane of the motoneuron to the ultimate contractile process, was, so to speak, under observation by micromethods relating microanatomy to electrochemical reactions at the microlevel. In addition, visualization at that level was rapidly improved by the electron microscope.

Considering this development merely from the specific point of view of motor control, it was essential knowledge at all stages, but the major line of research on control problems remained concentrated on Sherrington's final common path as the final neuronal executive. The impact of the parallel work on γ-motoneurons (see the section BACK TO MUSCULAR END ORGANS, p. 6) did not make itself felt until the midfifties.

Much, perhaps even most, work on motor control at the unitary level is still being carried out by extracellular microrecording. What then was the asset of the intracellular approach? In the first instance, postsynaptic membrane potentials below the threshold of firing became measurable, making accessible the concealed world of cellular operations that previously had been explored merely by indirect methods (conditioning following by testing). The intracellular electrode also opened up new avenues to synaptic microphysiology, for example, differentiating chemically from electrically transmitted impulses and separating dendritic from somatic localization. This electrode provided the means for classifying motoneurons in terms of membrane properties and for correlating them with cell size and axonal conduction velocity. By extracellular means alone it would not have been possible to obtain unequivocal evidence for differentiating the four concepts: facilitation, disinhibition, inhibition, and disfacilitation, now familiar in neurophysiology.

The use of intracellular recording could be discussed from many other aspects, but the ones mentioned have been selected for their relevance in our attempts to understand motor control. From this point of view, it is significant whether a motor act is modified by facilitation or by disinhibition; whether it is transmitted chemically or electrically; or whether it is mainly dendritic or somatic in origin. For a review of synaptology, see Eccles (37). As to the difference between somatic and dendritic activation, see, for instance, Rall (146) and Burke (23).

At the segmental level the intracellular electrode opened up facilities for studying internuncial contributions to the control of motoneurons. The approach of Lundberg and his colleagues (see Lundberg (119) for summary) was indirect, by using the motoneuron as an indicator, as well as direct, i.e., by recording from interneurons. Of general interest in this context is that a large number of reflex afferents and supraspinal tracts were found to employ common interneuronal circuits to control the output of the final executive.

BACK TO MUSCULAR END ORGANS

Several important lines of advance specifically raising the issue of motor control took their origin in the late forties and early fifties. One of them led to an experimental renaissance for the sensory endings in the muscles, whose types of unitary discharges had been elucidated in a pioneer study by Bryan Matthews (125) in 1933. The new information on conduction velocities in relation to mono- and polysynaptic reflexes now had to be related also to both muscular tension and extension and to the nature of the endings responsible for the reflexes. At the same time the gamma motor fibers, first properly identified by Leksell (108), opened up new aspects on control problems.

It soon became clear that, on stimulating cut ventral root fibers, an increase of extrafusal tension by a contraction short-circuiting the intrafusal muscles unloaded the spindles and produced a fast, autogenetic inhibition of the motoneurons. In a preparation with tonically active spindles, disfacilitation would occur during the rising contraction, but it could be shown that there also is a real tension-sensitive inhibition attributable to the Golgi tendon organs. Anatomy and physiology agreed in referring the excitatory response of extension, the stretch reflex, to the large spindle afferents. Whatever else the spindle and tendon endings might do, they at least elicited these two negative feedback responses on their own muscles and some synergists. Muscle shortening in contraction was counteracted by lengthening; muscle extension or stretch was counteracted by a shortening contraction. It is not yet quite clear whether the smaller spindle afferents (Group II) really are important at the segmental level or whether their main task in motor control might be to carry messages to higher centers. During this early period new ideas on proprioceptive motor control began to take shape and these are found in *Receptors and Sensory Perception. Silliman Lectures.* (62).

Through the γ-loop the spindles influence motoneurons, spinal interneurons, and supraspinal stations, but, then, from where and under what conditions are the small γ-motoneurons activated? Both these problems were well understood and had been approached experimentally at the time. Single-fiber techniques were used to show that the γ-fibers took part in a large number of reflexes (40, 89, 101) as well as in motor responses from several sites in the brain, most easily from the brain stem (70). Clearly, there were now two "final common paths" controlled from above, but because they were connected in the periphery through the γ-loop, supreme "finality" returned to the α-motoneuron. The early observations provided arguments for a general and common reply to our two questions: the small γ-motoneurons are mostly activated in such close relationship to the alpha executive that their exciting or inhibiting mechanisms somehow must be linked also in the neuraxis. Coactivation by α-γ linkage (62) implied the introduction of a new mechanism into the physiology of motor activity. Part of the gamma problem was thereby pushed into the ancient and vast complex of modes of alpha control, but there remained the separate, intriguing question of how the linkage is organized at different levels (67). The main interest, however, became at first devoted to the functional problem of what coactivation implied for motor control.

The acquisition of new physiological information on the muscle spindles was reflected in histology by a rapidly rising interest in their complex anatomy. In this field, collaboration between anatomists and physiologists became exemplarily intimate. Responding to their own needs, many neurophysiologists also undertook histological work (e.g., S. Cooper, I. A. Boyd, and R. S. Smith). Progress was reported in a number of symposia and conferences (8, 15, 63), and this trend of publication continues to the present time.

Single rat muscle spindles responding to stretch or electrical stimulation were observed under the microscope by R. S. Smith (166) and his pioneer experiment was repeated and expanded by others, in particular by Ian Boyd (16). The γ-motoneurons were subdivided by P. B. C. Matthews (126) into two components: one static and the other dynamic. In addition, much experimentation became concerned with the projections of the two fiber types on the different kinds of intrafusal muscles described by the histologists. These problems are dealt with in the chapter by Matthews in this *Handbook*.

IMPACT OF CYBERNETICS
ON MOTOR PHYSIOLOGY

Weiner's book, *Cybernetics or Control of Communication in the Animal and the Machine* (178), first appeared in 1947. For neurophysiologists studying circuits engaged in motor control, it had the appeal of offering general rules for types of activity with which they were familiar. To this categeory belonged, for instance, the two negative feedback responses to tension and extension mentioned in the previous section. These now became specimens of a general type of control, subjected to the definitions and constraints defined by regulation science.

At the moment, the early hope that cybernetics would provide the ultimate solution to the problems facing students who study integration in the central nervous system has lost much of its first appeal. The wealth of possible combinations and the hierarchical nature of the nervous system have prevented the discovery of parameters for mathematical applications, except in some simplified circuits lifted out of their context in integrative interaction. Two good examples of such exceptions are the pupillary reflex, as analyzed quantitatively by Stark (168) and Ito's (92) theory of the cerebellum as a "computer" linked with open-loop control systems. But it is no exaggeration to state that the many discoveries in the field of stretch reflex, γ-neuron, and spindle physiology owed little if anything to cybernetics. I have discussed this elsewhere in greater detail (68).

The great value of cybernetics lay in the concepts that it bequeathed to the expanding neurophysiology of the fifties. A new mode of thinking about certain types of problems followed when the physiologists accepted and began to apply concepts such as "gain," "redundancy," "feedback," "feedforward," and "stability." Cybernetics also drew attention to servomechanisms as good models for biological comparisons with machinery (129). To the credit of cybernetics should ultimately be added its role in contributing to establish the permanent position of "bioengineers" in the physiological laboratories.

It is clear, however, that although cybernetic thinking in the field of motor control may provide a formal description of an interacting chain of neural events, major physiological interest is likely to be differently directed. The main concerns extend, for example, to principles of neural re-representation, to questions of synaptic chemistry in relation to histology and function, to the organization of long-distance, mono- and polysynaptic effects from definite sites, to the nature of what is being localized (its "what," "how," and "why"), to the organization of voluntary activity, and to the influence of attention. Aspects of synaptic chemistry in relation to developmental physiology and specificity are likely to become even more important problems than they have been until now (93, 104).

FEEDBACK PROBLEMS IN
MOTOR CONTROL

The organization of recurrent inhibition of motoneurons is one of the best examples from the field of motor control illustrating both the advantages and the limitations of cybernetic thinking. Historically the interest in recurrent fibers began with their discovery, which Cajal rightly ascribed to Golgi (59) but their universal occurrence in nervous centers was demonstrated by Cajal, himself. Antidromic stimulation of motoneurons was an obvious experimental approach to their physiology and it was tried at an early date (see ref. 62 for historical notes) but proper analysis had to await techniques based on fiber splitting and microelectrodes.

In Renshaw's early, decisive paper of 1946 (153) he found that the antidromic inhibition of motoneurons coincided with a peculiar high-frequency discharge picked up by a microelectrode located among internuncial cells adjacent to the motoneurons. The next decisive step came from Eccles and his co-workers (39) who recorded intracellularly from single motoneurons. They found that an antidromic shock to the motoneurons caused a hyperpolarizing type of inhibition, whose time course was notched by the firing pattern of the interneurons discovered by Renshaw (the Renshaw cells). Timing and other lines of convergent evidence established the Renshaw cell as a kind of "commutator" reducing the outgoing excitatory discharge from the motoneurons by postsynaptic inhibition. There is today a considerable literature on recurrent inhibition such as the review by Haase et al. (73). From this literature some examples are chosen to illustrate the way in which increasing experimental insight, achieved by circuit analysis, reveals complexities of an organization that at the outset of investigation seemed simple.

A quantitative approach to the recurrent control of motoneuron firing served to establish two facts: *1*) that up to a saturation point the recurrent inhibitory effect was proportional to the firing rate of the antidromic stimulation, and *2*) that a constant antidromic input had a constant inhibitory effect on the firing (test) motoneuron. This was independent of the firing rate of the latter (see ref. 65 for summary). A cortical recurrent inhibition was found to have the same properties (22). These facts could be sensibly interpreted as implicating a mechanism for the stabilization of a discharge by negative feedback from its output, leading in addition to a useful suppression of feebly discharging motoneurons.

When all this had been demonstrated, complications began to mount. First, the Renshaw cell proved to be under the influence of a large number of reflex and supraspinal pathways determining whether it should be accessible to the recurrent input or blocked out by inhibition. Second, the recurrent inhibition in the cat was shown to act more powerfully on the small tonically discharging motoneurons than on their large phasic partners. Third, the Renshaw cell turned out to have an inhibitory effect also on the Ia inhibitory interneuron (see ref. 119 for review) which is the cell mediating the reciprocal inhibition from the large spindle afferents. Eccles (37) described this interneuron, and it has since been identified also by injection into it of Procion yellow (95). Fourth, some of the Renshaw cells have also been found to inhibit a number of γ-motoneurons (see ref. 73 for a summary).

In elaborate studies Lundberg (119) and his colleagues in Gothenburg (88, 95, 111) have described in detail the extensive supraspinal influences on the Ia inhibitory interneuron. These serve to emphasize or to suppress reciprocal activity according to the largely unknown needs of the animal. The same may be said about the effect of the Renshaw cell, also controlled from above, on the Ia inhibitory interneuron.

This expansion of the theme of segmental, recurrent control illustrates the likely final result of any sufficiently detailed analysis of a circuit including interneurons. Their role obviously is to make the functions of whatever they control adaptable to the numerous needs of the organism. The final criterion for understanding these roles is that we should be able to fit our factual disclosures into purposive integrations. Many of the workers active in this field have also tried to do so, but in the context of this chapter it is impossible to review the interpretations available for motor control by recurrent fibers, because it would require a large-scale presentation of the evidence on which they are founded. In the section COMMENTS ON CORTICAL LOCALIZATION, p. 10, I shall return to the general role of segmental control.

ADVENT OF STEREOTAXIS: SUBCORTICAL MOTOR CENTERS

The existence of subcortical centers for the regulation of posture and movement was well known by the workers who at the end of the last century studied the effects of cortical ablations as well as of pyramidal and brain stem transections. Decerebrate rigidity has a still older history (109). It was understood to be a release of centers in the lower pons from inhibiting influences at a higher level of the brain stem.

Much interest was devoted to the "extrapyramidal" system. This term was based on the finding that the stimulation of cortical motor fields in the dog and in the monkey also produced leg movements after severance of the pyramidal path in the medulla oblongata (144, 156, 169). A long list of later experimenters repeating and expanding the work on section of the pyramids or destruction of the motor area is found in Fulton's *Physiology of the Nervous System* (54) and later discussions are presented in Hassler (76) and Jung and Hassler (96). Accepting evidence of this nature Denny-Brown (33) pointed out that righting and tilting reactions also remain after transection of the cerebral peduncle interrupting direct corticobulbar fibers and the pyramid. The complex subcortical mechanisms of motor control, such as pallidocortical loops, corticoreticular connections, and clinical states (124) involving, for example, the basal ganglia, belong to a world of isolated observations, some functionally controversial. Their presentation and interpretation should be referred to special papers scrutinizing the evidence. For the early work of the anatomists, one can see Fulton (54) and Kappers et al. (97). My intention here, however, is to indicate some lines of development leading up to the present standardized use of stereotaxis.

The Dutch school at Utrecht (Magnus and de Kleijn) began with Sherrington's observations on "reflex figures" in the decerebrate animal and described the now familiar patterns of orientation and posture, summarized by Magnus (121) and Camis (25), using mostly thalamic rabbits. Precise localization could not be obtained by their methods based on ablations and transections. Rademaker (145), for instance, was wrong in ascribing to the red nucleus a major role in decerebrate rigidity, but this was a minor miss among many careful observations. More surprising is that the Dutch workers did not take up stereotaxis. Already in 1908, Horsley and Clarke (86) had designed the technique known by their joint names. It remained for Ranson (148) and Hess (79) to realize the value of the stereotactic approach and to perfect the necessary head holders and needle electrodes. Soon the revived technique was applied also for recording inside the brain, and stereotactic maps for the laboratory animals then began to appear in print. When stereotaxis became highly perfected for the human head, it was used to relieve Parkinsonian rigor by a local destruction within the thalamus.

Although Ranson's very active group made observations over a wide range, they became best known for their work on hypothalamic regulation of temperature, sleep, and wakefulness. Hess who discovered "stereotactic sleep" also took up problems of motor function roughly at the point where the Dutch workers had given up, perhaps because of the premature death of Magnus in 1927. Hess described a considerable number of higly specific, functional patterns in subcortical sites. Of interest for the localization of automatic compensatory mechanisms were the diencephalic directional movements in space such as lowering or raising of the head, rotation of it around the longitudinal axis, and contra- or ipsiversive turning. Cartographic accuracy of localization was a major aim of his work, but this block of solid functional information on motor patterns in the cat has so far proved difficult to evaluate, except in terms other than those concerned with mapping. These patterns are likely to be essential components of what we nowadays tend to call "programs" or "schemas."

Chemical points of view may in the end prove helpful in attempts to make systematic use of Hess's material, that is, if some motor patterns could be shown to be organized in chemically homogeneous sites. This is the case with the nigrostriatal system that gained so much in significance when it was proved to depend on dopamine and to be lacking this substance in cases of Parkinson's disease [Hassler (77), Hornykiewicz (85), Martin (124), and Ungerstedt (174)]. Also at the level of the spinal segments and tracts, the chemical approach has proved its value. There is evidence of monoaminergic control of the effects of the grouped flexor-reflex afferents (118) and of tonic-stretch reflexes (72).

In the prolific stereotactic experimentation of the forties, the reticular formation in the brain stem acquired a prominent position, largely owing to the initiative of Magoun and his co-workers (122, 123). This structure had long attracted the anatomists (137).

Although known from the great era of anatomical discoveries at the end of last century, it had never received an equal amount of attention on the part of the physiologists. The striking ascending effects of reticular stimulation on the whole cortex, discovered by Moruzzi and Magoun (131) in 1949, suddenly threw the reticular formation into the forefront of neurophysiological research. This, however, is not our present concern.

Magoun had participated in Ranson's laboratory in the experiments of Pitts et al. (140) localizing the respiratory center in the reticular formation. A more direct cue to motor control implied his participation in the discovery of pathological lesions in the brain stem in cases of human poliomyelitis (9). Then followed the work that disclosed two generalized effects on motoneurons: an inhibition from a medially located bulbomedullary region and an excitation from surrounding and somewhat higher, localized lateral sites. This finding was an unexpected exception from the more common reciprocal effects of supraspinal stimulation, but soon these, too, were obtained from the reticular formation by others (e.g., ref. 167). The controversy, general vs. specific effects, that ensued is well reviewed by Rossi and Zanchetti (155) in their balanced presentation of the anatomy and physiology of the reticular formation. In retrospect, it hardly seems necessary to speak of a controversy knowing as we do that the spinal cord has mechanisms for segmental redistribution of activity (described in the section FEEDBACK PROBLEMS IN MOTOR CONTROL, p. 7) and several centrifugal tracts in the cord to control them.

The concept of generalized excitation and inhibition was strengthened by the discovery that the γ-motoneurons are excited or inhibited by reticular stimulation (70) according to the topographical coordinates of the two effects, as given by Magoun and his colleagues. At the same time the findings introduced the possibility that the reticular effects, at least in part, might be mediated by the γ-loop. Again taking a retrospective view, the concept of coactivation of α- and γ-motoneurons by neural linkages has vindicated itself so well that the topographical agreement between the properties of the reticular α- and γ-responses is best interpreted as one of its consequences.

The impact of all this work made itself felt in physiology as a renewal of the interest in the problems of tone and posture. In anatomy extensive studies of the histology of the reticulum were performed. The early background in this field was discussed in 1932 by Bremer (18), and Brodal (19) summarized anatomical knowledge in 1957, relating it to functional studies.

As so often happens in neurophysiology, the experimental activity suddenly turned away from the pursuit of generalized motor effects on the spinal cord. The ascending aspect of reticular stimulation exercised a greater, more durable appeal because it generated the problem of arousal and emphasized the significance of nonspecific afferent inputs. The motor interest now settled for experiments on the components of the γ-loop: α's, γ's, spindles, and recurrent fibers, and the role of these factors in posture and movement also was examined.

STRETCH REFLEX IN MOTOR CONTROL

By regarding decerebrate rigidity as a state of pathologically exaggerated tonus, Sherrington had given it a central position in postural activity. The basic idea was his precybernetic notion of negative feedback. This interpretation, however, needed the work on the γ-loop to mature into full significance. For this section, detailed references to the early work are found in Granit (62) and to the later work in references 65, 67, 84, and 127. An early finding was that the extensor γ-motoneurons are hyperactive in decerebrate rigidity. This suggested that abolishment of the rigid state by deafferentation was caused by severance of the loop, even though it was known that other factors contributed as was summarized by Dow and Moruzzi (34). The released excitation that maintains rigidity is likely, on the principle of α-γ linkage, to have befallen both kinds of motoneurons. Nevertheless, the dramatic effect of deafferentation favors the notion that the activity across the loop is the decisive factor that makes the alpha executive spill over into the hyperactivity of the rigid state.

By the same principle the stretch reflex ceases to be merely a pathological oddity and instead acquires the status of an accompaniment to virtually every muscular act as a controlling element in contraction. By direct recording from human spindle afferents, Vallbo (175) has found that even fast movements of the finger muscles are accompanied by spindle outbursts of coactivation. The stretch reflex, given time, would fire the α-motoneurons or would raise their excitability during any muscular extension brought about by a load. Despite coactivation, some unloading of the spindles will always antagonize the rising excitation during the contraction that follows. In the long-lasting postural contractions it is easily observed that a balanced oscillatory state occurs as a consequence of slight unloading, which excites the spindles by stretch to reestablish the contraction. This again unloads the spindles that are reexcited, and the process continues in this manner. In the absence of gamma bias the spindles can act neither in load compensation nor to sustain tonic activity. Only phasic activity such as tendon jerks is possible. Sufficient extension would, however, compensate for the lack of gamma bias. In addition, there are pure alpha rigidities such as those seen after anemic decerebration in which one-half the cerebellum and a considerable part of the pons is destroyed (141, 142).

Much experimental work has shown that in the laboratory animals, including monkeys, spindle activity tends to precede the discharge of α-motoneurons both in reflex and supraspinal activation. This observation seemed to fit the follow-up-length hypothesis of Merton (129) according to which the excited γ-loop first establishes an intrafusal length-setting to drive the α-motoneurons. This continues until extra- and intrafusal length become equalized and the spindles are unloaded. In 1927 Rossi (154) had advanced a similar idea when he made the spindles' motor system responsible for the maintenance of tone. This paper (in Italian) was unknown to the experimenters of the early fifties whose results are being discussed here. Merton's hypothesis has neither found favor with other interpreters of the role of the γ-loop nor has it been finally ruled out. The most general argument against it has been that the gain in the loop is too low to fulfill such a role. This criticism is based on experiments with otherwise denervated hindlimbs in which only soleus or gastrocnemius were studied in isolation. Gain is, however, an adjustable quantity, dependent on the temporary requirements of the animal. Precise measurements have shown in the cat that every 10 mV of postsynaptic potential in high-gain motoneurons may raise 23 impulses/s and that stretch, by no means excessive, may produce up to 11 mV (65). It is being argued here that the limited number of experimentally testable situations does not permit final conclusions as to the nonexistence of follow-up cases.

The early work on the γ-loop also raised the question of whether all α-motoneurons participate equally in the stretch reflex. This proved not to be the case (69). In deafferented animals only the small α-motoneurons could be made to fire tonically by natural stimulation (repeated stretching), and only phasic responses were obtained from the large ones. In most motor acts, the small α-motoneurons are the first to be mobilized (78).

The essential role of the stretch reflex in motor control is based on recruitment of fresh motoneurons rather than on a rise in frequency of the individual participants (5, 32). A recruiting reflex works its way against both the afferent inhibition and the recurrent inhibition to which the small α-motoneurons are especially exposed. This means that the firing rate of the discharging motoneuron does not reflect the actual efficiency of a rising input frequency to raise excitatory impulses in proportion. The output is held down to a nearly constant firing rate. To this net result, its long-lasting afterhyperpolarization may add an essential contribution (100). For these reasons the recruited motoneurons are operating with a varying degree of supporting surplus excitation, measurable by testing with a constant inhibitory stimulus. From these early results, work has ramified into different directions, and these developments are reviewed in other chapters of this *Handbook*. Some points may be cursorily alluded to here.

Thus, considerable interest has been devoted to the cortical and cerebellar projections of the muscular afferents (105, 135, 139). These findings, and later ones supplementing them, have suggested the presence of cortical loops contributing to the stretch reflex.

Another interesting line of research began with Ranvier's (149) observations in 1880 on the anatomical and functional differences between red and white muscle. This work developed rapidly in the sixties: anatomically by histochemical methods and functionally by parallel studies of differential contractility, innervation, and vascularization of red and white motor units. An unexpected range of variation of capacities in terms of force, sustenance of a contraction, and vascularization has been demonstrated (24).

Vibratory stimulation of muscles, once tried in 1921 in Paul Hoffmann's laboratory (75), is another field that has expanded rapidly, both as a study of spindle properties and as observations on the tonic reflex elicited by the spindle afferents responding to vibration. Both Hagbarth and his colleagues at Uppsala and Lance and his group in Sydney have pioneered a revival of interest in the vibratory reflexes in human beings (see ref. 177).

COMMENTS ON CORTICAL LOCALIZATION

As a "battle of giants," Liddell (109) described the fight between Goltz and Ferrier at the Seventh International Medical Congress held in London in 1881. Although Goltz's operations on dogs gave no evidence in favor of the localization of motor functions in the cortex, Ferrier's monkeys with localized cortical lesions had localized effects in the limbs. Apparently, Polyak (143) was right in speaking of the "glaring inadequacies of Goltz's technique" as the probable explanation of his adherence to the old sterilizing concept of the functional equivalence of the cortex. By this time, Fritsch and Hitzig (52) had discovered the motor area and Jackson (171) had described the localized epilepsies known by his name. The development of ideas and techniques in the matter of cortical control of movement from those days up to the present era of microelectrodes and electronic instrumentation has been so well described by Phillips and Porter (138) that repetition by a less expert writer seems superfluous. I shall therefore restrict myself to some comments on the concept of localization and its significance and changing content over the years. The current leading experiments on cortical control of movement are considered by several authors in this volume. For a review of the early work (1902) on localization, see von Monakow (130).

The classic concept of localization referred to a representation of the senses and of movement in the cortex. In essence it dealt with what might be called the cartographic appurtenance of the cortical regions, which nowadays are defined by evoked potentials and local stimulation wherever these procedures can be applied. The problem of determining what is localized apparently originated with Jackson's question of whether muscles or movements are represented in the motor area. Clearly movements cannot be localized without a basic pattern of detailed muscular representation. Recently, this was studied extensively by Asanuma (see ref. 7 for summary) and his colleagues, and their findings would certainly have been accepted by Jackson. His comment would have been that his question really was concerned with the meaning or significance of a motor area. In this matter his answer was that the motor area is an organization for joining muscles into movements "in thousands of different combinations" (171). Essentially this point of view has been vindicated during 100 years of skillful experimentation. Almost as a corollary it follows that this organization must be accessible to numerous influences capable of evoking movements. A large portion of recent work has been devoted to the study of influences such as those from muscular end organs and from visual receiving areas. Linked α- and γ-operations, so characteristic for controlled motor events, even voluntary ones [Hagbarth and Vallbo (74)], are a feature of responses elicited from the motor area.

In comparison with a sensory projection such as the visual receiving area 17, the motor output area is a mechanism for synthesizing or integrating information for action, in primates even direct or monosynaptic to α- and γ-motoneurons, while area 17 is an analyzer of visual information that is re-represented elsewhere for various purposes. Despite these fundamental differences, both the motor and the visual (or any other) primary sensory area obey the same general rule that I have formulated elsewhere (e.g. ref. 68). "The greater the elaboration required for a percept or a motor act, the greater the number of cells engaged in it." To define elaboration, I gave examples such as the delicate manipulation of objects or a high degree of sensory discrimination. Attention was drawn to the well-known figurines of Penfield and Rasmussen and, also, of Woolsey and to the enormous cortical expansion of the foveal projection, as such, as well as by comparison with that of the peripheral retina. This rule, therefore, adds another dimension to the meaning or significance of localization. It may be said to be well documented by the experiments referred to in this section.

The classic concept of localization does not quite cover the recent results of microelectrode studies of single cells in the motor area. The general aim of these studies has been to produce a picture of the properties of sampled units within a localized area. In the end this will contribute to answering the question of what is being localized. It has been found that the cells are highly diversified, both with respect to output and input, the latter tending to be polymodal in character. The rule is that elaborated acts are represented in larger fractions of the motor area than simple movements. Therefore, this means that the key to their control function resides in the combinations of highly diversiform properties laid down in a large number of cooperating units. Diversity is likely to be greater in the input than in the output, whose final stage can rely also on important controls in the spinal cord.

The concept of localization, inasmuch as it refers to properties localized in sampled units or in columns of such units, thus has a functional precision reaching beyond the purely cartographic allocation of a motor area to a cortical site. There remains the task of discovering by which rules the differentiated, split-up properties of single cells combine to achieve the versatility and agility of animals in purposive action.

The electronic summation technique, originated by Dawson (29), when applied to voluntary movement (30, 57, 102), has shown in human beings and monkeys that complex bilateral changes of potential over large parts of the brain precede the "motor potential" that is related to the discharge of the pyramidal neurons as described by Evarts (42, 43). A replica of this behavior is seen in the local changes of cortical blood flow, which is studied by the methods elaborated by Ingvar and Lassen (91). The "consultation" of a very much larger bed of neurons than the motor area, itself, would indeed presuppose the great diversity of input into the units in that area that has been demonstrated experimentally.

The motor area is executive in character and partly monosynaptically connected to spinal motoneurons, which are placed by this connection, as a real extension of their cortical partners. In this sense, the spinal cord in primates is part of the motor area and associated also indirectly by its more numerous polysynaptic connections. It helps to understand the significance of the close relationship between motor area and spinal mechanisms if one compares action at the motor end station with the percept that is the final product of a sensory message from the eye.

The visual image may rest steadily in the focus of consciousness. The motor act is openly time dependent in a different and highly decisive way, and it is generally composed of swift transitions from one combined action of acting muscles to another. For this reason it stands in need of an efficient local exchange capable of fast execution of changing commands. In the section FEEDBACK PROBLEMS IN MOTOR CONTROL, p. 7, it was pointed out that there actually exist supraspinally controlled "switchboards" in the spinal segments capable of responding to such instant needs. These local feedback operations are Nature's answer to a desideratum.

There are many aspects of localization still to be discovered. Consider, for instance, a demanded ballistic movement such as typewriting or piano playing. The original voluntary demand must have included both a choice of motor units and a decision as to their sequence of entry and exit in a pattern of changing positions, forces, accelerations, velocities, and durations of activity. In the beginning, such a movement was guided by visual feedback. Then there followed a process of learning that led to automatization of a program or schema that for running control in the end is chiefly dependent on the feedback from the proprioceptive sphere (2, 56).

It does not seem likely that an automatized motor act is a purely cortical affair. Well-known observations point to participation of subcortical mechanisms. Thus, there are extremely fast and well-coordinated movements in animals without a prominent motor area. The latter, at its best, is a development for special purposes such as the precision grip and other delicate movements of the hand and the touching fingers. The observations (144, 156, 169, 172, 173) on section of the pyramids in the cat and the monkey, often repeated, reveal a large number of remaining "extrapyramidal" movements and good recovery of many motor acts. In addition, there are the observations by Hess (79) mentioned in the section ADVENT OF STEREOTAXIS, p. 8, on highly specific motor patterns obtainable by stereotactic stimulation in the diencephalon, and also quite recent experiences with animals after ablation of the motor area (33). An automatized program almost certainly includes decisive subcortical components of localization (21). There is a good anatomical basis for this statement in the findings reviewed by Kemp and Powell (99) of somatotopic, corticostriatal projections from all cortical regions. A review of earlier work is presented by Hassler (76, 77).

A complex automatic movement or a simple voluntary act can be carried out at varying rates over a great range of velocities. Greater velocity will generally be combined with an increase of acceleration, automatically involving force. This process of stepping up the speed of a motor act would seem to require a separate organization of neurons to control it. Would such a center be in the pallidum, in the cerebellum, or in several sites? For the first two alternatives there are suggestions in the work of DeLong (31) and Brooks and his colleagues (21). Because we know too little about the principles of "consultation" and "decision" of the brain, there is the possibility that my postulate of a separate velocity control also could be a reply to a wrongly formulated question. Nevertheless, well-known clinical observations show that when movements are pathologically slowed down they are still executed as purposive sequences. Thus, this suggests a differentiation between the design of a program fitted into the body image and the speed of its execution. Moreover, did not Lashley's rats (107), deprived of the cerebellum, virtually roll themselves through the maze guided merely by the retained program?

REORIENTATION IN CONCEPTS AND INTERESTS

If I now, finally, ask myself in what way the general outlook on the work and aims in the motor field has changed since the early twenties, the answer would be that experimenters now are trying to understand motor phenomena in terms of a predominant interest in the mechanisms of control. The traditional line of experimentation in this field was more concerned with effects as such and with the sites from which these could be elicited. Much descriptive work of this type is still being published, but more and more the purposive and organizational element in the term motor control has come to the fore. The term itself began to be generally used as late as in the sixties.

It goes without saying that the new techniques based on amplification, microelectrodes, and electron microscopy have played a major role in the reorientation of our attitudes to all motor problems. The isolated fiber or neuron had an uncanny ability for stirring up "why" and "what for" questions. One came, as it were, closer to the intimate workings of the nervous system. The advent of cybernetic thinking met a breeding ground prepared. Not only did cybernetics formulate rules for controlled processes, but it also emphasized the distinction between "hardware" and the program instilled into a purposive design making use of the "hard" components. The parallel experimentation on the centrifugal control of the muscle spindles was another influence that led straight into questions of why the spindles were controlled and what were the reasons for this control. Personally, I recall being much excited by seeing spontaneously active gastrocnemius spindles in the decerebrate cat completely silenced by electrical stimulation of the surface of the cerebellum, while the animal itself, a bit rigid, was lying quietly in its frame. Clearly, the effect could not be called a reflex even though in the end it did influence one.

Ultimately, we have arrived at the stage when the need for understanding the neural aspects of programming looms large across the frontiers of our field. I need not take up here the work of leading schools (e.g., Brooks, Evarts, Phillips, Porter, and Terzuolo, and the Moscow group of Gelfand, Gurfinkel, Orlowsky, and others). This is largely dealt with elsewhere. But I would like to draw attention to some less well-known research on the predictive element of a program in the hope that it would stimulate the study of factors such as genesis, structure, localization, stability, and plasticity of programming.

Anticipation was analyzed by Adams and Creamer (2) in order to discover whether it contained proprioceptive variables. Some evidence favored this view [see Christina (26) for criticism]. In the human tracking experiment with its roots in psychotechnics (see ref. 1 for summary) anticipation has always played a large role, and very recently Flowers (45, 46) has shown that normal subjects soon learn to follow a sinusoidal tracking course by switching to a predictive mode of control. Nevertheless, his Parkinsonian patients were incapable of doing this or did the switch with a deficit suggesting that the disease had attacked the capacity for creating the internal model, program or schema in the sense of Schmidt (160), required in prediction.

The operation of a predictive program is seen also

in the work of Melvill Jones and Watt (128). They demonstrated that human subjects in unexpected falls make preparatory muscular adjustments in anticipation of landing, although these, partly at least, may be direct reflexes from the vestibular end organs. Easier to develop might be the experiments (43a, 73a) on humans in which an event, as far down in the neuraxis as the monosynaptic component of the stretch reflex, tended to respond as it had done under an instruction and did so long after this instruction had been reversed to its opposite. Thus the stretch reflex behaved as if mere repetition of one kind of command had created a semipermanent program that predicted the continuance of the established mode of responding and prohibited annulment of it by a reversal of the intended aim.

In concluding with these remarks on "anticipation", I am fully aware of having left out facts, notions, and approaches that should have a place in an introduction to a history of motor control. Advances in the neurophysiology of the cerebellum, of the eye movements, and of respiratory motor mechanisms are such omissions. These, however, will be fully treated by other authors in this *Handbook* and so little is to be gained by overlapping at a lower level of knowledge with the specialists in these fields. My neglect of presynaptic inhibition and of dorsal root potentials is motivated by difficulties in assessing their precise significance for motor acts. On the whole, controlled motor operations have been best analyzed when it has been possible to deal with them in terms of the linked actions of α- and γ-motoneurons, the final executives.

REFERENCES

1. ADAMS, J. A. Human tracking behavior. *Psychol. Rev.* 58: 55–79, 1961.
2. ADAMS, J. A., AND L. R. CREAMER. Proprioception variables as determiners of anticipatory timing behavior. *Hum. Factors* 4: 217–222, 1962.
3. ADRIAN, E. D. *The Basis of Sensation*. London: Christophers, 1928.
4. ADRIAN, E. D. *The Mechanism of Nervous Action. Electrical Studies of the Neurone*. London: Oxford Univ. Press, 1932.
5. ADRIAN, E. D., AND D. W. BRONK. The discharge of impulses in motor nerve fibers. Part II. The frequency of discharge in reflex and voluntary contractions. *J. Physiol. London* 67: 119–151, 1929.
6. ADRIAN, E. D., AND Y. ZOTTERMAN. The impulses produced by sensory nerve-endings. Part II. The responses of a single end-organ. *J. Physiol. London* 61: 151–171, 1926.
7. ASANUMA, H. Recent developments in the study of the columnar arrangement of neurons within the motor cortex. *Physiol. Rev.* 55: 143–156, 1975.
8. BARKER, D. (editor). *Symposium on Muscle Receptors*. Hong Kong: Hong Kong Univ. Press, 1962. (Hong Kong. Univ., 1961.)
9. BARNHART, M., R. RHINES, J. C. MCCARTER, AND H. W. MAGOUN. Distribution of lesions of the brain stem in poliomyelitis. *Arch. Neurol. Psychiatry* 59: 368–377, 1948.
10. BASTIAN, C. The "muscular sense"; its nature and cortical localisation. *Brain* 10: 1–89, 1887.
11. BELL, C. On the nervous circle which connects the voluntary muscles with the brain. *Philos. Trans. R. Soc. London* 116: 163–173, 1826.
12. BELL, C. *The Hand*. London: Pickering, 1833.
13. BIEDERMANN, W. *Elektrophysiologie II*. Jena: Fischer, 1895.
14. BOER, S. DE. Die Bedeutung der tonischen Innervation für die Funktion der quergestreiften Muskeln. *Z. Biol. Munich* 65: 239–354, 1914–15.
15. BOYD, I. A. The structure and innervation of the nuclear bag muscle fibre system and the nuclear chain muscle fibre system in mammalian muscle spindles. *Philos. Trans. R. Soc. London Ser. B* 245: 81–136, 1962.
16. BOYD, I. A. The response of fast and slow nuclear bag fibres and nuclear chain fibres in isolated cat muscle spindles to fusimotor stimulation, and the effect of intrafusal contraction on the sensory endings. *Q. J. Exp. Physiol.* 61: 203–254, 1976.
17. BRAIN, R. The neurology of language. *Brain* 84: 145–166, 1961.
18. BREMER, F. Le tonus musculaire. *Ergeb. Physiol.* 34: 678–740, 1932.
19. BRODAL, A. *The Reticular Formation of the Brain Stem: Anatomical Aspects and Functional Correlations*. Edinburgh: Oliver & Boyd, 1957.
20. BRONDGEEST, P. J. Untersuchungen über den Tonus der willkürlichen Muskeln. *Arch. Anat. Physiol. Physiol. Abt.* 703–704, 1860.
21. BROOKS, V. B. Roles of cerebellum and basal ganglia in initiation and control of movements. *Can. J. Neurol. Sci.* 2: 265–277, 1975.
22. BROOKS, V. B., K. KAMEDA, AND R. NAGEL. Recurrent inhibition in the cat's cerebral cortex. In: *Inhibitory Neuronal Mechanisms*, edited by C. von Euler, S. Skoglund, and U. Söderberg. Oxford: Pergamon, 1968, p. 327–331.
23. BURKE, R. E. Composite nature of the monosynaptic excitatory postsynaptic potential. *J. Neurophysiol.* 30: 1114–1137, 1967.
24. BURKE, R. E., AND P. TSAIRIS. The correlation of physiological properties with histochemical properties in single muscle units. *Ann. NY Acad. Sci.* 228: 145–158, 1974.
25. CAMIS, M. *The Physiology of the Vestibular Apparatus*. Oxford: Clarendon, 1930. [Transl. by R. S. Creed].
26. CHRISTINA, R. W. Proprioception as a basis of anticipatory timing behavior. In: *Motor Control: Issues and Trends*, edited by G. E. Stelmach. New York: Academic, 1976, p. 187–199.
27. COHEN, LORD OF BIRKENHEAD. *Sherrington: Physiologist, Philosopher, and Poet. Sherrington Lectures*. Liverpool: Liverpool Univ. Press, 1958.
28. CREED, R. S., D. DENNY-BROWN, J. C. ECCLES, E. G. T. LIDDELL, AND C. S. SHERRINGTON. *Reflex Activity of the Spinal Cord*. Oxford: Clarendon, 1932.
29. DAWSON, G. D. Cerebral responses to nerve stimulation in man. *Br. Med. Bull.* 6: 326, 1950.
30. DEECKE, L., P. SCHEID, AND H. H. KORNHUBER. Distribution of readiness potential, pre-motion positivity, and motor potential of the human cerebral cortex preceding voluntary finger movements. *Exp. Brain Res.* 7: 158–168, 1969.
31. DELONG, M. R. Activity of pallidal neurons during movement. *J. Neurophysiol.* 34: 414–427, 1971.
32. DENNY-BROWN, D. B. On the nature of postural reflexes. *Proc. R. Soc. London Ser. B* 104: 252–301, 1929.
33. DENNY-BROWN, D. B. *The Cerebral Control of Movement. Sherrington Lectures*. Liverpool: Liverpool Univ. Press, 1966.
34. DOW, R. S., AND G. MORUZZI. *Physiology and Pathology of the Cerebellum*. Minneapolis: Univ. Minnesota Press, 1958.
35. DUCHENNE, G. B. *Physiologie des Mouvements*. Paris: Baillière, 1867, [*Physiology of Motion*, transl. by E. B. Kaplan. Philadelphia: Lippincott, 1949.]
36. ECCLES, J. C. *The Neurophysiological Basis of Mind*. Oxford: Clarendon, 1953.
37. ECCLES, J. C. *The Physiology of Synapses*. Berlin: Springer-Verlag, 1964.
38. ECCLES, J. C. *Physiology of Nerve Cells*. Baltimore: Johns Hopkins Univ. Press, H 1957.
39. ECCLES, J. C., P. FATT, AND K. KOKETSU. Cholinergic and

inhibitory synapses in a pathway from motor-axon collaterals to motoneurones. *J. Physiol. London* 126: 524-562, 1954.
40. ELDRED, E., AND K.-E. HAGBARTH. Facilitation and inhibition of gamma efferents by stimulation of certain skin areas. *J. Neurophysiol.* 17: 59-65, 1954.
41. ERLANGER, J., AND H. S. GASSER. *Electrical Signs of Nervous Activity*. Philadelphia: Univ. Pennsylvania Press, 1937.
42. EVARTS, E. V. Pyramidal tract activity associated with a conditioned hand movement in the monkey. *J. Neurophysiol.* 29: 1011-1027, 1966.
43. EVARTS, E. V. Representation of movements and muscles by pyramidal tract neurons of the precentral motor cortex. In: *Neurophysiological Basis of Normal and Abnormal Motor Activities*, edited by M. D. Yahr and D. P. Purpura. New York: Raven, 1967, p. 215-251. (Symp. Parkinson's Disease, 3rd, Columbia Univ., 1966).
43a. EVARTS, E. V., AND R. GRANIT. Relations of reflexes and intended movements. In: *Progress in Brain Research. Understanding the Stretch Reflex*, edited by S. Homma. Amsterdam: Elsevier, 1976, vol. 44, p. 1-14.
44. FICK, A. *Mechanische Arbeit und Wärmeentwicklung bei der Muskelthätigkeit*. Leipzig: Brockhaus, 1882.
45. FLOWERS, K. Some frequency response characteristics of Parkinsonism on pursuit tracking. *Brain* 101: 19-34, 1978.
46. FLOWERS, K. Lack of prediction in the motor behaviour of Parkinsonism. *Brain* 101: 35-52, 1978.
47. FOSTER, M. *A Textbook of Physiology*. London: Macmillan 1879.
48. FREY, M. VON. Studien über den Kraftsinn. *Z. Biol. Munich* 63: 129-154, 1914.
49. FREY, M. VON. Die Vergleichung von Gewichten mit Hilfe des Kraftsinns. *Z. Biol. Munich* 65: 203-238, 1915.
50. FREY, M. VON. Über Bewegungswahrnehmungen und Bewegungen in resezierten und in anästhetischen Gelenken. *Z. Biol. Munich* 68: 339-350, 1917-18.
51. FREY, M. VON Fortgesetzte Untersuchungen über die sinnesphysiologichen Grundlagen der Bewegungswahrnemungen. *Z. Neurol. Psychol.* 104: 821-831, 1926.
52. FRITSCH, G., AND E. HITZIG. Ueber die elektrische Erregbarkeit des Grosshirns. *Arch. Anat. Physiol. Physiol. Abt.*: 300-302, 1870.
53. FULTON, J. F. *Muscular Contraction and the Reflex Control of Movement*. Baltimore: William & Wilkins, 1926.
54. FULTON, J. F. *Physiology of the Nervous System* (3rd ed.). New York: Oxford Univ. Press, 1949.
55. GASKELL, W. H. On the action of muscarine upon the heart, and on the electrical changes in the non-beating cardiac muscle brought about by stimulation of the inhibitory and augmentor nerves. *J. Physiol. London* 8: 404-415, 1887.
56. GIBBS, C. B. The continuous regulation of skilled response by kinaesthetic feed back. *Brit. J. Psychol.* 45: 24-39, 1954.
57. GILDEN, L., H. G. VAUGHAN, JR., AND L. D. COSTA. Summated human EEG potentials with voluntary movement. *Electroencephalogr. Clin. Neurophysiol.* 20: 433-438, 1966.
58. GOLDSCHEIDER, A. *Gesammelte Abhandlungen II, Physiologie des Muskelsinnes*. Leipzig: Barth, 1898.
59. GOLGI, C. La cellula nervosa motrice. In: *Opera Omnia Ch. XVII*. Milano: Hoepli, 1903, vol. II., p. 537-542.
60. GOLTZ, F. Ueber die Funktionen des Lendenmarks des Hundes. *Pflueger's Arch. Gesamte Physiol. Menschen Tiere* 8: 460-498, 1874.
61. GRAHAM, J., AND R. W. GERARD. Membrane potentials and excitation of impaled single muscle fibers. *J. Cell. Comp. Physiol.* 28: 99-117, 1946.
62. GRANIT, R. *Receptors and Sensory Perception. Silliman Lectures*. New Haven: Yale Univ. Press, 1955.
63. GRANIT, R. (editor). *Muscular Afferents and Motor Control*. Stockholm: Almqvist & Wiksell, 1966. (Proc. Nobel Symp. I, Stockholm, 1965.)
64. GRANIT, R. *Charles Scott Sherrington, an Appraisal*. London: Nelson, 1966.
65. GRANIT, R. *Basis of Motor Control*. London: Academic, 1970.
66. GRANIT, R. Constant errors in the execution and appreciation of movement. *Brain* 95: 649-660, 1972.
67. GRANIT, R. The functional role of the muscle spindles—facts and hypotheses. *Brain* 98: 531-556, 1975.
68. GRANIT, R. *The Purposive Brain*. Cambridge: MIT Press, 1977.
69. GRANIT, R., H.-D. HENATSCH, AND G. STEG. Tonic and phasic ventral horn cells differentiated by post-tetanic potentiation in cat extensors. *Acta Physiol. Scand.* 37: 114-126, 1956.
70. GRANIT, R., AND B. R. KAADA. Influence of stimulation of central nervous structures on muscle spindles in the cat. *Acta Physiol. Scand.* 27: 130-160, 1952.
71. GRANIT, R., AND G. STRÖM. Autogenetic modulation of excitability of single ventral horn cells. *J. Neurophysiol.* 14: 113-132, 1951.
72. GRILLNER, S. The influence of DOPA on the static and the dynamic fusimotor activity to the triceps surae of the spinal cat. *Acta Physiol. Scand.* 77: 490-509, 1969.
73. HAASE, J., S. CLEVELAND, AND H.-G. ROSS. Problems of postsynaptic autogenous and recurrent inhibition in the mammalian spinal cord. *Rev. Physiol. Biochem. and Pharmacol.* 73: 73-129, 1975.
73a. HAGBARTH, K.-E. EMG studies of stretch reflexes in man. In: *Recent Advances in Clinical Neurophysiology*, edited by L. Widén. Amsterdam: Elsevier, 1967, p. 74-79.
74. HAGBARTH, K.-E., AND Å. B. VALLBO. Single unit recordings from muscle nerves in human subjects. *Acta Physiol. Scand.* 76: 321-334, 1969.
75. HANSEN, K., AND P. HOFFMANN. Über durch Vibration erzeugte Reflexreihen am Normalen und am Kranken. *Z. Biol. Munich* 74: 229-236, 1921.
76. HASSLER, R. Die extrapyramidalen Rindensysteme und die zentrale Regelung der Motorik. *Dtsch. Z. Nervenheilkd.* 175: 233-258, 1956.
77. HASSLER, R. Thalamic regulation of muscle tone and the speed of movement. In: *The Thalamus*, edited by M. D. Yahr and D. P. Purpura. New York: Columbia Univ. Press, 1966, p. 419-438.
78. HENNEMAN, E. Relation between size of neurons and their susceptibility to discharge. *Science* 126: 1345-1347, 1957.
79. HESS, W. R. *Das Zwischenhirn*. Basel: Schwabe, 1949.
80. HILL, A. V. The maximum work and mechanical efficiency of human muscles, and their most economical speed. *J. Physiol. London* 56: 19-41, 1922.
81. HODGKIN, A. L., AND A. F. HUXLEY. A quantitative description of membrane current and its application to conduction and excitation in nerve. *J. Physiol. London* 117: 500-544, 1952.
82. HOFFMANN, P. Demonstration eines Hemmungsreflexes im menschlichen Rückenmark. *Z. Biol. Munich* 70: 515-524, 1919-20.
83. HOFFMANN, P. *Untersuchungen über die Eigenreflexe (Sehnenreflexe) menschlicher Muskeln*. Berlin: Springer-Verlag, 1922.
84. HOMMA, S. (editor). *Progress in Brain Research. Understanding the Stretch Reflex*. Amsterdam: Elsevier, 1976, vol. 44.
85. HORNYKIEWICZ, O. Parkinson's disease: from brain homogenate to treatment. *Federation Proc.* 32: 183-190, 1973.
86. HORSLEY, V., AND R. H. CLARKE. The structure and functions of the cerebellum examined by a new method. *Brain* 31: 45-124, 1908.
87. HOWARD, I. P., AND W. B. TEMPLETON. *Human Spatial Orientation*. New York: Wiley, 1966.
88. HULTBORN, H. Convergence of interneurones in the reciprocal Ia inhibitory pathway to motoneurones. *Acta Physiol. Scand. Suppl.* 375: 1-42, 1972.
89. HUNT, C. C. The reflex activity of mammalian small-nerve fibres. *J. Physiol. London* 115: 456-469, 1951.
90. HUXLEY, A. F., AND H. E. HUXLEY. A discussion on the physical and chemical basis of muscular contraction. *Proc. R. Soc. London Ser. B* 160: 433-542, 1964.
91. INGVAR, D. H., AND N. A. LASSEN (editors). *Brain Work*. Copenhagen: Munksgaard, 1975.
92. ITO, M. Neural design of the cerebellar motor control system. *Brain Res.* 40: 81-84, 1972.

93. JACOBSON, M. *Developmental Neurobiology.* New York: Holt, Rinehart, Winston, 1970. (Developmental Biol. Ser.)
94. JAMES, W. *The Principles of Psychology.* New York: Macmillan, 1891.
95. JANKOWSKA, E., AND S. LINDSTRÖM. Morphology of interneurones mediating Ia reciprocal inhibition of motoneurones in the spinal cord. *J. Physiol. London* 226: 805–823, 1972.
96. JUNG, R., AND R. HASSLER. The extrapyramidal motor system. In: *Handbook of Physiology. Neurophysiology,* edited by J. Field and H. W. Magoun Washington, DC: Am. Physiol. Soc., 1960, sect. 1, vol. II, chapt. 35, p. 863–927.
97. KAPPERS, C. U. A., G. C. HUBER, AND E. C. CROSBY. *The Comparative Anatomy of the Nervous System of Vertebrates Including Man.* New York: Macmillan, 1936.
98. KATZ, B. *The Release of Neural Transmitter Substances. Sherrington Lectures,* Liverpool: Liverpool Univ. Press, 1969.
99. KEMP, J. M., AND T. P. S. POWELL. The connections of the striatum and globus pallidus: synthesis and speculation. *Philos. Trans. R. Soc. London Ser. B* 262: 441–457, 1971.
100. KERNELL, D. The repetitive discharge of motoneurones. In: *Muscular Afferents and Motor Control.* edited by R. Granit. Stockholm: Almqvist & Wiksell, 1966, p. 351–362. (Proc. Nobel Symp. I., Stockholm, 1965.)
101. KOBAYASHI, Y., K. OSHIMA, AND I. TASAKI. Analysis of afferent and efferent systems in the muscle nerve of the toad and cat. *J. Physiol. London* 117: 152–171, 1952.
102. KORNHUBER, H. H., AND L. DEECKE. Hirnpotentialänderungen beim Menschen vor und nach Willkürbewegungen, dargestellt mit Magnetbandspeicherung und Rückwärtsanalyse. *Pfluegers Arch.* 281: 52, 1964.
103. KRIES, J. VON. *Allgemeine Sinnesphysiologie.* Leipzig: Vogel, 1923.
104. KRNJEVIĆ, K. Chemical nature of synaptic transmission in vertebrates. *Physiol. Rev.* 54: 418–540, 1974.
105. LANDGREN, S., AND H. SILFVENIUS. Projection to cerebral cortex of Group I muscle afferents from the cat's hindlimb. *J. Physiol. London* 200: 353–372, 1969.
106. LASHLEY, K. S. The accuracy of movement in the absence of excitation from the moving organ. *Am. J. Physiol.* 43: 169–194, 1917.
107. LASHLEY, K. S. In search of the engram. In: *Brain Physiology and Psychology,* edited by C. R. Evans and A. D. J. Robertson. Berkeley: Univ. Calif. Press, 1966.
108. LEKSELL, L. The action potential and excitatory effects of the small ventral root fibres to skeletal muscle. *Acta Physiol. Scand.* 10: (Suppl. 31) 1945.
109. LIDDELL, E. G. T. *The Discovery of Reflexes.* Oxford:Clarendon, 1960.
110. LIDDELL, E. G. T., AND C. S. SHERRINGTON. Reflexes in response to stretch (myotatic reflexes). *Proc. R. Soc. London Ser. B* 96: 212–242, 1924.
111. LINDSTRÖM, S. Recurrent control from motor axon collaterals of Ia inhibitory pathways in the spinal cord of the cat. *Acta Physiol. Scand. Suppl.* 392: 1–43, 1973.
112. LING, G., AND R. W. GERARD. The normal membrane potential of frog sartorius fibers. *J. Cell. Comp. Physiol.* 34: 383–396, 1949.
113. LLOYD, D. P. C. Neuron patterns controlling transmission of ipsilateral hind limb reflexes in cat. *J. Neurophysiol.* 6: 293–315, 1943.
114. LLOYD, D. P. C. Conduction and synaptic transmission of the reflex response to stretch in spinal cats. *J. Neurophysiol.* 6: 317–326, 1943.
115. LLOYD, D. P. C., AND A. K. MCINTYRE. Monosynaptic reflex responses of individual motoneurons. *J. Gen. Physiol.* 38: 771–787, 1955.
116. LORENTE DE NÓ, R. The synaptic delay of the motoneurons. *Am. J. Physiol.* 111: 272–282, 1935.
117. LORENTE DE NÓ, R. Limits of variation of the synaptic delay of motoneurons. *J. Neurophysiol.* 1: 187–194, 1938.
118. LUNDBERG, A. Integration in the reflex pathway. In: *Muscular Afferents and Motor Control,* edited by R. Granit. Stockholm: Almqvist & Wiksell, 1966, p. 275–305. (Proc. Nobel Symp. I, Stockholm, 1965.)
119. LUNDBERG, A. Control of spinal mechanisms from the brain. In: *The Nervous System. Basic Neurosciences,* edited by D. B. Tower. New York: Raven, 1975, vol. I, p. 253–265.
120. MAGLADERY, J. W., AND D. B. MCDOUGAL JR. Electrophysiological studies of nerve and reflex activity in normal man. I. Identification of certain reflexes in the electromyogram and the conduction velocity of peripheral nerve fibres. *Bull. Johns Hopkins Hosp.* 86: 205–290, 1950.
121. MAGNUS, R. *Körperstellung.* Berlin: Springer-Verlag, 1924.
122. MAGOUN, H. W. *The Waking Brain.* Springfield, IL: Thomas, 1958.
123. MAGOUN, H. W., AND R. RHINES. *Spasticity: Stretch-Reflex and Extrapyramidal Systems.* Springfield, IL: Thomas, 1947.
124. MARTIN, J. P. *The Basal Ganglia and Posture.* London: Pitman, 1967.
125. MATTHEWS, B. H. C. Nerve endings in mammalian muscle. *J. Physiol. London* 78: 1–33, 1933.
126. MATTHEWS, P. B. C. The differentiation of two types of fusimotor fibre by their effects on the dynamic response of muscle primary endings. *Q. J. Exp. Physiol.* 47: 324–333, 1962.
127. MATTHEWS, P. B. C. *Mammalian Muscle Receptors and their Central Action.* London: Arnold, 1972.
128. MELVILL JONES, G., AND D. G. D. WATT. Muscular control of landing from unexpected falls in man. *J. Physiol. London* 219: 729–737, 1971.
129. MERTON, P. A. Speculations on the servo-control of movement. In: *The Spinal Cord,* edited by J. E. W. Wolstenholme. London: Churchill, 1953, p. 247–255. (Ciba Symp.)
130. MONAKOW, C. VON. Über den gegenwärtigen Stand der Frage nach der Lokalisation im Grosshirn. *Ergeb. Physiol.* 1: 534–665, 1902.
131. MORUZZI, G., AND H. W. MAGOUN. Brain stem reticular formation and activation of the EEG. *Electroencephalogr. Clin. Neurophysiol.* 4: 455–473, 1949.
132. MÜLLER, J. *Handbuch der Physiologie des Menschen. Band II.* Coblenz: Hölscher, 1838.
133. NASTUK, W. L., AND A. L. HODGKIN. The electrical activity of single muscle fibers. *J. Cell. Comp. Physiol.* 35: 39–74, 1950.
134. NATHAN, P. W., AND T. A. SEARS. Effects of posterior root section on the activity of some muscles in man. *J. Neurol. Psychiatry* 23: 10–22, 1960.
135. OSCARSSON, O. The projection of Group I muscle afferents to the cat cerebral cortex. In: *Muscular Afferents and Motor Control,* edited by R. Granit. Stockholm: Almqvist & Wiksell, 1966, p. 307–316. (Proc. Nobel Symp. I, Stockholm, 1965.)
136. PAILLARD, J., AND M. BROUCHON. Active and passive movement in the calibration of position sense. In: *The Neurophysiology of Spatially Oriented Behavior,* edited by S. J. Freedman. Homewood, IL: Dorsey, 1968, p. 37–55.
137. PAPEZ, J. W. Reticulo-spinal tracts in the cat. *J. Comp. Neurol.* 41: 365–399, 1926.
138. PHILLIPS, C. G., AND R. PORTER. *Corticospinal Neurones: Their Role in Movement.* London: Academic, 1977.
139. PHILLIPS, C. G., T. P. S. POWELL, AND M. WIESENDANGER. Projections from low-threshold muscle afferents of hand and forearm to area 3a of baboon's cortex. *J. Physiol. London* 217: 419–446, 1971.
140. PITTS, R. F., H. W. MAGOUN, AND S. W. RANSON. Localization of the medullary respiratory centers in the cat. *Am. J. Physiol.* 126: 673–688, 1939.
141. POLLOCK, L. J., AND L. DAVIS. The influence of the cerebellum upon the reflex activities of the decerebrate animal. *Brain* 50: 277–312, 1927.
142. POLLOCK, L. J., AND L. DAVIS. Studies in decerebration. V. The tonic activities of a decerebrate animal exclusive of the neck and labyrinthine reflexes. *Am. J. Physiol.* 92: 625–629, 1930.
143. POLYAK, S. *The Vertebrate Visual System,* Chicago: Univ. Chicago Press, 1947.
144. PRUS, J. Ueber die Leitungsbahnen und Pathogenese der Rin-

denepilepsie. *Wien. Klin. Wochenschr.* 857–863, 1898.
145. RADEMAKER, G. G. J. *Die Bedeutung der roten Kerne und des übrigen Mittelhirns für Muskeltonus, Körperstellung und Labyrinthreflexe.* Berlin: Springer-Verlag, 1926.
146. RALL, W. Distinguishing theoretical synaptic potentials computed for different soma-dendritic distributions of synaptic input. *J. Neurophysiol.* 30: 1138–1168, 1967.
147. RAMÓN Y CAJAL, S. *Histologie du Système Nerveux (Fr.ed.).* Madrid: Instituto Ramón y Cajal, 1952.
148. RANSON, S. W., AND H. W. MAGOUN. The hypothalamus. *Ergeb. Physiol.* 41: 56–163, 1939.
149. RANVIER, L. *Leçons d'Anatomie Générale sur le Système Musculaire.* Paris: Delahaye, 1880.
150. RENQVIST, Y. Über die den Bewegungswahrnehmungen zugrunde liegenden Reize. *Skand. Arch. Physiol.* 50: 52–96, 1926.
151. RENQVIST, Y. Ueber die Reizschwelle der Kraftempfindungen. *Z. Biol. Munich* 85: 391–405, 1926.
152. RENSHAW, B. Activity in the simplest spinal reflex pathways. *J. Neurophysiol.* 3: 373–387, 1940.
153. RENSHAW, B. Central effects of centripetal impulses in axons of spinal ventral roots. *J. Neurophysiol.* 9: 191–204, 1946.
154. ROSSI, G. Asimmetrie toniche posturale, ed asimetrie motorie. *Arch. Fisiol.* 25: 146–157, 1927.
155. ROSSI, G. F., AND A. ZANCHETTI. The brain stem reticular formation. *Arch. Ital. Biol.* 95: 199–435, 1957.
156. ROTHMANN, M. Über die physiologische Wertung der corticospinalen (Pyramiden-) Bahn. *Arch. Anat. Physiol. Physiol. Abt.* 217–275, 1907.
157. RUFFINI, A. Observations on sensory nerve-endings in voluntary muscles. *Brain* 20: 368–374, 1897.
158. RUFFINI, A. On the minute anatomy of neuromuscular spindles of the cat, and on their physiological significance. *J. Physiol. London* 23: 190–208, 1898–99.
159. SCHIFF, J. M. *Lehrbuch der Physiologie des Menschen I.* Lahr: Schauenburg, 1859.
160. SCHMIDT, R. A. The schema as a solution to some persistent problems in motor learning theory. In: *Motor Control: Issues and Trends,* edited by G. E. Stelmach. New York: Academic, 1976, p. 41–65.
161. SETCHENOV, J. *Physiologische Studien über die Hemmungsmechanismen für die Reflexthätigkeit des Rückenmarks im Gehirne des Frosches.* Berlin: Hirschwald, 1863.
162. SHERRINGTON, C. S. The muscular sense. In: *Textbook of Physiology,* edited by E. A. Schäfer. London: Pentland, 1900, vol. 2, p. 1002–1025.
163. SHERRINGTON, C. S. *Integrative Action of the Nervous System. Silliman Lectures.* New Haven: Yale Univ. Press, 1906.
164. SHERRINGTON, C. S. *Selected Writings of Sir Charles Sherrington,* edited by D. Denny-Brown. London: Hamish Hamilton, 1939.
165. SKAVENSKI, A. A. Inflow as a source of extraretinal eye position information. *Vision Res.* 12: 221–229, 1971.
166. SMITH, R. S. Properties of intrafusal muscle fibres. In: *Muscular Afferents and Motor Control,* edited by R. Granit. Stockholm: Almqvist & Wiksell, 1966, p. 69–80. (Proc. Nobel Symp. I, Stockholm, 1965.)
167. SPRAGUE, J. M., AND W. W. CHAMBERS. Control of posture by reticular formation and cerebellum in the intact, anesthetized and unanesthetized and in the decerebrated cat. *Am. J. Physiol.* 176: 52–64, 1954.
168. STARK, L. *Neurological Control Systems: Studies in Bioengineering.* New York: Plenum, 1968.
169. STARLINGER, J. Die Durchschneidung beider Pyramiden beim Hunde. *Neurol. Zentralbl.* 14: 390–394, 1885.
170. SWAZEY, J. P. *Reflexes and Motor Integration: Sherrington's Concept of Integrative Action.* Cambridge: Harvard Univ. Press, 1969.
171. TAYLOR, J. (editor). *Selected writings of Hughlings Jackson.* London: Hodder and Stoughton, 1931.
172. TOWER, S. The dissociation of cortical excitation from cortical inhibition by pyramid section, and the syndrome of that lesion in the cat. *Brain* 58: 238–255, 1935.
173. TOWER, S. Pyramidal lesion in the monkey. *Brain* 63: 36–90, 1940.
174. UNGERSTEDT, U. Stereotaxic mapping of the monoamine pathways in the rat brain. *Acta Physiol. Scand. Suppl.* 367: 1–48, 1971.
175. VALLBO, Å. B. Discharge patterns in human muscle spindle afferents during isometric voluntary contractions. *Acta Physiol. Scand.* 80: 552–556, 1970.
176. VULPIAN, E. F. A. *Leçons sur la Physiologie Générale et Comparée du Système Nerveux.* Paris: 1866.
177. WATANABE, S. (editor). *Vibratory Stimuli and the Tonic Vibration Reflex.* Tokyo: Saikon, 1977.
178. WEINER, N. *Cybernetics or Control of Communication in the Animal and the Machine* (2nd ed.). Cambridge: MIT Press, 1961.
179. WOODBURY, J. W., AND H. D. PATTON. Electrical activity of single spinal cord elements. *Cold Spring Harbor Symp. Quant. Biol.* 17: 185–188, 1952.

CHAPTER 2

Mechanics of skeleton and tendons

R. McNEILL ALEXANDER | *Department of Pure and Applied Zoology, University of Leeds, England*

CHAPTER CONTENTS

Basic Kinematics
Kinematics of Joints
Number of Muscles Required to Work Joints
Muscle Attachments
Moment Arms and Pennation Patterns
Properties of Skeletal Materials
Statics of Skeleton
Dynamics of Skeleton
Dynamics of Body
Stresses and Strains in Tendons
Stresses and Strains in Bones
Engineering Design of Bones
Conclusion

A PHYSIOLOGIST CONCERNED with coordination needs to be able to describe movements precisely. He needs to know how the ranges and variety of possible movements depend on the structure of joints and the arrangement of muscles. He may wish to know the forces that muscles must exert or that the skeleton must withstand in particular activities. He may wish to know which of several alternative coordination patterns enable an animal to move with the least expense of energy. For all these reasons, a volume about coordination needs a chapter about mechanics.

The title of this chapter refers only to the skeleton and tendons, but muscles are also mentioned frequently because they move the skeleton and exert forces on it. This chapter considers the numbers of muscles needed to move joints; it shows how muscles attach to the skeleton; and it shows how differences in the fiber arrangement of muscles are functionally equivalent to differences of lever arm. Other topics in muscle mechanics are dealt with in the chapter by Partridge and Benton in this *Handbook*.

BASIC KINEMATICS

Kinematics is the branch of mechanics concerned with the description of movement; therefore it is particularly useful to physiologists who are interested in the coordination of movement. This section gives a brief account of some of the principals of kinematics, which are used later in this chapter. Fuller accounts can be found in engineering textbooks (e.g., refs. 41, 56). Animals and other mechanisms move in three-dimensional space, but three-dimensional movements are rather difficult to describe and to represent on a two-dimensional page. Fortunately many movements of machines and some movements of animals can be treated as plane (two-dimensional) motion. The movement of a machine is plane motion if the velocity of every point on every part of it is always parallel to a single, fixed plane. Many machines are designed for plane motion. Animals seldom or never practice true plane motion, but it is sometimes convenient to treat their movements as plane motion. For instance, it is sometimes sufficiently accurate to treat human walking as plane motion, since all the limb segments move more or less parallel to the sagittal plane. It is often convenient to describe plane motion as if all the movements were occurring in the same plane, although the left and right arms (for instance) move in different, parallel planes.

Any plane movement of a rigid body can be described as a rotation about an axis at right angles to the planes in which the movement occurred. If the movement is treated as occurring in a single plane, this axis becomes a point in the plane and is known as the instantaneous center. Figure 1A shows two successive positions of a body in the plane defined by the axes 0X and 0Y. Movement from one position to the other can be described as a rotation through an angle ϕ about the instantaneous center (x_0, y_0). This center can be located by a construction dependent on the fact that when a body rotates about an axis, every point on the body moves at right angles to the radius on which it lies. Select two readily identifiable points, A and B, on the body. They are initially at A_1, B_1 and move to A_2, B_2. Draw lines A_1, A_2 and B_1, B_2 and their perpendicular bisectors. The latter intersect at the instantaneous center.

In general, movements in three-dimensional space cannot be described simply as rotation about a single axis. They can always be described, however, as a combination of rotation about an axis and displace-

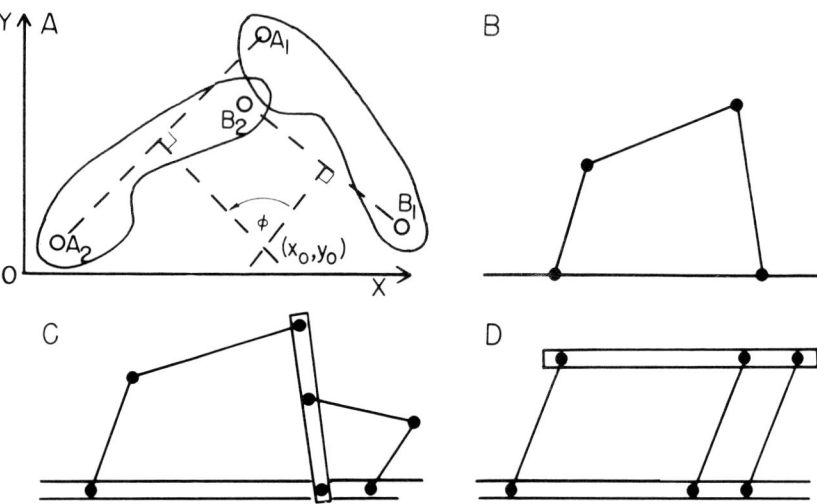

FIG. 1. *A*: two positions of a body moving in a plane, showing how instantaneous center (x_0, y_0) can be located. *B–D*: mechanisms consisting of rigid bars joined by hinges with axes perpendicular to paper. Each of these mechanisms has 1 degree of freedom.

ment along the same axis. This axis is called the screw axis because tightening a screw rotates the screw about its axis and moves it along its axis. There seems to be no simple construction capable of locating the screw axis, but Kinzel et al. (43) have shown how its location can be obtained by computation.

There are many conceivable alternative ways of describing a particular movement, and confusion may arise if different investigators describe the same movement in different ways. A description using the screw axis (or instantaneous center, for plane motion) has the advantage of being unique and is often to be preferred.

Any plane motion of a rigid body (Fig. 1*A*) can be described by specifying just three quantities, for instance, the angle of rotation about the instantaneous center (ϕ) and the two coordinates of the instantaneous center (x_0, y_0). Hence a body that is restricted to plane movement but is otherwise free is said to have three degrees of freedom of movement.

A rigid body moving freely in space has six degrees of freedom, for six quantities are needed to describe a movement. These can be, for example, the angle of rotation around the screw axis, the displacement along the screw axis, and four additional quantities which are needed to define the screw axis. If mutually perpendicular axes 0X, 0Y, and 0Z are used as a frame of reference, the screw axis can be defined by stating the X and Y coordinates of its intersection with the XY plane and the X and Z coordinates of its intersection with the XZ plane.

To specify the position of a rigid body in space we need information about the location of at least three points on it. These three points must not be in line. Two points are not enough because the body could be rotated about the axis through them without changing their positions.

We have to consider next the effects of joints. Consider two rigid bodies and regard one as fixed since we are concerned only with relative movement between them. If the bodies are not connected, the movable one has six degrees of freedom. If they are connected by a joint, the movable body has fewer degrees of freedom. If it has F degrees of freedom, F quantities suffice to describe its current position.

Figures 2*A*–*C* show examples of joints allowing just one degree of freedom of relative movement. Figure 2*A* represents a door hinged to a wall. The only movement the hinge allows is rotation about its axis, so any position of the door can be specified by a single quantity such as the angle θ or the distance x. In Figure 2*B* the only possible movement is sliding of the block along the bar so its position can be specified by a single quantity such as y. In Figure 2*C* the position of the nut can be specified either by the distance z or by the number of turns needed to tighten it. The hinge, the sliding joint, and the screw joint are the only joints that restrict movement to a single degree of freedom.

Figure 2*D* shows a universal joint, as used in the transmission systems of automobiles. It is in effect two hinges with their axes (AA and BB) mutually perpendicular. Two quantities (such as the angles of flexion at both joints) are needed to specify a position unambiguously, so one shaft has two degrees of freedom of movement relative to the other. In Figure 2*E* the block can rotate on the rod or slide along it, so two quantities (e.g., a distance and an angle) are needed to specify a position and the joint allows two degrees of freedom of relative movement. A ball-and-socket joint (Fig. 2*F*) allows rotation about any axis but a position can be specified by three quantities (for instance angles of flexion around AA, BB, and CC). It allows three degrees of freedom of relative movement.

Only a perfectly made joint would have its degrees of freedom strictly limited to the number intended; a

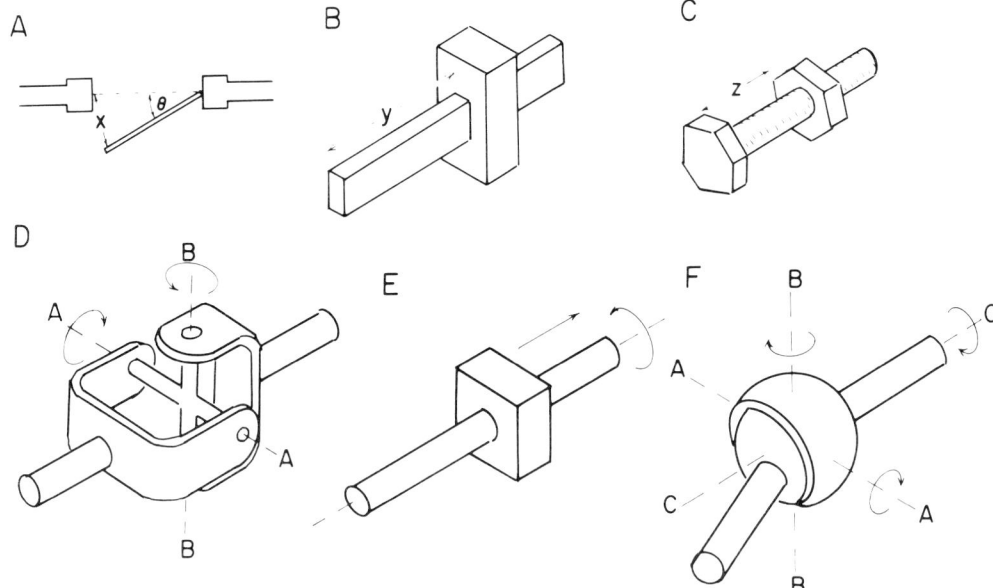

FIG. 2. *A–C*: examples of joints that allow 1 degree of freedom; *x*, *y*, and *z* are distances; θ is an angle. *D*, *E*: 2 degrees of freedom. *F*: 3 degrees of freedom of relative movement.

loosely fitting hinge, for instance, might allow some sliding as well as rotation. The degrees of freedom associated with such trivial movements are largely ignored in this chapter.

Now consider a system of rigid bodies connected by joints. Such a system is called a mechanism if relative movement between its parts is possible, and a structure if movement is not possible. A triangle of three bars hinged together is a structure, but four bars (Fig. 1*B*) form a mechanism if the axes of their connecting hinges are all parallel. The relative positions of the bars are defined by the angle between any two of them, so this mechanism has only one degree of freedom of relative movement. The hinged mechanism shown in Figure 1*C* also has one degree of freedom. These particular mechanisms are capable only of plane motion. Let a plane mechanism consist of n rigid bodies connected by j joints (each connecting just two bodies). Let j_1 of these joints be hinges or sliding joints allowing only one degree of freedom of relative movement in the plane. Let j_2 of the joints allow two degrees of freedom of relative movement in the plane ($j_1 + j_2 = j$). The system has F degrees of freedom of relative movement where

$$F = 3(n - 1) - 2j_1 - j_2 \qquad (1)$$

(If F is zero or negative the system is a structure, not a mechanism.) More generally for a three-dimensional mechanism, which has j_1 joints allowing one degree of freedom, j_2 joints allowing two degrees of freedom and so on

$$F = 6(n - 1) - \Sigma(6 - r)j_r \qquad (2)$$

(j_r is the number of joints allowing r degrees of freedom).

Equations 1 and 2 are generally reliable, but there are special cases of systems with more degrees of freedom than they predict. For example, the plane mechanism shown in Figure 1*D* consists of five bars connected by six hinges. Equation 1 predicts that it will have $3(5 - 1) - (2 \times 6) = 0$ degrees of freedom, but it actually has one degree of freedom because of the parallel arrangement of the bars.

KINEMATICS OF JOINTS

Man and other animals have a great variety of joints, but all of these cannot be discussed in this section. It is necessary to select a few examples that have been particularly well studied or that illustrate particular points. Some of the terms used in describing these movements require definition. In this chapter, flexion means the bending of a joint and extension means straightening a joint. The terms are used in these senses by many kinesiologists, but many human anatomists use different, more complex definitions (see ref. 70). These two terms are sufficient to describe the normal movements of joints such as the knee, but a third term is needed in some cases. If the movement of extension can be continued beyond the straight position, this further movement is called hyperextension. For instance the wrist can be flexed through about 90° (making the palm approach the forearm) or hyperextended through about 50° (making the back of the hand approach the forearm). Abduction generally means movement away from the medial plane, but is also used to describe movements of the hand and foot that spread the digits; adduction means the reverse. Protraction means movement in an anterior direction, and retraction means movement in a posterior direction. Rotation, if not further qualified, means rotation of a segment about its own long axis. There are additional terms, which are introduced as needed, that are peculiar to particular joints.

It has long been customary to describe the joint between the humerus and ulna as a hinge, and the joint between the ulna and radius as another hinge. The former allows flexion and extension of the elbow and the latter allows the hand to be turned to the prone or to the supine position (e.g., Fig. 9). The recent work of Youm and colleagues (75) has given new precision to this account. An arm was removed from a cadaver and three spark gaps each were attached rigidly to the ulna and to the radius. The humerus was clamped in a fixed position and the forearm was moved. A sonic digitizer system was used to obtain the three-dimensional Cartesian coordinates of each spark gap, at each position of the forearm. The positions relative to the spark gaps of the screw axes for different movements were computed from these coordinates. Finally the positions of the spark gaps relative to the bones were determined by taking X-radiographs in two mutually perpendicular directions, so that the positions of the screw axes could be related to the bones. It was found that the screw axis for flexion-extension was as shown in Figure 3A and that the screw axis for pronation-supination was as shown in Figure 3C, throughout the ranges of these movements. Little or nor movement occurs along the screw axes so the joints are, essentially, hinges.

These properties of the joints are easily explained in terms of their anatomy. Sections through the humerus and ulna, cut perpendicular to the screw axis, show the articulating surfaces as arcs of circles. If these surfaces were cylindrical and there were no ligaments to prevent it, the ulna could slide laterally on the humerus as well as flexing and extending, so the joint would behave like the one shown in Figure 2E. In fact, the articulating surfaces are more like a hyperboloid of one sheet than a cylinder; that is to say, the humerus is grooved like a pulley and the ulna is shaped to fit it. Because ligaments hold the two bones tightly together, sliding along the axis of the joint is effectively prevented. Figure 3B shows the main ligaments of the medial side of the joint. They radiate from attachments close to the axis of the joint so flexion and extension do not change the distance between the ends of each ligament very much. The ligaments neither become excessively slack at any position of the joint nor become so taut as to check its movement.

The proximal end of the radius has a short cylindrical head which fits a concavity in the ulna, and the distal end of the ulna has a convex surface, which fits a concavity in the radius. The two bones are held together by a sheet of collagen fibers (the interosseous membrane) and various ligaments including the annular ligament (Fig. 3C), which loops around the radius but is attached to the ulna at both ends.

The human wrist is a complex structure containing the eight carpal bones; nevertheless, it behaves essentially as a universal joint (Fig. 2D). All its movements can be described as combinations of flexion or extension and deviation to the radial or ulnar side. Andrews and Youm (13) studied the mobility of the wrists of living people while the arm was held stationary with the forearm pronated. A stiff plastic plate attached to the hand made the palm move as a rigid body. Attached spark gaps and a sonic digitizer system were used to locate the screw axes for flexion-extension and deviation. In each case the axis had a more or less constant position throughout the range of movement. Both axes passed through the capitate bone, but they did not quite intersect. The schematic diagrams in Figure 7 show that the superficially simple movements of flexion-extension and deviation involve movement both at the radiocarpal joint and at the intercarpal joint (see also ref. 76). There is a much simpler example of a universal joint at the bases of the fin rays of teleost fish (35).

Ball-and-socket joints occur in mammals at the hip and shoulder. The eye is also a ball that moves in a socket. A tightly fitted joint between two bones cannot allow three degrees of freedom of rotation unless the articulating surfaces are spherical. Neither the head of the femur nor the acetabulum is precisely spherical; nevertheless, they allow three degrees of freedom of relative movement because they do not fit each other tightly (18).

The joints described so far allow only rotary movements. There are others that allow linear movements. An example is the joint between the human tibia and fibula, which allows the fibula to slide proximally or distally. Small movements occur at this joint in running (71).

The jaw articulations of mammals allow both sliding and rotation. The jaws of cats and other carnivores have transversely elongated, roughly cylindrical condyles, which articulate in transverse grooves in the

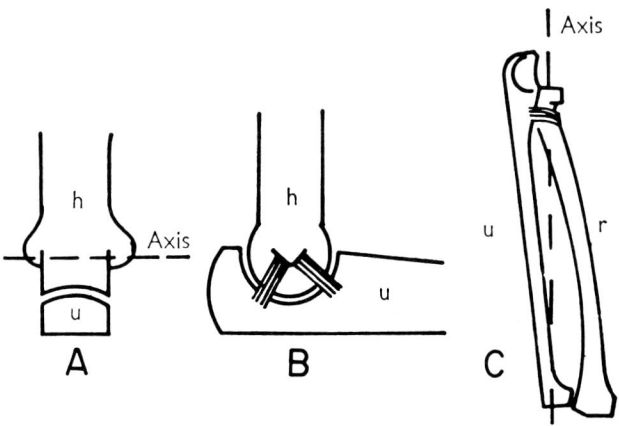

FIG. 3. Diagrams of bones and some of the ligaments of a human elbow and forearm: h, humerus; r, radius; u, ulna. A: section. B: medial view. [From Alexander (2).]

skull. They can slide transversely along the grooves as well as rotate in the grooves, so their movements are comparable to those of the joint shown in Figure 2E. [Scapino (58) has drawn attention to a third degree of freedom of movement in dogs: each half of the jaw can rotate a little about its own long axis.] The transverse-sliding movement is needed for the effective action of the carnassial teeth (Fig. 14), which cut food with a scissorlike action. These are the teeth dogs use when gnawing a bone with the side of the mouth. In carnivores as in other mammals, the lower jaw is narrower than the upper one, but carnivores can slide the lower jaw to the left or right. Therefore the cutting edges of the upper and lower carnassial teeth of one side are pressed tightly together and can cut effectively.

Rodents have a different jaw action which requires a different joint structure (39). The action is again a combination of rotation and sliding, but the direction of sliding is different. In carnivores the sliding is transverse, parallel to the axis of rotation. In rodents it is longitudinal, at right angles to the axis of rotation. The jaws can move forward so that the incisors bite against each other, as required for gnawing (Fig. 4, *top outlines*). Alternatively they can move back so that the lower incisors lie posterior to the upper ones, and the molars can be brought into contact with each

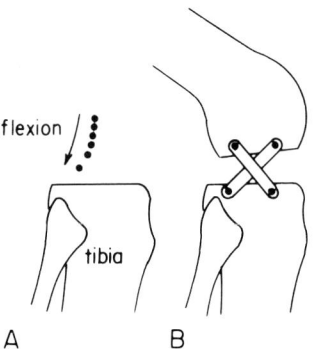

FIG. 5. *A*: outlines of a human tibia and fibula. *Dots* show successive positions of the instantaneous center of a normal knee during bending from 20° flexion. *B*: mechanism representing a knee joint. Further explanation is given in the text. [*A* data from Soudan et al. (66).]

other for chewing (Fig. 4, *bottom outlines*). Figure 4 shows that some anterior-posterior sliding is involved in both the gnawing and the chewing action as well as in the transition between them. The condyles of the lower jaw are knobs, which slide and rock in longitudinal grooves in the skull (not transverse grooves as in carnivores).

Many joints like those of the human forearm and wrist behave like hinges or universal joints with fixed axes. The human knee behaves like a hinge with a moving axis, and some ingenuity is needed to imitate it with man-made joints (40). The most complex part of the knee's motion is the three-dimensional "screw-home," which occurs in the last few degrees of extension (38). Over the rest of its range of movement, the knee exhibits very nearly plane motion and its instantaneous center can be located graphically using X-radiographs of successive positions (see Fig. 1A). Soudan et al. (66) have discussed the practical difficulties and have recommended a computational method in preference to the graphical one. They found that the instantaneous center moved during knee bending as shown in Figure 5A. Other investigators have found rather different paths for the instantaneous centers of normal knees (e.g., ref. 62).

The articulating surfaces of the knee do not fit closely, because the convex condyles of the femur rest on the relatively flat articular surface of the tibia. Movement is largely restricted to a single degree of freedom by ligaments, but since the ligaments are elastic, they also allow very limited movement in other degrees of freedom (48). With the femur held stationary the tibia can be adducted, abducted, or rotated through a few degrees, or displaced a few millimeters anteriorly or posteriorly.

There are ligaments on either side of the knee that connect the tibia to the femur. There is also a pair of cruciate ligaments in the gap between the two condyles of the femur (Fig. 6). If the shapes of the articulating surfaces and the positions of attachment of the cruciate ligaments were perfectly matched, flexion and

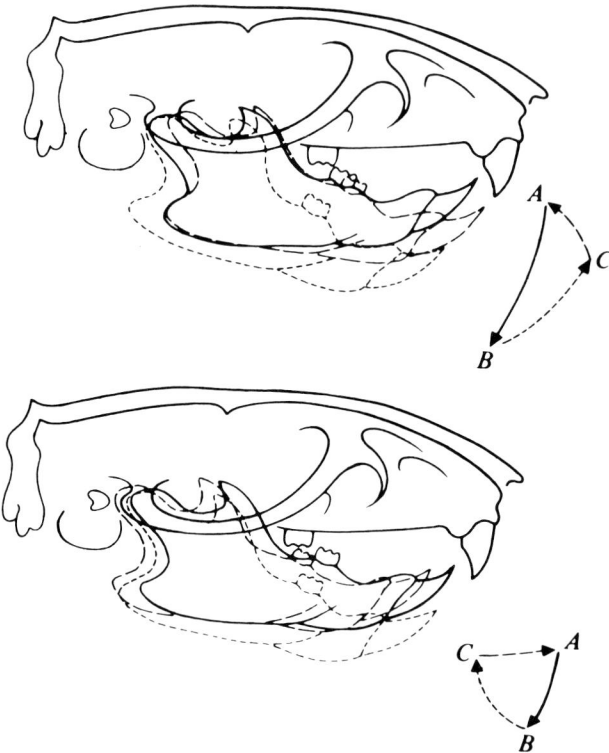

FIG. 4. Outlines of skull drawn from X-radiographs of rats (*Rattus norvegicus*) feeding. *Top outlines* show sequence of jaw positions involved in biting with incisors. *Bottom outlines* show sequence involved in chewing. *Arrows* A, B, C indicate sequence of movement in each case. [From Hiiemae (39) with permission from *Zool. J. Linn. Soc.*, vol 50, © 1971 Linnean Society of London.]

extension of the knee would neither stretch nor slacken the ligaments. Such an arrangement is represented in Figure 6 in which the ligaments have the same lengths in all three diagrams.

To keep both ligaments constant in length throughout its movement, the knee would have to move like the mechanism shown in Figure 5B. This diagram represents the ligaments as rigid bars hinged to the femur and tibia. It shows four bodies (two bones and two ligaments) connected by four parallel hinge joints (one at each end of each ligament). Equation 1 shows that this is a mechanism with only one degree of freedom so the tibia has only one possible path relative to the femur. The articulating surfaces (not represented in Fig. 5B) would need to be shaped in an appropriate way to maintain contact in all positions without changes of ligament length.

This is not the situation. The ligaments change in length as the joint moves. Wang and Walker (69) measured ligament lengths from X-radiographs of the knees of fresh cadavers with pins in the bones marking the ends of the ligaments. They found that bending the knee shortened the distance between the attachments of the posterior cruciate ligament by 9% but lengthened the anterior cruciate ligament by 7%. Investigators using different methods have reached other conclusions (27). It seems clear, however, that many of the ligaments on the outer surfaces of the knee become taut at full extension of the knee and serve to limit its range of movement.

The knee was treated as a mechanism rather than as a single joint in this discussion and Equation 1 was applied to it. Comparative anatomy presents other and more obvious examples of mechanisms. There are particularly elaborate examples in the skulls of teleost fish, which consist of numerous bones connected by hinges and sliding joints. Many teleosts such as the goldfish have mechanisms enabling them to protract the upper jaw, forming the open mouth into a tube. Equation 1 has been used to confirm that some schematic, planar models of teleost skull mechanisms have the required number of degrees of freedom (1). The human shoulder region has also been treated as a mechanism in three dimensions (34).

So far this section has dealt with the variety of movements that are possible at joints, rather than with ranges of movement. The range is often limited by ligaments becoming taut, as in the case of knee extension. This particular limit is exploited in man to save energy when standing. When people stand with their knees straight, the center of mass of the parts of the body above the knees lies anterior to the knees. Consequently the weight of the body tends to keep the knees fully extended and there is no need to maintain tension in knee muscles. The quadriceps muscles (the extensors of the knee) remain slack, which is obvious from the ease with which the patella can be moved from side to side. Electromyography confirms that they are inactive as are most or all of the flexor muscles of the knee (42).

Figure 7A, B illustrates how bone shape can affect ranges of movement. The carpal bones are bound closely together by ligaments. In primates (Fig. 7A1) they are so shaped that both flexion (Fig. 7A2) and hyperextension are possible. The very different shape in ungulates (Fig. 7B1) allows rather more flexion (Fig. 7B2), but hyperextension is prevented by stop facets. Apes often walk on their knuckles (67), but monkeys place their palms flat on the ground when they walk (see ref. 52). This requires hyperextension

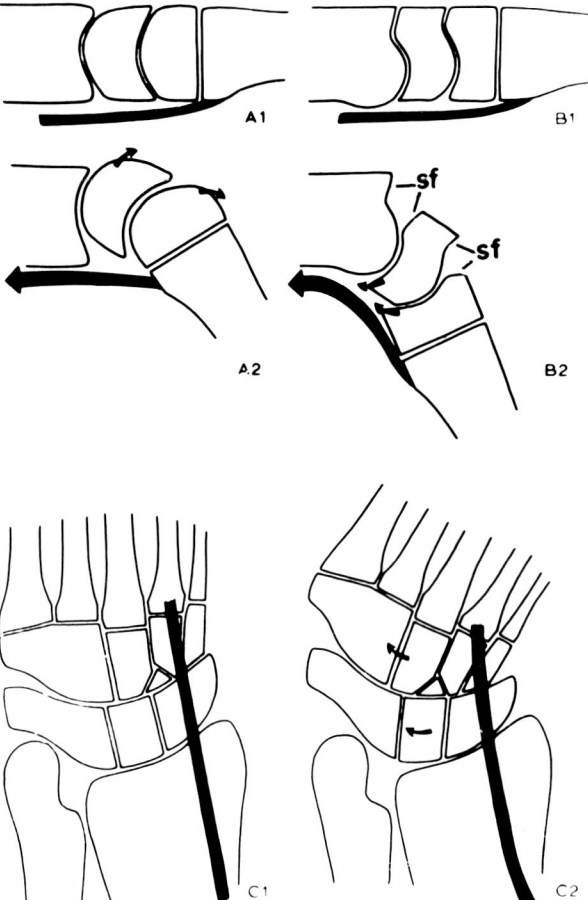

FIG. 7. Diagrammatic sections through bones of the wrist. A: primate. B: ungulate. Forearm is on *left* and hand on *right* in each case. Wrists are shown extended (A1, B1) and flexed (A2, B2). C: diagram of bones of a mammalian wrist. Wrist is extended (C1) and shows radial deviation (C2). sf, Stop facet. [From Yalden (74).]

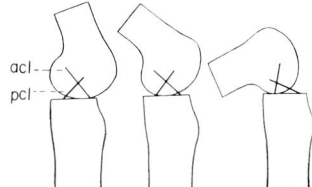

FIG. 6. Diagrams of human knee joint; acl, pcl, anterior and posterior cruciate ligaments, respectively. [From Barnett et al. (14).]

of the wrist. Ungulates walk on the hooves on their distal phalanges. There is no need for the wrist to hyperextend, and it remains straight while the foot is on the ground (again see ref. 52; the fetlock joint, which is hyperextended, is the metacarpophalangeal joint).

Figure 8 illustrates another way that the range of movement of a joint may be altered in the course of evolution (59, 60). In typical mammals including most monkeys (Fig. 8A), the rib cage is elliptical in transverse section with the long axis dorsoventral. The scapulae lie against the sides of the rib cage with the glenoid cavity, in which the humerus articulates, directed ventrally. This allows free movement of the forelimbs in a sagittal plane, as in running, but only allows restricted abduction. Brachiating monkeys and humans (Fig. 8B) have the glenoid cavity pointing more laterally, allowing the wider abduction that is useful in grasping branches and other objects. To attain this position without separating the scapula from the rib cage, the rib cage has become much broader.

NUMBER OF MUSCLES REQUIRED TO WORK JOINTS

A hinge joint normally needs two muscles to work it, a flexor and an extensor, but one muscle can suffice if it works against a spring. The two valves of clamshells are fastened together by an elastic hinge ligament. An adductor muscle closes the shell, but there is no antagonistic abductor muscle. The hinge ligament is strained while the shell is closed and its elastic recoil opens the shell when the adductor relaxes.

Two muscles are needed to work a nonelastic hinge joint and it might be supposed that four would be needed for two hinge joints. Three would do, however, as can be shown by considering the human elbow and forearm. The two hinge joints already described (Fig. 3) allow flexion-extension and pronation-supination. Suppose these joints were moved by three muscles: *1)* an extensor of the elbow, which had no tendency to pronate or supinate the forearm, *2)* a flexor-pronator, which tended both to flex the elbow and to pronate the forearm; and *3)* a flexor-supinator.

Extension could be performed by muscle 1; flexion by muscles 2 and 3 working together (the pronating effect of one counteracting the supinating effect of the other); pronation by muscles 1 and 2 together (the extending effect of 1 counteracting the flexing effect of 2); and supination by 1 and 3 together. Three muscles would suffice to produce all possible movements of the joints. These joints allow two degrees of freedom of relative movement. More generally it can be shown that $(n + 1)$ muscles suffice to produce all possible movements of a nonelastic system with n degrees of freedom of relative movement.

The elbow and forearm are worked by far more than three muscles. Some of them are shown in Figure 9. The biceps is a flexor-supinator muscle (it tends to supinate the forearm as well as flexing the elbow because of the position of its insertion on the radius). The brachioradialis is a flexor, which tends to pull the forearm to a position intermediate between prone and supine. The two pronator muscles are simply pronators; the supinator is simply a supinator. Several more muscles are present, which are not shown in Figure 9. The brachialis is a flexor of the elbow, and the triceps

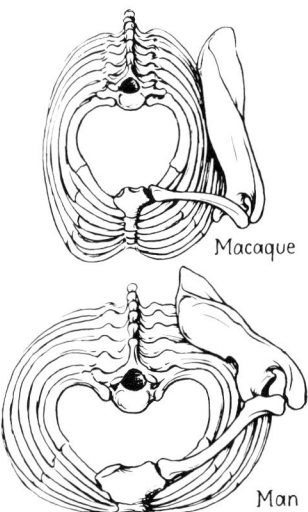

FIG. 8. Anterior views of skeleton of thorax. *A*: monkey (*Macaca*). *B*: man. [From Schultz (59).]

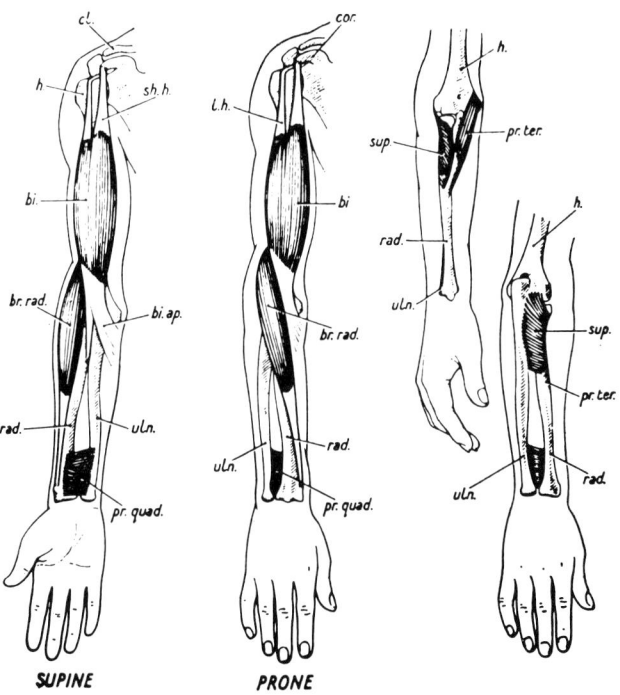

FIG. 9. Skeleton and some of the muscles of human arm. Labels include *bi.*, biceps; *br. rad.*, brachioradialis; *h.*, humerus; *pr. quad.*, pronator quadratus; *pr. ter.*, pronator teres; *rad.*, radius; *sup.*, supinator; *uln.*, ulna. [From Young (77).]

and anconeus are extensors. (All three of these insert on the ulna and so have neither pronating nor supinating effect). In all, there are eight muscles doing a job that could be done by three.

The different roles of the muscles have been demonstrated by electromyography (16). The brachialis is active whenever the elbow is flexed. The biceps is used as well when the elbow is flexed with the forearm in the supine position but generally not when the forearm is in the prone position. If it were used in the latter case, another muscle would have to be used as well to prevent supination. When the forearm is supinated with the elbow extended (for instance, in tightening a screw), the biceps is not used unless a large force is required. If the biceps were used, the triceps would need to be active as well to prevent it bending the elbow. Gentle supination is done by the supinator alone. Muscles seem to be selected for particular tasks in such a way as to avoid having two muscles with partly opposed effects acting simultaneously. This saves energy, for metabolic energy is needed merely to develop tension in muscles even when they are doing no work. If only the supinator has to be activated, less energy is needed to do a given amount of work by supination than if both the biceps and the triceps are used. Although such considerations seem to explain why there are more than three muscles to move the elbow and forearm, they do not seem capable of explaining why there are as many as eight.

MUSCLE ATTACHMENTS

Figure 10 shows some of the bones and muscles of the hindleg of a typical mammal. This illustrates the ways that muscles attach to bones and some of the ways that muscle fibers are arranged within muscles. The muscles shown have not been selected for their importance but simply to illustrate the range of structure that is found. Further examples are given in the chapter by Partridge and Benton in this *Handbook*.

In this discussion, it is convenient to call the proximal attachment of each muscle the origin and the distal attachment the insertion, although some anatomists feel these terms have undesirable functional implications. The adductor femoris is a large muscle with several distinct parts, which originates on the pelvic girdle and inserts on the femur. It is an extensor and adductor of the hip. The semitendinosus muscle crosses two joints and is an extensor of the hip and a flexor of the knee. It is one of the group of muscles at the back of the thigh, which are known collectively as the hamstrings. In contrast the vastus intermedius is an extensor of the knee. It is one of the group of four knee extensors known collectively as the quadriceps muscles, which insert by a common tendon. The gastrocnemius lateralis is a flexor of the knee and extensor of the ankle. It shares a tendon of insertion with the gastrocnemius medialis and (in mammals that possess it) the soleus.

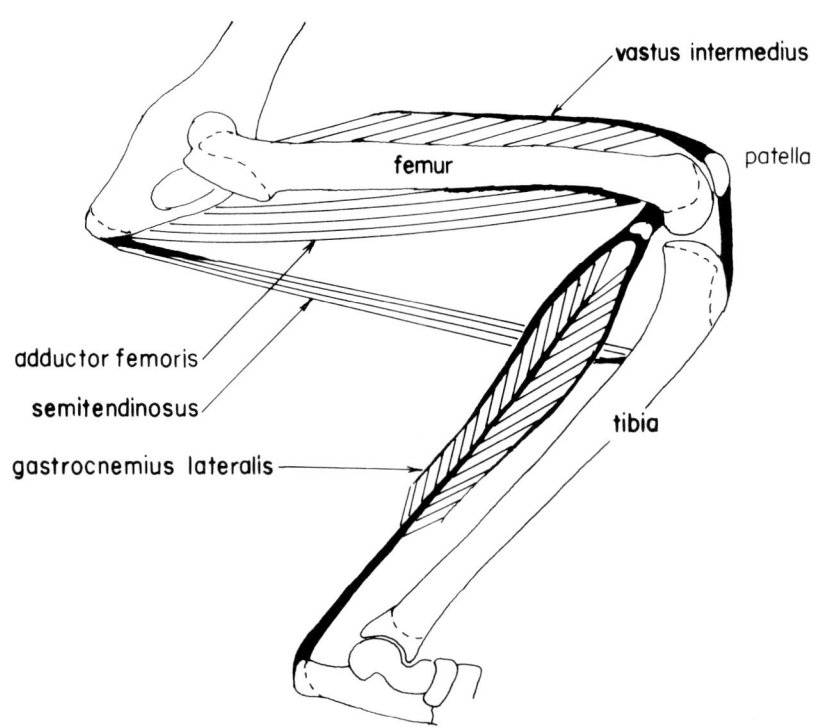

FIG. 10. Diagram showing some of the bones and muscles of a hind leg of a typical mammal. *Broken lines* separate epiphyses from diaphyses. *Dark areas* show tendons and aponeuroses.

Many and perhaps most attachments of muscles to bones are by way of tendons. The semitendinosus and gastrocnemius, for example, have tendons of both origin and insertion. These are typical cordlike tendons, but the tendon of insertion of the adductor femoris is a thin, wide sheet of collagen fibers, an aponeurosis. Some muscles attach directly to bone without an intervening tendon. The vastus intermedius and adductor (Fig. 10) originate directly on bone although they insert by tendons.

Some tendons have sesamoid bones embedded in them. There is a small sesamoid bone in the tendon of origin of the gastrocnemius lateralis. There is a much larger one, the patella, in the tendon of insertion that the vastus intermedius shares with the other quadriceps muscles. The patella slides up and down a groove in the distal end of the femur as the knee extends and flexes. The articulating surfaces of femur and patella are covered by articular cartilage, and it is possible that more satisfactory lubrication can be obtained in this way than if there were no sesamoid bone in the tendon. Lubrication must be important here, for tension in the tendon must press the patella against the femur. The small sesamoid bone in the origin of the gastrocnemius lateralis has no obvious function. The femur does not seem to deflect the tendon from a straight line, so there is no tendency for the tendon to be pressed against it. Indeed, the sesamoid bone does not seem to be in contact with the femur in X-radiographs of dog's knees in various positions.

Many bones in the young of higher vertebrates consist of a main shaft or diaphysis with small separate epiphyses. Diaphysis and epiphyses consist of bone, but they are connected by cartilaginous epiphysial plates (Fig. 31). When the animal becomes adult the epiphysial plates become ossified so that the epiphyses are no longer distinct from the diaphysis. This happens in man at about the age of 18 years. The articulating surfaces of bones are commonly on epiphyses: for instance, a distal epiphysis of the femur and a proximal epiphysis of the tibia articulate together at the knee (Fig. 10). Other epiphyses, called traction epiphyses, occur where tendons attach to bones, for example, at the origin of the semitendinosus and other hamstring muscles on the pelvic girdle and at the insertion of the gastrocnemius on the heel. It has been suggested that traction epiphyses evolved from sesamoids (15). Evidence for this is provided by the observation that traction epiphyses occur in some animals when sesamoids occur in others. For instance, the cormorant (*Phalacrocorax*) has a patella but the diving petrel (*Pelecanoides*) has a traction epiphysis protruding proximally from the tibia in the same position.

Tendons in the distal parts of the legs of some birds are ossified, as slender bands of bonelike tissue. Most readers will have encountered such tendons when eating domestic turkeys (*Meleagris*). These tendons are rather stiff, but have unossified sections interpolated in them where they round joints.

As well as illustrating how muscles attach, Figure 10 shows some of the ways that muscle fibers are arranged within muscles. The semitendinosus and the adductor femoris are parallel-fibered muscles: the muscle fibers run lengthwise along them from origin to insertion. (The muscle fibers of the semitendinosus are often interrupted by a narrow band of collagen halfway along the muscle, but this peculiar feature is not shown in Figure 10.) The muscle fibers of the semitendinosus are all approximately equal in length. Those of the adductor femoris are not of uniform length, but the longest fibers are furthest from the hip joint so that a movement that requires, for instance, 10% shortening of the longest fibers will probably also require about 10% shortening of the shortest fibers.

The vastus and gastrocnemius are pennate with muscle fibers running at an angle to the direction in which the muscle as a whole pulls. The vastus intermedius is unipennate with a single layer of muscle fibers fibers running obliquely from their origin on the femur to the aponeurosis on the superficial face of the muscle, which merges with the tendon of insertion. Many other unipennate muscles originate on an aponeurosis as well as inserting on one. The gastrocnemius lateralis is bipennate with two layers of muscle fibers converging on a central tendon of insertion. There are aponeuroses on the superficial and deep faces of the muscle, which merge into a single tendon of origin. Some pennate muscles are more complex with three, four, or even more layers of muscle fibers.

Two complex pennate muscles are illustrated in Figure 11. The plantaris muscle is very small in man but is one of the major leg muscles in antelopes. It lies alongside the gastrocnemius, but its tendon of insertion runs around the heel and along the foot to the phalanges. It not only flexes the knee and toes but also extends the ankle. In a 160-kg wildebeest (*Connochaetes*) the muscle (excluding the long tendon of insertion) had a mass of 95 g and was very roughly 200 mm long, but its muscle fibers were only 5 mm long.

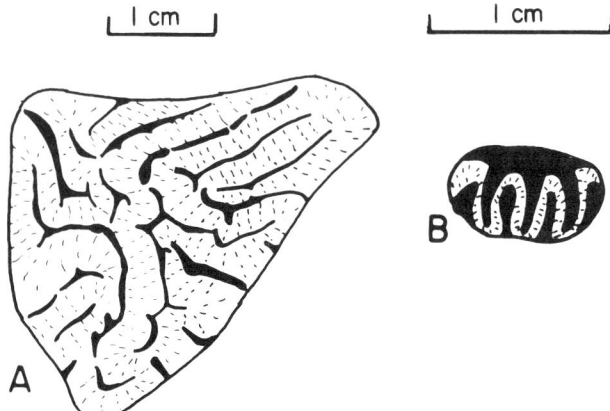

FIG. 11. *A*: section through the plantaris muscle of a wildebeest (*Connochaetes*). *B*: section through the interosseous muscle of forelimb of a sheep (*Ovis*). *Dark areas* show aponeuroses.

Figure 11A shows the very complex arrangement of aponeuroses required to pack such short muscle fibers into a reasonably compact muscle (see also ref. 6). The interosseous muscle of the forefoot of the sheep runs from the wrist to the digits. Its length (excluding tendons) is nearly 100 mm, but its muscle fibers are only about 1 mm long. They join the stout tendon of origin to the stout tendons of insertion but can have no significant contractile function. Even if these fibers could shorten by an amount equal to their own length, they could not flex the digits through more than 6° (28).

The plantaris and interosseus muscles in wildebeest, sheep, and other Bovidae probably have less functional importance than their tendons. The elasticity of their tendons has a major role in locomotion (see the section DYNAMICS OF BODY, p. 33). In the camel (*Camelus dromedarius*) both muscles have lost their muscle fibers entirely so that a stout, continuous band of collagen fibers runs from the origin to the insertion.

MOMENT ARMS AND PENNATION PATTERNS

In this section the quantitative details of muscle attachments and muscle fiber arrangements are discussed. Suppose a volume V of muscle is to be used to extend a joint. Suppose first that it is a parallel-fibered muscle with fibers of length l_0. This length is neither the maximum nor the minimum length of the fibers but the intermediate length at which they can exert most force. Since the cross-sectional area of the muscle is V/l_0, the maximum force (P_{max}) it can exert in isometric contraction is given by

$$P_{max} = \sigma V/l_0 \qquad (3)$$

when σ is the maximum isometric stress, which has been shown to be around 300 kN/m² for many vertebrate striated muscles (72).

The muscle is capable of exerting force actively (as distinct from the passive, elastic response to stretching) over a limited range of lengths, from a maximum l_{max} to a minimum l_{min}. We can write

$$l_{max} - l_{min} = \epsilon l_0 \qquad (4)$$

where ϵ has been shown to have values between 0.5 and 1.1 for various striated muscles (72).

The maximum rate of shortening of the muscle (u_{max}) can be written

$$u_{max} = \eta l_0 \qquad (5)$$

where η is the maximum rate of shortening expressed as muscle fiber lengths per unit time. This rate varies greatly between muscles (25).

Suppose a muscle of given volume (V) is constructed from muscle tissue with particular values of the properties σ, ϵ, and η. If the muscle is made long (given a large value of l_0), it is able to work over a large range of lengths ($l_{max} - l_{min}$ is large) and it is able to shorten

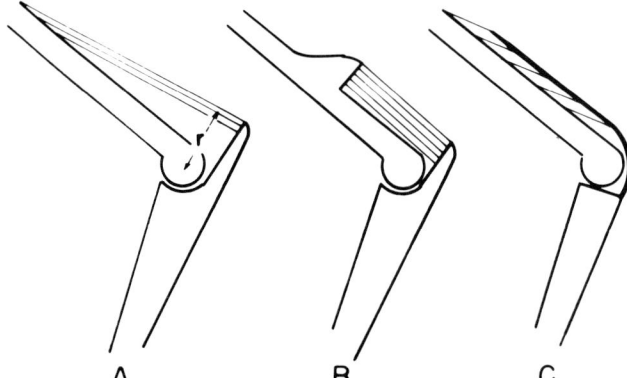

FIG. 12. Diagrams of a hinge joint with 3 alternative but equivalent extensor muscles. These diagrams are explained further in text. *r*, Moment arm of muscle about joint.

fast (u_{max} is large), but it is not able to exert large forces (P_{max} is small). If, however, the muscle is made shorter (and so fatter) it can exert more force but cannot contract so far or as fast.

Now imagine this muscle working a hinge joint (Fig. 12A). The moment arm of the muscle about the joint is r (this is the perpendicular distance from the line of action of the muscle to the instantaneous center of the joint). It is assumed for simplicity that the joint is so constructed that flexion and extension of the joint do not alter r. The maximum moment M_{max} that the muscle can exert about the joint is

$$M_{max} = rP_{max} = r\sigma V/l_0 \qquad (6)$$

The maximum angle θ_{max} (expressed in radians) through which the joint can be moved is

$$\theta_{max} = (l_{max} - l_{min})/r = \epsilon l_0/r \qquad (7)$$

The maximum angular velocity ω_{max} at which the joint can be moved is

$$\omega_{max} = u_{max}/r = \eta l_0/r \qquad (8)$$

Thus a large value of l_0/r enables the muscle to move the joint fast and through a large angle but not to exert large moments. A small value of l_0/r enables it to exert large moments but not to move the joint fast or far. Note that l_0 and r appear in Equations 6–8 solely as the ratio l_0/r. Figure 12A, B shows two muscles that are supposed to have equal volumes and to consist of muscle tissue of identical properties σ, ϵ, and η. Figure 12A shows a long slender muscle with a long moment arm and Figure 12B a short fat one with a short moment arm, but if (l_0/r) is the same for both, the two muscles are identical in their effects; they exert equal maximum moments and extend the joint at equal maximum rates through the same range of angles.

Suppose that the joint shown in Figure 12 is a knee. Both Figure 12A and B seem clumsy arrangements for an extensor muscle. In the former the moment arm is so long that an empty gap is left between the muscle and the femur. In the latter the short fat muscle makes an awkward bulge on the thigh. These disadvantages could be avoided in this particular case by adopting the pennate arrangement shown in Figure 12C. This is the arrangement actually found in the vastus intermedius (Fig. 10).

Consider a pennate muscle of volume V. Let its muscle fibers have length l'_0 (this is the length at which they can exert maximum force) and be set at an angle α (known as the angle of pennation) to the direction in which the muscle pulls. It makes no difference to the calculations whether the muscle is unipennate, bipennate, or more complex, provided that l'_0 and α each have the same value throughout the muscle. The total force the muscle fibers can exert in isometric contraction is $\sigma V/l'_0$ but this acts at an angle α to the direction in which the muscle as a whole pulls, so its component in the latter direction is only $\sigma V \cos \alpha / l'_0$. Thus the maximum moment that the pennate muscle shown in Figure 12C can exert is

$$M'_{max} = \sigma V r \cos \alpha / l'_0 \qquad (9)$$

The angle of pennation is not constant but increases as the muscle shortens. Precise calculation of the angle through which the muscle can move the joint would take account of this, but if α is not too large, little error is introduced by writing

$$\theta'_{max} \simeq \epsilon l'_0 / r \cos \alpha \qquad (10)$$

This follows from Eq. 4B of ref. 19. Note that the quantity w used in ref. 19 is equal to $2\, l'_0 \sin \alpha$ so that $\sin 2\alpha / w = 2 \sin \alpha \cos \alpha / w = \cos \alpha / l_0$).

Similarly

$$\omega'_{max} = \eta l'_0 / r \cos \alpha \qquad (11)$$

If $r \cos \alpha / l'_0$ for the muscle shown in Figure 12C has the same value as r/l_0 for the muscles shown in Figure 12A, B, all three muscles are equivalent in their effects. All exert the same moment and are capable of moving the joint through the same maximum angle at the same maximum angular velocity. Nevertheless, one muscle may tend to evolve rather than the others if it can be packed more conveniently into the body. Also, the elastic properties of tendons, which have not been considered in this section, confer important advantages in some situations (see the section DYNAMICS OF BODY, p. 33). Pennate structure generally involves long tendons.

Few muscles have angles of pennation greater than 30° (e.g., refs. 11, 19, 24). Consequently $\cos \alpha$ generally lies in the narrow range 0.87–1.00. Variations of angle of pennation thus have relatively little effect on muscle properties: variations of muscle fiber length l'_0 are much more important.

The effects of fiber length on the forces muscles can produce are illustrated by two muscles, which lie close to each other in the thigh of the frog, the gracilis major and the semitendinosus. Both run from the ischium to the tibiofibula so their overall lengths are similar, but their muscle fiber lengths are very different. The gracilis is a parallel-fibered muscle. In the frogs measured by Calow and Alexander (19), it had a mass of 165 mg, its muscle fibers were 28 mm long, and it exerted 2.0 N in isometric contraction. The semitendinosus is a much more slender muscle and is pennate. In Calow and Alexander's frogs it had a mass of only 60 mg but its muscle fibers were only 6 mm long and it exerted 2.5 N. Although much smaller than the gracilis, it exerted more force.

PROPERTIES OF SKELETAL MATERIALS

This section provides a brief account of the properties of tendon, bone, and some other skeletal materials. Much fuller accounts are given by Wainwright et al. (68).

Before beginning this discussion, a few engineering terms require explanation. Words such as "stress" and "strain" are often used by laymen as if they were synonyms but they have very different technical meanings. Stress is the force acting on unit area in a material. For instance, if a force F pulls lengthwise on each end of a bar of cross-sectional area A, there is a tensile stress F/A in the bar. If the forces were pushing instead of pulling on the ends of the bar, there would be a compressive stress F/A. Strain is a measure of deformation under stress. If a bar is stretched from its initial length l to a new length $l + \delta l$, it has undergone strain $\delta l / l$. Young's modulus relates stress to strain for elastic materials: it is tensile stress divided by the resulting strain, or $(F/A)/(\delta l/l)$. The tensile strength of a material is the stress needed to break it in tension, and the compressive strength is the stress needed to break it in compression. The terms explained briefly in this paragraph are defined by Alexander (2) and by Wainwright et al. (68).

The principle constituent of tendon is the protein collagen, which is present as fibers running lengthwise along the tendon and accounts for 70% to 80% of the dry weight of the tendon. Tendons are strong and flexible and can be stretched by about 10% (i.e., to strains around 0.1) before breaking. Fresh tendons have Young's modulus around 1.2 GN/m^2 and tensile strengths around 80 MN/m^2 (0.8 tonne wt/cm^2). Nylon thread has about the same modulus but is much stronger.

Most ligaments, like tendons, consist mainly of collagen. A notable exception is the ligamentum nuchae of the necks of ungulates, which consists mainly of elastin, a protein with properties like those of soft rubber. Its Young's modulus is only about 0.6 MN/m^2 and it stretches to double its initial length before breaking.

Bone consists mainly of roughly equal volumes of collagen and impure calcium phosphate. It is hard and stiff and stretches only 2% to 3% before breaking. Compact bone from the principal leg bones of mammals, stressed parallel to the length of the bone, has a Young's modulus of about 18 GN/m^2, a tensile strength of about 180 MN/m^2, and a rather higher compressive strength. These properties are quite similar to those of timber stressed parallel to the grain. Bone is weaker and has a lower Young's modulus when stressed in other directions.

Cartilage is a mucopolysaccharide gel reinforced by collagen fibers. It is markedly viscoelastic: the strain continues to increase for a long time after a stress has been applied. The strain eventually attained by human rib cartilage corresponds to a Young's modulus in the range 5–20 MN/m^2.

The more mobile joints of mammals are synovial joints (73). Their articulating surfaces are covered by a layer of cartilage and their cavities are filled by synovial fluid, which is a fluid containing protein and the polysaccharide hyaluronic acid. Such joints are remarkably well lubricated with coefficients of friction of 0.01 or less. These values are so low as to be difficult to explain. Recent theories include those of weeping lubrication (46) and of boosted lubrication (32).

STATICS OF SKELETON

Statics is the branch of mechanics that considers the forces on bodies at rest. A few examples will show how it can be applied to man and other animals.

The first example has historical interest, for it is taken from Borelli's *De Motu Animalium* (17), which was published in 1680 and is by far the earliest textbook of biomechanics. Borelli observed that a man can support a mass of 20 libra (probably 6.8 kg) from the tip of his thumb (Fig. 13A). What forces does this require in the thumb muscles? The problem will be tackled in a more rigorous and modern manner than Borelli's but the conclusion will be the same as his.

Figure 13B is a diagram of the type known as free-body diagrams. It shows the terminal phalanx of the thumb and the external forces that act on it. These forces are *1)* F_1, the weight of the load (67 N); *2)* F_2, the weight of the phalanx; *3)* F_3 and F_4, the forces exerted on the phalanx by the only two muscles that attach to it, the flexor pollicis longus and extensor pollicis longus, respectively; *4)* F_5, the reaction at the joint. The lines of action of these forces are distant (e.g., x_1) from the instantaneous center of the joint where F_5 is assumed to act. The F_1 and F_2 are vertical; F_3, F_4, and F_5 act at angles θ_3, θ_4, and θ_5 to the vertical. All these forces act approximately in the same plane so the problem can be treated as a planar one. The conditions for equilibrium of the phalanx are therefore *1)* The total of the vertical components of the forces must be zero

$$F_3 \cos \theta_3 + F_4 \cos \theta_4 - F_1 - F_2 - F_5 \cos \theta_5 = 0 \quad (12)$$

2) The total of the horizontal components of the forces must be zero

$$F_3 \sin \theta_3 + F_4 \sin \theta_4 - F_5 \sin \theta_5 = 0 \quad (13)$$

3) The total of the moments of the forces about any point must be zero

$$F_1 x_1 + F_2 x_2 - F_3 x_3 + F_4 x_4 = 0 \quad (14)$$

The force F_1 is known, and F_2 could be obtained by weighing the corresponding phalanx of a cadaver, but this is obviously so small compared to F_1 that it can be ignored. The instantaneous center of the joint could be located by taking X-radiographs of the joint in different positions and by applying the method indicated in Figure 1A. Force F_1 acts along the cord supporting the weight, and F_3 and F_4 act along the tendons of the muscles so the distances x_1, x_3, and x_4 could be obtained from an X-radiograph of the thumb supporting the weight (x_2 is not required if F_2 is ignored). Both θ_3 and θ_4 could be measured from the same radiograph. This leaves four unknowns: F_3, F_4, F_5, and θ_5. Because there are only three equations, there is no unique solution. Fortunately one of the unknowns can be eliminated with reasonable confidence. It seems unlikely that the extensor muscle would be active in these circumstances, so we can assume $F_4 = 0$. This assumption could be checked by electromyography. Equation 14 can thus be rewritten

$$F_1 x_1 - F_3 x_3 \simeq 0 \quad (15)$$

Borelli (17) estimated $x_1 = 3x_3$, so that $F_3 \simeq 3F_1$. Because F_1 was 67 N the flexor muscle must have exerted about 200 N. The remaining unknowns, F_5 and

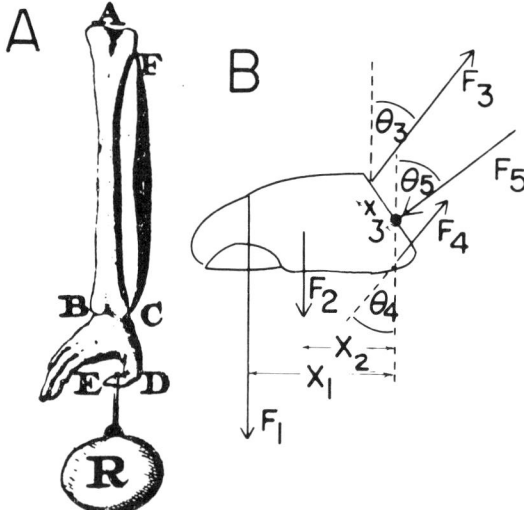

FIG. 13. *A*: diagram of a human arm with weight hanging from thumb. *B*: free-body diagram of distal phalanx of thumb in *A*. F_1, weight of load (67 N); F_2, weight of phalanx; F_3, F_4, forces exerted on phalanx by the 2 muscles attached to it, the flexor pollicis longus and extensor pollicis longus; F_5, reaction at joint. Lines of action of these forces are distant (e.g., x_1) from instantaneous center of joint where F_5 is assumed to act. F_1 and F_2 are vertical; F_3–F_5 act at angles θ_3–θ_5 to vertical. [*A* from Borelli (17).]

θ_5, could be obtained from Equations 12 and 13, if required.

This simple and rather trivial problem illustrates a method applicable to more complex problems, which are apt to arise in the study of muscular coordination. As an example of such a problem, consider the statics of human standing. What force must act in each of the many leg muscles in various postures? Seireg and Arvikar (61) tackled this problem, which like many other problems in human mechanics cannot be treated realistically as a plane problem. The conditions for equilibrium in three dimensions of a free body provide six equations. Seireg and Arvikar assumed that similar forces acted in both legs so they only had to examine the equilibrium of one of them. They considered four free bodies (foot, lower leg, thigh, and trunk) and would have obtained 24 equations, were it not that the symmetry of the forces on the trunk reduced the number by three. Unfortunately, 29 muscles seemed to require consideration. There were also unknown reactions at the joints and unknown moments exerted by ligaments (for instance, forces tending to bend the knee laterally would be resisted by such a moment). There were thus far more unknowns than equations and no unique solution was possible.

This recurring difficulty in biomechanics arises because joints generally have more muscles than degrees of freedom (see the section NUMBER OF MUSCLES REQUIRED TO WORK JOINTS, p. 23). Seireg and Arvikar (61) tried to overcome it by a method that has also been used in various forms by others. They specified (realistically) that no muscle could exert negative tension and then they chose the solution that minimized the quantity ($\Sigma F + k\Sigma M$). Here ΣF is the sum of the muscle forces and ΣM is the sum of the moments exerted by ligaments. They tried various values of the constant k to see which gave solutions consistent with electromyographic data and found that large values were most successful. If k was large enough the solutions were insensitive to its precise value and gave $\Sigma M = 0$.

The usefulness of electromyographic data in such problems is strictly limited, because of the difficulty of relating the electrical activity of a muscle to the force it is exerting (50). This method can, however, show whether a particular muscle is active in a particular posture and whether a change to another posture increases or decreases its activity.

The rationale of Seireg and Arvikar's approach (61) is that man may have evolved or learned to minimize the metabolic power required to maintain tension in muscles and to avoid imposing unnecessary stresses on ligaments. This approach can be refined by assigning different weighting factors to different muscles (54), although this raises the difficulty of choosing the factors.

It is sometimes useful to use other, quite distinct, criteria to eliminate improbable solutions. Vertebrate striated muscle generally exerts maximum isometric stresses around 300 kN/m^2 (e.g., ref. 72), so it seems reasonable to specify that no muscle will exert more stress than this in an acceptable solution. Oxidative muscle fibers are probably used preferentially in maintaining posture (see the chapter by Partridge and Benton in this *Handbook*), and a criterion that expressed this might be useful.

A further example of a problem in statics that illustrates another principle is that muscles may be arranged and used so as to minimize the danger of dislocating joints. The marten (*Martes*) is a carnivorous mammal, which feeds on squirrels and other prey. It has two main jaw-closing muscles, which pull in very different directions (Fig. 14A). Which muscle is likely to be more important in particular feeding activities? Consider first the situation when the marten is using its canine teeth to tear flesh (63). A force must act on the front of the lower jaw, which has a component forward (since the animal is tugging at the prey) and a component downward (since the upper jaw is pressing down on the lower one). This force must act more or less as shown by the free-body diagrams in Figure 14B, C. In Figure 14B it is assumed that only the temporalis muscle is acting, exerting the force T. The jaw must be in equilibrium under P, T, and the reaction R at the jaw articulation. It is easily shown that this can be the case only if the magnitudes of the forces are in the same proportion as the lengths of the arrows and R acts in the direction shown. This direction is forward and slightly downward, implying that the condyle of the jaw is being pushed backward and slightly upward into its socket. In contrast, Figure 14C shows the masseter as the only active muscle. The reaction is much larger and acts backward, implying that the jaw is being pulled forward out of its socket and must be restrained by tension in ligaments. If martens used only the masseter muscle when tugging their prey they would be apt to dislocate their jaws, but if they used only the temporalis muscles they would not.

Figure 14D, E shows a different use of the jaws. When the carnassial teeth are cutting flesh, a vertical force acts on the lower carnassial tooth. In Figure 14D only the temporalis muscle is being used, and analysis again shows that a large upward and forward reaction is required; there must be a tendency for the jaw to be pushed backward and downward out of its socket. Figure 14E, however, shows that if the masseter acts as well as the temporalis then equilibrium can in principle be achieved without any reaction at all at the jaw articulation.

Figure 14 shows that the temporalis is much better placed than the masseter for use when the marten is tugging at prey with its canines, but that the masseter has a particularly useful role in cutting flesh with the carnassials. The two jaw-closing muscles, running in different directions, are probably better than any single muscle of their total mass could be.

In Figures 13 and 14, the reactions F_5 and R were

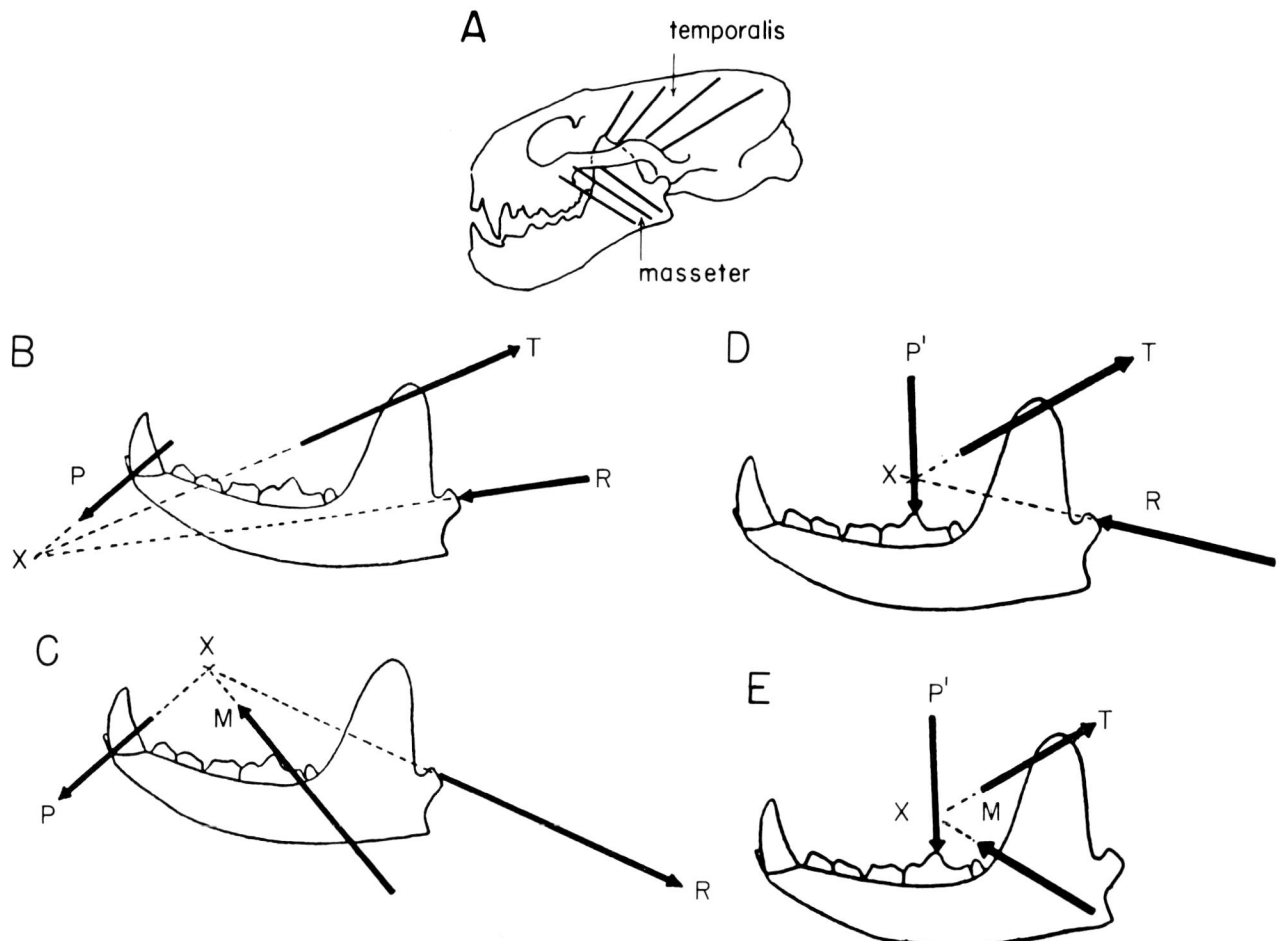

FIG. 14. *A*: diagram of skull of a mammal, showing temporalis and masseter muscles. *B–E*: lower jaws of *Martes*, showing the forces (P, P', T, M) that act on it in various circumstances described in text. Force P' acts on lower carnassial tooth. R, reaction at jaw articulation. [From Smith and Savage (63).]

each considered to act at a single point. How far is this justifiable? Figure 15*A* shows in more detail the forces that may act at a joint. This figure resembles a knee, but the conclusions that are drawn from it have wider validity. An external force F is supposed to act on the tibia exerting a clockwise moment about the knee. This is balanced by the counterclockwise moment of the force T exerted by the quadriceps muscles. A normal force C_N and a small tangential (frictional) force C_F are exerted on the tibia by the condyles of the femur. These forces alone are not in equilibrium. Since F is pulling to the left, a ligament must be taut, exerting a force L with a component to the right. Together forces C_N, C_F, and L represent the reaction that has hitherto been considered as a single force.

Further thought shows that it can be justifiable to treat the reaction as if it were a single force. Assuming that the taut ligament is practically inextensible, it is mechanically equivalent to a rigid bar with hinges at its ends (Fig. 15*B*, P and Q). The tibia can both roll and slide on the condyles of the femur, and the point

R is at present in contact with the femur. Suppose that the femur remains stationary and the knee extends so that the tibia rotates counterclockwise. Point Q can only move perpendicular to PQ; R can only move tangentially. Hence the point O where PQ intersects the perpendicular from the articulating surfaces at R must be the instantaneous center of the joint. Thus, L and C_N are in line with the instantaneous center. The frictional force C_F is at a distance OR from the instantaneous center, but is so small in healthy joints that it can usually be neglected. If the coefficient of friction in the joint is 0.003 (a likely value), C_F is only 0.003 C_N. Thus L and C_N are the only components of the reaction at the joint that have to be considered. Because both components are in line with the instantaneous center, they can be replaced in calculations by a single force acting at the instantaneous center.

It is often difficult to decide whether the ligaments of a joint are in tension or not. If they are not, $L = 0$ and the reaction at the joint acts at the point of contact between the articulating surfaces. Very little

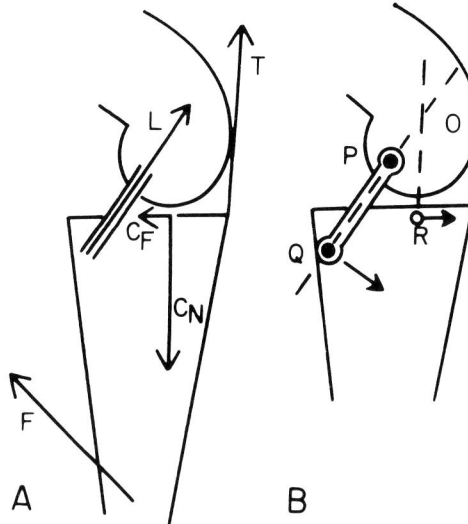

FIG. 15. A: diagram of a knee showing forces acting on tibia. Forces are F, external; T, exerted by quadriceps; C_N and C_F, normal and tangential, exerted by condyles of femur; L, exerted by ligaments. B: mechanism equivalent to the joint. At point O, PQ (*rigid bar*) intersects perpendicular from articulating surfaces. Hence O must be instantaneous center of joint. [From Alexander (8).]

error will result, however, from regarding it as acting at the instantaneous center because C_N is in line with the center and C_F is small.

These arguments tend to justify the practice of regarding the reaction at a joint as a single force acting at the instantaneous center, but they do not constitute a rigorous justification because ligaments are not wholly inextensible.

DYNAMICS OF SKELETON

Analysis of forces on the skeleton is more complicated for movements that involve accelerations. Consider a particle of mass (m) that has an acceleration $\ddot{x}$. This implies that the forces acting on it are not balanced but have a resultant $m\ddot{x}$. If an additional force $-m\ddot{x}$ were applied (i.e., a force $m\ddot{x}$ in the opposite direction to the acceleration) the particle would be in equilibrium. The usual method for analyzing such situations is to draw in this additional (fictitious) "inertia force" and to apply the equations for equilibrium. The inertia force on a body must be applied at the center of mass. A body may have angular acceleration as well as linear acceleration, and this is accounted for by drawing in a fictitious inertial torque. If the body has moment of inertia I (about an axis through its center of mass) and angular acceleration $\ddot{\theta}$ (about a parallel axis), the inertial torque is $-I\ddot{\theta}$. The minus sign indicates that this torque is in the opposite sense to the angular acceleration.

Many problems in biodynamics require three-dimensional treatment, but most of this section is devoted, for simplicity, to problems that can be treated with acceptable accuracy in two dimensions.

Consider a soccer player kicking a ball. How can we investigate the forces that act in the leg just before the foot strikes the ball? Figure 16A is a free-body diagram of the shank and foot. It shows the weight (mg) of this segment of the leg (acting at the center of mass of the segment), the force F exerted by the quadriceps muscles which are extending the knee, and the reaction R at the joint. Also it shows the inertia force $-m\ddot{x}$ and the inertial torque $-I\ddot{\theta}^2$. Figure 16B is a similar free-body diagram of the whole leg, showing forces at the hip.

There are methods for determining m, I, and the position of the center of mass in living subjects (49). Alternatively, measurements made on cadavers may be used (31, 33). The position and direction of the patellar tendon (and so of F in Fig. 16A) can be determined from X-radiographs. The reaction R is considered to act at the instantaneous center, which can also be located from X-radiographs (Fig. 1A). The acceleration $\ddot{x}$, its direction (given by the angle α), and the angular acceleration $\ddot{\theta}$ can be determined from a film. Conspicuous adhesive markers, attached to known points on the leg before the film was taken, make this easier. Small errors in measurements from films lead to large errors in the accelerations calculated from them unless smoothing techniques are used (37). These procedures provide the data needed to determine F, R, and the angle γ by solving the equations for equilibrium.

Analysis along these lines of films of good soccer players led Zernicke and Roberts (79) to the conclu-

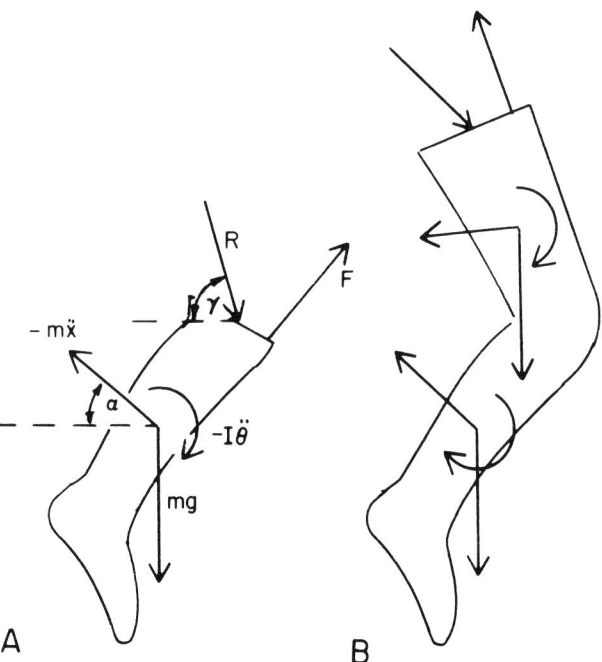

FIG. 16. Free-body diagrams of a soccer player's leg just before the foot kicks a ball. A: lower leg and foot. F, force exerted by quadriceps muscles extending knee; R, reaction at joint acting at angle γ; $-m\ddot{x}$, inertia force; $-I\ddot{\theta}$, inertial torque; mg, leg segment weight. Angle α gives acceleration direction. B: similar diagram of whole leg.

sion that the muscles must exert moments up to 122 N·m about the knee and 274 N·m about the hip, before the foot hits the ball. It is shown later in this section that larger moments act about the knee in running.

The rest of this section is about legs with their feet in contact with the ground. It is in principle possible to calculate the force on a foot by film analysis, taking account of the accelerations of all the segments of the body. This is laborious and apt to be inaccurate, although appropriate approximations sometimes make it possible to obtain realistic results without too much trouble (see ref. 12 for calculations of the forces on the feet of a kangaroo). It is generally far more convenient to use a force platform, if one is available, to measure the force exerted by the foot on the ground (37). A force platform is an instrumented panel, which can be set into the floor and which gives an electrical output indicating any force that acts on it. The most useful models give outputs representing the three components (vertical, longitudinal, and transverse) of the force, the two coordinates of its point of application on the platform, and its moment about a vertical axis through the center of the platform.

Figure 17A shows a force-platform record of a trained dog taking off for a running long jump. A series of low hurdles were placed just beyond the platform so that when the dog jumped over them, the final footfalls before takeoff were on the platform. The record shows that the vertical component of force rose to a maximum of about 1,000 N while the forepaws were on the platform, fell almost to zero, and then rose to a little more than 1,100 N while the hindfeet were on the platform. At the instant shown in Figure 17B, the vertical and longitudinal components of the force on the platform were 1,114 and 118 N, respectively. The resultant of these is 1,120 N, at 84° to the horizontal. (This is 3.2 times the weight of the dog.) There are two feet on the platform but they are symmetrically placed, and it seems reasonable to assume that each exerts one-half the total force, i.e., that each exerts 560 N at 84° as indicated. The line of action of the force is 0.13 m from the ankle joint so it must exert a moment of 560 × 0.13 = 73 N·m about the joint. This must be counteracted by muscles pulling on the Achilles tendon, which has a moment arm of 300 mm about the joint. Hence a force of 2,400 N (0.24 tonne wt) must act in the Achilles tendon. Figure 17C shows both this force and the components of the reaction at the ankle joint, which is required for equilibrium.

In an accurate analysis Figure 17C should have been made as complicated as Figure 16A. The weight of the foot, the inertia force, and the inertial torque would need to be considered. Rough calculations showed, however, that these were all small enough to be ignored. For instance, the weight of the foot was only about 3.4 N.

Because dogs have small paws, there was little possibility of error from drawing the force acting at the center of the paw (Fig. 17). Man has relatively large feet, and a given force has a very different moment about the ankle if it acts on the toes than if it acts on the heel. Force platforms that register the point of application of the force are particularly useful in studies of man. This refinement was not available for the investigation from which Figure 18 is taken, but there is relatively little room for error in the positions illustrated as the heels are off the ground.

In the investigation of Alexander and Vernon (11), it was found that a man running quite slowly exerted on the ground forces up to 1,800 N (2.7 times his weight). This involved moments up to 200 N·m acting both about the knee and the ankle. The same man was asked to make standing jumps from the platform,

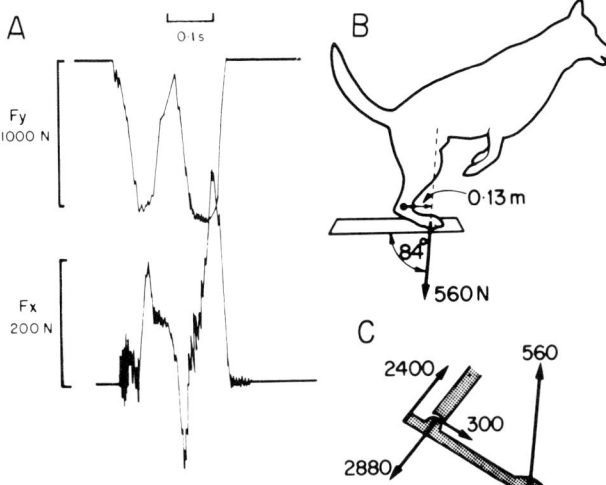

FIG. 17. A: force-platform record of a 36-kg dog taking off for a running long jump. Only the vertical (F_Y) and longitudinal (F_X) components of force are shown. An upward displacement of F_X record represents a backward force exerted by dog on the platform (i.e., a forward force exerted by platform on the dog). B: outline traced from film of same jump, showing force exerted by 1 foot at the instant when it was greatest. C: forces (in Newtons) acting on 1 foot at the instant shown in B. [A from Alexander (3); B and C from Alexander (4).]

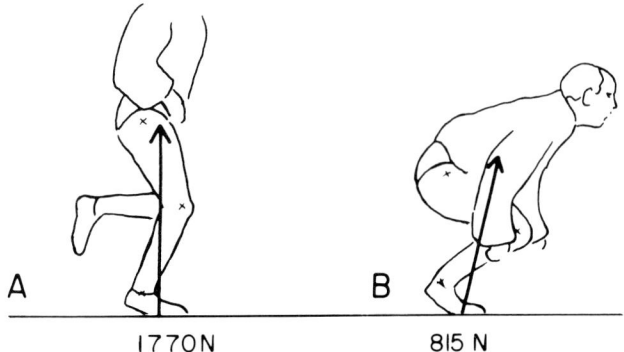

FIG. 18. Two outlines traced from films of the same 68-kg man. In A: running across force platform. B: taking off for a standing jump from the force platform. Force acting on right foot is represented by an arrow. The instant illustrated in each case is the one at which the moment of this force about the knee was greatest.

jumping as far as possible. The maximum force registered by the platform at takeoff was 1,630 N in this case, and because there were two feet on the platform, this represents only 815 N on each foot. The maximum moments about both knee and ankle were only about 120 N·m. Why were the moments so much smaller in jumping than in running, although the man was trying to jump as far as possible and was presumably exerting as much force as he could on the ground?

An explanation was obtained by considering the force required of the quadriceps muscles. The moment arm of the quadriceps muscles about the knee falls as the knee extends, because the condyles of the femur have a spiral profile. It falls from about 47 mm when the leg is relatively straight (e.g., Fig. 18A) to about 38 mm when the knee is bent at right angles (62) and probably about 35 mm when it is bent to the angle shown in Figure 18B. Hence a moment of 120 N·m in the bent position requires as much force in the quadriceps as one of 120 × (47/35) = 161 N·m in the straighter position. Furthermore much larger moments act about the hip in the standing jump than in running. They are balanced in part by the hamstring muscles, including the semitendinosus (Fig. 10), which also tend to flex the knee, increasing the force required of the quadriceps muscles. The quadriceps muscles may be exerting as much force in Figure 18B as in Figure 18A.

Some problems in biodynamics cannot be tackled realistically in two dimensions, so a three-dimensional analysis is necessary. This was the case in a recent study of forces at the human hip in walking and climbing stairs (26). Three light-emitting diodes each were attached to the subject's foot, lower leg, thigh, and trunk and were made to flash. The subject walked across a force platform in a darkened room with two cameras pointing at him from mutually perpendicular directions. The camera shutters were kept open so that photographs were obtained showing the paths of the flashing diodes as lines of dots. The position and linear and angular accelerations of each body segment of each flash were obtained from the photographs, and equations of motion were written for each segment. There were many more unknowns than equations, but this problem was dealt with in much the same way as in Seireg and Arvikar's (61) analysis of standing (see the section STATICS OF SKELETON, p. 28). The stages of the stride when the analysis showed each muscle exerting force corresponded reasonably well with the stages when electromyography indicated activity. This analysis produced estimates of forces at the hip, which were required by designers of artificial hip joints.

DYNAMICS OF BODY

Different patterns of coordination of the leg muscles can make the body as a whole travel in different ways, with different energy costs. This section shows how dynamics can be used to estimate the metabolic energy costs of different styles of locomotion. It deals both with human walking and running and kangaroos hopping.

The human walk differs from the run in many ways. It is performed at lower speeds and it involves a different pattern of foot placement. In walking each foot is set down before the other is lifted so that there are dual-support phases when both are on the ground. These occupy 10% to 40% of the duration of the stride (calculated from duty factors in ref. 10). In running there are floating phases with neither foot on the ground, which may occupy 40% or more of the stride.

Force-platform records of human walking and running show that the force a foot exerts on the ground has a forward component at first (while the foot is in

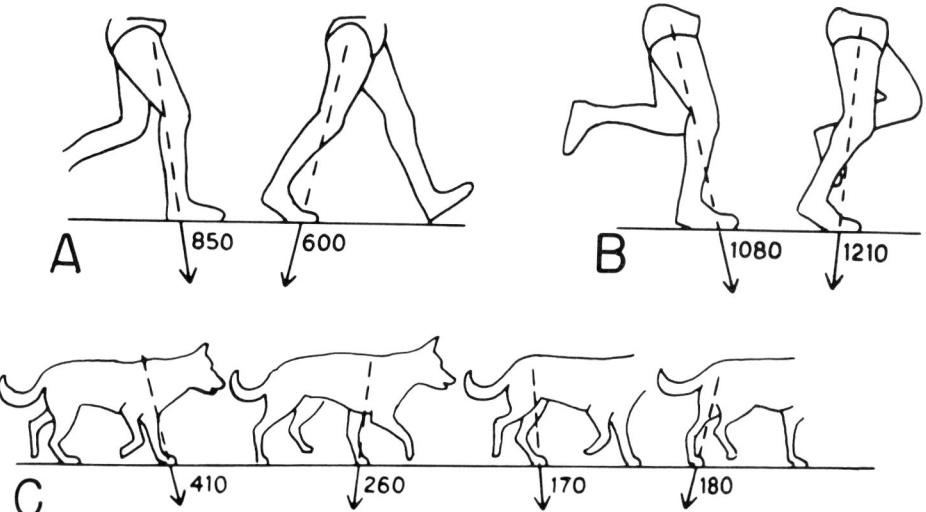

FIG. 19. Outlines traced from films of a 68-kg man and a 35-kg dog on a force platform, showing the magnitude (in Newtons) and direction of the force exerted by 1 foot. A: man walking. B: man running. C: dog trotting. [From Alexander and Goldspink (7).]

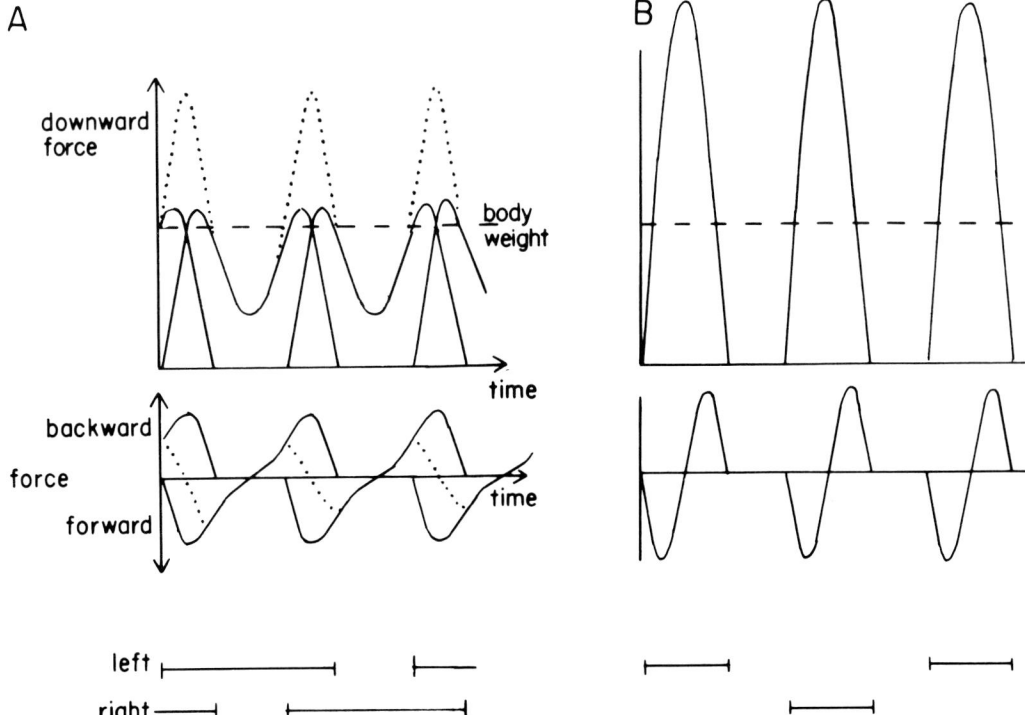

FIG. 20. Schematic graphs based on force-platform records, showing vertical and longitudinal components of force on the ground plotted against time. A: man walking. B: man running. *Continuous lines* show forces exerted by individual feet. *Dotted lines* during double-support phases in A show total force exerted by the 2 feet. *Bars* under graphs show when feet are on ground.

front of the hip) and a backward component later in the step (Figs. 19, 20). The initial forward force on the foot implies a backward, decelerating force on the body. The later backward one implies a forward, accelerating force on the body. Thus the velocity and kinetic energy of the body fluctuate in every step. They have minimum values as the hip passes over the supporting foot and maximum values in the double-support phase (of walking) and the floating phase (of running). These fluctuations can in principle be determined by analysis of film but are more easily calculated from force-platform records (21). It will be shown that the fluctuations of kinetic energy account for much of the energy cost of running, but it has been argued that more energy would be expended in other ways if the forces on the ground were kept vertical (7). Walking on ice requires near-vertical forces because of the low coefficient of friction and tends to be tiring.

The feet of dogs, sheep, horses, kangaroos, and presumably other animals exert forces that act forward and then backward in each step, like the feet of humans (see ref. 7).

The potential energy of the body, as well as the kinetic energy, fluctuates in each step. Figure 21 shows how a person's trunk rises and falls as he walks. It is highest as the hips pass over a supporting foot and lowest in the double-support phase. In running, however, the trunk is lowest as it passes over a supporting foot and highest in the middle of the floating phase.

Consider a body that is oscillating up and down. It has an upward acceleration at the bottom of each oscillation and a downward acceleration at the top of each oscillation. Next, consider what happens in walking (Fig. 20A). The vertical component of the force on the ground is less than body weight as the hip passes over a supporting foot so the center of mass of the body must have a downward acceleration at this stage. The total of the vertical components of force exerted by the two feet in the double-support phase is greater than body weight, so the body must have an upward acceleration at this stage. Thus the fluctuations of force are consistent with the observation that the body is highest as the hip passes over the supporting foot and lowest in the double-support phase. Cavagna (21) has shown how fluctuations of potential energy, like fluctuations of kinetic energy, can be calculated from force-platform records.

In running, the vertical component of the force exerted by each foot rises above body weight, approaching 3 times body weight even at quite low speeds (11). Thus, the center of mass has upward acceleration and minimum height while a foot is on the ground. Because the body falls freely under the influence of gravity during the floating phase, it has downward acceleration then and its height passes through a maximum.

If people moved on frictionless wheels, the only energy needed to keep them moving at a constant velocity over level ground would be the small amount needed to overcome air resistance. Human movement, however, is neither level nor at constant velocity. Whenever the total mechanical energy (kinetic and potential) of the body rises, the additional energy must be supplied by positive muscular work. Whenever the total falls, the excess energy must be degraded to heat by muscles performing negative work. Both positive and negative work performance consume metabolic energy (47). The metabolic energy needed for locomotion will be least if the fluctuations of mechanical energy are kept as small as possible.

In walking, energy is conserved by the principle of the pendulum (22). A pendulum has maximum kinetic energy and minimum potential energy at the bottom of its swing, but maximum potential energy and no kinetic energy at the ends of its swing. Energy is shuttled back and forth between the kinetic and potential forms. Similarly, in walking, the fluctuations of kinetic energy are out of phase with the fluctuations of gravitational potential energy so that the fluctuations of total mechanical energy are relatively small (Fig. 22).

In walking, unlike running, the vertical component of the force exerted by a foot has two maxima at about the one-fourth and three-fourths points of its period on the ground (Fig. 20). These are scarcely distinct in slow walking but are separated by a very deep minimum in fast walking so that the total vertical force on the body fluctuates much more in fast than in slow walking. This affects the amplitude of the potential energy changes, tending to make it match the amplitude of the kinetic energy changes at all speeds (10). It is impossible to make it match the kinetic energy changes at high speeds, and there is a critical speed above which running needs less energy than walking. People change from walking to running and quadrupedal mammals change from walking to trotting at speeds around $0.8\sqrt{gh}$, where g is the acceleration of free fall and h is the height of the hip joint from the ground (7). This is about 2.4 m/s for typical men, who have the hip about 0.9 m from the ground.

In running, kinetic and gravitational potential energy fluctuate in phase with each other (23). The same is true of kangaroos hopping (Fig. 22B). Both in running and in hopping, however, another form of potential energy assumes an importance it does not have in walking. This is elastic strain energy. The Achilles tendon and other tendons are stretched when the feet press on the ground, storing elastic strain energy. These tendons recoil elastically as the feet leave the ground and reconvert the strain energy to kinetic and potential energy. The principle is that of a bouncing ball which loses its kinetic energy as it hits the ground and is deformed elastically, storing strain energy which is reconverted to kinetic energy in the elastic recoil. Figure 22B shows strain energy stored in the Achilles tendons of a hopping wallaby, calculated by a method explained in the next section, STRESSES AND STRAINS IN TENDONS. The fluctuations of strain energy greatly reduce the fluctuations of total mechanical energy and would be seen to reduce them still more if the strain energy stored in other tendons were included. (Strain energy is also stored in the tendons of the quadriceps and interosseus muscles.) Some strain energy must be stored in the muscles themselves as well as in their tendons, but the amount is trivial (9, 51).

The kinetic energy fluctuations of the limbs, moving forward and back relative to the center of mass of the body, have been ignored in this account and so has

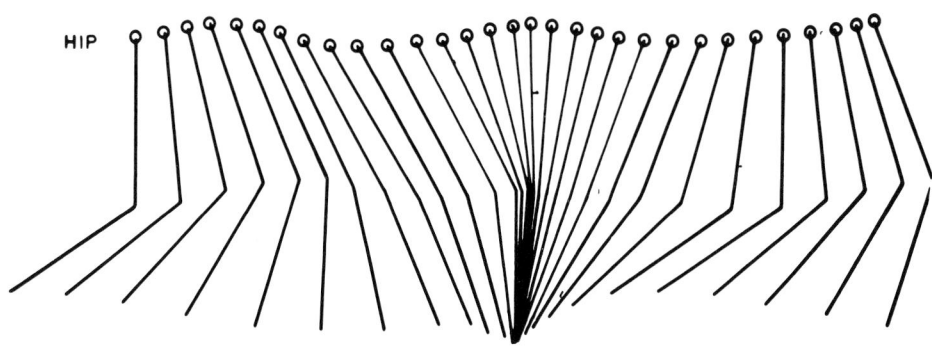

FIG. 21. Diagram showing how right leg and shoulder move in human walking. [From Carlsöö (20).]

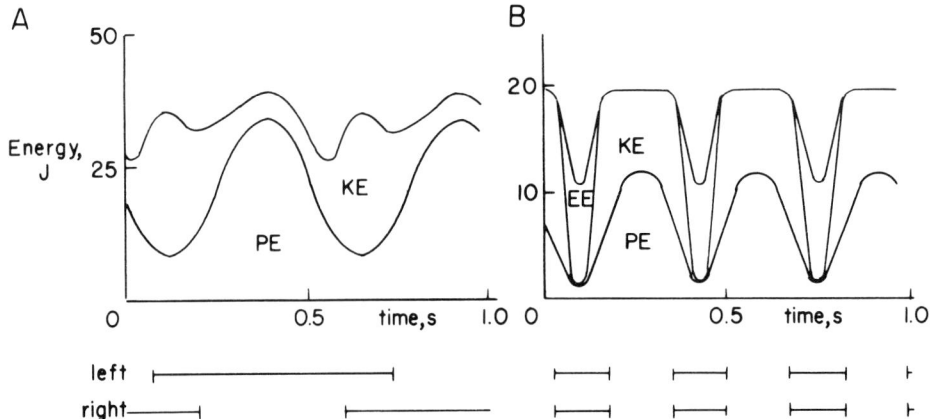

FIG. 22. Schematic graphs of mechanical energy against time. *A*: 70-kg man walking at 1.4 m/s. *B*: 10.5-kg wallaby (*Protemnodon*) hopping at 2.4 m/s. *PE*, potential energy; *KE*, kinetic energy; *EE*, elastic strain energy in Achilles tendons. *Bars* under graphs show when feet are on ground. [Data for *A* from Cavagna and Margaria (22); data for *B* from Alexander and Vernon (12).]

the work done against air resistance. Both are small at low speeds, but limb kinetic energy becomes important at high speeds (7).

STRESSES AND STRAINS IN TENDONS

Figure 17 shows a force of 2,400 N acting in the Achilles tendon of a dog. The stress in the tendon is obtained by dividing this force by the cross-sectional area of the tendon (3). It amounts to 110 MN/m^2, which is a little higher than most published values for the tensile strength of tendon, but the dog did not break the tendon. Published values of tensile strength may tend to be somewhat too low because of the difficulty of attaching tendons to testing equipment in such a way that they are evenly loaded. Also, a tendon may withstand briefly stresses which would break it if they were maintained.

Young's modulus for tendon is about 1.2 GN/m^2, so a stress of 110 MN/m^2 should stretch it by about 10% of its length, that is by about 25 mm in this case. Similar calculations for a running man and a hopping wallaby show that their Achilles tendons were probably stretched by 18 mm and 11 mm, respectively (9, 51).

In the case of the hopping wallaby, each Achilles tendon exerted a maximum force of 850 N, which stretched it by an estimated 11 mm. The elastic strain energy stored in a stretched material is 1/2 (force) × (extension) or 4.7 J in this case, so the two Achilles tendons together store 9.4 J. This is how the elastic strain energy shown in Figure 22*B* was calculated.

Zernicke et al. (78) estimated that the force on an athlete's patellar ligament was 14.5 kN at the instant when it broke in a weight-lifting competition.

STRESSES AND STRAINS IN BONES

Figure 17 shows that the reaction exerted by the tibia on the foot of a jumping dog had components 2,880 N parallel to the long axis of the tibia and 300 N at right angles to it. This implies that equal but opposite forces acted on the distal end of the tibia. These forces can be used to calculate stresses in the tibia using the methods devised by engineers to calculate stresses in beams (see ref. 3 and textbooks on the strength of materials).

Consider a cross section halfway along the tibia. This is 0.11 m from the distal end in the 36-kg dog. The 300 N component acts at right angles to the tibia and tends to bend it, compressing the posterior face of the bone and stretching the anterior face. Its tendency to bend the bone is measured by the bending moment 300 × 0.11 = 33 N·m. It is easily calculated that to resist this bending moment graded stresses must develop in the cross section, ranging from a compressive stress of 80 MN/m^2 at the posterior face through zero to a tensile stress of 80 MN/m^2 at the anterior face. The axial component of force of 2,880 N tends, however, to set up a uniform compressive stress throughout the cross section. This increases the compressive stress at the posterior face to 100 MN/m^2 and reduces the tensile stress at the anterior face to 60 MN/m^2. Similar stresses have been calculated for the humerus and various leg bones in kangaroos and antelopes, hopping and galloping (6, 12). They are about one-third to one-half of the tensile and compressive strengths of bone (68).

Simple beam theory seems adequate in cases like these for estimating stresses in the shafts of bones. The much more laborious technique of finite-element analysis is preferable when stresses near joints or muscle attachments are required (55, 57).

Stresses in bones have also been measured by means of strain gauges glued to the bones of living animals. In one experiment a strain gauge was glued to a man's tibia, immediately under the skin of the shin (45). Tensile strains up to 8.5×10^{-4} were registered when the man ran. Because Young's modulus for bone is about 18 GN/m^2 (68), this implies stresses around 15

MN/m². Greater stresses must have been developed nearer the anterior edge of the tibia.

ENGINEERING DESIGN OF BONES

This section is about the shapes and structure of bones and how they are adapted to the forces they must withstand. It is taken as axiomatic that it is generally desirable for bones to be as light as possible, consistent with the required strength and stiffness. Unnecessarily heavy bones would increase the mass of the body and the moments of inertia of the limbs so that more energy would be needed for locomotion.

The long bones of mammals' limbs are generally hollow with a central marrow-filled cavity. The principal leg bones of the rhinoceros (*Diceros*) and the humerus of the elephant (*Loxodonta*), however, have cancellous bone instead of soft marrow at their centers. Tubes are stiffer than solid rods made of the same quantity of the same material and are also stronger in bending. This is why tubes rather than solid rods are used for making bicycles and scaffolding. Tubular bones have presumably evolved for the same reason.

Bending moments set up graded stresses in a beam, ranging from maximum tensile stresses near the face, which is on the outside of the bend, to maximum compressive stresses near the opposite face. There must be an intermediate layer in the beam (or rather a surface, for it is infinitely thin) in which bending moments set up no stress at all. This is known as the neutral surface. Material near the neutral surface contributes very little to the strength of the beam in bending. The core of a rod lies near the neutral surface for bending moments in any direction. Consequently, the core may be omitted (making the rod a tube) with very little effect on the strength in bending.

Figure 23 illustrates a rod and three tubes that are all equally strong in bending. They are conveniently described by the ratio (internal diameter):(external diameter), which is called k. The external diameter of the tube with $k = 0.3$ is not perceptibly different from that of the solid rod $k = 0$, but it is equally strong. This shows how little the core contributes to strength in bending.

Figure 24 shows how the weight of a tube of given bending strength depends on the value of k. The lower line refers to an empty tube which is taken as a model of the air-filled bones of birds. The upper line refers to a tube with a filling which adds nothing to its strength but has a density one-half that of the tube wall. This is intended as a model of marrow-filled bones: the density of bone is about 2,000 kg/m³ and the density of marrow must be about the same as that of water 1,000 kg/m³. The figure suggests that it is advantageous for air-filled bones to have very high values of k, the higher k is the lighter the bone can be for given strength. Marrow-filled bones are, however, lightest with $k \simeq 0.6$, and bones with high values of k would be very heavy because they contained a large mass of marrow. The air-filled bones of birds have, appropriately, relatively thinner walls than the marrow-filled bones of mammals. For instance, k is about 0.9 for the humerus of a swan (*Cygnus*) but only 0.65 for the humerus of a sheep. Many mammal bones have values of k close to the ideal of 0.6, which is suggested by Figure 24.

The value of k cannot be greater than 1 for the cavity in a bone cannot be wider than the bone itself. Figure 24 suggests that for air-filled bones it is advantageous to have k as near to 1 as possible. This is misleading: the calculations on which the figure is based took account only of the danger of a tube breaking and ignored the possibility that it might fail by kinking like a plastic drinking straw. When a straw is bent it does not break in two but collapses suddenly with a kink in it. Tubes fail by breaking if k is low, but they fail by kinking if k is very high. There is a critical value of k that makes a tube equally likely to fail by breaking or kinking, and it can be shown that this is the optimum value for strength with lightness (2). It is difficult to calculate the value accurately, but it is probably not much more than 0.9 for tubes made of bone. The swan humerus with $k \simeq 0.9$ has struts running across its cavity, which reduce the danger of kinking.

A cylindrical tube with a wall of uniform thickness

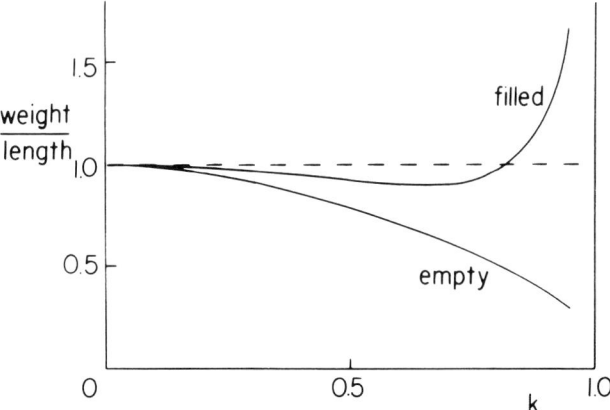

FIG. 24. Graphs of weight/unit length against k, (internal diameter):(external diameter), for cylindrical tubes of equal strength in bending. *Bottom line* shows the weight of empty tube. *Top line* shows weight of the same tube filled with a substance that has one-half the density of the tube wall.

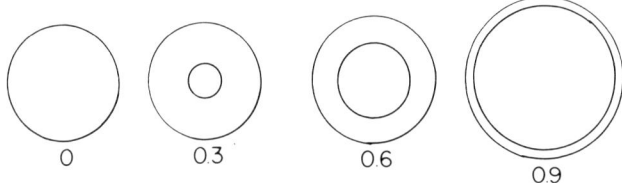

FIG. 23. Cross sections drawn to same scale. Rod and 3 tubes would all be equally strong in bending if made of same material. Numbers indicate k, ratio of internal diameter to external diameter.

has the same strength for all directions of bending. Many bones have highly asymmetrical cross sections, which must make them better able to withstand bending moments in some directions than in others. There is an intriguing difference between the fore and hind cannon bones of cattle and other ruminant mammals. (The cannon bones are the fused second and third metapodials.) The fore cannon bone has a greater transverse diameter than sagittal diameter and so must be better able to withstand transverse bending than fore-and-aft bending. The hind cannon bone tends to have greater sagittal than transverse diameter, so that the reverse is true (Fig. 25). Both the fore and hind cannon bones are subject to large bending moments in the sagittal plane during straight galloping and jumping, but large transverse forces may act on the forefeet and cause large bending moments in the fore cannon bones when the animal swerves.

Consider next whether bones should taper or have uniform thickness. In the simple situation shown in Figure 26A the bending moment is zero at the distal end of the bone, rises to a maximum at the muscle insertion, and falls to zero again at the joint. In Figure 26B an extensor muscle instead of a flexor is active so the bending moments act in the opposite direction (and so are shown as negative). The bending moment has its maximum numerical value at the joint. The numerical value of the bending moment increases from distal to proximal along most of the length of the bone (Fig. 26A, B).

Figure 26 shows only forces at right angles to the bone, which tend to bend it. In a more typical situation the forces would also have axial components tending to compress or (less likely) to stretch it. In a case considered in the section STRESSES AND STRAINS IN BONES, p. 36, the maximum stresses in a dog's tibia were only a little different from the stresses that would have acted in the absence of axial components of force, although the axial component of the force on the distal end of the bone was far greater than the component at right angles. This is a typical situation: stresses due to bending moments in long bones are usually much more important than stresses due to axial forces, except near the end of the bones where bending moments are small. Long bones and other long slender structures are more vulnerable to bending moments than axial forces; it is easier to break a stick by bending it than by pulling on its ends.

If a bone is to be made as light as possible, to withstand particular forces, it should be built in such a way that those forces set up equal stresses all along its length. Otherwise there is unnecessary weight in the less highly stressed parts. For most of the length of typical bones, bending moments tend to be proportional to the distance from the distal end and stresses due to axial components of force tend to be relatively unimportant, as has been shown. Hence for most of the length of a bone, ability to withstand bending moments should be proportional to distance from the distal end.

The ability of a bone to withstand bending moments at a particular cross section is indicated by a quantity called the section modulus, which is easily calculated from the dimensions of the cross section. The method of calculation is explained in engineering textbooks. Section modulus is defined in such a way that for a particular cross section

$$\text{maximum stress} = \frac{\text{bending moment}}{\text{section modulus}}$$

The arguments of the last few paragraphs indicate that for most of the length of a bone the section modulus should be proportional to the distance from the distal end. Figure 27 shows that this is approximately true for most of the length of a dog tibia; this bone tapers in almost ideal fashion for withstanding bending moments. Note that the sections measured for Figure 27 exclude the extreme distal end of the bone where the bending moment may be less important than the axial component of force and the shearing effect of the component at right angles to the bone. They also exclude the proximal end of the bone where forces at the joint and at muscle insertions cause abrupt changes in the gradient of the bending moment (see Fig. 26).

Stresses are reduced in some bones by the principles

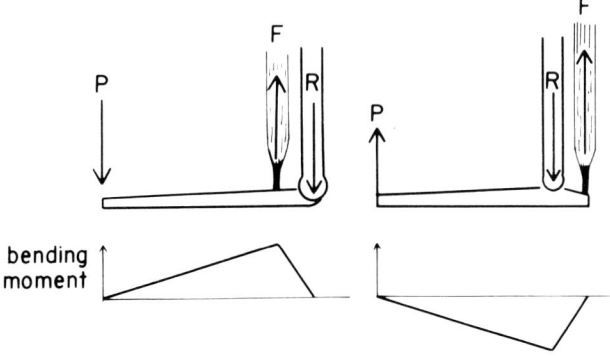

FIG. 26. *Top*, diagrams of 2 bones on which vertical forces act. *F*, force exerted by a muscle; *P*, external force; *R*, reaction at a joint. *Bottom*, graphs showing distribution of bending moments along the same bones. Bending moment is shown as positive if it tends to rotate distal part of bone counterclockwise.

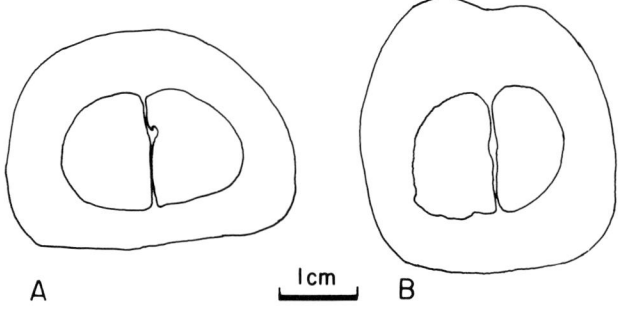

FIG. 25. Transverse sections of a fore (*A*) and a hind (*B*) cannon bone of an ox. Sections were cut halfway along the bones.

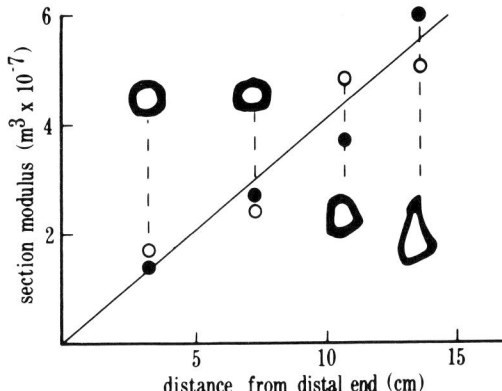

FIG. 27. Graph of section modulus against distance from distal end of the bone (tibia of a 24-kg dog). Overall length of bone was 17 cm. Values refer to bending moments in sagittal plane. Two points are given for each cross section because due to asymmetry the maximum tensile stress was not numerically equal to maximum compressive stress at opposite face of bone. Cross sections are also shown, with anterior edges uppermost. [From Alexander (5).]

of balanced loads and of bracing, which are illustrated in Figure 28. Figure 28A represents a pillar with a crosspiece. A load F on one arm of the crosspiece tends to set up compressive stresses in the pillar, since it acts parallel to the pillar. It also exerts a bending moment Fx tending to bend the pillar to the right. The bending moment can be eliminated by applying a balancing force (indicated by a broken arrow) to the other arm. This increases the total load on the pillar but makes the stress uniform across the pillar. The uniform (compressive) stress is less than the maximum stress acting in the unbalanced situation provided x is greater than 1/4 to 1/2 the radius of the pillar, depending on whether the pillar is solid or hollow (2). This illustrates the principle of balanced loads.

Figure 28B illustrates the principle of bracing. The force F acts on a pole, setting up bending moments in the pole and possibly breaking it. The danger of breakage can be reduced by fitting a guy rope, which exerts an oblique force F' and thereby reduces the bending moments.

Pauwels (53) drew attention to applications of these principles in the human body. Figure 28C shows part of the skeleton of a man who is either standing on one leg or taking a step. The force F represents the weight of the body (excluding the supporting leg) plus the inertia force due to any vertical acceleration of the body. It exerts a moment about the hip joint that may be balanced by the muscles indicated by thin continuous lines, which insert on the proximal end of the femur. In this case F will set up large bending moments in the shaft of the femur. Alternatively the moment about the hip may be balanced by tension in the iliotibial tract, a strong fascia (indicated by a broken line) near the lateral surface of the thigh. In this case the bending moments in the femur will be smaller (see also ref. 57). The effect of tension in the iliotibial tract is like that of the balancing load in Figure 28A.

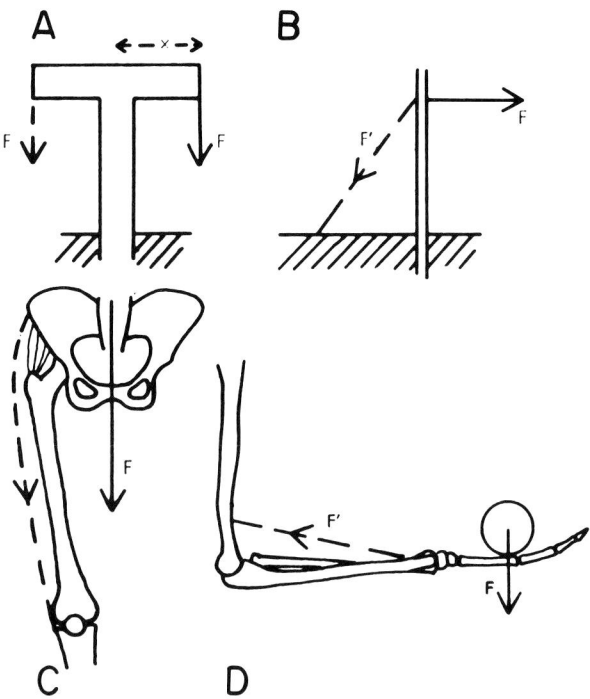

FIG. 28. A, B: diagrams illustrating principles of stress reduction by balanced loads and by bracing, respectively. C: pelvic girdle and part of skeleton of supporting leg of a man who has the other leg off the ground. D: arm skeleton of man holding a heavy object on his palm. Arrows represent forces. Further explanation is given in the text. [From Alexander (2).]

Figure 28D represents the arm of a man who is holding a heavy weight on his palm. If the moment about the elbow were balanced solely by the biceps and brachialis muscles (which insert near the elbow) large bending moments would act on the radius and ulna. If, however, it were balanced partly by a force F' exerted by the brachioradialis muscle, the bending moments would be smaller: the brachioradialis muscle would act like the guy rope in Figure 28B. It has been shown by electromyography that the brachioradialis is used, as well as the biceps and brachialis, when the elbow is bent against a large moment (16). Although the brachioradialis reduces stresses in the radius and ulna, in this situation it sets up additional stresses in the humerus so its effect is not wholly beneficial (53).

The ends of bones must be fairly large to provide articular surfaces of appropriate area, but if they were solid they would in many cases be unnecessarily heavy. They tend to consist of cancellous bone, a delicate three-dimensional network of fine strands (trabeculae) of bone. It is generally possible to see a clear pattern in the arrangement of trabeculae (Fig. 29). To understand the significance of the patterns, we need to understand the relationship between direct (tensile and compressive) stresses and shearing stresses.

Figure 30A shows a square block which is distorted in Figure 30B to a tall rectangle with tensile stresses acting vertically and compressive stresses running horizontally. In Figure 30C the block has been distorted

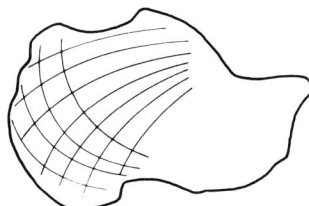

FIG. 29. A vertical longitudinal section of a human calcaneum, with *lines* showing directions in which trabeculae run.

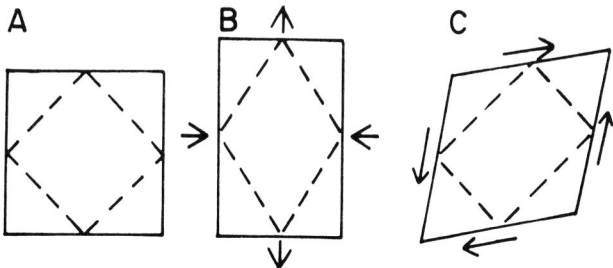

FIG. 30. Diagram of relationship between stresses. When direct stresses act vertically and horizontally, shear stresses act at 45°, and vice versa. *A*: block enclosing broken outline, which is square but tilted at 45°. *B*: square deformed to rhombus is sheared. *C*: square stretched to rectangle. [From Alexander (2).]

to a rhombus. Such deformation is called shearing and sets up shearing stresses parallel to the faces of the block. In Figure 30*A* the block encloses a broken outline. This part is itself square but is tilted at 45°. In Figure 30*B* this part is deformed to a rhombus: it is sheared. In Figure 30*C* it is stretched to a rectangle. These diagrams show that when direct stresses act vertically and horizontally shear stresses act at 45°, and vice versa.

Larger stresses act in the human heel during running than in walking or standing. Figure 31 shows how they probably act. Tensile stresses act along the Achilles tendon and round the heel to the plantar aponeurosis. Compressive stresses act radially in the heel, everywhere at right angles to the tensile stresses. Shear stresses (not shown in Fig. 31) act at 45° to the tensile and compressive stresses. A comparison of Figure 29 with Figure 31 shows that the trabeculae tend to be aligned with the tensile and compressive stresses and so to avoid the directions of the shear stresses. Alignment of trabeculae with direct stresses has also been demonstrated in other bones and seems to be a usual arrangement.

The directions of stresses in Figure 31 were obtained by photoelastic analysis of a plastic model. The directions of the strains in the heel of a sheep have been determined by a more direct method using strain gauges attached to the bone (44). The directions of the direct strains at the surface of the bone, at the stage of the stride when they were largest, coincided with the directions of the trabeculae within the bone.

The heel is capped by an epiphysis, which is separated from the main body of the bone, in children, by a cartilaginous epiphysial plate (Fig. 31). Shear stresses parallel to the epiphysial plate would be apt to shear the epiphysis off the bone, but the cartilage is well able to withstand compression or moderate tension. Figure 31 shows that most of the epiphysial plate is parallel to the tensile stresses, so that the compressive stresses tend to hold the epiphysis firmly in place. At the posterior end, the epiphysial plate crosses some of the lines of tensile stress. It does so in a series of steps so as always to be parallel either to the tensile stresses or to the compressive stresses, and never parallel to the shear stresses.

Such finesse of design is not universal. For example, there is an epiphysis at the insertion of the quadriceps muscles on the human tibia (Fig. 10). Part of its epiphysial plate is subject to shear. This part is reinforced by a dense array of collagen fibers (65).

Even small holes tend to weaken bones, because they give rise to localized stress concentrations when the bone is stressed. In some circumstances they reduce the forces that bones can withstand, but in others they merely reduce the energy that the bone can absorb in an impact before it breaks (68). Notches would have similar effects, but bones generally have smooth surfaces, remarkably free of notches. They are necessarily pierced by holes, but these are generally arranged so that they weaken the bone very little. The hole that admits blood vessels to the marrow generally runs obliquely, at only a small angle to the long axis of the bone. The fine canals around which Haversian systems form run lengthwise along bones. Even the orientation of bone cells seems arranged to weaken the bone as little as possible (29).

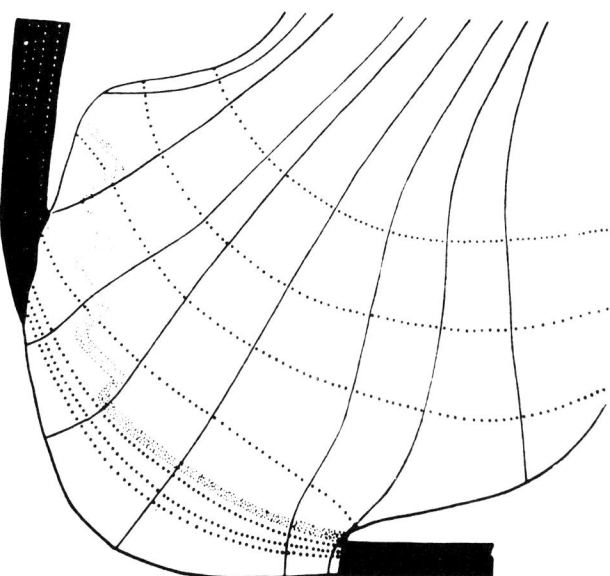

FIG. 31. Pattern of stresses acting in heel of a person standing on his toes, or running with toes on ground and heel off the ground. Diagram is based on data obtained by photoelastic analysis of a model. *Continuous lines* show directions of principal compressive stresses. *Dotted lines* show directions of principal tensile stresses. *Black areas* represent Achilles tendon and plantar aponeurosis. *Stippled band* represents epiphysial plate. [From Smith (64).]

A dropped cup is less likely to break on a carpeted floor because some of its kinetic energy is absorbed by the carpet. Similarly, soft tissues give bones some protection from impacts. Currey (30) measured the energy needed to break rabbit metatarsals by impact. In some experiments he left the bones bare, but in others he laid on them the piece of furry skin that covers them in life. When the skin was in place, 37% more energy was needed to break the bones. The skin apparently gives quite a useful degree of protection and the muscles, which cover many bones, must give much more.

CONCLUSION

This chapter shows some of the ways in which skeletal mechanics contribute to our understanding of the bodies of man and other animals. It shows how capability of movement depends on the structure of the skeleton and the arrangement of muscles. It shows how the mechanical consequences of different patterns of coordination can be assessed. Readers who wish to know more may like to consult the books by Alexander (2), Carlsöo (20), Gordon (36), Margaria (47), and Wainwright et al. (68).

REFERENCES

1. ALEXANDER, R. McN. Mechanisms of the jaws of some atheriniform fish. *J. Zool.* 151: 233-255, 1967.
2. ALEXANDER, R. McN. *Animal Mechanics*. London: Sidgwick & Jackson, 1968. (Biol. Ser.)
3. ALEXANDER, R. McN. The mechanics of jumping by a dog (*Canis familiaris*). *J. Zool.* 173: 549-573, 1974.
4. ALEXANDER, R. McN. *Biomechanics*. London: Chapman & Hall, 1975.
5. ALEXANDER, R. McN. Evolution of integrated design. *Am. Zool.* 15: 419-425, 1975.
6. ALEXANDER, R. McN. Allometry of the limbs of antelopes (Bovidae). *J. Zool.* 183: 125-146, 1977.
7. ALEXANDER, R. McN. Terrestrial locomotion. In: *Mechanics and Energetics of Animal Locomotion*, edited by R. McN. Alexander and G. Goldspink. London: Chapman & Hall, 1977, p. 168-203.
8. ALEXANDER, R. McN. Analysis of force platform data to obtain joint forces. In: *An Introduction to the Biomechanics of Joints and Joint and Joint Replacements*, edited by D. Dowson and V. Wright. London: Mech. Eng. Publ. In press.
9. ALEXANDER, R. McN., AND H. C. BENNET-CLARK. Storage of elastic strain energy in muscle and other tissues. *Nature London* 265: 114-117, 1977.
10. ALEXANDER, R. McN., AND A. S. JAYES. Optimum walking techniques for idealized animals. *J. Zool.* 186: 61-81, 1978.
11. ALEXANDER, R. McN., AND A. VERNON. The dimensions of knee and ankle muscles and the forces they exert. *J. Hum. Movement Stud.* 1: 115-123, 1975.
12. ALEXANDER, R. McN., AND A. VERNON. The mechanics of hopping by kangaroos (Macropodidae). *J. Zool.* 177: 265-303, 1975.
13. ANDREWS, J. G., AND Y. YOUM. A biomechanical investigation of wrist kinematics. *J. Biomech.* 12: 83-93, 1979.
14. BARNETT, C. H., D. V. DAVIES, AND M. A. MACCONNAILL. *Synovial Joints: Their Structure and Mechanics*. London: Longmans, 1961.
15. BARNETT, C. H., AND O. J. LEWIS. The evolution of some traction epiphyses in birds and mammals. *J. Anat.* 92: 593-601, 1958.
16. BASMAJIAN, J. V. *Muscles Alive: Their Functions Revealed by Electromyography*. (2nd ed.). Baltimore: Williams & Wilkins, 1967.
17. BORELLI, G. A. *De Motu Animalium*. Rome: Bernabo, 1680-1681.
18. BULLOUGH, P., J. GOODFELLOW, A. S. GREENWALD, AND J. O'CONNOR. Incongruent surfaces in the human hip joint. *Nature London* 217: 1290, 1968.
19. CALOW, L. J., AND R. McN. ALEXANDER. A mechanical analysis of a hind leg of a frog (*Rana temporaria*). *J. Zool.* 171: 293-321, 1973.
20. CARLSÖO, S. *How Man Moves: Kinesiological Studies and Methods*. London: Heinemann, 1972.
21. CAVAGNA, G. A. Force platforms as ergometers. *J. Appl. Physiol.* 39: 174-179, 1975.
22. CAVAGNA, G. A., AND R. MARGARIA. Mechanics of walking. *J. Appl. Physiol.* 21: 271-278, 1966
23. CAVAGNA, G. A., F. P. SAIBENE, AND R. MARGARIA. Mechanical work in running. *J. Appl. Physiol.* 19: 249-256, 1964.
24. CLARK, J., AND R. McN. ALEXANDER. Mechanics of running by quail (*Coturnix*). *J. Zool.* 176: 87-113, 1975.
25. CLOSE, R. I. Dynamic properties of mammalian skeletal muscles. *Physiol. Rev.* 52: 129-197, 1972.
26. CROWNINSHIELD, R. D., R. C. JOHNSTON, J. G. ANDREWS, AND R. A. BRAND. A biomechanical investigation of the human hip. *J. Biomech.* 11: 75-85, 1978.
27. CROWNINSHIELD, R. D., M. H. POPE, AND R. J. JOHNSON. An analytical model of the knee. *J. Biomech.* 9: 397-405, 1976.
28. CUMING, W. G., R. McN. ALEXANDER, AND A. S. JAYES. Rebound resilience of tendons in the feet of sheep (*Ovis aries*) *J. Exp. Biol.* 74: 75-81, 1978.
29. CURREY, J. D. Stress concentrations in bone. *Q. J. Micros. Sci.* 103: 111-33, 1962.
30. CURREY, J. D. The effect of protection on the impact strength of rabbit's bones. *Acta Anat.* 71: 87-93, 1968.
31. DEMPSTER, W. T. *Space Requirements of the Seated Operator*. Washington, DC: U.S. Dept. Commerce, Off. Tech. Serv., 1955. (WADC Tech. Rep. 55-159.)
32. DOWSON, D., A. UNSWORTH, AND V. WRIGHT. Analysis of 'boosted lubrication' in human joints. *J. Mech. Eng. Sci* 12: 364-369, 1970.
33. DRILLIS, R., AND R. CONTINI. *Body Segment Parameters*. New York: New York Univ., Sch. Eng. Sci., 1966. (Tech. Rep. 1166.03.)
34. DVIR, Z., AND N. BERME. The shoulder complex in elevation of the arm: a mechanism approach. *J. Biomech.* 11: 219-225, 1978.
35. GEERLINK, P. J., AND J. J. VIDELER. Joints and muscles of the dorsal fin of *Tilapia nilotica* L. (fam. Cichlidae). *Neth. J. Zool.* 24: 270-290, 1974.
36. GORDON, J. E. (editor). *Structures: Or Why Things Don't Fall Down*. Harmondsworth: Penguin, 1978.
37. GRIEVE, D. W., D. I. MILLER, D. MITCHELSON, J. P. PAUL, AND A. J. SMITH. *Techniques for the Analysis of Human Movement*. London: Lepus, 1975.
38. HALLEN, L. G., AND O. LINDAHL. The 'screw-home' movement of the knee joint. *Acta Orthop. Scand.* 37: 97-106, 1966.
39. HIIEMAE, K. The structure and function of the jaw muscles in the rat (*Rattus norvegicus* L.) III. The mechanics of the muscles. *Zool. J. Linn. Soc.* 50: 111-132, 1971.
40. HOBSON, D. A., AND L. E. TORFASON. Optimization of four-bar knee mechanisms—a computerized approach. *J. Biomech.* 7: 371-376, 1974.
41. HUNT, K. H. *Kinematic Geometry of Mechanisms*. Oxford: Clarendon, 1978.
42. JOSEPH, J., AND A. NIGHTINGALE. Electromyography of muscles of posture: thigh muscles in males. *J. Physiol. London* 126: 81-85, 1954.

43. KINZEL, G. L., A. S. HALL, AND B. M. HILLBERRY. Measurement of the total motion between two body segments. I. *J. Biomech.* 5: 93-105, 1972.
44. LANYON, L. E. Experimental support for the trajectorial theory of bone structure. *J. Bone Jt. Surg. Br. Vol.* 56: 160-166, 1974.
45. LANYON, L. E., W. G. J. HAMPSON, A. E. GOODSHIP, AND J. S. SHAH. Bone deformation recorded in vivo from strain gauges attached to the human tibial shaft. *Acta Orthop. Scand.* 46: 256-268, 1975.
46. LEWIS, P. R., AND C. W. MCCUTCHEN. Experimental evidence for weeping lubrication in mammalian joints. *Nature London* 48: 1285, 1959.
47. MARGARIA, R. *Biomechanics and Energetics of Muscular Exercise.* Oxford: Clarendon, 1976.
48. MARKOLF, K. L., J. S. MENSCH, AND H. C. AMSTUTZ. Stiffness and laxity of the knee—the contributions of the supporting structures. *J. Bone Jt. Surg. Am. Vol.* 58: 583-594, 1976.
49. MILLER, D. I., AND R. C. NELSON. *Biomechanics of Sport.* Philadelphia: Lea & Febiger, 1973. (Health Educ. Phys. Educ. Recreation Ser.)
50. MILNER-BROWN, H. S., AND R. B. STEIN. The relation between the surface electromyogram and muscular force. *J. Physiol. London* 246: 549-569, 1975.
51. MORGAN, D. L., U. PROSKE, AND D. WARREN. Measurements of muscle stiffness and the mechanism of elastic storage of energy in hopping kangaroos. *J. Physiol. London* 282: 253-261, 1978.
52. MUYBRIDGE, E. *Animals in Motion* (2nd ed.), edited by L. S. Brown. New York: Dover, 1957.
53. PAUWELS, F. Die Bedeutung der Bauprinzipien fur Beanspruchung der Röhrenknochen. *Z. Anat. Entwicklungsgesch.* 114: 129-166, 1948.
54. PENROD, D. D., D. T. DAVY, AND D. P. SINGH. An optimization approach to tendon force analysis. *J. Biomech.* 7: 123-129, 1974.
55. PIZIALI, R. L., T. K. HIGHT, AND D. A. NAGEL. An extended structural analysis of long bones—application to the human tibia. *J. Biomech.* 9: 695-701, 1976.
56. PRENTIS, J. M. *Dynamics of Mechanical Systems.* London: Longman, 1970.
57. RYBICKI, E. F., F. A. SIMONEN, AND E. B. WEIS. On the mathematical analysis of stress in the human femur. *J. Biomech.* 5: 203-215, 1972.
58. SCAPINO, R. P. The third joint of the canine jaw. *J. Morphol.* 116: 23-50, 1965.
59. SCHULTZ, A. H. Man and the catarrhine primates. *Cold Spring Harbor Symp. Quant. Biol.* 15: 35-53, 1950.
60. SCHULTZ, A. H. *The Life of Primates* London: Weidenfeld & Nicholson, 1969.
61. SEIREG, A., AND R. J. ARVIKAR. A mathematical model for evaluation of forces in lower extremeties of the musculo-skeletal system. *J. Biomech.* 6: 313-326, 1973.
62. SMIDT, G. L. Biomechanical analysis of knee flexion and extension. *J. Biomech.* 6: 79-92, 1973.
63. SMITH, J. M., AND R. J. G. SAVAGE. The mechanics of mammalian jaws. *Sch. Sci. Rev.* 40: 289-301, 1959.
64. SMITH, J. W. Observations on the postural mechanism of the human knee joint. *J. Anat.* 90: 236-260, 1956.
65. SMITH, J. W. The relationship of epiphysial plates to stress in some bones of the lower limb. *J. Anat.* 96: 58-78, 1962.
66. SOUDAN, K., R. VAN AUDEKERCKE, AND M. MARTENS. Methods, difficulties and inaccuracies in the study of human joint kinematics and pathokinematics by the instant axis concept. Example: the knee joint. *J. Biomech.* 12: 27-33, 1979.
67. TUTTLE, R. H. Knuckle-walking and the problem of human origins. *Science* 166: 953-961, 1969.
68. WAINWRIGHT, S. A., W. D. BIGGS, J. D. CURREY, AND J. M. GOSLINE. *Mechanical Design in Organisms.* London: Arnold, 1976.
69. WANG, C. J., AND P. S. WALKER. The effects of flexion and rotation on the length patterns of the ligaments of the knee. *J. Biomech.* 6: 587-596, 1973.
70. WARWICK, R., AND P. L. WILLIAMS (editors). *Gray's Anatomy* (35th ed.). London: Longman. 1973.
71. WEINERT, C. R., J. H. MCMASTER, AND R. J. FERGUSON. Dynamic function of the human fibula. *Am. J. Anat.* 138: 145-150, 1973.
72. WEIS-FOGH, T., AND R. MCN. ALEXANDER. The sustained power output from striated muscle. In: *Scale Effects in Animal Locomotion*, edited by T. J. Pedley. London: Academic, 1977, p. 511-525.
73. WRIGHT, V., D. DOWSON, AND J. KERR. The structure of joints. *Int. Rev. Connect. Tissue Res.* 6: 105-125, 1973.
74. YALDEN, D. W. The functional morphology of the carpal bones in carnivores. *Acta Anat.* 77: 481-500, 1970.
75. YOUM, Y., R. F. DRYER, K. THAMBYRAJAH, A. E. FLATT, AND B. L. SPRAGUE. Biomechanical analyses of forearm pronation-supination and elbow flexion-extension. *J. Biomech.* 12: 245-255, 1979.
76. YOUM, Y., R. Y. MCMURTRY, A. E. FLATT, AND T. E. GILLESPIE. Kinematics of the wrist. I. An experimental study of radial-ulnar deviation and flexion-extension. *J. Bone Jt. Surg. Am. Vol.* 60: 423-431, 1978.
77. YOUNG, J. Z., AND M. J. HOBBS. *The Life of Mammals: Their Anatomy and Physiology* (2nd ed.). Oxford: Clarendon, 1975.
78. ZERNICKE, R. F., J. GARHAMMER, AND F. W. JOBE. Human patellar-tendon rupture. *J. Bone Jt. Surg. Am. Vol.* 59: 179-183, 1977.
79. ZERNICKE, R. F., AND E. M. ROBERTS. Lower extremity forces and torques during systematic variation of non-weight bearing motion. *Med. Sci. Sports* 10: 21-26, 1978.

CHAPTER 3

Muscle, the motor

L. D. PARTRIDGE | Center for Health Sciences, University of Tennessee, Memphis, Tennessee

L. A. BENTON | Neuromuscular Engineering, Rehabilitation Engineering Center, Rancho Los Amigos Hospital, Downey, California

CHAPTER CONTENTS

Representation of Muscle Properties
  Dimensions used
  Models
  Real motor systems
  Summary
Properties of the Contractile Unit
  Passive mechanical contributions
  Response to neural signals
  Interaction between neural and other inputs
  Functional variations
  Summary
Multiple Units of Muscle
  The unit of muscle function
  Relationships in multiunit function
  Summary
Some Measures of Muscle Function
  Summary
Motor Functions of Muscles
Final Summary
Epilogue

Um nun näher zu erfahren, was vorgeht, wenn die Muskeln in Thätigkeit treten und badurch die Ursache der Bewegung der Glieder werden, wollen wir folgende drei Fragen behandeln:
  I. Auf welche Weise werden die Muskeln zur Thätigkeit angeregt?
  II. Welche Erscheinungen bieten die Muskeln bei ihrer Thätigkeit dar?
  III. In welchem Zusammenhange stehen diese Erscheinungen unter einander?

Handwörterbuch der Physiologie, edited by R. Wagner, vol. III, sect. 2, 1846 (537)

MUSCLE WAS ONE OF THE EARLIEST subjects of quantitative and graphic investigation in the history of physiology (173, 182, 183, 238, 247, 440, 444). First studies were concerned with the role of muscle in movement, but later emphasis turned to study of processes of contraction at the chemical and molecular level. Introduction of concepts of control systems after World War II (367, 547) revived a limited interest in mechanical aspects of gross muscle action. These studies re-asked the questions of a century earlier, as found at the head of this presentation (537), but this time they emphasized dynamic properties and descriptive forms that would allow synthesis of information about parts (393, 394, 396, 418, 420, 434, 500) into representation of larger systems (233, 234, 260, 392, 443). It was hoped that muscle could be characterized in a simple model of function which, with scaling adjustment, would be widely applicable.

This chapter deals with information about muscle as a transformer of nerve signals into actions in the Newtonian world of motor function. Although contractile theories have changed repeatedly (20, 113, 119, 151, 250, 271, 276, 277, 374, 384, 494, 519, 520, 544, 566) and are still debated (162, 163, 265, 388, 450), many phenomena to be discussed in this chapter were well known to early workers (247) from surprisingly sophisticated measurements and have not changed with the theories used to explain them. Some additional mechanical details that have been learned in recent control system studies are described. Other observations used here to describe gross function were derived from attempts to elucidate molecular processes within fibers. None of the muscle properties described in this chapter are recognized to be clearly incompatible with the cross-bridge theories of contraction, and several are widely accepted as supportive [(450); see also the chapter by Houk and Rymer in this *Handbook*]. The fitting of some of these observations with the theory is, however, based on subsidiary hypotheses (388) that have had little or no critical evaluation.

From a literature on mechanical aspects of muscle function, which we estimate to contain in the order of 10^5 items, only a very limited portion can be covered in this chapter. Each of the molecular processes in muscle, which in some cases seem to be closely related to motor properties, is a major topic in itself and cannot be reviewed adequately here. (See ref. 450 for a list of review papers up to 1970.) These processes include activation [(119, 401); and see the chapter by Krnjevic in this *Handbook*], contraction mechanism (131, 271, 275–277, 388, 450, 520), membrane activity (119, 305), muscle chemistry [(374, 388, 390, 565); and see the chapter by Burke in this *Handbook*], and the

44   HANDBOOK OF PHYSIOLOGY ~ THE NERVOUS SYSTEM II

ultrastructure of muscle (16, 275). These topics, which are at an analytical level different from motor control, can be reviewed in standard textbooks if desired (242, 445, 551, 560, 570). We describe instead a variety of phenomena that can be related directly to the mechanical action of muscle.

REPRESENTATION OF MUSCLE PROPERTIES

Dimensions Used

During the two centuries in which muscle and motor function have been studied quantitatively a wide range of terms have been used to describe the measures used. The interpretation of these terms is a considerable problem that is encountered in current literature almost as much as in older work (224). Several factors contribute to the complexity of terminology, and the result is more than an inconvenience. It can even become impossible to determine what measure of muscle action is reported in otherwise important papers.

That multiplicity of nomenclature, which developed naturally with the historical changes in mensuration, can be dealt with in old literature; in future work it should be a disappearing problem with international standardization of units (15, 150, 324, 344, 536). Grams weight, newtons, and pounds—all of which have been used to report muscle force—are dimensionally equivalent and can be compared by the use of a simple conversion factor. Nevertheless, there is no certain way to correct nomenclature that is dimensionally faulty and that, unfortunately, still appears regularly in current literature. Force is often meant when the term used is *power, strength, work, resistance,* or *effort*. Only occasionally is it possible to extract enough information from such presentations to be sure what was measured and, with only partial information, intuitive judgments can be wrong. For example, in the graphs by Levine and Wyman (331), frequently cited as the first report of the force-velocity effect, the abscissa is labeled *work*. From the shape of the curves this seems to be a mislabeling of the force scale, but

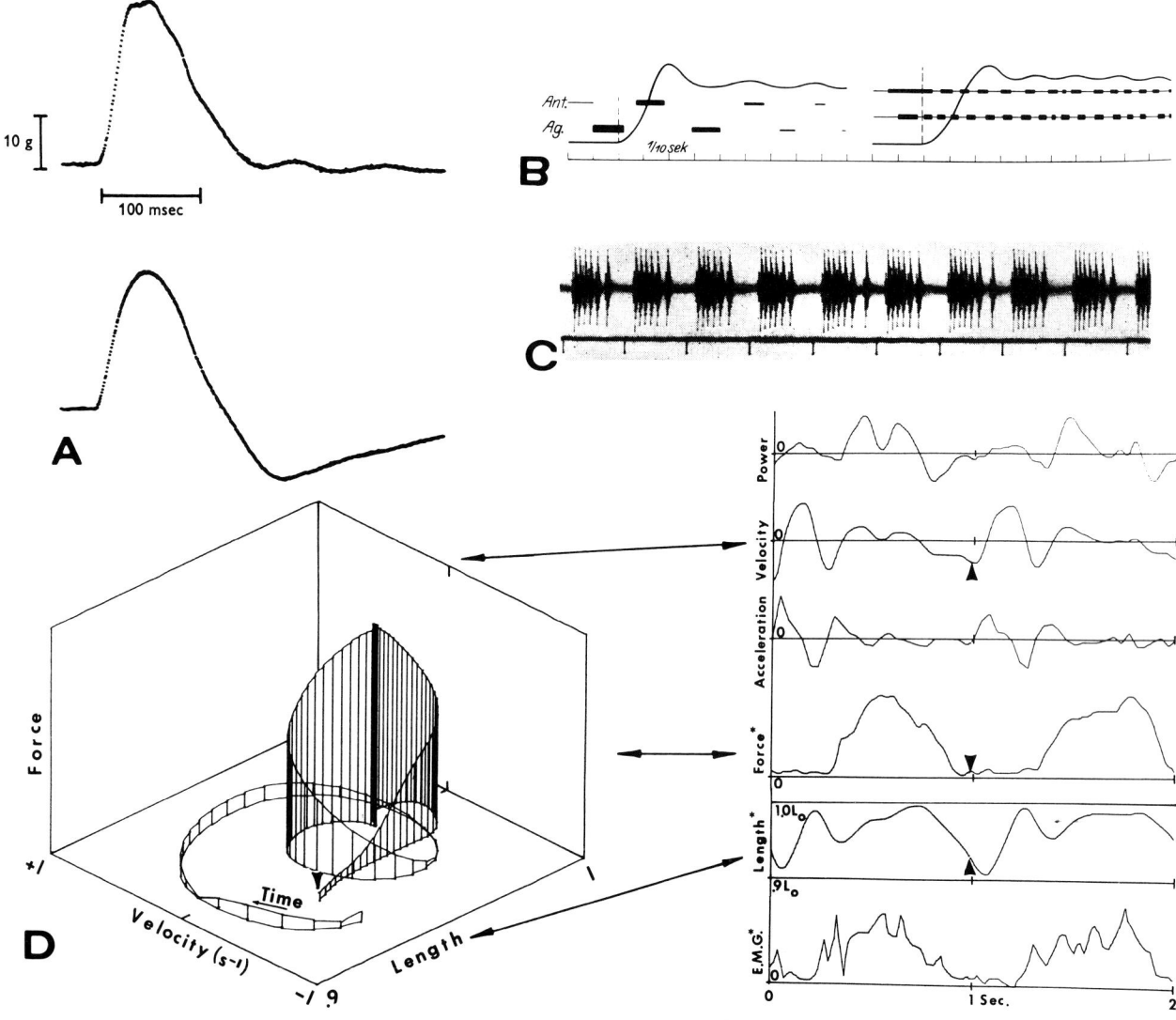

the text reveals that work indeed was measured. (What is not entirely obvious is the fact that total work was proportional to average force over the tested range, since work was measured each time over the same distance. The usual interpretation of force and the unusual label of work are in this case nearly equal, and the appearance of dimensional error is not supported by fact in either case.) Even after conversion of terms a complex nomenclature still remains because of the many dimensions involved in the study of muscle function (for examples see Table 1 in APPENDIX and Fig. 1). Different dimensions are inescapable in dealing with the clearly different topics of force, length, velocity, power, and work. Muscle response also may be measured in dimensions of a functional response (e.g., pressure in Fig. 18A); yet such basic dimensions are not always enough. Force properly may be reported in terms of total force, of force per unit cross-sectional area (stress), or as a dimensionless value relative to the force delivered by a twitch, a maximal tetanic contraction, or a maximal voluntary contraction. It is of no help that each of these three-dimensionally different measures sometimes is labeled simply *force*.

For this presentation many data are given in the form of graphs. Because of uncertainties with respect to conversion we have left labels on the coordinates in the units of the original presentation. In some cases additional information is given in the legends to allow the reader to normalize the graphs, but in other cases normalizing factors in the original papers have not been indicated. At least in the measurement of muscle rest length, however, an appreciable variability exists in the definitions of that measure as used in different studies, and we have not found a way to unify the data. Because of the complexity, inconsistency, and importance of measurement dimensions in quantifying motor activity, the investment of appreciable time in the study of measurement seems to be an inescapable requirement for careful work in motor control (see refs. 14, 76, 150, 214, 323, 324, 344, 431, and 536 and APPENDIX).

Models

Information about muscles has not been important in reductionist reviews of motor control physiology, but knowledge of muscle rules is essential to an integrative approach to motor control. When combining the parts of the system, both the result of the neural activity and the cause of sensory inputs that affect the neural part of motor control are dependent on muscle

FIG. 1. Examples of physiological actions of various muscles. *A*: twitch response to excitation of a few motor nerve fibers of human muscle obtained as ensemble average of output force from whole arm. *Upper record*, response during weak contraction of whole muscle; *lower record*, response from same motor units stimulated when remainder of muscle was strongly contracted. In the twitch during strong contractions, averaged force contribution rose to an appreciably lower peak than in the other series; then the average decreased to a value less than background level. In this measure both the primary or direct effect of excitation of the test unit and any consistent secondary effects that modify the activity of other units are combined in the total recorded response. *B*: two voluntary movements of human arm. Thickness of *horizontal bars*, periods of high, low, and no electromyograph (EMG) activity in agonist and antagonist muscles. First record made during a relaxed movement, second with a stiff arm. Periods of agonist and antagonist activities in first record show alternation with complete separation. In 2nd record the periods are completely overlapping with a rapid cycling of intensity of EMG. In spite of differences in electrical activity, however, the two movements follow similar time courses of position. *C*: sound produced by vibration of locust tympanum by tymbale muscle when artificially stimulated at 22.5 pulses/s. Stimulus points shown on *lower record*. Compare Fig. 7B, which shows isometric response of a similar muscle stimulated at 22 pulses/s. *D*: measures of triceps sura muscle action in 2 steps of a uniformly walking cat (399). All of the data originated in measurements (∗) of length, force, and EMG by Yager (563). Continuous approximations of length, velocity, and acceleration were derived by applying spline functions (408, 559) to 128 photographically determined point values of length. Power calculated as product of velocity and force (measured by transducer on tendon). EMG is shown as rectified and filtered interpretation of direct record. Ratio of force to acceleration does not represent changing inertia of load, in part because system is not free of external forces and also because acceleration is not measured in an inertial reference frame. For 1st step (ending at *arrowheads*) force, velocity, and length are plotted also in a pseudo-3-dimensional form, starting in swing phase and progressing continuously in direction of *time arrow*; pickets mark 10-ms intervals and eliminate ambiguity of 4-dimensional points as graphed on a plane. This trajectory over the phase plane (length vs. velocity) shows that in swing phase large velocities and displacements are associated with small forces, while largest forces occur at midlengths and lengthening velocities during stance phase of step. Rest length, $l = 1$, is near long end of lengths involved in walking, as also described in ref. 483. The EMG trajectory for this same step can be seen in ref. 393. For separated soleus and gastrocnemius records of force in walking cat, see refs. 285, 286, and 531. Note that 2 steps shown in this figure to have similar length patterns have appreciably more variation in acceleration, velocity, and EMG (278). As is most apparent on phase plane graph, when muscle returns to the starting length for 1st step, 2nd step is initiated at a different velocity and therefore cannot follow a course identical to the first. [*A*: from Milner-Brown et al. (373), with permission of Cambridge Univ. Press. *B*: from Wacholder (521). *C*: from Pringle (411), with permission of Cambridge Univ. Press. *D*: from Partridge (399), with permission of Raven Press.]

properties. To integrate muscle contributions into a concept of motor control requires a selected type of information about muscle. The mechanical response of muscle to neural signals is essential information, but the theoretical mechanism of generating that response is of indirect importance. Although it is not yet possible to construct a full description (model) of the functional relationships in motor control, we have organized this chapter to contribute to that goal. Because models and modeling are so central to the effort, some comments on our interpretation of models are necessary.

GENERAL FUNCTIONAL MODELS. The developing understanding of muscle has produced since antiquity a succession of models: verbal; pictorial [Figs. 2, 3; (273, 327)]; physical (135, 392, 409); graphical (40, 153, 201); and mathematical (124, 132, 146, 190, 196, 280, 298, 388, 407, 479). The current extent of modeling activity, however, is difficult to estimate. In the papers reviewed while preparing this chapter, it was found incidentally that at least 15% used some mathematical representation of muscle properties that might be called a formal model. (The percentage would be lower if restricted to those papers with equations using coefficients that were determined statistically.) A few other papers defined muscle models as physical systems composed of contractile proteins (409). Some papers dealt with systems containing real muscle, modeling some functional muscle situation (135, 190, 396). When one muscle is studied and the discussion deals with either muscles in general or the action of any other muscle (135, 190), the concept of modeling (165) is involved. If a model is defined as a man-made representation of some characteristic of a particular system, most physical arrangements used in muscle research, together with most of the forms in which the results are reported, can be classified as muscle models. The use of the term muscle model in different laboratories is, however, so varied that individual definitions sometimes fail to overlap. Yet by definition any model represents only part of the system and consequently will fail to match the real system in tests that require other parts. Special care is required in applying information about muscle (a model) to the larger context of motor control to avoid unjustified extrapolation. This chapter brings together the muscle properties usually recognized in motor control studies, but it also reviews some of the many situations in which that simple model is inappropriate.

It is recognized that most responses of most muscles are determined by the action of multiple components (Fig. 2) and multiple excitation impulses in each component, as well as by several physical factors affecting

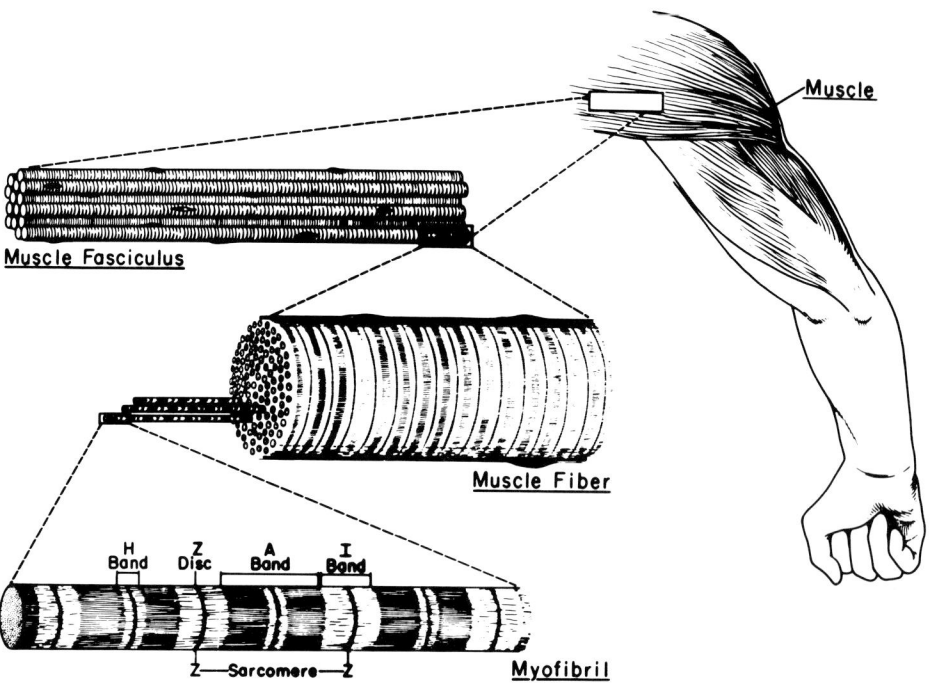

FIG. 2. Conventional nomenclature of successive structural subdivisions of vertebrate skeletal muscle down to sarcomere level. Functional motor unit does not correspond to any of these divisions. (For examples of diffuse distribution of a motor unit within a muscle, see Fig. 13 in the chapter by Burke in this *Handbook* and refs. 90, 94, 148, 155, 313, 319. It also should be noted that individual fibers may cross from one fasciculus to another (267, 268) or end within a fasciculus (6, 32, 33, 127, 255). Furthermore, the densely packed organization of fibers seen in histological section and in this schematic diagram of a fasciculus may represent a shift of extracellular fluid after loss of blood pressure (64, 123, 312). Normally, adjacent fibers may float separately within the muscle. [Adapted from Bloom and Fawcett (55).]

the muscle. The response of a single unit can be measured following a single pulse, however, and that impulse response can be described mathematically (191). In linear descriptions of motor control such equations for component responses are combined additively to describe response over the whole operating range. In fact, by the models used it can be seen that linear thinking is common (234). Many relationships in muscle, however, are nonlinear. The effect of each nerve impulse on a muscle nerve fiber does not add a fixed (quantal) increment of mechanical response (Figs. 1A, 4B, 8C). The increment added depends on other activity in the excited unit as well as in surrounding units and may range from appreciably larger than its contribution in isolation down to immeasurably small, depending on the conditions under which it is added (92, 135, 191, 501). Moreover, repetition of activation of a single unit also causes the contribution to change (Figs. 7C and D, 8C). For study of muscle summation action, linear models are then only useful under such restricted conditions that this failure of superposition introduces only tolerable error (234). Not only do unit responses not superimpose, but the effects of such factors as muscle length, velocity, stimulus, and temperature are not additive. Linear models are therefore of limited usefulness in these dimensions as well.

In the dynamic conditions characteristic of many motor activities in which muscle length or the stimulus to muscle, or both, is changing, the effects do not follow the exciting cause instantaneously. To describe the effects of a changing input requires a dynamic description, and static models can be totally misleading. If instantaneous stimulus rate is compared to muscle response using a rapidly cycling stimulus rate (Fig. 9C), for example, the dynamic lag can cause the maximum stimulus rate to correspond in time with minimal response (190, 394, 518). In linear systems either time- or frequency-based equations often are used to describe such dynamic properties (360, 453).

The combination of nonlinear and dynamic properties as found in muscle is not represented as easily (211, 325, 360, 546). The results of separate sinusoidal tests of different amplitudes and different biases have been used to provide an approximation to a variety of conditions. Similar data can be extracted from randomly modulated stimulus (354). Unfortunately, the simplicity and the accuracy of Fourier synthesis available in linear systems are lost in these cases (354). The derivation of Wiener kernels from analysis of results of tests using white noise inputs is a general approach that provides a specific description of nonlinear and dynamic systems (325, 360). Yet here too a problem develops in that the memory or hysteretic property of muscle response (Fig. 15A and C) to either neural or mechanical input is incompatible with the basic assumptions of this approach, at least in its simple form (227).

Thus a number of models exist that approximate parts of muscle function, but all of the models inescapably have appreciable defects. Deficiencies lie both in the formal models available and in defects in our understanding of the rules of the biological muscle as it responds to mechanical and neural actions. Most of the remainder of this chapter describes the mechanical function of muscle in terms of individually measured properties. Some of the properties then are combined into multifactored descriptions, but no unified model is offered that is complete enough even to predict quantitatively a muscle's mechanical response to neural drive under unconstrained conditions. Under restricted conditions, on the other hand, some very limited models not only produce good fits to physiological function but probably are important to the intuitive appreciation of functional relationships. Nevertheless, at the present stage of development the user of available models must be particularly cognizant of the limitations of the model used. The more formal models have the advantage of providing an unambiguous statement of what is included or excluded and are subject to rigorous rules of manipulation, thus reducing the risk of undetected internal inconsistencies. Yet the most formal (mathematical) models are not unique, have significant defects, and usually can be used only in the range from which they were derived. Consequently we have chosen an intermediate approach, giving preference to graphs over either verbal description or equations. Graphs allow a specific identification of the range and detail of the original data but sacrifice the ease of manipulation offered by the approximating equations.

A number of equations that have been used to fit individual functional properties can be found in the literature cited in this chapter. For any particular function the more complex equations tend to give a better fit to the particular source data. At the same time, however, they become too specific to represent the same property in other muscles or even in the same muscle under different conditions. We feel that the most useful models of muscle for study of motor control at the present time originate in empirical data instead of in contractile theory, not because of known conflict, but because more is known about muscle performance from experiment than can be predicted readily from current contractile theory. In any case, the ability of the nervous system to control complex muscle functions in an open loop mode indicates that the nervous system has discovered some sort of functional representation, from which one might infer that a good operational model of muscle probably is possible.

SPECIFIC MODELS. Historically, when a separate factor affecting muscle action has been studied in near isolation, the discussion of its implications to motor control often has involved a much simplified representation of other parts of the system. Some of these convenient fictions are important devices to isolate issues in muscle function and have been used enough to constitute significant models. These models, however, tend to have been defined by omissions and have not remained constant. To clarify the particular forms that are used repeatedly here, some of our assumptions are defined.

Idealized joint. Although the loads upon which most muscles act tend to be quite complex [(185, 215, 216); see the chapter by Alexander in this *Handbook*], many meaningful effects can be discussed most conveniently for those cases involving a simple load and joint. Incidentally, Leonardo da Vinci recognized that not all muscle effects are tensile [(327); quoted in ref. 461]. Frequently the simplifications from actual loads are recognizable only by the corrections that are not made in the calculation or discussion of effects. The joint often is inferred to be a hinge and devoid of significant friction, viscous impedance, or elastic restrictions. (See the chapter by Alexander in this *Handbook* for a more complete analysis of some special joints and see the chapters by Luschei and Goldberg and by Robinson for description of other pivoting joints.) The load in the common model is treated as a rigid body with a constant center of mass and constant moment of inertia around the joint axis. No correction is made for known movement of rotation axes (100, 157, 159, 213, 378, 473) or movement of the joint with respect to the inertial reference (exceptions may be found in refs. 100 and 233). Thus all movement is presumed to occur as simple rotation of a constant load. The ideal joint model is found in two variants. In both, the moment arm for the muscle remains essentially constant, and the muscle is a simple linear structure with no significant internal mass between two sharply localized tendons. In the first case, however, a single muscle operates against gravity, as in a common muscle lever experiment. Unlike the isotonic lever experiment, though, the distribution of the load gives it a significant moment of inertia. In the second case gravity plays no part, because the plane of movement has been chosen to be horizontal. Two identical muscles with equal moment arms act to produce torque of opposite sign on the inertial load. For this case the velocity of one muscle is equal in magnitude and opposite in sign to that of the other. Adjustment of simultaneous activity of antagonists [Fig. 1*B*; (117, 185, 262)] can allow more than one excitation pattern to produce the same torque response. Differences in torque contributions from the two muscles produce angular acceleration of the load but produce a new position only indirectly. With artificial loads attached to one or two real muscles, the ideal joint model can be produced experimentally (190, 396). It also has been possible to approximate the models for some human experiments by using selected limb positions [Figs. 1*B*, 19*B*; (246, 391, 438, 489)].

Free muscle system. Mechanical effects sometimes can be studied using a formalism called the *free body diagram* [(136, 355); and see the chapter by Alexander in this *Handbook* for an example of application to motor control], in which a rigid structure and all of the forces acting on that structure are isolated conceptually with an inertial frame of reference in order to simplify determination of the effects of the combined forces. In the free body diagram it is unnecessary to consider what other structures are associated with the free body or what action its movement accomplishes externally; only the resulting forces need be considered. A similar but less formalized isolation of muscle frequently is involved in the design and interpretation of muscle experiments related to motor control. By analogy to the free body diagram the conceptually isolated muscle is called a *free muscle system*. It is presumed that muscle obeys rules such that its response is characteristic of the combination of neural drive, force, movement, circulation, temperature, and other physical factors acting on it, without reference to how it is related to other body structures or to what external actions it is accomplishing. Thus it would not make any difference to the muscle whether it moved a limb with respect to the body, the body with respect to a fixed limb, or an artificial load, except as these actions affect balance of forces. Muscle action studied in isolation likewise would be the same as in situ if input conditions were the same. The response to a particular nerve impulse pattern would be independent of where or how that pattern was generated. In the probable event that some operating conditions differ, however, responses might not match (contrast Fig. 1*C* with Fig. 7*B*). The conceptual isolation equally might be applied to a single muscle fiber, a motor unit, or a whole muscle if the stimulus distribution, as well as pattern, were appropriate. Most of the data about muscle presented here have been learned from partially or completely isolated muscles; their application to motor control therefore assumes the validity of the free muscle concept.

Elastic matrix model. Morphological as well as functional evidence indicates that the stress-strain relationships in muscle are dependent in part on the viscoelastic framework in which the contractile units are embedded. Connective tissue, seen easily in histological examination of muscle, is located in the sarcolemma, between muscle fibers, connected to the ends of fibers, and in the tendons and aponeuroses by which muscles are connected to bones [Fig. 2*C* and *D*; (47, 55, 127, 268)]. Unstimulated muscle also reveals obvious elastic properties when stretched and released. The elasticity that appears to act in parallel to the contractile part of the muscle quite naturally has acquired the name *parallel elastic element*. More indirect evidence has led to the term *series elastic element* for the source of elastic properties of muscle which, in certain tests, seem to act in series with the contractile part of muscle (Fig. 4*C*). While series elastic elements must include tendons, the definitions of both parallel and series elastic elements are operational rather than anatomical (288) and may arise from appreciably different anatomical arrangements in different muscles (Fig. 3). In spite of a basis for question (273, 274), however, the usual representation of muscle clearly separates the two elastic elements and assumes no interaction between the elastic and the contractile elements except at their ends (340). Both the elastic and contractile parts nevertheless are presumed to contribute to observed properties of excited muscle. The delay of mechanical spread of force or displacement over the length of such a viscoelastic structure (458) is not ordinarily included in this muscle model.

Active state. Active state is a model of muscle contraction that actually is composed of a mixture of two models, a conceptual one and an operationally defined model. The concept presumes a process that is initiated by stimulus and is independent of movement. The measurement-based form was intended to define the same process, but in fact this definition of active state simply follows force in a specified test procedure. This procedure was designed to eliminate the effect on contraction force resulting from internal movement caused by what was presumed to be a simple series elastic element (550). In the conceptual model, brought forth by Gasser and Hill (186, 253, 254), the internally produced force acts on the load through an internal mechanical impedance, dissipating part of the force (446). Together the concept and the measurements have generated much research and discussion. The conceptual model has been criticized on various grounds (412, 529), and its value has been questioned even by its original author (259). Furthermore, the active state concept is descriptive and not related to current understanding of contractile theory. By contrast, in the sliding filament model the force generator is directly modified by length and velocity resulting from previous activity (131, 265, 274, 277), a feedback model. Nevertheless the operational version of the model of active state is now an extensive and useful collection of data on the dependence of muscle response on external mechanical factors.

Separate from active state, two related models have been suggested to fill somewhat different roles. The first, *activation* (412), describes a tension-dependent response to excitation for study of motor control from the response side. The second, a related function, probably should be called *relative activation* (399); the name originally suggested, *state of activation*, seems unduly confusing. This relative activation function is based on a linear comparison of actual muscle force to the minimum and maximum forces that excitation changes can produce in the muscle under operating conditions that are otherwise the same. Its range is 0–1 or 0%–100%. Relative activation provides a way to express the intensity of the final effect of neural drive without going into the details of dynamic and amplitude relations that would be needed to express the measured result in terms of actual neural excitation (Fig. 13*E*).

Real Motor Systems

Under limited conditions and for a few muscles, individual fibers acting in parallel deliver energy into a constant load involving a simple hinge joint. The neural control of such action has been studied intensively. This may, however, apply to only a small minority of actual motor control operations, either in humans or across the animal kingdom. Yet nervous control is also important over the wide range of variations. Consequently these different functions of muscle, although not as well known or as easily analyzed, must be included in the description of the controlled motor. In the chapter by Alexander in this *Handbook*, several of the well-defined mechanisms within which muscles operate have been analyzed. We introduce several other types of muscle operations, but generally without the benefit of careful analysis of the mechanics. These examples are presented either as the basis of possible tests of schemes advanced as general descriptions of motor control or as indicators of influences that have shaped the development of the controlling system.

RESPONSE DIMENSIONS. In contrast to the isometric or isotonic conditions under which muscle usually is tested, physiological muscle action is commonly auxotonic (440, 451), with length and force both changing (Fig. 1*D*). In addition inertial, elastic, and viscous loads (such as found in jumping, archery, and swimming) each involve different rules relating force and position (223, 523). The load size changes in the course of many motor activities (185, 321, 351, 473). With shoulder muscles, for example, elbow joint changes alter the inertia and gravity force of the arm. In the knee extensors of standing man, positioning force varies greatly between slight flexion and locked extension (292). For ankle muscles, contact with the ground changes the load from that of a freely moving foot referenced to the leg to the mass of the whole body moved against the earth reference (Fig. 1*D*). Even the same structure may be seen by a particular muscle to have different inertias depending on the motor action involved, as in the case of rotation of the forearm around the elbow hinge versus rotation around its long axis [(152); both are represented in Fig. 3 of the chapter of Alexander in this *Handbook*]. Additionally, the physical dimension controlled by a particular muscle is quite commonly subject to variability (71, 351, 480).

The energy function of muscle was recognized by Helmholtz to involve both mechanical (240) and thermal outputs (237). The mechanical output can reach almost 0.1 hp/kg (70 W/kg) of muscle (248). From Newtonian mechanics Duchenne recognized the need of muscle to stop movement (152), and Fenn described this energy-absorbing action as a lengthening contraction (169). In this function the muscle is acting as an impedance element (218). Elftman added the muscle role of energy transfer with conservation of mechanical

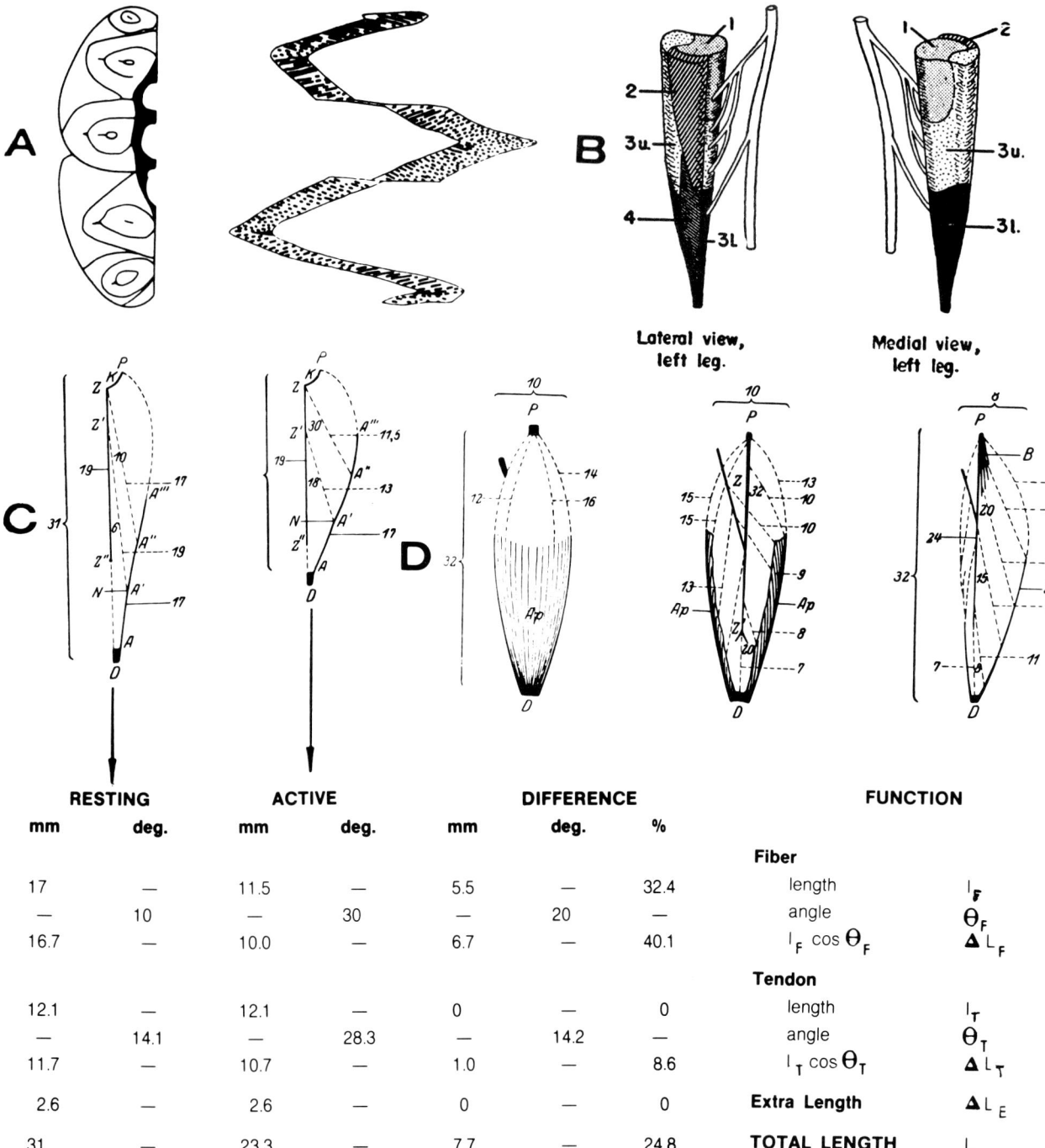

FIG. 3. Details of structure in gross muscles. *A*: primitive vertebrate muscle arrangement as seen in a single myomere in cartilagenous fish. Longitudinal and cross-sectional views show pattern that may be approximated as alternating concentric cones made up of these segmentally innervated muscle units. *B*: regional organization of major innervation divisions (arbitrarily numbered) as projected on two surface views of anterior tibial muscle of dog, showing mixtures of series and parallel relationships. *C*: conformation change in simple pennate frog muscle as result of total contraction (47). Table summarizes measured length and angle changes associated with A' fasciculus produced by contraction of whole muscle. The 40% shortening contribution by muscle fasciculus exceeded the 32% shortening of that fasciculus itself and includes effect of increase in angle of these active fibers. An added 13% decrease of total length resulted from the changing angle of connective tissue. Due to changing angles, as well as fiber shortening, total shortening of 7.7 mm is greater, not less, than 5.5-mm shortening of involved fibers in spite of angled orientation of fibers. *D*: organization of fasciculi (*dashed lines*) in the frequently studied frog gastrocnemius, as seen from superficial and deep surfaces and from a longitudinal section. *Solid lines* and locations Ap, Z, D, and P all mark major connective tissue structures. Sample fasciculus lengths, overall length and width, and a few pennation angles are marked. [*A*: from Alexander (10). *B*: from Wilder et al. (548). *C* and *D*: from Beritoff (47).]

energy [Fig. 4D; (156, 159)]. A pure example of this energy transfer involves an isometric muscle passing over two moving joints, absorbing energy at one end and mechanically transferring it to be put out at the other end. Energy production, transfer, and absorption can occur in rapid sequence within a particular muscle in the course of taking a step [Fig. 1D; (377)]. Even when maintaining a nearly constant position against varying external forces, the muscle alternates between the impedance and the force delivery functions (185). This alternately might be described in terms of elastic behavior (see the chapter by Houk and Rymer in this *Handbook*). The delivery of thermal from chemical energy (129) is an additional function of importance that is under neural control. In this connection it is well to remember that the 25%–50% maximal efficiency described for mechanical energy output (97, 414, 506) implies a 75%–50% minimal efficiency for output of heat energy, and one is inclined to suspect that shivering may represent a form of motor control in which efficiency for thermal output approaches 100% of the metabolic cost.

GEOMETRIC RELATIONSHIPS. The relationship between muscle action and motor effect is defined rigidly for a muscle acting on a hinge joint through a sharply localized tendon (see the chapter by Alexander in this *Handbook*); a muscle producing sliding action in a single degree of freedom also can use a well-defined (but different) relationship. When the muscle involvement includes more than one muscle head, a distributed muscle attachment, or compound internal organization [Fig. 3B; (472)], the relationships are describable either as multiple or as continuously varying functions with different lever ratios and muscle lengths. In these more complex mechanisms the lever arm and muscle length can be proportioned so that all parts of the muscle experience the same relative change in length. With other geometric arrangements (10, 426) the relation between length and lever can lead equally well to increased differences in relative velocities and the percentage of shortening in different parts of the muscle. When the load is elastic instead of rigid, the relationship between muscle force and muscle shortening changes with load stiffness [Fig. 4A; (436, 523)]. The relative relationships in different parts of a muscle also may be affected by elastic deformation, as would occur in a central tendon when subject to muscle fiber action distributed along its length. When muscles such as the cutaneous maximus, which is found in many mammals (428), or facial expression muscles in humans (472) work in a distributed way on a sheet of elastic material (the skin), the boundaries of a single action become indistinct. In addition, the muscle of unified function may change with the specific function involved, as when a cow flicks a small area of skin under a single fly or ripples large areas of skin in response to a swarm.

A muscle with a curved course between attachments converts a tensile force into a force normal to the length of the fiber, causing compression of underlying structures or structural displacement (215, 252, 353, 440, 472). Such a muscle action may be involved in producing the intramuscular pressure that, in spite of vasodilation in active muscle (176, 269, 317), reduces blood flow during sustained contraction (269, 326, 557). Examples of curved muscles include the diaphragm, human platysma, circular muscle of the upper esophagus, buccinator, and the bulbo cavernosus and ischio cavernosus muscles. The latter muscles apparently act similarly to the circular muscle of the earthworm to compress a closed hydraulic skeleton, which in penises of the dog and stallion produces the remarkable recorded pressures of 5,000 and 10,000 mmHg, respectively (41, 419). In spite of textbook attribution of the human erectile process to filling from arterial pressure (385, 445), which is almost always less than 200 mmHg, recognition of the inadequacy of a bicycle tire filled to an internal pressure of 4 lb/in.^{2} (200 mmHg) leads us to suggest, without data from cannulation, that skeletal muscle compression of the hydraulic system is important in the human being as well. For these curved muscles the relationship between successful motor function and fiber length is not obviously equivalent to the corresponding relationship in a hinge joint, and the control might be expected to be organized around different criteria of success.

It is well known that individual muscles operate as systems with nearly constant volume (182, 252, 327), but the changes in diameter D (538), which would be associated inversely with changes in length l seldom has been examined as a motor response, although it was known as early as 304 B.C. (Erasistratus, cited in ref. 440; other exceptions are referred to in refs. 47, 102, 454, 524, 571). It can be shown easily, however, that for a cylinder of fixed volume $dD/dl = 2D/l$, thus indicating that short cylinders, such as in muscle fibers in a pennate muscle, will have a diameter more sensitive to change in absolute length than will long cylinders of the same diameter. The outward bulging of a contracting limb muscle is a familiar sight and has been used to measure mechanical activity of muscles (102, 327, 426, 486, 571, 572)—as well as by competitors in body building contests. The neural control of a space-occupying muscle affects both length and diameter, and in some cases the change of conformation may be the important motor action (as in the tongue and the muscles of facial expression). The combination of longitudinal, transverse, and vertical muscles in the tongue seems to provide an ideal structural basis for conformation control (472). In any muscle, nevertheless, lateral (pushing) force, as well as displacement, can be developed with shortening (a vital fact for the rock climber depending for support on the use of a finger, arm, or leg "jammed" in a rock crevice). More generally important, the thickening of muscle fibers will change the angle of muscle pennation to the extent that the total shortening may be greater than the shortening of individual fibers [Fig. 3C; (47)]. The action on the skin tendon (524) of the complex myomere (Fig. 3A) of primitive vertebrates must include thickening effects in muscle. The total mechanical work done by any muscle fiber would be the sum of the work done by pushing and that done by pulling. Correspondingly, a muscle that curves over another would appear to be capable of an antagonistic action by compression. A bulging muscle similarly might interact with an exoskeleton. In all, lateral pushing by muscle has had little study, but it does appear to be one of the outputs of muscle that is used and, therefore, controlled in motor function. Again, criteria for success would not be identical with those usable for pure tensile actions.

As with any mechanism, geometric details of relationships between parts (e.g., motor units) are important to the determination of characteristics of the whole. The chapter by Alexander in this *Handbook* examines in some detail the trade-offs between lever ratios and fiber orientation for a jointed load. Here, too, motor control must deal with a variety of muscle geometries; fan-shaped muscles, for example, introduce a new complication. The human trapezius, temporalis, and deltoid have fibers that act on loads in different directions (108, 472). If a load can move in varied directions, as in these cases, the actions of different parts of a single muscle can be antagonistic (96, 133, 427, 472) or can vary over more than one degree of freedom (21, 96, 213, 434, 437, 540, 553). In a muscle with a continuum of fiber angles, recruitment of additional units is additive only in a vector sense (181) for the mechanical action. As Lombard and Abbott (341) found, the effect of changing joint angle can alter and even reverse the direction of torque produced by a muscle. When incrementally recruited units are involved in actions that differ in small steps through some dimension (e.g., fiber angle or, in spinal muscles, location along the spinal column), the result resembles the digital approximation to a continuous function. Questions arise about whether the control is organized digitally, continuously, or in some combined form.

In muscle actions not constrained by a joint [e.g., the scapula moving with respect to the trunk in aclavicular animals (21, 185)], the force couples generated

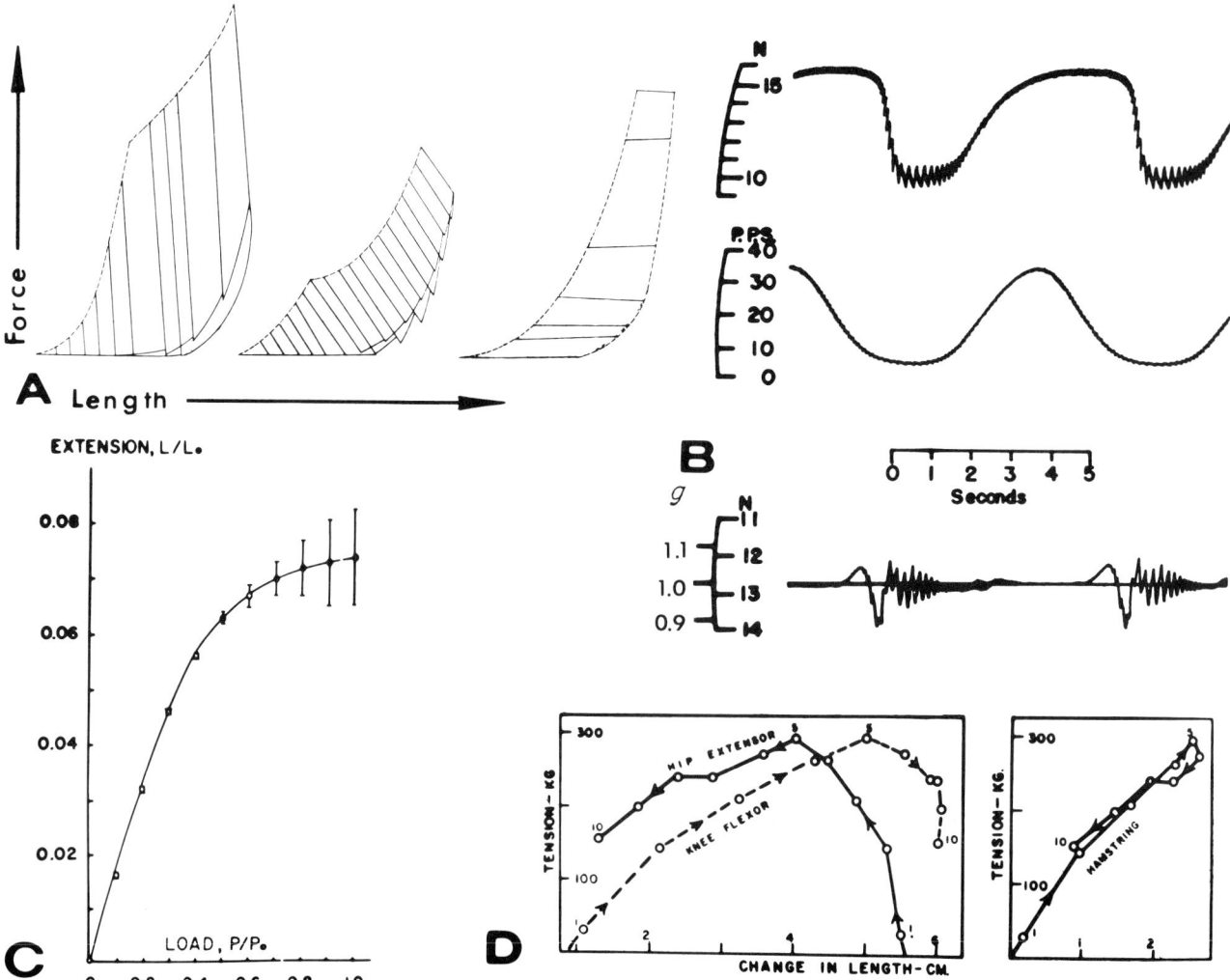

do not fall into clear classes of synergistic and antagonistic actions (21, 309). Muscles that are synergists for one degree of freedom simultaneously may be antagonists in another degree of freedom (472, 553), as is the case in some articulated systems described in the chapter by Alexander in this *Handbook*. In another case of muscle in a nonarticular relationship it is not clear to us that the degrees of freedom involved in the action of the lumbricales muscles, which connect to bone through other muscles (310, 311, 472), have been defined fully. The presence of complex (Fig. 3D; see also Fig. 11 in the Alexander chapter) and elastic connective tissue within muscles can result in such structural deformations that stretch of the whole muscle may lead to local shortening in parts of that muscle (359, 455). This connective tissue also is a major factor accounting for the great differences in the passive properties of some muscles [Fig. 5A; (412); and see the chapter by Alexander].

Muscles with fibers connected in series (6, 33, 102, 327, 359, 383, 446, 460, 472, 517, 525) introduce the analytic problem of the load impedance on one fiber involving the neurally adjustable properties of another fiber. In some muscles, including rectus abdominus and several neck and limb muscles (127, 268, 359, 432, 472), tendinous inscriptions divide the muscle into sections innervated by different spinal segments, making clear the separation of excitation of series elements. It is not evident, however, whether or not this separability is used functionally (for example, in adjusting the range of length over which the muscle could operate). Myomerically innervated muscles in fish are connected in a complex way, partly in series, through myosepta to adjacent muscle segments [Fig. 3A; (10, 220)], but it is not certain that the body movement generated is as much a tensile operation as it is an action changing the conformation (219, 524). In the common situation in which single fibers terminate within the fasciculus (127, 268, 525) the connective tissue carrying the load is described in a way suggesting that a combination of both series and series-parallel relationships occur among fibers. If fibers in such an organization serve a common motor unit, however, they might function as a longer single element rather than as individual, series-connected elements. Further study is needed.

EXTREME RESPONSES. While it is obvious that motor actions are restricted to the range of responses attainable by the involved muscle, there are some actions that give the appearance of falling outside that range and that should be explained either as representing an unusual muscle capability or as a misinterpretation. Some movements, for example, involve actions that are faster than seem compatible with muscle: *1*) The momentary closing of a hole in a bagpipe chanter is faster than the rise and fall of muscle contraction in a twitch. *2*) The rise of tension in a voluntary step

FIG. 4. Effects of load modify muscle responses. *A*: twitches of muscle from different initial lengths in frog gastrocnemius muscle operating on nearly isometric load (*left*), compliant spring load (*middle*), and isotonic load (*right*). These loads determine force-length slope through course of any contraction and thereby influence the pattern of maxima reached in the twitches. Passive length-force relationship (*right border*, each record) also differs slightly between stretching sequence (*upper passive curve*, each record) and release sequence. Load-dependent length-tension curves for twitch maxima are joined by *dashed lines*. *B*: cat triceps sura muscle responses to modulated stimulus. Cyclic modulation of rate of stimulus used for both tests is shown as *middle graph*. *Upper graph*, isometric force, measured in newtons. *Lower graph*, force from the identical muscle, subjected to the same stimulus sequence, but attached to an inertial load. Response was measured with an accelerometer in gravity units *g* from which the newton scale N was calculated. Mean force and length were similar in both cases, and isometric force changed smoothly with period of stimulus. Inertial load was moved against gravity with the same period, but change in force producing that load movement does not have a simple period. Actually only a small fraction of maximum isometric force (and that delivered intermittently) is required to move physiological-sized loads at moderate frequencies. *C*: calculated stretch of "series elastic component" with changes of the load on rat gracilis anticus muscles. Compliance (slope of curve) decreases as force increases. *Bars*, standard deviation of values measured from 5 muscles. This stretch represents the part of an overall length change that is considered not to occur in the contractile components. *D*: energy exchanges occurring with complex load on a 2-joint muscle (human hamstrings) through part of a running step. The 2-joint load allows separation of muscle length change (*right graph*) from that due to individual joint movement (two curves on *left graph*). Contributions to muscle length deviations, produced separately by hip movement and by knee movement, are plotted against force, as is total resulting change in muscle length. Numbered points identify correspondence of time on the 3 lines. Energy exchange at individual joint need not represent just energy produced or absorbed by the muscle. Area under curves is work done (integral of force with respect to distance). From 1–10 at knee, work is done on muscle by the load, whereas work is done by muscle at hip. *Right*: combined effect or net exchange in muscle energy for same points in time. Area under *right* curve from 1st to 6th point shows energy actually absorbed by muscle, and area under curve from 6th to 10th point shows mechanical energy delivered by muscle (part of delivered energy probably was from series elastic structures that shortened as tensile force was decreasing; if lengthening parallel elastic elements were under tension in this period they would have been absorbing energy). Comparison of areas under 3 curves shows that energy is conserved by transfer through muscle from knee to hip joint. [*A*: from Blix (54). *B*: from Partridge (394). *C*: from Bahler (24). *D*: from Elftman (158).]

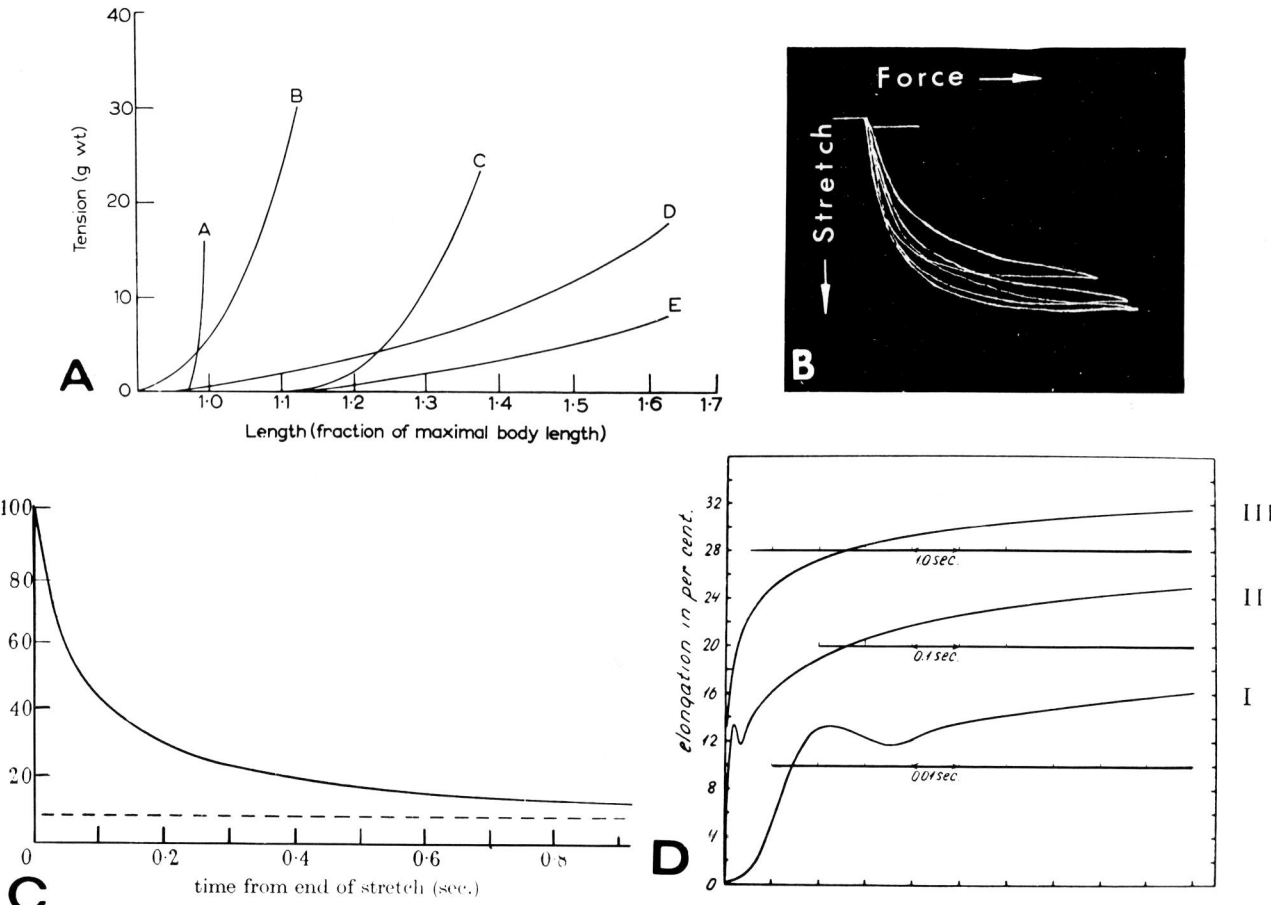

FIG. 5. Static and dynamic properties of unstimulated muscles. *A*: variations in relationships between muscle length and measured force in unstimulated muscles of several species. Abscissa lengths are normalized at maximum body lengths. In some muscles no force is generated passively within lengths attainable in situ, but for other muscles passive tension in normal operating range of lengths exceeds active contribution (see also Fig. 16B). *Curve A*, bumblebee flight muscle; *curve B*, locust flight muscle; *curve C*, frog sartorius; *curve D*, clam (*mytilus*) anterior byssal retractor; *curve E*, snail (*Helix*) pharynx retractor muscle. Other muscle curves can also be seen in part B and Figs. 4A; 11C and D; and 16B. *B*: length-tension relationship in an unstimulated frog gastrocnemius muscle measured at different rates of loading and unloading, using mercury to produce smooth force changes. Less stretch occurred with force increase, and particularly with fast increase, than with unloading. Force vs. displacement graphs were recorded directly using a special mechanical linkage. Dynamic aspect of passive response of muscle represented by difference between stretch and shortening curves commonly is ignored in dealing with muscle properties (compare Fig. 13.). *C*: "stress relaxation" after a step change in length of an unstimulated ileotibialis muscle of tortoise. *Unbroken curve*, force change in period immediately after stretch; *dashed line*, level at which force finally stabilized. *D*: three different time expansions of a record of "creep" of length after a step change in load on a single unstimulated frog fiber. *Time marks* in curve III, 10 s; *time marks* in curves II and I, 0.1 s and 0.01 s, also show initial oscillatory transient details as well as creep. Stretch scaled in percentage of equilibrium length (just taut). [*A*: from Hanson and Lowy (229). *B*: from Blix (54). *C*: from Hill (254). *D*: from Buchthal and Kaiser (82).]

response in some cases is faster than the rise of tension in a tetanic response. *3*) The movements of some insect wings or locust tympana (Fig. 1C) are driven by muscles at frequencies of 200–1,000 Hz (248, 411, 413, 440, 477, 520), although the same muscle stimulated at even lower rates results in smooth contraction, not oscillation (Fig. 7B). *4*) In the delivery of power in jumps of the spring beetle and grasshopper, energy is delivered faster than muscle is known to release power. Even the simple action of snapping the fingers involves movement velocities that are unusually high (173, 235). These examples of fast actions have different types of explanations, each of which represents a different aspect of motor control function. The brief musical note on the bagpipe is accomplished by sliding a finger past the hole, avoiding the need of reversing the movement, but in the case of rapidly rising tension a burst of impulses at a high rate has been found to bring the muscle quickly to a contraction level that later is maintained with a lower firing rate (202, 334,

464, 555); artificial stimulus can produce the same effect (395). Examination of the insect muscles during oscillation at high rates reveals that the loaded muscle is not following the pattern of nerve excitation (Fig. 1C) but instead is using an internal chemomechanical oscillatory process that may be a specialization restricted to a class of muscle called fibrillary (101, 352, 502). An appreciable part of the rapidly delivered power in jumps comes from energy stored in elastic structures by previous slow contraction (45, 173, 194, 235, 236), a more extreme case of use of elastically stored energy than is known in vertebrates [(98, 113–115, 209, 524); see the chapter by Alexander in this *Handbook*]. The finger-snapping movement is accomplished by releasing the movement only after contraction has already been fully developed (235).

Limits other than speed also appear to be exceeded by muscle action. A patient with neural damage, for example, sometimes can still make movements previously accomplished by a muscle now paralyzed (152, 472). Remaining members of the original excess number of muscles operating on the degrees of freedom involved (described in the Alexander chapter) can be used to produce the action. Tortoise muscle, on the other hand, delivers energy with an efficiency approaching 60%, in spite of the limit of 20%–40% ordinarily described in muscle (99, 350). This appears to be the result of a muscle specialization utilizing a trade-off between speed and efficiency (558).

These examples illustrate the difficulty of recognizing the relationship between unusual motor responses and their muscular bases. In a few cases the muscle involved exhibits a special capability. In other cases the surprising result arises from unusual application of muscle. In still others it is just a situation in which accurate observation of the response reveals that no extreme aspect actually is involved.

Summary

In addition to producing the isometric tensile force that usually is studied as muscle response, motor function involves a wide range of other actions. Likewise, the usual theoretical treatment of a motor system deals with a fixed load on a simple joint, although most loads actually deviate from this simple relationship in ways that appreciably affect interpretation. The internal structure in most body muscles is not one of fibers running in parallel the full distance between sharply localized tendon attachments. A complex connective tissue structure within the muscle also can contribute forces as important as the active muscle force. Curved muscles produce compressive forces at right angles to fiber direction. A shortening muscle expands in diameter and in that way may accomplish an important pushing action. Muscle loads may not have articular constraints, may tend to vary in size, and may change rapidly in form among inertial, elastic, viscous, and externally generated forces. Not only can a muscle produce force and deliver energy, but it is also called upon to absorb energy, transfer energy unchanged, or simply change shape with little energy effect. These varied structures and actions are all controlled through muscle. In some cases the simplifications that have been chosen to aid us in dealing with the concept of muscle in motor control instead may have distorted our understanding.

PROPERTIES OF THE CONTRACTILE UNIT

In normal activity the contractile proteins, muscle fibers, and entire motor unit each act within and on viscoelastic matrices. The final muscle action combines passive and active components. Subunits of excitable elements are identified readily (Fig. 2), but passive elements do not have clearly distinguishable subunits at levels below the whole muscle. Overlapping of connective tissue between separate muscles also occurs. Externally applied forces can demonstrate properties of the passive elements alone if the unexcited contractile structures show no mechanical effects, as is usually assumed. The addition of muscle excitation then superimposes an active response. In normal muscle activity only part of the contractile components are excited (9, 179, 188). To model normal muscle function it follows that actions of passive structures and excited and unexcited contractile elements all must be considered, as well as the way their actions combine.

Passive Mechanical Contributions

UNEXCITED MUSCLE. It has been known since Weber (537) that the unstimulated muscle has elastic properties. This nonlinear, perhaps exponential, relationship between stress and strain (Figs. 4C and 5A and B) is well documented (54, 76, 82, 161, 301, 352, 363, 380, 400, 423, 424, 537), varies among muscles in a single animal (541), and varies even more among different animals (Fig. 5A). It has been measured in isolated fibers (76, 82, 424, 469), empty sarcolemma (174, 424, 470), and in whole muscle [Fig. 5A and B; (537)]. In muscles in which the structure includes fibers that do not run simply from tendon to tendon (10, 47, 525) the separation of elastic elements into uncomplicated series and parallel parts is not clear. In some muscles a complex internal connective tissue system complicates the mechanical relationships (Fig. 3; see also Fig. 11 in the chapter by Alexander in this *Handbook*). Recently both theoretical and experimental bases have been brought forward in support of the proposition that part of what has been measured as series elasticity actually is within the contractile system at the molecular level within the individual sarcomeres (273, 274, 290, 542, 544). In several ways the identification of the functional elastic elements with particular morphological detail still is quite incomplete, and perhaps many real structures cannot be defined in the usual terms of parallel and series.

An unstimulated muscle is unlike a pure elastic structure (121, 380, 400, 541). Blix (54) demonstrated quite simply that when a loaded muscle is suddenly freed of part of its load the resulting oscillation is quickly damped. Buchthal (76) showed a similar damped oscillation in a single muscle fiber (Fig. 5D). If these unstimulated muscles had been purely elastic structures, as they often are described, these tests would have produced instead a sustained oscillation without the damping caused by energy loss. An alternate demonstration of this damping or energy absorption in the unstimulated muscle appears in a graph of length vs. tension recorded from an unstimulated muscle subjected to cyclic stretching (Fig. 5B). On such a graph of force vs. length the area under a curve is a measure of work. The stretching curve shows the work done on the muscle, and the release curve demonstrates the work done by the passive muscle. In unexcited muscle the curve on the release part of the cycle does not retrace the curve on the stretch half of the cycle but exhibits less force [Fig. 5B; (76, 400, 420, 424)]. The system is not energy conservative (541), and the area between the two curves measures energy absorbed by the muscle per cycle—the reason that oscillation is damped. Two other types of tests have revealed similar dissipative effects in unstimulated muscle. The force produced in a suddenly stretched muscle tends to decay slowly and, because velocity (and therefore power) is zero, without output of work. This decaying force, called *stress relaxation* or *yield* [Fig. 5C; (76, 82, 340, 529, 530)], indicates a loss of some of the energy stored by stretch. Likewise, after an initial abrupt stretch produced by a step increase of load, the stretch gradually increases with time (54, 304), while additional but nonrecoverable energy enters the muscle, a process called creep [Fig. 5D; (82, 83)]. These slow processes also represent energy absorption in muscle, but it is unclear to us whether all of these different observations are due to one or more than one process, each with a different time constant (82). In any case the unstimulated muscle is demonstrated to possess an energy-dissipating property that for some purposes might be modeled as viscosity (331, 380) or plasticity (13, 431, 504). Our own unpublished observations, however, lead us to favor a nonlinear model in which dissipation increases as passive tension F_p increases. This is seen, for example, incorporated in Coulter's model of passive muscle (121) with the notation changed slightly to be consistent with this chapter

$$F_p = A \exp \alpha l, + B \exp (\beta l + \gamma V)$$

A, α, B, β, and γ are constants for a particular muscle. The failure to include dissipative elements (37, 331, 380, 541) in a testable model of unstimulated muscle leads to unrealistic predictions of oscillatory interaction between any inertial load and either the series elastic (134) or the parallel elastic structure.

EXCITED MUSCLE. The total output of a muscle is the resultant of the passive and the active contributions, but the contributions are not independent. In some cases of physiological function the passive elastic force in parallel structures is larger than the active force (e.g., over part of range in Fig. 16B), but in other activities and muscles the operating range may not include lengths long enough even to produce passive force (Fig. 5A). When a passive element shortens at the same speed as an active element, the power output of each is proportional to the force in each. This leads to situations in which the passive element exchanges more power than the active element, although changes in the force added by the active element may be what determines direction of movement and, therefore, whether the power exchange is positive or negative. The compliance of series elastic elements (Fig. 4C) generally is presumed to affect the length and velocity of length changes in the contractile element (255). The stretching of the series elastic element by the contractile system stores energy in the series elastic structures and also would tend to unload parallel elastic elements, so that at a particular total length the force contributed by parallel elastic elements would decrease as the active force increased (205). The usual calculation of active force as the difference between total force and unstimulated force at the same length ignores this complication [Fig. 11C; (424, 537)]. From simple mechanical considerations it follows that in a period of decreasing muscle force, energy stored in series elastic elements is delivered to the load (82). The relationships among active forces, passive force, and total force are more complex when only part of the muscle is active because of the distributed and partially overlapping forces within the elastic matrix (33, 47, 369, 410). In terms of energy exchange, if some elements are stretched while others shorten, part of the power from the shortening components will be taken up by the stretching ones instead of being delivered to the load. Of course, that energy stored in stretched structures may be delivered to the load after the original muscle contraction has ended (12). Moreover, the action of a muscle may be transferred to a remote joint by way of the elastic coupling of fascia (285). It appears that any representation of the combination of passive and active components in physiological activity must be more complex than a simple additive series and/or parallel model. A realistic model to represent functional effects in a complex muscle structure, however, may be too cumbersome to be useful. Different simplifications may be needed in different modeling applications.

Response to Neural Signals

The active contribution of muscle is initiated through a series of processes finally delivering excitation to the contractile substance. The conduction of excitation over polarized membranes and the excitation across the neuromuscular junction recently were reviewed in the first volume of this *Handbook* section on the nervous system (119). Because of the long-known all-or-none phenomenon (208, 348, 410), it usually is assumed that in vertebrates the individual nerve impulses determine whether or not the muscle is excited, but they carry no further information. That is to say, the all-or-none character of the individual muscle unit response implies not constancy of response but only independence of stimulus once the threshold has been exceeded. Evidence that the muscle part of motor units cannot be assumed to act always in a strictly all-or-none and independent manner is indicated in the sections that follow. However, it is still reasonable to presume that the form of the information delivered to muscle by a single nerve is restricted to impulse patterning.

SINGLE STIMULUS. The simplest controlling action of the nervous system determining motor response is the single nerve impulse. After the arrival of the nerve impulse at the junction there is a delay during the spread along the muscle at 1–5 m/s and a brief local latent period; then several mechanical changes occur in the muscle. This total latency varies, depending on the measure of responses used [Figs. 6B, 7A, 10A, 14A; (54, 95, 238, 439)]. The time courses of a number of these constituent processes have been studied in considerable detail since the first published records in 1850 (Fig. 6A; see also ref. 239).

A variety of mechanical responses of muscle to a single exciting impulse have been studied. Usually the mechanical response to a stimulus pulse is a transient that is brief compared to the period of normal motor actions of the muscle. (Thus this minimal unit of response is less than the usual functional response.) For any muscle the time course of a recorded response depends both on what function is measured and the conditions of the test; some of these variations can be seen in Figures 1A and 6. Effects of differences in conditions may be represented in a number of observations: *1*) the oscillations shown in the first graphic record of muscle contraction, which were associated with the elastic elements in the load used [Fig. 6A; (239)]; *2*) the more extreme case of "ringing" of a muscle with its load, which is seen in the normal action of the tympanum muscle of the locust [Fig. 1C; (411)]; *3*) the flat-topped force record and delayed shortening record in the afterloaded contraction [Fig. 6B; (54, 289)], which resulted from the afterloaded operation; *4*) the changes in response with variations in load size [Fig. 6C; (54, 59)] and properties (Fig. 4A and B); *5*) the changes in shortening response associated with different initial muscle lengths (54); *6*) the changes in response of a muscle as a result of its previous activity (Figs. 7 and 14; (147)]; *7*) the change in time course of a motor unit response depending on activity level of the muscle within which the tested unit is located [Fig. 1A; (142, 373)]; *8*) the differences in force delivered by a muscle when it is isometric or when it is stretched or released after stimulus [Fig. 11A, 16A and C; (54, 254)]. The comparison of graphs of length (54), force (54, 142, 373), electrical response (Fig. 18), and volume [Fig. 6D; (34, 161, 456)] among functions recorded from related tests shows differences among the time courses of these various measures of the single response. The range in twitch responses that are found among various types of muscles are discussed under UNUSUAL MUSCLE PROPERTIES, p. 75 (also see the chapter by Burke in this *Handbook*). Both the noise inherent in the molecular nature of contraction (503, 544) and the relaxation that precedes contraction (3, 449) are probably too small to be of significance in motor control. Relatively little information is available about the nontwitching slow muscles (349) found even in mammals (249, 364). At first inspection there appears to be no unity in what muscle does within normal conditions.

The sources of "artifacts," which have been carefully avoided because they cause complications in muscle response, are in most cases factors with which ordinary muscle must on occasion deal, such as changing load inertia. One might even propose that the improved control of test conditions, which was needed to advance study of muscle response, separated muscle investigation from the conditions encountered by working muscle. Helmholtz's first record [Fig. 6A; (238)] shows an oscillation of the shortening muscle that was eliminated in his later records (240) by removing an elastic element in his equipment. The normal sound-producing function of the tympanum muscle of the locust, however, involves a similar interaction between muscle, load, and elastic structures that is necessary to produce the oscillation of singing. Since different loads are so complex and variable in motor activity, no particular condition can represent normal muscle load generally. In fact, the details of all of the records just described can be considered to be artifacts of the recording conditions. With respect to those actions that can be called normal motor function, the most unrealistic artifacts may be those in which experimental conditions have been simplified most effectively, so that variation of factors influencing the muscle response has been almost eliminated. If muscle were a linear system, the total response being the simple sum of several separately measured effects without interactions among components, such tests of isolated effects would provide full and sufficient descriptions of the whole system. The resulting simplicity of form would contribute to the usefulness of these descriptions. Interaction of effects, however, can be studied only in tests including variable combinations of the factors. The most important combinations probably would be those resembling actual conditions encountered in motor control, even if quite unsuitable for extracting information about the inner workings of

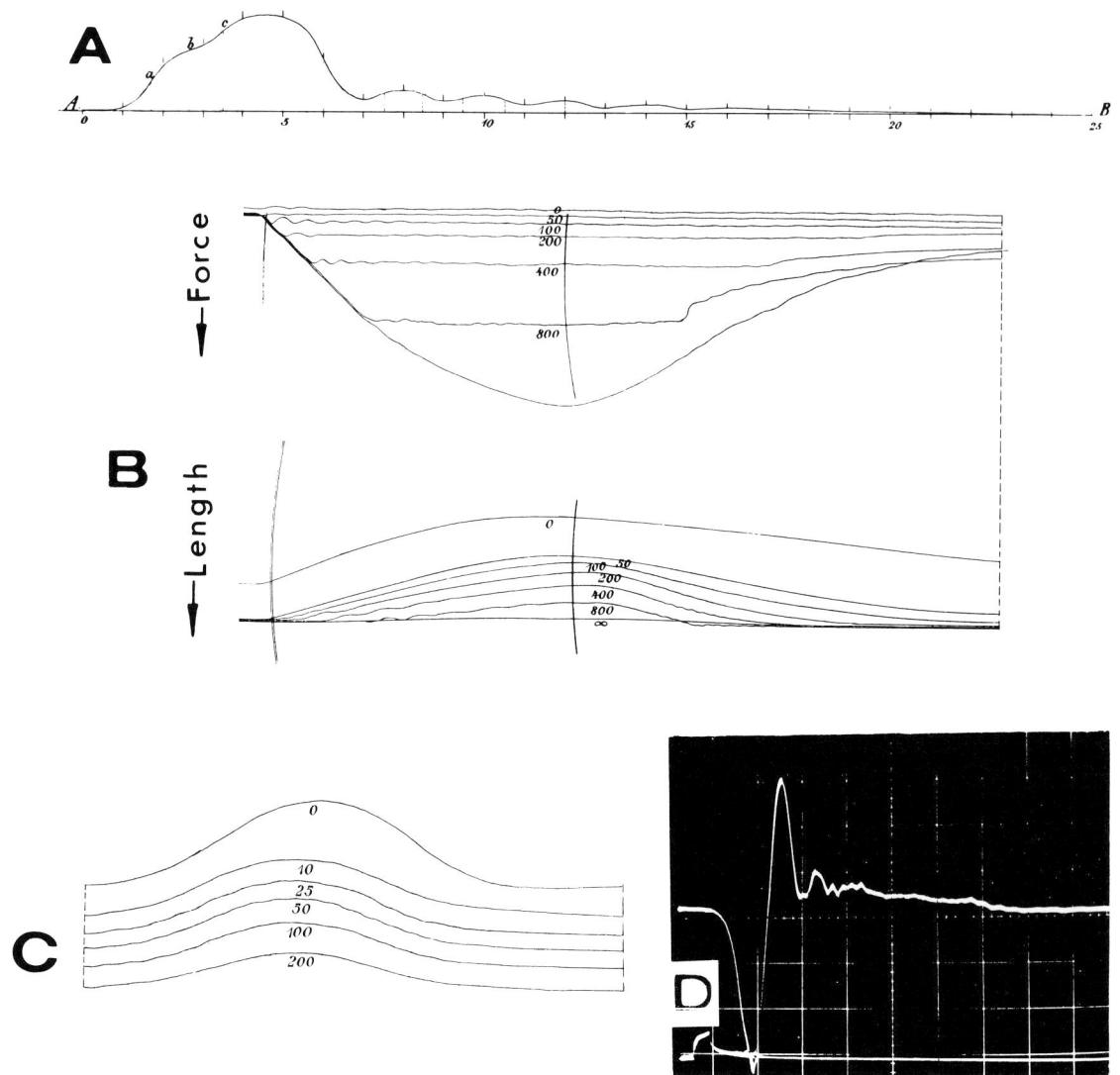

FIG. 6. Various responses of muscles to single stimulus pulses. *A*: first published record of muscle twitch (238). Frog gastrocnemius was attached to a complex inertial and elastic load, and record was made by a steel point scratching on a lightly smoked, moving glass plate. Oscillatory detail is characteristic of the particular combination of load and muscle and is avoided in most modern muscle experiments by reducing both inertia and elastic compliance of loads. *B*: Simultaneous force and length records through a series of twitches with different isotonic loads. Frog gastrocnemius muscle was afterloaded; that is, load was mechanically supported at a fixed position before and after muscle tension exceeded force required to lift the load. Characteristically the latent period for load movement increased with load size (weight marked in g), and movement period decreased. The shorter latent period for force development was unchanged. (The same 1893-1895 ref. 54 contains a large number of other records of twitches made with different types of load and load transients; both time-based records and force vs. length records are included.) *C*: effect of preload on muscle twitch (weight in g marked on lines). Weights were hung near the fulcrum to minimize effect of inertia, thus approximating an isotonic load. Stretch of loaded muscle before stimulus as well as changes in response can be seen. *D*: volume change in frog sartorius during isometric twitch. Major divisions on abscissa, 10 ms. Detail of volume change is highly sensitive to load conditions (34). Peak volume decrease is about $5 \times 10^{-3}\%$ of total muscle volume. [*A*: from Helmholtz (238). *B* and *C*: from Blix (54). *D*: from Baskin (34).]

muscle. The analysis of multidimensional data in a nonlinear system is difficult (165, 211, 360). The development of better tools for these more complex studies remains a challenge.

The independent response variations do have a pattern. An isometric load results in an almost pure force response by a muscle. With the same kind of stimulus and a light isotonic load, an almost pure length response is produced; with a spring load, length and force change together (Fig. 4*A*). Because of internal elastic and inertial elements, isotonic and isometric loads do not produce truly isotonic or isometric contractions. Sudden changes in load within the response period (54), such as the sudden change occurring in walking when the foot strikes or leaves the ground, alter the relative importance of force, impedance, and displacement in the response. Changes in size and initial position of the load modify the response generated by a simple stimulus (54). The response of a motor unit within an intact muscle likewise would change with loading introduced by activity in other muscle units (135). By modifying a high level of activity in other units the twitch record even can include a late phase in total force that falls below the base-line level (Fig. 1A). With an application of external force sufficient to stretch a contracting muscle the force delivered as a result of that stretch is different from that which would occur at the same length without the stretch (254, 289). The mechanical impedance so demonstrated also changes over time. In all of these tests contraction develops and decays after stimulus, but the form in which it is manifested depends on load (54, 172).

REPETITIVE STIMULUS. In addition to what can be learned about motor control from the response of muscle to a single stimulus pulse, it is also instructive to study effects of sustained excitation. In 1847, from experiments using a hand-cranked electromagnetic generator, Weber concluded that nerve produced sustained response in muscle by delivering a discontinuous excitatory process (537). In 1928 Adrian and Bronk (7–9) obtained electrical evidence in physiologically activated nerves of that discontinuous process acting on single units of muscle.

After a short refractory period (78) a new stimulus can initiate an additional response. In frog hindlimb muscle at room temperature a depolarization accompanied by refractoriness to stimulus passes over the fiber at a velocity of 3–5 m/s (283), followed in a few milliseconds by repolarization and recovery of excitability. With a mechanical response that lasts in the order of 100 ms, a new excitation response cycle therefore can be initiated well before the peak of the earlier mechanical response. Several responses resulting from repeated stimuli are shown in Figures 1, 7, 8C, 9A, 14C, 15A and C, 16, and 17B. Successive stimuli ordinarily result in a total response exceeding that occurring with a single impulse. The increment added by the second impulse may, however, be larger or smaller than that contributed by the first, depending on the muscle (Fig. 7C), the temperature (425, 526), the interval between stimuli [Fig. 8C; (92, 302)], and previous stimulation (Fig. 14A). With a train of impulses each impulse adds to the total response, and at a relatively high rate of stimulation successive responses blend into a nearly constant tetanic response (Fig. 7B). The increments of response added by successive stimuli are not constant, but they decrease, particularly at high rates of stimulus (Fig. 7D). Thus the response is not, as sometimes suggested (191, 241, 440, 452), the sum of fixed quantal responses (68, 92, 95, 231) to individual stimuli. Nevertheless, at low repetition rates the isometric or isotonic response of a number of muscles can be approximated to be the sum of simple twitches, each of which may be modeled by either a second- or third-order differential equation [Fig. 7D, left; (88, 116, 191, 231, 354)]. These properties are found in single fibers (76, 424), in single motor units (22, 51, 91, 144, 366, 379, 513, 561), and in whole muscle when stimulated as a single unit (54, 120, 153, 182, 247, 318, 426).

The application of trains of stimuli at various repetition rates to produce tetanic (58, 318, 440, 537) response has traditionally been used to investigate the means available for neural grading of response in single units (9, 76, 82, 153, 372, 505, 561). Whole muscle (Figs. 7B,D, 14C, 16A,C,D), single fibers (76), and motor units (89, 91, 366, 429, 430) have been tested with tetanic trains of stimuli. In the early quantitative study of tetanic responses (537), the hand-cranked electromagnetic generator used must have produced on occasion both unfused response trains and recruitment-modulating stimulus, but the lack of graphic recordings left with us no details until later studies provided them. A variety of mechanical devices, such as the adjustable "Wagner hammer" that was used to interrupt the primary current in DuBois-Reymond's induction coils, produced repetitive stimuli and relatively smooth responses (247). Complete tetanic fusion of response commonly requires rates near the limit or above those found in physiological function (120, 433, 495, 541). Kronecker and Stirling (318) reviewed the available means and presented a new device for producing rapidly repeated stimulus, thus extending the available range up to 22 kHz. Using sound as a criterion of movement, Kronecker found contraction was not smooth below 1 kHz. As a consequence of all of this study, muscle response to tetanic stimulus is now well known.

These response records allow an estimate of the effect of firing rate on response. Fig. 8A shows several different measurements of force response that have been used. Although not a common choice, the average force (see curve e in Fig. 8A) would seem to represent best the effective contribution to physiological action, and it approaches zero in the same way as do the curves that relate measured physiological force to electrical activity in muscle (281, 342, 568). All muscle response measures do not have the same relationship to firing rate; this is illustrated by the continuing increase of the rate of development of tension at stimulus levels above those producing maximal tension [Fig. 8B; (88)]. Muscle shortening also can be related to firing rate and, as shown in Figure 8C, the relationship is dependent on the load under which it is tested. It is probably of considerable importance to an understanding of neural control of muscle to recognize that muscle response is typically most sensitive to change in stimulus rate R (either $\partial L/\partial R$ or $\partial F/\partial R$)

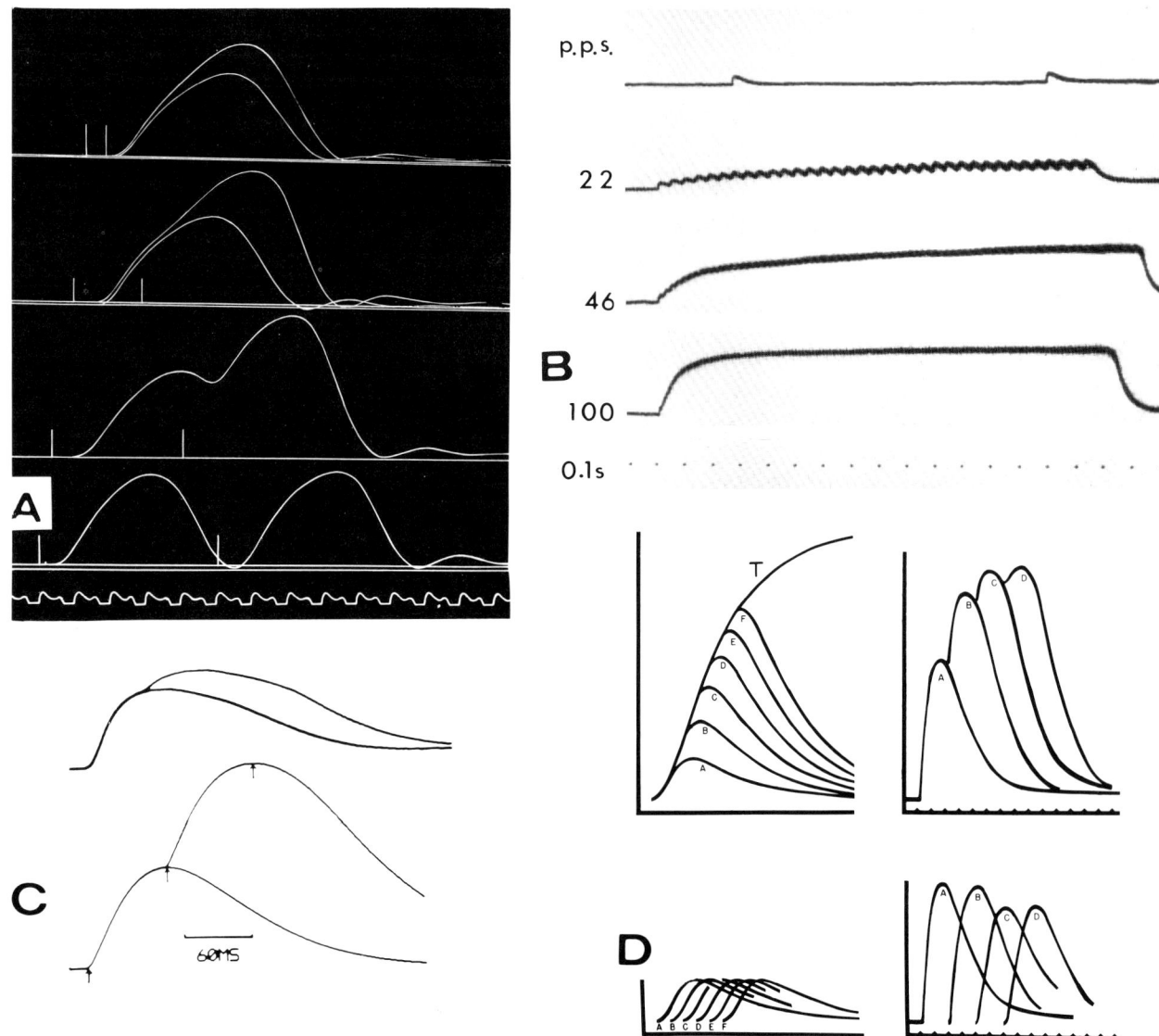

FIG. 7. Time graphs of muscle response to 2 or more stimuli in succession. *A*: traditional student laboratory demonstration (1905) of wave summation for 2 stimuli in nearly isotonic contractions of frog gastrocnemius. Stationary ordinates mark stimulus points. *Lower line*, time at 50 periods/s. *Upper 2 records*, response to 2 stimuli superimposed on record produced following a single stimulus. *B*: typical isometric response of striated muscle to trains of stimulus pulses delivered at 0.9, 22, 46, and 100 pulses/s. At 100 pulses/s response approaches a fused tetanus. The muscle used for this record was tymbal muscle of locust. Compare to physiological response of a similar muscle when attached to its normal load in Fig. 1C. *C*: isometric records of wave summation. *Lower records*, from cat soleus with 2 stimuli delivered at a 70 ms-interval at 37°C. Area added to record (mechanical impulse) by second stimulus is greater than that produced by 1st stimulus. *Upper record*, from frog sartorius with stimulus interval of 120 ms. (Time scale of frog muscle record is 77% as fast as that shown for cat record.) Impulse added by 2nd stimulus in this case is less than that contributed by 1st. In both records time from stimulus to peak of contributed force is longer for 2nd twitch than for 1st. *D*: successive contributions of individual stimuli in a sequence. *Upper graphs*, superimposed records of responses with different total number of stimuli in trains. *Lower graphs*, contribution of individual stimuli calculated by subtracting responses to trains differing by one pulse. *Left graphs*: theoretical linear summation, each impulse producing same contribution. *Right graphs*: actual frog sartorius responses, 5 pulses/s. Contribution and rate of rise of successive pulses decreased markedly, especially at higher rate. See Fig. 8C for a measure of isotonic contribution in displacement time product resulting from a pulse as a function of stimulus rate at which it is added. [*A*: from Beddard et al. (42). *B*: from Pringle (411), with permission of Cambridge Univ. Press. *C*: from Ranatunga (425). *D*: from Gilson et al. (191).]

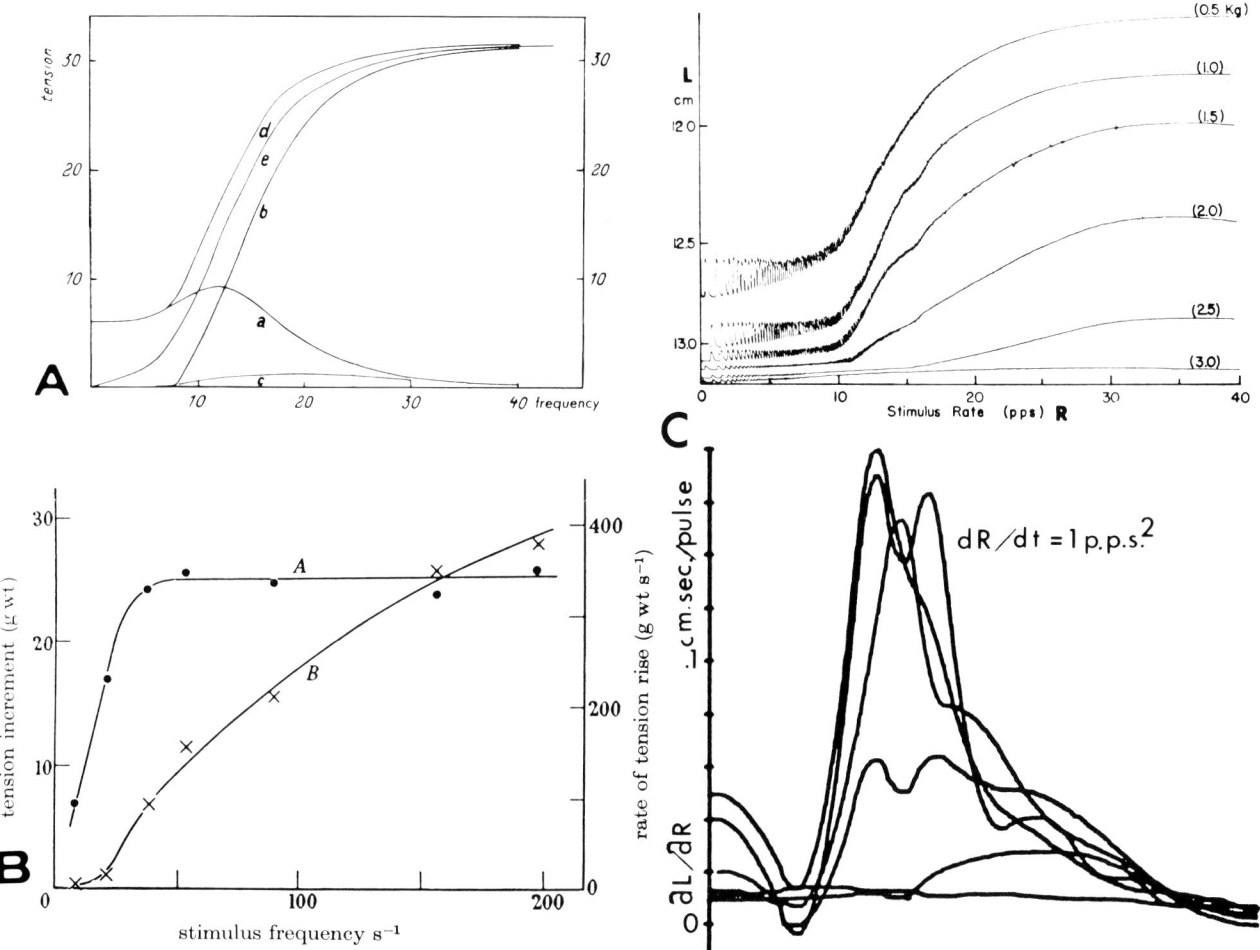

FIG. 8. Effects of stimulus rate on muscle response. *A*: several different ways of representing the same results. For these graphs a single fiber from frog semitendinosis was used, and isometric response was measured from periods of steady stimulus. Curve a, force differences in individual responses; curve b, contraction remainder at low point in response between stimuli; curve c, ratio of contraction remainder to stimulus rate; curve d, force peak (a + b); curve e, mean tension over time. All curves are plotted as functions of stimulus rate. *B*: rate of rise of tension (right ordinate and × values) at beginning of a stimulus train continues to increase through appreciably higher stimulus rates than does contractile tension (left ordinate and ● values). This is an additional example of measures of muscle response that are not equally sensitive to stimulus rate. *C*: family of nearly isotonic responses of cat triceps surae muscle to slowly increasing stimulus rate (1 pulse/s^2). Separate lines are made with different loads. At low stimulus rates and with small loads the responses to individual stimuli are particularly apparent (compare twitches in Fig. 6*C*). *Lower graphs* show derivative of average (negative) length with respect to stimulus rate ($-dl/dR$), which was calculated using spline functions (408, 559) on mean (smoothed) values of the *upper graphs*. These superimposed curves indicate that the principal sensitivity to stimulus rate for this muscle falls in the range of 8–25 pulses/s over a variety of loads. Separate peaks could represent populations of fast and slow muscle units within this muscle. [*A*: from Buchthal (76). *B*: from Machin and Pringle (352). *C*: from Partridge (395).]

in intermediate ranges of stimulus rate (8–25 pulses/s in Fig. 8*C*; see ref. 397). In different muscles calculation of the sensitivity curve shows variation in detail, including peaking at higher rates for fast muscles than for slow ones (120), sometimes remaining above zero at relatively high rates (421), and in some cases even becoming negative at high rates (48).

DYNAMIC STIMULUS. In most unit actions measured in physiological activity both the excitation to the unit and its response have been modulated rather than constant (e.g., Fig. 1*D*). Adrian and Bronk (8) first made records of activity of muscle nerves confirming that firing rate was modulated in motor control. Since then, supporting evidence of muscle control by changes of firing rate has been found in muscles dealing with a wide range of functions [e.g., Fig. 1*B* and *D* and Fig. 18; (82, 199, 202, 203, 212, 220, 228, 244, 339, 372, 416, 463, 467, 487, 518)].

Static description must be supplemented with dynamic data in order to deal with the processing of changing signals. Several types of test inputs can be applied to evaluate muscle dynamics. These include approximations to pulses, steps, sine waves, and even randomly distributed pulses. As early as 1944, linear differential equations were fitted to the twitch responses of muscle, allowing twitches of different muscles to be compared in terms of three coefficients (191). Although the integral of a pulse is a step, the corresponding operation on the twitch response did not predict observed tetanic responses and indicated that a nonlinearity was involved, as has been shown repeatedly since then (92, 95, 476, 563). In spite of the limitations introduced by this nonlinearity, both the twitch and tetanus responses (Figs. 6, 7, 14) nevertheless are informative about muscle dynamics, and both reveal a lag or low-pass filter (361) between neural drive and mechanical response of muscle. The evaluation is further complicated by the fact that all response measures do not change together; e.g., ability to resist stretch starts before and persists after termination of force for shortening or power delivery (253, 254, 289) and also is produced at lengths where no static force is generated (299).

Sinusoidal tests often provide convenient and accurate definitions of dynamic properties of linear systems (295, 453, 535). The introduction of sinusoidally modulated pulse rates for stimulus made frequency response tests possible for the mechanical response of muscle to neural inputs (393). Graphs of frequency vs. amplitude ratio and phase define the results of such tests and can be converted easily to a mathematical approximation (453, 573). For many muscles either force or displacement response is nearly constant over low frequencies and decreases over higher frequencies, a pattern characteristic of what is called a lag system [Fig. 9A and B; (95)]. At all frequencies the sinusoidal component of the response lags the stimulus cycle (Fig. 9C). The time difference decreases with frequency, but the fraction of a cycle of lag increases with frequency. (This dynamic lag in muscle causes temporal effects larger than many conduction delays on nerve fibers and needs to be considered in calculations that deal with timing of mechanical responses from neural events.) The same general pattern of response dynamics with quantitative variations has been found in a variety of muscles. Using a more complex analysis, similar frequency-response information has been derived from human muscles in voluntary activation (373, 476) and in cats with random stimulation tests (354).

The particular value of frequency-response data lies in the associated theoretical basis for application. Insofar as the linear approximation is valid the response of a system to any input pattern can be predicted by Fourier synthesis from the frequency components of the input combined with the measured frequency response of the system. Additionally, both mathematical and graphic methods are available to predict the overall frequency response of a system composed of parts with known frequency-response properties (for muscle application see refs. 398 and 443). An example of the latter type of calculation involving muscle has revealed an unexpected muscle action described here to illustrate a use of dynamic information about muscle. The frequency response between nerve firing rate and isometric contraction of muscle has been measured (393). The frequency response for rotation of an inertial mass in response to a torque-producing force can be derived from elementary mechanics (181). If muscle produces force in response to a neural signal, and if that force produced the torque that rotates the load, it might be expected that the combined properties could be calculated directly. The phase-shifts of the parts would add, as would the logs of the amplitude ratios, to produce the combined frequency responses. Conveniently, the frequency response for muscle force to stimulus has been measured (393). From Newtonian mechanics the dynamic relationship between force and movement shows a constant 180° phase lag and an amplitude ratio inversely proportional to frequency squared. Actual data for load-moving muscle, however, deviate dramatically from those predicted from isometric muscle and load (38, 394). Neither the phase nor the amplitude effect of inertia can be found in the response of inertially loaded muscle. This failure led to recognition of an almost complete compensation of effects of inertia by the exchange between shortening and force in muscle (395). The frequency-response measurements made this important, but previously overlooked, effect rather obvious.

Linear models of muscle ranging from equations of second-order lag to fifth-order lead-lag type (37, 38, 190, 191, 193, 373, 443, 453, 476, 481, 518) all describe similar dynamics and in fact include considerable lag. Models have been derived to represent isometric and isotonic response, but those derived from twitches have frequency-response curves that differ consistently from those from more continuous stimulation (190, 483, 563). Some of the nonlinearities can be represented as changes in coefficients that depend on the stimulus rate used in the test (Fig. 9D). Yet all of the models appear inadequate to represent ordinary auxotonic (451) activity unless supplemented by representation of the trade-off between force and length. It is important, however, that while recognizing the limitations of these formal linear models, one should not discard them in favor of an alternative that avoids the limitations by evading them.

Interaction Between Neural and Other Inputs

It is impossible to examine the response of muscle to stimulus variation without dealing with other factors, but in the typical experiment these factors are kept constant at some usually arbitrary level (for historic examples see refs. 182 and 440). In another type of experiment stimulus is held constant while one

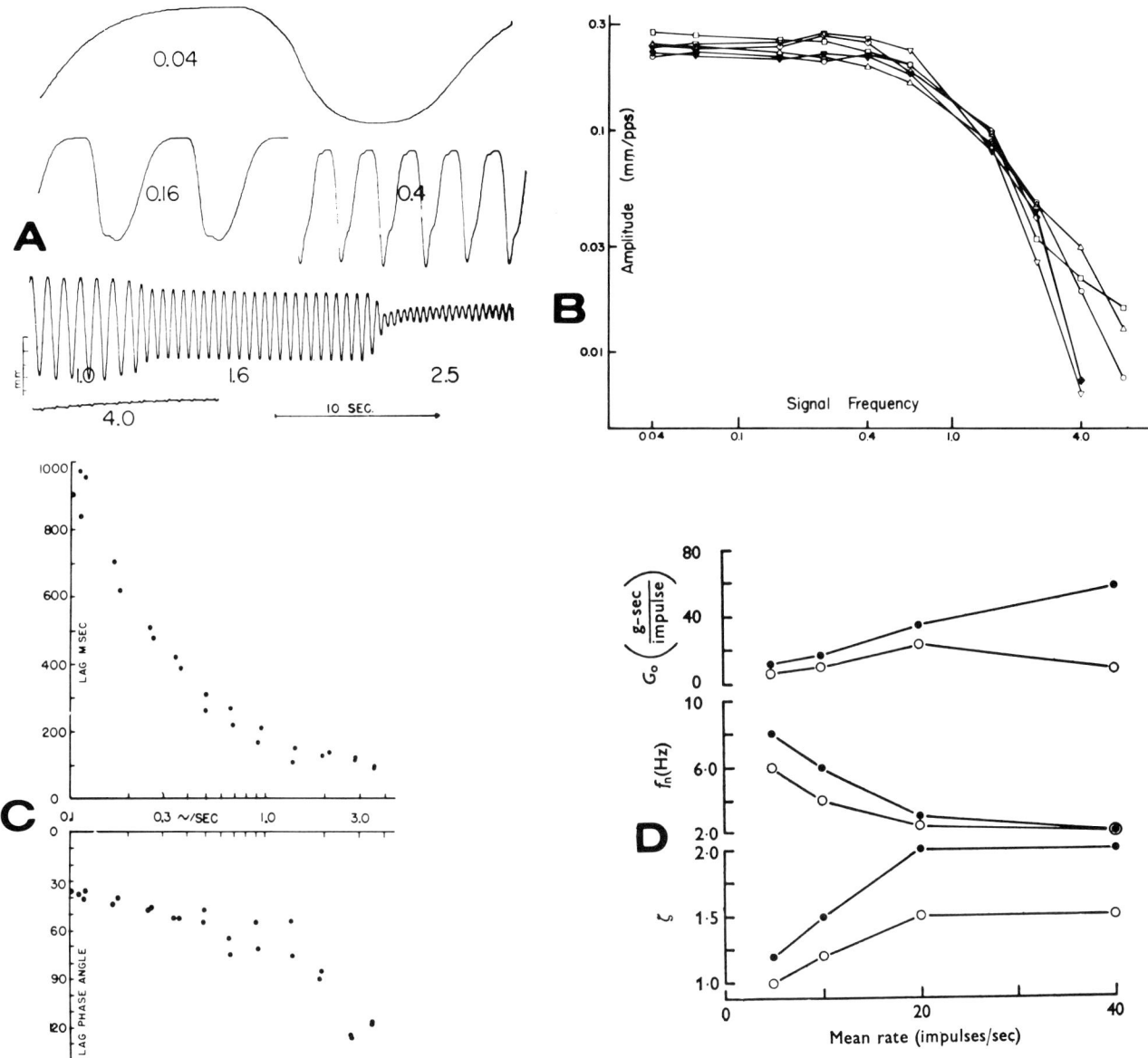

FIG. 9. Dynamic effects of modulated stimulation. *A*: time graphs of response of load moving by cat triceps sura muscle driven with a sinusoidally modulated stimulus rate, 5–25 pulses/s, and at modulation frequencies marked on graphs. Amplitude of modulation was constant, but response amplitude changed with frequency of modulation. *B*: change in movement amplitude with frequency of modulation cycle. All stimulus cycles ranged from 5 to 35 pulses/s. Although the gravity part of loads was constant, each line represents a different load inertia, spanning a 28-fold variation within the physiological range (394). Periodic force required for sinusoidally moving an inertial load increases proportional to inertia and proportional to the square of the frequency or, for this range $28 \times (6.3/0.04)^2 \simeq 7 \times 10^5$, which is the ratio of force cycles for a constant amplitude movement. Considering the proportionality of force cycle to movement amplitude, this graph represents an actual 8×10^3 range of amplitudes of response cycles of force produced by a constant amplitude of modulation of stimulus rate. *C*: temporal displacement between stimulus cycle and response cycle in isometric records of cat triceps sura force as a function of cyclic frequency. *Upper graph*, lag of response in ms; *lower graph*, same data in fractions of a 360° cycle. *D*: representation of muscle properties combining both nonlinear and dynamic aspects. Each set of 3 coefficients (G_0, f_n, and ζ) define one 2nd-order differential equation approximating data similar to that shown in parts in *C* and *B*. These coefficients when inserted in the equation specify dynamic properties of the muscle in one operating range of stimulus rates. Changes of coefficients with firing rate range represent some of the nonlinearities. ●, ○, Values obtained from different muscles. [*A* and *B*: from Partridge (394). *C*: from Partridge (393). *D*: from Mannard and Stein (354), with permission of Cambridge Univ. Press.]

of these other factors is varied. Such studies have revealed large changes in muscle response to stimulus within the physiological range as a result of change in the value of the tested variable. In normal function, however, most of the factors that affect muscle are subject frequently to simultaneous variations. Obviously the infinity of possible combinations of these factors cannot be tested, although varied combinations are important. Because muscle properties are nonlinear these effects are not independent, and a general description must deal with the ranges of combinations. If the rules change smoothly, however, a limited sampling may be representative of the whole range.

A few of the unidimensional descriptions are reviewed in the following discussion. Combinations of changes over two dimensions are less commonly tested and have been derived using several stepwise changes in one dimension while testing another (Figs. 4A, 6C, 8C, 9B, 11D, 12, 15A and C, 19). We also attempt to relate length, velocity, and stimulus rate to muscle force, although the data were obtained under restricted conditions (Fig. 13). It can only be hoped that the still higher order combinations involved in physiological function operate in a space represented by these restricted conditions, or at least that they are not subject to rules entirely different from those studied.

CHEMICAL INTERACTION. From activity at the neuromuscular junction to the generation of mechanical response in muscle fibers, most of the important processes occur at the molecular and submolecular levels (345, 374, 384, 565, 570). It would be no surprise that muscle function might be modified drastically by change of concentration of a number of chemicals. The all-or-none nature of muscle response (348) reduces some effects to a change in threshold, however, by eliminating further grading of muscle properties. The safety factor in neuromuscular transmission then may eliminate all effects on the muscle response. Internal storage and the ability in muscle to derive energy in anaerobic processes reduces the sensitivity of motor control to the immediate oxygen and metabolite supply of muscle (383, 384). Still many chemical effects are known. A large part of the literature, however, deals with alterations in chemical concentration so great that the studies must be considered pharmacological. Furthermore, much of the study of chemical effects in muscle has been designed to elucidate the metabolic processes of muscle (384) instead of evaluating the functional implications of changes in the chemical situation. In sports medicine, on the other hand, there is a long history of attempts to modify motor performance of muscle by hormonal (322) or metabolic means (14). The differences in chemical properties of fibers of different types are left for discussion in the chapter by Burke in this *Handbook*.

We have the impression from a scattered and inconsistent literature that within physiological operation it is likely that some chemical agents contribute meaningful signals to the determination of muscle response (e.g., refs. 175, 384), but we are not prepared to produce an organized exposition beyond a reminder of the potential involvement.

THERMAL INTERACTION. The quantitative dependence of muscle response on operating temperature is well documented [Fig. 10; (19, 107, 112, 231, 407, 425, 456, 528)] but seldom discussed in the context of motor control. Furthermore, the heat production of muscle [Fig. 10E; (18, 164, 251)] is seldom discussed as a general motor action. Yet in mammalians, as well as in poikilothermic animals, the thermal range of operation is great enough to have major effects on muscle properties (107, 194). Mammalian muscles operate over the whole range from hypothermia to fever (307, 534), individual muscles being subjected to self-heating as well [Fig. 10E; (18)]. Large thermal gradients occur, especially within limb muscles of arctic mammals (178), and in some muscles the gradients can be steep (107), rapidly changing, and particularly severe, as in a small fish penetrating a thermocline. Large, fast, and nonuniform thermal variations therefore are found in functioning muscle. Both timing and intensity of a variety of muscle responses to excitation are quite sensitive to temperature. As might be expected, heating decreases latent period [Fig. 10A; (440)], refractory period (78), contraction time [Fig. 10A; (111, 231, 407)], relaxation time [Fig. 10A; (231)], energy exchange (26), twitch time (Fig. 10A and D), and duration of post-tetantic potentiation (118). Temperature also affects twitch height in a complex way (Fig. 10A and C). Since relaxation and contraction are changed with different temperature coefficients, the twitch shape is altered with temperature [Fig. 10A; (231)]. Static and dynamic stiffness are reported to change differently with temperature [Fig. 10B; (226)], while the damping coefficient related to these factors changes inversely with temperature (380). The tension opposing stretch is reported to increase with cooling, while isometric tension decreases under the same conditions (180). At least one three-way interaction has been described between stimulus, temperature, and stretch (231). Some changes, however, are much more sensitive to temperature than others. For example, membrane potential varies only in proportion to absolute temperature (445), or about 1.03:1 for a change of 10°C. Rate of rise of tension changes 2.5:1 (231), yet relaxation speeds change 3.6:1 for the same change in temperature (231). Although these thermal effects should be expected to modify motor control significantly (18), little has been done beyond speculation (399) to determine how the complications of these interactions are compensated in the normal control of muscles.

MECHANICAL INTERACTION. Length is one of many dimensions that characterize muscle. Diameter or the general coordinates of advanced mechanics (195), while applicable, have not often been used (exception

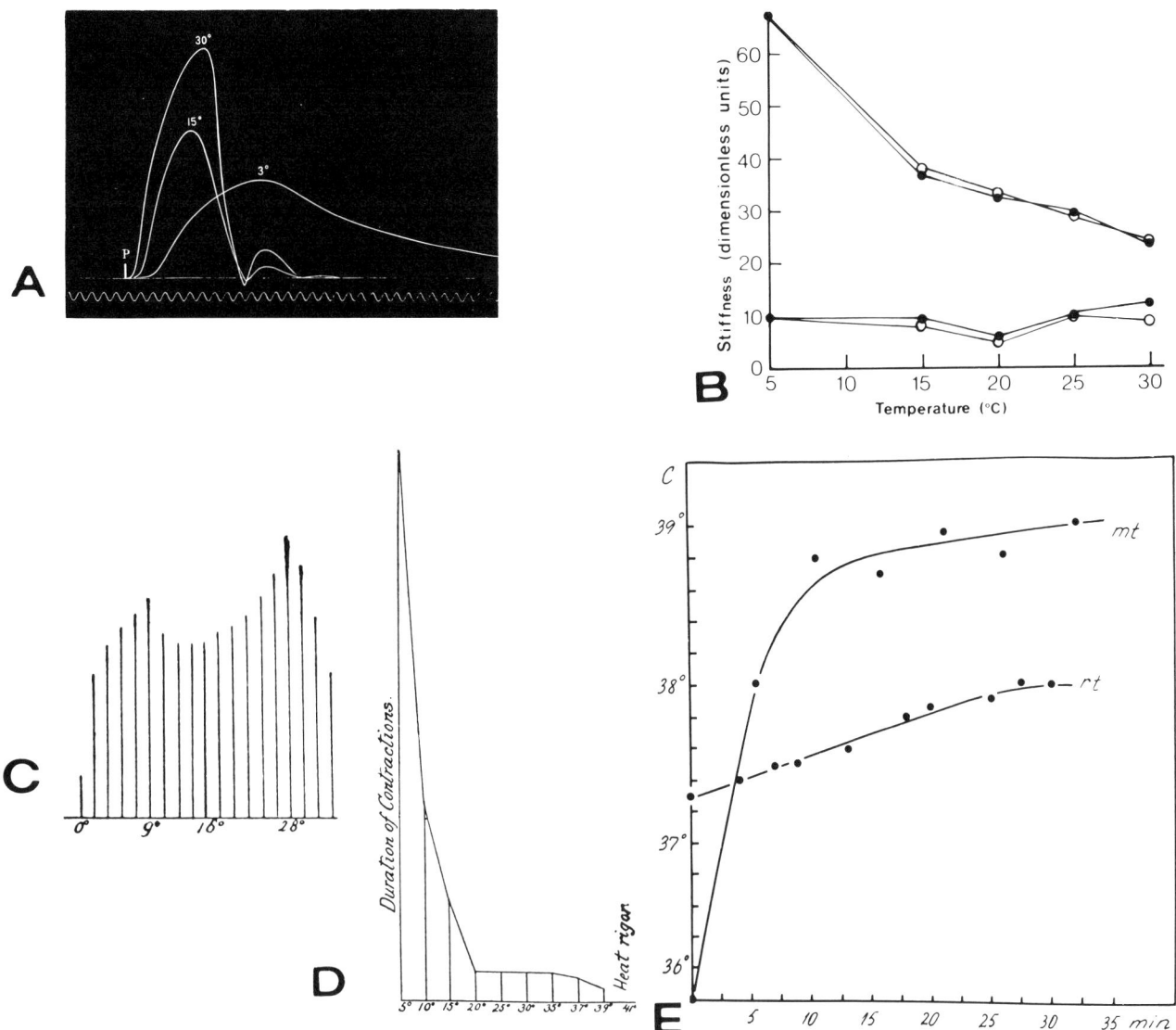

FIG. 10. Relations between muscle actions and temperature. *A*: twitch variations in frog muscle at 3 different temperatures. Time reference, 100 Hz. *B*: effect of temperature on tortoise muscle stiffness. *Lower lines*, static stiffness; *upper lines*, dynamic stiffness. Pairs of points are measured from one sequence of increasing and one sequence of decreasing temperature. *C*: height of frog muscle twitches at a sequence of temperatures between 0°C and 36°C. *D*: effect of temperature on duration of twitch. Temperature ranges between 5°C and 41°C, at which point response failed completely. *E*: change in temperature of body core, rt, and of muscle, mt, as a result of muscle activity in human. Crossing of the two curves shows a reversal of direction of heat transfer between muscle and relatively constant body core. Externally observable motor performance also changed in speed with temperature in this study, which may be related to "warm up" before athletic activity. [*A*: from *Handbook of Physiology*, by W. D. Halliburton, © 1911, used with permission of McGraw-Hill Book Co. *B*: from Fowler and Crowe (180). *C* and *D*: from Howell (263). *E*: from Asmussen and Bøje (18).]

in ref. 233). The first time derivative of length (velocity) is often evaluated, but acceleration and the higher derivatives that would make up a phase description (459, 545) are seldom considered. We describe relations between contraction and either length or velocity and then various combinations of these effects before considering a number of observations that might be described profitably with respect to the higher time derivatives of length or to a completely different set of dimensions. At best, however, these relationships are incompletely analyzed. In current muscle theory the effects of length are explained in terms of structure (201, 270, 297), and the effect of velocity is explained as related to reaction rate (31, 406). Still the chemical description is not a convenient basis to describe motor activity. In contrast, if properties that determine the mechanical action of muscle are describable in a theory-free form, it is possible that description could be fully adequate to deal with the mechanical action in motor control. Since muscle theory has been derived from observed mechanical properties, rather than mechanical properties from muscle theory, we consequently have developed this description in the direct mechanical form without appending theory of contraction. Nevertheless, the reader may find it useful as a mnemonic aid to relate observed muscle properties to a contractile theory.

Length. In excited muscle a nonlinear but complete trade-off occurs between force delivered and shortening produced and is described by the length-tension curve. Fick recognized this as a dependence of work output on muscle lengths (172). Total force, either for a twitch or for a tetanic response, generally increases with muscle length (Fig. 11). This exchange between length and force is comparable to the length feedback effect of the stretch reflex (210, 395), except that it does not involve the conduction delay. The ratio of $\Delta F/\Delta l$ compares to but is larger than the response ratio (gain) of the stretch reflex (e.g., see Fig. 1A in reference 186a, in which the contribution of the length-tension effect is almost four times that of a stiff reflex). In some cases a local maximum in force occurs near rest length for the muscle [Fig. 11B; (164)]. (Different definitions exist for rest length, although in some muscles they all give approximately the same value, as in Figure 11. In different papers this value may be defined as the muscle length when all slack is removed, the length at which maximal active contribution to tension occurs, the maximal functional length, or the length found in the body when relaxed. In some muscles, however, the indices differ—e.g., ref. 567—and have led some authors to use different terms.) The springlike relationship shown in length-tension curves was emphasized by Weber [Fig. 11A; (537)] and led to an extended study of this property. One of the most thorough examinations of relationships between length and force was published in 1893-1895 by Blix (54), who directly recorded quantitatively different graphs of certain relationships: *1*) isometric contractions; *2*) spring-loaded contractions (Fig. 4A); *3*) isotonic contractions (approximated by hanging weights near the fulcrum to minimize the effects of inertia; see Figs. 6C and 4A); *4*) afterloaded isotonic contractions (Fig. 6B); and *5*) contraction against abruptly changing loads. Blix also accomplished smoothly changing loads by adding or removing mercury in the load pan. He additionally recorded the velocity-dependent relationships between length and force in both passive and tetanically active muscle for both stretch and release conditions.

With quantitative differences (Fig. 11B), the relationship between length and active force shows a similarity of shape among the different preparations of whole muscles (30), single fibers [Fig. 11D; (424, 561, 567)], and single sarcomeres (200, 201). In simple muscles the forces in the length-tension curve rise with stimulus rate (Fig. 11D). In more complex muscle, however, activity in different sections of the muscle may produce force curves of a different shape (548). Muscle length also may affect relaxation time (495) and contraction rise time in both twitch and tetanic stimulation (424, 551). Initial muscle lengths also affect power and work delivered by the loaded muscle by affecting some or all of the components of contraction force, distance, or velocity.

Several mechanical properties of muscle can be determined from length-tension curves. With cyclic movement the area between the length-tension curve obtained on stretching and that on shortening usually has been described in a way that defines energy dissipation into the muscle. In vertebrate muscles where comparison has been made this energy absorption per cycle is greater in the active than in the passive muscle (76, 257, 296, 362). Similarly, when length is scaled with respect to rest length and force is scaled to cross-sectional area of muscle [Fig. 11A; (11, 537)], the coordinates of the graph become *stress* and *strain* (see APPENDIX). In linear regions the slope of such a curve is comparable with the modulus (Young's) of elasticity. Because the curves are nonlinear the point chosen for measurement can affect conclusions. Thus at constant force the stiffness defined as $\partial F/\partial l$ often decreases with excitation when compared with passive stiffness (537), while at constant length the same measure may increase, decrease, or even become negative with progressively increased excitation [Fig. 11C and D; (421, 423)]. (Today this use of stiffness does not infer that muscle is a simple elastic structure; for example, energy absorbed in the excited muscle when subjected to stretch is no longer recoverable after the stimulus ends.) In curves with a local maximum, force decreases when the active muscle is stretched beyond the length at force maximum in a length-dependent way ($\partial F/\partial l < 0$), but independent of any reflex (knife clasp) action.

Velocity. The differences between the length-tension curve developed in a lengthening active muscle and that developed with shortening [Fig. 12; (54, 76, 83, 143, 170, 527, 528, 549, 562)] might be related to the difference in velocity, as was noted (54) at least 30 years before graphs of the force-velocity effect were published. Using controlled velocity the relationship was determined for both lengthening and shortening velocities in a variety of animals [Fig. 12; (331, 562)]. Later it became conventional to place a series of loads on muscle and to plot the velocities at which the muscle drove the loads, with coordinates reversed from controlled velocity experiments (171, 251, 549). Only shortening velocities were studied in this form. Force is reduced to zero at high shortening velocities and increases with lengthening velocities. Isometric force is usually described as greater than one-half the maximal force, but in some muscles it is less (331). Several different equations have been fitted to the relationship for shortening velocities in a variety of muscles (20, 154, 171, 251, 407). Except for Pollisar's

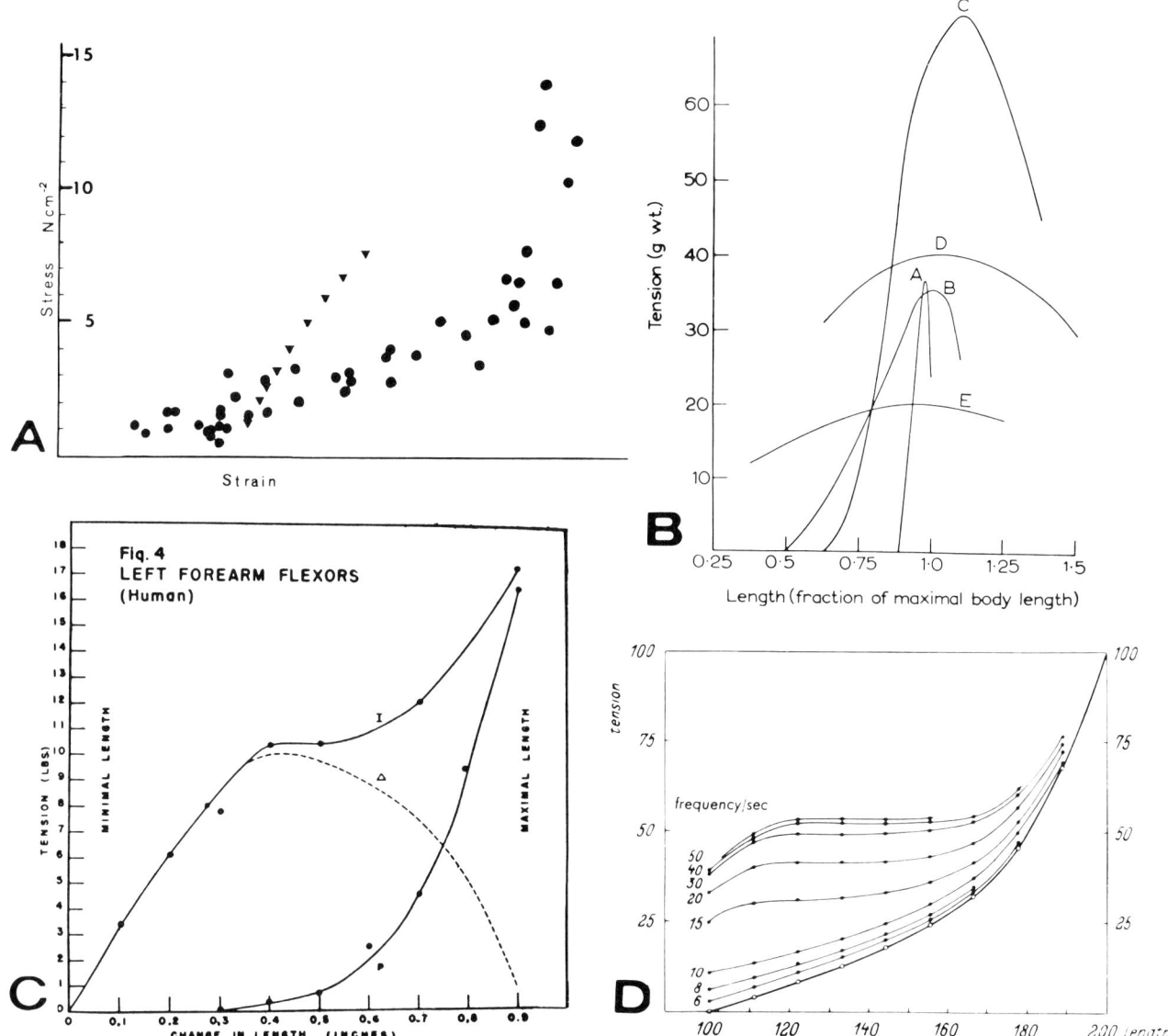

FIG. 11. Muscle contraction as modified by length. *A*: relationship between stress and strain in 12 tetanically stimulated glossopharyngeal muscles of frog. Data are from tables made by Weber in 1847 (537). Eleven muscles, ●, were loaded before stimulus. One muscle, ▼, was stimulated before loading. Normalization to stress and strain from length and tension, as described by Weber, allows comparison of muscles of quite different sizes. (We have crudely confirmed Weber's description of the very long range of lengths over which this muscle can respond.) *B*: comparison of active contribution to length-tension effect in several different muscles. (For passive contributions of the same muscles, see Fig. 5*A*.) A, bee flight muscle; B, locust flight muscle; C, frog sartorius; D, anterior byssal retractor of clam. Ordinates are not normalized to compensate for muscle size differences. *C*: conventional measurement of active contribution to length-tension effect. Passive response and maximal voluntary force were measured directly in human forearm flexor muscle with cineplastic tunnel prepared to allow external action of the tendon. Developed tension is calculated as difference between passive and maximal forces with no correction for result of local stresses within muscle and tendon. See Fig. 4*A* for similar data from twitches. *D*: family of length-tension curves for single fiber of frog semimembranous muscle. Parameter distinguishing individual curves is stimulus rate. Note nonuniform increments of stimulus rate and compare Fig. 8. Values were calculated as mean of 2 values measured with increasing and with decreasing stimulus rate. [*B*: from Hanson and Lowry (229). *C*: from Ralston et al. (423). *D*: from Buchthal (76).]

equation (407), however, the usual models fit only over shortening velocities and cannot be extrapolated for lengthening (412). Although normalized in both length and cross-sectional area, different muscles, even in the same animal (541), do not have the same force-velocity relationship (31, 229, 478). Even within a single muscle the contribution of velocity to force delivered varies with length (28, 29, 57, 154, 361), stimulus rate (Fig.

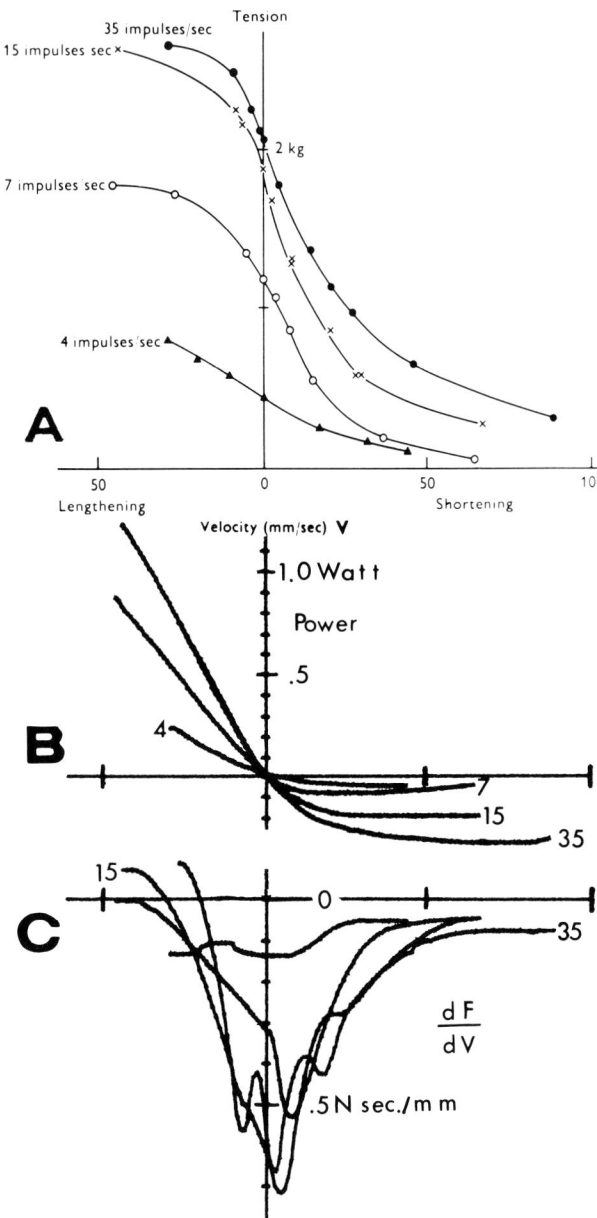

FIG. 12. Effect of velocity on muscle response, measured at constant velocities while passing through a test length. All sets of curves are drawn on same abscissa. A: Force-velocity effect at several different stimulus rates in cat soleus muscle using rotation of stimulus among 5 nerve branches. (Also see ref. 296 for differences introduced by slightly different test conditions.) B: rate of exchange of energy between muscle and load, or power, is equal to product of force F and velocity V. Negative power indicates output of energy by the muscle. (Energy delivered by each impulse, i.e., power ÷ pulse rate, varies with stimulus rate but is nearly independent of velocity over an appreciable range.) C: slope $\partial F/\partial V$ calculated from force-velocity curves in A, a measure of sensitivity of force to velocity, or mechanical impedance (as in ref. 397). Negative values are proportional to a viscosity-like measure. The value of this measure is greatest at low shortening velocities with high stimulus rates. Graphs B and C were calculated for this review from data points on force-velocity graph (A) using spline interpolation (408, 559). Spline fit lines pass through same data points, but they differ slightly from lines joining points in A. [A: from Joyce and Rack (294), with permission of Cambridge Univ. Press.]

12), and both mechanical and stimulus history (296). (Most force-velocity curve have been derived under conditions where passive force is near zero.)

The simple viscosity model of the force-velocity effect (186, 250, 331, 562) has been rejected in muscle studies, but the mathematical equivalent still is used when muscle is represented linearly in a control model. For a small range this linear mathematical model may introduce only small errors (38, 362, 512). While force in muscle varies with velocity V, this effect actually is not proportional (as in a viscous system) to velocity. In muscle the sensitivity of force to velocity, $\partial F/\partial V$, is greatest near zero velocity (Fig. 12C), decreasing with both more positive and more negative velocities. The rate of energy exchange (power = $F \cdot V$) between muscle and load also changes with velocity. Power absorption changes nearly proportionally with velocity in lengthening; but the power output for the nearly hyperbolic force-velocity curve for shortening muscles (154) is almost a constant (544), the value of which is dependent on activation (Fig. 12B). Clearly, maximum power output ($P < 0$) does not occur at the velocity producing either maximum force or maximum shortening. Overall power exchange depends, however, on velocity in a way that results in energy absorption or damping of oscillatory movement by muscles subject to constant activation.

Force-Length-Velocity-Excitation. While a simple muscle can produce at any moment only one output of tensile force, the state of the muscle must involve a length, velocity, and particular level of activation. That output force, then, must be the force generated: *1)* at a specific point on a length-tension curve; *2)* at a specific point on a force-velocity curve; *3)* at a particular point on a curve relating force to excitation; and *4)* at a particular point on a curve relating force to rate of change of excitation. Figure 11D relates force to length and excitation; Figure 12A relates force, velocity, and excitation. Figure 13A shows at the intersection of two curves the single force that defines an instantaneous combination of length, velocity, and excitation consistent with the separate relationships. (The effects of variation of such factors as rate of change of stimulus, acceleration, and temperature are not included.) One red line represents a constant high level of excitation, a single length, and various velocities. The other red line depicts the same excitation, but only one velocity and various lengths. The green line represents this latter velocity, zero excitation, and the same series of lengths. Changes in excitation would produce response forces moving between the red and green intersection points. At any other moment a new combination of length, velocity, and excitation would define a new pair of curves and a new point of intersection at the corresponding force. For a single level of excitation, then, a combination of all of the possible curves becomes a surface relating the three dimensions of length, velocity, and force (Fig. 13B). This surface would be different, of course, for muscles having different length-tension or force-velocity curves (e.g., Figs. 5A, 11B). Parts B and C of Figure 13 differ only in the relationship of the active force to the passive force. These theoretical surfaces were derived first from curve shapes found in limited experimental data. To these were added parallel response curves related in form, as inferred in experiments and mathematical models (4, 25, 232, 403, 569). It was assumed that the force-velocity effect proportionately modifies a contractile system, the effectiveness of which is mirrored in the length-tension curves. The part of this surface related to shortening velocities also has been derived directly from experimental data (25, 27).

By definition, all movements in the negative velocity half of this surface are in the direction of decreasing length l as indicated by the arrows. Increasing length falls on the other half surface. All movements can be represented as trajectories on the phase plane with these constraints on direction and a slope related to acceleration a as $(dV/dl) = (dV/dt)/(dl/dt) = a/V$. Similarly, movements of a muscle at constant excitation can be described on a force surface. Finally, activity with changing excitation would move through the length-velocity-force space. Thus an isometric twitch would move vertically above a single-length point at zero velocity, changing in both the excitation and the force dimension. A constantly excited muscle attached to an isotonic load can only move in length and velocity on the response surface along an isopleth of one force (25). Other loads would define other paths. In fact, any movements of a muscle, whether driven mechanically, neurally, or both, could be described by a trajectory moving through this four-dimensional space. The three-dimensional graph of Figure 1D describes the mechanical part of a physiological movement that was accompanied by the excitation sequence sampled in the associated time graph of the electromyogram (EMG). The relationships between the physiological movement and described muscle properties might be represented by the insertion of a properly scaled version of Figure 1D into the response space of a graph similar to Figure 13B and C, chosen to represent the particular muscle.

The trajectories taken by sinusoidal movements over a response surface illustrate several implicit expectations in the nature of the response surface. A sinusoidal length change, $l = A \sin \omega t$, defines the associated cyclic velocity as $V = dl/dt = A\omega \cos \omega t$. The trajectory over the phase plane that forms the base of these graphs is an ellipse with the length axis equal to $2A$ and the frequency-dependent velocity axis equal to $2A\omega$. Two frequencies of cyclic movement shown in Figure 13D represent relationships between the movement and the idealized response surface of a muscle. Projection of the ellipses from the phase plane upward to the response surface defines, at their intersections, two trajectories over the response surface, one for each frequency of movement. Because of the curvature of the response surface the forces so defined would not be sinusoidal; correspondingly, frequency would affect force bias, amplitude, and shape. The force is likely also to have a fundamental that is shifted in phase with respect to the stimulus cycle in a complex, frequency-dependent way. If the theoretical force is plotted against the length (on the work plane; see ref. 562), a loop is produced with time running clockwise. For a single cycle the work W done on the muscle is greater than the work done by the muscle, and energy proportional to the loop area is absorbed. There can be no patterns in which a movement and its return on this surface can occur without work ($W = \oint F \, dl$) being done on the muscle, because: 1) $F = dW/dl$; 2) moving from and returning to any length requires moving through all intermediate lengths; and 3) $\Delta F/\Delta V > 0$. The theoretical work curve shows a positive area, or energy absorption, as seen in animal studies (54, 72, 76, 282, 291, 422). It also shows the shift of mean force with frequency, as demonstrated by Brown (72) in cat muscle and by Buchthal (76) and by Blix (54) with slow stretch and release of frog muscle. Such an energy-absorbing surface describes a muscle that would support a load without sustained oscillation, even after a mechanical or neural transient. In a muscle with a response surface such as in Figure 13B or C, a cyclic movement of a constant load could be driven by the muscle only with a changing activation exposing a higher activation surface during the shortening period than the one describing the muscle during lengthening.

RELATIVE ACTIVATION. In controlling a single muscle the nervous system must operate between the lower limit of no excitation and an upper limit of maximal excitation, as might be represented by the red and green surfaces in Fig. 13B. The space between maximal and minimal surfaces corresponds to the range available to neural control. When, as in this figure, the bounded space is defined in Newtonian based dimensions, excitation does not bear a simple relationship to force response. Thus a horizontal plane that represents a particular force in different regions would intersect the passive surface as well as the maximal surface, fall within the controllable region, and yet be located in other ranges both above and below the attainable limits. Within the controllable range the relationship of any point can be described in its position between maximal and minimal force in terms of relative activation (399). Giving relative activation the value 0% on the passive surface and 100% on the maximal response surface at any length-velocity combination, the position of an attainable force between these surfaces can be scaled linearly to express the relationship of the end result of excitation without reference to what particular nonlinear and dynamic stimulus details were involved. Maximal and minimal attainable forces are functions of length and velocity as well as of such other dimensions as temperature and fatigue.

Figure 13E illustrates the calculation of the time

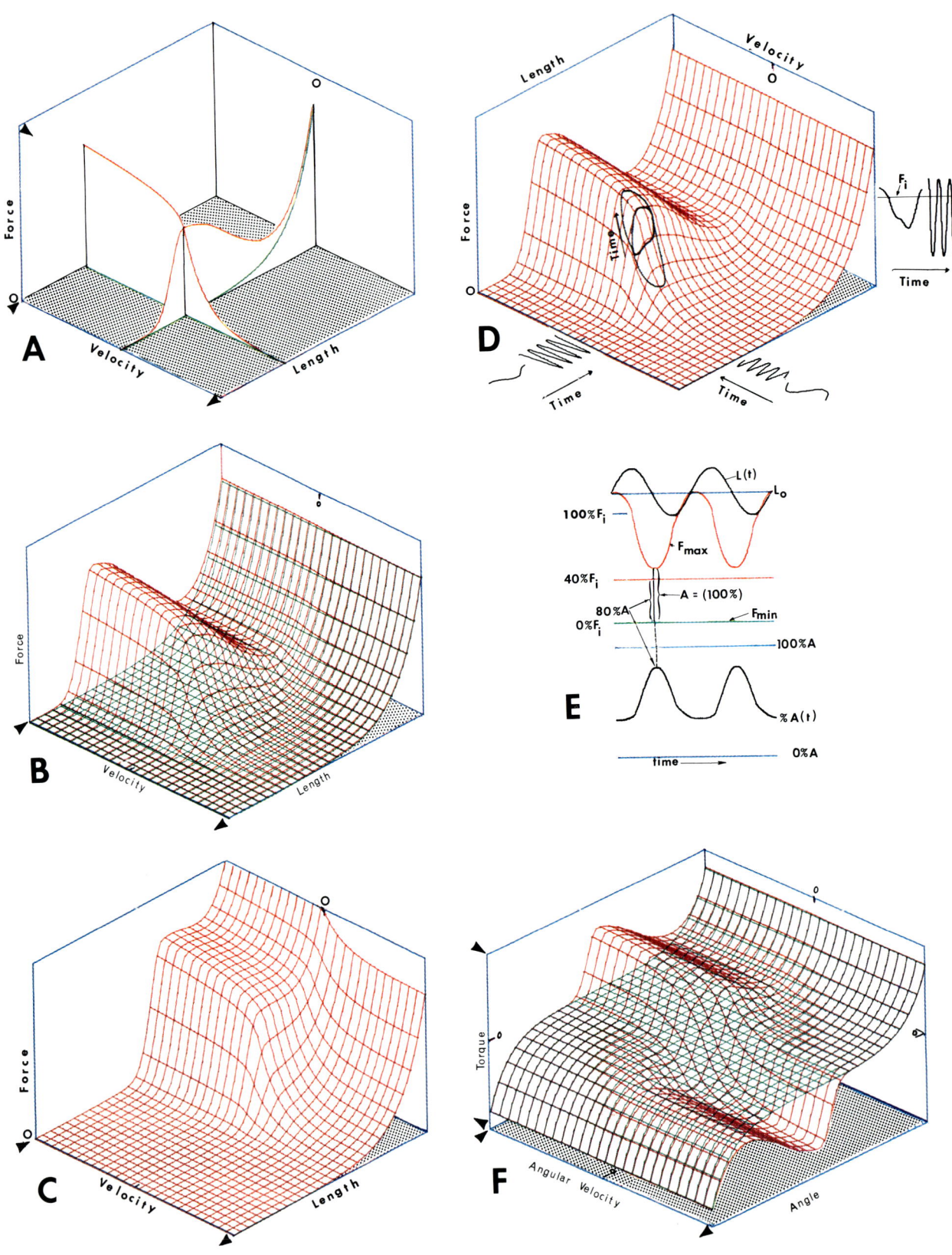

sequence of one relative activation pattern for a muscle (with response surfaces similar to that in Fig. 13*B*) plotted over two cycles of sinusoidal length change. The considerable force fluctuation at 100% activation is shown by the red curve in Figure 13*E*. Passive force, shown on the green line, remains almost zero. For this movement to occur at a constant force equal to 40% of maximal isometric force requires activation to vary from 80% to 35%. The time course of the relative activation required to produce that constant force through the cyclic movement also is cyclic, phase shifted, and not proportional to any simple measure of the movement. The changing relationship between excitation (activation) and force as a result of operating length and velocity is also represented in Figure 19*A* and *B*.

A MUSCLE MODEL. To this point we have assembled well-known information about muscle function that constitutes one muscle model. (Some implications of this model, however, are not conventionally discussed.) The graphic model is based on data (Figs. 5–12) obtained under carefully controlled and thus quite restricted conditions. A number of known complica-

FIG. 13. Expected 3-dimensional mechanical relationship in response of muscle. Muscle force as related to length, velocity, and excitation drawn by combining usual descriptions (for related experimental data, see Figs. 8*C*, 9*B*, 10, 11*D*, 12*A*). *Arrows* on velocity axes show relationship between velocity sign and change of length (angle). *Arrows* on torque axis in *F* relate torque to corresponding direction of change of velocity. *A*: one 3-dimensional description of response properties of a single muscle at a particular moment. Excitation of the muscle defines length-tension-velocity relationships in that muscle. At a single length this relationship is described as a force-velocity curve, and at a single velocity it is a length-tension curve. For length and velocity at some moment, instantaneous force falls at intersection of 2 such curves in length-velocity-force space. *Red* and *green* lines might correspond to 2 curves from a stimulus rate family, such as shown in Fig. 11*D* for length axis and Fig. 12*A* along velocity axis. At any other moment force output could be defined in terms of intersection of an appropriate stimulus-determined pair of intersecting length-tension and force-velocity curves, at least a 4-dimensional relationship. (Note: No dynamic component is represented in the passive response, although one is known to exist; see Fig. 5*B–D*.) *B*: the 26 different *red* graphs of active length-tension curves intersect in this diagram with each of the 26 *red* force-velocity curves to define 676 of the points to which a particular excitation level might bring a muscle. Same number of intersections in *green* represent passive muscle. (The different individual curves were derived from assumption that at any length the nonlinear velocity effect is proportional to isometric active force at that length.) Inclusion of all possible points between samples drawn here would produce a "response surface". If *red* surface designates the possible responses of maximally active muscle, then neural control would operate in space between *red* and *green* surfaces. (See ref. 25 for an experimentally derived half-surface drawn with a different orientation of the axes.) *C*: another variation of a response surface differing from *B* by a simple shift in relationship between passive and active length effects. Different muscles have properties that range between and beyond these types. *D*: representation of a sinusoidal movement as a trajectory over a response surface. A sinusoidal change in length, $l = A \sin \omega t$, defines a cyclic velocity, $V = A \omega \cos \omega t$, that varies in amplitude with frequency. Such pairs of curves trace eliptic paths on phase (base) plane and define complex closed loop trajectories over response surface. Time-varying force traced by such trajectories is periodic but not sinusoidal. This transformation from movement into force is inferred by the accepted length and velocity properties of maximally and constantly activated muscle. Response cycle has a phase-shift based on shape of response surface; it changes with movement frequency, amplitude, and bias. (Nonsinusoidal patterns of movement similarly can be graphed over this theoretical surface. As illustrated in Figs. 15 and 16, more complex stimulus and movement patterns tend to produce deviations from response surface predicted by the usual muscle description and represented by these graphs.) *E*: time graphs for one movement over response surface of *D*. Two cycles of sinusoidal length change centered around rest length, L_0, are shown by *black* curve at top of figure. Corresponding but phase-shifted force cycle for a maximally activated muscle is shown by the periodic, nonsinusoidal, *red* curve marked F_{max}. In some stretching parts of the cycle that force exceeds maximum isometric force, 100% F_i. At the specified lengths passive forces are all near 0 (0% F_i), as shown by line marked F_{min}. Any constant force (e.g., 40% of F_i) falls at different relative positions with respect to minimum and maximum force for velocity-length combinations as values change through the movement. If such a constant force can be produced through a movement, then a variation of activation of the muscle would be required. Here activation A is defined for any particular force as the relative position of that force between F_{max} and the passive force for existing physical conditions at the moment. In this example in order to maintain the constant 40% F_i force through the described movement, the neural drive would have to provide a time-varying activation (from 33% to 80% of maximal), as plotted on line marked % A. *F*: theoretical response surfaces for a pair of matched antagonist muscles. *Green* lines represent surface expected while both muscles are unexcited. *Red* lines represent the response surface expected when both muscles are maximally active. This surface does not show a simple cancellation of force; i.e., coactive surface is not a horizontal plane equal to passive surface. For the slopes, $\partial T/\partial \theta$ relates to stiffnesslike properties, and $\partial T/\partial V$ relates to a viscosity-like property. Lengths, velocities, and forces that describe linear action of a single muscle are replaced here by angles, angular velocities, and torques, which describe combined action of antagonist muscles on a hinge joint. [Adapted from Partridge (399).]

tions also have been avoided. Where variations of muscle properties are continuous, these functions still approximate operation in a region around the tested points.

If the regions in which muscle functions are known are within the conditions for most frequent operation, the resulting limited model may be applicable over much larger parts of the total operating time of many muscles than it is over the total descriptive space of potential function. This is suggested by the frequency with which a linear second-order model of a motor function closely approximates the actual function (e.g., ref. 391), in spite of the obvious involvement of a number of nonlinearities and individual components that would require a much higher order for complete description. The model assembled from these data is thus a first approximation of some simple tensile actions of familiar vertebrate muscles, but it is not a functional model of general application.

Stating the model simply: Neural signals affect activation of muscle in a nonlinear, history-dependent, and lagging way. The interpretation of relative activation as total force is then dependent on temperature, length, and velocity. The changing force applied to the equations of motion of the load defines a vector (contraction) that specifies the instantaneous rate of movement of the muscle unit through the length-velocity-force space. For any combination of activation and location in that space there is a characteristic muscle impedance (77). Experiments provide only local tests of the quantitative rules for this model.

The model described is entirely deterministic, with no stochastic component, and represents our belief that at or beyond the level of the whole fiber a muscle is a complex but well-defined operator. At the molecular level the basic process is presumably stochastic (56, 67, 503). With very careful control of conditions in a single muscle, simple tests produce almost identical responses over a period of hours. Furthermore, we also find consistency of response to precisely repeated but complex sequences of stimuli and mechanical input (L. A. Benton, T. M. Hamm, and L. D. Partridge, unpublished observations; this is also recognizable in the results in ref. 226). It therefore is suggested that most of the error in the model presented is, in fact, owing to error in the model and not to some random biological variability.

The description of this model is multidimensional, both dynamic and nonlinear, and does not define in usual dimensions a fixed responsiveness to stimulus. For an input measured in firing rate the nonlinear transformation has minimal sensitivity to stimulus at both low and high rates and shows a maximal sensitivity that falls between the two and in the ordinary physiological range (Fig. 8C). The dynamic lag introduces an appreciable time delay (Fig. 9C) for a variety of reflex actions. The inclusion of temperature (and probably other dimensions) in the input to muscle makes that input a vector through several conventional dimensions. In this vector form activation is entirely determined by input, but part of the input is not under direct and immediate neural control. Likewise, contraction is multidimensional in Newtonian space and can rotate in that space with load changes [Fig. 4; (59, 60, 223)] and operating region. If muscle output is a single dimension, that dimension would be a nonlinear function mapping the result of internal trades among force, length, and velocity. The contraction vector then could be a consistent transformation on the whole input vector and have rules dependent on the existing mechanical state and load. Because of the exchange possible in this output vector the displacements produced by a given nerve signal are much less dependent on load than they would be if the muscle were a simple force generator.

This model was chosen in order to use available data stated in familiar dimensions, but it represents only one of an infinity of equally correct descriptions (459). Various mathematical representations of combinations of such muscle properties have been published (e.g., refs. 234, 443). By addition of further terms in the input or in the rules determining state trajectory this model can be extended to deal with more complex but still deterministic muscle properties when these properties are adequately defined.

Functional Variations

In addition to the properties included in this tensile muscle model based on long-accepted mechanical properties of muscle, a variety of observations indicate the presence of other complications. Some of the deviations in tensile actions are associated with abrupt transients in either stimulus or movement. Other deviations relate to a memorylike effect. A third category of deviations concerns unusual muscles. For nontensile actions of muscle and response to less studied inputs the nature of any first-order dynamic properties is essentially unknown. Nontrivial effects of some of these extra inputs include force deviations as large as maximal isometric force and changes of muscle properties that invert certain relationships. Some normal functions even depend on these deviations from the conventional model.

As far as the model predicts observed muscle responses, these responses are inferred by those well-known muscle properties that make up the model. Prediction failures, then, indicate muscle properties that have not been included. The model implies that returning a muscle to the same length, velocity, temperature, and steady excitation will always result in the same force. This force would always be greater in a muscle being stretched than during shortening through the same length. Repeated stimulation at short intervals would produce summation of response. The nonlinear dynamic properties of the model predict other response patterns (although less obviously), and failures of these predictions might reveal additional defects in the model.

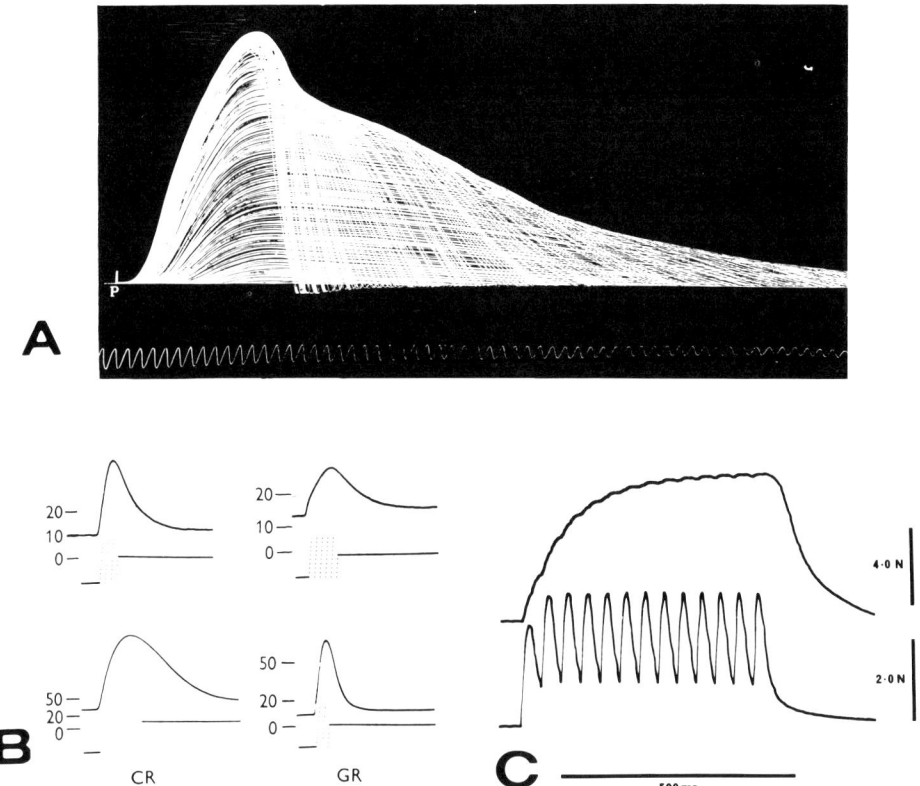

FIG. 14. Effects of excitation history on dynamics of muscle response. *A*: sequence of afterload frog muscle twitches recorded as fatigue develops. Increased height over first few trials (treppe) is followed by decreased amplitude (fatigue) as well as by increased latent period, increased time to peak, and slowed relaxation. This latter effect is known as contracture. *B*: change of response in 2 cat limb muscles as a result of surgically crossed innervation. *Upper two graphs*, normal muscle twitches in crureus and gracilis muscles. *Lower records*, altered response under influence of reinnervation by crossed nerves—slow muscle becoming faster and fast muscle becoming slower. Line below twitch record shows a digital measure of contraction time in ms arranged in series of *dots*, each column with a maximum of 10 1-ms points. *C*: adaptation of response of anterior tibial muscle of rabbit to long-term activity pattern. Two isometric responses to stimulus trains of 25 pulses/s. *Lower record*, response of normal muscle; *upper record*, muscle modified by stimulation at 10 pulses/s over a 5-month period. [*A*: from *Handbook of Physiology* by W. D. Halliburton, © 1911. Used with permission of McGraw-Hill Book Co. *B*: from Buller et al. (87), with permission of Cambridge Univ. Press. *C*: from Salmon (447).]

STIMULUS HISTORY. Alterations of muscle response with long-term excitation patterns are well known but seldom considered in the context of motor control; yet nerve signals must be adjusted for response rules. The mechanical response of muscle to excitation can be affected by many factors—for example: *1*) changes in fiber size in disuse atrophy (192, 285), exercise (207) or extension hypertrophy (192); *2*) addition of fibers with hypertrophy (122, 207); and *3*) changes of muscle length with prolonged limitation of movement (207). Clinical procedures also might change muscle response, as in the alteration of muscle dynamics that can be produced by surgically crossed innervation (Fig. 14*B*) or by long-term artificial stimulation [Fig. 14*C*; (447, 478)]. Additionally, relatively short term activity can markedly alter muscle response through fatigue [(Fig. 14*A*; (54, 177, 263, 279, 303, 537)]. The early fatigue of response in fast fibers [(90); see the chapter by Burke in this *Handbook*] in a mixed muscle might affect the dynamic and geometric function of that muscle. At least with artificial stimulus the length-tension pattern for a muscle can vary with fatigue (548). A number of alterations of muscle by nerve have been described under the name trophic actions (230, 442), some of which probably are determined by the excitation arriving by way of the nerve.

Stimulation at moderate to high rates can affect the response characteristics of muscle to subsequent stimuli. Different experimental protocols have produced information that has been described as hysteresis (82, 199, 221, 394, 396, 508, 555), latch or catch (266, 554), fused state (287), crystallization (161), consolidation, thixotropic action (83), treppe (143, 348, 451), post-tetanic potentiation (73, 168), and enhancement (222). In each case the contraction to a stimulus pattern is increased by effects of the previous stimulus. Each of

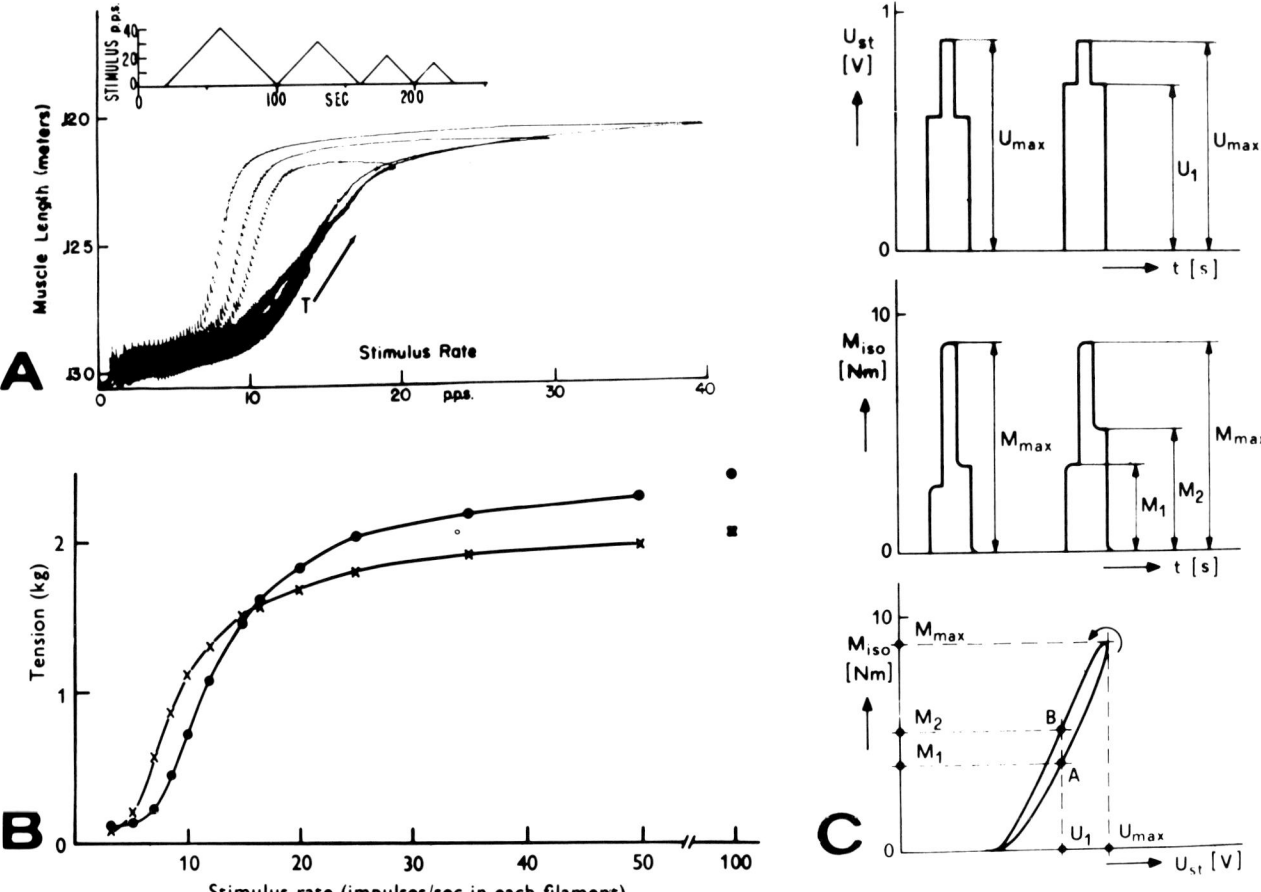

FIG. 15. Deviations of muscle response to stimulus from that of a simple, response surface model with lag. Examples show that muscle responses vary with stimulus history and past activity in other units and that mechanical effects are variable with stimulus level. A: hysteresis in cat triceps sura muscle response to rate modulation of stimulus. *Insert*, time sequence of stimulus. In graph of length vs. stimulus rate, time progresses in a counterclockwise direction. After a high stimulus rate, contraction is sustained even at appreciably lower stimulus rate. Similar hysteresis patterns are also found in isometric responses. Hysteresis did not occur in cycle with lowest maximum rate. B: difference in relationships between stimulus rate and force in lengthening and in isometric muscle. At high stimulus rates lengthening muscle, ●, produced more force than isometric muscle, ×, a relationship represented in the response surface diagrams of Fig. 13. At low stimulus rates, however, the relationship is reversed, suggesting a locally reversed slope for the force-velocity curve at such stimulus rates. C: hysteresis in muscle response to recruiting type of stimulus modulation in human peroneus muscle at constant rate of 50 pulses/s. U_{st}, time graphs of stimulus intensity; M_{iso}, isometric responses to stimulus. *Lowest graph*, force vs. stimulus, derived by combining data of type shown in the 2 time graphs and as labeled for point A and point B. [A: from Partridge (396). B: from Joyce et al. (296), with permission of Cambridge Univ. Press. C: from Trnkoczy (508).]

the first few stimuli at the beginning of a train of stimuli at a low rate leaves a residual effect, increasing response to the next stimulus, or treppe (Fig. 14A). A brief tetanic train of stimuli can produce even greater increase of response to single stimuli, i.e., posttetanic potentiation or enhancement (73, 168, 222). This increases both contraction peak and duration, and it decays slowly with time (336, 485). Contraction in response to a particular stimulus rate can be appreciably greater if it follows a period of higher stimulus rate than if it follows low stimulus rates [Fig. 15A; (92, 221, 346, 392, 394, 396, 522, 554, 555)]. Such hysteresis, catch, or latch effects may even occur when the high rate spans only two pulses (92, 221). In invertebrates it has been suggested that this property allows sustained contraction with minimal energy expenditure (266), and generally it also may allow a noisy nerve signal to control a smooth contraction. Another related observation is the familiar smoothing of contraction that develops through the first few responses to a train of stimuli delivered at a near-tetanic rate. Such terms as crystallization apply to the observation that in similar conditions muscle develops a decreasing sensitivity to changes of force as well as to excitation. Although these diverse observations have been consolidated here as hysteretic behavior of muscle responding to neural signals, the basis for this behavior probably involves more than one internal process. In addition, different observations have historically been explained in different ways.

In muscle the various responses to excitation do not always progress in parallel to the force response. For example, the rate of development of tension increases with stimulus rate quite differently than does the maximal tension developed (Fig. 8B), and stiffness changes differently than does force (555). Further, in a restricted range, the sign of the viscosity-like property, $\Delta F/\Delta V$, can be dependent on stimulus rate (Fig. 15B).

While vertebrate muscle control ordinarily, but not always, is described to involve only a single and excitatory nerve fiber for each motor unit, multiple innervation of muscle fibers may be the primitive form (23, 74, 283, 284, 306, 308, 349, 364, 448, 515, 516). In invertebrates, however, single muscle fibers often are supplied with as many as eight (264, 514, 515) even functionally different nerve fibers. Invertebrate nerves modify and inhibit as well as excite contraction (236, 264, 266, 308, 314, 474, 488, 514–516), and simultaneous activity of more than one type of fiber occurs naturally (474, 514, 515). It is clear that the neural input to such muscle fibers, based on the separate nerve signals, could be described as multidimensional or as a vector.

MECHANICAL HISTORY. Movement is necessary to test the response surface, but movement details affect the shape of that surface. The slope of the length-tension curves depends markedly on whether load is changed before or after the beginning of stimulus [Figs. 11A, 16A; (54, 527)], usually being stiffer when loaded after stimulus, except in "Weber's paradox" (see ref. 225). Also, a rapid loading of an excited muscle can cause more lengthening than that caused by an equal amplitude but slower loading (Fig. 16C), the different length remaining after the transients have ended. Furthermore, vibratory stretching of an excited muscle can decrease the force (82) and increase the compliance of that muscle, but the amount of that change depends on the stimulus rate (296) and on the amplitude of the oscillation (227). The stiffness measured by small amplitude vibration seems to be a different function from the slope, $\partial F/\partial l$, of the length-tension curve (227). The term *short-range stiffness* describes what may be an alternate demonstration of this muscle property (295, 387, 417). One approach subjects an excited and stationary muscle to a ramp of length change (see Fig. 16 in the chapter by Houk and Rymer in this *Handbook*) and relates measured increments of force, ΔF, and length, Δl, taken over brief time intervals. The ratio $\Delta F/\Delta l$ is larger at the beginning of the ramp than in midramp, which is interpreted as showing that the muscle is stiffer in the first part of the stretch than it is during the greater displacement that follows. This test might be related to the characteristics of the response surfaces in our Figure 13, raising questions about possible artifacts. For a small movement on that surface, $\Delta F \simeq \Delta l \cdot \partial F/\partial l + \Delta V \cdot \partial F/\partial V$. Since in a time period including the beginning of a ramp $\Delta V \neq 0$ and in the middle of a ramp $\Delta V = 0$, the initial, but not midramp, measurement of $\Delta F/\Delta L$ will include a velocity component in addition to the stiffness component $\Delta l \cdot \partial F/\partial l$, and any short-range stiffness effect will be mixed with a velocity effect, $\Delta V \cdot \partial F/\partial V$. This problem is particularly obvious at the end of the ramp, where $\Delta l \simeq 0$, $\Delta V < 0$, $\Delta F < 0$, implying that $\Delta F/\Delta l = -\infty$. However, in this period $\Delta F \simeq \Delta V \cdot \partial F/\partial V$, and $\Delta l \cdot \Delta F/\Delta l$ is not an appropriate value to calculate. Correspondingly it appears that short-range stiffness is difficult to determine by the ramp method. (Incidentally, $\partial F/\partial l$ on the response surface diagrams changes as a function of velocity as well as of length.)

Movement may affect the development of oscillation damping properties in muscle. Mechanical oscillation at the beginning of excitation, for example, seems to limit the development of the damping action (396). Similarly, a tetanic stimulus rate, which produces a fused contraction, can become subtetanic when the muscle is subjected to an abrupt length change (Fig. 16D). Both of these observations seem to represent flattening of the force-velocity curve consequent to the movement and would be consistent with a reduction of relative activation by the mechanical displacement. (The repeated stretch sometimes used to initiate a clinical clonus test may act on the muscle damping in the same way.)

Muscle also shows a memorylike retention of effects of mechanical history. Recent movement affects rate of change of force (65). A muscle stimulated at a moderate to high rate while at a stationary length becomes stiff, its equilibrium length being set by the length at which it was held. Small random or patterned displacements from that length do not disturb the memorylike properties during sustained stimulus, and force depends on the length at start of stimulus (Fig. 16A). Large transients embedded in a random displacement tend to reset the operating characteristics of the muscle with a "jump" discontinuity in the response, however, and this new state then persists (227). This memory of mechanical history is reset by either large or fast transient changes in length, a single twitch in a rest period (1, 245), or by brief interruption of steady stimulus [Fig. 16C; (1)]. It is tempting to consider the possibility that the jumps are related in part to the instability suggested by negative slope regions of the response surface (256) shown in Figure 13B but missing in Figure 13C.

UNUSUAL MUSCLE PROPERTIES. Some muscles appear to have unique properties, but simple quantitative differences can masquerade as qualitative variations. For example, the latch effect, once described only in clam muscles (266), now has been demonstrated in

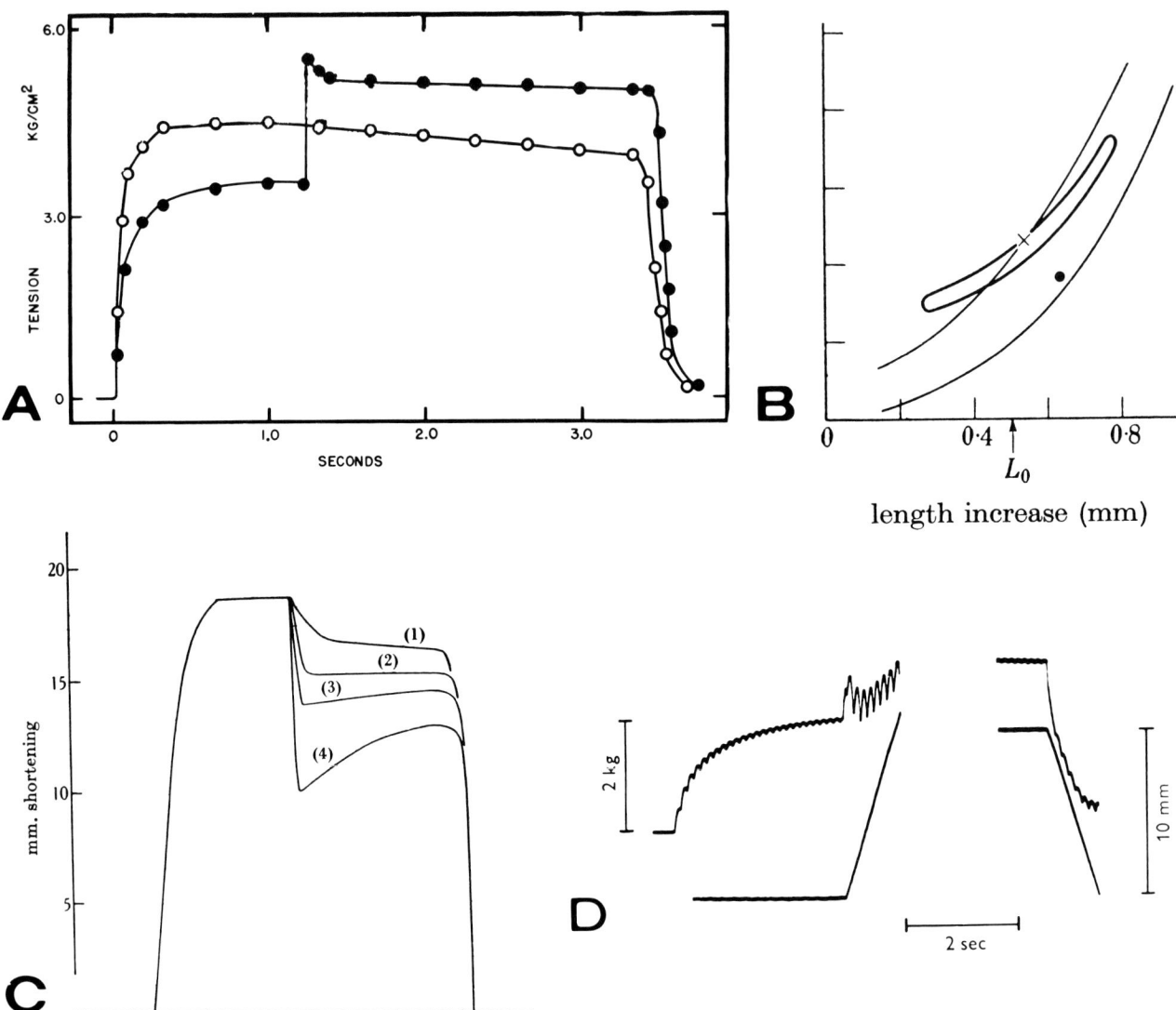

FIG. 16. Responses to mechanical inputs that deviate from response prediction implied by a simple version of the type of model illustrated in Fig. 13. *A*: response of stimulated triceps sura muscle to stretch showing mechanical hysteresis. In both lines stimulus was 120 pulses/s and velocity 0 at the same final lengths. In response marked by ●——● stimulus was started with muscle at a shorter length followed by a quick stretch to test length, producing a persistent increase of force over that in other response, with test length used throughout stimulus period. (See also Fig. 11*A*.) *B*: length-tension relationship in flight muscle of water beetle. *Lower curve*, passive muscle; *upper curve*, active muscle; *loop*, trajectory plotted on work plane with tetanized muscle subjected to cyclic stretch. Response travels around loop in an energy-delivering, counterclockwise direction, in contrast to energy-absorbing, clockwise loops ordinarily described with other muscles. In this case, unlike the diagramed force surfaces, force at shortening velocities is greater than those at the same length and lengthening velocities. This relationship allows these muscles to drive an oscillatory movement without a corresponding oscillating excitation pattern. *C*: length of a tetanically stimulated muscle before, during, and after a transition from one force to a larger force. In each line, muscle shortened at beginning of stimulus, stretched as load increased, then lengthened again at the end of stimulus. Initial and final forces were the same for each load increase, but rate of change of force varied, increasing from line (1) to line (4). Effect of different rates of loading persisted in terminal periods of constant and equal load. Greatest stretch occurred with fastest loading. *D*: disruption of fusion of tetanus during mechanical movement. *Left* part of record shows a stretch; *right* part shows a subsequent release of cat soleus while stimulated at 8.5 pulses/s. *Upper lines*, force; *lower lines*, muscle length. [*A*: from Walker (528). *B*: from Machin and Pringle (352). *C*: from Katz (304), with permission of Cambridge Univ. Press. *D*: from Joyce et al. (296), with permission of Cambridge Univ. Press.]

vertebrate muscles (394) and in a variety of other invertebrate muscles (554) under selected test ranges. Moreover, even in vertebrates there are slow muscle fibers (249, 265, 349, 364) that do not twitch and have a graded response, but this seems to be only a quantitative variation from that of the better known twitch muscles of vertebrates. Some other unusual properties that have been described in special muscles and in pathologically altered muscles also may be only quantitative variations.

Special muscles. The wave summation of responses to successive stimuli is reported to be absent in the white muscle of the carp (564). It would appear, then, that sustained contraction could not be achieved in units of such muscle. Fibrillary muscles in insects, on the other hand, have been found to interact with inertial or elastic loads to produce an oscillatory response that is independent of the stimulus detail and much higher in frequency than the stimulus (Fig. 1C). While these muscles show typical isometric responses in tetanic tests (Fig. 7B), an oscillatory mechanical movement causes the muscle to deliver energy in each cycle [Fig. 16B; (101, 413, 502, 503)]; thus the force in shortening is greater than the force during lengthening, and a reversal of slope of the force-velocity curve on the dynamically sampled response surface is revealed. In another variation some earthworm muscles have selectively activated fast and slow responses (490, 491).

Functionally the thoracic intervertebral muscles of turtle seem unrelated to any recognizable motor role typical of that described in an ideal joint. Perhaps the most extreme case of deviation of function in specialized muscle is that of electric organs of some fishes in which all contractile action has been lost and motor control produces only an electrical response (520).

Pathological muscle. In some cases the muscle in motor control has a function altered by pathological conditions. Direct disorders range from gross trauma to hereditary deficiencies of a single enzyme. Muscle function also may be altered due to modified operating conditions arising secondary to extramuscular pathologies.

Simple variation in the passive elastic matrix surrounding the contractile elements changes the relationship between neural drive and the total force delivered by the muscle at a particular length, as found in the pathological reduction of muscle fiber content that produces fibrous contracture (69, 472, 533). This is not the same phenomenon as the contracture of fatigued muscle described in older physiology texts (42, 263, 440). While fibrous contractures occur in muscular dystrophy, myositis, myosclerosis, Addison's disease, and chronic denervation, even immobilization of a normally innervated muscle can result in an effectively similar myostatic contracture (5).

Neuromuscular junction. Pathology involving the neuromuscular junction changes the usual one-to-one transfer of impulses from nerve to muscle. Alteration of acetylcholine (ACh) release, or receptor response to it, or its inactivation can all occur. Various neurotoxins, such as botulism toxin, block terminal nerve release of ACh (5, 126, 457, 499, 533). Resulting paralysis initially affects bulbar muscles and can lead to respiratory failure. In contrast, black widow spider venom causes a massive, spontaneous release of ACh, rapidly depleting the transmitter (126) and effecting general muscle cramping, spasm, and rigidity (5). Wood tick poison also causes defective ACh release, although its mechanism is debated (5, 69). Continuous production of toxin by an imbedded tick is thought, however, to be necessary for maintaining the resultant paralysis (5, 69).

Endogenous agents also can impede the normal delivery of acetylcholine. The Eaton-Lambert myasthenic syndrome seems to involve deficient release of ACh. Symptoms of limb muscle weakness subside with repeated stimulation or successive attempts to voluntarily perform motor activity. Some unknown substance is postulated to be interfering with presynaptic utilization of calcium, upon which ACh release is dependent (69, 140).

Myasthenia gravis also involves a deficit in neuromuscular transmission, although explanation of its etiology has been suggested in various hypotheses (5, 128). Most recently it has been described as an autoimmune disorder in which an antibody against the receptor protein at the motor end plate is produced, thus blocking action of ACh (5, 69, 533). Plasma exchange has been shown to improve the myasthenic condition, an effect presumed due to an immediate reduction of the concentration of the antibody (386). Myasthenia is characterized clinically by variable and abnormal weakness of voluntary muscles especially after repetitive or sustained contraction, with notable recovery of power after a period of rest (5, 533).

Partial denervation. Denervation eliminates central control of muscle fibers and also may lead to abnormal relationships between remaining functions of nerve and muscle. Either spinal or peripheral lesions may be involved (5). Following denervation ACh sensitivity develops beyond the motor end plate (370, 533), and spontaneous fibrillary twitching occurs throughout the muscle (138). The stimulus of these continual, asynchronous contractions is presumed to be circulating ACh (5, 441). These changes are discussed in some detail in the first volume of this *Handbook* section on the nervous system (442). In partial denervation remaining intact nerve fibers form sprouts that innervate the abandoned muscle fibers (138, 139). The result is a muscle with unusually large motor units among those remaining after the partial denervation (109).

Membrane. Some muscle pathologies involve altered excitatory properties beyond the end plate region. Myotonia, for example, appears as a sustained contraction of muscle fibers caused by repetitive membrane depolarization (533). The relaxation process is gradual and may be prolonged over several seconds (69). Myotonic response not only occurs after voluntary contractions but also can be set off by mechanical percussion of the muscle and by brief electrical stimulation (5). Some evidence suggests myotonia to be due to a decreased membrane permeability to chloride, which is important in inactivating the contractile process (5, 69). Myotonia accompanies several hereditary disorders, and it also may be induced experimentally by drugs and chemicals (5, 69, 533). Distinctive differences among the various myotonias are described. Another membrane disorder, familial periodic paralysis, is commonly associated with potassium deficiency and loss of membrane excitability (365).

Contractile protein. Functional alterations in the contractile protein system also are a known source of motor control pathology. A simple change in muscle bulk can vary the mechanical response available to a particular neural signal. Roughly, the maximum power output available from a muscle is proportional to the mass of the contractile system that produces the chemomechanical conversion. Muscle hypertrophy, atrophy, agenesis, and degeneration dystrophy are examples of conditions effecting functional change secondary to a volume change of muscle.

True hypertrophy is an increase in the number or size of constituent muscle fibers (207) and can result normally from voluntarily increased muscle activity, or pathologically from the increased activity caused either by a muscle fiber disease (5) or by excessive neural activity. Whether hypertrophy involves added fiber volume or greater fiber number is debated (5, 122, 207), but the possible force that can be produced by the muscle is increased concomitantly with cross-sectional size. On the other hand, length changes wth muscle growth clearly involve addition of new sarcomeres of normal length (86, 207), except in crayfish, where sarcomeres themselves have been shown to grow in length (207).

Degeneration implies destruction of tissue or an irreversible alteration in appearance, including replacement of muscle fibers by fat cells and collagen. The pseudohypertrophy evident in the early stages of muscular dystrophy is an interesting variation of degeneration (5, 140). Despite the appearance of increased muscle bulk and a feeling of firmness, muscle force actually is progressively decreased due to degeneration and loss of contractile fibers.

Frequently muscle degeneration is due to a circulatory deficiency. It has been suggested that venous occlusion is more severe than arterial occlusion and leads to fibrosis and muscle shortening not seen after arterial occlusion (5). The level of vascular lesion and collateral circulation decide the distribution of final necrosis. Arterial occlusion may be among intramuscular vessels (polyarteritis nodosa), in peripheral arteries (atherosclerosis), or in a main artery (Volkmann's contracture).

Muscle atrophy, however, describes a loss of muscle volume that can be reversible (5). Although neuromuscular pathologies effect various degrees of both simple atrophy and degeneration, atrophies due to disuse [occurring in periods as short as 3 days (285)] are here considered representative. The principal effect of disuse atrophy, when imposed by skeletal immobilization, by paralysis due to an upper neuron lesion, or by severed tendon, is reduction in muscle bulk and volume by sarcoplasmic and myofibril diminution. Prevention or retardation of size atrophy by electrical stimulation or by static stretch of the affected muscle has been described (482).

Deficiency of muscle volume may result from congenital agenesis or other defect of formation. While any muscle group may be affected, with or without additional structural and functional abnormalities, the pectoral and trapezius muscles are deficient in human beings more frequently than other muscle groups (5).

Metabolism. Muscle function may be altered as a secondary result of metabolic disorders. Glycogen storage disease, for example, results from lack of an enzyme necessary for carbohydrate metabolism and not only deprives muscle of an energy source but also leads to deposition of a large mass of glycogen within the muscle (5, 147). Endocrine gland abnormalities act more indirectly through modification of enzyme actions and membrane phenomena. Correction of the hormonal problem usually restores muscle function (5, 69).

Hyperthyroidism with increased metabolism depletes high-energy phosphate stores within the muscle (5, 533) and causes muscle weakness and increased fatigability. Hypothyroidism, on the other hand, seems to slow those metabolic processes that affect the contractile mechanism of the muscle fiber (5). Weakness and fatigue again result and may be accompanied by muscular aches, cramps, and a slowed relaxation following contraction, although electromyography docs not suggest a true myotonia (5, 69, 147).

Pathology of the parathyroid glands, which are important in mobilizing calcium from bone and in decreasing renal reabsorption of phosphate, produces abnormality ranging from hypocalcemic muscle tetany to muscle weakness, fatigability, pain, and atrophy (5).

Acromegaly, Cushing's disease, and Addison's disease are adrenal and pituitary abnormalities in which there is a rather nonspecific muscle weakness, usually in proximal limbs (69).

These alterations in muscle with pathology not only constitute a nonneural basis for abnormal function but are a problem with which the nervous system deals except in the most severe cases. A relatively normal muscle changes to a muscle that still functions but in either a quantitatively or a qualitatively different way. For such a muscle the result of a nerve impulse has changed, and particular actions that can still be accomplished must be produced by altered intensity and pattern of neural drive.

Summary

A unit of muscle subjected to neural excitation produces motor responses in a physiological environment. Muscle responses have been studied when the single varying input is either stimulus, length, velocity, or temperature. Less commonly the response of particular muscles has been examined while two or more of these inputs are varied. Several measures of muscle response are affected by the instantaneous firing rate of the nerve (an input), but excitation-response relationships also are dependent on how fast excitation is changing and on both excitation and mechanical history. The total output of muscle involves a combination of force, velocity, position, mechanical impedance, and heat. The rules by which muscle transforms neural signals into mechanical output vary widely among animals, among different muscles in a single animal, among motor units in a single muscle, and even in different actions of the same units. These rules also change with long-term history of the muscle, with pathology, and with the immediate environment. Although information about these properties was important in the development of current contractile theory, that application has not been discussed here. One general description defines muscle as a device that transforms an input vector into a mechanical output vector in a nonlinear, time-dependent way, with the relationship including a memory. The input vector includes both neural and environmental factors. The moving output vector is defined in the space of the various response dimensions, but its trajectory through that space (i.e., the changes in proportions of force, velocity, length, and other dimensions that make up the contraction) depends on the load upon which the muscle acts.

MULTIPLE UNITS OF MUSCLE

The single unit of muscle, which was considered in the previous section, is defined by being excited as an entity. Whether that unit is as small as a fiber or as large as an assembly of a few muscles, there nevertheless is a similarity of properties. With invertebrate exceptions (264), however, almost no motor acts are accomplished by single muscle units. Normally multiple units are involved and exhibit some degree of independence (17, 106, 117, 188, 199, 451, 462, 464, 467, 468, 507, 543). The combination of unit actions is an issue separate from the generation of excitation patterns (see the chapters by Houk and Rymer, Stein and Lee, Henneman and Mendell, and Robinson in this *Handbook*) and partially separate from joint kinematics (see the chapter by Alexander). In the discussion that follows we confine our treatment almost entirely to tensile functions in joint-based systems.

The Unit of Muscle Function

The minimal unit of physiological activation, the motor unit (347), is an obvious candidate for an independent functional unit, and in spite of changes in definition (89, 335) it has always included all of the muscle fibers served by a single axon. A motor unit that comprises a whole arthropod muscle (264) or that acts isometrically through independent attachments to a load (as in intercostal muscles) might function reasonably as an independent unit. On the other hand a motor unit that shares in the movement of a load (135), or that acts on common elastic connections with other motor units, deals with a load that is subject to change by those other units. Since the contraction vectors are in part determined by the load, such units do not operate independently (332). When small numbers of units are involved (515) each unit contributes a relatively large portion of the action on the load; as a consequence, individual interactions are great. (During cocontraction of two equal units attached in parallel to a load, each acts on only half of the load it would have if active alone.) When large numbers of units have overlapping action, cumulative (but not individual) interactions are large (368, 507). In general it appears that motor units are functionally interacting units (135, 368) rather than independent units. The minimal unit of independent function, therefore, would appear ordinarily to be larger than a single motor unit.

A whole anatomical muscle also might act as a minimal independent unit. At least in some cases the orderly recruitment and derecruitment of motor units [(93, 141, 155, 219, 220, 244, 320); and see the chapter by Henneman and Mendell in this *Handbook*] gives whole muscle a unity and consistency of action, in spite of the noise introduced by independence of timing of impulses in different motor units (104, 467, 468, 492, 493). With constant order, recruitment is only a fixed part of intensity grading. Whole muscles, like motor units, often have combined actions on loads that are sometimes complex, such as the energy-exchanging actions between the respiratory functions of abdominal, thoracic, and diaphragm muscles (353). Use of the same argument that is applied to the motor unit leads to the conclusion that only those whole muscles that have neither synergists nor antagonists (e.g., the adductor of some bivalves) are likely to work as completely independent units. On the other hand, this independence then does not apply to most muscles.

A single degree of freedom, in the mechanical sense, likewise usually cannot be isolated functionally, because single muscles can act on more than one movement of a single joint [(152, 157, 197, 206); and see Fig.

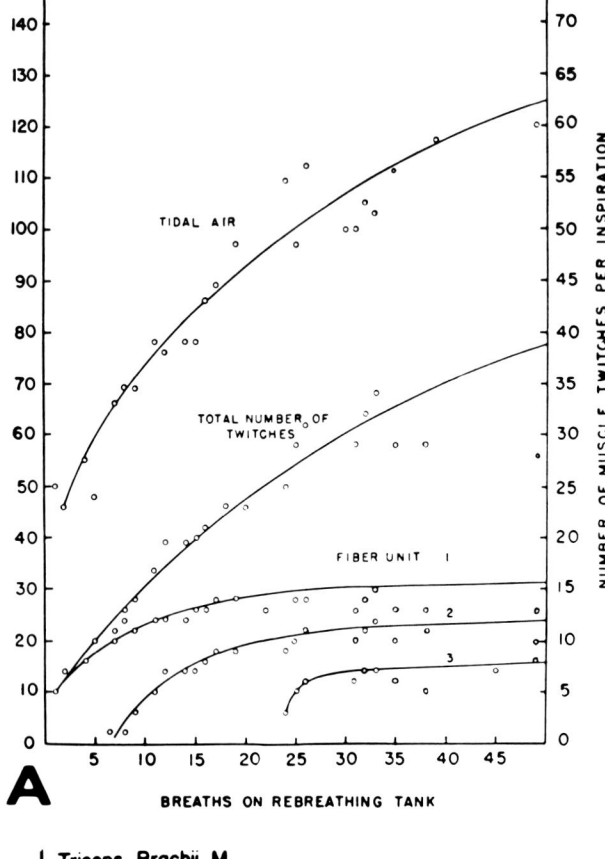
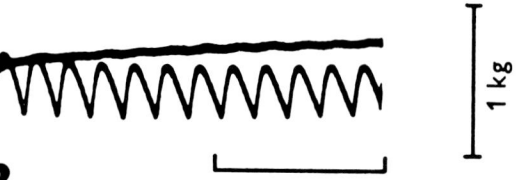
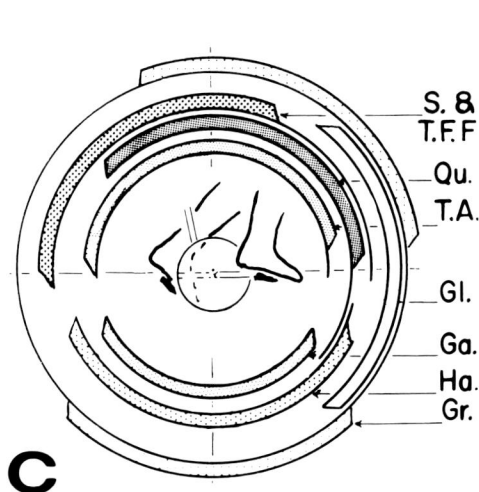
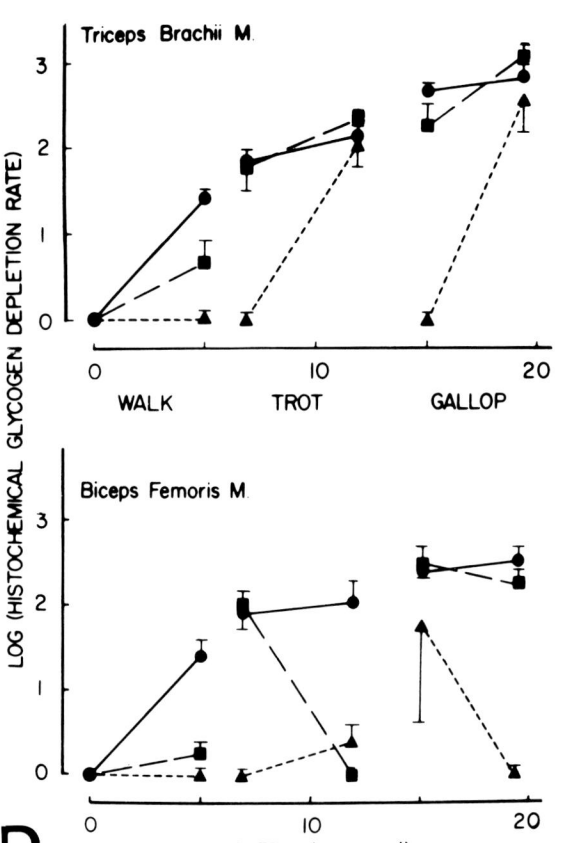

FIG. 17. Combinations of independent units of muscle. (See also Figs. 1B, 13F, and 15C.) A: recruitment of 3 separate respiratory motor units and accompanying increase of firing in individual units (measured from unit electromyogram (EMG) records) as total response intensity increases. Measured motor response is tidal air moved as it increased with rebreathing. B: smoothing of soleus isometric response by alternation of excitation among groups of motor units. Muscle nerve was divided into 5 branches, and each was provided with separate stimulus electrodes. Responses to individual stimuli can be distinguished in record made with synchronous stimulus to all branches. Rotating of branch stimulus (with each division stimulated in turn at same rate) produced response that was not only smoother but greater in magnitude than average of synchronous response. (Normal recruitment produces asynchronous instead of rotating excitation, presumably a less effective means of smoothing.) C: combination of activity of several muscles during bicycling. Weak and strong EMG activity are shown by single and broad lines, respectively. Note variable overlap between muscle activity periods, as well as two separated phases of strong activity in gracilis, Gr. D: recruitment of 3 types of motor units in 2 muscles of lion as speed of locomotion increases. Discontinuities in graphs represent change in type of gait. As seen in histochemical evidence, relative intensity of activity of different types of units does not change in the same order through all gaits and muscles. [A: from Gesell et al. (188). B: from Rack and Westbury (421), with permission of Cambridge Univ. Press. C: from Houtz and Fischer (262). D: from Armstrong et al. (17).]

14 of the chapter by Alexander in this *Handbook*]. Others cross more than one joint (Fig. 4D; and see Fig. 10 in the chapter by Alexander) and cause interaction (158, 216, 472). Remote movements that change the gravity or inertia seen by a muscle also provide another form of load modification. Within an animal, in fact, muscle units that would produce contraction vectors independent of action of any other muscle unit appear to be the exception, not the rule. While considering either vector or scalar combination of the mechanical actions of multiple units of muscle, it therefore must be recognized that by that combination the responses of the units probably are modified. The nature of this interaction is such that the nerve signal to a unit of muscle will produce variable mechanical contribution, depending on how it is combined with activity of other units; nevertheless, in the unlikely event of identically repeated total motor acts, that signal should produce nearly identical results.

Relationships in Multiunit Function

The combination of results of unit excitations that have been determined by interaction is not a trivial mechanical issue. The easy description that the action of synergists (whole muscles or motor units) adds, whereas that of coactive antagonists cancels, is seriously deficient. Such approximations, however, often have been accepted but not experimentally tested. Yet to a great extent, evidence of the deficiency of these approximations is indirect and theoretical. Fortunately this theory is based on mechanical rather than biological assumptions, and it is subject to rigorous rules of internal consistency.

ANTAGONISTS. Antagonists, defined to be a combination of muscles with opposite directions of action, are analyzed kinematically in the chapter by Alexander; we emphasize instead the muscle role. In addition to subtraction of torque contributions (223, 260, 261) when one muscle stretches its tense antagonist, energy is transferred into the stretched muscle and lost for immediate external action. Basmajian (35, 36), Cohen and Gans (117), Houtz and Fisher (262), Lestienne and Bouisset (328–330), Stetson and Bouman (486), Townsend (506), and Wacholder (521) are among those who have used electromyography to demonstrate both the alternate and overlapping activation of antagonist muscles. In cyclic limb movement (515), of course, one might argue that sequentially active antagonists together can replace the energy lost in each cycle and are, from the energy standpoint, synergists. Wacholder also demonstrated that a variety of strategies are used in exciting an antagonist pair to produce a movement. Weak contractions separated in time and fluctuating simultaneous contraction are both used to produce similar movements, but the two involve differing amounts of cancellation (Fig. 1B). Ordinary motor actions include coordination of more complex groups of muscles with less easily defined relationships [e.g., Fig. 17C and D; (35, 36, 109, 117, 160, 185, 216, 220, 262, 353, 427, 507)]. The elbow extensor-flexor antagonists allow a convenient demonstration of torque cancellation in a static case. When held in a gravity-free orientation, a constant position represents zero torque of the elbow joint, and with torque cancellation stationary position can be produced with varying degrees of activity in the antagonists. Torque cancellation is not a cancellation of all muscle effects, however. During cocontraction these muscles produce a' stiff elbow, while the same zero torque with relaxed antagonists is associated with a compliant joint. This simple demonstration is expanded in two ways, mathematically and graphically, in the discussion that follows.

Force F in each muscle generates torque, T, in proportion to its moment arm r, but the torque of antagonists has opposite sign. In the static torque balance situation, the torque produced by one muscle, $T_1 = F_1 r_1$, cancels that of the other muscle, $T_2 = -F_2 r_2$, and $T = T_1 + T_2 = 0$. For a small angular movement $\Delta\theta$ one muscle would be stretched (Δl_1) while the other shortens ($-\Delta l_2$) and

$$r_1 \Delta\theta \simeq \Delta l_1 \quad \text{and} \quad r_2 \Delta\theta \simeq -\Delta l_2$$

If both muscles are stiff, $(\partial F/\partial l) > 0$, then the angular stiffness

$$(\partial T/\partial \theta) \simeq (\partial F_1/\partial l_1)\, r_1^2 + (\partial F_2/\partial l_2)\, r_2^2$$

is the combined effects of the two muscles. In words: while torques subtract, stiffnesses add, and length changes are opposite and proportional. A parallel argument shows that the individual contributions also add for the viscosity-like property relating torque to angular velocity.

Let us digress to examine broader implications of this relationship. In an individual muscle neural control of force and control of mechanical impedance are inseparable. As just demonstrated, however, independent innervation of antagonists provides the ability to separate control of the important motor functions of torque and mechanical impedance (218). Incidentally, patients with parkinsonism show a separation of these functions, in that they are found to have an impedance property that is increased more than their tonic muscle force (170, 539). It is also well known that the nervous system, through muscles, can independently control other functions such as force, velocity, and position (70, 480). Just as the independent control of antagonist muscles allows separation of the control of the dimensions of force and mechanical impedance, it would seem necessary that the neural control of the other dimensions also involves independence of activation of muscles that contribute dimensionally different actions to their combined effect. No greater number of independent dimensions of control would seem possible than the number of functionally different and separably activated motor units.

Graphic combination of the torque effects of two muscles can display the antagonist relationship as a torque surface (Fig. 13F) comparable to the force surface drawn for one muscle (Fig. 13B-D). In such graphs the points of static or dynamic balancing of an external force would fall on a single torque isopleth for the muscle combination. Stationary equilibrium could occur where this nulling isopleth crosses zero velocity. The slopes of the surface, even on the null isopleth, represent the mechanical impedance of the muscle part of the system. Had the two muscles produced a complete cancellation of effects, however, the surface would have been a horizontal plane. A change in activation of either muscle would alter the combined surface, relocate the null isopleth in length and velocity, and change the local mechanical impedances.

Both passive and active stiffness of muscle are functions of muscle length. For antagonist muscles this makes the overlap of lengths (75) important. Thus, without some adjustment, a different geometric relationship between bone and muscle (as after surgery or a malaligned fracture) would affect both static and dynamic function. In addition, when one two-joint muscle is involved in an antagonist pair the antagonist relationship is variable, as it is when a member of an antagonist pair deals in a single joint with two degrees of freedom (152, 157, 472).

SYNERGISTS. Of all of the types of synergist actions, only the cases of common action on a load are considered here. A number of other muscle combinations are called synergists but are not treated separately. They include units acting on neighboring joints in a similar way (465), muscles that select one of two actions of another muscle (152) by opposing the alternate action, muscles that brace a body part so that a movement becomes effective (375, 427, 472), or those muscles that by cocontraction (39, 521) produce joint immobilization (36, 328, 427, 472). Such muscles act physically in the same way, either as antagonists or as part of the load. On the other hand, motor units acting in parallel within a muscle are included here as synergists. This arbitrary division, however, is for economy of space and is not an attempt to deal with the general and even conflicting uses of the term synergist.

The combined action of motor units within a muscle is described conventionally as *summation*. With asynchrony of unit activity this provides a smoothing of response beyond that produced by lag in individual units [Fig. 17B; (204)]. Gradation of the number of active units (188, 347), as well as graded firing rate (8, 9, 188), adjusts response intensity (Fig. 17A), and this recruitment spreads over anatomically separate synergists (187).

The term summation is used here in the colloquial rather than the technical sense. From the first law of thermodynamics, however, it is clear that summation must be used correctly in the technical sense with respect to power P and work. The total mechanical energy output is equal to the sum of the mechanical outputs of all muscle components (observing proper sign to distinguish absorption from production). This requirement for conservation of energy dictates, however, that for any geometric arrangement the total output of a muscle cannot also involve the sum of both component forces F_i and component movements (lengths or velocities V_i). Therefore, for n structural components

$$P = \sum_{i=1}^{n} P_i = \sum_{i=1}^{n} F_i V_i \neq \left(\sum_{i=1}^{n} F_i\right) \cdot \left(\sum_{i=1}^{n} V_i\right)$$

Thus both forces and velocities cannot sum. If force and velocity cannot both sum, then force cannot sum in combination with either acceleration or length changes. Therefore it is necessary to define what is meant by summation before determination can be made of the proper application of the term in the technical sense.

The heterogeneity of real muscles further complicates the process of summation [(11, 50, 85, 185, 243, 366, 389, 484); and see the chapters by Burke and by Henneman and Mendell in this *Handbook*]. Conversely, the diversity of unit properties broadens the range available to control. Returning to the definition of unit contractions as vectors specifying the trajectories of responses in the physically defined space, summation must be some type of vector summation. (Under limited conditions this is equivalent to scalar summation, and the equations of motion provide the adjustments for energy conservation.) For a muscle like the human trapezius the fan-shaped arrangement of fibers gives the result that forces have a direction as well as magnitude that is variable. If the load is not constrained, dimensions are added because velocity and length become directionally variable with units activated. Furthermore, when units are connected partly or wholly in series (3, 32, 102, 127, 167, 432, 525), one unit becomes a variable part of the load for another. This is also true of sarcomeres in a single fiber where response also may not be homogeneous over the whole length (272). Units with different activation dynamics or response surfaces (11, 212, 371, 435, 451, 496, 509, 552) also would give the whole muscle a response in dynamics that varies with the organization of unit activations (17, 389, 507). Insofar as neural control can select from functionally different motor units, total motor response can be steered within this response hyperspace. The multiplicity of motor units therefore can add dimensions instead of just magnitude to the control.

Even sequentially activated units would be expected to interact (134, 135, 332) because of length and velocity dependence of force. On the parts of a response surface where $\partial F/\partial l > 0$, muscle shortening due to previous activity of other units would reduce a unit's response force. In effect the load-dependent contraction of one unit is a signal that adjusts the contraction of subsequent activity in other units on the basis of the impedence encountered by the earlier action (399).

Under most circumstances the more compliant the load, the less will be the force generated with succeeding activations. Thus the contractile system provides an automatic adjustment for load size, and this adjustment does not involve nerve conduction delay. For a load involving an appreciable viscous or inertial component, however, velocity or displacement, or both, will lag delivered force due to the laws of mechanics; and the time one twitch will most influence another will be similarly delayed. When multiple units are active, one unit then might be expected first to deliver force, which would result in a cumulative displacement of load and muscle, and thereby finally reduce the force delivered by other units. Biphasic muscle force following unit activation has been recorded with a late phase of force decrement [Fig. 1A; (142, 373)], presumably due not to muscle pushing but to reduction of average force in background units. It might be predicted that as recruitment progresses the increasing interaction of more active units would alter the response wave shape progressively more. By predominantly reducing the latter part of the twitch, this interaction would make a faster effective response wave and therefore may be a factor in the difference observed between the dynamics of single twitches and the dynamic relationships between electromyogram (EMG) and physiological muscle responses (95, 226, 476, 563).

Quantitative differences in motor units are important if unit selection can be used to determine response properties. Since Ranvier in 1874 (426) described the different speed of red and white muscle it has been presumed that these dynamic properties are selectively used for differing function. In pectinate bivalves, for example, the separate fast and slow adductor muscles have been specialized to extremes of a function. The fast part closes the shell cyclically during swimming, while the slow part provides prolonged shell closure. On the velocity axis there is no apparent overlap of function of these synergists (345). One then might question whether the two adductor muscles are properly synergists if their function does not overlap on one dimension, velocity. Cephalopods similarly use slow and fast muscles separately for breathing and swimming functions (509). Among vertebrates, fishes have evolved a similar but less extreme separation on the velocity axis. A laterally placed band of red fibers is used in slow, sustained swimming, while the bulk of the musculature is white, fast, more medially placed, rapidly fatiguing, and used for quick spurts of movement (11, 426). In this case the location of the fast and slow muscles would appear to be such that their intrinsic difference in speed could be augmented by the effect of different local movement velocities. Since the magnitude (or velocity) of muscle movements varies both with joint movement and with moment arm of the muscles' points of action (as analyzed in the chapter by Alexander), geometric differences in muscle arrangement can affect the effective speed and range of muscles as related to final action. Consideration of these mechanical factors leads to the question, Do some of the complex arrangements of fasciculi (e.g., Fig. 3D) within muscles provide the nervous system with extra controllable dimensions along the axes of either space or dynamics? At least in some mammalian muscles part of this potential for control nevertheless appears to be unused. Fixed patterns of recruitment [see the chapter by Henneman and Mendell in this *Handbook*; (93, 142)] do not provide the basis for use of other dimensions by motor unit selection, but variable activity patterns in other cases [e.g., Fig. 17D; (50, 103, 464, 475)] leave open the possibility of selective use.

Summary

Motor activities ordinarily involve multiple motor units. These units are not fully independent in either activation or response. Larger associations of units are flexible, however, and the organization of muscle function is not classified readily into an organization of fixed functional units. Two motor units associated in a particular geometric action may be functionally almost identical, have overlapping but not identical dynamic range and direction of action, or even have opposing direction of action or nonoverlapping dynamic range. Combined action needs to be described in terms of vector summation of individual responses. Selective control of multiple units provides a basis for separation of control in dimensions not independently controllable in single motor units (i.e., with antagonist muscles, force and stiffness can each be controlled). The minimal system capable of such dimensional separability therefore must include more than one motor unit.

SOME MEASURES OF MUSCLE FUNCTION

The action of an individual muscle in motor function involves a variety of physical changes, several of which are a source of useful measures (Fig. 18). All indicate muscle activity, but in details the measures are as diverse as the underlying processes. Relationships among the measures are neither linear nor related one to one [Fig. 19; (95)]. The electromyogram (EMG) originates in depolarization of surface membranes of muscle fibers with almost undetectable contamination from nerve fibers and neuromuscular junctions (63). The rustling myosonogram (Fig. 18C), easily detectable at the surface with a stethoscope or the ear, probably originates largely in the abrupt volume changes in individual fibers [Fig. 6D; (161, 456)]. Additional components are due to vibration set up between moving structures, but there is probably mini-

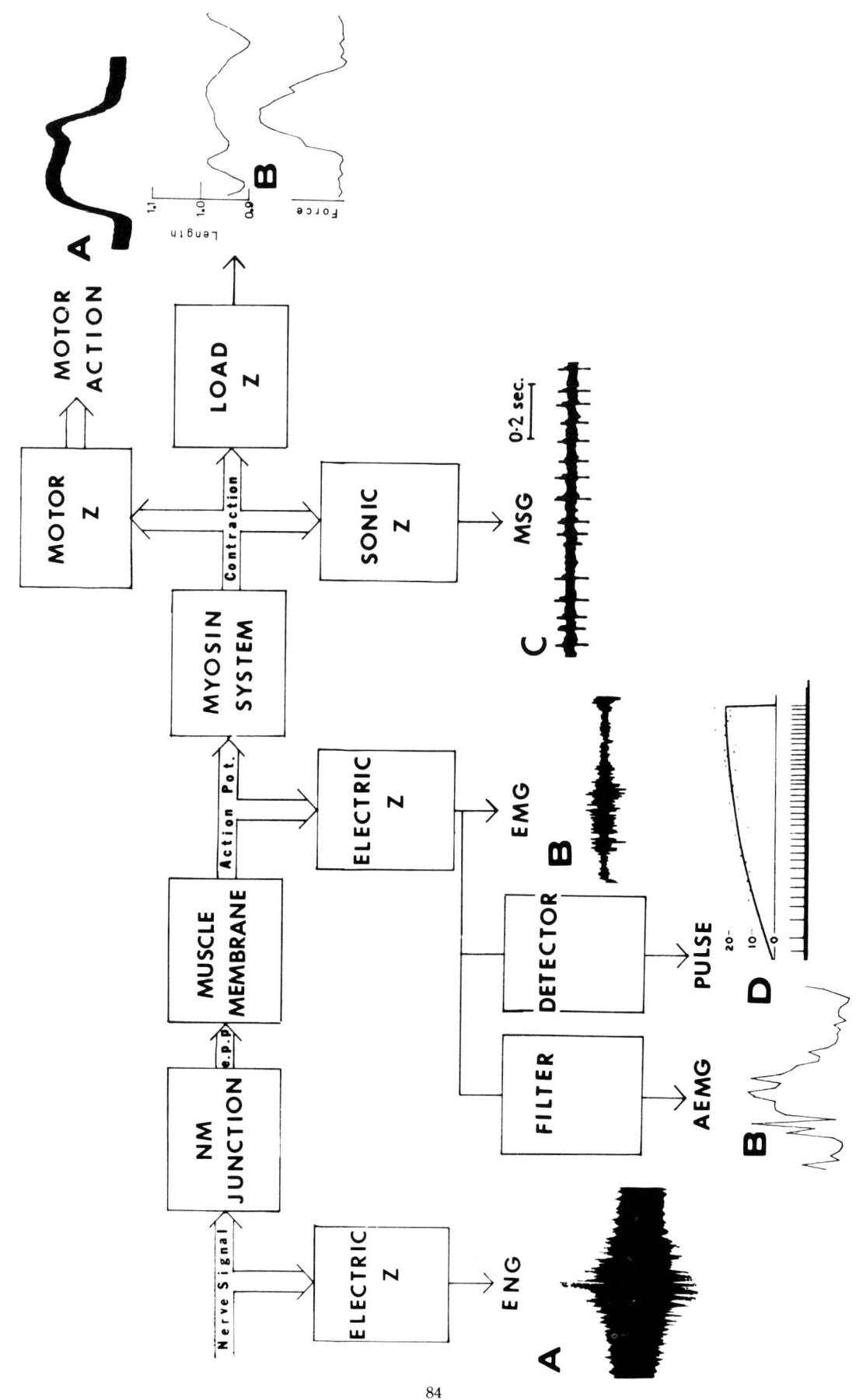

mal contribution from the subsonic frequency components of the ordinary twitch. In physiological activity muscle tension is important but only rarely has been measured in sufficient isolation (exceptions: refs. 285, 286, 423, 462, 532, 563) to define the contribution of a single muscle. Although easily observed the lateral displacement of contracting muscle (Fig. 3C) is of complex origin. In addition to the exchange between fiber length and diameter it also involves longitudinal movement of tapered muscle, straightening of curved muscle, shape changes in complex muscles, and deformation due to actions of other muscles. Muscle length and velocity, which can be well measured in some muscles but are undefinable in others, may be either active or passive. The transmission of sound through muscle changes with excitation (510–512), but this property appears not to have been used to study physiological function.

Most methods of measuring muscle activity today are adaptations of older procedures. The use of electrical activity of muscle, first reported by Galvani (184), slowly developed as an esoteric laboratory tool (53, 138, 333, 405, 521); then after advances in electronics it abruptly became the EMG in routine use for clinical neurology (35, 109, 137, 197, 198, 333, 358, 471, 513). The scientific investigations in 1665 by the Jesuit priest Francisco Maria Grimbaldi (quoted in ref. 61) demonstrated that muscle sound originated in vibrations of the body structure against the ear instead of in spirits trying to escape from the ear canal. Modern instrumentation has not been used to add appreciably to knowledge of the myosonogram beyond that developed up to the first third of the twentieth century (61, 62, 129); in fact, muscle sound is seldom mentioned in modern textbooks. Lateral displacement of muscle, on the other hand, is a measure that has been recorded occasionally for a century (102, 426, 454, 572), and evaluation by manual palpation is a well-established clinical tool (43, 152). Tendon force, which has been used to study isolated muscle, also has been measured in human amputees having surgically produced arrangement for external attachment of tendons [Fig. 11C; (281, 423)]. Implanted tendon transducers have been used to measure the dynamic force of ankle extensors in cat (285, 286, 531, 532, 563). For a few muscles, special limb positioning allows clinical isolation of force from a single muscle in external measurement (e.g., refs. 109, 110). On the other hand, muscle length information as shown by limb position has existed for more than a century. Ordinary sequential photographs by Marey (356, 357) and Muybridge (381, 382) have been refined to radiocinematographs (100, 133) and automatically measured video records (100, 145, 556). Mechanical measurements now also are available from multiangular goniometers (100). Torques generated by muscles have been calculated by combining data about inertia of body parts with photographic and other records of movement (66, 156, 356). Force plate information also has been used to calculate joint torques with or without photographic data (99, 125, 355, 402, 415, 416).

All measures of muscle activity introduce special selection and modifications of information. Single-unit responses are recognizable in EMG and sonograms [Fig. 18; (46, 62, 166, 404)], but total response is poorly represented. The response picked up is local, it decays (79–81, 84, 105, 343), and it is modified (40, 60, 63, 80, 337) with distance from the source. When activity is not uniformly distributed through the muscle this localization can be important [(452, 472); see the chapter by Robinson in this *Handbook*]. Special calculation is needed to deal with signal loss by interference (52, 376). Processing through pulse count [Fig. 19B–D; (35, 46, 109)], rate measure (Fig. 18D), or rectification and filtration [Figs. 18B, 19A and C; (338)] is needed to extract information about the changing intensity of overall activity (35, 52, 518). Both treatments involve arbitrary decisions concerning filter choice: *1)* Should

---

FIG. 18. Relationships between several measures of muscle action. *Broad arrows* represents the multiple signals carried in the signal pathway within the biological system. Mechanical and electrical impedances through which biological signals are coupled to recorder system are marked Z. Electromyogram (EMG) signal may be further processed to some form of pulse signal or to an averaged EMG. Functional output may be measured as any of a variety of motor actions, as well as in form of direct muscle responses. *A*: nerve activity (ENG) and motor action as measured from phrenic nerve and as tracheal pressure show examples of entry of nerve signal into a muscle system and a motor consequence. *B*: direct EMG, averaged EMG (AEMG), muscle force, and length—measured during one step of walking, from cat triceps surae muscle. Non-phase-shifting digital filter was used to average EMG signal. Force was sampled from tendon in situ and length measured from slow motion movie films. These signals differ as a result of transformations that have occurred in instrumentation as well as in biological components. *C*: muscle sound pulses recorded from auricularis superior muscle. Myosonogram (MSG) pulses are related one to one to EMG pulses of same unit. Little systematic information is available about how effects of length, velocity, and temperature are represented in the sonogram. *D*: 3 pulse-based measures from a unit of respiratory muscle. *Bottom line*, time of visually identified unit pulses; *points* on graph, pulse-by-pulse calculation of firing rates (inverse interval); *solid line*, smoothed pattern of firing rate. Accepted methods include variations in derivation of each of these measures of muscle activity, and these variations introduce noticeable differences in the way a particular action is displayed. [*A*: from Gesell (187). *B*: from Yager (563). *C*: from Gordon and Holbourn (203), with permission of Cambridge Univ. Press. *D*: from Gesell et al. (189).]

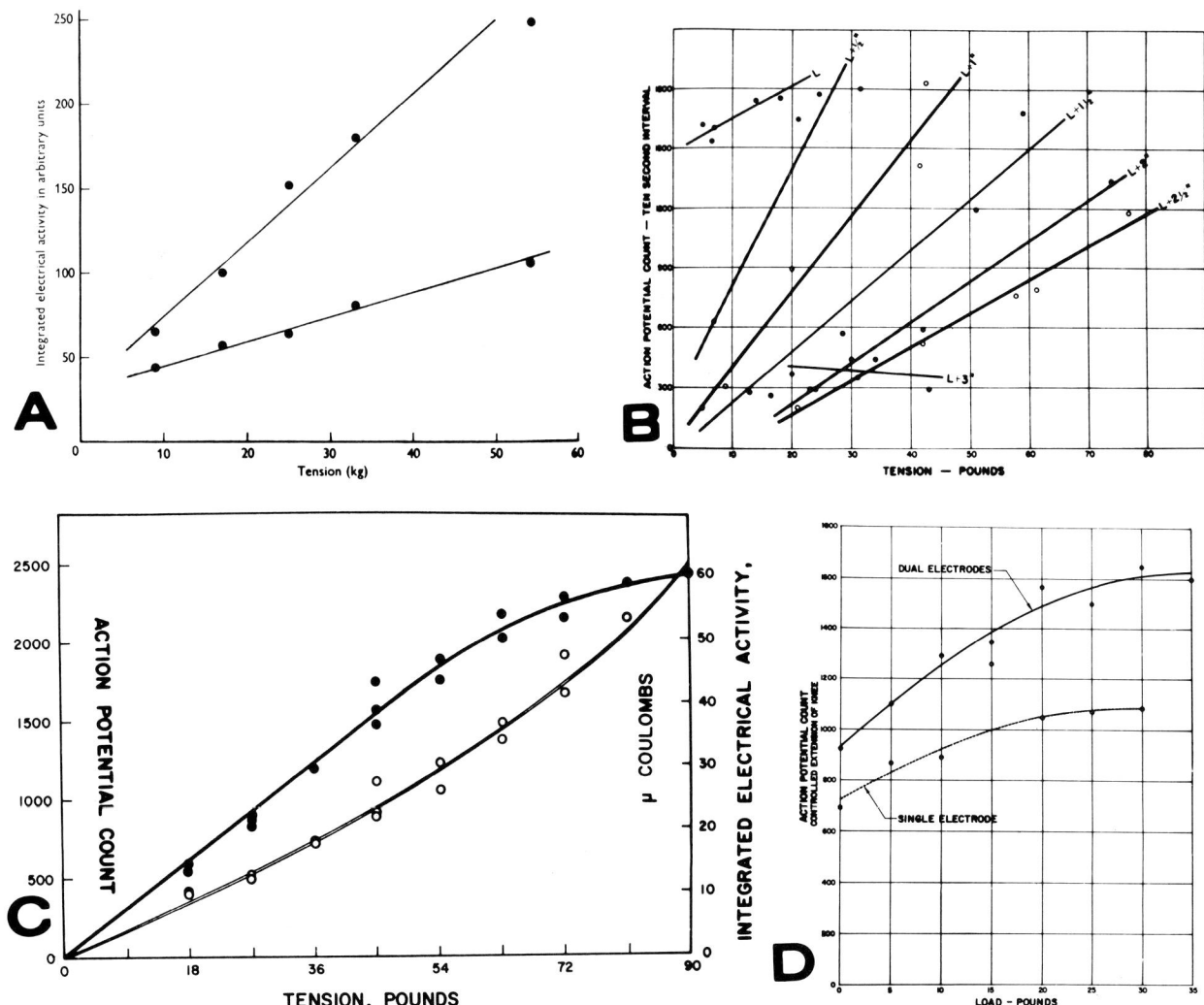

FIG. 19. Variation of relations between measures of physiological muscle activity with type of measurement and mechanical conditions. *A*: relationship between muscle force and integrated electromyogram (EMG). Each measurement on *upper* line made from the muscle while shortening; measurements on *lower* line made during lengthening of same muscle, showing velocity effect on force-EMG relationship. *B*: effect of muscle length on force-EMG relation in human soleus. *Separate lines*, lengths determined by ankle position in 0.5-in. increments of muscle length. Mechanical action of gastrocnemius was avoided by bending the knee. *C*: different nonlinear functions relating force to integrated EMG and to action potential count from same EMG (scaled to match at high and low ends of samples). *D*: effect of different electrode arrangements on relationship between force and EMG recorded in same tests. Monopolar and bipolar electrodes were used, and spike count was measured. Electrode placements also affects voltage and frequency distributions of EMG (337). [*A*: from Bigland and Lippold (49), with permission of Cambridge Univ. Press. *B*: from Close et al. (110). *C* and *D*: from Close (109).]

a filter introduce lag (337), as does muscle contraction? *2)* What form of digital filters is best (44, 149, 360, 408)? and *3)* For all filters, what division should be made between signal to be retained and noise to be suppressed? On repetition of voluntary movement of EMG smoothed by ensemble averaging shows a consistency of that fine structure (497, 498) that in the past seems to have been dismissed as noise. Special computation, however, is required to restore continuous function or to extract time derivatives from point samples of data (408, 559) provided by video or cinematographic measurements. While the remaining methods produce continuous functions, what they measure may be affected by surgical preparation.

Differences among the various measures of muscle activity (Fig. 18) can be useful for extracting special information from the muscle and also can limit the transferability of information from one particular measure to substitution for another. The source of normal EMG is in a one-to-one relationship to nerve drive (9,

132), whereas the other measures are all derived from mechanical responses. Electromyogram magnitude changes with recording details (Fig. 19D), however, and different representations of EMG are not proportional to each other (Fig. 19C). The mechanical output, as might be expected, is related to excitation and to EMG in a velocity-dependent (Fig. 19A), length-dependent (Fig. 19B), and nonlinear [Fig. 19C; (300, 316, 574)] way. The continuous functions give information about the end result of the combinations of factors and of unit contraction and relate more closely to final motor response. Both types of discrete responses show rate of firing of individual units (189, 404). It appears that the sonogram might be usable to record unit activity without interference from electrical stimulus, and it also may indicate alterations in mechanical response of units. Of all of the measures, however, EMG currently is the most effective tool to isolate activity of almost any chosen muscle (35, 109, 117, 166, 262, 292). The wave form of the unit EMG response changes with contraction intensity (316) and also has been related to specific pathological changes of muscle and its innervation (35, 109, 137, 138).

Summary

For various reasons a number of measures of muscle activity have been used in motor control studies, including several versions of EMG, mechanical measures, and sound. Because the functions in muscle that are evaluated by these indicators are partially independent, these measures are not fully interchangeable. Equivalence must be considered, particularly when an indirect measure of some muscle function may be more convenient than a direct measure. For example, it is important that muscle force may be nearly proportional to integrated EMG under restricted conditions, but under other conditions the two measures may be almost completely independent. Although sound has not been a frequently used measure in recent studies of muscle, its characteristics may be advantageous for some uses. The EMG also may contain more meaningful information about muscle control than is commonly recognized; i.e., rather than noise, the fine structure of the EMG may represent the necessary signal that compensates the complexity of muscle response.

MOTOR FUNCTIONS OF MUSCLES

... far from being merely as passive recipients and transmitters of impulses, [the structures] modify as well as transmit what they receive.

C. S. Sherrington (466)

All controlled motor acts are generated by response of muscle to neural signals, without regard to how those signals are produced. Furthermore, the quotation that introduces this section describes the operation of muscle as much as it describes that of the motoneurons to which Sherrington applied it. Thus for that part of muscle's output contraction, which is the result of the input of nerve firing rate, the muscle action changes the signal dimensions (transduction). If, in a group of motor units, control is somewhat separable and unit responses differ in relative weighting of motor dimensions, then each muscle unit also is a transducer of a vector signal. Both independence and redundancy of the response controlled through the muscle units then can exist as defined in a vector form, with or without a unit-by-unit equality or independence (315, 545). When expressed in usual dimensions muscle input is converted nonlinearly and with a time shifting transformation to output (i.e., isometric force is related to stimulus rate nonlinearly and with lag). Additionally, muscle response is a function not only of the neural signal but also of mechanical and other signals, and it includes effects of both stimulus and mechanical history. Muscle combines these signals in determining output (computation). In this view, gross muscle is a transducer, transformer, and computer, controlling a vector output from multiple inputs. Alternately, muscle was described in the subsection A MUSCLE MODEL, p. 71, as producing a one-to-one transduction and transformation on the input, the input being defined as a vector function on several factors. By extending the description to multiple motor nerves, including muscle history and internal mechanics, the vector description applies to whole muscle systems. In either the vector or the multiple input form the muscle not only provides mechanical capability for the motor system but shares with the nervous system in combining the factors determining the form of the motor response. By itself neural drive to muscle can control a consistent effect of the face of variation of muscle conditions only if the neural signal is provided in some way with adjustments that are inversely equivalent to the muscle variation. On the other hand, signals on multiple and nonidentical motor units can call upon the muscle computation to produce controlled response that partially overrides the influence of load in determining the direction of contraction of individual units (395).

FINAL SUMMARY

Ordinary motor responses are delivered through contributions of multiple units of active and passive muscle. Neural signals control activation of the muscle in a history-dependent, lagging, and nonlinear way. How that activation is transduced into tensile and lateral forces depends on the mechanical state of the muscle. Interaction between these forces and the rules of the load establish how that state of the system will change over time—whether the muscle delivers or receives power from the load, or sometimes whether it transfers energy from one part of the load to another.

Multiple motor units interact through the load mechanics to determine the changing vector describing the state of the system, which over time returns to effect the response characteristics of the muscle units. With muscle units having different geometric or functional properties, combinations of their graded activity on the total contraction vector give a means of adjusting control of more than one contraction dimension, such as system stiffness, length, force, or velocity. Distributed muscle systems work with, not for, the nervous system in the determination of motor response in the face of existing conditions and exhibit their full character only when unit actions are combined.

EPILOGUE

What muscle does in motor control is an issue separate from this chapter's consideration of how it does it.

At any particular moment the motor system finds the body and environment in some state (459). Together the nervous system with the muscles can manipulate chemical, mechanical, and thermal energy (172) to bring the system to a new state (217, 399). The transition often appears to allow different trajectories (70). If more than one trajectory is possible toward desired future states, the attainment of state goals at minimal cost takes on biological importance. An ideal motor controller would provide an optimal distribution of nerve impulses with consideration of the state goals, transition costs, and state-dependent rules. The interaction between muscle and load powers the transition of physical state, regardless of what form it takes. Over the long term the measure of merit for this state controller would seem to be the probability that it regularly enhances the attainment of the evolutionary reward in individual and species survival, a function which on short intervals sometimes may be correlated with joint angles or muscle lengths.

There may be a special reason why a close examination of muscle properties could provide a useful approach to the general study of motor control. The nonlinear, dynamic, and hysteretic properties of single muscle units predated the evolution of most of the neural system that controls motor activity in higher forms. In effect, then, these muscle properties may contain design specifications upon which much of the nervous system was developed. On the other hand, the geometric and functional complexity appearing in muscles with the development of higher animals may represent, in part, solutions to problems that were inadequately handled by the computational algorithms chosen in the evolution of nervous systems. Thus the study of muscle not only can clarify the meaning of signals that are generated by the nervous system but also may become a powerful tool to further the understanding of the principles of design of the nervous system.

APPENDIX

Units for Measure of Motor Function

A significant problem in motor function data lies in the complexity of the units used. Tabulation of results or comparison of different measurements requires a matching of units, but this often is impossible. Three problems are involved: *1*) Different well-defined units have been used over history (e.g., dynes, grams force, pounds, and newtons). Such data are usually easily brought to a compatible form by using simple conversion factors [(323, 536); for discussion of special problems in the conversion consult ref. 15]. *2*) Particularly in dynamic measures, units may not be convertible among studies. For example, cm/s and length/s deal with muscle shortening but are not dimensionally equivalent. Furthermore, special coefficients expressing change in some function are frequently dimensionless ratios between the values of some measure taken at two arbitrarily chosen points in time. Even when two such coefficients represent the same process, they may not have one-to-one equivalence (90, 429). *3*) The most limiting problem is where the unit of measure cannot be recognized; for example terms such as *work* frequently have a common use that conflicts with the technical definition, but the colloquial term may be used to describe subjective observations in clinical usage (375). In experimental activities, on the other hand, some terms or symbols are carefully but differently defined in separate laboratories. Thus, the capital letter P is used to represent some load dimension in mechanics, in muscle, and for motor control. Apparently originating as an abbreviation for poise (293) or *pois* or *pensum* before 1850 (537), it refers to a static load compressing or hung on a structure (229, 251, 301, 504, 537). In muscle studies it also is used for maximal contractile tension (161, 251), tension/cm^2 (161), where its dimensions correspond to pressure and the proper unit is the pascal (Pa, refs. 15, 161), shortening force as contrasted to force opposing lengthening (2). In classic mechanics, P conventionally represents momentum (195), while P is also the symbol for mechanical power (344). When diversely used symbols are used without identification, confusion is encouraged.

For essentially qualitative description, unit convertibility is optional. Yet for comparison of separate data or the increasingly common analytic or synthetic operation of relating component action to results in larger systems, unit compatibility is essential.

The definitions, names, and dimensions in the appended table provide an abbreviated collection of SI units (La Systeme International d'Unités) applicable to mechanical measurements in motor control.[1] Any other mechanical measure can be derived from the three base units. The information represents the coherent units, which are adopted as official by many countries, are the basis for the U.S. legal definitions, and are the official technical standards for several private and government organizations (15, 150, 324, 344). They are not official for the American Physiological Society, which has never formally adopted any specific standards for measurement usage. In addition to those functions which are rigidly and consistently defined in the various standards, a

---

[1] An approved English translation of the SI document is now available from Her Majesty's Stationery Office in the United Kingdom or from the National Bureau of Standards in the United States as "The International System of Units (SI)." Partial or complete translations are also available in Bulgarian, Czech, German, Japanese, Portuguese, and Spanish.

TABLE A1. *Dimensions of Mechanical Functions and SI Units**

Function	SI Unit	Dimension	Other Units and Terms†	Definition or Conversion	Notes
BASE UNITS					
Length (l)	meter (15) metre (m)	m	[Angstrom unit (Å) (temporary use)] Position	Definition of m is based on wavelength of one line in ^{86}Kr spectrum. 10^{10} Å = 1 m	
Mass (M)	kilogram (kg)	kg	[gram] [pound (lb)]	Defined as the mass of a platinum iridium cylinder preserved in Sèvres, France. 2.205 lb = 1 kg	
Time (t)	second (s)	s	[minute] [hour] [day] [σ, old symbol]	Defined in terms of one characteristic frequency of ^{133}Cs or "cesium clock." 1 σ = 1 ms	The use of double prefixes, e.g., mμm, should be avoided; use nm (15, 324, 344).

					Prefix	SI Abbreviation	Multiplier Equivalent
					giga	G	10^9
					mega	M	10^6
					kilo	k	10^3
					centi	c	10^{-2}
					milli	m	10^{-3}
					micro	μ	10^{-6}
					nano	n	10^{-9}
					pico	p	10^{-12}

DERIVED UNITS (DEFINED ONLY IN TERMS OF SI BASE UNITS)

Rectilinear Measures

Function	SI Unit	Dimension	Other Units and Terms	Definition or Conversion	Notes
Force (F)	newton (N)	m·kg·s^{-2}	[gram force] [gram weight (g_w)] [dyne (dyn)] [poundal] linear energy transfer (L) tension ($F > 0$)	$F = M \cdot a$ $102.0 \pm 0.3\ g_w = 1$ N 7.233 poundal = 1 N 10^5 dyn = 1 N	In muscle studies, force generated by the muscle is ordinarily plotted upward. On relating this force to muscle length, its action would produce a negative acceleration. For antagonist muscles, operating sign must be chosen carefully and used consistently. With more than one degree of freedom, force becomes a vector function.
Velocity (V)		m·s^{-1}	meter/second (speed)	$V = \dfrac{dl}{dt} = \dot{l}$	Speed is the magnitude of velocity without directional information; velocity is a directed vector.
Acceleration (a)		m·s^{-2}	meter/second^2 [acceleration due to gravity (g)]	$a = \dfrac{dV}{dt} = \ddot{l}$ $1\ g \cong 9.8$ m·s^{-2}	Lowercase letter g is used as abbreviation for both the acceleration of gravity and the gram unit; it can be a source of confusion if the italic form for gravity is not observed.
Force rate‡ ($\dot{F}$)		m·kg·s^{-3}	newton/second	$\dfrac{dF}{dt} = \dot{F}$	Related to rate of stretch of series elastic structures or velocity for a spring load.

TABLE A1.—Continued

Function	SI Unit	Dimension	Other Units and Terms†	Definition or Conversion	Notes
Power (P_m)	watt (W)	$m^2 \cdot kg \cdot s^{-3}$	[horsepower (hp)] joule/second	1.34×10^{-3} hp = 1 W 1 J/s = 1 W $P_m = \dfrac{dW}{dt} = F \cdot V$	Abbreviation P_m specifically designates mechanical power (150), but the use of such subscripts is rejected by other authorities (15). The positive sign conventionally is used to designate the absorption of energy in the system being studied. W = work.
Work (W) Energy (E)	joule (J)	$m^2 \cdot kg \cdot s^{-2}$	[gram-centimeter] newton-meter [erg] watt-second [calorie] [large calorie, or kilocalorie (kcal)] kinetic energy (K)	10.2×10^3 g·cm ≅ 1 J 1 N·m = 1 J 10^7 erg = 1 J 1 W·s = 1 J 0.239×10^{-3} kcal ≅ 1 J $K = \tfrac{1}{2} M \cdot V^2$	Total work done by muscle is the sum of potential energy, kinetic energy, and heat energy produced. Although classical measures from muscle often considered the potential energy of the load lifted, many studies have included all three parts. In spite of the definition, the term *work* has been applied in clinical situations to describe functions of force in an attempt to reconcile the fact that whereas isometric force does no work, it can be associated with production of fatigue (375).
Impulse (g)		$m \cdot kg\ s^{-1}$	[gram-centimeter/second] newton-second momentum (P)	$\int_{t_0}^{t_1} F\,dt = M \cdot \Delta V = P$	This measure often has been expressed as simply the area under a graph of force vs. time in actions that are usually isometric. When acting on a pure inertial load, impulse produces a momentum change equal in size to the impulse. (See comment on use of P in APPENDIX text.)
Area (A)		m^2	[cm^2]	$10^4 \times cm^2 = 1\ m^2$	
Frequency (f)	hertz (Hz)	s^{-1}	reciprocal seconds cps (old symbol) rotational frequency (n) firing rate (R) [angular frequency (ω) in radians × second^{-1}]	1 cps = 1 Hz $\omega/2\pi = f$	The abbreviation cps (cycles per second) can be confused with counts per second. The letter n is used for rotational frequency. The abbreviation Hz is used particularly for sinusoidal frequency. Firing or stimulus rate can be used to designate repetition of stimulus pulses or nerve or muscle responses to reduce confusion between periodic impulses in nerve and muscle and the frequency of a resulting cyclic movement (393, 480).
Angular Measures Angle (θ)	radian (rad)	1	[degree] [grade]	For a circle (distance on curve/radius of curvature) = radians spanned $57.3° ≅ 1$ rad ½ π rev = 1 rad $(200/\pi)$ grade = 1 rad	For many joints, the axis of rotation changes with position, complicating the angle measurement. In a periodic process, defining one cycle as 2π allows points in the cycle or differences between cycles to be described in terms of corresponding angle. Inverse trigonometric functions of angles are designated by the prefix *arc*, e.g., arc sin θ, but the notation $\sin^{-1}\theta$ also is used frequently (536).

TABLE A1.—Continued

Function	SI Unit	Dimension	Other Units and Terms†	Definition or Conversion	Notes
Moment of inertia (I)		$m^2 \cdot kg$	kilogram-meter^2		Tables exist for calculating I for a variety of geometric structures composed of uniform material. The moment of inertia of a biological structure often changes because of conformation changes.
Torque (T)		$m^2 \cdot kg \cdot s^{-2}$	newton-meter newton-meter/radian moment of force moment of a couple	$F \cdot \text{lever arm} = T$	The lever arm for a muscle may change with joint position. This newton-meter measure is distinct from the newton-meter = joule measure of energy, since the orientation of the distance component with respect to the force directions differs in the two cases.
Angular velocity (ω)		s^{-1}	angular frequency radian/second [frequency (f)]	$\dfrac{d\theta}{dt} = \omega$ $2\pi \cdot f = \omega$	See notes for angle.
Angular acceleration (α)		s^{-2}	radian-second^{-2}	$d\omega/dt = \alpha$ $T/I = \alpha$	Many animal movements involve both rotation of inertial structures and displacement of their centers of mass. Insofar as the structures can be represented as rigid bodies the two aspects of their movement easily can be calculated separately. The total energy and energy changes, however, are the sum of the rotational and the translational parts (344).
Rotational power (P_r)	watt (W)	$m^2 \cdot kg \cdot s^{-3}$	joule/second	$T \cdot \omega = P_r$	
Rotational kinetic energy (K_r)	joule (J)	$m^2 \cdot kg \cdot s^{-2}$	watt-second	$\tfrac{1}{2} I \cdot \omega^2 = K_r$	
Angular momentum (L)		$m^2 \cdot kg \cdot s^{-1}$	moment of momentum	$\int T dt = L$ $I \cdot \omega = L$	
Mechanical Impedance Measures					Impedance measures are calculated representations of system properties and are not directly measured.
Stiffness (k)‡		$kg \cdot s^{-2}$	newton/meter spring constant	$\Delta F / \Delta l = k$	In non-Hookian range, k has only local meaning. The term *elasticity* often is used incorrectly; it properly refers to the ability to return to the original dimensions after deforming stress is removed.
Modulus of elasticity (E)	pascal (Pa)	$m^{-1} \cdot kg \cdot s^{-2}$	Young's modulus (Y) stress/strain	$Y = E$ $\dfrac{d\sigma}{d\epsilon} = E$	The value $1/E$ is designated coefficient of extensibility (527).

TABLE A1.—Continued

Function	SI Unit	Dimension	Other Units and Terms†	Definition or Conversion	Notes
Coefficient of internal viscosity (η_{approx})‡		$m^{-1} \cdot kg \cdot s^{-1}$	pascal-second newton-second/meter^2 [centipoise (cP)] stress/strain rate	$\sigma/\dot{\epsilon} = \eta_{approx}$ $10^3 \cdot cP = 1\ Pa \cdot s$	Found in the slope of the normalized force-velocity curve (393). This is clearly not Newtonian viscosity but is dimensionally equivalent.
Mechanical resistance (R_m)		$kg \cdot s^{-1}$	newton-second/meter [mechanical ohm] (viscous resistance)	$F/V = R_m$	The real part of mechanical impedance.
Mechanical reactance (X_m)		$kg \cdot s^{-1}$	newton-second/meter (inertial and elastic resistance)	$F/V = iX_m$ (quadrature)	The imaginary part of mechanical impedance.
Mechanical impedance (Z_m)‡		$kg \cdot s^{-1}$	newton-second/meter	$Z_m = R_m + iX_m$	The complex ratio of a sine wave force acting on a system to the sine-wave velocity resulting from that force. This dependence on frequency may be symbolized as $Z_m(\omega)$. These terms can be used to describe either the load upon which muscle acts or the way muscle responds to external force.
Relaxation time constant (τ)		s^{-1}	stress (or creep) relaxation time		Time required for decay of tension (or length) to $1/e$ of original increment after step of length (or force) has been applied. Properly used only when decay is exponential.
Damping coefficient (δ)‡		s^{-1}	damping factor		The ratio of the logarithmic decrement of a damped harmonic oscillation to its undamped period. In nonlinear system can only be approximated.
NORMALIZED UNITS					Various attempts have been made to produce normalized measures of motor activity to allow comparison between cases. In some cases, the resulting unit is dimensionally equivalent to standard mechanical units. The listing of units in this section is not a recommendation for use as much as an indication of past use.
Relative length (l_r)‡		1	lengths	l/l_0	Definitions of rest length of a muscle, l_0: 1) muscle length in body when relaxed (423); 2) length beyond which passive tension increases (530); 3) length at which maximum twitch or tetanic contractile force occurs (22, 94); or 4) maximum length in body (229, 541). Value of l_0 is sometimes corrected for tendon effects.
Strain (ϵ)		1	relative elongation	$(l - l_0)/l_0$	
Relative velocity (V_r)‡		1	velocity	V/V_0	Abbreviation V_0 = maximum shortening velocity without load. (Compare strain rate.)

CHAPTER 3: MUSCLE, THE MOTOR   93

TABLE A1.—*Continued*

Function	SI Unit	Dimension	Other Units and Terms[†]	Definition or Conversion	Notes
Normal stress (σ)	pascal (Pa)	$m^{-1} \cdot k \cdot s^{-2}$	newton/meter² [millimeters Hg (Torr)] [dyne/centimeter²] [pound/inch², or psi] "pressure" force/muscle area	$1 \text{ N/m}^2 = 1 \text{ Pa}$ $7.5 \times 10^{-3} \text{ mmHg} = 1 \text{ Pa}$ $10 \text{ dyn/cm}^2 = 1 \text{ Pa}$ $0.145 \times 10^{-3} \text{ psi} = 1 \text{ Pa}$ $F/A = \sigma$	After correction for geometric differences, this function allows comparison of internal stresses in contractile parts of diverse muscles.
Relative force (F_r)[‡]		1	twitch tension tetanic tension $[P/P_0]$	$F/F_t = F_r$	Abbreviations F_t is maximal force of a reference twitch, but also maximal tetanic force is used as a normalizing value (251). P_{ob} has been extensively used as the symbol for maximum tetanic force (258).
Accelerating force ratio[‡]		$m \cdot s^{-2}$	"acceleration"	F/animal mass	In limb muscle this function relates response to relative load for animals of same shape but different size. It fails, however, to correct for moment of inertia ratios.
Specific power (P_s)		$m \cdot s^{-3}$	watt/kilogram	P/muscle mass $= (P_s)$	Relates power output to metabolic mass of contractile system. Also, in impact loading of a homogeneous structure, internal strain for a given absorption of energy is proportional to volume or mass of the loaded structure (504). Thus, normalization to muscle mass may be appropriate for discussion in cases of impact loading, such as in jumping, gait, ball-catching.
Modulus of elasticity (E)	pascal (Pa)	$m^{-1} \cdot kg \cdot s^{-2}$	stress/strain	$\dot{\sigma}/\dot{\epsilon} = E$	A normalization of both length and cross-sectional area in determining force. The term "elasticity" does not define the mechanism of generating the force-length relationship but represents only the observed relationship.
Strain rate ($\dot{\epsilon}$)[‡]		s^{-1}	length/second	$l_0^{-1} \cdot \dfrac{dl}{dt} = \dot{\epsilon}$	Strain rate, a relative velocity, allows comparison between muscles of different lengths.
Stress rate ($\dot{\sigma}$)[‡]		$m^{-1} \cdot kg \cdot s^{-3}$	pascal/second	$\dfrac{d\sigma}{dt} = \dot{\sigma}$	Useful for evaluating series elastic effects and for comparison of force-velocity effects (529).

Reference numbers in parentheses.   * See paragraph 3 of the APPENDIX for an elaboration of values and definitions included in table.   ‡ Units included in brackets are dimensionally equivalent measures but differ in size by a conversion coefficient.   † Terms without brackets are alternate terms for the same unit.   ‡ Suggested function name in absence of an established term or a dimensionally equivalent term from mechanics. These should be used in motor system measurement with reservation.

number of additional functions are needed or have been used repeatedly in the study of muscle and motor activity, but they do not have either consistent or official names except as produced by combining SI terms. The authors have added several of these functions (marked‡) in the table, specified their dimensions, defined them in SI units, and, with an attempt at consistency, identified them with one of their arbitrary names. For derived units, more than one correct SI name may be possible for the same unit (15). A few of the complications of nomenclature and definitions in common usage as well as conversions from a few old units are given in the table and notes.

The dimension column in Table A1 can help to identify the functions and units resulting from calculations. In preparation for any calculation, however, colloquial terms like *acceleration* and *deceleration* must be reduced to the corresponding technical terms, e.g., acceleration with definition of positive or negative direction. The anatomical and clinical term *flexion* requires separation into clearly distinct dimensions of angle and angular velocity, whereas the usual terms of adduction-abduction, flexion-extension-hyperextension, and circumduction as applicable to the wrist reduce to quantitative values in only two degrees of freedom. No effort is made here, however, to provide the forms needed to deal with the complex joint mechanics or with the six degrees of freedom that might exist in each movable structure (see ref. 195 and the chapter by Alexander in this *Handbook*).

Whereas unnecessary addition of new units or the use of vaguely defined dimensions is undesirable, it is inevitable that some motor relationships require additional derived dimensions. Table A1 then can be only a guide, not a rule.

The following notes have been compiled from recommendations in the standards documents and represent frequently encountered issues in motor control measurement. (More details of definitions, usage, precise, values, conversion factors, and notation are available in refs. 15, 82, 195, 324, 344, 431, and 536; ref. 150 provides also the technically equivalent words in English, French, and German.) The use of special type faces is partially standardized (15, 324) and may provide the only clue to symbols with distinctly different meanings. In general, italic type is used for symbols of functions. Unit names should always be printed in roman (upright) type. When the unit is named for a person, the symbol (but not the name) takes a capital letter. Boldface type ordinarily represents vectors. Abbreviations for units are not changed in the plural, and periods are not part of the symbols. Where no special unit name is provided, standard names are combined, a process that can produce more than one correct name for a particular value. For an index of previously established names for dimensionless numbers (in addition to those identified in Table A1 by the designation 1 in the dimension column) see "Tables for Identifying Dimensionless Groups" in reference 536. The unit of weight is the newton, but because the term is often misused to mean mass, it has been recommended that the functional name *weight* be avoided (15, 150). (The 0.3% variation of the magnitude of 1 kg force with location on the earth is a trivial error compared with the variability in aerospace situations.) For large or small values, either suffixes or multipliers (e.g., m or $\times 10^{-3}$) may be used. To reduce errors, the steps in multipliers should ordinarily be restricted to increments of 10^3, arranged to give significant figures ranging between 0.1 and 9,999, except when this causes varying multipliers in tabular or similar data (15, 344). The unit and its prefix constitute a single symbol. Thus, $cm^2 = (.01 m)^2$ and not $.01 (m^2)$. The number of digits carried in the mantissa should reflect the precision of the values given (15). Thus in a particular case, 300×10^3 may be a more correct form than the 285,714 actually obtained by calculation.

Attempts (15, 344, 536) to minimize confusion arising in the differences between European and American usage of commas and periods in mensuration have resulted in the following recommendations:

1. A raised dot (not available on some automatic printers) or space between symbols represents multiplication (prefixes are not separated by a space).

2. In Europe, and where the dot is used to indicate multiplication, the decimal point should be marked with a comma.

3. A dot over a symbol invariably represents differentiations with respect to time.

4. Long numbers can be separated in groups of three digits by spaces (but not by commas).

The mechanical impedance description for the way a motor system or muscle opposes external forces has not been used with uniform definitions, particularly with respect to dynamic aspects. The terms for mechanical impedance used in the table were obtained from mechanical engineering usage (324, 504). A number of rheological terms, such as friction, plasticity, and thixotropy, which may eventually prove important in motor control measurements, have been omitted, in spite of limited use (82, 431) and specific definition (504). Thus, the opposition of a muscle or limb to external force now described as a nonlinear viscosity-like property may eventually be better described as a specific rheological property separated from the true viscous effect (20, 82, 161).

We wish to express our appreciation to staff members of the libraries at Stanford University, University of California Los Angeles, and Rancho Los Amigos Hospital for assistance with the bibliographical search, to Jin Emerson for patiently deciphering a series of revisions of the text, and to Roy Kneller for instruction on graphic arts methods used for preparing the figures.

REFERENCES

1. ABBOTT, B. C., AND X. M. AUBERT. The force exerted by active striated muscle during and after change of length. *J. Physiol. London* 117: 77–86, 1952.
2. ABBOTT, B. C., B. BIGLAND, AND J. M. RITCHIE. The physiological cost of negative work. *J. Physiol. London* 117: 380–390, 1952.
3. ABBOTT, B. C., AND J. M. RITCHIE. Early tension relaxation during a muscle twitch. *J. Physiol. London* 113: 330–335, 1951.
4. ABBOTT, B. C., AND D. R. WILKIE. The relation between velocity of shortening and the tension-length curve of skeletal muscle. *J. Physiol. London* 120: 214–223, 1953.
5. ADAMS, R. D. *Diseases of Muscle: A Study in Pathology* (3rd ed.). Hagerstown, MD: Harper & Row, 1975.
6. ADRIAN, E. D. The spread of activity in the tenuissimus muscle of the cat and in other complex muscles. *J. Physiol. London* 60: 301–315, 1925.
7. ADRIAN, E. D. *The Mechanism of Nervous Action: Electrical Studies of the Neurone*. Philadelphia: Univ. of Pennsylvania Press, 1932.
8. ADRIAN, E. D., AND D. W. BRONK. The discharge of impulses in motor nerve fibres. Part 1. Impulses in single fibres of the phrenic nerve. *J. Physiol. London* 66: 81–101, 1928.
9. ADRIAN, E. D., AND D. W. BRONK. The discharge of impulses in motor nerve fibres. Part 2. The frequency of discharge in

reflex and voluntary contraction. *J. Physiol. London* 67: 119–151, 1929.
10. ALEXANDER, R. McN. The orientation of muscle fibres in the myomeres of fishes. *J. Mar. Biol. Assoc. UK* 49: 263–290, 1964.
11. ALEXANDER, R. McN. Muscle performance in locomotion and other strenuous activities. In: *Comparative Physiology*, edited by I. Bolis, K. Schmidt-Nielsen, and S. H. P. Maldrell. Amsterdam: North Holland, 1973, p. 1–20.
12. ALEXANDER, R. McN., AND A. VERNON. The mechanics of hopping by kangaroos (Macropodidas). *J. Zool.* 117: 265–303, 1975.
13. ALEXANDER, R. S. Viscoelastic determinants of muscle contractility and "cardiac tone." *Federation Proc.* 21: 1001–1005, 1962.
14. AMERICAN COLLEGE OF SPORTS MEDICINE. *Encyclopedia of Sport Sciences and Medicine*. New York: Macmillan, 1971.
15. AMERICAN SOCIETY FOR TESTING AND MATERIALS. *Standard for Metric Practice*. Philadelphia, PA: Am. Soc. Testing Materials, 1976. Document ANSI/ASTM E 380-76. (Also available as Institute of Electrical and Electronics Engineers document IEEE Std 268-1979. New York: Inst. Elec. Electron. Eng., 1979.)
16. ANDERSSON-CEDERGREN, E. Ultrastructure of motor end plate and sarcoplasmic components of mouse skeletal muscle fibers as revealed by three dimensional reconstructions from serial sections. *J. Ultrastruct. Res. Suppl.* 1: 1–191, 1959.
17. ARMSTRONG, R. B., P. MARUM, C. W. SAUBERT IV, H. J. SEEHERMAN, AND C. R. TAYLOR. Muscle fiber activity as a function of speed and gait. *J. Appl. Physiol.: Respirat. Environ. Exercise Physiol.* 43: 672–677, 1977.
18. ASMUSSEN, E., AND O. BØJE. Body temperature and capacity for work. *Acta Physiol. Scand.* 10: 1–22, 1945.
19. ASMUSSEN, E., F. BONDE-PETERSEN, AND K. JØRGENSEN. Mechano-elastic properties of human muscles at different temperatures. *Acta Physiol. Scand.* 96: 83–93, 1976.
20. AUBERT, X. La relation entre la force et la vitesse d'allongement et de raccourcissement du muscle strié. *Arch. Int. Physiol. Biochim.* 64: 121–122, 1956.
21. BADOUX, D. M. An introduction to biomechanical principles in primate locomotion and structure. In: *Primate Locomotion*, edited by F. A. Jenkins, Jr. New York: Academic, 1974. p. 1–43.
22. BAGUST, J., S. KNOTT, D. M. LEWIS, J. C. LUCK, AND R. A. WESTERMAN. Isometric contractions of motor units in a fast twitch muscle of the cat. *J. Physiol. London* 231: 87–104, 1973.
23. BAGUST, J., D. M. LEWIS, AND R. A. WESTERMAN. Polyneural innervation of kitten skeletal muscle. *J. Physiol. London* 229: 241–255, 1973.
24. BAHLER, A. S. Series elastic component of mammalian skeletal muscle. *Am. J. Physiol.* 213: 1560–1564, 1967.
25. BAHLER, A. S. Modeling of mammalian skeletal muscle. *IEEE Trans. Biomed. Eng.* 15: 249–257, 1968. (Correction 16: 159, 1969.)
26. BAHLER, A. S. Mechanical properties of relaxing frog skeletal muscle. *Am. J. Physiol.* 220: 1983–1990, 1971.
27. BAHLER, A. S., AND J. T. FALES. Dynamics of mammalian muscle contractile component. *Physiologist* 9: 133, 1966.
28. BAHLER, A. S., J. T. FALES, AND K. L. ZIERLER. The active state of mammalian skeletal muscle. *J. Gen. Physiol.* 50: 2239–2253, 1967.
29. BAHLER, A. S., J. T. FALES, AND K. L. ZIERLER. The dynamic properties of mammalian skeletal muscle. *J. Gen. Physiol.* 51: 369–384, 1968.
30. BANUS, M. G., AND A. M. ZETLIN. The relation of isometric tension to length in skeletal muscle. *J. Cell. Comp. Physiol.* 12: 403–420, 1938.
31. BÁRÁNY, M. ATPase activity of myosin correlated with speed of muscle shortening. *J. Gen. Physiol.* 50: Suppl.: 197–216, 1967.
32. BARDEEN, C. R. Variation in the internal architecture of the m. obliquus abdominis externus in certain mammals. *Anat. Anz.* 23: 241–249, 1903.
33. BARRETT, B. The length and mode of termination of individual muscle fibers in the human sartorius and posterior femoral muscles. *Acta Anat.* 48: 242–257, 1962.
34. BASKIN, R. J. Changes of volume in striated muscle. *Am. Zool.* 7: 593–601, 1967.
35. BASMAJIAN, J. V. Muscles Alive: Their Functions Revealed by Electromyography (4th ed.). Baltimore, MD: Williams & Wilkins, 1978.
36. BASMAJIAN, J. V., AND M. A. MACCONNALL. *Muscles and Movements: A Basis for Human Kinesiology* (2nd ed.). Huntington, NY: Krieger, 1977.
37. BAWA, P., A. MANNARD, AND R. B. STEIN. Predictions and experimental tests of a visco-elastic muscle using elastic and inertial loads. *Biol. Cybern.* 22: 139–145, 1976.
38. BAWA, P., AND R. B. STEIN. Frequency response of human soleus muscle. *J. Neurophysiol.* 39: 788–793, 1976.
39. BEAUNIS, H. Recherches physiologiques sur la contraction simultanée des muscles antagonistes. *Arch. Physiol. Norm. Pathol. Ser. 5* 1: 55–69, 1889.
40. BECKER, R. O. The electrical response of human skeletal muscle to passive stretch. *J. Bone Jt. Surg.* 42A: 1091–1103, 1960.
41. BECKETT, S. D., R. S. HUDSON, D. F. WALKER, T. M. REYNOLDS, AND R. I. VACHON. Blood pressure and penile muscle activity in the stallion during coitus. *Am. J. Physiol.* 225: 1072–1075, 1973.
42. BEDDARD, A. P., J. S. EDKINS, L. HILL, J. J. R. MACLEOD, AND M. S. PEMBREY. *Practical Physiology*. London: Arnold, 1905.
43. BEEVOR, C. E. Croonian lectures on muscular movements and their representations in the central nervous system. *Br. Med. J.* 1: 1357–1360, 1417–1421, 1480–1484; 2: 12–16, 1903.
44. BEKEY, G. A., C-W. CHANG, J. PERRY, AND M. M. HOFFER. Pattern recognition of multiple EEG signals applied to the description of human gait. *Proc. IEEE* 65: 674–681, 1977.
45. BENNET-CLARK, H. C. The energetics of the jump of the locust, *Schistocerca gregaria*. *J. Exp. Biol.* 63: 53–83, 1975.
46. BERGSTRÖM, R. M. The relationship between number of impulses and the integrated electrical activity in electromyogram. *Acta Physiol. Scand.* 45: 97–101, 1959.
47. BERITOFF, J. Über die Kontraktionsfähigkeit der Skelettmuskeln. IV. Über die physiologische Bedeutung des gefiederten Baues der Muskeln. *Pflügers Arch. Ges. Physiol.* 209: 763–778, 1925.
48. BIGLAND, B., AND O. C. J. LIPPOLD. Motor unit activity in the voluntary contraction of human muscle. *J. Physiol. London* 125: 322–335, 1954.
49. BIGLAND, B., AND O. C. J. LIPPOLD. The relation between force, velocity and integrated electrical activity in human muscles. *J. Physiol. London* 123: 214–224, 1954.
50. BINDER, M. D., W. E. CAMERON, AND D. G. STUART. Speed-force relations in the motor units of the cat tibialis posterior muscle. *Am. J. Phys. Med.* 57: 57–65, 1978.
51. BINDER, M. D., J. S. KROIN, G. P. MOORE, AND D. G. STUART. The response of Golgi tendon organs to single motor unit contractions. *J. Physiol. London* 271: 337–349, 1977.
52. BIRÓ, G., AND L. D. PARTRIDGE. Analysis of multiunit spike records. *J. Appl. Physiol.* 30: 521–526, 1971.
53. BISHOP, G. H., AND A. S. GILSON, JR. Action potentials accompanying the contractile process in skeletal muscle. *Am. J. Physiol.* 82: 478–495, 1927.
54. BLIX, M. Die Länge und Spannung des Muskels. *Skand. Arch. Physiol.* 3: 295–318, 1892; 4: 399–409, 1893; 5: 150–172, 173–206, 1895.
55. BLOOM, W., AND D. W. FAWCETT. *A Textbook of Histology* (10th ed.). Philadelphia, PA: Saunders, 1975.
56. BOREJDO, J., AND M. F. MORALES. Fluctuations in tension during contraction of single muscle fibers. *Biophys. J.* 20: 315–334, 1977.
57. BORNHORST, W. J., AND J. E. MINARDI. A phenomenological theory of muscular contraction. II. Generalized length variations. *Biophys. J.* 10: 155–171, 1970.
58. BOUDET (DE PARIS). Recherches sur le bruit musculaire. *C. R. Soc. Biol.* 32: 40–44, 1880.
59. BOUISSET, S., AND F. GOUBEL. Relation entre l'activité élec-

tromyographique intégrée et la vitesse d'exécution de mouvements monoarticulaires simples. *J. Physiol. Paris* 59: *Suppl.* 19: 359, 1967.
60. BOUISSET, S., AND B MATON. Comparaison des activités électromyographiques globale élémentaire au cours du mouvement volontaire. *Rev. Neurol.* 122: 427–429, 1969.
61. BOUMAN, H. D., AND G. VAN RIJNBERK. Die akustischen Erscheinungen der Muskeln (Muskelgeräusch, Muskelton). *Arch. Néerl. Physiol.* 23: 441–507, 1938.
62. BOUMAN, H. D., AND G. VAN RIJNBERK. On muscle sound produced during voluntary contraction in man: an experimental study. *Arch. Néerl. Physiol.* 23: 34–55, 1938.
63. BOYD, O. C., P. O. LAWRENCE, AND P. J. A. DRATTY. On modeling the single motor unit action potential. *IEEE Trans. Biomed. Eng.* 25: 236–243, 1978.
64. BOYLE, P. J., E. J. CONWAY, F. KANE, AND H. L. O'REILLY. Volume of interfibre spaces in frog muscle and the calculation of concentrations in the fibre water. *J. Physiol. London* 99: 401–414, 1941.
65. BOZLER, E. Mechanical control of the rising phase of contraction of frog skeletal and cardiac muscle. *J. Gen. Physiol.* 70: 697–705, 1977.
66. BRAUNE, C. W., AND O. FISHER. Der Gang des Menschen. I. Versuche unbelasten und belasten Menschen. *Abh. Math. Phys. Kl. Koenigl. Saeschs. Ges. Wiss.* 21: 153–322, 1895.
67. BROKAW, C. J. Computer simulation of movement-generating cross bridges. *Biophys. J.* 16: 1013–1041, 1976.
68. BRONK, D. W. The energy expended in maintaining a muscular contraction. *J. Physiol. London* 69: 306–315, 1930.
69. BROOKE, M. H. *A Clinician's View of Neuromuscular Diseases.* Baltimore, MD: Williams & Wilkins, 1977.
70. BROOKS, V. B. Motor programs revisited. In: *Posture and Movement,* edited by R. E. Talbott and D. R. Humphrey. New York: Raven, 1979, p. 13–49.
71. BROOKS, V. B., AND S. D. STONEY, JR. Motor mechanisms: the role of the pyramidal system in motor control. *Annu. Rev. Physiol.* 33: 337–392, 1971.
72. BROWN, A. C. *Analysis of the Myotatic Reflex* (Ph.D. thesis). Seattle: Univ. of Washington, 1959. (Abstr. in *Diss. Abstr.* 20: 60-4277, 1960.)
73. BROWN, G. L., AND U. S. VON EULER. The after effects of a tetanus on mammalian muscle. *J. Physiol. London* 93: 39–60, 1938.
74. BROWN, M. C., AND P. B. C. MATTHEWS. An investigation into the possible existence of polyneuronal innervation of individual skeletal muscle fibers in certain hind-limb muscles of the cat. *J. Physiol. London* 151: 436–457, 1960.
75. BRUMLIK, J. *The Quantitation of Muscle Tone in the Spastic State: an Analysis of Increased Muscle Tone, Comparing Spasticity and Rigidity* (Ph.D. thesis). Evanston, IL: Northwestern Univ., 1961. (Abstr. in *Diss. Abstr.* 22: 61-5296, 1961.)
76. BUCHTHAL, F. The mechanical properties of the single striated muscle fibre at rest and during contraction and their structural interpretation. *Dan. Biol. Medd. Kbh.* 17: 1–140, 1942.
77. BUCHTHAL, F. The rheology of the cross striated muscle fibre and its minute structural interpretation. *Pubbl. Staz. Zool. Napoli* 23: 115–146, 1951.
78. BUCHTHAL, F., AND L. ENGBECK. Refractory period and conduction velocity of striated muscle fiber. *Acta Physiol. Scand.* 59: 199–220, 1963.
79. BUCHTHAL, F., F. ERMINIO, AND P. ROSENFALCK. Motor unit territory in different human muscles. *Acta Physiol. Scand.* 45: 72–87, 1959.
80. BUCHTHAL, F., C. GULD, AND P. ROSENFALCK. Multielectrode study of the territory of a motor unit. *Acta Physiol. Scand.* 39: 83–104, 1957.
81. BUCHTHAL, F., C. GULD, AND P. ROSENFALCK. Volume conduction of the spike of the motor unit potential investigated with a new type of multielectrode. *Acta Physiol. Scand.* 38: 331–354, 1957.
82. BUCHTHAL, F., AND E. KAISER. The rheology of the cross striated muscle fiber with particular reference to isotonic conditions. *Dan. Biol. Medd. Kbh.* 21: 1–318, 1951.
83. BUCHTHAL, F., AND P. ROSENFALCK. Elastic properties of striated muscle. In: *Tissue Elasticity,* edited by J. W. Remington. Washington, DC: Am. Physiol. Soc., 1957, p. 73–97.
84. BUCHTHAL, F., AND P. ROSENFALCK. On the structure of motor units. In: *New Developments in Electromyography and Clinical Neurophysiology,* edited by J. E. Desmedt. Basel, Switzerland: Karger, 1973, vol. 1, p. 71–85.
85. BUCHTHAL, F., AND H. SCHMALBRUCH. Contraction times and fibre types in intact human muscle. *Acta Physiol. Scand.* 79: 435–452, 1970.
86. BULLER, A. J. The physiology of skeletal muscle. In: *Neurophysiology,* edited by C. Hunt. Baltimore, MD: Univ. Park, 1975, p. 279–302. (*Int. Rev. Physiol. Ser.,* vol. 3.)
87. BULLER, A. J., J. C. ECCLES, AND R. M. ECCLES. Interactions between motoneurones and muscles in respect of the characteristic speeds of their responses. *J. Physiol. London* 150: 417–439, 1960.
88. BULLER, A. J., AND D. M. LEWIS. The rate of tension development in isometric tetanic contractions of mammalian fast and slow skeletal muscle. *J. Physiol. London* 176: 337–354, 1965.
89. BURKE, R. E. Motor unit types of cat triceps surae muscle. *J. Physiol. London* 193: 141–160, 1967.
90. BURKE, R. E., D. N. LEVINE, P. TSAIRIS, AND F. E. ZAJAC III. Physiological types and histochemical profiles in motor units of the cat gastrocnemius. *J. Physiol. London* 234: 723–748, 1973.
91. BURKE, R. E., D. N. LEVINE, F. E. ZAJAC III, P. TSAIRIS, AND W. K. ENGEL. Mammalian motor units: physiological-histochemical correlation in three types in cat gastrocnemius. *Science* 174: 709–712, 1971.
92. BURKE, R. E., P. RUDOMIN, AND F. E. ZAJAC III. The effect of activation history on tension production by individual muscle units. *Brain Res.* 109: 515–529, 1976.
93. BURKE, R. E., W. Z. RYMER, AND J. V. WALSH, JR. Relative strength of synaptic input from short-latency pathways to motor units of defined type in cat medial gastrocnemius. *J. Neurophysiol.* 39: 447–458, 1976.
94. BURKE, R. E., AND P. TSAIRIS. Anatomy and innervation ratios in motor units of cat gastrocnemius. *J. Physiol. London* 234: 749–765, 1973.
95. CALVERT, T. W., AND A. E. CHAPMAN. The relationship between the surface emg and force transients in muscle: simulation and experimental studies. *Proc. IEEE* 65: 682–689, 1977.
96. CARLSÖÖ, S. Eine electromyographische Untersuchung der Muskelaktivität im Musculus deltoideus. *Acta Morphol. Neerl. Scand.* 2: 346–429, 1959.
97. CATHCART, E. P., D. T. RICHARDSON, AND W. CAMPBELL. Studies in muscle activity. II. The influence of speed on the mechanical efficiency. *J. Physiol. London* 58: 355–361, 1924.
98. CAVAGNA, G. M. Storage and utilization of elastic energy in skeletal muscle. *Exercise Sport Sci. Rev.* 5: 89–129, 1977.
99. CAVAGNA, G. A., H. THYS, AND A. ZAMBONI. The source of external work in level walking and running. *J. Physiol. London* 262: 639–657, 1976.
100. CHAO, E. Y. Experimental methods for biomechanical measurements of joint kinematics. In: *CRC Handbook of Engineering in Medicine and Biology,* edited by B. N. Feinberg and D. G. Fleming. West Palm Beach, FL: CRC Press, 1978, vol. 1B, p. 385–411.
101. CHAPLAIN, R. A. On the contractile mechanism of insect fibrillar flight muscle. IV. A quantitative chemo-mechanical model. *Biol. Cybern.* 18: 137–153, 1975.
102. CHAUVEAU, A. De l'enervation partielle des muscles. *Arch. Physiol. Norm. Pathol. Ser. 5* 1: 124–140, 1889.
103. CLAMANN, H. P. Statistical analysis of motor unit firing patterns in a human skeletal muscle. *Biophys. J.* 9: 1233–1251, 1969.
104. CLAMANN, H. P. Activity of single motor units during isometric tension. *Neurology* 20: 254–260, 1970.
105. CLARK, J. W., JR., E. C. GRECO, AND T. L. HARMAN. Experience with a Fourier method for determining the extracellular potential fields of excitable cells with cylindrical geometry. *CRC*

Crit. Rev. Bioeng. 3: 1-22, 1978.
106. CLARK, R. W., AND E. S. LUSCHEI. Short latency jaw movement produced by low intensity intracortical microstimulation of the precentral face area in monkeys. *Brain Res.* 70: 144-147, 1974.
107. CLARKE, R. S. J., R. F. HELLEN, AND A. R. LIND. The duration of sustained contractions of the human forearm at different muscle temperatures. *J. Physiol. London* 143: 454-473, 1952.
108. CLEMENTE, C. D. *Anatomy: A Regional Atlas of the Human Body.* Philadelphia, PA: Lea & Febiger, 1975.
109. CLOSE, J. R. *Functional Anatomy of the Extremities: Some Electronic and Kinematic Methods of Study.* Springfield, IL: Thomas, 1973.
110. CLOSE, J. R., E. D. NICKEL, AND F. N. TODD. Motor-unit action-potential counts (their significance in isometric and isotonic contractions). *J. Bone Jt. Surg.* 42A: 1207-1222, 1960.
111. CLOSE, R. The relation between intrinsic speed of shortening and duration of the active state of muscle. *J. Physiol. London* 180: 542-559, 1965.
112. CLOSE, R. I. Dynamic properties of mammalian skeletal muscles. *Physiol. Rev.* 52: 129-197, 1972.
113. CNOCKAERT, J. C. Comparaison électromyographique du travail en allongement et en raccourcissement au cours de mouvements de va-et-vient. *Electromyogr. Clin. Neurophysiol.* 15: 477-489, 1975.
114. CNOCKAERT, J. C., AND F. GOUBEL. Rôle de l'énergie potentielle élastique dans le travail musculaire. *Eur. J. Appl. Physiol. Occup. Physiol.* 34: 131-140, 1975.
115. CNOCKAERT, J. C., AND E. PERTUZON. Sur la géometrie musculo-squelettique du triceps brachii: application à la détermination dynamique de sa compliance. *Eur. J. Appl. Physiol. Occup. Physiol.* 32: 149-158, 1974.
116. COGGSHALL, J. C., AND G. A. BEKEY. EMG-force dynamics in human skeletal muscle. *Med. Biol. Eng.* 8: 265-270, 1970.
117. COHEN, A. H., AND C. GANS. Muscle activity in rat locomotion: movement analysis and electromyography of the flexors and extensors of the elbow. *J. Morphol.* 146: 177-196, 1975.
118. CONNOLLY, R., W. GOUGH, AND S. WINEGRAD. Characteristics of the isometric twitch of skeletal muscle immediately after tetanus. *J. Gen. Physiol.* 57: 697-709, 1971.
119. COOPER, S., AND J. C. ECCLES. The isometric responses of mammalian muscles. *J. Physiol. London* 69: 377-385, 1930.
120. COSTANTIN, L. L. Activation in striated muscle. In: *Handbook of Physiology. The Nervous System,* edited by J. M. Brookhart and V. B. Mountcastle. Bethesda, MD: Am. Physiol. Soc., 1977, sect. 1, vol. I, pt. 1, chapt. 7, p. 215-259.
121. COULTER, N. A., JR., AND J. C. WEST. Nonlinear passive mechanical properties of skeletal muscle. *Wright Air Dev. Div. Tech. Rep.* 60-636: 1-7, 1960.
122. CRAIG, E. S. *Morphology of Human Skeletal Muscle Cells: Ultrastructural Observations Which Challenge the Concept of Stability in the Definitive State of These Cells* (Ph.D. thesis). Memphis: Univ. of Tennessee, 1970. (Abstr. in *Diss. Abstr.* 32B: 673, 1971.)
123. CREESE, R., N. W. SCHOLES, AND W. J. WHALEN. Resting potentials of diaphragm muscle after prolonged anoxia. *J. Physiol. London* 140: 301-317, 1958.
124. CROWE, A. A mechanical model of muscle and its application to the intrafusal fibers of the mammalian muscle spindle. *J. Biomech.* 3: 583-592, 1970.
125. CROWNINSHIELD, R. D., AND R. A. BRAND. Kinematics and kinetics of gait. In: *CRC Handbook of Engineering in Medicine and Biology,* edited by B. N. Feinberg and D. G. Fleming. West Palm Beach, FL: CRC Press, 1978, p. 413-429.
126. CULL-CANDY, S. G., H. LUNDH, AND S. THESLEFF. Effects of botulinum toxin on neuromuscular transmission in the rat. *J. Physiol. London* 260: 177-203, 1976.
127. CULLEN, T. S., AND M. BRÖDEL. Lesions of the rectus abdominus muscle simulating an acute intra-abdominal condition. I. Anatomy of the rectus muscle *Bull. Johns Hopkins Hosp.* 61: 295-316, 1937.
128. DAHLBÄCK, O., D. ELMQVIST, T. R. JOHNS, S. RADNER, AND S. THESLEFF. An electrophysiologic study of the neuromuscular junction in myasthenia gravis. *J. Physiol. London* 156: 336-343, 1961.
129. D'ARSONVAL, A. Sur un appareil destiné à measurer la conductibilité des tissus vivants pour le son. *C. R. Soc. Biol.* 38: 103-104, 1886.
130. D'ARSONVAL, A. Production de chaleur dans les muscles. *C. R. Soc. Biol.* 38: 124-125, 1886.
131. DAVIES, R. E. A molecular theory of muscle contraction: calcium-dependent contractions with hydrogen bond formation plus ATP-dependent extensions of part of the myosin-actin cross-bridges. *Nature* 199: 1068-1074, 1963.
132. DELUCA, C. J. Physiology and mathematics of myoelectric signals. *IEEE Trans. Biomed. Eng.* 26: 313-325, 1979.
133. DEDUCA [sic], C. J., AND W. J. FORREST. Force analysis of individual muscles acting simultaneously on the shoulder joint during isometric abduction. *J. Biomech.* 6: 385-393, 1973.
134. DEMIÉVILLE, H. N. *Existence and Nature of Mechanical Interactions Between Motor Units: Experimental and Theoretical Evidence* (Ph.D. thesis). Memphis: Univ. of Tennessee, 1973. (Abstr. in *Diss. Abstr.* 34B: 4001-4002, 1973.)
135. DEMIÉVILLE, H. N., AND L. D. PARTRIDGE. Probability of peripheral interaction between motor units and implications for motor control. *Am. J. Physiol.*: 238: (*Regulatory, Integrative Comp. Physiol.* 7): R119-R137, 1980.
136. DEMPSTER, W. T., AND J. C. FINERTY. Relative activity of wrist moving muscles in static support of the wrist joint: an electromyographic study. *Am. J. Physiol.* 150: 596-606, 1947.
137. DENNY-BROWN, D. Interpretation of the electromyogram. *Arch. Neurol. Psychiatry Chicago* 61: 99-128, 1949.
138. DENNY-BROWN, D., AND J. B. PENNYBACKER. Fibrillation and fasciculation in voluntary muscle. *Brain* 61: 311-334, 1938.
139. DESMEDT, J. E., AND S. BORENSTEIN. Collateral innervation of muscle fibres by motor axons of dystrophic motor units. *Nature London* 246: 500-501, 1973.
140. DESMEDT, J. E., B. EMERYK, H. HAINAUT, H. REINHOLD, AND S. BORENSTEIN. Muscular dystrophy and myasthenia gravis. In: *New Developments in Electromyography and Clinical Neurophysiology,* edited by J. E. Desmedt. Basel, Switzerland: Karger, 1973, vol. 1, p. 380-399.
141. DESMEDT, J. E., AND E. GODAUX. Critical evaluation of the size principle of human motoneurons recruitment in ballistic movements and in vibration-induced inhibition or potentiation. *Trans. Am. Neurol. Assoc.* 102: 104-108, 1977.
142. DESMEDT, J. E., AND E. GODAUX. Fast motor units are not preferentially activated in rapid voluntary contractions in man. *Nature London* 267: 717-719, 1977.
143. DESMEDT, J. E., AND K. HAINAUT. Kinetics of myofilament activation in potentiated contraction: staircase phenomenon in human skeletal muscle *Nature London* 217: 529-532, 1968.
144. DEVANANDAN, M. S., R. M. ECCLES, AND R. A. WESTERMAN. Single motor units of mammalian muscle. *J. Physiol. London* 178: 359-367, 1965.
145. DIJKSTRA, S., AND J. J. DENIER VAN DER GON. An analog computer study of fast, isolated movements. *Kybernetik* 12: 102-110, 1973.
146. DIJKSTRA, S., J. J. DENIER VAN DER GON, T. BLANGÉ, J. M. KAREMAKER, AND A. E. J. L. KROMER. A simplified sliding-filament muscle model for simulation purposes. *Kybernetik* 12: 94-101, 1973.
147. DOWNEY, J. A., AND R. C. DARLING. *Physiological Basis of Rehabilitative Medicine.* Philadelphia, PA: Saunders, 1971.
148. DOYLE, A. M., AND R. F. MAYER. Studies of the motor unit in the cat. *Bull. Univ. Md. Sch. Med.* 54: 11-17, 1969.
149. DRAPER, N. R., AND H. SMITH. *Applied Regression Analysis.* New York: Wiley, 1966.
150. DRAZIL, J. V. *Dictionary of Quantities and Units.* Cleveland, OH: CRC Press, 1971.
151. DUBUISSON, M. *Muscular Contraction.* Springfield, IL: Thomas, 1954.
152. DUCHENNE, G. B. *Physiology of Motion,* transl. by E. B. Kaplan. Philadelphia, PA: Saunders, 1959. (From *Physiologie des Mouvements,* Paris, 1867.)
153. ECCLES, J. C., AND C. S. SHERRINGTON. Numbers and contraction-values of individual motor-units examined in some mus-

cles of the limb. *Proc. R. Soc. London Ser. B* 106: 326-357, 1930.
154. EDMAN, K. A. P., L. A. MULIERI, AND B. SCUBON-MULIERI. Non-hyperbolic force-velocity relationship in single muscle fibers. *Acta Physiol. Scand.* 98: 143-156, 1976.
155. EDSTRÖM, L., AND E. KUGELBERG. Histochemical composition, distribution of fibers and fatigueability of single motor units. Anterior tibial muscle of the rat. *J. Neurol. Neurosurg. Psychiatry* 31: 424-433, 1968.
156. ELFTMAN, H. The function of muscles in locomotion. *Am. J. Physiol.* 125: 357-366, 1939.
157. ELFTMAN, H. The transverse tarsal joint and its control. *Clin. Orthop.* 16: 41-46, 1960.
158. ELFTMAN, H. Biomechanics of muscle with particular application to studies of gait. *J. Bone Jt. Surg.* 48A: 363-377, 1966.
159. ELFTMAN, H. Dynamic structure of the human foot. *Artificial Limbs* 13: 49-58, 1969.
160. ENGBERG, I., AND A. LUNDBERG. An electromyographic analysis of muscular activity in the hindlimb of the cat during unrestrained locomotion. *Acta Physiol. Scand.* 75: 614-630, 1969.
161. ERNST, E. *Biophysics of the Striated Muscle.* Budapest: Hungarian Acad. Sci., 1963.
162. ERNST, E., K. KOVÁCS, G. METZGER-TÖRÖK, AND C. TROMBITÁS. Longitudinal structure of the striated fibril. *Acta Biochim. Biophys. Acad. Sci. Hung.* 4: 177-186, 1969.
163. ERNST, E., K. KOVÁCS, G. METZGER-TÖRÖK, AND C. TROMBITÁS. Transverse structure of the striated fibril. *Acta Biochim. Biophys. Acad. Sci. Hung.* 4: 187-194, 1969.
164. EVANS, C. L., AND A. V. HILL. The relation of length to tension development and heat production on contraction in muscle. *J. Physiol. London* 49: 10-16, 1914.
165. EYKHOFF, P. *System Identification: Parameter and State Estimation.* London: Wiley, 1974.
166. FAABORG-ANDERSEN, K. Electromyographic investigation of intrinsic laryngeal muscles in humans. *Acta Physiol. Scand. Suppl.* 140: 1-149, 1957.
167. FEINSTEIN, B., B. LINDEGÅRD, E. NYMAN, AND G. WOHLFART. Morphologic studies of motor units in normal human muscles. *Acta Anat.* 23: 127-142, 1955.
168. FENG, T. P., L-Y. LEE, C-W. MENG, AND S-C. WANG. Studies on the neuromuscular junction. IX. The after effects of tetanization on N-M transmission in cat. *Chinese J. Physiol.* 13: 79-108, 1938.
169. FENN, W. O. Contractility. In: *Physical Chemistry of Cells and Tissues,* edited by R. Höber. Philadelphia, PA: Blackiston, 1945, sect. 7, p. 445-522.
170. FENN, W. O., AND P. H. GARVEY. The measurement of elasticity and viscosity of skeletal muscle in normal and pathological cases; a study of so-called "muscle tonus". *J. Clin. Invest.* 13: 383-397, 1934.
171. FENN, W. O., AND B. S. MARSH. Muscular force at different speeds of shortening. *J. Physiol. London* 85: 277-297, 1935.
172. FICK, A. *Untersuchungen über Muskel-Arbeit.* Basel, Switzerland: H. Georg, 1867.
173. FICK, A. Specielle Bewegunugslehre. In: *Handbuch der Physiologie,* edited by L. Hermann. Leipzig, Germany: 1879, vol. I, pt. 2, p. 239-346.
174. FIELDS, R. W., AND J. J. FABER. Biophysical analysis of the mechanical properties of the sarcolemma. *Can. J. Physiol. Pharmacol.* 48: 394-404, 1970.
175. FINERTY, J. C., AND R. GESELL. The effect of cH on humoral stimulation of striated muscle and its application to the chemical control of breathing. *Am. J. Physiol.* 145: 1-15, 1945.
176. FIXLER, D. E., J. M. ATKINS, J. H. MITCHELL, AND L. D. HORWITZ. Blood flow to respiratory, cardiac, and limb muscles in dogs during graded exercise. *Am. J. Physiol.* 231: 1515-1519, 1976.
177. FLETCHER, W. M. The relation of oxygen to the survival metabolism of muscle. *J. Physiol. London* 28: 474-498, 1902.
178. FOLK, G. E. *Textbook of Environmental Physiology* (2nd ed.). Philadelphia, PA: Lea & Febiger, 1974.
179. FORBES, A., L. R. WHITAKER, AND J. F. FULTON. The effect of reflex excitation and inhibition on the response of a muscle to stimulation through its motor nerve. *Am. J. Physiol.* 82: 693-716, 1927.
180. FOWLER, W. S., AND A. CROWE. Effect of temperature on resistance to stretch of tortoise muscle. *Am. J. Physiol.* 231: 1349-1355, 1976.
181. FRENCH, A. P. *Newtonian Mechanics.* New York: Norton, 1971.
182. FULTON, J. F. *Muscular Contraction and the Reflex Control of Movement.* Baltimore, MD: Williams & Wilkins, 1926.
183. FULTON, J. F., AND L. G. WILSON. *Selected Readings in the History of Physiology* (2nd ed.). Springfield, IL: Thomas, 1966.
184. GALVANI, L. *Commentary on the Effects of Electricity on Muscular Motion* (transl. by M. G. Foley). Norwalk, CT: Burndy Library, 1954. (*De Viribus Electricitatis in Motu Musculari Commentarius.* Bologna: 1791.)
185. GAMBARYAN, P. P. *How Mammals Run: Anatomical Adaptations* [transl. from Russian]. New York: Wiley, 1974. (Leningrad: Mlekopitaiuschikh-Prisposobitel'nye, 1972.)
186. GASSER, H. S., AND A. V. HILL. The dynamics of muscular contraction. *Proc. R. Soc. London. Ser. B* 96: 398-437, 1924.
187. GESELL, R. A neurophysiological interpretation of the respiratory act. *Ergeb. Physiol. Biol. Chem. Exp. Pharmakol.* 42: 477-639, 1940.
188. GESELL, R., A. K. ATKINSON, AND R. C. BROWN. The gradation of intensity of inspiratory contractions. *Am. J. Physiol.* 131: 659-673, 1941.
189. GESELL, R., C. S. MAGEE, AND J. W. BRICKER. Activity patterns of the respiratory neurons and muscles. *Am. J. Physiol.* 128: 615-628, 1940.
190. GESINK, J. W. *Transfer Characteristics of Load Moving Skeletal Muscle* (Ph.D. thesis). Ann Arbor: Univ. of Michigan, 1973. (Abstr. in *Diss. Abstr.* 34B: 3764 3765, 1973.)
191. GILSON, A. S., JR., S. M. WALKER, AND G. M. SCHOEPFLE. The forms of the isometric twitch and isometric tetanus curves recorded from the frog's sartorius muscle. *J. Cell. Comp. Physiol.* 24: 185-199, 1944.
192. GOLDBERG, A. L., J. D. ETLINGER, D. F. GOLDSPINK, AND C. JABLECKI. Mechanism of work-induced hypertrophy of skeletal muscle. *Med. Sci. Sports* 7: 248-261, 1975.
193. GOLDBERG, S. J., G. LENNERSTRAND, AND C. D. HULL. Motor unit responses in the lateral rectus muscle of the cat: intracellular current injection of abducens nucleus neurons. *Acta Physiol. Scand.* 96: 58-63, 1976.
194. GOLDSPINK, G. Design of muscles in relation to locomotion. In: *Mechanics and Energetics of Animal Locomotion,* edited by R. McN. Alexander and G. Goldspink. London: Chapman & Hall, 1977. p. 1-22.
195. GOLDSTEIN, H. *Classical Mechanics.* Reading, MA.: Addison-Wesley, 1950.
196. GOODALL, M. C. Kinetics of muscular contraction. *Yale J. Biol. Med.* 30: 224-243, 1957.
197. GOODGOLD, J. *Anatomical Correlates of Clinical Electromyography.* Baltimore, MD: Williams & Wilkins, 1974.
198. GOODGOLD, J., AND A. EBERSTEIN. *Electrodiagnosis of Neuromuscular Diseases* (2nd ed.). Baltimore, MD: Williams & Wilkins, 1978.
199. GOODWIN, G. M., AND E. S. LUSCHEI. Discharge of spindle afferents from jaw-closing muscles during chewing in alert monkeys. *J. Neurophysiol.* 38: 560-571, 1975.
200. GORDON, A. M., A. F. HUXLEY, AND F. J. JULIAN. The length-tension diagram of single vertebrate striated muscle fibers. *J. Physiol. London* 171: 28P-30P, 1964.
201. GORDON, A. M., A. F. HUXLEY, AND F. J. JULIAN. The variation of isometric tension with sarcomere length in vertebrate muscle fibres. *J. Physiol. London* 184: 170-192, 1966.
202. GORDON, G., AND A. H. S. HOLBOURN. A simultaneous study of the action potentials and movements of single motor units in the tonic stretch reflex. *J. Physiol. London* 107: 18P, 1948.

203. GORDON, G., AND A. H. S. HOLBOURN. The sounds from single motor units in a contracting muscle. *J. Physiol. London* 107: 456–464, 1948.
204. GORDON, G., AND A. H. S. HOLBOURN. The mechanical activity of single motor units in reflex contractions of skeletal muscle. *J. Physiol. London* 110: 26–35, 1949.
205. GOSLOW, G. E., JR., R. M. REINKING, AND D. G. STUART. Physiological extent, range and rate of muscle stretch for soleus, medial gastrocnemius and tibialis anterior. *Pfluegers Arch.* 341: 77–86, 1973.
206. GOSLOW, G. E., JR., E. K. STAUFFER, W. C. NEMETH, AND D. G. STUART. Digit flexor muscles in the cat: their action and motor units. *J. Morphol.* 137: 335–352, 1972.
207. GOSS, R. J. *The Physiology of Growth*. New York: Academic, 1978.
208. GOTCH, F. The submaximal electrical response of nerve to a single stimulus. *J. Physiol. London* 28: 395–416, 1902.
209. GOUBEL, F. Évaluation de l'énergie élastique emmagasinée par le muscle lors d'une contraction isométrique. *J. Physiol. Paris* 65: 238A, 1972.
210. GOUBEL, F., F. LESTIENNE, AND S. BOUISSET. Détermination dynamique de la compliance musculaire in situ. *J. Physiol. Paris* 60: 255, 1968.
211. GRAHAM, D., AND D. MCRUER. *Analysis of Nonlinear Control Systems*. New York: Wiley, 1961.
212. GRANIT, R. Neuromuscular interaction in postural tone of the cat's isometric soleus muscle. *J. Physiol. London* 143: 387–402, 1958.
213. GRANT, P. G. Biomechanical significance of the instantaneous center of rotation: the human temporomandibular joint. *J. Biomech.* 6: 109–113, 1973.
214. GRAY, D. E. (editor). *American Institute of Physics Handbook* (3rd ed.). New York: McGraw-Hill, 1972.
215. GRAY, J. Studies in the mechanics of the tetrapod skeleton. *J. Exp. Biol.* 20: 88–116, 1944.
216. GRAY, J. *How Animals Move*. Cambridge, England: Cambridge Univ. Press, 1960.
217. GREENE, P. H. Problems of organization of motor systems. *Quart. Rep., Inst. Computer Res.*, Univ. of Chicago, 1971, ser. II C, no. 29, p. 1–66.
218. GRILLNER, S. The role of muscle stiffness in meeting the changing postural and locomotor requirements for force development by the ankle extensors. *Acta Physiol. Scand.* 86: 92–108, 1972.
219. GRILLNER, S. On the generation of locomotion in the spinal dogfish. *Exp. Brain Res.* 20: 459–470, 1974.
220. GRILLNER, S., AND S. KASHIN. On the generation and performance of swimming in fish. In: *Neural Control of Locomotion*, edited by R. M. Herman, S. Grillner, P. S. G. Stein, and D. G. Stuart. New York: Plenum, 1976, p. 181–201.
221. GURFINKEL', V. S., AND YU, S. LEVIK. Dependence of contraction of the muscle on the sequence of stimulating pulses. *Biophysics USSR* 18: 121–127, 1973.
222. GUTTMAN, S. A., R. G. HORTON, AND D. T. WILBER. Enhancement of muscle contraction after tetanus. *Am. J. Physiol.* 119: 463–473, 1937.
223. GYDIKOV, A. *Microstructure of the Voluntary Movements in Man* [Engl. summary and legends]. Sofia: Bulgarian Acad. Sci., 1970.
224. HALL, V. M. D. The role of force or power in Liebig's physiological chemistry. *Med. Hist.* 24: 20–59, 1980.
225. HALLIBURTON, W. D. *Handbook of Physiology* (10th ed.). Philadelphia, PA: Blakistons, 1911.
226. HALPERN, W., AND N. R. ALPERT. A stochastic signal method for measuring dynamic mechanical properties of muscle. *J. Appl. Physiol.* 31: 913–925, 1971.
227. HAMM, T. M. *Identification of the Mechanical Properties of Skeletal Muscle* (Ph.D. thesis). Memphis: Univ. of Tennessee, 1979. (Abstr. in *Diss. Abstr.* 40: 5556B, 1980.)
228. HAMMOND, P. H., P. A. MERTON, AND G. G. SUTTON. Nervous gradation of muscular contraction. *Br. Med. Bull.* 12: 214–218, 1956.
229. HANSON, J., AND J. LOWY. Structure and function of the contractile apparatus in the muscles of invertebrate animals. In: *Structure and Function of Muscle*, edited by G. H. Bourne. New York: Academic, 1960, vol. I, p. 265–335.
230. HARRIS, A. J. Inductive functions of the nervous system. *Annu. Rev. Physiol.* 36: 251–305, 1974.
231. HARTREE, W., AND A. V. HILL. The nature of the isometric twitch. *J. Physiol. London* 55: 389–411, 1921.
232. HATZE, H. A myocybernetic control model of skeletal muscle. *Biol. Cybern.* 25: 103–119, 1977.
233. HATZE, H. A complete set of control equations for the human musculo-skeletal system. *J. Biomech.* 10: 799–805, 1977.
234. HATZE, H. A general myocybernetic control model of skeletal muscle. *Biol. Cybern.* 28: 143–157, 1978.
235. HAYCRAFT, J. B. Upon the production of rapid voluntary movements. *J. Physiol. London* 23: 1–9, 1898.
236. HEITLER, W. J., AND M. BURROWS. The locust jump. I. The motor programme. *J. Exp. Biol.* 66: 203–219, 1977.
237. HELMHOLTZ, H. VON. Ueber die Wärmeentwickelung bei der Muskelaction. *Arch. Anat. Physiol.* 144–164, 1848.
238. HELMHOLTZ, H. VON. Messungen über den zeitlichen Verlauf der Zuckung animalischer Muskeln und die Fortpflanzungsgeschwindigkeit der Reizung in den Nerven. *Arch. Anat. Physiol.* 276–364, 1850.
239. HELMHOLTZ, H. VON. Verlaütige, Bericht über die Fortpflanzungsgeschwindigkeit der Reizung. *Arch. Anat. Physiol.* 71–73, 1850.
240. HELMHOLTZ, H. VON. Messungen über Fortpflanzungsgeschwindigkeit der Reizung in den Nerven. *Arch. Anat. Physiol.* 199–216, 1852.
241. HELMHOLTZ, H. VON. *Monatsber. d Berliner Acad.* P328, 1854. Cited in *Handbuch der Physiologie*, by L. Hermann. Leipzig, Germany: 1879, vol. 1.
242. HENNEMAN, E. Peripheral mechanisms involved in the control of muscle. In: *Medical Physiology* (13th ed.), edited by V. B. Mountcastle. St. Louis, MO: Mosby, 1974, p. 617–635.
243. HENNEMAN, E., AND C. B. OLSON. Relations between structure and function in the design of skeletal muscles. *J. Neurophysiol.* 28: 581–598, 1965.
244. HENNEMAN, E., G. SOMJEN, AND D. O. CARPENTER. Functional significance of cell size in spinal motoneurons. *J. Neurophysiol.* 28: 560–580, 1965.
245. HERMAN, R. The myotatic reflex: clinico-physiological aspects of spasticity and contracture. *Brain* 93: 273–312, 1970.
246. HERMAN, R., H. SCHAUMBERG, AND S. REINER. A rotational joint apparatus: a device for study of tension-length relations of human muscle. *Med. Res. Eng.* 6: 18–20, 1967.
247. HERMANN, L. Allgemeine Muskelphysik. In: *Herman's Handbuch der Physiologie*, by L. Hermann. Leipzig, Germany: 1879, vol. I, pt. 1, p. 3–260.
248. HERTEL, H. *Structure, Form and Movement* (transl. by M. S. Katz). New York: Reinhold, 1966.
249. HESS, A. Vertebrate slow muscle fibers. *Physiol. Rev.* 50: 40–62, 1970.
250. HILL, A. V. The maximum work and mechanical efficiency of human muscles, and their most economical speed. *J. Physiol. London* 56: 19–41, 1922.
251. HILL, A. V. The heat of shortening and the dynamic constants of muscle. *Proc. R. Soc. London Ser. B* 126: 136–195, 1938.
252. HILL, A. V. The pressure developed in muscle during contraction. *J. Physiol. London* 107: 518–526, 1948.
253. HILL, A. V. The abrupt transition from rest to activity in muscle. *Proc. R. Soc. London Ser. B* 136: 399–420, 1949.
254. HILL, A. V. The development of the active state of muscle during the latent period. *Proc. R. Soc. London Ser. B* 137: 320–329, 1950.
255. HILL, A. V. The effect of series compliance on the tension developed in a muscle twitch. *Proc. R. Soc. London Ser. B* 138: 325–329, 1951.
256. HILL, A. V. The mechanics of active muscle. *Proc. R. Soc.*

London Ser. B 141: 104–117, 1953.
257. HILL, A. V. Production and absorption of work by muscle. *Science* 131: 897–903, 1960.
258. HILL, A. V. *Trails and Trials in Physiology.* Baltimore, MD: Williams & Wilkins, 1965.
259. HILL, A. V. *First and Last Experiments in Muscle Mechanics.* London: Cambridge Univ. Press, 1970.
260. HOUK, J., AND E. HENNEMAN. Feedback control of skeletal muscles. *Brain Res.* 5: 433–451, 1967.
261. HOUK, J. C., JR. A study of human postural control. *NEREM Rec.* 138–139, 1963.
262. HOUTZ, S. J., AND F. J. FISCHER. An analysis of muscle action and joint excursion during exercise on a stationary bicycle. *J. Bone Jt. Surg.* 41A: 123–131, 1959.
263. HOWELL, W. H. *A Text-Book of Physiology* (5th ed.). Philadelphia, PA: Saunders, 1913.
264. HOYLE, G. *Comparative Physiology of the Nervous Control of Muscular Contraction.* London: Cambridge Univ. Press, 1957.
265. HOYLE, G. Diversity of striated muscle. *Am. Zool.* 7: 435–449, 1967.
266. HOYLE, G., AND J. LOWY. The paradox of *Mytilus* muscle. A new interpretation. *J. Exp. Biol.* 33: 295–310, 1956.
267. HUBER, E. Über das Muskelgebiet des N. facialis bei Katze und Hund nebst allgemeinen Bemerkungen über die Fascialismuskulatur der Säuger. *Anat. Anz.* 51: 1–17, 1918.
268. HUBER, G. C. On the form and arrangement in fasciculi of striated voluntary muscle fibers. *Anat. Rec.* 11: 149–168, 1917.
269. HUDLICKÁ, O. *Muscle Blood Flow: Its Relation to Muscle Metabolism and Function.* Amsterdam: Swets & Zeitlinger, 1973.
270. HUXLEY, A. F. Interpretation of muscle striation: evidence from visible light microscopy. *Br. Med. Bull.* 12: 167–170, 1956.
271. HUXLEY, A. F. Muscle structure and theories of contraction. *Prog. Biophys. Biophys. Chem.* 7: 255–318, 1957.
272. HUXLEY, A. F., AND L. D. PEACHEY. The maximum length for contraction in vertebrate striated muscle. *J. Physiol. London* 156: 150–165, 1961.
273. HUXLEY, A. F., AND R. M. SIMMONS. Proposed mechanism of force generation in striated muscle. *Nature London* 233: 533–538, 1971.
274. HUXLEY, A. F., AND R. M. SIMMONS. Mechanical transients and the origin of muscular force. *Cold Spring Harbor Symp. Quant. Biol.* 37: 669–680, 1972.
275. HUXLEY, H. E. The ultra-structure of striated muscle. *Br. Med. Bull.* 12: 171–173, 1956.
276. HUXLEY, H. E. Muscle cells. In: *The Cell,* edited by J. Brachet and A. E. Mirsky. New York: Academic, 1960, vol. 4, 365–481.
277. HUXLEY, H. E. Structural organization and the contraction mechanism in striated muscle. In: *Biology and the Physical Sciences,* edited by S. Devons. New York: Columbia Univ. Press, 1969, p. 114–138.
278. HYNDMAN, R. W., JR., AND R. K. BEACH. The transient response of the human operator. *IRE Trans. Med. Electron.* 12: 67–71, 1958.
279. IKAI, M., K. YABE, AND K. ISCHII. Muskelkraft und muskuläre Ermüdung bei willkürlicher Anspannung und elektrischer Reizung des Muskels. *Sportarzt Sportmed.* 5: 197–204, 1967.
280. INBAR, G. F., AND D. ADAM. Estimation of muscle active state. *Biol. Cybern.* 23: 61–72, 1976.
281. INMAN, V. T., H. J. RALSTON, J. B. DE C. M. SAUNDERS, B. FEINSTEIN, AND E. W. WRIGHT, JR. Relation of human electromyogram to muscular tension. *Electroencephalogr. Clin. Neurophysiol.* 4: 187–194, 1952.
282. JANSEN, J. K. S., AND P. M. H. RACK. The reflex response to sinusoidal stretching of soleus in the decerebrate cat. *J. Physiol. London* 183: 15–36, 1966.
283. JARCHO, L. W., C. EYZAGUIRRE, B. BERMAN, AND J. L. LILIENTHAL, JR. Spread of excitation in skeletal muscle: some factors contributing to the form of the electromyogram. *Am. J. Physiol.* 168: 446–457, 1952.
284. JARCHO, L. W., C. L. VERA, C. G. MCCARTHY, AND P. B. WILLIAMS. The form of motor unit and fibrillation potentials. *Electroencephalogr. Clin. Neurophysiol.* 10: 527–540, 1958.
285. JEDWAB, J. D. *Telemetry of Force, Length and EMG From Individual Muscles of the Triceps Surae During Unrestrained Locomotion* (Thesis). Clayton, Victoria, Australia: Monash Univ., 1977.
286. JEDWAB, J. D., R. A. WESTERMAN, AND S. P. ZICCONE. Telemetry of force, length and EMG in the soleus muscle of the freely moving cat. *Aust. Physiol. Pharmacol. Soc. Proc.* 8: 181P, 1977.
287. JEWELL, B. R. The nature of the phasic and the tonic responses of the anterior byssal retractor muscle of *Mytilus. J. Physiol. London* 149: 154–177, 1959.
288. JEWELL, B. R., AND D. R. WILKIE. An analysis of the mechanical components in frog's striated muscle. *J. Physiol. London* 143: 515–540, 1958.
289. JEWELL, B. R., AND D. R. WILKIE. The mechanical properties of relaxing muscle. *J. Physiol. London* 152: 30–47, 1960.
290. JI, S. A general theory of ATP synthesis and utilization. *Ann. NY Acad. Sci.* 227: 211–226, 1974.
291. JÍMENEZ-PABÓN, E., AND R. A. NELSON. Quantitative measurements of muscle tone in cats. *Neurology* 15: 1120–1126, 1965.
292. JOSEPH, J. Electromyographic studies on muscle tone and the erect posture in man. *Br. J. Surg.* 51: 616–622, 1964.
293. JOURNAL OF PHYSIOLOGY. Suggestions to authors. *J. Physiol. London* 182: 1–33, 1966.
294. JOYCE, G. C., AND P. M. H. RACK. Isotonic lengthening and shortening movements of cat soleus muscle. *J. Physiol. London* 204: 475–491, 1969.
295. JOYCE, G. C., P. M. H. RACK, AND H. F. ROSS. The forces generated at the human elbow joint in response to imposed sinusoidal movements of the forearm. *J. Physiol. London* 240: 351–374, 1974.
296. JOYCE, G. C., P. M. H. RACK, AND D. R. WESTBURY. The mechanical properties of cat soleus muscle during controlled lengthening and shortening movements. *J. Physiol. London* 204: 461–474, 1969.
297. JULIAN F. J. Activation in a skeletal muscle contraction model with a modification for insect fibrillar muscle. *Biophys. J.* 9: 547–570, 1969.
298. JULIAN, F. J., K. R. SOLLINS, AND M. R. SOLLINS. A model for the transient and steady-state mechanical behavior of contracting muscle. *Biophys. J.* 14: 546–562, 1974.
299. JULIAN, F. J., AND M. R. SOLLINS. Variation of muscle stiffness with force at increasing speeds of shortening. *J. Gen. Physiol.* 66: 287–302, 1975.
300. KADEFORS, R., I. PETERSÉN, AND H. BROMAN. Spectral analysis of events in the electromyogram. In: *New Developments in Electromyography and Clinical Neurophysiology,* edited by J. E. Desmedt. Basel, Switzerland: Karger, 1973, vol. 1, p. 628–637.
301. KAISER, K. Ueber die Elasticität des thätigen muskels. *Z. Biol. Munich* 38: 1–15, 1899.
302. KAMADA, T. The supernormal phase in muscular contraction. *J. Physiol. London* 76: 187–192, 1932.
303. KARPOVICH, P. V., P. H. COHAN, AND M. IKAI. Study of endurance of various muscle groups. *Res. Q. Am. Assoc. Health Phys. Educ. Recreat.* 35: 393–397, 1964.
304. KATZ, B. The relation between force and speed in muscular contraction. *J. Physiol. London* 96: 45–64, 1939.
305. KATZ, B. The role of the cell membrane in muscular activity. *Br. Med. Bull.* 12: 210–213, 1956.
306. KATZ, B., AND S. W. KUFFLER. Multiple motor innervation of the frog's sartorius muscle. *J. Neurophysiol.* 4: 209–223, 1941.
307. KEATINGE, W. R. *Survival in Cold Water.* Oxford, England: Blackwell, 1969.
308. KENNEDY, D., AND W. J. DAVIS. Organization of invertebrate motor systems. In: *Handbook of Physiology. The Nervous System,* edited by J. M. Brookhart and V. B. Mountcastle. Bethesda, MD: Am. Physiol. Soc., 1977, sect. 1, vol. I, pt. 2, chapt. 27, p. 1023–1087.
309. KENT, B. E. Functional anatomy of the shoulder complex: a

review. *Phys. Ther.* 51: 867–887, 1971.
310. KERNELL, D., A. DUCATI, AND H. SJÖHOLM. Properties of motor units in the first deep lumbrical muscle of the cat's foot. *Brain Res.* 98: 37–55, 1975.
311. KERNELL, D., AND H. SJÖHOLM. Recruitment and firing rate modulation of motor unit tension in a small muscle of the cat's foot. *Brain Res.* 98: 57–72, 1975.
312. KLEEMAN, F. J., L. D. PARTRIDGE, AND G. H. GLASER. Resting potential and distribution of muscle fibers in living mammalian muscle. *Am. J. Phys. Med.* 40: 183–191, 1961.
313. KNOTTS, D., M. LEWIS, AND J. C. LUCK. Motor unit areas in a cat limb muscle. *Exp. Neurol.* 30: 475–483, 1971.
314. KNOWLTON, F. P., AND C. J. CAMPBELL. Observations on peripheral inhibition in arthropods. *Am. J. Physiol.* 91: 19–26, 1929.
315. KOLMAN, B. *Elementary Linear Algebra.* Toronto, Canada: Macmillan, 1970.
316. KOMI, P. V., AND J. H. T. VIITASALO. Signal characteristics of EMG at different levels of muscle tension. *Acta Physiol. Scand.* 96: 267–276, 1976.
317. KROGH, A. The supply of oxygen to the tissues and the regulation of the capillary circulation. *J. Physiol. London* 52: 457–474, 1919.
318. KRONECKER, H., AND W. STIRLING. Die Genesis des Tetanus. *Arch. Anat. Physiol. Physiol. Abt. Leipzig* 2: 1–40, 1878.
319. KUGELBERG, E. Properties of the rat hind-limb motor units. In: *New Developments in Electromyography and Clinical Neurophysiology,* edited by J. E. Desmedt. Basel, Switzerland: Karger, 1973.
320. KUGELBERG, E., AND C. R. SKOGLUND. Natural and artificial activation of motor units—a comparison. *J. Neurophysiol.* 9: 399–412, 1946.
321. LAMARRE, Y., AND J. P. LUND. Load compensation in human masseter muscles. *J. Physiol. London* 253: 21–35, 1975.
322. LAMB, D. R. Androgens and exercise. *Med. Sci. Sports* 7: 1–5, 1975.
323. LANDOWNE, M., AND R. W. STACY. Glossary of terms. In: *Tissue Elasticity,* edited by J. W. Remington. Washington, D.C.: Am. Physiol. Soc., 1957, p. 191–203.
324. LAPEDES, D. N. (editor). *Dictionary of Scientific and Technical Terms.* New York: McGraw-Hill, 1974.
325. LEE, Y. W., AND M. SCHETZEN. Measurement of the Wiener kernels of a non-linear system by cross-correlation. *Int. J. Control* 2: 237–254, 1965.
326. LEEUWENHOEK, A. VAN. Letter to Royal Society of London, 7 September, 1688. In: *Collected Letters,* edited by J. J. Swart. Amsterdam: Swets & Zeitlinger, 1967, vol. 8, no. 110, p. 2–57.
327. LEONARDO DA VINCI. *On the Human Body* (facsimile and transl. by C. D. O'Malley and J. B. de C. M. Saunders). New York: Schuman, 1952.
328. LESTIENNE, F. Rôle des forces d'origine visco-élastique dans l'activité freinatrice exercée par le groupe musculaire antagoniste. *J. Physiol. Paris* 65: 263A, 1972.
329. LESTIENNE, F., AND S. BOUISSET. Pattern temporel de la mise en jeu d'un agoniste et d'un antagoniste en fonction de la tension de l'agoniste. *Rev. Neurol.* 118: 550–554, 1968.
330. LESTIENNE, F., AND S. BOUISSET. Quantification of the biceps-triceps synergy in simple voluntary movements. In: *Visual Information Processing and Control of Motor Activity Symposium.* Sofia: Bulgarian Acad. Sci., 1969, p. 445–449.
331. LEVIN, A., AND J. WYMAN. The viscous elastic properties of muscle. *Proc. R. Soc. London Ser. B.* 101: 218–243, 1927.
332. LEWIS, D. M., J. C. LUCK, AND S. KNOTT. A comparison of isometric contractions of the whole muscle with those of motor units in a fast-twitch muscle of the cat. *Exp. Neurol.* 37: 68–85, 1972.
333. LICHT, S. *Electrodiagnosis and Electromyography* (3rd ed.). New Haven, CT: Licht, 1971.
334. LIDDELL, E. G. T., AND C. S. SHERRINGTON. A comparison between certain features of the spinal flexor reflex and of the decerebrate extensor reflex respectively. *Proc. R. Soc. London Ser. B.* 95: 299–339, 1924.
335. LIDDELL, E. G. T., AND C. S. SHERRINGTON. Recruitment and some other features of reflex inhibition. *Proc. R. Soc. London Ser. B* 97: 488–518, 1925.
336. LILEY, A. W., AND K. A. K. NORTH. An electrical investigation of effects of repetitive stimulation on mammalian neuromuscular junction. *J. Neurophysiol.* 16: 509–527, 1953.
337. LINDSTRÖM, L. H., AND R. I. MAGNUSSON. Interpretation of myoelectric power spectra: a model and its applications. *Proc. IEEE* 65: 653–662, 1977.
338. LIPPOLD, O. C. J. The relative between integrated action potentials in a human muscle and its isometric tension. *J. Physiol. London* 117: 492–499, 1952.
339. LIPPOLD, O. C. J., J. W. T. REDFEARN, AND J. VUČO. The rhythmical activity of groups of motor units in the voluntary contraction of muscle. *J. Physiol. London* 137: 473–487, 1957.
340. LITTLE, R. C., AND W. B. WEAD. Diastolic viscoelastic properties of active and quiescent cardiac muscle. *Am. J. Physiol.* 221: 1120–1125, 1971.
341. LOMBARD, W. P., AND F. M. ABBOTT. The mechanical effects produced by the contraction of individual muscles of the thigh of the frog. *Am. J. Physiol.* 20: 1–60, 1907.
342. LOOFBOURROW, G. N. Electrographic evaluation of mechanical response in mammalian skeletal muscle in different conditions. *J. Neurophysiol.* 11: 153–167, 1948.
343. LORENTE DE NÓ, R. A study of neurophysiology, Part II. *Studies from the Rockefeller Institute.* 132: 1946.
344. LOWE, D. A. *A Guide to International Recommendations on Names and Symbols for Quantities and on Units of Measurement.* Geneva, Switzerland: World Health Organiz., 1975.
345. LOWY, J. Contraction and relaxation in the adductor muscles of *pecten maximus*. *J. Physiol. London* 124: 100–105, 1954.
346. LOWY J., AND B. M. MILLMAN. Contraction and relaxation in smooth muscle of lamellibranch molluscs. *Nature London* 183: 1730–1731, 1959.
347. LUCAS, K. On the gradation of activity in a skeletal muscle fibre. *J. Physiol. London* 33: 125–137, 1905.
348. LUCAS, K. The "all or none" contraction of the amphibian skeletal muscle fibre. *J. Physiol. London* 38: 113–133, 1909.
349. LUFF, A. R., AND U. PROSKE. Properties of motor units of the frog iliofibularis muscle. *Am. J. Physiol.* 236 (*Cell Physiol.* 5): C35–C40, 1979.
350. LUPTON, H. An analysis of the effects of speed on the mechanical efficiency of human muscular movement, (with Appendix by A. V. Hill). *J. Physiol. London* 57: 336–353, 1923.
351. LUSCHEI, E. S., AND G. M. GOODWIN. Patterns of mandibular movement and jaw muscle activity during mastication in the monkey. *J. Neurophysiol.* 37: 954–966, 1974.
352. MACHIN, K. E., AND J. W. S. PRINGLE. The physiology of insect fibrillar muscle. II. Mechanical properties of a beetle flight muscle. *Proc. R. Soc. London Ser. B* 151: 204–225, 1959.
353. MACKLEN, P. T. Respiratory mechanics. *Annu. Rev. Physiol.* 40: 157–184, 1978.
354. MANNARD, A., AND R. B. STEIN. Determination of the frequency response of isometric soleus muscle in the cat using random nerve stimulation. *J. Physiol. London* 229: 275–296, 1973.
355. MANTER, J. T. The dynamics of quadrupedal walking. *J. Exp. Biol.* 15: 522–540, 1938.
356. MAREY, E. J. De la locomotion terrestre chez les bipèdes et les quadrupèdes. *J. Anat. Physiol.* 9: 42–80, 1873.
357. MAREY, E. J. *La Machine Animale.* Paris: F. Alcan, 1886.
358. MARINACCI, A. A. *Applied Electromyography.* Philadelphia, PA: Lea & Febiger, 1968.
359. MARKEE, J. E., W. W. THOMPSON, AND S. O. THORNE, JR. The relation of separately innervated areas of muscle to amount of shortening and strength of contraction. *Anat. Rec.* 97: 355, 1947.
360. MARMARELIS, P. Z., AND V. Z. MARMARELIS. *Analysis of Physiological Systems: The White-Noise Approach.* New York: Plenum, 1978.
361. MARSHALL, J., AND E. G. WALSH. Physiological tremor. *J. Neurol. Neurosurg. Psychiatry* 19: 260–267, 1956.

362. Mashima, H., K. Akazawa, H. Kushima, and K. Fujii. The force-load-velocity relation and the viscous-like force in the frog skeletal muscle. *Jpn. J. Physiol.* 22: 103–120, 1972.
363. Matthews, P. B. C. The dependence of tension upon extension in the stretch reflex of the soleus muscle of the decerebrate cat. *J. Physiol. London* 147: 521–546, 1959.
364. Matyushkin, D. P. Motor innervation of tonic muscle fibers of the oculomotor system. *Federation Proc.* 22: T728–T731, 1963. (Transl. from *Fiziol. Zh. SSSR Im. I. M. Sechenova* 48: 534, 1962.)
365. McArdle, B. Familial periodic paralysis. *Br. Med. Bull.* 12: 226–229, 1956.
366. McPhedran, A. M., R. B. Wuerker, and E. Henneman. Properties of motor units in a homogeneous red muscle (soleus) of the cat. *J. Neurophysiol.* 28: 71–84, 1965.
367. Merton, P. A. Speculations on the servo-control of movement. In: *The Spinal Cord*, edited by J. L. Malcolm, J. A. B. Gray, and G. E. W. Wolstenholme. Boston, MA: Little, Brown, 1953, p. 247–260. (Ciba Found. Symp.)
368. Merton, P. A. Interaction between muscle fibers in a twitch. *J. Physiol. London* 124: 311–324, 1954.
369. Meyer-Lohmann, J., W. Riebold, and D. Robrecht. Mechanical influence of the extrafusal muscle on the static behaviour of deefferented primary muscle spindle endings in cat. *Pfluegers Arch.* 352: 267–278, 1974.
370. Miledi, R. The acetylcholine sensitivity of frog muscle fibres after complete or partial denervation. *J. Physiol. London* 151: 1–23, 1960.
371. Millman, B. M. Mechanism of contraction in molluscan muscle. *Am. Zool.* 7: 583–591, 1967.
372. Milner-Brown, H. S., R. B. Stein, and R. Yemm. Changes in firing rate of human motor units during linearly changing voluntary contractions. *J. Physiol. London* 230: 371–390, 1973.
373. Milner-Brown, H. S., R. B. Stein, and R. Yemm. The contractile properties of human motor units during voluntary isometric contractions. *J. Physiol. London* 228: 285–306, 1973.
374. Mommaerts, W. F. H. M. The molecular transformation of actin. Parts I, II, III. *J. Biol. Chem.* 198: 445–457, 459–467, 469–475, 1952.
375. Monod, H. How muscles are used in the body. In: *The Structure and Function of Muscle* (2nd ed.), edited by G. H. Bourne. New York: Academic, 1972, vol. 1, p. 23–74.
376. Moore, A. D. Synthesized EMG waves and their implications. *Am. J. Phys. Med.* 46: 1302–1316, 1967.
377. Morrison, J. B. The mechanics of muscle function in locomotion. *J. Biomech.* 3: 431–451, 1970.
378. Morrison, J. B. The mechanics of the knee joint in relation to normal walking. *J. Biomech.* 3: 51–61, 1970.
379. Mosher, C. G., R. L. Gerlach, and D. G. Stuart. Soleus and anterior tibial motor units of the cat. *Brain Res.* 44: 1–11, 1972.
380. Moss, R. L., and W. Halpern. Elastic and viscous properties of resting frog skeletal muscle. *Biophys. J.* 17: 213–228, 1977.
381. Muybridge, E. *The Human Figure in Motion* [1887]. (Reprint.) New York: Dover, 1955.
382. Muybridge, E. *Animals in Motion* [1887]. (Reprint, edited by L. S. Brown.) New York: Dover, 1957.
383. Myrhage, R. Microvascular supply of skeletal muscle fibers. *Acta Orthop. Scand. Suppl.* 168: 1–46, 1977.
384. Needham, D. M. *Machina Carnis: The Biochemistry of Muscular Contraction in Its Historical Development*. Cambridge, England: Cambridge Univ. Press, 1971.
385. Newman, H. F., J. D. Northrup, and J. Devlin. Mechanism of human penile erection. *Invest. Urol.* 1: 350–353, 1964.
386. Newson-Davis, J., A. J. Pinching, A. Vincent, and S. G. Wilson. Function of circulating antibody to acetylcholine receptor in myasthenia gravis: investigation by plasma exchange. *Neurology* 28: 266–272, 1978.
386a. Nichols, T. R. Reflex and non-reflex stiffness of soleus muscle in the cat. In: *Control of Posture and Locomotion*, edited by R. B. Stein, K. G. Pearson, R. S. Smith, and J. B. Redford. New York: Plenum, 1974, p. 407–410. (Adv. in Behav. Biol., vol. 7.)
387. Nichols, T. R., and J. C. Houk. Reflex compensation for variation in the mechanical properties of a muscle. *Science* 181: 182–184, 1973.
388. Noble, M. I. M., and G. H. Pollack. Molecular mechanisms of contraction. *Circ. Res.* 40: 333–342, 1977.
389. Norris, F. H., Jr., and E. L. Gasteiger. Action potentials of single motor units in normal muscle. *Electroencephalogr. Clin. Neurophysiol.* 7: 115–126, 1955.
390. Pantin, C. F. A. Comparative physiology of muscle. *Br. Med. Bull.* 12: 199–202, 1956.
391. Partridge, L. D. Motor control and the myotatic reflex. *Am. J. Phys. Med.* 40: 96–103, 1961.
392. Partridge, L. D. A simulation approach to analysis of muscle control reflexes. *Digest Int. Cong. on Med. Electron., New York, 1961*, p. 105.
393. Partridge, L. D. Modifications of neural output signals by muscles: a frequency response study. *J. Appl. Physiol.* 20: 150–156, 1965.
394. Partridge, L. D. Signal-handling characteristics of load-moving skeletal muscle. *Am. J. Physiol.* 210: 1178–1191, 1966.
395. Partridge, L. D. Intrinsic feedback factors producing inertial compensation in muscle. *Biophys. J.* 7: 853–863, 1967.
396. Partridge, L. D. Interrelationships studied in a semibiological "reflex." *Am. J. Physiol.* 223: 144–158, 1972.
397. Partridge, L. D. Some consequences of nonlinear properties of a motor system. *Wiss. Z. Karl Marx Univ. Leipzig* 21: 156–165, 1972.; also *Biocybernetics* 4: 156–165, 1972.
398. Partridge, L. D. Integration in the central nervous system. In: *Engineering Principles in Physiology*, edited by J. H. U. Brown and D. S. Gann. New York: Academic, 1973, vol. 1 p. 47–98.
399. Partridge, L. D. Muscle properties: a problem for the motor controller physiologist. In: *Posture and Movement: Perspective for Integrating Sensory and Motor Research on the Mammalian Nervous System*, edited by R. E. Talbott and D. R. Humphrey. New York: Raven, 1979, p. 189–229.
400. Partridge, L. D., and G. H. Glaser. Adaptation in regulation of movement and posture. A study of stretch responses in spastic animals. *J. Neurophysiol.* 23: 257–268, 1960.
401. Peachey, L. D., and R. H. Adrian. Electrical properties of the transverse tubular system. In: *The Structure and Function of Muscle* (2nd ed.), edited by G. H. Bourne. New York: Academic, 1973, vol. 3, p. 1–30.
402. Pedotti, A. A study of motor coordination and neuromuscular activities in human locomotion. *Biol. Cybern.* 26: 53–62, 1977.
403. Pertuzon, E., and G. Comyn. Étude, sur un modèle muscle-movement, de la forme du signal de commande du muscle. *J. Physiol. Paris* 65: Suppl.: 284A, Oct. 1972.
404. Pierce, D. S., and I. H. Wagman. A method of recording from single muscle fibers or motor units in human skeletal muscle. *J. Appl. Physiol.* 19: 366–368, 1964.
405. Piper, H. Über die Rhythmik der Innervationsimpulse bei willkürlichen Muskelkontraktionen und über verschiedene Arten der künstlichen Tetanisierung menschlicher Muskeln. *Z. Biol. Munich* 53: 140–156, 1910.
406. Podolsky, R. J., A. C. Nolan, and S. A. Zaveler. Cross-bridge properties derived from muscle isotonic velocity transients. *Proc. Natl. Acad. Sci. USA* 64: 504–511, 1969.
407. Polissar, M. J. Physical chemistry of contractile process in muscle, I–IV. *Am. J. Physiol.* 168: 766–781, 782–792, 793–804, 805–811, 1952.
408. Pollard, J. H. *A Handbook of Numerical and Statistical Techniques*. London: Cambridge Univ. Press, 1977.
409. Portzehl von Hildegard, H. Der Arbeitszyklus geordneter Aktomosinsysteme (Muskel und Muskelmodelle). *Z. Naturforsch. Teil B* 7: 1–10, 1952.
410. Pratt, F. H. The all-or-none principle in graded response of skeletal muscle. *Am. J. Physiol.* 44: 517–542, 1917.
411. Pringle, J. W. S. The mechanism of the myogenic rhythm of certain insect striated muscles. *J. Physiol. London* 124: 269–291, 1954.

412. PRINGLE, J. W. S. Models of muscle. *Symp. Soc. Exp. Biol.* 14: 41–68, 1960.
413. PRINGLE, J. W. S. The contractile mechanism of insect fibrillar muscle. *Prog. Biophys. Mol. Biol.* 17: 1–60, 1967.
414. PRINGLE, J. W. S. Evidence from insect fibrillar muscle about the elementary contractile process. *J. Gen. Physiol. Suppl.* 50: 139–156, 1967.
415. PROCHAZKA, V. J., K. TATE, R. A. WESTERMAN, AND S. P. ZICCONE. Remote monitoring of muscle length and EMG in unrestrained cats. *Electroencephalogr. Clin. Neurophysiol.* 37: 649–653, 1974.
416. PROCHAZKA, A., R. A. WESTERMAN, AND S. P. ZICCONE. Discharges of single hindlimb afferents in the freely moving cat. *J. Neurophysiol.* 39: 1090–1104, 1976.
417. PROSKE, U., AND P. M. H. RACK. Short-range stiffness of slow fibers and twitch fibers in reptilian muscle. *Am. J. Physiol.* 231: 449–453, 1976.
418. PRYOR, M. G. M. Mechanical properties of fibres and muscles. In: *Progress in Biophysics and Biophysical Chemistry*, edited by J. A. V. Butler and J. T. Randall. New York: Academic, 1950, vol. 1, p. 216–268. Also in: *Deformation and Flow in Biological Systems*, edited by A. Frey-Wyssling. Amsterdam: North-Holland, 1950, p. 157–193.
419. PUROHIT, R. C., AND S. D. BECKETT. Penile pressure and muscle activity associated with erection and ejaculation in the dog. *Am. J. Physiol.* 231: 1343–1348, 1976.
420. RACK, P. M. H. The behavior of a mammalian muscle during sinusoidal stretching. *J. Physiol. London* 183: 1–14, 1966.
421. RACK, P. M. H., AND D. R. WESTBURY. The effects of length and stimulus rate on tension in the isometric cat soleus muscle. *J. Physiol. London* 204: 443–460, 1969.
422. RACK, P. M. H., AND D. R. WESTBURY. The short range stiffness of active mammalian muscle and its effect on mechanical properties. *J. Physiol. London* 240: 331–350, 1974.
423. RALSTON, H. J., V. T. INMAN, L. A. STRAIT, AND M. D. SHAFFRATH. Mechanics of human isolated voluntary muscle. *Am. J. Physiol.* 151: 612–620, 1947.
424. RAMSEY, R. W., AND S. F. STREET. The isometric length-tension diagram of isolated skeletal muscle fibers of the frog. *J. Cell. Comp. Physiol.* 15: 11–34, 1940.
425. RANATUNGA, K. W. Influence of temperature on the characteristics of summation of isometric mechanical responses of mammalian skeletal muscle. *Exp. Neurol.* 54: 513–532, 1977.
426. RANVIER, L. De quelques faits relatifs à l'histologie et à la physiologie des muscles striés. *Arch. Physiol. Norm. Pathol. Ser. 2*, 1: 1–15, 1874.
427. RASCH, P. J., AND R. K. BURKE. *Kinesiology and Applied Anatomy* (3rd ed.). Philadelphia, PA: Lea & Febiger, 1967.
428. REIGHARD, J., AND H. S. JENNINGS. *Anatomy of the Cat* (2nd ed.). New York: Holt, 1901.
429. REINKING, R. M., J. A. STEPHENS, AND D. G. STUART. The motor units of cat medial gastrocnemius: problem of their categorisation on the basis of mechanical properties. *Exp. Brain Res.* 23: 301–313, 1975.
430. REINKING, R. M., J. A. STEPHENS, AND D. G. STUART. The tendon organs of cat medial gastrocnemius: significance of motor unit type and size for the activation of Ib afferents. *J. Physiol. London* 250: 491–512, 1975.
431. REMINGTON, J. W. Introduction to muscle mechanics, with a glossary of terms. *Federation Proc.* 21: 954–963, 1962.
432. RICHMOND, F. J. R., AND V. C. ABRAHAMS. Morphology and enzyme histochemistry of dorsal muscles of the cat neck. *J. Neurophysiol.* 38: 1312–1321, 1975.
433. RITCHIE, J. M. The duration of the plateau of full activity in frog muscle. *J. Physiol. London* 124: 605–612, 1954.
434. ROBERTS, T. D. M. Rhythmic excitation of a stretch reflex, revealing (a) hysteresis, (b) difference between the responses to pulling and to stretching. *Q. J. Exp. Physiol. Cogn. Med. Sci.* 48: 328–345, 1963.
435. ROBINSON, D. A. The mechanics of human saccadic eye movement. *J. Physiol. London* 174: 245–264, 1964.
436. ROBINSON, D. A. A quantitative analysis of extraocular muscle cooperation and squint. *Invest. Ophthalmol.* 14: 801–825, 1975.
437. ROBINSON, M. The temporomandibular joint: theory of reflex controlled nonlever action of the mandible. *J. Am. Dent. Assoc.* 33: 1260–1271, 1946.
438. ROHMERT, W. Ermittlung von Erholungspausen für statische Arbeit des Menschen. *Int. Z. Angew. Physiol. Einschl. Arbeitsphysiol.* 18: 123–164, 1960.
439. ROOS, J. The latent period of skeletal muscle. *J. Physiol. London* 74: 17–33, 1932.
440. ROSEMANN, R. *Landois' Lehrbuch der Physiologie des Menschen* (17th ed.). Berlin: Urban-Schwarzenberg, 1921.
441. ROSENBLUETH, A. *The Transmission of Nerve Impulses at Neuroeffector Junctions and Peripheral Synapses*. New York: Wiley, 1950.
442. ROSENTHAL, J. Trophic interactions of neurons. In: *Handbook of Physiology. The Nervous System*, edited by J. M. Brookhart and V. B. Mountcastle. Bethesda, MD: Am. Physiol. Soc., 1977, sect. 1, vol. I, pt. 2, chapt. 21, p. 775–801.
443. ROSENTHAL, N. P., T. A. MCKEAN, W. J. ROBERTS, AND C. A. TERZUOLO. Frequency analysis of stretch reflex and its main subsystems in triceps surae muscles of the cat. *J. Neurophysiol.* 33: 713–749, 1970.
444. ROTHSCHUH, K. E. *History of Physiology* (transl. and edited by G. B. Risse). Huntington, NY: Krieger, 1973.
445. RUCH, T. C., AND H. D. PATTON. *Physiology and Biophysics*. Philadelphia, PA: Saunders, 1965.
446. RUSHTON, W. A. H. Nerve supply to Lucas's alpha substance. *J. Physiol. London* 74: 231–261, 1932.
447. SALMONS, S. Letter to Editor. *Med. Biol. Eng.* 13: 608–609, 1975.
448. SAMOJLOFF, A., AND W. WASSILJEWA. Zur Frage der plurisegmentellen Innervation. IV. Mitteilung. *Pfluegers Arch. Gesamte Physiol. Menschen Tiere* 213: 723–734, 1926.
449. SANDOW, A. Studies on the latent period of muscular contraction. Method. General properties of latency relaxation. *J. Cell. Comp. Physiol.* 24: 221–256, 1944.
450. SANDOW, A. Skeletal muscle. *Annu. Rev. Physiol.* 32: 87–138, 1970.
451. SANTESSON, C. G. Studien über die allgemeine Mechanik des Muskels. *Scand. Arch. Physiol.* 3: 381–436, 1892; 4: 46–97, 98–134, 135–193, 1893.
452. SASSA, K., AND C. S. SHERRINGTON. On the myogram of the flexor-reflex evoked by a single break-shock. *Proc. R. Soc. London Ser. B* 92: 108–117, 1921.
453. SAVANT, C. J. *Basic Feedback Control System Design*. New York: McGraw-Hill, 1958.
454. SCHÄFER, E. A., H. E. L. CANNEY, AND J. O. TUNSTALL. On the rhythm of muscular response to volitional impulses in man. *J. Physiol. London* 7: 111–117, 1886.
455. SCHÄFER, S. S., AND S. KIJEWSKI. The dependence of the acceleration response of primary muscle spindle endings on the mechanical properties of the muscle. *Pfluegers Arch.* 350: 101–122, 1974.
456. SCHÄFFER, B., AND J. ÖRKÉNYI. Time-relations of initial volume decrease and contraction in frog muscles. *Acta Biochim. Biophys. Acad. Sci. Hung.* 7: 255–261, 1972.
457. SCHILLER, H. H., AND E. STRÅLBERG. Human botulism studied with single-fiber electromyography. *Arch. Neurol. Chicago* 35: 346–349, 1978.
458. SCHOENBERG, M., J. B. WELLS, AND R. J. PODOLSKY. Muscle compliance and the longitudinal transmission of mechanical impulses. *J. Gen. Physiol.* 64: 623–642, 1974.
459. SCHULTZ, D. G., AND J. L. MELSA. *State Function and Linear Control Systems*. New York: McGraw-Hill, 1967.
460. SCHWARZACHER, H. G. Über die Länge und Anordnung der Muskelfasern in menschlichen Skeletmuskeln. *Acta Anat.* 37: 217–231, 1959.
461. SEIREG, A. Leonardo da Vinci—The bio-mechanician. In: *Biomechanics*, edited by D. Bootzin and H. C. Muffley. New York: Plenum, 1969, p. 65–74.
462. SEIREG, A., AND R. J. ARVIKAR. A mathematical model for evaluation of forces in lower extremities of the musculo-skeletal

system. *J. Biomech.* 6: 313-326, 1973.
463. SEVERIN, F. V., M. L. SHIK, AND G. N. ORLOVSKII. Work of the muscles and single motor neurons during controlled locomotion. *Biophysics USSR* 12: 762-772, 1967. (Transl. from *Biofizika* 12: 660-668, 1967.)
464. SEYFFARTH, H. The behavior of motor units in healthy and paretic muscles in man. Parts I and II. *Acta Psychiat. Neurol.* 16: 79-109, 261-278, 1941.
465. SHERRINGTON, C. S. Experiments in examination of the peripheral distribution of the fibres of the posterior roots of some spinal nerves. Part II. *Phil. Trans. R. Soc. London Ser. B* 190: 45-186, 1898.
466. SHERRINGTON, C. S. Some functional problems attached to convergence. *Proc. R. Soc. London Ser. B* 105: 332-362, 1930.
467. SHIAVI, R. G. *Control of and Interaction Between Motor Units in a Human Skeletal Muscle During Isometric Contractions* (Ph.D. thesis). Philadelphia, PA: Drexel Univ., 1972. (Abstr. in *Diss. Abstr.* 33: 72-24-563, 1972.)
468. SHIAVI, R., AND M. NEGIN. Multivariate analysis of simultaneously active motor units in human skeletal muscle. *Biol. Cybern.* 20: 9-16, 1975.
469. SICHEL, F. J. M. The elasticity of isolated resting skeletal muscle fibres. *J. Cell. Comp. Physiol.* 5: 21-42, 1934.
470. SICHEL, F. J. M. The relative elasticity of the sarcolemma and of the entire skeletal muscle fiber. *Am. J. Physiol.* 133: P446-P447, 1941.
471. SIMPSON, J. A. Terminology of electromyography. *Electroencephalogr. Clin. Neurophysiol.* 26: 224-226, 1969.
472. SINCLAIR, D. C. Muscles and fasciae. In: *Cunningham's Textbook of Anatomy* (11th ed.), edited by G. J. Romanes. London: Oxford Univ. Press, 1972, p. 259-397.
473. SMIDT, G. L. Biomechanical analysis of knee flexion and extension. *J. Biomech.* 6: 79-92, 1973.
474. SMITH, D. O. Central nervous control of excitatory and inhibitory neurons of opener muscle of the crayfish claw. *J. Neurophysiol.* 37: 108-118, 1974.
475. SMITH, J. L., B. BETTS, V. R. EDGERTON, AND R. F. ZERNICKE. Rapid ankle extension during paw shakes: selective recruitment of fast ankle extensors. *J. Neurophysiol.* 43: 612-620, 1980.
476. SOECHTING, J. F., AND W. J. ROBERTS. Transfer characteristics between EMG activity and muscle tension under isometric conditions in man. *J. Physiol. Paris* 70: 779-793, 1975.
477. SOTAVALTA, O. Some studies on the flying tones of insects and the determination of the frequency of the wing strokes. *Ann. Entomol. Fenn. Suom. Hyonteistiet Aikak.* 7: 32-52, 1941. (Abstr. in *Biol. Abstr.* 21: 23712, 1947.)
478. SRÉTER, F. A., A. R. LUFF, AND J. GERGELY. Effect of cross-reinnervation on physiological parameters and on properties of myosin and sarcoplasmic reticulum of fast and slow muscles of the rabbit. *J. Gen. Physiol.* 66: 811-821, 1975.
479. STARK, L. *Neurological Control Systems: Studies in Bioengineering.* New York: Plenum, 1968.
480. STEIN, R. B. Peripheral control of movement. *Physiol. Rev.* 54: 215-243, 1974.
481. STEIN, R. B., A. S. FRENCH, A. MANNARD, AND R. YEMM. New methods for analysing motor function in man and animals. *Brain Res.* 40: 187-192, 1972.
482. STEINBERGER, W. W., AND E. M. SMITH. Maintenance of denervated rabbit muscle with direct electrostimulation. *Arch. Phys. Med. Rehabil.* 49: 573-577, 1968.
483. STEPHENS, J. A., R. M. REINKING, AND D. G. STUART. The motor unit of cat medial gastrocnemius: electrical and mechanical properties as a function of muscle length. *J. Morphol.* 146: 495-512, 1975.
484. STEPHENS, J. A., AND D. G. STUART. The motor units of cat medial gastrocnemius: speed-size relations and their significance for the recruitment order of motor neurons. *Brain Res.* 91: 177-195, 1975.
485. STEPHENS, J. A., AND D. G. STUART. The motor units of cat medial gastrocnemius: twitch potentiation and twitch-tetanus ratio. *Pfluegers Arch.* 356: 359-372, 1975.
486. STETSON, R. H., AND H. D. BOUMAN. The coordination of simple skilled movements. *Arch. Neerl. Physiol.* 20: 177-254, 1935.
487. SUZUKI, J-I., AND B. COHEN. Integration of semicircular canal activity. *J. Neurophysiol.* 29: 981-995, 1966.
488. TAKEUCHI, A., AND N. TAKEUCHI. A study of the inhibitory action of γ-amino-butyric acid on neuromuscular transmission in the crayfish. *J. Physiol. London* 183: 418-432, 1966.
489. TARDIEU, C., P. COLBEAU-JUSTIN, M. D. BRET, A. LESPARGOT, E. HUET DE LA TOUR, AND G. TARDIEU. An apparatus and a method for measuring the relationship of triceps surae torques to tibiotarsal angles in man. *Eur. J. Appl. Physiol. Occup. Physiol.* 35: 11-20, 1976.
490. TASHIRO, N. Mechanical properties of the longitudinal and circular muscle in the earthworm. *J. Exp. Biol.* 54: 101-110, 1971.
491. TASHIRO, N., AND T. YAMAMOTO. The phasic and tonic contraction in the longitudinal muscle of the earthworm. *J. Exp. Biol.* 55: 111-122, 1971.
492. TAYLOR, A. Grouping of action potentials in voluntary muscle. *J. Physiol. London* 157: 55P-56P, 1961.
493. TAYLOR, A. The significance of grouping of motor unit activity. *J. Physiol. London* 162: 259-269, 1962.
494. TAYLOR, C. P. S. Isometric muscle contraction and the active state: an analog computer study. *Biophys. J.* 9: 759-780, 1969.
495. TEIG, E. Force and contraction velocity of the middle ear muscles in the cat and the rabbit. *Acta Physiol. Scand.* 84: 1-10, 1972.
496. TEIG, E. Tension and contraction time of motor units of the middle ear muscles in the cat. *Acta Physiol. Scand.* 84: 11-21, 1972.
497. TERZUOLO, C. A., J. F. SOECHTING, AND R. PALMINTERI. Studies on the control of some simple motor tasks. III. Comparison of the EMG pattern during ballistically initiated movements in man and squirrel monkey. *Brain Res.* 62: 242-246, 1973.
498. TERZUOLO, C. A., J. F. SOECHTING, AND P. VIVIANI. Studies on the control of some simple motor tasks. I. Relations between parameters of movement and EMG activities. *Brain Res.* 58: 212-216, 1973.
499. THESLEFF, S. Supersensitivity of skeletal muscle produced by botulinum toxin. *J. Physiol. London* 151: 598-607, 1960.
500. THOMAS, J. G. The torque angle transfer function of the human eye. *Kybernetik* 3: 254-263, 1967.
501. THOMSON, J. D. Dimensional and dynamic features of mammalian gastrocnemius muscle. *Am. J. Physiol.* 200: 951-954, 1961.
502. THORSON, J., AND D. C. S. WHITE. Distributed representations for actin-myosin interaction in the oscillatory contraction of muscle. *Biophys. J.* 9: 360-390, 1969.
503. THORSON, J., AND D. C. S. WHITE. Dynamic force measurement at the microgram level, with application to myofibrils of striated muscle. *IEEE Trans. Bio.-Med. Eng.* 22: 293-299, 1975.
504. TIMOSHENKO, S. P., AND J. M. GERE. *Mechanics of Materials.* New York: Van Nostrand, 1972.
505. TOKUMASU, K., K. GOTO, AND B. COHEN. Eye movements produced by the superior oblique muscle. *Arch. Ophthalmol.* 73: 851-862, 1965.
506. TOWNSEND, M. A. A relationship between muscle performance when producing and absorbing work. *J. Biomech.* 6: 261-265, 1973.
507. TOWNSEND, M. A., S. P. LAINHART, R. SHIAVI, AND J. CAYLOR. Variability and biomechanics of synergy patterns of some lower-limb muscles during ascending and descending stairs and level walking. *Med. Biol. Eng.* 16: 681-688, 1978.
508. TRNKOCZY, A. Static hysteresis loop of electrically stimulated muscles. *Med. Biol. Eng.* 12: 182-187, 1974.
509. TRUEMAN, E. R., AND A. PACKARD. Motor performances of some cephalopods. *J. Exp. Biol.* 49: 495-507, 1968.

510. TRUONG, X. T. Extensional wave-propagation characteristics in striated muscle. *J. Acoust. Soc. Am.* 51: 1352-1356, 1972.
511. TRUONG, X. T. Visco-elastic propagation of longitudinal waves in skeletal muscle. *J. Biomech.* 5: 1-10, 1972.
512. TRUONG, X. T. Viscoelastic wave propagation and rheologic properties of skeletal muscle. *Am. J. Physiol.* 226: 256-264, 1974.
513. TWAROG, B. M. The regulation of catch in molluscan muscle. *J. Gen. Physiol.* 50: (Suppl.) 157-168, 1967.
514. TYRER, N. M. Innervation of the abdominal intersegmental muscles in the grass-hopper. I, II. *J. Exp. Biol.* 55: 305-314, 315-324, 1971.
515. USHERWOOD, P. N. R. Insect neuromuscular mechanisms. *Am. Zool.* 7: 553-582, 1967.
516. USHERWOOD, P. N. R., AND H. GRUNDFEST. Peripheral inhibition in skeletal muscle of insects. *J. Neurophysiol.* 28: 497-518, 1965.
517. VAN HARREVELD, A. On the force and size of motor units in the rabbit's sartorius muscle. *Am. J. Physiol.* 151: 96-106, 1947.
518. VIVIANI, P., J. F. SOECHTING, AND C. A. TERZUOLO. Influence of mechanical properties on the relation between EMG activity and torque. *J. Physiol. Paris* 72: 45-58, 1976.
519. VOLKMANN, A. W. Versuche und Betrachtungen über Muskelcontractilität. *Arch. Anat. Physiol. Wiss. Med.* 215-288, 1858.
520. VON BUDDENBROCK, W. *Vergleichende Physiologie. Physiologie der Erfolgsorgane.* Basel, Switzerland: Birkhäuser, 1961, vol. V.
521. WACHOLDER, K. Willkürliche Haltung und Bewegung inbesondere im Lichte elektrophysiologisher Untersuchungen. *Ergeb. Physiol. Biol. Chem. Exp. Pharmakol.* 26: 568-775, 1928.
522. WAGNER, R. Muskeltonus und Aktionsstrom im Umklammerungsreflex. *Z. Biol. Munich* 82: 21-26, 1924.
523. WAGNER, R. Arbeitsdiagramme bei der Willkürbewegung I and II. *Z. Biol. Munich* 86: 367-396, 397-426, 1927.
524. WAINWRIGHT, S. A., F. VOSBURGH, AND J. H. HEBRANK. Shark skin: function in locomotion. *Science* 202: 747-749, 1978.
525. WALKER, L. B., JR. Multiple motor innervation of individual muscle fibers in the m. tibialis anterior of the dog. *Anat. Rec.* 139: 1-11, 1961.
526. WALKER, S. M. Failure of potentiation in successive, posttetanic, and summated twitches in cooled skeletal muscle of the rat. *Am. J. Physiol.* 166: 480-484, 1951.
527. WALKER, S. M. Tension and extensibility changes in muscle suddenly stretched during tetanus. *Am. J. Physiol.* 172: 37-41, 1953.
528. WALKER, S. M. The relation of stretch and of temperature to contraction of skeletal muscle. Parts I, II. *Am. J. Phys. Med.* 39: 191-215, 234-258, 1960.
529. WALKER, S. M. Lengthening contraction and interpretations of active state tension in the isometric twitch response of skeletal muscle. *Am. J. Phys. Med.* 55: 192-204, 1976.
530. WALKER, S. M., AND A. G. THOMAS. Changes in twitch tension induced by quick stretch and stress relaxation. *Am. J. Physiol.* 198: 523-527, 1960.
531. WALMSLEY, B., J. A. HODGSON, AND R. E. BURKE. The forces produced by hind limb muscles in freely moving cats. *Soc. Neurosci. Abstr.* 3: 280, 1978.
532. WALMSLEY, B., J. A. HODGSON, AND R. E. BURKE. Forces produced by medial gastrocnemius and soleus muscles during locomotion in freely moving cats. *J. Neurophysiol.* 41: 1203-1216, 1978.
533. WALTON, J. N. (editor). *Disorders of Voluntary Muscle* (3rd ed.). London: Churchill Livingstone, 1974.
534. WARD, M. *Mountain Medicine, a Clinical Study of Cold and High Altitude.* New York: Van Nostrand, 1975.
535. WATKINS, B. O. *Introduction to Control Systems.* New York: MacMillan, 1969.
536. WEAST, R. C. (editor). *Handbook of Chemistry and Physics* (56th ed.). Cleveland, OH: CRC Press, 1975.
537. WEBER, E. Muskelbewegung. In: *Handwörterbuch der Physiologie,* edited by R. Wagner. Brunswick, Germany: Bieweg, 1846, vol. III, pt. 2, p. 1-122.
538. WEBER, E. H. Ueber Eduard Weber's Entdeckungen in der Lehre von der Muskelcontraction. *Arch. Anat. Physiol. Wiss. Med.* 483-527, 1846.
539. WEBSTER, D. D. A method of measuring the dynamic characteristics of muscle rigidity, strength, and tremor in the upper extremity. *IRE Trans. Med. Electron.* 6: 159-164, 1959.
540. WEIJS, W. A., AND R. DAMTUMA. Electromyography and mechanics of mastication in the albino rat. *J. Morphol.* 146: 1-34, 1975.
541. WELLS, J. B. Comparison of mechanical properties between slow and fast mammalian muscles. *J. Physiol. London* 178: 252-269, 1965.
542. WELLS, J. B. Relationship between elastic and contractile components in mammalian skeletal muscle. *Nature* 214: 198-199, 1967.
543. WELTMAN, G., H. GROTH, AND J. LYMAN. A myoelectric system for training functional dissociation of muscles. *Arch. Phys. Med. Rehabil.* 43: 534-537, 1962.
544. WHITE, D. C. S., AND J. THORSON. The kinetics of muscle contraction. *Prog. Biophys. Mol. Biol.* 27: 173-255, 1973.
545. WHITE, H. J., AND S. TAUBER. *Systems Analysis.* Philadelphia, PA: Saunders, 1969.
546. WIENER, N. Response of nonlinear device to noise. *MIT Radiation Lab Report* 5: 16S (129), 1942.
547. WIENER, N. *Cybernetics: Control and Communications in the Animal and the Machine.* New York: Wiley, 1948.
548. WILDER, B. J., T. C. KENASTON, P. A. MABE, JR., T. L. DULIN, J. A. GERGAN, F. R. HOOK, JR., M. WILLIAMS, AND J. E. MARKEE. Observations on fatigue patterns of anterior tibial muscles. *Am. J. Phys. Med.* 32: 331-337, 1953.
549. WILKIE, D. R. The relation between force and velocity in human muscle. *J. Physiol. London* 110: 249-280, 1950.
550. WILKIE, D. R. The mechanical properties of muscle. *Br. Med. Bull.* 12: 177-182, 1956.
551. WILKIE, D. R. The contractile system. In: *Starling's Principles of Human Physiology* (14th ed.), edited by H. Davson and M. G. Eggleton. London: Lea & Febiger, 1968, p. 812-831.
552. WILLS, J. H. Speed of responses of various muscles of cats. *Am. J. Physiol.* 136: 623-628, 1942.
553. WILSON, D. M. Bifunctional muscles in the thorax of grasshoppers. *J. Exp. Biol.* 39: 669-677, 1962.
554. WILSON, D. M., AND J. L. LARIMER. The catch property of ordinary muscle. *Proc. Natl. Acad. Sci. USA* 61: 909-916, 1968.
555. WILSON, D. M., D. O. SMITH, AND P. DEMPSTER. Length and tension hysteresis during sinusoidal and step function stimulation of arthropod muscle. *Am. J. Physiol.* 218: 916-922, 1970.
556. WINTER, D. A., R. K. GREENLAW, AND D. A. HOBSON. Television-computer analyses of kinematics of human gait. *Comput. Biomed. Res.* 5: 498-504, 1972.
557. WISNES, A., AND A. KIRKEØ. Regional distribution of blood flow in calf muscles of rat during passive stretch and sustained contraction. *Acta Physiol. Scand.* 96: 256-266, 1976.
558. WOLEDGE, R. C. The energetics of tortoise muscle. *J. Physiol. London* 197: 685-707, 1968.
559. WOOD, G. A., AND L. S. JENNINGS. On the use of the spline function for data smoothing. *J. Biomech.* 12: 477-479, 1979.
560. WOODBURY, J. W., A. M. GORDON, AND J. T. CONRAD. Muscle. In: *Physiology and Biophysics* (19th ed.), edited by T. C. Ruch and H. D. Patton. Philadelphia, PA: Saunders, 1965, p. 113-152.
561. WUERKER, R. B., A. M. MCPHEDRAN, AND E. HENNEMAN. Properties of motor units in a heterogeneous pale muscle (m. gastrocnemius) of the cat. *J. Neurophysiol.* 28: 85-99, 1965.
562. WYMAN, J., JR. Studies on the relation of work and heat in tortoise muscle. *J. Physiol. London* 61: 337-352, 1926.
563. YAGER, J. G. *The Electromyogram as a Predictor of Muscle Mechanical Response in Locomotion* (Ph.D. thesis). Memphis, Univ. of Tennessee, 1972. (Abstr. in *Diss Abstr.* 33B: 3909-3910, 1972.)
564. YAMAMOTO, T. Electrical and mechanical properties of the red

and white muscles in the silver carp. *J. Exp. Biol.* 57: 551–567, 1972.
565. YOUNG, M. Molecular basis of muscle contraction. *Annu. Rev. Biochem.* 38: 913–950, 1969.
566. ZACHAR, J. *Electrogenesis and Contractility in Skeletal Muscle Cells.* Bratislava, Czechoslovakia: Slovak Acad. Sci., 1971.
567. ZACHAR, J., AND D. ZACHAROVÁ. The length-tension diagram of single muscle fibres of the crayfish. *Experientia* 22: 451–452, 1966.
568. ZAHALAK, G. I., J. DUFFY, P. A. STEWART, H. M. LITCHMAN, R. H. HAWLEY, AND P. R. PASLAY. Force-velocity-EMG data for the skeletal muscle of athletes. *National Science Found. Report* GK 40010X-32, 1973.
569. ZIERLER, K. L. Some aspects of the biophysics of muscle. In: *The Structure and Function of Muscle* (2nd ed.), edited by G. H. Bourne. New York: Academic, 1973, vol. 3, p. 117–183.
570. ZIERLER, K. I. Mechanism of muscle contraction and its energetics. In: *Medical Physiology* (13th ed.), edited by V. B. Mountcastle. St. Louis, MO: Mosby, 1974, vol. 1, p. 77–120.
571. ZIMKIN, N. V., AND T. G. PAKHOMOVA. The interrelationship between hardness, viscosity, strength, and bioelectric activity in human muscles [in Russian]. *Fiziol. Zh. SSSR im. I. M. Sechenova* 58: 1099–1108, 1972. (Abstr. in *Biol. Abstr.* 56: 50058, 1973.)
572. ZIMKIN, N. V., V. G. PANOV, AND V. T. RAIKOV. Fast and slow fibers in human muscles. *Neurosci. Behav. Physiol.* 6: 1–8, 1973. (Transl. from *Fiziol. Zh. SSSR im. I. M. Sechenova* 57: 1259–1266, 1971.)
573. ZUBER, B. L. Eye movement dynamics in the cat: the final motor pathway. *Exp. Neurol.* 20: 255–260, 1968.
574. ZUNIGA, E. N., AND D. G. SIMONS. Nonlinear relationship between averaged electromyogram potential and muscle tension in normal subjects. *Arch. Phys. Med. Rehabil.* 50: 613–620, 1969.

For additional selected references on muscle mechanical function, see references 182, 308, and 384, each of which cites between 950 and 3,000 items. For early German language sources see reference 400. We should like to suggest that the extensive early muscle literature is best read with the aid of a nineteenth century German dictionary and an old anatomy text (e.g., ref. 428) to clarify spelling and nomenclature changes.

CHAPTER 4

Transmitters in motor systems

K. KRNJEVIĆ | *Departments of Anesthesia Research and Physiology, McGill University, Montreal, Quebec, Canada*

CHAPTER CONTENTS

Chemical Transmitters
  Definition
    Varieties of transmitters
      Intracellular mediators
      Intercellular communication
  Identification of transmitters
    Theory
    Practical considerations
    Conclusions
Transmitters in Peripheral Motor Systems
Transmitters in Spinal Motor Mechanisms
  Spinal motoneurons and their synaptic control
    Monosynaptic reflex
    Other excitatory inputs on motoneurons
    Inhibitory inputs on motoneurons
    Presynaptic inhibition
    Other relevant spinal mechanisms
Transmitters in Supraspinal Motor Systems
  Brain stem
    Cranial motoneurons
    Red nucleus
    Reticulospinal cells
    Vestibulospinal cells
  Cerebellum
    Cerebellar output (Purkinje cells)
    Cerebellar inhibitory interneurons
    Excitatory interneurons: the granule cells
    Cerebellar inputs
  Basal ganglia
    Transmitters in various striatal pathways
    Nigrostriatal pathway
    Other striatal afferents
    Striatonigral pathways
    Other striatal efferent pathways
    Pallidosubthalamic projection
    Striatal interneurons
  Motor cortex
    Pyramidal tract neurons
    Cortical inhibitory mechanisms
    Other transmitters in the cortex

THIS CHAPTER deals principally with synaptic mechanisms in vertebrates, especially mammals. Many of the basic mechanisms, however, are widely distributed. The essential steps in reflex movement are beautifully illustrated by their simplest expression, the coupling of external stimulus to motor response in a single-celled animal, Paramecium. This inhabitant of pond water is propelled by the activity of cilia. If it meets an obstacle the ciliary movements are reversed, and the animal backs away (Fig. 1). How is this done? Of course there are no separate sensory and motor cells, so here transmission is entirely intracellular. According to Eckert (119), the messenger is Ca^{2+}: the mechanical stimulus initiates a depolarization, which increases the membrane permeability to Ca^{2+}. Because pond water is usually rich in Ca^{2+}, this depolarization is followed by an influx of Ca^{2+} that triggers the reversal of ciliary beating; but the reversal persists only a short time, because active removal of Ca^{2+} soon returns the internal free Ca^{2+} to its normal low level.

What makes this example particularly illuminating is that it summarizes, in an abbreviated version, some important features of motor control in Metazoa. Muscle contraction is also triggered by a rise in intracellular free Ca^{2+}, and the primary sensory stimulus activates synaptic transmission in a reflex pathway by initiating a depolarization that spreads to the central terminals of the afferent fibers and increases their permeability to Ca^{2+}: in this case, however, internal Ca^{2+} triggers the secretion of an intercellular transmitter [the analogy may be even closer if contractile proteins are involved in the mechanism of transmitter release (28)], which tends to depolarize the next cell in the reflex arc, and so on. But even the simplest vertebrate reflex (the stretch reflex) involves three separate kinds of cells in series and correspondingly two sets of cellular junctions; and, of course, far greater populations of cells and synapses are involved in other reflexes and various types of motor behavior.

Perhaps the most realistic way of looking at neurons is to think of them primarily as secretory cells whose main function is to receive and convey information. Their ability to release chemical agents for purposes of intercellular communication may well be the only property that all neurons have in common. [Of course, they must also be able to recognize such agents and make appropriate responses, but this is a more general property of body cells, without which no integrated organism could exist (172).] As in the case of other secretory cells, secretion is activated by Ca^{2+} entry (101, 175, 235, 347, 425). Because depolarization generally tends to raise the membrane permeability to

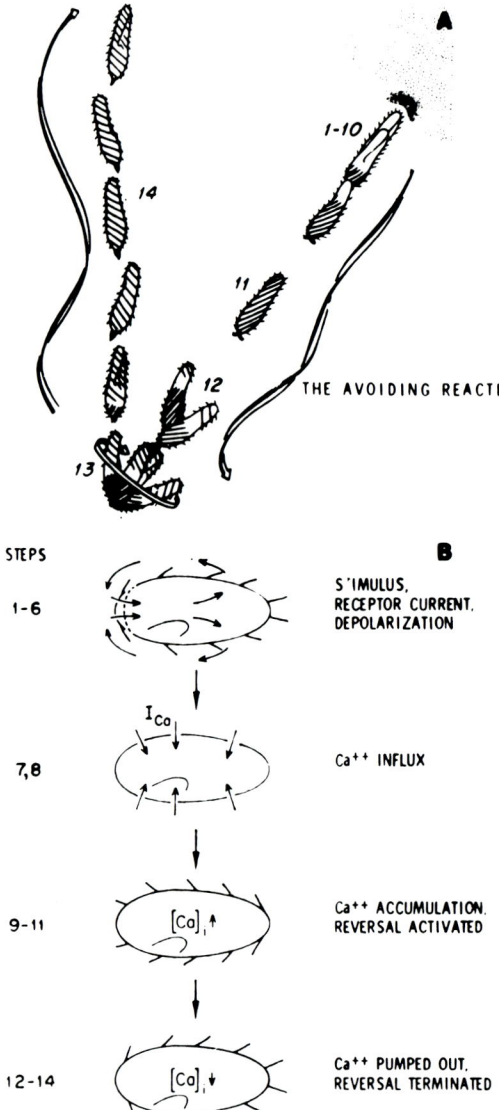

FIG. 1. The avoiding reaction of Paramecium. *A*: retreat from stimulus and resumption of forward locomotion. *B*: sequence of steps corresponding to numbers in *A*. *Step 1*, stretch of anterior membrane upon collision with obstacle; *step 2*, local increase in membrane conductance; *step 3*, inward receptor current through stimulated membrane; *step 4*, electrotonic spread of receptor current produces *step 5*, outward current through rest of membrane (*arrows* show current flow). *Step 6*, depolarization of cell membrane (receptor potential) produces *step 7*, increase in calcium conductance; *step 8*, inward Ca^{2+} current; *step 9*, rise in intracellular Ca^{2+} concentration; *step 10*, cilia reverse beat; and *step 11*, cell swims backward. *Step 12*, Ca^{2+} is pumped out; *step 13*, intracellular concentration of Ca^{2+} drops, cilia resume normal orientation; and *step 14*, cell swims forward. [From Eckert (119). Copyright 1972 by the American Association for the Advancement of Science.]

secretory function appears to be concentrated at the nerve endings. These are more or less closely related to other cells and therefore any secreted material can be used to transfer information particularly efficiently and selectively, as well as with minimum latency. By far the most important determinant of the time course of transmission is distance, because diffusion times vary as the square of the distance: hence for distances of less than 1 μm length, diffusion delays are less than 1 ms; for distances of 1 cm or more, diffusion times are measured in years! This explains why nerve fibers had to be developed in larger organisms to conduct rapid electrical signals—for short distances by electrotonic spread, for greater distances by action potentials. Only animals with a nervous system would be capable of reacting quickly to changes in their environment. It is therefore not surprising that rapid purposeful movements are characteristic only of Protozoans and Metazoans that possess nerve fibers (and not plants or sponges).

CHEMICAL TRANSMITTERS

Definition

Any product of cell activity that can initiate a significant change in cellular function (in the same or another cell) is a potential transmitter. This general definition evidently covers a tremendous range of agents. On the one hand it includes electricity and some inorganic ions. Electric transmission, though once favored as the predominant synaptic mechanism, is now believed to be restricted to relatively few sites in the central nervous system of the mammal (315). Its characteristics have been fully described earlier (26). It is not discussed further here, except where it is particularly relevant for motor control (as in subsection MONOSYNAPTIC REFLEX, p. 115).

On the other hand, any substance that is a substrate for an enzyme or can regulate its activity could also be a transmitter. Indeed, receptors for transmitters such as acetylcholine (ACh) have many of the attributes of enzymes (179, 408): they are largely protein in nature, and the specific receptor sites correspond to allosteric sites, the activation of which causes a conformational change in the protein macromolecule, thus altering its functional state (351). In the case of receptors, however, the typical result is a change in membrane ionic permeability rather than in enzymatic activity. Some transmitters may act on membrane-held enzymes, as has been suggested for the activation of adenylate cyclase by catecholamines (475).

Varieties of Transmitters

INTRACELLULAR MEDIATORS. Though often called "messengers," these are effectively transmitters. The most important may well be Ca^{2+}, as already indicated. Its intracellular functions include the initiation of var-

Ca^{2+} (12, 13), the transfer of information from cell to cell is mediated by the secretion of substances that initiate (or facilitate) depolarization (these are usually excitatory) or that prevent depolarization (usually inhibitory).

In most central neurons that we know about, the

ious effector processes, e.g., muscle contraction (61); glandular secretion, as well as the secretion of hormones and other transmitters from endocrine and nerve cells (425); the activation of several enzymes such as adenylate cyclase, phosphodiesterase, protein kinases, and ATPase (54a, 411); and a variable component of membrane potassium permeability (268, 344, 345). Some other agents are also believed to play a comparable important role as intracellular mediators, such as cyclic nucleotides (164, 474) and prostaglandins (199, 432).

INTERCELLULAR COMMUNICATION. *Slowly and diffusely acting hormones, growth factors, etc.* These are relatively complex molecules, being peptides, proteins, or steroids. They should probably be classed into two main groups.

1. The first group consists of the hormones released into the general circulation by the nonneural endocrine glands, such as the pituitary, thyroid, pancreas, and gonads. Some of these hormones, such as adrenocorticotrophins and the gonadotrophins, act on specific targets that are outside the nervous system, though they may also alter the excitability of certain brain cells and thus affect behavior (97). Others, like insulin, thyroxin, and calcitonin, directly or indirectly influence the metabolic or ionic exchanges of cells throughout the body, including those of the brain. Hormones typically produce changes in RNA synthesis and enzyme activity and in general act on intracellular targets (335, 378, 399) that are reached either directly or by internalization of the surface-receptor: hormone complex (52). Any actions on the nervous system are therefore likely to be relatively slow and inconspicuous and perhaps most important for the growth of cells and synapses during development (335, 405). But there are more striking immediate effects, such as the marked depression of neuronal excitability induced by progesterone and related molecules (438). Thus the isomer of pregnanediol, commercially known as Althesin or Alphathesin, is a powerful, rapidly acting general anesthetic (385). Cyclic variations in secretion of such hormones may influence to a significant extent motor activity and therefore need to be kept in mind in long-term studies of motor behavior.

2. In the second group we have peptides that are released by neural, endocrine, and paracrine cells, especially in the gut and the brain. They may act as typical hormones, carried by blood and operating at some distance on endocrine or exocrine glands or smooth muscle; or they may be local hormones and perhaps even synaptic transmitters, exciting or inhibiting adjacent nerve cells or muscle cells at synapses (167, 413, 456). The longest known peptides of this type, such as substance P, cholecystokinin, gastrin, and secretin, were first isolated from the gut and were long believed to be purely intestinal hormones. In recent years they have all been shown to exist in the central nervous system in specific groups of nerve fibers (123, 188, 305, 314, 413).

TABLE 1. *Chemical Messengers*

Intracellular
  Ca^{2+}
  Cyclic nucleotides
  Prostaglandins
  H^+
  Substrates for various enzymes
Intercellular
Hormones
  With widespread actions, possibly on many tissues, controlling cellular growth, metabolism, and ionic environment
    Insulin
    Thyroxin
    Calcitonin
    Antidiuretic hormone
    Growth hormone
    Adrenocorticosteroids
    Estrogens
    Nerve growth factor, etc.
  Acting mainly on other endocrine glands
    Hypothalamopituitary
      Thyrotropin-releasing hormone
      Gonadotropin-releasing hormones
      Somatostatin
    Released by anterior pituitary
      Adrenocorticotropin
      Thyrotropin
      Gonadotropins, etc.
  Neurointestinal hormones
    Substance P
    Secretin
    Cholecystokinin
    Opioid hormones, etc.
Synaptic transmitters (with rapid actions at synapses)
  Excitatory
    Well established or highly probable
      Acetylcholine (nicotinic)
      L-Glutamate
      L-Aspartate
    Mostly hypothetical
      ATP
      Noradrenaline
      Dopamine
      Serotonin
      Histamine
      Peptides: substance P, somatostatin
  Inhibitory
    Well established
      GABA
      Glycine
    Largely hypothetical
      β-Alanine
      Taurine, imidazole acetic guanidine derivatives
      Acetylcholine
      ATP
      Norepinephrine, dopamine, serotonin, histamine
      Peptides
Neuromodulators
  Mostly hypothetical
    Acetylcholine, muscarinic
    Monoamines: norepinephrine, dopamine, serotonin
    Peptides: substance P, somatostatin, enkephalins, etc.

Overlapping this group are the neuropeptides of the hypothalamopituitary complex (434), including the "releasing factors" or hormones that are secreted by hypothalamic cells into the hypothalamopituitary portal system and that control the release of hormones from the pituitary. Several of these peptides, as well as angiotensin and opioids (enkephalin and endorphin), have been found in various central and peripheral nerve fibers (188). Because they have proved to have significant excitatory or inhibitory actions on nerve cells (100, 218, 414), they may also operate as synaptic transmitters or modulators (see next subsection).

Synaptic transmitters. It must be emphasized that the most generally accepted theories about synaptic transmitters and how they operate are based on information obtained at neuromuscular junctions. Thus, according to the model of the vertebrate nerve-muscle junction (Fig. 2), the transmitter (ACh) is synthesized from its precursor (choline) and prepackaged in multimolecular "quanta" in the presynaptic nerve endings, from which it is released by Ca^{2+} influx upon the arrival of an action potential; the released transmitter diffuses with minimal delay (<1 ms) across the minute junctional gap and reacts with specific receptors situated in the immediately adjacent postsynaptic membrane: this reaction leads to a selective increase in permeability (especially for Na^+ as well as for K^+) resulting in Na^+ influx, depolarization, and therefore excitation; the reaction is extremely fast and reversible, and the transmitter action is almost immediately terminated by removal of the transmitter through hydrolysis of ACh, mediated by a specific acetylcholinesterase (240, 241, 481). Unfortunately most of these features are not typical of central synapses. Nicotinic cholinergic synapses are very rare in the central nervous system; there is little evidence of quantal transmission; central transmitters are probably removed from the extracellular medium by uptake into cells; and conductance changes are often difficult to detect (at least at excitatory synapses).

The most conspicuous synaptic actions in the CNS are inhibitory and are generated by large increases in Cl^- permeability. A more realistic and therefore useful model is that of the crustacean neuromuscular system, where a double innervation provides both excitatory and inhibitory control, mediated by the release of glutamate and γ-aminobutyric acid (GABA), respectively (481). The parallel is made particularly relevant by the fact that glutamate and GABA may well be the most important excitatory and inhibitory transmitters in the mammalian central nervous system. However, since we still know so little about the mechanisms of most central synapses (except for inhibitory synapses), it is better not to place too many restrictions on the use of the term synaptic transmitter, though most authors would agree that it is particularly appropriate for any agent released from nerve ending at synapses that have a brief excitatory or inhibitory action on the immediately adjacent postsynaptic nerurons. Whether the same term should be used to describe agents that act more diffusely and at a somewhat greater distance (because they are released from "varicosities" or other unconventional synapses) or because their action is relatively slow and prolonged is less clear. There is some reason for considering them as a separate category, discussed in the next subsection.

Neuromodulators. This is a somewhat nebulous

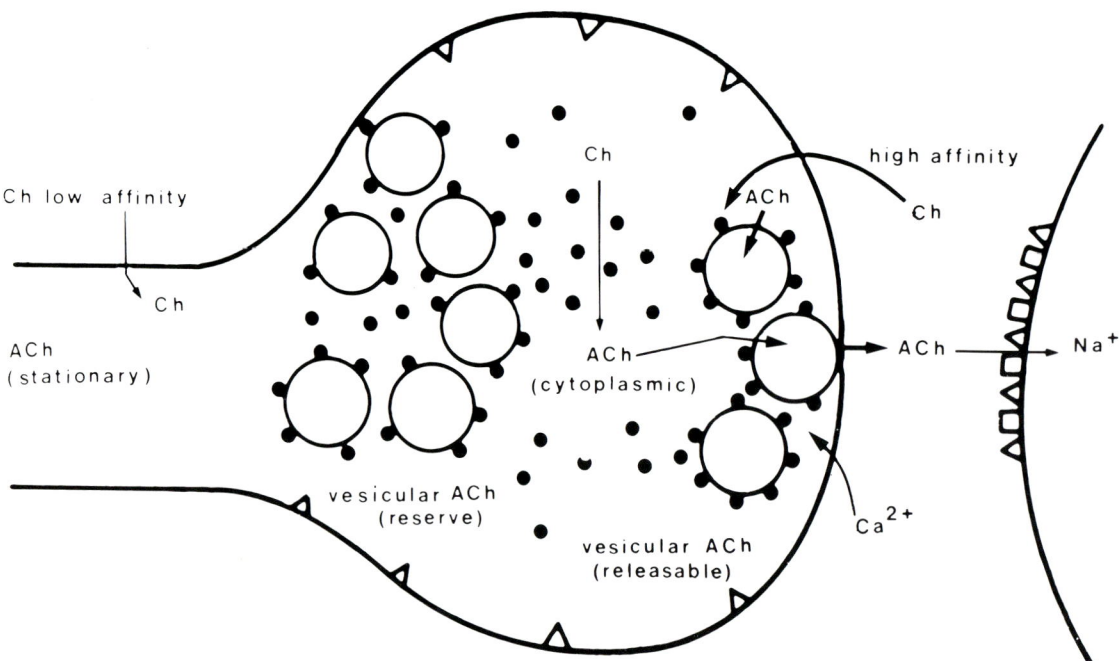

FIG. 2. Scheme illustrating synthesis, storage, and release of ACh in a model cholinergic nerve terminal. Choline acetyltransferase is represented by *filled dots* inside terminal, acetylcholinesterase by *open triangles* both inside terminal and on surface of postsynaptic cell, and receptors on latter by *open squares*. Ch, choline. [From MacIntosh and Collier (323).]

category into which are often placed agents that are not clearly either hormones or synaptic transmitters (though the same agent, e.g., ACh, may be a typical transmitter at one site and a "modulator" at another). To some extent this reflects our ignorance about their precise mode of action. On the other hand we know that certain substances that are released in the brain have prolonged facilitatory effects on other synaptic actions, which are most easily described as modulation. Thus acetylcholine, acting as a muscarinic substance, does not produce very quick excitatory effects through an increase in membrane conductance, but rather produces a prolonged activation of other synaptic inputs whose mechanism appears to be a decrease in potassium currents (282, 284, 501). Comparable effects may be mediated by a variety of peptides, including substance P (18, 259, 262, 264); generally peptides are more likely to be modulators than transmitters. There is also reason to believe that monoamines operate as modulators rather than synaptic transmitters (333, 511). The modulating effect could also occur at a presynaptic site by producing changes in transmitter release (as in presynaptic inhibition): several agents are believed to act in this way, including GABA, ACh, and enkephalin (see ref. 297 for a recent discussion of modulatory actions). Modulation could play a crucial role in learning processes, but there is still little more than suggestive evidence that it is an important mechanism in the vertebrate central nervous system.

Identification of Transmitters

THEORY. Only two criteria are absolutely fundamental: *1*) the action of the postulated transmitter must be identical in every respect to the natural synaptic action, and *2*) the substance in question must be released during synaptic activity in amounts fully adequate to account for the observed synaptic action.

As pointed out by Werman (502), the first criterion (identity of action) is of particular importance, and it is amenable to rather critical testing. Evidently all aspects of the action transmitter must be considered: changes in excitability, membrane potential, and conductance. Not only should these changes be identical with what is observed during synaptic activity, but they should be changed identically by altering the membrane potential and the internal or external ionic environment. Another point of importance (that was not mentioned by Werman) is the time course of action, which clearly must be consistent with the speed and duration of synaptic action. The new technique of noise or fluctuation analysis (88, 242), by providing a means of measuring both the magnitude and the duration of the elementary conductance changes evoked by single molecules of transmitter, is likely to be another important tool for establishing the identity of action.

Further criteria provide useful additional evidence that is less obviously critical: *1*) The agent in question is present in the tissue in substantial amounts; this criterion is not critical, because the transmitter could conceivably be rapidly synthesized from a precursor as needed for release. *2*) The enzymes necessary for synthesizing the transmitter are present at the synapse; this also is not absolutely critical, because the transmitter could be synthesized some distance away and then diffuse or be transported to the nerve endings. *3*) Specific mechanisms of removal of the released transmitter are also present, either by uptake into cells or by enzymatic degradation; this criterion is not critical because the transmitter could well diffuse away from the synapse fast enough to ensure a short-lasting effect. *4*) Transmission can be blocked by a specific pharmacological antagonist; though useful, this is also not fully critical, because antagonists are only relatively specific and there is no way of absolutely ensuring the specificity of a given agent.

PRACTICAL CONSIDERATIONS. In practice the identification of transmitters depends on the accuracy and reliability of techniques used in assessing the theoretical criteria listed above.

Criterion of identity of action. The technique that revolutionized this field was the microiontophoretic application of chemicals in the close vicinity of excitable cells (70, 92, 261, 431). By accurately localizing the application both in space and in time, it is reasonably certain that the substance in question is acting on a particular cell, and its time course of action can be studied with some precision. When intracellular recording (permitting measurements of membrane potential, conductance, and reversal potentials) is combined with extracellular iontophoresis, the criterion of identity of action can be applied quite rigorously (e.g., Fig. 3).

On the other hand the iontophoretic technique can generate serious artifacts (spurious potential and conductance changes), especially when very brief pulses of current are applied (261). Moreover, being relatively difficult and very time consuming, it cannot yield quick results. It has been applied especially to cells that are easily identified by activation of clearly defined pathways, such as spinal and cranial motoneurons, Deiters' neurons, pyramidal tract neurons, and Purkinje cells. Most central neurons are relatively small and fragile and therefore do not readily withstand intracellular penetrations; but as techniques improve and the investigators' skill improves (and their inhibitions diminish), more and more cells are proving to be amenable to this form of investigation [e.g., striatal neurons (30, 256)], and iontophoretic studies with intracellular recording are now being made even in awake, unparalyzed animals (513).

Studies in vitro. In recent years there has been a great increase in studies of possible transmitters in mammalian central neurons in vitro. Although in 1966 Yamamoto and McIlwain (520) had already demon-

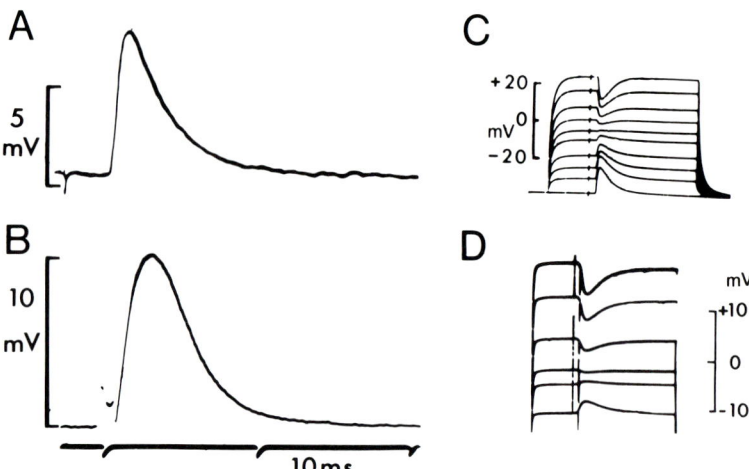

FIG. 3. Acetylcholine action at muscle end plate. *A*: end-plate potential in Mg-paralyzed rat diaphragm. *B*: ACh-evoked potential; ACh was released by 1-ms pulse of current (35 nA) through ACh-containing micropipette. Thus when released near end plate, ACh can closely reproduce effect of natural transmission. *C, D*: ACh potentials and end-plate potentials evoked in frog sartorius muscle have similar reversal potentials. *C*: nerve-activated end-plate potentials are superimposed on long depolarizing pulses of increasing intensity. *D*: ACh potentials superimposed on long depolarizing pulses. [*A, B* from Krnjević and Miledi (270); *C, D* from Katz and Miledi (244).]

strated that electrical activity could be recorded from isolated thin slices of brain, until recently Yamamoto was the only author to exploit this technique systematically (518, 519, 521).

Now, however, slices prepared from practically every region of the CNS are being investigated in numerous laboratories [e.g., especially hippocampus (8a, 100, 506, 517), cerebellum (372), and spinal cord (480)]. Important advantages of the slice include its mechanical stability (because it is not subject to respiratory and circulatory pulsations), the possibility of changing the external ionic concentration, and direct visualization of a given cell and its processes. The ability to see the cell permits a systematic survey of the chemical responsiveness of its different components (such as soma and dendrites). Of course, there are also disadvantages: a slice cannot be made very thin without cutting the processes of many cells, some essential tissue factors may be lost into the superfusate, and the supply of oxygen and substrates may be significantly impaired by the diffusion distance.

Another type of in vitro preparation is that of mammalian neurons grown in vitro, for example, in dissociated tissue cultures. This is anything but a new technique, but its popularity has increased vastly in the last few years. It is now extensively used for studies of transmitter mechanisms (320, 410). Perhaps even more than "acute" slices, cultured cells are liable to have properties that differ significantly from those of neurons in situ. Nevertheless the possibility of recording from a homogenous and predictable population is an enormous advantage, especially for studies of the development of synaptic mechanisms. Thus, although these in vitro preparations are not full substitutes, they do help to elucidate observation made in situ: they are likely to prove more directly useful and realistic "models" of brain than are invertebrate preparations.

Criterion of adequate release. The technical difficulties involved here are even more serious and indeed until now have been largely insuperable: at no synapse has the criterion of adequate release been entirely fulfilled. Even at the peripheral neuromuscular junction there has been only an approximate agreement between the amounts of ACh demonstrated to be released and the amount needed for excitation (271, 294). For the central nervous system, of course, the evidence available is at best merely suggestive.

The reasons for this paucity of evidence are not the lack of precision and specificity of techniques used in detecting even minute amounts of organic chemicals. Gas chromatography–mass spectrometry makes possible the determination of even attomolar (10^{-18} mol) amounts of substances (53, 209). Measurements of extremely small quantities (pmol or less) of hormones and peptides have become possible by the combination of immunological techniques (to obtain specific antibodies) with radiolabeling in the method of radioimmunoassay (515). It is therefore no longer necessary to rely on quite sensitive but seldom fully specific methods of bioassay (325).

Another powerful tool is the use of radioisotopes as precursors of likely transmitters through the natural pathway of synthesis, thus ensuring that the endogenous pool of transmitter is labeled and not a quite different pool of exogenous transmitter (taken up from extracellular space). If the label in the released material is properly identified by the use of chromatographic techniques, amino acid analysis, etc., the release of endogenous transmitters evoked by synaptic activation can be measured with precision, e.g., endogenous excitatory and inhibitory amino acids labeled through such natural substrates as glucose (Fig. 27) or glutamine (85, 173, 401). Similarly, labeled choline is commonly used to study the release of acetylcholine in the brain (323), and tyrosine and other precursors of monoamines are used for studies of the release of dopamine and other possible monoamine transmitters in the striatum and other parts of the brain (156).

One of the principal difficulties in this kind of research is to ensure that the released transmitter is collected before its removal by powerful physiological mechanisms of uptake. Unless they can be inactivated, one can scarcely expect to collect more than a small fraction of the released transmitter. Really effective blockers of uptake are seldom available. Because most transport systems are driven by Na⁺ influx, in principle one should be able to block uptake by removing Na⁺, but this would probably also abolish transmitter release. Another source of uncertainty is the extent to which material is released via the transport system, since this is probably reversible [for example, when the driving force, the Na⁺ electrochemical gradient, is outward instead of inward (231, 308)]. Apparent release owing to exchange is of course likely to be particularly marked in studies using exogenous radioisotopes. A further problem is the possibility that large amounts of transmitter may leak from nerve fibers in a nonpackaged form (243); it is not clear whether this occurs only, or even mainly, from nerve terminals and whether it is Ca dependent (the usual criterion of synaptically significant release).

Presence of possible transmitter in tissue under physiological conditions. Various techniques already mentioned have been used to measure relevant agents in tissues, such as bioassay, amino acid analysis, gas chromatography, mass fragmentography (a form of mass spectrometry), radioimmunoassay, and labeling through precursors. The principal difficulties arise from the fact that one seldom deals with a single population of cells, and therefore the precise location of the material may be open to question, though with painstaking microscopic techniques it is possible to isolate single cells or even the contents of individual cells [Fig. 4; (371)]. Alternatively, various fractions or subfractions of brain homogenates, consisting mainly of nerve endings or even synaptic vesicles, can be obtained by differential centrifugation (507).

A further problem is that transmitter levels appear to be quite labile, and special precautions are necessary to avoid marked postmortem changes caused by continued enzymatic activity. Various more or less complicated techniques of rapid freezing have been developed for this purpose (494). The quickest and most effective method now available is microwave hyperthermia (464).

Selective localization can be demonstrated by subtraction, that is, by making specific lesions that destroy the neurons in question, thus causing the loss of any substances concentrated in these cells; for example, in the spinal cord by cutting the dorsal roots and thus removing primary afferent terminals (422) or in the cerebellum by x-irradiation or genetic selection that removes granule cells (424, 527). Of course in such experiments it is assumed that the removal of a given population of fibers or cells does not significantly alter the neurochemistry of the remaining tissue.

More direct localization of possible transmitters in nerve cells and fibers can be achieved by combining histological and histochemical, immunological, or autoradiographic techniques. Particularly successful examples of histochemical methods include the Falck-Hillarp histofluorescence technique for demonstrating various monoamines (79) and the use of specific antisera to demonstrate the cellular distribution of various peptides (188, 394). Of course the presence of a given substance in a nerve cell does not prove that it is involved in synaptic (or some other form of) transmission. Nevertheless this is a useful pointer, and the histochemical findings have undoubtedly had a dramatic impact, partly because they provide such a graphic illustration of the distributions of populations of cells having distinct chemical characteristics.

Presence of enzymes. The presence of synthetic enzymes is particularly valuable for the identification of probable transmitters. The technology of identifying and estimating enzyme activity has developed tremendously, and even minute amounts of tissue can now be made to yield precise data (514). Enzyme activity can also be detected in situ by the use of specific substrates and radioautography (or some other marker) and thus localize enzymes involved in the synthesis of GABA or monoamines in certain regions (Fig. 13*B*) or even in nerve endings [Fig. 21; (394, 417)]. Attempts at a histochemical demonstration of choline acetyltransferase, the enzyme that acetylates choline to form ACh, have until now been much less successful. The much easier demonstration of acetylcholinesterase activity (451) is unfortunately less useful because this enzyme may be present in noncholinergic cells.

Mechanisms of removal. Most transmitters appear to be rapidly taken up by perisynaptic cellular elements: nerve terminals (Fig. 12*A*), postsynaptic cells, and neuroglia (217, 458, 496). In a somewhat circular argument the presence of uptake mechanisms is often considered crucial evidence that a given agent must be a transmitter. But this is not very compelling, considering the widespread mechanisms of uptake of many substances, including most amino acids (55, 231). Because these are typically sodium coupled, sodium dependence of such uptake cannot be of great significance for the identification of transmitters (458).

Pharmacological antagonists. Drugs that selectively block certain kinds of synaptic transmission operate by either competing with the transmitter for its specific membrane receptors (like curare, atropine, strychnine, and bicuculline) or by preventing its release from presynaptic terminals [like tetanus (71, 83), botulinum toxin (41), and perhaps baclofen (400)]. Such drugs are increasingly used to identify possible transmitters released by various pathways. Classic blockers of acetylcholine, such as curare, dihydro-β-erythroidine, and atropine, operate effectively in the central nervous system (78, 115, 275); but with peripheral blockers of monoamines the situation is far from simple. There is very little consensus about their effectiveness and specificity in the central nervous system (33, 39, 171, 388), except for dopamine antagonists, such as haloperidol, which are relatively well defined (197).

Some amino acid blockers are now well known.

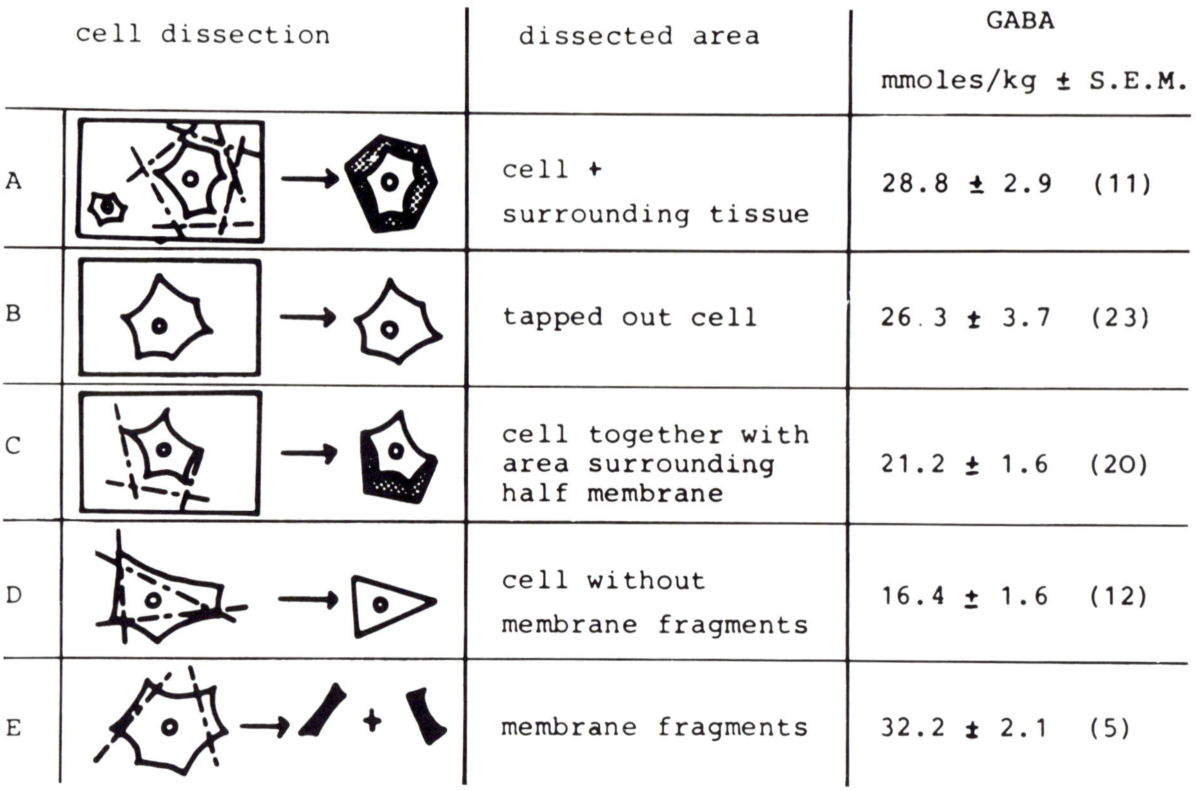

cell dissection	dissected area	GABA mmoles/kg ± S.E.M.
A	cell + surrounding tissue	28.8 ± 2.9 (11)
B	tapped out cell	26.3 ± 3.7 (23)
C	cell together with area surrounding half membrane	21.2 ± 1.6 (20)
D	cell without membrane fragments	16.4 ± 1.6 (12)
E	membrane fragments	32.2 ± 2.1 (5)

FIG. 4. Diagram demonstrating technique for measuring γ-aminobutyric acid (GABA) content inside Deiters' neurons and in their immediate surroundings in thin sections of frozen tissue. [From Okada and Shimada (371).]

Strychnine has long been familiar as a convulsant that acts especially on the spinal cord (442). It is now clear that strychnine is an effective antagonist of glycine but is usually not an antagonist of GABA [Figs. 11, 17; (508)]. Because strychnine also interferes with other "glycinelike" inhibitory amino acids, including β-alanine and taurine (229a, 372), its effectiveness at a given synapse demonstrates only that the transmitter is probably a glycinelike agent.

Antagonists of GABA are even less specific or powerful. Picrotoxin interferes mainly with GABA-mediated inhibition (Figs. 20 and 24) both post- and presynaptic (229, 229a), probably not by blocking the GABA receptor, but rather the Cl⁻ ionophores (374, 375, 455). Bicuculline, on the other hand, has a more direct action on post- and presynaptic GABA receptors [Figs. 13 and 17; (72, 229, 229a, 374, 375)]. Having a relatively low affinity for the receptors, bicuculline must be applied in relatively large amounts; this creates some difficulty because of its low solubility and poor stability in solution. The methiodide or methochloride derivative is therefore more useful, being both more stable and more soluble. A further problem is that bicuculline appears to have some direct excitatory actions of its own, which complicate the interpretation of the results (280). Most peptides do not yet have any well-established antagonists, except for the naturally-occurring opioids that are blocked by naloxone (205), though even this classical specific antagonist of morphine may also antagonize the effects of GABA (169).

More or less irreversible antagonists, labeled either radioactively or with a fluorescent dye, are used increasingly to study the localization and distribution of cells possessing receptors for specific transmitters (257, 522).

CONCLUSIONS. It must be kept in mind that studies of central neurotransmitters have progressed significantly only in the last 10–20 years. As recently as 1964 a leading expert could write "an even greater disappointment to all interested in synaptic physiology has been the failure to elucidate the nature of any chemical transmitter in the mammalian nervous system other than acetylcholine" (45). We now have strong indications of the most likely transmitters at many synapses, though curiously enough acetylcholine is probably *not* one of the most important central transmitters. All the same, the information available for any one synapse is often fragmentary and in no case could one claim that both principal criteria *identity of action* and *adequate release* are even close to being fulfilled. This should be neither surprising nor discouraging, remembering the long time and the effort that were needed to identify ACh as the transmitter at the much more accessible neuromuscular junction (where ACh indeed still does not fulfill all the main criteria).

Any statements about chemical transmitters in motor pathways must therefore be read with appropriate reservations. There is little of the certainty that one has come to expect from morphological demonstrations of connections between groups of nerve cells, or even (though to a somewhat lesser degree) from measurements of orthodromic or antidromic electrical responses.

In the past, studies of motor control have been largely dominated by electrophysiological investigations, with good reason, because these are more practicable and lend themselves to greater precision. But it is clear that at most synapses transmission is mediated chemically. Not to know about these transmitters and how they operate is a serious drawback, since the characteristics of the junctions set the limits within which the whole system can operate. Moreover, some knowledge of the relevant neurochemistry and pharmacology provides great opportunities for modifying the overall performance.

Mechanisms of synaptic transmission, including the chemical transmitters used in peripheral and invertebrate junctions, have been extensively reviewed in the first volume of this *Handbook* section on the nervous system (26, 328, 481), and readers are referred to them for further information.

TRANSMITTERS IN PERIPHERAL MOTOR SYSTEMS

A systematic survey of transmitter mechanisms in motor function must include at least a mention of the various links in the chain of transmission from the executive cells in the central nervous system, the motoneurons, to the process of muscle contraction. There are three gaps across which the motor command must be transmitted in this pathway: *1*) between the motor nerve ending and the muscle fiber, *2*) between the muscle fiber membrane (the sarcolemma) and the sarcoplasmic reticulum, and *3*) between the reticulum and the contractile proteins.

The system appears to operate as follows. The electrically conducted action potential of the motor axon triggers a release of acetylcholine (ACh) from the nerve terminal: ACh excites the muscle fiber by interacting with specific receptors concentrated in the closely adjacent end plate [Fig. 2; 179, 240, 293, 328, 481)]. Depolarization spreads from the sarcolemma into the interior of the muscle fiber along the polarized membrane of the transverse tubular system (48, 61, 211, 483). The manner in which the signal is then transmitted to the adjacent sarcoplasmic reticulum, which releases the Ca^{2+} that initiates contraction by interacting with the troponin component of myofilaments, is still uncertain (48, 61, 125). Various suggested mechanisms include direct electrical transmission, the liberation of a chemical transmitter, gating by the movement of a charged membrane component (54, 445), and influx of extracellular Ca^{2+} (from the T tubules). The latter is perhaps the most likely, because Ca^{2+} does trigger Ca^{2+} release from the sarcoplasmic reticulum (125), but whether influx of Ca^{2+} is a prerequisite for excitation-contraction coupling is still a matter of controversy (20, 463).

TRANSMITTERS IN SPINAL MOTOR MECHANISMS

The spinal cord is extensively involved in motor control, in the first place because motoneurons are part of the "final common path" through which the central nervous system evokes and controls movement (162, 442). Second, it contains all the mechanisms needed for simple reflexes as well as for some quite elaborate organized activity, such as the scratch reflex and even locomotion (165, 442). We now have available a great deal of information about the electrophysiology of synaptic transmission in the spinal cord, much of which was obtained by Eccles and his collaborators (111–113) and was fully reviewed in his monographs [for more recent comprehensive surveys, see Burke and Rudomin (46) and Redman (412)].

Spinal Motoneurons and Their Synaptic Control

MONOSYNAPTIC REFLEX. The simplest reflex mediated by motoneurons is that evoked by activation of Ia-afferent fibers from muscle spindles of the homonymous muscle. Though extensively studied since its discovery by Renshaw (415), this reflex remains largely obscure as far as its synaptic mechanism is concerned. The Ia-synapses make up less than 1% of all synapses on motoneurons. They are situated mostly within one space constant of the soma and show no particular morphological specialization, including no gap junctions (46, 412).

As originally described by Eccles (111, 112), the monosynaptic excitatory postsynaptic potential (EPSP) in cat motoneurons was voltage sensitive and could be reversed at a potential near zero. It was therefore readily explained by a brief chemical transmitter action that evoked a transient short circuit of the membrane resistance. It looked very much like the muscle end-plate potential; indeed these pioneering intracellular studies on motoneurons definitively converted Eccles to the belief that central synapses operate mainly by chemical rather than purely electrical mechanisms.

This simple picture has not stood up to further experimentation. The first major attack came from Rall et al. (406). They emphasized that conductance changes were not regularly detectable in cat motoneurons and that most EPSPs could not be reversed by depolarization (especially their initial phase). Hence there was no clear evidence against electrical transmission, especially by a low-resistance junction that would permit presynaptic conductance changes to be "seen" post synaptically. These observations were confirmed by Shapovalov and Kurchavyi [Fig. 5A; (441)]

and Werman and Carlen (503). Werman and Carlen suggested a dual mechanism for the Ia EPSP, initially electrical (mediated by a high-resistance junction) and then chemical. Such a dual junctional process would not be without precedent: EPSPs in ciliary ganglia of the chick also have both electrical and chemical components (329).

An important recent study by Edwards et al. (121, 122) has cast serious doubt on previous evidence (296) that a quantal mechanism operates at the Ia-synapses, as it does in muscle (92). The successful "quantal analysis" of Ia EPSPs recorded under a variety of conditions had seemed to confirm the chemical character of this synapse. Very different results, however, are obtained from cat motoneurons, if exceptional precautions are taken to improve the signal-to-noise ratio. Edwards, Redman, et al. (121, 412) thus found that unitary EPSPs (evoked by activating a single Ia-afferent fiber) occurred in an all-or-none manner, which showed no indication of quantal fluctuations (Fig. 5B–D) and could not be reversed by depolarization (122). The nonquantal character of the unitary EPSP was by no means incompatible with a chemical synapse, but it was just as consistent with an electrical mode of transmission and inevitably reinforced the doubts that had been raised by Rall et al. (406).

In the amphibian spinal cord, monosynaptic EPSPs are also untypical, judging by their resistance to lack of Ca^{2+} or applications of Mg^{2+}, Mn^{2+}, and Co^{2+} (4, 440). This appears to indicate a significant component of electrical transmission, at least in some amphibians. Some authors have observed an effective block of transmission in amphibians by Mg^{2+}, Mn^{2+}, and Co^{2+} (19, 131); the conflicting reports may reflect difficulties of ion penetration or species-linked (or perhaps seasonal) variations in electrical coupling.

There is positive evidence in favor of a mainly or purely chemical mechanism for the Ia EPSP in the cat spinal cord. According to recent observations, monosynaptic EPSPs are depressed or even abolished by low Ca^{2+} or by Mn^{2+} and Co^{2+} [Fig. 6; (87, 266, 439)]. Although these do not totally exclude electrical transmission, because ionic changes could conceivably prevent terminal invasion, nevertheless this is strong ev-

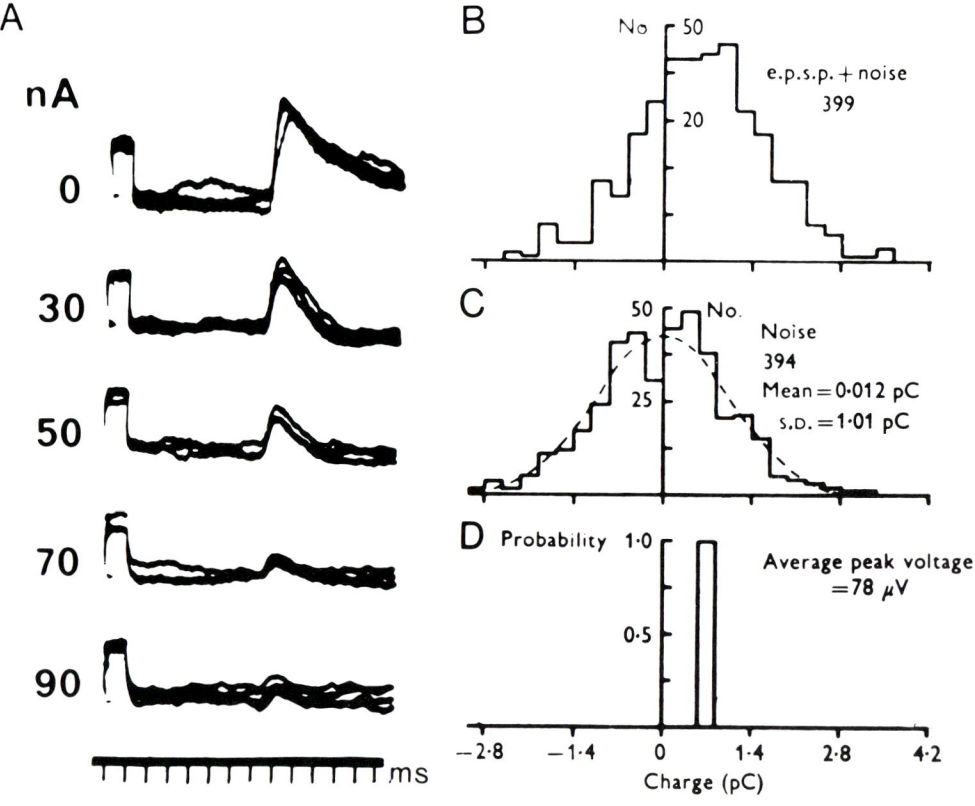

FIG. 5. Unlike end-plate potentials, monosynaptic excitatory postsynaptic potentials (EPSPs) in spinal motoneurons are seldom easily reversed and do not show quantal properties. A: monosynaptic group Ia EPSP in cat motoneurons diminishes with progressive depolarization (increasing depolarizing currents are indicated), but there is no true reversal by even the largest currents. Calibration pulses indicate 2 mV and time marks indicate ms. B–D: charge fluctuations recorded in cat spinal motoneuron during stimulation of single Ia-fiber. B shows fluctuations caused by unitary EPSP as well as background noise; C shows fluctuations caused by noise alone; D indicates charge variations due to EPSP alone (computed). Note all-or-none character indicating no quantal components. [A from Shapovalov and Kurchavyi (441). B–D from Edwards et al. (121).]

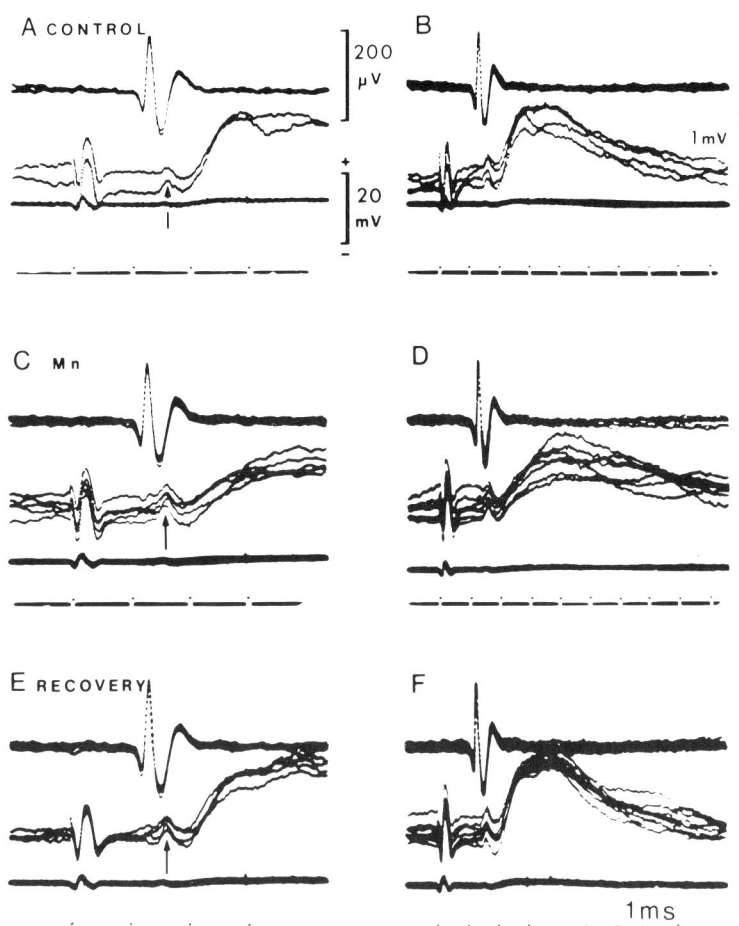

FIG. 6. Depression of monosynaptic excitatory postsynaptic potentials (EPSP) in spinal cord of cats by extracellular Mn^{2+}. Intracellular recording from sacral motoneuron, and EPSP evoked by stimulating posterior biceps-semitendinosus nerve at intensity 1.25 × threshold for evoking detectable response from dorsal root fibers. *Traces* show, from above down, afferent volley monitored from dorsal roots near point of entry into spinal cord, EPSP at high-gain AC amplification (see calibration bar in *B*), resting potential, and EPSP at lower gain DC amplification (see calibration bar in *A*), and time signal. In each instance two or more traces are superimposed during stimulation at 2/s. *A, B*: control EPSPs on fast and slow time base, respectively. *C, D*: EPSPs evoked by same intensity of stimulation after 2 min of Mn^{2+} release (from extracellular micropipettes). Note hyperpolarizing shift of DC trace. *E, F*: substantial recovery of EPSP between 7 and 8 min after end of release of Mn^{2+}. Arrows in *A*, *C*, and *E* indicate small potential, apparently reflecting presynaptic fiber or terminal activity. [From Krnjević et al. (266).]

idence for chemical transmission. Moreover Engberg and Marshall (129a), by injecting polarizing currents through a separate intracellular microelectrode, were able to show that Ia EPSPs of cat motoneurons can be symmetrically reversed at membrane potentials between 0 and +10 mV. Because of the large coupling artifacts of double-barreled electrodes, previous authors could not monitor the membrane potential while polarizing motoneurons.

Other evidence in keeping with a chemical process is more circumstantial, but by no means negligible. Both in cats and in amphibians, motoneurons are sharply depolarized by the naturally occurring dicarboxylic amino acids L-glutamate and aspartate [Figs. 7 and 8; (44, 77, 126, 440, 530)]. Glutamate excites even more effectively other neurons receiving a primary afferent input (153, 223, 529). Hence glutamate or aspartate would undoubtedly be effective transmitters if they were released by primary afferent terminals. It is significant that the drug baclofen, which is the most effective pharmacologic blocker of primary afferent synapses in the spinal cord of the cat (146, 395) and the cuneate nucleus (146) and which probably acts by suppressing transmitter release, has recently been shown to depress selectively glutamate and aspartate release in guinea pig cerebral cortex (400). On the other hand there is only limited direct evidence (from experiments on rats) that glutamate is actually released by primary afferent activity (421, 423). Glutamate is certainly present in dorsal root fibers, however, and its distribution (especially that of free glutamate) is fully consistent with a role as transmitter released by afferent terminals (161, 227).

The mechanism of excitation by glutamate remains unclear. Zieglgänsberger and Puil (530) recorded a large conductance increase in cat motoneurons during depolarization by glutamate (Fig. 9*B*), but in more recent experiments on cats (126) and frogs (440, 459) there were no consistent changes in motoneuron conductance (Fig. 7*A*, *B*). According to a detailed study by Engberg et al. (126), a fall in conductance tends to accompany the initial depolarizing action; but if glutamate is applied in large and prolonged doses there is a progressive rise in conductance, which may be due to glutamate uptake or an indirect action mediated by other neurons. Furthermore the depolarization induced in amphibian motoneurons by glutamate shows no real reversal potential even when the membrane potential is raised to +60 mV [Fig. 7*C*; (440)]. This raises some doubts about the significance of the difference between the extrapolated reversal potentials for glutamate and EPSPs reported in studies of mouse

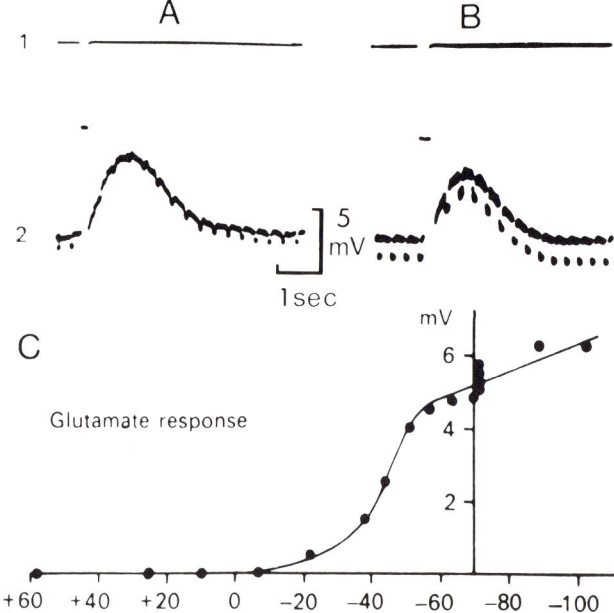

FIG. 7. Effect of glutamate on spinal motoneurons in isolated frog spinal cord. *A, B*: depolarizing effect evoked by brief application of glutamate. Iontophoretic current pulse is monitored in traces labeled 1 (110 nA for *A*, 130 nA for *B*). Superimposed constant current pulses, repeated at regular intervals, indicate marked reduction in input resistance of cell *A*, but little or no change in that of cell *B*. *C*: plot of peak amplitude of glutamate response against membrane potential. Note highly nonlinear relation and absence of reversal. [From Shapovalov et al. (440).]

spinal cells in culture (410). Hösli et al. (201) observed that the depolarizing action of glutamate on spinal neurons in culture disappears if external Na$^+$ is replaced with Li$^+$. Since Li$^+$ usually blocks Na$^+$-active transport more readily than Na$^+$ channels, this is also consistent with a mechanism of depolarization related to Na$^+$-linked glutamate uptake (126, 273b). Whatever the precise mechanism of action of glutamate is, its ambiguous characteristics show a curious parallel with those of the Ia EPSP.

Some other possible transmitters have been proposed for the primary afferent pathway: *1*) ATP (194), which has a substantial though variable excitatory effect on cuneate neurons (307) and *2*) the 11 amino acid peptide substance P (305). The presence of the latter in many dorsal roots and the strong depolarizing action on amphibian and cat motoneurones (379) as well as the absence of a clear conductance increase (264, 532) are certainly in agreement with this idea. The effect of substance P is characteristically so prolonged (182, 264, 272, 361), however, that it is difficult to see how it could mediate the sharp and brief synaptic actions typical of many primary afferent inputs (Fig. 8*A*, *B*). On the other hand, we now know that substance P is present mainly in afferent fibers of small diameter and that it is particularly effective in exciting nociceptive dorsal horn cells (181, 189, 191); therefore it is likely to be a specific transmitter or modulator in the nociceptive pathway.

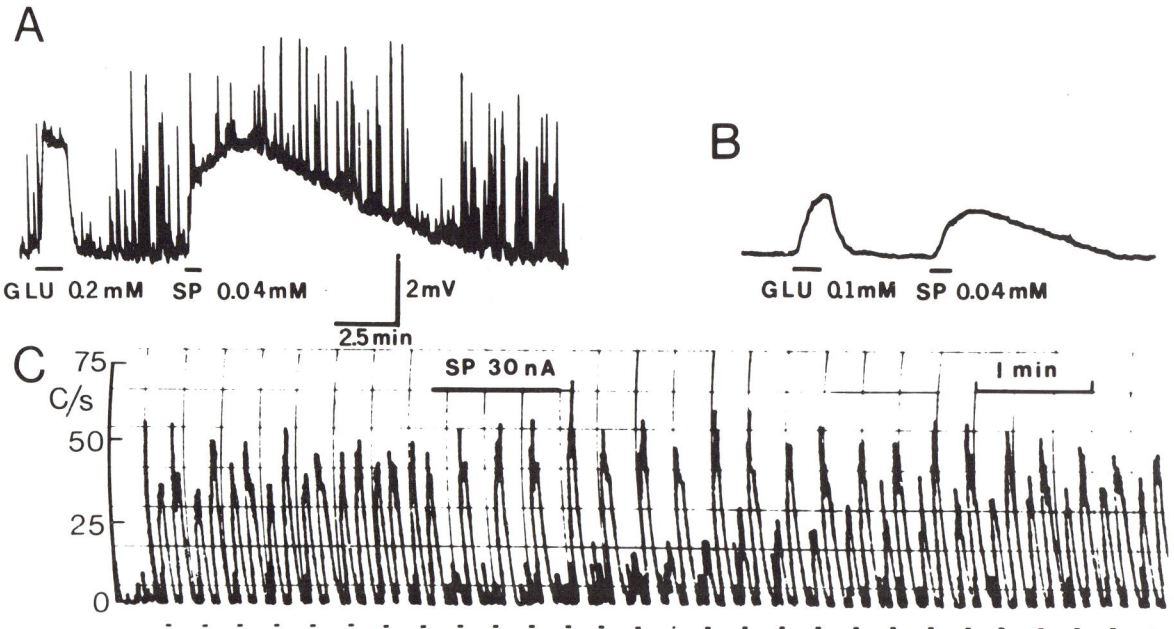

FIG. 8. Some effects of substance P on spinal neurons. *A*: depolarizing action of glutamate (GLU) or substance P (SP) on frog motoneurons; note much longer effect of substance P. Responses obtained by sucrose-gap technique from ventral root of isolated frog cord. *B*: after treatment with tetrodotoxin to prevent action potentials in adjacent cells and indirect excitation of motoneurons. *C*: selective block of ACh action on Renshaw cell, excited alternatively with glutamate, aspartate, or ACh (*dots* below *traces* indicate ACh applications). [*A, B* from Nicoll (361); *C* from Krnjević and Lekić (267). Reproduced by permission of the Natl. Res. Counc. Can. from the *Can. J. Physiol. Pharmacol.* 55: 958–961, 1977.]

Summary. Overall, the weight of evidence is more in favor of a chemical rather than electrical mode of generation of the Ia EPSP. The unusual features of this EPSP may reflect technical difficulties or perhaps the "unorthodox" action of the most likely transmitter, glutamate. But a firm conclusion would be premature without more compelling evidence about the identity and mode of action of the presumed transmitter. The Ia-synapse provides an excellent illustration of the problems and uncertainties that investigators have to face when they try to identify the mechanisms and the transmitters that operate at central excitatory synapses.

OTHER EXCITATORY INPUTS ON MOTONEURONS. Many other multisynaptic pathways converge on motoneurons, some originate from the periphery, others from the spinal cord or higher regions of the CNS.

It has been suggested that spinal excitatory interneurons are more likely to liberate aspartate than glutamate, because ischemic lesions of the cord, which selectively destroy the interneuronal population, cause a greater depletion of aspartate than glutamate (161). Motoneurons are sensitive to aspartate, whose action is comparable to that of glutamate (77), so aspartate may well be a physiological transmitter in some multisynaptic pathways.

As far as we know, there are no other excitatory transmitter systems intrinsic to the spinal cord, with the exception of some substance P-containing neurons (314) and of course probably many cholinergic ones. Many cells, especially in the dorsal horn, are rich in acetylcholinesterase and choline acetyltransferase (237, 451, 452), and motoneurons are sensitive to ACh (278, 531). This has a slow depolarizing action, probably mediated by a fall in membrane conductance to K^+ (Fig. 9), and therefore resembles the muscarinic action on cortical neurons (284). Hence a facilitatory cholinergic action may have a significant function. It remains to be determined whether the recent demonstration (68) that collateral branches of motor axons can form synapses on motoneurons (including their cells of origin) indicates a functionally significant positive feedback or a nonfunctional morphological curiosity.

Little is known about transmitters released by excitatory inputs of supraspinal origin. There is little information about the excitatory transmitter released by corticospinal fibers that generate monosynaptic EPSPs in motoneurons of primates (222, 300, 403), except for negative evidence that the pyramidal tracts are neither cholinergic (134) nor monoaminergic (79). These EPSPs are similar to the EPSPs evoked by Ia-afferents; the only significant difference is a striking "frequency potentiation" seen during tetanic stimulation. According to the neurochemical evidence (141), however, many corticofugal pathways probably operate by releasing glutamate, and no other powerful and rapidly acting excitant has been discovered in the

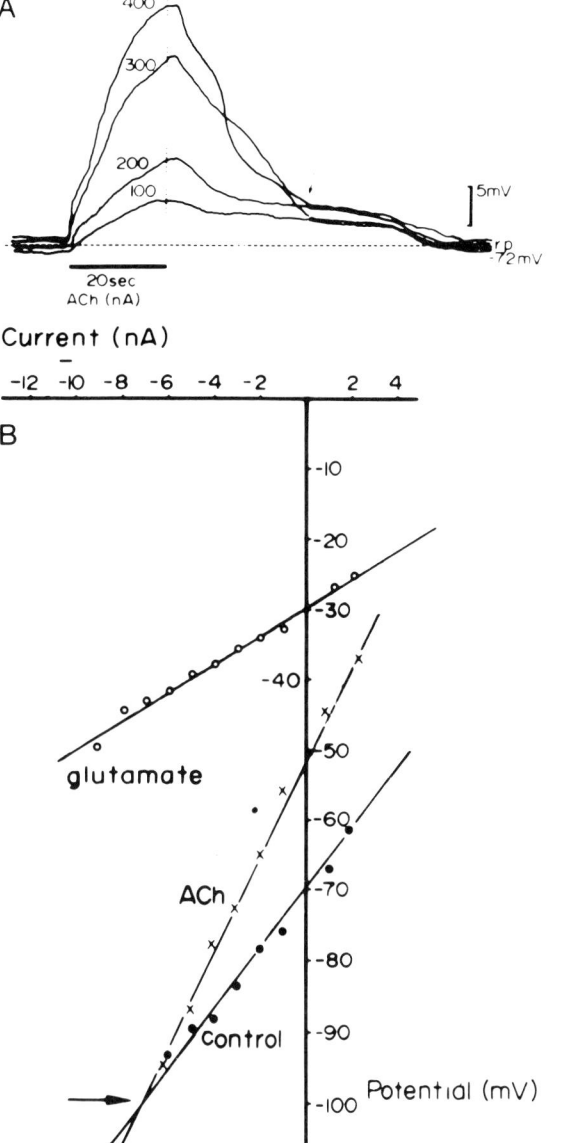

FIG. 9. Depolarizing action of acetylcholine on spinal neurons in cats. *A*: superimposed *traces* show slow and prolonged depolarizing effect of increasing iontophoretic doses of acetylcholine, each applied for 20 s. *B*: current-voltage plot obtained from interneuron in control state (*filled circles*) and during applications of ACh (250 nA) and glutamate (200 nA). Note that ACh causes resistance to increase, and depolarizing action has negative reversal potential. By contrast, depolarizing action of glutamate causes resistance to fall, and extrapolated reversal potential appears to be much more positive than resting potential. [From Zieglgänsberger and Reiter (531), © 1974, with permission of Pergamon Press, Ltd.]

cortex; therefore it is reasonable to suspect that corticospinal fibers also release glutamate (or perhaps aspartate) from their terminals (see also refs. 472 and 472a).

A facilitatory cholinergic influence originating from the brain stem may be present, as in other parts of the central nervous system. Descending monoaminergic facilitatory pathways are believed to be of importance, but because monoamines have mainly depressant effects when tested directly on motoneurons (129, 130, 232, 392), the effects of monoamines on locomotor performance (discussed in subsection OTHER RELEVANT SPINAL MECHANISMS, p. 123) are likely to be mediated indirectly.

Summary. On the basis of mostly circumstantial evidence, other excitatory inputs into motoneurons are thought to include: *1*) aspartate-releasing terminals of spinal interneurons; *2*) cholinergic pathways of segmental and/or supraspinal origin—these would have a slow and prolonged muscarinic, facilitatory action; *3*) monoaminergic (norepinephrine-, dopamine-, and serotonin-releasing) descending pathways, which appear to have a facilitatory effect, though possibly mediated indirectly; *4*) peptidergic fibers of spinal origin may also be significant (especially some releasing substance P); *5*) corticospinal fibers that may liberate glutamate.

INHIBITORY INPUTS ON MOTONEURONS. *Glycine-mediated inhibitions.* The two best-defined pathways (because they can be elicited most readily in pure form) are the Ia inhibitory pathway from antagonist muscles and the motor axon–recurrent collateral–Renshaw cell pathway extensively studied in cats by Eccles and collaborators (116). The corresponding inhibitory interneurons have been clearly identified: the Renshaw cells of the recurrent pathway (116, 220) and the Ia-interneurons (112, 207, 221, 223). There is general agreement that these inhibitory synapses probably operate by liberating glycine. The principal evidence for this is that glycine has a strong inhibitory action when applied iontophoretically to lumbosacral motoneurons in cats (75, 279, 504, 505). As shown in Figure 10, this action is characterized by a large conductance increase and a hyperpolarization with a reversal level that is highly sensitive to the internal Cl^- concentration. In all these respects, it resembles the IPSPs generated by these pathways (112); and since both the IPSP and the glycine action are readily antagonized by strychnine [Fig. 11; (69, 75, 303, 318)], glycine is clearly the leading candidate for the inhibitory transmitter released by Renshaw cells and the Ia inhibitory interneurons.

Admittedly, direct evidence of glycine release by inhibitory terminals is lacking, but *1*) glycine is certainly present in the mammalian cord, especially in the ventral horn [Fig. 12; (10)] and it is selectively taken up by some nerve endings (192); *2*) there is high-affinity glycine uptake (230, 359); *3*) strychnine binding sites (likely to be glycine receptors) are abundant in the cord (89); and *4*) there is even some evidence that glycine can be released from slices of rat spinal cord in vitro (174, 196). Hence, although some other related amino acids such as β-alanine or taurine act much like glycine and are also antagonized by strychnine, they are relatively scarce in the spinal cord and therefore less likely to be important inhibitory transmitters.

Gamma-aminobutyric acid-mediated inhibitions. GABA also inhibits most spinal neurons, but its action

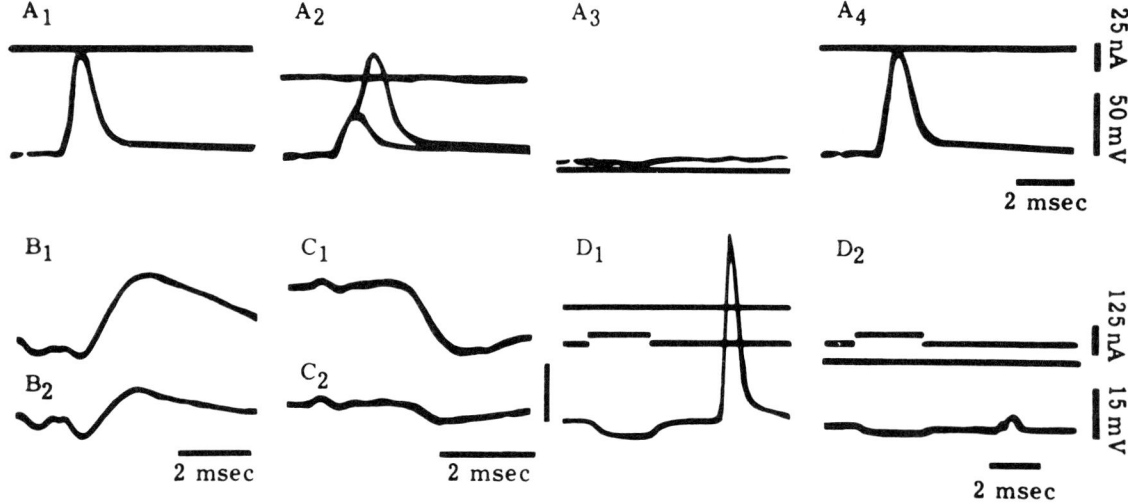

FIG. 10. Effects of glycine on membrane potentials and conductance of cat spinal motoneuron. A_1–A_4, progressive block of antidromic action potential by increasing amounts of glycine (iontophoretic current of 31 nA in A_2 and 90 nA in A_3). A_1 and A_4 are initial and final control potentials. Iontophoretic current monitored by additional trace. Note also hyperpolarization in A_3. Glycine also markedly depresses postsynaptic potentials (PSPs): compare excitatory PSPs in B_1 and B_2, the latter obtained while applying glycine (155 nA), similarly compare inhibitory PSPs in C_1 and C_2 (control and during glycine release of 69 nA). Finally, traces D_1 and D_2 show reduction in membrane resistance (as well as block of antidromic invasion) during application of glycine (189 nA), again monitored by extra trace. [From Aprison and Werman (11). With permission from M. H. Aprison and R. Werman. In: *Neurosciences Research*, edited by S. Ehrenpreis and O. C. Solnitsky. New York: Academic, 1968, vol. 1, p. 143–174. Copyright by Academic Press Inc. (London) Ltd.]

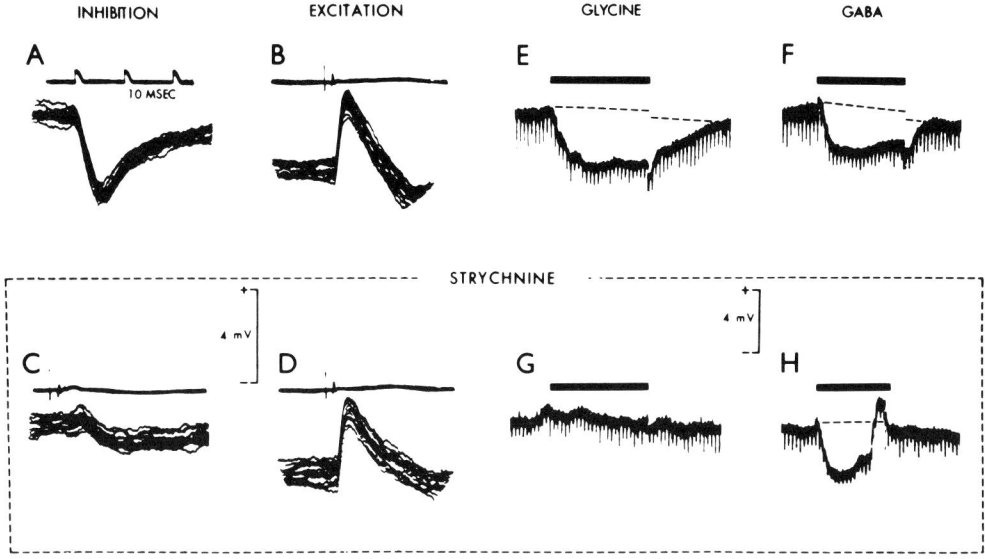

FIG. 11. Intracellular potentials recorded in two spinal motoneurons in cat demonstrate action of strychnine. A, B: control IPSP and EPSP evoked in gastrocnemius motoneuron by stimulating peroneal and gastrocnemius nerves, respectively. C, D: same PSPs after release of strychnine by diffusion from extracellular electrode for 3 min. Note marked reduction of IPSP, but little change in EPSP. E, F: hyperpolarizing responses evoked in another motoneuron by 30 nA glycine and 60 nA γ-aminobutyric acid (GABA). Much briefer IPSPs are superimposed on DC trace. G, H: same responses during extracellular iontophoresis of strychnine. Note selective block of glycine response. [From Curtis (71).]

is not regularly antagonized by strychnine (75) and, when tested on motoneurons, it is consistently much weaker than glycine (279, 505). Nevertheless, according to Kellerth (248), several types of inhibition acting on cat motoneurons are insensitive to strychnine, but are clearly antagonized by picrotoxin, which has long been known to antagonize the inhibitory action of GABA in crustacean systems (419) and appears to have a comparable effect in the mammalian central nervous system (152, 250, 486, 487). Thus Kellerth (248) was led to conclude that about one-half of the various inhibitory inputs on cat motoneurons could be mediated by GABA: some of these appeared to be "remote," not unlike inhibitions that have been ascribed to a presynaptic depolarizing action on primary afferent fibers (see subsection PRESYNAPTIC INHIBITION, p. 122). But Kellerth was able to show that these inhibitory inputs were associated with a clear depression of motoneuronal excitability and therefore are probably postsynaptic inhibitions. Strychnine-insensitive but bicuculline-sensitive inhibitions of motoneurons have also been described in later reports (72, 229). As far as the action of GABA on motoneurons is concerned, the conductance change appears to be identical to that produced by glycine, being essentially a marked increase in G_{Cl} (75, 279); the GABA and glycine reversal potentials are therefore identical. But, unlike glycine, GABA shows a marked fading of its action (279), which may be due to the rapid removal of GABA by uptake, true desensitization of GABA receptors, or inactivation of Cl^- channels.

Another significant feature of the postulated GABA-mediated inhibitions (in the spinal cord and elsewhere) is that they have a slower time course than the probable glycine-mediated inhibitions (98). This is seen even when unitary conductance changes are measured by the method of fluctuation analysis (17), indicating that for some reason the molecular events resulting from the interaction of GABA and its receptors have a relatively prolonged time course. It is now believed that the antispastic action of benzodiazepine drugs is caused by an increased sensitivity of GABA receptors involved in various inhibitory pathways, not through a direct action of the drugs but one mediated by distinct, presumably closely associated benzodiazepine receptors (60a).

Like glycine, GABA is readily found in the spinal cord, being especially concentrated in the dorsal horn (132, 350). The specific synthesizing enzyme, glutamate decarboxylase (GAD), which manufactures GABA from glutamate (420), is also present in large amounts, especially in the substantia gelatinosa (15, 132); some GAD-containing terminals have even been found synapsing with motoneurons (509). Both high- and low-affinity GABA uptake are also features of the spinal cord (330); GABA release has been demonstrated in vitro (423). Most of the data do not show that GABA is necessarily involved in inhibitory pathways acting directly on motoneurons, because it is now likely that GABA is the transmitter that depolarizes primary afferents during presynaptic inhibition (311); nevertheless the slower acting picrotoxin- or bicuculline-sensitive inhibitory inputs on motoneurons are probably mediated by GABA.

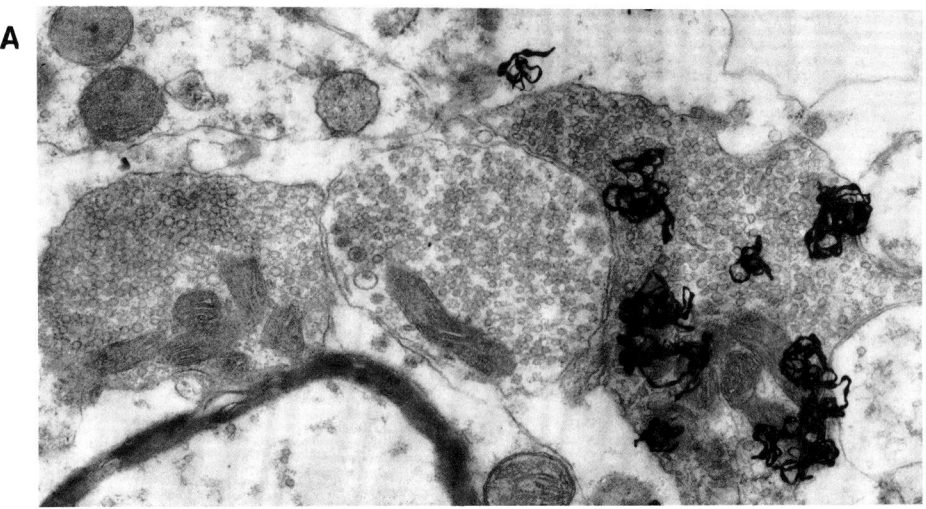

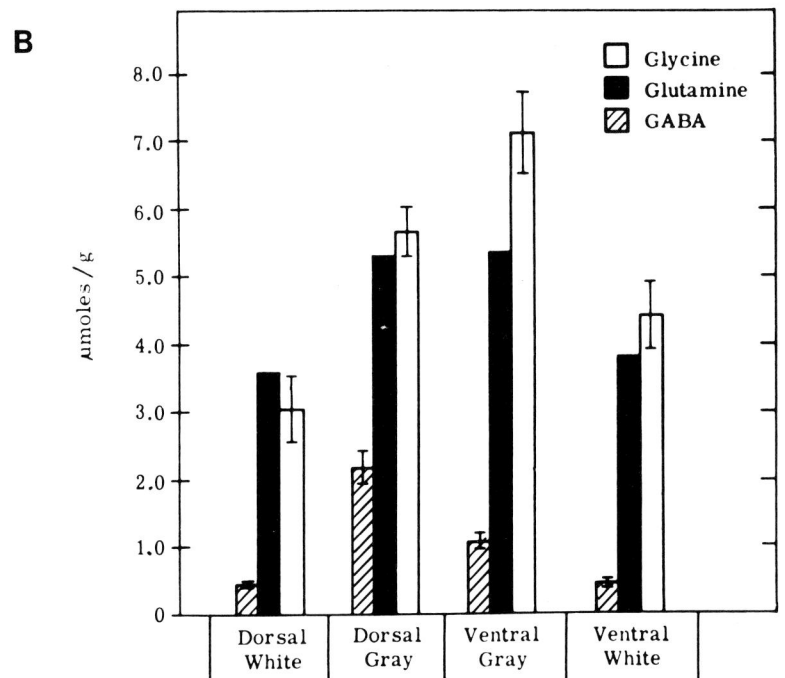

FIG. 12. *A*: electron-microscopic autoradiograph from rat spinal cord slice incubated with [^{3}H]-glycine. Note strong radioactivity over presumed glycinergic bouton (×30,000). *B*: concentrations of glycine and γ-aminobutyric acid (GABA) in four areas of cat spinal cord; distribution of glutamine included for comparison. [*A* from Hökfelt and Ljungdahl (192); *B* from Aprison and Werman (11). With permission from M. H. Aprison and R. Werman. In: *Neurosciences Research*, edited by S. Ehrenpreis and O. C. Solnitsky. New York: Academic, 1968, vol. 1, p. 143–174. Copyright by Academic Press Inc. (London) Ltd.]

PRESYNAPTIC INHIBITION. The best-known presynaptic inhibitory mechanism in the spinal cord is that associated with "primary afferent depolarization" (113). Although originally proposed some 15 years ago, the involvement of GABA in the mechanism of presynaptic depolarization has only been convincingly demonstrated in the past 5 years (311). Sensory neurons are readily depolarized by GABA, not only at their terminals (81, 309, 363) but also in peripheral nerves (310, 353) and in the dorsal root ganglia (95, 154). The predominant mechanism is an increase in Cl$^-$ conductance (as for the postsynaptic action), but depolarization occurs because of the relatively high internal Cl$^-$ content in sensory neurons and fibers. The presynaptic inhibitory action is probably exerted by small neurons of the substantia gelatinosa containing GABA and GAD [Fig. 13*B*; (15, 16, 339, 350, 509)], which are activated by various afferent and descending inputs (113, 435). Pharmacologically both the inhibition and primary afferent depolarization resemble other GABA-mediated mechanisms in showing antagonism by picrotoxin and bicuculline (Fig. 13) and potentiation by barbiturates and tranquilizers (311, 435).

A later component of the primary afferent depolarization probably has a different mechanism, and is caused by an extracellular accumulation of K^+ released by afferent volleys (21, 260, 271, 273, 273a).

Presynaptic inhibition may also be mediated by presynaptic norepinephrine and serotonin receptors (176) or by opiate receptors (186, 321, 457); the former could be activated by descending monoaminergic fibers (311) and the latter by opioid-releasing cells of the substantia gelatinosa (295).

Any kind of presynaptic depolarizing mechanism would tend to depress synaptic transmission at the first synapse in the afferent pathway by reducing the amount of transmitter released by afferent impulses, presumably through voltage-dependent inactivation of Ca^{2+} inward currents; though recent observations by Dunlap and Fischbach (109) suggest that GABA, norepinephrine, serotonin, and enkephalin operate by interfering directly with Ca^{2+} influx into sensory terminals (independently of depolarization). Such an inhibitory system therefore would operate as a more or less selective sensory gate that could play an important role in the control of pain (346, 354, 497) as well as various motor responses (see subsection OTHER RELEVANT SPINAL MECHANISMS, this page).

Summary. The most conspicuous inhibitory pathways acting on motoneurons (e.g., Ia inhibitory interneurons and Renshaw cells) probably liberate glycine. This is indicated especially by the excellent agreement between inhibitory postsynaptic potentials (IPSPs) and the action of glycine (hyperpolarization due to high Cl^- permeability, similar reversal potential), both being selectively blocked by strychnine as well as by the localization of glycine in the spinal cord and its uptake into nerve endings. Gamma aminobutyric acid is also a significant inhibitor which may be responsible for almost as many inhibitory actions as glycine. Both transmitters produce identical increases in Cl^- permeability, but GABA actions are slower, and they are more susceptible to block by picrotoxin or bicuculline. Dorsal horn interneurons liberate GABA onto primary afferent terminals by axoaxonal synapses causing primary afferent depolarization and presynaptic inhibition (unlike central neurons, afferent fibers are relatively rich in Cl^- and are therefore depolarized when their Cl^- permeability is raised by GABA). Extracellular (periterminal) accumulations of K^+, following afferent activity, probably also contribute to primary afferent depolarization.

OTHER RELEVANT SPINAL MECHANISMS. *Renshaw cells.* As pointed out in more detail in several other chapters in this *Handbook*, the Renshaw cells are of real significance in motor control, not only because they exert a negative feedback on motoneuronal output (112, 416), but even more importantly because they strongly inhibit the Ia-interneurons [Fig. 14; (208, 224)].

From the point of view of chemical transmission, Renshaw cells are also of special interest: first, for a historical reason, because the cholinergic motor axon–Renshaw cell synapse was the first central chemical

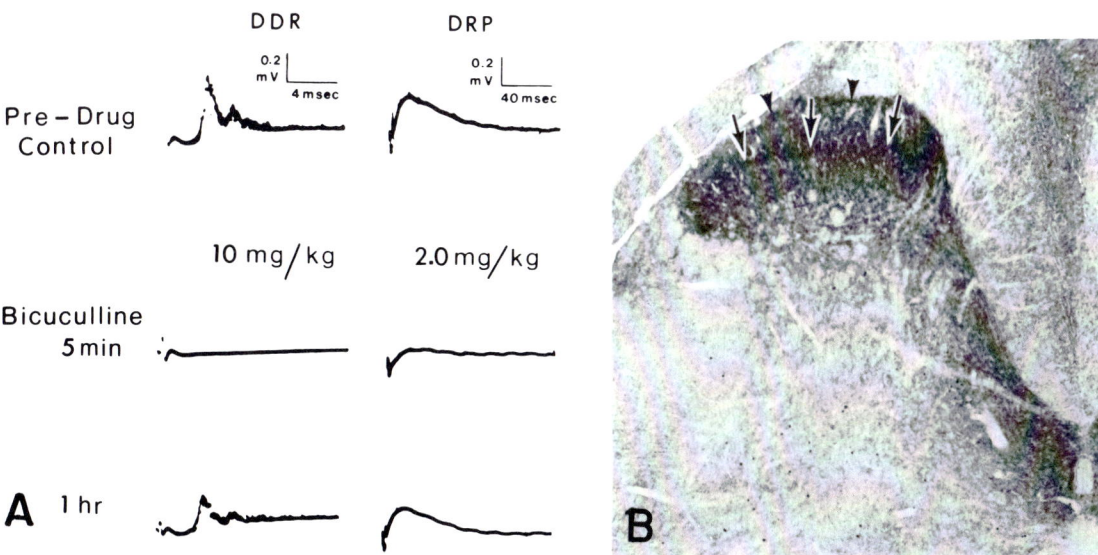

FIG. 13. Evidence indicating involvement of γ-aminobutyric acid (GABA) in spinal presynaptic inhibition. *A*: dorsal root reflex (DDR) and dorsal root potential (DRP) recorded in unanesthetized spinal cat practically eliminated by intravenous bicuculline. Note only partial recovery 1 h later. *B*: photomicrograph of dorsal horn from rat lumbosacral spinal cord. *Arrows* point to site of intense glutamic acid decarboxylase activity in marginal layer and in substantia gelatinosa. × 70. [*A* from Levy (311), *B* from McLaughlin et al. (339).]

transmitter mechanism to be identified with reasonable certainty; second, because it has remained a unique example of a well-established nicotinic cholinergic synapse in the central nervous system. Its discovery followed from the logical deduction that because motor axons excited muscle fibers by a cholinergic process, comparable cholinergic excitation was likely at the intraspinal terminals of the recurrent collateral branches of the same axons (116). Renshaw cells indeed proved to be highly sensitive to cholinomimetics, injected intra-arterially (115, 116) or in the spinal cord by microiontophoresis (73); and both transmission and the effects of ACh could be blocked by nicotinic antagonists. The resemblance to neuromuscular transmission, however, was partly misleading. The most effective blocking agents are not curare and related compounds [α-bungarotoxin is indeed quite ineffective (108)], but rather ganglionic blockers such as dihydro-β-erythroidine and mecamylamine (490). Moreover, it turned out that Renshaw cells have significant muscarinic receptors (78) so that they can be activated in two cholinergic modes, one having a rapid time course (phasic) and one a much slower time course (tonic). Clearly, Renshaw cells resemble sympathetic ganglion cells rather than skeletal muscle fibers.

If the most important function of Renshaw cells is to provide an inhibitory control over Ia inhibitory interneurons, then the Renshaw tonic activity may be functionally of particular significance, which may explain why in the rat a significant contribution of Renshaw cells to reflex activity is more easily demonstrated by injecting a muscarine antagonist than a nicotine antagonist (427).

Renshaw cells receive other inputs. Noncholinergic excitations (78) are likely to be mediated by excitatory amino acids; in the cat Renshaw cells are consistently more sensitive to aspartate than to glutamate (106, 267), but the reverse is found in rats (210). They are also inhibited by some other inputs, notably a mutually inhibitory one from other Renshaw cells [Fig. 14; (428)]. But unlike the other inhibitory actions of Renshaw cells, which are probably all mediated by the release of glycine (71), this mutual inhibition is not readily blocked by strychnine [(23), but compare ref. 74]. Renshaw cells also appear to have receptors for monoamines, which are predominantly inhibitory (130, 499), but there is no convincing evidence of a monoaminergic innervation.

Another curious feature is that Renshaw cells are not excited by substance P; instead, this peptide produces a selective block of the action of ACh [Fig. 8C; (24, 267)]. In contrast to most other spinal neurons, Renshaw cells are excited by morphine as well as endogenous opioids (82, 107).

Summary. The cholinergic innervation of Renshaw cells by motor axon collaterals remains the only well-established example of a rapidly acting, nicotinic synapse in the CNS. Renshaw cells, however, resemble sympathetic ganglion cells rather than muscle end

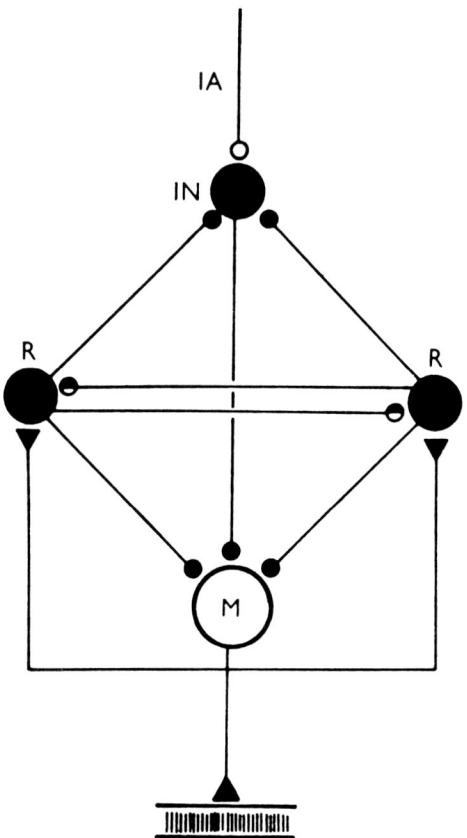

FIG. 14. Diagram of connections between motoneurons (M), Renshaw cells (R), and interneuron mediating Ia inhibition (IN). Cholinergic terminals represented by *filled triangles*, glycinergic terminals by *filled circles* (strychnine sensitive) or *half-filled circles* (strychnine resistant). [From Belcher et al. (23).]

plates because *1*) they have dual cholinergic receptors, fast-acting nicotinic and slower acting muscarinic; and *2*) the nicotinic receptors are particularly sensitive to ganglionic blocking agents (such as dihydro-β-erythroidine and mecamylamine) and not at all to α-bungarotoxin. The nicotinic excitation is antagonized by substance P. On the other hand, Renshaw cells receive noncholinergic excitatory inputs that are probably mediated by aspartate or glutamate, and they are excited by opioid peptides. The inhibitory actions of Renshaw cells on motoneurons, Ia inhibitory interneurons, and other Renshaw cells are probably all mediated by glycine.

Monoaminergic descending facilitation of spinal motor mechanisms. A major series of papers from the Lundberg laboratory has led to the present great interest in the role of descending monoaminergic pathways in the initiation and control of integrated motor behavior by the spinal cord. Originally these studies were triggered by tentative evidence that L-dopa and serotonin potentiate the flexor reflex in the acutely spinalized rabbit (49). Less attention might have been paid to this brief report had it not been followed by extensive histochemical investigations that convincingly demonstrated the presence in the spinal cord of a widespread innervation by fibers containing norepinephrine and serotonin, with terminals concentrated especially in the ventral horn, which evidently originated from the brain stem, because these monoamines (and presumably the corresponding fibers) vanished after spinal transection (50, 79).

The first studies by Lundberg and his collaborators (6, 7) confirmed that the overall stretch reflex was enhanced by systemic injections of dopa, but there was a somewhat paradoxical simultaneous depression of the short-latency reflex and the concomitant depolarization of afferent terminals (Fig. 15). Thus dopa did not simply facilitate discharges, but it exerted a kind of switching action, which was interpreted as a release of long-latency, prolonged activity from a background of inhibition exerted by the short-latency pathway (the two systems being mutually inhibitory). Because the effects of dopa could be blocked by a dopa-decarboxylase inhibitor, by reserpine (which depletes nerve endings of norepinephrine but not dopamine), or by drugs that antagonize the postsynaptic action of norepinephrine (e.g., phenoxybenzamine), it was concluded that dopa must act mainly by releasing norepinephrine from noradrenergic neurons, and that through such neurons supraspinal centers exert a significant influence on the mode of activity prevalent in the spinal cord.

The functionally significant reciprocal organization of extensor and flexor motoneurons becomes evident in the isolated spinal cord after an injection of dopa, which presumably releases this system from tonic inhibition by the short-latency flexor-reflex system (219). Further studies on effects of dopa on γ-motoneurons (166) revealed in particular differential effects on static and dynamic components of the fusimotor systems (27), as well as the possibility of α-γ-coactivation even in the fully isolated spinal cord (454). Later observations reinforced the idea that noradrenergic terminals are involved in the action of dopa by demonstrating comparable effects of a drug that was said to release norepinephrine more specifically (133). But other evidence indicated (127) that serotonin-releasing pathways may also modulate spinal reflexes, because 5-hydroxytryptophan (the precursor of serotonin) proved to have quite a potent, dopa-like effect [as already suggested by the preliminary observations of Carlsson et al. (49)]. Moreover, when reserpine was injected to release monoamines from nerve terminals, the resulting dopa-like action on spinal reflexes was blocked not by phenoxybenzamine (an antagonist of norepinephrine), but by methysergide (a serotonin antagonist).

The existence of a tonic descending monoaminergic inhibition in decerebrate cats seemed to be confirmed by the further depression of tone produced by nialamide, a monoamine oxidase (MAO) inhibitor (MAO is one of the enzymes that catabolize norepinephrine). Because phenoxybenzamine had no effect, however

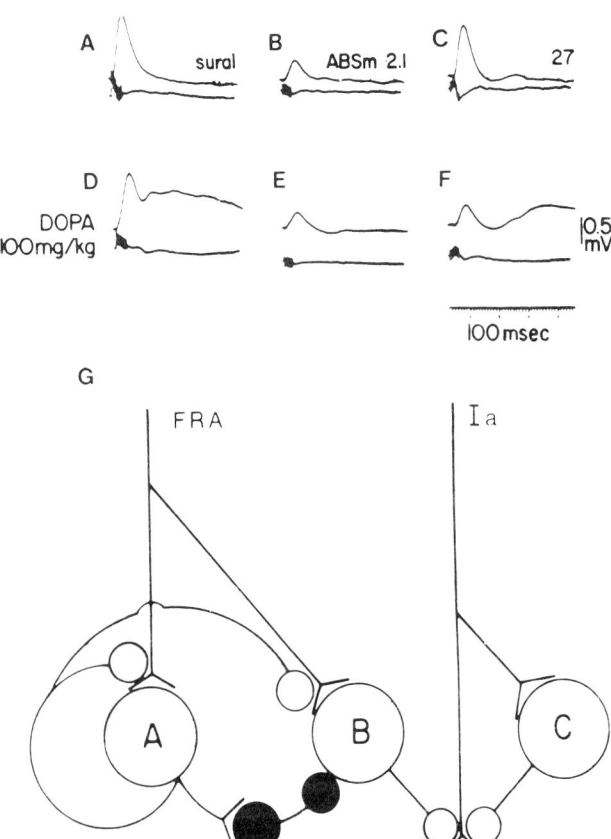

FIG. 15. A–F: effect of L-dopa on dorsal root potentials evoked from flexor-reflex afferents. Upper traces show dorsal root potentials recorded from most caudal dorsal root in L_6. Lower traces recorded from L_7 dorsal root entry zone. A–C are initial control traces. In A, sural nerve was stimulated with intensity of about 10 × threshold. In B and C, anterior biceps–semimembranous nerves were stimulated at 2.1 and 27 × threshold intensity. D–F: corresponding records obtained after injection of dopa. Note depression of early dorsal root potential and appearance of late component evoked by high-threshold stimulation. G: diagram of postulated neuronal pathways involved in depolarization of Ia-afferent terminals by activity in flexor reflex afferents (such as sensory pathways activated in A–F above). In spinal cat, activity in pathway through A normally prevents dorsal root potential evoked in Ia-afferent through pathway B. By suppressing pathway through A, dopa would permit long-latency depolarization of Ia-terminals through pathway B. Filled circles represent postsynaptic inhibitory neuron. [From Anden et al. (8).]

(indicating little or no noradrenergic synaptic action), although methysergide caused a partial diminution of tone (128), the authors had to conclude that the tonic control in decerebrate cats was significantly mediated by a serotonergic, facilitatory pathway; though some other pathways must also be active because total destruction of the raphe nuclei (the origin of descending serotonin-containing tracts) did not abolish the descending tonic influence. There is an abundance of other data indicating a facilitatory action of serotonin on spinal reflexes (and also some inhibitory effects); they are mostly based on studies of topical applications of serotonin or the effects of agents such as 5-

hydroxytryptophan that increase the tissue levels of serotonin, and complementary studies of the effects of electrical stimulation of raphe nuclei, controlled by the administration of serotonin antagonists (9).

Iontophoretic studies with monoamines. There have been many such studies of the actions of monoamines on spinal neurons (130, 232, 426, 498). By far predominant is an inhibitory action (Fig. 16), especially on motoneurons (129, 327, 392), though Jordan et al. (232) believe that this is probably an indirect effect. Marshall and Engberg's (327) demonstration that the hyperpolarizing effect of norepinephrine has a reversal potential near −20 mV and is associated with a fall in conductance indicated a reduction in Na$^+$ and K$^+$ conductance, which is not inconsistent with the suppression of an excitatory input. Most authors have assumed that the postulated descending aminergic pathways, which probably include a significant dopaminergic component (59), exert their excitatory effects by a release phenomenon.

More recent studies showing monoaminergic facilitation of locomotion in the spinal animal (145, 165, 443) logically continue from previous investigations. The well-known initiation of walking by electrical stimulation of the midbrain locomotor area ("cuneiform nucleus") in mesencephalic, thalamic, or even lightly anesthetized animals has been interpreted as being due to activation of a monoaminergic descending system that can convert the spinal interneuronal network into an autonomous system generating stepping (165, 443). Although both noradrenergic and tryptaminergic systems might be involved, injections of dopa or clonidine (a norepinephrine agonist) do not raise the excitability of α-motoneurons, whereas 5-hydroxytryptophan injections do. Because midbrain stimulation does not make motoneurons more excitable, its effects are more likely to be mediated by a noradrenergic pathway.

These observations are very impressive, but their interpretation needs some caution. An important criterion used (7) in interpreting the effects of dopa was the blocking action of phenoxybenzamine. In fact, there is little satisfactory evidence that this drug blocks α-actions of norepinephrine in the central nervous system; several iontophoretic studies of spinal interneurons have failed to reveal any such consistent and specific antagonism (33, 130, 498, 499).

Other puzzling features include the dopa-like effect of reserpine (127), which was expected to act by releasing norepinephrine from aminergic terminals, but proved to be insensitive to phenoxybenzamine; and the substantial effects produced by dopa and other norepinephrine-releasing agents (as well as 5-hydroxytryptophan) in chronic spinal preparations that have presumably lost all monoaminergic terminals (7, 9, 127, 133). Similarly according to Jordan and Steeves (233, 464a), injections of 6-hydroxydopamine, which also cause most of the spinal norepinephrine to disappear, do not prevent the activation of locomotion by midbrain stimulation. They concluded that de-

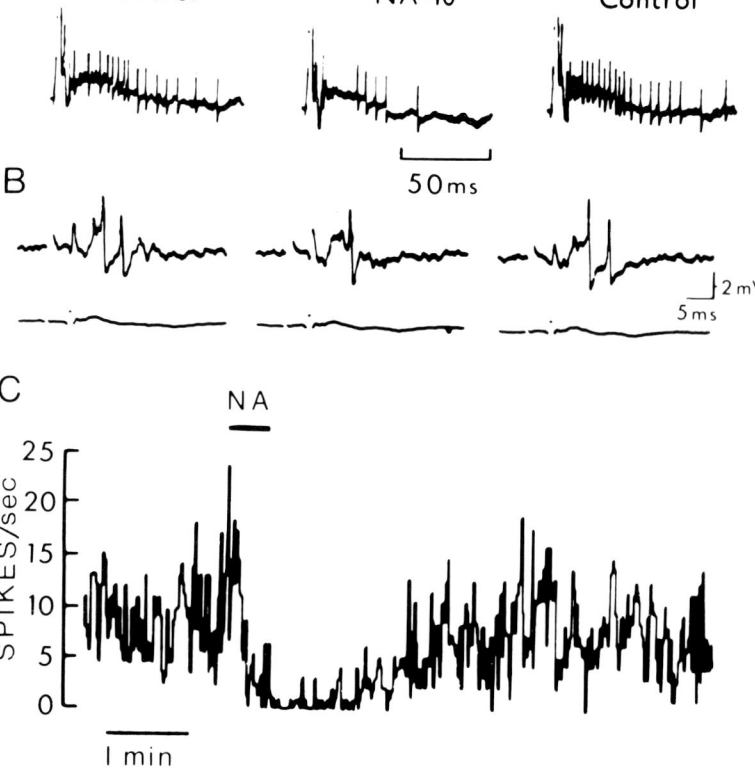

FIG. 16. Inhibitory actions of norepinephrine (NA) in cat spinal cord. *A*: repetitive firing of spinal interneuron excited by single shock to peroneal nerve. *B*: ventral horn interneuron also firing repetitively in response to stimulation of gastrocnemius nerve. Iontophoretic applications of norepinephrine (14 nA in *A*, 25 nA in *B*) depress synaptic response. *C*: spontaneous firing of another ventral horn interneuron markedly reduced by short application of norepinephrine (50 nA); calibration shows frequency of firing in spikes per second. [*A* from Engberg and Ryall (130); *B*, *C* from Jordan et al. (232). Reproduced by permission of the Natl. Res. Counc. Can. from the *Can. J. Physiol. Pharmacol.* 55: 399–412, 1977.]

scending monoaminergic pathways cannot be the sole mediator of the effects of midbrain stimulation.

One should also bear in mind that if there is enough intraneuronal decarboxylase activity, systemic injections of dopa or 5-hydroxytryptophan could lead to substantial accumulations of monoamines inside various neurons (especially after inhibition of MAO). These could result in significant changes in neuronal excitability (265) that are unrelated to the activity or even presence of monoaminergic pathways.

Summary: monoaminergic facilitation. The well-known facilitation of spinal reflexes and locomotor activity by systemic injections of precursors of norepinephrine or serotonin (such as dopa or 5-hydroxytryptophan) is still not readily explainable in terms of increased transmitter release from monoaminergic terminals. Serotonin-, norepinephrine-, and dopamine-containing fibers of supraspinal origin are undoubtedly present; but dopa and 5-hydroxytryptophan do not lose their effectiveness after the disappearance of such descending fibers. Some other mechanisms of action must therefore be at least partly involved.

TRANSMITTERS IN SUPRASPINAL MOTOR SYSTEMS

Brain Stem

CRANIAL MOTONEURONS. From the limited evidence available, it appears that cranial motoneurons do not differ greatly from spinal motoneurons in synaptic mechanisms and the effects of various possible transmitters. Judging by their sensitivity to intracellular Cl⁻, IPSPs are generated by an increase in Cl⁻ conductance (214, 316, 352, 487). They are inhibited by both glycine and GABA, but the importance of glycine in the brain stem diminishes as one proceeds in the rostral direction. In the hypoglossal nucleus, motoneurons are sensitive to both glycine and GABA (487), GABA being more effective when applied to the dendrites and glycine more effective at the soma (3), though IPSPs are blocked by strychnine (135, 352). By contrast in the more rostral nuclei, inhibition is sensitive to picrotoxin rather than strychnine (214, 365). This agrees with a general trend for glycine synthesis, content, receptors, high-affinity uptake, and inhibitory actions to be maximal in the spinal cord and lower brain stem and to diminish toward the forebrain, where GABA seems predominant as an inhibitory agent (compare refs. 10, 76, 80, 89, 262).

There is little information about excitatory synaptic mechanisms and transmitters acting on cranial motoneurons. According to McCall and Aghajanian (333), trigeminal motoneurons are readily excited by glutamate. Perhaps the most interesting point is that the effectiveness of glutamate can be greatly potentiated by serotonin and norepinephrine, so there is a possibility of monoaminergic modulation of motor control by a form of postsynaptic facilitation reminiscent of some facilitatory actions of norepinephrine in the cerebellum (187, 511).

RED NUCLEUS. Cells in the red nucleus receive at least two kinds of excitatory input: one at the dendrites comes from the cerebral cortex; the other, at the soma, comes from the interpositus nucleus of the cerebellum (compare ref. 489). Possible transmitters have been tested systematically by Davis and Vaughan (84) and Huffman and Davis (204), using extracellular recording in cats and baboons, respectively, and by Altmann et al. (1, 2), mainly recording rubral potentials intracellularly in cats. These authors are agreed that the dicarboxylic amino acids glutamate and aspartate are the only strong and consistent excitants of rubral cells (Fig. 17A, B), aspartate being slightly more potent than glutamate (1). Sometimes when large amounts of amino acids were applied, the depolarization was associated with a modest rise in input conductance. Judging by the maximum depolarizations that could be achieved with glutamate as well as extrapolated current-voltage data, the reversal potential for the action of glutamate could be near −30 mV. Two postulated glutamate antagonists [1-hydroxy-3-aminopyrrolidone-2 (HA-966) and glutamate diethyl ester] depressed glutamate-evoked responses, whereas HA-966 also reduced corticorubral and interpositorubral EPSPs; but both drugs appeared to have some direct hyperpolarizing effects, raising some doubts about their specificity as glutamate antagonists.

The possibility that corticorubral fibers release glutamate would agree with some neurochemical evidence indicating that other corticofugal pathways operate by releasing glutamate (141). Tsukahara and Fuller (488) assumed that the absence of conductance increase during EPSPs of cortical origin could be ascribed to their generation at a remote dendritic site, but this may be a characteristic of the action of glutamate.

According to Davis and Vaughan (84), in the cat spontaneous firing of rubral cells, as well as EPSPs evoked by stimulating the brachium conjunctivum, are sharply inactivated by intravenous LSD but not by the cholinergic antagonists dihydro-β-erythroidine or atropine. Because LSD had little effect on firing evoked by amino acids, they concluded that the natural excitatory transmitter was neither a dicarboxylic amino acid nor ACh and suggested that it may be identical with the transmitter released by optic nerve terminals in the lateral geniculate (where LSD also produces a striking block of synaptic transmission). Their tests did not exclude another explanation, however, that LSD prevents the release of the transmitter from the terminals of the brachium conjunctivum, in which case the transmitter could still be aspartate or glutamate. This seems to be the more reasonable alternative, because none of the several other agents tested (monoamines and ACh) had the required excitatory effect. On the other hand, the excitation of small rubral cells by ACh (204) would be consistent with the existence of some kind of cholinergic facilitatory input.

Norepinephrine, dopamine, serotonin, and less reg-

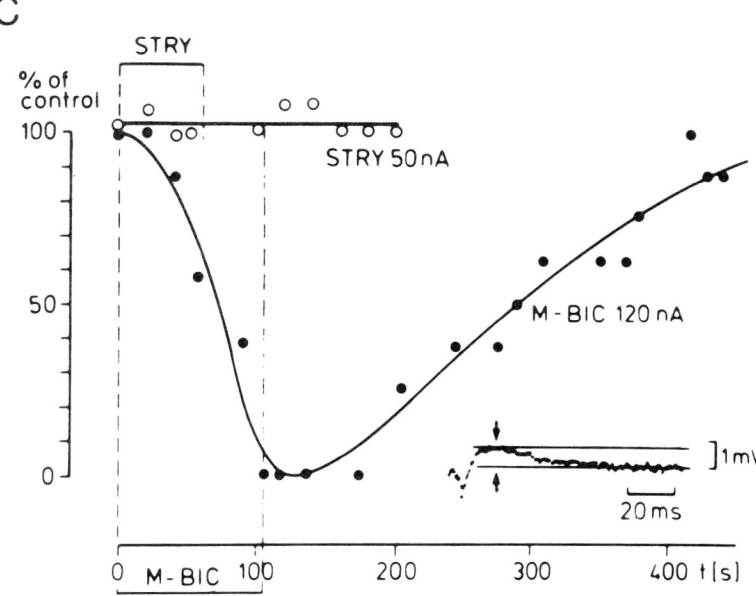

FIG. 17. Effects of possible transmitters and antagonists on synaptic responses in red nucleus of cat. *A, B*: intracellular records show that aspartic acid, applied iontophoretically, reduces amplitude of EPSPs evoked from cortex (*A*) or interpositus nucleus (*B*). Diminished amplitude of resistance-measuring pulses in *B* also indicates marked increase in membrane conductance. *C*: iontophoretic application of bicuculline methochloride (120 nA for 100 s) abolished positive field potential (compare *inset trace*), reflecting inhibition evoked in red nucleus by cortical stimulation. Lack of effect of strychnine also indicates GABAergic nature of this inhibition. [*A, B* from Altmann et al. (2); *C* from Altmann et al. (1).]

ularly ACh tended to inhibit many rubral cells; but the most potent inhibitors were GABA and glycine. Both had a hyperpolarizing effect (with a reversal potential 5-15 mV more negative than the resting potential) associated with a large increase in conductance (2). Short-latency IPSPs, which can be evoked in these cells by cortical stimulation (488), had the same reversal level as the amino acid-evoked hyperpolarizations. Because GABA was consistently more powerful than glycine, and IPSPs and the action of GABA could be greatly diminished by bicuculline methochloride or picrotoxin (but not by strychnine; see Fig. 17C), Altmann et al. (2) concluded that the corticorubral inhibition was probably mediated by the release of GABA, presumably from inhibitory interneurons activated by corticofugal fibers. In agreement with this conclusion is the presence of substantial amounts of GABA and GAD in the nucleus (132).

RETICULOSPINAL CELLS. According to a systematic microiontophoretic study (202), these cells in the cat are readily excited by glutamate, the responses having the usual rapid time course. Strong excitatory effects of norepinephrine and serotonin (but not dopamine) were also seen consistently (Fig. 18). They are of interest because other unidentified medullary reticular cells showed much more variable responses to monoamines. Their slow time course was in sharp contrast to the quick excitations produced by glutamate.

The strongest inhibitory effects were those of glycine, which was regularly more powerful than GABA (484). Its Cl⁻-sensitive hyperpolarizing action was associated with a conductance increase and was therefore comparable to the effects of glycine in the spinal cord (505). In agreement with these findings the inhibitory synaptic inputs to the same neurons were blocked by strychnine, indicating that they are probably mediated by glycine (484). Because these appear to be conducted via recurrent collaterals of inhibitory reticular spinal cells, it has been argued that the spinal endings of the same cells also operate by releasing glycine (484).

VESTIBULOSPINAL CELLS. Most of the relevant infor-

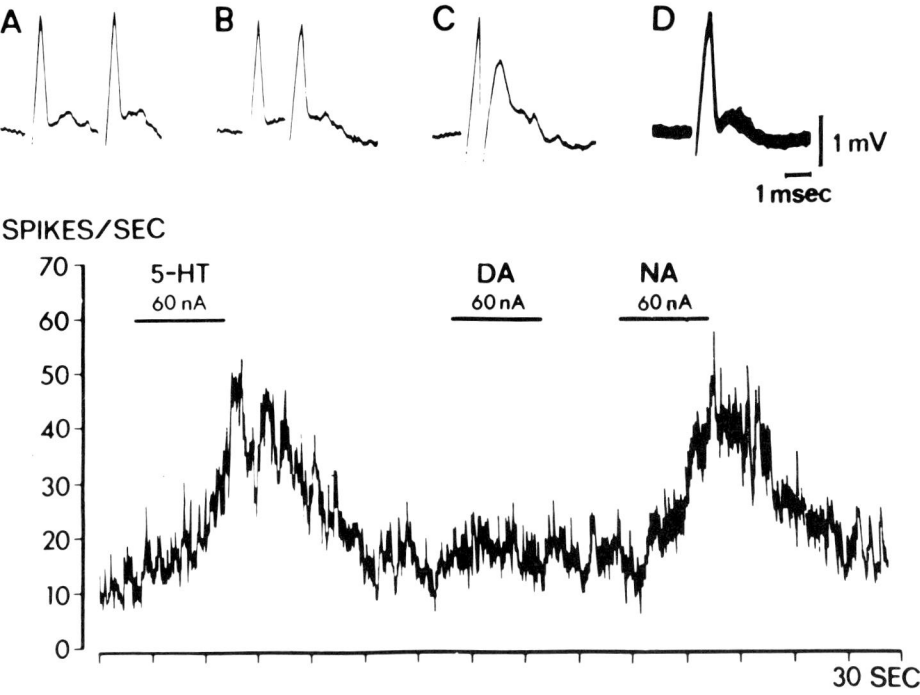

FIG. 18. Action of serotonin (5-HT), dopamine (DA), and norepinephrine (NA) on spontaneous firing of reticulospinal neuron, identified by antidromic activation from cervical spinal cord in decerebrated cat. Note short refractory period when 2 pulses were applied (A–C) and good following at high frequency of stimulation (110/s) and constant latency in D. Note also strong firing evoked by serotonin and norepinephrine. [From Hösli et al. (202).]

mation has been obtained from Deiters' nucleus. A particularly significant feature was the demonstration by Ito and Yoshida (215) that Deiters' neurons in the cat receive a direct monosynaptic inhibitory input from the cerebellar cortex; this feature helped to establish the exclusively inhibitory nature of the output of the cerebellar cortex as well as the identity of the inhibitory transmitter released by cerebellar Purkinje cells, the only efferent cells of the cerebellar cortex.

A systematic investigation of the effects of GABA (366, 369) showed that in every respect GABA and the monosynaptic IPSP evoked by cerebellar stimulation produced identical changes in membrane conductance and potential; the effects of GABA and the IPSP have practically identical reversal levels (Fig. 19). These observations were fully confirmed by Ten Bruggencate and Engberg (485, 486). Although glycine proved to be of comparable potency with effects hardly distinguishable from those of GABA, the ready block of both the cerebellar IPSPs and the effects of GABA (but not glycine) by picrotoxin and bicuculline—and their insensitivity to strychnine, which blocked the effects of glycine—provide strong evidence that in the cat at least the natural transmitter released by the Purkinje cell terminals is GABA rather than glycine (72, 369, 486). Neurochemical studies in rodents have shown that the part of Deiters' nucleus directly innervated by cerebellofugal fibers has a relatively high content in GABA and GAD, both being selectively diminished by cerebellar lesions (144). Finally, Obata and Takeda (368) were able to show that cerebellar stimulation in the cat leads to a release of GABA into the 4th ventricle in the vicinity of Deiters' nucleus. These data provide an unusually strong case for identifying GABA as the transmitter mediating the inhibition of Deiters' neurons by cerebellofugal (Purkinje cell) axons.

The high sensitivity of these neurons to glycine would seem to indicate the presence of a significant glycinergic input, but until now there has been little evidence of such an input, with the possible exception of an inhibitory input from collateral branches of inhibitory reticulospinal cells (484).

The manner in which vestibular inputs excite Deiters' neurons has not been elucidated. As some other bulbospinal neurons (compare subsection RETICULO-SPINAL CELLS, p. 128), Deiters' cells are strongly excited by norepinephrine (516). Although the action of norepinephrine was blocked by a norepinephrine antagonist (dichlorisoprenaline), this drug did not affect the excitation produced by vestibular activation. Similarly, although ACh often excites these cells (466, 516) in the slow and prolonged manner typical of muscarinic effects, the activation evoked by a vestibular input was not blocked by atropine (516). If these cells indeed receive a cholinergic input, it is more likely to have a modulatory (facilitatory) role (466).

The nature of the transmitter that mediates the vestibular excitation thus remains unsolved. These cells are readily excited by glutamate (369, 516), so glutamate or aspartate could be the transmitter in

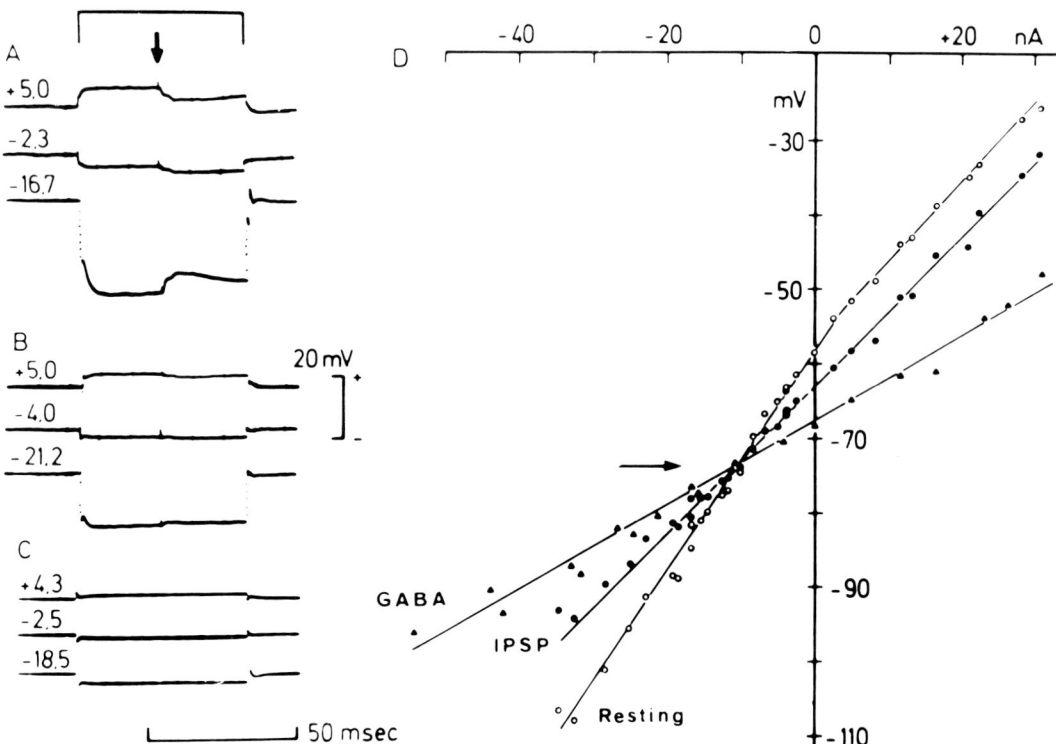

FIG. 19. Identification of γ-aminobutyric acid as inhibitory transmitter responsible for IPSPs evoked in Deiters' neurons of cat by cerebellar stimulation. A–C: examples of experimental data. In A, reversal potential for IPSP (evoked at *arrow*) demonstrated by applying depolarizing or hyperpolarizing current, indicated in nA. B: similar series during iontophoretic administration of GABA (270 nA). C: control runs performed extracellularly. D: graph of voltage current data showing fall in resistance during IPSP (*filled circles*) and GABA application (*triangles*), and common reversal level at horizontal *arrow*. [From Obata et al. (369).]

question, but stronger evidence is needed to make this more than a reasonable possibility.

Summary. The limited evidence available (including the lack of any serious alternative) suggests that the rapid excitatory synaptic actions observed in the brain stem motor nuclei could be mediated by glutamate or aspartate. Some neurons (especially the reticulospinal) are consistently excited by norepinephrine and serotonin in a relatively slow and prolonged manner that is consistent with a possible modulatory function of some monoaminergic pathways. Similarly the slow excitation produced by ACh points to the possibility of a cholinergic modulatory influence. The clearest synaptic inhibitions are generated by increases in Cl⁻ permeability; the most likely transmitters are glycine and GABA, glycine being more prominent in the caudal region (e.g., hypoglossal nucleus, reticulospinal neurons) and GABA more prominent rostrally (oculomotor nuclei, red nucleus). GABA is also probably the transmitter released in Deiters' nucleus by the projection from the cerebellar cortex.

Cerebellum

Because it is relatively accessible and its neuronal circuitry has been substantially worked out (114, 117, 380), the cerebellum has been a favorite target for investigation of chemical synaptic mechanisms.

CEREBELLAR OUTPUT (PURKINJE CELLS). That Purkinje cells are exclusively inhibitory was first demonstrated in cats by Ito and his collaborators (117, 213, 215, 216). The chemical transmitter that mediates this inhibitory action is probably GABA.

Various neurochemical data are certainly consistent with this idea. The cerebellar cortex is rich in GABA and also in glutamic acid decarboxylase (GAD), the enzyme that forms GABA from glutamate (132, 298, 420). Studies of Purkinje cells obtained from tissue slices by microdissection (367) have shown a substantial GABA content. Admittedly much of this could have been due to GABA-releasing inhibitory endings that remain attached to the Purkinje cell; in keeping with this is the finding that the absence of Purkinje cells in certain mice ("nervous" mutants), albeit associated with a clear reduction in the GABA content of deep cerebellar nuclei, is not reflected in a corresponding loss of GABA from the cerebellar cortex (424). Presumably the Purkinje cell bodies have only a relatively low content of GABA.

As already mentioned, the Purkinje cell terminals on Deiters' and interpositus neurons contain both GABA (Fig. 4) and GAD (15, 144, 340, 371); and Obata

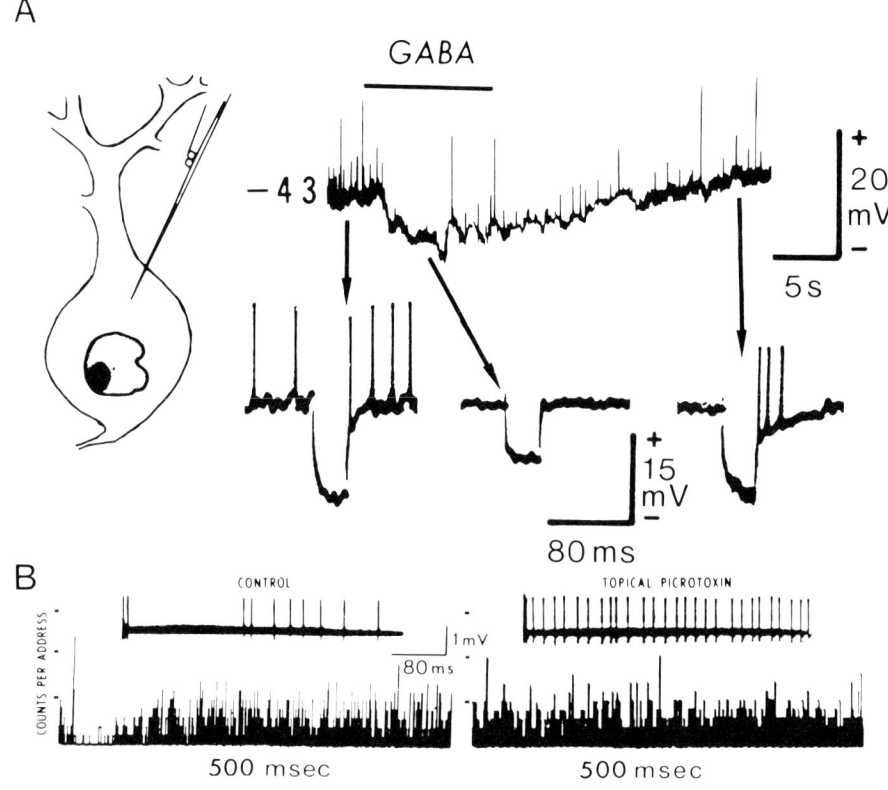

FIG. 20. Gamma aminobutyric acid (GABA) and inhibition of frog cerebellar Purkinje cells. *A*: iontophoretic application of GABA causes hyperpolarization (*upper trace*) and marked reduction in resistance as shown by diminution of resistance-testing pulses (*below*). Calibrations indicate 5 s and 20 mV (*top*) and 80 ms and 50 mV (*bottom*). *B*: synaptic inhibitory action evoked by local stimulation of parallel fibers blocked by topical application of picrotoxin (5×10^{-5} M). At *left*, controls show inhibitory pause in extracellularly recorded unit firing (*above*) and corresponding poststimulus time histogram (*below*). Traces at *right* illustrate disappearance of inhibition during application of picrotoxin. [From Woodward et al. (510).]

and Takeda (368) have shown that stimulation of the cerebellar vermis of the cat leads to a release of GABA into the fourth ventricle near the site of termination of Purkinje cell axons. It is curious, however, that Purkinje cell terminals in the deep nuclei show little evidence of high-affinity GABA uptake (193, 473). But there is pharmacological evidence that the inhibitory actions of the Purkinje cells can be blocked relatively selectively by GABA antagonists (72, 369).

CEREBELLAR INHIBITORY INTERNEURONS. The cerebellum provides an excellent illustration of the predominant role of inhibition in central neural networks: not only is its output via the Purkinje cell axons exclusively inhibitory, but this output can itself be modulated by a set of inhibitory cells, providing for a remarkably flexible system of control by disinhibition. There are two varieties of such cells: *1*) the basket cells, whose terminals make synapses on Purkinje cell bodies; and *2*) the stellate cells, whose endings synapse mainly with Purkinje cell dendrites (117, 380).

Basket cells. That GABA is the main transmitter released by basket cells is suggested by the following. Purkinje cells are readily inhibited by GABA (Fig. 20) much more so than by other amino acids (including glycine) or any other known physiological agent (72, 245, 273b, 510). Moreover the relatively prolonged IPSPs evoked by the interneurons are insensitive to strychnine but can be blocked by picrotoxin (Fig. 20*B*) and bicuculline (35, 72, 510). Immunohistochemical evidence of particularly strong GAD activity in axosomatic terminals on Purkinje cells further supports the idea that the basket cells are GABAergic (340).

Stellate cells. Most of the information available about basket cells also applies to the stellate cells and their terminals on Purkinje cell dendrites [Fig. 21; compare ref. 340]. Thus GABA is probably their main transmitter; but there is some reason to believe that taurine may be released by some stellate cells (though not by basket cells). This is largely based on the findings that taurine is most highly concentrated in the molecular layer and that the taurine content of the cerebellar cortex (356) is substantially reduced by X irradiation, which selectively destroys stellate cells. Because Purkinje cells are not insensitive to taurine (372), especially in the region of the dendrites (147), taurine could be an inhibitory transmitter at some stellate cell synapses.

Golgi cells. These inhibitory interneurons act predominantly at the level of granule cells, partly by a presynaptic action and partly by a postsynaptic action (117). Much evidence supports the idea that Golgi cells are GABAergic: they contain GAD (340) and take up GABA (193), and their inhibitory action is blocked by relatively large doses of picrotoxin or bicuculline but is resistant to strychnine (35). There is also evidence, however, that some Golgi cells contain choline acetyltransferase and acetylcholinesterase (AChe), at least in small rodents, so Kasa and Silver (238) have proposed that they may inhibit by a cholinergic mechanism [though there is no evidence that ACh inhibits granule cells (334)]. It may be relevant

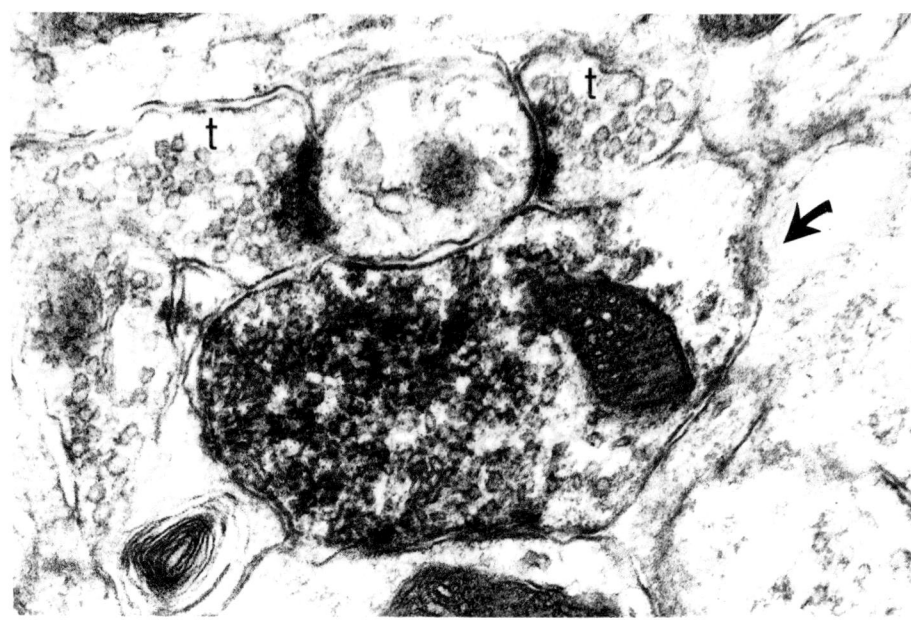

FIG. 21. Glutamate decarboxylase (GAD) reaction product indicates presumed GABAergic synaptic terminal (*arrow*) in molecular layer of rodent cerebellar cortex. Two adjacent terminals (*t*) not labeled. ×43,000. [From Wood et al. (509).]

that some granule cells are inhibited by low doses of glutamate (521).

EXCITATORY INTERNEURONS: THE GRANULE CELLS. These are the only known excitatory neurons in the cerebellar cortex. They receive a large input from the spinal cord and brain stem (via mossy fibers), and they relay excitation to the Purkinje cells via parallel fibers: these travel horizontally in the molecular layer, where they make synapses on dendrites of numerous Purkinje cells.

Everything now points to L-glutamate as the excitatory transmitter released by parallel fibers: *1*) the high sensitivity of Purkinje cells to glutamate (155, 245, 273b), particularly in the region of the dendrites (56); *2*) the similar reversal potential for the effect of glutamate and the parallel fiber-evoked EPSP (170a); *3*) the high concentration of glutamate (132), especially in the molecular and granule cell layers (356); as well as *4*) the selective reduction in glutamate content and synaptosomal glutamate uptake in cerebellar tissue of animals lacking granule cells, either following a viral infection (527) or owing to a genetic defect (424).

CEREBELLAR INPUTS. *Climbing fibers.* These fibers originate solely from the inferior olive (96, 117, 380). They activate Purkinje cells in a highly unusual manner: in contrast to its innervation by many parallel fibers, each Purkinje cell receives only one climbing fiber; but this makes multiple synapses with the cell body and dendrites. The excitatory action is also virtually unique. It is so powerful that each volley leads to a high-frequency repetitive discharge of the Purkinje cell followed by spike inactivation (117). Another remarkable feature is that the EPSP evoked by climbing fiber activity is highly sensitive to the postsynaptic (Purkinje cell) membrane potential (Fig. 22) and is thus readily reversed by depolarization (118).

These properties of the response evoked by climbing fibers should make it particularly suitable for studies of transmitter mechanisms; unfortunately, there is still little evidence as to the nature of the transmitter. All that can be said is that both in rats treated with 3-acetylpyridine (355), which causes a rapid and selective destruction of climbing fibers, and in human beings suffering from olivopontocerebellar atrophy (382), there is no change in cerebellar content in glutamate, but aspartate is reduced; so the transmitter could be aspartate. That glutamate is probably not involved is further indicated by observations of Hackett et al. (170a) that the climbing fiber-evoked EPSP has a more positive reversal potential than the depolarizing effect of glutamate or the parallel fiber-evoked EPSP. It may be relevant that climbing fiber terminals are rich in large, dense-core vesicles (302), suggesting a possible monoaminergic mechanism. But again, the predominant effect of monoamines on most Purkinje cells is inhibitory (245, 449, 516), which argues strongly against norepinephrine, dopamine, or serotonin being the main excitatory transmitter released by climbing fibers. Similarly the relatively weak and irregular excitatory action of ACh (64, 334) is hardly consistent with a cholinergic mechanism of excitation. Although ergothioneine has been proposed as a physiological excitatory agent in the cerebellum (66, 67), iontophoretic applications of ergothioneine show only minimal excitatory effects in the cerebellum (64, 285), and further biochemical studies by Briggs (40) have not confirmed the original studies of Crossland et al. (67).

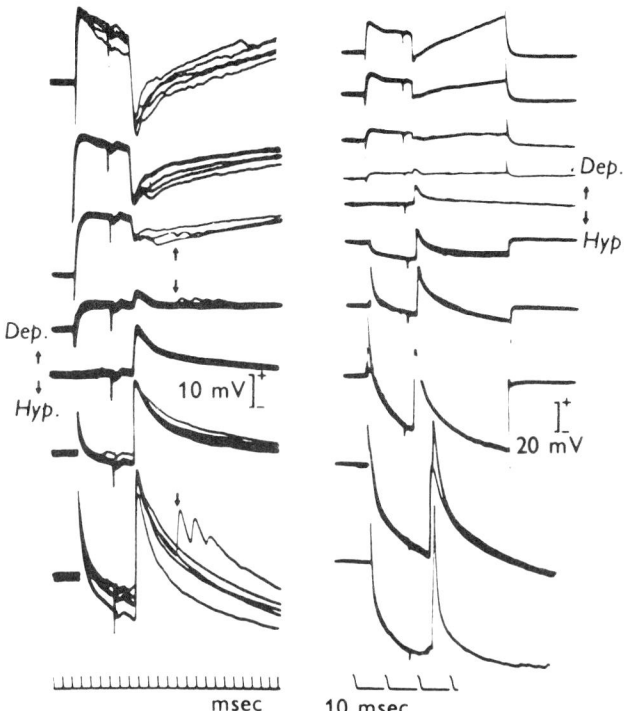

FIG. 22. Climbing fiber–evoked EPSPs in Purkinje cell of cat cerebellum are easily reversed by depolarization. Both sets of records obtained from same cell, those at *right* with slower sweeps and lower amplification. [From Eccles et al. (118).]

Mossy fibers. There has been a good deal of controversy about a possible cholinergic action of mossy fibers. The middle cerebellar peduncle and the granular layer of the cerebellar cortex contain substantial amounts of choline acetyltransferase (134, 178, 234, 238), as well as acetylcholinesterase (387, 450); and ACh is present in isolated mossy fiber terminals (212). McCance and Phillis (334), who applied ACh at various depths in the cerebellum of the cat, concluded that ACh strongly excites many granule cells but has little effect on most Purkinje cells. This might seem to provide further evidence that at least a significant proportion of mossy fibers (perhaps especially those originating from midbrain reticular nuclei) are indeed cholinergic.

There is much evidence to the contrary, however. A striking feature of cerebellar ACh and its related enzymes is their marked variability in different species. Although abundant in guinea pigs and rats, they are very much less prominent in cats and pigeons (212, 450, 451). Moreover, chronic isolation of the cerebellar cortex does not lead to a great reduction in cortical AChe (387); therefore it is unlikely that this enzyme is present mainly in cerebellar afferents and their terminals. Finally, systematic tests of various kinds of cerebellar units by Crawford et al. (64) led them to conclude that neither granule cells nor basket cells were affected by ACh; only the Purkinje cells regularly showed a slow excitation (often preceded by a phase of depression), which proved to be predominantly muscarinic in character.

Thus there is insufficient evidence for any definitive statements about the cholinergic nature of mossy fibers: in spite of a variety of suggestive data, it seems unlikely that most mossy fibers could be cholinergic. Which other transmitter(s) might be released is a matter of conjecture. Because granule cells are sensitive to excitatory amino acids [(64, 334); but compare ref. 521], glutamate or a related amino acid may be the transmitter. Some mossy fibers contain serotonin, and it seems that serotonin may also excite some granule cells (37); but without stronger evidence, it can only be said that some mossy fibers could be tryptaminergic.

Monoaminergic inputs. Norepinephrine-containing fibers from the locus coeruleus project to the cerebellar cortex, as they seem to project to many other parts of the brain and spinal cord (79, 148, 376). As already mentioned, in the cat, neocerebellar neurons are mainly depressed by norepinephrine, but cells in the archicerebellum tend to be excited (245, 516). In the rat, norepinephrine apears to have an exclusively depressant action (449). The time course of the depressant action is relatively slow in cats but fast in rats. It has been proposed that its mechanism is by a reduction in Na^+ conductance, mediated by cyclic AMP (449). Other observers have failed to observe any significant depressant effects of cyclic AMP, however (160, 299). According to a more recent report (187, 511), it appears that the postulated noradrenergic system may actually potentiate the effects of various transmitter agents on Purkinje cells. A particularly careful analysis of norepinephrine-containing terminals in other parts of the brain by Descarries et al. (94) has shown that these terminals do not form typical synapses, but rather form varicosities that are not closely apposed to postsynaptic cells (as in many parts of the peripheral autonomic system). The noradrenergic innervation could thus be involved in diffuse modulation of nerve cell activity, perhaps through changes in local blood flow (91) rather than by synaptic inhibition. Its significance for normal function, however, is not clear, because this innervation can be totally and selectively removed by chemical lesions (with 6-hydroxydopamine) without any evidence of significant impairment of cerebellar function (326).

Some serotonin-containing fibers, possibly originating from raphe nuclei, are also present in the cerebellar cortex (190). Serotonin has a predominantly inhibitory action on Purkinje cells (37, 245), which may reflect a significant inhibitory role of a tryptaminergic innervation.

Summary. The most prominent cortical neurons, the Purkinje cells, are exclusively inhibitory: they are the only output cells of the cerebellar cortex and they probably inhibit other neurons by releasing GABA. The two major inputs into the cerebellar cortex are the mossy fibers and the climbing fibers. Mossy fibers have a very wide origin from the spinal cord and brain stem. It has been suggested that they activate the granule cells by a cholinergic mechanism, but there is significant evidence against this. The climbing fibers probably originate exclusively from the inferior olive [(117); confirmed by ref. 96]; they directly excite Purkinje cells through especially powerful multiple synaptic connections that may operate by releasing aspartate. Of the main intracerebellar neurons, only the granule cells are excitatory, and there are now strong indications that they excite the dendrites of Purkinje cells by releasing glutamate. The other interneurons are inhibitory: the three main types, the basket, stellate, and Golgi cells, most likely release GABA, but some other inhibitory amino acids may also be involved, for example, taurine in the case of stellate cells. Finally, Purkinje cells tend to be inhibited by norephinephrine and excited by ACh: it has been postulated that inhibitory monoaminergic (noradrenergic) and facilitatory cholinergic pathways also play a significant part in the control of cerebellar neural activity; but the evidence is mostly fragmentary and permits little more than some tentative conclusions.

Basal Ganglia

The basal ganglia are exceptionally rich in neurotransmitters and the associated enzymes (132). Thus the striatum (caudate putamen) contains more dopamine and ACh than does any other part of the CNS, as well as relatively large amounts of GABA, glutamate, and serotonin; it is also rich in some neuroactive peptides, including substance P (42, 433) and enkephalin (180). There are even higher concentrations of GABA and substance P in the substantia nigra. Considering the clear association between deficiency of dopamine and clinical manifestations of extrapyramidal motor disorders (198, 460), one can presume that dopamine plays some important part in synaptic transmission and modulation in this region of the brain, which is the most prominent portion of the extrapyramidal motor system.

TRANSMITTERS IN VARIOUS STRIATAL PATHWAYS. Biochemical and histochemical evidence at first seemed to indicate important cholinergic and dopaminergic afferent pathways originating from the substantia nigra (compare refs. 5, 396, 446). Because ACh had a predominantly excitatory action (36, 342) and dopamine a predominantly inhibitory action (36, 343) on caudate neurons, it appeared that the substantia nigra exerted both an excitatory (cholinergic) and an inhibitory (dopaminergic) control over caudate function. In spite of a great deal of further investigation, however, the role played by dopamine or acetylcholine in the caudate neurons is still not certain: there is no general agreement as to whether these agents act mainly as excitatory or inhibitory transmitters, and it is unlikely that ACh is released by a nigrostriatal pathway. The following sections summarize the salient points about transmitters and related mechanisms in the basal ganglia; for a more detailed review, see reference 101a.

NIGROSTRIATAL PATHWAY. Anatomical and electrophysiological evidence of a direct monosynaptic excitatory connection between the substantia nigra and the caudate nucleus is very strong (51, 138, 256). This agrees with other evidence (206, 251) that all of the inputs to the caudate nucleus are excitatory, caudate IPSPs being mediated secondarily by intrinsic cells. It is of interest that EPSPs in caudate neurons can be readily reversed by depolarization (Fig. 23). But how does the nigrostriatal dopaminergic input fit into this picture, considering the inhibitory action of dopamine repeatedly observed on striatal cells (25, 60, 139, 183, 528)?

A possible resolution of this paradoxical situation was recently provided by Kitai et al. (256). During intracellular recording they found that "brief" iontophoretic applications of dopamine tend to depolarize many caudate neurons (Fig. 23) showing monosynaptic EPSPs in response to nigral stimulation. They suggested that the depressant effects of dopamine previously reported might be explained if long applications of dopamine activate inhibitory interneurons. On the other hand, Kitai's observations are not easily reconciled with the fact that almost total depletion of nigrostriatal dopamine by 6-hydroxydopamine (139) does not abolish the nigrostriatal monosynaptic excitation. It thus may be necessary to postulate a second nigrostriatal excitatory pathway (258) having a different transmitter, which could be a dicarboxylic amino acid, as well as perhaps the presence of both inhibitory and excitatory receptors for dopamine (137). Until further experiments have fully confirmed Kitai's observations (for example, ref. 418), the problem of the precise nature of the nigrostriatal dopaminergic influence cannot be considered definitively solved.

An important reason for the great interest in the role of dopamine in the striatum is the pronounced diminution in striatal dopamine that is a characteristic feature of Parkinsonism, and the notably successful treatment with the dopamine precursor L-dopa (62): this can be said to have initiated a new era of neurochemical treatment of neurological disorders, a domain previously notorious for the lack of any rational therapy. Although the striking effectiveness of L-dopa fully justified its use, this should not blind us to the present inadequate understanding of its precise mode of operation.

Parkinsonism is believed to be caused by degeneration of nigrostriatal dopaminergic cells (198). This idea is supported by the remarkably high positive correlation between the number of surviving dopamine-containing cells and corresponding tissue levels of dopamine after administration of 6-hydroxydopamine on the one hand, and the quality of motor performance of rats on the other (409). If, however, in Parkinson patients the relevant cells have disappeared

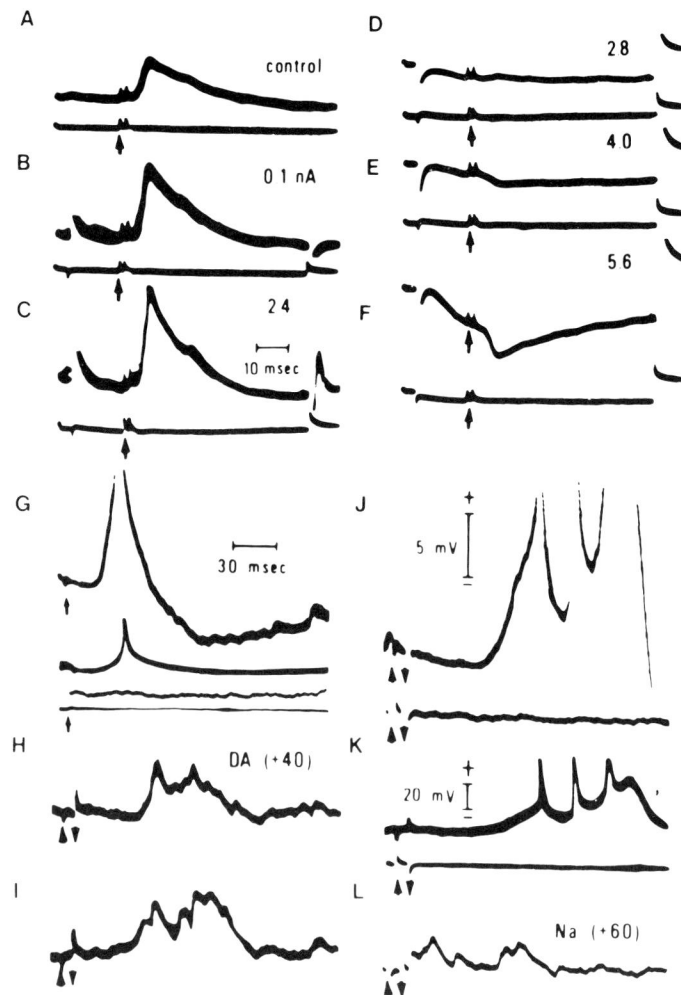

FIG. 23. Properties of EPSPs and effects of dopamine recorded in caudate neurons. *A-F*: EPSP, evoked from median forebrain bundle, was enhanced by hyperpolarization (*A-C*) and then depressed or reversed by depolarization (*D-F*); *lower trace* of each pair is an extracellular control. *G*: action potential evoked by nigral stimulus recorded on high-gain AC and low-gain DC *traces* (*above* and *below*); *lowest trace* is an extracellular control. *H*: depolarizing response evoked by extracellular dopamine (DA) release (14 nA for 10 ms). Repeated applications of same dopamine pulse evoked progressively greater responses (compare *I* and *J* at same gain, and *K* at much lower gain). *L*: control recorded while applying pulse of Na$^+$ instead of dopamine. [From Kitai et al. (256).]

and are not simply unable to manufacture enough dopamine, how does L-dopa restore normal function? Perhaps it boosts the activity of a small number of remaining dopaminergic neurons. Alternatively, L-dopa may be taken up and converted to dopamine in neurons that are not normally dopaminergic (110, 491). Recent evidence that intraneuronal injections of dopamine can markedly alter neuronal excitability (265) suggests a further possibility: that large doses of L-dopa may significantly influence the firing of various neurons by raising their intracellular dopamine level. It should also be remembered that the nigrostriatal pathway may be important for the regulation of striatal blood flow (304).

There has been much speculation about the possibility that the striatal receptor for dopamine is an adenylate cyclase (247) or is closely related to such an enzyme (246, 437). The functional significance of this apparent association between dopaminergic activity and cyclic AMP formation is not very clear. Cyclic nucleotides may phosphorylate protein kinases that are of importance for cell function (163, 200), though perhaps more for long-term regulation than for synaptic activation.

OTHER STRIATAL AFFERENTS. The important direct excitatory projection from the cerebral cortex (43, 51, 251, 255) may well operate by liberating L-glutamate in the striatum. This is indicated by the high sensitivity of caudate neurons to the dicarboxylic amino acids (29, 36, 462), the marked diminution in striatal glutamate levels (141, 254) and in high-affinity glutamate uptake (99) after cortical lesions, as well as the high sensitivity of striatal neurons to kainic acid, which is thought to depend on the presence of a glutamate-releasing innervation (47, 336).

McLennan and York (342) suggested that the other major striatal input, from the intralaminar thalamic nuclei, is cholinergic, but this has not been corroborated by histochemical and neurochemical investigations. The prevalent belief is that cholinergic cells are mainly intrinsic to the striatum (see subsection STRIATAL INTERNEURONS, p. 137).

STRIATONIGRAL PATHWAYS. More recently, there has been a surge of interest in the efferent pathways from the striatum. The substantia nigra is known to contain particularly high concentrations of GABA and substance P, and much work has been done to establish a possible synaptic role for these agents.

This has been done most successfully for GABA, which appears to be the agent released by a direct inhibitory pathway projecting from the caudate nucleus to the substantia nigra. This is indicated by electrophysiological demonstrations of the monosynaptic character of this inhibition (136, 525), its abolition by picrotoxin (402), and the high sensitivity of nigral cells to GABA but not glycine [Fig. 24; (136)]. Further confirmation is given by the presence in the substantia nigra of GAD-containing terminals and their disappearance after striatal lesions (142, 436, 473); the results of Schwarcz and Coyle (436) are particularly convincing, because the caudate lesions were made with kainic acid, which appears to destroy only local neurons, leaving "fibres de passage" and terminals intact. These studies have not confirmed an earlier suggestion that the descending GABAergic pathway originates mainly from the globus pallidus (338).

The discovery that Huntington's chorea is accompanied by a large loss of striatal GABA and GAD (31, 383) is clearly relevant in this context, and a parallel has been drawn between the action of kainic acid and the pathological process responsible for neuronal death in Huntington's disease (47, 336).

Substance P is highly concentrated in the substantia nigra (305), where it can be released by depolarizing stimulation (226). It has a strong excitatory action on nigral neurons (103), with the prolonged time course characteristic of its action in other parts of the CNS (264). Judging by the effects of striatal lesions (42), especially those produced by kainic acid injections into the caudate nucleus (195), many substance P-containing terminals in the substantia nigra probably originate from cells in the caudate nucleus, especially in its anterior portion, and also perhaps the pallidum. These caudate cells are probably distinct from the presumed GABAergic striatonigral cells, which tend to be situated more posteriorly in the caudate nucleus (see also refs. 150, 151, 433). These data thus seem to indicate the presence of a separate, substance P-releasing and excitatory striatonigral pathway, projecting especially to the pars reticulata.

The situation in the substantia nigra seems to be even more complicated. There is evidence that dopamine is released from dendrites of the presumed dopaminergic neurons (situated in the pars compacta) and that it may act on the same population of cells and provide a negative feedback that reduces their activity. Dopamine may act as well on neurons in the pars reticulata (through dendrodendritic synapses), and perhaps also on striatonigral terminals that release GABA and/or substance P (358, 362). Moreover, GABAergic intrinsic neurons may also be present in the substantia nigra (358). In addition, there are many afferent terminals rich in norepinephrine (495) and serotonin (381), which originate from the lower brain stem, including the raphe nuclei. These afferent

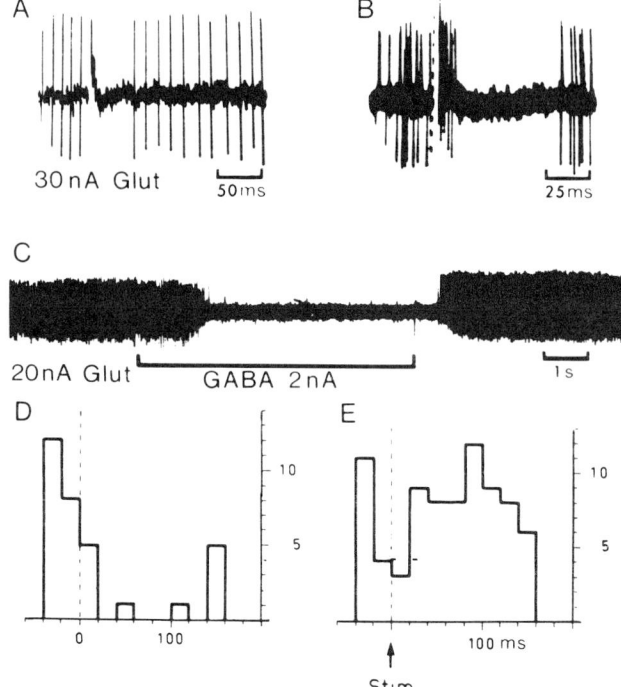

FIG. 24. Inhibition of nigral unit in cat by caudate stimulation. A, B: ongoing firing of unit in substantia nigra maintained by slow release of glutamate; single shock stimulation in caudate was 1.5 × threshold in A and 2 × threshold in B. C: strong inhibitory effect of γ-aminobutyric acid on glutamate-evoked discharge of same unit. D–E: poststimulus time histograms of firing of nigral unit inhibited by caudate stimulation, before and after injection of 2.5 mg/kg picrotoxin. [A–C from Feltz (136). Reproduced by permission of the Natl. Res. Counc. Can. from the Can. J. Physiol. Pharmacol. 49: 1113–1115, 1971. D–E from Precht and Yoshida (402).]

terminals are more likely to have inhibitory than excitatory effects (102, 103).

Although the striatonigral inhibitory pathway may act partly as a negative feedback on the activity of the nigrostriatal dopaminergic system, its main function is probably to inhibit the cells of the pars reticulata, which provide significant nigrothalamic and nigrostriatal efferent pathways for the output of the striatum [Fig. 25; (170, 254)]. According to Olianas et al. (373), unilateral intranigral injections of muscimol [the powerful GABA agonist (229, 364)] induce turning movements precisely opposite to those seen following intrastriatal injections of dopamine agonists (see ref. 491). This effect cannot be mediated via the striatal dopaminergic system, because it is insensitive to dopamine antagonists. Moreover, a chronic muscimol-like effect was obtained by injecting kainic acid into the substantia nigra. Olianas et al. (373) therefore argue that the nigral pars reticulata cells, which are destroyed by kainic acid, must be in the nigral efferent pathway that initiates the characteristic turning movements. If the nigrothalamic pathway is itself made up of inhibitory neurons (524), there are two inhibitory systems in series in this striatal output (as in the caudate-pallidum-subthalamus pathway, see subsection PALLIDOSUBTHALAMIC PROJECTION, this page). This can operate effectively only if the second (nigrothalamic) link is tonically excited by some other input. One may speculate that the required background of excitation is provided by the substance P–releasing striatonigral fibers, whose role otherwise is not particularly clear.

OTHER STRIATAL EFFERENT PATHWAYS. The principal efferent pathways from the corpus striatum thus appear to be inhibitory. The largest of these, the projection to the globus pallidus (51), is clearly inhibitory (526): judging by the high GAD content of the pallidum (including the entopeduncular nucleus) and its decline after lesions of the striatal afferent fibers, this pathway is probably GABAergic (142).

There is a close parallel between the striatum and the cerebellum: in both cases, the neuronal inputs are predominantly (and perhaps exclusively) excitatory, whereas the efferent pathways are mainly inhibitory and GABAergic. The only known exception is the striatonigral substance P–containing pathway, which is presumably excitatory; but because its major target is probably the nigrothalamic and nigrotectal system, the overall output via the substantia nigra is also mediated by inhibition.

PALLIDOSUBTHALAMIC PROJECTION. An important pathway in the striatal output system is the projection from the pallidum to the subthalamic nucleus (51, 253). This also appears to be an inhibitory pathway (370); according to a recent study by Fonnum et al. (143), it is rich in GAD and therefore also likely to be GABAergic. This striatal output therefore operates through multiple GABAergic inhibitory pathways arranged in series, and therefore it may have a net excitatory action (through "disinhibition"). If the postulated GABAergic projection from the entopeduncular nucleus to the lateral habenula (357) indeed inhibits an inhibitory pathway to the dorsal raphe nucleus, one may have three inhibitory systems in series, with inhibition of disinhibition giving an overall inhibition!

STRIATAL INTERNEURONS. The striatum contains very large numbers of interneurons (51, 251), some of which must be responsible for the widespread IPSPs generated by various forms of activation (30, 43). Because the effect of GABA on caudate neurons are comparable with IPSPs (30), and blockage of GABA receptors by intracaudate injections of picrotoxin induces myotonic manifestations (482), it is likely that many of these interneurons are GABAergic.

On the other hand, the presence of many cholinergic cells is suggested by the very high concentrations of ACh, AChe, and choline acetyltransferase in the striatum (132, 178, 319, 322, 451), as well as ACh receptors (522). At one time this was thought to indicate an ascending cholinergic innervation (446). But the present consensus is that the presumed cholinergic neurons are intrinsic (337, 433). Except in barbiturate-anesthetized animals, the action of ACh on caudate neurons is predominantly excitatory (36, 342, 462). According to Bernardi et al. (29), this slow depolarizing action (Fig. 26) is not associated with a fall in membrane resistance and therefore resembles other slow muscarinic excitatory actions (263, 284).

Recent observations by Takagi and Yamamoto (479) indicate a specific depressant action of ACh on input from the corticostriate pathways (but not the nigrostriatal pathway). This is of some significance, because a presynaptic depression of transmitter

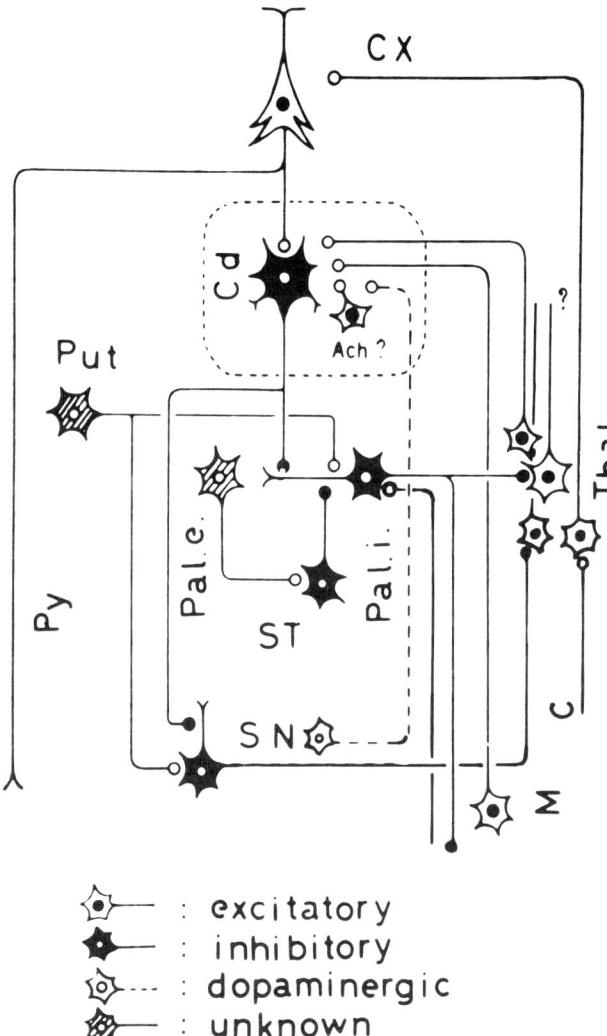

FIG. 25. Schematic diagram of basal ganglia showing main connections between various nuclei as well as probable function. Cx, cerebral cortex; Cd, caudate; Thal, thalamus; Pal i. and Pal e., internal and external segments of globus pallidus; ST, subthalamic nucleus; SN, substantia nigra; Py, pyramidal tract; Put, putamen; M, midbrain. [From Yoshida and Obata (524).]

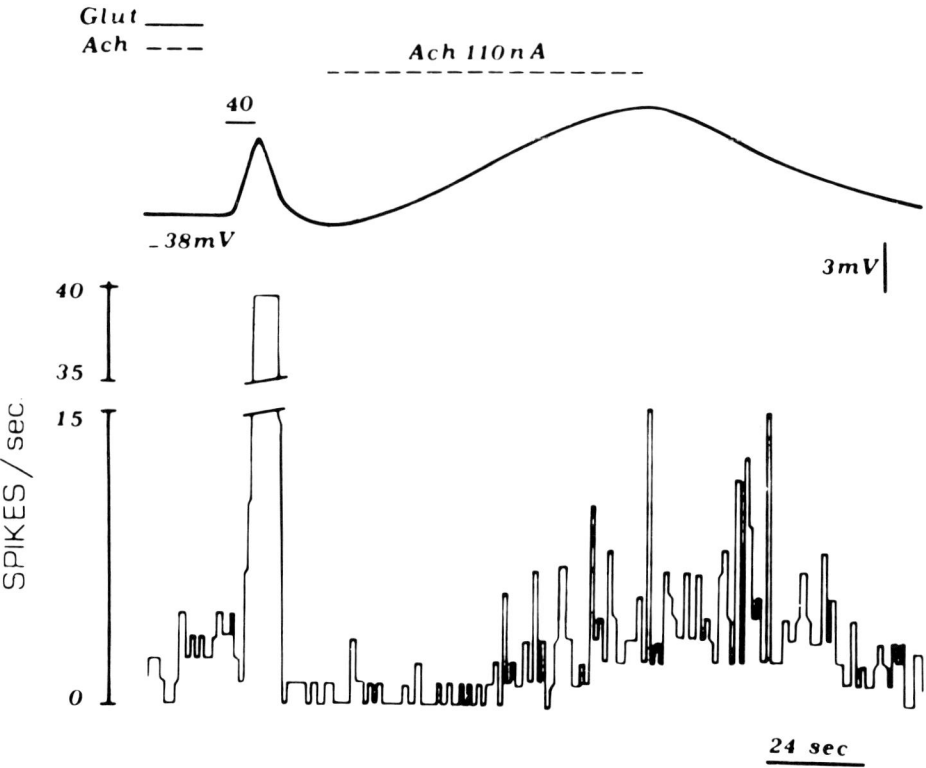

FIG. 26. Excitatory action of glutamate and ACh on caudate neuron in cat: *above*, DC trace showing quick depolarization caused by glutamate and slow depolarization caused by ACh (resting potential −38 mV). Discharge frequency indicated on same time base by histogram *below*. [From Bernardi et al. (29).]

release would explain the initial inhibition of spontaneous firing that so often precedes the excitatory action of ACh, not only in the caudate nucleus (for example, ref. 29) but also in the cortex (274, 284) and other parts of the CNS (263). A similar presynaptic mechanism would also account for the otherwise puzzling depression of IPSPs observed during applications of ACh in the caudate nucleus (29). Presynaptic receptors for ACh also appear to be present on striatal dopaminergic nerve endings; according to De Belleroche and Bradford (86) these receptors may be either nicotinic or muscarinic, the former promoting and the latter inhibiting dopamine release. They were less prominent in the experiments of Takagi and Yamamoto (479).

The particularly high level of enkephalin in the striatum and pallidum (453) suggests the possibility of a significant role of opioid peptides in striatal function.

Summary. It appears that the main inputs into the striatum are excitatory, and at least one of them, that from the cortex, is probably mediated by glutamate-releasing terminals. The main striatal output, to the pallidum and substantia nigra, is inhibitory and probably GABAergic, and the further pallidosubthalamic and nigrothalamic efferent connections are probably also inhibitory. Striatal activity appears to be modulated by a dopaminergic input from the substantia nigra, but it is still not fully certain whether this is mainly excitatory or inhibitory. Intrinsic interneurons probably include many GABAergic inhibitory cells, cholinergic cells that have "modulatory" as well as presynaptic inhibitory actions, and probably some peptidergic neurons: these include cells that release enkephalin, as well as a substance P-releasing efferent excitatory pathway to the substantia nigra. The main function of the cholinergic and peptidergic neurons may be to provide the background of tonic excitation needed for the effective operation of chains of inhibitory cells.

Motor Cortex

PYRAMIDAL TRACT NEURONS. There is no direct evidence about the transmitters released by pyramidal tract cells; but considering some neurochemical evidence, which favors L-glutamate as the transmitter released by other corticofugal neurons, including the corticostriatal (99), corticothalamic (141), corticogeniculate, and corticocollicular (236), one may reasonably expect that pyramidal tract cells also release glutamate (or perhaps aspartate) from their terminals in the spinal cord, as well as from other terminals in the cortex itself (472), in the red nucleus, the pontine nuclei, the dorsal column nuclei (472a), and so on.

Excitatory amino acids. Pyramidal tract neurons are themselves readily excited by L-glutamate and aspartate (63, 273b, 274). No other agents known to be normally present in the cortex have such a powerful, rapid, and reproducible excitatory action. Indeed the cerebral cortex has the highest content in glutamate (≫10 mM) of all parts of the central nervous system (132). Effective uptake mechanisms are also present for the removal of these excitatory amino acids (14, 141, 470), and the Ca^{2+}-dependent release of glutamate (and to a lesser extent aspartate) from the cerebral cortex in vivo, or cortical slices (Fig. 27) or synaptosomes in vitro, is now well established (38, 57, 225, 401). Although most of the criteria for a transmitter function of glutamate are thus fulfilled, there is still inadequate information about its precise mechanism of excitation. Krnjević and Schwartz (288) reported that in some instances the depolarizing effect of glutamate was associated with increased conductance, but it is not certain whether the conductance change is a primary effect of glutamate or one secondary to the large depolarization; moreover there is no reliable information about the reversal potential for this depolarizing action. Hence it is by no means clear whether the depolarization is mediated by an increase in membrane permeability to Na^+ (and/or Ca^{2+}), as in crustacean muscle (377), or is related to a Na^+-linked active transport of glutamate into nerve cells (126, 273b).

There is great interest in finding a specific pharmacological antagonist for the dicarboxylic amino acids (compare refs. 34, 184a, 341, 364, 472, 493). No agent proposed so far has proved wholly reliable: the most promising is perhaps D-α-aminoadipic acid, as a relatively specific blocker of aspartate effects (34, 184). These studies indicate that aspartate and glutamate act on distinct receptors rather than a general dicarboxylic amino acid receptor.

Acetylcholine. A significant characteristic of pyramidal tract cells is that they are also readily excited by ACh (63, 274, 430, 461, 471). This is by no means a universal feature of cortical neurons, ACh-sensitive cells being rare in superficial layers of the cortex; even in the deeper layers, random sampling yields a proportion of ACh-sensitive neurons that is usually well under 50% (274, 471).

This action of ACh differs markedly from that of glutamate. It is slower in onset and is always much more prolonged, outlasting the application by some tens of seconds (Fig. 28). The depolarizing effect is often associated with an increase in cell resistance (284, 513), and its reversal potential is negative even after intracellular injections of Cl^-. Krnjević et al. (284) therefore concluded that it was mainly due to a fall in K^+ permeability. Its pharmacological properties indicate muscarinic receptors that are strikingly similar to those classically described in the gut and elsewhere (275). This conclusion is confirmed by in vitro observations on the binding properties of brain muscarinic receptors (32).

A curious feature of this excitatory action is that it is often preceded by a reduction in ongoing discharges. When background firing is pronounced, the depression may be the most obvious effect of ACh. A comparable depression is the only effect of ACh on cells in more superficial cortical layers (393, 407). It is not certain whether this reflects a postsynaptic inhibitory mechanism, as suggested by Phillis et al. (391), or perhaps more likely a presynaptic interference with ongoing transmitter release comparable to the inhibitory effects of ACh observed in slices of pyriform cortex (519), hippocampus (203), and striatum (479).

It is well known that ACh is present and can be synthesized in the cerebral cortex (178, 322), probably in terminals of subcortical nerve cells (177), and that it is continually released (58, 105, 324) at a rate that bears some relation to the degree of wakefulness (58)

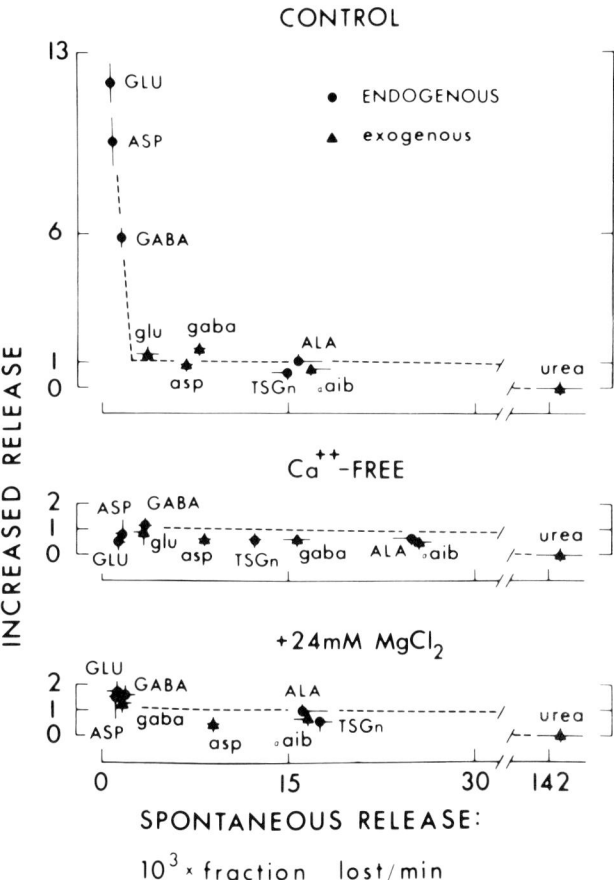

FIG. 27. Electrical stimulation of guinea pig cortical slices causes selective enhancement of release of endogenous putative transmitter amino acids: glutamate (GLU), aspartate (ASP), and γ-aminobutyric acid (GABA); in contrast to alanine (ALA), threonine, serine, and glutamine (TSGn), and also α-aminoisobutyric (aib). Selective release clearly seen in control graph *above* is totally abolished in absence of calcium or in presence of high concentration of magnesium (compare two graphs *below*). Endogenous amino acids labeled by superfusion with radioactive glucose; exogenous ones by superfusion with radioactive amino acids. Increase in release during electrical stimulation (ordinates) expressed as multiple of spontaneous release [From Potashner (401), © 1978, with permission of Pergamon Press, Ltd.]

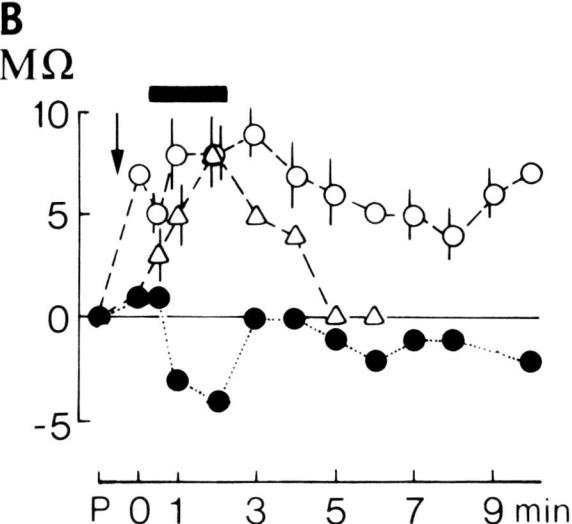

FIG. 28. *A*: excitation of cortical neuron in cat by acetylcholine shows typical slow time course of depolarization and firing. *B*: changes in resistance of motor cortex neuron evoked by ACh with and without simultaneous electrical excitation (*heavy bar* indicates period of ACh release). *Open triangles*, mean values of resistance increase from 21 cells (with standard errors) in absence of other stimulation; *open circles*, corresponding data from 24 cells made to fire throughout period of ACh application by intracellular injection of depolarizing current; note longer persisting increase in resistance. *Filled circles*, control data from 15 cells made to discharge by depolarizing current but without application of ACh. [*A* from Krnjević et al. (284); *B* from Woody et al. (513).]

and can be raised by sensory or brain stem (reticular) stimulation (390, 477). Because ACh release is depressed by physostigmine and enhanced by atropine [Fig. 29; (105, 324, 478)], there is evidently a negative feedback control of ACh release, at least part of which must be mediated in the cortex itself (397, 478), most likely via the presynaptic muscarinic receptors already discussed.

Significance of the cholinergic excitatory action. As originally emphasized by Krnjević et al. [(284); compare also ref. 263], the reduction in pyramidal tract cell K^+ permeability evoked by ACh provides a particularly effective facilitation of other excitatory inputs by tending to depolarize the cell, by reducing the braking action of K^+ outward current, and also by increasing the electrotonic space constant of the cell membrane. All these factors make it more likely that a given excitatory input generates action potentials. In addition, the reduction in delayed K^+ currents would promote repetitive discharges in response to a brief input. It has therefore been postulated that cortical "arousal" is caused by such cholinergic facilitation (263), mediated by ACh release from terminals of the diffuse network of AChe-containing nerve fibers that can be demonstrated in the cortex (290, 291). These fibers appear to ascend from a wide region of the base of the brain (290, 291, 447), and they may well correspond to the direct connections between the frontal cortex on the one hand and the hypothalamus and basal ganglia on the other, demonstrated more recently by the use of horseradish peroxidase (252, 312).

Is the suggestion that arousal is caused by cholinergic facilitation compatible with the observed behavior of neurons in the motor cortex? At first sight the answer seems to be negative. Recordings from single pyramidal tract cells do not show a marked tendency for firing to increase during arousal and, indeed, fast conducting pyramidal tract cells "appear" to be inhibited at the onset of arousal because their finding is reduced (467, 468). It can be shown, however, that in spite of this reduction in firing, pyramidal tract cells become more responsive to antidromic invasion (468). Hence all pyramidal tract cells indeed become more excitable during arousal, as would be expected if arousal is mediated by cholinergic pathways. The latter may operate not only directly, by releasing ACh near the pyramidal tract cells, but also indirectly, by inhibiting cortical inhibitory interneurons (468). The pause in firing of fast pyramidal tract cells may well be a form of disfacilitation, which can be explained not only by inhibition of excitatory interneurons and other excitatory inputs, but also by a presynaptic cholinergic depressant action, which would reduce the effectiveness of any ongoing excitatory input (compare ref. 519).

In any case there are reasonable grounds for believing that large numbers of cortical cells (including pyramidal tract neurons) are under the influence of a facilitatory cholinergic system, which may be important not just as a quantitative but also as a qualitative control of cortical activity. A lowered responsiveness of corticofugal neurons consequent on diminished cholinergic activation could provide the "de-efferentation" that may be required for sleep, or for loss of consciousness more generally. It has been suggested that a similar effect would be produced by conditions that selectively suppress the facilitatory action of ACh, such as hypoxia or narcosis, which by slowing down intracellular Ca^{2+} sequestration allow intracellular Ca^{2+} to raise K^+ permeability (157, 263, 268, 476).

Another possible role for ACh is indicated by the studies of Woody and his collaborators (512). They have shown that the formation of a conditioned reflex in the cat (eye blink or nose twitch) is associated with a persistent increase in the excitability of motor cortex neurons that project to the relevant brain stem motor nucleus. After confirming that ACh induces a comparable, but normally only temporary, increase in excitability [as in the experiments of Krnjević et al. (284)], Woody et al. (513) further reported that when the application of ACh was combined with direct stimulation of the observed neuron, the increase in

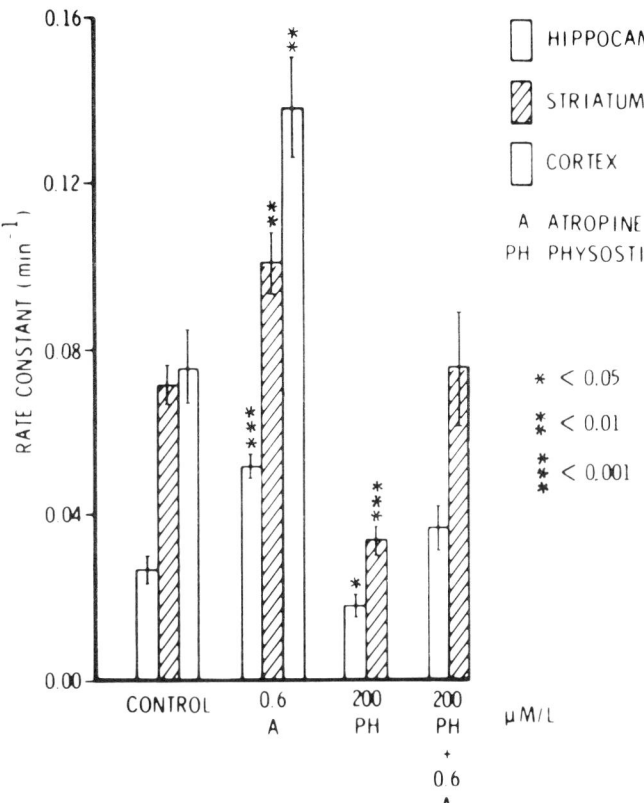

FIG. 29. Effects of muscarinic agents on rate constants of [^{3}H]acetylcholine release evoked by 25 mM K$^+$ in 3 different cerebral tissues. Note enhancement of release by atropine and depression by physostygmine. [From Szerb (478).]

excitability and input resistance persisted much longer (Fig. 28). In other words, the effect produced was much like that seen during conditioning. Thus, if during conditioning a reflex neuronal discharge is combined with cholinergic activation, this conjunction could lead to a long-lasting enhancement of excitability in a selected neuronal population. In such a way ACh could play a significant role in learning.

CORTICAL INHIBITORY MECHANISMS. Inhibitory processes are prevalent in the cortex, most forms of neural activity being accompanied by inhibition of neighboring cells and followed by inhibition of the previously active cells. These inhibitions are clearly manifested by a large reduction of excitability, typically lasting 100 ms or more, as well as hyperpolarizing IPSPs associated with a large increase in membrane conductance (65, 104, 286, 386, 398, 404, 465). The very strong and consistent inhibitory action of GABA first led to the suggestion that GABA is an inhibitory transmitter in the cortex (273b). Later intracellular experiments (104, 289) revealed a striking similarity between the effects of GABA and the IPSPs: in both cases there was a hyperpolarization and increase in conductance, as well as similar reversal levels sensitive to intracellular injections of Cl$^-$. Thus synaptic inhibition and GABA both appeared to act by enhancing the neuron's membrane permeability to Cl$^-$.

Unlike spinal cells, cortical neurons were mostly insensitive to glycine (249, 273b), so there was little likelihood that inhibition could be mediated principally by glycine. This is supported by the ineffectiveness of strychnine as a blocker of cortical inhibition (287).

A major inhibitory role of GABA is indicated by other data, showing that the cortex of various mammals contains large amounts of GABA (132) and glutamate decarboxylase (GAD) (15); that GABA is released from the cortex as a result of stimulation, both in vivo (225, 348) and in vitro [Fig. 27; (38, 401, 492)]; and that GABA is actively taken up by nerve endings, neuroglia, and probably postsynaptic cells (124, 192). Judging by the number of terminals that contain GAD or take up GABA, it appears that one-third to one-half of all terminals may be GABAergic. This obviously agrees well with the ubiquity of inhibitory effects recorded in the cortex.

Pharmacological evidence that GABA mediates inhibition of cortical cells has been more controversial; the main antagonists that have been proposed, picrotoxin and bicuculline (229), appear to be either not very effective or not very selective when applied in the cortex (159, 185, 287), possibly because cortical GABA receptors belong to a less susceptible population than GABA receptors in some other regions of the central nervous system (364). Some other convulsant agents, including benzyl penicillin and tubocurarine (72, 185), have also been suggested as GABA antagonists.

Although GABA is probably the most important inhibitory transmitter in the cortex, it would be premature to dismiss altogether some other related inhibitory agents, such as glycine or taurine, though they are usually much weaker than GABA (273b, 277); β-alanine (90), guanidine propionic acid (273b), and some imidazole derivatives (158, 276) are also strong inhibitors; one or more of these agents could be released by a certain proportion of inhibitory interneurons.

OTHER TRANSMITTERS IN THE CORTEX. *Monoamines.* Monoamines are present in the cortex, apparently in fibers that form a diffuse network, more or less evenly distributed throughout the various regions, but which account for only a small fraction of all nerve terminals (301). They include norepinephrine, dopamine, and serotonin.

The norepinephrine-containing system probably originates exclusively from the locus coeruleus (148, 313, 376); its terminals in the cortex do not form typical synapses on neurons but rather free varicosities (94), not unlike those seen in the sympathetic innervation of peripheral blood vessels. The dopamine-containing fibers have a different origin from the brain stem, from groups of cells in or close to the substantia nigra (313). The serotonin-containing fibers probably originate from the raphe nuclei (148), but they also end in varicosities rather than clear synapses (93).

It therefore seems that the monoaminergic pathways exert a relatively diffuse influence on cortical neurons. What is its nature? On the whole, monoamines have mainly depressant effects on cortical neurons, including pyramidal tract cells (63, 276, 389, 391, 429), though excitatory effects have been reported to be more conspicuous under certain conditions (228). Some other kind of synaptic or modulatory action may be important. For example, is it possible that monoamines facilitate other synaptic inputs, as they do at the neuromuscular junction (269, 292) or in molluscan ganglia (444) mainly by enhancing transmitter release? There is some evidence from studies in the cerebellum that norepinephrine might have a postsynaptic facilitatory action on the responses evoked by various transmitters (187, 511).

It has been suggested that monoamines are involved in mechanisms of learning; but this has received little support from studies of the effects of selective destructions of the monoaminergic pathways (140, 331, 332). The most impressive evidence obtained until now is that of Kasamatsu and Pettigrew (239). Young kittens treated with 6-hydroxydopamine showed a greatly diminished capacity for reorganizing synaptic connections after monoocular deprivation. Moreover the defect could be reversed by local superfusion of the visual cortex with norepinephrine (384). Thus it seems that noradrenergic activity may be essential for the maintenance of synaptic plasticity, at least during certain stages of development. Although the mechanism of this action is entirely speculative, the possibility should be kept in mind that it is somehow linked to changes in cerebral blood flow and water permeability that can be elicited by stimulation of the locus coeruleus (22, 91, 168).

Adenosine derivatives. Although there has been much speculation regarding a possible transmitter function of adenosine derivatives (46a), there is little evidence of this function in the cortex. Adenosine triphosphate (ATP) is only a weak excitant of cortical cells (273b). Adenosine monophosphate (AMP), on the other hand, appears to have a substantial presynaptic effect, depressing transmitter release [(120); compare also ref. 306], which could be of functional significance if AMP is released in the cortex.

Peptides. Any statement about the function of peptides in the cortex would be premature. But considering the relatively large amounts of peptides that are present in some cortical cells (188, 413), for example, some of the highest levels of cholecystokinin are found in the cortex (413), as well as the significant excitatory or inhibitory effects produced by some peptides (100, 414), these may provide to be important cortical transmitters or, perhaps more likely, modulators.

Summary. So far as one can tell, the most important excitatory and inhibitory transmitters in the motor cortex are glutamate and GABA, respectively; but there are also significant modulatory cholinergic (muscarinic) actions, both facilitatory and depressant, that are probably of importance for mechanisms related to arousal, consciousness, and learning; the functional role of the diffuse monoaminergic and peptidergic innervations is at present less clear.

REFERENCES

1. ALTMANN, H., G. TEN BRUGGENCATE, P. PICKELMANN, AND R. STEINBERG. Effects of glutamate, aspartate, and two presumed antagonists on feline rubrospinal neurones. *Pfluegers Arch.* 364: 249–255, 1976.
2. ALTMANN, H., G. TEN BRUGGENCATE, P. PICKELMANN, AND R. STEINBERG. Effects of GABA, glycine, picrotoxin and bicuculline methochloride on rubrospinal neurones in cats. *Brain Res.* 111: 337–345, 1976.
3. ALTMANN, H., G. TEN BRUGGENCATE, AND W. SONNHOF. Differential strength of the action of glycine and GABA in hypoglossus nucleus. *Pfluegers Arch.* 331: 90–94, 1972.
4. ALVAREZ-LEEFMANS, F. J., A. DE SANTIS, AND R. MILEDI. Effects of some divalent cations on synaptic transmission in frog spinal neurones. *J. Physiol. London* 294: 387–406, 1979.
5. ANDEN, N.-E., A. DAHLSTRÖM, K. FUXE, AND K. LARSSON. Further evidence for the presence of nigro-neostriatal dopamine neurons in the rat. *Am. J. Anat.* 116: 329–333, 1965.
6. ANDEN, N.-E., M. G. M. JUKES, A. LUNDBERG, AND L. VYKLICKY. The effect of DOPA on the spinal cord. 1. Influence on transmission from primary afferents. *Acta Physiol. Scand.* 67: 373–386, 1966.
7. ANDEN, N.-E., M. G. M. JUKES, AND A. LUNDBERG. The effect of DOPA on the spinal cord. 2. A pharmacological analysis. *Acta Physiol. Scand.* 67: 387–397, 1966.

588, 1975.
94. DESCARRIES, L., K. C. WATKINS, AND Y. LAPIERRE. Noradrenergic axon terminals in the cerebral cortex of rat. III. Topometric ultrastructural analysis. *Brain Res.* 133: 197–222, 1977.
95. DESCHENES, M., P. FELTZ, AND Y. LAMOUR. A model for an estimate *in vivo* of the ionic basis of presynaptic inhibition: an intracellular analysis of the GABA-induced depolarization in rat dorsal root ganglia. *Brain Res.* 118: 486–493, 1976.
96. DESCLIN, J. C. Histological evidence supporting the inferior olive as the major source of cerebellar climbing fibers in the rat. *Brain Res.* 77: 365–384, 1974.
97. DE WIED, D. Pituitary-adrenal system hormones and behaviour. In: *The Neurosciences: Third Study Program*, edited by F. O. Schmitt and F. G. Worden. Cambridge: MIT Press, 1974, p. 653–666.
98. DIAMOND, J., AND S. ROPER. Analysis of Mauthner cell responses to iontophoretically delivered pulses of GABA, glycine and L-glutamate. *J. Physiol. London* 232: 113–128, 1973.
99. DIVAC, I., F. FONNUM, AND J. STORM-MATHISEN. High affinity uptake of glutamate in terminals of corticostriatal axons. *Nature London* 266: 377–378, 1977.
100. DODD, J., AND J. S. KELLY. Is somatostatin an excitatory transmitter in the hippocampus? *Nature London* 273: 674–675, 1978.
101. DOUGLAS, W. W. Stimulus-secretion coupling: the concept and clues from chromaffin and other cells. *Brit. J. Pharmacol.* 34: 451–474, 1968.
101a.DRAY, A. The striatum and substantia nigra: a commentary on their relationships. *Neuroscience* 4: 1407–1439, 1979.
102. DRAY, A., J. DAVIES, N. R. OAKELY, P. TONGROACH, AND S. VELLUCCI. The dorsal and medial raphe projections to the substantia nigra in the rat: electrophysiological, biochemical and behavioural observations. *Brain Res.* 151: 431–442, 1978.
103. DRAY, A., AND D. W. STRAUGHAN. Synaptic mechanisms in the substantia nigra. *J. Pharm. Pharmacol.* 28: 400–405, 1976.
104. DREIFUSS, J. J., J. S. KELLY, AND K. KRNJEVIĆ. Cortical inhibition and γ-aminobutyric acid. *Exp. Brain Res.* 9: 137–154, 1969.
105. DUDAR, J. D., AND J. C. SZERB. The effect of topically applied atropine on resting and evoked cortical acetylcholine release. *J. Physiol. London* 203: 741–762, 1969.
106. DUGGAN, A. W. The differential sensitivity to L-glutamate and L-aspartate of spinal interneurones and Renshaw cells. *Exp. Brain Res.* 19: 522–528, 1974.
107. DUGGAN, A. W., AND D. R. CURTIS. Morphine and the synaptic activation of Renshaw cells. *Neuropharmacology* 11: 189–196, 1972.
108. DUGGAN, A. W., J. G. HALL, AND C. Y. LEE. Alpha-bungarotoxin, cobra neurotoxin and excitation of Renshaw cells by acetylcholine. *Brain Res.* 107: 166–170, 1976.
109. DUNLAP, K., AND G. D. FISCHBACH. Neurotransmitters decrease the calcium component of sensory nerve action potentials. *Nature London* 276: 837–839, 1978.
110. DUVOISIN, R. C., AND C. MYTILINEOU. Where is L-dopa decarboxylated in the striatum after 6-hydroxydopamine nigrotomy? *Brain Res.* 152: 369–373, 1978.
111. ECCLES, J. C. *The Neurophysiological Basis of Mind*. Oxford: Clarendon, 1953.
112. ECCLES, J. C. *The Physiology of Nerve Cells*. Baltimore: Johns Hopkins Press, 1957.
113. ECCLES, J. C. *The Physiology of Synapses*. Berlin: Springer-Verlag, 1964.
114. ECCLES, J. C. The cerebellum as a computer: patterns in space and time. *J. Physiol. London* 229: 1–32, 1973.
115. ECCLES, J. C., R. M. ECCLES, AND P. FATT. Pharmacological investigations on a central synapse operated by acetylcholine. *J. Physiol. London* 131: 154–169, 1956.
116. ECCLES, J. C., P. FATT, AND K. KOKETSU. Cholinergic and inhibitory synapses in a pathway from motor-axon collaterals to motoneurones. *J. Physiol. London* 126: 524–562, 1954.
117. ECCLES, J. C., M. ITO, AND J. SZENTAGOTHAI. The cerebellum as a neuronal machine. New York: Springer-Verlag, 1967.

118. ECCLES, J. C., R. LLINAS, AND K. SASAKI. The excitatory synaptic action of climbing fibres on the Purkinje cells of the cerebellum. *J. Physiol. London* 182: 268–296, 1966.
119. ECKERT, R. Bioelectric control of ciliary activity (locomotion in the ciliated protozoa is regulated by membrane-limited calcium fluxes). *Science* 176: 473–481, 1972.
120. EDSTROM, J. P., AND J. W. PHILLIS. The effects of AMP on the potential of rat cerebral cortical neurones. *Can. J. Physiol. Pharmacol.* 54: 787–790, 1976.
121. EDWARDS, F. R., S. J. REDMAN, AND B. WALMSLEY. Statistical fluctuations in charge transfer at Ia synapses on spinal motoneurones. *J. Physiol. London* 259: 665–688, 1976.
122. EDWARDS, F. R., S. J. REDMAN, AND B. WALMSLEY. The effect of polarizing currents on unitary Ia excitatory post-synaptic potentials evoked in spinal motoneurones. *J. Physiol. London* 259: 705–723, 1976.
123. ELDE, R., AND T. HÖKFELT. Localization of hypophysiotropic peptides and other biologically active peptides within the brain. *Annu. Rev. Physiol.* 41: 587–602, 1979.
124. ELLIOTT, K. A. C., AND N. M. VAN GELDER. Occlusion and metabolism of γ-aminobutyric acid of brain tissue. *J. Neurochem.* 3: 28–40, 1958.
125. ENDO, M. Calcium release from the sarcoplasmic reticulum. *Physiol. Rev.* 57: 71–108, 1977.
126. ENGBERG, I., J. A. FLATMAN, AND J. D. C. LAMBERT. The actions of excitatory amino acids on motoneurones in the feline spinal cord. *J. Physiol. London* 288: 227–261, 1979.
127. ENGBERG, I., A. LUNDBERG, AND R. W. RYALL. The effect of reserpine on transmission in the spinal cord. *Acta Physiol. Scand.* 72: 115–122, 1968.
128. ENGBERG, I., A. LUNDBERG, AND R. W. RYALL. Is the tonic decerebrate inhibition of reflex paths mediated by monoaminergic pathways? *Acta Physiol. Scand.* 72: 123–133, 1968.
129. ENGBERG, I., AND K. C. MARSHALL. Mechanism of noradrenaline hyperpolarization in spinal cord motoneurones of the cat. *Acta Physiol. Scand.* 83: 142–144, 1971.
129a.ENGBERG, I., AND K. C. MARSHALL. Reversal potential for Ia excitatory post synaptic potentials in spinal motoneurons of cats. *Neuroscience* 4: 1583–1591, 1979.
130. ENGBERG, I., AND R. W. RYALL. The inhibitory action of noradrenaline and other monoamines on spinal neurones. *J. Physiol. London* 185: 298–322, 1966.
131. ERULKAR, S. D., G. E. DAMBACH, AND D. MENDER. The effect of magnesium at motoneurons of the isolated spinal cord of the frog. *Brain Res.* 66: 413–424, 1974.
132. FAHN, S. Regional distribution studies on GABA and other putative neurotransmitters and their enzymes. In: *GABA in Nervous System Function*, edited by E. Roberts, T. N. Chase, and D. B. Tower. New York: Raven, 1976, p. 169–186.
133. FEDINA, L., A. LUNDBERG, AND L. VYKLICKY. The effect of a noradrenaline liberator (4, α-dimethyl-tyramine) on reflex transmission in spinal cats. *Acta Physiol. Scand.* 83: 495–504, 1971.
134. FELDBERG, W., AND M. VOGT. Acetylcholine synthesis in different regions of the central nervous system. *J. Physiol. London* 107: 372–381, 1948.
135. FELPEL, L. P. Effects of strychnine, bicuculline and picrotoxin on inhibition of hypoglossal motoneurons. *J. Neurosci. Res.* 3: 289–294, 1977.
136. FELTZ, P. γ-Aminobutyric acid and a caudato-nigral inhibition. *Can. J. Physiol. Pharmacol.* 49: 1113–1115, 1971.
137. FELTZ, P. Pharmacological considerations about establishing true actions of dopamine on striatal neurones with nigral inputs. In: *Iontophoresis and Transmitter Mechanisms in the Mammalian Central Nervous System*, edited by R. W. Ryall and J. S. Kelly. Amsterdam: Elsevier/North-Holland, 1978, p. 25–38.
138. FELTZ, P., AND D. ALBE-FESSARD. A study of an ascending nigro-caudate pathway. *Electroencephalogr. Clin. Neurophysiol.* 33: 179–193, 1972.
139. FELTZ, P., AND J. DE CHAMPLAIN. Persistence of caudate unitary responses to nigral stimulation after destruction and

functional impairment of the striatal dopaminergic terminals. *Brain Res.* 43: 595-600, 1972.
140. FIBIGER, H. C. Drugs and reinforcement mechanisms: a critical review of the catecholamine theory. *Annu. Rev. Pharmacol. Toxicol.* 18: 37-56, 1978.
141. FONNUM, F. Comments on localization of neurotransmitters in the basal ganglia. In: *Amino Acids as Chemical Transmitters*, edited by F. Fonnum. New York: Plenum, 1978, p. 143-153.
142. FONNUM, F., Z. GOTTESFELD, AND I. GROFOVA. Distribution of glutamate decarboxylase, choline acetyltransferase and aromatic amino acid decarboxylase in the basal ganglia of normal and operated rats. Evidence for striatopallidal, striatoentopeduncular and striatonigral GABAergic fibres. *Brain Res.* 143: 125-138, 1978.
143. FONNUM, F., I. GROFOVA, AND E. RINVIK. Origin and distribution of glutamate decarboxylase in the nucleus subthalamicus of the cat. *Brain Res.* 153: 370-374, 1978.
144. FONNUM, F., J. STORM-MATHISEN, AND F. WALBERG. Glutamate decarboxylase in inhibitory neurons. A study of the enzyme in Purkinje cell axons and boutons in the cat. *Brain Res.* 20: 259-275, 1970.
145. FORSSBERG, H., AND S. GRILLNER. The locomotion of the acute spinal cat injected with clonidine i.v. *Brain Res.* 50: 184-186, 1973.
146. FOX, S., K. KRNJEVIĆ, M. E. MORRIS, E. PUIL, AND R. WERMAN. Action of baclofen on mammalian synaptic transmission. *Neuroscience* 3: 495-515, 1978.
147. FREDERICKSON, R. C. A., M. NEUSS, S. L. MORZORATI, AND W. J. McBRIDE. A comparison of the inhibitory effects of taurine and GABA on identified Purkinje cells and other neurons in the cerebellar cortex of the rat. *Brain Res.* 145: 117-126, 1978.
148. FUXE, K., T. HÖKFELT, AND U. UNGERSTEDT. Morphological and functional aspects of central monoamine neurons. *Int. Ref. Neurobiol.* 13: 93-126, 1970.
150. GALE, J. S., E. D. BIRD, E. G. SPOKES, L. L. IVERSEN, AND T. JESSELL. Human brain substance P: distribution in controls and Huntington's chorea. *J. Neurochem.* 30: 633-634, 1978.
151. GALE, K., J.-S. HONG, AND A. GUIDOTTI. Presence of substance P and GABA in separate striatonigral neurons. *Brain Res.* 136: 371-375, 1977.
152. GALINDO, A. GABA-picrotoxin interaction in the mammalian central nervous system. *Brain Res.* 14: 763-767, 1969.
153. GALINDO, A., K. KRNJEVIĆ, AND S. SCHWARTZ. Microintophoretic studies on neurones in the cuneate nucleus. *J. Physiol. London* 192: 359-377, 1967.
154. GALLAGHER, J. P., H. HIGASHI, AND S. NISHI. Characterization and ionic basis of GABA-induced depolarizations recorded in vitro from cat primary afferent neurones. *J. Physiol. London* 275: 263-282, 1978.
155. GELLER, H. M., AND D. J. WOODWARD. Responses of cultured cerebellar neurons to iontophoretically applied aminoacids. *Brain Res.* 74: 67-80, 1974.
156. GLOWINSKI, J. Storage and release of monoamines in the central nervous system. In: *Handbook of Neurochemistry*, edited by A. Lajtha. New York: Plenum, 1970, vol. 4, p. 91-114.
157. GODFRAIND, J. M., H. KAWAMURA, K. KRNJEVIĆ, AND R. PUMAIN. Actions of dinitrophenol and some other metabolic inhibitors on cortical neurones. *J. Physiol. London* 215: 199-222, 1971.
158. GODFRAIND, J. M., K. KRNJEVIĆ, H. MARETIĆ, AND R. PUMAIN. Inhibition of cortical neurones by imidazole and some derivatives. *Can. J. Physiol. Pharmacol.* 51: 790-797, 1973.
159. GODFRAIND, J. M., K. KRNJEVIĆ, AND R. PUMAIN. Doubtful value of bicuculline as a specific antagonist of GABA. *Nature London* 228: 675-676, 1970.
160. GODFRAIND, J. M., AND R. PUMAIN. Cyclic adenosine monophosphate and norepinephrine: effect on Purkinje cells in rat cerebellar cortex. *Science* 174: 1257-1258, 1971.
161. GRAHAM, L. T., R. P. SHANK, R. WERMAN, AND M. H. APRISON. Distribution of some synaptic transmitter suspects in cat spinal cord: glutamic acid, aspartic acid, γ-aminobutyric acid, glycine, and glutamine. *J. Neurochem.* 14: 465-472, 1967.
162. GRANIT, R. *The Basis of Motor Control.* New York: Academic, 1970.
163. GREENGARD, P. Cyclic nucleotides, protein phosphorylation and neuronal function. *Adv. Cyclic Nucleotide Res.* 5: 585-601, 1975.
164. GREENGARD, P. Possible role for cyclic nucleotides and phosphorylated membrane proteins in postsynaptic actions of neurotransmitters. *Nature London* 260: 101-108, 1976.
165. GRILLNER, S. Locomotion in vertebrates: central mechanisms and reflex interaction. *Physiol. Rev.* 55: 247-304, 1975.
166. GRILLNER, S., T. HONGO, AND A. LUNDBERG. The effect of DOPA on the spinal cord. 7. Reflex activation of static γ-motoneurones from the flexor reflex afferents. *Acta Physiol. Scand.* 70: 403-411, 1967.
167. GROSSMAN, M. I. Chemical messengers: a view from the gut. *Federation Proc.* 38: 2341-2343, 1979.
168. GRUBB, R. L., M. E. RAICHLE, AND J. O. EICHLING. Peripheral sympathetic regulation of brain water permeability. *Brain Res.* 144: 204-207, 1978.
169. GRUOL, D. L., J. L. BARKER, L. M. HUANG, AND T. G. SMITH. Is naloxone a specific opiate antagonist (Abstract)? *Federation Proc.* 38: 1401, 1979.
170. GUYENET, P. G., AND G. K. AGHAJANIAN. Antidromic identification of dopaminergic and other output neurons of the rat substantia nigra. *Brain Res.* 150: 69-84, 1978.
170a. HACKETT, J. T., S.-M. HOU, AND S. L. COCHRAN. Glutamate and synaptic depolarization of Purkinje cells evoked by parallel fibers and by climbing fibers. *Brain Res.* 170: 377-380, 1979.
171. HAIGLER, H. J., AND G. K. AGHAJANIAN. Peripheral serotonin antagonists: failure to antagonize serotonin in brain areas receiving a prominent serotonergic input. *J. Neural. Transm.* 35: 257-273, 1974.
172. HALDANE, J. B. S. La signalisation animale. *Annee Biol.* 58: 89-98, 1954.
173. HAMBERGER, A., G. CHIANG, E. S. NYLÉN, S. W. SCHEFF, AND C. W. COTMAN. Stimulus evoked increase in the biosynthesis of the putative neurotransmitter glutamate in the hippocampus. *Brain Res.* 143: 549-555, 1978.
174. HAMMERSTAD, J. P., J. E. MURRAY, AND R. W. P. CUTLER. Efflux of amino acid neurotransmitters from rat spinal cord slices. II. Factors influencing the electrically induced efflux of [^{14}C]glycine and ^{3}H-GABA. *Brain Res.* 35: 357-367, 1971.
175. HARVEY, A. M., AND F. C. MACINTOSH. Calcium and synaptic transmission in a sympathetic ganglion. *J. Physiol. London* 97: 408-416, 1940.
176. HEADLEY, P. M., A. W. DUGGAN, AND B. T. GRIERSMITH. Selective reduction by noradrenaline and 5-hydroxytryptamine of nociceptive responses of cat dorsal horn neurones. *Brain Res.* 145: 185-189, 1978.
177. HEBB, C. O., K. KRNJEVIĆ, AND A. SILVER. Effect of undercutting on the acetylcholinesterase and choline acetyltransferase activity in the cat's cerebral cortex. *Nature London* 198: 692, 1963.
178. HEBB, C. O., AND A. SILVER. Choline acetylase in the central nervous system of man and some other mammals. *J. Physiol. London* 134: 718-728, 1956.
179. HEIDMANN, T., AND J.-P. CHANGEUX. Structural and functional properties of the acetylcholine receptor protein in its purified and membrane-bound states. *Annu. Rev. Biochem.* 47: 317-357, 1978.
180. HENDERSON, G., J. HUGHES, AND H. W. KOSTERLITZ. *In vitro* release of Leu- and Met-enkephalin from the corpus striatum. *Nature London* 271: 677-678, 1978.
181. HENRY, J. L. Effects of substance P on functionally identified units in cat spinal cord. *Brain Res.* 114: 439-451, 1976.
182. HENRY, J. L., K. KRNJEVIĆ, AND M. E. MORRIS. Substance P and spinal neurones. *Can. J. Physiol. Pharmacol.* 53: 423-432, 1975.
183. HERZ, A., AND W. ZIEGLGÄNSBERGER. The influence of microelectrophoretically applied biogenic amines, cholinominetics and procaine on synaptic excitation in the corpus striatum.

Int. J. Neuropharmacol. 7: 221-230, 1968.
184. HICKS, T. P., J. G. HALL, AND H. MCLENNAN. Ranking of excitatory amino acids by the antagonists glutamic acid diethylester and D-α-aminoadipic acid. *Can. J. Physiol. Pharmacol.* 56: 901-907, 1978.
184a.HICKS, T. P., AND H. MCLENNAN. Amino acids and the synaptic pharmacology of granule cells in the dentate gyrus of the rat. *Can. J. Physiol. Pharmacol.* 57: 973-978, 1979.
185. HILL, R. G., M. A. SIMMONDS, AND D. W. STRAUGHAN. A comparative study of some convulsant substances as γ-aminobutyric acid antagonists in the feline cerebral cortex. *Br. J. Pharmacol.* 49: 37-51, 1973.
186. HILLER, J. M., E. J. SIMON, S. M. CRAIN, AND E. R. PETERSON. Opiate receptors in cultures of fetal mouse dorsal root ganglia (DRG) and spinal cord: predominance in DRG neurites. *Brain Res.* 145: 396-400, 1978.
187. HOFFER, B. J., R. FREEDMAN, D. PURO, AND D. J. WOODWARD. Interaction of norepinephrine with cerebellar neuronal circuitry. *Neurosci. Abstr.* 1: 204, 1975.
188. HÖKFELT, T., R. ELDE, O. JOHANSSON, A. LJUNGDAHL, M. SCHULTZBERG, K. FUXE, M. GOLDSTEIN, G. NILSSON, B. PERNOW, L. TERENIUS, D. GANTEN, S. L. JEFFCOATE, J. REHFELD, AND S. SAID. Distribution of peptide-containing neurons. In: *Psychopharmacology: A Generation of Progress*, edited by M. A. Lipton, A. Di Mascio, and K. F. Killam. New York: Raven, 1978, p. 39-66.
189. HÖKFELT, T., R. ELDE, O. JOHANSSON, R. LUFT, G. NILSSON, AND A. ARIMURA. Immunohistochemical evidence for separate populations of somatostatin-containing and substance P-containing primary afferent neurons in the rat. *Neuroscience* 1: 131-136, 1976.
190. HÖKFELT, T., AND K. FUXE. Cerebellar monoamine nerve terminals, a new type of afferent fibers to the cortex cerebelli. *Exp. Brain Res.* 9: 63-72, 1969.
191. HÖKFELT, T., J. O. KELLERTH, G. NILSSON, AND B. PERNOW. Substance P: localization in the central nervous system and in some primary sensory neurons. *Science* 190: 889-890, 1975.
192. HÖKFELT, T., AND A. LJUNGDAHL. Light and electron microscopic autoradiography on spinal cord slices after incubation with labelled glycine. *Brain Res.* 32: 189-194, 1971.
193. HÖKFELT, T., AND A. LJUNGDAHL. Autoradiographic identification of cerebral and cerebellar cortical neurons accumulating labeled gamma-aminobutyric acid (^{3}H-GABA). *Exp. Brain Res.* 14: 354-362, 1972.
194. HOLTON, F. A., AND P. HOLTON. The capillary dilator substances in drug powders of spinal roots; a possible role of adenosine triphosphate in chemical transmission from nerve endings. *J. Physiol. London* 126: 124-140, 1954.
195. HONG, J. S., H. Y. T. YANG, G. RACAGNI, AND E. COSTA. Projections of substance P containing neurons from neostriatum to substantia nigra. *Brain Res.* 122: 541-544, 1977.
196. HOPKIN, J., AND M. J. NEAL. Effect of electrical stimulation and high potassium concentrations on the efflux of [^{14}C]glycine from slices of spinal cord. *Br. J. Pharmacol.* 42: 215-223, 1971.
197. HORNYKIEWICZ, O. Dopamine: its physiology, pharmacology and pathological neurochemistry. In: *Biogenic Amines and Physiological Membranes in Drug Therapy*, edited by J. H. Biel and L. B. Abood. New York: Dekker, 1971, pt. B, p. 173-258.
198. HORNYKIEWICZ, O. Parkinson's disease: from brain homogenate to treatment. *Federation Proc.* 32: 183-190, 1973.
199. HORTON, E. W. Hypotheses on physiological roles of prostaglandins. *Physiol. Rev.* 49: 122-161, 1969.
200. HOSEY, M. M., AND M. TAO. Protein kinases and membrane phosphorylation. *Curr. Top. Membr. Transp.* 9: 233-320, 1977.
201. HÖSLI, L., P. F. ANDRES, AND E. HÖSLI. Ionic mechanisms associated with the depolarization by glutamate and aspartate on human and rat spinal neurones in tissue culture. *Pfluegers Arch.* 363: 43-48, 1976.
202. HOSLI, L., A. K. TEBECIS, AND H. P. SCHONWETTER. A comparison of the effects of monoamines on neurones of the bulbar reticular formation. *Brain Res.* 25: 357-370, 1971.

203. HOUNSGAARD, J. Inhibition produced by iontophoretically applied acetylcholine in area CA1 of thin hippocampal slices from the rat. *Acta Physiol. Scand.* 103: 110-111, 1978.
204. HUFFMAN, R. D., AND R. DAVIS. Pharmacology of the brachium conjunctivum: red nucleus synaptic system in the baboon. *J. Neurosci. Res.* 3: 175-192, 1977.
205. HUGHES, J. Isolation of an endogenous compound from the brain with pharmacological properties similar to morphine. *Brain Res.* 88: 295-308, 1975.
206. HULL, C. D., G. BERNARDI, D. D. PRICE, AND N. A. BUCHWALD. Intracellular responses of caudate neurons to temporally and spatially combined stimuli. *Exp. Neurol.* 38: 324-336, 1973.
207. HULTBORN, H. Convergence on interneurones in the reciprocal Ia inhibitory pathway to motoneurones. *Acta Physiol. Scand. Suppl.* 375: 5-42, 1972.
208. HULTBORN, H., E. JANKOWSKA, AND S. LINDSTRÖM. Recurrent inhibition of interneurones monosynaptically activated from group Ia afferents. *J. Physiol. London* 215: 613-636, 1971.
209. HUNT, D. F., AND F. W. CROW. Electron captive negative chemical ionization mass spectrometry. *Analyt. Chem.* 50: 1781-1784, 1978.
210. HUTCHINSON, G. B., H. MCLENNAN, AND H. V. WHEAL. The responses of Renshaw cells and spinal interneurones of the rat to L-glutamate and L-aspartate. *Brain Res.* 141: 129-136, 1978.
211. HUXLEY, A. F., AND R. E. TAYLOR. Local activation of striated muscle fibres. *J. Physiol. London* 144: 426-441, 1958.
212. ISRAEL, M., AND V. P. WHITTAKER. The isolation of mossy fibre endings from the granular layer of the cerebellar cortex. *Experientia* 21: 325-327, 1965.
213. ITO, M. Neurophysiological aspects of the cerebellar motor control system. *Int. J. Neurol.* 7: 162-176, 1970.
214. ITO, M., S. M. HIGHSTEIN, AND T. TSUCHIYA. The postsynaptic inhibition of rabbit oculomotor neurones by secondary vestibular impulses and its blockage by picrotoxin. *Brain Res.* 17: 520-523, 1970.
215. ITO, M., AND M. YOSHIDA. The origin of cerebellar-induced inhibition of Deiters' neurones. 1. Monosynaptic initiation of the inhibitory postsynaptic potentials. *Exp. Brain Res.* 2: 330-349, 1966.
216. ITO, M., M. YOSHIDA, K. OBATA, N. KAWAI, AND M. UDO. Inhibitory control of intracerebellar nuclei by the Purkinje cell axons. *Exp. Brain Res.* 10: 64-80, 1970.
217. IVERSEN, L. L. Role of transmitter uptake mechanisms in synaptic neurotransmission. *Br. J. Pharmacol.* 41: 571-591, 1971.
218. JAN, Y. N., L. Y. JAN, AND S. W. KUFFLER. A peptide as a possible transmitter in sympathetic ganglia of the frog. *Proc. Natl. Acad. Sci. USA* 76: 1501-1505, 1979.
219. JANKOWSKA, E., M. G. M. JUKES, S. LUND, AND A. LUNDBERG. The effect of DOPA on the spinal cord. 5. Reciprocal organization of pathways transmitting excitatory action to alpha motoneurones of flexors and extensors. *Acta Physiol. Scand.* 70: 369-388, 1967.
220. JANKOWSKA, E., AND S. LINDSTRÖM. Morphological identification of Renshaw cells. *Acta Physiol. Scand.* 81: 428-430, 1971.
221. JANKOWSKA, E., AND S. LINDSTRÖM. Morphology of interneurones mediating Ia reciprocal inhibition of motoneurones in the spinal cord of the cat. *J. Physiol. London* 226: 805-823, 1972.
222. JANKOWSKA, E., Y. PADEL, AND R. TANAKA. Projections of pyramidal tract cells to α-motoneurones innervating hind-limb muscles in the monkey. *J. Physiol. London* 249: 637-667, 1975.
223. JANKOWSKA, E., AND W. J. ROBERTS. Synaptic actions of single interneurones mediating reciprocal Ia inhibition of motoneurones. *J. Physiol. London* 222: 623-642, 1972.
224. JANKOWSKA, E., AND R. TANAKA. Neuronal mechanism of the disynaptic inhibition evoked in primate spinal motoneurones from the corticospinal tract. *Brain Res.* 75: 163-166, 1974.
225. JASPER, H., AND I. KOYAMA. Rate of release of amino acids from the cerebral cortex in the cat as affected by brainstem and thalamic stimulation. *Can. J. Physiol. Pharmacol.* 47:

889-905, 1969.
226. JESSELL, T. M. Substance P release from the rat substantia nigra. *Brain Res.* 151: 469-478, 1978.
227. JOHNSON, J. L. Glutamic acid as a synaptic transmitter candidate in the dorsal sensory neuron: reconsiderations. *Life Sci.* 20: 1637-1644, 1977.
228. JOHNSON, E. S., M. H. T. ROBERTS, A. SOBIESZEK, AND D. W. STRAUGHAN. Noradrenaline sensitive cells in cat cerebral cortex. *Int. J. Neuropharmacol.* 8: 549-566, 1969.
229. JOHNSTON, G. A. R. Physiologic pharmacology of GABA and its antagonists in the vertebrate nervous system. In: *GABA in Nervous System Function*, edited by E. Roberts, T. N. Chase, and D. B. Tower. New York: Raven, 1976, p. 395-411.
229a. JOHNSTON, G. A. R. Neuropharmacology of amino acid inhibitory transmitters. *Annu. Rev. Pharmacol. Toxicol.* 18: 269-289, 1978.
230. JOHNSTON, G. A. R., AND L. L. IVERSEN. Glycine uptake in rat central nervous systems slices and homogenates: evidence for different uptake systems in spinal cord and cerebral cortex. *J. Neurochem.* 18: 1951-1961, 1971.
231. JOHNSTONE, R. M. Electrogenic amino acid transport. *Can. J. Physiol. Pharmacol.* 57: 1-15, 1979.
232. JORDAN, L. M., D. A. MCCREA, J. D. STEEVES, AND J. E. MENZIES. Noradrenergic synapses and effects of noradrenaline on interneurones in the ventral horn of the cat spinal cord. *Can. J. Physiol. Pharmacol.* 55: 399-412, 1977.
233. JORDAN, L. M., AND J. D. STEEVES. Chemical lesioning of the spinal noradrenaline pathway: effects on locomotion in the cat. In: *Neural Control of Locomotion*, edited by R. M. Herman, S. Grillner, P. S. G. Stein, and D. G. Stuart. New York: Plenum, 1976, p. 769-773.
234. KAN, K.-S. K., L.-P. CHAO, AND L. F. ENG. Immunohistochemical localization of choline acetyltransferase in rabbit spinal cord and cerebellum. *Brain Res.* 146: 221-229, 1978.
235. KANNO, T., D. E. COCHRANE, AND W. W. DOUGLAS. Exocytosis (secretory granule extrusion) induced by injection of calcium into mast cells. *Can. J. Physiol. Pharmacol.* 51: 1001-1004, 1973.
236. KARLSEN, R. L., AND F. FONNUM. Evidence for glutamate as a neurotransmitter in the corticofugal fibres to the dorsal lateral geniculate body and the superior colliculus in rats. *Brain Res.* 151: 457-467, 1978.
237. KASA, P., S. P. MANN, AND C. HEBB. Localization of choline acetyltransferase. *Nature London* 226: 812-816, 1970.
238. KASA, P., AND A. SILVER. The correlation between choline acetyltransferase and acetylcholinesterase activity in different areas of the cerebellum of rat and guinea pig. *J. Neurochem.* 16: 389-396, 1969.
239. KASAMATSU, T., AND J. D. PETTIGREW. Depletion of brain catecholamines: failure of ocular dominance shift after monocular occlusion in kittens. *Science* 194: 206-208, 1976.
240. KATZ, B. *Nerve, Muscle and Synapse*. New York: McGraw-Hill, 1966.
241. KATZ, B. *The Release of Neural Transmitter Substances*. Liverpool: University Press, 1969.
242. KATZ, B., AND R. MILEDI. The characteristics of 'end-plate noise' produced by different depolarizing drugs. *J. Physiol. London* 230: 707-717, 1973.
243. KATZ, B., AND R. MILEDI. Transmitter leakage from motor nerve endings. *Proc. R. Soc. London Ser. B* 196: 59-72, 1977.
244. KATZ, B., AND R. MILEDI. The reversal potential at the desensitized end-plate. *Proc. R. Soc. London Ser. B* 199: 329-334, 1977.
245. KAWAMURA, H., AND L. PROVINI. Depression of cerebellar Purkinje cells by microiontophoretic application of GABA and related amino acids. *Brain Res.* 24: 293-304, 1970.
246. KEBABIAN, J. W. Venom of Russell's viper uncouples the dopamine receptor from striatal adenylyl cyclase. *Brain Res.* 144: 194-198, 1978.
247. KEBABIAN, J. W., G. L. PETZOLD, AND P. GREENGARD. Dopamine-sensitive adenylate cyclase in caudate nucleus of rat brain, and its similarity to the "dopamine receptor." *Proc. Natl. Acad. Sci. USA* 69: 2145-2149, 1972.
248. KELLERTH, J. O. Aspects on the relative significance of pre- and postsynaptic inhibition in the spinal cord. In: *Structure and Function of Inhibitory Neuronal Mechanisms*, edited by C. von Euler, S. Skoglund, and V. Söderberg. Oxford: Pergamon, 1968, p. 197-212.
249. KELLY, J. S., AND K. KRNJEVIĆ. The action of glycine on cortical neurones. *Exp. Brain Res.* 9: 155-163, 1969.
250. KELLY, J. S., AND L. P. RENAUD. On the pharmacology of the γ-aminobutyric acid receptors on the cuneo-thalamic relay cells of the cat. *Br. J. Pharmacol.* 48: 369-386, 1973.
251. KEMP, J. M., AND T. P. S. POWELL. The synaptic organization of the caudate nucleus. *Philos. Trans. R. Soc. London Ser. B* 262: 403-412, 1971.
252. KIEVIT, J., AND H. G. J. M. KUYPERS. Basal forebrain and hypothalamic connections to frontal and parietal cortex in the rhesus monkey. *Science* 187: 660-662, 1974.
253. KIM, R., K. NAKANO, A. JAYARAMAN, AND M. B. CARPENTER. Projections of the globus pallidus and adjacent structures: an autoradiographic study in the monkey. *J. Comp. Neurol.* 169: 263-290, 1976.
254. KIM, J. S., R. HASSLER, P. HAUG, AND K.-S. PAIK. Effect of frontal cortex ablation on striatal glutamic acid level in rat. *Brain Res.* 132: 370-374, 1977.
255. KITAI, S. T., J. D. KOCSIS, AND J. WOOD. Origin and characteristics of the cortico-caudate afferents: an anatomical and electrophysiological study. *Brain Res.* 118: 137-141, 1976.
256. KITAI, S. T., M. SUGIMORI, AND J. D. KOCSIS. Excitatory nature of dopamine in the nigro-caudate pathway. *Exp. Brain Res.* 24: 351-363, 1976.
257. KOBAYASHI, R. M., M. PALKOVITS, R. E. HRUSKA, R. ROTHSCHILD, AND H. I. YAMAMURA. Regional distribution of muscarinic cholinergic receptors in rat brain. *Brain Res.* 154: 12-23, 1978.
258. KOCSIS, J. D., AND S. T. KITAI. Dual excitatory inputs to caudate spiny neurons from substantia nigra stimulation. *Brain Res.* 138: 271-283, 1977.
259. KRIVOY, W. A., J. R. COUCH, J. L. HENRY, AND J. M. STEWART. Synaptic modulation by substance P. *Federation Proc.* 38: 2344-2347, 1979.
260. KRIZ, N., E. SYKOVA, AND L. VYKLICKY. Extracellular potassium changes in the spinal cord of the cat and their relation to slow potentials, active transport and impulse transmission. *J. Physiol. London* 249: 167-182, 1975.
261. KRNJEVIĆ, K. Microiontophoresis. In: *Methods of Neurochemistry*, edited by R. Fried. New York: Dekker, 1971, p. 129-172.
262. KRNJEVIĆ, K. Chemical nature of synaptic transmission in vertebrates. *Physiol. Rev.* 54: 418-540, 1974.
263. KRNJEVIĆ, K. Acetylcholine receptors in vertebrate CNS. In: *Handbook of Psychopharmacology*, edited by L. L. Iversen, and S. H. Snyder. New York: Plenum, 1975, vol. 6, p. 97-125.
264. KRNJEVIĆ, K. Effects of substance P on central neurons in cats. In: *Substance P*, edited by U. S. von Euler and B. Pernow. New York: Raven, 1977, p. 217-230.
265. KRNJEVIĆ, K., Y. LAMOUR, J. F. MACDONALD, AND A. NISTRI. Intracellular actions of monoamine transmitters. *Can. J. Physiol. Pharmacol.* 56: 896-900, 1978.
266. KRNJEVIĆ, K., Y. LAMOUR, J. F. MACDONALD, AND A. NISTRI. Depression of monosynaptic EPSPs by Mn and Co in cat spinal cord. *Neuroscience* 4: 1331-1339, 1979.
267. KRNJEVIĆ, K., AND D. LEKIĆ. Substance P selectively blocks excitation of Renshaw cell by acetylcholine. *Can. J. Physiol. Pharmacol.* 55: 958-961, 1977.
268. KRNJEVIĆ, K., AND A. LISIEWICZ. Injections of calcium ions into spinal motoneurones. *J. Physiol. London* 225: 363-390, 1972.
269. KRNJEVIĆ, K., AND R. MILEDI. Some effects of adrenaline upon neuromuscular propagation in rats. *J. Physiol. London* 141: 291-304, 1958.
270. KRNJEVIĆ, K., AND R. MILEDI. Acetylcholine in mammalian neuromuscular transmission. *Nature London* 182: 805-806, 1958.

271. KRNJEVIĆ, K., AND J. F. MITCHELL. The release of acetylcholine in the isolated rat diaphragm. *J. Physiol. London* 155: 246-262, 1961.
272. KRNJEVIĆ, K., AND M. E. MORRIS. An excitatory action of substance P on cuneate neurones. *Can. J. Physiol. Pharmacol.* 52: 736-744, 1974.
273. KRNJEVIĆ, K., AND M. E. MORRIS. Extracellular accumulation of K$^+$ evoked by activity of primary afferent fibers in the cuneate nucleus and dorsal horn of cats. *Can. J. Physiol. Pharmacol.* 52: 852-871, 1974.
273a. KRNJEVIĆ, K., AND M. E. MORRIS. Correlation between extracellular focal potentials and K$^+$ potentials evoked by primary afferent activity. *Can. J. Physiol. Pharmacol.* 53: 912-922, 1975.
273b. KRNJEVIĆ, K., AND J. W. PHILLIS. Iontophoretic studies of neurones in the mammalian cerebral cortex. *J. Physiol. London* 165: 274-304, 1963.
274. KRNJEVIĆ, K., AND J. W. PHILLIS. Acetylcholine-sensitive cells in the cerebral cortex. *J. Physiol. London* 166: 296-327, 1963.
275. KRNJEVIĆ, K., AND J. W. PHILLIS. Pharmacological properties of acetylcholine-sensitive cells in the cerebral cortex. *J. Physiol. London* 166: 328-350, 1963.
276. KRNJEVIĆ, K., AND J. W. PHILLIS. Actions of certain amines on cerebral cortical neurones. *Br. J. Pharmacol. Chemother.* 20: 471-490, 1963.
277. KRNJEVIĆ, K., AND E. PUIL. Electrophysiological studies on actions of taurine. In: *Taurine*, edited by R. Huxtable and A. Barbeau. New York: Raven, 1976, p. 179-189.
278. KRNJEVIĆ, K., E. PUIL, AND R. WERMAN. Is cyclic guanosine monophosphate the internal "second messenger" for cholinergic actions on central neurons? *Can. J. Physiol. Pharmacol.* 54: 172-176, 1976.
279. KRNJEVIĆ, K., E. PUIL, AND R. WERMAN. GABA and glycine actions on spinal motoneurones. *Can. J. Physiol. Pharmacol.* 55: 658-669, 1977.
280. KRNJEVIĆ, K., E. PUIL, AND R. WERMAN. Bicuculline, benzyl penicillin and inhibitory amino acids in the spinal cord of the cat. *Can. J. Physiol. Pharmacol.* 55: 670-680, 1977.
281. KRNJEVIĆ, K., E. PUIL, AND R. WERMAN. EGTA and motoneuronal after-potentials. *J. Physiol. London* 275: 199-223, 1978.
282. KRNJEVIĆ, K., R. PUMAIN, AND L. RENAUD. Excitation of cortical cells by barium. *J. Physiol. London* 211: 43P-44P, 1970.
284. KRNJEVIĆ, K., R. PUMAIN, AND L. RENAUD. The mechanism of excitation by acetylcholine in the cerebral cortex. *J. Physiol. London* 215: 247-268, 1971.
285. KRNJEVIĆ, K., M. RANDIĆ, AND D. W. STRAUGHAN. Ergothioneine and central neurones. *Nature London* 205: 603-604, 1965.
286. KRNJEVIĆ, K., M. RANDIĆ, AND D. W. STRAUGHAN. Inhibitory process in the cerebral cortex. *J. Physiol. London* 184: 16-48, 1966.
287. KRNJEVIĆ, K., M. RANDIĆ, AND D. W. STRAUGHAN. Pharmacology of cortical inhibition. *J. Physiol. London* 184: 78-105, 1966.
288. KRNJEVIĆ, K., AND S. SCHWARTZ. Some properties of unresponsive cells in the cerebral cortex. *Exp. Brain Res.* 3: 306-319, 1967.
289. KRNJEVIĆ, K., AND S. SCHWARTZ. The action of γ-aminobutyric acid on cortical neurones. *Exp. Brain Res.* 3: 320-336, 1967.
290. KRNJEVIĆ, K., AND A. SILVER. A histochemical study of cholinergic fibres in the cerebral cortex. *J. Anat.* 99: 711-759, 1965.
291. KRNJEVIĆ, K., AND A. SILVER. Acetylcholinesterase in the developing forebrain. *J. Anat.* 100: 63-89, 1966.
292. KUBA, K. Effects of catecholamines on the neuromuscular junction in the rat diaphragm. *J. Physiol. London* 211: 551-570, 1970.
293. KUFFLER, S. W. Specific excitability of the end-plate region in normal and denervated muscle. *J. Neurophysiol.* 6: 99-110, 1943.
294. KUFFLER, S. W., AND D. YOSHIKAMI. The number of transmitter molecules in a quantum: an estimate from iontophoretic application of acetylcholine at the neuromuscular synapse. *J. Physiol. London* 251: 465-482, 1975.
295. KUHAR, M. J. Histochemical localization of opiate receptors and opioid peptides. *Federation Proc.* 37: 153-157, 1978.
296. KUNO, M. Quantum aspects of central and ganglionic synaptic transmission in vertebrates. *Physiol. Rev.* 51: 647-678, 1971.
297. KUPFERMANN, I. Modulatory actions of neurotransmitters. *Annu. Rev. Neurosci.* 2: 447-465, 1979.
298. KURIYAMA, K., B. HABER, B. SISKEN, AND E. ROBERTS. The γ-aminobutyric acid system in rabbit cerebellum. *Proc. Natl. Acad. Sci. USA* 55: 846-852, 1966.
299. LAKE, N., AND L. M. JORDAN. Failure to confirm cyclic AMP as second messenger for norepinephrine in rat cerebellum. *Science* 183: 663-664, 1974.
300. LANDGREN, S., C. G. PHILLIPS, AND R. PORTER. Minimal synaptic actions of pyramidal impulses on some alpha motoneurones of the baboon's hand and forearm. *J. Physiol. London* 161: 91-111, 1962.
301. LAPIERRE, Y., A. BEAUDET, N. DEMIANCZUK, AND L. DESCARRIES. Noradrenergic axon terminals in the cerebral cortex of rat. II. Quantitative data revealed by light and electron microscope radioautography of the frontal cortex. *Brain Res.* 63: 175-182, 1973.
302. LARRAMENDI, L. M. H., AND T. VICTOR. Synapses on the Purkinje cell spines in the mouse. An electron microscopic study. *Brain Res.* 5: 15-30, 1967.
303. LARSON, M. D. An analysis of the action of strychnine on the recurrent IPSP and amino acid induced inhibitions in the cat spinal cord. *Brain Res.* 15: 185-200, 1969.
304. LAVYNE, M. H., W. A. KOLTUN, J. A. CLEMENT, D. L. ROSENE, K. S. PICKREN, N. T. ZERVAS, AND R. J. WURTMAN. Decrease in neostriatal blood flow after D-amphetamine administration or electrical stimulation of the substantia nigra. *Brain Res.* 135: 76-86, 1977.
305. LEEMAN, S. E., AND E. A. MROZ. Substance P. *Life Sci.* 15: 2033-2044, 1974.
306. LEKIĆ, D. Presynaptic depression of synaptic response of Renshaw cells by adenosine 5'-monophosphate. *Can. J. Physiol. Pharmacol.* 55: 1391-1393, 1977.
307. LEMBECK, F. Zur Frage der centralen Übertragung afferenter Impulse. III. Das Vorkommen und die Bedeutung der Substanz P in den dorsalen Wurzeln des Ruckenmarks. *Arch. Exp. Pathol. Pharmakol.* 219: 197-213, 1953.
308. LEVI, G., AND M. RAITERI. Modulation of γ-aminobutyric acid transport in nerve endings: role of extracellular γ-aminobutyric acid and of cationic fluxes. *Proc. Natl. Acad. Sci. USA* 75: 2981-2985, 1978.
309. LEVY, R. A. GABA: a direct depolarizing action at the mammalian primary afferent terminal. *Brain Res.* 76: 155-160, 1974.
310. LEVY, R. A. The effect of intravenously administered γ-aminobutyric acid on afferent fiber polarization. *Brain Res.* 92: 21-34, 1975.
311. LEVY, R. A. The role of GABA in primary afferent depolarization. *Prog. Neurobiol. Oxford* 9: 211-267, 1977.
312. LEWIS, P. R., AND Z. J. SELIM. A combination of two histochemical techniques for tracing putative cholinergic central neurones. *J. Physiol. London* 284: 29P-30P, 1978.
313. LINDVALL, O., A. BJORKLUND, AND I. DIVAC. Organization of catecholamine neurons projecting to the frontal cortex in the rat. *Brain Res.* 142: 1-24, 1978.
314. LJUNGDAHL, A., T. HÖKFELT, AND G. NILSSON. Distribution of substance P-like immunoreactivity in the central nervous system of the rat. 1. Cell bodies and nerve terminals. *Neuroscience* 3: 861-943, 1978.
315. LLINAS, R. Electrical synaptic transmission in the mammalian central nervous system. In: *Golgi Centennial Symposium Proceedings*, edited by M. Santini. New York: Raven, 1975, p. 379-386.
316. LLINAS, R., AND R. BAKER. A chloride-dependent inhibitory postsynaptic potential in cat trochlear motoneurons. *J. Neurophysiol.* 35: 484-492, 1972.

318. LODGE, D., D. R. CURTIS, AND S. J. BRAND. Pharmacological study of the inhibition of ventral group Ia-excited spinal interneurones. *Exp. Brain Res.* 29: 97–105, 1977.

319. LYNCH, G. S., P. A. LUCAS, AND S. A. DEADWYLER. The demonstration of acetylcholinesterase containing neurones within the caudate nucleus of the rat. *Brain Res.* 45: 617–621, 1972.

320. MACDONALD, R. L., AND J. L. BARKER. Enhancement of GABA-mediated postsynaptic inhibition in cultured mammalian spinal cord neurons: a common mode of anticonvulsant action. *Brain Res.* 167: 323–336, 1979.

321. MACDONALD, R. L., AND P. G. NELSON. Specific opiate-induced depression of transmitter release from dorsal root ganglion cells in culture. *Science* 199: 1449–1451, 1978.

322. MACINTOSH, F. C. The distribution of acetylcholine in the peripheral and the central nervous system. *J. Physiol. London* 99: 436–442, 1941.

323. MACINTOSH, F. C., AND B. COLLIER. Neurochemistry of cholinergic terminals. *Handb. Exp. Pharmacol.* 42: 99–228, 1976.

324. MACINTOSH, F. C., AND P. E. OBORIN. Release of acetylcholine from intact cerebral cortex. *Abstr. 19th Int. Physiol. Congr. Montreal, 1958,* p. 580–581.

325. MACINTOSH, F. C., AND W. L. M. PERRY. Biological estimation of ACh. *Methods Med. Res.* 3: 78–92, 1950.

326. MALMFORS, T., AND H. THOENEN. *6-Hydroxydopamine and Catecholamine Neurons.* New York: Elsevier, 1971.

327. MARSHALL, K. C., AND I. ENGBERG. Reversal potential for noradrenaline-induced hyperpolarization of spinal motoneurons. *Science* 205: 422–425, 1979.

328. MARTIN, A. R. Junctional transmission II. Presynaptic mechanisms. In *Handbook of Physiology. The Nervous System,* edited by J. M. Brookhart and V. B. Mountcastle. Bethesda, MD: Am. Physiol. Soc., 1977, sect. 1, vol. I, pt. 1, chapt. 10, p. 329–355.

329. MARTIN, A. R., AND G. PILAR. Transmission through the ciliary ganglion of the chick. *J. Physiol. London.* 168: 464–475, 1963.

330. MARTIN, D. L. Carrier-mediated transport and removal of GABA from synaptic regions. In: *GABA in Nervous System Function,* edited by E. Roberts, T. N. Chase, and D. B. Tower. New York: Raven, 1976, p. 347–386.

331. MASON, S. T., AND S. D. IVERSEN. Learning in the absence of forebrain noradrenaline. *Nature London* 258: 422–424, 1975.

332. MASON, S. T., AND S. D. IVERSEN. Reward, attention and the dorsal noradrenergic bundle. *Brain Res.* 150: 135–158, 1978.

333. MCCALL, R. B., AND G. H. AGHAJANIAN. Serotonergic facilitation of facial motoneuron excitation: a modulatory effect. *Brain Res.* 169: 11–27, 1979.

334. MCCANCE, I., AND J. W. PHILLIS. Cholinergic mechanisms in the cerebellar cortex. *Int. J. Neuropharmacol.* 7: 447–462, 1968.

335. MCEWEN, B. S. Steroid hormone receptors in developing and mature brain tissue. In: *Neuroscience Symposia,* edited by J. A. Ferrendelli, B. S. McEwen, and S. H. Snyder. Bethesda, MD: Soc. Neurosci., 1976, vol. 1, p. 50–66.

336. MCGEER, E. G., P. L. MCGEER, AND K. SINGH. Kainate-induced degeneration of neostriatal neurons: dependency upon corticostriatal tract. *Brain Res.* 139: 381–383, 1978.

337. MCGEER, P. L., D. S. GREWAAL, AND E. G. MCGEER. Influence of noncholinergic drugs on rat striatal acetylcholine levels. *Brain Res.* 80: 211–217, 1974.

338. MCGEER, P. L., E. G. MCGEER, J. A. WADA, AND E. JUNG. Effects of globus pallidus lesions and Parkinson's disease on brain glutamic acid decarboxylase. *Brain Res.* 32: 425–431, 1971.

339. MCLAUGHLIN, B. J., R. BARBER, K. SAITO, E. ROBERTS, AND J. Y. WU. Immunocytochemical localization of glutamate decarboxylase in rat spinal cord. *J. Comp. Neurol.* 164: 305–322, 1975.

340. MCLAUGHLIN, B. J., J. G. WOOD, K. SAITO, R. BARBER, J. E. VAUGHN, E. ROBERTS, AND J.-Y. WU. The fine structural localization of glutamate decarboxylase in synaptic terminals of rodent cerebellum. *Brain Res.* 76: 377–391, 1974.

341. MCLENNAN, H. Actions of excitatory amino acids and their antagonism. *Neuropharmacology* 13: 449–454, 1974.

342. MCLENNAN, H., AND D. H. YORK. Cholinergic mechanisms in the caudate nucleus. *J. Physiol. London* 187: 163–175, 1966.

343. MCLENNAN, H., AND D. H. YORK. The action of dopamine on neurones of the caudate nucleus. *J. Physiol. London* 189: 393–402, 1967.

344. MEECH, R. W. Intracellular calcium injection causes increased potassium conductance in *Aplysia* nerve cells. *Comp. Biochem. Physiol.* 42A: 493–499, 1972.

345. MEECH, R. W. Calcium-dependent potassium activation in nervous tissues. *Annu. Rev. Biophys. Bioeng.* 7: 1–18, 1978.

346. MELZACK, R., AND P. D. WALL. Pain mechanisms: a new theory. *Science* 150: 971–979, 1965.

347. MILEDI, R. Transmitter release induced by injection of calcium ions into nerve terminals. *Proc. R. Soc. London Ser. B* 183: 421–425, 1973.

348. MITCHELL, J. F., AND V. SRINIVASAN. Release of ^{3}H-γ-aminobutyric acid from the brain during synaptic inhibition. *Nature London* 224: 663–666, 1969.

350. MIYATA, Y., AND M. OTSUKA. Quantitative histochemistry of γ-aminobutyric acid in cat spinal cord with special reference to presynaptic inhibition. *J. Neurochem.* 25: 239–244, 1975.

351. MONOD, J., J. WYMAN, AND J.-P. CHANGEUX. On the nature of allosteric transition: a plausible model. *J. Mol. Biol.* 12: 88–118, 1965.

352. MORIMOTO, T., M. TAKATA, AND Y. KAWAMURA. Effect of lingual nerve stimulation on hypoglossal motoneurons. *Exp. Neurol.* 22: 174–190, 1968.

353. MORRIS, M. E., G. DI COSTANZO, S. FOX, J. F. MACDONALD, AND R. WERMAN. Actions of GABA, glycine and baclofen on afferent fibres and their central synapses. *Soc. Neurosci. Abstr.* 4: 582, 1978.

354. MUDGE, A. W., S. E. LEEMAN, AND G. D. FISCHBACH. Enkephalin inhibits release of substance P from sensory neurons in culture and decreases action potential duration. *Proc. Natl. Acad. Sci. USA* 76: 526–530, 1979.

355. NADI, N. S., D. KANTER, W. J. MCBRIDE, AND M. H. APRISON. Effects of 3-acetylpyridine on several putative neurotransmitter amino acids in the cerebellum and medulla of the rat. *J. Neurochem.* 28: 661–662, 1977.

356. NADI, N. S., W. J. MCBRIDE, AND M. H. APRISON. Distribution of several amino acids in regions of the cerebellum of the rat. *J. Neurochem.* 28: 453–455, 1977.

357. NAGY, J. I., D. A. CARTER, J. LEHMANN, AND H. C. FIBIGER. Evidence for a GABA-containing projection from the entopeduncular nucleus to the lateral habenula in the rat. *Brain Res.* 145: 360–364, 1978.

358. NAGY, J. I., S. R. VINCENT, J. LEHMANN, H. C. FIBIGER, AND E. G. MCGEER. The use of kainic acid in the localization of enzymes in the substantia nigra. *Brain Res.* 149: 431–441, 1978.

359. NEAL, M. J. The uptake of [^{14}C]glycine by slices of mammalian spinal cord. *J. Physiol. London* 215: 103–117, 1971.

360. NELSON, P. G., B. R. RANSOM, M. HENKART, AND P. N. BULLOCK. Mouse spinal cord in cell culture. IV. Modulation of inhibitory synaptic function. *J. Neurophysiol.* 40: 1178–1187, 1977.

361. NICOLL, R. A. Promising peptides. In: *Neuroscience Symposia,* edited by J. A. Ferrendelli, B. S. McEwen, and S. H. Snyder. Bethesda, MD: Soc. Neurosci., 1976, vol. 1, p. 99–122.

362. NIEOULLON, A., A. CHERAMY, AND J. GLOWINSKI. Release of dopamine *in vivo* from cat substantia nigra. *Nature London* 266: 375–377, 1977.

363. NISHI, S., S. MINOTA, AND A. G. KARCZMAR. Primary afferent neurones: the ionic mechanism of GABA-mediated depolarization. *Neuropharmacology* 13: 215–219, 1974.

364. NISTRI, A., AND A. CONSTANTI. Pharmacological characterization of different types of GABA and glutamate receptor in vertebrates and invertebrates. *Prog. Neurobiol. Oxford* 13: 117–235, 1979.

365. OBATA, K., AND S. M. HIGHSTEIN. Blocking by picrotoxin of both vestibular inhibition and GABA action on rabbit oculo-

motor neurones. *Brain Res.* 18: 538–541, 1970.
366. OBATA, K., M. ITO, R. OCHI, AND N. SATO. Pharmacological properties of the post-synaptic inhibition by Purkinje cell axons and the action of γ-aminobutyric acid on Deiters' neurones. *Exp. Brain Res.* 4: 43–57, 1967.
367. OBATA, K., M. OTSUKA, AND Y. TANAKA. Determination of γ-aminobutyric acid in single nerve cells of cat central nervous system. *J. Neurochem.* 17: 697–698, 1970.
368. OBATA, K., AND K. TAKEDA. Release of γ-aminobutyric acid into the fourth ventricle induced by stimulation of the cat's cerebellum. *J. Neurochem.* 16: 1043–1047, 1969.
369. OBATA, K., K. TAKEDA, AND H. SHINOZAKI. Further study on pharmacological properties of the cerebellar-induced inhibition of Deiters' neurones. *Exp. Brain Res.* 11: 327–342, 1970.
370. OHYE, C., C. LE GUYADER, AND J. FEGER. Responses of subthalamic and pallidal neurons to striatal stimulation: an extracellular study on awake monkeys. *Brain Res.* 111: 241–252, 1976.
371. OKADA, Y., AND C. SHIMADA. Gamma-aminobutyric acid (GABA) concentration in a single neuron—localization of GABA in Deiters' neuron. *Brain Res.* 107: 658–662, 1976.
372. OKAMOTO, K., D. M. J. QUASTEL, AND J. H QUASTEL. Action of amino acids and convulsants on cerebellar spontaneous action potentials *in vitro*: effects of deprivation of Cl$^-$, K$^+$ or Na$^+$. *Brain Res.* 113: 147–158, 1976.
373. OLIANAS, M. C., G. DE MONTIS, G. MULAS, AND A. TAGLIAMONTE. The striatal dopaminergic function is mediated by the inhibition of a nigral non-dopaminergic neuronal system via a strio-nigral GABAergic pathway. *Eur. J. Pharmacol.* 49: 233–241, 1978.
374. OLSEN, R. W., M. BAN, AND T. MILLER. Studies on the neuropharmacological activity of bicuculline and related compounds. *Brain Res.* 102: 283–299, 1976.
375. OLSEN, R. W., M. K. TICKU, P. C. VAN NESS, AND D. GREENLEE. Effects of drugs on γ-aminobutyric acid receptors, uptake, release and synthesis *in vitro*. *Brain Res.* 139: 277–294, 1978.
376. OLSON, L., AND K. FUXE. On the projections from the locus coeruleus noradrenaline neurons: the cerebellar innervation. *Brain Res.* 28: 165–171, 1971.
377. ONODERA, K., AND A. TAKEUCHI. Permeability changes produced by L-glutamate at the excitatory post-synaptic membrane of the crayfish muscle. *J. Physiol. London* 255: 669–685, 1976.
378. OPPENHEIMER, J. H. Thyroid hormone action at the cellular level. *Science* 203: 971–979, 1979.
379. OTSUKA, M., AND T. TAKAHASHI. Putative peptide neurotransmitters. *Annu. Rev. Pharmacol. Toxicol.* 17: 425–439, 1977.
380. PALEY, S. L., AND V. CHAN-PALEY. *Cerebellar Cortex*. New York: Springer-Verlag, 1974.
381. PALKOVITS, M., M. BROWNSTEIN, AND J. M. SAAVEDRA. Serotonin content of the brain stem nuclei in the rat. *Brain Res.* 80: 237–249, 1974.
382. PERRY, T. L., R. D. CURRIER, S. HANSEN, AND J. MACLEAN. Aspartate-taurine imbalance in dominantly inherited olivo-ponto cerebellar atrophy. *Neurology* 27: 257–261, 1977.
383. PERRY, T. L., S. HANSEN, AND M. KLOSTER. Huntington's chorea. Deficiency of γ-aminobutyric acid in brain. *N. Engl. J. Med.* 288: 337–342, 1973.
384. PETTIGREW, J. D., AND T. KASAMATSU. Local perfusion of noradrenaline maintains visual cortical plasticity. *Nature London* 271: 761–763, 1978.
385. PHILLIPPS, G. H. Structure-activity relationships in steroidal anaesthetics. In: *Molecular Mechanisms in General Anaesthesia*. edited by M. J. Halsey, R. A. Millar, and J. A. Sutton. New York: Churchill Livingston, 1974, p. 32–47.
386. PHILLIPS, C. G. Actions of antidromic pyramidal volleys on single Betz cells in the cat. *Q. J. Exp. Physiol.* 44: 1–25, 1959.
387. PHILLIS, J. W. Acetylcholinesterase in the feline cerebellum. *J. Neurochem.* 15: 691–698, 1968.
388. PHILLIS, J. W. *The Pharmacology of Synapses*. London: Pergamon, 1970.
389. PHILLIS, J. W. Neomycin and ruthenium red antagonism of monoaminergic depression of cerebral cortical neurones. *Life Sci.* 15: 213–222, 1974.
390. PHILLIS, J. W., AND G. C. CHONG. Acetylcholine release from the cerebral and cerebellar cortices: its role in cortical arousal. *Nature London* 207: 1253–1255, 1965.
391. PHILLIS, J. W., N. LAKE, AND G. YARBROUGH. Calcium mediation of the inhibitory effects of biogenic amines on cerebral cortical neurones. *Brain Res.* 53: 465–469, 1973.
392. PHILLIS, J. W., A. K. TEBECIS, AND D. H. YORK. Depression of spinal motoneurones by noradrenaline, 5-hydroytryptamine and histamine. *Eur. J. Pharmacol.* 4: 471–475, 1968.
393. PHILLIS, J. W., AND D. H. YORK. Cholinergic inhibition in the cerebral cortex. *Brain Res.* 5: 517–520, 1967.
394. PICKEL, V. M. Immunocytochemical localization of neuronal antigens: tyrosine hydroxylase, substance P, [Met^5]-enkephalin. *Federation Proc.* 38: 2374–2380, 1979.
395. PIERAU, F.-K., AND P. ZIMMERMAN. Action of a GABA-derivative on postsynaptic potentials and membrane properties of cats' spinal motoneurones. *Brain Res.* 54: 376–380, 1973.
396. POIRIER, L. J., AND T. L. SOURKES. Influence of the substantia nigra on the catecholamine content of the striatum. *Brain* 88: 181–192, 1965.
397. POLAK, R. L. An analysis of the stimulating action of atropine on release and synthesis of acetylcholine in cortical slices from rat brain. In: *Drugs and Cholinergic Mechanisms in the CNS*, edited by E. Heilbronn and A. Winter. Stockholm: Forsvarets Forskningsanstalt, 1970, p. 323–338.
398. POLLEN, D. A., AND H. D. LUX. Conductance changes during inhibitory post-synaptic potentials in normal and strychninized cortical neurons. *J. Neurophysiol.* 29: 369–381, 1966.
399. POSNER, B. I., AND J. M. MCKENZIE. Hormone receptors: general considerations and clinical significance. *Clin. Invest. Med.* 1: 81–85, 1978.
400. POTASHNER, S. J. Baclofen: effects on amino acid release. *Can. J. Physiol. Pharmacol.* 56: 150–154, 1978.
401. POTASHNER, S. J. The spontaneous and electrically evoked release, from slices of guinea-pig cerebral cortex, of endogenous amino acids labelled via metabolism of D- U-^{14}C glucose. *J. Neurochem.* 31: 177–186, 1978.
402. PRECHT, W., AND M. YOSHIDA. Blockage of caudate-evoked inhibition of neurons in the substantia nigra by picrotoxin. *Brain Res.* 32: 229–233, 1971.
403. PRESTON, J. B., AND D. G. WHITLOCK. Intracellular potentials recorded from motoneurons following percentral gyrus stimulation in primate. *J. Neurophysiol.* 24: 91–100, 1961.
404. PURPURA, D. P., AND R. J. SHOFER. Cortical intracellular potentials during augmenting and recruiting responses. I. Effects of injected hyperpolarizing currents on evoked membrane potential changes. *J. Neurophysiol.* 27: 117–132, 1964.
405. RABIÉ, A., C. FAVRE, M. C. CLAVEL, AND J. LEGRAND. Sequential effects of thyroxine on the developing cerebellum of rats made hypothyroid by propylthiouracil. *Brain Res.* 161: 469–479, 1979.
406. RALL, W., R. E. BURKE, T. G. SMITH, P. G. NELSON, AND K. FRANK. Dendritic location of synapses and possible mechanism for the monosynaptic EPSP in motoneurons. *J. Neurophysiol.* 39: 1169–1193, 1967.
407. RANDIĆ, M., R. SIMINOFF, AND D. W. STRAUGHAN. Acetylcholine depression of cortical neurones. *Exp. Neurol.* 9: 236–242, 1964.
408. RANG, H. P. Acetylcholine receptors. *Q. Rev. Biophys.* 7: 283–399, 1975.
409. RANJE, C., AND U. UNGERSTEDT. High correlations between number of dopamine cells, dopamine levels and motor performance. *Brain Res.* 134: 83–93, 1977.
410. RANSOM, B. R., P. N. BULLOCK, AND P. G. NELSON. Mouse spinal cord in cell culture. III. Neuronal chemosensitivity and its relationship to synaptic activity. *J. Neurophysiol.* 40: 1163–1177, 1977.
411. RASMUSSEN, H., AND D. B. P. GOODMAN. Relationships between calcium and cyclic nucleotides in cell activation. *Physiol. Rev.* 57: 422–509, 1977.

412. REDMAN, S. Junctional mechanisms at group Ia synapses. *Prog. Neurobiol. Oxford* 12: 33–83, 1979.
413. REHFELD, J. F., N. GOLTERMANN, L.-I. LARSSON, P. M. EMSON, AND C. M. LEE. Gastrin and cholecystokinin in central and peripheral neurons. *Federation Proc.* 38: 2325–2329, 1979.
414. RENAUD, L., AND A. PADJEN. Electrophysiological analysis of peptide actions in neural tissue. In: *Centrally Acting Peptides*, edited by J. Hughes. London: Macmillan, 1978, p. 59–84.
415. RENSHAW, B. Activity in the simplest spinal reflex pathways. *J. Neurophysiol.* 3: 373–387, 1940.
416. RENSHAW, B. Influence of discharge of motoneurons upon excitation of neighboring motoneurons. *J. Neurophysiol.* 4: 167–183, 1941.
417. RIBAK, C. E., J. E. VAUGHN, K. SAITO, R. BARBER, AND E. ROBERTS. Immunocytochemical localization of glutamate decarboxylase in rat substantia nigra. *Brain Res.* 116: 287–298, 1976.
418. RICHARDSON, T. L., J. J. MILLER, AND H. MCLENNAN. Mechanisms of excitation and inhibition in the nigrostriatal system. *Brain Res.* 127: 219–234, 1977.
419. ROBBINS, J. The excitation and inhibition of crustacean muscle by amino acids. *J. Physiol. London* 148: 39–50, 1959.
420. ROBERTS, E., AND S. FRANKEL. Glutamic acid decarboxylase in brain. *J. Biol. Chem.* 188: 789–795, 1951.
421. ROBERTS, P. J. The release of amino acids with proposed neurotransmitter function from the cuneate and gracile nuclei of the rat *in vivo*. *Brain Res.* 67: 419–428, 1974.
422. ROBERTS, P. J., AND P. KEEN. Effect of dorsal root section on amino acids of rat spinal cord. *Brain Res.* 74: 333–337, 1970.
423. ROBERTS, P. J., AND J. F. MITCHELL. The release of amino acids from the hemisected spinal cord during stimulation. *J. Neurochem.* 19: 2473–2481, 1972.
424. ROFFLER-TARLOV, S., AND R. L. SIDMAN. Concentrations of glutamic acid in cerebellar cortex and deep nuclei of normal mice and weaver, staggerer and nervous mutants. *Brain Res.* 142: 269–283, 1978.
425. RUBIN, R. P. *Calcium and the Secretory Process*. New York: Plenum, 1974.
426. RYALL, R. W. Neuropharmacology of the spinal cord. In: *The Spinal Cord*, edited by G. Austin. Springfield, IL: Thomas, 1972, p. 113–146.
427. RYALL, R. W., AND H. L. HAAS. On the physiological significance of muscarinic receptors on Renshaw cells: a hypothesis. In: *Cholinergic Mechanisms*, edited by P. G. Waser. New York: Raven, 1975, p. 335–341.
428. RYALL, R. W., M. F. PIERCEY, AND C. POLOSA. Intersegmental and intrasegmental distribution of mutual inhibition of Renshaw cells. *J. Neurophysiol.* 34: 700–707, 1971.
429. SALMOIRAGHI, G. C., AND C. N. STEFANIS. Patterns of central neurons responses to suspected transmitters. *Arch. Ital. Biol.* 103: 705–724, 1965.
430. SALMOIRAGHI, G. C., AND C. N. STEFANIS. A critique of iontophoretic studies of central nervous system neurons. *Int. Rev. Neurobiol.* 10: 1–30, 1967.
431. SALMOIRAGHI, G. C., AND F. WEIGHT. Micromethods in neuropharmacology: an approach to the study of anesthetics. *Anesthesiology* 28: 54–64, 1967.
432. SAMUELSSON, B., M. GOLDYNE, E. GRANSTRÖM, M. HAMBERG, S. HAMMARSTRÖM, AND C. MALMSTEN. Prostaglandins and thromboxanes. *Annu. Rev. Biochem.*, 47: 997–1029, 1978.
433. SCALLY, M. C., I. H. ULUS, R. J. WURTMAN, AND D. J. PETTIBONE. Regional distribution of neurotransmitter-synthesizing enzymes and substance P within the rat corpus striatum. *Brain Res.* 143: 556–560, 1978.
434. SCHALLY, A. V., D. H. COY, AND C. A. MEYERS. Hypothalamic regulatory hormones. *Annu. Rev. Biochem.* 47: 89–128, 1978.
435. SCHMIDT, R. F. Presynaptic inhibition in the vertebrate central nervous system. *Ergeb. Physiol. Biol. Exp. Pharmacol.* 63: 20–101, 1971.
436. SCHWARCZ, R., AND J. T. COYLE. Neurochemical sequence of kainate injections in corpus striatum and substantia nigra of the rat. *Life Sci.* 20: 431–436, 1977.
437. SEEMAN, P., J. L. TEDESCO, T. LEE, M. CHAU-WONG, P. MULLER, J. BOWLES, P. M. WHITAKER, C. MCMANUS, M. TITTLER, P. WEINREICH, W. C. FRIEND, AND G. M. BROWN. Dopamine receptors in the central nervous system. *Federation Proc.* 37: 130–136, 1978.
438. SELYE, H. Anesthetic effect of steroid hormones. *Proc. Soc. Exp. Biol. Med.* 46: 116–121, 1941.
439. SHAPOVALOV, A. I., V. I. SHIRIAEV, AND Z. A. TAMAROVA. Synaptic activity in motoneurons of the immature cat spinal cord *in vitro*. Effects of manganese and tetrodotoxin. *Brain Res.* 160: 524–528, 1979.
440. SHAPOVALOV, A. I., B. I. SHIRIAEV, AND A. A. VELUMIAN. Mechanisms of postsynaptic excitation in amphibian motoneurones. *J. Physiol. London* 279: 437–455, 1978.
441. SHAPOVALOV, A. I., AND G. G. KURCHAVYI. Effects of transmembrane polarization and TEA injection on monosynaptic actions from motor cortex, red nucleus, and group Ia afferents on lumbar motoneurons in the monkey. *Brain Res.* 82: 49–67, 1974.
442. SHERRINGTON, C. *The Integrative Action of the Nervous System*. New Haven: Yale Univ. Press. 1906.
443. SHIK, M. L., AND G. N. ORLOVSKY. Neurophysiology of locomotor automation. *Physiol. Rev.* 56: 465–501, 1976.
444. SHIMAHARA, T., AND L. TAUC. Heterosynaptic facilitation in the giant cell of Aplysia. *J. Physiol. London* 247: 321–341, 1975.
445. SHLEVIN, H. H. Effects of external calcium concentration and pH on charge movement in frog skeletal muscle. *J. Physiol. London* 288: 129–158, 1979.
446. SHUTE, C. C. D., AND P. R. LEWIS. Cholinesterase-containing systems of the brain of the rat. *Nature London* 199: 1160–1164, 1963.
447. SHUTE, C. C. D., AND P. R. LEWIS. The ascending cholinergic reticular system: neocortical, olfactory and subcortical projections. *Brain* 90: 497–520, 1967.
448. SIGGINS, G. R., B. J. HOFFER, AND F. E. BLOOM. Cyclic adenosine monophosphate: possible mediator for norepinephrine effects on cerebellar Purkinje cells. *Science* 165: 1018–1020, 1969.
449. SIGGINS, G. R., A. P. OLIVER, B. J. HOFFER, AND F. E. BLOOM. Cyclic adenosine monophosphate and norepinephrine: effects on trans-membrane properties of cerebellar Purkinje cells. *Science* 171: 192–194, 1971.
450. SILVER, A. Cholinesterases of the central nervous system with special reference to the cerebellum. *Int. Rev. Neurobiol.* 10: 57–109, 1967.
451. SILVER, A. *The Biology of Cholinesterases*. Amsterdam: North Holland, 1974.
452. SILVER, A., AND J. H. WOLSTENCROFT. The distribution of cholinesterases in relation to the structure of the spinal cord in the cat. *Brain Res.* 34: 205–227, 1971.
453. SIMANTOV, R., M. J. KUHAR, G. W. PASTERNAK, AND S. H. SNYDER. The regional distribution of a morphine-like factor enkephalin in monkey brain. *Brain Res.* 106: 189–197, 1976.
454. SJOSTROM, A., AND P. ZANGGER. Muscle spindle control during locomotor movements generated by the deafferented spinal cord. *Acta Physiol. Scand.* 97: 281–291, 1976.
455. SNODGRASS, S. R. Use of ^{3}H-muscimol for GABA receptor studies. *Nature London* 273: 392–394, 1978.
456. SNYDER, S. H., AND R. B. INNIS. Peptide neurotransmitters. *Annu. Rev. Biochem.* 48: 755–782, 1979.
457. SNYDER, S. H., AND R. SIMANTOV. The opiate receptor and opioid peptides. *J. Neurochem.* 28: 13–20, 1977.
458. SNYDER, S. H., A. B. YOUNG, J. P. BENNETT, AND A. H. MULDER. Synaptic biochemistry of amino acids. *Federation Proc.* 32: 2039–2047, 1973.
459. SONNHOF, U., P. GRAFE, D. W. RICHTER, N. PAREKH, G. KRUMNIKL, AND M. LINDER. Investigations of the effects of glutamate on motoneurons of the isolated frog spinal cord. In: *Iontophoresis and Transmitter Mechanisms in the Mammalian Central Nervous System*, edited by R. W. Ryall and J. S. Kelly. Amsterdam: Elsevier, 1978, p. 391–393.

460. SOURKES, T. L. Central actions of DOPA and dopamine. *Rev. Can. Biol.* 31: (Suppl.) 153-168, 1972.
461. SPEHLMANN, R. Acetylcholine and prostigmine electrophoresis at visual cortical neurons. *J. Neurophysiol.* 26: 127-139, 1963.
462. SPENCER, H. J., AND V. HAVLICEK. Alterations by anesthetic agents of the responses of rat striatal neurons to iontophoretically applied amphetamine, acetylcholine, noradrenaline, and dopamine. *Can. J. Physiol. Pharmacol.* 52: 808-813, 1974.
463. SPIECKER, W., W. MELZER, AND H. C. LÜTTGAU. Extracellular Ca^{2+} and excitation-contraction coupling. *Nature London* 280: 158-160, 1979.
464. STAVINOHA, W. B., J. FRAZER, AND A. T. MODAK. Microwave fixation for the study of acetylcholine metabolism. In: *Cholinergic Mechanisms and Psychopharmacology*, edited by D. J. Jenden. New York, Plenum, 1978, p. 169-179.
464a. STEEVES, J. D., B. J. SCHMIDT, B. J. SKOVGAARD, AND L. M. JORDAN. Effect of noradrenaline and 5-hydroxytryptamine depletion on locomotion in the cat. *Brain Res.* 185: 349-362, 1980.
465. STEFANIS, C., AND H. JASPER. Recurrent collateral inhibition in pyramidal tract neurons. *J. Neurophysiol.* 27: 855-877, 1964.
466. STEINER, F. A., AND G. WEBER. Die Beeinflussung labyrinthär erregbarer. Neurone des Hirnstammes durch Acetylcholin. *Helv. Physiol. Pharmacol. Acta* 23: 82-89, 1965.
467. STERIADE, M., M. DESCHÊNES, AND G. OAKSON. Inhibitory process and interneuronal apparatus in motor cortex during sleep and waking. 1. Background firing and responsiveness of pyramidal tract neurons and interneurons. *J. Neurophysiol.* 37: 1062-1092, 1974.
468. STERIADE, M., AND J. A. HOBSON. Neuronal activity during the sleep-waking cycle. *Prog. Neurobiol. Oxford* 6: 155-376, 1976.
469. STERIADE, M., P. WYZINSKI, M. DESCHENES, AND M. GUERIN. Disinhibition during waking in motor cortex neuronal chains in cat and monkey. *Brain Res.* 30: 211-217, 1971.
470. STERN, J. R., L. V. EGGLESTON, R. HEMS, AND H. A. KREBS. Accumulation of glutamic acid in isolated brain tissue. *Biochem. J.* 44: 410-418, 1949.
471. STONE, T. W. Cholinergic mechanisms in the rat somatosensory cerebral cortex. *J. Physiol. London* 225: 485-499, 1972.
472. STONE, T. W. Cortical pyramidal tract interneurones and their sensitivity to L-glutamic acid. *J. Physiol. London* 233: 211-225, 1973.
472a. STONE, T. W. Blockade by amino acid antagonists of neuronal excitation mediated by the pyramidal tract. *J. Physiol. London* 257: 187-198, 1976.
473. STORM-MATHISEN, J. High affinity uptake of GABA in presumed GABAergic nerve endings in rat brain. *Brain Res.* 84: 409-427, 1975.
474. SUTHERLAND, E. W. Studies on the mechanism of hormone action. *Science* 177: 401-408, 1972.
475. SUTHERLAND, E. W., AND G. A. ROBISON. Metabolic effects of catecholamines. A. The role of cyclic-3',5'-AMP in responses to catecholamines and other hormones. *Pharmacol. Rev.* 18: 145-161, 1966.
476. SWEETMAN, A. J., AND A. F. ESMAIL. Evidence for the role of calcium ions and mitochondria in the maintenance of anaesthesia in the rat. *Biochem. Biophys. Res. Commun.* 64: 885-890, 1975.
477. SZERB, J. C. Cortical acetylcholine release and electroencephalographic arousal. *J. Physiol. London* 192: 329-343, 1967.
478. SZERB, J. C. Characterization of presynpatic muscarinic receptors in central cholinergic neurons. In: *Cholinergic Mechanisms and Psychopharmacology, Advances in Behavioural Biology*, edited by D. J. Jenden. New York: Plenum, 1978, vol. 24, p. 49-60.
479. TAKAGI, M., AND C. YAMAMOTO. Suppressing action of cholinergic agents on synaptic transmissions in the corpus striatum of rats. *Exp. Neurol.* 62: 433-443, 1978.
480. TAKAHASHI, T. Intracellular recording from visually identified motoneurones in rat spinal cord slices. *Proc. R. Soc. London Ser. B* 202: 417-421, 1978.
481. TAKEUCHI, A. Junctional transmission 1. Postsynaptic mechanisms. In: *Handbook of Physiology. The Nervous System*, edited by J. M. Brookhart and V. B. Mountcastle. Bethesda, MD: Am. Physiol. Soc., 1977, sect. 1, vol. I, pt. 1, chapt. 9, p. 295-327.
482. TARSY, D., C. J. PYCOCK, B. S. MELDRUM, AND C. D. MARSDEN. Focal contralateral myoclonus produced by inhibition of GABA action in the caudate nucleus of rats. *Brain* 101: 143-162, 1978.
483. TAYLOR, S. R., AND R. E. GODT. Calcium release and contraction in vertebrate skeletal muscle. *Symp. Soc. Exp. Biol. Cambridge* 30: 361-380, 1976.
484. TEBĒCIS, A. K., AND A. DI MARIA. Strychnine-sensitive inhibition in the medullary reticular formation: evidence for glycine as an inhibitory transmitter. *Brain Res.* 40: 373-383, 1972.
485. TEN BRUGGENCATE, G., AND I. ENGBERG. Effects of GABA and related amino acids on neurones in Deiters' nucleus. *Brain Res.* 14: 533-536, 1969.
486. TEN BRUGGENCATE, G., AND I. ENGBERG. Iontophoretic studies in Deiters' nucleus of the inhibitory actions of GABA and related amino acids and the interactions of strychnine and picrotoxin. *Brain Res.* 25: 431-448, 1971.
487. TEN BRUGGENCATE, G., AND U. SONNHOF. Effects of glycine and GABA, and blocking actions of strychnine and picrotoxin in the hypoglossus nucleus. *Pfluegers Arch.* 334: 240-252, 1972.
488. TSUKAHARA, N., AND D. R. G. FULLER. Conductance changes during pyramidally induced postsynaptic potentials in red nucleus neurons. *J. Neurophysiol.* 32: 35-42, 1969.
489. TSUKAHARA, N., K. TOYAMA,, AND K. KOSAKA. Electrical activity of red nucleus neurones investigated with intracellular microelectrodes. *Exp. Brain Res.* 4: 18-33, 1967.
490. UEKI, S., K. KOKETSU, AND E. F. DOMINO. Effects of mecamylamine on the Golgi recurrent collateral-Renshaw cell synapse in the spinal cord. *Exp. Neurol.* 3: 141-148, 1961.
491. UNGERSTEDT, U. Post-synaptic supersensitivity after 6-hydroxy-dopamine induced degeneration of the nigro-striatal dopamine system. *Acta Physiol. Scand. Suppl.* 367: 69-93, 1971.
492. VALDÉS, F., AND F. ORREGO. Electrically induced, calcium-dependent release of endogenous GABA from rat brain cortex slices. *Brain Res.* 141: 357-363, 1978.
493. VAN HARREVELD, A., AND E. FIFKOVA. Effects of amino acids on the isolated chicken retina, and on its response to glutamate stimulation. *J. Neurochem.* 20: 947-962, 1973.
494. VEECH, R. L., AND R. A. HAWKINS. Brain blowing: a technique for in vivo study of brain metabolism. In: *Research Methods in Neurochemistry*, edited by N. Marks and R. Rodnight. New York: Plenum, 1974, vol. 2, p. 171-182.
495. VERSTEEG, D. H. G., J. VAN DER GUGTEN, W. DE JONG, AND M. PALKOVITS. Regional concentrations of noradrenaline and dopamine in rat brain. *Brain Res.* 113: 563-574, 1976.
496. VON EULER, U. S. Synthesis, uptake and storage of catecholamines in adrenergic nerves, the effect of drugs. *Handb. Exp. Pharmakol. New Ser.* 33: 186-230, 1972.
497. WALL, P. D. The gate control theory of pain mechanisms. An examination and re-statement. *Brain* 101: 1-18, 1978.
498. WEIGHT, F. F., AND G. C. SALMOIRAGHI. Responses of spinal cord interneurons to acetylcholine, norepinephrine and serotonin administered by microelectrophoresis. *J. Pharmacol. Exp. Ther.* 153: 420-427, 1966.
499. WEIGHT, F. F., AND G. C. SALMOIRAGHI. Adrenergic responses of Renshaw cells. *J. Pharmacol. Exp. Ther.* 154: 391-397, 1966.
500. WEIGHT, F. F., AND G. C. SALMOIRAGHI. Motoneurone depression by norepinephrine. *Nature London* 213: 1229-1230, 1967.
501. WEIGHT, F. F., AND J. VOTAVA. Slow synaptic excitation in sympathetic ganglion cells: evidence for synaptic inactivation of potassium conductance. *Science* 170: 755-758, 1970.
502. WERMAN, R. Criteria for identification of central nervous system transmitter. *Comp. Biochem. Physiol.* 18: 745-766, 1966.
503. WERMAN, R., AND P. CARLEN. Unusual behavior of the Ia EPSP in cat spinal motoneurons. *Brain Res.* 112: 395-401, 1976.
504. WERMAN, R., R. A. DAVIDOFF, AND M. H. APRISON. Inhibition of motoneurons by iontophoresis of glycine. *Nature London*

214: 681-683, 1967.
505. WERMAN, R., R. A. DAVIDOFF, AND M. H. APRISON. Inhibitory action of glycine on spinal neurons in the cat. *J. Neurophysiol.* 31: 81-95, 1968.
506. WHITE, W. F., J. V. NADLER, AND C. W. COTMAN. The effect of acidic amino acid antagonists on synaptic transmission in the hippocampal formation in vitro. *Brain Res.* 164: 177-194, 1979.
507. WHITTAKER, V. P. The application of subcellular fractionation techniques to the study of brain function. *Progr. Biophys.* 15: 39-96, 1965.
508. WOJTOWICZ, J. M., K. C. MARSHALL, AND W. J. HENDELMAN. Electrophysiological and pharmacological studies of the inhibitory projection from the cerebellar cortex to the deep cerebellar nuclei in tissue culture. *Neuroscience* 3: 607-618, 1978.
509. WOOD, J. G., B. J. MCLAUGHLIN, AND J. E. VAUGHN. Immunocytochemical localization of GAD in electron microscopic preparations of rodent CNS. In: *GABA in Nervous System Function*, edited by E. Roberts, T. N. Chase, and D. B. Tower. New York: Raven, 1976, p. 133-148.
510. WOODWARD, D. J., B. J. HOFFER, G. R. SIGGINS, AND A. P. OLIVER. Inhibition of Purkinje cells in the frog cerebellum. II. Evidence for GABA as the inhibitory transmitter. *Brain Res.* 33: 91-100, 1971.
511. WOODWARD, D. J., H. C. MOISES, B. D. WATERHOUSE, B. J. HOFFER, AND R. FREEDMAN. Modulatory actions of norepinephrine in the central nervous system. *Federation Proc.* 38: 2109-2116, 1979.
512. WOODY, C. D. Aspects of the electrophysiology of cortical processes related to the development and performance of learned motor responses. *Physiologist* 17: 49-69, 1974.
513. WOODY, C. D., B. E. SWARTZ, AND E. GRUEN. Effects of acetylcholine and cyclic GMP on input resistance of cortical neurons in awake cats. *Brain Res.* 158: 373-395, 1978.
514. WU, J.-Y. Microanalytical methods for neuronal analysis. *Physiol. Rev.* 58: 863-904, 1978.
515. YALOW, R. S. Radioimmunoassay: a probe for the fine structure of biological systems. *Science* 200: 1236-1245, 1978.
516. YAMAMOTO, C. Pharmacologic studies of norepinephrine, acetylcholine and related compounds on neurons in Deiters' nucleus and the cerebellum. *J. Pharmacol. Exp. Ther.* 156: 39-47, 1967.
517. YAMAMOTO, C. Activation of hippocampal neurons by mossy fiber stimulation in thin brain sections in vitro. *Exp. Brain Res.* 14: 423-435, 1972.
518. YAMAMOTO, C. Electrical activity recorded from thin sections of the lateral geniculate body, and the effects of 5-hydroxytryptamine. *Exp. Brain Res.* 19: 271-281, 1974.
519. YAMAMOTO, C., AND N. KAWAI. Presynaptic action of acetylcholine in thin sections from the guinea pig dentate gyrus in vitro. *Exp. Neurol.* 19: 176-187, 1967.
520. YAMAMOTO, C., AND H. MCILWAIN. Electrical activities in thin sections from the mammalian brain maintained in chemically defined media in vitro. *J. Neurochem.* 13: 1333-1343, 1966.
521. YAMAMOTO, C., H. YAMASHITA, AND T. CHUJO. Inhibitory action of glutamic acid on cerebellar interneurones. *Nature London* 262: 786-787, 1976.
522. YAMAMURA, H. I., M. J. KUHAR, AND S. H SNYDER. In vivo identification of muscarinic cholinergic receptor binding in rat brain. *Brain Res.* 80: 170-176, 1974.
523. YORK, D. H. Possible dopaminergic pathway from substantia nigra to putamen. *Brain Res.* 20: 233-249, 1970.
524. YOSHIDA, M., AND K. OBATA. Actions of putative neurotransmitters on cat pallidal neurons. In: *Iontophoresis and Transmitter Mechanisms in the Mammalian Central Nervous System*, edited by R. W. Ryall and J. S. Kelly. Amsterdam: Elsevier, 1978, p. 71-74.
525. YOSHIDA, M., AND W. PRECHT. Monosynaptic inhibition of neurons of the substantia nigra by caudato-nigral fibers. *Brain Res.* 32: 225-228, 1971.
526. YOSHIDA, M., A. RABIN, AND M. ANDERSON. Monosynaptic inhibition of pallidal neurons by axon collaterals of caudato-nigral fibres. *Exp. Brain Res.* 15: 333-347, 1972.
527. YOUNG, A. B., M. L. OSTER-GRANITE, R. M. HERNDON, AND S. H. SNYDER. Glutamic acid: selective depletion by viral induced granule cell loss in hamster cerebellum. *Brain Res.* 73: 1-13, 1974.
528. ZARZECKI, P., D. J. BLAKE, AND G. G. SOMJEN. Interactions of nigrostriate synaptic transmission, iontophoretic O-methylated phenethylamines, dopamine, apomorphine and acetylcholine. *Brain Res.* 115: 257-272, 1976.
529. ZIEGLGÄNSBERGER, W., AND A. HERZ. Changes of cutaneous receptive fields of spino-cervical-tract neurones and other dorsal horn neurones by microelectrophoretically administered amino acids. *Exp. Brain Res.* 13: 111-126, 1971.
530. ZIEGLGÄNSBERGER, W., AND E. PUIL. Actions of glutamic acid on spinal neurones. *Exp. Brain Res.* 17: 35-49, 1973.
531. ZIEGLGÄNSBERGER, W., AND C. REITER. A cholinergic mechanism in the spinal cord of cats. *Neuropharmacology* 13: 519-527, 1974.
532. ZIEGLGÄNSBERGER, W., AND I. F. TULLOCH. Effects of substance P on neurones in the dorsal horn of the spinal cord of the cat. *Brain Res.* 166: 273-282, 1979.

CHAPTER 5

Motor prostheses

J. THOMAS MORTIMER | *Applied Neural Control Laboratory, Biomedical Engineering Department, Case Western Reserve University, Cleveland, Ohio*

CHAPTER CONTENTS

History
Perspective
Electrochemical Aspects of Stimulation
  Metal-tissue interface without applied field
  System for electrical excitation
  Relationship between electrode potential and charge density
  Regulated voltage vs. regulated current
  Monophasic stimulation
  Biphasic stimulation
    Reversible region
    Irreversible region
    Experimental note
    Imbalanced biphasic stimulation
    Expanding capacitive region
    Balanced biphasic stimulator
  Summary
Tissue Damage
  Electrode materials
    Passive properties
  Brain (surface electrodes)
    Passive implants
    Active implants
  Nerve (cuff electrode)
  Muscle (coiled wire electrode)
    Passive implants
    Active implants
  Summary
Nerve Excitation
  Membrane response to applied electrical field
    First-order membrane model
    Pulse amplitude–pulse duration relationship
    Pulse charge–pulse duration relationship
    Effect of secondary pulse
  Excitation of myelinated nerve
    Threshold dependence on fiber diameter
    Threshold dependence on axon-electrode separation
  Threshold relationship between nerve and muscle
  Effects of electrode configuration on threshold
      and excitation site
    Cuff electrode
    Surface electrode
  Neural fatigue
  Summary
Electrical Activation of Skeletal Muscle
  Brief review of muscle physiology
    Muscle fiber type
    Motor unit properties
  Electrical excitation of normal muscle
    Nerve cuff electrode
    Surface electrode
    Intramuscular electrode

  Conclusion
Muscle alterations induced by electrical activation
  Changes in contractile properties
  Metabolic changes
  Time course of changes
  Fatigue resistance
  Reversibility of changes
Force modulation
  Recruitment
  Frequency modulation
  Sequential stimulation
Summary
Clinical Applications
  Paralyzed muscle
    General considerations
    Hemiplegia
    Spinal cord injury
    Respiration
  Scoliosis
    Animal experiments
    Human experiments
  Summary
Summary

A PROPAGATED ACTION POTENTIAL can be effected by subjecting a nerve to a rapidly changing electrical field. This phenomenon is known as electrical excitation, activation, or stimulation. An action potential so evoked is indistinguishable, by the end organ, from an action potential appearing in the natural control signal. This fact leads logically to the conclusion that by electrically generating a transmitted neural signal, we can effect external control over any given end organ that is under neural control. Therefore functional electrical stimulation (FES), or functional neural stimulation (FNS), is potentially a powerful tool for the restoration of lost or impaired body function. Its potential and limits have not yet been realized, but work already performed suggests that FES is worth pursuing. For instance, it has been shown that visual sensation can be electrically evoked in the blind (8, 17), auditory sensation can be electrically evoked in the deaf (18, 45, 71), and paralyzed muscle can be made to contract (6, 39, 55). (An excellent collection of papers on the general subject can be found in ref. 30c.)

HISTORY

Application of the neuroelectric phenomenon to nontherapeutic clinical problems is rather recent, beginning sometime in the early 1960s. The studies of that decade generally involved placing electrodes on or near certain neural structures, turning on the electrical current, and observing the response. Generally the desired response was more or less attained, but it was accompanied by problems that precluded the clinical use of the technique, such as unpredictable response, tissue destruction, accommodation or fatigue (over time the system's response diminished), activation of other body systems, and frequent hardware failure. This initial period yielded a catalogue of possible applications, but, with the exception of the cardiac pacemaker, virtually no usable clinical systems have resulted. I believe that this general lack of success probably is due more to a lack of understanding of basic mechanisms related to the technique than to a failure of the concept. During the 1970s more emphasis has been placed on basic aspects in the hope of overcoming unwanted side effects. The Neural Prostheses Program, initiated in the Laboratory for Neural Control in the National Institute of Neurologic Diseases and Stroke (now the National Institute of Neurological Communicative Diseases and Stroke) can be credited with pioneering this direction in the research.

PERSPECTIVE

Restoration of body function through FES at best only approaches the function of the normal system. The degree of success most probably depends on the degree of interaction required between the restored system and the conscious person (closed-loop operation). Open-loop systems that come close to reproducing the normal function (i.e., the cardiac pacemaker) are apt to provide clinical utility sooner than systems requiring closed-loop control.

The material in this chapter helps the investigator exploit the application of the neuroelectric phenomenon. It is presented here in five major sections. The first three are basic in nature and are concerned with electrochemistry, damage, and the mechanism of electrical excitation. These three sections are generally applicable to the nervous system. The fourth section concerns the basic aspects effecting electrical control of the motor system. In the last section a review of current efforts in clinical application of the neuroelectric phenomenon to the motor system is given.

ELECTROCHEMICAL ASPECTS OF STIMULATION

The application of an electrical field in a typical stimulation system involves electron flow in the metal components and ion flow in the tissue medium. Conversion between the two processes occurs at the metal-tissue interface. Knowledge of the processes that occur at this interface is critical in formulating the electrical characteristics of the excitation waveform (stimulus). At present, many if not most of the reaction processes that occur in the conversion cannot be precisely defined. Likewise the effects of the resulting reaction products on body tissues (even those far removed from the electrode) cannot be precisely defined. Thus as a practical matter, the recommended approach to stimulation is to seek conditions under which no net reaction products are generated.

Metal-Tissue Interface Without Applied Field

When the surface of a metal electrode and an electrolyte medium (such as exists in the body) come into contact, thermodynamic forces operate to bring the metal and solution into equilibrium (see Fig. 1). The surface properties of the electrode and the ionic composition of the solution affect the equilibrium conditions of the system. Metal ions may migrate away from the metal in solution, resulting in a potential difference between the solution and the metal. This potential difference in turn provides an attractive force for ions in the solution. The process, which involves the net motion of charge carriers, continues until an equilibrium condition is achieved. For a stimulation electrode to be of practical use, the metal-tissue equilibrium must be at a point where the net metal-ion loss is essentially zero. If it is not, the electrode is eventually lost due to corrosion. Inhomogeneities on the metal surface, which exist in all practical electrodes, may produce local potential differences that favor continued loss of metal ions (pitting or crevice corrosion). Some metals or alloys have a greater tendency than others to exhibit this type of corrosion and are therefore less suitable for use as stimulating electrodes.

The overall result of the processes leading to equilibrium is an ordering of charge (or ions) on the metal surface and at the solution-metal interface. The total amount of charge of either polarity generally depends on the real surface area of the electrode. (Real surface area is distinguished from geometric surface area because at the atomic level the surface area can be substantially greater than the geometric area.) Surface conditions of the metal, e.g., oxide films and organic contaminants, can alter the charge ordering. Oxide films can be firmly bonded to the metal surface and act to protect the metal surface from further ion loss, as in the case of stainless steel, and may also serve as insulators. Organic contaminants, on the other hand, appear to add to instability or variability in charge distribution under passive conditions.

The charge ordering or separation that occurs at the surface of the metal and solution medium resembles that occurring on the two plates of a capacitor.

This charge-separating property is of critical importance because it means an electrical stimulus can be applied to an electrode without generating potentially toxic reaction products.

System for Electrical Excitation

Figure 2 shows a typical system used to study electrode behavior. This system includes, in addition to a stimulating electrode, a reference electrode that is used in test situations (but not necessarily in a practical stimulation system) to make in vitro measurements. The test or stimulating electrode is the electrode of primary interest; the indifferent electrode is required to complete the electrical circuit. The reference electrode is usually a standard electrode, such as a saturated calomel or hydrogen electrode. Potential measurements (V'_E) made between the test and reference electrodes are dependent on the reactions taking place on the test electrode and the ohmic drop in the solution medium but independent of the reactions at the indifferent electrode. The ohmic drop can be eliminated by adjusting the resistor and subtracting a potential corresponding to the ohmic component of V'_E, V_R, from V'_E, yielding V_E, the electrode potential. System potential V_S includes all potential drops in the system.

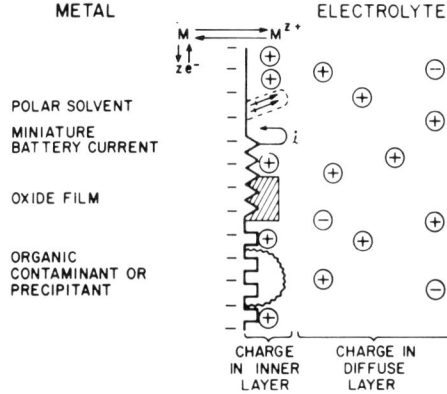

FIG. 1. Cross-sectional representation of metal-electrolyte interface. Charge in inner layer is more highly organized than in outer or diffuse layer, but because of inhomogeneities in surface conditions, it is not necessarily uniformly distributed. Surface deformations and coatings or contaminants on surface produce local potential differences that can support current flow or modify charge transfer properties of electrode under active conditions. [From Dymond (19).]

Relationship Between Electrode Potential and Charge Density

The application of an external potential source to a metal electrode forces electron flow in the metal, which alters the charge distribution (from equilibrium) at the metal-solution interface. The altered charge distribution is reflected in the electrode potential V_E. The change in V_E varies directly with the amount of charge moved and inversely with the electrode surface area. For metal-stimulating electrodes such as those in current use, the relationship between V_E and charge density (Q/A) takes the general form shown in Figure 3. The resting or equilibrium potential of the electrode is located in the region labeled reversible. Here charge can be added to or subtracted from the metal surface in a reversible manner. In this region the metal-solution interface reacts to transient field changes like an electrical capacitor. On either side of this region (beyond points I or II in Fig. 3), the reactions supporting the charge transfer are not readily reversible by changing the polarity of the externally applied potential. As positive charge is added to the metal, the potential rises along the curve to point I. Above point I, when sufficient energy is available, irreversible reactions may occur; i.e., metal ions are released, metal compounds are formed, saline is oxidized, and/or water is electrolyzed. The following are examples of reactions that can occur when platinum becomes sufficiently anodic (11)

electrolysis of water
$$2H_2O \rightarrow O_2 + 4H^+ + 4e^- \tag{1}$$

oxidation of saline
$$Cl^- + H_2O \rightarrow ClO^- + 2H^+ + 2e^- \tag{2}$$

oxidation of metal
$$Pt + 4Cl^- \rightarrow PtCl_4^{2-} + 2e^- \tag{3}$$

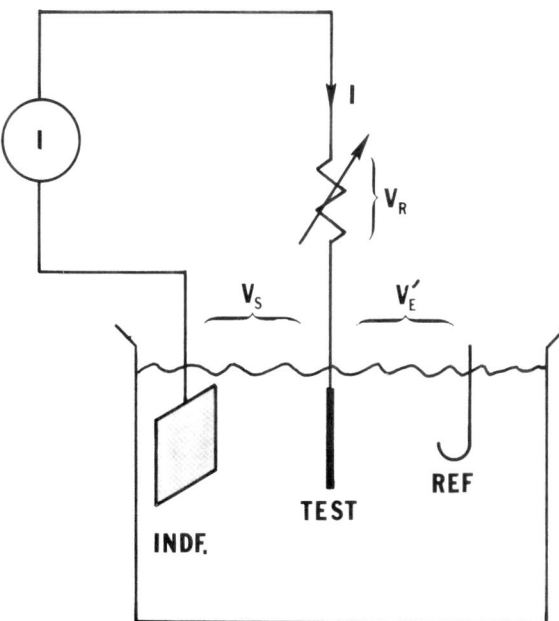

FIG. 2. Schematic representation of electrode test configuration. The potential V_S represents system potential and includes surface potential of both test and indifferent (INDF.) electrodes. The potential V'_E is electrode potential V_E plus ohmic potential of electrode and component of the ohmic potential of electrolyte medium. Value of resistor can be adjusted to yield value of V_R that equals ohmic component of V'_E. Subtracting V_R from V'_E approximates V_E, electrode potential. REF, reference electrode.

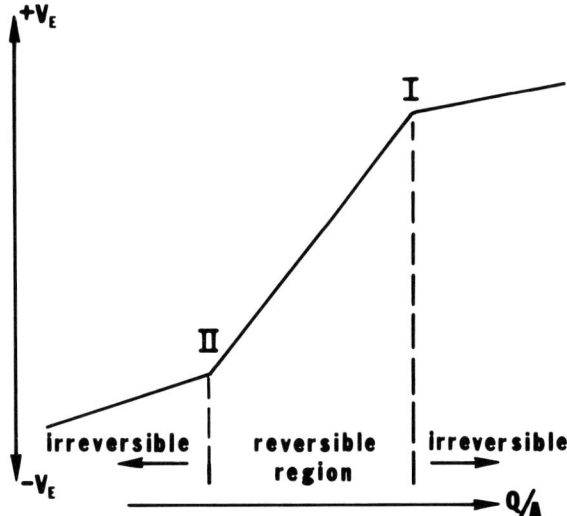

FIG. 3. Idealized representation of relationship between electrode potential V_E and charge density (charge per unit of real electrode area, Q/A). Charge injection in reversible region involves processes that are completely reversible and do not result in net change in chemical species. Charge injection in irreversible regions (to right of point I or left of point II) involves electrochemical reactions that cannot be reversed by driving current in opposite direction.

oxidation of organics
$$C_6H_{12}O_6 + 6H_2O \rightarrow 6CO_2 + 24H^+ + 24e^- \quad (4)$$

For stainless steel the most probable reaction is the dissolution of iron (43)

$$Fe \rightarrow Fe^{2+} + 2e^- \quad (5)$$

In Equations 1, 2, and 4, the hydrogen ion concentration is increased, causing the local pH to become acidic. The platinum and chloride compounds formed in Equations 2 and 3 are powerful oxidizing agents and could cause cell death in the vicinity of the electrode. If Equation 5 occurs, the electrode may be lost to corrosion.

The application of an external potential that increases the negative charge on the electrode forces the electrode potential V_E to move from the resting level toward or beyond point II. In this region the most probable reaction is H_2 deposition (43)

$$2H_2O + 2e^- \rightarrow H_2 + 2OH^- \quad (6)$$

By increasing the electrode potential in the negative direction beyond that at which Equation 6 occurs (increasing the negative charge per unit area), the following reaction may occur

$$O_2 + H_2O + 2e^- \rightarrow OH^- + O_2H^- \quad (7)$$

When H^+ is available, as it is in a saline medium, O_2H^- proceeds to O_2H_2 (the strong oxidizing agent hydrogen peroxide). In Equations 6 and 7 the production of OH^- results in a local increase in pH. As is discussed in subsection *Muscle (Coiled Wire Electrode)*, p. 163,

changes in pH can interrupt local blood flow, possibly resulting in tissue necrosis. It should also be kept in mind that blood can buffer and therefore some change in the hydrogen ion concentration may be accommodated without damage to the adjacent cells.

Regulated Voltage vs. Regulated Current

A typical waveform used to excite neural tissue is a rectangular pulse. The pulse can be either voltage controlled or current controlled. In the voltage-controlled case, the current I injected into the medium decreases as the charge Q injected increases because of the voltage buildup at the electrode surface: $It = Q$, where t is time. The injected charge or the electric field in tissue medium cannot be controlled because of the variability in surface conditions. Therefore repeatability is not reliable. In the case of the regulated-current pulse, current is maintained during the pulse and is independent of changes in the electrode potential. Also when the voltage response to a regulated-current pulse is examined, one sees that the applied field, in the medium containing the excitable tissue, remains contant during the pulse. This latter aspect, illustrated in Figure 4, is important for reproducibility. In this figure three aspects of the voltage waveform V'_E are distinguished. *1)* The V_O component is the ohmic drop in the tissue medium. *2)* The V_E component (often referred to as the polarization potential) reflects the voltage change at the electrode-tissue interface in response to the change in surface charge and any other local changes in potential (e.g., those due to transient changes in the concentration of ion species). *3)* The transient change V_O at the rising edge and that at the falling edge are equal and purely resistive in nature. Therefore maintaining a constant current during the stimulus pulse yields a constant electrical field in the medium containing the excitable tissue. The trailing portion of the waveform (V_{RX}) reflects a transient return of the potential at the metal-tissue interface toward equilibrium or rest conditions. In general this relaxation time is substantially greater than the width of the stimulus pulse and may be greater than the rest period between pulses.

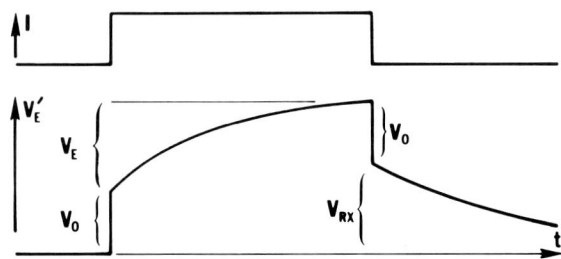

FIG. 4. Voltage waveform observed between test electrode and reference electrode in response to regulated-current pulse. See text for explanation.

Monophasic Stimulation

The application of a pulsed, unidirectional field (polarity of only one sign, positive or negative), as shown in Figure 4, is termed monophasic stimulation. In many practical situations the interpulse interval is less than the time required for the electrode to reestablish equilibrium or to return to the original prepulse electrode potential. When this situation occurs, the peak electrode potential V_E increases with each successive pulse. Therefore, even though the charge density (charge per area) of a single pulse is within the reversible region (Fig. 3), the nth pulse in a train can result in an electrode potential that favors the occurrence of irreversible reactions beyond points I or II. This situation is illustrated in Figure 5 for a series of anodic pulses. For platinum all pulses occurring in the train beyond the fourth pulse can result in the potentially damaging reactions shown in Equations 1, 2, 3, and 4. For stainless steel the electrode begins to corrode, shown in Equation 5.

The results for a series of cathodic pulses are similar to those for anodic pulses, but the electrode potential V_E creeps into the region to the left of point II (Fig. 3). Beyond point II sufficient energy is available for the reactions of Equations 6 and 7 to occur. In this case, if the OH^- generation rate exceeds the buffering capacity of the medium, the local pH becomes basic.

Biphasic Stimulation

Charge accumulation at the electrode-tissue interface can be reduced during a train of stimuli by adding a pulse of opposite polarity after each stimulus pulse (biphasic stimulation). To facilitate this discussion we call the first pulse in the cycle the primary pulse, P,

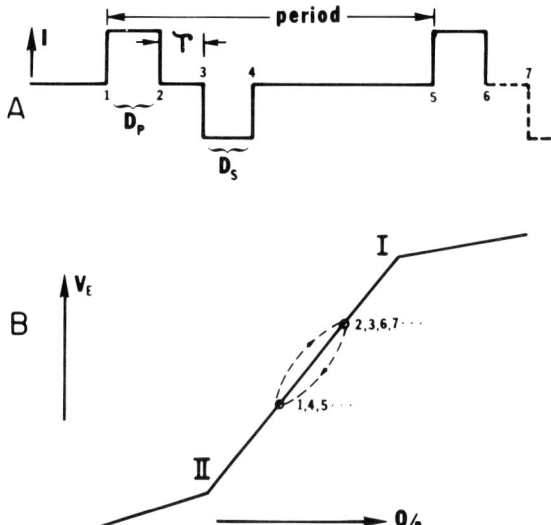

FIG. 6. Balanced-charge biphasic stimulation. *A*: stimulus waveform with zero net charge transfer per cycle. *B*: variation in electrode potential, for conditions where charge is accommodated entirely within reversible region. *I* and *D* refer to current pulse amplitude and pulse duration. Subscripts P and S refer to primary and secondary stimulus pulses, respectively. Parameter τ is time delay between end of primary pulse and beginning of secondary pulse. Points 1–7 in *A* correspond to points in *B*.

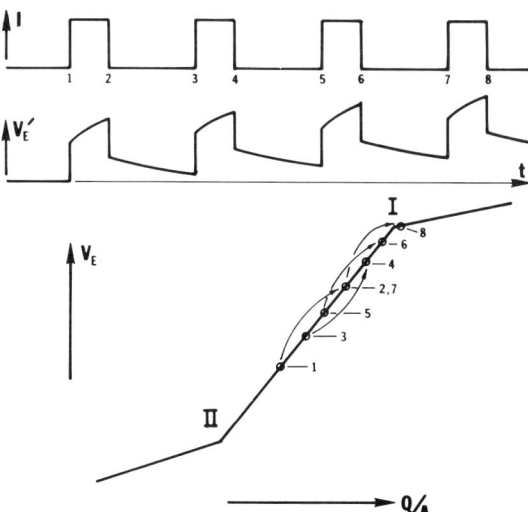

FIG. 5. Electrode response to monophasic regulated-current stimulation. Current waveform is shown in *upper part* of figure, and voltage waveform is shown in *middle*. Points 1–8 shown in electrode potential–charge density plot correspond to points listed on time axis of current waveform. See text for details.

and the second pulse the secondary pulse, S (Fig. 6*A*). The function of the primary pulse is to effect a conducted action potential; the function of the secondary pulse is to reverse the electrochemical process that resulted during the primary pulse. A delay, τ, is introduced between the end of the primary pulse and the beginning of the secondary pulse. In our initial discussion we treat τ as zero; however, in EFFECT OF SECONDARY PULSE, p. 167, the need for a nonzero delay becomes apparent.

REVERSIBLE REGION. When the charge injected (per unit area) during the primary pulse is less than the limits of the reversible region of the electrode, and the charge injected in the primary and secondary pulses are identically equal $[I_P D_P \equiv I_S D_S$ (I is current pulse amplitude, D is pulse duration) or $Q_P \equiv Q_S$; see Fig. 6*A*], the waveform is termed balanced-charge biphasic. The behavior of the metal-tissue interface under balanced conditions is shown in Figure 6*B*, where we have assumed that *1*) the delay τ between pulses is short and no change in the electrode potential occurs before the onset of the secondary pulse, and *2*) the kinetics of the electrochemical processes are sufficiently fast to reverse completely the processes that occurred during the primary pulse. Under these conditions no net change occurs in the ionic species in the vicinity of the electrode; this is considered the ideal mode of operation.

IRREVERSIBLE REGION. In the event that a slight charge imbalance between the two phases exists, or that the above assumptions are not met, the base point may drift toward one end of the reversible region. For example, if $Q_P > Q_S$ or the reversal kinetics are not fast enough, the base point drifts in the direction of point I during a train of stimuli. Under the same conditions, but with the polarity reversed (I_P is negative and I_S is positive), the drift of the base point is toward point II. This drift continues with each successive pulse until the charge injected in the irreversible region equals the charge imbalance. The point is illustrated in Figure 7 for a pulse waveform satisfying the two above assumptions, but $Q_P = 5 > Q_S = 4$ (Q is given in coulombs per unit area). The base point is initially at 1. The electrode potential V_E moves to point 2 in response to Q_P (5 units on the Q/A axis), and then to point 3 in response to Q_P (4 units back). The base point for the next cycle (point 4) coincides with point 3 (1 unit above point 0 on the Q/A axis). During the time interval 4–5, the Q_P injected yields an electrode potential at point 5. The last portion of charge injected results in an electrode potential that could support irreversible reactions. During the time period 5–6, the Q_S injected is accommodated by the reversible region, and point 6 lies 4 units to the left of the right-hand limit of the reversible region. The next pulse moves 5 units to the right, or 1 unit into the irreversible region (point 8); the following Q_S pulse moves the operating point to 6, 7, 9, 10..., the new base point. All further pulsing moves the operating point between points 6 and 8. The net result is that the charge dissipated in irreversible processes is equal to the charge imbalance between Q_P and Q_S.

When relatively large primary pulses are used, the electrode is forced to operate in the irreversible region even though the charge is balanced. This case is illus-

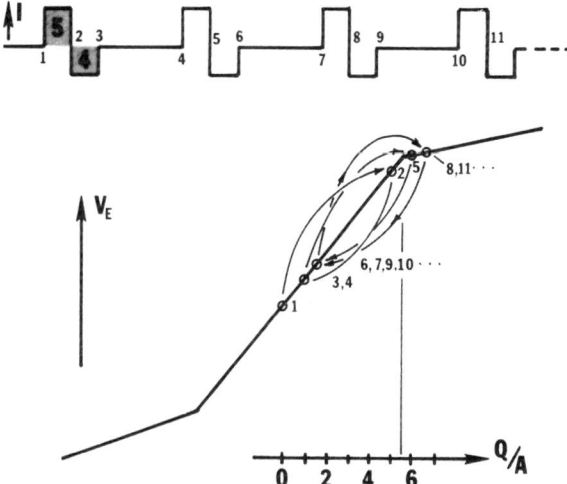

FIG. 7. Electrode-potential behavior for biphasic stimulation under conditions of charge imbalance. In case illustrated, anodic charge injected per unit area in primary pulse is 1 unit greater than that injected during secondary cathodic pulse. Numbers appearing on current waveform correspond to numbers appearing on plot of V_E vs. Q/A.

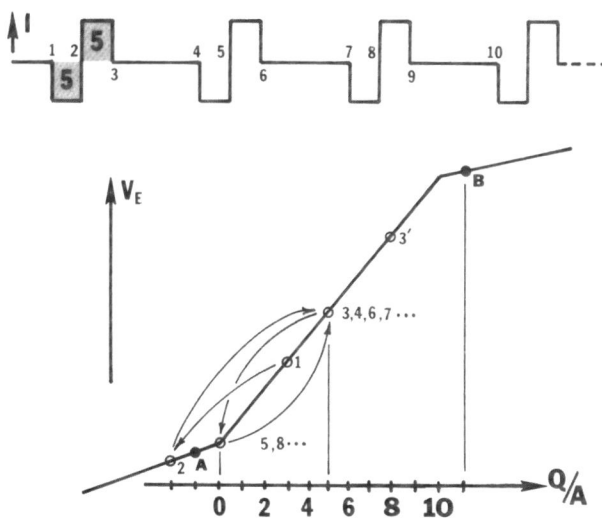

FIG. 8. Electrode-potential variation for relatively large stimulus pulses under balanced charge conditions. See text for details.

trated in Figure 8 for a cathodic primary pulse (typical of many practical systems). The initial base point is labeled 1. The first primary pulse drives the electrode potential into the irreversible region, beginning at the left-hand limit. Therefore at time 3 the operating point is at point 3, which is 5 units to the right of the left-hand limit of the reversible region. The second primary pulse, also of 5 units, is handled entirely in the reversible region and moves the operating point to point 5. Each succeeding pulse moves the operating point between points 3 (base point) and 5. Increasing the charge density by 3 units (to 8 units) results in a further positive shift in the base point to point 3′, but there is no change in the maximum negative excursion of the operating point (under steady-state conditions). In this example, when Q_P equals 10 units, the operating point moves between the two limits of the reversible region in steady state. A further increase in charge forces the maximum excursion of the operating point into the irreversible regions of both I and II. For example, when Q_P and Q_S equal 11 units each, the limits of the operating point are A and B. At either of these points the potentially damaging reactions of Equations 1–7 may occur. When the electrode is stainless steel, it corrodes during the anodic cycle and its usefulness as an electrode is eventually lost.

EXPERIMENTAL NOTE. With 316 stainless steel and balanced biphasic current stimulation, it has been found that at 50 Hz, 20 mA, and 10 mm^2 of surface area, pulse widths less than 200 μs do not result in corrosion. At pulse widths greater than 400 μs, electrode corrosion is frequently observed. These results indicate that the width of the reversible region is between 0.4 and 0.8 μC/mm^2.

IMBALANCED BIPHASIC STIMULATION. To avoid operating in the irreversible anodic region, one can limit the magnitude of the anodic phase so that it does not exceed the capacity of the reversible region. For instance, in Figure 8, the maximum allowed charge density during the anodic phase is 10 units. Therefore, for an 11-unit cathodic pulse and a 10-unit anodic pulse, the limits of the operating point are point A during the cathodic cycle and the right-hand edge of the reversible region during the anodic cycle. The imbalance of the charge in the two phases has been discussed by McHardy et al. (43) as a means of avoiding corrosion when stainless steel electrodes are used. Note that if the imbalance favors the anodic pulse, then the limits of the operating point become B and the left-hand edge of the reversible region.

EXPANDING CAPACITIVE REGION. An alternative method of expanding the "safe" region of the electrode is to coat the surface of the metal with a nonconducting film, thus forming a true capacitive region. In 1974 Guyton and Hambrecht (29) reviewed earlier attempts to design the "capacitor electrode." The major problem encountered was achieving adequate charge storage, in an acceptable electrode volume, to stimulate excitable tissue. This problem was overcome by using anodized sintered tantalum (29). The sintering process yields a real surface area 10–100 times larger than the geometrical area of the electrode. A tantalum pentoxide film is formed by passing an anodic current through the electrode in an oxygen-containing electrolyte solution. The thickness of the film is controlled by the so-called anodizing voltage. Advantages of this electrode are that the electrode film is self-healing under in vivo anodic conditions, and that under proper operating conditions the surface reactions are, electrochemically, totally reversible. The disadvantages are that the sintered material is brittle and cannot be formed into configurations that require bending, and that the system can only be operated in the anodic region ($V_E > 0$) because a cathodic current destroys the insulating film when $V_E < 0$. The latter is a minor limitation, but the brittleness eliminates the use of electrodes at implant sites where flexible materials are required to avoid mechanical damage.

BALANCED BIPHASIC STIMULATOR. Perfect charge balance with two rectangular (positive and negative) pulses is practically impossible. Slight drift to the positive or negative is inevitable. The circuit diagram shown in Figure 9 is a relatively simple way to achieve a balanced-charge waveform at the stimulating electrodes. The switch is an electronic one. The charge injected during the primary pulse is stored on the capacitor C, which is discharged during the interpulse interval. The value of C is chosen as small as possible but must not exceed the power supply capacity of the regulated-current supply. For example, if the maximum supply voltage of the stimulator is V_{max} volts, and Q_{Pmax} is the maximum charge to be injected, then $C > Q_{Pmax}/V_{max}$.

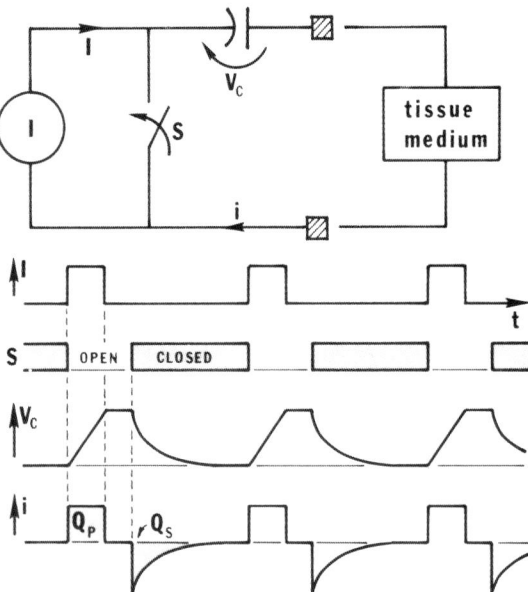

FIG. 9. Schematic diagram for practical balanced-charge biphasic stimulator with timing diagrams. I, stimulator current; S, switch, closed during indicated period; V_C, voltage developed across capacitor C; i, electrode current. Circuit operation is described in text.

Summary

The process of effecting an electrical field in an ionic medium requires a transformation in the charge carrier at the metal-tissue interface. In the metal, charge is carried by electrons, whereas in the tissue medium, charge is carried by ions. The transformation at the metal-tissue interface may be reversible or irreversible, depending on the electrode potential. The safest transformation process in terms of tissue injury appears to involve the reactions in the reversible region. The broader this region, the more charge can be transformed reversibly. In the reversible region the electrode acts as a charge integrator. Therefore to avoid the eventual irreversible processes that are inevitable with monophasic stimulation, the reversible region must be discharged between stimulus pulses. In order to assure operation within the reversible region, the positive and negative charges must be balanced in each cycle or period. A net imbalance forces the transformation process to be irreversible, in the direction of the net imbalance.

TISSUE DAMAGE

A major consideration in designing a system to effect external control over the nervous system by electrical excitation is the avoidance of tissue injury or destruction that results from the stimulus and/or the presence of the electrode. The stimulus may cause damage through the effects of the applied field, heating, and the electrochemical process at the metal-tissue interface. The electrode may cause damage due to the poor biocompatibility of its material, and mechanical damage may result from the physical presence of the electrode.

Electrode Materials

The material chosen for the electrode is critical for the long-term success of a stimulation system. The most important considerations are *1)* passive compatibility of the material with tissue, *2)* storage capacity of the electrode's reversible region, and *3)* the mechanical compatibility of the material with tissue.

PASSIVE PROPERTIES. Implant materials initiate a foreign-body response that usually leads to encapsulation of the foreign body. The more compatible the material, the thinner is the encapsulation layer. As the encapsulation layer thickens, the separation between the excitable tissue and the electrode increases. Thus the electrode moves away from the excitable tissue, and greater stimulus currents (more charge) are required to effect excitation of the neural tissue.

The foreign-body response is a function of both the chemical compatibility (inert surface properties) and the mechanical compatibility of the electrode.

Chemical compatibility. The recommended materials at present are platinum, platinum-iridium (alloy), and 316 stainless steel. Platinum is listed first because more is known about it and because the passive tissue response to it is considered acceptable for use in both the central nervous system and the peripheral motor system. Platinum-iridium alloys are also acceptable but show a greater tendency toward surface erosion when subjected to high pulsing currents (10). Stainless steel (316) is commonly used in surgical implants. It is acceptable for electrode use in the peripheral motor system, but insufficient data are available to recommend it for electrode use in the central nervous system. Other materials under current investigation are pure iridium, pure rhodium, platinum-rhodium alloys, tungsten "bronzes," tantalum-tantalum pentoxide (Ta-Ta$_2$O$_5$), and cobalt-chromium alloys. Much less is known about these materials, and they are less readily available to the investigator than platinum, platinum-iridium, and stainless steel.

Storage capacity of reversible region. In general it is desirable to minimize the physical size of an electrode, thereby limiting its surface area. For the electrode to operate effectively and remain within the safe region, it must have a relatively large reversible region. Its capacity is a function of its real, not geometric, area and the material of which it is made. Roughening the surface, e.g., by sand blasting, can increase the capacity of the electrode by increasing the real area 3–5 times without altering its geometric size.

The relative storage capacity of the materials mentioned above cannot be precisely stated, but there are rough estimates. For platinum, Brummer and McHardy (10) indicate a capacity of 2.1 μC/mm^2. This estimate takes into account the operation of the electrode in a region where electron transfer takes place but is presumed to be totally reversible. Based on the data of Pudenz et al. (63) for blood-brain barrier, the safe region, which is presumed reversible, is 0.30–0.45 μC/mm^2 for platinum in cerebral cortex. At the author's laboratory, 316 stainless steel has a storage capacity of 0.4–0.8 μC/mm^2 (geometric area).

Mechanical compatibility. The foreign-body response observed around metal implants is an encapsulation by fibrous tissue. The fibrous tissue does not physically bond to the metal, and therefore relative motion is possible between the electrode and tissue. This relative motion can induce cell trauma, which in turn leads to further fibrous tissue growth. Morrison (47) found that tissue growth into a porous material acts to mechanically stabilize the material (i.e., substitute for tissue attachment). He also noted that this mechanical stabilization reduces the thickness of the fibrous encapsulation layer, a finding that supports use of the porous tantalum pentoxide electrode (29).

Flexible materials are less likely than stiff materials to cause trauma in body areas where the relative motion can be high. Therefore electrodes and lead wires formed from flexible small-diameter wire (25 μm–200 μm) are most often used. The biggest problem with small wires that undergo repeated bending is that they work-harden and fracture. When the electrode or lead wire fractures, an open electrical circuit results and the electrode is no longer effective. Mechanical strength is thus very important; platinum is weaker in this regard than the steel and the chromium alloys (Table 1).

In order to prolong the time until wire fracture, the wire can be coiled into a helix. A coiled helix is less stiff than a straight wire over the same length. Furthermore the bending of the helix is accommodated by the wire in torsional rotation rather than in transverse bending, which reduces stress on the material. Caldwell and Reswick (13) used this concept to design a very effective electrode for intramuscular use, discussed in subsection *Muscle (Coiled Wire Electrode)*, p. 163.

Stranded wires (many wires twisted together) have

TABLE 1. *Mechanical Properties of Selected Electrode Materials*

Material	Ultimate Tensile Strength in Fully Annealed State		% Elongation
	psi	kN/m^2	
Platinum*	24,000	165,000	55
90% Pt-10% Ir*	45,000	310,000	30
316 Stainless steel*	90,000	620,000	45
HS-25 (Co-Cr-W)†	130,000	900,000	
MP-35 (Co-Cr-Ni-Mo)‡	135,000	930,000	70

Values are given for fully annealed state to allow direct comparison. In actual use, material is in a hardened state and tensile strength is greater. * *ASM Metals Handbook,* vol. 1. † *ASTM Standard Specification #F-90.* ‡ Latobe Steel Co.

also been used as both lead wires and electrodes. The advantage of stranded wires is the redundancy afforded by many wires in physical contact: although some wires may break, the conduction properties of the whole electrode are not lost.

Brain (Surface Electrodes)

PASSIVE IMPLANTS. The tissue reaction in the vicinity of a subdural-epipial electrode can be strongly affected by the surgical implant procedure. If great care is taken it appears that surface electrodes can be placed on the brain with minimal trauma. Gross observation of the implant site has shown a fibrous encapsulation of the electrode (usually an array of three or more electrodes on a silicone rubber carrier). The capsule is thicker on the superficial side than on the side in contact with the brain surface: average outer thickness (including the dura mater) is 400 μm, and average inner thickness is 160 μm (65). If the electrode is not flush with the surface of the carrier (i.e., it protrudes toward the brain), a dimple or depression in the brain surface occurs (23). In both of the above studies no neuronal damage was found beneath the electrode (1, 23).

ACTIVE IMPLANTS. Platinum has been the most commonly used material in brain stimulation studies to date. Systematic studies of the effects of stimulation on brain tissues are few; the most complete are those reported by Pudenz et al. (63, 64). Damage was assessed in these studies by breakdown of the blood-brain barrier and by light microscopy. Ultrastructural changes were reported in a few of the studies by Agnew et al. (1). This group found direct coupled monophasic stimulation far more injurious than biphasic stimulation. Only with the lowest value tested (0.3 μC/mm^2) was biphasic stimulation found safe, as judged by the absence of the breakdown of blood-brain barrier and by light microscopy.

Tantalum pentoxide electrodes, proposed by Guyton and Hambrecht (29, 30), can be operated in a region where all pulsed charge is accommodated by completely reversible reactions. Initial in vivo results showed no significant changes in threshold for motor response except an apparent increase in pore resistance, attributed to tissue ingrowth. A more complete test of the porous electrode has been reported by Bernstein et al. (4). These authors state that under their test conditions Ta-Ta$_2$O$_5$ "was one of the best materials thus far tested for chronic long-term stimulation of the central nervous system." Their tests lasted approximately 1 mo and involved a total of 40 h of stimulation at 3 mA, 250 μs (primary pulse width), and 50 Hz. The electrodes had a geometric area of 0.8 mm^2 and a real area of 8.0 mm^2. These parameters reduced to 0.75 μC/phase, 0.935 μC/geometric mm^2 phase, and 0.00935 μC/real mm^2 phase.

A comparison of the results obtained with Ta$_2$O$_5$ to those obtained with platinum yields a very encouraging picture for the porous-capacitive electrode. The tissue response appears, at least for 1 mo, to be acceptable, and the charge handling capacity of the Ta$_2$O$_5$ electrode is at least three times greater (on a geometric-area basis) than that of the platinum electrode.

Nerve (Cuff Electrode)

Systematic studies of the effects of stimulus current on peripheral nerves have not been performed to date. However, data are available supporting the safe use of cuff electrodes in patients for many years (25). The information available (25, 31, 80) suggests that the major source of injury is mechanical trauma resulting from the method of application and fixation, rather than trauma induced by the stimulus current. Mechanical trauma can be reduced by the inclusion of connective tissue with the nerve; placing the nerve in direct contact with a close-fitting cuff should be avoided.

Muscle (Coiled Wire Electrode)

Implanting the stimulating electrode directly into a muscle avoids possible injury to the peripheral nerve and provides a degree of selective muscle excitation not possible with peripheral nerve excitation. The implantation of a metal conductor in a muscle places more emphasis on metal strength and mechanical durability than in the cases of the surface and cuff electrodes. Large excursions in the muscle can result in the electrode bending through 180°. A straight wire fractures within a few days when subjected to repeated bending; however, a coiled wire electrode, such as that described by Caldwell and Reswick (13), functions for many months without failure.

The coiled wire electrode is fabricated by winding single or stranded wire around a mandril, usually 100 μm in diameter. The resulting helix can be loaded into a hypodermic needle, leaving a small barb outside the canula (Fig. 10). Electrode implantation is accomplished by driving the tip of the needle into the muscle to the desired position; withdrawal of the needle leaves behind the coiled wire electrode. Implantation of these electrodes through the skin has a very definite experimental advantage because it permits many experiments on humans that would not be feasible if a surgical procedure were required.

The small coiled wire electrode and the electrode exit site from the skin must be protected from mechanical abuse. We have found that a cover over the electrode exit site provides adequate shielding from outside contact and also provides a stable connector for the large electrical wires leading to the stimulator. The electrodes, covered by the protector cap, can remain through the skin for over a year without infection. Tissue appears to grow into the coils and provide sufficient mechanical stability to eliminate wire motion at the exit site. Cultures taken from electrode segments below the skin have been consistently negative. Infection has not been a problem in any of the over 1,000 implants we have performed to date.

PASSIVE IMPLANTS. Passive implantation of the coiled wire electrode into normal muscle results in a mild foreign-body response that should have no detectable effect on muscle performance. A typical reaction site is shown in Figure 11, where the electrode is encapsulated with fibrous tissue. Capsule thickness varies with the size of the electrode. For a 200-μm coil formed from 45-μm 316 stainless steel, the thickness of the capsule ranges from 50 to 300 μm, with a mean around 100 μm. For a 1,000-μm coil formed from a stranded wire (10 wires, each 25 μm in diameter in a teflon tube), the capsule thickness varies from 100 to 500 μm, with a mean around 300 μm.

ACTIVE IMPLANTS. *Monophasic stimulation.* The results we have obtained from tissue stimulated with monophasic current pulses indicates that some irreversible electrochemical reactions in the cathodic directions can be tolerated. Figure 12 shows the area occupied by damaged muscle cells as a function of the stimulus parameters. At monophasic charge densities less than or equal to 0.2 μC/mm^2 per pulse, the tissue reaction in the area of the electrode was indistinguishable from that of the control tissue. However, at charge densities greater than or equal to 1.0 μC/mm^2, we found large areas of necrotic muscle tissue. Microscopic observation of the damaged areas consistently showed damaged blood vessels, suggesting that primary damage was to the vessels, and that muscle-tissue damage was secondary to the vascular damage.

The most probable electrochemical reaction in the cathodic direction results in hydrogen formation and an increase in local pH. Because the charge in each pulse is accommodated by irreversible reactions and the lower charge densities were tolerated whereas the upper were not, we concluded that the charge injected per unit time (OH$^-$ generation) was a critical factor in determining muscle-tissue damage. Time rate of charge injection is, by definition, current, and blood is a reasonably good buffer. Therefore, in a normally perfused muscle, hydroxyl ion–generation rates corresponding to 10 μA/mm^2 or less appear to be adequately buffered. The application of direct current (not pulsed) to the muscle and pulsed currents at frequencies and charge densities at and above 10 μA/mm^2 has confirmed this conclusion.

Balanced-charge biphasic stimulation. Tissue damaged because of the application of a balanced-charge biphasic pulse was statistically indistinguishable from control tissue over the entire region evaluated (0.1–2.0 μC/mm^2, charge density of primary pulse; Fig. 12). In a few experiments, however, we did observe electrode corrosion at charge densities equal to or greater than 1.0 μC/mm^2. As discussed in subsection EXPERIMENTAL NOTE, p. 160, the corrosion potential may be reached (during the anodic secondary pulse) at primary pulse charge densities as low as 0.4 μC/mm^2.

The maximum charge density during the primary pulse may be increased by limiting the charge in the anodic phase to the capacity of the reversible region (see section IMBALANCED BIPHASIC STIMULATION, p. 159). The maximum acceptable imbalance is determined by the buffering capacity of the perfused muscle. One can predict from existing data that minimal tissue damage occurs when a charge density of 0.6 μC/mm^2 is injected during the primary (cathodic) pulse phase and a charge density of 0.4 μC/mm^2 is applied during the secondary (anodic) pulse phase using a

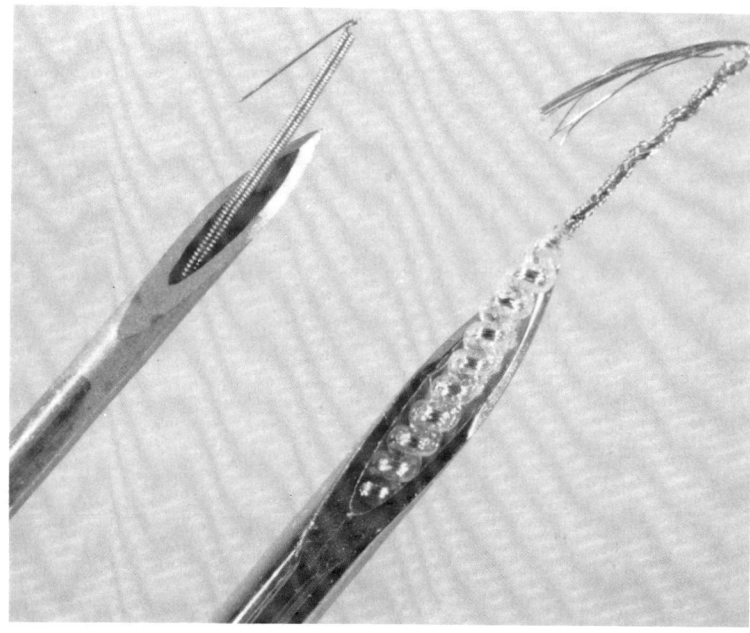

FIG. 10. Coiled wire stimulating electrode. *Right*: electrode formed from stranded wire loaded in 19-gauge hypodermic needle. *Left*: electrode formed from insulated stainless steel wire (45-μm diam) loaded in 23-gauge hypodermic needle. Light-colored areas of coil are deinsulated. These electrodes are similar to those described by Caldwell and Reswick (13).

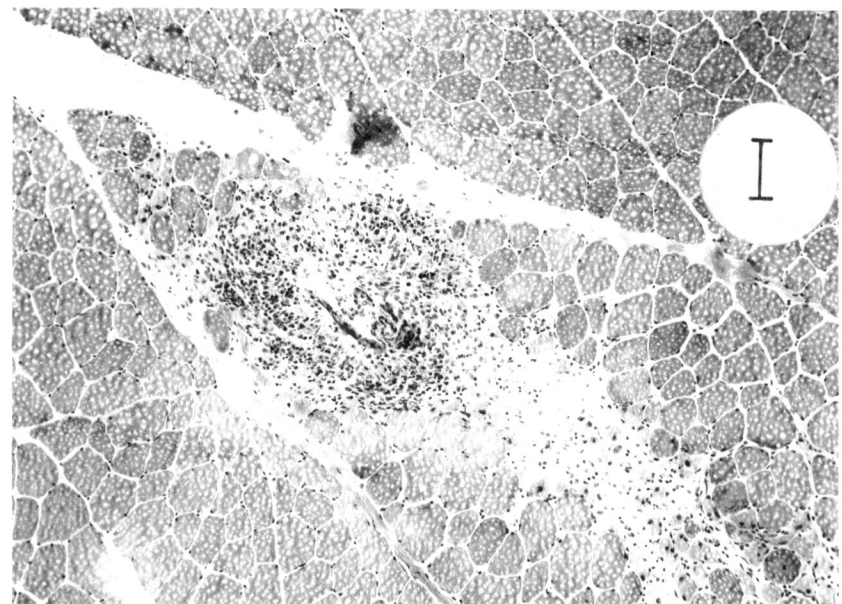

FIG. 11. Typical muscle-tissue reaction to passive implant of single-strand coiled wire electrode. Section was taken from cat triceps brachii muscle 5 days after electrode insertion. Implanted electrode was identical to electrode formed from 45-μm stainless steel wire shown in Figure 10. Section shown is stained with hematoxylin and eosin. *Vertical bar*, 100 μm long. (J. T. Mortimer, D. Kaufman, and U. Roessmann, unpublished data.)

stainless steel electrode operating at 50 Hz. For the coiled wire electrode standardly used (10 mm²), this involves 20 mA and 300 μs for the primary pulse and 20 mA and 200 μs for the secondary pulse. A motor axon within approximately 10–20 mm of the electrode would probably be activated with little difficulty at this magnitude.

Summary

Brain tissue and muscle tissue can be stimulated safely for prolonged periods of time, provided caution is taken when choosing the stimulus parameters and electrode material. Balanced-charge biphasic stimulation is required for brain stimulation. Brain stimulation with platinum electrodes should not exceed charge densities of 0.3 μC/mm² during the primary pulse. Preliminary investigations with the Ta-Ta₂O₅ capacitor electrodes suggest that charge densities greater than 0.3 μC/mm² (geometric area) may be safely injected into brain tissue with these electrodes. Note that this assumes a real area 100 times greater than the geometric area.

Healthy muscle tissue can tolerate monophasic stimulation, provided the average current density over a cycle does not exceed 10 μA/mm²; however, biphasic stimulation is recommended. With balanced-charge biphasic stimulation, the corrosion limits are reached when the charge density reaches 0.4 μC/mm² per phase. An imbalance of charge may extend the magnitude of the primary pulse. (To avoid corrosion, the secondary pulse cannot exceed the above limit.) To avoid tissue damage, however, the net imbalance must not exceed a net average cathodic current of 10 μA/mm².

NERVE EXCITATION

The excitability of neural tissue is dependent on the physical properties of the membrane, position of the tissue relative to stimulating electrodes, and the elec-

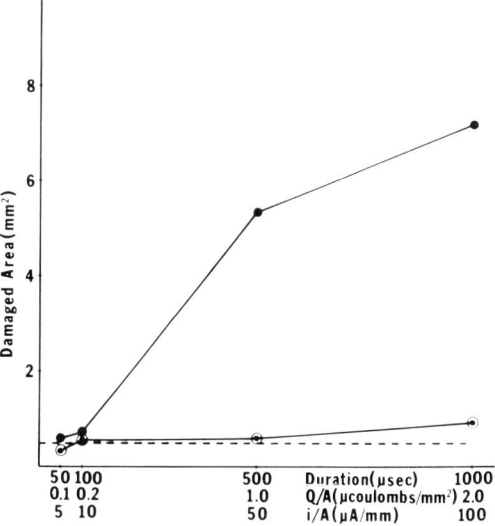

FIG. 12. Tissue reaction to active implant as function of stimulus parameters. *Closed circles* represent data taken from muscle stimulated with monophasic current pulses. Open circles indicate data based on balanced-charge biphasic stimulation. Tissue reaction is measured in terms of area occupied by abnormally staining tissue (damaged area). *Dotted line* indicates average reaction area for passive coiled wire electrode implant of single-strand type. Stimulus amplitude was fixed at 20 mA and frequency was 50 Hz for all tests. Horizontal axis is given in units of pulse duration, charge density in the primary pulse, and average current density (for monophasic stimulation). (J. T. Mortimer, D. Kaufman, and U. Roessmann, unpublished data.)

trical parameters of the stimulus. (Excitability is the relative ease with which one can effect a conducted action potential. It has the units of the electrical parameters and is the reciprocal of the threshold (e.g., high excitability–low threshold.) Through this dependency the possibilities for selective excitation of specific structures without concomitant excitation of neighboring tissues are expanded (for discussion, see ref. 21).

Membrane Response to Applied Electrical Field

FIRST-ORDER MEMBRANE MODEL. A first-order approximation of an axon is shown by the ladder network in Figure 13. Pulsed current (positive charge) is injected into the membrane at the anode and returns to the source through the cathode. The membrane response under the anode (left-hand side) and the cathode (right-hand side) is shown as a function of time and increasing current in the lower portion of Figure 13. The resting potential is lower on the inside than on the outside of the membrane (i.e., the outside is positive with respect to the inside). Positive charge injected through the node beneath the anode increases the potential difference between the inside and outside for all stimulus amplitudes. At the cathode, current flows in the opposite direction, and the potential difference between the inside and the outside of the axon decreases. For a subthreshold current I_1, the membrane is only slightly depolarized, and no propagated action is initiated. Increasing the current to threshold (I_2) results in a self-propagating depolarization that

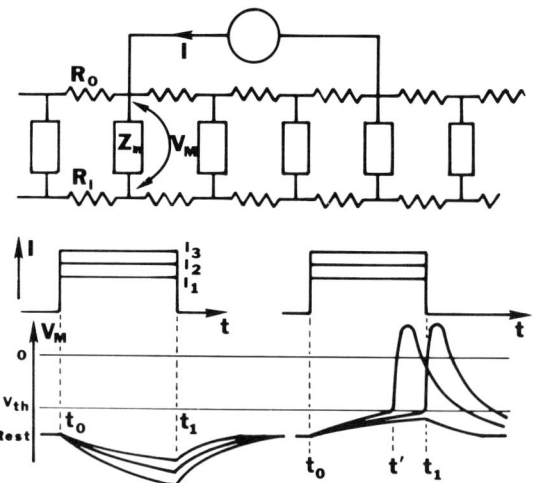

FIG. 13. Ladder-network model for nerve-fiber excitation. In upper part of figure is axon model; R_O is extracellular internodal impedance, Z_M is transmembrane impedance, and R_I is the intracellular internodal impedance. V_M is transmembrane potential; under conditions of rest, inside is negative relative to outside. Membrane response to 3 current pulses of different magnitude (I_1, I_2, and I_3), at anode in lower left and at cathode in lower right. See text for details.

reverses the membrane potential temporarily. This response, the so-called all-or-none response or action potential, is capable of producing a depolarizing current in adjacent nodes, thus propagating the injected response along the axon to termination. Once initiated this propagated response is indistinguishable from the naturally occurring action potential.

PULSE AMPLITUDE–PULSE DURATION RELATIONSHIP. Increasing the current amplitude (see Fig. 13) beyond the threshold value to I_3 results in an earlier activation. At time $t' < t_1$, threshold has been reached, and the membrane is capable of sustaining the depolarization. Therefore all charge passed between t' and t_1 is of no consequence, and for membrane depolarization purposes the excitation pulse could have been terminated at t'. Alternately the threshold at t' is I_3, where $t' < t_1$ and $I_3 > I_2$. The relationship between threshold current (linearly related to the applied electrical field) and pulse duration is the well-known strength-duration curve exhibited by excitable membrane. The experimentally derived amplitude-duration relationship is quite well fitted to the mathematical equation

$$I_{th} = \frac{I_R}{1 - e^{-Kt}} \quad (8)$$

where I_{th} is the threshold current, t is the pulse duration, I_R is the rheobase current, and K is a constant, characteristic of the particular membrane. The rheobase current is the theoretical current required for a pulse of infinite duration. In practice it is difficult to measure because the membrane tends to accommodate to the applied electrical field for long-duration pulses. Furthermore I_R is sensitive to the separation between the excited membrane and the electrode (a parameter usually not known). For these reasons a second term, chronaxie, is frequently used. Chronaxie is defined as the pulse duration for a threshold pulse twice the magnitude of the rheobase current. Chronaxie times are tissue dependent; for instance, a value less than 10 ms is characteristic of motor nerves, and a value greater than 10 ms is characteristic of muscle tissue.

PULSE CHARGE–PULSE DURATION RELATIONSHIP. In the previous sections the importance of minimizing charge injection during stimulation was emphasized. The relationship between injected charge and threshold can be obtained from Equation 8. The charge injected during depolarization with a rectangular current pulse is the product of the stimulus amplitude and pulse duration. Therefore

$$Q_{th} = I_{th}t = \frac{I_R t}{1 - e^{-Kt}} \quad (9)$$

As the pulse duration t becomes very large, the threshold charge approaches the asymptote

$$Q_{th} = I_R t \quad (10)$$

As the pulse duration approaches zero, the exponential term can be replaced by the approximation

$$e^{-Kt} = 1 - Kt \quad (11)$$

This substitution yields

$$Q_{th} \to Q_{min} = \frac{I_R}{K} \text{ as } t \to 0 \quad (12)$$

This is the theoretical minimum charge required to excite the tissue.

Insight into the practical significance of Equation 9 can be gained by normalizing it to the minimum value (Eq. 12)

$$\frac{Q_{th}}{Q_{min}} = \frac{Kt}{1 - e^{-Kt}} \quad (13)$$

Solving Equation 8 for K when the threshold current is at $2I_R$ and the pulse width is at the chronaxie t_c yields

$$K = \frac{1}{t_c} \ln 2 \quad (14)$$

Substituting Equation 14 into Equation 13 yields

$$\frac{Q_{th}}{Q_{min}} = \frac{\dfrac{t}{t_c} \ln 2}{1 - \dfrac{1}{2^{t/t_c}}} \quad (15)$$

Subtracting 1 from both sides of Equation 15 and multiplying both sides by 100 yields the percent charge injected over the absolute theoretical minimum

$$\% \text{ extra charge} = \frac{\dfrac{t}{t_c} \ln 2}{1 - \dfrac{1}{2^{t/t_c}}} - 1 \times 100 \quad (16)$$

Equation 16 is plotted as a function of the normalized pulse duration in Figure 14. This plot suggests that one must inject approximately 38% more charge at chronaxie than is absolutely necessary and that the excess charge may be reduced to 18% by halving the pulse duration of the stimulus. Note that as one seeks to minimize the amplitude of the current pulse (t/t_c becomes large as $I_{th} \to I_R$), the excess charge increases very rapidly. Therefore in an effort to minimize charge injection at the electrode-tissue interface, narrow (short-duration) pulse widths are recommended. These results have been confirmed (44) using the Frankenhaeuser-Huxley model (22); they have been corroborated experimentally in motor axon excitation (15).

EFFECT OF SECONDARY PULSE. To utilize the reversible region of the metal-tissue interface, the charging effect

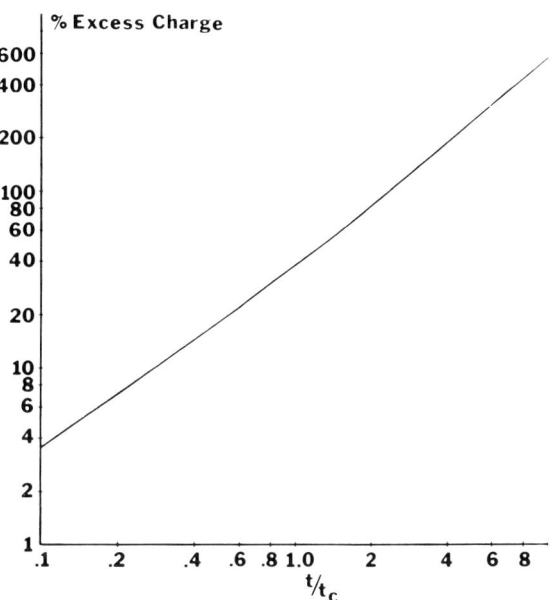

FIG. 14. Charge injected to reach membrane threshold in excess of theoretical minimum as function of pulse duration. Pulse duration (t) has been normalized to the chronaxie value (t_c).

of the primary stimulus pulse must be reversed by the addition of a secondary current pulse. Experimentally we have found that the introduction of the secondary pulse (e.g., opposite polarity) immediately following the primary pulse decreases the evoked response achieved with only the primary pulse (monophasic stimulation).

Experiments conducted on single-fiber myelinated axons revealed a "vulnerable period" following the lagging edge of the stimulus. At short pulse widths the membrane potential (at threshold) transiently increased (returning toward resting levels) before decreasing again to complete depolarization (Fig. 15A). Introducing the secondary pulse immediately after the primary pulse extinguished the regenerative depolarization process and canceled the effects of the primary (depolarization) pulse (76). Figure 15B shows the effect of increasing the magnitude of the secondary pulse when the primary pulse amplitude is slightly over threshold. Note that the area under the secondary pulse is much less than that of the primary pulse.

The problem of extinguishing the depolarization process was eliminated by introducing a delay between the lagging edge of the primary pulse and the leading edge of the secondary pulse. The effect of increasing the delay between the two pulses is shown in Figure 15C.

In a practical system one does not drive all neurons at threshold or suprathreshold values. The neural tissue close to the electrode is often at suprathreshold, whereas tissue farther away is always at threshold. To illustrate the effect of the delay between pulses, the experiment documented in Figure 16 was conducted with intramuscular electrodes on cat tibialis anterior muscle. The magnitude and duration of the secondary pulse were insufficient to effect any measurable twitch force. The results of this experiment suggest a practical value for the delay between the two pulses. At a 100-μs delay, only 10% of the monophasic force was lost. The addition of the 100-μs delay between pulses is not expected to have any significant effect on the electrochemical reactions that would occur without the delay. The 100-μs value also corresponds to the experimentally derived value obtained by Lilly (40) when he proposed the balanced pulse-pair waveform as the safest and most effective stimulus.

An alternative method of reducing unwanted repolarization is to decrease the amplitude of the secondary pulse. By employing the circuit shown earlier in Figure 9 and varying the value of the capacitor, one can suppress the neural effects of the secondary pulse. Figure 17 shows the effect of the peak amplitude of the secondary pulse on evoked twitch. (Increasing the value of the capacitor lowers the peak anodal current and increases the time constant.)

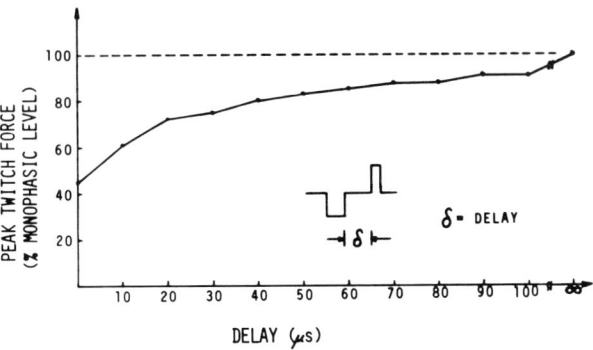

FIG. 16. Reduction in evoked muscle force resulting from effects of secondary stimulus pulse. Force is shown as function of increasing delay between end of primary pulse and onset of secondary pulse. Secondary pulse in this experiment was insufficient to effect a measurable force. [From van den Honert and Mortimer (76).]

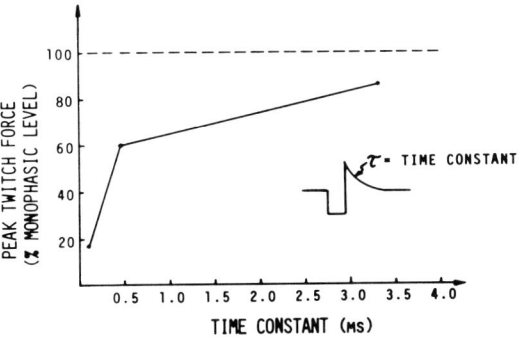

FIG. 17. Effect of altering amplitude of secondary pulse on evoked muscle force. Circuit used to generate balanced-charge biphasic waveform is shown in Figure 9. See text for explanation. [From van den Honert and Mortimer (76).]

Excitation of Myelinated Nerve

Employing the Frankenhaeuser-Huxley equations (22) to model the nodal (transmembrane) current, McNeal (44) analyzed the response of myelinated nerve to monophasic stimuli. A myelinated axon was placed in an infinite, isotropic medium; the point source electrode was 1 mm from the center node. The material presented in the following sections was derived from a McNeal-type model. It gives the reader insight into threshold dependence of a nerve on axon diameter and position with respect to the electrode.[1]

THRESHOLD DEPENDENCE ON FIBER DIAMETER. The strength-duration curves for four fiber diameters are plotted in Figure 18A. The center node of each fiber is located 1 mm from the point source electrode. Note here the rate at which the curves diverge (the amplitude difference between curves increases as the pulse duration decreases). This divergence is shown more clearly in Figure 18B, in which the current threshold

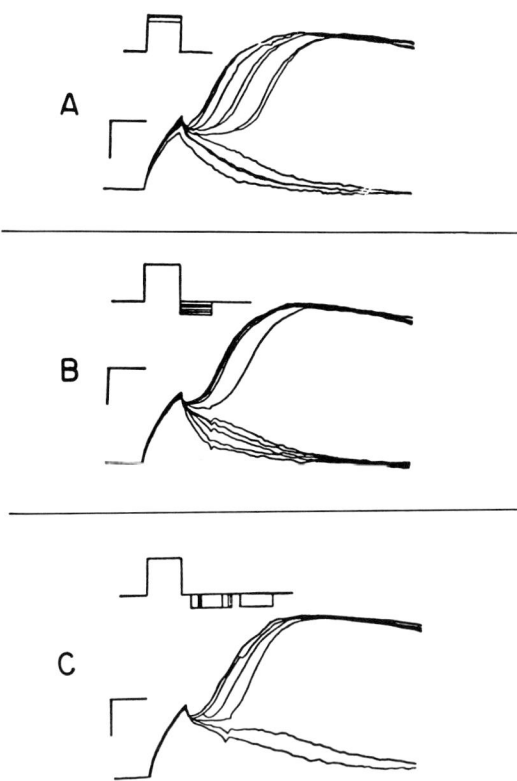

FIG. 15. Transmembrane voltage response of myelinated nerve to short pulse stimuli. A: effect of increasing primary pulse amplitude. B: effect of increasing secondary pulse amplitude. C: transmembrane voltage response of myelinated nerve to increasing delay between primary and secondary pulses. Vertical calibration bar is 20 mV, and horizontal bars are 50 μs. [From van den Honert and Mortimer (76).]

---

[1] I am indebted to Christopher Van Den Honert for his assistance in performing these calculations.

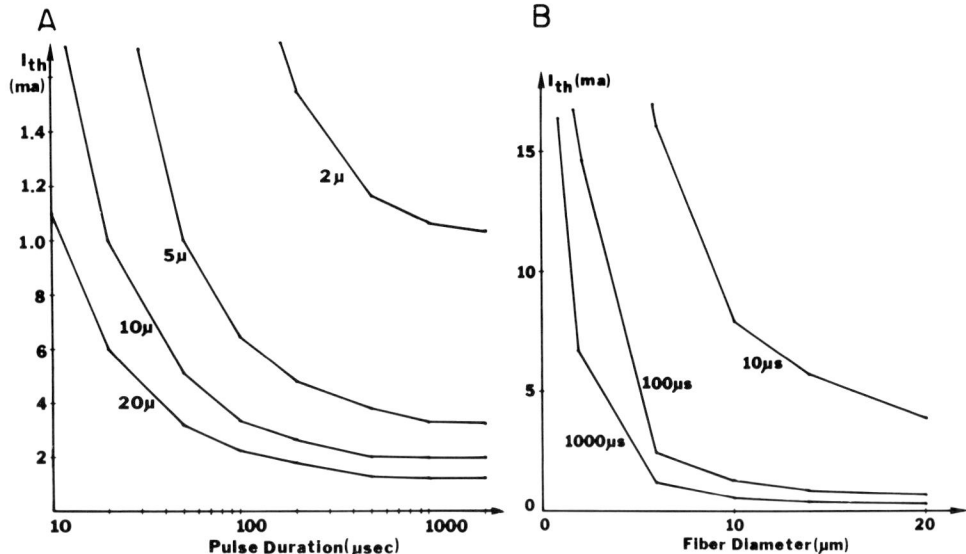

FIG. 18. Relationship among stimulus amplitude, pulse width, and fiber diameter derived from Frankenhaeuser-Huxley equations of myelinated axon. A: strength-duration curves for nerve fibers with diameters ranging from 2 μm to 20 μm. B: stimulus threshold as function of nerve diameter and stimulus pulse width. [Curves were generated in our laboratory using mathematical model described by McNeal (44).]

has been plotted as a function of fiber diameter. The three curves shown are for three separate pulse durations (10 μs, 100 μs, and 1,000 μs). At long pulse durations (1,000 μs), the threshold differences between fibers of varying diameters (particularly at the large axon end) are very little. However, as the pulse duration is decreased, the threshold separation becomes more pronounced. This indicates that one may achieve a greater degree of selectivity with shorter pulse widths (excitation of large fibers without excitation of small fibers in the same physical space). This is particularly useful when motor nerves are physically accompanied by sensory nerves and one wishes to excite the motor nerves without evoking an uncomfortable sensation.

THRESHOLD DEPENDENCE ON AXON-ELECTRODE SEPARATION. Holding the pulse width fixed and calculating the threshold-diameter relationship for varying separation distances between the axon and electrodes yields the plots shown in Figure 19. Increasing the separation between axon and electrodes causes an increased threshold (as seen by the stimulator) and an increased separation between thresholds of axons of different sizes. From these curves one can also gain a sense of relative excitability for different fibers at different physical positions. Take as an example a stimulus current of 5 mA and pulse width 100 μs (Fig. 19, dashed horizontal line). All axons greater than 1.5 μm in diameter and located 1 mm from the electrode are excited. At 2 mm from the electrode all axons greater than 5 μm in diameter are excited, and at 5 mm only axons with diameters greater than 18 μm are excited.

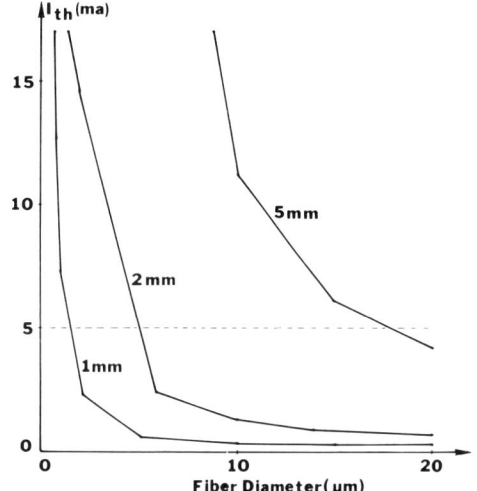

FIG. 19. Effect of increasing separation between electrode and axon on stimulus threshold. In these calculations stimulus pulse width was fixed at 100 μs. [Curves were generated in our laboratory using mathematical model described by McNeal (44).]

Threshold Relationship Between Nerve and Muscle

The electrical excitability of skeletal muscle is substantially lower (higher threshold) than that of motor nerve. The relationship is illustrated in Figure 20. At short pulse durations (< 100 μs), direct muscle excitation requires a much greater stimulus amplitude than indirect muscle excitation (direct excitation of the motor nerve).

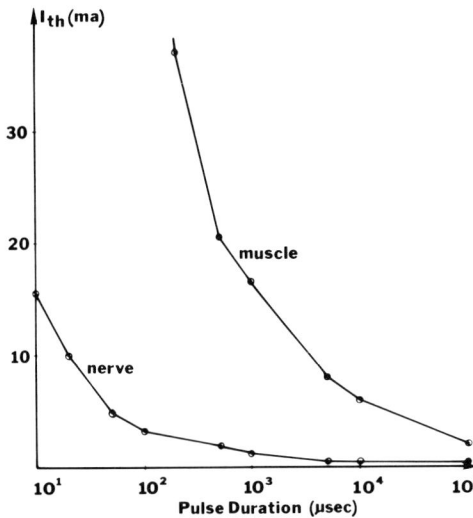

FIG. 20. Strength-duration relationship for nerve excitation (indirect muscle excitation) and direct muscle excitation. During these experiments evoked muscle response was held constant at small fraction of total possible muscle force. Stimulus was delivered through intramuscular electrode before and after administration of curare. (Data are representative of data collected from many experiments in our laboratory and are, in principle, identical to type of curves classically presented for innervated and denervated muscle.)

Effects of Electrode Configuration on Threshold and Excitation Site

The site at which critical (threshold) depolarization of the membrane occurs can be modified or controlled by the electrode configuration. For the model depicted in Figure 13, critical depolarization is first reached at the node closest to the cathode where the maximum outward flow of current occurs. Inward current flows in the vicinity of the anode, resulting in membrane hyperpolarization rather than depolarization. However, in some electrode configurations, the point at which excitation occurs may actually be in the vicinity of the anode. Two basic configurations are discussed in this subsection, the cuff electrode and the surface electrode.

CUFF ELECTRODE. *Bipolar configuration.* A bipolar cuff electrode implanted in a conducting medium is approximated by the model in Figure 21A. Positive charge or current flows from the positive electrode (anode) to the negative electrode (cathode) by two basic pathways. Current I_{int} flows only within the electrode and I_{ext} flows through the external conducting medium. The effects of I_{int} are described by the model in Figure 13. However, to accommodate the external current flow, the model must be modified by adding the additional current paths shown in Figure 21B. When current is allowed to flow in the external medium, a portion of the axoplasmic current flows away from the anode, eventually exiting the membrane and returning via the external medium to the cathode. Similarly current may enter the membrane

to the right of the cathode. In the region to the left of the anode, one can speak of an apparent cathode and to the right of the cathode, an apparent anode. Current at the apparent cathode flows in a direction so as to effect membrane depolarization. Current-flow calculations have been carried out in a model containing discrete components that approximate the nerve and tissue medium (37). Results are shown for two electrode spacings in Figure 22. In the case of the closely spaced pair of electrodes, the action potential occurs at the lowest amplitude immediately adjacent to the cathode. However, with the presence of an apparent cathode to the left of the anode, one could eventually reach a stimulus amplitude where depolarization could occur to the left of the anode. The shift in excitation points would show up as a latency change when recording from a position left of the anode. Increasing separation between the two electrodes decreases the difference between the peak current at the real cathode and the apparent cathode. This implies that the current flowing at the apparent cathode increases with increasing electrode separation. Thus in a very long electrode, current flow in the external medium would be favored as the path of least resistance. In such a case one would see only the effects of the apparent cathode.

Monopolar configuration. Making the electrode very long has an effect similar to moving one electrode away from the nerve (indifferent electrode). Thus the transmembrane current distribution along the length of the axon to the left of the electrode is similar to that shown to the left of the anode in Figure 22. Current flow in the nodes to the right mirrors the flow in the nodes to the left. In the monopolar case, current enters the membrane in the hyperpolarization direction and flows to the left and right in the axoplasm. It then exits the membrane at some distance from the electrode. The exit nodes become the virtual cathodes

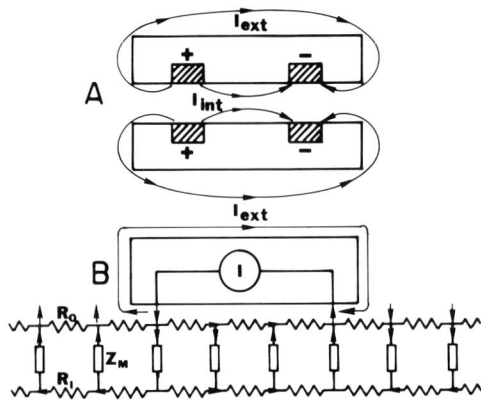

FIG. 21. Bipolar nerve cuff electrode. *A*: electrode in longitudinal section. Nerve courses from right to left through center of electrode; possible stimulus current pathways are indicated by *arrows*. *B*: ladder-network model of system, including current pathways external to electrode cuff. See Figure 13 for details of model. *Arrows* indicate direction of local current flow.

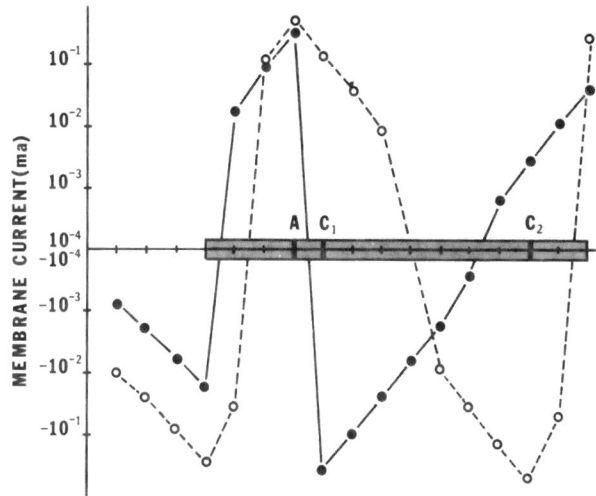

FIG. 22. Transmembrane current distribution for axon in cuff-type electrode. Negative current results in local depolarization of axon. *Shaded region* represents insulator portion of electrode with axon located along horizontal axis of graph. Nodes of Ranvier, for ladder-network model, are located at tic marks along horizontal axis. Node separation in model was 2.5 mm. Anode electrode was located at point indicated by A, and for closely spaced case (2.5 mm), cathode was located at point C_1. Cathode was located at C_2 for 20-mm separation case. *Solid line*, current distribution for case C_1. *Dashed line*, current distribution for case C_2. [Adapted from Karkar (37).]

and the sites for action-potential activation. The magnitude of the transmembrane current flowing at the apparent cathodes is generally less than the magnitude of the current at the real anode because of the diffusion in both directions along the axon. If the polarity of the active electrode were reversed, one would find depolarization under the active electrode, also the region of highest relative current density. Therefore the magnitude of the stimulus would be less for cathodic activation than for anodic excitation (when the axon lies in a plane parallel to the plane of the active electrodes). However, this does not mean that the anodic threshold is always higher than the cathodic threshold, as is shown in subsection SURFACE ELECTRODE, this page.

Tripolar configuration. Current flow in the external medium can be eliminated in the cuff electrode by forcing the potentials on both sides of the active electrode to be identical in value. Placing three electrodes in the cuff and connecting the two outer electrodes eliminates current flow outside the cuff. The field and resulting current flow are shown in Figure 23 for the tripolar electrode. All depolarization current flows in the vicinity of the real cathode, and all hyperpolarizing current flows in the vicinity of the two anodes. This configuration eliminates the possibility of exciting structures (excitable tissue) extraneous to the inside of the cuff electrode.

SURFACE ELECTRODE. When an electrode is placed on the surface of the brain, skin, or muscle, the plane of the electrode surface is frequently perpendicular to the axon. In many such instances the terminal end of the axon, i.e., the end nearest the surface, is a receptor cell body or a structure that is excited less readily than an axon by an electrical stimulus. Marks (42) has calculated the change in transmembrane potential for a simulated descending cortical neuron (see Fig. 24). The interesting aspect of this calculation is that the direction of the change in membrane potential far from the electrode can be opposite that calculated near the electrode. Therefore if the less-excitable terminal lies within a distance r of the electrode, the lowest observed threshold can occur when the polarity of the stimulating electrode is positive (anodic).

Neural Fatigue

Neural fatigue, or loss of electrical excitability, is not expected to be a major problem in the clinical application of electrical stimulation. In most applica-

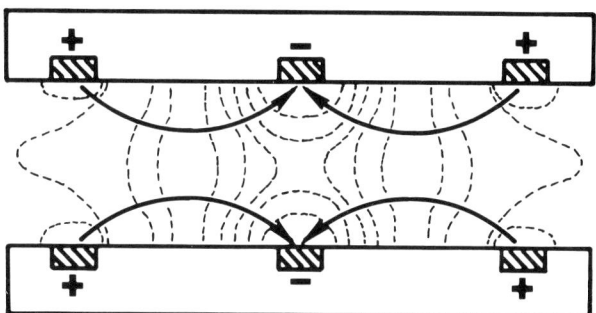

FIG. 23. Electrical field map (*dashed lines*) and resultant current flow (*solid lines*) for tripolar cuff electrode. Electrode shown in longitudinal section. [Adapted from Testerman et al. (75).]

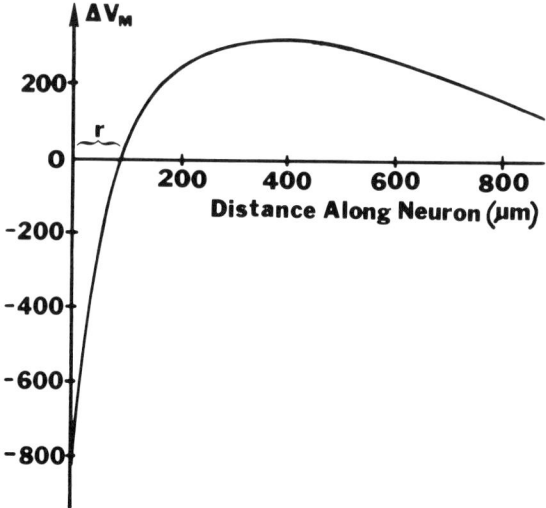

FIG. 24. Transmembrane potential change along nerve cell. Stimulating electrode is located at zero, and indifferent electrode is located a great distance to right. Note that change in transmembrane potential reverses sign at distance r to right of stimulating electrode. [Adapted from Marks (42).]

tions the nerve is not driven for long periods without rest. There is, however, some suggestion that the nerve may fatigue if driven electrically for many hours. Glenn and his colleagues (26) reported that after 12 h of stimulation of the phrenic nerve with unidirectional current, induced ventilation became less effective. They found that alternating the polarity of every-other stimulus pulse greatly extended the time of effective stimulation. The effect of alternating the polarity of every-other stimulus pulse has two effects, both of which are local to the electrode. First, the electrochemical reactions in the vicinity of the electrodes are reversed and second, the site of action-potential initiation is alternated (see *Bipolar configuration*, p. 170). Therefore the fatigue that Glenn et al. observed must have occurred at the site of electrical activation and not at some point along the transmission path distal to the electrode.

Summary

Membrane depolarization occurs when an applied electrical field effects a net outward flow of current (positive-charge flow). When the plane or surface of the electrode(s) is parallel to the axis of the axon, one can expect to find a lower threshold for cathodic excitation than for anodic excitation. If a nonexcitable terminal structure is nearest the electrode, anodic excitation may yield a lower stimulus threshold value. This latter situation is most commonly encountered with surface electrodes, as opposed to cuff-type electrodes.

The injected charge required to effect threshold depolarization in a nerve decreases with decreasing pulse width. The threshold difference between axons of different diameters increases with decreasing pulse width.

In order to avoid the suppressive effects of the secondary pulse, i.e., suppression of the action-potential generation, a delay of approximately 100 µs is recommended between the lagging edge of the primary pulse and the leading edge of the secondary pulse.

ELECTRICAL ACTIVATION OF SKELETAL MUSCLE

Electrical excitation of skeletal muscle may effect externally controlled muscle contraction in patients unable to execute the desired contraction voluntarily. To effect a functional contraction, the muscle must apply the precise force required to move or maintain the limb as desired. The concept of precise control of force and position suggests the use of a feedback-control system. In principle feedback control compensates for any error in the muscle. The study of automated feedback control of muscle is relatively new and future success depends on the development of transducers and control schemes. Although present systems employ visual feedback, for practical purposes they are open-loop systems. Under open-loop conditions, the control problem is simplified when the electrically activated muscle can produce repeated and/or sustained contractions without significant fatigue. The material discussed in this section focuses on what is currently known about muscle fatigue in the electrically activated muscle and techniques that have been developed to minimize the rate of force decay.

Brief Review of Muscle Physiology

A brief review of muscle physiology is offered here for the sake of continuity. (Thorough discussions of this material can be found in this *Handbook* in the chapters by Burke, Henneman and Mendell, and Partridge and Benton.)

MUSCLE-FIBER TYPE. Current convention differentiates muscle fibers into three groups, depending on physiological and metabolic properties. In reality the designated types may only reflect three points or regions of a continuous spectrum of muscle properties. The first group is designated as fast twitch, glycolytic (FG). Burke, in this *Handbook*, refers to this group as FF. These fibers usually appear large in cross section, have a low capacity for oxidative metabolism and a high capacity for glycolytic metabolism, exhibit a twitch contraction of relatively short duration, and under repeated stimulation fatigue rapidly and recover slowly. In mixed muscle this group of fibers is often more heavily distributed in the region of the muscle closest to the skin surface (Fig. 25). In cat gastrocnemius, FG fibers generate a peak force of between 1.5 and 2.0 kg/cm^2 (12).

At the opposite end of the spectrum is the group designated as slow twitch, oxidative (SO). Burke refers to this group as S. These fibers are smaller in cross-sectional area than the FG group and have a high capacity for oxidative metabolism and a low capacity for glycolytic metabolism. The twitch contraction is relatively slow and long in duration and hence exhibits fusion at a relatively low stimulus frequency. Under repeated stimulation these fibers do not fatigue rapidly and are quick to recover from a prolonged contraction. In mixed muscle this group of fibers is often seen in the deeper portions of the muscle. In cat gastrocnemius these fibers generate a peak force of 0.6 kg/cm^2 (12).

The middle group of fibers is designated as fast twitch, oxidative (FO). Burke refers to this group as FR. These fibers have a high capacity for both oxidative and glycolytic metabolism. The contraction time of this group is much faster than that of the SO group but may be slightly slower than that of the FG group. Subjected to repeated stimulation, the force produced by this group is maintained much longer than that of the FG group but decays more rapidly than that in the SO group. Force recovery in this group appears to

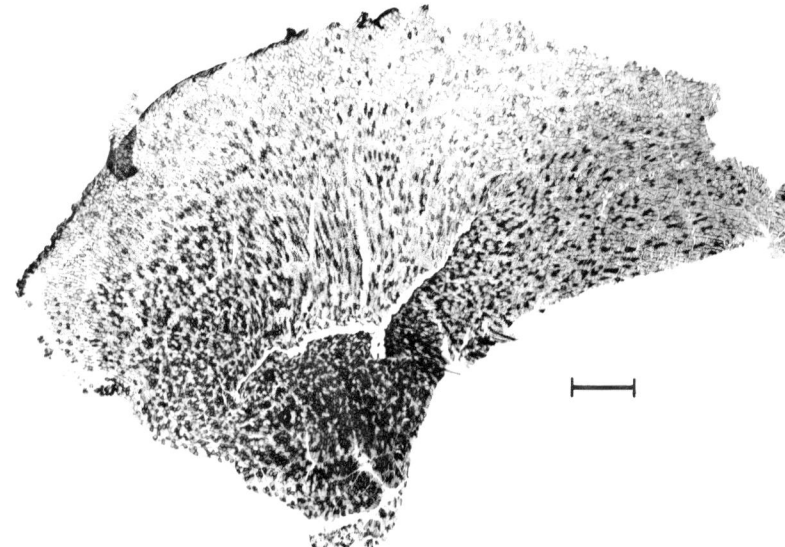

FIG. 25. Cross section of rat tibialis anterior muscle. Fibers have been stained for NAD diaphorase. Dark-staining fibers are classified as oxidative. Superficial portion of muscle is in *upper part* of figure. Calibration, 1 mm. (Compare with Fig. 2 in ref. 51).

be faster than in the FG group. The cross-sectional area of FO fibers is similar to that of SO fibers. In cat gastrocnemius this group develops a force between 2.6 and 2.9 kg/cm^2 (12).

Representative force-time characteristics of these three fiber groups are shown in Figure 26. The force-time characteristics of the FG group are the least desirable for patient-oriented systems under current investigation: current systems generally are required to produce a sustained force output for prolonged or repeated contractions.

MOTOR UNIT PROPERTIES. All muscle fibers innervated by the same axon have been found to be of the same histochemical type (12, 20). The force developed by the FG motor units is greater than that developed by the FO units, which in turn is greater than that developed by the SO units (12, 20). Motor units producing the greatest force are innervated by axons of large diameter, and motor units producing a small force are innervated by axons of small diameter (32). Small motor units are recruited before the large motor units under natural conditions (33). The presumed natural recruitment order for steady-state contraction begins at low forces with the small SO units recruited first and ends at maximal muscle force with recruitment of the large FG motor units (32). The FO fibers are recruited in the midforce range.

Electrical Excitation of Normal Muscle

The force-time characteristics of the electrically excited mixed-fiber muscle are controlled by the fatigue properties of the active fibers, which are those with the lowest relative electrical excitability. The relative electrical excitability depends both on motor-axon diameter (Fig. 18) and axon-electrode geometry (Fig. 19). The latter is the only parameter under the control of the investigator. The excited fibers and the expected force-time relationship are discussed in the following sections for three commonly used stimulation configurations: nerve cuff electrode, surface electrode, and intramuscular electrode.

NERVE CUFF ELECTRODE. The electrical field is approximately uniform within the cuff of an electrode encircling a nerve. Under such conditions the largest motor axons have the lowest electrical threshold. Since the large axons innervate the large motor units, and because the large motor units are commonly FG, the force-time characteristics of the muscle activated with a cuff electrode are, at low stimulus amplitudes, those of the FG motor fibers. At higher amplitudes the force-time characteristics continue to be dominated by the FG fibers if the muscle contains a reasonable FG population.

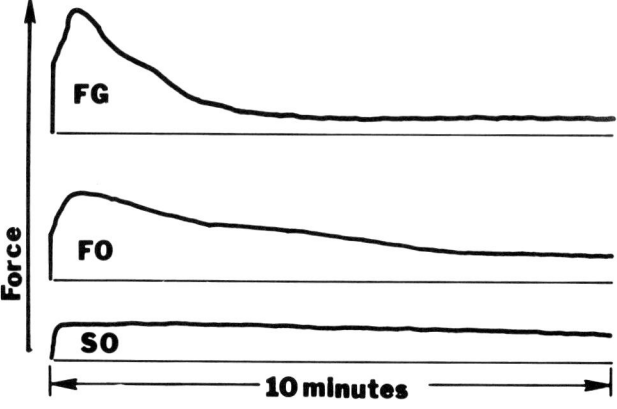

FIG. 26. Fatigue characteristics of 3 motor unit types: FG, fast twitch, glycolytic; FO, fast twitch, oxidative; and SO, slow twitch, oxidative. [Adapted from Edström and Kugelberg (20).]

SURFACE ELECTRODE. Placing the stimulating electrode on the skin over a muscle yields an electrical field that decreases with increasing separation between nerve fiber and electrode. Therefore the electrode current required to reach threshold for superficial fibers is lower than that required for deeper nerve fibers.

The general path of the motor axons is from deep to superficial. Thus one can expect to excite the fast-fatiguing FG fibers before the threshold for the deeper but more fatigue-resistant fibers is reached.

INTRAMUSCULAR ELECTRODE. The electrical field generated by an intramuscular electrode (as in Fig. 10) has roughly circular symmetry, with the axis of symmetry along the axis of the electrode. Figure 27A shows a muscle in cross section; the axis of the electrode is perpendicular to the page. The border of the circular area represents the hypothetical threshold limits. At distances greater than these limits, the intensity of the stimulus field is less than threshold for nerve excitation. All motor nerves within the circular area become active upon stimulation, and these nerve fibers in turn excite their respective muscle fibers (shaded region of Figure 27A). Figure 27B shows a normal muscle excited by an intramuscular electrode. The section was stained for glycogen; the lighter region has been depleted due to repeated activation. The muscle fibers excited include a large number of superficial FG fibers in addition to the fatigue-resistant oxidative fibers deeper in the muscle. This distribution is a consequence of the innervation geometry.

CONCLUSION. Electrical excitation of motor nerve with conventional electrode schemes unavoidably recruits the FG motor fibers. These muscle fibers characteristically fatigue more rapidly than do fibers belonging to the oxidative groups. In terms of a functional patient system, this means that if the force-time profile of the FG population is not adequate to meet the needs of the patient, then a normal muscle that is electrically driven probably will not prove useful.

Muscle Alterations Induced by Electrical Activation

Electrically induced exercise, as well as voluntarily performed exercise, can enhance the ability of the muscle to sustain repeated contraction. In this section the physiological and metabolic changes resulting from electrically induced exercise are discussed.

CHANGES IN CONTRACTILE PROPERTIES. *Contraction time.* Electrically induced exercise has been found to prolong the duration of twitch contraction (58, 62, 69). This increase in contraction time appears to occur even with relatively short periods of exercise (as little as 15 min/day). Figure 28 shows the change in twitch duration in cat tibialis anterior muscle for various periods of exercise induced daily over a 4-wk period. Twitch duration is closely related to the fusion frequency of the muscle: the longer the duration of the twitch, the lower the fusion frequency. Fusion frequency for a normal muscle is about 40 Hz; after 4 wk of 24 h/day, 10-Hz stimulation, it is near 10 Hz (see Fig. 28). In terms of effecting a functional contraction, the decrease in fusion frequency could improve the ability of the muscle to sustain a given force.

Contractile protein changes. Electrophoretic analysis of stimulated mixed-fiber muscles shows a myo-

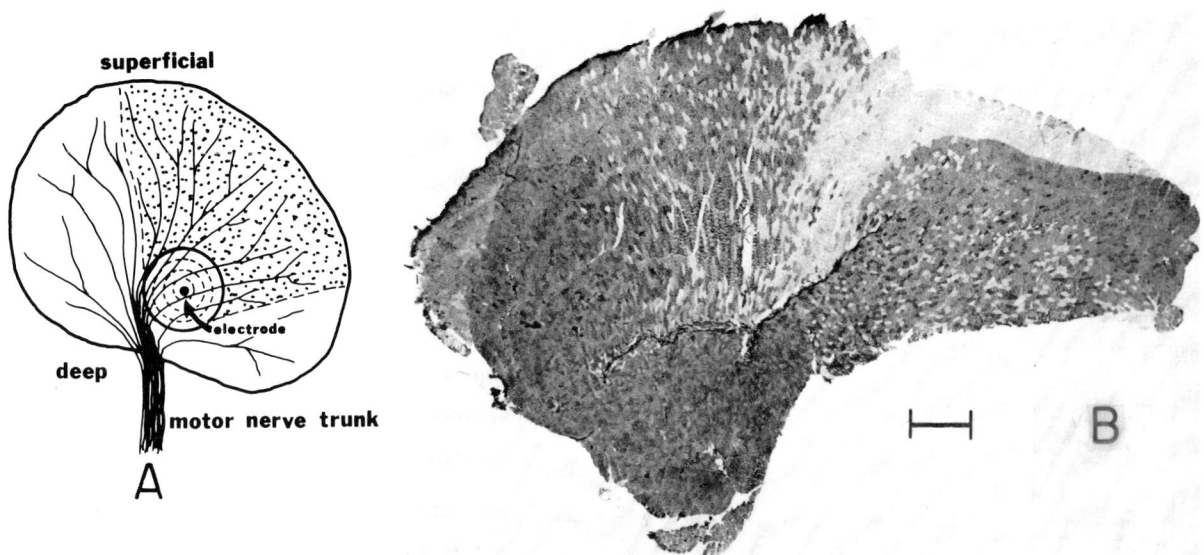

FIG. 27. Cross section of muscle A: innervation pattern and electrode location. *Circular area* around electrode represents region of muscle subjected to threshold or suprathreshold stimulus pulse. *Shaded area* represents region of muscle activated. B: cross section of rat tibialis anterior muscle stained for glycogen (PAS, periodic acid Schiff). Light-staining area has been depleted of glycogen by stimulation at 10 Hz for 10 min. (Compare with ref. 51.) Calibration bar is 1 mm long.

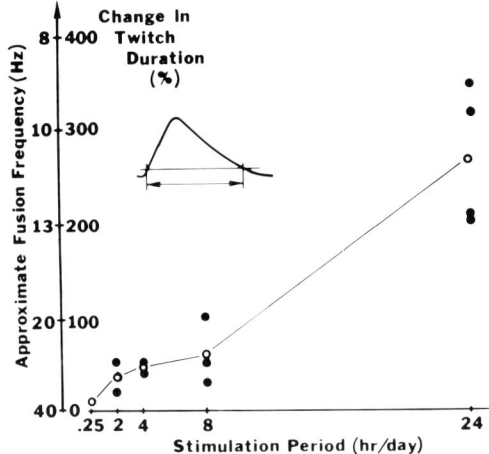

FIG. 28. Changes in duration of twitch contraction as function of daily period of stimulation, measured after 4 wk of stimulation. Assuming fusion frequency in unstimulated control muscle is 40 Hz, new fusion frequency can be estimated by change in twitch duration. (J. T. Mortimer and U. Roessmann, unpublished data.)

fibrillar protein pattern consistent with that in muscle fibers undergoing a transition or conversion from fast twitch to slow twitch (60, 68). The stimulated tibialis anterior muscle shows a decrease in the light-chain, fast-type myosin. The changes were more pronounced with longer periods of stimulation, both in terms of hours per day and total number of days. In one animal stimulated for 56 days (10 Hz, 24/day), the myosin-protein profile for the stimulated tibialis anterior muscle differed only slightly from that seen in the control soleus muscle.

Change in force. In muscles stimulated for 24 h/day, the exercised muscle produces less tetanic force than does the contralateral control muscle (69). For periods of 8 h/day or less, the results are not as clear. Pette et al. (62) reported an increase in twitch force for some rabbit fast muscles stimulated 8 h/day; our results, on the other hand, showed a decrease in muscle force for cat tibialis anterior muscle for both 4 h/day and 8 h/day stimulation periods. The cause and significance of the force decrease are not known. However, evidence strongly suggests that the force decrease is a consequence of a conversion from FG to FO and FO to SO. As mentioned earlier regarding cat gastrocnemius, the FG group produces 1.5–2.0 kg/cm^2, the FO produces 2.6–2.9 kg/cm^2, and the SO yields 0.6 kg/cm^2 (12). In cat tibialis anterior muscle, the FO and SO fibers have the same cross-sectional areas in both the normal muscle and the stimulated muscle. These fibers also have half the cross-sectional area of the FG fibers. The effect of induced exercise, histochemically, is an apparent decrease in FG fibers and a concomitant increase in FO and SO fibers (58, 60–62, 67). Assuming fiber conversion does occur and taking into account the previously mentioned force-production properties of the respective fiber types, one can see that the maximal force generated by the converted muscle can be less, without loss of muscle fibers.

Change in muscle mass. A muscle that has been stimulated for 24 h/day at 10 Hz appears smaller and weighs less than the contralateral control. Muscles stimulated for shorter periods per day also usually weigh less than the controls. The mass change, the fiber-diameter change, and the myosin-protein change are probably associated with, if not part of, the same phenomenon.

METABOLIC CHANGES. *Histochemical changes.* The histochemical changes observed in a muscle subjected to a prolonged period of electrically induced exercise (repeated contraction) are consistent with the idea that a muscle fiber can adapt to the working demands placed on it. There is, in fact, experimental evidence supporting the idea that a fast-twitch, glycolytic fiber can be changed to a fast-twitch, oxidative fiber by repeated electrical activation and that similarly, a fast-twitch, oxidative fiber can be converted to a slow-twitch, oxidative fiber.

Our experiments have shown that when muscle is subjected to daily periods of exercise lasting for 4 wk, the rate at which conversion occurs appears to increase with work demand. A muscle subjected to 10 pulses/s for 15 min/day develops an increased number of oxidative fibers, as evidenced by increased staining intensity (the depth of staining increases as the induced exercise period is increased from 2–4 h/day to 8–24 h/day). In the 24 h/day studies, fibers in the stimulated area show a much higher capacity for oxidative metabolism (darker staining) than do the darkest staining fibers in the unstimulated region (Fig. 29).

On the basis of sections stained for myofibrillar ATPase, it appears that there is no increase in the number of SO fibers when the daily periods of exercise are 4 h or less. At 8 h/day, there may be an increased number of SO fibers. However, there is an obvious increase in SO fibers for daily periods of induced exercise of 24 h/day at 10 Hz (Fig. 29).

In the animals stimulated for 24 h/day in our studies, there was an increase in fat deposits and a decreased staining intensity in sections stained for phosphorylase. Both these changes are consistent with a decreased dependence on glycolytic metabolism and an increased dependence on aerobic metabolism.

Capillary density and changes in blood flow. Microscopic examination of a normally fast-type muscle that has been electrically activated at 10 Hz for 4 wk shows a marked increase in the number of capillaries per fiber. In normal rabbit extensor digitorum longus muscle, the average number of capillaries per muscle fiber ranges from 1.1 to 1.4, and in the stimulated muscle, the average is 2.1 (9).

Measurements of blood flow and oxygen consumption show changes in the stimulated muscle that are consistent with increased capillary density and increased capacity for aerobic metabolism (35). Mea-

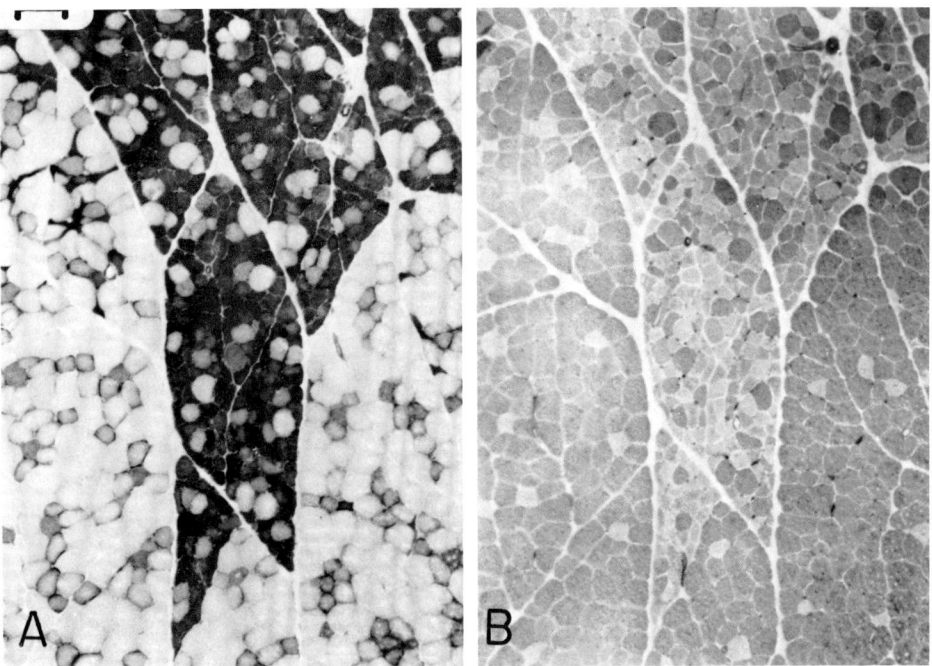

FIG. 29. Histochemical changes seen in electrically stimulated muscle. Muscle had been stimulated at 10 Hz, 24 h/day, for 28 days. *A*: section stained for NADH. *Darker area* is stimulated region. *B*: section stained for myofibrillar ATPase; light-staining fibers are classified as slow twitch, oxidative. Calibration bar is 100 μm long. (J. T. Mortimer and U. Roessmann, unpublished data.)

surements made in rabbit muscle are shown in Figure 30.

TIME COURSE OF CHANGES. In muscles stimulated at 10 Hz, 24 h/day, measurable changes have been found as early as 4 days after the onset of stimulation. The staining patterns for oxidative enzymes (62) and capillary density (9) have both been observed to change in this short period. These changes occur both in continuously and intermittently stimulated muscles. The rate of change in histochemical staining pattern appears to depend on the daily period of induced exercise (60). The changes occur at a greater rate with longer daily periods of induced exercise. Data presently available provide little insight into the ultimate or steady-state pattern for different daily periods of exercise. Changes in muscles that have been stimulated continuously (24 h/day) appear to continue even after 60 days of continuous stimulation (60). These changes indicate increased capacity for aerobic metabolism and decreased capacity for anaerobic metabolism.

Changes in contraction time have been reported as early as 4 days after the onset of stimulation (62). The largest change in contraction time occurs when the changes in contractile protein become apparent [about 3 wk with continuous stimulation; (60)]. With 10-Hz continuous stimulation, the contraction time shows a continuous slowing through the first 3 mo of stimulation [Fig. 31; (52)]. Histochemically a muscle stimu-

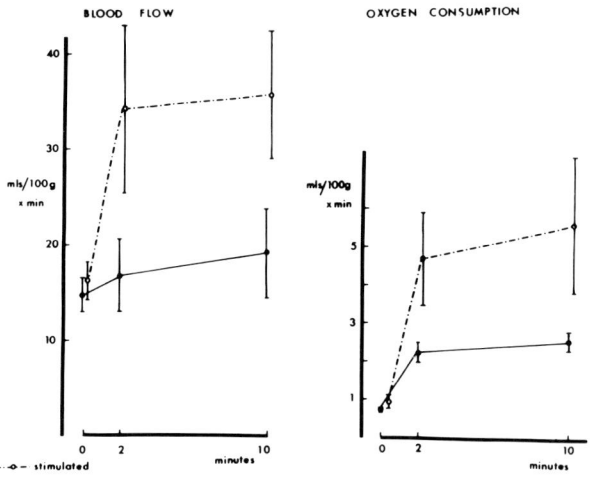

FIG. 30. Blood flow (*left*) and oxygen consumption (*right*) in rabbit muscles stimulated for 28 days (*broken lines*) and in contralateral control muscles (*solid lines*), at rest (time 0) and during a 10-min period of isometric contractions [From Hudlická et al. (35).]

lated for 3 mo, 24 h/day, appears as a muscle dominated by slow-twitch, oxidative fibers.

FATIGUE RESISTANCE. The increased capacity for aerobic metabolism, proliferation of capillaries, and slowing of the twitch contraction improves the ability of the muscle to sustain repeated contraction, often a critical factor for human applications. The rate of improvement increases with longer daily periods of induced exercise, and the degree of improvement becomes greater with an increased number of days of induced exercise (35, 58, 62).

Figure 32 shows the force-time characteristics for a control and a stimulated tibialis anterior muscle of cat. Note the resemblance of the curves to those shown for the FG and SO fibers in Figure 26.

REVERSIBILITY OF CHANGES. Experiments we have performed indicate that a converted muscle returns to its original state if the electrical stimulus is removed. The rate at which it returns to that state appears to be much slower than the rate at which it is altered when subjected to continuous stimulation. In one animal stimulated continuously for 41 days, histochemical evidence of conversion existed 91 days after the electrical stimulus was removed. In another animal stimulated continuously for 30 days, no histochemical evidence was noted of the prior conversion at 173 days after the stimulus was stopped (unpublished observations, J. T. Mortimer and U. Roessmann).

Force Modulation

Force modulation can be accomplished in the electrically activated muscle in much the same manner as it is in the normal muscle, i.e., by increasing the number of active fibers (recruitment) and their rate of firing.

RECRUITMENT. The threshold value for nerve excitation and the spatial separation between the fibers and the electrode make it possible to grade the number of active nerve fibers, either by amplitude modulation (increasing the intensity of the stimulus amplitude and fixing the pulse width) or by pulse-width modulation (fixing the amplitude and extending the pulse width). A plot of force vs. amplitude or pulse width would show a threshold and an irregularly shaped curve. The characteristics of the curve differ for each electrode because the threshold is different for individual nerve fibers and is dependent on the separation between the electrode and the fibers. The irregular shape of the curve is a result of the nonuniform distribution of nerve fiber within a muscle. Considering only the shape of the curves, there is no distinct advantage of one method of modulation over the other. Pulse-width modulation is superior, however, both in terms of minimizing the amount of charge injected and with respect to the simplicity with which an implant system can be made dependable (independent of variations in antennae separation). With pulse-width modulation, assuming the stimulator is operating at the maximum stimulus amplitude, the charge injection is automatically minimized. By comparison, the charge can be decreased by decreasing the pulse duration at any submaximal point in amplitude modulation (Fig. 33).

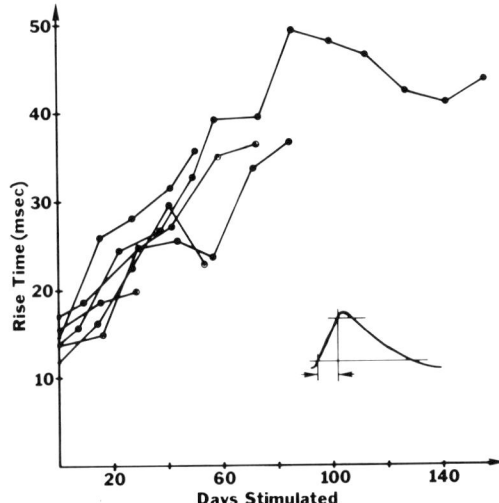

FIG. 31. Rise time of twitch contraction recorded from 6 cats. Each curve represents 1 animal, and each animal was stimulated at 10 Hz, 24 h/day. [From Murphy (52).]

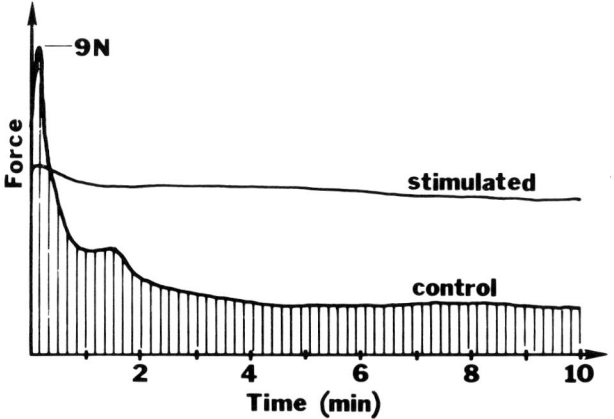

FIG. 32. Fatigue characteristics of stimulated cat tibialis anterior muscle. Stimulus frequency was 10 Hz. *Shaded region* of control indicates muscle force returned to resting level between successive stimuli. Stimulated muscle was virtually fused at 10 Hz. Muscle force is given in newtons. [Data were obtained in our laboratory from normal muscle and muscle that had been stimulated at 10 Hz, for 24 h/day, for 250 days (49).]

FREQUENCY MODULATION. Decreasing the interpulse interval between successive stimuli brings the twitch contractions closer together so that they begin to fuse. As the overlap increases, the peak force begins to rise, and the difference between the peak (maximum) and valley (minimum) forces begins to decrease (Fig. 34). The envelope or shape of this curve is relatively smooth compared to a recruitment-type curve. In addition the shape is independent of electrode position and stimulus amplitude, assuming neither varies. From the practical point of implementation, frequency modulation, like pulse-width modulation, is relatively independent of antenna displacement in an implanted system.

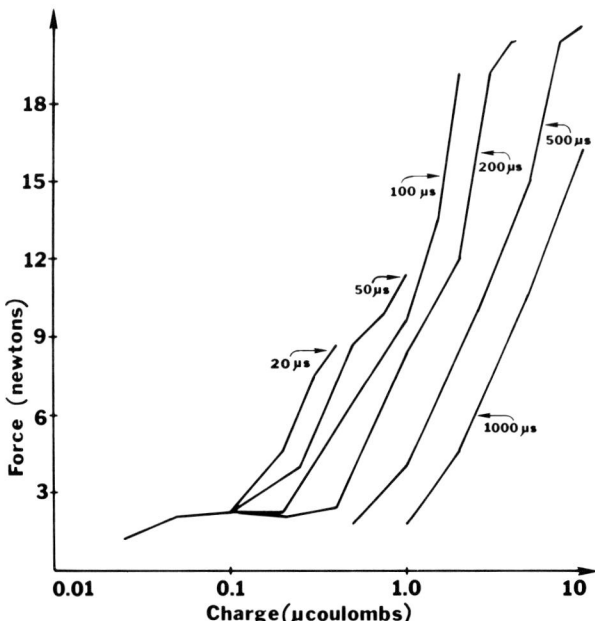

FIG. 33. Muscle force as function of charge injected during monophasic stimulation in cat tibialis anterior muscle. Each curve was obtained at fixed pulse width. [Unpublished data from our laboratory. They convey essentially the same information presented by Crago, Mortimer, et al. (15).]

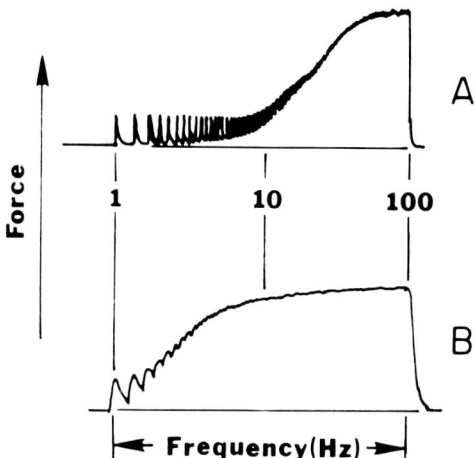

FIG. 34. Force-frequency characteristics. A: fast muscle (cat tibialis anterior). B: slow muscle (cat soleus). Horizontal axis is shown as natural log frequency. Force is in arbitrary units.

SEQUENTIAL STIMULATION. Excitation of a single muscle through multiple electrodes individually activating separate portions of the muscle in a sequential time pattern is termed sequential stimulation (59). The technique allows one to excite a muscle at a relatively low driving rate (below the fusion frequency) and yet produce a smooth muscle force at the tendon. For example, if the fusion frequency for a specific muscle is f_f, and n electrodes are used to activate n separate portions of the muscle, then a fused contraction can be obtained for an electrode stimulus rate of f_f/n when the phase shift between each electrode is $360°/n$.

Figure 35 shows a three-electrode system, each electrode driven 120° out of phase with the others. Each compartment of the muscle is activated at a rate below the fusion frequency, whereas the tendon exerts a force like that of a fused contraction. When the individual compartments are activated sequentially at frequencies below the fusion frequency, the result is a force that is fused and a muscle that fatigues less rapidly than when stimulated at the fusion frequency. To take advantage of the improved fatigue resistance with sequential stimulation, overlap in the excited regions must be avoided. Muscle fibers driven by two electrodes out of phase fatigue at a rate greater than those driven by only one.

Excitation of nonoverlapping regions. Overlap results when the same muscle fibers are excited by two separate electrodes. The amount of overlap can be estimated by measuring the difference between the force effected when two electrodes are separately and simultaneously driven. This is illustrated in Figure 36. The forces F_1 and F_2 are measured as functions of stimulus magnitude I_1 and I_2 when each electrode is separately activated. The subliminal fringe area (shaded region of Fig. 36) around F_1 and F_2 represents motor nerve fibers that were partially depolarized by I_1 and I_2, but because the nerve was not fully depolarized, no force contribution was recorded. The dotted area common to both F_1 and F_2 represents the region of overlap, which is excited by both electrodes. The small crosshatched areas common to the fringe areas of F_1 and F_2 represent the locations where the stimulus strengths of both I_1 and I_2 acting simultaneously are

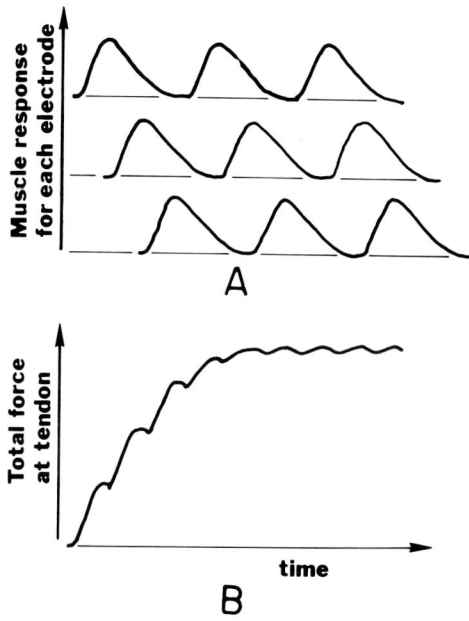

FIG. 35. Sequential stimulation. A: force contribution of 3 compartments of muscle, each stimulated 120° out of phase with the others. B: summed force as seen by common muscle tendon. [Adapted from Peckham et al. (59).]

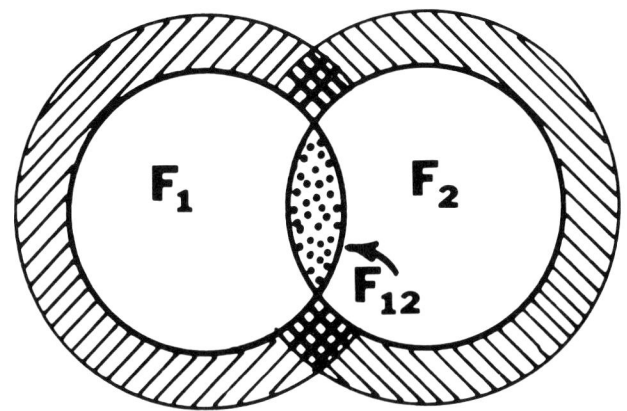

FIG. 36. Idealized representation of compartment overlap. F_1 and F_2, forces measured as functions of stimulus strength; F_{12}, force effected by I_1 or I_2 and common to both (see text).

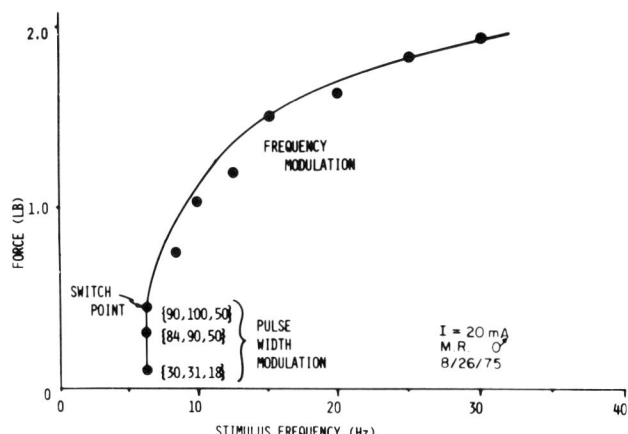

FIG. 37. Force characteristics of muscle controlled by stimulus-amplitude modulation and pulse-rate modulation. Numbers shown in brackets indicate pulse width, in μs, for each of 3 electrodes at that particular force level. [From Peckham and Mortimer (55).]

sufficient to effect a force contribution to F_{12}. Without the existence of the subliminal fringe area

$$\frac{F_1 + F_2 - F_{12}}{\frac{1}{2}(F_1 + F_2)} \cdot 100$$

yields the percent overlap. However, with the subliminal fringe area, overlap might not be accurately calculated because the crosshatched area adds to the actual overlap region. Possible error can be compensated for by adding a delay between I_1 and I_2 sufficient to allow recovery from the partial depolarization of I_1 and short enough to be within the absolute refractory period of those fibers contributing to F_1. Using such a delay the subliminal fringe area of F_1 is eliminated. The appropriate delay is obtained by comparing the force effected by a single pulse to that resulting from a pair of like amplitude pulses as a function of delay between the paired pulses. This yields a value between 500 μs and 900 μs for the appropriate delay.

Force modulation with sequential stimulation. Amplitude and frequency modulation can be effectively used with sequential stimulation to grade the contraction force. Amplitude (or pulse-width) modulation grades the force from the lowest levels to the point where the overlap between electrodes exceeds an acceptable limit. At that point the entire muscle is assumed to be active, and further force increases are effected by increasing the stimulus rates to the respective electrodes. The technique is illustrated in Figure 37 with a muscle that has a fusion frequency of approximately 18 Hz. The minimum stimulus frequency for this three-electrode sequential activation system was 6 Hz. Pulse width was modulated to effect the increased force (values given in μs) to the switch point. From the switch point the pulse duration was fixed and the frequency increased.

Summary

Rapid fatigue of muscle has been a major problem in effecting electrically induced, functional muscle contractions. The problem stems from the relatively low electrical threshold of the large motoneurons innervating the fast-twitch, glycolytic muscle fibers. Experiments have shown that with long-term electrically induced exercise, the contractile and metabolic properties of these fibers can be converted to a fatigue-resistant fiber with properties of the fast-twitch, oxidative or slow-twitch, oxidative muscle fiber. Converted muscles are able to produce sustained contractions for prolonged periods of time. The muscle may produce less force and have less mass; these changes appear to be inherent in the conversion of fiber type.

CLINICAL APPLICATIONS

Electrical activation of the nervous system makes it possible to externally control the motor system, thus providing the opportunity to restore impaired body function (e.g., posture, locomotion, respiration). Until now most research in functional stimulation has involved intervention at the peripheral level of the motor system rather than at more central areas such as spinal cord and brain. The material discussed in this section concentrates on experimental work at the peripheral level.

Paralyzed Muscle

GENERAL CONSIDERATIONS. *Upper and lower motoneuron lesion.* The existence of the lower motoneuron is critical to any system dealing with paralyzed muscle. Without a functional lower motoneuron the muscle cannot be driven by nerve excitation; direct electrical activation of muscle requires a much higher stimulus amplitude (see Fig. 20). In addition the higher magnitudes required for direct activation most likely exceed the maximum allowed values to avoid tissue damage. In paralysis resulting from lesions in the central nervous system, the lower motoneuron is almost always preserved except in the immediate vicinity of a cord lesion. (This latter situation is further discussed in subsection SPINAL CORD INJURY, p. 181.)

Disuse atrophy. Loss of voluntary motor control frequently renders a muscle inactive. In time the inactivity results in muscle-fiber atrophy (36), yielding a muscle that produces a weak force and fatigues rapidly. The effects of disuse atrophy have been found to be reversible in the human through a program of electrically induced exercise (27, 56, 80). Figure 38A shows the electrically activated force recorded from forearm muscles of quadriplegic patients before and after an induced exercise program. Figure 38B shows the change in fatigue resistance recorded from the muscle. The exercise program consisted of 10-Hz stimulation, 2.5 s on, 2.5 s off, for daily periods of exercise ranging from 4 to 6 h. Although one would expect a relationship to exist between the stimulus paradigm and the force/fatigue-resistance properties of the muscle, the knowledge available is insufficient to recommend a specific exercise program to achieve a particular characteristic in a given period of time.

Surface stimulation. Surface stimulation is generally restricted to situations where the neural tissue is located in the superficial layer of the body rather than in the deeper layers. When one scans the surface of the skin with an electrode, a point of lowest threshold is usually apparent for a specific muscle. This point is the motor point.

The most common problem encountered in surface stimulation of patients retaining skin sensation in the area of the stimulating electrodes is a painful or uncomfortable sensation. This uncomfortable sensation is a result of excitation of the sensory fibers in the skin, and it can be minimized by the use of narrow pulse widths (see Fig. 18B). Practically speaking, pulse widths on the order of 50–100 µs are the smallest that can be used for motor system activation. Another cause of discomfort to the patient is poor contact between the electrode and the skin, resulting in locally high current densities that can effect small sensory-fiber excitation. The problem of poor contact can be minimized by using well-wetted electrodes or conducting gels. The use of a regulated voltage source rather than a current source minimizes the possibility of locally high current densities. As the effective area decreases, the impedance increases, and therefore the local current density is less sensitive to area changes. In many applications percutaneous intramuscular electrodes should be considered because discomfort resulting from stimulation of skin afferents is avoided.

HEMIPLEGIA. A cerebral vascular accident generally renders all or a portion of one side of the body paralyzed. Patients retain an intact lower motoneuron on the affected side and normal control on the opposite side. The development of acceptable assistive devices for this patient population has been slow because the systems require frequent maintenance and high gadget tolerance by patients. Also, even though the loss of control of one extremity handicaps the patients, passive bracing and normal control of the other extremity permit them to adapt and continue to perform most of the essential tasks required in everyday living.

Upper extremities. Applications of electrical stimulation to the upper extremities have focused on excitation of the wrist and finger extensors in patients who retain control over the flexor compartment (66, 78). The systems employ surface electrodes with the control command initiated by shoulder movement and

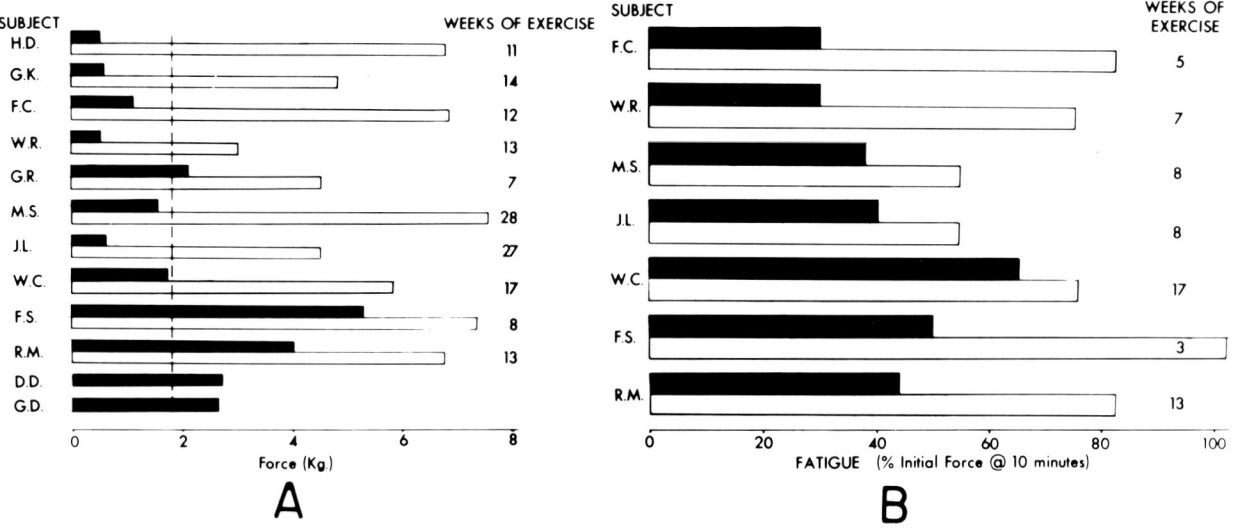

FIG. 38. Force and fatigue characteristics for patients with spinal cord injury before and after program of electrically induced exercise. *A*: force before exercise (*solid bar*) and after exercise (*open bar*). *Dotted line* indicates minimum force level generally considered necessary for performing functions of daily living. *B*: fatigue resistance is indicated by percent of maximum force remaining after 10 min of 10-Hz stimulation. *Solid bar* indicates fatigue before exercise and *open bar* shows fatigue after exercise. [From Peckham, Mortimer, and Marsolais (56).]

electromyograms from nonaffected muscles. Clinical acceptance to date has been limited, probably for reasons similar to those previously mentioned.

Lower extremities. Applications of electrical stimulation to facilitate impaired lower extremity function have ranged from relatively simple single-channel systems to multichannel systems that attempt to coordinate the contractions of several muscles during walking. The simplest one-channel system, designed to dorsiflex the ankle during the swing phase of gait, was one of the earliest patient applications of electrical stimulation investigated (39). This early version was technically modified by a group in Ljubljana, Yugoslavia (79) and was evaluated by that group as well as by others. In 1976 it was estimated that 2,000 patients had used electrical stimulation to correct "foot drop" (79). A comprehensive evaluation of results obtained with these systems has yet to be published.

An interesting side effect has been reported in some patients using electrical activation of the dorsiflexors to correct foot drop: certain facilitatory or therapeutic effects persist after the stimulus has been removed (78). In some patients, voluntary force has been found to increase after stimulation and to be elevated for many minutes (> 60 in some cases) after cessation of the conditioning stimulus (79). Altered reflex patterns have also been reported to persist after stimulation (14).

Attempts to correct more complex gait anomalies by patterned excitation of as many as six muscles during the gait cycle have recently begun (72). These preliminary investigations indicate more success in achieving correction of those anomalies that occur during the swing phase of gait than in those that occur during the stance phase.

SPINAL CORD INJURY. A traumatic injury to the spinal cord generally eliminates virtually all transmission of neural information between the peripheral nervous system and the central nervous system for body regions subserved by the spinal cord below the level of the lesion. In such cases motor and sensory losses are frequently similar on both sides of the body but are usually not identical. Therefore the loss of control of one extremity is usually accompanied by a similar loss of control of the opposite extremity. With the loss of function in both extremities, any small improvement in limb function achieved with an assistive device can make significant differences in the ability of the patient to perform the tasks of everyday living. Under these conditions the technical inconveniences of a system are more likely to be tolerated by the patient. This is particularly true for the quadriplegic patient who can regain rudimentary hand functions with such a system.

Upper extremity considerations. When considering systems to be used by the patient with spinal cord injury, it is important to establish the existence of an intact lower motoneuron. In order to make use of surviving voluntary control, the investigator should be concerned with muscles innervated by nerves originating from spinal cord segments very near the area of the cord lesion. For example, it is useless to provide hand function to a patient without elbow control, but for a patient with elbow control, hand control can be a significant improvement. A cord lesion may be variable in extent and may involve lower motoneuron damage (7). Fortunately many muscles derive their innervation from several spinal roots, and therefore some intact lower motoneurons are likely to be found in muscles subserved by nerve fibers originating in the region of the lesion. Due to distributed innervation and the possibility of intact axons sprouting and reinnervating the muscle fibers (38), wholly denervated muscles are not common. Clinical experience with the C_5 (fifth cervical segment) quadriplegic patient supports this suggestion (57).

In patients with paralyzed muscles, low contractile force and rapid fatigue are observed. As discussed in subsection CHANGES IN CONTRACTILE PROPERTIES, p. 174, these muscles can be conditioned by a program of electrically induced exercise to produce the required properties.

Restoration of hand function in the C_5 quadriplegic patient. The functional C_5 quadriplegic patient retains voluntary control over elbow flexion and some control over forearm supination (via musculus biceps) but no control over wrist and hand function.

An elementary form of hand function can be effected in the C_5 quadriplegic patient by a combination of passive bracing and electrical stimulation of the forearm muscles. Electrically activating the finger flexors (musculus flexor digitorum profundus and/or musculus flexor digitorum superficialis) brings the tips of the index and middle fingers into contact with the thumb. The musculus flexor digitorum superficialis provides, in addition to finger flexion, forearm pronation (absent in the C_5 quadriplegic patient). The induced pronation can be countered by voluntary supination effected by musculus biceps. Wrist and thumb positions are maintained with a lightweight polypropylene splint, and hand opening is effected by excitation of the finger extensor muscles (musculus extensor digitorum communis and/or musculus extensor indicus).

In general, hand opening is a transient action (not likely to be affected by fatigue) and can be effected by a single-electrode system. Finger closing, however, is intended for grasping and holding objects for extended periods of time. Muscle-force decay, or fatigue, is minimized by altering the contractile and metabolic properties of the muscle through an electrically induced exercise program (see subsection CHANGES IN CONTRACTILE PROPERTIES, p. 174) and by using three-electrode sequential stimulation (see subsection SEQUENTIAL STIMULATION, p. 178). The grasping force is under patient control and is modulated by fiber recruitment and fiber firing rate (see Fig. 37).

Patient control of the orthotic device is mediated

through a portion of the body retaining voluntary control. When choosing the control site, care must be taken to avoid interfering unnecessarily with any voluntary control the patient retains (48). Transduction of the shoulder position (relative to the sternum) is an adequate method of providing a proportional signal, under voluntary control, to the stimulator (3, 50). With shoulder control, elevation of the shoulder provides the control signal for finger flexion, and shoulder depression causes finger extension.

This system has been used by eight patients for periods of up to 4 yr. The results demonstrate that functional hand motions can be effected by electrical excitation of the paralyzed muscles. Future efforts must focus on closed-loop control of force and length, so as to ease the control demands placed on the patient; implantable systems that are free of mounting problems and electrode migration; performance feedback to conscious levels; and acquisition of control signals from the body in a manner that does not interfere with the remaining natural function of the patient. Close coupling to the nervous system by implant recording and stimulating electrodes should certainly help achieve many of these goals. Recent reports concerning long-term recording from cortical cells (70), spinal ganglia (41), and peripheral nerve (16, 34, 73) suggest that close coupling to the nervous system may soon be practical. For further discussion of the information in this subsection, see reference 55.

RESPIRATION. Pulmonary dysfunction resulting from the loss of higher central nervous system control has been overcome in humans by electrical activation of the phrenic nerve (24, 26). Applications include patients with lesions located very high on the spinal cord and patients with respiratory center malfunction (e.g., Ondine's curse; ref. 25).

The stimulation systems used have been subcutaneous implants powered by radio frequency with leads attached to cuff electrodes located on the phrenic nerve in the region of the lower neck (24). In general, unilateral implants have been used in patients with Ondine's curse; bilateral implants are generally used in quadriplegic patients. Activation of a single phrenic nerve provides adequate ventilation for an 8- to 12-h period per 24-h period. The electrode systems employed have been bipolar, tripolar, and more recently monopolar.

Damage to the phrenic nerve by the cuff electrodes has been observed in both animals and humans and appears to be related to mechanical trauma rather than to electrical stimulation (25). With bipolar electrodes Glenn et al. (25) reported that 16% (11 nerves in 37 patients) of the implanted phrenic nerves showed impaired or absent function.

Fatigue, or decreasing efficacy, has been a problem with most of the patients using electrophrenic respiration. The fatigue takes two forms, one with rapid onset (1 or 2 h) and the other with a more gradual onset (12 h). In quadriplegic patients the tidal volume decreases within a few minutes during the days first following implant but disappears after weeks of stimulation (28). It is probable that a disuse-type atrophy of the diaphragm is reversed by electrically induced exercise, like it is for forearm muscles of patients with spinal cord injury (see subsection *Disuse atrophy*, p. 180). The second, more slowly developing form of fatigue has been observed as a decreasing efficacy of phrenic nerve stimulation over an 8- to 12-h period. This phenomenon has been seen uniformly in both animals and humans. Tanae and colleagues (74) studied the decreased efficacy of phrenic nerve pacing in animals as a function of stimulus waveform. Their studies showed a significant improvement in efficacy when the polarity of the stimulating pulse was reversed between pulses (Figs. 39 and 40). The increased efficacy of the alternating-pulse form must be related to a form of neural fatigue at the electrode location rather than to physiological fatigue at a more distal location (see discussion in subsection *Neural Fatigue*, p. 171).

Technical problems related to stimulator malfunction have been the primary source of failure in systems used by pulmonary patients. The problem appears to be related to fluid leakage into the implant. It is likely that this problem will be solved in the near future as new encapsulation methods become available.

Scoliosis

Electrical activation of muscles acting on the spinal column can, in principle, apply a corrective force to the deformed, scoliotic spine (5, 54). Conventional methods of scoliosis treatment include bracing (for a developing curve in a growing child) and spinal fusion (for severe curves). Bracing is cosmetically undesirable and is felt by many to be psychologically damaging to the child. Electrical stimulation of spinal musculature offers the possibility of treating scoliosis in the growing

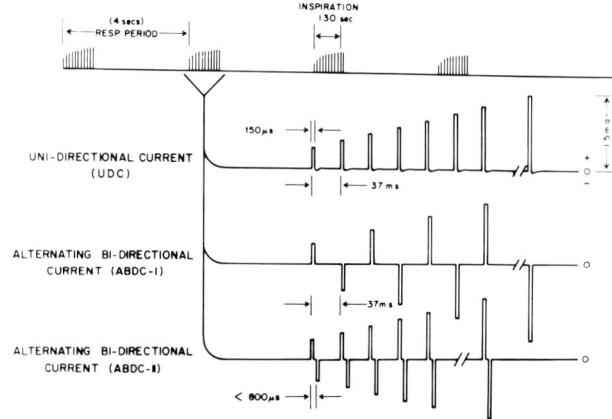

FIG. 39. Three types of stimulus waveforms applied to phrenic nerve through bipolar electrodes. [From Tanae et al. (74).]

child while avoiding the undesirable cosmetic effects of the brace.

The spinal muscle stimulation technique is presently considered experimental. The following material covers animal experiments and preliminary experience with human patients.

ANIMAL EXPERIMENTS. Mammalian animal models for idiopathic scoliosis as seen in the human have not been found to date. Therefore experimentation with electrical stimulation has been limited to first effecting an abnormal spinal curvature by stimulating muscles on one side of the spinal column and then attempting to reverse the curve by moving the electrodes to the opposite side of the spine. Such studies have been performed in dogs (53, 54), pigs (M. A. Herbert and W. P. Bobechko, personal communication), rabbits (5, 46), and sheep (in my laboratory). The results of these studies are summarized in Table 2. From these data one can conclude that it is difficult to create curves greater than 15° and that the curves can be induced by both a series of twitches (0.5 Hz) and fused tetanic contractions. The difficulty in achieving curves greater than 15° may reflect a mechanical property of the quadruped spine, which is somewhat different from the human spine. However, it is more likely that the difficulty reflects the fact that gravity cannot contribute to the generation of a scoliotic curve in the quadruped.

Examination of the paraspinal muscles in the pig has shown that the stimulated muscles appear atrophic after daily periods of stimulation exceeding 8 h. Considering the material presented in subsection CHANGES IN CONTRACTILE PROPERTIES, p. 174, it is likely that these investigators were observing fiber conversion rather than a deleterious "wasting." Examination of sheep paraspinal muscles in our experiments has shown changes that are consistent with fiber-type conversion.

HUMAN EXPERIMENTS. The pioneering efforts of Bobechko and Herbert at the Hospital for Sick Children in Toronto have precipitated the most extensive clinical population studies to date. The system they employ utilizes three electrodes: a parallel pair of cathodes and a single anode. The anode is placed in the deep paraspinal musculature at the apex of the curve, and the cathodes are located approximately two spinal segments rostral and caudal to the apex, also in the deep paraspinal musculature. The system is powered by a totally implantable receiver powered by radio frequency. Stimulation is applied during the sleeping period at a rate of 30 Hz, 1 s on, 10 s off.

The number of patients studied by Bobechko and Herbert is greater than 70. About half this group have experienced a technical malfunction in the equipment that now appears to have been corrected. Among those experiencing no technical problems, approximately

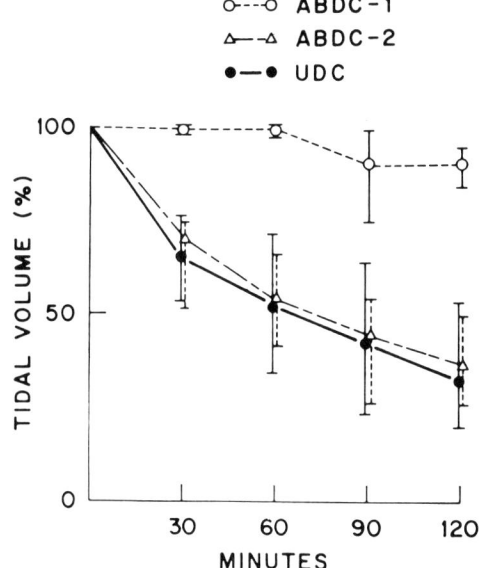

FIG. 40. Average tidal-volume changes during 2 h of stimulation using the stimulus waveform shown in Figure 39. [From Tanae et al. (74).]

TABLE 2. *Scoliosis Studies in Animals*

Animal	Stimulation Paradigm	Period of Stimulation, days	Mean Induced Curve	Reference Number
Dog	2 electrode pairs, 2-22 Hz	7-70	6°±5° (2°-20°)	54
Pig	3 electrodes, 30 Hz, 1 s on, 9 s off, 14-16 h/day	42-56	12°±5° (3°-23°)	Unpublished data
Rabbit	0.67 Hz, 24 h/day	42	Structural curve	5
Rabbit	6-10 electrodes, 0.5 Hz, 24 h/day	45-102	22°±15° (3°-40°)	46
Sheep	3 active electrodes, 10 Hz, 2 h on, 1 h off, 24 h/day	170-246	12°±1° (11°-13°)	48a

Values in parentheses are ranges.

60% have demonstrated either no progression in the curve or a decrease in the curve.

Percutaneous electrode system. The percutaneous electrode system we have worked with is based on the implant system of Bobechko and his colleagues and on experience gained with percutaneous electrodes in restoration of hand function. With percutaneous electrodes one can stimulate deep paraspinal muscle (primary multifidusand longissimus) without causing uncomfortable skin sensation and without using a surgical procedure (required for the system powered by radio frequency).

The primary concern when using a percutaneous system is possible infection at the electrode entry site. In the five patients we have studied (four for more than a year), no infections have been observed around the electrode track. The patients have led normally active lives. Occasionally superficial granulomas have formed (3-5 mm in diameter and 2 mm in height) at the electrode entry site, but these have been easily controlled by a topical application of silver nitrate. The life expectancy of the multistrand coiled wire is approximately one year. The patient population is too small for evaluation of correction efficacy, but it is expected that results would be similar to those obtained with the totally implantable system.

Surface electrode system. Axelgaard and his colleagues (2) have reported preliminary results with transcutaneous (surface electrode) electrical activation of trunk musculature. In a screening procedure of 27 scoliosis patients, these investigators found that the greatest acute correction was obtained with a pair of surface electrodes placed on the axillary line (lateral thorax) on the convex side of the curve. The least effect was noted when the electrodes were placed 30 mm lateral to the spinous processes. Intermediate results were obtained when the electrode pair was placed between the most medial and the most lateral locations.

Preliminary evaluation of lateral-musculature stimulation in patients with idiopathic scoliosis shows results that appear compatible with the implant and percutaneous methods just described. The stimulation paradigm under study is a 25-Hz train, 4 s on and 8 s off, applied during sleep.

Summary

Functional muscle contraction can be electrically evoked in normal and paralyzed muscle. The results of studies using electrical stimulation in correcting posture and restoring limb motion and respiration have demonstrated the feasibility of a motor prosthesis. However, many technical problems that often inconvenience the patient and limit public acceptance of many devices remain to be solved.

SUMMARY

Electrical activation of the nervous system offers a potentially powerful tool to aid in the restoration of lost or impaired motor function. The close proximity of the stimulating electrode to the excitable tissue requires that careful consideration be given to the use of processes that could cause irreversible damage to living cells; electrochemical reactions at the electrode surface and incompatibility of the materials with the tissue both present possible hazards. The damaging processes related to electrochemical reaction may be minimized by restricting the stimulus parameters (charge per unit area) to the limits of the reversible region of the electrode. For multipulse stimulation this requires charge-balanced biphasic stimulation, i.e., the net charge driven through the electrodes is zero during a stimulus cycle. The efficiency of electrical activation, based on charge injection required to effect nerve excitation, increases as the magnitude of the stimulus pulse width decreases. Therefore narrow stimulus pulse widths (50-100 μs) are recommended. As the pulse width decreases, the difference between threshold increases for axons of different diameters, enabling larger axons to be selectively excited. With biphasic, regulated-current stimulation, the secondary or reversal pulse can suppress the excitatory effects of the primary pulse. Adding a delay of 100 μs between the lagging edge of the primary pulse and the leading edge of the secondary pulse reduces the suppressive effects of the secondary pulse.

Rapid fatigue of the electrically activated muscle, often a problem in clinical applications, stems from the relatively low electrical threshold of the large motoneurons innervating the fast-twitch, glycolytic muscle fibers. Long-term electrically induced exercise can "convert" the contractile and metabolic properties of these fibers such that a fatigue-resistant fiber with properties of the fast-twitch, oxidative or slow-twitch, oxidative muscle fiber is formed. Converted muscles are able to produce sustained contractions for prolonged periods of time. They may produce less force and have less mass; these changes appear to be inherent properties of the conversion of fiber type.

Clinical studies using electrical stimulation to correct posture and to restore limb motion and respiration indicate the feasibility of a motor prosthesis. However, many technical problems often inconveniencing the patient and limiting public acceptance of the devices remain to be solved.

The National Institute of Neurological Communicative Diseases and Stroke Neural Prosthesis Program, and particularly the workshops of this program, provided the germination medium for much of the material presented here. For this, recognition is given to Drs. F. T. Hambrecht and K. Frank. The Alexander von Humboldt-Stiftung provided partial support during the writing of this manuscript while the author was a guest at the Institute fur Biokybernetik, Universität Karlsruhe. We also acknowledge Ms. Barbra Good, medical editor; Ms. Mary Buynack, secretary; and Mrs. Nancy Caris, photography, for assistance in the preparation of this manuscript.

REFERENCES

1. AGNEW, W. F., T. YUEN, R. H. PUDENZ, AND L. S. BULLARA. Electrical stimulation of the brain. *Surg. Neurol.* 4: 438–448, 1975.
2. AXELGAARD, J., D. R. MCNEAL, AND J. C. BROWN. Lateral electrical surface stimulation for the treatment of progressive scoliosis. *Proc. Int. Symp. External Control of Human Extremities, 6th, Dubrovnik, Yugoslavia, 1978.*
3. BAYER, D. M., R. H. LORD, J. W. SWANKER, AND J. T. MORTIMER. A two-axis shoulder position transducer for control of orthotic/prosthetic devices. *IEEE Trans. Ind. Electron. Control Instrum.* 19: 61–64, 1972.
4. BERNSTEIN, J. J., L. L. HENCH, P. F. JOHNSON, W. W. DAWSON, AND G. HUNTER. Electrical stimulation of the cortex with tantalum pentoxide capacitive electrodes. In: *Functional Electrical Stimulation*, edited by J. B. Reswick and F. T. Hambrecht. New York: Dekker, 1977, p. 465–477.
5. BOBECHKO, W. P. Electrical stimulation in scoliosis. *Program, Functional Neuromuscular Stimulation, Natl. Acad. Sci. Workshop, Apr. 1972*, p. 145–146.
6. BRADLEY, W. E., L. E. WITTMERS, S. N. CHOU, AND L. A. FRENCH. Use of a radio transmitter receiver unit for the treatment of neurogenic bladder. *J. Neurosurg.* 19: 782–786, 1962.
7. BRANDSTATER, M. E., AND S. M. DINSDALE. Electrophysiological studies in the assessment of spinal cord lesions. *Arch. Phys. Med. Rehabil.* 57: 70–74, 1976.
8. BRINDLEY, G. S., AND W. S. LEWIN. The sensations produced by electrical stimulation of the visual cortex. *J. Physiol. London* 196: 479–493, 1968.
9. BROWN, M. D., M. A. COTTER, O. HUDLICKÁ, AND G. VRBOVÁ. The effects of different patterns of muscle activity on capillary density, mechanical properties and structure of slow and fast rabbit muscles. *Pfluegers Arch.* 361: 241–250, 1976.
10. BRUMMER, S. B., AND J. MCHARDY. Current problems in electrode development. In: *Functional Electrical Stimulation*, edited by J. B. Reswick and F. T. Hambrecht. New York: Dekker, 1977, p. 499–514.
11. BRUMMER, S. B., AND M. J. TURNER. Electrical stimulation of the nervous system: the principle of safe charge injection with noble metal electrodes. *Bioelectrochem. Bioenergetics* 2: 13–25, 1975.
12. BURKE, R. E., AND P. TSAIRIS. Anatomy and innervation ratios in motor units of cat gastrocnemius. *J. Physiol. London* 234: 749–765, 1973.
13. CALDWELL, C. W., AND J. B. RESWICK. A percutaneous wire electrode for chronic research use. *IEEE Trans. Biomed. Eng.* 5: 429–432, 1975.
14. CARNSTAM, B., L. E. LARSSON, AND T. S. PREVEC. Improvement of gait following functional electrical stimulation. *Scand. J. Rehabil. Med.* 9: 7–13, 1977.
15. CRAGO, P. E., P. H. PECKHAM, J. T. MORTIMER, AND J. P. VAN DER MEULEN. The choice of pulse duration for chronic electrical stimulation via surface, nerve, and intramuscular electrodes. *Ann. Biomed. Eng.* 2: 252–264, 1974.
16. DELUCA, C. J., AND L. D. GILMORE. Voluntary nerve signals from several mammalian nerves: long-term recording. *Science* 191: 193–195, 1976.
17. DOBELLE, W. H., AND M. G. MLADEJOVSKY. Phosphenes produced by electrical stimulation of human occipital cortex, and their application to the development of a prosthesis for the blind. *J. Physiol. London* 243: 553–576, 1974.
18. DOBELLE, W. H., S. S. STENSAAS, M. G. MLADEJOVSKY, AND J. B. SMITH. A prosthesis for the deaf based on cortical stimulation. *Ann. Otol. Rhinol. Laryngol.* 82: 445–463, 1973.
19. DYMOND, A. M. Characteristics of the metal-tissue interface of stimulation electrodes. *IEEE Trans. Biomed. Eng.* 23: 274–280, 1976.
20. EDSTRÖM, L., AND E. KUGELBERG. Histochemical composition, distribution of fibers and fatiguability of single motor units. *J. Neurol. Neurosurg. Psychiatry* 31: 424–433, 1968.
20a. FIELDS, W. S. (editor). *Neural Organization and Its Relevance to Prosthetics*. New York: Intercontinental Med. Book, 1973.
21. FINKELSTEIN, A., AND A. MAURO. Physical principles and formalisms of electrical excitability. In: *Handbook of Physiology. The Nervous System*, edited by E. Kandel. Bethesda, MD: Am. Physiol. Soc., 1977, sect. 1, vol. I, pt. 1, chapt. 6, p. 161–213.
22. FRANKENHAEUSER, B., AND A. F. HUXLEY. The action potential in the myelinated nerve fiber of *Xenopus laevis* as computed on the basis of voltage clamp data. *J. Physiol. London* 197: 302–315, 1964.
23. GILMAN, S., G. W. DAUTH, V. M. TENNYSON, AND L. KREMZNER. Chronic cerebellar stimulation in the monkey. Preliminary observations. *Arch. Neurol.* 32: 474–477, 1975.
24. GLENN, W. W. L., W. G. HOLCOMB, J. B. L. GEE, AND R. RATH. Central hypoventilation: long-term ventilatory assistance by radiofrequency electrophrenic respiration. *Ann. Surg.* 172: 755–774, 1970.
25. GLENN, W. W. L., W. G. HOLCOMB, J. F. HOGAN, T. KANEYUKI, AND J. KIM. Long-term stimulation of the phrenic nerve for diaphragm pacing. In: *Functional Electrical Stimulation*, edited by J. B. Reswick and F. T. Hambrecht. New York: Dekker, 1977, p. 97–112.
26. GLENN, W. W. L., W. G. HOLCOMB, J. HOGAN, I. MATANO, J. B. L. GEE, E. K. MOTOYAMA, C. S. KIM, R. S. POIRIER, AND G. FORBES. Diaphragm pacing by radio frequency transmission in the treatment of chronic ventilatory insufficiency: present status. *J. Thorac. Cardiovasc. Surg.* 66: 505–520, 1973.
27. GLENN, W. W. L., W. G. HOLCOMB, A. J. MCLAUGHLIN, J. M. O'HARE, J. F. HOGAN, AND R. YASUDA. Total ventilatory support in a quadriplegic patient with radiofrequency electrophrenic respiration. *N. Engl. J. Med.* 286: 513–516, 1972.
28. GLENN, W. W. L., W. G. HOLCOMB, R. K. SHAW, J. F. HOGAN, AND K. R. HOLSCHUH. Long-term ventilatory support by diaphragm pacing in quadriplegia. *Ann. Surg.* 183: 566–577, 1976.
29. GUYTON, D. L., AND F. T. HAMBRECHT. Capacitor electrode stimulates nerve or muscle without oxidation-reduction reactions. *Science* 181: 74–76, 1973.
30. GUYTON, D. L., AND F. T. HAMBRECHT. Theory and design of capacitor electrodes for chronic stimulation. *Med. Biol. Eng.* 7: 613–622, 1974.
30a. HAMBRECHT, F. T. Neural prostheses *Annu. Rev. Biophys. Bioeng.* 8: 239–267, 1979.
30b. HAMBRECHT, F. T., AND K. FRANK. The future possibilities for neural control. In: *Advances in Electronics and Electron Physics*, edited by L. Marton. New York: Academic, 1975, vol. 38, p. 55–81.
30c. HAMBRECHT, F. T., AND J. B. RESWICK (editors). *Functional Electrical Stimulation*, New York: Dekker, 1977.
31. HERSHBERG, P. I., S. SHON, G. P. ARGAWAL, AND A. KANTROWITZ. Histologic changes in continuous, long-term electrical stimulation of a peripheral nerve. *IEEE Trans. Biomed. Eng.* 14: 109–114, 1967.
32. HENNEMAN, E., AND C. B. OLSON. Relations between structure and function in the design of skeletal muscles. *J. Neurophysiol.* 28: 581–598, 1965.
33. HENNEMAN, E., G. SOMJEN, AND D. O. CARPENTER. Excitability and inhibitibility of motoneurons of different sizes. *J. Neurophysiol.* 1965, 28: 599–620, 1965.
34. HOFFER, J. A., AND W. B. MARKS. Long-term peripheral nerve activity during behavior in the rabbit. *Adv. Behav. Biol.* 18: 767–768, 1976.
35. HUDLICKÁ, O., M. BROWN, M. COTTER, M. SMITH, AND G. VRBOVÁ. The effect of long-term stimulation of fast muscles on their blood flow, metabolism and ability to withstand fatigue. *Pfluegers Arch.* 369: 141–149, 1977.
36. KARPATI, G., AND W. K. ENGEL. Correlative histochemical study of skeletal muscle after suprasegmental denervation, peripheral nerve section and skeletal fixation. *Neurology* 18: 681–692, 1968.
37. KARKAR, M. N. *Nerve Excitation With a Cuff Electrode—A Model* (M. S. thesis). Cleveland, OH: Case Western Reserve Univ., 1975.
38. KUGELBERG, E., L. EDSTRÖM, AND M. ABBRUZZESE. Mapping

of motor units in experimentally reinnervated rat muscle. *J. Neurol. Neurosurg. Psychiatry* 33: 319–329, 1970.
39. LIBERSON, W. T., H. J. HOLMQUEST, AND D. SCOTT. Functional electrotherapy stimulation of the peroneal nerve synchronized with swing phase of the gait of hemiplegic patients. *Arch. Phys. Med. Rehabil.* 1961, 42: 101–105, 1961.
40. LILLY, J. C. Injury and excitation by electric currents: A. The balanced pulse-pair waveform. In: *Electrical Stimulation of the Brain,* edited by D. E. Sheer. Austin: Univ. of Texas Press, 1961, chapt. 6.
41. LOEB, G. E., M. J. BAK, AND J. DUYSENS. Long-term unit recording from somatosensory neurons in the spinal ganglia of the freely walking cat. *Science* 197: 1192–1194, 1977.
41a. LOEB, G. E., J. MCHARDY, E. M. KELLIHER, AND S. B. BRUMMER. Neural prosthesis. In: *Biocompatibility.* West Palm Beach, FL: CRC, vol. 6, in press.
42. MARKS, W. B. Polarization changes of stimulated cortical neurons caused by electrical stimulation at the cortical surface. In: *Functional Electrical Stimulation,* edited by J. B. Reswick and F. T. Hambrecht. New York: Academic, 1977.
43. MCHARDY, J., D. GELLER, AND S. B. BRUMMER. An approach to corrosion control during electrical stimulation. *Ann. Biomed. Eng.* 5: 144–149, 1977.
43a. MCNEAL, D. R., AND J. B. RESWICK. Control of skeletal muscle by electrical stimulation. In: *Advances in Biomedical Engineering,* edited by J. H. U. Brown and J. F. Dickson III. New York: Academic, 1976, vol. 6.
44. MCNEAL, R. Analysis of a model for excitation of myelinated nerve. *IEEE Trans. Biomed. Eng.* 23: 329–337, 1976.
45. MICHELSON, R. P. The results of electrical stimulation of the cochlea in human sensory deafness. *Ann. Otol. Rhinol. Laryngol.* 80: 914–919, 1971.
46. MONTICELLI, G., E. ASCANI, V. SALSANO, AND A. SALSANO. Experimental scoliosis induced by prolonged minimal electrical stimulation of the para-vertebral muscles. *Ital. J. Orthop. Traumatol.* 1: 39–54, 1975.
47. MORRISON, S. J. *Tissue Reaction to Three Ceramics of Porous and Nonporous Structures* (M.S. thesis). Clemson, SC: Clemson Univ., 1975.
48. MORTIMER, J. T. Man-machine communication: a major problem in the restoration of limb function. *J. Dyn. Syst. Meas. Control* 97: 217–219, 1975.
48a. MORTIMER, J. T. Intramuscular electrical stimulation of skeletal muscle. *Prog. Rep. Neural Prostheses Program, 12th, NIH-NINCDS, 1978.*
49. MORTIMER, J. T. Intramuscular electrical stimulation of skeletal muscle. *Prog. Rep. Neural Prostheses Program, 14th, NIH-NINCDS, 1979.*
50. MORTIMER, J. T., D. M. BAYER, R. H. LORD, AND J. W. SWANKER. Shoulder position transduction for proportional two axis control of orthotic/prosthetic systems. In: *The Control of the Upper-Extremity Prostheses and Orthoses,* edited by P. Herberts, R. Kadefors, R. Magnusson, and I. Petersén. Springfield, IL: Thomas, 1974, p. 131–145.
51. MORTIMER, J. T., AND P. H. PECKHAM. Intramuscular electrical stimulation. In: *Neural Organization and Its Relevance to Prosthetics,* edited by W. S. Fields. New York: Intercontinental Medical Book, 1973, p. 131–146.
52. MURPHY, T. *Physiologic Changes in Electrically Stimulated Skeletal Muscle; Chronic Evaluation in Cat* (M.S. thesis). Cleveland, OH: Case Western Reserve Univ. 1977.
53. OLSEN, G. A., H. ROSEN, R. B. HOHN, AND B. SLOCUM. Electrical muscle stimulation as a means of correcting induced canine scoliotic curves. *Clin. Orthop.* 125: 227–235, 1977.
54. OLSEN, G. A., H. ROSEN, S. STOLL, AND G. BROWN. The use of muscle stimulation for inducing scoliotic curves. A preliminary report. *Clin. Orthop.* 113: 198–211, 1975.
55. PECKHAM, P. H., AND J. T. MORTIMER. Restoration of hand function in the quadriplegic through electrical stimulation. In: *Functional Electrical Stimulation,* edited by J. B. Reswick and F. T. Hambrecht. New York: Dekker, 1977, p. 83–95.
56. PECKHAM, P. H., J. T. MORTIMER, AND E. B. MARSOLAIS. Alteration in the force and fatiguability of skeletal muscle in quadriplegic humans following exercise induced by chronic electrical stimulation. *Clin. Orthop.* 114: 326–334, 1976.
57. PECKHAM, P. H., J. T. MORTIMER, AND E. B. MARSOLAIS. Upper and lower motor neuron lesions in the upper extremity muscles of tetraplegics. *Paraplegia* 14: 115–121, 1976.
58. PECKHAM, P. H., J. T. MORTIMER, AND J. P. VAN DER MEULEN. Physiologic and metabolic changes in white muscle of cat following induced exercise. *Brain Res.* 50: 424–429, 1973.
59. PECKHAM, P. H., J. P. VAN DER MEULEN, AND J. B. RESWICK. Electrical activation of skeletal muscle by sequential stimulation. In: *The Nervous System and Electrical Currents,* edited by N. Wulfson and A. Sances, Jr. New York: Plenum, 1970, p. 45–50.
60. PETTE, D., W. MULLER, E. LEISNER, AND G. VRBOVÁ. Time dependent effects on contractile properties, fiber population, myosin light chains and enzymes of energy metabolism in intermittently and continuously stimulated fast twitch muscles of the rabbit. *Pfluegers Arch.* 364: 103–112, 1976.
61. PETTE, D., U. RAMIREZ, W. MUELLER, R. SIMON, U. EXNER, AND R. HILDEBRAND. Influence of intermittent long-term stimulation on contractile, histochemical and metabolic properties of fiber populations in fast and slow rabbit muscles. *Pfluegers Arch.* 361: 1–7, 1975.
62. PETTE, D., M. E. SMITH, H. W. STAUDTE, AND G. VRBOVÁ. Effects of long-term electrical stimulation on some contractile and metabolic characteristics of fast rabbit muscles. *Pfluegers Arch.* 338: 257–272, 1973.
63. PUDENZ, R. H., L. A. BULLARA, D. DRU, AND A. TALALLA. Electrical stimulation of the brain. II. Effects of the blood brain barrier. *Surg. Neurol.* 4: 265–270, 1975.
64. PUDENZ, R. H., L. A. BULLARA, S. JACQUES, AND F. T. HAMBRECHT. Electrical stimulation of the brain. III. The neural damage model. *Surg. Neurol.* 4: 389–400, 1975.
65. PUDENZ, R. H., B. A. BULLARA, AND A. TALALLA. Electrical stimulation of the brain. I. Electrodes and electrode arrays. *Surg. Neurol.* 4: 37–42, 1975.
66. REBERSEK, S., AND L. VODOVNIK. Proportionally controlled functional electrical stimulation of hand. *Arch. Phys. Med. Rehabil.* 54: 378–382, 1973.
67. RILEY, D. A., AND E. F. ALLIN. The effects of inactivity programmed stimulation and denervation on the histochemistry of skeletal muscle fiber types. *Exp. Neurol.* 40: 391–413, 1973.
68. SALMONS, S., AND F. A. SRÉTER. Significance of impulse activity in the transformation of skeletal muscle type. *Nature London* 263: 30–34, 1976.
69. SALMONS, S., AND G. VRBOVÁ. The influence of activity on some contractile characteristics of mammalian fast and slow muscles. *J. Physiol. London* 201: 535–549, 1969.
70. SCHMIDT, E. M., M. J. BAK, AND J. S. MCINTOSH. Long-term chronic recording from cortical neurons. *Exp. Neurol.* 52: 496–506, 1976.
71. SIMMONS, F. B. Electrical stimulation of the auditory nerve in man. *Arch. Otolaryngol.* 84: 1–54, 1966.
72. STANIC, U., R. ACIMOVIC-JANEZIC, N. GROS, A. TRNKOCZY, T. BAJD, AND M. KLJAJIC. Multichannel electrical stimulation for correction of hemiplegic gait. *Scand. J. Rehab. Med.* 10: 75–92, 1978.
73. STEIN, R. B., J. A. HOFFER, T. GORDON, L. A. DAVIS, AND D. CHARLES. Long term recordings from cat peripheral nerve during degeneration and regeneration: implications for human nerve repair and prosthetics. In: *Nerve Repair: Its Clinical and Experimental Basis,* edited by D. L. Jewett and H. R. McCarroll. St. Louis, MO: Mosby, 1978.
74. TANAE, H., W. G. HOLCOMB, R. YASUDA, J. F. HOGAN, AND W. W. L. GLENN. Electrical nerve fatigue: advantages of an alternating bidirectional waveform. *J. Surg. Res.* 15: 14–21, 1973.
75. TESTERMAN, R. L., N. R. HAGFORS, AND S. I. SCHWARTZ. Design and evaluation of nerve stimulating electrodes. *Med. Res. Eng.* 10: 6–11, 1971.

76. VAN DEN HONERT, C., AND J. T. MORTIMER. The response of the myelinated nerve fiber to short duration biphasic stimulating currents. *Ann. Biomed. Eng.* 7: 117–125, 1979.
77. VODOVNIK, L., AND S. REVERSEK. Improvements in voluntary control of paretic muscles due to electrical stimulation. In: *Neural Organization and Its Relevance to Prosthetics*, edited by W. S. Fields. New York: Stratton Intercontinental, 1973, p. 101–115.
78. VODOVNIK, L., AND S. REBERSEK. Myoelectric and myomechanical prehension systems using functional electrical stimulation. In: *The Control of the Upper-Extremity Prostheses and Orthoses*, edited by P. Herberts, R. Kadefors, R. Magnusson, and I. Petersén. Springfield, IL: Thomas, 1974, p. 151–165.
79. VODOVNIK, L., U. STANIC, A. KRALJ, R. ACIMOVIC, F. GRACANIN, S. GROBELNIK, P. SUHEL, C. GODEC, AND S. PLEVNIK. Functional electrical stimulation in Ljubljana. In: *Functional Electrical Stimulation*, edited by J. B. Reswick and F. T. Hambrecht. New York: Dekker, 1977, p. 39–54.
80. WATERS, R. Electrical stimulation of the peroneal and femoral nerves in man. In: *Functional Electrical Stimulation*, edited by J. B. Reswick and F. T. Hambrecht. New York: Dekker, 1977, p. 55–64.

CHAPTER 6

Muscle spindles: their messages and their fusimotor supply

PETER B. C. MATTHEWS | *University Laboratory of Physiology, Oxford, England*

CHAPTER CONTENTS

Tendon Organs
Structure of Muscle Spindles
   Classic view
   Recognition of motor duality
   Subdivision of nuclear-bag fibers
Functional Properties of Primary and Secondary Spindle Afferent
     Endings
   Different responses to various stimuli
   Mode of summation of signal components
   Amplitude nonlinearity
   Linear responses to sinusoidal stretching
   Assessment
   Possible intermediate endings
Motor Supply to Muscle Spindle
   Gamma motor axons
   Delimitation of static and dynamic fusimotor axons
     Main differences
     Speed of action
     Recent reexamination
   Intrafusal destination of static and dynamic axons
     Initial ideas
     Histological tracing of individual fusimotor fibers
     Glycogen depletion analysis
     Studies on single living spindles: visual observation,
       intracellular recording
     Assessment of position
   Properties of intrafusal muscle fibers
     Differences in contractility
     Creep
     Membrane potentials
   Beta or skeletofusimotor axons
Possible Functional Roles for the Fusimotor System
   Maintenance of sensitivity
   Central regulation of spindle sensitivity (parameter control)
     Position sensitivity
     Dynamic measurements of position sensitivity
     Velocity sensitivity
     Relation of velocity sensitivity to position sensitivity
     Gain of spindle to dynamic stimuli
   Fusimotor biasing and suggested role as servo input
     Servo hypothesis
     Coactivation
     Assessment
     Servo assistance and modeling of movement
Summary
   Structure
   Functional differences between primary and secondary endings
   Static and dynamic fusimotor axons
   Possible functional roles for the fusimotor system

IN TERMS of the quantity of nervous traffic, the sensory receptors embedded in a muscle at least equal the extrafusal muscle fibers that make up its main bulk. For example, about 150 α-motor fibers to the cat soleus are outnumbered by some 240 fibers, both afferent and efferent, concerned with the sensors and their regulation rather than with the direct command for motor action (approximately 140 group I plus group II afferents, and 100 γ-efferents). The processing and elaboration of all this regulatory impulse traffic by the central nervous system (CNS) undoubtedly requires considerable neural attention. Thus a detailed understanding of the central mechanisms of motor control in the intact animal seems likely to be bound up with the elucidation of the normal functional role of so much afferent feedback, even though many motor structures may be able to continue to act in its absence, as shown by the ability of a deafferented animal to demonstrate a wide range of motor activity. The afferent information on the state of affairs at the periphery appears to be utilized to interact with motor command signals at many levels of the nervous system, from the motoneurons upward, so that no motor center should be considered without paying attention to the possibility of sensory feedback. Indeed, in some cases it may merely be a matter of verbal definition or of history whether a given central structure is thought of as sensory or motor; for example, a structure such as the Ia inhibitory interneuron may be thought of as sensory by virtue of its lying on a reflex arc, or as motor by virtue of its lying on a route to the motoneurons from a higher center. Neuron types or even whole nuclei may well only reveal their function when appropriate experiments can be designed to study the interplay upon them of processed sensory messages and coded motor commands. Thus a knowledge of the muscle receptors themselves and, more particularly, the messages that they send to the CNS and how these depend on fusimotor activity is widely accepted as an essential prelude to the understanding of much of the central side of motor control.

Only the periphery is discussed in this chapter.

Before turning to detail it should be emphasized that there is no single function for the muscle afferents, and that the CNS may well use the same message simultaneously for several quite different purposes; for example, both for reflex load compensation and for sensory awareness. Moreover, much the same sort of information provided by the receptors in different muscles or in different species may be utilized rather differently by a given level of the CNS. A particular challenge is provided by the occurrence of a wealth of spindles in the extraocular muscles of certain species, including humans. These spindles seem to have nothing to do with the load compensation which is so ubiquitous a function of spindles in limb muscles, because this does not occur for the eye (116). Instead, it must be assumed that they provide for regulatory mechanisms, possibly cerebellar, upon which we can only speculate but which hint at their importance by the very high density of spindles in these muscles.

In the past 20 years the structure and function of muscle receptors has received almost continuous attention in symposia, monographs, handbooks, and reviews. Therefore particular attention has been given to the more recent work and how it has grown out of earlier views. Reviews of the earlier work that reveal the progressive evolution of thinking can be found in the following sources: The Hong Kong Symposium of 1961 (14); Matthews' review of 1964 (135); the Stockholm Symposium of 1965 (86); Granit's book of 1970 (87); Matthews' book of 1972 (137); Stein's review of 1974 (171); Hunt's book of 1974 (103); the Tokyo symposium of 1975 (96); and Murthy's review of 1978 (144), which contains references on the reflex and central excitation of γ-motoneurons, but is not discussed in this chapter (but see the chapter by Baldissera, Hultborn, and Illert in this *Handbook*). The recent contributions provided by human microneurography were reviewed in 1979 by Vallbo et al. (182a), the originators of the technique. A remarkably comprehensive bibliography of some 2,500 references relating to muscle receptors, but not to their central actions, has been prepared for work up to 1975 by Eldred and his colleagues (70, 71), without text but with the full title of each paper. A more selective approach is taken in this chapter, but certain key ideas are developed in the context of background information to set the scene and to make the current position comprehensible to those who come with little previous detailed reading of the subject.

TENDON ORGANS

In this chapter discussion is devoted to the muscle spindles and, except for the following few comments, ignores the tendon organs because the scene is changing slowly and there is little serious controversy. Excellent reviews are available (87, 103, 137). But the neglect in this chapter should not be taken to disparage the role of the tendon organs in motor control, which on the basis of their number and the large size of their afferent fibers must be as essential as that of the spindles. The role of the tendon organs has been further emphasized by the recognition in the past decade that, viewed in terms of muscle action, their mechanical threshold is very low. They are excited to discharge quite briskly by the tetanic contraction of single motor units and, indeed, probably by the contraction of just a single one of the 10–20 muscle fibers that insert upon a fascicle bearing a tendon organ (98, 111, 176). The older view that they had a high threshold was based simply on their responses to passive stretch of the whole muscle, when many fail to be excited by a stretch falling within the physiological range of movement, especially under static conditions (99, 173, 174). As simple mechanical considerations show, a passive stretch of the cat soleus muscle producing some 500 g in the whole tendon would produce no more tension on a tendon organ fascicle than the 50 mg produced by a single contracting muscle fiber (29).

The sampling provided by the array of tendon organs in a limb muscle is probably wide enough to include virtually every motor unit at least once (111, 159). It can therefore be assumed that the summed output of the Ib-afferents from the tendon organs provides the CNS with a continuous averaged measure of the tension in a muscle. There is, however, no simple general relation between the tension provided by a motor unit and the increase in tendon organ discharge (90, 110, 169, 176). The summed Ib discharge from a contracting muscle, however, can be confidently presumed to provide a statistically acceptable signal related to mean tension, though not necessarily on a linear scale. Preference is possibly given to the recruitment of new motor units rather than to increasing the development of tension by the motor units that are already active (173). This overall measure, like the signal provided by individual Golgi tendon organs, sums the tension produced by muscle fibers of widely differing contractile properties (111, 159). The tendon organs show a comparatively low sensitivity to large dynamic stimuli over and above that shown to the same tension applied in the steady state (132, 170), so to a first approximation they signal tension per se rather than the rate of change of tension. For small signals the transfer function of the tendon organs seems to be rather similar to that of the spindle endings (2). Thus for practical purposes the tendon organs may be thought of as contraction receptors with a low enough threshold to be involved in the continuous signaling of the effect of muscle contraction in developing tension, and hence in the control of this essential facet of muscle action (see the chapter by Houk and Rymer in this *Handbook*). Because of the force-velocity properties of muscle, as well as the occurrence of fatigue, there is no constant 1:1 relation between motor firing and the development of contractile tension, so the tendon organs provide a unique source of information to the CNS in this respect. There is no longer any support for the older view that the main function of tendon organs is to provide the afferent limb of an inhibitory safety mechanism that reflexly shuts off muscle contraction whenever tension becomes dangerously high; indeed, there is little firm evidence that this ever occurs at all.

STRUCTURE OF MUSCLE SPINDLES

Classic View

What may be termed the classic picture of spindle structure was provided largely by Sherrington (167) and by Ruffini (161) working independently but along congruent lines in the 1890s. Their view of the internal functional "wiring" of the muscle spindle was accepted virtually without modification for over half a century, throughout which it sufficed as the basis for thought about what was known of the physiology of the muscle spindle and its role in motor regulation. Change was initiated around 1960 as it came to be recognized that the intrafusal muscle fibers should be divided into two distinct groups, the nuclear-bag and nuclear-chain fibers, and that these might be controlled somewhat independently by the CNS. The position is now one of considerably greater complexity than the classic picture and one in which agreement on all the details is yet to be reached.

The classic picture, which still provides a secure starting point for understanding, is epitomized in Ruffini's drawing of the central region of the muscle spindle, which is shown in Figure 1 (161). Some 4–6 intrafusal muscle fibers run in parallel along the length of the spindle; they are enclosed by a capsule in the heavily innervated central region where they are separated from the spindle by fluid. The centrally placed primary ending in the cat has such prominent spirals around the intrafusal fibers that Ruffini named it the annulospiral ending; this is much less pronounced in humans (59, 178). Sherrington in 1894 (167) showed that the primary ending survived deefferentation and was thus an afferent terminal. The secondary ending, or endings, for there may be more than one in a spindle, are supplied by slightly finer medullated fibers than the primary ending, and lie to the side of it; however, on average there is only about one secondary ending per primary ending because some spindles contain none. They also were considered to be afferent terminals on the basis of their morphology, which was quite unlike that of any known motor ending. To emphasize their difference from the primary ending they were named flower-spray endings. In addition, plate endings were recognized that were, in general, like the end plates on extrafusal muscle fibers, but were rather larger and showed sufficient points of difference for Ruffini to suggest that they too were sensory. Ruffini's view was fortified by Sherrington's finding that unlike the extrafusal muscle fibers the spindle persisted with remarkably little change after section of the motor nerve, and so might perhaps not receive a motor innervation at all. A few years later, however, with the tracing of branches of ordinary motor nerve fibers to endings on the intrafusal muscle fibers of certain lower animals (lizard, snake, frog), it became accepted that the plate endings of the mammal were also motor, as has since been amply confirmed. The final lease of life of the classic picture was provided by a well-documented reiteration by Barker in 1948 (13), which attracted widespread attention because the γ-efferent system was just then becoming amenable to direct electrophysiological investigation.

Recognition of Motor Duality

The limitations of the classic picture suddenly became apparent in the late 1950s as a result of several new observations. Within a few years it was evident that the classic view needed to be altered to incorporate additional features on the motor side. First, Cöers and Durand (57) studied histochemically the location of cholinesterase within the spindle and found that the stained segments of the intrafusal fibers far exceeded the regions where the plate endings mainly lay; they suggested that some or all of Ruffini's fine flower-spray terminals might be motor rather than sensory. Second, Boyd (30) and Cooper and Daniel (59) independently stressed that the difference of both diameter and nuclear arrangement of different intrafusal fibers was so great that it seemed appropriate to divide them into two separate morphological categories; these were named the nuclear-bag fibers and the nuclear-chain fibers on the basis of the arrangement of the nuclei in the central equatorial regions of the fibers. Third, in deafferented spindles Boyd (30) found that some motor fibers, which were not sympathetic in origin, terminated in a fine "network" arrangement, which was quite distinct from the classic plate endings that were also present.

By 1964 the diagram of Figure 2 provided a coherent

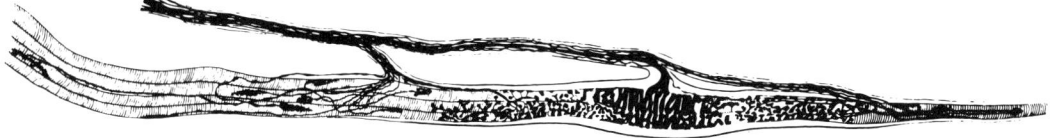

PLATES   SECONDARY PRIMARY   SECONDARY

FIG. 1. Classic picture of muscle spindle as seen by Ruffini in 1898 (161). Retouched.

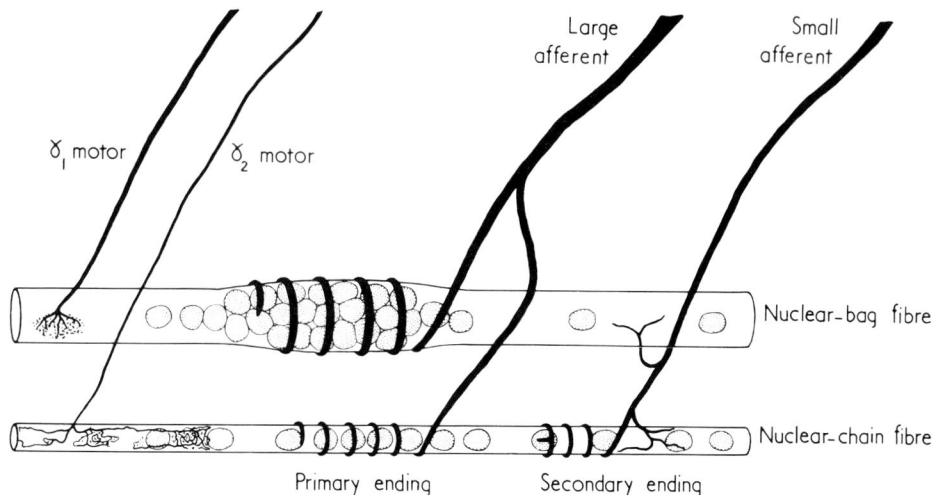

FIG. 2. Simplified diagram of central region of muscle spindle as it was recognized in 1964, largely on the basis of Boyd's work (30), with 2 types of intrafusal muscle fiber, each with its own motor innervation, and 2 kinds of afferent axon. [From Matthews (137).]

simplification of the new anatomy, with two types of intrafusal muscle fiber instead of one; but disagreement persisted as to whether the motor innervation to the bag and chain fibers was provided by separate axons, as held by Boyd (30), or whether it was commonly shared, as held by Barker (14). Debate also continued as to whether the plate endings and the diffuse motor endings were each restricted to one type of intrafusal muscle fiber, as in Figure 2, or whether either kind of termination might be found on either kind of fiber. The uncertainties resulted from the near impossibility of using conventional light microscopy to trace the course of individual fine axons throughout their length because they intermingled with so many other axons. It should be realized that Figure 2 is grossly simplified in a number of respects: it shows only the central millimeter or so of the spindle out of a total of 5-6 mm; it shows only one intrafusal fiber of either kind, whereas there are commonly 2-3 bag fibers and 4-6 chain fibers; it shows only 2 motor fibers, whereas there may be 10 or more motor axons entering the spindle and then branching, though some of these may be derived from stem axons that branch before the spindle is reached.

For the next decade debate continued along essentially the same lines, sharpened by the desire to relate the morphological arrangements to the newly established functional dichotomy of the static and dynamic fusimotor axons. The diffuse motor ending was, with general agreement at a symposium (14), renamed the trail ending as proposed by Barker and Ip (20), and its appearance was more fully described along with that of the plate ending. Careful tracing of motor axons within the muscle nerve (1) showed that there was no clear relation between their diameter in the nerve trunk and that at the point of entry to the spindle, so that the latter could not provide a basis for classifying motor axons into two different groups as had been hoped (30). The plate endings were subdivided morphologically into p_1 and p_2 plates (22). The p_1 plates resembled extrafusal motor end plates in having a well-nucleated sole plate and marked extrajunctional folding, and on a few occasions were shown to be derived from branches of the motor axons supplying extrafusal muscle fibers possibly corresponding to the terminations of the β- and γ-axons, respectively (15, 22). The p_2 plates were rather larger than the p_1 plates, lacked a sole plate, and had appreciably less junctional folding. The trail endings consist of nonmedullated ramifications varying in length from 10 to 200 μm and with a variety of points of possible synaptic contact. The sharpness of the morphological division of these terminations remains open to debate; the extremes are certainly distinct, but intermediate forms may give rise to confusion, and the appearance of an ending may perhaps be related partly to the type of intrafusal fiber upon which it lies. Thus for the time being it seems best to eschew categorical statements about the precise statistical distribution of the different types of endings on the different types of intrafusal fiber. However, it seems that all three types of ending may be found on either bag or chain intrafusal fibers (15), and on occasion a given intrafusal fiber—whether bag or chain—may receive both a plate ending and a trail ending (see Fig. 70 in ref. 15). The matter is currently being investigated electron microscopically and is further complicated by the realization that it now has to be examined in light of the existence of two separate types of nuclear-bag fiber, as discussed in the next subsection.

Subdivision of Nuclear-Bag Fibers

In the early 1960s the chief interest was to establish that the bag and chain fibers were distinct morphological entities and thus likely to have different functional roles. Once this had been largely agreed on, attention shifted to the question of whether there were intermediate types of fiber, because histochemical techniques in particular showed a range of staining reactions. Yellin (184), for example, divided intrafusal fibers into four types on the basis of their staining for phosphorylase and succinic dehydrogenase. The question that then arose was whether such subdivisions were of functional significance; the initial reaction was usually one of caution. But over the past few years the evidence has strengthened that the bag fibers should be divided into two types, both morphologically and functionally separate. These are now usually called the bag_1 and bag_2 fibers. These terms, introduced by Ovalle and Smith in 1972 (146), were based on the density of the staining in cat and monkey of intrafusal myofibrillar ATPase after preincubation for 15 min with mild solutions of acid (pH 4.4) or alkali (pH 10.4). The chain fibers behaved homogenously and all had an ATPase that resisted alkali incubation (alkali stable), but that was inactivated by acid pretreatment (acid labile). Some bag fibers (the bag_1 fibers) showed the inverse pattern, with an ATPase that was alkali labile but acid stable, while others (the bag_2 fibers) contained an ATPase that survived pretreatment at either pH (acid and base stable); in addition, after acid treatment when the ATPase of both survived, that of the bag_2 fibers stained much more strongly than that of the bag_1 fibers.

Two further points of morphological difference between the bag_1 and bag_2 fibers have now been established. First, in the cat the bag_2 intrafusal fibers have prominent thick elastic fibers that run longitudinally along the polar regions and continue past the ends of the intrafusal fibers into the main muscle; the bag_1 fibers have rather few elastic fibers (80), and the chain fibers contain fewer still (60). Aside from the mechanical interest, the density of elastic fibers also provides a rapid and convenient way of identifying the fiber type. Thus after an electrophysiological experiment on an isolated spindle, neither detailed histochemistry nor electron microscopy is necessary for fiber identification. Second, Banks et al. (12) have examined the two types of bag fiber electron microscopically and correlated their findings with the histochemical identification of the fibers made on separate serial sections of the same spindles from rabbit, rat, and cat. The difference lay in the strength of development of the M line (the dark band in the center of the H zone in the middle of the sarcomere), which in a given section is always much more prominent in the bag_2 than in the bag_1 fibers. They distinguished a fully developed M line, termed M-type appearance, which is the characteristic of the nuclear-chain fibers throughout their length, from "an M line consisting of two faint parallel lines," which was termed dM-type appearance. The bag_2 fibers had M appearance in the polar regions, indistinguishable from that of the chain fibers, but this shaded off to dM appearance in the equatorial region of the fibers. All the bag_1 fibers were the dM type in rat spindles, but in rabbit and cat they showed a region of M-type appearance well out at the poles of the spindle. The regional variation in the strength of the line along the length of a given intrafusal fiber complicates comparison of the two kinds of fiber and raises the interesting possibility that the contractility of the fibers might also change along their length. Nonetheless, the differences appear consistent and place the bag_2 fibers closer than the bag_1 fibers to the chain fibers, which is consistent with the finding that both bag_2 and chain fibers possess a high activity of alkali-stable ATPase. Again, longitudinal variations in the intensity of various histochemical reactions was noted. Banks et al. (12) compared their findings with others in the literature and noted that in many papers prior to 1977 the terminology was irresolvably self-contradictory in terms of the present classification, a situation related to the fact that previously it had not been possible to correlate histochemical and electron microscopic (EM) observations on one and the same spindle. For example, in earlier work on the rabbit (21) what was then called an intermediate fiber on general morphological and histochemical grounds would now be classified as a bag_1 fiber, whereas on EM study the same term was then applied to what would now be classified as a bag_2 fiber. Thus the literature on the early attempts to subdivide the bag fibers is fraught with pitfalls for the unwary reader. The morphological evidence for the subdivision of the bag fibers is supported by physiological experiments showing differences in their contractility and in their innervation, which are discussed in subsection *Intrafusal Destination of Static and Dynamic Axons*, p. 203.

FUNCTIONAL PROPERTIES OF PRIMARY AND
SECONDARY SPINDLE AFFERENT ENDINGS

Different Responses to Various Stimuli

The morphological division made in 1898 by Ruffini achieved functional meaning in 1961 when Cooper (58) found that the well-known sensitivity of primary endings to large dynamic stimuli was not present to nearly the same extent in the equally numerous secondary endings. The classification of the endings was made according to the conduction velocity of their afferent fibers; fibers conducting at over 72 m/s were ascribed to primary endings and those below to secondary endings. The basis for this division was Hunt's (102) demonstration for the cat hindlimb of a bimodality of the distribution of conduction velocities of spindle afferent fibers (distinguished from those from tendon organs on the basis of their behavior during muscle contraction), coupled with the classic observation that at the point of entry to the spindle the axons of primary endings are usually considerably thicker than those of secondary endings. Cooper's findings with ramp stretches were soon amply validated under a wide range of conditions (92, 134, 160). The essential result is that for any large movement the absolute change in firing of the primary ending when movement starts or stops is much greater than that of the secondary ending, even though both endings may be firing at much the same rate under the static conditions that precede or follow movement. A particular example is illustrated in Figure 3, and there can be little doubt that this difference in behavior is an important feature in the signaling of the same peripheral event provided by the two endings. In general, it is tempting to suppose that the difference in relative sensitivity of the two endings to static and to dynamic stimuli enables the central nervous system (CNS), by comparison of the discharges, to decide on the instantaneous value of the length of the muscle, whether it is moving or still, and on the velocity and direction of any movement. If only a single channel of sensory information were available none of this could be decided without making very considerable demands, either upon the memory of previous conditions (as done in inertial navigation) or upon freedom from noise in the neural signals (as would be required if a velocity signal were to be obtained by differentiating a length signal).

One way of assessing the dynamic sensitivity of an ending is to measure the so-called dynamic index, which is defined as the drop in the firing rate that occurs between the terminal part of the dynamic phase of a ramp stretch at constant velocity and that found 0.5 s later on the subsequent "hold" phase of the stretch (62, 114, 134). For a given velocity of stretching this measure is regularly larger for primary than for secondary endings; its absolute value also increases more rapidly for the primary ending when the velocity of stretching is increased. In contrast, under static conditions measurement of either the absolute value of firing or of the position sensitivity (impulses/s firing per mm increase in stretch) shows relatively little difference for the two kinds of ending for large stretches (115, 123, 134). As might be expected from the effect of stretching, the inverse effect of releasing

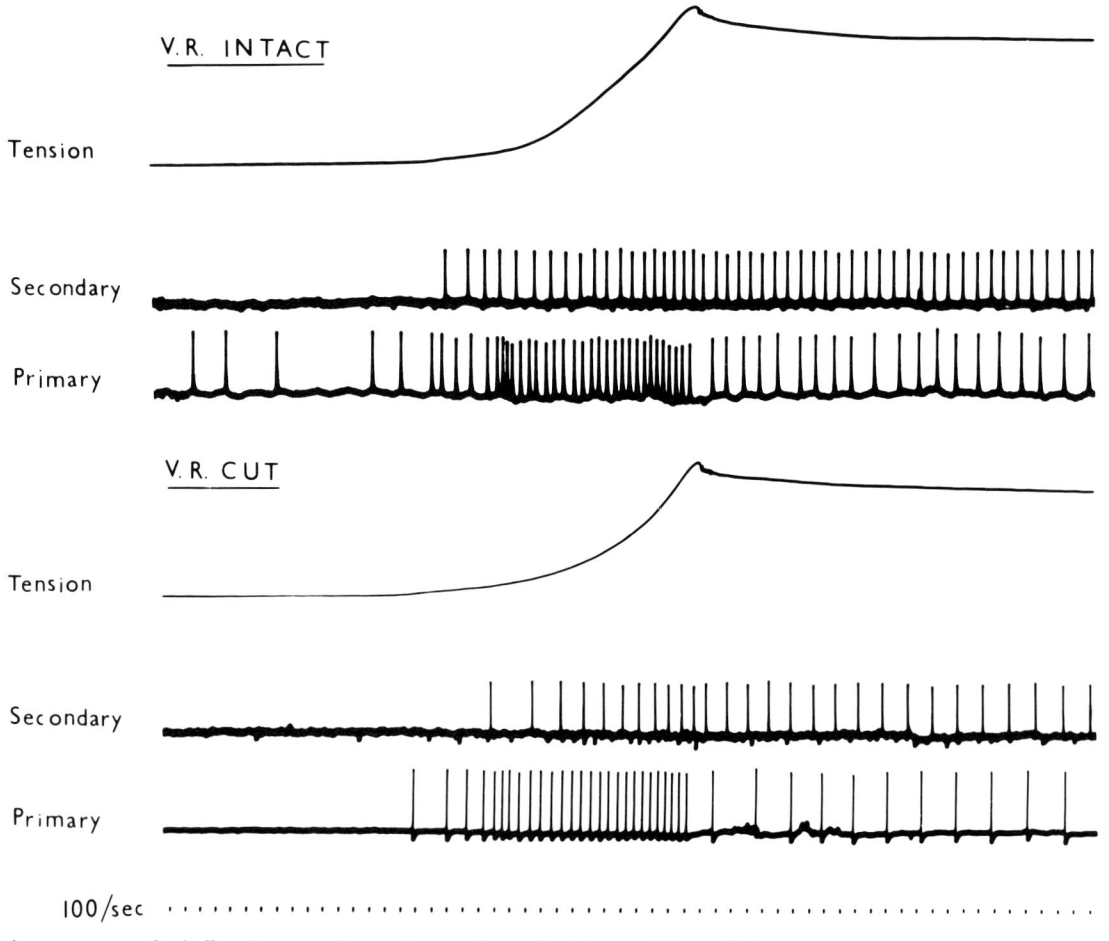

FIG. 3. Contrasting responses of spindle primary and secondary endings of cat to a rapidly applied stretch to the soleus (approximately 14 mm at 70 mm/s). Responses shown in both presence and absence of tonic fusimotor activity of decerebrate cat. *Bottom*, responses of endings when deefferented by ventral root (V.R.) section. *Top*, responses of the same endings when ventral roots were intact and were tonically biased by spontaneous fusimotor activity. [From Matthews (137).]

a muscle is greater for the primary ending than for the secondary ending, and the former falls silent much more readily than the latter. Likewise, sinusoidal stretching of whatever amplitude elicits a much greater difference in firing during the stretch and release phases of the cycle for the primary than for the secondary ending. Again, a brief tap of the type used to elicit a tendon jerk induces a much brisker burst of firing from the primary ending than from the secondary ending which may remain almost unaffected and simply continue with its preexisting discharge. These contrasting forms of behavior are illustrated diagrammatically in Figure 4.

Of particular interest from the practical point of view of studying synaptic connectivity is that the parameters of a brief stretch can be set to selectively excite the primary ending and to have relatively little action on the secondary ending or the Golgi tendon organ; this is accomplished by applying the stretch to a noncontracting muscle and making the pulse both sufficiently brief (about 5 ms) and sufficiently small (about 30–50 μm) (131, 175, 177). Rather similarly, high frequency vibration at 100–500 Hz applied longitudinally by attaching a severed tendon to a vibrator can produce highly selective activation of primary endings and, in a well-stretched muscle, amplitudes of 25–50 μm can induce the majority of the primary endings of the cat soleus to follow the vibration with 1 spike/cycle (driving) without significantly increasing the mean frequency of firing of secondary endings or Golgi tendon organs (39). However, selectivity of action is not nearly so well achieved when the muscle is contracting; the Golgi tendon organs may then show an appreciable response to vibration. Secondary endings may be excited when the vibrator is placed on the belly of the muscle directly over the spindle (28), though there is every reason to believe that their threshold is still a good deal higher than that of the primary endings. Thus it is scarcely surprising that in the normal human subject microneuronography shows that muscle vibration, quite apart from its action on cutaneous afferents, may not be completely selective among the muscle afferents for the Ia endings (47). In line with this differential sensitivity of the primary and secondary endings to discharge extra impulses on vibrating at some 10–50 μm amplitude, even smaller amplitudes of vibration modulate the time of firing of impulses of the primary endings much more than that of the secondary endings. This can be assessed quantitatively by computer analysis and is 30 or more times greater for the primary ending [Fig. 6; (64, 138)]; indeed, an amplitude of movement of only 0.1 μm at frequencies of 100–500 Hz applied to the 5-cm-long soleus of the cat gives measurable modulation of the probability of firing of the primary ending in relation to the phase of the cycle.

Another intriguing and unexplained difference between the two kinds of ending, which might perhaps be related to their differential sensitivity to high frequency transients, is that the secondary ending fires its impulses in a much more regular stream than does the primary ending, even though the latter has long been noted as an example of a rather regularly firing sense organ. When the spindle is deefferented and the muscle held at a constant length, the coefficient of variation of the interspike-interval distribution is 0.02 and 0.06 for the secondary and primary endings, respectively (139); the value for each is increased about fourfold in the presence of the tonic fusimotor activity of the decerebrate cat. Because the variability may be considered to be noise, the secondary ending must provide an appreciably more accurate signal of the length of the muscle. However, the variability of the discharge of the primary may be advantageous as it may help improve the signaling of dynamic events; when these events contain a rhythmic component comparable to the mean frequency of firing of the spike train then variability decreases the tendency of the spikes to become "phase-locked" upon this component of the stimulus with consequent interference with the signaling of the other components of the stimulus (172).

The simplest view of all these findings is that the secondary ending provides a signal that chiefly indicates the instantaneous value of the length of the muscle, albeit with a bias and probably a calibration set by fusimotor activity (see subsection GAIN OF SPINDLE TO DYNAMIC STIMULI, p. 216). The primary ending, on the other hand, provides a signal that combines components relating to the instantaneous values of both the length and the velocity of stretching and possibly also to the acceleration, with the precise proportions of each of these values in the signal varying with the degree and type of fusimotor activity. It has been clear since the earliest studies (136) that the velocity signal, as assessed crudely by the dynamic index, increases far less rapidly than in direct proportion to velocity, and that an appreciable dynamic

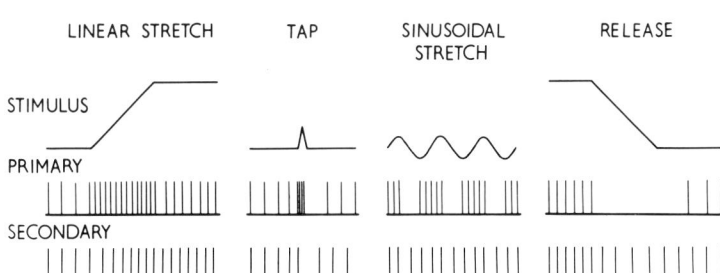

FIG. 4. Diagrammatic comparison of responses of "typical" primary and secondary endings to various stimuli of large amplitude applied in the absence of fusimotor activity. [From Matthews (135).]

index persists with velocities of stretching as low as 0.1 mm/s; this relation is illustrated in log-log plots of dynamic index against velocity, which have the effect of further linearizing the response (164). It seems possible for a physiologist equipped with a suitable calibration table to use prerecorded spindle discharges to deduce retrospectively the mechanical parameters of ramp and other stimuli, but it is still far from certain that this is how the CNS looks at the spindle discharges from the point of view of motor control; it should be especially noted that the dynamic index is not a measure that can assist in ongoing motor regulation because it can only be determined after the event.

Mode of Summation of Signal Components

A current issue is whether spindle firing is best viewed as representing the arithmetic sum of a number of components related to physically separate parameters of the stimulus (i.e., length, velocity). Dissent has recently been voiced by Rymer et al. (162) on the basis of measurement of the firing of both kinds of afferent during a prolonged ramp stretch applied to the soleus muscle of the decerebrate cat with spontaneous fusimotor bias. Under these conditions the instantaneous frequency of firing of either kind of ending was considered best expressed by an equation of the form

$$\text{frequency} = K(x - x_o) V^f$$

where x and V are the instantaneous values of length and velocity, and K, x_o, and f are constants. The difference between primary and secondary endings was then found to reside in differences in the gain constant K, rather than differences in the velocity exponent f as might have been expected. In other words, viewed in this way there is no difference between the two kinds of ending in their relative sensitivity to velocity and to length. They also noted that the velocity dependence of the primary ending was "quite modest" because the value of f was about 0.3; however, these results are in line with previous findings and need not prevent determination of the velocity at a given length, provided the calibration of the ending is known (nonlinear compression extends the range of values that can be signaled). But the suggestion that in the messages from the spindles the relation between velocity and length is multiplicative rather than additive considerably increases the difficulty of considering the situation in common-sense mechanical terms. However, the above equation has yet to be tested under a wide variety of conditions and until then it may be suspected to have a limited applicability and to be inadequate to support wide generalizations on the roles of the endings. For example, the equation completely fails to describe the continued firing of a spindle ending during release of a muscle, however slow, because the velocity is then negative. Nor does it describe the firing that occurs when a muscle is simply held at a constant length when the velocity is zero. The subjective experience of steadily continuing limb movement when vibration is applied to a stationary muscle in conscious humans (85, 141) strongly suggests that at some levels the CNS may interpret high frequency Ia firing in terms of movement (velocity) and separately from position. Using large-amplitude triangular wave forms of stretch and release, Lennerstand and Thoden (123, 125) subdivided the response into various components (length and two velocity responses with different time constants), which they treated as additive rather than multiplicative although one of them (the slow velocity response) was related to both length and velocity. It seems unlikely that the last word has been said, and formal mathematical descriptions of behavior are of limited value, because normal biological variability is such that the same data could well be fitted by equations of different form and thus of considerably different theoretical significance.

Amplitude Nonlinearity

The more fundamental difficulty in comprehensively describing the relation between the frequency of firing of the afferents and the parameters of the stimulus is that the endings, particularly the primary endings, behave nonlinearly in yet another respect and markedly change their behavior with increased amplitude of the stimulus. In 1969 two separate groups (138, 148) showed that, although the primary ending did respond in a reasonably linear fashion to small sinusoidal stretches (below about 100 μm at 1 Hz), it became much less sensitive and the phase of the response changed when the amplitude of movement was further increased. Within the linear range the depth of afferent modulation increases in direct proportion to the stimulus, but beyond this the increase becomes progressively smaller. The departure from linearity with increasing amplitude has since been studied in more detail both with sinusoidal stretching (100) and with ramp stretches of progressively increasing amplitude (94). The sensitivity of the primary ending within the linear range (expressed as impulses/s firing per unit extension) may be one or two orders of magnitude (i.e., 10–100 times) greater than that shown with larger stretches; for example, for small stretches applied dynamically the sensitivity of the passive primary ending may be 100–800 impulses/s per mm whereas for static stretches of several millimeters the position sensitivity of the primary ending is typically below 5 impulses/s per mm. Because of this high sensitivity of the primary ending within its linear range, a movement of 50 μm at 1 Hz of a 5-cm soleus may lead to very appreciable modulation of its firing (e.g., 20–30 impulses/s, around a similar resting discharge). Thus the nonlinear behavior of the primary ending seems to be a design feature of interest; it allows the primary ending to increase its versatility by signaling the occurrence of small stretches without being prevented, by saturation of its limited firing range, from also signaling the magnitude of large stretches. Moreover, it is especially important from the functional point of view that after a stretch of large amplitude the primary ending can reset itself so that the high value of sensitivity manifests itself again within a few seconds of the achievement of a new length; it seems quite likely that the resetting could also take place continuously during sufficiently slow movements, but the matter has yet to be tested experimentally.

The termination of the linear range of primary endings is probably brought about mechanically by the sudden yielding of the poles of the intrafusal fibers so that the stretch is no longer so fully transmitted to the sensory terminals. The poles of the fibers are thought to show a static friction type of behavior (stiction) with a high rigidity until movement suddenly begins because, it is suggested (40, 94, 137), of the existence of relatively stable bonds between the actin and myosin filaments in the sarcomere. Such stiction also seems implicated in the "initial burst" of higher frequency firing that a primary ending may show at the beginning of a period of dynamic stretching as in Figure 5 (40, 114, 134) and which, by careful analysis of the response to ramps of different velocity, Hasan and Houk (94) showed to occur at a given degree of stretch rather than at a given time from the beginning of stretching. The peak frequency that occurs in the initial burst increases with the velocity of stretching and thus, under most experimental conditions, with the initial acceleration. Whether this initial response should be thought of as an acceleration response has thus been hotly debated (94, 126, 163, 166), but in the absence of knowledge of how commonly it occurs under physiological conditions and what the CNS makes of it the matter seems largely semantic. The initial burst is still shown by isolated spindles separated from all extrafusal muscle fibers (104, 105) and so cannot be attributed solely to the nonlinear behavior of the main muscle as has been suggested (166), though this may perhaps contribute to the effect (156). An ending under steady fusimotor drive shows a less marked initial burst than a passive ending (114). The burst of the passive ending can be greatly enhanced by a preceding period of fusimotor stimulation applied with the muscle at the initial length (40, 155), which may also lead to a prolonged increase in the mean rate of Ia firing at the initial length (40, 107, 108). Thus it seems possible that the burst seen in some spindle afferents in the conscious animal at the beginning of their being stretched by the antagonistic muscle, such as during chewing and walking, may represent just such a potentiation by preceding fusimotor activity and thus make the whole matter of functional importance (84). A relatively slow intrafusal relaxation could, however, equally contribute to such effects (89).

Linear Responses to Sinusoidal Stretching

Studies with sinusoidal stretching restricted to their linear range of movement have demonstrated two further points of interest in the relative behavior of primary and secondary endings (138, 148). These are illustrated in Figure 6, which compares the frequency-response curves of primary and secondary endings that are influenced by steady fusimotor activity in the decerebrate cat. First, the absolute value of the sensitivity of the primary ending is much greater than that of the secondary ending at all frequencies of stretching, including at the low frequencies where the curves are approximately flat. The flatness suggests that in this range the endings are responding predominantly to the stimulus of length and that the absolute value of the stimulus of velocity is functionally unimportant; a significant sensitivity to an increase in velocity should be shown by an increase in the value of sensitivity with an increase in frequency, because the sensitivity is expressed in terms of the length change and for a

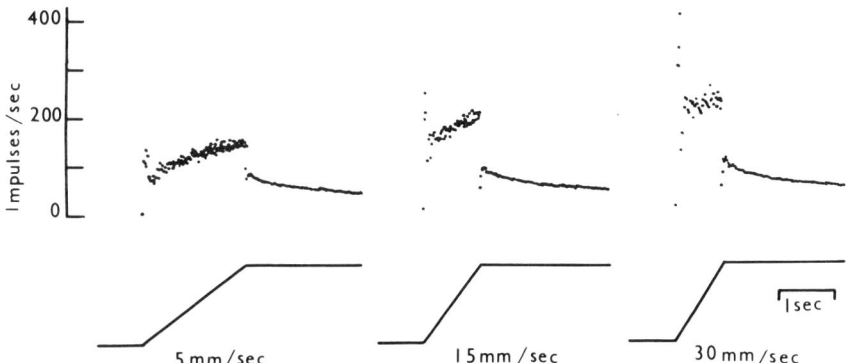

FIG. 5. Effect of increasing the velocity of stretching on the initial burst given by a primary ending at beginning of stretch and on the more prolonged velocity response. A 6-mm stretch was applied to a deefferented soleus muscle of cat. Time calibration applies only to the static phases of the response; dynamic phases are on slightly expanded time scales, which may be deduced from the parameters of stretching. [From Matthews (137).]

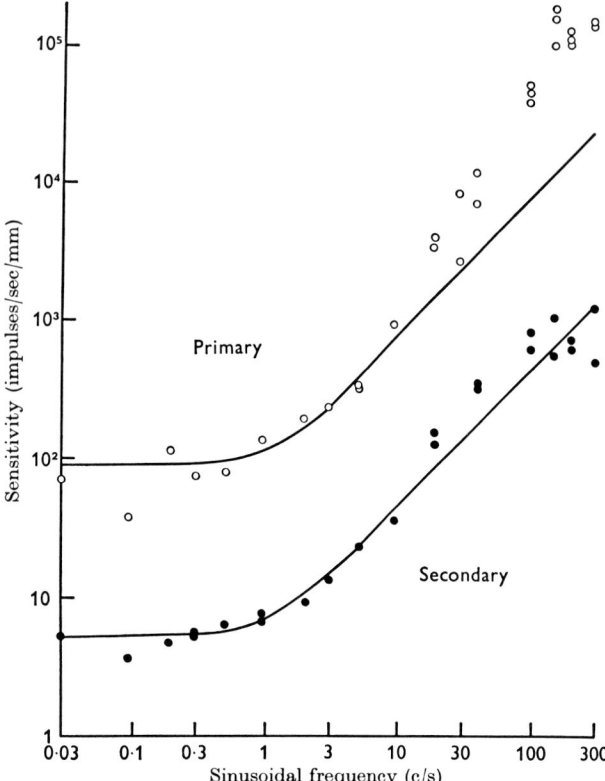

FIG. 6. Comparison of the sensitivity to sinusoidal stretching within the linear range of a primary and a secondary ending studied together over a wide range of frequencies of stretching measured in cycles per second (Hz). The sensitivity at any frequency is defined as the amplitude of the afferent response, considered as a sinusoidal modulation of firing (measured in impulses per second) divided by the amplitude of stretching (measured in millimeters). The endings were being tonically biased by the spontaneous fusimotor activity of the decerebrate cat. The continuous lines represent the vector sum of responses to the length component of the stimulus (dominant for the horizontal portion at low frequencies) and to the velocity component (dominant for the diagonal portion of the line at high frequencies). The same curve transposed vertically approximately fits both endings over a considerable region. This shows that in the linear range they differ in their absolute sensitivity, rather than in the ratio of their length to their velocity sensitivity. The upward deviation of the points for the primary ending above 10–20 Hz can be taken as showing an "acceleration sensitivity," but at these frequencies the linear range is only a few μm in extent so the finding cannot be transferred to stretches of appreciable extent. As a very rough approximation the linear range at any frequency can be deduced from the graphs by assuming that it corresponds to a modulation of firing of some 15 impulses/s, so that at 1 c/s it was around 150 μm for the primary and 2 mm for the secondary ending. [From Matthews and Stein (138).]

given amplitude of movement the velocity increases with frequency. But it should be immediately noted that the response of the endings at these low frequencies is still phase-advanced on the stimulus by some 30°; moreover, such phase-advances persist for the deefferented endings down to frequencies of 0.001 Hz, i.e., 1 cycle/16 min (93). Thus the endings remain very aware that some movement is still occurring and that the conditions are not truly static. In deefferented endings the difference in sensitivity of primary and secondary endings tends to be less marked than in the decerebrate preparation (64, 93); this is because the sensitivity of the secondary ending in the linear range is rather greater than in Figure 6; the lower value in the decerebrate preparation may be presumed to be the result of fusimotor activity distributed among several different axons and thus may perhaps be regarded as the more normal. Figure 7 illustrates the great effect this difference in sensitivity of the two kinds of ending has on their response to the small irregularities of movement that occur during a reflexly induced isotonic contraction.

The second point to be noted in Figure 6 is that the sensitivity for both the primary and the secondary ending begins to rise upward with frequency at much the same region, namely at 1–2 Hz. Treated most simply the value of this "corner frequency" provides an indication of the relative sensitivity of an ending to the stimulus of increasing length and increasing velocity when both are applied dynamically. Thus according to this data, within their linear range the primary and secondary endings do not show gross differences in relative sensitivity to length and velocity for frequencies up to 5–10 Hz. However, at higher frequencies the sensitivity of the primary ending does increase more rapidly than that of the secondary ending, showing that they are not identical in their sensitivity to the higher differentials of the length stimulus. Moreover, at frequencies above 2 Hz the primary ending shows appreciably more phase-advance in its response (148). These qualitative observations are entirely borne out and formalized by fitting transfer functions with a number of constants to the data (148, 149), which, incidentally, are remarkably similar for cat and for isolated human spindles (150). Thus all the data for small stretches applied over a physiologically important frequency range show that the primary and secondary endings differ principally in the absolute value of their sensitivity rather than in their relative sensitivity to length and to velocity. This finding contrasts the simpler view of their responses to large ramp stretches, but as already indicated the interpretation is surrounded by pitfalls so there is not necessarily a conflict in the findings. Attempts to deduce the large signal responses from the small signal responses by application of a linear attenuation factor have met with frustration (51, 93), showing that the nonlinearities indeed play a crucial part in determining the precise neural response to any input wave form of appreciable amplitude.

It seems likely that the form of the small signal frequency-response curves reflects largely upon the transducing properties of the nerve terminals rather than upon any differences in the mechanical properties of the relevant intrafusal muscle fibers. The difference in absolute sensitivity may be partly related to the effectiveness with which the mechanical stimulus is transmitted to the nerve terminals, by virtue of the fact that the primary ending lies on a specialized

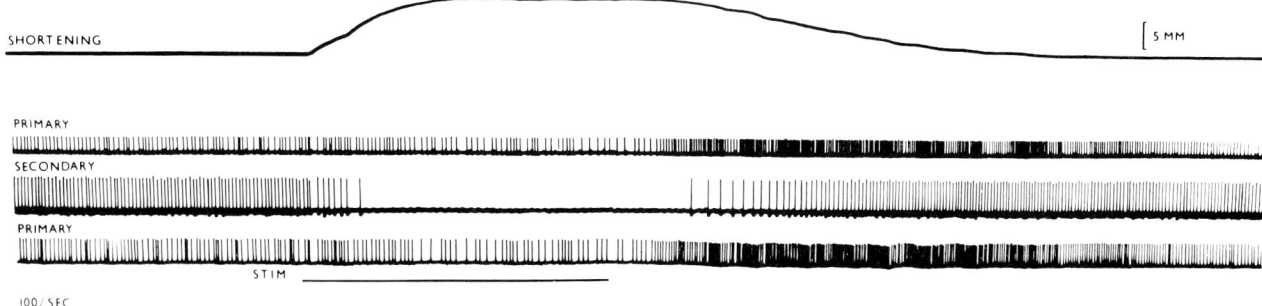

FIG. 7. Soleus muscle of decerebrate cat contracting in response to stimulation of contralateral peroneal nerve. Physiological manifestation of a high sensitivity of primary ending, but not of secondary ending, to small stretches. Sensitivity of primary ending is demonstrated by the fact that both of the 2 primary endings can be seen to respond in synchrony to the small irregularities occurring in a reflexly induced muscle contraction, which occurred under approximately isotonic conditions. Discharges of the 3 afferents were recorded simultaneously. [From Matthews (137).]

region of intrafusal fiber that lacks myofilaments (and thus any stable "stuck" bonds), while the secondary ending lies on an intrafusal region that is more nearly homogeneous with the rest of the fiber. This whole matter awaits detailed study in the isolated spindle. The marked nonlinear responses of the primary ending are, however, fairly generally felt to depend additionally on the mechanical factors introduced by the yielding of the intrafusal poles with larger stretches.

Assessment

In conclusion, from the point of view of the CNS, what seems to matter is that any truly static stimulus is signaled with approximately similar sensitivity by the two kinds of afferent ending, but the moment an element of movement is introduced the primary ending invariably demonstrates more sensitivity, irrespective of whether the movement is small or large and signaled linearly or nonlinearly. Moreover, under dynamic conditions the firing level of the primary ending signals the extent of a movement as well as indicating the fact of its occurrence. All these facts are relevant to understanding the role of the two kinds of ending in the higher regulation of movement and posture. What remains under debate is how far it remains useful or meaningful to talk of a difference in velocity sensitivity of the endings: whether, for example, the greater absolute effect of increasing the velocity of large stretches on the frequency of firing of the primary ending should be seen as a meaningfully greater velocity response, or whether attention should be focused on the fact that the proportional increase in the velocity response with increasing velocity is much more similar for the two kinds of ending, because such a large component of the dynamic response of the primary ending is attributable simply to the occurrence of movement and the resulting offset in its discharge (94). Given the complexities and the inherent nonlinearity of the behavior of the endings such problems do not appear close to resolution; they too easily become lost in semantics when they are pursued. But it remains appropriate to consider the primary ending more dynamically sensitive than the secondary ending and, in light of current restricted evidence, it probably remains helpful to continue to say that part of the difference in dynamic sensitivity to large stretches may be attributed to a greater velocity sensitivity of the primary ending, remembering that there may be a better way to express such a complex situation. The fact, already mentioned, that the subjective experience of muscle vibration, and thus a presumed excess Ia-afferent input, is one of movement, the velocity of which varies with the experimental conditions, is a cogent reason for feeling that the CNS can indeed extract the speed of muscle movement from the spindle messages quite independently of its assessment of muscle length (85, 141).

Possible Intermediate Endings

The differences so far described between primary and secondary endings have largely been based on the study of the cat soleus, particularly of endings that have been selected to show reasonably typical behavior with afferents lying well away from the putative dividing line of conduction velocity of 72 m/s. The question of to what extent endings with afferents conducting near the dividing line behave typically or whether they show intermediate types of behavior remains unanswered; equally, it requires to be established that primary and secondary endings in other muscles and in other species behave similarly and to be determined for each case where the dividing line between the conduction velocities of primary and secondary afferents should be placed. From a variety of studies it appears that the responses of the endings of the cat soleus have proved to be a good example on which to base the general case of an essential difference in the sensitivity of primary and secondary endings to dynamic stimuli, usually as assessed by measurement of the dynamic index. The same responses have been found for too many other cat muscles to require documentation, for human spindles both isolated from the body (145, 150) and in situ (47, 181), though the latter is without measurement of conduction velocity, for baboon spindles (52, 117, 118), and for sheep extraocular spindles (43). Some deviations from typical behavior appear attributable to the location of the spindle in question in relation to the region of a complex muscle that is only slightly extended by the applied stretch (183). The demonstration of bimodality in the afferent fiber spectrum (histogram of number of fibers vs. their diameter) usually shows the appropriate place to draw the line between primary and secondary afferents. Invariably, when it has proved possible to measure the afferent conduction velocity, the measured properties of the ending (notably the dynamic index) have proved to be graded more or less continuously with the conduction velocity of the axon so that those near the dividing line may show intermediate properties, as has been long appreciated for the soleus (134). However, provided that the fiber spectrum does show a well-marked bimodality it follows that the majority of spindle afferents come from endings with well-differentiated properties so that the minority with intermediate behavior may be held to be of lesser functional significance. Moreover it seems that in some cases endings that show intermediate behavior in the passive state (with fusimotor activity in abeyance), which is how they have normally been studied, should be considered to be "really" primary or "really" secondary endings on the basis of their behavior once the intrafusal muscle fibers are induced to contract. In the cat soleus, the intrafusal contraction elicited by the injection of succinylcholine (SCh) induces virtually all intermediate endings to declare themselves as either primary with a large dynamic index or as secondary with a small dynamic index (158); SCh preferentially excites the bag$_1$ fibers (80). The same result was obtained for spindles in the jaw-closing muscles of the cat (56), though in this case in the passive state there was no sign of bimodality in the histogram relating the number of endings observed to the value of their dynamic index, though bimodality appeared after the injection of SCh (in these experiments it was not feasible to measure afferent conduction velocity).

Spindles in the sheep extraocular muscles, however, prove to be something of an exception (43). There is the usual continuous statistical relation between dynamic index and conduction velocity, but there is no bimodality in the distribution of afferent conduction velocity. Intermediate fibers are thus in the majority whether they are classified on the basis of their behavior or on the basis of their conduction velocity. Moreover, in this case SCh did not bring out any bimodality of behavior as elsewhere, although the interpretation of the experiments is complicated by the fact that the SCh concurrently produced a contraction of the slow extrafusal muscle fibers that are present in this muscle. It may be concluded that for the usual limb muscles it remains proper to think in terms of well-differentiated populations of primary and secondary endings and to neglect intermediate endings. But for other muscles there may be a significant number of intermediate forms of behavior, even though the endings might be histologically classifiable as primary or secondary. The question that then arises is whether their synaptic connections are such that the CNS could treat their information in any special way. Indeed, going further, when there is no clear bimodality either of behavior or of numbers it could even be asked how far the subdivision into primaries and secondaries is helpful in functional terms because they then seem merely to represent the extremes of a continuum.

MOTOR SUPPLY TO MUSCLE SPINDLE

Gamma Motor Axons

The existence of a group of small diameter (4–8 μm) medullated motor axons to skeletal muscle was fully documented by histological counting by Eccles and Sherrington in 1930 (66). They assumed, apparently without significant self-questioning, that the slimness of these axons simply reflected upon their supplying motor units with a below average number of ordinary muscle fibers, although the idea that they might supply the muscle spindles had already been broached (121). However, the means to establish this experimentally only became available in the 1940s when it was shown *1*) that stimulation of these small fibers produces no overt tension in the muscle, and *2*) that it does cause considerable excitation of the muscle spindle afferents, both primary and secondary. Thus these motor axons were shown to be devoted exclusively to supplying the muscle spindles. This achievement was initiated by Leksell in 1945 (122) using multifiber techniques and was brought to fruition by Kuffler, Hunt, and Quilliam (102, 120) using single fiber techniques both for recording and stimulating. The fibers are now called by various names: γ-efferents (122), small motor fibers (120), or fusimotor fibers (106). The proposition that all γ-efferents are specifically fusimotor remains without challenge, though the precise diameter at which a motor fiber is judged to be a γ-efferent varies with the muscle as well as with the species. But the converse proposition that the whole of the motor supply to the muscle spindle is necessarily derived from the γ-efferents does not hold, for on occasion there may also be a significant β-innervation from branches of the larger motor axons which also supply extrafusal muscle fibers (see subsection *Beta or Skeletofusimotor Axons*, p. 210).

Delimitation of Static and Dynamic Fusimotor Axons

MAIN DIFFERENCES. With the subdivision of the intrafusal muscle fibers into the morphologically distinct bag and chain fibers, particularly with the suggestion that they might be independently innervated, it became natural to search for functional differences in the action of different fusimotor axons on the spindle. Almost at once, following a lead given by Jansen and Matthews (114), a difference was found by the author of this chapter, which has stood the test of time, namely in the effect of repetitive stimulation of a single fusimotor axon on the response of a spindle primary ending to a large ramp-and-hold stretch (133). Some fibers, the then-named dynamic fusimotor axons, had the usual excitatory effect on the primary ending, albeit a weak one, with the muscle held at a constant length; they also strikingly sensitized the ending to the dynamic phase of the stimuli so that the normal change in firing at the beginning and end of the rising phase of the ramp was markedly enhanced. In contrast, other fibers—the static fusiomotor axons—while having a more powerful excitatory action at a constant length diminished the sensitivity of the primary ending to the dynamic phase of the ramp, making its behavior much more like that of the secondary ending. These effects are illustrated in Figure 8 and were shown systematically by measurement of the dynamic index, which was increased on dynamic fusimotor stimulation and decreased on static fusimotor stimulation for all velocities of stretch (62, 63). A similar subdivision of efferents into static and dynamic axons has been demonstrated in the baboon (53, 54, 117), in the rabbit (79), and in the rat (4), as well as being confirmed for a variety of muscles in the cat. Parenthetically, it may be noted that the original choice of a large ramp as the mechanical stimulus to use in searching for a difference in fusimotor action proved to be a fortunate one, for no other situation has yet been charted in which the action of the two kinds of axon can be so readily and reliably distinguished; it is probably significant that under the same circumstances a difference in behavior of the primary and secondary endings is so well displayed.

The functional distinctiveness of the static and dynamic axons has been further established by the following findings.

1. When a given fusimotor axon is found to influence more than one primary ending, its action always runs true to type and it retains its static or dynamic specificity. Because there is only one primary ending in each muscle spindle the specificity must be a property of the axon and does not arise from any chance relation that it enters into with one particular spindle (37, 63, 78). Also when two axons of the same type are stimulated simultaneously, their combined action shows no sign of any change of character (41, 124).

2. Stimulation at different sites within the CNS may have either a predominantly static or a predominantly dynamic action, showing that at least some motor centers can exert an independent control on the two types of fusimotor fiber and thus enter into differential connections with their motoneurons. Sporadic observations of such events by Jansen and Matthews (114) encouraged the search for the two types of fusimotor axon. Subsequent work, particularly that of Appelberg and his colleagues on the red nucleus has amply validated the idea [(7); see the chapter by Baldissera, Hultborn, and Illert in this *Handbook*].

3. Study of the effects on a primary and a secondary ending lying within the same muscle showed that static axons regularly have a considerable excitatory action on secondary endings as well as on primary endings, but that dynamic axons have little or no action on the secondary ending even though it lies within a spindle in which the same dynamic axon is producing a considerable excitatory action on the primary ending. In their original demonstration, Appelberg et al. (6) found that one out of nine secondary endings was influenced by a dynamic axon to slightly increase its dynamic sensitivity; a few other examples have been illustrated (65).

The static-dynamic dichotomy of fusimotor axons has since been observed and commented on in a large number of papers. Various other differences between their actions have been noted in specific circumstances but none seems as clear-cut or as important as those emphasized above. Unfortunately, there is no absolute difference between the conduction velocities of static and dynamic fusimotor axons, a condition that would greatly assist experimentation; in the tibialis posterior of the cat the slowest fusimotor axons are predominantly static (37), but this is not so for all muscles. In the cat, static axons outnumber dynamic axons by between two and four to one (37, 78). However, the ratio probably varies with both the muscle and the species. Spindles in the baboon soleus seem particularly well supplied with dynamic axons (1.5 static to 1 dynamic; ref. 53); those in the rabbit soleus seem rather badly supplied (6 static to 1 dynamic; ref 79). The branching pattern of efferents has not been sufficiently studied to decide whether the ratio of the numbers of the two kinds of fiber to a given spindle can be applied to the absolute numbers of each type of axon to a given muscle.

When a preexisting stretch is released the normal silence of the passive primary ending is very much

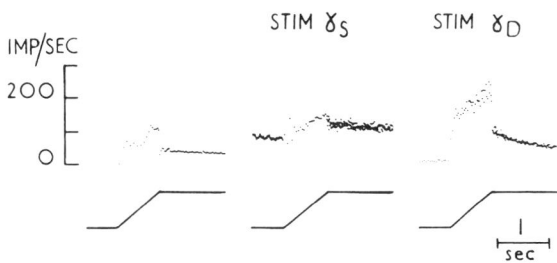

FIG. 8. Contrasting effects of static (γ_S) and dynamic (γ_D) fusimotor axons on responsiveness of a primary ending to large amplitude ramp stretching in cat. Records of instantaneous frequency, *a*, in absence of fusimotor stimulation; *b*, during repetitive static axon stimulation; *c*, during repetitive dynamic axon stimulation. Stretch was 6 mm at 30 mm/s. Time scale expanded during dynamic phase of stretch. [From Brown and Matthews (42).]

more effectively counteracted by static stimulation than by dynamic stimulation. Likewise, during the releasing phase of low-frequency sinusoidal stretching the primary ending shows a pause much more readily during dynamic than during static axon stimulation. During the rising phase of sinusoidal stretching dynamic stimulation augments the firing above the corresponding level for constant stretch much more than does static stimulation. Thus, fitting a sine curve to the responses shows that dynamic stimulation leads to a much greater depth of afferent modulation by the sinusoidal movement than does static stimulation (82, 100). However, during high-frequency sinusoidal vibration of the muscle (order of 100 Hz), stimulation of either kind of fusimotor fiber increases the ease with which the already sensitive primary ending shows 1:1 driving (39); 5 μm peak-to-peak movement of the soleus tendon may then be sufficient, implying a very much smaller stretch of the spindle itself. Analytic studies of the sensitivity to such high frequencies of stretching, but of amplitudes far below that required to elicit vibrator driving, confirm the sensitizing action of both kinds of axon on the responsiveness of the primary ending to movement of very high frequency [see Fig. 19; (82)].

SPEED OF ACTION. The intrafusal contractions elicited by the two kinds of fusimotor axon appear to differ; those elicited by static activation are appreciably faster. This difference was first apparent from the study of the phenomenon of fusimotor driving, in which each stimulus to the isolated fusimotor axon is followed by an afferent spike so that the afferent rhythm becomes the same as the stimulus rhythm (120); weaker tendencies may be shown by 1:2 driving with an afferent spike for every alternate stimulus. The same underlying intrafusal action may manifest itself, particularly with low frequency stimulation, by the occurrence of more than one spike per stimulus so that afferent discharge becomes grossly irregular. These effects are most readily attributed to the ripples of an unfused intrafusal contraction providing a powerful dynamic stimulus to the primary ending, and thus argue for a fast intrafusal contraction. Secondary endings rarely show appreciable signs of driving, probably because of their much lower sensitivity to high-frequency movement. The important observation is that driving and its related phenomena are quite commonly seen when static axons are stimulated, but not when dynamic axons are stimulated (37, 63, 78), thus suggesting that the former typically supply a more rapidly contracting intrafusal system. A few static axons, however, are as free from driving actions as the dynamic axons. These effects can be studied in more detail by assessing the extent of modulation to be seen in the frequencygram in which superimposed records are made of the response of the ending, expressed as an instantaneous frequency, to successive repetitions of the same stimulus pattern (25), and in the post-stimulus histogram in which the timing of the afferent spikes is related to the time of the stimuli applied to the fusimotor axon (73, 82). Both methods show that usually with static axon stimulation the endings tend to fire at certain particular times with regard to the stimulus and to avoid firing at other times.

The rise in the frequency of afferent firing at the beginning of a period of repetitive fusimotor stimulation is commonly more abrupt when static axons are stimulated, and the afferent firing may briefly overshoot its subsequent steady level (53, 63, 130). But these effects are so variable for different fusimotor axons of the same kind, and so influenced by the initial length of the muscle and the frequency of stimulation that they have so far provided little help in fusimotor classification. Quite surprisingly in light of the foregoing evidence, and of some interest in considering the significance of the central biasing of fusimotor firing, it has been found that the transfer function relating changes in the mean frequency of fusimotor stimulation to the frequency of afferent firing is the same for the two types of fusimotor axon when the frequency of their stimulation is modulated sinusoidally at frequencies up to about 10 Hz (3, 51, 99a). This finding remains puzzling in relation to intrafusal mechanisms, because the rest of the evidence favors the idea that static axons supply the more rapidly contracting intrafusal fibers; perhaps part of the answer may be that the static system is working through the dual contractile system of the bag_2 and the chain fibers and that with different tests one or the other may predominate.

RECENT REEXAMINATION. The sharpness of the division of fusimotor axons into functionally well-separated static and dynamic axons was recently reexamined to see whether it might have arisen from some bias in the selection of axons for study, or from the application of rather limited criteria for classification, such as an excessive reliance on the dynamic index (78). The outcome has been to reaffirm the validity of the division of axons into quite separate static and dynamic axons with distinct effects which, for a given axon, remain consistent from spindle to spindle. It was found, however, that the action of a given axon on a given spindle sometimes gave rise to suspicion that a pure static action had been contaminated by a degree of dynamic action, or vice versa, but there was no tendency for any such suspected admixture of actions to recur when the same axon was tested on another spindle. The template for suspecting a degree of admixture of actions was provided by simultaneously stimulating a static and a dynamic axon influencing the same spindle, as illustrated in Figure 9. The dynamic contribution to the overall mixed responses is best shown by the characteristic slow decay of firing at the end of the dynamic phase of the ramp stretch, and the static contribution leads to firing when the stretch is released, and to a general elevation of the level of firing. Sometimes, however, the dynamic con-

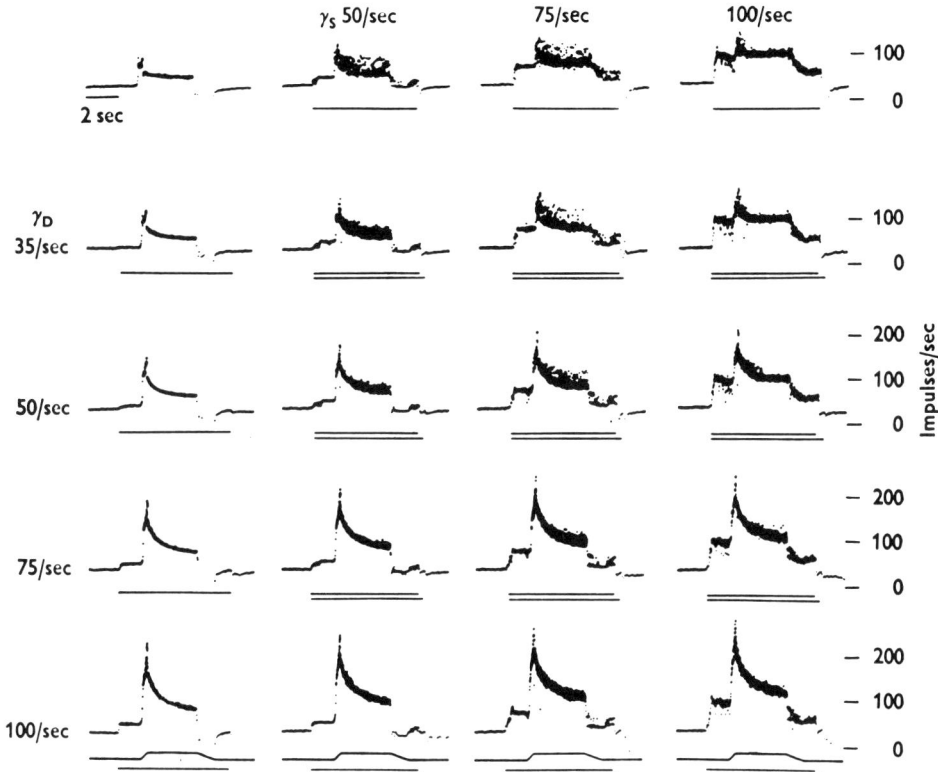

FIG. 9. Simultaneous stimulation of a pair of single fusimotor axons (1 static, γ_S; 1 dynamic, γ_D), of cat. Each axon stimulated at several frequencies to show effect on responsiveness of a primary ending to a ramp stretch as the balance between them is shifted. [From Emonet-Dénand, Matthews, et al. (78).]

tribution was almost obscured by a powerful static contribution. One-third of the responses elicited by single axons showed some suspicion of admixture, and of these a suspected dynamic contribution to static action was far commoner than the other way around. These findings are thus of some relevance to the problem of the precise distribution of the motor axons within the spindle without interfering with the acceptance of a duality of the fusimotor outflow.

Intrafusal Destination of Static and Dynamic Axons

INITIAL IDEAS. The functional separation of the static and dynamic axons raised the question of how they achieve their different actions upon the primary ending. There are two distinct aspects to the problem, namely, how the two sorts of axon differ in their intrafusal distribution and mode of termination, such as by selecting a particular kind of intrafusal fiber or a particular longitudinal segment, and just how any such anatomic difference leads to the observed effects on the behavior and stretch responsiveness of the afferent terminals. Attention has largely concentrated on the first aspect of the matter and in particular on the hypothesis, which was introduced at the outset, that the dynamic axons supply the bag fibers and the static axons supply the chain fibers (114, 133). This hypothesis had its roots in Boyd's (30) suggestion, based on his own histological observations, that the bag and chain fibers had independent motor supplies and the hypothesis simply related the observed functional duality to this supposed structural duality. The choice for the bag fibers rather than the chain fibers as the destination of the dynamic axons, and vice versa for the static axons, was initially based on little more than a hunch, for the arguments used were agreed to be tenuous. By 1972, however, evidence had accumulated to suggest that if a 1:1 correspondence were accepted between the static-dynamic and the bag-chain dualities then the relation should indeed be between dynamic axons and bag fibers, and static axons and chain fibers (137). The evidence, which remains pertinent and has been brought up to date with additional references, is as follows.

1. Direct observation on isolated spindles (31, 86) shows, on the one hand, that in accordance with their ultrastructural appearance the chain fibers contract more rapidly than the bag fibers; on the other hand, various techniques show that stimulation of static axons activates a more rapidly contracting system than does stimulation of dynamic fibers, as already discussed.

2. Histological observation shows that the secondary

ending lies predominantly on the chain fibers and electrophysiological experiment shows that static axons have a powerful excitatory action on the secondary ending, but the dynamic axons are usually without influence although they are known to supply the spindle in question (6). Excitation seems most likely to arise from the contraction of the intrafusal fiber on which the ending lies rather than from contraction of other fibers lying in parallel with it.

3. Succinylcholine and acetylcholine mimic the effect of dynamic fusimotor stimulation on the primary ending, but observations of their effects on isolated spindles show that the bag fibers are led to contract strongly whereas the chain fibers appear to be paralyzed (80, 86, 158).

All these observations fall into place if it is the dynamic axons that supply the bag fibers and the static axons that supply the chain fibers, but it would be self-contradictory if the relation were the other way around. But when a consensus seemed imminent, turmoil was reintroduced. Several completely independent lines of evidence showed that static axons commonly supply the bag fibers as well as the expected chain fibers, and sometimes even to the exclusion of the chain fibers. The dynamic axons, however, continued to "behave themselves" under this further scrutiny and have continued to be found to restrict their innervation to bag fibers—albeit usually to only a single one of the two or three bag fibers in a spindle. There was a brief period of confusion while this fresh evidence was accumulating, because it was initially deployed solely to contradict the only existing hypothesis rather than to create a new one.

The uncertainty, however, was short-lived as evidence was being gathered indicating that the bag fibers themselves should be subdivided into two types, distinct both morphologically and functionally, with one responsible for dynamic action and the other, along with the chain fibers, responsible for static action. This development, in its current form, is illustrated diagrammatically in Figure 10, which helps indicate that in the essentials the transformation in thought has been relatively slight. The experiments leading to this new view and the allocation of dynamic action to the bag$_1$ rather than the bag$_2$ fibers are discussed in detail in the next subsection.

HISTOLOGICAL TRACING OF INDIVIDUAL FUSIMOTOR FIBERS. Barker (14, 15) has long contended that tracing an individual fusimotor fiber within the spindle shows that it can supply both bag fibers and chain fibers, but the complexity of the neural tangle is such that only isolated examples could be illustrated and the frequency of such occurrence remained in doubt. The view was put on a solid footing by operatively simplifying the spindle so that its motor supply was reduced to a single γ-axon following the degeneration of all other α- and γ-fibers to the muscle as a result of cutting the axons in the ventral roots a few days

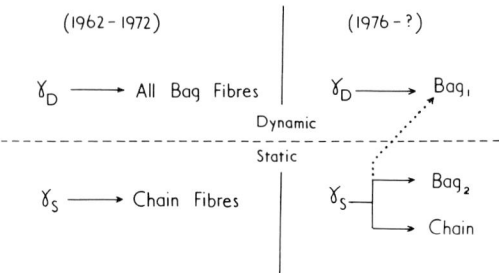

FIG. 10. Developing views on relation between functional classification into static (γ_S) and dynamic (γ_D) axons, and morphological classification of intrafusal muscle fibers. *Dotted line* from static axon to bag$_1$ fiber represents the chief matter of current controversy.

beforehand (19). In this simplified spindle it proved possible to trace the remaining fiber convincingly throughout its course using normal histological methods. In the first stage of the operation a single γ-motor fiber to the tenuissimus muscle of the cat was identified in an intact ventral root filament. All the rest of the ventral root supply to the muscle was then severed. At this stage, it was not feasible for technical reasons to identify the remaining γ-fiber as static or dynamic. This was done in a second operation, 7–12 days after the first, when it was also confirmed electrophysiologically that only one γ-fiber was still surviving. These operations were performed in Toulouse by Emonet-Dénand, Laporte, and Proske. The muscle was then removed and examined histologically with silver staining in Durham by Barker and Stacy. For reasons that remain obscure, in the only published series of experiments (19), all 10 surviving γ-axons proved to be static fibers and none were dynamic; thus the experiment is as yet incomplete. But two major points were established, as illustrated in Figure 11, namely, that static axons commonly terminate on bag fibers as well as on chain fibers and that all their terminations are trail type, irrespective of the kind of intrafusal muscle fiber on which they lie. The authors were confident that these findings were not dependent on any sprouting from the terminations of the remaining fiber that might result from denervation of most of the intrafusal fibers; such sprouting of ordinary α-motor fibers begins on the third postoperative day (95).

A particular study was made of 30 spindles from 6 preparations, each supplied by a single static axon. The single γ-axon supplied chain fibers on their own in only 8 of these spindles, while in 15 spindles it supplied both bag and chain fibers, and in 7 spindles it supplied solely a bag fiber. Thus it became quite untenable to believe that static axons had any sort of exclusive relation with the chain fibers. At that time there was no attempt to subdivide the bag fibers into two types. With hindsight it may be noted that for 18 of the 22 spindles with bag fiber innervation it is certain from the published account that a single bag fiber only was supplied by the static axon; for 2 of the remaining spindles 1 bag fiber was seen to have ter-

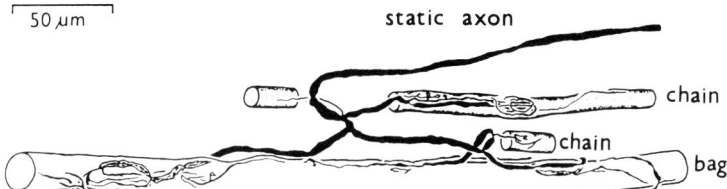

FIG. 11. Drawing of the way in which a sole surviving static axon following degeneration of the rest of the motor innervation in cat was seen to distribute itself between a bag fiber and 2 chain fibers. All the terminations are trail-type ending. [From Barker et al. (19).]

minations upon it at either pole, but it is uncertain whether it was the same or a different fiber; for only 2 spindles were 2 bag fibers seen to be innervated and it is not stated whether or not there was a third bag fiber in these spindles to provide a dynamic contribution. Thus, though it was unrecognized at the time, these important experiments are entirely in line with the scheme of Figure 10.

GLYCOGEN DEPLETION ANALYSIS. Edström and Kugelberg (68) showed that the constituent fibers of a single motor unit could be made to declare themselves histologically by stimulating their motor axon in isolation from others and then staining the muscle for glycogen by the periodic acid-Schiff (PAS) method. The activated muscle fibers then stand out from their neighbors because they are paler by virtue of having consumed much of their glycogen in the preceding tetanic contraction; the depletion of preexisting glycogen is encouraged by forcing the muscle to metabolize anaerobically by occluding its circulation. This method was first applied to the muscle spindle by Brown and Butler (35) using the tenuissimus muscle. They found that while, as expected, dynamic axons depleted bag fibers and not chain fibers, static axons regularly depleted bag fibers in addition to the expected chain fibers; this is shown diagrammatically in Figure 12 where a fiber is shown as fully depleted although depletion only occurred along part of its length, presumably that part of it that underwent a local contraction. Thus once again the preferred hypothesis on the distribution of the static axons was contradicted, though this time the dynamic axons had proved amenable to study and had "behaved" themselves. In this work, which was performed before the subdivision of the bag fibers, it is slightly puzzling that there was no sign of any such dichotomy and a given dynamic axon might deplete all the bag fibers in a spindle, as also might a given static axon in addition to its depletion of the chain fibers. A more recent repetition of the same experiment by Barker et al. (17), combined with identification of the type of intrafusal muscle fiber influenced, showed that the dynamic axons deplete solely the bag$_1$ fibers and not the bag$_2$ fibers (Fig. 13). It is possible that in the earlier experiments some bag fibers were falsely characterized as depleted. Such a situation might arise if both kinds of bag fiber normally contain less glycogen than the chain fibers, because

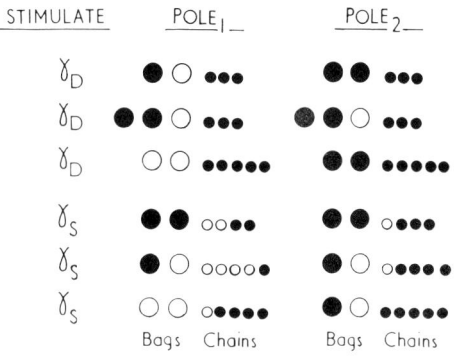

FIG. 12. Examples from the first study of the intrafusal depletion of glycogen after stimulation of single γ-fibers. Static axon, γ$_S$; dynamic axon, γ$_D$. Each *horizontal row* represents a spindle, with its several intrafusal muscle fibers shown by *circles*. Presence of glycogen is shown by *solid circle*, and its depletion following neural activation of the fiber is shown by *open circle*. The bag fibers were not then subdivided. [Rearranged from Brown and Butler (35).]

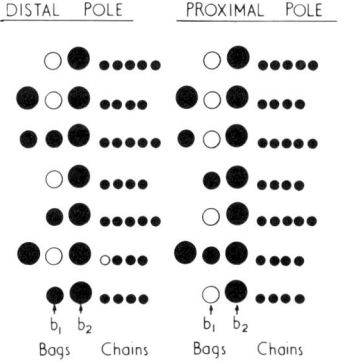

FIG. 13. Recent examples that glycogen depletion, after stimulation of single dynamic axons, is restricted to bag$_1$ intrafusal fibers. Each *row* represents a spindle with its intrafusal muscle fibers shown by *circles*. Solid circle, glycogen presence; open circle, glycogen depletion. [Adapted from Barker et al. (17).]

they would look paler, thus suggesting glycogen depletion. But recent work shows that static axons to tenuissimus (17) or to peroneus brevis (75) may deplete either the bag$_1$ fiber or the bag$_2$ fiber, as well as chain fibers. The occasional depletion of bag$_1$ fibers on their own that was reported in the recent tenuissimus experiments seems likely to have been accompanied by some chain fiber activation, because with their initial high glycogen content chain fibers are difficult to deplete entirely and a partial depletion was suspected in some cases (ref. 17, p. 66). In peroneus longus, in contrast, Brown and Butler (36) found that static axons depleted only a single bag fiber in the spindle, and because it was always the largest fiber it is likely to have been the bag$_2$ fiber. The association of bag$_1$ fibers with dynamic action has been further consolidated by experiments in which β-axons (skeletofusimotor) with a pronounced dynamic action were studied and found to produce a selective depletion of the bag$_1$ fibers (17).

STUDIES ON SINGLE LIVING SPINDLES: VISUAL OBSERVATION, INTRACELLULAR RECORDING. The groups led by Boyd in Glasgow (32) and Bessou in Toulouse (10, 27) have both successfully isolated the muscle spindle from its surrounding muscle fibers while preserving its afferent and its efferent innervation intact and in connection with the spinal roots for separation of single units. Therefore any fusimotor axon can be identified as static or dynamic by the only means currently available, namely, by its action on the afferent responsiveness to stretch. This has permitted much greater insight into what is happening (34). The effect of an identified axon on the various intrafusal fibers can then be studied rather directly by watching to see which fibers move when it is stimulated and, more particularly, whether a local contraction with sarcomere shortening can be detected in cine photographs or video recordings. Intracellular recording provides a further and possibly more discriminating way of demonstrating that a particular intrafusal fiber has been activated by a particular axon. Chain fibers can be recognized by virtue of their size. Desirably, any bag fiber studied requires labeling in some way so that it can be subsequently characterized, by histochemistry or by elastic fiber content, as a bag$_1$ or a bag$_2$ fiber, but this was not done in the earlier experiments. More recently still, the greater sensitivity of the bag$_1$ fiber to locally applied acetylcholine provides an indicator at the time of the experiment (80).

When dynamic axons are stimulated a weak contraction of one of the bag fibers unaccompanied by any contraction of the chain fibers has been observed (10, 27, 32). When static axons are stimulated a bag fiber may often be seen to contract in addition to the chain fibers, and the contraction is appreciably more powerful (greater movement) and faster than that elicited by dynamic axon stimulation; moreover, sometimes one of the bag fibers may contract on its own without the chain fibers (10, 27, 32). However, the same bag fiber was never seen to be activated by both a static axon and a dynamic axon in those experiments in which it proved possible to isolate both types of axon. Figure 14 shows some of these findings diagramatically. The Glasgow group (32) were so impressed by these differences that they subdivided the bag fibers into two types depending on which kind of axon elicited their contraction, and termed them the static nuclear bag and the dynamic nuclear bag; because

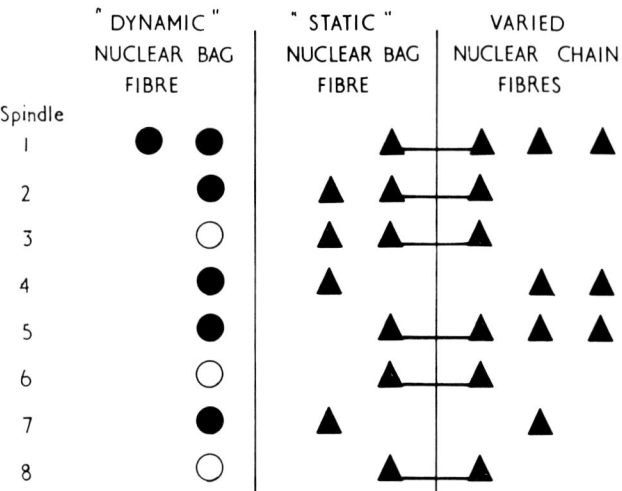

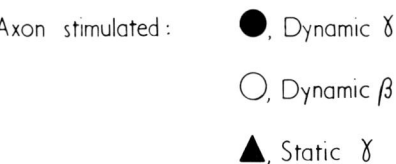

FIG. 14. Diagrammatic representation of the particular intrafusal muscle fibers that were seen to contract by Boyd and his colleagues in isolated spindles after stimulation of single fusimotor axons. Each *row* represents a spindle and each *symbol* represents an intrafusal muscle fiber that was seen to move with fusimotor stimulation. The symbol is varied with the type of axon that was found to activate the fiber in question. ●, Dynamic γ; ○, dynamic β; ▲, static γ. When a given axon influenced 2 different types of intrafusal fiber the symbols are joined by a *horizontal line*. It may be seen that a bag fiber influenced by a dynamic axon (dynamic nuclear bag) was never influenced by a static axon or in combination with a chain fiber, but that other bag fibers were activated by static axons (static nuclear bag) and that this was commonly in conjunction with chain activation. [Adapted from Boyd et al. (32).]

they then proceeded to show that this functional classification corresponded to the histological classification into bag$_1$ and bag$_2$ fibers these provisional names have now been largely abandoned. Thus in current terminology Boyd and his colleagues (32) suggested that dynamic axons activate bag$_1$ fibers and that static axons activate bag$_2$ fibers, the latter usually in conjunction with chain fibers but sometimes on their own. In a limited sample, the use of microelectrode recording of synaptic and/or action potentials as the indicator of intrafusal activation has largely supported this view (16). Of 9 intrafusal muscle fibers activated by dynamic axons, 7 were bag$_1$ fibers, 1 a bag$_2$ fiber, and 1 a chain fiber. Of 13 intrafusal fibers activated by a static axon, 5 were chain fibers, 8 were bag$_2$ fibers, and none were bag₁ fibers (the paucity of chain fibers is probably attributable to their smaller size and consequent greater difficulty of impalement).

ASSESSMENT OF POSITION. These various lines of evidence have led to general agreement with the view that bag₁ activation underlies and provides the essential feature of dynamic action, while static action is based on a variable combination of bag₂ and chain activation. Disagreement persists concerning whether bag₁ excitation commonly occurs along with bag₂ and chain excitation during static action. The view of Boyd's group is that this does not occur, because they never observed what they regarded as a significant bag₁ contraction when static axons were stimulated; their scheme of innervation is shown in Figure 15. The view of Barker's group, in association with their collaborating physiologists, is that it does occur, because they regularly observed glycogen depletion of bag₁ fibers when static axons were stimulated, as shown in Figure 16. As already portrayed, Figure 10 shows the uncertainty in the current position narrowed to the presence or absence of the dotted line. The conflict can only be resolved by faulting one or the other of the techniques, or by developing yet another line of attack which is generally agreed to be more reliable. Visual observation could conceivably overlook a weak but physiologically significant bag₁ contraction occurring at the same time as the stronger bag₂ and chain contractions, and this would be especially likely if the bag₁ contraction were chiefly important for the effect it has on the mechanical responses of the intrafusal fiber to stretching. On the other hand glycogen depletion might perhaps be too sensitive an indicator of metabolic change in the bag₁ fibers, because they normally stain palely, and it is perhaps subject to vagaries that have yet to be charted; for example, individual extrafusal muscle fibers show a patchy longitudinal distribution of depletion even though they would be presumed to be activated by a propagated action potential traveling along their full length (16).

But if it occurs, the bag₁ contribution to static action is likely to remain a dynamic-type contribution and under many circumstances to be submerged under the more powerful static-type actions of the other two types of intrafusal muscle fiber, because this is what is observed experimentally when a dynamic axon, providing a known bag₁ contribution, is stimulated at the same time as a moderately powerful static axon (78, 101).

The dynamic fusimotor system emerges from this prolonged period of controversy much as it entered, namely, as a motor system operating via a specialized set of axons and terminating on a single specialized type of intrafusal muscle fiber, albeit it is now the bag₁ fiber rather than all the bag fibers. The static fusimotor system, however, is now seen to possess a multiple motor apparatus, with two functionally distinct types of intrafusal muscle fiber under its control. This raises two questions of considerable interest for motor control as a whole. First, should static axons be subdivided into two or more classes depending on the distribution of their terminals to the two types of

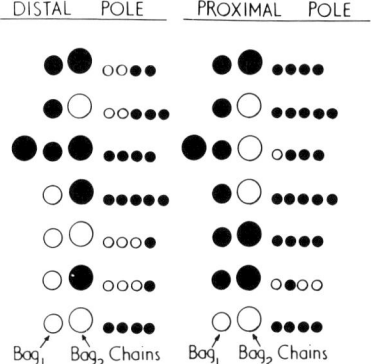

FIG. 16. Recent examples of varied patterns of glycogen depletion involving all 3 types of intrafusal fiber seen when single static axons are stimulated. Each *row* represents a spindle with its intrafusal muscle fibers shown by *circles*. *Solid circle*, glycogen presence; *open circle*, glycogen depletion. [Adapted from Barker et al. (17).]

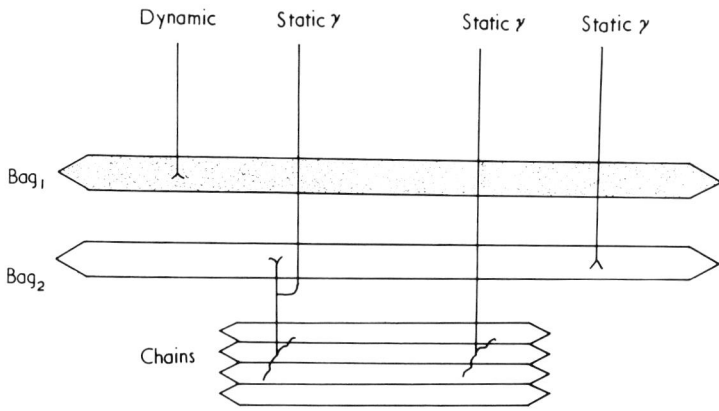

FIG. 15. Motor innervation of spindle as described by Boyd et al. in 1977 with a completely independent innervation of bag₁ and bag₂ intrafusal muscle fibers, but with the innervation of bag₂ and chain fibers partly in common. [Redrawn from Boyd et al. (32).]

intrafusal muscle fibers? Second, what functionally advantageous properties are conferred on static action by its using two types of intrafusal fiber instead of just one? This remains an enigma except to restate the fact that the chain fibers contract more rapidly and could thus provide for faster activation of the afferent terminals. The functional role of any bag_1 contribution to static action remains even less understood.

The answer to the first question, whether static axons should be subdivided, hangs on the experimental determination of the localization of the terminations within different spindles of individual static axons, but as yet the evidence is fragmentary. Within a given spindle three variants of static axon distribution may be distinguished with general agreement, namely to chain fibers alone, to bag_2 fibers on their own, and to both these types of fiber in variable combination—ignoring for the time being any distribution of bag_1 fibers. In glycogen-depletion experiments 7 static axons were studied, each of which acted on 2 or more spindles (31 γ-spindle combinations; ref. 17) with the finding that there was no constancy in their distribution; for example, the same static axon could activate only a bag_2 fiber in one spindle, only chain fibers in another, and both bag_2 and chain fibers in a third spindle. In isolated spindle experiments two separate spindles were studied in a given cat on two occasions (32). In each of these experiments an axon was seen to have a different effect in the two members of the pair of spindles studied; in each experiment for one spindle of the pair, chain fibers were activated on their own, but in the other of the pair the presumed bag_2 fiber was activated—in one case on its own, and in the other in combination with chain fibers. Two further axons studied in one of the experiments were found to have the same action in both spindles.

Less direct evidence of a variable distribution of a given static axon is provided by the varied effect it may have in producing 1:1 driving in different spindles, because driving seems likely to be related to the innervation of chain fibers (32, 78). It may be concluded that there is no possibility that the bag_2 and chain fibers comprise independent effector systems, each under private motor control, because they are obligatorily activated together by many of the static axons. There are, however, two hints in the literature that the CNS may perhaps be able to exert a degree of selectivity in the activation of bag_2 and chain fibers. First, in the glycogen-depletion experiments just described (17) the three slowest conducting static axons studied had no effect on the bag_2 fibers in the nine spindles they influenced, although the five faster conducting static axons affected bag_2 fibers in three-quarters of the spindles they influenced. Second, the direct microscopic observation of semi-isolated spindles that remained under the influence of the CNS in anesthetized cats with intact ventral roots showed that the bag_2 fibers contracted on their own, without the chain fibers, on a number of occasions when the anesthesia was lightened or the motor cortex was stimulated electrically (81). It remains to be seen whether these are chance observations or prove to be significant.

Properties of Intrafusal Muscle Fibers

It seems likely that the major functionally significant difference between the various intrafusal fibers lies in their contractile properties. However, there are various other differences that might prove to be equally significant: *1*) the length of the fibers, with both bag fibers running far outside the capsule, while the chain fibers terminate approximately with the capsule (15, 30); this might produce differences in their mechanical interactions; *2*) the relationship of the secondary ending to the intrafusal fiber in question; the secondary ending has long been known to lie predominantly on the chain fibers; limited recent evidence suggests that when it does send a branch to bag fibers it has no special predilection for bag_2 as opposed to bag_1 fibers (11); *3*) the transducing properties might differ among the different primary afferent terminations lying on the various fibers; although these are all derived from one and the same Ia-fiber there is as yet no direct evidence to show if they all behave in the same way, particularly with regard to their relative sensitivity to static and to dynamic stimuli; *4*) the longitudinal localization of the motor terminals may vary on the different fibers (15) and this could lead to local contractions in different regions of the spindle, and thus possibly to different mechanical effects.

DIFFERENCES IN CONTRACTILITY. Direct observation of isolated spindles shows that chain fibers contract more rapidly than the bag_2 fibers, which are themselves faster than the bag_1 fibers (27, 31, 32). Calculation of the mean values of contraction and relaxation times, all obtained with repetitive stimulation (see Table 3 in ref. 32), gives ratios of 1.4 and 2.6 for the relative time course of the contraction of the bag_2 and the bag_1 fibers, respectively, in relation to that of the chain fibers. Associated with this somewhat greater speed, and probably also reflecting their ability to show all-or-none spikes, the chain fibers give oscillatory contractions in time with the stimulus; this effect is especially marked at low frequencies but may still persist even at frequencies above 100 Hz. This rapid mechanical response of the chain fibers appears to be the basis of driving by static axons, for bag_2 fibers do not show any such oscillation at frequencies above 10–20 Hz, and static axons, which excite only a bag_2 fiber in an isolated spindle, do not produce driving. Bag_1 fibers show no sign of such oscillatory contraction (31) and likewise dynamic axons never produce driving. Interesting differences between the contractions of the various types of intrafusal fiber are seen as the frequency of fusimotor stimulation is progressively increased. At frequencies of 10 Hz and below the chain fibers show a rapid quivering while the bag fibers usually appear to remain quiescent, although some bag$_2$ fibers may show some movement, including twitches with single shocks. At 10–20 Hz both types of bag fiber usually begin to show a smooth contraction, which increases with the frequency to reach a maximum for frequencies around 75 Hz for bag$_1$ fibers and slightly higher for bag$_2$ fibers. Appreciable maintained shortening of chain fibers, however, does not occur until the frequency of stimulation approaches 50 Hz and the contraction does not reach a maximum until the frequency approaches 150 Hz. These values are largely based on observations made at room temperature and should not be treated as absolute.

All these contractions observed in isolated spindles, whether of bag or chain fibers, are localized to a part of the length of the spindle, with shortening in this region matched by extension of other regions. The contraction focuses are of variable length, but never include the central region of the spindle innervated by the primary ending. Commonly a given fusimotor axon elicits a contraction in only one pole of the spindle. The spirals of the primary ending can fortunately be reliably recognized in the living spindle, and it is found that contraction of the bag$_2$ and chain fibers produces an appreciably greater elongation of these spirals than does contraction of the bag$_1$ fibers. It should be noted that the chain fibers move as a bunch yet they move independently of the bag fibers, which can also move freely past each other. Thus contraction of a given type of intrafusal fiber influences only its own spirals by direct action. As an approximation, when excited by a single fusimotor axon at optimum frequency, bag$_1$ contraction extends its primary spirals by only about 5% whereas both bag$_2$ and chain fibers can open their own spirals by about 20% (31). The association of this greater contractile activity with a faster speed of contraction means that fusimotor activation of both bag$_2$ and chain fibers produces a four- to sixfold greater velocity of extension of the primary terminals than do the bag$_1$ fibers.

CREEP. It thus appears unlikely that when the bag$_1$ fiber is neurally activated it plays a significant role in producing a direct excitation of the primary terminals by stretch. Instead, the bag$_1$ fiber seems likely to have a special role in determining the response of the primary ending to a dynamically applied stretch of appreciable amplitude. The well-known effects of dynamic fusimotor stimulation can now be recognized to be attributable to selective activation of the bag$_1$ fibers. In addition, the bag$_1$ fibers are alone in showing the interesting mechanical effect named intrafusal creep by Boyd (31). This effect consists of a slow creep or shortening of the central innervated region of the intrafusal fiber when the dynamic phase of a ramp and hold stretch is completed, so that over a period of 1–2 s part of the initial deformation of the terminals produced by the application of the stretch is annulled. Such creep removes about 25% of the initial stretch from the center of the bag$_1$ fiber when the spindle is passive. But the creep gets several times larger when the bag$_1$ fiber is stretched while it is being activated by simultaneous stimulation of a dynamic fusimotor axon, though as yet this effect has been achieved on very few occasions (31, 33); in contrast, neither bag$_2$ nor chain fibers showed any sign of creep during static axon stimulation. From the similarity of its time course it seems inevitable that this creep must be the origin of most if not all of the slow adaptive decay of firing of the primary afferent, which is such a prominent feature of its response to a ramp and hold stretch applied during dynamic fusimotor stimulation (63, 78), and which contributes importantly to the enhancement of the dynamic index during dynamic fusimotor stimulation. In simplistic mechanical terms the creep may be attributed to an increased viscoelastic resistance of the intrafusal poles so that they show a high stiffness under dynamic conditions but then yield with maintained stretch. But this begs the question of the biological origin of such behavior, which can only be determined by experiment. Among the alternatives are that the viscoelasticity simply relates to the mechanical properties of the intrafusal myofilaments, that it results from a temporary stretch-induced depolarization of the bag$_1$ plasma membrane with the consequent activation of additional contraction, and that it results from the stretch activation of the myofilaments so that their contractile activity is temporarily increased by the stretch as has been described for other types of muscle (151), though on a more rapid time scale.

MEMBRANE POTENTIALS. The localization of the contraction to a part of the length of a bag$_1$ fiber during dynamic fusimotor stimulation is to be expected, because dynamic axons invariably produce a local depolarization without any sign of an all-or-none action potential. This effect was first indicated by extracellular recording (24) and has since been fully validated by intracellular recording from bag fibers, some of which were definitively identified as bag$_1$ fibers (16, 26). Extracellular recording indicates that static axon stimulation may elicit partially propagated action potentials in some intrafusal fibers, but that propagation does not occur across the central region of the spindle from one pole to the other. The first intracellular recordings showed that in 50% of the penetrations static axons produced an all-or-none potential (26), but the type of intrafusal fiber affected was not then identified. In recent work on identified intrafusal muscle fibers (16) static axons elicited action potentials from four of the five chain fibers studied, and the fifth was thought to be damaged. In contrast, static axons elicited junction potentials, without any sign of all-or-none behavior, from seven of eight bag$_2$ fibers; because these are larger than the chain fibers and easier to penetrate, the likelihood of systematic damage can be largely excluded. Thus, it may be concluded that as a general rule static axons elicit action potentials from chain fibers and junction potentials from bag$_2$ fibers, but in the absence of knowledge of the length constants and other properties of the two kinds of intrafusal fiber the relative effects on the contractile machinery of partially propagated action potentials and nonpropagated junction potentials remain unknown. The chief difference between the two modes of activation may reside in the way effects summate during the activation of several fusimotor axons that supply the same intrafusal fiber. A recent paradox is that during dynamic axon stimulation the focus of the contraction as observed microscopically does not invariably correspond to the location of an end plate, and thus to the site of presumed maximal depolarization (8–10); one possibility is that this situation arises because of a change of mechanical properties of the intrafusal muscle fibers along their length and associated with their longitudinal variations in the histological and ultrastructural appearance of one and the same fiber as mentioned in subsection *Subdivision of Nuclear-Bag Fibers*, p. 192 (12). Thus it can be seen that a large number of interesting but painstaking microexperiments, both mechanical and electrical, remain to be performed on the intrafusal muscle fibers before we can get a clear idea of just how they work.

Beta or Skeletofusimotor Axons

With increasing evolutionary complexity the motor supply to the muscle spindle has become separated from that to the main muscle fibers with the development of efferent axons that are specifically fusimotor. This simpler more primitive arrangement is still found in lizards, snakes, and amphibians where the spindles are supplied exclusively by branches of the ordinary motor axons (157). Because these species may have both fast and slow extrafusal muscle fibers, they also possess scope for a dual type of control (140), though when the spindle contains only a single intrafusal muscle fiber control may well be obtained by specialization between different muscle spindles. It is now becoming apparent that in mammals mixed skeletofusimotor or β-axons may persist alongside the specialized fusimotor axons. When first detected, the β-fibers seemed likely to be so infrequent that they could be considered as an evolutionary remnant (23); but as more cases are reported for a wider variety of muscles the idea is emerging that they have persisted to provide some definite functional advantage. Among the possibilities are *1*) the obligatory provision of an entirely hard-wired coactivation of intrafusal and extrafusal muscle fibers to keep the behavior of the spindle in line with that of the main muscle and to prevent it from slackening during muscle contraction without the need for additional neural control; *2*) the provision of a more rapid activation of the spindle than would be achieved by the more slowly conducting γ-efferents (though the saving in conduction time is slight); and *3*) the provision of a measure of positive feedback if the increased afferent firing produced by the intrafusal contraction should then reflexly activate the β-motoneurons themselves (97). They may also perhaps persist as a measure of economy for certain small muscles that receive only a very limited number of nerve fibers. For example, in the rat certain small muscles of the tail usually receive only a single γ-efferent, which is invariably static in its action, while the dynamic supply to its spindle or spindles is derived from one or two of its few faster motor fibers, which also have an extrafusal action (5). For its much larger soleus muscle, however, the rat achieves a dynamic action on spindles by the use of slow axons that are specifically fusimotor and are present in addition to the purely static axons (4). The full functional significance of β-innervation will become apparent only with further experiments directed toward charting the frequency of its occurrence and the strength of its action. To provide a basis for thought, the present knowledge of β-innervation in the cat is outlined below.

The difficulty of establishing the occurrence of a mixed skeletofusimotor innervation resides in the difficulty in proving that any action on the spindle arises from contraction of its intrafusal fibers, rather than merely from the mechanical effects of the contraction of nearby extrafusal fibers. This condition tends to rule out mass methods in which a number of large motor fibers are stimulated together. Instead attention has concentrated on the effects of stimulating single motor axons isolated in ventral root filaments. A major problem then is how to separate for intensive study those motor axons that are likely to have a genuine intrafusal action from the far more numerous large axons which simply influence the spindle via the extrafusal muscle fibers. In the earlier work attention was concentrated on certain small muscles such as the first deep lumbrical (23) or the abductor digiti quinti medius or tenuissimus (142), where virtually every motor fiber can be isolated and tested for the effects of its stimulation on single spindle afferents; when a sufficiently small number of both afferents and efferents are involved the chances of success become reasonably high. The demonstration of a specific intrafusal action is achieved partly by progressively increasing the frequency of stimulation and showing that the afferent discharge continues to increase with frequencies for which the extrafusal contraction has reached a maximum (because the "fusion" frequency of intrafusal fibers is much higher than that of extrafusal fibers), or by largely abolishing the extrafusal contraction while allowing a degree of intrafusal contraction to persist. The latter may be achieved by graded curarization or by fatigue induced by high-frequency stimulation, to both of which the intrafusal fibers appear to be the more resistant (23, 74, 77). There is, however, no certainty that these methods provide a comprehensive test for the occurrence of motor innervation of the spindle by axons that also supply extrafusal muscle fibers, because there is no necessity for the intrafusal effect to always be able to manifest itself under such relatively unfavorable circumstances.

Nonetheless in addition to the small muscles just mentioned it has proved possible to demonstrate the regular occurrence of β-fibers to a number of large muscles such as the peroneus brevis, the tibialis anterior, and the flexor hallucis longus (74); this innervation was demonstrated by reducing the large muscle to what was effectively a small muscle by section of all but a very small portion of its nerve close to the muscle. For the peroneus brevis it was estimated that about 70% of its spindles received some β-innervation as well as four or more γ-efferents (77). It should be noted that in spite of an exhaustive single fiber search no sign has been found of fast axons that are exclusively fusimotor and do not supply extrafusal muscle fibers (72). When tested appropriately, virtually all the β-axons that have been isolated by these means have proved to have a dynamic action, and one that can be quite powerful (18). However, even when the action of a β-fiber is not particularly powerful in itself the action may well be potentiated when the fiber is activated in conjunction with a fusimotor axon, and so it need not be written off as functionally insignificant. All these β-fibers have usually proved to have conduction velocities in the lower part of the α-fiber range for the muscle in question and appear to supply the weaker more slowly contracting motor units with fibers of the slow oxidative type (18).

Thus until 1976 or so the pattern of action of β-fibers that seemed to be emerging was that they provided a dynamic control of the spindle in association with relatively slow muscle contraction. Moreover, glycogen-depletion experiments confirmed that the spindle action was achieved by selective activation of bag$_1$ fibers (18). However, a new complexion has been put on all this by the recent demonstration that for both peroneus tertius and tenuissimus, activation of a number of the faster α-axons (conduction velocity > 80 m/s) that is reasonably guaranteed to be unaccompanied by any γ-efferent activation may produce glycogen depletion in nuclear-chain fibers; thus there is a strong argument that they have been activated (91, 109). Interestingly the degree of specificity of depletion of the chain fibers is much greater than that produced by stimulating static fusimotor axons in comparable experiments where bag$_2$ and/or bag$_1$ fibers are also affected. The effects of these fast β-axons on the afferent discharge of spindles may be presumed to be static and appear to have hitherto passed unnoticed in the cat, although it had been seen in the rabbit (76); perhaps the difficulty in demonstrating a "fast" action of β-fibers arises from a much greater strength of the accompanying extrafusal action of the fast motor units concerned. As yet there is no clear guide to the frequency of occurrence of this fast action nor has it yet been studied with single fiber methods, but stimulation of 60% to 80% of the "fast" α-fiber supply to the part of muscle studied showed depletion in one or two of the chain fibers in nearly one-third of the spindles examined. Notably, depletion usually occurred in the longest of the chain fibers in each spindle. Clearly the story of the β-fibers has further to unfold, but for the usual large mammalian muscles there is no question of the fusimotor system being supplanted by the β-fibers. Rather, we must adapt to the idea that both the static and the dynamic control of the spindle by specific fusimotor axons is commonly supplemented by an obligatory coactivation with the extrafusal fibers by the action of β-fibers.

POSSIBLE FUNCTIONAL ROLES FOR THE FUSIMOTOR SYSTEM

The advantages conferred upon the body by the possession of a specific system for the selective motor control of the muscle spindles continues to be the subject of debate. Understanding of the fusimotor system is naturally bound up with the larger problem of the nature of the roles that spindles themselves can play in the body, and so it is premature to attempt a final judgment. Rather one should rest content with the broad view obtained by balancing various suggestions against each other. Three main strands of thought may be distinguished in successive attempts to read functional meaning into the existence of the fusimotor system. These blend into each other so that even though in their extreme forms they might appear to be irreconcilable, in practice parts of each can be believed without creating a contradiction. The three ideas are *1)* that fusimotor activity provides a way of maintaining the sensitivity of the spindle endings under different conditions, particularly in the face of contraction of the main muscle; *2)* that they provide for the adjustment of the sensitivity of the spindle so as to suit its responsiveness to the prevailing mechanical conditions (this may be called parameter control); *3)* that they comprise the input to some sort of servomechanism, which reflexly elicits contraction of the main muscle via the stretch reflex, though insofar as this ever occurs the fusimotor system is recognized to act in collaboration with the α-fiber system to produce "servoassistance" rather than to provide a pure "follow-up length servo." These suggestions are expanded upon in the next subsections.

Maintenance of Sensitivity

In the absence of intrafusal contraction the primary ending falls silent during contraction of the main muscle fibers because the resulting slight yielding of the tendon leads to slackening of the spindle. Likewise, during muscle shortening the measuring properties of the passive spindle primary fall into abeyance. In the first single fiber study of fusimotor action Kuffler et al. (120) immediately recognized that such silence could be largely counteracted by appropriate fusimotor activity and suggested that under normal circumstances such "activity would enable the same muscle stretch to cause a similar increment of sensory discharge at different initial tensions, thus providing a peripheral adjustment for maintaining the constancy of the reflex arc in the face of different conditions." It was further suggested that fusimotor action could be "interpreted as a compensatory mechanism to adjust for mechanical change and to ensure a more constant response to given amounts of stretch" (119). In essence, it was suggested that the fusimotor system existed to maintain the constancy of calibration of the muscle spindle, viewed as a measuring instrument, and to overcome the "design defect" that led to its silence during an important range of physiological conditions; this position was, however, never explicitly formulated.

The weakness of the above case in light of the then current information was seized upon by Eldred et al. (69) who, on the basis of their single fiber recordings in the decerebrate cat, saw the spindle "at the behest of the higher centres" which regardlessly switch it "up and down even to the extremes of its range," and independently of the length of the muscle or its degree of contraction. They also noted that "since the relation between spindle frequency and muscle length is a straight line . . . there will be no part of the range which is more sensitive than another and thus to which it requires to be biassed." Instead, they took their experiments to show that enhanced fusimotor activity contributed by reflex action "a decisive fraction of its excitation" to the α-motoneuron and they discussed this finding in terms of the then newly promulgated servo hypothesis. Thus the earlier idea of calibration maintenance was overshadowed, and no attempt seems to have been made at the time to rescue it.

The recognition of the considerable nonlinearity of the response of the primary ending, however, now puts a new complexion on the matter. The high sensitivity that is shows to small stretches in comparison to large stretches (see subsection *Amplitude Nonlinearity*, p. 196) is only moderately well maintained at different lengths of the muscle when the spindle is passive and is much more so in the presence of tonic fusimotor activity (82). Tonic fusimotor discharge can also be expected to "reset" the high sensitivity that occurs when the muscle is shortened to a new length more rapidly than occurs in the passive spindle. So it seems possible that the development of the functionally favorable region of high sensitivity may have been supported by the development of a dynamic fusimotor system that assisted in resetting and maintaining a constancy of calibration of the spindle's response to small stretches. During static fusimotor action the response to small stretches is also maintained approximately constant with muscle length, albeit at a rather low value.

Central Regulation of Spindle Sensitivity (Parameter Control)

Once it was established that the fusimotor system comprised the functionally separable static and dynamic axons it became immediately obvious that they must be performing different roles and the search for a unitary functional action for the γ-efferents was over. Not only are the effects of the two kinds of axon on the spindle different, there is also substantial evidence that they may on occasion be activated independently by the CNS (see the chapter by Baldissera, Hultborn, and Illert in this *Handbook*). The static axons then inherited the role that had hitherto been that of all the γ-efferents, namely, to produce an excitation of the afferent terminals that was not so very different from that produced by an externally applied stretch. But such a view is quite inapplicable to dynamic fusimotor action in which there is relatively little direct excitation of the primary ending and virtually none of the secondary ending, yet there is a powerful sensitization of the primary ending in its responsiveness to large dynamic stimuli. Moreover, dynamic action was further shown to be unsuited to act as a command signal for muscle shortening in a length servo, because it was incapable of preventing the Ia-afferent from falling silent during releases of quite moderate velocity (corresponding to the effect of muscle contraction) and in spite of an increasing frequency of fusimotor activation (129). Thus dynamic action was seen to have as its raison d'être the control of the dynamic responsiveness of the spindle primary ending, rather than any simple biasing action on spindle discharge. It followed that static action was also seen as important for its role in setting the dynamic responsiveness of the primary and secondary endings to a low value, as well as for its action in biasing their firing by direct excitatory action.

Thus was born the idea that a major function of the fusimotor system is to regulate the responsiveness of the spindle endings to suit the requirements of the prevailing motor act, and by so providing the spindle with a variable calibration make it a much more versatile recording instrument than it could ever be with any particular fixed value of sensitivity. This may be called parameter control because fusimotor action changes the parameters of response of the afferent endings to a fixed mechanical stimulus. The idea differs from earlier views in that the central regulation of the parameter in question in the light of current requirements is seen as the essential, rather than just the maintenance of the spindle calibration at some single constant value in the face of disturbing factors. The term parameter control also has value in that it immediately leads one to ask for a more precise description of the parameter or parameters that are under control. Unfortunately, however, we still lack precise answers largely because of the difficulty of describing the nonlinear behavior of the endings by a relatively simple equation with a limited number of separable parameters. Indeed, for the time being the attempt to do so with the precision of mathematics may even tend to obscure physiological meaning, which at the present stage of understanding may in some respects be better approached qualitatively. Nonetheless some partial answers are discussed in the next subsection, though it should be emphasized that for many purposes it remains quite sufficient to say simply that dynamic fusimotor action enhances, or at least maintains at a high value, the responsiveness of the primary ending to stimuli of any and every kind that contain a component of actual movement, whereas static fusimotor action tends to lower such dynamic sensitivity.

POSITION SENSITIVITY. The simplest parameter of the afferent response of an ending is its position sensitivity measured under static conditions. The position sensitivity is the slope of the line relating the frequency of firing to the length of the muscle, which is altered over an appreciable part of the physiological range (i.e., over at least 2-3 mm for most muscles); the relation usually proves to be tolerably linear over most of its range (69, 92, 123). Dynamic axon stimulation usually has little or no effect on the value obtained; put another way, their weak direct excitatory effect is fairly constant at different muscle lengths (63, 127). Static axon stimulation is likewise often without effect on the position sensitivity, but sometimes it is definitely increased for both primary and secondary endings (41, 63, 112, 127, 130). For example, in one particular case the value increased from 5 to 12 impulses/s per mm for a primary ending during stimulation at 150/s (41). The effect can be even more marked when several axons are stimulated simultaneously, which in some cases potentiates their action in this respect (41). For the secondary endings such an increase in the position sensitivity is the only appreciable "parameter control" action of static stimulation, as this has little effect on their already low dynamic sensitivity. In the conscious cat, an increase of position sensitivity of secondary endings in the jaw closing muscles has been noted during lapping (55). But just how and when any such increase in position sensitivity is physiologically relevant remains an open question. There is no tendency for a given static axon to run true to type in its action in this respect when it is tested upon more than one ending (41, 112, 127), though at one time it was suggested that this might be the case (125).

DYNAMIC MEASUREMENTS OF POSITION SENSITIVITY. The ensuing question is how best to describe the progressive increase in spindle firing that occurs during the rising phase of a large ramp or triangular stretch at constant velocity. As illustrated in Figure 17 after an initial rapid rise in firing at the beginning of the stretch the relation between the instantaneous frequency of firing and the length is often remarkably linear; this linearity is found during either static or dynamic axon stimulation. Crowe and Matthews (62) using ramp stretch regarded the slope of the relation as providing another value for the position sensitivity of the ending, though now measured under dynamic conditions; this is equivalent to regarding the firing at

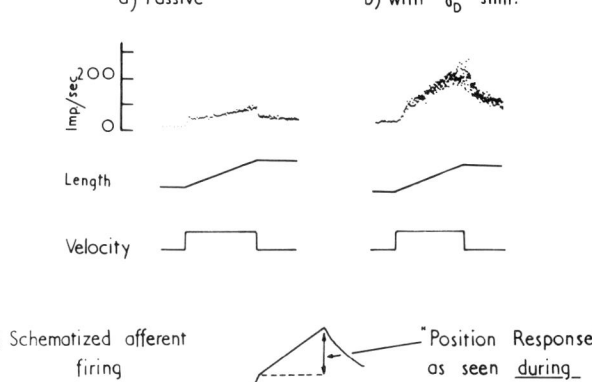

FIG. 17. Position response of a primary ending as seen during dynamic stretching, assuming that length and velocity components of response are approximately additive. Dynamic fusimotor (γ_D) stimulation appears to have a specific action in augmenting this dynamically determined position response without appreciably affecting the position response determined under truly static conditions; the latter then has a much lower value than the former. [Redrawn from Crowe and Matthews (62).]

any moment as made up of the sum of responses to the instantaneous values of the length of the muscle and the velocity of its stretching. They considered that to a first approximation its value was independent of the velocity of stretching, though it tended to increase slightly with increasing velocity in the range of 5-100 mm/s. During static axon stimulation the dynamically obtained position sensitivity agreed with that obtained under static conditions. But during dynamic axon stimulation the dynamically obtained position sensitivity was markedly greater than the same index measured under truly static conditions. The difference was, moreover, progressively enhanced when the frequency of dynamic axon stimulation was increased, as also was the increase of the dynamically measured value above the passive value. This somewhat paradoxical finding on the difference between static and dynamic measurements seems likely to be related to the slow adaptive decay of firing that occurs after completion of the dynamic phase of a ramp stretch applied during dynamic stimulation, which in its turn seems related to the "creep" shown by the bag$_1$ fibers alone of the intrafusal muscle fibers after completion of a stretch (33). Thus the paradox appears to be related to the fundamentals of dynamic action as currently recognized rather than a nonsensical observation to be put aside.

Substantially the same observations were made by Lennerstrand and Thodén (127) using triangular stretching at velocities of 0.5-32 mm/s. They called the same measure of slope the slow velocity response (still expressed in impulses/s per mm). Again, it was described as being very considerably increased during dynamic axon stimulation, and in spite of the constancy of the statically determined position response. But they described it as increasing with increasing velocity of stretching during dynamic stimulation though not for the passive ending, thus further complicating understanding. The effect of velocity on the dynamically determined "position response" may perhaps be related to the use of triangular rather than ramp stretches, because this form of stretching would seem to lead to higher values for the measurement under otherwise similar conditions (see illustrations in refs. 41, 78), probably through the response to the rising phase of the triangular stretch being conditioned by the immediately preceding release. In any case, for the higher velocities of stretch the effect of velocity was sufficiently small for Lennerstrand and Thoden to suggest also that "the slow velocity response by its time course serves to 'integrate' the response to the dynamic part of the length change" and so signal position, although with a "gain" somewhat dependent on velocity. The behavior with lower velocities may perhaps be largely irrelevant for functional consideration because they might fall outside the "working range" of the conditions the spindle primary is designed to signal in the body when it is tuned up by dynamic fusimotor action. By analogy, in instrumentation practice the response to a particular direct current variable such as length may often be most expeditiously provided by an alternating current device with a time constant that is sufficiently long not to obtrude itself under normal working conditions, although it would grossly deform any measurement made under slowly changing or truly static conditions. At any rate, the whole problem of the dynamic measurement of position sensitivity seems of sufficient interest for it to attract further study and is very relevant to the role of dynamic fusimotor action in influencing the responsiveness of the primary ending to any dynamic stretch of appreciable amplitude such as sinusoidal stretching.

VELOCITY SENSITIVITY. As already amply noted the nonlinearities of the spindle prevent any single measure providing a full and proper indication of the sensitivity of its afferent endings to the conceptually distinct stimulus of velocity. It is agreed, of course, that for a given length of the muscle the frequency of firing is higher while the muscle is being stretched than when it is not, and that the excess under dynamic conditions increases with the velocity of stretching. As shown in Figure 18 the crude measure of the dynamic index is systematically increased by dynamic fusimotor stimulation and systematically decreased by static fusimotor stimulation (62). Part of this excess during dynamic axon stimulation depends on the extent to which the "dynamic position response" is boosted above the "static position response" by the fusimotor stimulation and thus should not in any way be taken as a simple velocity response. The working simplification of the past few years in considering the dynamic index as a direct measure of velocity sensitivity now seems best avoided, because it readily becomes potentially misleading in attempting the more precise understanding to which we now aspire. But after allowing for this slow component there is a rapid component of response that is also increased by dynamic axon stimulation and decreased by static axon stimulation. The same is true for the "quick velocity response" of Lennerstrand and Thoden (127, 128) observed in triangular stretching. In both cases the slope of the relation may be altered by fusimotor stimulation. Thus current evidence suggests that dynamic stimulation increases and static stimulation decreases the absolute size of the response of the spindle primary ending to the stimulus of velocity.

But whatever measure is used, the relation between the index of velocity sensitivity and velocity departs from a straight line on a linear plot, as in Figure 18. Moreover, any linear approximation fails to pass through zero so that an estimate of the average slope still does not provide a single full measure of "velocity sensitivity" because the intercept also needs to be stated; hence, two parameters and not just one appear to be required. It is thus important to note that, as in Figure 18, dynamic stimulation has a strong tendency to shift the curve of dynamic index against velocity upward, and that a change of slope is only marked for the lower velocities of stretching and the higher frequencies of stimulation; for other muscles, the change of slope during dynamic axon stimulation may be less pronounced than it is for the cat soleus (cat tibialis posterior, ref. 37; baboon soleus, ref. 54).

The same relation is found for the quick velocity response observed with triangular stretching (127). The usual effect of static axon stimulation is a uniform reduction of its value with little or no change of slope. On log-log plots, however, which straighten out the normal curvature of the linear plots (cf. Fig. 18), static axon stimulation has been reported to increase the slope and dynamic axon stimulation to reduce it (164). Thus while it may be concluded that from at least some points of view dynamic axon stimulation does increase velocity responsiveness and static axon stimulation does reduce it, the matter is far from simple when one attempts to characterize the effect in detail.

RELATION OF VELOCITY SENSITIVITY TO POSITION SENSITIVITY. In a linear system subjected to a sinusoidal mechanical input the phase angle of the output relative to the input gives a direct measurement of relative sensitivity to length and to velocity; pure velocity sensitivity gives a phase advance of 90°, pure length sensitivity gives a phase angle of 0°, and intermediate values give intermediate phase angles. At 1 Hz the passive spindle primary shows a phase advance of 35° or more, indicating that it is indeed responding to some compound of length and velocity stimuli. Whatever the complications in precisely measuring the velocity sensitivity, because the peak spindle firing occurs before the peak of the extension there is no question of it responding to length alone. The value of

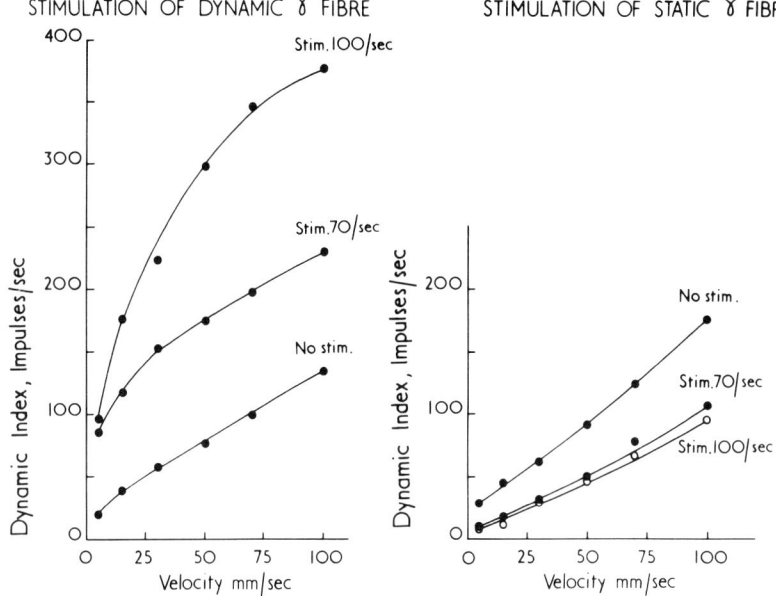

FIG. 18. Effects of fusimotor stimulation on the relation for a primary ending between dynamic index and velocity of stretching for large amplitude stretching (6-mm stretch of cat soleus). Dynamic index is difference between frequency of discharge just before end of dynamic phase of a ramp stretch and that occurring 0.5 s later with the muscle held at the final length. [From Crowe and Matthews (62).]

the phase angle is also interesting from another point of view, namely that of reflex stability and the tendency for a muscle to develop any reflexly initiated tremor. In an engineered system the tendency to oscillate can often be damped by causing some element of the system, such as a length transducer, to respond with appreciable phase advance on its input. It is thus natural to inquire whether the dynamic sensitivity of the primary ending could be performing such a function. (See the chapters by Rack and by Stein and Lee in this *Handbook*.) It was indeed speculatively suggested at the very outset that the control of the dynamic sensitivity of the spindle by fusimotor action might perhaps represent a control of the phase advance of the spindle and thus the damping of the stretch reflex arc (113, 114). But the detailed studies of Crowe and Matthews (62) showed that no conclusion could be reached solely on the observation of an increase of velocity sensitivity, especially as assessed simply on the dynamic index, because among other things the position sensitivity measured dynamically was also increased by dynamic action.

Recent direct measurements of the response of the spindle to sinusoidal stretching strongly suggest that any effect of fusimotor stimulation on the phase of the spindles' response is too small and too erratic to be considered functionally significant for motor control. Thus the suggestion of such a role for any fusimotor-induced regulation of spindle phase founders for the want of evidence. When the stretching is made suitably small the spindle behaves linearly, thus permitting the categorical statement that at the low frequencies important for motor control its phase does not change with fusimotor stimulation, as illustrated in Figure 19 (50, 51, 82). In accordance with this, the form of the low-frequency–response curve is not altered but merely depressed by a constant amount, which is large for static action and very small for dynamic action. The effects above 20 Hz seem of considerable interest from the point of view of the internal working of the spindle, but seem to have little relevance to the problems of muscle control in the body. When the stretching is of larger amplitude (up to several millimeters) the modulation of afferent firing can still be fitted with a sine and its phase angle determined, but there are now various signs of nonlinearity in the response so that the parameters of this single sinusoid no longer provide a comphrensive assessment of the afferent behavior, and less significance can be attached to small changes in phase angle. For example, with increased amplitude of stretching the phase advance of the passive primary ending increases by as much as 20°–30°. The spindle may show about 15° greater advance during dynamic than during static stimulation but there seems little reason to attach major significance to this measurement, which might be due to nonlinearities. Moreover, if the stimulation of a static and of a dynamic fiber are combined, the phase of the spindle response shows no systematic alteration of the relative balance of action of the two kinds of fiber by altering their relative rates of stimulation (101), though this should occur if the action on phase was of prime physiological significance. Similar measurements on the response of the secondary ending in its linear range

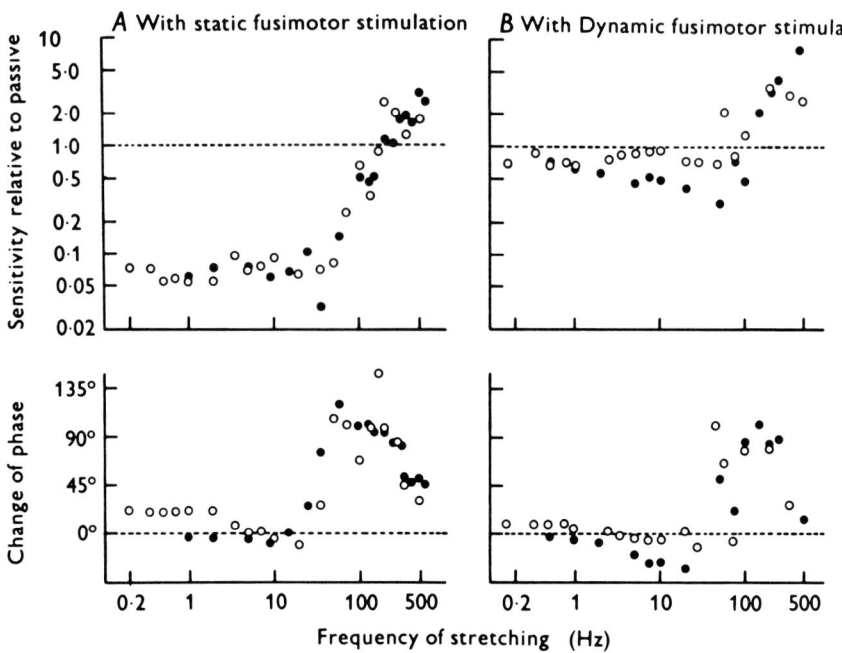

FIG. 19. Change induced by fusimotor stimulation in responsiveness of spindle primary ending to small amplitude sinusoidal stretching of a wide range of frequencies. *Top*, logarithmic plots of ratio of sensitivity of activated spindle (cf. Fig. 6) to that of passive spindle. *Bottom*, linear plots of arithmetic difference between the phases in the 2 states. For motor control purposes, only the effects below 20–30 Hz appear relevant. At each frequency the amplitude of stretching was restricted to the linear range. ○, Obtained from a single spindle; ●, static and dynamic effects from separate spindles. [From Goodwin, Hulliger, and Matthews (82).]

again show no effect of static axon stimulation on the phase of its response. Thus from present evidence it may be concluded that fusimotor action does not function as a controller of the phase of the spindle and thus of the damping of the stretch reflex arc.

GAIN OF SPINDLE TO DYNAMIC STIMULI. An important finding arising from the quantitative studies with sinusoidal stretching is that the sensitivity or gain of the primary ending to the stretching, expressed as impulses per second of firing per unit extension, is about tenfold greater during dynamic than during static axon stimulation. This applies whatever the amplitude of movement and for frequencies up to about 30 Hz, which may be considered the physiological limit for the purposes of motor control (though when the movement is large the matter has yet to be studied in detail at the higher frequencies). For static action the sensitivity is always reduced far below the value obtained for the passive spindle with the same parameters of stretching. For dynamic action the sensitivity may be slightly reduced from or maintained at the passive value when the movement is small (up to about 200-μm amplitude at 1 Hz), but is increased above the passive value when the amplitude of movement is large; this slightly paradoxical observation need not distract attention from what may be judged the functionally much more important observation of the great

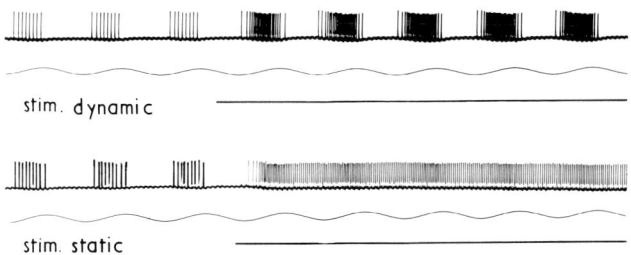

FIG. 20. Effect of fusimotor stimulation on response of a primary ending to sinusoidal stretching of appreciable amplitude (1 mm peak to peak at 3 Hz.) γ_D, Dynamic axon; γ_S, static axon. [From Crowe and Matthews (63).]

difference in sensitivity found during the two types of fusimotor action. Figure 20 illustrates this difference qualitatively by a direct display of spikes, which suffices to demonstrate the gross difference in modulation of the afferent firing produced by the same stretch applied during stimulation of each type of axon. Intermediate values of sensitivity to large stretches may be obtained with continuous gradation by controlling the relative balance of static to dynamic action, by altering their relative frequencies of activation when the two types of axon are stimulated simultaneously (101). It should be noted that even when dynamic action does not change the sensitivity from the passive value, it may have the beneficial action of holding this value relatively much more constant with changes of muscle length than would occur for the passive response. For the secondary ending, static fusimotor action leads to only a relatively small reduction in sensitivity, to about 50% of the passive value, when the action of single axons on the response to small stretches is tested. However, on the basis of experiments on decerebrate cats it seems possible that the reduction may perhaps be appreciably more pronounced when several static axons are active simultaneously (64, 138). During stimulation of single static axons the sensitivity of primary and secondary endings becomes remarkably similar for a wide range of amplitudes and for frequencies up to about 10 Hz; the primary ending, however, is still expected to show appreciably more phase advance than the secondary ending.

There seems to be nothing special about sinusoidal movement for the assessment of the dynamic sensitivity of the spindle and similar results are to be expected with triangular or any other wave form incorporating an element of motion. Indeed, so far, exact measurement of sinusoidal responses has done rather little other than to put on a sound footing what is immediately apparent from displays of instantaneous frequency on spike trains, namely that dynamic action sets the responsiveness of the primary ending to a high level for any and every dynamic stimulus, whereas static action turns the sensitivity down to a much lower level. The new feature obtained by quantitative analysis is that this should be viewed as a general action on sensitivity, as measured dynamically, and not as a specific sensitizing action of the response to the stimulus of velocity independently of the stimulus of progressive length change. All in all, the terms dynamic and static continue to be appropriate labels for the two types of fusimotor action for both of which parameter control can be seen to be one of their essential features, and probably the only one for the dynamic axons.

It is worth noting as a final twist that the effect of dynamic activity in promoting a high sensitivity to small disturbances, as might be advantageous in postural holding reactions, only occurs in the virtual absence of static activity. Any static activity that is sufficient to increase the mean firing of the primary ending appreciably leads to complete occlusion of the effect of dynamic axon stimulation, so that the response of the ending to small stretches is simply like that obtained when the static axon is stimulated on its own (101, 124, 165). Thus if it desires to produce a high spindle sensitivity to small movements the CNS needs to activate the dynamic fusimotor neurons rather selectively. For large movements, however, dynamic fusimotor action can break through and sum with static action to produce an effect on sensitivity that is intermediate between that produced by either on their own. This is also of interest in relation to the functional role of any static axon activation of bag$_1$ intrafusal muscle fibers.

Fusimotor Biasing and Suggested Role as Servo Input

When other factors remain unchanged an increase in fusimotor activity leads to an increased firing of both primary and secondary afferent endings. Expressed in terms of impulses per second, the effect of static axon stimulation is about twice as great for primary endings as it is for secondary endings (41, 127, 128). The effect of dynamic stimulation on primary endings at constant length is often comparatively weak in spite of a powerful dynamic sensitizing action. However, in two published series the excitation produced by dynamic axons was reported on average to be about the same as that produced by static axons (37, 62), but some of the excitation may have been provided by activation of bag$_2$ or chain fibers along with the essential bag$_1$ fiber to give a response that might perhaps be more properly described as mixed. Pure dynamic axons have a considerably weaker direct excitatory action than static axons (78). Because the static axons to a given spindle considerably outnumber the dynamic axons (see subsection *Delimitation of Static and Dynamic Fusimotor Axons*, p. 200), there seems little doubt that virtually all the direct excitatory action of primary endings must originate with the static fusimotor system, as also, of course, does that of the secondary endings.

A major question from the functional point of view is whether the direct excitatory action of the fusimotor system should be seen as meaningful in itself, in the sense that such an increased afferent firing occurs normally in the body during motor acts and leads to some desired motor consequence. Alternatively, it might be in some senses a by-product of providing the spindle with a contractile system so as to enable it to adjust itself to movements of the whole muscle and be brought into unnatural prominence by the use of unphysiologically high frequencies of stimulation of individual fusimotor axons, or the use of "pathological" preparations such as the decerebrate cat. Thought on this matter has been dominated for the last quarter of a century by the servo hypothesis in which increased Ia-afferent firing resulting from fusimotor activation was seen as the essential and necessary link in eliciting contraction via the "γ-route"; thus until quite recently independent thought on the matter has been largely in abeyance, and attention has been concentrated on the servo hypothesis as a whole.

SERVO HYPOTHESIS. The servo hypothesis as originally introduced by Merton in 1953 (143) contained two separate elements, *1*) that a voluntarily contracting muscle remains under autogenetic stretch reflex control throughout the course of a movement, and *2*) that fusimotor activity commonly provides the whole of the command signal, which resets the preexisting equilibrium of the stretch reflex and therefore automatically guides the muscle to a new length. It was implicitly supposed that the gain of the stretch reflex was sufficiently high for a comparatively modest increase in spindle firing to elicit a sufficiently powerful contraction to deal with most eventualities, and also that the stretch reflex was sufficiently well focused on individual motoneuron pools to ensure contraction only of closely synergistic muscles; later work cast doubt on both points (67, 137, 147). Initially the hypothesis was supported slightly indiscriminately by evidence favoring either of its two basic elements, for it tended quite erroneously to be supposed that the use of only the γ-route, and not the α-route, to command contraction would permit the self-regulating properties of the stretch reflex to remain continuously in action during the course of a movement. In fact, provided the spindles do not fall completely silent the muscle can equally remain under reflex control during a movement that is mediated solely by direct activation of the motoneurons so long as the command signal is made sufficiently powerful to allow for the partial withdrawal of reflex support from the spindles (135, 137); approximately steady fusimotor activity related weakly or not at all to the progress of the contraction might well suffice to prevent total spindle silencing during movement. Thus the steady accumulation of evidence over the years, with recent highlights, demonstrating the existence of servo or reflex control during the course of voluntary movement and muscle contraction throws little or no light on the functional role of any concurrent γ-bias and on the extent of its modulation during muscular acts. This can only be determined by recording from the γ-efferents and/or the spindle afferents themselves during the course of various acts, preferably in the intact unanesthetized state. Here the evidence is currently equivocal.

In the earliest experiments on anesthetized cats the prominent findings were that γ-motoneurons were commonly activated in advance of the α-motoneurons as a result of central stimulation or reflex activation and, likewise, that increased spindle firing might precede overt muscle contraction (69, 88); both observations fitted in with the suggestion that an increased γ-bias served to initiate muscle action reflexly. In addition, interruption of the feedback reflex pathway by local dorsal root section could abolish gross muscle contraction without influencing the central modulation of γ-bias, as required by the servo hypothesis, though again not sufficient to prove it. As a result of this work the servo hypothesis was widely accepted from about 1953 to 1973, though sometimes in such a loose form as to be almost unrecognizable. The demise of the follow-up servo hypothesis was brought about by three main factors. The first was the progressive recognition that selective fusimotor activation was uncommon and that coactivation of α- and γ-fibers was the usual rule, as had been equally emphasized with the earliest recordings but without the implications for the follow-up servo hypothesis being especially noted. The second factor was the fuller demonstration than before that chronic deafferentation in no way prevented a wide range of movements such as in chewing (83), showing at the least that the body could switch rapidly out of the follow-up servo mode. Third, recordings of Ia activity in progressively more natural situations showed no signs of γ-fiber activity and Ia firing regularly preceding α-fiber firing as was required if the former were to be the sole cause of the latter. Thus probably none would now argue that the biasing action of fusimotor axons should be seen as giving them a uniquely essential role in the initiation and mediation of muscle contraction.

COACTIVATION. The ensuing problem, which is still with us, is to inquire into the meaning that should be attached to the normal occurrence of a central coactivation of γ-motoneurons with α-motoneurons. Particular points at issue are how commonly such coactivation leads to an appreciable increase in spindle firing above preexisting levels, and whether any such increased afferent input produces a significant increase in α-motoneuron firing. Concerning the latter, there is little information available for the intact state, as opposed to the decerebrate cat, and it is tied up with the uncertainty about the reflex role of the group II afferents from the spindle secondary endings. If these exert a predominantly inhibitory action on their own motoneurons, then the net outcome of an increase in static fusimotor activity could prove to be either excitatory or inhibitory depending on the relative potencies of the group Ia and the group II pathways; this in its turn might depend on whether either pathway was being switched on or switched off by higher action on its interneurons or incoming afferent fibers (see the chapter by Baldissera, Hultborn, and Illert in this Handbook). At any rate, the days are past when it was enough simply to demonstrate increased Ia firing for significant servo action to be accepted. The degree to which coactivation of the α-motoneurons along with the γ-motoneurons actually increases spindle firing seems to vary from preparation to preparation. Assessment is further complicated by the use of Ia recording to indicate the behavior of the γ-efferents, for when the spindle slows during muscle contraction it may be very hard to decide whether the γ-motoneurons escaped being activated and coactivation was absent, or whether the simultaneous activation of the γ-motoneurons was just at too low a level to enable the spindles to keep up fully with the shortening of the main muscle.

Under isometric conditions central coactivation of the γ-motoneurons along with the α-motoneurons commonly leads to an increase in spindle firing above its preexisting level; this has been seen, for example, in the decerebrate cat for the triceps surae muscle (69), in the conscious human for forearm muscles making steady contractions as shown in Figure 21 (180–182), and in the human during standing (44). For humans it is notable that the fusimotor-induced in-

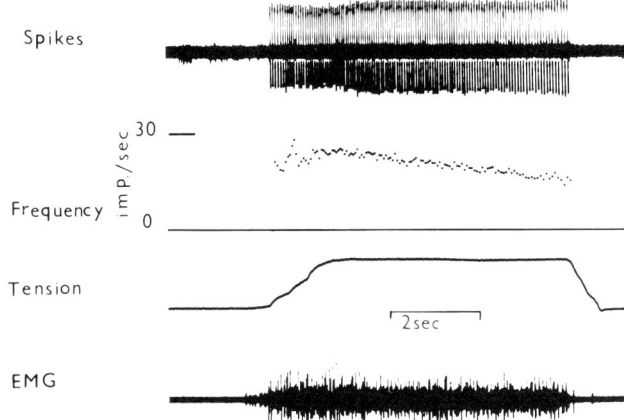

FIG. 21. Discharge in the human of a presumed primary spindle afferent during a weak, voluntary isometric contraction of the muscle it supplied (flexor of index finger). EMG, electromyogram. [From Vallbo (179).]

crease in the frequency of Ia discharge is very modest in comparison with that in the cat (20/s as opposed to 100/s), reminding one of the necessity of remaining awake to the possibility of the existence of other, more significant differences between the species; for example, with increased peripheral conduction distance, and hence reflex delay, the operation of a servo might be expected to face more serious difficulties in large animals. In human voluntary contraction the Ia firing and hence, presumably, the intensity of γ-motoneuron activation is closely graded with the strength of the contraction (182), suggesting that the input coupling for the two types of motoneurons is fairly tight; nerve pressure block experiments exclude the possibility that the fusimotor action might be mediated solely by β-axons (49). Except for the selective activation of α-motoneurons in the tonic vibration reflex (48) there has yet to be a demonstration of the independent activation of α- and of γ-motoneurons in the human, and there is still no human experimental evidence for the selective activation of the spindle that might be expected to occur under some set of conditions simply by virtue of its possessing its own private motor supply.

Once strict isometricity is abandoned and moderately rapid movement is allowed, then in all preparations so far studied the signs of coactivation become far less prominent and the pattern of spindle discharge may become dominated by the effect of change of length, with increased firing during stretch of a muscle by the action of its antagonist and with slowing during the shortening produced by its own contraction; Figure 22 shows a particular example. This state of affairs has been described for chewing movements in the cat (55) and in the monkey (84), where the recording is made intracranially from the cell bodies of the mesencephalic nucleus of the fifth nerve, and for walking and other movements in the conscious cat, where the unitary recording was achieved by fine mobile electrodes placed in the dorsal roots (153, 154). Signs of coactivation can, however, usually be detected when the muscle contracts provided that its length changes only slowly. In other cases, as during walking in the decerebrate cat, the fusimotor action on the Ia-afferents may take precedence over the effects of stretch so that the firing is modulated in phase with the muscle contraction rather than with the stretch (168). This action is particularly marked for spindles in the inspiratory intercostal muscles of the anesthetized cat (61). Figure 23 illustrates a particular case of a unit similar to that of Figure 22, but one for which the variation of fusimotor bias more or less compensated for the effect of the movement as its firing remained approximately constant during most of the movement. In humans, where the unitary recording is achieved with intraneural tungsten electrodes, only rather slow movements have so far been studied. For these the Ia firing is remarkably similar while the muscle is shortening and while the muscle is lengthening against an approximately steady load as illustrated in Figure 24 (46), and there is little sign of the additional γ-motoneuron-induced firing, which might have been suggested by the servo theory to occur during the shortening and so provide its cause.

Assessment

Thus while in some situations, particularly isometric ones, the α-motoneurons may well be provided with part of their drive reflexly via the γ-route there remain many other situations where it seems unlikely that the γ-route contributes anything of consequence, if indeed it contributes any direct drive at all. But this is not to say that the spindles do not assist in the reflex regulation of movement when a muscle shortens or that the usual coactivation is irrelevant. As recently emphasized (45, 46), any irregularities that occur in the course of a movement or any minor obstacles lead to a recordable change in human spindle firing, which may then lead to the appropriate reflex compensatory change in motoneuron firing. Similarly, in human isometric contraction the spindle may on occasion be very sensitive to small tension fluctuations that occur in a nominally steady force development in which increased tension unloads the spindle (182); these results again suggest that the spindle, assisted by its fusimotor bias, plays a part in fine regulation. In certain movements of the conscious cat, however, any coactivation left the spindles behaving in response to obstruction of the movement very much as they did when all γ-bias was abolished by anesthesia and the same movement was imposed by the experiments (152). More detailed and preferably quantitative studies of spindles during a variety of musclar acts are greatly needed to help cast more light on all this.

At present two views remain at least partially acceptable and to some extent complementary as schematically illustrated in Figure 25. The first view is

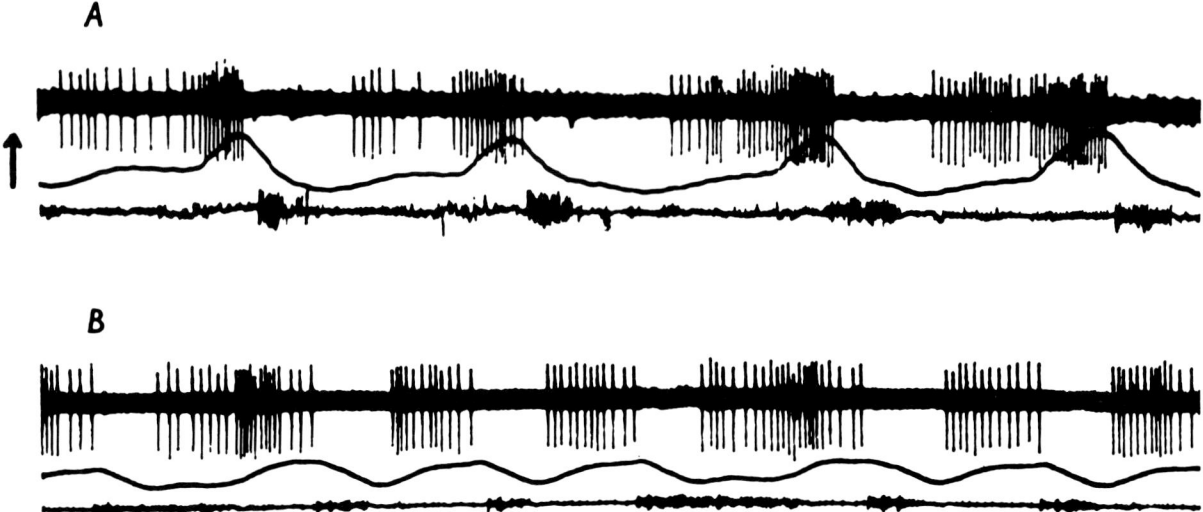

FIG. 22. Responses of a presumed spindle primary afferent from a jaw closing muscle of conscious cat. *A*: during eating. *B*: during lapping. *Top*, spindle spikes; *middle*, jaw movement with jaw opening upward, length of *arrow* indicates 25°; *bottom*, gross electromyogram recorded from masseter muscle in which the spindle lay. [From Cody et al. (55).]

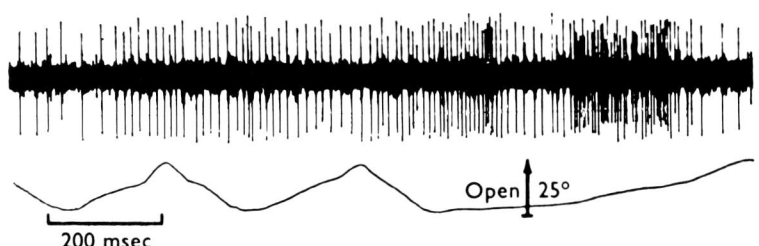

FIG. 23. Example of a period of movement in the conscious cat. Degree of fusimotor activity was such that the discharge of a presumed spindle primary afferent remained approximately constant. Records taken during licking of lips from a jaw-closing spindle that behaved similarly to that of Figure 22*A*. Length of *arrow* indicates 25°. [From Cody et al. (55).]

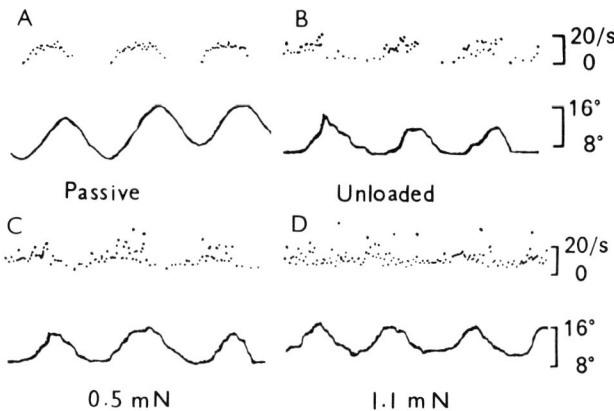

FIG. 24. Behavior of a presumed primary spindle afferent in the human during slow rhythmic voluntary movement. Spindle lay in the tibialis anterior. *A*: foot was moved passively. *B–D*: foot was moved actively either unloaded or against a load (expressed as torque in Newton meters) produced by a rubber band opposing flexion, and thus augmenting contraction of the tibialis anterior. *Top*, instantaneous frequency of firing; *bottom*, ankle movement. [From Burke et al. (46).]

that, as in the earliest tradition, the fusimotor bias serves simply to set the calibration and sensitivity of the spindle throughout the course of any movement for which the CNS wishes to receive continuous information about its course. The two kinds of fusimotor axon would then be seen as having "parameter regulation" as their special function. A high dynamic sensitivity would, however, probably be beyond achievement during the course of a rapid shortening because the bag$_1$ fibers would be unable to contract rapidly enough to keep up. But as an escape clause it should be remembered that, of course, virtually all muscle action involves two opposing muscles so that for rapid movements the CNS might find it simplest to obtain information about what is happening by analyzing the high-frequency firing of the relaxing muscle that is being stretched; and it might abandon the attempt to provide sufficient γ-bias to keep the spindles of the contracting muscle firing during its rapid shortening. This would probably also entail temporary switching off of the reflex connections that normally provide for

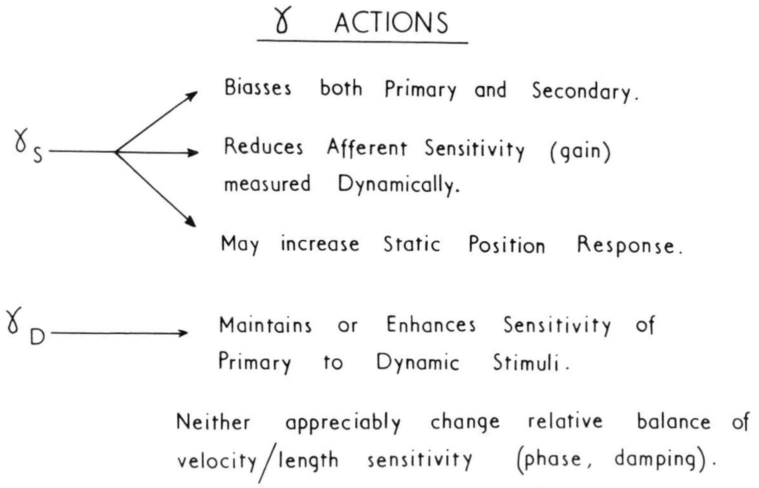

γ ACTIONS

γ_S
- Biasses both Primary and Secondary.
- Reduces Afferent Sensitivity (gain) measured Dynamically.
- May increase Static Position Response.

γ_D → Maintains or Enhances Sensitivity of Primary to Dynamic Stimuli.

Neither appreciably change relative balance of velocity/length sensitivity (phase, damping).

FIG. 25. Summarizing diagram of static (γ_S) and dynamic (γ_D) fusimotor actions that may be currently deemed to be of functional importance.

continuous stretch reflex control, but it would be quite appropriate for such a ballistic movement to be performed without the occurrence of feedback. The information from spindles is probably also of value in a variety of other ways for a variety of levels of the CNS.

SERVO ASSISTANCE AND MODELING OF MOVEMENT. The second view is that spindles provide a degree of servo assistance of movement. This rather loose term can be used to cover two or more slightly separate ideas. As used before (136, 137, 171) it tended to be directed primarily toward describing coactivation of sufficient strength to increase Ia firing and thereby reflexly supplying part of the drive to the motoneurons, in addition to that portion reaching them directly. This mode of operation would avoid the delay inherent in using the γ-loop on its own while equally preserving feedback control. However, the specification of the final position of the muscle would then no longer be provided by knowing the length of the muscle at which the fusimotor-enhanced Ia firing would be restored to normal as in the original follow-up hypothesis, for when the reflex drive had been thereby annulled the direct drive on the α-motoneurons would cause the muscle to shorten still further; the degree of further shortening would depend on the gain of both the Ia and II reflex feedback loops. A slight modification of the idea, which avoids this difficulty and which can still pass under the term of servo assistance, was suggested in 1964 by Matthews (135) and later given formal illustration by Phillips in 1969 (147). It is that the fusimotor discharge is tailored to reproduce within the spindle the extent and time course of the movement that it is planned that the extrafusal fibers should perform, so that if the trajectory of the movement occurs as desired then the spindle firing changes rather little throughout its course. But any deviation from the planned movement would then lead to a change in spindle firing, either an acceleration or a slowing, and this would provide for an immediate reflex compensation to bring the movement back onto target. Such a mode of operation would entail coactivation of α- and γ-fibers not in a fixed ratio, but in proportions adjusted to suit the prevailing mechanical conditions. The planned performance of a given movement against a known load would entail more α-motoneuron firing but the same amount of γ-motoneuron firing as the performance of the same movement without a load. Because the spindle firing would remain constant when the movement proceeded correctly there would then never be any conflict between the central and the reflex drives upon the motoneurons, such as at the final desired equilibrium length, and the reflex would only be called into play if and when things went wrong. In the servo context all this would make sense of the anatomical independence of the γ-motoneurons from the α-motoneurons and would provide for a superiority of this system over the simple obligatory coactivation of lower animals with their fixed ratio of action upon the extra- and the intrafusal muscle fibers. Moreover, following this way of thinking a small degree of obligatory coactivation would provide no obstacle to understanding because an essential degree of independence of the spindle could still be assured by the central manipulation of the behavior of the purely fusimotor fibers.

From this point of view what is asked of γ-motoneuron firing is that it should lead to the setting up of a model within the spindle to mirror the intended movement. Such an idea retains considerable validity if the function of the spindle messages is simply to signal how well the movement has been performed throughout its course, irrespective of whether or not this information is used for immediate corrective action at the spinal or any other level. This is similar to viewing the γ-efferent discharge as an "efference copy" or a "corollary discharge" sent from a motor center to a sensory center to be used as a template of the expected state of affairs for comparison with the afferent discharge returning during the execution of a motor act; but, in this case, the comparison would be made before rather than after the generation of the afferent signal. The detection and measurement of an unexpected small signal that occurs in the presence of a large, but predictable, signal can be achieved most effectively by using a suitable backing signal to hold a highly sensitive measuring instrument within its working range and thus prevent it being saturated by the large signal, which under these circumstances contains no information. To achieve the same precision with an instrument that would measure throughout the full range of the large signal would make tremendously greater demands upon its performance and freedom from noise. For such a mode of operation there would be no necessity for the spindle firing to be held precisely at the particular null value of the preexisting level before the movement; the requirement is simply that the spindle should not be allowed at any stage to fall too near either silence or saturation, and that to read full meaning into the spindle messages the analyzing centers should have independent access to the level of fusimotor bias, conceived equally as a backing signal and as a gain control. But because the backing signal would, presumably, normally be provided by static axon activity, the gain during any such mode of operation would seem to be reduced obligatorily from the very high values it may have with the muscle at a constant length when passive or with dynamic activation. However, neither such mode of operation nor effective servo assistance appears to apply to movements that are so rapid that the spindles in the contracting muscles fall quite silent as they shorten.

Finally, it should be emphasized in all such considerations that the role of the secondary ending seems likely to be as crucial as that of the primary ending. The primary ending, with its nonlinearity of response and great sensitivity to dynamic stimuli, seems best suited to signaling small sudden deviations with a view to their immediate correction. The secondary ending is much better at signaling quasi-steady states and the relation between muscle length and static fusimotor bias with a view to longer term regulation. However, they are not independent channels of information, but rather are both exposed to the same external stretch and are both influenced by the same static fusimotor bias, with only the dynamic axons to provide a variable degree of coupling between their behavior. Acting together they may be presumed to provide for a versatility of muscle control that neither could supply on its own, and possibly to provide information that could be obtained only by the analysis of their discharges in relation to each other.

SUMMARY

Structure

The mammalian muscle spindle is now thought to contain three morphologically distinct types of intrafusal muscle fiber. The nuclear-chain fibers, of which there are several in a given spindle, are thinner and shorter than the nuclear-bag fibers, have their nuclei arranged in a longitudinal chain in the equatorial region of the spindle, and have a well-developed M line in the middle of the sarcomere. The nuclear-bag fibers are now divided into bag_1 and and bag_2 fibers. These fibers are generally similar in their gross appearance with a collection of nuclei (bags) in the equatorial region of the spindle, but they differ histochemically in their staining reactions for myofibrillar ATPase and in the appearance of the M line, which may be absent in the bag_1 fiber and which is only moderately developed in the bag_2 fiber. Such criteria place the bag_2 fibers closer than the bag_1 fibers to the chain fibers. There is usually one bag fiber of each kind within a spindle. Three types of motor terminal are currently recognized, though their precise delimitation, their efferent axons of origin, and the extent to which each may be found on each type of intrafusal fiber awaits resolution. They are the trail endings, which extend an appreciable distance along the intrafusal muscle fibers, and the discretely localized p_1 and p_2 plate endings; the p_1 plates are smaller and have more junctional infolding than the p_2 plates. The afferent endings are subdivided into only two kinds, as they have been since the turn of the century. The primary ending, of which there is only one in a given spindle, lies in the poorly striated equatorial region of the spindle and usually has terminations on every one of the intrafusal fibers. The secondary endings, of which there may be none, one, or more than one, flank the primary ending along the length of the intrafusal fibers and are more densely distributed to chain fibers than to bag fibers; their afferent fibers are thinner than those from the primary endings.

Functional Differences Between Primary and Secondary Endings

Under static conditions the primary and secondary endings discharge at similar rates, though the discharge of the secondary ending is more regular. To any kind of dynamic stimulus the primary ending gives an appreciably greater response. This can be seen with ramp stretches of large extent, with tendon taps, with low-frequency sinusoidal stretching, and with high-frequency vibration. It seems possible that the CNS may use these contrasting signals from the two endings of one sensory event to determine both the amplitude and the velocity of a disturbance, but this has yet to be established and the CNS may have other ways of integrating these two parallel channels of information signaling the same thing after different transformations. Recently, the primary ending has been shown to behave rather nonlinearly in response to stimuli of graded amplitude, being relatively more sensitive to small stimuli than to large stimuli; it is thereby enabled to pick up changes of muscle length of the order of 10 μm without being prevented by saturation from signaling the extent of large stretches. The functional dichotomy between primary and secondary endings is well established for limb muscles of a variety of species and here there is also a pronounced bimodality in the spectrum of afferent-fiber diameter; but there are hints that there may be a continuous gradation of afferent responsiveness with fiber size, and thus the dichotomy of function may be less clear for muscles where a bimodality of spindle afferent diameter is less pronounced.

Static and Dynamic Fusimotor Axons

The small diameter γ-efferent axons have long been established as exclusively fusimotor, because their stimulation leads to an increase of afferent discharge of both primary and secondary spindle endings without overt change in muscle tension. Since 1962 it has been accepted that they can be subdivided on functional grounds into static and dynamic axons. The dynamic axons have a relatively weak excitatory action on the primary ending when the length of the muscle is held constant, but they greatly sensitize the primary ending to dynamic stimuli and thus accentuate the specific features of its mechanical responsiveness. A minor exception is that for very small stretches dynamic axon stimulation simply maintains the already high sensitivity of the primary ending at approximately the passive value seen when the muscle is well stretched. The secondary endings are rarely significantly influenced by dynamic axons. The static axons excite both primary and secondary endings to fire under static conditions and reduce the sensitivity of both types of ending to dynamic stimuli. Studies with sinusoidal stretching suggest that these changes in the responsiveness of the endings to dynamic stimuli should be viewed as changes in gain to all stimuli applied under dynamic conditions rather than as specific changes in the level of velocity sensitivity, because the phase of the response to a sinusoidal stretch does not change systematically with the level of fusimotor activation. When static and dynamic axons are stimulated simultaneously then the static action occludes the dynamic action for small imposed stretches; for large stretches the response obtained is intermediate between that for static and for dynamic action on their own. This might provide for a further regulation of gain, though it should be noted that the very highest levels of gain can only be obtained by selective activation of the dynamic system, as might be involved in the regulation of posture rather than of movement.

The static axons are more numerous than the dynamic axons and appear to act via a more rapidly contracting intrafusal system.

A combination of physiological and morphological work has now produced a consensus that the dynamic axons produce their specific effects by virtue of supplying the bag$_1$ intrafusal muscle fibers and that the static axons produce their contrasting effects by virtue of supplying the bag$_2$ and/or the chain fibers, either separately or in combination. A challenging question is why the apparently functionally homogeneous effector system of the static axons should be provided with the dual effector apparatus of the bag$_2$ and the chain fibers; perhaps a sufficient answer is provided by the fact that the contractile properties of these two types of fiber differ, with the chain fibers being "faster." Controversy continues as to how far the static and dynamic axons restrict their distribution to those intrafusal muscle fibers that are responsible for the specificity of their actions as given above; certain evidence suggests that the static axons may also quite frequently supply the bag$_1$ intrafusal muscle fibers.

Skeletofusimotor axons (β-axons) are found in increasing numbers as the search intensifies, so that it now seems improper to look upon them as an evolutionary remnant. However, in large muscles they are an addition to the purely fusimotor axons, which are still believed to provide the major motor supply to the spindle. Both dynamic and static actions now seem to be mediated by β-axons; the former are mediated by slower conducting axons that supply weaker, slower units, and the latter are mediated by faster conducting axons that supply faster, stronger motor units.

Possible Functional Roles for the Fusimotor System

Three reasons have been adduced at various times to explain the existence of a specific fusimotor system; these shade into each other and can still all be accepted in some degree, although in their extreme forms they are exclusive. First, fusimotor activity may provide for the maintenance of the sensitivity of the spindle in the face of externally imposed changes, most notably prolonged change of muscle length or phasic effects of muscle contraction acting to unload the spindle. The former may well apply to the sensitizing action of the dynamic axons in maintaining a high sensitivity to small stimuli. Second, fusimotor activity seems to provide for the regulation of the sensitivity of the spindle to suit the prevailing mechanical conditions, rather than simply holding it at some universally appropriate value. This may be dubbed parameter control, leading to the question of which parameters of spindle responsiveness should be viewed as the ones under control. As just noted, on the basis of sinusoidal stretching it no longer seems appropriate to believe that the dynamic axons exert a specific action on the velocity sensitivity of the primary ending independently of its position sensitivity, because when measured under dynamic conditions the latter also is raised by dynamic action. Rather, the gain of the ending seems to be under control, being high during dynamic action and low during static action irrespective of the size of the stimulus under consideration. Third, fusimotor activity biases the spindle and increases the firing rate of both primary and secondary endings for a given length of the muscle. In the now defunct follow-up servo hypothesis such increased firing of Ia-afferents from primary endings was supposed to be responsible for reflexly initiating and maintaining muscle contraction, but it is now recognized that the coactivation by descending pathways of α- and γ-motoneurons is the rule. This may perhaps still provide for a degree of servo assistance of movement, either by reflexly providing some additional drive to the α-motoneurons by any increase in Ia discharge, or by virtue of holding the Ia firing at an approximately constant level during contraction and muscle shortening so that the spindle is ready to signal any disturbance to the movement. The uncoupling of intrafusal contraction from extrafusal contraction that is provided by a specific γ-fusimotor system (but not by a skeletofusimotor β-system) would allow the α-motor firing to be set centrally to be appropriate for the anticipated load while the fusimotor firing could be made appropriate to the planned trajectory of the movement. Indeed, from this point of view there is no need for the spindle signals to be restricted to, or even used for, immediate reflex compensation. The fusimotor action could equally be viewed as providing a continuously modulated backing signal to maintain a sensitive recording instrument in the appropriate part of its range ready to detect external signals, without its being saturated by much larger internally generated signals of known time course and thus without information content. During rapid movements, however, spindles in the contracting muscle may fall silent and therefore have little opportunity of contributing to any form of regulation. The role of the equally numerous secondary endings in regulatory responses has attracted much less attention than that of the primary ending, though it seems likely that acting together they provide for a versatility of muscle control that neither could supply on its own.

REFERENCES

1. ADAL, M. N., AND D. BARKER. Intramuscular branching of fusimotor fibres. *J. Physiol. London* 177: 288-299, 1965.
2. ANDERSON, J. H. Dynamic characteristics of Golgi tendon organs. *Brain Res.* 67: 531-537, 1974.
3. ANDERSSON, B. F., G. LENNERSTRAND, AND U. THODEN. Response characteristics of muscle spindle endings at constant length to variations in fusimotor activation. *Acta Physiol. Scand.* 74: 301-318, 1968.
4. ANDREW, B. L., G. C. LESLIE, AND N. J. PART. Some observations on the efferent innervation of rat soleus muscle spindles. *Exp. Brain Res.* 31: 433-443, 1978.
5. ANDREW, B. L., AND N. J. PART. The division of control of muscle spindles between fusimotor and mixed skeletomotor fibres in a rat caudal muscle. *Q. J. Exp. Physiol.* 57: 213-225, 1974.
6. APPELBERG, B., P. BESSOU, AND Y. LAPORTE. Action of static and dynamic fusimotor fibres on secondary endings of cat's spindles. *J. Physiol. London* 185: 160-171, 1966.
7. APPELBERG, B., AND A. MOLANDER. A rubro-olivary pathway. I. Identification of a descending system for control of dynamic sensitivity of muscle spindles. *Exp. Brain Res.* 3: 372-381, 1967.
8. ARBUTHNOTT, E. R., I. A. BOYD, M. H. GLADDEN, AND P. N. MCWILLIAM. Real and apparent γ axon contraction sites in intrafusal fibres. *J. Physiol. London* 268: 25P-26P, 1977.
9. BANKS, R. W., D. BARKER, P. BESSOU, B. PAGES, AND M. J. STACEY. Serial-section analysis of cat muscle spindles following observation of the effects of stimulating dynamic fusimotor axons. *J. Physiol. London* 263: 180P-181P, 1976.
10. BANKS, R. W., D. BARKER, P. BESSOU, B. PAGES, AND M. J. STACEY. Histological analysis of muscle spindles following direct observation of effects of stimulating dynamic and static motor axons. *J. Physiol. London* 283: 605-619, 1978.
11. BANKS, R. W., D. BARKER, AND M. J. STACEY. Intrafusal branching and distribution of primary and secondary afferents. *J. Physiol. London* 272: 66P-67P, 1977.
12. BANKS, R. W., D. W. HARKER, AND M. J. STACEY. A study of mammalian intrafusal muscle fibres using a combined histochemical and ultrastructural approach. *J. Anat.* 123: 783-796, 1977.
13. BARKER, D. The innervation of the muscle spindle. *Q. J. Microsc. Sci.* 89: 143-186, 1948.
14. BARKER, D. (editor). *Symposium on Muscle Receptors. Proceedings.* Hong Kong: Hong Kong Univ. Press, 1962.
15. BARKER, D. The morphology of muscle receptors. In: *Handbook of Sensory Physiology. Muscle Receptors,* edited by C. C. Hunt. Berlin: Springer-Verlag, 1974, vol. 3, pt. 2, p. 1-190.
16. BARKER, D., P. BESSOU, E. JANKOWSKA, B. PAGÈS, AND M. J. STACEY. Identification of intrafusal muscle fibres activated by single fusimotor axons and injected with fluorescent dye in cat tenuissimus spindles. *J. Physiol. London* 275: 149-165, 1978.
17. BARKER, D., F. EMONET-DÉNAND, D. W. HARKER, L. JAMI, AND Y. LAPORTE. Distribution of fusimotor axons to intrafusal muscle fibres in cat tenuissimus spindles as determined by the glycogen-depletion method. *J. Physiol. London* 261: 49-69, 1976.
18. BARKER, D., F. EMONET-DÉNAND, D. W. HARKER, L. JAMI, AND Y. LAPORTE. Types of intra- and extrafusal muscle fibre innervated by dynamic skeletofusimotor axons in cat peroneus brevis and tenuissimus muscles, as determined by the glycogen depletion method. *J. Physiol. London* 266: 713-726, 1977.
19. BARKER, D., F. EMONET-DÉNAND, Y. LAPORTE, U. PROSKE, AND D. W. STACEY. Morphological identification and intrafusal distribution of the endings of static fusimotor axons in the cat. *J. Physiol. London* 230: 405-427, 1973.
20. BARKER, D., AND M. C. IP. The motor innervation of cat and rabbit muscle spindles. *J. Physiol. London* 171: 27P-28P, 1965.
21. BARKER, D., AND D. W. STACEY. Rabbit intrafusal muscle fibres. *J. Physiol. London* 210: 70P-72P, 1970.
22. BARKER, D., M. J. STACEY, AND M. N. ADAL. Fusimotor innervation in the cat. *Philos. Trans. R. Soc. London Ser. B.* 258: 315-346, 1970.
23. BESSOU, P., F. EMONET-DÉNAND, AND Y. LAPORTE. Motor fibres innervating extrafusal and intrafusal muscle fibres in the cat. *J. Physiol. London* 180: 469-672, 1965.
24. BESSOU, P., AND Y. LAPORTE. Potentials fusoriaux provoqués par la stimulation de fibres fusimotrices chez le chat. *C. R. Acad. Sci.* 260: 4827-4830, 1965.
25. BESSOU, P., Y. LAPORTE, AND B. PAGÈS. Frequencygrams of spindle primary endings elicited by stimulation of static and

dynamic fusimotor fibres. *J. Physiol. London* 196: 47-63, 1968.
26. BESSOU, P., AND B. PAGÈS. Intracellular potentials from intrafusal muscle fibres evoked by stimulation of static and dynamic fusimotor axons in the cat. *J. Physiol. London* 227: 709-727, 1972.
27. BESSOU, P., AND B. PAGÈS. Cinematographic analysis of contractile events produced in intrafusal muscle fibres by stimulation of static and dynamic fusimotor axons. *J. Physiol. London* 252: 397-427, 1975.
28. BIANCONI, R., AND J. P. VAN DER MEULEN. The response to vibration of the end organs of mammalian muscle spindles. *J. Neurophysiol.* 26: 177-190, 1963.
29. BINDER, M. D., J. S. KRONIN, G. P. MOORE, AND D. G. STUART. The response of Golgi tendon organs to single motor unit contractions. *J. Physiol. London* 271: 337-349, 1977.
30. BOYD, I. A. The structure and innervation of the nuclear bag muscle fibres and the nuclear chain muscle fibre system in mammalian muscle spindles. *Philos. Trans. R. Soc. London Ser. B.* 245: 81-136, 1962.
31. BOYD, I. A. The response of fast and slow nuclear bag fibres and nuclear chain fibres in isolated cat muscle spindles to fusimotor stimulation, and the effect of intrafusal contraction on the sensory endings. *Q. J. Exp. Physiol.* 61: 203-254, 1976.
32. BOYD, I. A., M. H. GLADDEN, P. N. MCWILLIAM, AND J. WARD. Control of dynamic and static nuclear bag fibres and nuclear chain fibres by gamma and beta axons in isolated cat muscle spindles. *J. Physiol. London* 265: 133-162, 1977.
33. BOYD, I. A., M. H. GLADDEN, AND J. WARD. The contribution of intrafusal creep to the dynamic component of the Ia afferent discharge of isolated muscle spindles. *J. Physiol. London* 273: 27P-28P, 1977.
34. BOYD, I. A., AND J. WARD. Motor control of nuclear bag and nuclear chain intrafusal fibres in isolated living muscle spindles from the cat. *J. Physiol. London* 244: 83-112, 1975.
35. BROWN, M. C., AND R. G. BUTLER. Studies on the site of termination of static and dynamic fusimotor fibres within muscle spindles of the tenuissimus muscle of the cat. *J. Physiol. London* 233: 553-573, 1973.
36. BROWN, M. C., AND R. G. BUTLER. An investigation into the site of termination of static gamma fibres within muscle spindles of the cat peroneus longus muscle. *J. Physiol. London* 247: 131-143, 1975.
37. BROWN, M. C., A. CROWE, AND P. B. C. MATTHEWS. Observations on the fusimotor fibres of the tibialis posterior muscle of the cat. *J. Physiol. London* 177: 140-159, 1965.
38. BROWN, M. C., I. ENGBERG, AND P. B. C. MATTHEWS. Fusimotor stimulation and the dynamic sensitivity of the secondary ending of the muscle spindle. *J. Physiol. London* 189: 545-550, 1967.
39. BROWN, M. C., I. E. ENGBERG, AND P. B. C. MATTHEWS. The relative sensitivity to vibration of muscle receptors of the cat. *J. Physiol. London* 192: 773-800, 1967.
40. BROWN, M. C., G. M. GOODWIN, AND P. B. C. MATTHEWS. After-effects of fusimotor stimulation on the response of muscle spindle primary afferent endings. *J. Physiol. London* 205: 677-694, 1969.
41. BROWN, M. C., D. G. LAWRENCE, AND P. B. C. MATTHEWS. Static fusimotor fibres and the position sensitivity of muscle spindle receptors. *Brain Res.* 14: 173-187, 1969.
42. BROWN, M. C., AND P. B. C. MATTHEWS. On the subdivision of the efferent fibres to muscle spindles into static and dynamic fusimotor fibres. In: *Control and Innervation of Skeletal Muscle*, edited by B. L. Andrew. Dundee: Thomson, 1966, p. 18-31.
43. BROWNE, J. S. The responses of muscle spindles in sheep extraocular muscles. *J. Physiol. London* 251: 483-496, 1975.
44. BURKE, D., AND G. EKLUND. Muscle spindle activity in man during standing. *Acta Physiol. Scand.* 100: 187-199, 1977.
45. BURKE, D., K.-E. HAGBARTH, AND L. LÖFSTEDT. Muscle spindle responses in man to changes in load during accurate position maintenance. *J. Physiol. London* 276: 159-164, 1978.
46. BURKE, D., K.-E. HAGBARTH, AND L. LÖFSTEDT. Muscle spindle activity in man during shortening and lengthening contractions. *J. Physiol. London* 277: 131-142, 1978.
47. BURKE, D., K.-E. HAGBARTH, L. LÖFSTEDT, AND B. G. WALLIN. The responses of human muscle spindle endings to vibration of non-contracting muscles. *J. Physiol. London* 261: 673-693, 1976.
48. BURKE, D., K.-E. HAGBARTH, L. LÖFSTEDT, AND B. G. WALLIN. The responses of human muscle spindle endings to vibration during isometric contraction. *J. Physiol. London* 261: 695-711, 1976.
49. BURKE, D., K.-E. HAGBARTH, AND N. F. SKUSE. Voluntary activation of spindle endings in human muscles temporarily paralysed by nerve pressure. *J. Physiol. London* 287: 329-336, 1979.
50. CHEN, W. J., AND R. E. POPPELE. Static fusimotor effect on the sensitivity of mammalian muscle spindles. *Brain Res.* 57: 244-247, 1973.
51. CHEN, W. J., AND R. E. POPPELE. Small-signal analysis of response of mammalian muscle spindles with fusimotor stimulation and a comparison with large-signal responses. *J. Neurophysiol.* 41: 15-27, 1978.
52. CHENEY, P. D., AND J. B. PRESTON. Classification and response characteristics of muscle spindle afferents in the primate. *J. Neurophysiol.* 39: 1-8, 1976.
53. CHENEY, P. D., AND J. B. PRESTON. Classification of fusimotor fibers in the primate. *J. Neurophysiol.* 39: 9-19, 1976.
54. CHENEY, P. D., AND J. B. PRESTON. Effects of fusimotor stimulation on dynamic and position sensitivities of spindle afferents in the primate. *J. Neurophysiol.* 39: 20-30, 1976.
55. CODY, F. W. J., L. M. HARRISON, AND A. TAYLOR. Analysis of activity of muscle spindles of jaw-closing muscles during normal movements in the cat. *J. Physiol. London* 253: 565-582, 1975.
56. CODY, F. W. J., R. W. H. LEE, AND A. TAYLOR. A functional analysis of the components of the mesencephalic nucleus of the fifth nerve of the cat. *J. Physiol. London* 226: 249-261, 1972.
57. COËRS, C., AND J. DURAND. Données morphologiques nouvelles sur l'innervation des fuseaux neuromusculaires. *Arch. Biol.* 67: 685-715, 1956.
58. COOPER, S. The responses of the primary and secondary endings of muscle spindles with intact motor innervation during applied stretch. *Q. J. Exp. Physiol.* 46: 389-398, 1961.
59. COOPER, S., AND P. M. DANIEL. Muscle spindles in man; their morphology in the lumbricals and the deep muscles of the neck. *Brain* 86: 563-586, 1963.
60. COOPER, S., AND M. H. GLADDEN. Elastic fibres and reticulin of mammalian muscle spindles and their functional significance. *Q. J. Exp. Physiol.* 59: 367-385, 1974.
61. CRITCHLOW, V., AND C. VON EULER. Intercostal muscle spindle activity and its γ-motor control. *J. Physiol. London* 168: 820-847, 1963.
62. CROWE, A., AND P. B. C. MATTHEWS. The effects of stimulation of static and dynamic fusimotor fibres on the response to stretching of the primary endings of muscle spindles. *J. Physiol. London* 174: 109-131, 1964.
63. CROWE, A., AND P. B. C. MATTHEWS. Further studies of static and dynamic fusimotor fibres. *J. Physiol. London* 174: 132-151, 1964.
64. CUSSONS, P. D., M. HULLIGER, AND P. B. C. MATTHEWS. Effects of fusimotor stimulation on the response of the secondary ending of the muscle spindle to sinusoidal stretching. *J. Physiol. London* 270: 835-850, 1977.
65. DURKOVIC, R. G., AND J. B. PRESTON. Evidence of dynamic fusimotor excitation of secondary muscle spindle afferents in soleus muscle of cat. *Brain Res.* 75: 320-323, 1974.
66. ECCLES, J. C., AND C. S. SHERRINGTON. Numbers and contraction-values of individual motor-units examined in some muscles of the limb. *Proc. R. Soc. London Ser. B* 106: 326-357, 1930.
67. ECCLES, R. M., AND A. LUNDBERG. Integrative pattern of Ia synaptic actions on motoneurones of hip and knee muscles. *J. Physiol. London* 144: 271-298, 1958.

68. EDSTRÖM, L., AND E. KUGELBERG. Histochemical composition, distribution of fibres and fatiguability of rat soleus motor units. *J. Neurol. Neurosurg. Psychiatry* 31: 424–433, 1968.
69. ELDRED, E., R. GRANIT, AND P. A. MERTON. Supraspinal control of the muscle spindle and its significance. *J. Physiol. London* 122: 498–523, 1953.
70. ELDRED, E., H. YELLIN, L. GADBOIS, AND S. SWEENEY. Bibliography on muscle receptors; their morphology, pathology and physiology. *Exp. Neurol. Suppl.* 3: 1–154, 1967.
71. ELDRED, E., H. YELLIN, M. DESANTIS, AND C. M. SMITH. Supplement to bibliography on muscle receptors: their morphology, pathology, physiology and pharmacology. *Exp. Neurol.* 55: 1–118, 1977.
72. ELLAWAY, P. H., F. EMONET-DÉNAND, M. JOFFROY, AND Y. LAPORTE. Lack of exclusively fusimotor α-axons in flexor and extensor leg muscles of the cat. *J. Neurophysiol.* 35: 149–153, 1972.
73. EMONET-DÉNAND, F., M. HULLIGER, P. B. C. MATTHEWS, AND J. PETIT. Factors affecting modulation in post-stimulus histograms on static fusimotor stimulation. *Brain Res.* 134: 180–184, 1977.
74. EMONET-DÉNAND, F., L. JAMI, AND Y. LAPORTE. Skeleto-fusimotor axons in hind-limb muscles of the cat. *J. Physiol. London* 249: 153–166, 1975.
75. EMONET-DÉNAND, F., L. JAMI, Y. LAPORTE, AND N. TANKOV. Glycogen depletion elicited in peroneus brevis by static α axons. *Neurosci. Lett. Suppl.* 1: 93, 1978.
76. EMONET-DÉNAND, F., E. JANKOWSAKA, AND Y. LAPORTE. Skeleto-fusimotor fibres in the rabbit. *J. Physiol. London* 120: 669–680, 1970.
77. EMONET-DÉNAND, F., AND Y. LAPORTE. Proportion of muscle spindles supplied by skeletofusimotor axons (β-axons) in peroneus brevis muscle of the cat. *J. Neurophysiol.* 38: 1390–1394, 1975.
78. EMONET-DÉNAND, F., Y. LAPORTE, P. B. C. MATTHEWS, AND J. PETIT. On the sub-division of static and dynamic fusimotor actions on the primary ending of the cat muscle spindle. *J. Physiol. London* 268: 827–861, 1977.
79. EMONET-DÉNAND, F., Y. LAPORTE, AND B. PAGÈS. Fibres fusimotrices statiques et fibres fusimotrices dynamiques chez le lapin. *Arch. Ital. Biol.* 104: 195–213, 1966.
80. GLADDEN, M. H. Structural features relative to the function of intrafusal muscle fibres in the cat. In: *Progress in Brain Research. Understanding the Stretch Reflex*, edited by S. Homma. Amsterdam: Elsevier, 1976, vol. 44, p. 51–59.
81. GLADDEN, M. H., AND P. N. MCWILLIAM. The activity of intrafusal fibres during cortical stimulation in the cat. *J. Physiol. London* 273: 28P–29P, 1977.
82. GOODWIN, G. M., M. HULLIGER, AND P. B. C. MATTHEWS. The effects of fusimotor stimulation during small amplitude stretching on the frequency-response of the primary ending of the mammalian muscle spindle. *J. Physiol. London* 253: 175–206, 1975.
83. GOODWIN, G. M., AND E. S. LUSCHEI. Effects of destroying spindle afferents from jaw muscles on mastication in monkeys. *J. Neurophysiol.* 37: 967–981, 1974.
84. GOODWIN, G. M., AND E. S. LUSCHEI. Discharge of spindle afferents from jaw-closing muscles during chewing in alert monkeys. *J. Neurophysiol.* 38: 560–571, 1975.
85. GOODWIN, G. M., D. I. MCCLOSKEY, AND P. B. C. MATTHEWS. The contribution of muscle afferents to kinaesthesia shown by vibration induced illusions of movement and by the effects of paralysing joint afferents. *Brain* 95: 705–748, 1972.
86. GRANIT, R. (editor). *Muscular Afferents and Motor Control*. Stockholm: Almqvist and Wiksell, 1966. (Proc. Nobel Symp. I, Stockholm, 1965.)
87. GRANIT, R. *The Basis of Motor Control*. London: Academic, 1970.
88. GRANIT, R., AND B. R. KAADA. Influence of stimulation of central nervous structures on muscle spindles in cat. *Acta Physiol. Scand.* 27: 130–160, 1952.
89. GREGORY, J. E., A. PROCHAZKA, AND U. PROSKE. Responses of muscle spindles to stretch after a period of fusimotor activity compared in freely moving and anaesthetized cats. *Neurosci. Lett.* 4: 67–72, 1977.
90. GREGORY, J. E., AND U. PROSKE. The responses of Golgi tendon organs to stimulation of different combinations of motor units. *J. Physiol. London* 295: 251–262, 1979.
91. HARKER, D. W., L. JAMI, Y. LAPORTE, AND J. PETIT. Fast-conducting skeletofusimotor axons supplying intrafusal chain fibers in the cat peroneus tertius muscle. *J. Neurophysiol.* 40: 791–799, 1977.
92. HARVEY, R. J., AND P. B. C. MATTHEWS. The response of de-efferented muscle spindle endings in the cat's soleus to slow extension in the muscle. *J. Physiol. London* 157: 370–392, 1961.
93. HASAN, Z., AND J. C. HOUK. Analysis of response properties of deefferented mammalian spindle receptors based on frequency response. *J. Neurophysiol.* 38: 663–672, 1975.
94. HASAN, Z., AND J. C. HOUK. Transition in sensitivity of spindle receptors that occurs when muscle is stretched more than a fraction of a millimeter. *J. Neurophysiol.* 38: 673–689, 1975.
95. HOFFMAN, H. Local re-innervation in partially denervated muscle: a histophysiological study. *Aust. J. Exp. Biol. Med. Sci.* 28: 383–392, 1950.
96. HOMMA, S. (editor). *Progress in Brain Research. Understanding the Stretch Reflex*. Amsterdam: Elsevier, 1976, vol. 44.
97. HOUK, J. C. The phylogeny of muscular control configurations. In: *Biocybernetics*, edited by H. Drischel and P. Dettmar. Jena: Fischer, 1972, vol. iv, p. 337–344.
98. HOUK, J. C., AND E. HENNEMAN. Responses of Golgi tendon organs to active contractions of the soleus muscle of the cat. *J. Neurophysiol.* 30: 466–481, 1967.
99. HOUK, J. C., J. J. SINGER, AND E. HENNEMAN. Adequate stimulus for tendon organs with observations on mechanics of ankle joint. *J. Neurophysiol.* 34: 1051–1065, 1971.
99a. HULLIGER, M. The responses of primary spindle afferents to fusimotor stimulation at constant and abruptly changing rates. *J. Physiol. London* 294: 461–482, 1979.
100. HULLIGER, M., P. B. C. MATTHEWS, AND J. NOTH. Effects of static and of dynamic fusimotor stimulation on the response of Ia fibres to low frequency sinusoidal stretching covering a wide range of amplitudes. *J. Physiol. London* 267: 811–838, 1977.
101. HULLIGER, M., P. B. C. MATTHEWS, AND J. NOTH. Effects of combining static and dynamic fusimotor stimulation on the response of the muscle spindle primary ending to sinusoidal stretching. *J. Phyiol. London* 267: 839–856, 1977.
102. HUNT, C. C. Relation of function to diameter in afferent fibres of muscle nerves. *J. Gen. Physiol.* 38: 117–131, 1954.
103. HUNT, C. C. (editor). *Handbook of Sensory Physiology. Muscle Receptors*. Berlin: Springer-Verlag, 1974, vol. 3, pt. 2.
104. HUNT, C. C., AND D. OTTOSON. Impulse activity and receptor potential of primary and secondary endings of isolated mammalian muscle spindles. *J. Physiol. London* 252: 259–281, 1975.
105. HUNT, C. C., AND D. OTTOSON. Initial burst of primary endings of isolated mammalian muscle spindles. *J. Neurophysiol.* 39: 324–330, 1976.
106. HUNT, C. C., AND A. S. PAINTAL. Spinal reflex regulation of fusimotor neurones. *J. Physiol. London* 143: 195–212, 1958.
107. HUTTON, R. S., J. L. SMITH, AND E. ELDRED. Postcontraction sensory discharge from muscle and its source. *J. Neurophysiol.* 36: 1090–1103, 1973.
108. HUTTON, R. S., J. L. SMITH, AND E. ELDRED. Persisting changes in sensory and motor activity of a muscle following its reflex activation. *Pfluegers Arch.* 353: 327–336, 1975.
109. JAMI, L., D. LAN-COUTON, K. MALMGREN, AND J. PETIT. "Fast" and "slow" skeletofusimotor innervation in cat tenuissimus spindles; a study with the glycogen-depletion method. *Acta Physiol. Scand.* 103: 284–298, 1978.
110. JAMI, L., AND J. PETIT. Frequency of tendon organ discharges elicited by the contraction of motor units in cat leg muscles. *J. Physiol. London* 261: 633–645, 1976.
111. JAMI, L., AND J. PETIT. Heterogeneity of motor units activating

single Golgi endon organs in cat leg muscles. *Exp. Brain Res.* 24: 485-493, 1976.
112. JAMI, L., AND J. PETIT. Fusimotor actions on sensitivity of spindle secondary endings to slow muscle stretch in cat peroneus tertius. *J. Neurophysiol.* 41: 860-869, 1978.
113. JANSEN, J. K. S., AND P. B. C. MATTHEWS. The dynamic responses to slow stretch of muscle spindles in the decerebrate cat. *J. Physiol. London* 159: 20P-22P, 1961.
114. JANSEN, J. K. S., AND P. B. C. MATTHEWS. The central control of the dynamic response of muscle spindle receptors. *J. Physiol. London* 161: 357-373, 1962.
115. JANSEN, J. K. S., AND P. B. C. MATTHEWS. The effects of fusimotor activity on the static responsiveness of primary and secondary endings of muscle spindles in the decerebrate cat. *Acta Physiol. Scand.* 55: 376-386, 1962.
116. KELLER, E. L., AND D. A. ROBINSON. Absence of a stretch reflex in extraocular muscles of the monkey. *J. Neurophysiol.* 34: 908-919, 1971.
117. KOEZE, T. H. The response to stretch of muscle spindle afferents of baboon's tibialis anticus and the effect of fusimotor stimulation. *J. Physiol. London* 197: 107-121, 1968.
118. KOEZE, T. H. Muscle spindle afferents in the baboon. *J. Physiol. London* 229: 297-317, 1973.
119. KUFFLER, S. W., AND C. C. HUNT. The mammalian small-nerve fibres; a system for efferent nervous regulation of muscle spindle discharge. *Res. Publ. Assoc. Res. Nerv. Ment. Dis.* 30: 24-37, 1952.
120. KUFFLER, S. W., C. C. HUNT, AND J. P. QUILLIAM. Function of medullated small-nerve fibres in mammalian ventral roots: efferent muscle spindle innervation. *J. Neurophysiol.* 14: 29-54, 1951.
121. LANGLEY, J. N. The nerve fibre constitution of peripheral nerves and of nerve roots. *J. Physiol. London* 56: 382-396, 1922.
122. LEKSELL, L. The action potential and excitatory effects of the small ventral root fibres to skeletal muscle. *Acta Physiol. Scand.* 10: (Suppl. 31) 1-84, 1945.
123. LENNERSTRAND, G. Position and velocity sensitivity of muscle spindles in the cat. I. Primary and secondary endings deprived of fusimotor activation. *Acta Physiol. Scand.* 73: 281-299, 1968.
124. LENNERSTRAND, G. Position and velocity sensitivity of muscle spindles in the cat. IV. Interaction between two fusimotor fibres converging on the same spindle ending. *Acta Physiol. Scand.* 74: 257-273, 1968.
125. LENNERSTRAND, G., AND U. THODEN. Fusimotor effects on position and velocity sensitivity of muscle spindles. *Experientia* 23: 205-206, 1967.
126. LENNERSTRAND, G., AND U. THODEN. Dynamic analysis of muscle spindle endings in the cat soleus using length changes of different length-time relations. *Acta Physiol. Scand.* 73: 234-250, 1968.
127. LENNERSTRAND, G., AND U. THODEN. Position and velocity sensitivity of muscle spindles in the cat. II. Dynamic fusimotor single-fibre activation of primary endings. *Acta Physiol. Scand.* 74: 16-29, 1968.
128. LENNERSTRAND, G., AND U. THODEN. Position and velocity sensitivity of muscle spindles in the cat. III. Static fusimotor single-fibre activation of primary and secondary endings. *Acta Physiol. Scand.* 74: 30-49, 1968.
129. LENNERSTRAND, G., AND U. THODEN. Muscle spindle responses to concomitant variations in length and in fusimotor activation. *Acta Physiol. Scand.* 74: 153-165, 1968.
130. LEWIS, D. M., AND U. PROSKE. The effect of muscle length and rate of fusimotor stimulation on the frequency of discharge in primary endings from muscle spindles in the cat. *J. Physiol. London* 122: 511-535, 1972.
131. LUNDBERG, A., AND G. WINSBURY. Selective activation of large afferents from muscle spindles and Golgi tendon organs. *Acta Physiol. Scand.* 49: 155-164, 1960.
132. MATTHEWS, B. H. C. Nerve endings in mammalian muscle. *J. Physiol. London* 78: 1-53, 1933.
133. MATTHEWS, P. B. C. The differentiation of two types of fusimotor fibre by their effects on the dynamic response of muscle spindle primary endings. *Q. J. Exp. Physiol.* 47: 324-333, 1962.
134. MATTHEWS, P. B. C. The response of de-efferented muscle spindle receptors to stretching at different velocities. *J. Physiol. London* 168: 660-678, 1963.
135. MATTHEWS, P. B. C. Muscle spindles and their motor control. *Physiol. Rev.* 44: 219-288, 1964.
136. MATTHEWS, P. B. C. The origin and functional significance of the stretch reflex. In: *Excitatory Synaptic Mechanisms,* edited by P. Andersen and J. K. S. Jansen. Oslo: Universitetsforlaget, 1970, p. 301-315.
137. MATTHEWS, P. B. C. *Mammalian Muscle Receptors and their Central Actions.* London: Arnold, 1972.
138. MATTHEWS, P. B. C., AND R. B. STEIN. The sensitivity of muscle spindle afferents to sinusoidal stretching. *J. Physiol. London* 200: 723-743, 1969.
139. MATTHEWS, P. B. C., AND R. B. STEIN. The regularity of primary and secondary muscle spindle afferent discharges. *J. Physiol. London* 202: 59-82, 1969.
140. MATTHEWS, P. B. C., AND D. R. WESTBURY. Some effects of fast and slow motor fibres on muscle spindles of the frog. *J. Physiol. London* 178: 178-192, 1965.
141. MCCLOSKEY, D. I. Differences between the senses of movement and position shown by the effects of loading and vibration of muscles in man. *Brain Res.* 61: 119-131, 1973.
142. MCWILLIAM, P. N. The incidence and properties of β axons to muscle spindles in the cat hind limb. *Q. J. Exp. Physiol.* 60: 25-36, 1975.
143. MERTON, P. A. Speculations on the servo-control of movement. In: *The Spinal Cord,* edited by G. E. W. Wolstenholme. London: Churchill, 1953, p. 247-255.
144. MURTHY, K. S. K. Vertebrate fusimotor neurones and their influences on motor behaviour. *Prog. Neurobiol. Oxford* 11: 249-307, 1978.
145. NEWSOM DAVIS, J. The response to stretch of human intercostal muscle spindles studied in vitro. *J. Physiol. London* 249: 561-579, 1975.
146. OVALLE, W. K., AND R. S. SMITH. Histochemical identification of three types of intrafusal muscle fibres in the cat and monkey based on the myosin ATPase reaction. *Can. J. Physiol. Pharmacol.* 50: 195-202, 1972.
147. PHILLIPS, C. G. Motor apparatus of the baboon's hand. *Proc. R. Soc. London Ser. B* 173: 141-174, 1969.
148. POPPELE, R. E., AND R. J. BOWMAN. Quantitative description of linear behavior of mammalian muscle spindles. *J. Neurophysiol.* 33: 59-72, 1970.
149. POPPELE, R. E., AND W. J. CHEN. Repetitive firing behavior of mammalian muscle spindle. *J. Neurophysiol.* 35: 357-364, 1972.
150. POPPELE, R. E., AND W. R. KENNEDY. Comparison between behaviour of human and cat muscle spindles recorded in vitro. *Brain Res.* 75: 316-319, 1974.
151. PRINGLE, J. W. S. Stretch activation of muscle: function and mechanism. *Proc. R. Soc. London Ser. B* 201: 107-130, 1978.
152. PROCHAZKA, A., J. A. STEPHENS, AND P. WAND. Muscle spindle discharges in normal and obstructed movements. *J. Physiol. London* 287: 57-66, 1979.
153. PROCHAZKA, A., R. A. WESTERMAN, AND S. P. ZICCONE. Discharges of single hindlimb afferents in the freely moving cat. *J. Neurophysiol.* 39: 1090-1104, 1976.
154. PROCHAZKA, A., R. A. WESTERMAN, AND S. P. ZICCONE. Ia afferent activity during a variety of voluntary movements in the cat. *J. Physiol. London* 268: 423-448, 1977.
155. PROSKE, U. Stretch-evoked potentiation of responses of muscle spindles in the cat. *Brain Res.* 88: 378-383, 1975.
156. PROSKE, U., AND J. E. GREGORY. The time-course of recovery of the initial burst of primary endings of muscle spindles. *Brain Res.* 121: 358-361, 1977.
157. PROSKE, U., AND R. M. A. P. RIDGE. Extrafusal muscle and muscle spindles in reptiles. *Prog. Neurobiol. Oxford* 3: 3-29, 1974.
158. RACK, P. M. H., AND D. R. WESTBURY. The effects of suxamethonium and acetylcholine on the behaviour of cat muscle

spindles during dynamic stretching, and during fusimotor stimulation. *J. Physiol. London* 186: 698–713, 1966.
159. REINKING, R. M., J. A. STEPHENS, AND D. G. STUART. The tendon organs of cat medial gastrocnemius: significance of motor unit type and size for the activation of Ib afferents. *J. Physiol. London* 250: 491–512, 1975.
160. RENKIN, B. Z., AND Å. B. VALLBO. Simultaneous responses of groups I and II cat muscle spindle afferents to muscle position and movement. *J. Neurophysiol.* 27: 429–450, 1964.
161. RUFFINI, A. On the minute anatomy of the neuromuscular spindles of the cat, and on their physiological significance. *J. Physiol. London* 23: 190–208, 1898.
162. RYMER, W. Z., J. C. HOUK, AND P. E. CRAGO. The relation between dynamic response and velocity sensitivity for muscle spindle receptors. *Proc. Int. Union Physiol. Sci.* 13: 1992, 1977.
163. SCHÄFER, S. S. The acceleration response of a primary muscle-spindle ending to a ramp stretch of the extrafusal muscle. *Experientia* 23: 1026–1027, 1967.
164. SCHÄFER, S. S. The characteristic curves of the dynamic response of primary muscle spindle endings in the absence and presence of stimulation of fusimotor fibres. *Brain Res.* 59: 395–399, 1973.
165. SCHÄFER, S. S. The discharge frequencies of primary muscle spindle endings during simultaneous stimulation of two fusimotor fibres. *Pfluegers Arch.* 350: 359–372, 1974.
166. SCHÄFER, S. S., AND S. KIJEWSKI. The dependency of the acceleration response of primary muscle spindle endings on the mechanical properties of muscle. *Pfluegers Arch.* 350: 101–122, 1974.
167. SHERRINGTON, C. S. On the anatomical constitution of nerves of skeletal muscles; with remarks on recurrent fibres in the ventral spinal nerve-root. *J. Physiol. London* 17: 211–258, 1894.
168. SHIK, M. L., G. N. ORLOVSKII, AND F. V. SEVERIN. Organisation of locomotor synergism. *Biophysics* 11: 1011–1019, 1966. (Transl. of *Biofizika* 11: 879–886, 1966.)
169. STAUFFER, E. K., AND J. A. STEPHENS. The tendon organs of cat soleus: static sensitivity to active force. *Exp. Brain Res.* 23: 279–291, 1975.
170. STAUFFER, E. K., AND J. A. STEPHENS. Responses of Golgi tendon organs to ramp-and-hold profiles of contractile force. *J. Neurophysiol.* 40: 681–691, 1977.
171. STEIN, R. B. Peripheral control of movement. *Physiol. Rev.* 54: 215–243, 1974.
172. STEIN, R. B., AND A. S. FRENCH. Models for the transmission of information by nerve cells. In: *Excitatory Synaptic Mechanisms,* edited by P. Andersen and J. K. S. Jansen. Oslo: Universitetsforlaget, 1970, p. 247–257.
173. STEPHENS, J. A., R. M. REINKING, AND D. G. STUART. Tendon organs of cat medial gastrocnemius: responses to active and passive forces as a function of muscle length. *J. Neurophysiol.* 38: 1217–1231, 1975.
174. STUART, D. G., G. E. GOSLOW, C. G. MOSHER, AND R. M. REINKING. Stretch responsiveness of Golgi tendon organs. *Exp. Brain Res.* 10: 463–476, 1970.
175. STUART, D. G., C. G. MOSHER, R. L. GERLAC, AND R. M. REINKING. Selective activation of Ia afferents by transient muscle stretch. *Exp. Brain Res.* 10: 477–487, 1970.
176. STUART, D. G., C. G. MOSHER, R. L. GERLACH, AND R. M. REINKING. Mechanical arrangement and transducing properties of Golgi tendon organs. *Exp. Brain Res.* 14: 274–292, 1972.
177. STUART, D. G., W. D. WILLIS, AND R. M. REINKING. Stretch-evoked excitatory postsynaptic potentials in motoneurons. *Brain Res.* 33: 115–125, 1971.
178. SWASH, M., AND K. P. FOX. Muscle spindle innervation in man. *J. Anat.* 112: 61–80, 1972.
179. VALLBO, Å. B. Slowly adapting muscle receptors in man. *Acta Physiol. Scand.* 78: 315–333, 1970.
180. VALLBO, Å. B. Discharge patterns in human muscle spindle afferents during isometric voluntary contractions. *Acta Physiol. Scand.* 80: 552–566, 1970.
181. VALLBO, Å. B. Afferent discharge from human muscle spindles in noncontracting muscles. Steady state impulse frequency as a function of joint angle. *Acta Physiol. Scand.* 90: 303–318, 1974.
182. VALLBO, Å. B. Human muscle spindle discharge during isometric voluntary contractions. Amplitude relations between spindle frequency and torque. *Acta Physiol. Scand.* 90: 319–336, 1974.
182a.VALLBO, Å. B., K.-E. HAGBARTH, H. E. TOREBJORK, AND B. G. WALLIN. Somatosensory, proprioceptive, and sympathetic activity in human peripheral nerves. *Physiol. Rev.* 59: 919–957, 1979.
183. WINDHORST, U., J. MEYER-LOHMANN, AND J. SCHMIDT. Correlation of the dynamic behaviour of deefferented primary muscle endings with their static behaviour. *Pfluegers Arch.* 357: 113–122, 1975.
184. YELLIN, H. A histochemical study of muscle spindles and their relationship to extrafusal fibre types in the rat. *Am. J. Anat.* 125: 31–37, 1969.

CHAPTER 7

Limitations of somatosensory feedback in control of posture and movement

PETER M. H. RACK | *Department of Physiology, University of Birmingham, Birmingham, England*

CHAPTER CONTENTS

Some Properties of Servomechanisms
   Loop gain
   Frequency transfer function
   Properties of different loads
   Vector representation of frequency transfer function
   Vector representation of a delay
   Combination of different vectors
   A velocity-sensitive transducer
   A low-pass filter
   Stability
   Nonlinear systems
Response of Limbs to Sinusoidal Movements
   Effects of limb mass
   Resistance of muscles to movement
   The two components of muscle force
   Muscles as low-pass filters
   Timing of reflex force
   Timing of muscle spindle afferent activity
   Reflex delay
   Summary
Negative Stiffness and Spontaneous Oscillations
   Factors affecting stability of stretch reflexes
   Nature of the external load
   Level of muscle activation
   Resistance to movements of different amplitudes
   Comparing the stretch reflex with a man-made control system
   Stability of a man-made system
   Stability and gain in the stretch reflex
   Summary
Reflex Responses or Precomputed Activity?
   Response to a sudden disturbance
   Tuning of the neuromuscular system
   Triggered responses to a disturbance
   Summary
Servo Assistance of Voluntary Movements
Precomputed Movements
   Summary
Feedback and Learning
Forward-Looking Control Systems
Conclusions

STRETCH REFLEXES HAVE often been regarded as servo-control mechanisms through which signals from muscle receptors contribute to the control of motoneuronal activity. They are often thought to control muscle length and limb position (37, 62) by comparing actual length with an instructed length and using the difference as an error signal to generate a correcting movement. Such a system might be expected to simplify the controlling functions of the higher parts of the nervous system and to provide some compensation for load changes and unexpected disturbances. The facts that the descending nerve fibers may act on the stretch-reflex pathway in more than one place and that the stretch reflex may involve pathways that extend far outside the spinal segments (18, 55, 68) complicate this simple view but do not necessarily contradict it.

Muscle length is not the only controllable quantity. Servo adjustment of force might be accomplished in a similar way by using signals from Golgi tendon organs and pressure receptors; or the signals from Golgi tendon organs and muscle spindles might be combined so as to lead to adjustments in the stiffness with which the limb meets a displacing force (64).

A motor system based on such mechanisms would appear to have great advantages for the animal, and it is hardly surprising that physiologists have often used these mechanisms as a framework within which to consider and model many features of the motor system.

There are, however, some serious difficulties. A servo-control system functions effectively when it has a high loop gain, so that a small error signal would give rise to a relatively large correction; but the gains of stretch-reflex pathways do seem low. Furthermore the transport of signals around the reflex pathways involves considerable delays, and it is well known to engineers that a combination of a high gain and a long transport delay can all too easily lead to oscillatory instabilities. Therefore one should not expect stretch reflexes to provide the precise servo control achieved by some engineering mechanisms. These constraints on the performance of the stretch reflex are much the same whether the controlled variable is position, force, or muscle stiffness.

There are some situations in which the combination of a long reflex delay and a high reflex gain does indeed lead to uncontrollable oscillations, and it is particularly interesting to consider how the animal usually manages to avoid these situations. The first parts of this chapter attempt to separate some of the different factors that have a bearing on the reflex "stability." The later part of the chapter considers some of the ways that animals may achieve rapid and effective control in spite of their rather slow neuromuscular apparatus. Some of the more complex forms of reflex behavior take on new significance when they are looked upon as methods of obtaining the best performance from this inherently slow system.

In any analysis of the stretch reflex as a servocontrol system, one has to remember that it is a highly nonlinear mechanism to which the elementary methods of systems analysis can only be applied with great caution. In particular it is generally unsafe to use information obtained from one sort of movement or disturbance (such as an impulsive one) to make predictions about some other pattern of movements. The most useful information regarding the stability of the stretch reflexes and their tendencies to spontaneous oscillations comes from situations in which spontaneous clonic oscillations actually occurred and from experiments in which muscles or limbs were driven through similar sinusoidal movements while measurements were made of their readiness or reluctance to follow these movements.

Since many of the arguments and conclusions of this chapter arise from consideration of the stability of stretch-reflex performance, spontaneous oscillations and imposed sinusoidal movements are considered at some length.

SOME PROPERTIES OF SERVOMECHANISMS

The following brief and simplified description is intended to highlight some points of particular importance in the subsequent consideration of biological systems and to introduce some of the terms used in this chapter. The properties of servomechanisms and the methods used in analyzing their performance are described in detail in many textbooks of engineering (76).

The elementary error-controlled servomechanism is usually designed to respond to a small error between the intended state and the actual state with a powerful correcting signal. In the language of the control engineer, it is said to have a high loop gain.

Figure 1A is a diagram of a simple system for controlling the position of some device or "load." The input signal is combined with a signal from the position transducer to give an error signal that is supplied to the motor to generate a force. This force then moves the load in a direction that decreases the signal from the position transducer and thus decreases the driving force. In such a system the amplifier and motor are usually designed so that a small movement at the sensor generates a correcting force that is large in relation to the load being moved. If this is so, then the movement follows the input signal, continuing to do so even though there may be some small changes in the load and even though it might encounter unexpected disturbing forces.

If we suppose that the system is an idealized linear one and that the load is a simple elastic resistance,

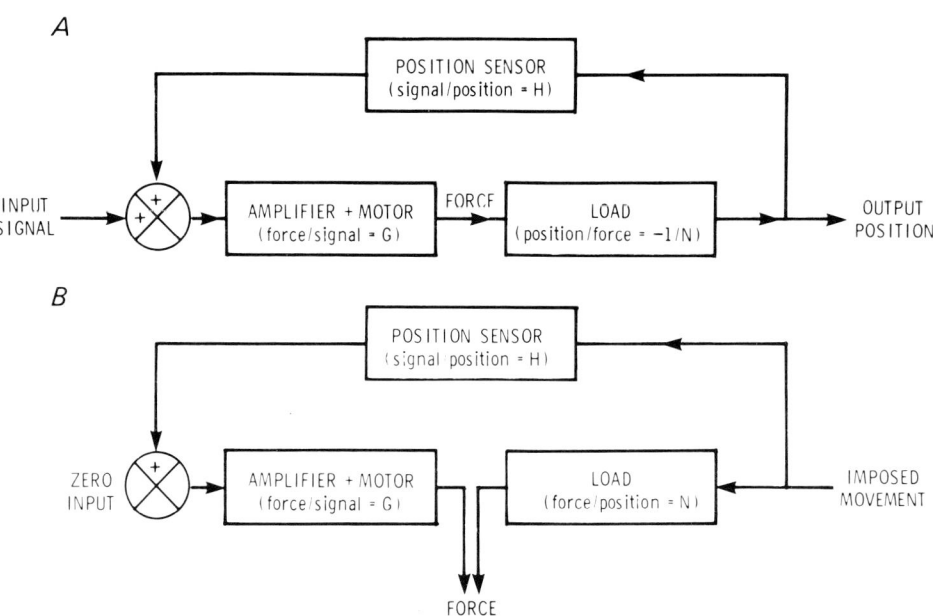

FIG. 1. A: schematic diagram of position-controlling servomechanism. Motor is assumed to generate a force proportional to its input, irrespective of movement. A positive force (tension) causes a negative length change (shortening). B: when same system is moved by forces applied to the load, the actual force required is the sum of forces required to move the load and forces necessary to overcome resistance generated in feedback pathway.

then the relation between the input signal and the output position is given by the equation

$$\frac{\text{output}}{\text{input}} = \frac{-G/N}{1 + HG/N} \quad (1)$$

where G describes the properties of the amplifier and motor, H describes the properties of the sensor, and the load has a stiffness N. In Figure 1A the load (position/force) has a negative sign, since a positive (pulling) force leads to a negative (shortening) change in length.

It is clear from Equation 1 that if G is made very large relative to N, then the output is related to the input signal by the equation output $\simeq$ −input/H, and this remains true even though there may be small changes in N. The system in fact compensates for changes in loading. (The difference in sign between input and output is correct since an increase in input causes a decrease in length.) As long as G is much larger than N, the output is also independent of the exact value of G, so that the system compensates for some nonlinearities and other deficiencies in the amplifier or motor.

If such a system were subjected to an external disturbance while the input remained constant (Fig. 1B), then it would resist displacement with a force that is the sum of the force due to the stiffness of the load and the force due to the operation of the servo loop

$$\text{force/displacement} = N + GH \quad (2)$$

Loop Gain

Engineers often measure the gain around their complete servo loop as a dimensionless quantity. In Figure 1A

$$\text{loop gain} = -HG/N \quad (3)$$

In man-made systems this loop gain can usually be measured directly after opening the loop at some point. In biological systems it may be impossible to open the reflex loops and directly measure the gain; the concept of loop gain is nevertheless important because it gives an index of the ability of the system to deal with load changes. Loop gain is also important when considering the stability of the system.

It is necessary to distinguish between the dimensionless loop gain (−HG/N in Fig. 1), the stiffness of the servo (HG), and the stiffness of the whole system including the load (HG + N), though it may not always be possible to measure all of these quantities. It is unfortunate that this distinction has not always been clearly made in the literature.

Frequency Transfer Function

In the preceding paragraph, Figure 1 was considered as a highly idealized system. In real systems the transducers, amplifiers, and motors seldom transmit or transduce signals without some distortion or delay, and different frequency components of the signal are subject to different changes in amplitude and phase. Furthermore such systems rarely work with simple elastic loads, and the presence of inertia or friction in the load introduces frequency-dependent phase differences between force and position.

Diagrams such as Figure 1 are still useful in describing real (linear) systems, however, and Equations 1, 2, and 3 remain true, but H, G, and N cease to be simple constants and become transfer functions modifying the amplitude and phase of the various frequency components of the signal presented to them. The output/input properties of the system, the stiffness, and the loop gain may still be computed, but they must be expressed as complex functions with phases and gains dependent on the frequency of the signal. The frequency transfer functions of some simple elements of servo systems are now described.

Properties of Different Loads

In the foregoing paragraphs we assumed the load was elastic. In practice our limbs (and many other control systems) usually act on loads that have a considerable mass. A mass resists disturbances with a force proportional to acceleration; it therefore resists a sinusoidal movement $r\sin\omega t$ with a force $-mr\omega^2 \cdot \sin\omega t$ (where r is the amplitude of movement and m the mass to be moved). The force required to drive a mass through a sinusoidal movement is thus opposite in sign to (180° out of phase with) the movement, and it increases in amplitude with the square of the movement frequency.

If a load includes some linear Newtonian viscous friction η, the friction will resist movement with a force that is proportional to the velocity of movement; such a load resists the movement $r\sin\omega t$ with a force $\eta r\omega \cdot \cos\omega t$. This force appears as a sinusoid that is 90° ahead of the movement, with an amplitude that increases in proportion to the frequency of movement. Other forms of friction also generate forces that are 90° ahead of the movement, though these may not increase with frequency in the same way. In most of the cases considered here, the load consists of a combination of elastic, frictional, and inertial (mass) components. The frequency transfer function of such a load may be displayed in a number of different ways. In this chapter these and other transfer functions are displayed as vectors; the method of vector representation is therefore briefly described.

Vector Representation of Frequency Transfer Function

Different workers have displayed transfer functions of components of the motor system in different ways. Each method has its own advantages, but for simplicity only one method is used in this chapter, and where necessary experimental results are redrawn in this form.

Figure 2 is a plot of the frequency transfer function of a load that combines elastic resistance to movement, viscous friction, and inertia. The point N defines the resistance to movement and with increasing frequency of movement, it moves along the path indicated. The distance of N from the origin gives the stiffness of the load (force/displacement), whereas ϕ indicates the angle by which the force sinusoid leads the position sinusoid. The points marked along the curve indicate equal increments of frequency.

At the very lowest frequencies the vectors lie on or close to the horizontal axis; the resistance is then dominated by the stiffness k of the elastic component, which gives rise to a force component $kr\sin\omega t$ in phase with the position sinusoid. With increasing frequency the viscous friction adds a progressively larger force $\eta r\omega \cdot \cos\omega t$, and the effect of the mass adds a force $-mr\omega^2 \cdot \sin\omega t$, which increases even more steeply. The effects of each of these can be seen in Figure 2; this ability to separate the different components is the main virtue of this type of display.

The position of the point N has been described in terms of an amplitude of stiffness and a phase. It is often useful to describe frequency-dependent stiffness as a combination of its elastic (horizontal) and viscous (vertical) components. The elastic stiffness then defines the component of force in phase with position; this is positive at low frequencies when the elastic resistance dominates, but it may be negative at high frequencies when the effect of the mass dominates. The viscous stiffness defines the component of force that is 90° out of phase with the movement; in Figure 2 this is always positive though other situations may arise in which it could become negative.

The Newtonian viscous friction considered above is the only type of frictional resistance that behaves in a linear way. Another type of friction is important, however, and must be mentioned here. Figure 3A shows the frequency transfer function of a load in which the friction is a type that resists movement with a stiffness β that is independent of velocity. The load may still be described as having a viscous stiffness, but this does not increase with increasing frequency. If there were no mass, then the vector would remain at the point y at all frequencies.

Vector Representation of a Delay

Figure 3B shows the frequency transfer function of a pathway involving a fixed delay; the signal may be amplified, but its shape is not altered in any other way. As the frequency of the input signal is increased, the delay amounts to a progressively larger fraction of the cycle, and the vector moves in a clockwise direction around the origin. The size of the circle indicates the gain of the pathway; if this were a diagram of the reflex stiffness (force/movement), then the larger circle would indicate the stiffer reflex.

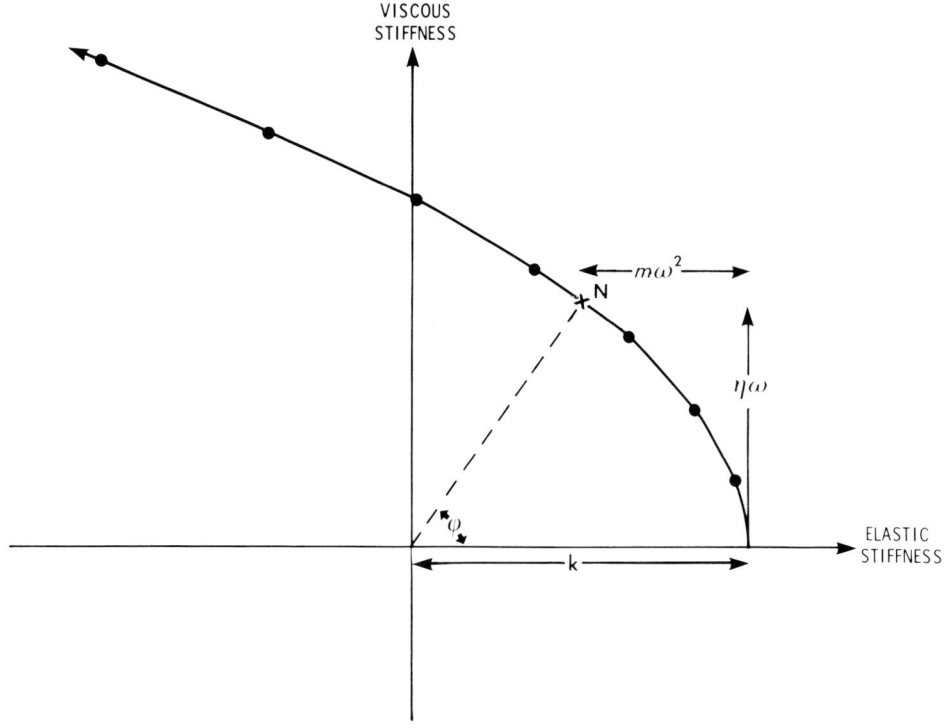

FIG. 2. Frequency transfer function of load that combines elastic resistance k, viscosity η, and mass m. Vector **N** follows path indicated as frequency of movement increases. Distance of **N** from origin gives its modulus, and the angle ϕ indicates phase lead of force on position. *Points* marked along path indicate equal increments in frequency; ω, angular velocity.

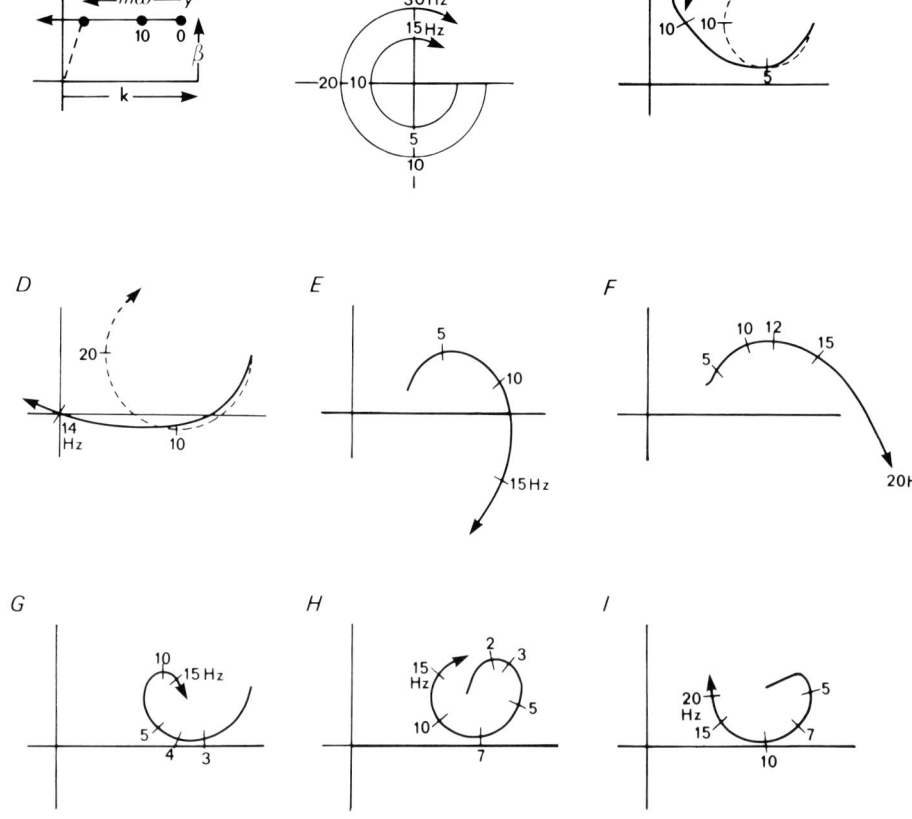

FIG. 3. Vector representations of numerous frequency transfer functions. *A*: mechanical load of elastic stiffness *k* and mass *m*, the frictional resistance of which does not change with frequency. When *m* is zero, the vector has the value y at all frequencies. *B*: 2 examples of feedback systems in which a force proportional to length occurs at some fixed interval after that length. For *smaller circle*, interval was 50 ms; for *larger*, 25 ms. *Larger circle* indicates greater force per unit displacement. *C*: combination of reflex stiffness and load stiffness obtained by geometrical addition of vector path in *A* to *smaller circle* in *B*. *Solid line* shows stiffness of system with its mass; *broken line* shows it without the mass. *D*: similar to *C*, but *larger circle* of *B* has been added to *A*. *E*: effect of velocity-sensitive transducer. Delay and load are same as in *D* (without mass), but reflex activity is assumed to be proportional to velocity of movement. *F*: again load and delay are same as in *D*, but reflex activity is assumed to be initiated by muscle spindles with transfer functions $Ks(s + 0.44)(s + 11.3)(s + 44.0)/(s + 0.04)(s + 0.816)$. See reference 69. *s*, Laplace operator. *G*, *H*, and *I*: diagrams of how vector paths in *D*, *E*, and *F* are modified by effects of low-pass filter [critically damped second-order filter with corner frequency 6 Hz (54)].

A 50-ms delay gives the frequency values marked on the smaller circle, whereas a 25-ms delay gives the frequencies marked around the larger circle.

Combination of Different Vectors

In describing reflex behavior it is often necessary to consider the effect of adding a reflex force to the force due to mechanical properties of the load. Each of these is a complex quantity, and they can only be combined by a process of vector addition. In Figure 3C and D this process is illustrated by the use of some highly simplified examples. Figure 3C (solid line) was obtained by adding the vectors of Figure 3A to the vectors following the smaller circular path in Figure 3B. Figure 3C thus describes the stiffness of a simplified system in which the stiffness of the load (Fig. 3A) is added (as in Eq. 2) to the reflex stiffness (Fig. 3B). The dashed line in Figure 3C shows how the same system would behave if the load included no mass.

Because mass moves the vectors to the left by an amount $m\omega^2$, it is a simple matter to calculate and sketch the effects of adding or subtracting mass: this is a facility that is used in the discussion of experimental results.

Figure 3D is a similar combination of Figure 3A and the vectors following the larger circular path in Figure 3B.

A Velocity-Sensitive Transducer

Figure 3E shows the behavior of a system in which the reflex response is assumed to be initiated by a transducer, the response of which is proportional to the velocity of movement. The load is assumed to have no mass and there is a 25-ms delay. Apart from the properties of the transducer, the situation is therefore the same as that illustrated by the dashed line in Figure 3D. Note that although the vectors pass far below the horizontal axis, they do so at higher frequencies than in Figure 3D, since the reflex activity is now initiated earlier in the cycle of movement.

In Figure 3F the transducer is assumed to combine position, velocity, and acceleration sensitivity (Poppele and Bowman's mathematical description of the muscle spindle primary afferent discharge); again there is a 25-ms delay. The reflex activity is now initiated even earlier in the cycle of movement, and it is at still higher movement frequencies that the vectors pass below the horizontal axis.

A Low-Pass Filter

Figure 3G, H, and I shows how the responses in Figure 3D, E, and F (immediately above) might be modified by the action of a low-pass filter. As the frequency of movement is increased, the reflex signal is progressively attenuated, and its contribution to the total stiffness becomes smaller; the signal is also subjected to further delays so that each frequency point is moved farther around the loop in a clockwise direction.

Filters with different characteristics attenuate the various frequency components by different amounts, but in each case the path of the vector eventually converges toward a central point as the effect of the reflex diminishes at high frequencies.

Stability

Feedback pathways usually involve delays. These may be simple transport delays due to slowly conducting pathways (Fig. 3B-D), or they may be phase lags involved in low-pass filtering or other processes. The corrections that are generated in response to a displacement may therefore be applied a significant time after the displacement has occurred. A powerful correction applied too late may lead to an overshoot and perhaps to a continuing oscillation.

In the simple linear system, the criteria for stability or instability can be stated quite definitely (76). Most of these systems are unstable if the loop gain ($-HG/N$ in Fig. 1A) has a positive sign and, at the same time, a value greater than 1. These values for the loop gain usually occur (if they do occur) in some definite frequency range where the frequency transfer function of the combined components $-HG/N$ has the appropriate amplitude and phase; the system can then be expected to undergo an oscillation of increasing amplitude at some frequency within that range.

It may not always be practical to interrupt the reflex pathway and measure the loop gain of the system. It is possible, however, to make some definite statements about the stability of the system from a knowledge of the way it resists an imposed sinusoidal movement. If there is any frequency at which the system offers no resistance whatever to a sinusoidal movement, then this is the frequency at which spontaneous oscillations may be expected to occur when the system is uncoupled from the driving mechanism; such a situation exists in Figure 3D (at 14 Hz) where the path of the vector passes through the origin. The force/displacement is then zero, so that in Equation 3, $N = -HG$ and the loop gain ($-HG/N$) takes the value $+1$. It is less obvious, though equally true, that when the path of the stiffness vectors passes below the zero point and encircles it in a clockwise direction, the system will be unstable and will usually break into an oscillation of increasing amplitude.

Note that the method of determining stability described in the preceding paragraph does not depend on separating the reflex component of stiffness from that due to the load; such a separation is not always possible or even real. The above discussion contains some simplifications. Engineering textbooks provide fuller descriptions of stability criteria that take into account the complex nature of the loop gain (76).

Nonlinear Systems

Most of the systems considered so far (except for the non-Newtonian friction of Fig. 3) have been linear in their behavior. More detailed information about the properties of linear systems can be found in elementary engineering textbooks.

In applying methods of linear analysis to the highly nonlinear biological systems, one must tread with great caution. The response to simple sinusoidal inputs cannot necessarily be used to predict the responses to other patterns of input in which the different frequency components are mixed together; nor can the response to a sinusoid of one amplitude be used to predict the response to a sinusoid of some other amplitude.

We can use only the analytical tools that we have, and there is useful information to be gained by sinusoidal analysis of the musculoskeletal system. When the response to a sinusoidal displacement is an approximately sinusoidal resisting force, we can make some predictions about the performance of the system. In particular we can identify the conditions under which spontaneous oscillations may occur.

RESPONSE OF LIMBS TO SINUSOIDAL MOVEMENTS

The previous section described the frequency transfer functions of some simple mechanical elements and showed how these might be combined together into slightly more complicated systems. If the transfer characteristics of individual components of the stretch reflex were known in detail (along with all their nonlinearities), it would be possible, though laborious, to compute how they would interact with each other and how the complete system would behave. In most experimental situations, however, we have the reverse situation: we examine the behavior of the whole limb and attempt to make deductions about the properties of the component parts. It is seldom possible to open the control loop, as an engineer might wish to do, and one has to draw what conclusions one can from the behavior of the system with its feedback loops in operation.

In analyzing the response of a limb to sinusoidal movements, we attempt to break down the resisting forces into those components that are due merely to the mass of the moving parts, those that are attributable to the mechanical properties of the muscles and other soft tissues, and those that are due to activity in stretch reflexes (47). The situation is depicted in the flow diagram of Figure 1B; the external force is the reflex force plus the forces required to overcome the inertia and the elastic and viscous resistances of the moving parts. The feedback pathway has not been opened, but because the movement is entirely determined by the external driving mechanism, the reflex activity no longer affects its course.

Figure 4 illustrates a method of driving the elbow joint; the forearm and hand are attached by a crank to an eccentric driving pin on a rotating wheel (71). A similar method may be used for other joints (72). The sinusoidal movement thus imposed on the limb is usually met by an approximately sinusoidal force, and at frequencies above 4 Hz or so, the subject can do little to alter its waveform. By voluntary effort, however, the subject can extend the limb with more or less mean force and thus alter the base line about which these force fluctuations occur. Most of the useful records are obtained at these higher frequencies where voluntary intervention is not a problem, and the most interesting records are obtained when the subject exerts a steady mean flexing force.

The inset in Figure 4 is a record of the force during sinusoidal movement. The force record is not a perfect sinusoid, but the departures from a pure sine wave are quite small. In analyzing the results these small departures are usually disregarded, and only the force component at the frequency of the movement is extracted and used (47).

It is important to confine the movement to a single joint and to maintain a very positive coupling between the driving mechanism and the limb so that all the parts intended to move do move, and do so through a known distance. It is then possible to calculate the fraction of the applied force that is taken up in overcoming the inertia of the limb and of its splints and coverings.

Figure 5 is a vector plot of the stiffness of the interphalangeal joint of the thumb, determined over a range of different frequencies. A mean flexing force that was about one-third of the subject's maximum

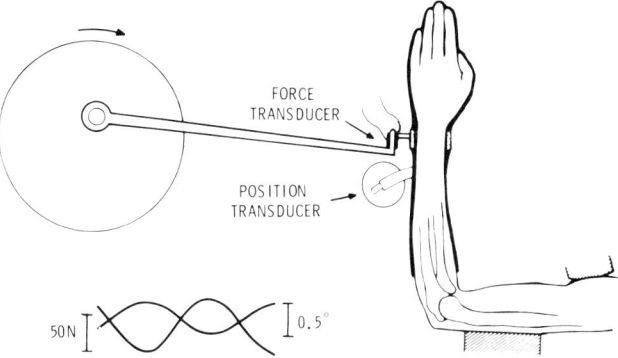

FIG. 4. Method of driving human elbow joint through sinusoidal flexion-extension movements. Forearm is fixed in splints and constrained to move about axis of joint. A crank couples the wrist to an eccentric pin on a rotating wheel. *Inset record*, frequency was 15 Hz, and tension in crank was highest in flexion. [From Rack (71).]

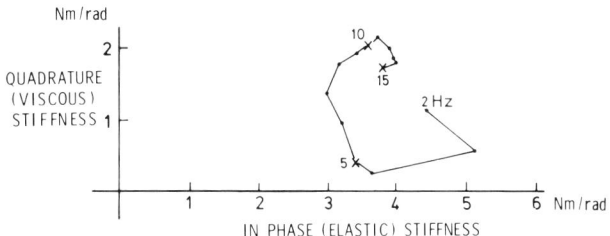

FIG. 5. Stiffness of interphalangeal joint of thumb. Joint was driven through sinusoidal movements of ± 1.3° while subject maintained a mean flexing torque of 0.75 N·m. Resistance to movements at 2–15 Hz is represented here as a series of vectors. Some frequencies are marked on figure. [From Brown, Rack, and Ross (10).]

was maintained to facilitate this; the mean level of force was displayed to the subject on a meter.

As in Figure 3, each point in Figure 5 represents the resistance to movement at a particular frequency; some of these frequencies are written on the figure. With increasing frequency the vector moves round in a clockwise direction, tracing out an approximately C-shaped path. One can immediately see that the result is very similar to the frequency transfer function diagrammed in Figure 3C, where a delayed reflex force is combined with the force required to move a load having elastic resistance and friction but no mass. Unlike the linear system, this figure describes the stiffness of the joint only for the particular amplitudes of movement that were used in the experiment; other amplitudes usually gave different results (as described in subsection *Resistance to Movements of Different Amplitudes*, p. 243).

The C-shaped or circular vector path of the type shown in Figure 5 is typical of results obtained from the human thumb or fingers (8, 72), and similar results have been obtained during imposed sinusoidal movements of the monkey mandible (28). At these joints the muscular forces are large compared to the mass that has to be moved; when, however, a similar experiment was performed at a more proximal joint, the effects of the extra mass made the results look (superficially) very different.

Effects of Limb Mass

In Figure 6, line **A** is the path of the vector that describes the resistance to a sinusoidal movement of the forearm. The movement was confined to the elbow joint, and again the subject exerted a steady mean flexing force. This record shows a large phase separation between position and force (also seen in Fig. 4) that is very different from the response to sinusoidal movement of the thumb or fingers. When, however, the mass of the forearm is measured and the forces required to move it are calculated and subtracted, one is left with the C-shaped vector path marked **B**, which has the same general shape as the vector path in Figure 5.

Although the response of the intact limb shown in record **A** is the important one for any analysis of overall behavior of that limb, the effect of the mass dominates the picture so as to obscure the other features, and it is the resistance remaining after the effect of the mass has been subtracted (record **B**) that is often most valuable in any attempt to analyze the reflex behavior.

Since neither the joints nor the other soft tissue offer much resistance to imposed movement (72), except at the extremes of their range, one can assume that the C-shaped vector paths seen when the mass is small (Fig. 5) or after its effect has been subtracted (**B** in Fig. 6) are mainly determined by the muscular resistance to movement.

For the actual experimental measurements of Figure 6 (47), the limb was encased in splints having a significant mass (equivalent to a 600-g wt held in the hand); the stiffness vector was then displaced even farther out to the left (**C** in Fig. 6).

Resistance of Muscles to Movement

If a limb is forcibly displaced, there is usually an increase in tension in the extended muscles. Some of this increase may be due to a reflex activation of motor units, but there is also an important component of the resisting force that does not depend on any increase in the level of motoneuronal activity.

Isolated muscles or muscle fibers subjected to continuous steady stimulation respond to changes in their lengths with changes in force. Shortening is accompanied by a decrease in tension, whereas lengthening usually leads to an increase (1, 52). This is a mechanical property of muscle tissue that can be observed either in a fully tetanized muscle or in a muscle that is activated at more physiological rates (48). The force depends on both the muscle length and the lengthening or shortening movement. The precise relationship between force and velocity has attracted the interest of muscle physiologists for many years (40); for our present purposes it is sufficient to describe it as a viscoelastic resistance (24), though this does not imply either linear elastic or Newtonian viscous behavior.

The actual processes within the muscle that determine its elasticity and viscous friction, are quite different from those determining the behavior of most physical viscoelastic systems (42): the energy absorbed by the viscous element does not necessarily appear as additional heat (22, 41), and its resistance does not change in a simple way with velocity of movement.

It has long been realized that the length-tension relation in the rigid extensor muscles of a decerebrate cat depends on an interaction between reflex activity

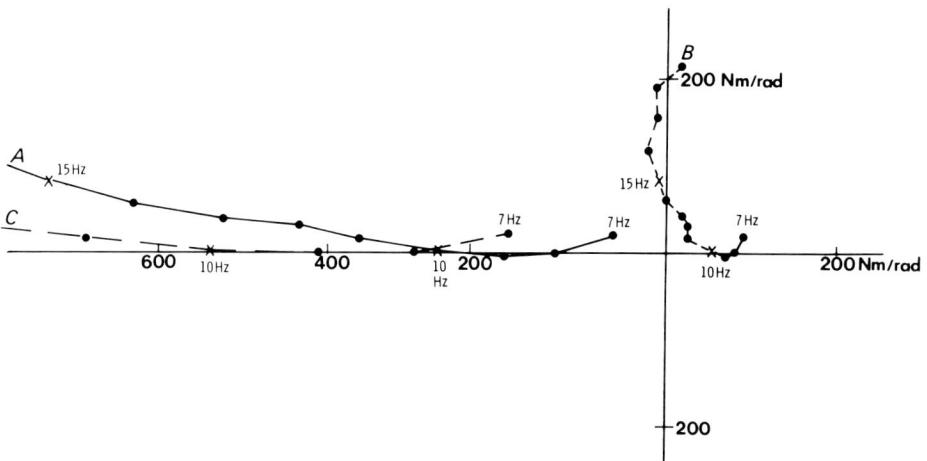

FIG. 6. Resistance to sinusoidal movement of human elbow. Joint was driven through movements of ± 0.24° (see Fig. 4) while subject maintained a mean flexing torque of 10 N·m. **A**: limb-stiffness vectors. **B**: component of stiffness remaining after subtraction of force required to move mass of forearm and hand. **C**: stiffness of limb when encased in splints that were equivalent to a mass of 600 g held in the hand. C is original experimental result from which **A** and **B** were obtained. [Replotted from Joyce, Rack, and Ross (47).]

and muscle properties. This has been demonstrated in a muscle under static conditions (32) and during slow extension movements (58). During faster movements the situation is considerably more complicated. The problem may be approached by comparing the behavior of reflex-controlled muscles with the behavior of muscles that are continuously activated though deprived of reflex control and employing the same sequence of movements on both occasions. Comparisons of this sort have been made on soleus muscles of decerebrate cats (45, 70) and on the jaw-closing muscles of conscious monkeys (28).

The Two Components of Muscle Force

Figure 7 shows the response of a cat soleus muscle to sinusoidal stretching. Figure 7A is a record of muscle length (above) and tension (below). Tetanic stimulation of the motor nerve was started partially through the record and, in the later cycles of the movement, the force exerted by the tetanized muscle varied approximately sinusoidally, with the peak force preceding the peak muscle length.

Figure 7B shows vector plots of muscle stiffness at three different amplitudes of sinusoidal movement. At all amplitudes and frequencies the muscle resisted with some combination of viscous and elastic stiffness, and at each amplitude elastic stiffness increased with increasing frequency. This type of response is to be expected from a viscoelastic muscle that is coupled through an elastic tendon (70).

This behavior of the tetanized muscle is very different from the behavior of the same muscle in a decerebrate cat whose stretch reflexes are active (45), and it is very different from the responses of a voluntarily contracting human muscle (Figs. 5 and 6). Thus one is led to suppose that the reflex modulation of motor activity may account for these differences.

Some useful and more precise confirmation comes from experiments on monkeys' jaw muscles (28). The particular arrangement of the afferent pathways from muscle spindles in the jaw-closing muscles makes it possible to interrupt them surgically without serious damage to either the motor fibers or other sensory pathways. By taking advantage of this anatomical arrangement, Luschei and his colleagues examined the response of the jaw-closing muscles in monkeys before and after interruption of the afferent feedback from the muscle spindles [(28); see also the chapter by Luschei and Goldberg in this *Handbook*]. The particular virtue of this experiment lies in being able to record from the same muscles, with and without their muscle spindle stretch reflexes, during contractions of similar force and with the same sequences of movements.

Figure 8 is a plot of the results of Goodwin et al. (28). Figure 8A shows the path of the stiffness vectors when the innervation of the muscles was intact. This vector follows a circular path that is similar in general

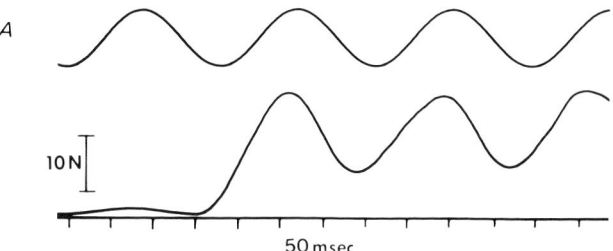

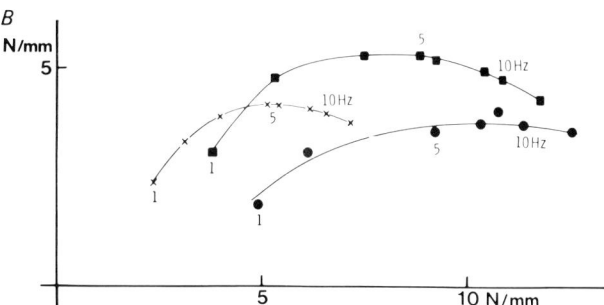

FIG. 7. Response of tetanized muscle to sinusoidal stretching. *A*: cat soleus muscle stretched through ± 0.8 mm at about 5 Hz. Tetanic stimulation (50 impulses/s) began during record. *B*: stiffness vectors plotted at 3 different amplitudes: × = ± 1.9 mm; ■ = ± 0.8 mm; ● = ± 0.35 mm. Some frequencies are marked on figure. [From Rack (70).]

shape to those obtained from human limbs (Figs. 5 and 6B). Figure 8B shows the very different vector path recorded from the same animal after interruption of the muscle afferents; this is similar in general shape and direction to the stiffness recorded in a tetanized cat muscle (Fig. 7B).

Figure 8B was taken to represent the stiffness of the muscle when it was essentially without reflex modulation of its activity; phasic modulation of the electromyogram at the movement frequency was reduced to a low level. By subtracting this nonreflex stiffness from the initial total stiffness, Goodwin et al. were able to obtain a record measuring the amount of resistance contributed by the action of the reflex (Fig. 8C).

The reverse of this process shows that the total stiffness may be regarded as the sum of a nonreflex stiffness (due to the mechanical properties of the muscles) and a stiffness due to the stretch reflex. There is then an obvious similarity between the total force seen in Figure 8A and the combination of a viscoelastic load and a delayed reflex resistance seen in Figure 3C-I.

It is not usually experimentally possible to separate the components of limb stiffness in humans the same way that it is done in monkeys, but the similarity between records obtained from human limbs (Figs. 5, 6B, 9, 11, 12, and 13) and from the monkey jaw strongly suggests that the former also represents a combination of a reflex force and a nonreflex muscle stiffness.

The resemblance between experimental results and the combination of a delayed reflex force with a viscoelastic load (Fig. 3C and D) does not depend on a

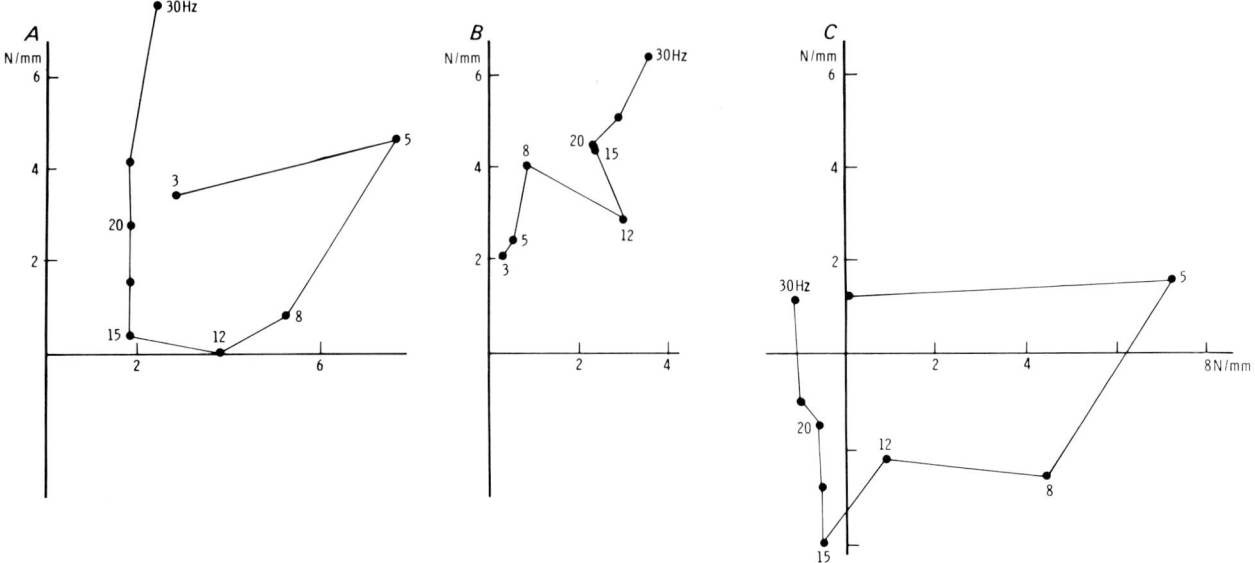

FIG. 8. Resistance to imposed sinusoidal opening-closing movement of a monkey mandible. Movement was ± 0.5 mm at incisors. Monkey maintained a mean biting force of 8 N. *A*: stiffness vectors in intact animal. *B*: stiffness vectors after interruption of afferents from jaw-closing muscles. *C*: vectors in *B* have been subtracted from those in *A* to demonstrate amount of stiffness that could be attributed to action of stretch reflex. [Replotted from Goodwin et al. (28).]

particular method of display; the similarity could also be inferred from results obtained from decerebrate cats (45), and these were displayed in quite different ways.

In the servo control of posture and movement, and in the block diagram of Figure 1, the muscle thus performs two different functions. It serves as an actuator through which the reflex signals give rise to forces, and it also acts as a viscoelastic load. The viscoelastic property of an active muscle contributes to the resistance to movement, and this is true whether the movement is externally imposed or generated by neural activity.

The separation of the resisting force into those components due to the viscoelastic properties and to reflex action is extremely useful, capturing some essential features of the system. One should not, however, push this analogy too far; the two functions are not really separate since the same muscle fibers may perform both, and the fluctuating activity generated by a reflex signal can modulate the viscoelastic resistance as well as the force.

Separation of jaw muscle stiffness into two components is beyond reproach so long as one defines the reflex component as the difference between the total stiffness and that part remaining when the muscle exerts the same force under nonreflex conditions. One cannot, however, assume a very simple relationship between this reflex stiffness and the amplitude of the reflex signal, since the same burst of reflex activity has different effects depending on whether it is delivered to the muscle during lengthening or shortening.

Muscles as Low-Pass Filters

Although the reflex component of force arises through a reflex modulation of motoneuronal activity, the relationship between the rate of motoneuronal discharge and the resulting force is not a simple one (see the chapter by Partridge and Benton in this *Handbook*).

The ability of muscle fibers to translate changing neural activity into muscular contraction has been most widely investigated under isometric conditions (54, 66), though some experiments have also been carried out on muscles where length was allowed to change (67). Muscles have been described as having the properties of a low-pass filter (6, 57): a slow train of pulses in the motor nerve leads to a similar train of force impulses, but a faster train of action potentials gives rise to a tetanus in which the intermittent nature of the stimulation is filtered out and does not give rise to an equivalent intermittent force.

This low-pass filtering may also be demonstrated under conditions that are more nearly physiological. When the muscle is stimulated by a continuing pulse train, but the rate of these pulses is slowly modulated up and down, then the muscle force increases and decreases in the same way. When, however, the modulation of the stimulus rate is made more rapid, the changes in force become progressively smaller (54, 66). The neural signal is thus subjected to a filtering process in which the lower frequency components are translated into equivalent forces and the higher frequency components filtered out. The correctness of this conclusion may be confirmed by comparing the frequency content of the rectified electromyogram with the corresponding force record (15, 28).

In the slow soleus muscle of the cat (5) and human (6), there is progressive attenuation of the force fluctuations as the frequency is increased, and this becomes significant at about 2 Hz. In the faster cat plantaris the attenuation is significant at a frequency of about 6 Hz, and in monkey jaw-closing muscles attenuation becomes significant above 10 Hz (28). These figures are only approximate, but they serve to illustrate the range of muscle performance.

This low-pass filtering property of muscles modifies the reflex response to movements. Whereas the relatively slow modulation of motoneuronal activity accompanying a slow sinusoidal movement leads to the corresponding reflex force fluctuations, higher frequency movements have less effect because the rapid changes in motoneuronal activation do not appear as force changes.

This effect may be seen in the diagram of Figure 3G, where progressive increases in frequency have smaller and smaller effects on the value of the stiffness vector. The path of the vector spirals inward toward a point where only the nonreflex component of the stiffness remains. A similar effect may be seen in the experimental results illustrated in Figures 5 and 11A.

Timing of Reflex Force

Although the resistance at different joints may be described by vectors that follow (after subtraction of forces due to the mass) similar C-shaped paths, the distribution of the various frequency points differs from joint to joint.

In the monkey jaw the reflex was sufficiently delayed to occur 90° after maximum muscle length at a frequency between 12 and 15 Hz (Fig. 8C). When the reflex pathway was intact this extra force in midshortening reduced the total viscous stiffness to a minimum at about that frequency (Fig. 8A).

At the human elbow joint, with its longer reflex pathway, the minimum viscous stiffness occurred at a lower frequency (9–10 Hz in Fig. 6), and the reflex component of force was presumably then maximal about 90° after maximum muscle length was reached. In the thumb, which is controlled by even slower stretch-reflex pathways (56), the minimum viscous stiffness occurred at still lower frequencies (4–5 Hz in Fig. 5).

The general trend of these results could have been expected: the faster the reflex pathway, the shorter is the interval between activation of the sensory receptors and the consequent reflex force and the higher the frequency of movement must be for the reflex response to lengthening to be delayed into the subsequent shortening movement; this is illustrated in Figure 3B–D.

Timing of Muscle Spindle Afferent Activity

A knowledge of the reflex delay does not by itself enable one to predict the responses to different frequencies of movement. One needs to know when in the cycle of movement the sensory receptors are most strongly activated and when therefore the most vigorous reflex activity is initiated.

Most, if not all, of the stretch-reflex activity probably arises from muscle spindles. These are described in detail in the chapter by Matthews in this *Handbook*; it is only necessary here to note that some of their afferent fibers are sensitive to the velocity of extension as well as to muscle length, and during sinusoidal movements they appear also to be sensitive to acceleration. The maximum afferent discharge may certainly precede maximum length by more than 90°, though the amount of this phase advance depends on the frequency of the movement (69).

Some of the effects of velocity- and acceleration-sensitive receptors are illustrated in the diagrams of Figure 3E and F; note that when the reflex activity is initiated earlier in the lengthening movement, the force does not spill over into the subsequent shortening until a higher frequency of movement is reached. When there is additional phase advancement of the reflex signal within the spinal cord, a still higher frequency must be reached before the reflex force occurs during the shortening movement (45, 81).

Reflex Delay

The reflex delay is in two parts. There is the time taken for conduction of the reflex signal through the neural pathways (both inside and outside the central nervous system), and there is the time required for activation of the muscle fibers and force generation.

The neural component of the delay may be measured from the electromyographic response to a sudden limb perturbation. In the human ankle a sudden extension of the Achilles tendon generates a reflex electromyogram (EMG) in the gastrocnemius after an interval of 30–40 ms, and this is assumed to be a result of activity in a spinal stretch-reflex pathway. This is followed by other waves of EMG activity, the timing of which varies under different experimental conditions. There is often, however, a major burst of activity as late as 120 ms after the displacement (61, 63). In the biceps brachii the EMG response begins at about 18 ms, but there is another major burst of activity at about 50 ms [(37); see also the chapter by Evarts in this *Handbook*]. In the thumb there is very little activity with timing that would correspond to that of a spinal stretch reflex, and the first major response to a perturbation begins after about 45 ms but does not peak until about 70 ms (56).

The delay between neural activation of a muscle and the resulting tension is well known when it is the time to peak tension of a muscle twitch. More interesting for our present purpose is the response to a continuously changing rate of neural activation. If the rate of stimulation is modulated up and down, then each rise or fall in the stimulus rate is followed after an interval by the corresponding rise or fall in tension. This interval is not necessarily the same as the time to peak of a twitch, nor does it remain the same when the stimulus rate is modulated at different frequencies (54, 66). This delay in muscle activation is often regarded as the phase lag that accompanies the low-pass filtering property of the muscle (6).

Summary

By driving a limb or part of a limb through sinusoidally alternating movements and measuring the alternating forces required to maintain the movements, one obtains a measure of the limb's mechanical resistance. This resistance is a complex quantity, since both the amplitude and phase of force change with frequency of movement.

The resistance of the limb may be divided into a component that is merely due to its mass and a component that is due to the resistance of its muscles to extension. The latter may be further subdivided into the resistance that is attributed to the viscoelastic nature of the active muscle fibers and a component that reflects the periodic activation of muscle fibers in a reflex response to the movement.

The timing of this reflex component of force depends on the point in the cycle of movement at which the reflex activity is initiated, on the delay around the reflex pathway, and on the frequency of movement. A reflex initiated relatively late in the lengthening movement, or one that is subject to long delays, may generate forces that do not occur until the subsequent shortening phase of the movement; the reflex then reduces the resistance to movement.

Although reflex assistance of the movement generally occurs at a lower frequency when the delay is longer, the actual relation between the frequency of movement and the timing of the reflex force is not a simple one because the timing of both the muscle spindle activity and the muscle component of the delay change with changing frequency. Therefore sinusoidal movements do not provide an easy method of determining exact values for the reflex delays.

Muscle tissue has the properties of a low-pass filter; although it readily translates a slowly changing motoneuronal discharge into a corresponding force change, it does not respond to a rapidly changing motoneuronal discharge rate in the same way. The reflex modulation of muscle force therefore becomes progressively smaller as the frequency of movement is increased.

NEGATIVE STIFFNESS AND SPONTANEOUS OSCILLATIONS

Figures 5, 6**B**, and 8*A* show how voluntarily contracting muscles resist a sinusoidal displacement. In each of these figures the stiffness vectors follow a roughly circular path, moving in a clockwise direction as the frequency of movement increases. Although this is the usual pattern of response, there are variations in the size and shape of the path, in the position it occupies with respect to the axes, and in the distribution of the different frequency points around it.

In particular there are occasions when the vectors pass below the horizontal axis, so that at some frequencies the muscle force lags behind the muscle length. Vector path **B** in Figure 9 and Figure 11*A* illustrate this situation for the human elbow joint and for the interphalangeal joint of the thumb; similar figures could be constructed from the responses of monkey jaw muscles (28).

The data of Figure 9 are from the same subject as those of Figure 6 and were obtained during movements of the same amplitude, but in Figure 9 the subject was exerting a much higher mean flexing force. Vector path **A** shows the response of the whole arm including the mass of the forearm; **B** depicts the stiffness that remains after subtraction of the force required to move the mass. Thus **B** is analogous to **B** in Figure 6.

Between 6 and 13 Hz, where the vectors of Figure 9 lie below the horizontal axis, the muscle force rose higher when the muscle was shortening than when it was lengthening, a situation quite opposite to the effect arising from any normal friction or viscous resistance. This muscle could be said to have a negative viscous resistance, which did not impede the movement (as would a normal viscous resistance) but assisted it. Under these circumstances the changing muscle force tends to permit each lengthening movement and assist each shortening. The muscle then actually does work on the driving mechanism in each cycle of movement, something than no passive mechanical system does. Further positive proof of a reflex response to the movement is that this negative viscous stiffness continued for many successive cycles (47).

Neither the mass of the forearm nor any additional mass that may be carried by it affects the viscous stiffness, so that vector path **A** in Figure 9, which includes forces due to the mass as well as to the stiffness of the muscles, makes exactly the same dip into the region of negative viscous stiffness. Since, however, the mass does have a large effect on the component of force that is in phase with the movement, this vector follows a path beneath the origin, and the phase relations between force and position are very different from those of the C-shaped or circular figures that represent the muscle forces only.

The addition of still more mass gives a result that is different again. With the particular mass used in Figure 9, path **C**, the path of the vectors actually passes through the origin (the zero stiffness point) at about 6 Hz. Therefore at this frequency the force on the crank remained the same whether the muscle was long, short, lengthening, or shortening. In this situation the rotation of the driving wheel and movement

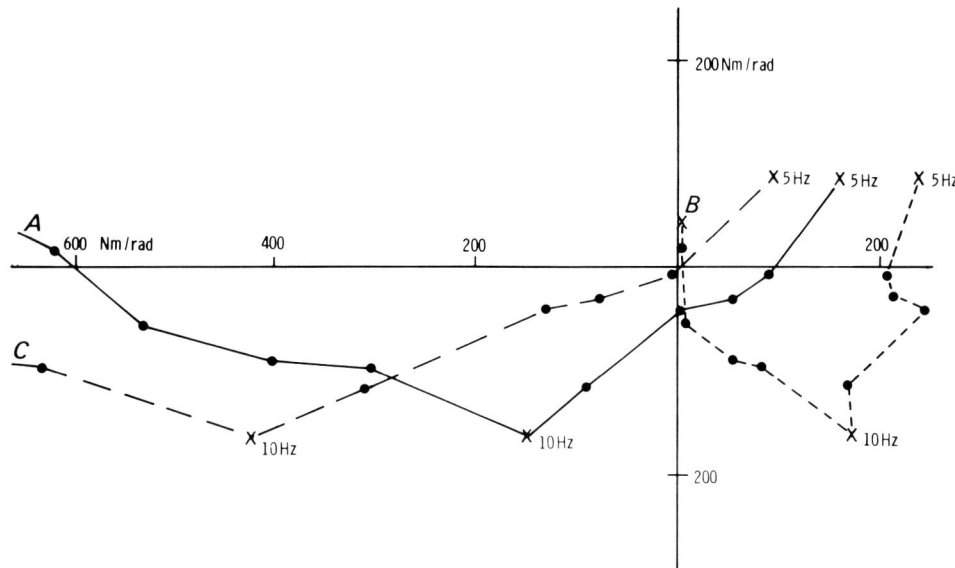

FIG. 9. Resistance to sinusoidal movement of human elbow. Same subject and amplitude of movement as Figure 6. Mean flexing torque was 32 N·m. **A**: resistance of limb to movements. **B**: component of stiffness remaining after subtracting component of force due to mass. **C**: stiffness that was actually measured when limb was encased in splints. [Replotted from Joyce, Rack, and Ross (47).]

of the crank did nothing that would either assist or prevent the movement, and decoupling the crank could be expected to leave the limb in a state of continuing free oscillation at about 6 Hz.

This prediction is in fact confirmed by Figure 10, which shows the same limb with the same mass in a state of uncontrollable oscillation (46). The subject was flexing against a compliant spring with a force similar to the mean force in Figure 9; so long as this force was maintained, the subject was quite unable to control the movement.

When during sinusoidal driving the stiffness vector actually encircles the origin, one would predict in a linear system spontaneous oscillations of progressively increasing amplitude (see subsection *Stability*, p. 234). In the present nonlinear situation, one would certainly expect the amplitude of spontaneous oscillation to rise above the amplitude of the driven movement, though one could not predict how large it would become.

The amplitude of the spontaneous oscillation in Figure 10 is larger than the amplitude of sinusoidal movement in Figure 9. This too is to be expected; if the sinusoidal driving had been done adding the spring of Figure 10, then the path of the vector **C** would have encircled the origin.

The actual frequency of the oscillation in Figure 10 is higher than the 6 Hz that might have been predicted from Figure 9, but this difference is also attributable to the elastic stiffness of the added spring.

Figure 11A shows the resistance of a thumb interphalangeal joint to sinusoidal movement. The actual mean flexing force was less than that in Figure 5, but the subject was not so strong, and this force was a larger fraction of her maximum. As in Figure 9, there

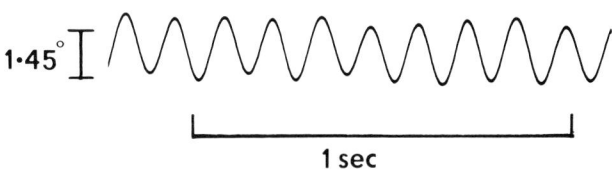

FIG. 10. Spontaneous oscillation at normal elbow joint (same subject as Figs. 6 and 9). Subject flexed with force of 32 N·m against a spring. Spring had a stiffness equivalent to 106 N·m and mass of forearm together with its enclosing splints was 0.149 kg·m².

is a range of frequencies (4–6 Hz) within which the viscous stiffness becomes negative. The dashed line in Figure 11A shows how the stiffness vectors are altered by the addition of a mass to the terminal phalanx so that their paths pass beneath and around the origin. With this mass the free moving joint undergoes a spontaneous oscillation at some frequency around 5 Hz; this is shown in Figure 11B for a subject exerting the same force against a compliant spring (9).

Spontaneous oscillations of this sort quite commonly occur when we exert a large force with our arms against an "awkward" load. The clear relation between these spontaneous movements and the response to sinusoidal driving leaves little doubt that the spontaneous movements are the self-sustaining oscillation of a stretch reflex, though not necessarily of a spinal stretch reflex. From the results of sinusoidal driving, one can predict the changes in frequency that accompany changes in load (46, 72). Spontaneous oscillations of normal joints appear to be analogous with the clonus that occurs in some patients with hyperactive stretch reflexes.

The spontaneous clonus that fairly often occurs at

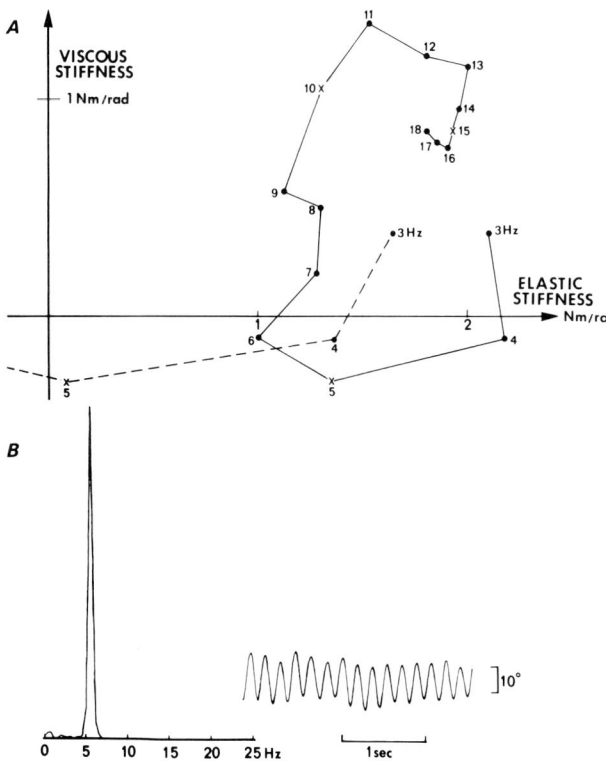

FIG. 11. *A*: resistance to sinusoidal movement at interphalangeal joint of thumb. Movement was through ± 1.3° while subject exerted a mean flexing torque of 0.5 N·m. *Solid line* joins vectors that denote stiffness of thumb alone. *Broken line* shows how these vectors are displaced by addition of a mass with moment of inertia 1.3 g·m². *B*: spontaneous tremor of same joint; thumb was loaded with a mass of inertia 1.3 g·m², and subject flexed with a force of 0.5 N·m against a compliant spring (spring stiffness equivalent to 0.08 N·m/rad).

the normal ankle joint probably also depends, at least in part, on similar activity (2, 31), though the situation is more complicated and may also involve some other mechanisms (73).

Factors Affecting Stability of Stretch Reflexes

The involuntary oscillations just described have very obvious disadvantages for an animal in a competitive environment, and it is pertinent to ask how we usually avoid this potentially dangerous situation.

These self-sustaining oscillations do not arise from some single defect in the stretch-reflex control but from the interaction of a number of different factors, including the timing and intensity of the reflex activity, the nature of the external load, and the level of muscle activation. In the succeeding paragraphs I separate and examine some of these factors.

The problem can best be approached through a knowledge of limb responses to imposed sinusoidal movements; we are particularly interested in whether or not the stiffness remains safely positive at all frequencies. In terms of the vector representation of stiffness, we want to know what it is that determines the relation of the vectors to the origin. There is some experimental information about the effects of external loads and different amounts of muscle force and about the behavior of the limbs during different amplitudes of movement. Some of the other parameters of the stretch reflexes, such as the duration of the conduction delays, the velocity sensitivity of the receptors, and the low-pass filtering function of the muscles, are less accessible to experimental manipulation. Their roles have to be inferred from a comparison of different stretch reflexes as well as a comparison of the stretch reflex with man-made servo-control systems.

Nature of the External Load

When at some frequency of movement the limb exhibits a negative viscous stiffness, the effect of the stretch reflex is to assist the movement. It is then possible to bring the stiffness vector beneath the origin by adding some suitable mass or spring; if that mass or spring is its only load, the limb will break into spontaneous oscillation (Figs. 9, 10, and 11). Adding an external load can be regarded as tuning a mechanical system, part of which is inside and part of which is outside the limb, so that it readily follows movements at a frequency at which the reflex activity provides the driving force (46).

Many of our limb joints operate on a wide variety of different loads. The joints of the lower limbs carry a variable proportion of the body weight, and the loads on the shoulder, elbow, and wrist joints depend on what we have in our hands. At a frequency where these joints have a negative viscous stiffness, they are in danger of uncontrolled oscillation with some load or another, a situation that presumably must be avoided. The load required for spontaneous oscillations may be an unusual one, however; neither the compliant spring that gave the violent elbow movements of Figure 10 nor the large mass that was attached to the terminal phalanx of the thumb in Figure 11*B* are loads often met. Thus one way of avoiding these troublesome oscillations is to avoid the particular loads with which they occur, and this amounts to keeping the natural frequency of the mechanical system well away from the frequencies at which the stretch reflex can sustain an oscillation.

Level of Muscle Activation

When a normal limb is at rest, and its muscles are inactive, it takes a rapid displacement to provoke any noticeable stretch reflex. When muscles are already voluntarily contracting, however, much less dramatic extensions may meet with considerable reflex resistance, which increases parallel to the contractile force (55).

A similar relationship between reflex activity and voluntary force may be inferred from the response to sinusoidal movements. Figure 12 shows the stiffness

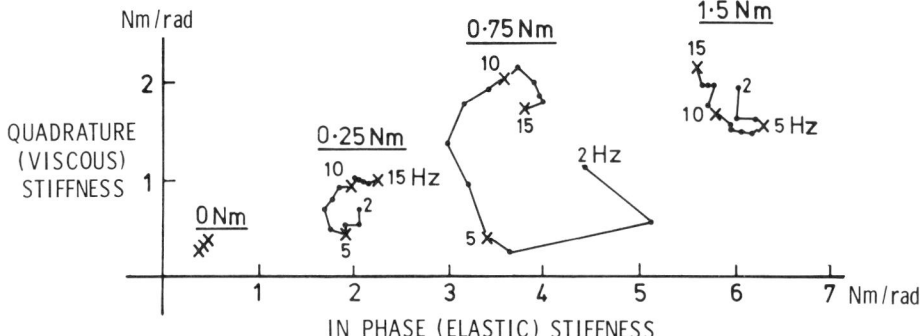

FIG. 12. Effect of mean flexing force on stiffness at thumb interphalangeal joint. The 0.75-N·m record is from Figure 5; with other mean flexing forces (marked on figure), stiffness vectors follow different paths. [From Brown, Rack, and Ross (10).]

of the interphalangeal joint of the thumb measured at a number of frequencies while the subject exerted four different mean flexing forces. When there was no flexing effort whatever, the resisting force was small and the different frequency points lie close together. The stiffness vectors do not follow the circular path characteristic of a delayed reflex force, and no EMG activity could be detected in flexor pollicis longus.

When a subject does exert a flexing force at the joint, the stiffness vectors follow the C-shaped path previously described, indicating that a component of the force is attributable to delayed stretch-reflex activity. Figure 12 shows how the stiffness of the same joint changed as the subject exerted a number of different mean forces: the C was largest when the force was about one-third maximal, and it became smaller when very large forces were exerted.

Taking the size of the C as a rough indication of the amplitude of the reflex force (by analogy with Fig. 3), one can conclude that reflex activity increases with flexing force, though it decreases when the muscles contract with near-maximal force. (Incoming reflex activity presumably causes little increase in force since the muscle is almost fully activated.)

The intensity of muscle contraction also affects the resistance to movement in another way. With each increase in mean force there is a concomitant increase in that component of muscle stiffness that is quite independent of the reflex activity (see subsection *Tuning of the Neuromuscular System*, p. 247). This increase in the nonreflex stiffness of the muscles appears in Figure 12 as a displacement of the whole C-shaped vector path away from the origin in a direction that implies a higher viscoelastic resistance.

With increasing muscle force there are thus changes in both the reflex and the nonreflex components of the resistance to movement, and these do not always change in the same direction. There is always some frequency at which reflex activity reduces the viscous stiffness, and the stiffness vectors are then at the lowest part of their C-shaped path (3–6 Hz in Fig. 12). This reduction is greater when, during a vigorous effort, the reflex is more active and the C is larger; but the increase in nonreflex stiffness accompanying a greater force includes an increase in viscous stiffness that lifts the C upward. In Figure 12 these two effects approximately balance each other for movements at 3–6 Hz. Hence with increases in force up to 0.75 N·m, any decrease in viscous resistance due to the reflex activity is offset by the positive viscous stiffness provided by the nonreflex properties of the muscle. As a result total viscous resistance to movements at this frequency range changes little.

There is not always this balance between the two opposing effects. A comparison of Figures 6 and 9 shows that the increase in reflex activity accompanying the higher force clearly caused the viscous stiffness to become negative (see specifically Figure 9 at 7–13 Hz); this effect was by no means counterbalanced by any increase in the muscle's viscous stiffness that may have occurred. In this example the increase in flexing force put the limb into a state where involuntary oscillations occurred.

Resistance to Movements of Different Amplitudes

Measurements of resistance to small movements cannot predict the resistance of limbs to larger movements as they do in a linear system.

Figure 13 shows the resistance of an elbow joint that was moved through three different amplitudes. If the system had been linear, then the vectors would have followed the same path on each occasion, since the force/displacement would have been independent of the displacement amplitude. The vectors of Figure 13 do in fact follow paths that are quite different: with small amplitudes of movement (**A** and **B**), there is a range of frequencies where the viscous stiffness is negative and the vectors lie below the origin. With larger amplitudes (**C**), however, the path of the vector is lifted upward and there is no frequency at which the viscous stiffness is negative.

Because the vectors of the response to movements of small amplitude (**A** and **B** in Fig. 13) encircle the origin, the limb would undergo a spontaneous oscillation at some frequency between 9 and 10 Hz if it were

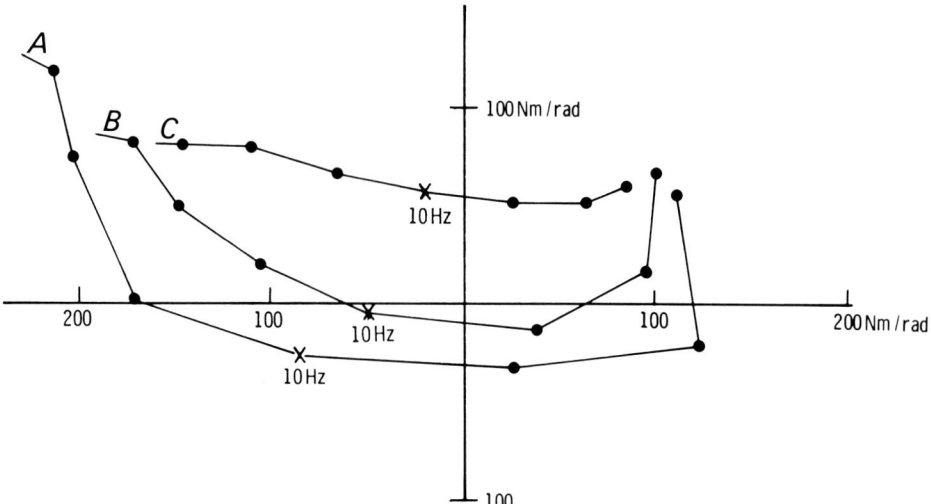

FIG. 13. Resistance of human elbow joint to different amplitudes of sinusoidal movement. Resistance includes forces required to overcome mass of forearm. Mean flexing torque, 26 N·m. Amplitude of movement for **A**, ±0.12°; **B**, ±0.25°; and **C**, ±1.2°. [Replotted from Joyce, Rack, and Ross (47).]

free to do so. The negative viscous stiffness would then actually assist the movement, which would therefore grow in amplitude. This growth, however, would change the properties of the limb, which would then no longer be described by records **A** and **B**, but by something between **B** and **C**.

In **C**, where there is a positive viscous resistance, any oscillatory movement that did begin would decay in amplitude due to the damping effect of this viscous stiffness. In a free movement the properties of the limb would therefore be described by one or another of these vector paths as the amplitude of the oscillation waxed or waned. With the load conditions of Figure 13, a stable oscillation should occur at about 9.5 Hz and at whatever amplitude of movement is needed to take the stiffness vector through the origin. Such an oscillation does indeed occur (46).

In summary one can say that although the delayed force arising from stretch-reflex activity may sometimes support a spontaneous oscillation, the properties of the neuromuscular system change with the amplitude of movement in a way that limits the growth of the oscillation. The oscillation therefore continues at some limited amplitude and can be described in engineering terms as a stable limit cycle.

There are two physiological mechanisms that probably contribute to the changes in limb stiffness accompanying changing amplitudes of movement. Muscle spindles are known to be less sensitive to large movements than to small ones [(38, 60); see also the chapter by Matthews in this *Handbook*], so doubling the movement amplitude does not double the rate of afferent fiber discharge. Therefore the reflex response is probably relatively reduced as the amplitude of movement increases (59). Since it is the reflex component of force acting after a delay that gives the negative viscous resistance, it is hardly surprising that the viscous stiffness is less negative when the reflex is less effective.

The viscous resistance that arises from the mechanical properties of active muscle fibers may increase as the amplitude increases from very small movements to larger ones. This probably also contributes to the alterations in the total limb stiffness.

It has been implied that these limit cycles amount to a defective operation of the system that the animal normally wishes to avoid. This is not necessarily so; there are activities such as running or hopping in which the limited oscillatory behavior may be employed to advantage. It is possible that the oscillatory tendencies of the stretch reflexes may be used in these situations, and the frequencies at which some of these repetitive movements usually occur are such that reflex activity could contribute to them (61).

Comparing the Stretch Reflex With a Man-Made Control System

The engineer who sets out to design a servo-control system usually wants it to have a high loop gain ($-HG/N$ in Fig. 1). Such a system faithfully translates an input into an equivalent output and is relatively immune to external disturbances and changes in load (see subsection *Loop Gain*, p. 231). Restating this in terms of the stretch reflex and assuming that this is a position controller, one might expect a reflex stiffness (HG in Fig. 1 and Eq. 3) that is high compared with the combined stiffness N of the muscles and the external loads against which the reflex usually operates. The stretch reflex might then achieve the load compensation that is often attributed to it, simplifying the task of the higher motor centers.

Experimental evidence suggests, however, that the stiffness of the stretch reflex is rather disappointingly small. This is true whether the measurements are made on muscles of a decerebrate cat (59), on the fingers of conscious human subjects (80), or on the neck muscles of a conscious monkey (7). This apparent shortcoming of the stretch reflex has sometimes puzzled physiologists—why such a feeble stretch reflex when there appear to be good reasons for a powerful one? Figures 9–11 may provide an answer: when the stiffness of the stretch reflex is high compared with the stiffness of the muscles and the external load, uncontrolled oscillations are likely to occur. Oscillatory instabilities are all too familiar to control engineers, and it is instructive to look at the methods they employ to avoid and prevent them in the systems they construct.

Stability of a Man-Made System

Whenever the transport of signals around the feedback loop takes a significant time, there are some frequencies of sinusoidal movement at which the correcting signal is applied too late, so that it assists and tends to perpetuate the movement. These resonant frequencies of the feedback loop are higher when the transport delay is short. They are also higher when the correcting signal arrives earlier through the action of phase-advancing mechanisms or, in the case of a position control, by a velocity-sensitive transducer.

By keeping the delays minimal and employing phase-advancing mechanisms, the engineer always tries to ensure that the resonant frequencies of the feedback loop are well above the range in which the system has to operate. A filter is then introduced into the loop that selectively attenuates these high-frequency signals but has little effect on the lower frequencies. Thus the filter reduces the loop gain at the resonant frequency to some low level (less than 1) while maintaining a high gain for the lower frequency signals that are to be preserved. In this way the risk of oscillatory instabilities is avoided, but lower frequency disturbances are still effectively managed by the servo-control system. It is worth emphasizing that this favorable situation can only be achieved when the resonant frequency of the control loop is brought well outside the working range of the system so that effective differential filtering is possible.

Stability and Gain in the Stretch Reflex

The same methods that an engineer might employ to improve the performance and ensure the stability of the control system are found in the stretch reflexes. The velocity sensitivity of muscle spindles and the additional phase advance imparted in the spinal cord both tend to mitigate the effects of the reflex delays, thus raising the resonant frequency of the reflex pathway. The low-pass filtering property of the muscles then reduces the loop gain for the higher frequency movements. When one tries to put these statements into more quantitative terms, however, the result is not quite what one might have expected of a servo-control system. The delays involved in the stretch-reflex pathways are often so long that their resonant frequencies remain low in spite of the phase-advancing effects. At the elbow joint, spontaneous oscillation occurs at frequencies as low as 6–7 Hz, and at joints where reflex control is dominated by slower pathways, such as the fingers and thumb, the resonant frequencies may be under 5 Hz. Some of the slower muscles attenuate the effects of reflex activity at these frequencies, but faster muscles are certainly capable of generating changing forces that may have important components at 6 Hz or higher (54). Indeed survival may often have required correspondingly fast movements.

It seems then that the resonant frequencies of many of these reflex pathways are either in or near the frequency range in which the limbs are regularly used. Under these circumstances there is little possibility of effective differential filtering that would reduce the gain to a low level at the resonant frequency while retaining a high gain in the normal working range of the system. Therefore it should be no surprise that experimental investigations suggest that the gain of the stretch-reflex loop is low. If it were otherwise, limbs would be in a state of continuing oscillation.

Although we cannot expect to see the stretch reflex operating with gains that would make it a very effective servomechanism, there are some features that might make it better than the above analysis suggests. By distributing the control among a number of pathways of different lengths, the animal might be able to avoid some of the problems that arise from the single simple control loop (65, 77). The dangers of spontaneous oscillation might be avoided if the different delays were distributed such that the frequency range within which some reflex pathway tended to support a spontaneous oscillation was one in which another reflex pathway had an opposite effect. The net gain would be low for signals at all frequencies where the actions of the different reflex pathways were opposed to each other, but combined activity in the different pathways could still provide an effective resistance to slow displacements.

If the stretch-reflex activity were confined to slow muscle fibers and the faster fibers were employed in voluntary movements, then a stiffer reflex (more reflex force/displacement) could probably be employed without danger of instability, since the low-pass filtering effect of these slow muscles would reduce the gain of the reflex to a safe level (in all but the lowest frequency ranges) without necessarily impairing fast voluntary movements. It does seem that the slower motoneurons are often more accessible to stretch-reflex afferents than are the faster ones (13), though most of the evidence presently available suggests that reflex responses and voluntary movements employ the same muscle fibers and recruit them in the same order [(39); see also the chapter by Henneman and Mendell in this *Handbook*)].

An interesting nonlinearity arises because the resistance to the velocity and extent of a movement depends on the level of muscle activation, and this in turn depends (through the stretch reflex) on the velocity and extent of the movement. The normal resistance of the muscles to extension is further multiplied by the sensitivity of the muscle spindles to give a force that increases very steeply as the speed and extent of movement increases. This property of the stretch reflex and the nonlinear properties of the muscles themselves are such that the animal may operate its stretch reflexes with gains that lead to occasional small-amplitude tremors without risking the disastrous instabilities that might occur in the (theoretical) linear system.

There is always the possibility (as yet unsupported by evidence) that a developing tremor might activate some higher part of the nervous system that would respond with sequences of discharge so timed that they would have a specific damping effect.

Summary

During sinusoidal stretching of a muscle there is some frequency range in which the response to lengthening is a reflex force that is delayed until the subsequent shortening movement. A force that is so timed tends to assist the movement; it has an effect that is the opposite of friction or viscosity and may therefore be described as a negative viscous resistance. If, through powerful reflex activity, this negative viscous resistance should outweigh the positive viscous resistance of the active muscle fibers, then at that frequency the whole limb will exhibit a negative viscous stiffness, and the muscles will assist the movement rather than resisting it.

A limb that assists its own sinusoidal movement at some frequency will break into spontaneous oscillation at that frequency if it is free to do so. In normal limbs, however, this spontaneous oscillation or clonus occurs only with a restricted range of loads and forces, and these can be confidently predicted from a knowledge of the responses to imposed sinusoidal movements.

Sinusoidal analysis of limb stiffness not only indicates whether a spontaneous oscillatory movement will occur, but it also helps to distinguish the many factors that combine and interact to permit or prevent the oscillation.

It is assumed that animals normally need to avoid uncontrolled oscillations of their limbs. The experimental evidence suggests that they do this by maintaining a low level of stretch-reflex activity. This sometimes surprises physiologists when they consider the improvements in performance that may follow the use of high-gain feedback pathways in man-made control systems. The stretch reflexes are different, however, from most man-made control systems. An engineer minimizes conduction delays and thereby raises the natural frequency of the feedback loop as high as possible. The loop gain is then reduced by differential filtering for signals close to the resonant frequency, whereas a usefully high gain is retained in the lower range of frequencies where the system will operate. In the stretch reflex the delays are so long that the resonant frequency of the reflex path is low and close to, if not actually within, the working range of the system. Differential filtering is thus impossible and the system cannot have a high gain for signals throughout its working range and still avoid spontaneous oscillation.

Therefore the stretch reflexes cannot have the high loop gains that an engineer might hope to achieve. A moderate gain may nevertheless be useful, and the combination of phase-advancing mechanisms in the reflex pathway and low-pass filtering in the muscles no doubt help toward that end.

REFLEX RESPONSES OR PRECOMPUTED ACTIVITY?

We have seen that the combination of reflex delays and fast-moving limbs precludes the existence of a high-gain, position-controlling servomechanism of the type usually designed by control engineers. This same reflex delay would have a similar unstabilizing effect on servomechanisms designed to control muscle force or stiffness, and therefore they too could have only a small gain.

Thus it first appears that the stretch reflex plays only a minor part in some of the slower postural adjustments and little or no part in shaping the faster voluntary movements. If this is so, then presumably we must confront many disturbing forces by switching on precomputed patterns of muscular activity; the faster voluntary movements must also be precomputed and then executed "ballistically," since there is not time for afferent activity to modify them.

Although the precomputation of motor activity is undoubtedly of great importance, too clear a distinction between precomputed actions and those carried out under feedback control should not be made. In this chapter I argue that there is a continuum of activity extending from the slow responses to entirely unexpected events to precomputed actions that depend on detailed information and planning; it has a wide intermediate range, however, within which the animal may set up relatively rapid responses to disturbances that it anticipates might occur.

Response to a Sudden Disturbance

An entirely unexpected disturbing force that catches us off guard meets with little effective resistance. The man who walks down a flight of stairs but misjudges the number of steps may find himself thrown badly off balance, and stretch reflexes give him no immediate help. Records of EMG activity during landing from a fall or jump confirm that all the initial resistance of the muscles is preprogrammed from a knowledge of when and how the impact will occur (33, 61).

If we were given only the two possibilities that the neuromuscular responses to a disturbance are either stretch-reflex responses or preprogrammed responses, we would conclude that only the latter effectively deal with the faster disturbances. It would follow that unexpected disturbances, for which no preprogramming had been done, would often meet with ineffective or inappropriate resistance. There is, however, mounting evidence of a range of reactions that are intermediate between the simple "hard-wired" reflex and the fully preprogrammed response. The intensity of a reflex response may be preset in anticipation of a disturbance that is known to be a possibility, although it cannot be precisely foreseen. In particular the reflex gain may be "turned up" to usefully high levels when the individual undertakes particular tasks or anticipates the need for a particular response. Adjusting the properties of the spinal cord to deal with a particular situation has been described in the Russian literature as "tuning" of the stretch reflex (4, 34).

To preset the gain of the reflex is different (in concept) from preprogramming the movement; in the former the response still depends on the timing and nature of the afferent input to the reflex, whereas in the latter the whole movement is executed as a result of the advance planning. (In a later section I suggest that the two processes may be less distinct than they first appear.)

In view of the oscillatory instabilities that result when the stretch-reflex gain is maintained at a high level, one must presume either that the gain is turned up to high levels only for periods that are brief compared with the time course of possible oscillations, or that there exists some other compensatory mechanism that reduces the oscillatory tendencies.

Thus the response to a sudden disturbance depends partly on the way the reflex pathways have been tuned in anticipation of a disturbance and partly on the nature of the disturbance itself. Therefore the response may often appear to be intermediate between a voluntary movement and a movement that is entirely reflex. Later in this chapter I argue that there is in fact a continuum of reponses extending from the pure reflex through the tuned reflex and triggered response to the fully preprogrammed voluntary movement. Along with this we have another continuum of events, ranging from disturbances that are entirely foreseen, to those that are partially anticipated, to those that are quite unexpected.

The next subsection discusses the part that this tuning process may play in the response of a limb to a sudden disturbance. These tuning or setting-up processes are not confined to the reflex behavior, and the section begins by describing how the muscles themselves are set up to meet a disturbance.

Tuning of the Neuromuscular System

Since the reflex response to a limb displacement only appears after some delay, any immediate resistance must be due to the properties of the limb itself. The physical properties of the muscles are important here.

Passive muscles present little resistance to movements within most of the joint range. Muscles that are activated by stimulation at physiological rates, however, do resist changes in length with large changes in force (32, 58, 74); particularly large changes in force occur during the first part of such a movement (48). Figure 14 shows records of the force generated by a muscle before and during controlled shortening and lengthening movements. The uppermost record shows the movements, and the lower records show the forces during stimulation of motor units at three different rates. During stimulation at 15 impulses/s, the tension fell abruptly at the beginning of the shortening movement and rose equally rapidly at the onset of the lengthening movement. This high level of muscle stiffness (change in force/change in length) does not persist, however; the later part of the shortening movement is met by only a gradual fall in force, whereas during the later part of lengthening, the force may not rise at all and may sometimes actually decrease.

This short-range stiffness can play an important part in the initial response of a limb to a disturbing force. Consider a joint that is held in some position by the cocontraction of a pair of antagonist muscles. At rest the pair of muscles creates a force balance; this is indicated in the first part of Figure 15, where the flexing force is upward and the extending force downward. A sudden extension of the joint thus leads to a steep increase in tension of the flexor muscle and a corresponding decrease in tension of the extensor muscle. The joint thereby resists the movement with a net force arising from the sum of the stiffnesses of the two muscles.

The resistance to the first part of a movement is a property of muscle tissue that does not depend on reflex activity. The amount of this stiffness is not the same on all occasions, however; it can be preset by altering the force of contraction of the muscles concerned. When opposing muscles are vigorously contracting, the limbs exhibit a high level of stiffness, but if the muscles are less completely activated (Fig. 14, 7 and 3 pps), then not only is the isometric tension in each muscle smaller, but the changes in force that accompany the first part of a movement are also correspondingly reduced (48, 64), and the limb is more compliant. It is common experience that we cocontract

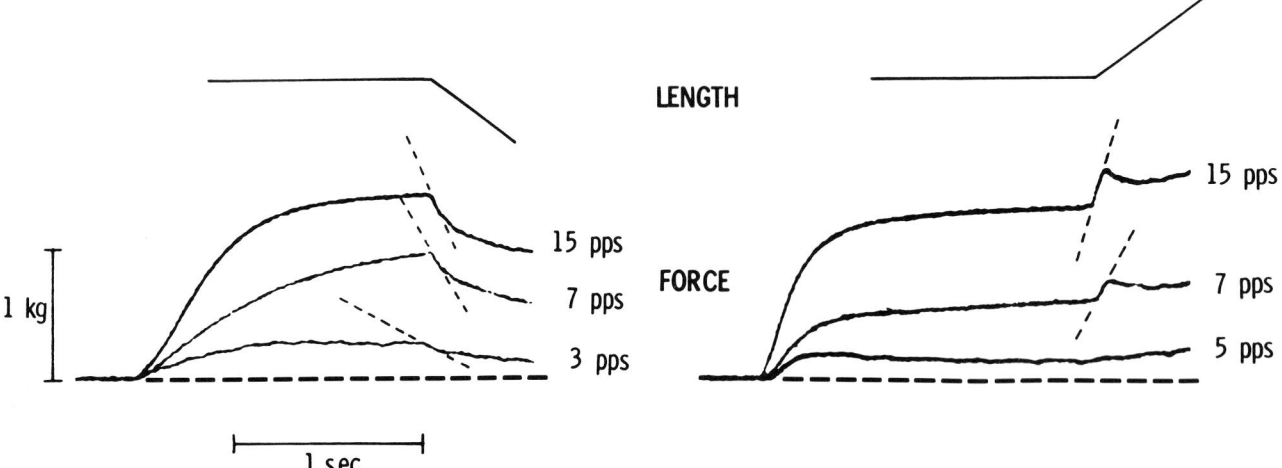

FIG. 14. Effect of movement on continuously stimulated muscle. Cat soleus muscle was stimulated by trains of pulses that were distributed sequentially among different groups of motor units so that while each muscle fiber was stimulated at only 3, 5, 7, or 15 pulses/s (pps), action potentials reached the muscle at 5 × that rate. *Dotted lines* indicate rapid changes in tension that accompanied first part of shortening or lengthening movement.

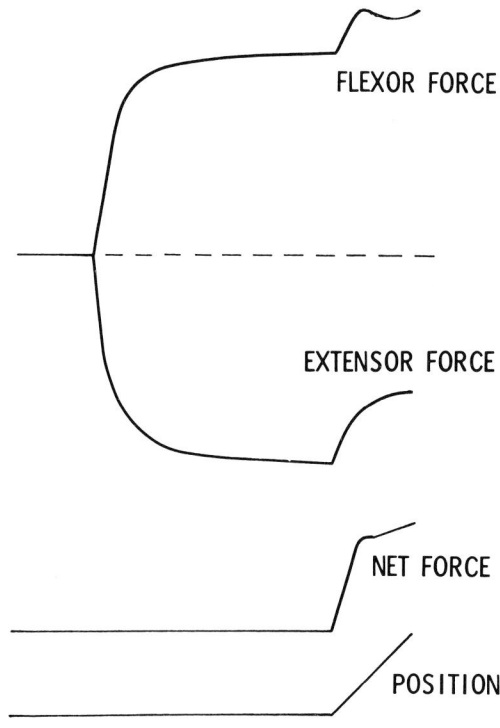

FIG. 15. Diagram showing effects of cocontraction of antagonist muscles. Forces developed by flexor and extensor muscles (similar to the 15 pps record of Fig. 14) act in opposite directions and so long as there is no movement of the joint, there is no external force. When, however, the joint is subjected to an extending movement, the force in the flexor muscle rises and the force in the extensor falls; the joint resists the displacement with a force that depends on the summed stiffnesses of the 2 muscles.

muscles to stiffen our limbs in anticipation of some disturbing force that we wish to resist; this cocontraction may be the preparation for a disturbance with a force and direction that we cannot exactly predict. We probably stiffen our joints like this when we carry a full glass in a crowded room, but the stiffness of our ankles as we walk on an uncertain, uneven surface, such as a grass-covered slope, may be quite different.

The reflex resistance to muscle extension is also subject to considerable modification, and the changes in reflex behavior accompanying many disorders of the motor system are very well known. Here we are more concerned with changes in reflex properties that occur from time to time in normal individuals.

It has long been known that the tendon reflex in a group of muscles may be facilitated by the forcible contraction of muscles elsewhere in the body (Jendrassek's maneuver). This is in itself evidence that the effectiveness of the spinal stretch reflex is subject to alteration. More precise experiments have shown that the H-reflex for a particular muscle is often facilitated when the subject is actively using that muscle (29, 34); this facilitation actually precedes the muscle effort by up to 100 ms (30, 34).

The increase in reflex stiffness that accompanies sustained muscular activity has been mentioned, and there is no doubt that forcible contraction of a muscle is often associated with a high level of stretch-reflex activity, though this need not amount to an enhancement of the reflex loop gain (see subsection *Level of Muscle Activation*, p. 242).

These increases in reflex activity occur either on a background of increased muscle activity or at a time when muscle activity has been instructed by higher parts of the nervous system. More interesting here are the changes in reflex gain that may be brought about by the prior intentions of the subject without any concomitant change in motoneuronal activation. These have been most clearly demonstrated in experiments recording the electromyographic responses to sudden imposed movements of human limbs. A sudden forcible movement of the elbow joint is followed by a reflex electromyographic response in the flexor or extensor muscles, the first part of which is undoubtedly a spinal stretch reflex. A number of workers (20, 35, 51) have shown that the magnitude of this reflex response may change according to the intentions of the subject. When the subjects were instructed to resist the movement there was a larger spinal stretch reflex than when they were instructed to relax and allow the displacement to happen. Similar responses have been obtained from the human tibialis anterior (43) and from the biceps brachii of trained monkeys (21).

This voluntary increase in the gain of the spinal stretch reflex has generally seemed small, and indeed some workers have doubted its existence (16). There is, however, a larger change in the effectiveness of the spinal stretch reflex in subjects who have been repeatedly subjected to the same disturbance and have practiced resisting it (20).

There are a number of mechanisms that may modify the gain of the spinal stretch reflex. An increase in static fusimotor activity might bring the mean discharge rate of muscle spindle afferents nearer to the motoneuron threshold, so that extension of the muscle or electrical stimulation of afferents more easily provokes a reflex discharge. An increase in dynamic fusimotor activity directly increases the sensitivity of the muscle spindles to a rapid extension. An increase in other inputs to the motoneuron or a decrease in presynaptic inhibition also brings the motoneurons nearer to their threshold and thus increases the probability of a burst of afferent activity initiating a reflex response. There is debate as to which parts these different mechanisms actually play in modifying the gain of the fast spinal stretch reflex (11, 12, 14, 43, 49). For our present purposes it is sufficient that the gain of the reflex may be modified.

The experiments of Hammond (37) demonstrated that the resistance to a sudden limb displacement consists of a number of different reflex components, and some of the later parts of the response often play a more important part than the faster spinal reflexes. These later responses probably involve a number of different pathways; some involve the cerebral cortex (18, 56, 68), whereas others do not (25). Here they are lumped together under the general term long-loop stretch reflexes.

The important point here is that these later reflex responses may be modified by the prior intention or training of the subject to a much greater extent than the fast spinal reflexes. In the simplest situation the intention to resist a displacement leads to a large resistance, the timing of which implies reflex activity, whereas the intention to "let go" may greatly diminish the long-loop component of the response or remove it entirely (20, 37, 79).

The prior intention of the subject (conscious or unconscious) thus acts at different levels to modify the response to a disturbance. Even though a subject might not know the direction of a disturbance, or the precise time at which it will occur, the neuromuscular system can be appropriately prepared by setting the muscle stiffness and the reflex gains to suitable levels. Reflexes that in the relaxed limb might seem to be too feeble to be useful thus have their gains increased to meet a particular situation.

It generally seems that the response to a disturbance improves (i. e., it becomes more appropriate) when the foreknowledge is more complete; in other words, a knowledge of the direction of the coming disturbance improves the reflex response to that disturbance (18).

In the previous paragraphs it has been useful to think of the stretch reflex in terms of a servo-control loop with a gain that is adjustable by training or voluntary intention. It is, however, equally reasonable to regard this as a system in which the motor activity depends on a combination of two signals, one that represents the peripheral events and another that represents the voluntary intention. In this particular situation the mode of interaction of these two inputs, wherever they meet, is such that the peripheral event determines the pattern of the motoneuronal activity, whereas the voluntary intention has something akin to a gating effect on it.

Under other circumstances, which are considered below, the relationship between these two inputs and the relative weighting of their effects on the motor activity may be quite different and may not in the least resemble conventional servo-control action.

Triggered Responses to a Disturbance

Subjects may be trained or instructed to meet a displacing force not merely with resistance, but with an active movement of the limb in either the same or the opposite direction as the force. The situation is then more complicated; as one might expect, the muscles that are stretched by the initial displacement first show a stretch reflex that is increased when the subject intends to make an opposing movement but decreased when the intent is to move in the same direction as the displacement. The later part of the movement, however, depends entirely on the previous intention of the subject, so that a subject instructed to flex the joint does so, whatever the direction of the initial disturbance (16, 20, 21, 79).

The response has been described as having two clear components, one that can properly be called a stretch reflex and the other that is regarded as a separate "triggered response" to the disturbance (16). Although this distinction is convenient because it allows us to retain the separate ideas of a stretch reflex and a voluntary response, the two components merge in all experimental results. There is no one point where one can say that the reflex response ends and the voluntary responses begin. Rather there is a gradual transition from the earlier (fast spinal) reflexes, which are subject to only partial voluntary control, to the long-loop reflexes, which are subject to considerable modification, to the triggered responses, where the incoming afferent activity merely initiates the predetermined movement, and finally to the conscious voluntary corrections.

When a joint is subjected to a sudden displacement, electromyograms from stretched muscles show a discharge that has an amplitude reaching a number of peaks at different intervals after the movement; these peaks are often assumed to reflect the activity of a number of different reflex pathways followed by voluntary responses (51). The earliest of these peaks, designated M1 by Lee and Tatton (51), is undoubtedly a fast spinal reflex, and some of the later reflex responses probably involve the sensorimotor parts of the cerebral cortex, though the detailed pathways have not yet been worked out and the separate natures of the different peaks are by no means established (see the chapters by Porter and by Evarts in this *Handbook*). For now we can only regard the transition from the reflex to the voluntary response as a gradual one with many intermediate stages.

Whereas the stretch reflex is a motor response, the nature of which is determined by the muscle extension (though its amplitude may be modified by voluntary intensions), the triggered response represents a different interaction between the voluntary intention and the incoming afferent activity (wherever they meet); it is now the afferent activity that has the gating effect, and the voluntary intention that determines the pattern of the response.

It is possible to envisage other forms of interaction between the voluntary intention and the afferent activity, and indeed there could be a continuum between situations where the response is a pure reflex and situations where it is entirely voluntary. Here the simpler concepts of control theory hinder rather than help; one can no longer identify which pathway is an input, which is an error signal, and which is a gain control. Attempts to force the biological system into some easily described pattern of servo loops are thus not useful.

Summary

The response of a limb to a sudden disturbing force involves different neuromuscular mechanisms operating after different time intervals.

The stiffness of actively contracting muscle provides an immediate resistance to movement that does not depend on any reflex response. Muscles are particularly resistant to small changes in length and are most effective in opposing the first part of a displacement.

Spinal stretch reflexes operate after some delay, and other longer loop reflexes operate after a longer interval; these responses merge into the triggered responses and the still slower voluntary reactions.

When a disturbing force is entirely unexpected, the resistance is usually slight. When, however, there is some foreknowledge that a disturbance may occur, the neuromuscular system may be tuned to deal with it; muscles may be cocontracted against each other to increase their stiffness, and the effective gains of stretch reflexes may be increased. Furthermore the nervous system may prepare a definite pattern of response that is triggered by the displacement. The response to a sudden disturbance thus depends on how clearly it is foreseen, and there is a whole range of intermediate possibilities between the reflex response to an entirely unexpected disturbance and the precomputed response to one that was entirely forseen.

Although it may often be useful to distinguish between reflexes, triggered responses, and voluntary reactions, these merge into each other, and it is neither practical nor helpful to separate them completely.

SERVO ASSISTANCE OF VOLUNTARY MOVEMENTS

A simple mechanical control system with a high feedback loop gain may compensate deficiencies or nonlinearities in the actuators and changes in the nature of the load. The task of the operator is then considerably simplified since the instructions are faithfully translated into limb positions or movements.

The delays involved in the stretch reflex limit the way that it assists and modifies a voluntary movement, just as they limit its usefulness in meeting an external disturbance. Very slow movements can certainly be made bit by bit under feedback control: the boy learning to play the violin moves his finger along the string until his ears tell him that he has the correct position; the mechanic turning a nut continues until sensory information from the wrist and hand indicate that it is tight enough. Faster movements cannot be made in this way. During a rapid passage, the nervous system of the skilled violinist is busy generating neural activity for the next note to be played and perhaps the one after that; thus sensory information from the ears or the fingers will certainly be too late to alter the tuning of a particular note while it is sounding. Similarly a mechanic using a hammer is hardly able to employ feedback to alter the velocity or trajectory of the hammer once it is fully in motion. This line of thought once again leads us to conclude that there are two different types of movement; the first is achieved slowly under feedback control, and the second is due to motoneuronal activity and is entirely precomputed and executed ballistically.

Since these ballistic movements are executed at speeds that do not permit any feedback control, it is not possible for immediate servo control to simplify the task of the controller. In fact there is no alternative to a full precomputation of the required motoneuronal activity, and this computation must take into account characteristics of the muscles such as the relation among stimulus rate, velocity, length, and tension, as well as the state of fatigue of the muscles, the loads to be moved, and the positions and velocities of all the moving parts.

In the course of normal spontaneous activities, there are many movements that are less clearly impulsive but that are nevertheless too fast for sensory feedback to mold their immediate progress; many of the movements of the skilled musician or sportsman are good examples. Very often these movements form part of some larger pattern of activity that may have been learned and that may depend on other forms of sensory information. In describing these as preprogrammed movements, we mean only that the programming is carried out prior to any control by a stretch-reflex loop. Such movements may be modified by other higher reflex pathways that are themselves quite adaptable. This aspect of feedback control is discussed in the next section.

The distinction between ballistic movements and movements that are reflex controlled becomes clearest when, under laboratory conditions, the experimenter calls for some impulsive movement and then suddenly alters the load or introduces a disturbing force (3, 23, 36). No reflex compensation for the disturbance is possible during the first part of such a movement, though reflex adjustments may appear later in its course (36).

Just as the reflex resistance to a sudden disturbance can be set up when the disturbance is anticipated, it seems likely that a similar process is involved in the execution of voluntary movements, though our information about this comes more from everyday experience than from formal laboratory experiments (see the chapter by Bizzi in this *Handbook*). Voluntary actions that meet with an unexpected load may go awry; attempts to lift an object that appears heavy but that is actually light usually end in an inaccurate movement, and reflexes are very slow to correct this. Everyday experience does suggest, however, that subjects who realize that their information about the load is incomplete may be able to use their limbs, muscles, and reflexes in ways that make the action less vulnerable to the unexpected obstacle. We can open doors that are very different in their weight without faltering or dissect tissues that are very different in their resistance. No doubt some of this improved control is achieved by using the inertia of the moving parts and setting the muscle stiffness to make the movement independent of the load. It also seems probable that the stretch reflexes are tuned to suitable levels in preparation for the movement so that their action, late though it is, has the optimal effect. The changes in H-reflex that precede a voluntary movement are presumably part of this tuning procedure (30).

PRECOMPUTED MOVEMENTS

Since delays in the neuromuscular system limit the speed and effectiveness of any simple and direct form of servo control, the nervous system can only make fast movements by computing the necessary motoneuronal activity ahead of time with as much accuracy as possible. Furthermore it always initiates and controls movements on the basis of sensory information that is distinctly out of date.

The control of many of these movements may be the end result of some other reflex process, and when we describe them as preprogrammed, this only means that they are carried out in circumstances where there is no time to monitor their progress. This vestibulo-ocular reflex (see the chapter by Robinson in this *Handbook*) provides a particularly straightforward example; here the function is to maintain the direction of gaze in spite of head movements, and this is accomplished by using information that comes not from the eyes themselves, but from the vestibular system that signals head movement. This then is not a servo-control loop of the type described thus far, since there is as yet no signal to indicate the error between the actual direction of gaze and the intended direction. The contractions of the oculomotor muscles depend on a prediction of what is probably necessary, without (as yet) any test of the result against the intention. This is a type of direct control in which vestibular input provides the basis for computations that may have been learned and perfected on earlier occasions (44). The results of these computations are then used to control the eye muscles. This procedure has sometimes been described as feedforward (44, 53), by analogy with engineering systems, in which a similar computed instruction may rapidly achieve an approximately correct result without utilizing the normal feedback pathways and error signals.

Such direct reflex control also occurs in the limbs, and many spinal reflexes are of this type; the flexor-withdrawal reflex is an obvious example. At a higher level a similar type of reflex places a motorist's foot on the brake pedal when a child is seen stepping into the road. Afferent information from a variety of different sources is involved, and this information is often used in ways that may be modified by previous experience, learned habits, and conscious intensions. A tennis player returning a fast service must control his limbs in a similar way; he must prepare his stroke long before the ball crosses the net, and to do this he must use what he can see and hear of the service and the ball's trajectory. He must then extrapolate from this to estimate where and when the ball will come within reach of his racket. While this information is coming in, his nervous system is computing and instructing the pattern of motoneuronal activity that will enable him to make the best return. Sensory information, learned reflex responses, and voluntary intentions are all combined together in computing the motor response.

These precomputed movements may later be modified by afferent activity generated during the movement itself, so that the final outcome depends on a combination of the precomputed instruction and any servo-control effect. Furthermore the same afferent discharges that are the error signals of the stretch reflexes provide some of the information on which future computations are based; indeed the stretch-reflex correction of errors may be regarded as a crude first part to the next round of precomputed movements. Once again we have a continuum in which the reflex correction of previous errors merges into the preparation for succeeding movements, and it is perfectly reasonable to view the afferent limb of the stretch reflex as providing just one particular type of information used in the ongoing process of computing future movements.

Even though we may not be able to completely separate preprogrammed and servo-controlled movements, the underlying strategies are very different, each method having its limitations and advantages. We have already seen that the functioning of an elementary servo system is very seriously impeded by delays around the loop and cannot be improved beyond a certain point for as long as these delays remain. The ability to predict a situation and initiate a correct movement is not limited by time delays in the same absolute way; given sufficient computing power and complete information about the internal and external environment, it would be theoretically possible to calculate when and how much each muscle must contract. This amounts to controlling movements by a process of dead reckoning, and the fact that all the sensory information is inevitably out of date is important only if the information is inaccurate or if unforeseen changes occur between the activation of the receptors and the execution of the movement.

In practice sensory information about the environment can never be complete; animals can only absorb a finite and limited amount of information, and some of it will be wrong. A surface that appears secure may be slippery, an object may be heavier than it looks, or an apparently safe place may conceal an enemy. The animal therefore uses the most recent sensory information available, keeping the computing time to a minimum and still building in various protective reflexes as contingency plans (flexor withdrawal, blink reflex, righting reflexes).

This method of control is very different from the simpler types of error-controlled servomechanism in which there is very rapid and effective feedback control of some particular variable. There are, however, other man-made systems that can be usefully compared with parts of the nervous system; some of these are considered in section FORWARD-LOOKING CONTROL SYSTEMS, p. 253.

Summary

Because they are limited in both speed and gain, the stretch reflexes can provide only a limited servo assistance, and that is solely for slow movements. For rapid movements the patterns of motoneuronal activity must be computed and sent without the benefit of immediate information about their effects.

If the motoneuronal discharge is inappropriate, or if the movement encounters some entirely unexpected obstacle, the result may be very different from what was intended. If the possibility of an error or disturbance can be foreseen, however, then its effects can probably be mitigated by setting up muscle forces, limb positions, and reflex gains to minimize any possible ill effects.

Executing a normal range of rapid and accurate movements with our relatively slow muscles and neural pathways requires a very highly developed ability to precompute the appropriate motoneuronal signals. Precomputations are based on prior information about the state (position, velocity) of the limbs to which they are directed, and there can be no absolute distinction between a precomputed response that relies heavily on this afferent information and a simpler reflex response to these same afferent signals. Simple stretch-reflex responses thus merge into the more elaborate patterns of movement, and any separation becomes somewhat artificial.

FEEDBACK AND LEARNING

The learning of motor skills is a subject in itself—whole volumes could undoubtedly be written on this alone. Here I merely relate some of the elementary reflex responses previously discussed to the wider patterns of learned behavior.

We are all familiar with the processes involved in acquiring a new manual skill such as writing, manipulating a new instrument, or tying a knot. Whenever possible we slow the movement down so that we can monitor each stage by direct observation, minimizing and correcting the errors as we go along. We are thus using feedback control in the most elementary way—in the way that it is used in simple mechanical control systems—and we are accepting the limitations imposed by the slowness of the neuromuscular system.

After repeating the movements a number of times, we have acquired sufficient experience to make the necessary sequence of motions with less reliance on the monitoring process and its attendant delays; hence the whole action can be executed more rapidly because the nervous system does not wait at each stage for information about what has actually happened and then take time to make corrections. The activity is therefore transferred from the servo-controlled category to the preprogrammed category (but remember that these two categories merge and interact).

Instead of saying that we have acquired sufficient experience, we might say that we have established the pattern of the movement, implying that somewhere within the brain the behavior of a group of neurons has been semipermanently modified so that a particular sensory input or voluntary intention now leads to a smooth performance of the learned action. How and where such patterns of movements are stored is a central problem of neurophysiology (44).

Skill continues to increase long after we have stopped looking at each fragment of the movement. A violinist continues to perfect a phrase by repetitive practice even though each individual movement of the fingers is executed so quickly that sensory information from the ear or the peripheral receptors plays no part in its immediate control. The overall sensory impression of one trial modifies the next attempt by updating the precomputed pattern of the movements involved. Hence this can be regarded as another form of feedback control in which a whole highly organized pattern of sounds is compared with some concept of the ideal pattern to yield a multidimensional error signal used to modify the pattern of finger, hand, and arm movements for the next run-through. A similar process is involved in learning ballistic skills (like hitting a golf ball) and other movements that by their nature cannot be taken slowly and broken down into their constituent parts. Animals learning a conditioned reflex in a deafferented limb (50, 78) presumably do so in this way.

It is particularly interesting that experience can also modify the vestibuloocular reflex (26, 27); this reflex is not consciously learned and until recently could have been regarded as a hard-wired reflex of the nervous system. It may change its properties and even its direction when, by the use of reversing prisms, an optical situation is created such that rotation of the head requires rotation of the eyes in the same direction to keep the retinal image stable (see the chapter by Robinson in this *Handbook*). The firmly established nature of this reflex is reflected in the fact that it takes weeks to reverse direction, whereas more recently learned responses might be altered by only a few practice runs.

The importance of these acquired patterns of movement and the extent to which they are molded and modified as a result of sensory feedback over long periods increase with the complexity of the vertebrate world. This process contrasts with the simple and immediate feedback control that forms the basis of the classic servo system.

FORWARD-LOOKING CONTROL SYSTEMS

Many of the differences between the animal's motor system and the simpler error-controlled servomechanisms appear to arise from delays involved in the biological processes. There are, however, other more sophisticated man-made systems that may be more similar to the biological motor-control systems.

Consider the situation of a spacecraft or satellite at a distance from the earth such that radio signals pass to and from it with significant delays. If it is to be controlled from the earth, then the controller will have problems akin to those facing the nervous system. Information received on earth will always be out of date, and correcting signals sent out from the earth will take effect only after appreciable delay. The controller therefore has the task of extrapolating from the information received and from knowledge of the behavior of the spacecraft to determine its state (position, velocity, attitude) at the time when the correcting signals will reach it. The corrections that must actually be used thus depend on the results of the extrapolation. The procedure may be simplified and improved by incorporating into the control system some analogue representation or model of the spacecraft and its trajectory and keeping this updated by computed extrapolations of position, velocity, and attitude. If sufficient knowledge of the properties of the craft are built into the model, these extrapolations can be very accurate, extending forward into the future.

We assume that within the brain there is a neural representation of the external world (17) that must also depend on out-of-date sensory information. This is clearly similar to the analogue representation of a spacecraft, though in the animal's environment, the number of variables to be considered and the repertoire of possible responses are so large that the problem becomes much more complex. This complexity is further increased because the animal learns from its experiences, and therefore its reactions to the same pattern of afferent activity are being continuously modified. This resembles the self-optimizing control systems now being investigated and developed by engineers.

Although extrapolations from previous information give a good picture of the present and future states of a spacecraft when it is subject only to external forces, it is clearly desirable to inform the analogue of any signals sent out to its motors so that their effects on the trajectory can be computed and immediately incorporated in the model without waiting for actual information about the new trajectory (see the chapter by Arbib in this *Handbook*).

Again there appears to be a similar mechanism within the nervous system where information is continuously fed back from lower to higher levels (19), and this is presumed (among other things) to keep the higher centers informed about movements that have been commanded even though they may not yet have been executed. Some of these pathways are described in "Anatomy of the Descending Pathways," by Kuypers, in this *Handbook*.

Experiments on animals and humans indicate that motor activity is frequently accompanied by corollary discharges that produce an illusion that the commanded movement has indeed been carried out, even though the peripheral motor apparatus may have been disabled in some way (see the chapter by McCloskey in this *Handbook*). Important here is that this form of internal feedback can supply a provisional estimate of the position and movement of a limb long before real sensory information is available and before the movement has actually occurred.

The hypothesis of an "ahead-of-time" analogue of movements may be extended in a number of directions to involve various anatomical structures and even to include conscious thoughts and intentions; but these extensions are too speculative to be included here. If, however, one accepts that the nervous system has probably developed so as to best do the job, then some ahead-of-time representation of movements is certainly expected.

CONCLUSIONS

In their struggle to survive, animals need to make fast, accurate, and complex movements that are often executed in a rapidly changing environment where unexpected disturbances are common. Their neuromuscular systems can act with only a limited speed, however, and only limited power is available; the larger the animal, the more serious become its difficulties.

During slow activities animals compare actual movements and forces with those intended and then make appropriate corrections. This type of servo control has a limited value, however, in shaping faster movements when the delays involved in correcting an error are a substantial fraction of the time available for the whole action. The animals can only make such movements by estimating what is needed and then getting on with it as best they can. These estimates are usually correct, or nearly correct (in the species that survive), but the animals also build in any safeguards they can against unexpected happenings or miscalculations.

The ability to look ahead, to predict coming situations, and to compute the appropriate responses has been developed to a remarkable degree. Some of the responses are virtually automatic, others are learned from past experience and are subject to continuous modification, and yet others depend on what we describe as voluntary decisions.

The patterns of motoneuronal activity required for rapid skilled movements are exceedingly complex, and feedback of sensory information from the periphery does little to simplify the immediate problems of the controller. Information about the success of a particular maneuver can, however, be used over a longer term to modify the reactions of the animal on future occasions.

The animal can take some precautions against an unexpected disturbance or a miscalculated movement, but the effectiveness of these safeguards depends a great deal on whether the animal has any foreknowledge that some dislocation of its plan might occur. If it has some warning, there are a number of ways it can prepare its neuromuscular system. When the animal anticipates a sudden disturbing force that it needs to resist, it can stiffen its limbs by holding its antagonist muscles in a state of contraction. It can also briefly increase the gain of its stretch reflexes to increase their resistance to movement. If the animal is able to anticipate the direction from which a disturbing force might come, it can further improve the reflex response, and if it knows that the best response to the disturbance is a jump or jerk in some particular direction, it can set up such a movement as a triggered response.

None of the reflex responses are very rapid, but they are the best that the nervous system can do, and the simpler reflex responses are a good deal faster than voluntary movements. The more complex triggered responses are not so rapid, however, and there is no clear demarcation between them and the voluntary responses.

The author is grateful to H. F. Ross for many useful discussions.

REFERENCES

1. ABBOTT, B. C., AND X. M. AUBERT. The force exerted by active striated muscle during and after change of length. *J. Physiol. London* 117: 77–86, 1952.
2. AGARWAL, G. C., AND G. L. GOTTLIEB. Oscillation of the human ankle joint in response to applied sinusoidal torque on the foot. *J. Physiol. London* 268: 151–176, 1977.
3. ANGEL, R. W. Myoelectric patterns associated with ballistic movements. *J. Hum. Movement Stud.* 1: 96–103, 1975.
4. ASATRYAN, D. G., AND A. G. FELDMAN. Functional tuning of the nervous system with control of movement and maintenance of posture. Mechanographic analysis of the work of the joint on execution of postural task. *Biophysics* 10: 925–935, 1965.
5. BAWA, P., A. MANNARD, AND R. B. STEIN. Effects of elastic loads on the contractions of cat muscles. *Biol. Cybern.* 22: 129–137, 1976.
6. BAWA, P., AND R. B. STEIN. Frequency response of human soleus muscle. *J. Neurophysiol.* 39: 788–793, 1976.
7. BIZZI, E., P. DEV, P. MORASSO, AND A. POLIT. Effect of load disturbances during centrally initiated movements. *J. Neurophysiol.* 41: 542–556, 1978.
8. BROWN, T. I. H., P. M. H. RACK, AND H. F. ROSS. Sinusoidal driving of finger joints. *J. Physiol. London* 263: 184P–185P, 1976.
9. BROWN, T. I. H., P. M. H. RACK, AND H. F. ROSS. Tremor in human thumb. *J. Physiol. London* 269: 3P–4P, 1977.
10. BROWN, T. I. H., P. M. H. RACK, AND H. F. ROSS. The thumb stretch reflex. *J. Physiol. London* 269: 30P–31P, 1977.
11. BULLER, A. J., AND A. C. DORNHORST. The reinforcement of tendon reflexes. *Lancet* 2: 1260–1262, 1957.
12. BURG, D., A. J. SZUMSKI, A. STRUPPLER, AND F. VELHO. Observations on muscle receptor sensitivity in the human. *Electromyogr. Clin. Neurophysiol.* 15: 15–28, 1975.
13. BURKE, R. E. Synaptic input to fast and slow twitch motor units of cat triceps surae. *J. Physiol. London* 196: 605–630, 1968.
14. BUSSEL, B., C. MORIN, AND E. PIERROT-DESEILLIGNY. Mechanism of monosynaptic reflex reinforcement during Jendrassik manoeuvre in man. *J. Neurol. Neurosurg. Psychiatry* 41: 40–44, 1978.

15. CALVERT, T. W., AND A. E. CHAPMAN. The relationship between the surface e.m.g. and force transients in muscle: stimulation and experimental studies. *Proc. IEEE* 65: 682-689, 1977.
16. CRAGO, P. E., J. C. HOUK, AND Z. HASAN. Regulatory actions of human stretch reflex. *J. Neurophysiol.* 39: 925-935, 1976.
17. CRAIK, K. J. W. *The Nature of Explanation*. Cambridge: Cambridge Univ. Press, 1943.
18. EVARTS, E. V. Motor cortex reflexes associated with learned movements. *Science* 179: 501-503, 1973.
19. EVARTS, E. V., E. BIZZI, R. E. BURKE, M. DELONG, AND W. T. THATCH. Central control of movement. *Neurosci. Res. Program Bull.* 9: 1-170, 1971.
20. EVARTS, E. V., AND R. GRANIT. Relations of reflexes and intended movements. In: *Progress in Brain Research. Understanding the Stretch Reflex*, edited by S. Homma. Amsterdam: Elsevier, 1976, vol. 44, p. 1-14.
21. EVARTS, E. V., AND J. TANJI. Gating of motor cortex reflexes by prior instruction. *Brain Res.* 71: 479-494, 1974.
22. FENN, W. O. A quantitative comparison between the energy liberated and the work performed by the isolated sartorius muscle of the frog. *J. Physiol. London* 58: 175-203, 1923.
23. GARLAND, H., AND R. W. ANGEL. Spinal and supraspinal factors in voluntary movement. *Exp. Neurol.* 33: 343-350, 1971.
24. GASSER, H. S., AND A. V. HILL. The dynamics of muscular contraction. *Proc. R. Soc. London Ser. B* 96: 398-437, 1924.
25. GHEZ, C., AND Y. SHINADA. Spinal mechanisms of the functional stretch reflex. *Exp. Brain Res.* 32: 55-68, 1978.
26. GONSHOR, A., AND G. MELVILLE-JONES. Short-term adaptive changes in the human vestibulo-ocular reflex. *J. Physiol. London* 256: 361-379, 1976.
27. GONSHOR, A., AND G. MELVILLE-JONES. Extreme vestibulo-occular adaptation induced by prolonged optical reversal of vision. *J. Physiol. London* 256: 381-414, 1976.
28. GOODWIN, G. M., D. HOFFMAN, AND E. S. LUSCHEI. The strength of the reflex response to sinusoidal stretch of monkey jaw closing muscles during voluntary contraction. *J. Physiol. London* 279: 81-112, 1978.
29. GOTTLIEB, G. L., G. C. AGARWAL, AND L. STARK. Interactions between voluntary and postural mechanisms of the human motor system. *J. Neurophysiol.* 33: 365-381, 1970.
30. GOTTLIEB, G. L., AND G. C. AGARWAL. Modulation of postural reflexes by voluntary movement. *J. Neurol. Neurosurg. Psychiatry* 36: 540-546, 1973.
31. GOTTLIEB, G. L., AND G. C. AGARWAL. Physiological clonus in man. *Exp. Neurol.* 54: 616-621, 1977.
32. GRANIT, R. Neuromuscular interaction in postural tone of the cat's isometric soleus muscle. *J. Physiol. London* 143: 387-402, 1958.
33. GREENWOOD, R., AND A. HOPKINS. Muscle responses during sudden falls in man. *J. Physiol. London* 254: 507-518, 1976.
34. GURFINKEL, V. S., AND YE. I. PAL'TSEV. Effects of the state of the segmental apparatus of the spinal cord on the execution of a simple motor reaction. *Biophysics* 10: 944-951, 1965.
35. HAGBARTH, K. E. EMG studies of stretch reflexes in man. *Electroencephalogr. Clin. Neurophysiol.* 25: (Suppl.) 74-79, 1967.
36. HALLETT, M., AND C. D. MARSDEN. Effect of perturbations on the EMG pattern of ballistic movements in man. *Electroencephalogr. Clin. Neurophysiol.* 43: P596, 1977.
37. HAMMOND, P. H. An experimental study of servo action in human muscular control. In: *Proc. Conf. Med. Electron., 3rd, London, 1960*, p. 190-199.
38. HASAN, Z., AND J. C. HOUK. Analysis of response properties of deefferented mammalian spindle receptors based on frequency response. *J. Neurophysiol.* 38: 663-672, 1975.
39. HENNEMAN, E., G. SOMJEN, AND D. O. CARPENTER. Excitability and inhibitibility of motoneurons of different sizes. *J. Neurophysiol.* 28: 599-620, 1965.
40. HILL, A. V. *Trails and Trials in Physiology*. London: Arnold, 1965.
41. HILL, A. V. AND J. V. HOWARTH. The reversal of chemical reactions in contracting muscle during an applied stretch. *Proc. R. Soc. London Ser. B* 151: 169-193, 1959.
42. HUXLEY, A. F. Muscular contraction. *J. Physiol. London* 243: 1-43, 1974.
43. ILES, J. F. Responses in human pretibial muscles to sudden stretch and to nerve stimulation. *Exp. Brain Res.* 30: 451-470, 1977.
44. ITO, M. Neurophysiological aspects of the cerebellar motor control system. *Int. J. Neurol.* 7: 162-176, 1970.
45. JANSEN, J. K. S., AND P. M. H. RACK. The reflex response to sinusoidal stretching of soleus in the decerebrate cat. *J. Physiol. London* 183: 15-36, 1966.
46. JOYCE, G. C., AND P. M. H. RACK. The effects of load and force on tremor at the normal human elbow joint. *J. Physiol. London* 240: 375-396, 1974.
47. JOYCE, G. C., P. M. H. RACK, AND H. F. ROSS. The forces generated at the human elbow joint in response to imposed sinusoidal movements of the forearm. *J. Physiol. London* 240: 351-374, 1974.
48. JOYCE, G. C., P. M. H. RACK, AND D. R. WESTBURY. The mechanical properties of cat soleus muscle during controlled lengthening and shortening movements. *J. Physiol. London* 204: 461-474, 1969.
49. KAWAMURA, T., AND S. WATANABE. Timing as a prominent factor of the Jendrassik manoeuvre on the H reflex. *J. Neurol. Neurosurg. Psychiatry* 38: 508-516, 1975.
50. KONORSKI, J. *Integrative Activity of the Brain*. Chicago, IL: Univ. of Chicago Press, 1967.
51. LEE, R. G., AND W. G. TATTON. Motor responses to sudden limb displacements in primates with specific CNS lesions and in human patients with motor system disorders. *Can. J. Neurol. Sci.* 2: 285-293, 1975.
52. LEVIN, A., AND WYMAN, J. The viscous elastic properties of muscle. *Proc. R. Soc. London Ser. B* 101: 218-243, 1927.
53. MCKAY, D. M. Conscious control of action. In: *Brain and Conscious Experience*, edited by J. C. Eccles. New York: Springer-Verlag, 1966, p. 422-445.
54. MANNARD, A., AND R. B. STEIN. Determination of the frequency response of isometric soleus muscle in the cat using random nerve stimulation. *J. Physiol. London* 229: 275-296, 1973.
55. MARSDEN, C. D., P. A. MERTON, AND H. B. MORTON. Servo action in human voluntary movement. *Nature London* 238: 140-143, 1972.
56. MARSDEN, C. D., P. A. MERTON, AND H. B. MORTON. Stretch reflex and servo action in a variety of human muscles. *J. Physiol. London* 259: 531-560, 1976.
57. MARSHALL, J., AND E. G. WALSH. Physiological tremor. *J. Neurol. Neurosurg. Psychiatry* 19: 260-267, 1956.
58. MATTHEWS, P. B. C. The dependence or tension on extension in the stretch reflex of the soleus muscle of the decerebrate cat. *J. Physiol. London* 147: 521-546, 1959.
59. MATTHEWS, P. B. C. *Mammalian Muscle Receptors and Their Central Actions*. London: Arnold, 1972.
60. MATTHEWS, P. B. C., AND R. B. STEIN. The sensitivity of muscle spindle afferents to small sinusoidal changes in length. *J. Physiol. London* 200: 723-743, 1969.
61. MELVILLE-JONES, G., AND D. G. D. WATT. Observations on the control of stepping and hopping movements in man. *J. Physiol. London* 219: 709-727, 1971.
62. MERTON, P. A. Speculations on the servo control of movement. In: *The Spinal Cord*, edited by G. E. W. Wolstenholme. London: Churchill, 1953, p. 247-255.
63. NASHNER, L. M. Adapting reflexes controlling the human posture. *Exp. Brain Res.* 26: 59-72, 1976.
64. NICHOLS, T. R., AND J. C. HOUK. Improvement in linearity and regulation of stiffness that results from actions of stretch reflex. *J. Neurophysiol.* 39: 119-142, 1976.
65. OGUZTORELI, M. N., AND R. B. STEIN. The effects of multiple reflex pathways on the oscillations in neuromuscular systems. *J. Math. Biol.* 3: 87-101, 1976.
66. PARTRIDGE, L. D. Modifications of neural output signals by

muscles: a frequency response study. *J. Appl. Physiol.* 20: 150–156, 1965.
67. PARTRIDGE, L. D. Signal-handling characteristics of load-moving skeletal muscle. *Am. J. Physiol.* 210: 1178–1191, 1966.
68. PHILLIPS, C. G. Motor apparatus of the baboon's hand. *Proc. R. S. London Ser. B* 173: 141–174, 1969.
69. POPPELE, R. E., AND R. J. BOWMAN. Quantitative description of linear behavior of mammalian muscle spindles. *J. Neurophysiol.* 33: 59–72, 1970.
70. RACK, P. M. H. The behaviour of a mammalian muscle during sinusoidal stretching. *J. Physiol. London* 183: 1–14, 1966.
71. RACK, P. M. H. The stretch reflex response to movement of human elbow joint. In: *Control of Posture and Locomotion*, edited by R. B. Stein, K. B. Pearson, R. S. Smith, and J. B. Redford. New York: Plenum, 1973, p. 245–255. (Adv. Behav. Biol. Ser., vol. 7.)
72. RACK, P. M. H., H. F. ROSS, AND T. I. H. BROWN. Reflex responses during sinusoidal movement of human limbs. In: *Cerebral Motor Control in Man: Long Loop Mechanisms*, edited by J. E. Desmedt. Basel: Karger, 1978, p. 216–228.
73. RACK, P. M. H., H. F. ROSS, AND D. K. W. WALTERS. Interactions between the stretch reflex and a 'repeat tendency' of the motoneurone pool in the human. *J. Physiol. London* 290: 21P–22P, 1979.
74. RACK, P. M. H., AND D. R. WESTBURY. The effects of length and stimulus rate on tension in the isometric cat soleus muscle. *J. Physiol. London* 204: 443–460, 1969.
75. ROBSON, J. G. The effects of loading on the frequency of muscle tremor. *J. Physiol. London* 149: 29P–30P, 1959.
76. SHINNERS, S. M. *Modern Control System Theory and Application*. Reading, MA: Addison-Wesley, 1972.
77. STEIN, R. B., AND M. N. OGUZTORELI. Reflex involvement in the generation and control of tremor and clonus. In: *Physiological Tremor, Pathological Tremor, Clonus*, edited by J. E. Desmedt. Basel: Karger, 1978, p. 28–50.
78. TAUB, E., AND A. J. BERMAN. Movement and learning in the absence of sensory feedback. In: *The Neuropsychology of Spatially Orientated Behavior*, edited by S. J. Freedman. Homewood, IL: Dorsey, 1968, p. 173–192.
79. THOMAS, J. S., J. BROWN, AND G. E. LUCIER. Influence of task set on muscular response to arm perturbations in normal subjects and Parkinson patients. *Exp. Neurol.* 55: 618–628, 1977.
80. VALBO, A. B. Human muscle spindle discharge during isometric voluntary contractions. Amplitude relations between spindle frequency and torque. *Acta Physiol. Scand.* 90: 319–336, 1974.
81. WESTBURY, D. R. The response of motoneurones of the cat to sinusoidal movements of the muscles they innervate. *Brain Res.* 25: 75–86, 1971.

CHAPTER 8

Neural control of muscle length and tension

JAMES C. HOUK | Department of Physiology, Northwestern University
W. ZEV RYMER | Medical and Dental Schools, Chicago, Illinois

CHAPTER CONTENTS

Control Theory Concepts
  Systems and models
  Control systems
  Feedback, feedforward, and adaptive systems
  Principle of negative feedback
  Regulated variables and properties
  Control configurations
  Summary
Hypotheses of Motor Servo Function
  Salient features of the available sensors
  Follow-up servo hypothesis
  Spindle receptors as model-reference error detectors
  Conditional feedback and servo assistance
  β-System and the possibility for zero sensitivity
  Stiffness regulation
  Summary model
  Adaptive models
  Summary
Muscle Mechanical Stiffness
  Stiffness definitions
  Length dependence
  Recruitment of motor units
  Rate modulation of motor units
  Instantaneous stiffness and short-range elasticity
  Instantaneous stiffness beyond the short-range region
  Ramp responses: transient properties and nonlinearity
  Natural combinations of recruitment and rate modulation
  Summary
Central Pathways
  Primary ending projections
  Tendon organ projections
  Projections from secondary endings and group II
      free nerve endings
  Projections from groups III and IV free nerve endings
  Clasp-knife reflex
  Long-loop reflexes
  Summary
Simplified Animal Models
  Decerebrate preparation
  Spinal preparation
  Summary
Tonic Stretch Reflex in Functionally Isolated Muscles
  Basic features of the stretch reflex
  Static force-length relations
  Normalized stiffness
  Mechanically and neurally mediated components
  Actions of control signals on the motor servo
  Dependence of incremental stiffness on initial force
  Loop gain of force feedback
  Summary
Static Regulatory Characteristics in Intact Subjects
  Skeletal mechanics and coordinate systems
  Steady-state responses to changes in load force
  Torque-angle relations
  Equivalent stiffness and the concept of composite motor servos
  Effect of instructional set
  Gain variation vs. gain control
  Summary
Dynamic Responses to Mechanical Disturbances
  Dynamic features of force development
  Dependence of transient responses on initial force
  Amplitude dependence and linearity
  Asymmetry of motor servo responses
  Compensation for yielding
  Predictive compensation: feedforward versus nonlinear
      feedback viewpoints
  Vibration and the stretch reflex
  Velocity dependence and damping
  Summary
Implementation of Movement Commands
  α-γ-Relations
  Positional stiffness deduced from spindle relations
  β-Innervation of muscle spindles
  Analytical approaches to actions of α-, β-, and γ-motoneurons
  Equilibrium point control
  Stiffness regulation vs. stiffness control
  Perturbations during movement
  Compliance, load compensation, and biological design
  Summary

THE FUNDAMENTAL FEATURES of skeletomotor control derive from the properties of muscles, motor units, muscle stretch receptors, and spinal neurons. Figure 1 is a simplified block diagram of the basic control system, called the *motor servo*. It consists of a mechanical portion (an individual muscle and the load upon which it acts) and a neuroregulatory portion (the set of autogenetic reflex pathways) discussed in the chapter by Baldissera, Hultborn, and Illert in this *Handbook*. The signals traversing these pathways originate from muscle stretch receptors, they are integrated by a neural network organized predominantly at a segmental level in the spinal cord, and the resultant skeletomotor output returns in motor axons to the same muscle from which the afferent signals originated. Thus autogenetic circuits are actually local feedback loops, which apparently function to regulate the mechanical variables monitored by the various muscle receptors. These variables are muscle length

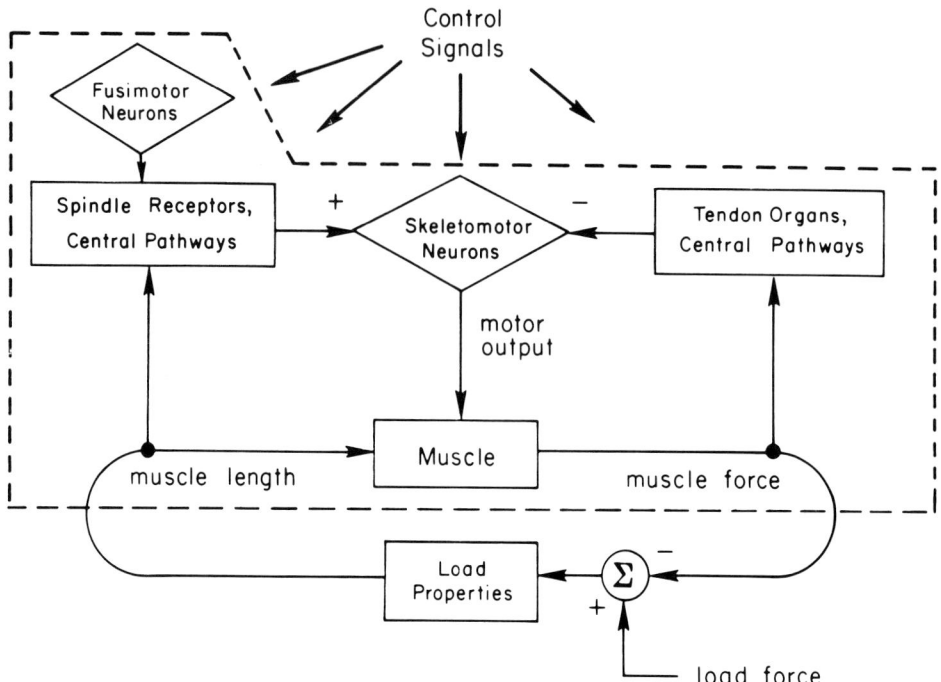

FIG. 1. Basic organizational plan of the motor servo. Muscle and load forces act on load properties (e.g., inertia) to produce length changes. Muscle force is regulated by motor output from skeletomotor neurons (reflex action) but also varies in response to changes in length (so-called mechanical response). Muscle length (and velocity) is monitored by spindle receptors and force by Golgi tendon organs. These signals provide excitation and inhibition, respectively, to skeletomotor neurons by way of central pathways (certainly segmental, and perhaps also suprasegmental). Neural control signals are sent to skeletomotor and fusimotor neurons and to interneurons in the reflex pathways.

(and its derivatives) sensed by muscle spindle receptors, and muscle force or tension sensed by Golgi tendon organs.

The motor servo is a particularly important topic in motor control, since it is involved, in one way or another, in all motor acts, whether these are simple responses to muscle stretch or complex movements produced by central motor commands. In effect, the motor servo functions as a *final common processor* of motor commands that are sent to it from other regions of the nervous system in ensembles of nerve fibers. This role is analogous, though on another hierarchical level, to the role of the motor unit, which serves as the final common pathway for motor integration at the cellular level. A productive approach to the understanding of how the motor servo translates central motor commands into changes in muscle length and force has been to study how these variables are controlled when mechanical disturbances, rather than central commands, act as inputs. Furthermore these responses to disturbances in mechanical load are intrinsically important themselves, since they represent the first line of defense, so to speak, in the continual interaction that occurs between an organism and its mechanical environment.

The operations of the motor servo have been the subject of extensive experimental investigation throughout the fifty some years since the stretch reflex was first subjected to detailed analysis by Liddell and Sherrington (170). Frequent attempts have been made to incorporate the empirical findings into the conceptual framework of feedback-control theory, and the hypotheses thus generated have helped to direct attention to important unresolved questions requiring further experimentation. This chapter lays out the major theoretical ideas and then reviews the experimental evidence regarding these hypotheses. In addition we include background sections on control theory, muscle mechanics, central pathways, and simplified animal preparations. The latter are arranged so that readers with experience in any of these particular topics can easily skim over the material.

CONTROL THEORY CONCEPTS

Systems and Models

A system can be defined as any assemblage of objects united by processes of physical interaction that relate measurable quantities one to another. The measurements of the relevant quantities are usually expressed as sets of values called signals, variables, or time functions. System theory deals primarily with the relations between such variables, rather than with the actual physical nature of the quantities they describe. One comes to view some of the variables as being determined independently, by causes extrinsic to the system, and others as being dependent on these, although this distinction is sometimes arbitrary. The independent variables are called inputs, the dependent ones are called states, and the outputs are variables that derive from the states. The system is defined to include all the processes that intervene to relate outputs to inputs. In this section only elementary aspects of system theory are summarized, and the reader is referred to the chapter by Arbib in this *Handbook* for a discussion of more advanced concepts.

A key concept in system theory is the notion of an *operator* or *transfer function*. These equivalent terms arise from an abstraction—a view of a system as a process that operates upon input variables to transform them into output variables. This notion provides a convenient way of thinking about a mathematical model of a system. The model is a set of rules such as an equation or graph that details the steps in the conversion process. Inputs are added, subtracted, multiplied, divided, integrated, and differentiated to convert them into outputs. The equation specifies which of these elementary mathematical operations are required, together with the particular order in which they must be performed. We are all accustomed to using the symbols $+$, $-$, $\times$, $\div$, $\int ( ) \, dt$, and $d( )/dt$ to represent these elementary operations; they are examples of elementary operators.

In other cases it is more convenient to write the equation characterizing a system in a more abstract manner. Then a single symbol, also called an operator, is used to represent a whole sequence of elementary mathematical operations. For example, a general equation characterizing any system is

$$y(t) = S[x(t)] \tag{1}$$

where $x(t)$, hereafter written simply as x, is the input, S is the system operator, and y is the output. If the system has more than one input, x will be a vector consisting of a set of input functions $(x_1, x_2, \ldots, x_n)$ and, similarly, the output y may also be a vector. Operator notation obviously saves space in writing equations, but more importantly it encourages abstract thinking about a system as being characterized by a single complex operation. As will be shown shortly, this abstract approach is particularly useful in demonstrating general properties of classes of systems, i.e., conclusions based on very few assumptions regarding the detailed characteristics of the component processes.

Another useful concept is that of inverse operations. The inverse of an operation S, written S^{-1}, is an operation that undoes the original one. Thus if S describes the conversion of an input x into an output y (Fig. 2A), S^{-1} describes a process that converts y back into x (Fig. 2B). As a simple example, division by a constant is an operation that is the inverse of multiplication by the same constant. On the other hand, inversion of an operation may be much more complex than this, and in some cases a unique inverse does not exist (a system that squares the input has no unique inverse), or it may exist but yet be impossible to

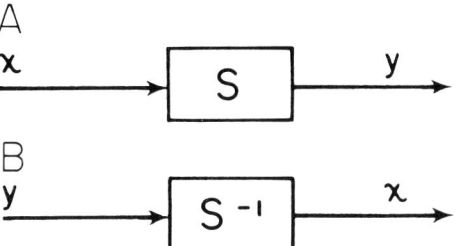

FIG. 2. System models and their inverses. *A*: the system operator S converts an input x into an output y. *B*: the inverse of S, written S^{-1}, converts y back into x. [Adapted from Houk (131). Systems and models. In: *Medical Physiology* (14th ed.), edited by V. B. Mountcastle. St. Louis, MO: The C. V. Mosby Co., 1980.]

construct, in which case it is called unrealizable (the inverse of a pure time delay, a predictor, is unrealizable, since it defies causality).

Models are hypotheses describing how a system actually functions. They can be expressed as equations, graphs, block diagrams, physical analogues, or simply as words. The advantage of using mathematics is that this mode of expression is both precise and concise. The disadvantage is that one generally must make simplifying assumptions in order to express the measured properties of a system in the form of equations, and further assumptions may be required to solve the equations. For example, ordinary linear differential equations with constant coefficients, or Laplace transforms of this class of equations, are often used to express models of systems. This is because general techniques for solving these equations are known and relatively easy to apply (131, 212, 215, 251). The use of these equations, however, involves the assumption that the salient properties of a system are captured by a compartmentalized (rather than distributed) model that is linear and has parameters that do not change with time. Alternatively one can explore models that include these complexities by using computer simulation techniques, and there are also some nice mathematical methods for studying the asymptotic behavior of nonlinear systems.

Control Systems

Figure 3 introduces a conventional view of the control problem and provides definitions of terms used in this chapter. The purpose of the overall system is to control the values of certain variables within prescribed limits. These controlled variables are a subset of the outputs of what is called the controlled system. An interacting set of physicochemical processes typically forms a controlled system, which is subject to the influences of two categories of input—disturbances and forcing functions. Disturbances are uncontrolled inputs that cause undesired changes of the state of the controlled system, and, hence, of controlled variables. Forcing functions are inputs that can be manipulated to cause (or force) desired changes in state. The function of the controller is to generate appropriate forcing functions, based on its inputs, called references, set points, or command signals that designate the desired behavior of the overall system.

Another category of input to the controller, not shown in Figure 3, derives from sensors that monitor the states of the controlled system and other variables. Information from sensors is required when disturbances are sufficiently large to produce unacceptable changes in controlled variables. Control systems designed primarily to compensate for these disturbances are called regulators, and the controlled variables may then be called regulated variables.

Feedback, Feedforward, and Adaptive Systems

The regulatory sensors can be situated to detect potential disturbances or to detect the effects the disturbances have on regulated variables (Fig. 4). The former configuration is called feedforward and the latter is called feedback. Each of these two control strategies has particular advantages and disadvantages.

Because responses of most controlled systems are not instantaneous, disturbances generally occur in advance of the disturbing effects they provoke. Thus the detection of disturbances by the sensors in a feedforward regulator provides predictive information about impending changes in regulated variables. The controller must then use this information to calculate the effects that measured disturbances are likely to have on the regulated variables and the forcing functions required to counteract these effects. To do this, the controller of a feedforward regulator must, in essence, contain a model of how the controlled system behaves. The precision of regulation clearly depends upon the accuracy of this model. Since the body's controlled systems are frequently nonlinear and time-varying, the models contained within the brain must be either highly complex or else simplified representations of these complex systems. The requirement of complex models for precise regulation is one of the major disadvantages of feedforward control. Another disadvantage derives from the fact that many variables must be monitored to specify all of the potential disturbances and to provide an up-to-date model of a controlled system, since its properties usually change with time. Sensors capable of monitoring all of these variables may not be available, in which case a feedforward regulator is bound to make errors.

One of the intriguing examples of feedforward regulation in body homeostasis concerns the classic conditioned reflex. Pavlov (235), who was one of the first to investigate this phenomenon, demonstrated that practically any sensory cue (the conditioned stimulus) can trigger a given physiological response, provided the former is presented in association with a stimulus (the unconditioned stimulus) that normally elicits the latter. Thus the controller for salivary secretion responds to the sounding of a bell after a period of training during which bell ringing is followed by the introduction of food into the mouth, the latter being a normal stimulus for salivation. In this example the

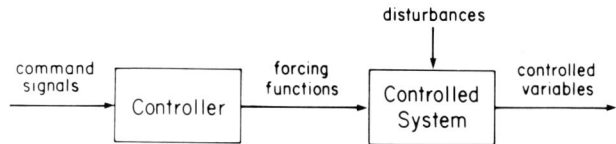

FIG. 3. Basic signals and components of a control system. Command signals designating desired performance are operated on by controller to produce forcing functions. These are inputs to the controlled system that produce desired changes in controlled variables. Uncontrolled inputs act as disturbances and produce undesired changes in controlled variables. [From Houk (131). Homeostasis and control principles. In: *Medical Physiology* (14th ed.), edited by V. B. Mountcastle. St. Louis, MO: The C. V. Mosby Co., 1980.]

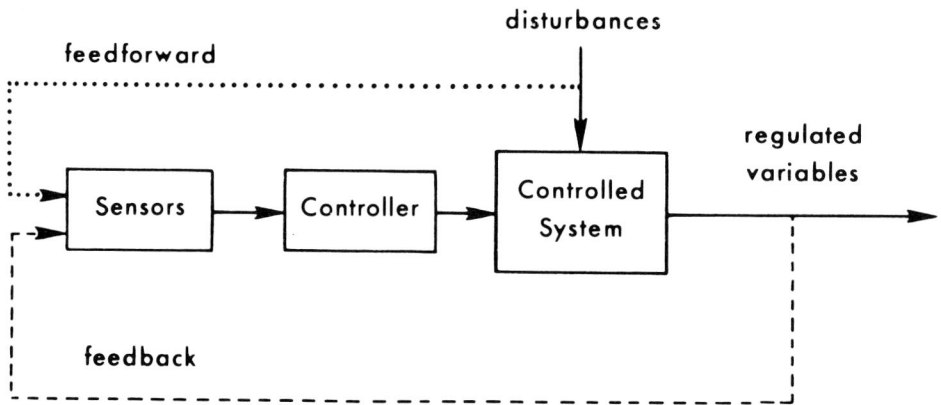

FIG. 4. Feedforward and feedback configurations for regulation. The function of a regulator is to diminish the effects that disturbances have on regulated variables. In a feedforward system regulatory actions are based on signals from sensors that detect potential disturbances, whereas in a feedback system regulatory actions are based on signals from sensors that detect the effects disturbances have on regulated variables. [From Houk (131). Homeostasis and control principles. In: *Medical Physiology* (14th ed.), edited by V. B. Mountcastle. St. Louis, MO: The C. V. Mosby Co., 1980.]

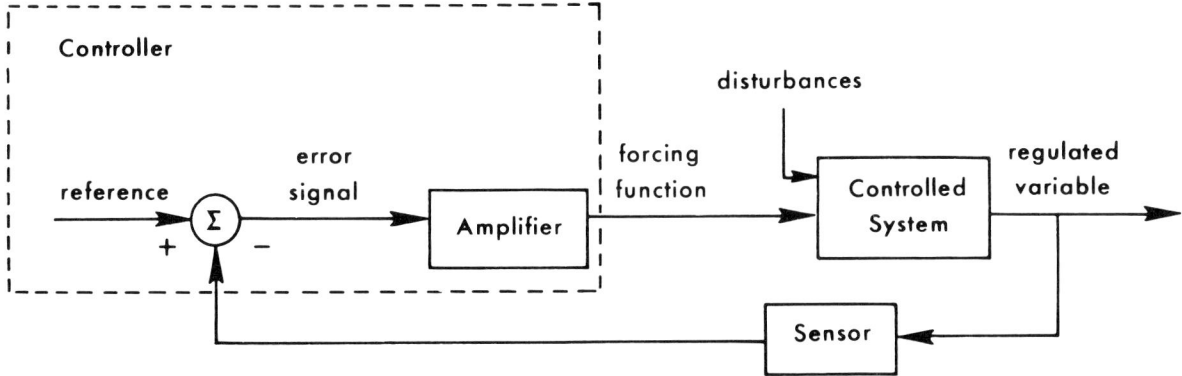

FIG. 5. Simple example of a negative-feedback system. Appropriate forcing functions are generated by 2 elementary operations—error detection (subtraction) and amplification. [From Houk (131). Homeostasis and control principles. In: *Medical Physiology* (14th ed.), edited by V. B. Mountcastle. St. Louis, MO: The C. V. Mosby Co., 1980.]

conditioned reflex provides a feedforward mechanism that prepares the mouth for food that is about to arrive. As is typical of feedforward systems, this mechanism is subject to errors in performance. The first time the bell is not followed by the presentation of food salivation occurs anyway, even though it is inappropriate.

Regulation based on the feedback configuration is free of the major disadvantages of feedforward control, but it has other disadvantages. The fact that feedback control is based on the current and past values of regulated variables eliminates the possibility of completely erroneous regulatory actions. Furthermore the variables that must be monitored are only the regulated ones, and the calculations performed by a feedback controller can be made extremely simple. There are three major disadvantages of feedback regulation: *1*) speed—the regulatory actions must await the consequences of the disturbances; *2*) stability—due to the presence of a closed loop of control, excessive corrective action can be propagated around the loop in an unending cycle of oscillation; *3*) error—the correction depends on the existence of an error and therefore is incomplete (except in special cases in which a perfect integrator is present in the control pathway).

While feedback and feedforward are the two basic strategies for controlling moment-to-moment regulatory actions, a third stategy, adaptive control, functions over longer time periods. Adaptive control is loosely defined as any control that changes to meet changing needs. All regulatory systems satisfy this definition. In the strict sense of the term, however, an adaptive modification is distinguished as a beneficial change in the moment-to-moment properties of a system that occurs over a long time period, one longer than that required for individual responses (3, 7). Biological examples include the hypertrophy of a muscle that occurs as a long-term response to physical training, the acquisition of a new conditioned reflex, or the learning of a new and better response through operant reinforcement.

An adaptive control system has, in addition to the component processes already described, a special subsystem that evaluates the quality of the responses to stimuli, either as they occur naturally or as they are evoked by internally generated test signals. This measure of quality is then used as a basis for adjusting the parameters or structure of the main regulatory system. Thus a well-designed adaptive system should continue to improve its performance based on past experience and readily adjust to new situations. For this reason adaptive control is equated with learning. Needless to say, the general theory of adaptive systems is presently at a rather primitive stage, although definite progress is being made (18, 216, 276, 277).

Principle of Negative Feedback

The essential feature of a negative-feedback system is the provision for a closed loop of control through which any disturbance in output is opposed. Figure 5 shows how this can be accomplished with the use of a few simple components. A sensor is situated so as to detect one of the outputs of the controlled system, the regulated variable. The output of the sensor, which is proportional to the actual value of the regulated variable, is subtracted from a reference signal, or set point, which represents a desired value of the regulated variable, to form an error signal. This step is called error detection. The error signal is then amplified and sent as a forcing function to the controlled system, thereby forcing the regulated variable back toward the reference value. For example, a disturbance that depresses slightly the value of the regulated variable will result in a small, positive error signal that, when amplified and delivered to the controlled system, will act to elevate (and hence restore) the value of the regulated variable.

The extent to which negative feedback reduces the errors caused by disturbances is uniquely determined by a single parameter (or function) called the loop gain of the system. The meaning of loop gain can be understood if one considers the output of a general type of feedback regulator to consist of two components as shown in Figure 6: *1)* a disturbance component y_d that represents the uncompensated response to a disturbance, obtained when feedback is absent and *2)* a compensatory component y_c that represents the portion of the output that is attributable to feedback. Loop gain G can then be defined as the relationship of the compensatory component to the net response y

$$y_c = G[y] \quad (2)$$

G is a composite operation that includes the gain and reference of the controller, the gain of the controlled system, and the sensitivity of the sensor, all lumped together. The loop gain may be a constant (in a linear, static system), but in general it includes lags and delays and therefore is a function of frequency (dynamic system). It may also be a function of amplitude (nonlinear system) and time (time-varying system).

The precise relation between error reduction and loop gain is easily derived as follows

$$y = y_d - y_c \quad (3)$$

$$y = y_d - G[y] \quad (4)$$

$$(1 + G)[y] = y_d \quad (5)$$

The quantity (1 + G) is itself an operator, and if its inverse exists, the attenuation operator A can be defined; no assumption of linearity is required

$$y = A[y_d] \quad (6)$$

where

$$A = (1 + G)^{-1} \quad (7)$$

The significance of this result is the following. The variable y_d represents the severity of a disturbance in terms of the alteration in the controlled variable it would provoke without feedback. Any response to a disturbance, and hence to y_d, can be considered an error. The operator A defines the extent to which feedback diminishes this error; error reduction thus depends in an inverse manner on the magnitude of the loop gain. What constitutes good attenuation is of course relative, but a loop gain of 9 yields a 10:1 reduction in error [A = 1/(1 + 9)]. Negative values for G represent positive feedback, which increases the error rather than decreasing it.

Regulated Variables and Properties

It is important to identify regulated variables, since this is one way of specifying the function of a biological feedback system. For cases in which only a single variable is sensed and fed back, it follows that this variable (or a variable derived directly from it) is the regulated one, since the best a negative-feedback system can do is minimize disturbances in the monitored variable. Physiological regulators, however, often receive feedback from several different types of sensors, each of which may monitor a different variable depending on the site of the sensor and its special properties. The latter situation is germane to the analysis of motor servo function, since several categories of muscle receptor serve as feedback sensors, and these receptors are responsive to different mechanical variables.

Given that more than one variable is available as feedback to a controller, the next question is how this additional information is used (cf. ref 131). The possibilities vary along a continuum between two extremes in strategy. One extreme is to use the information to control each of the monitored variables independently and simultaneously. The other is to combine the information about several variables to form a single regulated property. A first step in distinguishing between the alternative strategies is to determine the number of degrees of freedom available in the control of the system. If there is but a single degree of freedom in this control, there cannot be more than one regulated property. As the number of degrees of freedom increases, so does the potential for the simultaneous control of several variables or properties.

Control Configurations

A *servomechanism,* or servo for short, is a control system that operates on the principle of negative feedback. The difference between a regulator that uses negative feedback (also called a servoregulator) and a servomechanism is that the reference signal (cf. Fig. 5), previously assumed constant, is allowed to vary as a function of time and is often called a command signal. A derivation similar to that given in *Principle of Negative Feedback,* p. 261, can be used to demonstrate that the controlled variable y will respond to the command signal w according to

$$y = SC(1 + FSC)^{-1}[w] \quad (8)$$

where S, C, and F are operators representing the respective properties of the controlled system, controller, and feedback sensor. Equation 8 does not depend on linearity, but only on the assumption that the

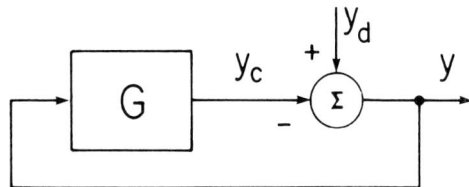

FIG. 6. Generalized negative-feedback system. The regulated variable y is expressed in terms of 2 components. Open loop (uncompensated) response to a disturbance (y_d) and the compensatory response (y_c) produced by the feedback system. The system is characterized by loop gain (G). [From Houk (131). Homeostasis and control principles. In: *Medical Physiology* (14th ed.), edited by V. B. Mountcastle. St. Louis, MO: The C. V. Mosby Co., 1980.]

inverse $(1 + FSC)^{-1}$ exists. Assuming a faithful sensor (with properties $F = 1$) and a high loop gain ($FSC \gg 1$), Equation 8 can be approximated by

$$y \cong SC(SC)^{-1}[w] = w \qquad (9)$$

The result $y \cong w$ means that the system output accurately reproduces the command signal, a condition representing ideal control. Accordingly ideal control can be approached if it is possible to raise the loop gain to very high values. Note that high values of loop gain also make system performance insensitive to nonlinearities and time variations in the properties of the controlled system.

In practice, the extent to which these desirable features can be achieved is limited by the fact that high gains can cause severe stability problems, particularly in loops with time delays. This certainly is a relevant limitation in visually guided tracking movements, due to the long latency in the control pathway associated with a reaction time. It is also a limitation in motor servo performance, and questions concerning stability in motor servo loops are discussed at length in chapters by Rack and by Stein and Lee in this *Handbook*.

Model-reference control systems are of several types, but all have in common the use of a component that represents a model of the actual controlled system (cf. refs. 127, 274). The forcing function is sent to both the models S_2 and the actual system S_1, as shown in Figure 7A, and a special type of error signal, called a reference error, is created by subtracting the actual output from the model output ($y_2 - y_1$). The reference error signal may then be put to different uses as shown by options 1, 2, and 3 in Figure 7A. The basic idea of model reference comparison was orginated by Helmholtz to explain the absence of a sensation of world movement during voluntary eye movement and later applied to a variety of biological problems by Von Holst and Mittelstaedt (285), MacKay and others (cf. 182; the chapter by McCloskey in this *Handbook*). Some of the engineering designs based on this principle are discussed in the following paragraphs.

In a *conditional-feedback* system, option 1, the error is processed (e.g., amplified) and summed with the original forcing function to provide a modified forcing function that is sent to the controlled system (166). This configuration is designed to cancel feedback under conditions in which the controlled system responds precisely as does the model, which is made to represent ideal performance. When disturbances interfere with ideal performance, an error signal is produced, amplified, and applied to the controlled system so as to reduce the error. The efficacy of error reduction depends on the loop gain of the negative-feedback pathway in the same manner discussed previously, and the system is also subject to instability if there is too much delay in the loop or if the gain is too high. The major engineering advantage of the conditional-feedback configuration is that feedforward and feedback features can be designed separately, the former by altering the dynamic properties of the controller (attempting to make C approach S_1^{-1}) and the latter by altering gain and dynamic properties of the feedback loop. This might be advantageous in biological design (evolution) as well.

Additional theoretical advantages result if the reference error is also fed back to the model system (option 2 in Fig. 7A). This creates a positive-feedback

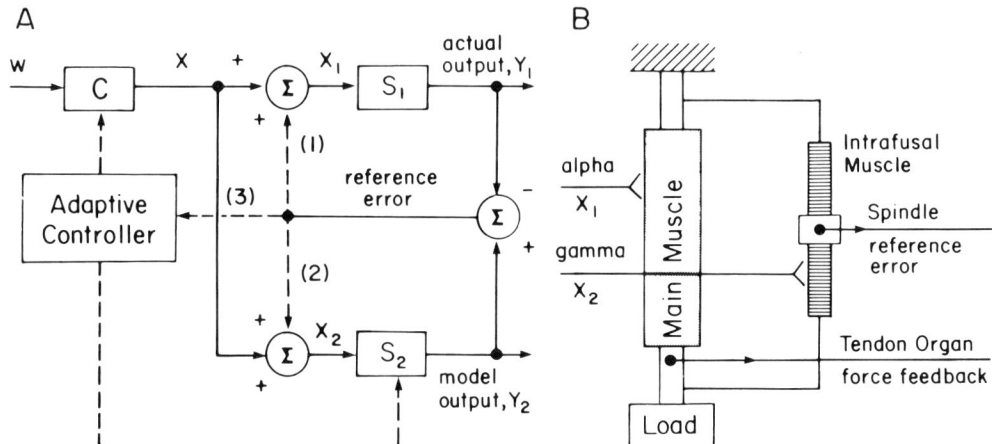

FIG. 7. Model-reference control systems. *A*: forcing functions are sent to both the controlled system S_1 and a model of the controlled system S_2. A reference error is computed as the difference between actual output y_1 and model output y_2. Options 1, 2, and 3 show different ways in which the reference error signal can be used. *B*: diagram to illustrate how the spindle receptor can be seen as a model reference error detector. The controlled system is main muscle and its load, intrafusal muscle is assumed to the model system, and the spindle afferent endings are situated to detect differences between main and intrafusal muscle shortening. [From Houk (131). Homeostasis and control principles. In: *Medical Physiology* (14th ed.), edited by V. B. Mountcastle. St. Louis, MO: The C. V. Mosby Co., 1980.]

loop, which, if appropriately tuned, can actually result in improved stability along with greater attenuation of errors. In fact errors may be reduced to zero if the gain of the positive-feedback loop is precisely 1, and this gives rise to what has been called a zero-sensitivity system, since it is insensitive to disturbances (274). The third option in Figure 7A involves an adaptive controller that uses the reference error as a basis for modifying the properties of the main controller C and/or the model S_2.

Summary

The basic terminology of control theory was introduced and applied to a discussion of the relative merits of several different types of control system. In the following section these ideas are applied to several models of motor servo function.

HYPOTHESES OF MOTOR SERVO FUNCTION

Salient Features of the Available Sensors

Since functional characteristics of feedback-control systems are to a considerable extent determined by the properties of its sensors (cf. *Regulated Variables and Properties*, p. 262), it is important to review briefly the salient features of the principle muscle stretch receptors before considering theories of motor servo function.

The specialized efferent innervation of the muscle spindle that was described in the chapter by Matthews in this *Handbook* has been the focus of several of the hypotheses that are described here. These ideas are based on the well-documented dual responsiveness of primary and secondary spindle receptors to muscle stretch and to contraction of the miniature intrafusal muscle fibers upon which the sensory endings lie (cf. Fig. 7B and Fig. 8). Since the central sensory zone of an intrafusal muscle fiber displays less contractile activity than do the poles, it is stretched when the fiber is activated. This stretch causes receptor discharge rate to rise, as is indicated in Figure 8 by the positive sign at the summing junction. Furthermore the whole structure lies functionally in parallel with the main (or extrafusal) muscle and, as a consequence, when the main muscle lengthens, the intrafusal fiber is also lengthened, again causing stretch of the sensory zone and increased discharge. Conversely, extrafusal shortening causes decreased afferent discharge, which is indicated in Figure 8 by the negative sign at the summing junction. In effect, the spindle receptor responds to the difference between the amounts of intrafusal and extrafusal shortening, where intrafusal length actually refers only to the contractile poles of the intrafusal fiber. The additional influence of γ-dynamic inputs in modifying the sensitivity of the receptor to stretch is shown as a potential adaptive control in Figure 8.

Both primary and secondary endings in muscle spindles show static responses that are approximately proportional to the amount of stretch; thus they are both length sensors. In addition, primary endings show a marked dynamic responsiveness that bears a superficial resemblance to velocity sensitivity, although the actual dependence of response on velocity is rather weak (137).

Golgi tendon organs are selectively sensitive to the force of contraction, more or less independently of the length of the muscle. They do not have high thresholds for discharge as was formerly believed, but instead are sensitive to force variations throughout most of the physiological range (cf. ref. 133).

Follow-up Servo Hypothesis

One of the first detailed theories concerning the function of the fusimotor system is the follow-up servo hypothesis proposed by Merton in 1951 (210) and elaborated more fully in his 1953 paper (211). Merton postulated that most movements are initiated by motor commands sent to γ-motoneurons, or fusimotor neurons (γ-command in Fig. 8), rather than directly via commands to α-motoneurons (α-command in Fig. 8). According to this hypothesis, the commands first travel to the periphery where they produce shortening of the polar zones of intrafusal muscle fibers. The resultant increase in spindle discharge is then conducted back to the spinal cord where it excites the α-motoneurons (or skeletomotor neurons) reflexly, leading to activation of the main muscle followed by extrafusal shortening.

The second major postulate in Merton's hypothesis is that the autogenetic reflex pathways function as a servomechanism that regulates muscle length. This is shown in Figure 8 by the negative-feedback loop from spindle receptors through α-motoneurons to the controlled system consisting of extrafusal muscle and the mechanical load upon which the muscle acts. Note that the only autogenetic reflex pathway included in this hypothesis is the one from spindle receptors.

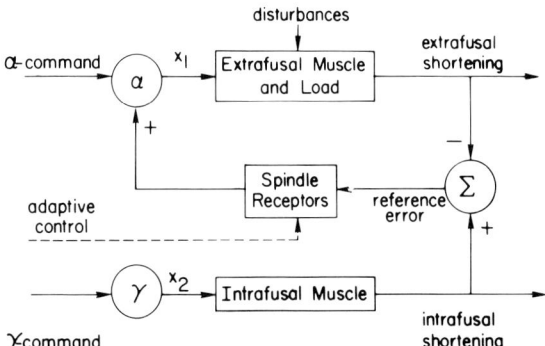

FIG. 8. Block diagram illustrating α-γ-relations. α-Commands produce shortening of extrafusal muscle and γ-commands produce shortening of intrafusal muscle. α-Commands reduce spindle discharge, whereas γ-commands increase it, suggesting that spindle receptors may function as reference error detectors as in Figure 7.

Merton assumed that autogenetic inhibition via tendon organs has a high threshold, serving only to protect the muscle from excessive strain.

The follow-up part of the hypothesis (commands are sent to fusimotor neurons) and the length-servo part (muscle length is the regulated variable of the motor servo) were combined as follows. The intrafusal shortening produced by the γ-command was supposed to establish a reference length, creating an error signal at the summing node, and the servo was then supposed to reduce this error toward zero by producing a controlled amount of extrafusal shortening. A high gain in the length-feedback pathway would make the amount of extrafusal shortening closely approximate the prior shortening of the intrafusal fibers and also be relatively independent of disturbances produced by changes in mechanical load. This supposed reduction of the dependence of movement on the loading conditions is generally referred to as *load compensation*. Both the follow-up part and the length-servo (or load compensation) part of Merton's hypothesis have been challenged by subsequent experimental data and by alternative hypotheses.

Spindle Receptors as Model-Reference Error Detectors

Experimental studies stimulated by Merton's hypothesis suggested that command signals for movement are sent to α- and γ-motoneurons more or less simultaneously (the evidence is reviewed briefly in α-γ-*Relations,* p. 308, and in more detail in the chapter by Matthews in this *Handbook*). This situation, termed α-γ-*linkage* by Granit (96) and α-γ-*coactivation* by Phillips (236), is captured by Figure 8 if it is assumed that α- and γ-commands arrive as a combined pair, either in parallel pathways or in branches of the same input fibers.

Given this pattern of motor command, the dual responsiveness of spindle receptors to intrafusal contraction and muscle stretch provides a natural mechanism for a model-reference calculation (see *Control Configurations,* p. 262), if one also postulates that the intrafusal muscle represents a model of the controlled system, consisting of the main muscle and its load. In this view the forcing function to the controlled system (x_1 in Fig. 7A and Fig. 8) is conveyed by action potentials in α-fibers innervating the main muscle, whereas the forcing function to the model (x_2) is conveyed by signals in γ-fibers that innervate intrafusal muscle. Movements are produced by sending signals in both alpha and gamma motor axons. If the subsequent shortening of the main muscle is equal to the shortening of the intrafusal muscle, the stretch applied to the sensory zone should not change nor should spindle discharge change. This represents the null condition described earlier in which actual output equals model output, and the reference error in Figure 7 is zero. In contrast, an unusually large load would interfere with the shortening of the main muscle, causing a reference error in the form of increased discharge of spindle afferents. Conversely, an unusually small load would lead to an excess of extrafusal shortening, causing a reference error expressed as a decrease in spindle firing. It is clear from this discussion that the null condition of no change in spindle discharge should occur for some particular intermediate value of load, and loads differing from this should result in reference errors.

The movement-control hypotheses described in the following two sections are based on the initial assumption that muscle spindles function to detect reference errors in muscle length.

Conditional Feedback and Servo Assistance

The concept of α-γ-linkage led to a revision of the follow-up servo hypothesis that Matthews (195) referred to as *servo assistance,* for reasons to be explained below in this section. Essentially the same idea had been outlined briefly in the classic paper on the reafference principle published by Von Holst and Mittelstaedt in 1950 (285), and it also conforms with the suggestions offered in 1952 by Kuffler and Hunt (163). In the engineering literature this mode of control has been called conditional feedback, which, as discussed in *Control Configurations,* p. 262, and illustrated by option 1 in Figure 7A, is a subcategory within the general class of control systems termed model reference. Let us consider the rationale for these basically similar ideas.

The term conditional feedback stems from the fact that feedback in a system of this type vanishes when there is no reference error—thus a nonzero feedback signal is conditional upon the occurrence of an error. Similarly, the term servo assistance implies that the servo loop is quiescent when there is no error and becomes operative as part of the response to an error. For example, movement against an unusually large load would produce a reference error in Figure 8, and the latter should excite motor neurons to produce an enhanced force in compensation for the added load. In contrast, movement against a normal load would result in equivalent intrafusal and extrafusal shortening, no reference error, and no servo assistance.

The condition of a vanishing reference error requires some explanation. What is really meant is that spindle receptor discharge remains constant at some finite level, rather than actually dropping to zero impulse/s. This biasing of discharge about some elevated level is important, since it permits the detection of bidirectional reference errors that result from unusually small versus unusually large loads.

One of the interesting consequences of the conditional-feedback configuration is that the effects of disconnecting the feedback signals, as for example in the dorsal rhizotomy procedure, should be much less devastating than they would be in a more conventional feedback system. Assuming there is some simple compensation for the withdrawal of excitatory bias provided by tonic spindle discharge, the rhizotomized subject should be able to make movements against usual loads without any modification in the α-commands (Fig. 8) sent from higher centers. Problems would result mainly when unusually large or small loads are encountered. Thus, the notion of conditional feedback may help to explain the considerable motor abilities that remain after dorsal rhizotomy.

β-System and the Possibility for Zero Sensitivity

The skeletofusimotor, or β-configuration, shown in Figure 9 also has the potential to operate as a model-reference system. The reader will recall that β-motoneurons branch to innervate both extrafusal and intrafusal muscle fibers. Until recently this type of innervation was thought to be prominent only in amphibians and reptiles, but more recent work discussed in IMPLEMENTATION OF MOVEMENT COMMANDS, p. 308, indicates that β-innervation probably occurs regularly in mammals as well, along with α- and γ-innervation.

In order for the β-configuration to provide conditional feedback one must again postulate that the intrafusal muscle functions as a model of the controlled system, the extrafusal muscle and its load. In this case the main forcing function is conveyed by the branches of β-motoneurons innervating extrafusal muscle fibers, whereas the forcing function to the model is conveyed by the branches innervating intrafusal muscle (compare Figs. 7A and 9). As with the α-γ-configuration shown in Figure 8, the reference error is assumed to be the difference between the amounts of intrafusal and extrafusal shortening. Feedback is "conditional," since under some ideal (presumably the usual) loading condition the resultant reference error registered during movement should be zero.

The β-configuration has another interesting feature

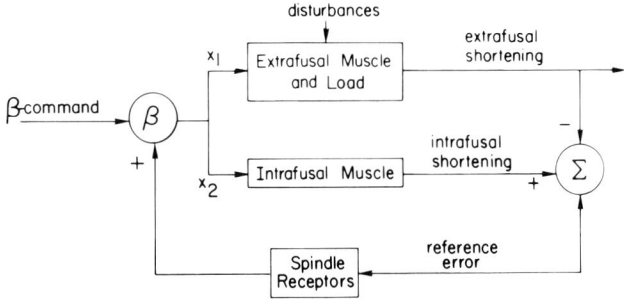

FIG. 9. Block diagram illustrating the organization of β-innervation. Forcing functions from β-motoneurons promote both extrafusal and intrafusal shortening. As in Figures 7 and 8, spindle receptors are shown detecting the difference between intrafusal and extrafusal shortening, a reference error. The positive-feedback loop from β-motoneurons through intrafusal muscle and spindle receptors back on β-motoneurons raises the possibility of zero-sensitivity operation.

built into its basic structure, a positive-feedback loop from β-motoneurons to intrafusal muscle through spindle receptors back to β-motoneurons. A theoretical analysis of the system (127) has demonstrated that with this positive-feedback pathway, zero-sensitivity operation (option 1 combined with option 2 in Fig. 7A) could be achieved, provided the gain of this loop is unity. At first sight this seems to be an advantage that the β-configuration has over separate α- and γ-innervation. It has also been shown (127), however, that zero-sensitivity operation could occur if spindles projected back on γ-motoneurons. Autogenetic γ-projections were once rejected but are now being reconsidered (cf. ref. 62, 227). Spindle afferents also project to the brain where reference errors might be used to compute adaptive modifications (option 3 in Fig. 7A, along the lines discussed in CONTROL THEORY CONCEPTS, p. 258.

Stiffness Regulation

A major assumption in each of the hypotheses discussed up to this point is that muscle length is the regulated variable of the motor servo. This assumption is not well supported by current experimental evidence, however, as reviewed later, nor does it fit well with the presence of negative force feedback from tendon organs (127). These considerations together with supporting data led Nichols and Houk (226) to propose instead that stiffness, which is a ratio of force change to length change, may be the regulated property of the motor servo. A simplified graphic analysis of a hypothetical stretch reflex will serve to introduce the concept of reflex stiffness in relation to its neural and mechanical origins.

Figure 10 illustrates the three major components of static response that occur when an added load lengthens a muscle to elicit a stretch reflex. The first, a muscular component, is purely mechanical and is associated with the positive slope of the muscle length–tension curve (shown dashed in Fig. 10). The second, a length-feedback component, is mediated by the spindle pathway and consists of a facilitation of motor output that tends to increase force. The third, a force-feedback component, is mediated by the tendon organ pathway and consists of an inhibition of motor output that tends to decrease force. The actual change in force is the result of these three components, as illustrated by point d in Figure 10. This overall motor servo response is characterized by the slope of the heavy line segment a-d, which is called *reflex stiffness* and is given by

$$\frac{\Delta f}{\Delta x} = \frac{F_1 - F_0}{L_1 - L_0} \qquad (10)$$

where Δf represents the resultant force increment produced by a stretch Δx.

It is apparent from Figure 10 that length feedback acts to increase reflex stiffness, which improves the

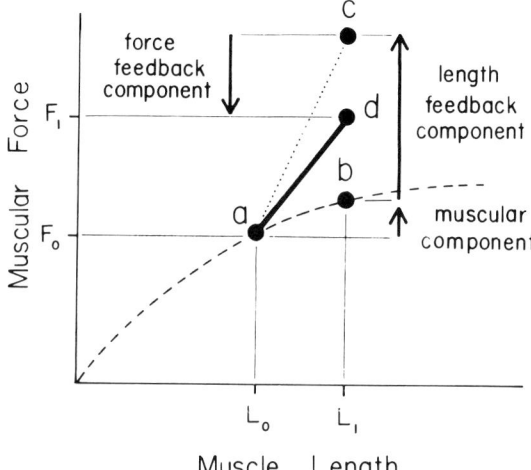

FIG. 10. Component analysis of hypothetical stretch reflex. Stretch from L_0 to L_1 causes force to increase from F_0 to F_1. Reflex stiffness is defined by the slope of the line segment a-d equal to $(F_1 - F_0)/(L_1 - L_0)$. The diagram dissects this overall response into 3 components: the muscular-mechanical component arises from the length-tension properties of the muscle (*dashed curve*), the length-feedback component originates in spindle discharge and increases stiffness, and the force-feedback component originates in tendon organ discharge and decreases stiffness. [From Houk (127a). Feedback control of muscle: a synthesis of the peripheral mechanisms. In: *Medical Physiology* (13th ed.), edited by V. B. Mountcastle. St. Louis, MO: The C. V. Mosby Co., 1974.]

rigidity of length regulation in analogy with a stiff spring. A given load disturbance causes less disturbance in length if stiffness is high. In contrast, force feedback acts to decrease reflex stiffness, which is the same as increasing the compliance. This improves force regulation but interferes with length regulation, since a given load disturbance causes a greater disturbance in length if compliance is high. It is clear from this example that length and force cannot both be well regulated at the same time. In analogy with the discussion in *Regulated Variables and Properties*, p. 262, it would appear that combinations of length and force feedback might serve to regulate some property rather than each variable independently, and the theoretical analysis of this problem provided by Nichols and Houk (226; also see 128) suggests that the regulated property should be stiffness. A simplified version of this derivation will be given here.

Load perturbations ordinarily provoke changes in both muscle length and muscle force. Whether or not this causes a change in motor output should depend on the balance between length and force feedback as shown in Figure 1 and summarized by the following equation

$$\Delta e = g_S \Delta x - g_T \Delta f \tag{11}$$

where Δe represents the change in motor output, which is taken to be the error signal of the motor servo. For simplicity we have used the constant parameters g_S and g_T to represent the respective gains of spindle afferent and tendon organ pathways, and we have assumed that control signals remain at constant values. It is particularly instructive to consider the null conditions under which there would be no need for a compensatory change in motor output, in which case Δe would remain equal to zero. Substituting $\Delta e = 0$ and solving for Δf

$$\Delta f_i = (g_S/g_T)\Delta x \tag{12}$$

where the subscript i designates that this is an ideal force change that results in no error signal. The special significance of g_S/g_T will become evident.

The actual force change is made up of mechanical and neurally mediated components

$$\Delta f = K \Delta x + A \Delta e \tag{13}$$

where K represents the mechanical stiffness, which in the example of Figure 10 is simply the slope of the length-tension curve, and A is an activation factor that converts the error signal into a neurally mediated component of force change referred to as reflex action (cf. *Dynamic Features of Force Development*, p. 297; and Fig. 35). To obtain Equation 12 we assumed an absence of any change in motor output, so we should also set $\Delta e = 0$ in Equation 13

$$\Delta f_m = K \Delta x \tag{14}$$

where the subscript m designates that this is a purely mechanical response. The postulated perfect cancellation of length feedback by force feedback ($\Delta e = 0$) will occur only if the mechanical force Δf_m happens to equal the ideal force Δf_i. Comparison of Equations 12 and 14 indicates that this condition is met if the mechanical stiffness of the muscle happens to be equal to the ratio g_S/g_T.

This ratio of gain factors has been called the *regulated stiffness*, since it represents a reference ratio that should determine the sign and magnitude of compensatory changes in motor output. Thus whenever the actual mechanical stiffness is less than this ratio, there is a deficit in force feedback, Δe in Equation 11 becomes positive, and the resultant input to the muscle tends to restore stiffness toward the reference ratio. Conversely, whenever mechanical stiffness is greater than this ratio, there is an excess of force feedback, Δe becomes negative, and the resultant decrease in motor output again tends to restore reflex stiffness toward the reference ratio. It is noteworthy that the regulation of this ratio property is predicted to result from a linear summation of excitatory and inhibitory signals at the level of the motoneuron. No fancy calculations are required.

The hypothesis for stiffness regulation does not eliminate the need for hypotheses concerning movement control. On the contrary, the two can be readily integrated (127). For example, the addition of a force-feedback loop to Figure 8 gives rise to a system in which stiffness is regulated while movements are controlled by α- and γ-commands, in any combination. The major modification of the movement hypotheses is that command signals now control the threshold of the stretch reflex rather than commanding a particular length. This, in fact, is quite consistent with the summary model of the motor servo described in the next section.

Summary Model

The participation of the motor servo in complex motor acts is best understood with the aid of an overall model that concisely summarizes input-output properties. While summary models can be derived by combining models of the component parts, the more direct approach is to formulate them on the basis of input-output data. The account given here derives mainly from the work of Fel'dman (72, 73), stimulated by the earlier experiments of Matthews (193, 194) and supported by numerous studies that are reviewed later in this chapter.

Although the mechanical load is an integral part of the motor servo (Fig. 1), system characterization is simplified by considering the neuromuscular components (enclosed by dashed lines in Fig. 1) and the mechanical load separately. Since the properties of the load are easily modeled by well-known equations, the main problem becomes one of discovering a mathematical expression of the form

$$f = F[x, c_i] \qquad (15)$$

that details the input-output properties of the neuromuscular portion. Here muscle force f is chosen as the output whereon muscle length x and a composite control signal c_i serve as the major inputs. The dependence of motor servo properties on velocity and acceleration is not exluded since the operator F can perform differentiation of x.

The composite control signal c_i is actually a set of neural commands that act on the motor servo at several points and are potentially capable of an independent control of several parameters. However, Fel'dman (72) proposed, on the basis of input-output data to be reviewed later, that the central control of this system ordinarily is much simpler than this. Specifically he postulated that the potential dependence on several variables (x and the various c_i's) in most cases reduces to a dependence on a single variable, the quantity ($x - x_0$) where x_0 represents the threshold of the stretch reflex established as the net result of the combined actions of the individual c_i's. Hence, Equation 15 can be rewritten as

$$f = \phi\,[x - x_0] \qquad (16)$$

ϕ is an operator having the units of stiffness that specifies an "invariant" relationship between muscle force and length. While Fel'dman's work has emphasized the static properties of this force-length relation, a dependence on velocity can be included by permitting ϕ to be a dynamic operator, representing the dynamic stiffness of the motor servo.

Since the actual dependence on velocity is rather weak (see *Velocity Dependence and Damping*, p. 306), the salient features of the force-length relations can be portrayed by a set of curves on a plot of muscle force versus muscle length. The solid curve in Figure 11 shows the typical dependence of force on length observed experimentally under conditions in which it is safe to assume that control signals remained constant. The intersection with the abscissa, labeled threshold length, is the length the muscle assumes when it is unloaded, i.e., when $f = 0$. According to Fel'dman's hypothesis, neural control signals act mainly by altering this threshold, x_0 in Equation 16, which has the effect of shifting the entire force-length relation along the abscissa, as shown by the dashed curve in Figure 11. The dotted curve is included to illustrate an alternative mode of control that is discussed in the next section.

The block diagram in Figure 12 indicates how Equation 16 can be combined with another equation

$$x = L[f_d - f] \qquad (17)$$

where L represents load properties and f_d is a disturbance force, to evaluate overall motor servo performance. The specific form of L depends on the nature of the load. For example, if the load is inertial, L becomes

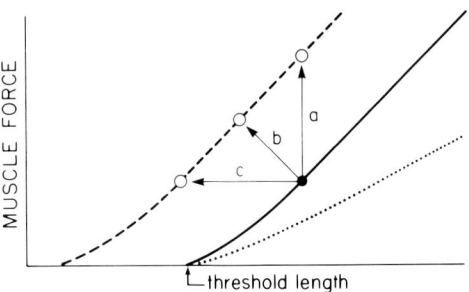

FIG. 11. Summary model of the motor servo. *Solid line* represents the static relationship between muscle force and length observed when control signals (cf. Fig. 1) remain constant. Control signals could act to change the threshold length (*dashed curve*) or to alter the slope of the force-length relation (*dotted curve*). The usual mode of control appears to be the former. Trajectories a, b, and c illustrate the load dependence of responses to a control signal. [From Houk (130). Reproduced, with permission, from Annu. Rev. Physiol., vol. 41. © 1979 by Annual Reviews, Inc.]

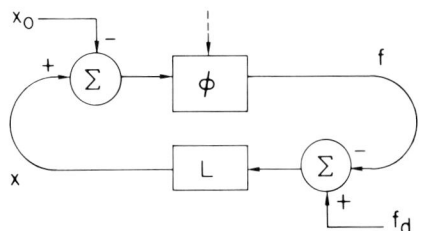

FIG. 12. Block diagram to illustrate the interaction between motor servo properties (represented by the operator ϕ) and the mechanical load. The operator L represents load properties, f_d is a disturbance force, f is muscle force, x is muscle length, and x_0 is the threshold length of the strength reflex (Fig. 11) established by central motor commands.

division by a constant, the mass, and double integration; in the case of a spring load, L is a constant multiplier, the compliance of the spring.

The trajectories labeled a, b, and c in Figure 11 provide a graphic example to illustrate an important point—both muscle length and force are determined by the properties of both the load and the neuromuscular portion. The assumed input is a neural control signal that causes the illustrated shift in the force-length relation. The trajectories show the resultant changes in muscle force and length under three loading conditions: a) when pulling on an immovable object, b) when pulling on a spring, and c) when pulling against a constant disturbance force. Note that it would be inaccurate to say that the neural signal controls either length or force. Instead it controls the threshold length, and the particular force and length that result depend on the interaction between the properties of the motor servo (ϕ) and the load (L and f_d).

Adaptive Models

It is well documented that a human subject can modify his responsiveness to mechanical disturbances based on prior instructions, such as "make your arm rigid" or "relax." The modifications are properly considered to be the product of an adaptive mechanism in the brain that controls the motor servo. The result is an alteration in the effective stiffness presented to mechanical loads that apparently meets changing requirements for reactions to the external environment (e.g., a compliant stiffness is advantageous for body suspension, whereas a rigid stiffness assists positional control). Two rather different models have been proposed to explain the neural mechanism for this type of adaptation.

Hammond (114) suggested that adaptation is achieved by altering the gain of transmission through length-servo pathways, a control strategy referred to as parametric adaptation. Coupling this idea with the hypothesis for stiffness regulation reviewed earlier, one can postulate that a controlled increase in the gain of length feedback (g_S in Eq. 12) would make the regulated stiffness more rigid, whereas an increase in force feedback (g_T) would make it more compliant. These gain changes could be produced by presynaptic modulation or by gating inputs to interneurons in reflex pathways. Another interesting possibility is a selective control of the dynamic component of stiffness by activating dynamic fusimotor neurons ("adaptive control" in Fig. 8).

The hypothesis for a parametric adaptive control of the motor servo is contrary to (though not completely excluded by) the summary model discussed in the previous section, since it involves a change in the shape of the force-length relation (a hypothetical example of which is shown by the dotted curve in Fig. 11) rather than a simple shift of an invariant curve along the length axis (the dashed curve). However, the possibility can be included in the summary model by postulating a second functional category of control signal, the unlabeled dashed input in Figure 11. This neural input is assumed to be an adaptive control that modifies ϕ, the dynamic stiffness of the motor servo, via the mechanisms discussed in the previous paragraph. To avoid confusion, throughout the remainder of this chapter we use the term *motor command* to provide specific reference to the first and more usual type of control signal, the one that sets the threshold length in Figure 11.

An alternative hypothesis concerning the mechanism that adaptively controls the motor output is the two-stage model shown in Figure 13 (129, 130). Here the autogenetic reflex pathways of the motor servo are collectively represented by the box labeled Continuous Processor, whereas motor commands sent to the motor servo are postulated to be generated by a stimulus-response (S-R) processor. According to this model, adaptive responsiveness resides in the S-R processor rather than in the motor servo.

Unlike the operations of the motor servo, those of the S-R processor presumably do not employ continuous feedback; instead, it is assumed that afferent signals are analyzed primarily to detect the occurrences of environmental stimuli. Once detection is achieved, the process is triggered to release open-loop motor commands that control the motor servos regulating the activities of individual muscles. In other words, the S-R processor represents a central mechanism that generates motor commands that control reaction-time movements.

The adaptive controls applied to the S-R processor are presumed to be capable of altering either the particular sensory cues required to trigger a given response or the quantity or quality of the response released by any given sensory cue. One imagines a set of neural detectors that can be tuned to respond to different sensory cues or to internal commands; the initiatory signals from these detectors might then be used to trigger transitions in the state of a neural network that controls the levels of descending motor commands.

One of the interesting possibilities contained in this type of model is the potential for operating on the basis of the feedforward principle discussed earlier (cf. Fig. 4). Environmental stimuli associated with mechanical disturbances could be detected before they have had a chance to modify posture or movement and so used to trigger a compensatory motor command that counteracts a disturbance as, or even before, it develops.

Summary

Several of the models of the motor servo reviewed in this section focus on alternative roles for the fusimotor input to muscle spindles in movement control. While these hypotheses have generally included the assumption that autogenetic feedback functions to

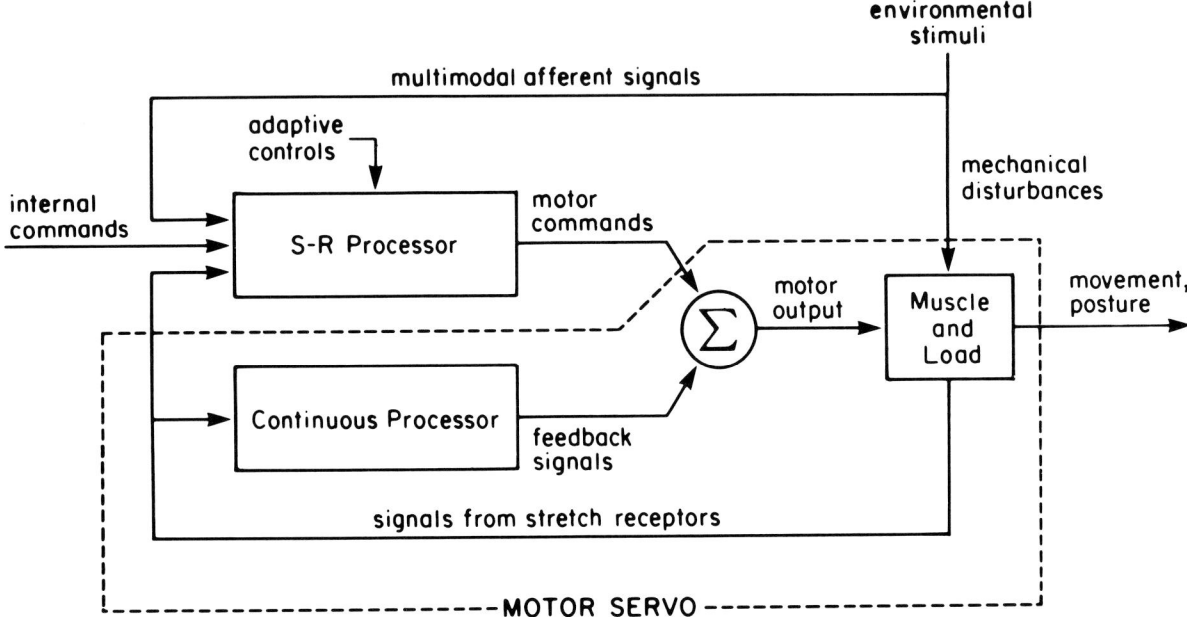

FIG. 13. Two-stage model of adaptive motor control. Motor output signals are assumed to be generated by 2 parallel processes that have rather different characteristic properties. Continuous Processor is assumed to operate in an analogue fashion, combining inputs from stretch receptors to produce continuous feedback compensation. The S-R (stimulus-response) Processor is assumed to operate more like a logical device, using sensory cues to trigger the release of preselected motor programs in a discontinuous fashion. Adaptive control is assumed to result mainly from the establishment of flexible S-R relations rather than from alterations in the gain of the continuous-feedback loops. [From Houk (129a). *Posture and Movement: Perspective for Integrating Sensory and Motor Research on the Mammalian Nervous System,* edited by R. E. Talbott and D. R. Humphrey. New York: Raven, © 1979.]

control muscle length, they can be modified to include other alternatives. One such alternative described here in some detail is the hypothesis that length and force feedback combine to regulate the stiffness of the motor servo. We also describe a summary model of the motor servo that is based on empirical input-output data, and we briefly discuss how the adaptive control of motor servo properties could be accomplished either by parametric gain control or by establishing versatile stimulus-response relations.

MUSCLE MECHANICAL STIFFNESS

An adequate assessment of the regulatory hypotheses discussed in the previous section requires knowledge of the manner in which a muscle responds to stretch and release in the absence of neuroregulation. There are deficiencies in muscle mechanical properties, and these deficiencies must be understood as a preface to an evaluation of the efficacy of the regulatory actions that compensate for them. The approach taken here is to describe the properties of skeletal muscle in terms of its mechanical stiffness and to review the dependence of stiffness on the initial conditions and on the parameters of length change. The reader is referred to the chapter by Partridge and Benton in this *Handbook* for a more general account of muscle physiology.

Stiffness Definitions

Stiffness is always represented by a force-to-length ratio, but since this ratio can be assessed in different ways, under either static or dynamic conditions, one needs to provide some alternative definitions. *Static stiffness* is the ratio of the increment (or decrement) in force divided by the corresponding increment (or decrement) in length measured under steady-state conditions. There are two useful measures of dynamic stiffness. *Incremental dynamic stiffness* ($\Delta f/\Delta x$) is the ratio of force increment to length increment measured under transient conditions, whereas *instantaneous stiffness* (df/dx) is a dynamic infinitesimal measure calculated from the slope of a force-length trajectory. Instantaneous stiffness (df/dx) is equivalent to the slope of a time plot of force (df/dt) during the constant velocity phase of ramp changes in length. In addition it is often convenient to use the term stiffness in a larger sense, with reference to an entire force-length relation. For example, the stiffness operator K in

$$f = K[x] \qquad (18)$$

converts a length variable x into a force f.

If K in Equation 18 were a constant multiplier, the properties would be like those of an ideal (linear and undamped) spring. In this case all of the above mentioned measures of stiffness would yield the same result, the value of the spring constant K. Furthermore none of the measures of stiffness would depend on the initial length or force or on other initial conditions. However, muscle is both dynamic and highly nonlinear, and as a consequence its stiffness varies considerably depending on the velocity and amplitude of length change and on the initial conditions. Correspondingly, the reader should not expect this chapter to provide any unique values for stiffness. Instead the purpose of the chapter is to document the various conditions under which muscle stiffness varies.

Length Dependence

Since length-tension curves are usually constructed from measurements of the steady force developed at each of several lengths, the slopes of these curves provide one way of assessing the static stiffness of the muscle. Figure 14 was prepared to provide a summary illustration of a typical set of length-tension curves for skeletal muscle. The active + passive curve represents a force-length relation for a maximally activated muscle—all motor units recruited and discharging at high rates. It is apparent from the slope of the curve that static stiffness is appreciable at intermediate lengths, but it decreases toward zero as the peak of the length-tension curve is approached, in spite of the fact that the force there is highest. In contrast the stiffness of the passive muscle is negligible at intermediate lengths but becomes significant toward the end of the normal physiological range of muscle lengths.

The shaded region between the active + passive and the passive curves in Figure 14 is labeled the control zone, since it represents the range over which the CNS can modulate force by controlling motor output. Within this zone force is graded by the recruitment of motor units in the order small to large and by the modulation of the discharge rates of active units (see the chapter by Henneman and Mendell in this *Handbook*). Whenever force is varied by recruitment and rate modulation, there are simultaneous alterations in mechanical stiffness that occur in an obligatory fashion.

Recruitment of Motor Units

The effect of recruitment on static mechanical stiffness has been studied by comparing the length-tension curves obtained when different numbers of motor units are electrically stimulated at physiological rates (138, 225). The results are in reasonable agreement with the simple hypothesis that recruitment adds contractile elements (muscle fibers) in parallel, although departures from this rule were noted for low levels of recruitment at short lengths.

The addition of contractile elements in parallel amounts to a scaling of the entire length-tension curve, in proportion to the level of recruitment. Thus if we let $P[x]$ represent the active length-tension curve for

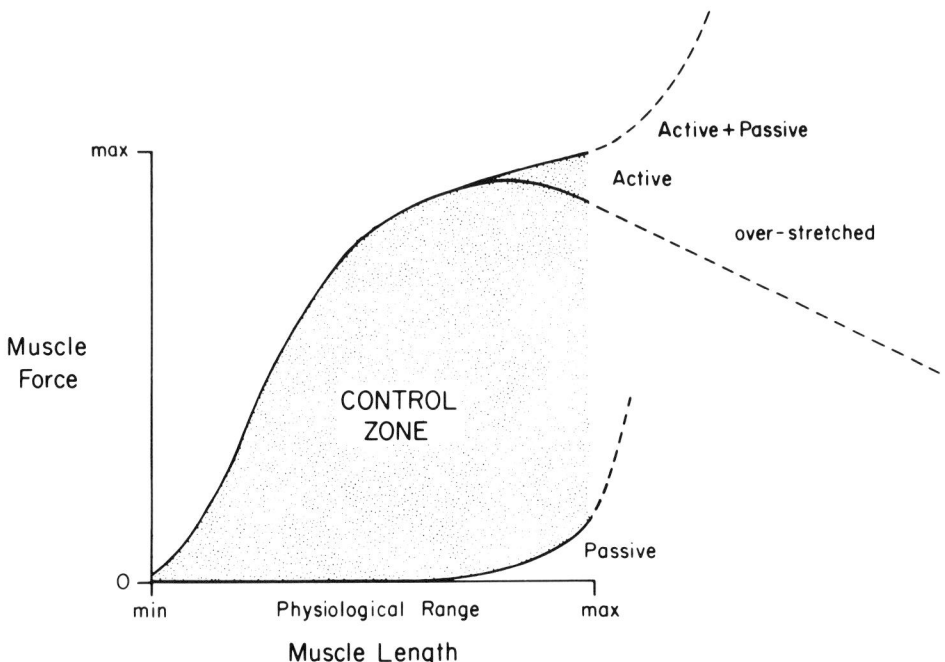

FIG. 14. Length-tension characteristic of skeletal muscle. *Active + Passive curve* shows the force produced by a typical muscle that is maximally activated, as a function of length throughout the physiological range. *Passive curve* shows the corresponding force when the muscle is entirely relaxed. *Shaded region* represents the control zone within which muscle force can be modulated by recruitment and rate modulation of motor units.

a fully recruited muscle, and if we use the ratio f_0/f_{max} as a measure of the level of recruitment, the active component of muscle force can be written

$$f_a(x) = \frac{f_0}{f_{max}} P[x] \quad (19)$$

where f_0 is the initial force at any given initial length, and f_{max} is the maximal force at that same length. In essence, the ratio f_0/f_{max} serves as a measure of the cross-sectional area of myofibrils that have been recruited to activity.

The active mechanical component of static stiffness (K_a) can be assessed from Equation 19 as follows

$$K_a(f_0, x_0) = \frac{\Delta f_a}{\Delta x} = \left(\frac{f_0}{f_{max}}\right) \cdot \left(\frac{\Delta P[x]}{\Delta x}\right)\Bigg|_{x_0} \quad (20)$$

K_a, like f_a in Equation 19, is directly proportional to the level of recruitment, and it also depends on the slope of the whole-muscle length-tension curve at the particular initial muscle length, x_0.

Total muscle force and total mechanical stiffness can be obtained by adding a passive component, whenever the latter is appreciable. Although the procedure of simply adding passive and active components to obtain total force is not precise, because the series elasticity of the tendon is commonly in series with both the passive parallel elasticity and the contractile mechanisms, errors that result from the simplification are seldom appreciable (cf. appendix in ref. 138, for an analysis that includes these corrections).

In conclusion, increases in force produced by the recruitment of motor units are closely analogous to adding prestretched springs in parallel. Consequently, recruitment produces an increase in mechanical stiffness that is approximately proportional to the increase in force.

Rate Modulation of Motor Units

The dependence of static stiffness on discharge rate has been studied by comparing length-tension curves obtained when a whole muscle is electrically stimulated at different rates within the physiological range (97, 103, 193, 225, 248). In several of these studies, distributed stimulation of ventral root filaments was used to mimic the asynchronous activity of motor units. Asynchrony normally insures smooth contractions even though discharge rates are well below the fusion frequencies of the individual units. The dashed curves in Figure 15 show the larger forces and the characteristic shifts of the length-tension curves to the left produced by higher rates of stimulation. The unbroken traces are dynamic trajectories that will be discussed in the next section.

Rack and Westbury (248) correlated their findings on whole muscle with the sliding filament model of contraction, based on histological measurements of sarcomere lengths. The curves obtained with stimulus rates of 50 impulses/s or higher correspond reasonably well with the clamped-sarcomere length-tension curves obtained by Gordon, Huxley, and Julian (89), provided the somewhat longer length of thin filaments in mammals, as opposed to amphibians, is taken into account (40). However, at lower and more physiological stimulus rates the force at any given length was considerably smaller. This finding was attributed to bond turnover caused by internal shortening and lengthening movements within individual sarcomeres, since the latter were activated at rates below their fusion frequencies. Regardless of the specific mechanism, it is quite clear that low activation rates yield length-tension peaks at points beyond the region of maximum cross-bridge overlap, and the steep ascending portion of the curve can occur quite independently of the degree of filament overlap (225, 248).

Inspection of the slopes of the length-tension curves in Figure 15 illustrates that increasing rate can either increase or decrease muscular stiffness, or it can leave stiffness unaltered, depending on the particular rates and on the initial length about which the slope is assessed. For example, at the length corresponding to a 105° ankle angle, stiffness is low at 5 impulses/s, increases to a substantial value at 10 impulses/s, and then decreases once more at 35 impulses/s. While the corresponding variations are somewhat less if one holds constant the initial force, rather than the initial length, clearly there is no simple relation between stiffness and motor unit discharge rate.

In spite of these complexities, a linear model fit to the family of curves may provide adequate accuracy under appropriately restricted conditions. Thus the effects of discharge rate are sometimes approximated by a shift in the slack length of a linear spring

$$f = K(x - x_1) \quad (21)$$

where f and x represent force and length, the constant K is the stiffness of the spring and x_1 is its slack length. Increasing discharge rate is treated as a reduction in x_1. As will be pointed out later, this model appears to be more accurate as a descriptor of the responses to slow, constant velocity stretches as employed by Grillner (103), than it is for static length-tension properties such as those illustrated in Figure 15.

Instantaneous Stiffness and Short-Range Elasticity

Instantaneous stiffness can be assessed from the slopes of the solid trajectories in Figure 15, which are plots of instantaneous force as a function of length during periods of stretch at constant velocity (152). These stretch responses followed an isometric period during which force built up to various initial values (the x's in Figure 15), dependent on initial muscle length and stimulus rate as discussed earlier. The slopes of the trajectories that take off from each initial point represent the instantaneous stiffness that prevails after different amounts of stretch. It is apparent

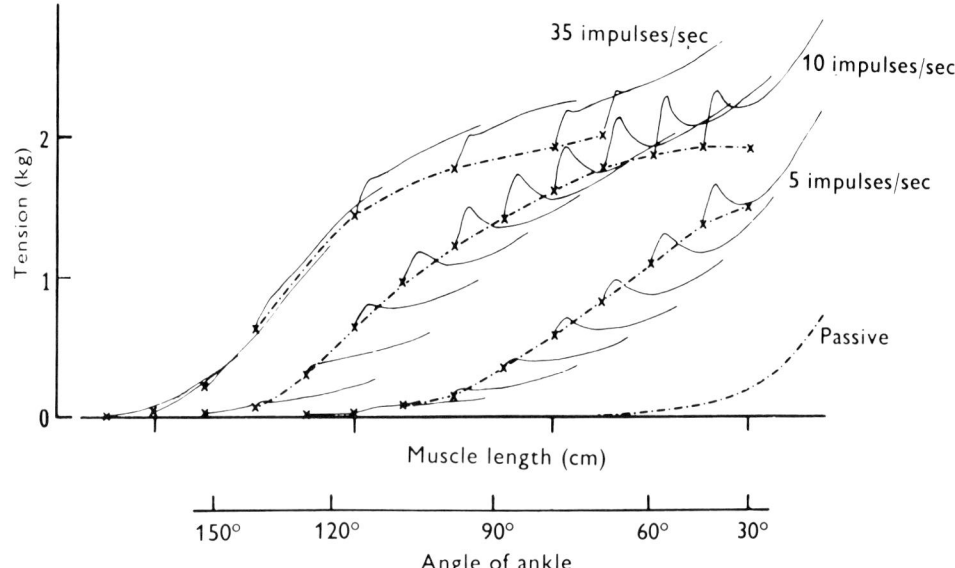

FIG. 15. Length-tension relations in cat soleus. The broken curves represent the length-tension plots obtained at different stimulus rates. The solid curves are the force-length trajectories obtained when the muscle was stretched at constant velocity (7.2 mm/s) beginning from each of the points (the x's) on the length tension curves. [From Joyce et al. (152).]

that stiffness is high initially, but beyond a certain point force yields and stiffness decreases abruptly. This quantity then undergoes some rather bizarre variations, including transient phases of negative stiffness at low stimulus rates, and it does not recover the high initial value for the remaining period of constant velocity stretch. If the muscle is shortened at constant velocity, stiffness is also higher initially than it is later, although the reduction is less prominent than it is with lengthening. The initial high stiffness, called *short-range elasticity*, and the transition to lower stiffness are best appreciated in terms of the sliding filament hypothesis (78, 143, 152, 218, 225, 249, 269). The reader should bear in mind, however, that the variations in stiffness described here are well-documented phenomena that will remain valid even if the sliding filament hypothesis is eventually discarded.

The total range (lengthening plus shortening) over which stiffness remains high during small cyclical perturbations corresponds approximately to a 4% change in muscle length at high velocities. (The smaller range at low velocities indicates that yielding depends on time as well as amplitude.) If a correction is made for the presence of a compliant tendon, this range amounts to a 2%-3% change in fiber length or a 25-35-nm movement in each half sarcomere, which is in agreement with the expected range of cross-bridge deformation (248). When the muscle shortens or lengths from an initial isometric contraction, high stiffness is present over only approximately half of this range, about 1.5% of fiber length or about 2% of the physiological range of length change. These correlations together with the marked change in diffraction spectra that accompany the yield in force (78) strongly support the hypothesis originally put forth by Joyce, Rack, and Westbury (152) that the reduction in stiffness is caused by a sudden increase in the rate at which cross bridges are broken down. Presumably the energy required for breaking actomyosin bonds is supplied by external forces during lengthening in contrast to being supplied by the hydrolysis of adenosine triphosphate (ATP) during shortening.

The series elastic element in Hill's (121) three-component model of muscle, which is equivalent to short-range stiffness, apparently consists of two portions in series with each other, the passive stiffness of the tendon and the active stiffness of the cross bridges. The former is a constant in any given muscle, whereas the latter is proportional to the magnitude of muscle force when this variable is altered by changing the stimulation rate, the level of recruitment, or muscle length (218, 226, 249). These procedures each alter the number of cross bridges per half sarcomere that pull on the tendon and, therefore, produce proportional changes in both force and the stiffness of short-range elasticity. Rack and Westbury (249) reported that the constant of proportionality between these variables in cat soleus and gastrocnemius muscles is approximately $1.3 \text{ N} \cdot \text{mm}^{-1} \cdot (\text{N mean force})^{-1}$, which agrees with Huxley and Simmons' (143) clamped-sarcomere data on amphibian fibers. The passive stiffness of the tendon is about three times the maximum cross-bridge stiffness in the cat soleus, although it is half this relative magnitude in the kangaroo gastrocnemius, presumably as an adaptation for storing elastic energy during hopping (219).

Instantaneous Stiffness Beyond the Short-Range Region

The transition from the short-range elastic region is marked not only by a reduction in stiffness but also by a qualitative change. Prior to the transition, muscle mechanical stiffness is approximately constant at a given initial force and it is predominantly elastic. In other words, force change is proportional to and in phase with the length change and essentially independent of velocity. In contrast, stiffness develops a complex dependence on length, velocity, and stimulus rate after the transition, as illustrated by the trajectories in Figure 15 subsequent to the point at which yielding occurs. There appears to be a transient phase, which lasts longer at lower stimulus rates, followed by a convergence of the trajectories on what can be recognized as a dynamic length-tension curve. The latter lies entirely above the static length-tension curve at high stimulus rates, as would be expected if a frictional force added to that static force. At lower stimulus rates, however, the dynamic curve falls below the static curve at short lengths, which on a phenomenological level represents negative friction, and rises above the static curve at longer lengths. These particular alterations tend to make the dynamic length-tension curve at stimulus rates in the vicinity of 10 impulses/s more linear than the static one, which may be why the curves reported by Grillner (103) appear more linear than those reported by other authors.

All of the trajectories in Figure 15 were obtained during stretch at the same velocity, one within the range encountered by this muscle during walking. Higher stretch velocities give rise to larger forces, although the differences are small and the dependence on lengthening velocity clearly falls short of being proportional (151, 152, 225). Shortening always results in a fall in force from the isometric value at any given length, even at low stimulus rates, and the change seen is typically larger than that associated with an equivalent velocity of lengthening. The results during shortening are approximately fitted by the well-known force-velocity equation of Hill (121), which has been repeatedly shown to be quite accurate for shortening during higher rates of stimulation.

Ramp Responses: Transient Properties and Nonlinearity

Transient responses to ramp-and-hold changes in length provide an effective means for studying both dynamic and static properties and the transition between the two that occurs during the plateau phase of the ramp. Figure 16 shows examples of transient responses to stretch, superimposed upon isometric contractions for three different rates of stimulation. Muscle linearity can also be assessed if ramp amplitude and direction are varied while holding the duration of the constant velocity phase fixed. Figure 17, which includes only the incremental portions of force records

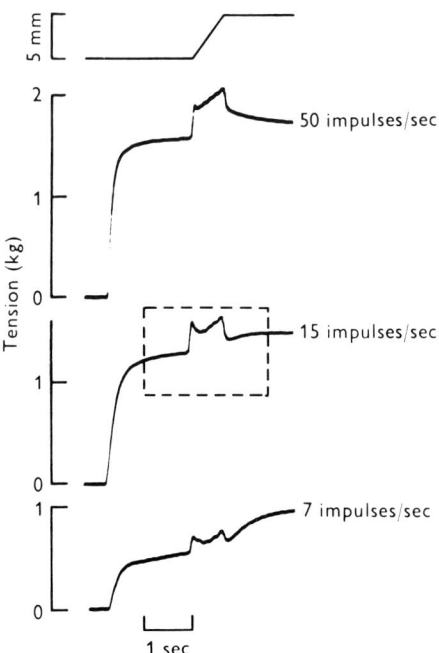

FIG. 16. Responses of cat soleus muscle to ramp-and-hold stretch (5 mm at 7.2 mm/s) applied while the muscle was being stimulated at each of 3 rates. *Dashed box* encloses the incremental transient response, shown as a function of ramp amplitude and direction in Figure 17. [Adapted from Joyce et al. (152).]

(the part enclosed within the dashed box in Fig. 16), illustrates the manner in which the transient response depends on the amplitude of stretch (records on left) and release (records on right) when the stimulus rate is 13.3 impulses/s. The release responses are easiest to understand and therefore are considered first.

Responses to release are dominated initially by the high dynamic stiffness of the cross bridges and later by the much lower static stiffness associated with the slope of the length-tension curve. The dynamic-to-static transition is a phase of tension redevelopment initiated by the breakdown of cross bridges and promoted by their reformation at somewhat shorter sarcomere lengths. It is apparent from Figure 17 that the time course of this transitional process is faster with larger amplitudes of release, which is a nonlinear feature. So although the response prior to ramp plateau (first vertical marker in Fig. 17) scales in direct proportion to the magnitude of the ramp, the criterion for linearity, the response evaluated 1 s after ramp onset (second vertical marker) does not. This is a slightly nonlinear feature. The 1-s response is more sensitive to amplitude for small ramps than it is for large ramps. Overall, responses to release demonstrate appreciable dynamic properties but only modest departures from linear behavior.

The responses to stretch are also dominated initially by the high stiffness of cross bridges and ultimately by the low stiffness associated with the length-tension curve. However, the transition between the two is complicated by the yield in force that occurs during stretch and by the dip in force that occurs just after ramp plateau. It is apparent from Figure 17 that the yield occurs earlier when the size (and also the velocity) of the ramp are increased. This is consistent with the notion that the range of high stiffness prior to cross-bridge turnover corresponds with a certain amplitude of stretch. The actual change in latency is somewhat less than predicted on this basis, which documents the secondary dependence of this range on velocity.

After yielding there must be a slippage between thick and thin filaments that continues for the remainder of the constant velocity phase of the ramp. Remarkably the force increment toward the end of this phase varies by less than a factor of 1.5 in the face of a 17-fold increase in the size of the ramp. Although performance up to the time of yield is quite linear, after the yield it is highly nonlinear as evidenced by the failure to scale in proportion to the amplitude of the input. In the period just after ramp plateau, slippage between thick and thin filaments apparently becomes particularly marked, giving rise to the dip in force that sets this variable to a value below the ultimate isometric force at the new length. Phenomenologically the dip corresponds to a phase of negative incremental stiffness and a continuation of highly nonlinear behavior.

The overall effect of stimulus rate on the transient response is best understood in terms of three component effects. The first is that higher rates promote more cross-bridge formation, which tends to make response scale in proportion to the initial force (Fig. 16). Proportional scaling is generally valid only for the region of short-range elasticity, but in special cases it may hold approximately for later phases of response (122, 226). A second effect concerns the changes in the shape of the length-tension curve produced by increasing rate (Fig. 15), which can either increase or decrease static stiffness as discussed previously. The third effect concerns the manner in which rate changes affect the transition from short-range elasticity to the static stiffness of the length-tension curve. As illustrated in Figure 16, lower rates result in a disproportionate fall in the force developed during the constant velocity phase after yielding and in the immediate postramp period, thus accentuating the yield and dip in responses to stretch and slowing the redevelopment of isometric force in responses to release. The latter effect also appears as a slowing of the initial development of isometric tension at lower stimulus rates in Figure 16.

The less drastic yield and the absence of a dip in the 50 impulses/s record in Figure 16 probably results from an enhancement of the rate of cross-bridge formation promoted by a higher sarcoplasmic calcium concentration. Though this degree of enhancement is atypical for the soleus muscle when activated at its normal tonic rates, it may actually be more typical for other muscles such as the cat gastrocnemius (249). High levels of activation reduce or eliminate the phases of negative stiffness noted earlier, but this does not alter the fact that the stretch response during the transitional period is highly nonlinear.

In contrast to these complex alterations in transient responses produced by rate modulation, the effect of recruitment is relatively simple. As with the static case

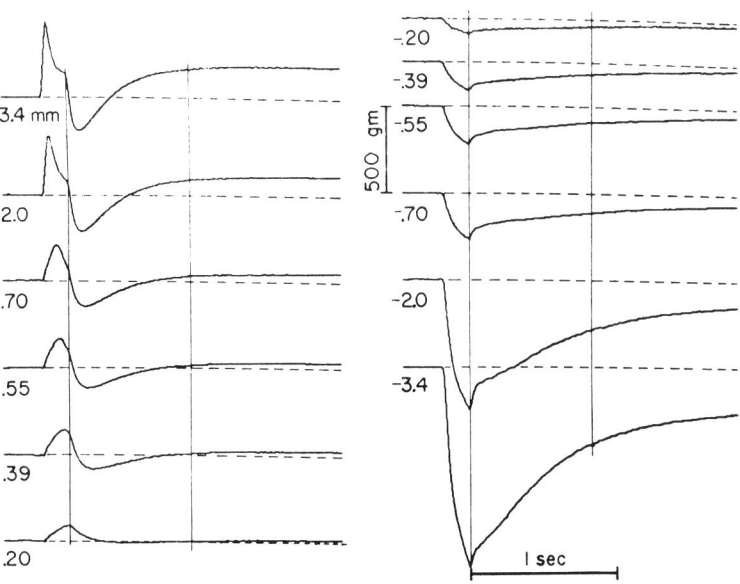

FIG. 17. Incremental transient responses of cat soleus muscle obtained with different amplitudes of stretch and release. Muscle was stimulated at 13.3 impulses/s before and throughout each force record. *First vertical marker* indicates the time of ramp plateau (160 ms) and the *second* indicates 1 s after ramp initiation. Note that the changes in force are not scaled versions of each other as they would be for a linear system. [From Nichols (225).]

discussed earlier, recruitment effects on transient responses are quite well accounted for by the assumption that the muscle fibers are functionally in parallel with each other, at least in the case of the soleus muscle where this has been tested (226). Thus the entire nonlinear transient response scales in proportion to the level of initial force.

Natural Combinations of Recruitment and Rate Modulation

Recruitment and rate modulation are ordinarily used in combination to grade muscle force. The available evidence suggests that recruitment is the more important mechanism at low levels of force, whereas rate modulation is more important at high force levels (214, 217). So one would expect appreciable variations in active muscle stiffness as force varies in the low range and perhaps less appreciable variations in the high force range. Nichols and Houk (226) evaluated the combined effects in the soleus muscle of the decerebrate cat by grading initial force with a crossed-extensor reflex after autogenetic reflexes had been abolished by transection of the ipsilateral dorsal roots. While there was a fair amount of scatter in the data, both dynamic and static phases of response varied approximately in proportion to the initial force throughout the lower half of the physiological range; it was not possible to study the upper half of the range of force gradation. This result suggests that Equations 19 and 20, though strictly applicable only to recruitment, may be sufficiently accurate for a first-order characterization of the variations in muscle force and mechanical stiffness that result from recruitment and rate modulation in combination, at least in the 0%–50% range of force gradation.

Summary

The inherent mechanical stiffness of skeletal muscle depends in a complex manner on the initial conditions and on the parameters of length change. Static stiffness is proportional to initial force when the latter variable is graded by recruitment. When force is graded by changing initial length or discharge rate, however, the dependence is more complex and is best summarized by the slopes of a family of length-tension curves. Within the short-range elastic region, dynamic stiffness (both incremental and instantaneous) is high in comparison with static stiffness, relatively independent of the direction and velocity of length change, and proportional to the initial force, whether the latter is graded by recruitment, rate modulation, or changes in initial length. This short-range elasticity yields, and stiffness decreases abruptly when the muscle is stretched at moderate to high velocities by more than about 2% of the physiological range of length change. The magnitude and time course of the decrease in stiffness depend in a complex manner on stimulus rate, initial length, and the velocity and amplitude of stretch; the dependence on the level of recruitment is simply proportional to initial force. Alterations in stiffness also occur in association with release beyond about 2%, but the changes are less marked than those associated with stretch.

These variations in mechanical stiffness appear to represent deficiencies in muscle performance, which are partially compensated by motor servo actions, as described in later sections.

CENTRAL PATHWAYS

The output of the motor servo depends upon sensory input from spindle receptors and tendon organs to derive the appropriate error signal and to issue the appropriate corrective response (see *Stiffness Regulation*, p. 266). A necessary step in these derivations is the passage of this sensory information across one or more intervening synapses in the spinal cord. The purpose of this section is to review briefly the pathways by which muscle afferents influence spinal motoneurons, concentrating largely upon autogenetic connections; these connections are summarized in Figure 18. A detailed description of the general electrophysiology and connection of spinal neurons has been presented in the first volume in this *Handbook* section on the nervous system (35) and in the chapter by Baldissera, Hultborn, and Illert in this volume. Reciprocal Ia inhibitory effects and the segmental actions of Renshaw cells are considered in the same chapter.

Primary Ending Projections

The primary spindle (Ia) afferent projection to homonymous motoneurons has been studied extensively, [see reviews of Redman, (250); Burke and Rudomín, (35)]. In relation to the problem of motor servo action, the Ia-afferent volley that originates with the onset of rapid muscle stretch appears to be important in initiating an early onset of motor output. It is also likely that this initial, predominantly monosynaptic Ia input causes motoneurons to be recruited in a sequence consistent with the size principle (see the chapter by Henneman and Mendell in this *Handbook*). The basis of continuing motor output remains uncertain when it is observed, for example, during the maintained phase of a stretch-reflex response. There is little doubt that the monosynaptic Ia-projection is an important source of excitation; nevertheless, there are suggestions that other sources of excitation probably exist.

Although the possibility of polysynaptic Ia-projections has been advanced intermittently, the evidence has remained largely indirect in nature (6, 101, 140, 142, 153, 228, 241, 275). The relevant arguments regarding Ia polysynaptic input are based on the results of intracellular recordings in motoneurons and on the time course of motoneuronal discharge and force change in whole muscle.

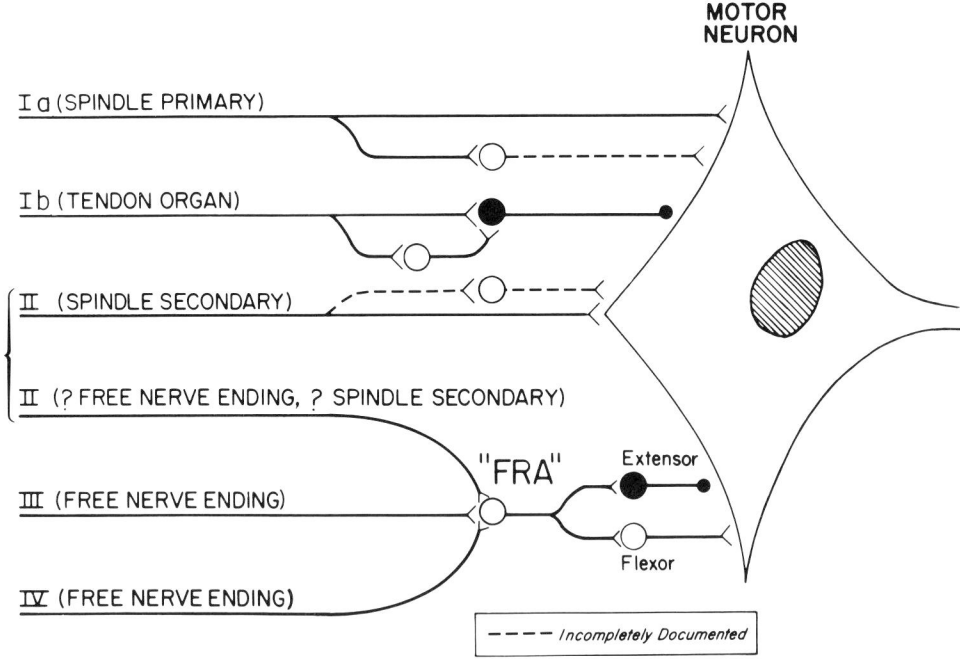

FIG. 18. Summary of the major autogenetic connections of muscle afferents to spinal motoneurons. Well-documented pathways such as Ia, Ib, and flexor-reflex afferents ("FRA") are shown as *continuous lines*. More speculative or incompletely documented connections are shown as *dashed lines*. ○, Excitatory interneurons; ●, inhibitory interneurons. Renshaw cells are omitted for simplicity.

To illustrate the findings derived from intracellular recordings, Ia excitatory postsynaptic potentials (Ia EPSPs) arising at polysynaptic latency have been reported in a cat model of spasticity (228) and during fictive locomotion elicited in the spinal cat (261). The existence of an excitatory interneuron is also supported by studies in which combined muscle stretch and stimulation of the pinna produced a prolonged period of increased excitability of the extensor motoneurons that far outlasted the duration of either excitatory stimulus. This augmented excitability was attributed to posttetanic potentiation at an interneuron receiving convergent input from Ia-afferent and other sensory fibers (101). Repetitive electrical stimulation of Ia-afferents can also give rise to prolonged electromyographic activity that far outlasts the stimulus duration (140–142), implying that reverberative activity of Ia-interneurons might exist. Alvord and Fuortes (6) and later Tsukahara and Ohye (275) showed that during stimulation of the Ia-afferent input, motoneuronal firing probability was increased at latencies that were consistent with a polysynaptic Ia-projection.

Perhaps the most convincing evidence in support of polysynaptic Ia-projections is that derived from studies using longitudinal tendon vibration. The slow rise time and decay time of the force output during tonic vibration (110, 196), the lack of dependence of force output upon the detailed temporal properties of afferent input (200), and the profound depression of the tonic vibration reflex (TVR) by minute doses of barbiturate that are insufficient to impair monosynaptic transmission (153) suggest that polysynaptic Ia-projections may be important. While these findings would seem to implicate a Ia-interneuron, no Ia-interneuron has yet been identified that provides direct excitatory projections to the homonymous motoneuron pool (hence the incompletely documented designation in Fig. 18). A group of interneurons has been described that receives Ia-afferent excitation, and that appears to lie more laterally in the intermediate spinal nucleus than the well-studied inhibitory Ia-interneuron pool (see ref. 149). These neurons would seem to be excellent candidates, but their efferent connections have not yet been studied.

In spite of the lack of direct verification, a potentially significant contribution from excitatory Ia-interneurons to motor servo action remains likely.

Tendon Organ Projections

The existence of inhibitory actions of Ib-fibers on motoneurons has been recognized for some time, largely on the basis of intracellular recordings that showed inhibitory postsynaptic potentials (IPSPs) arising at latencies consistent with the existence of one or more intervening interneurons (56; see Fig. 18). Activation of the Ib-projection to extensor motoneurons has been consistently recorded as inducing disynaptic or trisynaptic inhibition, but the effects on flexor motoneurons are less clearly defined. For example, Eccles et al. (56) found rather few examples of Ib synaptic effects on flexor motoneurons. This deficit appears to have been a consequence of a lack of appropriate descending bias, because quite strong inhibitory potentials are revealed when Ib-afferent stimuli are conditioned with tetanic stimulation of the red nucleus (126). The experiments cited also revealed that many actions of Ib-fibers are not just reciprocally organized. Coupled excitatory and inhibitory effects, extending to muscles acting at quite distant joints, have been reported (56, 126).

A number of studies have reported the existence of neurons in the intermediate nucleus of the spinal cord that are sensitive to electrical activation of muscle nerves at Ib strength—these neurons could correspond with those producing the electrically induced IPSPs (57, 125, 288). Relatively few attempts to characterize the putative Ib-interneuron have been made using adequate stimulation of tendon organs as a means for activating the Ib-afferent input. Granit et al. (100) showed that the silent period observed during muscle twitch is mediated partly by tendon organ–induced postsynaptic inhibition. The study by Lucas and Willis (175) verified that a small-amplitude tendon tap was a selective stimulus to Ia-afferents, (179, 268) and then showed that larger tap amplitudes activated both Ia- and Ib-afferent fibers. Using the sensitivity to large-amplitude taps as a criterion, a substantial number of interneurons in the intermediate nucleus of the cat lumbosacral spinal cord were reported to receive Ib-afferent input (175). However, given the nonselective nature of the input, some residual doubt regarding this identification must persist. To this date no method for selective activation of Ib-afferents has been used, although there is promise in techniques based upon the procedure described by Jack and Roberts (146), in which the threshold of Ia-afferent fibers was increased by prolonged tendon vibration, allowing subsequent relatively uncontaminated electrical stimulation of Ib-fibers. The efferent projection of interneurons receiving Ib input has not been investigated, and its correspondence (or lack of correspondence) with the properties anticipated on the basis of intracellular recordings remains to be established.

It has recently been reported that there is an inhibitory autogenetic Ia-projection (77) that may well arise from interneurons receiving convergent Ia and Ib input. The functional significance of such mixed convergence patterns has not yet been explored.

Projections From Secondary Endings and Group II Free Nerve Endings

The traditional view of the central actions of group II afferents was based on classic monosynaptic testing techniques (172, 173) and on intracellular recordings obtained during electrical stimulation of muscle nerves (27, 60). The consensus has been that group II fibers originate almost entirely in secondary endings, and that secondary spindle afferent effects are mediated through interneuron pools that are inhibitory to extensor motoneurons and excitatory to flexors, features shared with many other high-threshold muscle and cutaneous afferents. These apparently uniform central effects have led investigators to assign the group II afferent pathway to the broad class of flexor-reflex afferents [the "FRA" of Holmqvist and Lundberg, (124)] that is characterized by diffuse flexor activation and inhibition of extensors. Recently, this view has been challenged by a number of studies indicating that the central projections of group II afferents may not be uniform in their action, but may mediate two opposing types of effects.

The claim of dual excitatory and inhibitory actions of group II fibers is based largely on the results of innovative approaches to the central actions of muscle receptors. For example, several studies have utilized identified single spindle secondary afferent fibers, isolated in continuity from dorsal root fibers, in the manner of Mendell and Henneman (207, 208). The spike discharge on the single fiber is then used to synchronize an ensemble average of intracellular events—a spike-triggered average. Both Kirkwood and Sears (158, 159) and Stauffer et al. (266) have shown that distinct monosynaptic EPSPs can be extracted from background synaptic noise with this technique. The EPSPs are usually somewhat smaller than those generated by single Ia-afferent fibers (approximately 40–70 μV for primary afferents versus 8–30 μV for secondaries) but are of sufficient magnitude to provide a significant excitatory input. This monosynaptic projection is depicted as part of the group II secondary spindle input in Figure 18. Further evidence in support of excitatory group II projections has been derived recently using averages of synaptically mediated population potentials in the motor nuclei (180, 181). These potentials were measured using the proximal ends of sectioned ventral roots, and the averages were synchronized by the discharge of intact secondary afferent fibers. The latency and time course of the averaged potentials were not unlike those of monosynaptic EPSPs.

An earlier series of studies (197, 204) based largely on the use of vibration as a means of clamping the Ia-afferent input was the first to suggest that secondary spindle afferent fibers may contribute autogenetic excitation to extensor motoneurons. These studies depend on the finding that small-amplitude, longitudinal vibration of a muscle tendon acts as a selective stimulus to the primary ending, producing one-to-one driving of the ending for each cycle of vibration (24, 28). Under some conditions high-frequency tendon vibration induces a sustained muscle contraction, the TVR (196). Using this capacity of vibration to clamp Ia-afferent discharge, Matthews (197) reported that the vibration reflex and stretch reflex did not interact in a way that would have been predicted were they each to depend entirely on the Ia-afferent input. Specifically the increment in force evoked by vibration did not decline as the muscle length (and the resting discharge of the Ia-afferent) was increased. On the basis of these and other results, Matthews suggested that the stretch-induced central excitation was not mediated entirely by the Ia-afferent pathway. The secondary spindle pathway was advanced as a possible source of this excitation, entirely on indirect grounds.

Further evidence supporting the existence of a second source of afferent excitation for motoneurons was provided by Westbury (287), McGrath and Matthews (204), and Kanda and Rymer (154) on the basis of experiments in which vibration was used to control the Ia-afferent input. Although these various experiments provided suggestive results, they did not directly identify the source of the excitation. Furthermore Jack and Roberts (147) have reported that one-to-one driving of Ia-afferent fibers by each vibration cycle is disrupted when the muscle is contracting and then stretched over several millimeters. This disruption is especially prominent during states of varying dynamic fusimotor bias.

The hypothesis that group II afferents excite extensor motoneurons is further complicated by the long-standing observation of inhibition of extensor motoneurons when group II fibers in muscle nerves are stimulated electrically. Two broad hypotheses have been advanced to reconcile the various results.

The first hypothesis (197, 199, 259) suggests that two separate sets of group II fibers with separate central connections exist. Many muscle nerves are known to contain substantial numbers of group II fibers that might not originate in secondary spindle receptors (see, e.g., ref. 13, 183, 229). Since such fibers would also be activated by electrical stimulation of muscle nerves at group II strength, their central actions could confuse the overall picture. For example, these nonspindle group II fibers could project to a distinct set of inhibitory interneurons that might then make connections to homonymous extensor motoneurons. This possibility is incorporated in Figure 18 as the lower solid group II projection to the FRA interneurons. The central projections of secondary spindle afferents could then be quite separate and purely excitatory in nature.

The second hypothesis states that secondary ending projections may go to both excitatory and inhibitory interneurons (178). This hypothesis requires that excitatory interneurons be suppressed in the spinal and anesthetized cat (since inhibitory effects of electrical stimulation of muscle nerves predominate) and that excitatory interneuron activity predominate in the decerebrate preparation (in which excitatory effects predominate). This hypothesis necessarily implies that the net synaptic effects of afferent projections may be switched by descending pathways. Although no clear evidence of supraspinally mediated switching exists, there is now ample evidence of changing effects of peripheral stimulation during various phases of the locomotion cycle (see the chapter by Grillner in this *Handbook*), giving some credence to the general notion of switching.

One study (82) has reported the existence of interneurons in the intermediate nucleus of the spinal cord that are activated selectively by electrical stimulation of muscle afferents at group II strength—selective activation was achieved by electrical blockade of group I afferent fibers. These results provide a possible neural substrate for polysynaptic group II effects. Nevertheless, the receptor origins of these fibers were not established and, as with the prospective Ib-interneurons, the nature and strength of any efferent synaptic connections remain to be determined.

Projections From Groups III and IV Free Nerve Endings

The receptor origins of muscle afferents with group III or IV fiber diameters are not completely certain; however, it is likely that these fibers originate in free nerve endings (264). Regardless of origin, the synaptic effects of these spinal projections usually conform with the patterns established by many other high-threshold afferents (124), hence their inclusion in the "FRA" category. The functional consequences of activating such afferents are also consistent with this classification, since thermal (120), chemical (79, 80, 209, 260, 161), and nociceptive or high-threshold mechanical stimulation of muscle belly or tendon (162) all activate muscle afferent fibers and give rise to potent flexion reflexes (230). Finally, as discussed in the next section, activation of these afferents could be responsible for the clasp-knife reflex in situations where the appropriate inhibitory interneurons are accessible to excitatory input from the groups III and IV afferents (see Fig. 18).

Clasp-Knife Reflex

The clasp-knife reflex is an abrupt collapse in force that occurs when a spastic limb is moved beyond some threshold angle. The functional contributions of various muscle afferents to the clasp-knife reflex have been reappraised in recent studies (33, 259). In each study, the clasp-knife reflex was examined using the decerebrate cat preparation in which there was introduced a dorsal hemisection of the thoracic spinal cord. This hemisection appears to interrupt descending dorsal reticulospinal fibers that inhibit interneurons of the flexor-reflex pathway releasing many segmental inhibitory reflexes (Fig. 19). Under these conditions stretch of the soleus muscle can be shown to induce a profound inhibition that depends jointly on muscle length (33, 259) and muscle force (259).

In the past the clasp-knife reflex has been attributed variously to the central actions of Golgi tendon organ afferents (11), to inhibition of fusimotor neurons (61), and more recently to central inhibitory effects of secondary spindle afferents (33). An examination of the responses of primary and secondary spindle and tendon organ afferent fibers during clasp-knife responses, however, failed to establish a correlation between the

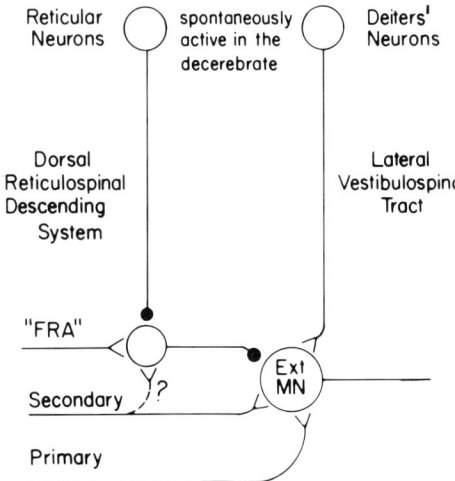

FIG. 19. Neural elements involved in clasp-knife reflex. Primary and secondary spindle afferents provide autogenetic excitation to extensor motoneurons. These neurons also receive tonic excitatory input from the vestibulospinal tract. In the decerebrate state, dorsal reticular neurons that inhibit segmental FRA interneurons are also active, reducing flexor-reflex activity. Section of the dorsolateral quadrants of the cord interrupts the dorsal reticulospinal pathway, thereby releasing segmental flexion reflexes. These include the clasp-knife reflex.

discharge of these muscle afferents and the quantitative features of the clasp-knife reflex (259). In addition a profound inhibition of soleus muscle force was induced by gentle mechanical stimulation of the muscle and tendon surface, at strengths insufficient to modulate primary or secondary afferent discharge to any significant degree. In sum, none of the established encapsulated receptors (spindle receptors and tendon organs) showed discharge patterns that were well correlated with the clasp-knife inhibition.

It has been known since the studies of Lloyd (172, 173) that electrical stimulation of groups III and IV muscle afferent fibers can induce inhibition of extensor motoneurons. It has also been determined that many groups III and IV fibers are activated by muscle stretch and contraction (80, 160). Moreover it is conceivable that a similar group of low-sensitivity muscle stretch receptors providing afferents with group II fiber diameter exists—in fact, several such group II fibers were isolated in the study of Rymer, Houk, and Crago (259). At the present time, the evidence with regard to stretch sensitivity of such afferents is quite fragmentary, and a more detailed study of nonspindle group II afferents is clearly warranted. In spite of the lack of direct evidence, on the basis of the joint length and force dependence of the clasp-knife reflex, the absence of detailed correlations between the clasp-knife characteristics and the discharge of identified spindle and tendon organ afferents, it seems likely that low-sensitivity stretch receptors (spanning groups II, III, and IV conduction velocity) may be responsible for the clasp-knife reflex. These low-sensitivity stretch receptors would presumably provide spinal projections to inhibitory interneurons belonging to the "FRA" group. This possibility is included as the free nerve ending source of group II fibers in Figure 18. This approach, which is in accord with the first hypothesis of group II central effects (i.e., separate spindle and nonspindle group II pathways) does not eliminate the possibility of supraspinally mediated interneuronal switching; the need for a switching hypothesis simply becomes much less compelling.

The remaining issue concerns the reasons for the release of inhibitory reflexes (such as the clasp-knife reflex) in the spastic state. The relevant evidence has been provided by Burke et al. (33) and is summarized in Figure 19. These authors showed that section of the spinal dorsolateral fasciculus transformed rigidity of the decerebrate cat preparation into a state characterized by clasp-knife inhibition and other manifestations of spasticity. It was further argued that the spinal lesion interrupts the descending dorsal reticulospinal projection (60), which appears to suppress activity in flexor-reflex interneurons (65). Transection of these pathways would then release activity in previously inactive reflex circuits, including several that could potentially inhibit extensor motoneurons. A parallel between the animal model of spasticity and the human state was drawn by showing that excitatory cortical projections to dorsal reticulospinal neurons may be necessary to maintain activity in these pathways (10).

Long-Loop Reflexes

To this point we have assumed that the pathways mediating motor servo actions are located in regional segments of the spinal cord. However, this position is contrary to the views expressed in several influential reports dealing with stretch reflexes in intact subjects (67, 69, 185, 186, 206, 271). According to these and many other sources, the spinal component of the stretch reflex is both brief and small and is dominated by a long-loop reflex characterized by medium-latency electromyographic responses to limb perturbations.

The evidence in support of long-loop contributions is derived partly from the patterns of electromyographic (EMG) response to limb perturbations in human and monkey preparations and partly from recordings in motor cortex and related structures in both anesthetized and conscious monkeys. With regard to the EMG responses, investigators in several laboratories have found that abrupt muscle stretch provokes a peaked pattern in the processed EMG, which has subsequently been characterized in terms of grouped discharges of motor units (17). The particular pattern obtained varies somewhat between laboratories, but in each case it consists of several short- and intermediate-latency peaks in the averaged rectified electromyogram. For example, Tatton and his collaborators have recognized the four peaks shown in Figure 20, the first of which (M1) begins at a latency consistent with an origin in the Ia monosynaptic path-

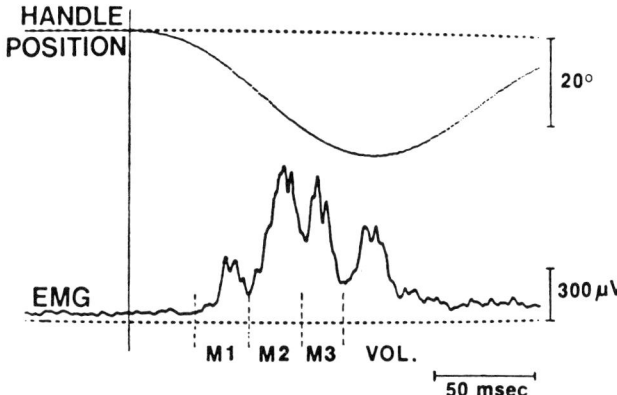

FIG. 20. Averaged rectified EMG response from wrist extensors of a normal subject following sudden flexor displacements of the wrist. The *vertical line* indicates when torque motor was turned on. Subject was instructed to actively return the handle to the central zone as soon as the displacement occurred. Onset latencies for the components of the response: M1 = 32 ms; M2 = 59 ms; M3 = 85 ms; "voluntary" activity = 107 ms. Downward deflection of handle position trace represents flexion at the wrist. [From Lee and Tatton (169).]

way and the last of which is attributed to the onset of a voluntary response. The other two peaks (M2 and M3) sometimes merge into a single response that appears to be similar to what other investigators have called the medium-latency component (5, 164) or the functional stretch reflex (206). The A- and B-waves described by Marsden and collaborators (186) may be analogous to the later half of Tatton's M1 component and his M2 component, respectively (190).

The common theme in all of this is the identification of medium-latency components in the EMG responses to abrupt stretch, components that follow the monosynaptic tendon-jerk response but occur before the presumed latency of a voluntary response. These medium-latency responses have been attributed to conduction through excitatory long-loop pathways between the segment and supraspinal structures because of an apparent correspondence between the timing of EMG response components and the calculated times required to traverse such (hypothetical) long-loop pathways. This emphasis on latency derived initially from a study of human stretch reflexes by Hammond (114) showing that medium-latency (50-60 ms) EMG components of response to biceps stretch are modifiable by prior instruction. Because of their delayed onset and their modifiability, these responses were assigned to long-loop pathways traversing supraspinal structures.

The notion of long-loop connections was subsequently reinforced and expanded by Phillips (236, 237) and Heath et al. (118), who described neurons in cortical area 3a that were responsive to activation of Ia-afferents. It was further suggested that these neurons acted as part of the afferent limb of a transcortical servo loop, the efferent limb being provided by the corticospinal projection. Recordings from motor cortex (42, 67, 70) provided evidence for such afferent connections and revealed that pyramidal tract neurons responded at short latency to limb perturbations that would certainly have activated spindle afferents. More direct evidence regarding the specific contributions of spindle afferents to the activation of corticospinal neurons in conscious primates has been provided recently by studies in which selective muscle stretch was induced without activating cutaneous afferents (290). In addition, electrophysiological evidence, derived from the cat, has supported the existence of connections between areas 3a and 4 (292) although a more direct pathway, from the ventralis posterior lateralis pars oralis (VPLo) nucleus of the thalamus appears to be the source of muscle afferent projections to area 4 in the monkey (8). Also it has been reported recently that pyramidal neurons responding to limb perturbation project back to the same muscles that are activated by limb perturbations (38).

The above results provide strong evidence for the existence of a transcortical loop. However, it remains unclear whether this pathway functions as a servoregulatory loop that should be included within the functional boundaries of the motor servo, or whether its main function is in the genesis of reaction-time movements [see Evarts and Vaughan (71) and Houk (128) for alternative views]. Furthermore if it does function as a motor servo loop, one would like to know what this pathway adds to the servoregulatory actions mediated by the segmental pathways discussed earlier.

Many investigators have discounted the possible contributions of segmental pathways to the medium-latency responses on the basis of the following arguments. First, when different muscles are compared, the latency of these EMG components was found to increase in proportion to the distance of the muscle from cortex (187). Second, it was claimed that medium-latency EMG waves were modifiable by prior instruction (67–71, 114, 191). Third, their magnitude was influenced selectively by lesions of the dorsal columns (168, 188) and sensorimotor cortex (2, 189). An example of a reduced intermediate-latency EMG response, taken from a subject with a unilateral brain stem lesion, is shown in Figure 21.

Although a transcortical loop could certainly provide delayed excitation to spinal motoneurons, it might not act in the production of the peaked pattern of EMG. The medium-latency EMG waves could equally arise from purely segmental mechanisms, such as strong synchronization of motor unit discharge, synchronization of afferent input, fluctuating inhibition, conduction through polysynaptic spinal pathways, or from oscillatory behavior of spinal neuronal networks (but cf. ref. 17). In fact, medium-latency peaks are seen in the EMG responses of decerebrate and spinal cats and monkeys (83, 213, 226, 273), all of which lack the transcortical loop. The close resemblance between the EMG components seen in comparisons of intact and spinal animals (83) appears to

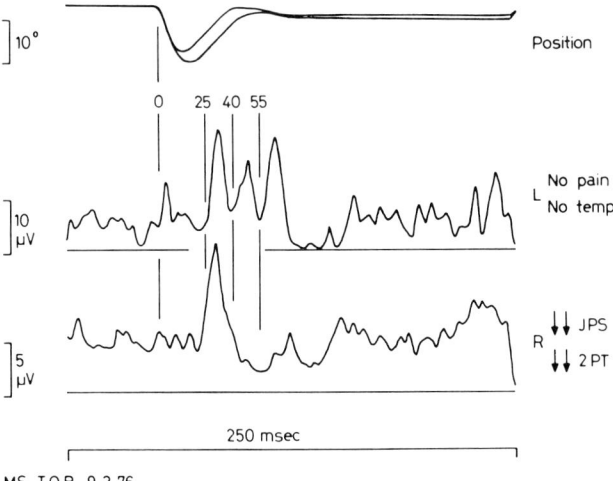

FIG. 21. Response to a fast brief stretch of the long thumb flexor in a patient with a lesion in the right brain stem (due to stroke), causing loss of pain and temperature sensation in the left arm and loss of appreciation of joint position, vibration, and tactile discrimination in the right arm, but no apparent motor deficit. The *upper records* show the angular position of the right and left thumbs. The *middle* and *lower* records show the full-wave rectified EMG recorded from flexor pollicis longus of the left and right hands. Subject held the thumb stationary against a standing force of 2 N. At time 0, indicated by the *vertical marker*, a force of 30 N was applied for 3 ms. Each *trace* is the average of 24 trials. In the EMG record from the left long thumb flexor there are clear responses at monosynaptic latency (25 ms), and later responses at 40 and 55 ms. In the record for the right long thumb flexor, the monosynaptic response is still evident, but the medium- and long-latency responses are not apparent. [From Marsden et al. (190).]

demonstrate that the segmentation of EMG responses into short-, medium-, and long-latency components is, in fact, attributable to spinal mechanisms. The finding does not exclude the possibility that the amplitudes of these waves are modulated by transcortical and other supraspinal loops. The previous findings of a disappearance of specific medium-latency components subsequent to various brain lesions appear to be attributable mainly to alterations in the central excitatory state of the spinal cord (213). In *Effect of Instructional Set*, p. 294, we review arguments suggesting that the supraspinal modulation of medium-latency EMG components, when present, has more to do with the generation of reaction-time movements than with motor servo actions.

Summary

The major autogenetic connections are summarized in Figure 18, which also reinforces the point that of the autogenetic reflex connections of muscle afferents (the solid lines) the monosynaptic are the best studied. This emphasis on monosynaptic connection is certainly an outcome of the technical difficulties associated with the study of interneurons and polysynaptic connections and has no bearing on the functional significance of interneuronal connections. The evidence supporting long-loop connections as components of the motor servo is reviewed and shown to be inconclusive at best.

SIMPLIFIED ANIMAL MODELS

A normal or near normal central excitatory state is one of the key requirements for productive studies of length and force control mechanisms. In other words motoneurons and interneurons in reflex pathways must receive appropriate tonic levels of background excitation and inhibition, since an absence or modification of this activity results in abnormal depression or an uncharacteristic enhancement of reflex transmission. A normal excitatory state is insured in studies of intact subjects, but the responses obtained may represent a complex hierarchy of control actions. For example, presumed motor servo actions may be contaminated by reaction-time movements, as discussed in *Effect of Instructional Set*, p. 294. Furthermore surgical procedures that simplify the experimental system are nearly always required to identify the afferent sources and specific neuronal pathways that mediate the observed responses. Because of these conflicting requirements, we must judiciously synthesize the results from intact subjects and from subjects in which transections and ablations have been used to create simplified experimental systems. This section reviews the characteristic features of two simplified systems that have been particularly useful in studies of the motor servo.

Decerebrate Preparation

The discovery of many basic motor reflexes and the analysis of their neural mechanisms has depended critically on several fortunate properties of the decerebrate state. This state of the spinal cord and lower brain stem is produced by a transection through the mesencephalon (263) or by an interruption of the cerebral circulation (239). Upon recovery from the anesthetic, a typical decerebrate animal makes few spontaneous movements (other than breathing and sometimes stepping) yet is highly responsive to a variety of natural stimuli. The responses thus provoked are simple motor patterns that appear to represent fragments of the more complex behavioral acts of the intact animal, some of which are reestablished if the animal is maintained for the long term (12). The decerebrate animal usually shows a depressed responsiveness to nociceptive stimuli that allows the experimenter to undertake surgical maneuvers (limb dissection, laminectomy) essential in the analysis of mechanism, without greatly disrupting the reflexes under investigation. Another useful feature is the tonic activity of the extensor motoneurons (extensor rigidity), which mimics tonicity during standing. These combined features made possible the discovery and analysis of the stretch reflex by Liddell and Sherrington in 1924 (170).

The characteristic loss of spontaneous movements in the decerebrate is the combined result of an interruption of neural circuits through the brain above the lesion and a depression of neural circuits, such as the spinal locomotor network (see the chapter by Grillner in this *Handbook*) and brain stem postural network (see the chapter by Wilson and Peterson in this *Handbook*), below the lesion. The depression of nociceptive reflexes is attributable, at least in part, to a tonic inhibition of the flexor-reflex pathway mediated by enhanced tonic discharge conducted in the dorsal reticulospinal descending system (65). This tonic inhibition is thought to contribute to extensor rigidity by blocking inhibitory transmission from the FRA to extensor motoneurons [cf. Grillner (102); Fig. 19].

Many of the properties of the released extensor tonus are the same as those associated with normal postural contractions. In both cases the recruitment of motor units follows the size principle [(119); see the chapter by Henneman and Mendell in this *Handbook*]. Also the tonic discharge of skeletomotor neurons depends partly on excitatory input from spindle receptors that derives from tonic activity in fusimotor neurons and partly on direct input to α-motoneurons (201, 262, 283). In the decerebrate a major source of the combined α-γ-input descends in the vestibulospinal pathway (cf. ref. 105), presumably mimicking a postural motor command. This activity results from spontaneous discharge of Deiters' neurons (Fig. 19).

The levels of tonus are independent of potential modifications in the gain in each of the autogenetic reflex pathways. An enhanced sensitivity to tendon taps (hyperreflexia) is associated with the decerebrate state, but this measure does not adequately assess gain. Hyperreflexia is caused by a general increase in motoneuron excitability that probably reflects changes in bias rather than authentic modifications in gain. For example, if the motoneuron pool is biased closer to threshold, the same gain in the Ia pathway will result in a larger motor volley and tendon jerk.

The gain of length versus force feedback (138) and the relative gain in primary and secondary spindle receptor pathways (197) have been estimated in the decerebrate cat, but there are no comparable measures available for intact subjects. There is qualitative indication (48), however, that the gain of force feedback via tendon organs is probably higher in human subjects than in the decerebrate cat. It is also known (59, 126) that IPSPs mediated by Ib volleys are depressed in the decerebrate cat, in contrast with the spinal cat, but no comparable measures in intact subjects are available.

Spinal Preparation

Acutely spinalized animals lack the requisite excitatory state of interneuronal pathways for well-developed stretch reflexes due to the interruption of tonic descending activity caused by the transection (37, 203). For example, it is apparent from Figure 19 that a spinal transection would interrupt tonic excitation from Deiters' neurons and would also release the inhibition of extensor motoneurons due to any spontaneous activity in the flexor-reflex pathway. Recovery from this depressed state (spinal shock) is slow and incomplete. Although deep tendon reflexes may return after a period of minutes to hours, they represent only a partial manifestation of authentic stretch reflexes, a portion mediated predominantly by the monosynaptic Ia pathway. In spite of this, profitable studies of stretch reflexes have been conducted on chronically maintained spinal animals (234) and on acute spinal animals after the administration of certain pharmacological agents that reverse the depressed excitability associated with spinal shock. Agents that have been used successfully are 5-HTP [5-hydroxytryptophan; (4)] and L-dopa [L-dihydroxyphenylalanine; (88)]. Since these substances are precursors of transmitters in descending fibers but not in fibers of intrinsic spinal neurons or of dorsal root afferents, one can reasonably assume that their actions substitute (partially) for the removal of tonic descending activity caused by the cord transection.

The importance of the experiments with spinal animals is that they demonstrate the sufficiency of segmental pathways in the mediation of motor servo actions. But for convenience, most of the studies on functionally isolated muscles have been conducted in the decerebrate animal, under the likely assumption that the responses obtained are also mediated by segmental reflex pathways.

Summary

The decerebrate animal appears to be a good preparation for the study of motor servo function and mechanism. The extensor rigidity of this preparation may suffer from a depressed gain in the Ib pathway, but it has a normal order of motor unit recruitment and a coactivity of α- and γ-motoneurons that is one of the characteristic features of motor servo activity in intact subjects.

TONIC STRETCH REFLEX IN FUNCTIONALLY ISOLATED MUSCLES

Basic Features of the Stretch Reflex

Liddell and Sherrington (170) and Denny-Brown (49) developed the basic procedures still used today for studying the stretch reflex of functionally isolated muscles in decerebrate and spinal animals. An individual muscle, usually an extensor since rigidity is best developed in extensors, is functionally isolated by transecting all (or most) of the cutaneous and motor nerves in the experimental limb, sparing the nerve to the muscle under study. This leaves intact the autogenetic reflex pathways to and from the muscle. The muscle is then attached to a mechanical or electromechanical stretching device that is fitted with transducers for measuring the force and length of the muscle and sometimes velocity and acceleration. Usually muscle length is controlled, thus serving as the input variable, while force is monitored as the output variable. Electromyographic (EMG) activity can also be monitored to provide a measure of motor output. The system thus available for experimental study is that portion of the motor servo enclosed by dashed lines in Figure 1.

The outstanding property of this neuromuscular system is a graded resistance to length change that to a first approximation resembles the properties of a spring. Figure 22, which reproduces one of the original records from Liddell and Sherrington (170), illustrates this and other characteristic features of the stretch reflex. Throughout the 1-s period during which the stretch was applied (dotted trace labeled T), the developed force (trace M) increased in a springlike manner approximately in proportion to the amount of stretch. However, unlike the behavior of a purely elastic system, force decayed slightly while the muscle was held at the longer length. The maintained component of force in response to a maintained stretch is called the tonic stretch reflex.

The degree of adaptation (i.e., the amount of decay in force) depends on several factors. In the first place it varies considerably between preparations and becomes greatest (adaptation to zero active force) in animals that for other reasons are judged to be in poor condition. In addition, however, nearly all preparations show some degree of adaptation, which is simply an expression of dynamic properties analogous to those of a mechanical system consisting of a spring plus a dashpot or some other frictional element in parallel. Thus, if the muscle is stretched to the same

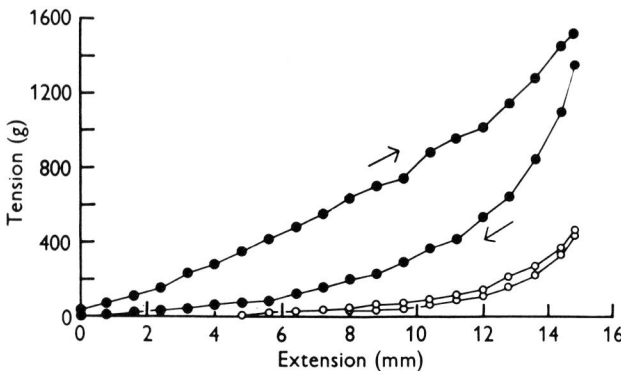

FIG. 23. Stretch reflex of the soleus muscle of decerebrate cat. *Upper curve* shows total tension during stretch at 1.7 mm/s. The stretch was maintained for 2 s before shortening muscle at the same velocity to obtain the descending curve. *Lower curves* show the passive tension obtained during stretch and release while the reflex was being inhibited. [From Matthews (193).]

length more rapidly, force rises more rapidly and to a higher value during stretch and correspondingly decays more at stretch plateau. Force typically decays to the same steady-state value independent of stretch velocity, as an expression of the static (or purely elastic) properties. Dynamic features of stretch reflexes will be given more detailed treatment in DYNAMIC RESPONSES TO MECHANICAL DISTURBANCES, p. 297.

The remaining trace in Figure 22 (the dashed trace labeled P) represents the passive component of the total force M. Liddell and Sherrington obtained it by applying the same stretch to the muscle after its nerve had been cut, and they interpreted the difference as a demonstration that a major component of the observed resistance is of reflex origin. Note that according to conventional terminology the term stretch reflex applies to the entire stretch response, even though its passive component is quite unrelated to reflex function. The difference between total force and its passive component is called the active component of the stretch reflex, which can be further broken down into an active muscle mechanical component and a neurally mediated component, as will be elaborated in *Mechanically and Neurally Mediated Components*, p. 285.

Static Force-Length Relations

A useful way of displaying the static properties of the motor servo is on a plot of force versus muscle length as illustrated in Figure 23, which is taken from an early study by Matthews (193). The muscle was stretched at a low velocity (→) to maximal physiological length, held at that length for a couple of seconds, and then shortened at the same low velocity (←). The closed points represent the total force, whereas the open points represent the passive forces observed during a stretch-release sequence applied to an inactive muscle. The fact that force (tension in Fig. 23) decayed slightly when the muscle was held at maximal length

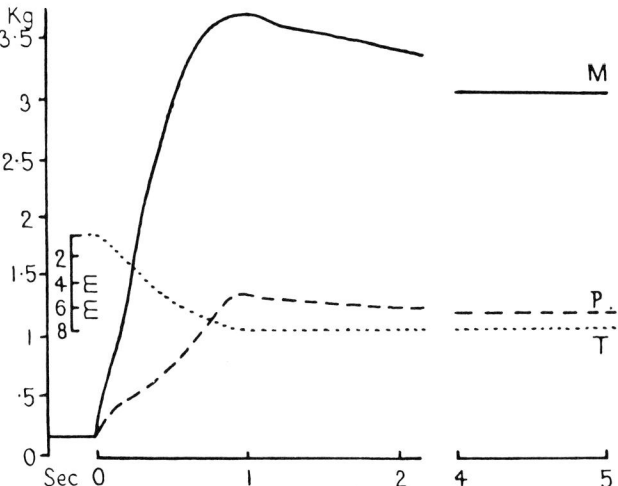

FIG. 22. Stretch reflex of quadriceps muscle of decerebrate cat. *Trace T* shows the time course of stretch, *M* shows the force produced in the muscle with autogenic reflexes intact, and *P* shows the passive muscle force produced after cutting the motor nerve. [From Liddell and Sherrington (170).]

and decreased along a lower curve when the muscle was shortened is again indicative of a dynamic component, in spite of the fact that the velocity was extremely slow (the stretch phase occurred over a 15-s time period). Although Figure 23 thus does not show the true static relation between force and length, one can imagine it as a curve located somewhere between the two curves showing response during slow stretch and slow release. In order to approximate more closely the truly static force-length relation, different amplitudes of stretch have been applied and maintained for 4–30 s (97, 225), at which time force has decayed to nearly its steady-state value. The heavy solid curve in Figure 24 shows a static relation obtained by Nichols (224) in a decerebrate cat that demonstrated strong rigidity.

Static force-length relations are usually approximately linear, although there may be a concave region near threshold and either saturation or upward curvature at longer lengths. Assuming an approximately linear relation, the slope of a straight line fit to the data will represent the static stiffness of the motor servo

$$f = K(x - x_0) \quad (22)$$

where f and x are muscle force and length, respectively, x_0 is the threshold of the stretch reflex, and K is the static stiffness. Equation 22 is a static, linear approximation to the more general expression for force-length relations considered earlier (Eq. 16).

For the soleus muscle of the cat, which has been most extensively studied, static stiffness may be as high as 3 N/mm (Newtons per millimeter; 1 N/mm is equivalent to 100 g·wt/mm). At the other extreme there may be essentially no static resistance to stretch. While zero stiffness is considered to be a sign of poor preparation, values in the range 0.2 to 0.5 N/mm are not uncommon (97, 150, 193). In contrast, the static stiffness of the cat's medial gastrocnemius is typically 2–3 N/mm and can be as high as 5 N/mm (45), but then the maximal force of this muscle is approximately 4 times greater than that of the soleus.

Normalized Stiffness

If values of static stiffness are to be compared between species or between different muscles in the same species, one should convert them to some normalized measure. Here it seems reasonable to express the force and length changes used to compute the slope of the force-length relation as fractions of the normal physiological ranges

$$K_n = \frac{\text{force change}}{\text{force range}} \bigg/ \frac{\text{length change}}{\text{length range}} \quad (23)$$

or

$$K_n = K \cdot \frac{\text{length range}}{\text{force range}} \quad (23a)$$

where K_n represents the normalized stiffness; a value of 1 would signify that stretching a muscle over its full range would result in a force modulation over its full range. For a cat soleus muscle the force range is 20–25 N and the length range is 25–30 mm. Thus, normalized stiffness ranges from 0.2 to 3 and a typical value in an animal with well-developed rigidity is in the vicinity of 1. For the cat gastrocnemius the force range is about 4 times greater whereas the length range is similar. This together with the absolute stiffness values given earlier yields a normalized stiffness in the vicinity of 0.7, only slightly less than that for soleus.

Mechanically and Neurally Mediated Components

The force-length curve of a tonic stretch reflex (Fig. 23) and the active length-tension curve of a muscle (Figs. 14 and 15) are similar in that both represent a springlike property that opposes stretch (97, 103, 193, 231). In addition, the slopes of the curves, which represent static stiffness, can be remarkably similar under certain selected conditions. Detailed comparisons using the soleus muscle in the decerebrate cat indicate that the stiffness of a typical tonic stretch reflex is approximately matched by the slope of the steepest portion of the length-tension curve of the stimulated muscle (103, 107, 225). In normalized units, the static stiffness of a fully recruited muscle can be as large as 2, although normalized stiffness is clearly less than this at nonoptimal initial lengths and stimulus rates (Fig. 15), and it decreases at lower levels of recruitment (Eq. 20). It seems clear that autogenetic reflexes do not greatly augment the stiffness of the motor servo over and above the stiffness that could be achieved by simply recruiting all of the motor units of a muscle.

It has also been shown (107, 240) that a level of spinal motor output capable of producing this maximal or near maximal muscular stiffness can occur spontaneously after the dorsal roots have been sectioned to eliminate the normal excitatory input from muscle spindles. The production of this high level of motor output without reflex involvement requires a strong central excitatory drive to the relevant motoneurons. Pompeiano (240) obtained the requisite excitation in forelimb motoneurons by combining a thoracic spinal transection to eliminate ascending inhibition with a traditional decerebration to produce descending excitation. Grillner and Udo (107) obtained it in lumbosacral motoneurons by decerebellation of decerebrate animals or by administering the excitatory pharmacological agent 5-HTP to spinal animals.

The former results demonstrate that a major portion of motor servo stiffness could be (but is not necessarily) of muscle mechanical, rather than neural, origin. However, electromyographic (EMG) recordings demonstrate that stretch and release do result in a prominent reflex modulation of motor output. This EMG response is monotonically related to muscle length and displays a distinct threshold (49, 97). The existence of a threshold value of muscle length below which the motoneuronal pool is quiescent suggests that rather different mechanisms are responsible for the production of motor servo force-length relations and muscle mechanical length-tension curves, even though the two often have the same exterior appearance. While muscle length-tension curves mimic motor servo curves by displaying an apparent threshold length below which the developed force is nearly zero (Fig. 15), this results from mechanical limitations rather than from the motoneuronal quiescence that characterizes actual motor servo performance. The modulation of the EMG observed above threshold is also contrary to a simple mechanical explanation, although the quantitative significance of this modulation requires evaluation.

Grillner and Udo (108) reported that a disproportionately large number of soleus motor units in the decerebrate are recruited during the first few millimeters of slow stretch beyond threshold, which led them to suggest that essentially the whole motor pool is recruited near threshold and muscle length-tension curves account for the stretch reflex beyond this point. An alternative interpretation of their data follows from the size principle (see the chapters by Burke and by Henneman and Mendell in this *Handbook*). The large number of units recruited near threshold are probably small ones, whereas the few recruited at longer lengths are probably large. The recruitment of a few large units at longer lengths could easily produce as much resistance as the recruitment of many small units of shorter lengths. The equation

$$f = F\left(\frac{n}{N}\right)^2 \qquad (24)$$

provides a quantitative expression for this phenomenon, called the recruitment nonlinearity, that was derived empirically from published motor unit data (138); f and n are force and the number of active motor units whereas F and N represent the maximal values of these variables. According to this expression, half of the motor units in the soleus pool should be recruited when the force is only 25% of maximum, which appears to be in accord with Grillner and Udo's (108) observations. A similar nonlinear relation between force and number of motor units applies to the medial gastrocnemius muscle (39) and to the triceps surae as a whole (see the chapter by Burke in this *Handbook*).

The difficult problem of deducing mechanical efficacy from electrical events can be circumvented if muscular and neural components are estimated myographically. Figure 24 shows an example of the results of a myographic analysis by Nichols (224), made possible by Grillner and Udo's (107) finding that all tonically active soleus motor units discharge at approximately 8 impulses/s in the decerebrate preparation. The heavy solid curve shows the static force-length relation of the intact motor servo, and the broken

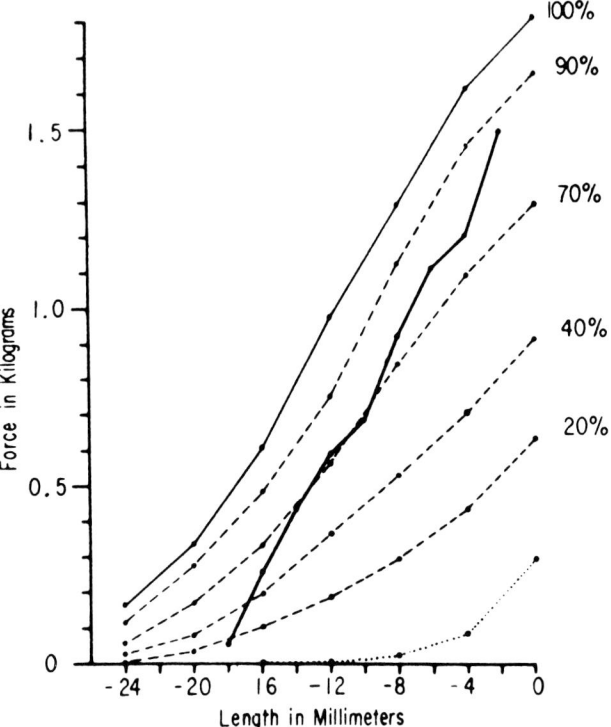

FIG. 24. Comparison of tonic stretch reflex with length-tension curves for the soleus muscle of decerebrate cat. The *heavy line* represents the static force-length relationship obtained by waiting 30 s for adaptation at each successive length. Other *curves* are length-tension curves obtained at the end of the experiment by stimulating different proportions of the cut ventral roots at 8 pulses/ s. The passive curve is *dotted*. [From Nichols (224).]

curves show the 8 impulses/s length-tension curves of the same muscle at different percentages of artificial recruitment. The mechanical component of the overall reflex can thus be gauged by comparing slopes at each point of intersection. It is apparent that mechanical stiffness was small near threshold and grew progressively to become approximately 50% of motor servo stiffness at the longest length studied, at which point approximately 90% of the muscle mass was recruited.

The results discussed in the previous paragraph support the proposal for a greater rate of motor unit recruitment near threshold. The example also shows that recruitment continues to be an important mechanism throughout the normal range of the reflex. What seems particularly remarkable is the relative constancy of overall reflex stiffness (the nearly constant slope of the heavy curve) as the origin of this property shifts gradually from a neural to a mechanical basis.

Actions of Control Signals on the Motor Servo

Electrophysiological studies have shown that pathways descending from the brain to the spinal cord have direct actions on α- and γ-motoneurons, as well as actions on interneurons in reflex pathways and on presynaptic terminals [cf. ref. (177)]. It is sometimes presumed that the interneuronal and presynaptic actions are particularly important in controlling reflex responsiveness and that movements, instead, are controlled by direct actions on motoneurons. Certainly, there is now good evidence that movement commands are sent to both skeletomotor and fusimotor neurons [(99); α-γ-*Relations*, p. 308.] and it is also clear that reflex transmission, as tested by electrophysiological techniques, can be altered by descending activity (see the chapter by Baldissera, Hultborn, and Illert in this *Handbook*). Changes in reflex transmission, however, only demonstrate the anatomical convergence of descending and reflex pathways; the normal actions of a descending input that converges on a reflex pathway might add to an ongoing input from the periphery and thus bias reflex threshold, rather than alter the gain of the reflex.

Studies in decerebrate animals in which control signals to the motor servo (cf. Fig. 1) are altered in a variety of ways have in most instances demonstrated a simple shift in the threshold of the force-length relation shown by the dashed curve in Figure 11, corresponding to a bias type of input, rather than a change in its slope as illustrated by the dotted curve in Figure 11, corresponding to gain control. Matthews (193) reported on the effects of activating synergistic, antagonistic, and crossed-extensor reflex pathways, and on the consequences of spontaneous variations in rigidity and the depression caused by a procaine paralysis of γ-fibers. The salient effect of each of these procedures was a shift of the force-length relation along the abscissa, i.e., an alteration in stretch reflex threshold with little change in the shape of the curve. Excitatory inputs lowered the threshold, whereas inhibitory inputs moved it to a longer muscle length. As shown in Figure 25, Fel'dman and Orlovsky (76) obtained the same result with tonic stimulation of descending pathways. Various excitatory and inhibitory combinations obtained by stimulating ipsilateral and contralateral Dieters' nucleus, the pyramidal tract, and the medial medullary reticular formation resulted simply in threshold changes. However, Kim and Partridge (157) reported that utricular nerve stimulation sometimes caused changes in shape (at low levels of central excitatory state) as well as shifts in the threshold. Even in these cases, the family of stretch-reflex curves was nonintersecting, which suggested that there was only one degree of freedom in the modulatory effect. In other words, there was no evidence that force and slope could be independently controlled.

The basic uniformity of these results is striking in view of the variable α- to γ-motoneuron contribution to the different simulated motor commands. Descending and crossed-extensor pathways are known to coactivate α- and γ-motoneurons, the synergistic and antagonistic pathways activate mainly α-motoneurons, and paralysis of the γ-motoneurons alters only the γ-

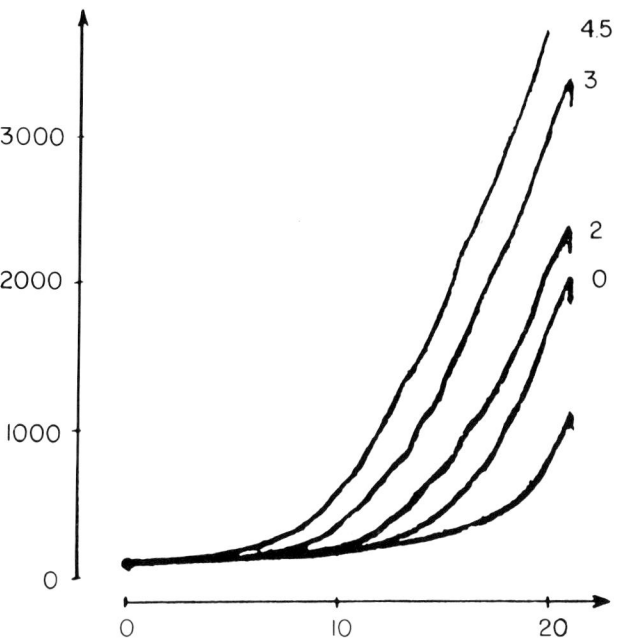

FIG. 25. Family of force-length relations obtained at different intensities of Deiters' nucleus stimulation. The ordinate is the force in g·wt and the abscissa is muscle extension in mm. Reflex force was registered while the muscle (gastrocnemius in decerebrate cat) was stretched slowly to its maximal physiological length. Deiters' nucleus stimulation at a fixed rate was delivered before and throughout the period of stretching, to mimic a constant level of central motor command. The numbers represent stimulus intensity (V) and the *unlabeled curve* is the response of the passive muscle. [From Fel'dman and Orlovski (76).]

signal. Apparently the static performance of the motor servo is rather independent of the α–γ-ratio.

More profound alterations in the slope or general shape of the force-length relation have also been described. Changes of this type sometimes characterize spontaneous variations in ridigity (97, 225), and they are regularly produced by spinal lesions of the dorsolateral columns that, as discussed earlier, convert a normal stretch reflex into a clasp-knife reflex. Such findings must be interpreted with caution, since they could be simply the result of pathological phenomena and play no role in normal motor servo function. This issue is better addressed in experiments with intact subjects (cf. subsection *Gain Variation vs. Gain Control*, p. 296).

Dependence of Incremental Stiffness on Initial Force

Often it is not feasible or practical to obtain complete force-length relations. Thus many investigators have studied the motor servo in terms of incremental responses to changes in muscle length applied about some initial length and initial level of reflex force. If the length changes are applied at a low velocity, or if they are maintained until a steady state is reached, the ratio of force change to length change provides a measure of static stiffness that can be compared with the slope of the static force-length relation, in analogy with the earlier discussion of incremental muscular stiffness.

It is apparent from an inspection of a family of typical force-length curves (Fig. 25) that the slope (representing stiffness) is not constant. Since the curves are generally nonintersecting, specification of an initial force and muscle length would be expected to define quite adequately the initial operating conditions for an incremental analysis. Furthermore the shapes of the different force-length curves in a family are quite similar, as if a single curve were simply translated along the abscissa. Correspondingly, one would expect that most of the variation in the stiffness determined from incremental measurements would be dependent on the initial force, with much less dependence on initial length. These expectations are well supported by a variety of studies with functionally isolated muscles (20, 76, 122, 138, 225, 226, 254). Typically one finds that incremental stiffness increases at low initial forces, flattens to become independent of initial force throughout a midrange, and may decrease once more at very high initial forces. This dependence on initial force is illustrated by the individual curves in Figure 26 for observations at each of several initial lengths. The basic similarity of the curves illustrates an absence of any major dependence on initial length.

Figure 27 compares several incremental stretch responses to illustrate the dependence of the reflex and its underlying mechanical component on the initial force. The mechanical component was small at low initial forces, due to the fact that only a few fibers were active, but with recruitment it grew to become approximately 3 N/mm, which represents essentially 100% of the total quasistatic reflex response estimated 1 s after ramp onset. In contrast with the simple proportionality between the mechanical component and the initial force, overall reflex stiffness rose steeply from a zero value when the reflex was modulated below threshold (not shown) to a high value at relatively low forces. It then remained stable at about 3 N/mm throughout the range illustrated, due to the fact that the neural component (indicated by the difference between R and M traces) decreased as the muscular component increased. The changes associated with the dynamic phase of the response are also intriguing, but discussion will be postponed until DYNAMIC RESPONSES TO MECHANICAL DISTURBANCES, p. 297.

Loop Gain of Force Feedback

The material presented to this point suggests that the contribution of muscle mechanical stiffness to the stretch reflex can be either large or small; it varies considerably depending on the initial conditions. Autogenetic reflexes appear to produce compensatory responses that reduce the dependence of overall reflex stiffness on initial muscle length and force. Although

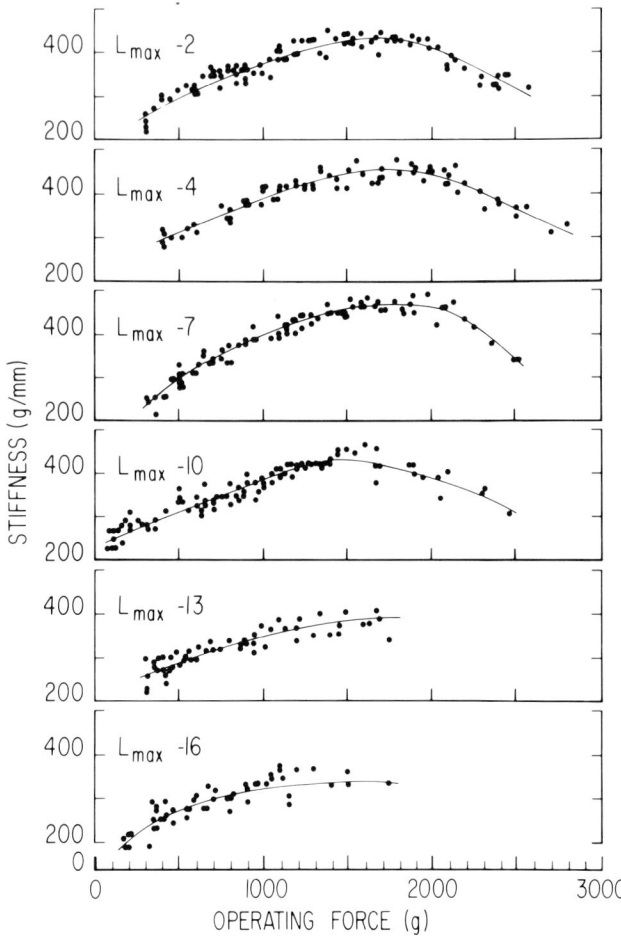

FIG. 26. Incremental stiffness of the stretch reflex in the decerebrate cat as a function of initial force and initial length. At each initial length the initial (or operating) force was modulated by eliciting a strong reflex, and stiffness was measured from responses to 1-mm pulses lasting 200 ms that were applied to the soleus muscle as force progressively decayed. Each *point* represents the incremental force-to-length ratio at the end of one pulse. [From Hoffer and Andreassen (122).]

these results support the hypothesis for stiffness regulation, they provide no information concerning the respective roles of spindle receptor and tendon organ pathways. A useful initial approach to this problem of partitioning regulatory actions between length and force-feedback pathways was developed by Houk and collaborators (138) on the basis of a linear analysis of the system. The simplified version of this analysis given here ignores the effects of tendon elasticity, although comment concerning these effects is made at an appropriate point.

An equation giving motor servo stiffness in terms of the three underlying components illustrated earlier in Figure 10 can be derived by substituting the expression for Δe in Equation 11 into Equation 13

$$\Delta f = K\Delta x + Ag_S\Delta x - Ag_T\Delta f \qquad (25)$$

$$\frac{\Delta f}{\Delta x} = \frac{K + Ag_S}{1 + Ag_T} \qquad (26)$$

where K is the mechanical stiffness of the muscle, Ag_S is the component of stiffness generated by length feedback from spindle receptors, and Ag_T is the dimensionless loop gain of force feedback. (The inclusion of series elasticity results in an additional component of force feedback produced by unloading of spindle receptors during contraction.) The attenuation factor $1/(1 + Ag_T)$ represents the inhibitory force-feedback component as shown in Figure 10.

Values of loop gain appreciably <1 clearly have no effect on overall stiffness ($\Delta f/\Delta x$), and it can also be shown that this is the condition for no beneficial effect aiding stiffness regulation. Assuming that Ag_T is ≪1, Equation 26 can be rewritten as

$$\frac{\Delta f}{\Delta x} = K + Ag_S \quad (27)$$

Thus with low loop gains, stiffness will simply be the sum of a mechanical component and a spindle feedback component.

At the other extreme, if the loop gain of force feedback were ≫1, Equation 26 could be written

$$\frac{\Delta f}{\Delta x} = \frac{K}{Ag_T} + \frac{g_S}{g_T} \quad (28)$$

Large values of loop gain would progressively reduce the dependence of motor servo stiffness on the mechanical stiffness (K/Ag_T would go to 0), leaving stiffness to be determined by the ratio of the gains in spindle and tendon organ pathways. This diminution of dependence on variations in mechanical stiffness could be an important mechanism for stiffness regulation. In view of these potential advantages, it is disappointing that measurements of the loop gain of force feedback in functionally isolated muscles have yielded rather low values.

Measurement of the loop gain of force feedback requires some way of injecting a disturbance within the force-feedback loop that goes from motoneurons to muscle to tendon organs back to motoneurons. It is also important to minimize spindle feedback effects either by keeping the muscle isometric or by using the same stretch amplitude for test and control observations. Houk and collaborators (138) held the cat soleus muscle isometric and studied the tendon organ pathway by stimulating small ventral root filaments to produce disturbance forces within the muscle. Loop gain, gauged from the extent of attenuation of the internal disturbance, was never greater than 1 and a typical value was 0.5. In a similar series of experiments Jack and Roberts (147) found values in the range 0–0.15. Rymer and Hasan (256) used dantrolene sodium to produce changes in soleus contractility that acted similarly as internal disturbances. The incremental EMG response to a standard test stretch was not significantly influenced by drug treatments that decreased contractility by 20%–65%, indicating that loop gain was negligibly small. Finally, Hoffer and Andreassen (122a) have used a stimulation-induced potentiation of soleus muscle contractility as an internal disturbance. They reported no appreciable attenuation of the potentiation by reflex action, which again suggests that loop gain is negligibly small in the functionally isolated soleus muscle of the decerebrate cat.

Although the gain of force feedback may very well be higher in other preparations, as discussed in SIMPLIFIED ANIMAL MODELS, p. 282, it would appear that the apparent regulation of stiffness observed in functionally isolated muscles is attributable by default to transmission through the spindle receptor pathway. Here it is important to note that linear feedback from spindle receptors cannot explain the compensatory effects. The component Ag_S in Equation 27 is a constant in a linear system and therefore cannot compensate for variations in K. This implication that nonlinear feedback from spindle receptors is an important mechanism in stiffness regulation is taken up again in *Compensation for Yielding*, p. 302.

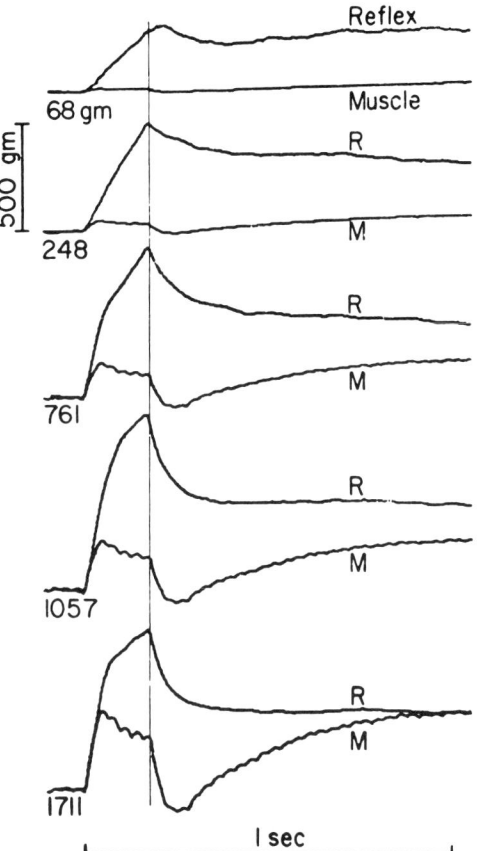

FIG. 27. Comparison of reflex and muscle mechanical responses at different levels of initial force. The input was a 2-mm ramp stretch applied at 12.5 mm/s to the soleus muscle. Initial force was modulated with a crossed-extension reflex to 5 different steady values in the case of the reflex responses. The muscle mechanical responses represent the force change recorded in an areflexive muscle that was electrically stimulated at 8 pulses/s. The mechanical response obtained was scaled (simulated recruitment) to watch the initial conditions. [From Nichols (225).]

Summary

The static properties of the motor servo are characterized by force-length curves that resemble muscle length-tension curves but are actually produced by a nonlinear pattern of motor unit recruitment. Many motor units are recruited as the muscle is first stretched past the threshold of the reflex, and most of the stiffness of the response in this region can be attributed to the neurally mediated component. At longer lengths, however, the mechanical stiffness of motor units that have already been recruited becomes progressively larger and tends to dominate the response at high force levels. The overall reflex stiffness is modestly dependent on initial force and relatively independent of muscle length. The fact that these appreciable dependencies are modest in comparison with the dependencies of muscle mechanical stiffness on initial force and length described in MUSCLE MECHANICAL STIFFNESS, p. 270, supports the hypothesis that autogenetic reflexes act to maintain the stiffness of the motor servo (*Stiffness Regulation*, p. 266). Since the loop gain of force feedback is small in functionally isolated muscles, the compensatory action must be attributed to nonlinear mechanisms in the spindle receptor pathway. The fact that the overall reflex stiffness is similar to and sometimes less than the stiffness of a maximally activated muscle is evidence against the length regulation hypothesis. If length were regulated, autogenetic reflexes should appreciably increase stiffness.

Experimental alterations in the control signals to the motor servo usually shift the threshold of the tonic stretch reflex without appreciably altering the slope (stiffness) of the force-length relation. In terms of the nomenclature introduced in *Adaptive Models*, p. 269, these effects resemble the actions of motor commands rather than adaptive controls, in support of the summary model described on p. 268.

STATIC REGULATORY CHARACTERISTICS IN INTACT SUBJECTS

Consideration of motor servo operations in intact subjects raises several new issues that were conveniently avoided in the previous section on functionally isolated muscles. These issues derive from the fact that muscles and their autogenetic regulatory loops are embedded within a complex motor system that engages in many control functions in addition to the local regulation of the length and force of individual muscles. Figure 28 summarizes some of the more basic features of added complexity, in this case arising from the mechanical and neural interactions between muscles that function as synergists or antagonists.

The mechanical linkage of the skeleton provides a mechanism for direct two-way interaction between muscles A and B (considered to be either synergists or antagonists), since both muscles apply forces on a common load and movement of the load affects the lengths of both muscles. Neural interaction arises from the projections of muscle proprioceptors onto synergistic and antagonistic motoneurons; these projections form closed feedback loops as a consequence of the mechanical linkages just mentioned. Since the signs of

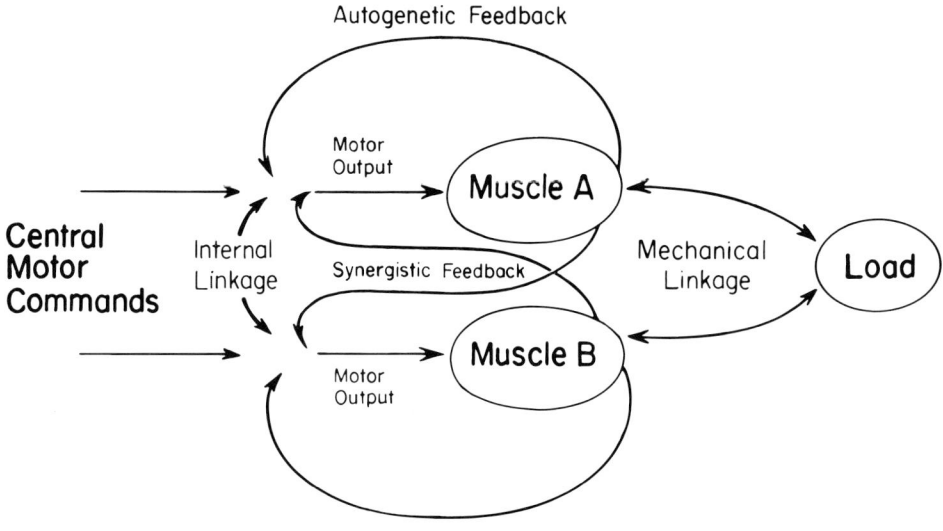

FIG. 28. Summary of relation between motor servos regulating contraction of single muscles (muscle A and muscle B) and their combined action as synergists. A given motor servo is represented by the *loop* that includes the muscle and its autogenetic feedback pathway. Factors that couple output from the two muscles are *1*) both muscles act on the same load, *2*) muscle afferent signals from one muscle are also distributed to the other muscle as synergistic feedback, *3*) connections between neural elements of each motor servo (internal linkage) may coordinate action between muscles, and *4*) central motor commands may be distributed to each motor servo.

the projections are the same as the signs of autogenetic projections for synergists and are in general opposite for antagonists [(58); see the chapter by Baldissera, Hultborn, and Illert in this *Handbook*], one would expect that the major effects would be to bolster the overall gain of length and force feedback as well as to facilitate spatial coordination among synergists, but these postulated functions have never been adequately evaluated. The internal linkages, such as the ones provided by Renshaw and Ia-interneurons (Baldissera, Hultborn, and Illert's chapter), provide additional channels for the coordination of muscle action about a joint.

Skeletal Mechanics and Coordinate Systems

Muscles insert at different distances from the center of rotation of a joint and the effective lever arm also varies with joint angle. Consequently, the forces developed by individual muscles cannot simply be summed to obtain a resultant force representing the combined actions of several agonists and antagonists. Summation is valid, however, if the forces are converted to torques (also called mechanical moments), which are the products of force times the effective lever arm for each muscle. A torque can be thought of as a force that promotes rotation, rather than linear motion, and the resultant torque is the sum of the individual contributions of agonists minus those of antagonists. The corresponding measure of rotational position is the angle of the joint, and the value that this angle assumes determines the lengths of each of the muscles via trigonometric equations. The fact that there can be only one joint angle guarantees that the lengths of muscles acting about a joint cannot be controlled individually, but only as a group.

Rotational movements about a single joint are relatively easy to analyze, but they are somewhat unnatural. Even the simplest movements generally involve several joints in some synergistic pattern, and there is evidence to suggest that the brain may control these multijoint synergies as facilely as it controls the synergies about a single joint (19). Hence, some investigators have chosen to study motor servo actions and movement-reflex interactions associated with multijoint synergies, and, as is shown by the examples in this section, the results appear to be quite compatible with ones obtained from experiments on single joints. Examples are the studies of head rotation by Bizzi, Polit, and Morasso (26) and of pushing and pulling movements of the arm by Evarts and Tanji (70) and by Crago, Houk, and Hasan (48).

Steady-State Responses to Changes in Load Force

Most investigators of functionally isolated muscles have studied force responses to imposed changes in muscle length as described in TONIC STRETCH REFLEX IN FUNCTIONALLY ISOLATED MUSCLES, p. 283, but investigators of stretch reflexes in intact subjects have more often chosen to study positional responses to changes in load force. Essentially the same information can be obtained with either approach, although the analysis of responses to force change is somewhat more complex due to the involvement of a mechanical load. As discussed earlier (*Summary Model*, p. 268), a mechanical load typically consists of both load properties and a load force (Figs. 1 and 12). In the simplest case the load properties are the inertia of the limb (or limb plus apparatus) and the load force is the result of gravity plus the force applied by the apparatus. The input consists of a change in load force, which, when applied to the inertial property of the load, causes an acceleration that progressively stretches the muscles and elicits a stretch reflex. A nontrivial problem addressed later (*Effect of Instructional Set*, p. 294) is that of insuring that subjects do not complicate their stretch reflexes by producing reaction-time movements.

Figure 29 shows the results obtained from the elbow musculature of two subjects using the protocol just outlined. The dashed step functions show the input changes in load force (positive forces tend to extend the arm) and the solid traces show, respectively, the arm forces resisting elbow extension, arm displacements, and the EMG responses of the biceps. Increases in load force accelerated the inertial load away from the subject, which elicited a stretch reflex in biceps. Decreases in load force permitted an excess of force of the elbow muscles to accelerate the inertia toward the body, which elicited an unloading reflex in biceps. In both cases the movement continued until arm force settled to a value appropriate to counterbalance the new load force, and this defined a new equilibrium state. The behavior of the arm as a whole was basically springlike, since a larger load force displaced it away from the body, whereas a smaller force permitted the arm to recoil toward the body.

The connection between these responses and the force-length relationship of the motor servo is elaborated in Figure 30, which is a simple adaptation of Figure 11. Imagine that the whole arm is replaced by a single muscle and that the solid force-length curve in Figure 30 represents the tonic stretch reflex of this muscle. The curve describes the reflex force that would be produced at any given length, whereas the force actually developed depends on an interaction with the mechanical load. At the initial load force designated, the muscle will be stretched, or will shorten to, the length indicated by the filled point, since only at this length will the reflex force be equal and opposite to the initial load force, insuring an equilibrium state. The responses to increases in load force shown in Figure 29 are approximately represented by trajectory a in Figure 30, which shows a transition to a new equilibrium. The muscle is stretched to a longer length at which it develops a larger reflex force, appropriate to counterbalance the larger force of the final load.

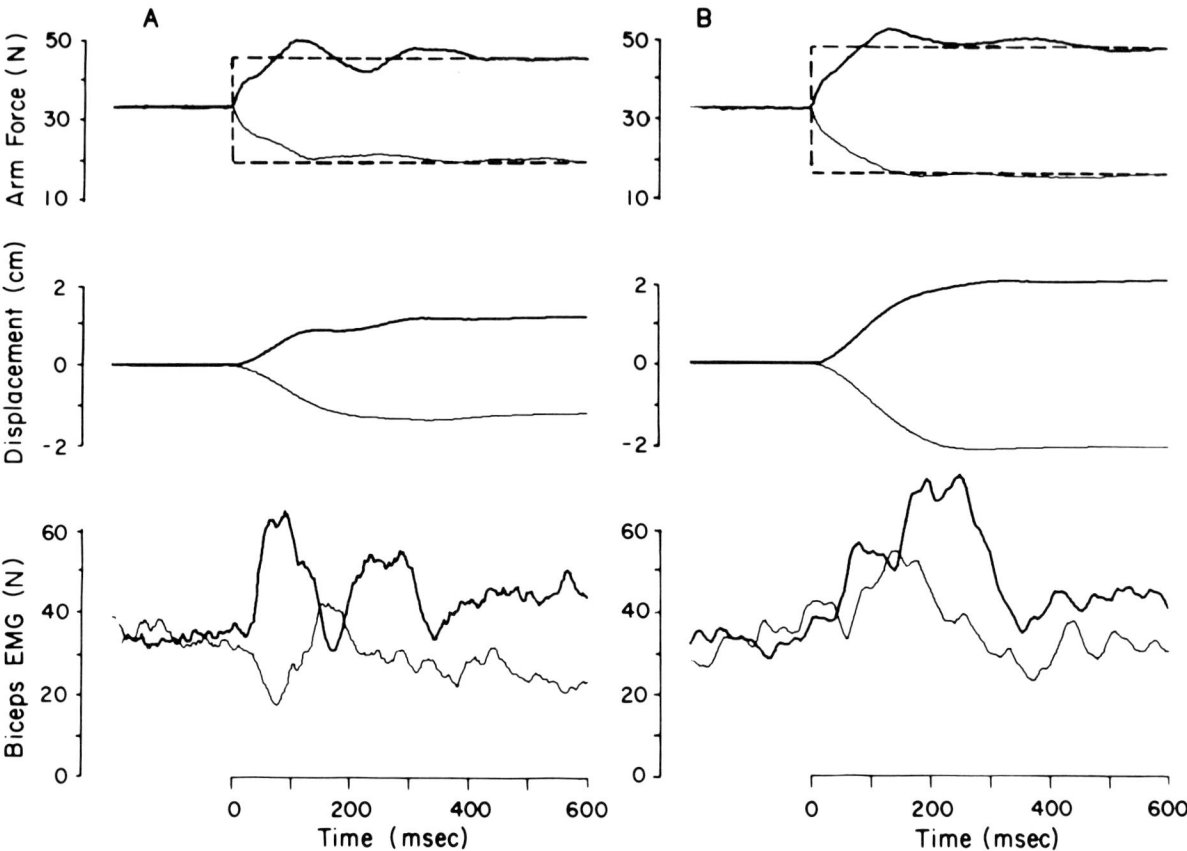

FIG. 29. Stretch and unloading reflexes in human arm. Symmetrical step increases or decreases in load force produce essentially symmetrical displacements of forearm, whereas biceps EMG responses are quite asymmetrical under these conditions. Step change in load force is depicted in *uppermost traces* as *dashed lines*, while resultant arm force, recorded by a load cell mounted within the apparatus, is a *continuous line. Heavy traces* represent responses to step increases in load force and *light traces* to equal but opposite decreases. EMG responses are full wave rectified and filtered (30 ms time constant) and calibrated in units of isometric force. Responses are ensemble averages taken from 2 different subjects using the no-intervention instruction (cf. Fig. 33). [From Crago, Houk, and Hasan (48).]

This example, though simplified, serves well to illustrate the interplay between the musculature and its mechanical load that determines the steady-state response to a change in load force. As such it provides a useful introduction to analogous interactions that have been characterized with torque-angle plots as described in the following section.

Torque-Angle Relations

Given that each of the motor servos regulating individual muscles acting about a joint is characterized by a force-length relation, the result of the combined regulations should be a torque-angle relation that serves to characterize the musculature of the joint as a whole (9, 72). The three solid curves in Figure 31 show a family of these torque-angle relations for the human elbow joint, analogous to the families of force-length curves described earlier. The positive slopes of the curves in both cases document a springlike restoring force. The particular joint angles at which torque is zero are analogous to the threshold lengths in Figure 25, and the modulating influence of central motor commands in both cases causes, to a first approximation, a simple shift of the curve along the abscissa. The negative torques are a new feature that results from the activity of antagonist muscles.

These curves were obtained by first having the subject establish one of three initial postures defined by the points $\alpha_6^{(1)}$, $\alpha_6^{(2)}$, or $\alpha_6^{(3)}$; in other words the subject had to flex the elbow against a load in order to achieve one of three joint angles corresponding to one of three different levels of central motor command. Then the load was abruptly reduced to one of several lower levels, which allowed the elbow to flex further (biceps unloaded). The subject was told not to intervene voluntarily in order to suppress reaction-time (secondary) movements (cf. *Effect of Instructional Set*, p. 294). Each of the open circles shows a new value of torque and angle to which the arm settled after being unloaded, and the solid curves through these points define the torque-angle relations that characterize the static properties of the elbow musculature under reflex control.

External loads can be characterized in terms of the static force or torque required to resist the load at each muscle length or position of the joint. For example, the line segments labeled a, b, and c in Figure 11 characterize the relation between force and length (Eq. 17) for an isometric load, a linear spring load, and a constant force load, respectively. Similarly the dashed curves in Figure 31 are a family of load lines that describe the elbow torque required to support different weights that were connected to the arm by way of pulleys. The required torque peaked at about 120° because the connecting cables were perpendicular to the arm, creating the greatest turning moment at this angle. Since the dashed curves represent the torque required at each angle and the solid curves described previously represent the torque actually produced by the musculature at each angle, a torque that is both required and available occurs only at joint angles corresponding to intersections of the relevant dashed and solid curves. Thus if the central motor command is at level (2) and the load is at level 3, the joint will settle to an angle of 110°, at which point the required and developed torque will both be 0.4 kg·m. This point of equilibrium, marked $\alpha_3^{(2)}$ in Figure 31, is stable, because at larger elbow angles the solid curve lies above the dashed curve insuring that the available torque will exceed the requirements for supporting the weight. Consequently the elbow will flex until the equilibrium between available and required torque is achieved.

Any change in load that occurs after the establishment of an initial equilibrium will cause a transition to a new equilibrium. Thus if the load in the previous example were increased to level 4, there would be a transition from $\alpha_3^{(2)}$ to the new equilibrium point $\alpha_4^{(2)}$. It is apparent from Figure 31 that this involves an extension of the elbow (stretch of the biceps muscle) and an increase in torque (due to a stretch reflex in biceps); the actual time course of motion would be like that shown by the stretch responses in Figure 29. In contrast, a reduction in load to level 2 would cause a transition from $\alpha_3^{(2)}$ to the new equilibrium point $\alpha_2^{(2)}$. In this case the elbow flexes (biceps shortens) and the torque decreases (due to an unloading reflex in biceps), which is similar to the unloading responses in Figure 29.

Equivalent Stiffness and the Concept of Composite Motor Servos

The former results indicate that a springlike resistance to stretch and release is a consistent property of neuromuscular systems ranging in complexity from single functionally isolated muscles (Figs. 22–25) to sets of several synergistic and antagonistic muscles operating to control joint rotation (Fig. 31) or even whole-arm movements (Fig. 29). In analogy with the stiffness of single-muscle systems, the rotational stiffness of the joint (change in torque divided by change in angle) or the overall stiffness of the arm (change in the pulling force of the arm divided by the change in distance between the shoulder joint and the hand) are appropriate and useful summary measures of static regulatory performance. These equivalent stiffnesses can be conceptualized as the result of replacing all of the active muscles by springs, representing individual motor servos. Correspondingly the overall system of muscles and proprioceptive feedback pathways can be thought of as a composite motor servo having qualitative features quite analogous to a functionally isolated muscle, though perhaps showing quantitative differences.

The data required for a complete synthesis of a composite motor servo in terms of the properties of its constituent motor servos is not presently available. Nevertheless, Fel'dman (72) has shown that the observed curvature of the torque-angle relations is well accounted for by the curvature of force-length relations seen in functionally isolated muscles when these curves are combined with the geometry of muscle attachment to the skeleton. Another type of comparison can be made by converting equivalent stiffness to a normalized value. The stiffness of the whole arm reported by Crago, Houk, and Hasan (48) was about 10 N/cm, which when multiplied by the length range (40 cm) and divided by the force range (500 N) yields a normalized stiffness of 0.9, which is within the range noted earlier for functionally isolated muscles in decerebrate cats. Although this apparent constancy of normalized stiffness may be fortuitous, it does seem

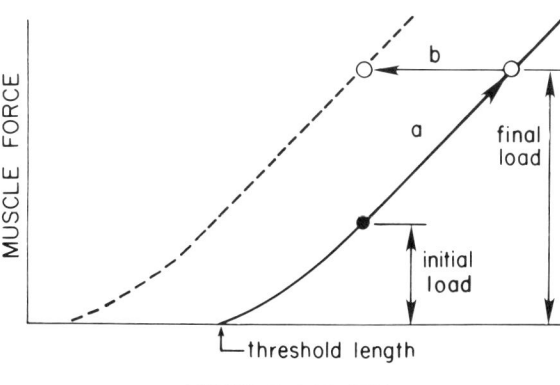

FIG. 30. Reflex (a) and reaction-time (b) components of response to a disturbance in force. Muscle length is determined by the interaction between the motor servo and the opposing load. ●, Initial equilibrium point, at which the force generated by the stretch reflex is equal and opposite to the initial load force. An increase in load force stretches the muscle along the force-length trajectory a, reaching a new equilibrium position (○), which is the point where final load is equal and opposite to stretch reflex force. The new equilibrium has been achieved at the expense of a significant length increase. The final load can be supported at the same length if the force-length relation is shifted to reach the position shown by *dashed line*. This shift may appear as a reaction-time movement causing shortening along trajectory b.

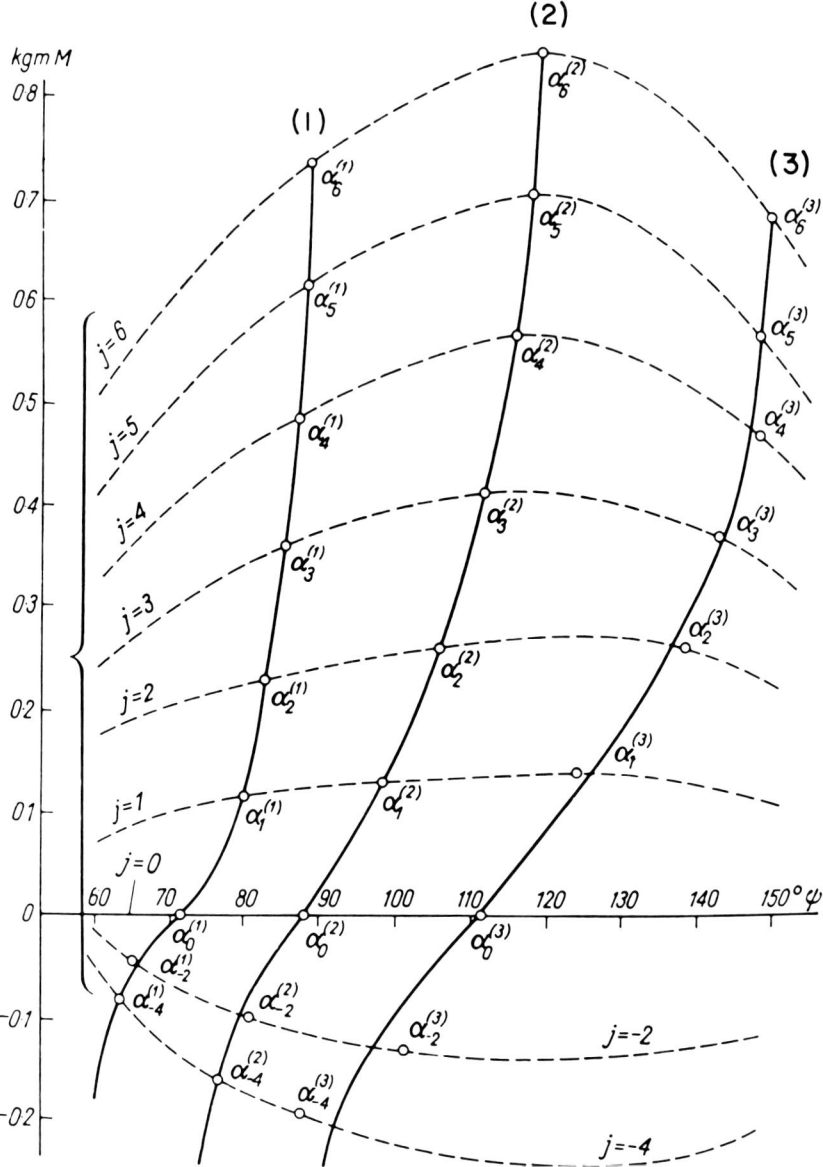

FIG. 31. Torque-angle curves relating the total moment developed by muscles at the elbow joint to the static joint angle, recorded following a series of load changes. ○, Joint positions reached following the change in load. *Solid lines* connect the angles achieved following load changes introduced from particular initial angles $\alpha_6^{(1)}$, $\alpha_6^{(2)}$, and $\alpha_6^{(3)}$. *Dashed lines* describe the external moments produced by the corresponding loads. [Adapted from Asatryan and Fel'dman (9).]

appropriate that muscle systems specialized to exert large forces also are endowed with a correspondingly large stiffness.

Effect of Instructional Set

The particular instructions given to the subject have an important influence on the responses obtained when a mechanical disturbance is applied to the limb or joint. An example of these effects of instructional set is shown in Figure 32, which is taken from a study of thumb responses to step increases in load force (191). In each of the three cases the initial effect of the change in load force was the same—an extension of the thumb and a medium-latency EMG response in the stretched flexor pollicis longus muscle. At latencies longer than 117 ms the responses differed considerably depending on the prior instructions given to the subject. The latency at which instruction-dependent differences in EMG responses occur can be longer than this and can also be as short as 50–60 ms (114, 128).

One obvious source of these instructional effects is the subject's "willful" reactions to the disturbance (variously called reaction-time movements, voluntary responses, intended responses, or triggered responses), and another potential source is a preset change in the

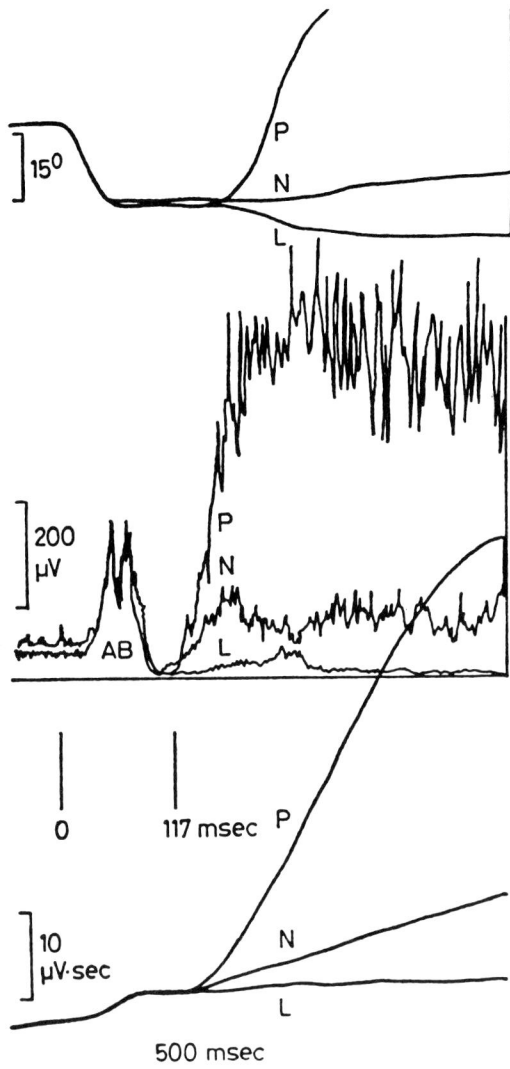

FIG. 32. The response to stretch of the long thumb flexor in human subjects depends upon prior instruction. At the outset, thumb is held flexed at 151°, supporting a force of 2 N, and it is then stretched abruptly at the point marked 0. Subject is instructed to either hold the thumb in a steady position (N), to relax (L), or to pull as hard as possible (P). The *upper records* show superimposed traces of angular position, the *center traces* show full wave rectified EMG (recorded from surface electrodes place over flexor pollicis longus), and the *lower traces* are fully integrated EMG records. [From Marsden et al. (191).]

sensitivity, or gain, of transmission through motor servo pathways. As discussed in *Adaptive Models*, p. 269, either or both mechanisms might contribute to the substantial adaptive capabilities of the motor system. It is important to distinguish between the two, since the underlying neural mechanisms are likely to be quite different. Furthermore there is the practical problem mentioned earlier that investigators studying the motor servo in intact subjects must be able to identify responses uncontaminated by reaction-time movements.

Hammond (114), who was one of the first to study these problems, reported no effects of instructional set on the short-latency responses of the human biceps muscle, but rather substantial effects on medium-latency and later components (using the terminology described in *Long-Loop Reflexes*, p. 280). Medium- and long-latency components were large when the subjects had been told to resist the disturbances and were sometimes completely inhibited when the subjects had been told to let go. Similar findings have been reported from several laboratories (48, 67–71, 93, 168, 191), although it should be noted that the instructional effects sometimes occur only in the long-latency components (as in Fig. 32). Some authors have reported that the short-latency component is also modulated by instructional set (67–70, 168), but these effects do not appear when the initial force of the limb is controlled. Variations in response associated with different initial forces probably result from system nonlinearities rather than from adaptive control mechanisms, as discussed in the following section.

The dependence of the medium-latency response on instructional set was originally interpreted as evidence for an adaptive gain-control mechanism (114). This conclusion was based on the assumption that reaction times are too slow to influence the amplitudes of medium-latency responses. By default the instructional effects on these components were attributed to adaptive changes in the gain of a length-feedback loop, and it was further postulated that gain control might be mediated by a transcortical servo loop (67, 236).

Distinguishing between a gain-control mechanism and a reaction-time process based on latency has two major disadvantages. One is that it relies heavily on a valid measure of a minimal reaction time and the other is that this approach is incapable of partitioning later components of response. Reaction times vary considerably with the modality and intensity of the stimulus and with several other parameters (see the chapters by Poulton and by Keele in this *Handbook*). The usual procedure in stretch-reflex studies has been to measure a reaction time to stimuli other than muscle stretch or to small tendon taps that provoke no appreciable reflex and to assume that the latency of a reaction in response to a large stretch would be no shorter (e.g. refs 114, 187, 206). Recent experiments in which alternative criteria were used to identify reaction-time mechanisms have demonstrated shorter latencies (48, 68), ones that in some cases are sufficiently fast to modulate the amplitude of medium-latency EMG responses (128). One of these alternative approaches is particularly well suited to partitioning the overall response into motor servo and reaction-time components, as illustrated in Figure 33.

This figure shows, for each of two subjects, six superimposed arm position responses to a standard step increase in load force, obtained with two different instructional sets. Simple, consistent, springlike responses were obtained with the no-intervention instruction, whereas more complex and more variable

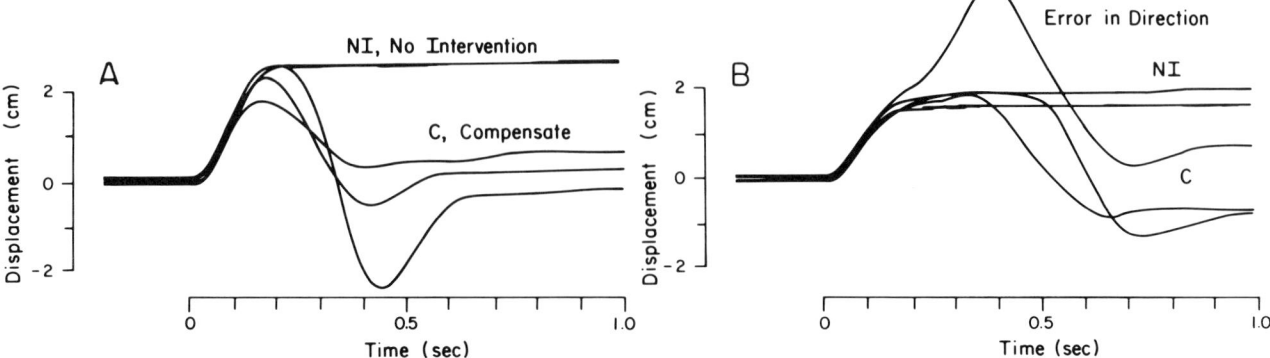

FIG. 33. Features of reaction-time movements of the arm, initiated in response to step change in load force. Force change occurs at time zero. The subject is told either to compensate (C) or "do not intervene voluntarily" (NI). In the latter case, both subjects (A, B) produced simple springlike response (NI *traces*). When the subject attempts to compensate for the perturbation (C), the initial trajectory is similar to that of NI but deviates at a point whose latency varies from trial to trial and with increasing choice (compensate vs. do not intervene). *Upper trace* in B depicts an inappropriate response, obtained with the compensate instruction. Records are of single trials, following ±18 N load changes in A and ±15 N change in B. [From Crago, Houk, and Hasan (48).]

responses were obtained with instructions to compensate or resist. The latter responses depart from the common initial phases of arm deflection at points that have been identified as the onsets of reaction-time movements based on three criteria. One is the variability of this latency, which was deliberately accentuated in these trials by introducing stimulus uncertainty. Subjects did not know whether the impending disturbance would deflect their arms away from the body (as in the trials shown) or toward the body (not illustrated). A second criterion is a shortening of the latency of the instructional effect that can occur when stimulus uncertainty is eliminated by using a single direction of disturbance. A third criterion is the presence of occasional errors in the direction of the compensatory response (Fig. 33, *right panel*). Stimulus uncertainty creates a choice situation that can have marked effects on the performance of a reaction-time process, whereas one would not expect any change in the operation of a servo loop in which the gain has been preset to increase the rigidity of the arm. Thus the increased latency, the variability, and the errors in direction observed are all indicative of a reaction-time mechanism. The absence of any fixed-latency instructional effect argues against the hypothesis for gain control. It would appear that the most recent experiments by the Marsden group (255) also favor this conclusion.

The instruction "do not intervene voluntarily" was first introduced by Asatryan and Fel'dman in 1965 (9) as a method for getting subjects to refrain from producing reaction-time movements, leaving relatively pure motor servo responses. The variability comparisons discussed in the previous paragraph lend support to the validity of this procedure and hence to the validity of the assumption that the torque-angle relations discussed on p. 292 represent motor servo properties. Nevertheless, some subjects are reported to have considerable difficulty in suppressing the superimposed reaction-time components, which suggests considerable automaticity in the underlying neural process (48, 128). The thumb-position responses obtained with the instruction "hold firm" (trace N in Fig. 32) appear to represent relatively pure motor servo responses; they are simple, springlike deflections that appear to be analogous to the no-intervention responses in Figure 33. Without evidence to the contrary, it seems reasonable to accept low variability and springlike properties as being indicative of motor servo responses in intact subjects.

Gain Variation vs. Gain Control

The results reviewed in the previous section suggest that effects of instructional set previously thought to demonstrate gain control instead may be attributable to short-latency reaction-time movements. Although these data do not exclude gain change as a mode of adaptive control, this possibility becomes less likely. Here we review other results in which there are apparent changes in gain, and we discuss whether or not the observations constitute evidence for gain control.

Several authors have demonstrated that the short- and medium-latency EMG responses to a standard disturbance undergo regular variation as the initial force is altered (91–95, 185, 186). Furthermore it is apparent from Figure 31 that the rotational stiffness of the elbow (slope of torque-angle curve) varies with initial torque in much the same way as the static incremental stiffness of a functionally isolated muscle varies with initial force (*Dependence of Incremental Stiffness on Initial Force*, p. 287). These variations are due at least in part to two major nonlinearities, the proportionality between the mechanical component and initial force (*Natural Combinations of Recruitment and Rate Modulation*, p. 276) and the recruitment nonlinearity (*Mechanically and Neurally Mediated Components*, p. 285). Gain variations associated with built-in nonlinear properties such as these cannot be controlled in any independent fashion and therefore do not constitute mechanisms for gain control. As discussed in *Adaptive Models*, p. 269, the adaptive control of gain requires a mechanism for adjusting gain independently of the central motor command that controls stretch reflex threshold. It follows that one should be able to demonstrate changes in stiffness while holding the initial mechanical conditions constant.

Changes in stiffness have been reported to occur without any change in the net initial torque or force of the limb in association with cocontraction of agonists and antagonists. Asatryan and Fel'dman (9) found that cocontraction increased the slopes of torque-angle curves in the vicinity of the zero net torque points, whereas the curves were not appreciably altered for torque values above about 10% of maximum. These changes can be accounted for by assuming that cocontraction is produced by adjusting the reflex thresholds of both agonists and antagonists to shorter muscle lengths, without altering the stiffness relations for either muscle group (72). Crago, Houk, and Hasan (48) reported that most subjects were not very effective at cocontracting when the arm was initially loaded with 10% maximal force. For those who succeeded, the stiffness of the arm was approximately doubled, apparently as a mechanical consequence of cocontraction, for the EMG changes observed during test stretch reflexes were not appreciably altered. These various results indicate that a limited degree of adaptive control over limb stiffness can be achieved by the mechanism of cocontraction. This mechanism is particularly important at low levels of initial force (i.e., in initially unloaded limbs).

There are many reports in the literature describing apparent changes in gain when stretch reflexes are elicited in initially inactive limbs. While it is true that the initial force is kept constant at zero in these cases, the inactive state fails to control the initial bias of the motoneuron pool. An identical afferent input can be expected to produce a larger response if the motor pool is biased near its threshold than if the pool is biased well below threshold, as would be the case in a totally relaxed state. Such effects may be important in preparing a subject for a transition from rest to activity, but they do not demonstrate an independent mechanism for gain control.

It is possible that gain-control mechanisms are activated subconsciously during appropriate postural tasks but are inaccessible to instructional set. Nashner (221) has described marked adaptive changes in the reflex responses to ankle rotation in free-standing subjects, but it is not certain whether these responses represent motor servo actions or triggered reactions (cf. ref. 94). The fact that the EMG activity occurs in fixed patterns of output to whole groups of leg muscles (222) is suggestive evidence for the involvement of a motor program, rather than a servoregulatory action.

Summary

The results reviewed in TONIC STRETCH REFLEX IN FUNCTIONALLY ISOLATED MUSCLES, p. 283, and in the present section suggest a great deal of similarity between the static properties of the motor servo in functionally isolated muscles and in muscle systems of intact subjects. In both cases the behavior is basically springlike, and control signals act mainly by altering the slack length of the equivalent spring, rather than by modifying the stiffness of the system. The major exception to this rule concerns the use of cocontraction to stiffen unloaded limbs in preparation for disturbances. Variations in motor servo gain occur in association with system nonlinearities, but there seem to be no clear examples to document gain control, which, in theory, could be an effective mechanism for modifying the rigidity of the limb. Although this negative result may simply reflect a failure to investigate appropriate situations, it does seem clear that this mode of adaptive control is not as prevalent as was once believed.

DYNAMIC RESPONSES TO MECHANICAL DISTURBANCES

In this section we describe the dynamic responses of the motor servo to imposed changes in muscle length and to changes in load, and we attempt to relate some of the characteristic features of these responses to specific afferent and efferent mechanisms. We show that some features derive from the response properties of muscle proprioceptors, whereas others relate more to muscle mechanical properties.

Dynamic Features of Force Development

As emphasized earlier, the increment in force produced by a muscle during a stretch reflex consists of a mechanical component, mediated by the mechanical properties of motor units that are initially active, and a reflex-action component, mediated by the recruitment of additional motor units and by increases in the discharge rates of units already recruited (cf. Eq. 13, and *Mechanically and Neurally Mediated Components*, p. 285). Recruitment and rate modulation represent the efferent mechanisms for the implementation of motor servo error signals. While we have discussed the mechanical responses to stretch and release in some detail (MUSCLE MECHANICAL STIFFNESS, p. 270), we have not yet given much attention to the effects of muscle mechanical properties on the translation of motor servo error signals into reflex action.

In many respects, muscle may be treated as a low-pass filter, which is to say that rapid fluctuations in the stimulus rate are smoothed and attenuated in the force output (see the chapter by Partridge and Benton in this *Handbook*). A clear example of this low-pass property is illustrated in Figure 13 in which the onset of a tetanic stimulus to the muscle nerve (which amounts to a step change in muscle excitation) induces a gradual and progressive increase in isometric muscle force. The time course of this smoothing effect is quite prolonged, since the final steady force may not be achieved until several hundred milliseconds after stimulus onset (depending upon the stimulus frequency). A comparable prolonged decline in force also follows stimulus cessation. These types of force prolongation would evidently smooth out fluctuations in motor output, but they must also limit the speed with which a motor servo correction can be executed.

In most published studies the low-pass properties of muscle have been quantified with frequency-response techniques, in which stimulus trains modulated over a wide range of sinusoidal frequencies are applied to motor axons, and the resultant force fluctuations are measured. To summarize some of the major results, when a train of stimulus pulses is subjected to sinusoidal rate modulation around a mean rate, the force output of the isometric muscle is also sinusoidal in time course, but peak-to-peak force modulation (which is a measure of system gain) declines steeply above a corner frequency (16, 66, 231, 242, 254). Similar findings were reported by Mannard and Stein (184) using a stimulus train whose rate was modulated by a random noise signal. The corner frequency varied among different muscles but lay in the range of 2-7 Hz in all cases. The results of these various frequency-response studies strongly support the low-pass filter analogy and show that the relation between isometric force change and stimulus input is well fitted by a linear second-order model whose properties may be defined by a low-frequency gain, natural frequency, and damping parameters (184). For the plantaris nerve-muscle preparation, typical values were: low-frequency gain 63 g·impulse^{-1}·s, natural frequency 5.0 Hz, and damping ratio 1.0.

Although the predictions provided by the linear models of isometric contraction are often close to the recorded force measurements, significant deviations from linearity do arise, particularly in response to high-frequency stimulus components. For example, very closely spaced stimuli, called doublets, give rise to unpredicted and sustained increases in isometric force. This phenomenon has been termed the catch property (289), and it is found in both mammalian (36, 109) and invertebrate muscle systems (289). Furthermore the relation between tetanic force and stimulus rate is not well fitted by any second-order linear model (233); during tetanic stimulation the magnitude of the force increase predicted by available models is considerably greater than that recorded under experimental conditions. In addition, the frequency-response function can also be shown to depend on the mean stimulus rate (184) and on absolute muscle length (248, 254), which is indicative of nonlinear behavior.

All of the latter studies deal with responses of isometric muscle, whereas, under most physiologically relevant conditions, changes in motoneuronal output arise in the course of ongoing variations in muscle length and tension. We have already described several important nonlinear features of the muscle response to lengthening; however, with some important exceptions [(232); cf. the chapter by Partridge and Benton in this *Handbook*], the response to joint variations in stimulus input and length has not been explored. Preliminary evidence indicates that one major nonlinearity, muscle yield, is minimized or even eliminated when muscle activation and stretch occur simultaneously (46, 47). In spite of the deficiencies of linear models (cited in previous paragraphs), a linear second-order transfer function for the stimulus-force relation remains a useful, if incomplete, description.

The low-pass features of the muscle response to neural input are not discernible in the reflex (242). When the functionally isolated muscle is subjected to sinusoidal length change, the rectified EMG shows a frequency-response curve in which gain rises rapidly above a corner frequency of 2 Hz. This EMG gain, which is analogous to that of a high-pass filter, counteracts the declining gain of muscle response to neural input at high frequency, so that the net gain remains essentially constant over much of the physiologically relevant frequency range. The high-pass feature of the EMG response appears to originate in the properties of muscle spindle receptors (242, 267).

Dependence of Transient Responses on Initial Force

In *Dependence of Incremental Stiffness on Initial Force*, p. 287, we reviewed the observation that the static incremental stiffness of the reflex response varies with the initial force level, rising at low initial forces, reaching an essentially stable value over much of the range of force modulation, and tapering off to somewhat lower values at near maximal forces (Fig. 26). It was pointed out that these variations are relatively minor in comparison with the approximately proportional dependence on initial force of the mechanical component. Figure 27 also displays broadly comparable changes in the *dynamic* incremental stiffness as the initial force is increased. When dynamic stiffness is measured at a constant point (ramp termination, for example), the stiffness is seen to increase with increasing initial force, being approximately 1.35 N/mm at the lowest initial force, then rising to a maximum of approximately 4 N/mm at an initial force of about 10.5 N. Even higher initial forces are associated with stable or falling stiffnesses, the latter resulting presumably from saturation of motor output mechanisms. These stiffness calculations also reveal that, although the increase in stiffness is substantial, it is not in proportion with initial force as would have been anticipated if the response were purely mechanical (cf. *Natural Combinations of Recruitment and Rate Modulation*, p. 276).

This difference between force and stiffness could result from a variety of factors. For example, as initial force rises, an increasing contribution from rate modulation of active motor units is to be expected, because the motor pool available for recruitment is progressively depleted; initial force increases resulting from rate modulation would not necessarily be associated with transient responses that scale with initial force, as was the case with recruitment. This relation between force and stiffness is as likely to be caused by nonlinearities in recruitment of new motor units, as by force-feedback contributions. These alternatives are evaluated at a later point; however, it is first necessary to further dissect the mechanical and reflex contributions to motor servo output.

To return to Figure 27, if we compare the total dynamic force output with the predicted muscle mechanical response, it becomes apparent that the mechanical contribution provides a greater and greater fraction of total force output as initial force is increased. In fact, the mechanical response provides the dominant contribution at the highest initial force level (1,711 g), contributing more than half the dynamic force increase, and essentially all of the static force. This increasing mechanical contribution is also accompanied by a progressive reduction in the magnitude of reflex action, which is probably responsible for the lack of scaling of the whole force response with initial force level. These data do not allow us to distinguish between reductions in reflex output arising from force feedback and reductions arising as a result of nonlinearities in the control of motor output.

The figure also shows that there are significant deviations in the time course of the reflex response that accompany increasing initial force. For example, the steepness of the initial rise in force increases at the higher force levels, but this region of high stiffness is then interrupted by a transition to a region of much lower stiffness. This two-phase dynamic response is most distinct at the highest initial force, as the mechanical component becomes more and more dominant. There are also interesting changes in the time course of postramp adaptation. The magnitude of adaptation is negligible at the lower force levels, but it becomes quite prominent at the highest force levels, presumably as a consequence of the larger adaptation in underlying muscle mechanical response.

In sum, it is evident that the stiffness of motor servo output is not constant in the face of changing initial force levels. The changes in stiffness appear to be relatively modest, however, and there are substantial regions of response in which changes in initial force induce negligible changes in stiffness. At the present time, the relative contributions of force feedback and output nonlinearities in this apparent stiffness regulation are unknown.

Amplitude Dependence and Linearity

In sections *Instantaneous Stiffness and Short-Range Elasticity*, p. 272, *Instantaneous Stiffness ... Region*, p. 274, and *Ramp Responses ... Nonlinearity*, p. 274, the stiffness of electrically stimulated muscle was shown to vary markedly with the amplitude, direction, and velocity of imposed length change. Comparison of these nonlinear properties with the dynamic response of muscle under reflex control illustrates that these dependencies are markedly reduced in the presence of reflex action. Figure 34 shows the response of normally innervated soleus to ramp stretches of varying amplitude, together with the predicted mechanical component. Stretch amplitudes varied from 0.2 mm to 3.4 mm, encompassing about 0.5%–10% of the maximum physiological range of movement, and were of fixed duration (160 ms). As in Figure 27, the predicted force output of that portion of the muscle that was active before the length change occurred (i.e., the muscle mechanical component) is superimposed on each reflex response. Estimates of the mechanical component were derived from measurements on electrically stimulated muscles, based on the assumptions that motor unit discharge rate was 8 pulses/s (107) and that increases in initial force resulted largely from activation of increasing fractions of the motoneuron pool. The accuracy of this approach to the prediction of muscle mechanical response is attested to by the superposition of the initial portions of the muscle and reflex responses.

A comparison of the reflex responses with the mechanical components reveals that the initial region of high stiffness in the reflex response extends smoothly beyond the point where yield would be expected to take place; no discontinuity is evident in the force records. This smooth force trajectory is not uniformly present in all responses, however. Under certain conditions such as very rapid stretch, very high initial force levels, or poorly functioning reflexes, discontinuities do appear on the force trace and these correspond quite closely in timing and magnitude with the predicted point of yield (226). These examples in which force discontinuities are detectable are useful because they provide strong evidence supporting the validity of the estimates of the underlying mechanical component of response.

In previous sections we have shown that motor servo action serves to minimize the dependence of responses to stretch on the initial force and length of muscle. Similarly, Figure 34 illustrates that in the presence of motor servo action the force change evoked during dynamic stretch or release is more closely proportional to the amplitude of length change than is the mechanical component. The relation be-

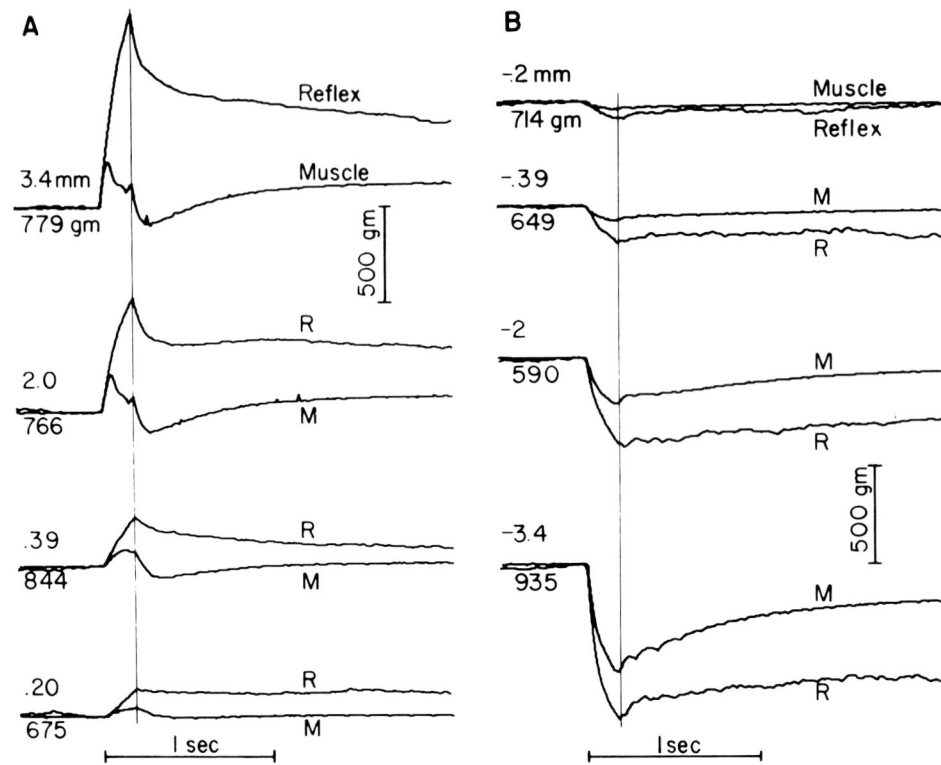

FIG. 34. Dependence of reflex (R) and mechanical (M) responses on the amplitude and direction of length change of soleus muscle in the decerebrate cat. Ramp changes in length had the same duration (160 ms) but were of differing amplitude. The amplitude of length change and the initial force are shown to the *left* of each record. The mechanical response (M) was derived from a different soleus muscle during stimulation of the ventral roots in a distributed manner at 8 pulses/s. Records in *A* represent responses to stretch, while those in *B* represent response to symmetrical release. [From Nichols and Houk (226).]

tween dynamic force and length becomes generally springlike, in that there is a roughly proportionate increase in force with increasing stretch amplitude. This relative constancy of stiffness is especially noteworthy during the dynamic phase of stretch when the stiffness of the mechanical response shows a marked reduction. A more precise assessment, however, provided by plots of force increment versus length increment (226) reveals that the stiffness is not quite constant, but is greatest for small amplitudes of stretch and release and then decreases moderately for increasing amplitudes of length change. Stiffness is also greatest during the dynamic phase of movement and then declines somewhat following ramp termination, particularly after large stretches (compare force response to 0.2 mm and 3.4 mm stretch in Fig. 34). However, these amplitude- and time-dependent variations in stiffness are minor when compared with the variations in stiffness of the underlying mechanical response discussed in *Ramp Responses: Transient Properties and Nonlinearity*, p. 274.

An analysis of linearity similar to that described for muscle in *Ramp Responses ... Nonlinearity*, p. 274, has been used to demonstrate that the initial region of high dynamic stiffness extends for about 400–500 μm

(226). This is about 1%–2% of the physiological range, a value commensurate with the amplitude of short-range stiffness observed in active areflexive muscle. If stretch amplitude exceeds this value, the stiffness shows a progressive 3- to 4-fold reduction. Similar amplitude dependence was first reported by Matthews (97), who showed that the soleus reflex stiffness associated with step changes in length remained high for up to 0.4 mm of stretch. While the high stiffness in the dynamic phase is probably attributable to muscle mechanics, high stiffness in the period following length change must be attributed largely to reflex action, because the static mechanical contribution is insignificant for these amplitudes of stretch. The enhanced sensitivity of primary endings to small amplitude stretch is undoubtedly a factor, although it is noteworthy that the region of high stiffness exceeds the small signal region of primary endings by a considerable margin (see below in this section). A secondary ending effect on spinal motor output may also be involved. In sum, while the initial transient region of high stiffness seems to be due to the mechanical properties of muscle, the augmentation that persists during small amplitude stretch is undoubtedly of reflex origin.

The linearity and amplitude dependence of the reflex response have also been studied with sinusoidal perturbations of muscle length or force in functionally isolated cat muscles (21, 242, 254) and in intact limbs of human and animal subjects [(20, 86); the chapter by Rack in this *Handbook*]. For example, Goodwin and colleagues (86) applied sinusoidal length perturbations to jaw-closing muscles in the primate and observed much larger stiffnesses for small movements (100 μm peak to peak) than for large movements (500 μm) over a wide range of sinusoidal frequencies. These amplitude-dependent variations were shown to depend on motor servo action, because they were eliminated by electrolytic lesions of the muscle afferent projection pathways. Similar amplitude-dependent changes in stiffness of reflexively activated cat muscles were noted by Berthoz and co-workers (20) in the course of sinusoidal variations in load force. In contrast, in the study by Rosenthal and colleagues (254), also performed in hindlimb muscles of the decerebrate cat preparation, the stiffness of reflex response to sinusoidal length change did not show comparable amplitude dependence. The force variation remained linearly dependent on amplitude for peak-to-peak movements of almost 3 mm over a wide range of frequencies. The reason for this difference in amplitude dependence is not known.

Finally, it is of some interest that the linear response region of muscle spindle receptors is even smaller than that of contracting areflexive muscle. For spindle receptors, the linear region is defined as the amplitude of stretch within which discharge rate remains proportional to the amplitude of length change—in the case of soleus primary endings, this amplitude is approximately 100 μm (116, 117, 202). It appears, therefore, that the motor servo is able to combine several nonlinear elements to provide an improved range of linear behavior. Some ways in which such cascaded nonlinearities might interact to increase the range of linear response is discussed in the next sections.

Asymmetry of Motor Servo Response

Although the force output in functionally isolated muscles recorded during stretch and release of equal amplitude is rather symmetrical, the EMG response assessed under the same conditions turns out to be quite asymmetrical (226). The existence of asymmetrical EMG response can be predicted from the fact that reflex action, which is equal to the difference between the mechanical component of response and the total reflex force, is much larger during stretch than it is during release (Fig. 35A). The EMG asymmetry should be opposite to that of the underlying muscle mechanical response to produce the observed asymmetry of reflex action. Similar results have been obtained in studies of the elbow musculature in humans (48). The EMG responses of biceps (Fig. 29) show greater increases during stretch, when muscle yield should be prominent, than decreases during release, when muscle shows less drastic reductions in stiffness. In fact, part B of this illustration shows that in some subjects the EMG may even increase substantially during release. Leaving the issue of mechanism aside for the moment, it should be noted that this type of asymmetry is not appropriate for a length servomechanism. During externally imposed muscle shortening, a length servo might be expected to withdraw muscle excitation, since persistent or increasing muscle excitation would assist further muscle shortening, rather than the restoration of the muscle to its original length. The pattern of the asymmetry is much more appropriate for a mechanism regulating stiffness, in that the EMG change appears tailored to preserve the symmetry in the mechanical stiffness of muscle.

The physiological basis of this asymmetrical EMG response has been subjected to little direct study; however, several possible mechanisms warrant consideration. First, it is conceivable that asymmetry of the muscle mechanical response gives rise to differences in the force-feedback signal during stretch and release, which in turn might be responsible for asymmetrical features of the motor output. This mechanism, however, is probably not the source of asymmetry, because calculations based on the estimated loop gain of force feedback in the decerebrate cat predict less regulation than is actually observed (226). Nevertheless, it has been pointed out that the augmentation of EMG during release of the human arm (depicted in Fig. 29B) could be a consequence of reduced activity of tendon organs; and, if so, this would suggest that force feedback has a higher gain in intact subjects than in the decerebrate subject.

A second possibility is that the EMG asymmetry could result from asymmetrical spindle receptor responses to stretch and release of muscle. During stretch, the primary ending responds by producing a substantial dynamic response, while during release it will often cease firing. In other words, asymmetry could develop because the shortening spindle receptor might drop below threshold producing a lower bound saturation (or rectification). This saturation would be most prominent when initial discharge rate is low and when shortening velocities and shortening amplitudes are large. The introduction of substantial levels of γ-static and γ-dynamic activity should only exacerbate the asymmetry, because γ-dynamic activity selectively augments the primary ending response to stretch (139), whereas γ-static activity reduces the rate decrease during muscle shortening (139). The postulated asymmetrical features of primary ending responsiveness have been observed, as shown in Figure 35B. Comparison of the reflex responses in part A with the spindle receptor responses in B, makes the point that the asymmetry of reflex action and the asymmetry of primary endings are broadly comparable. The response of secondary endings under these conditions is much more symmetrical, even in the presence of con-

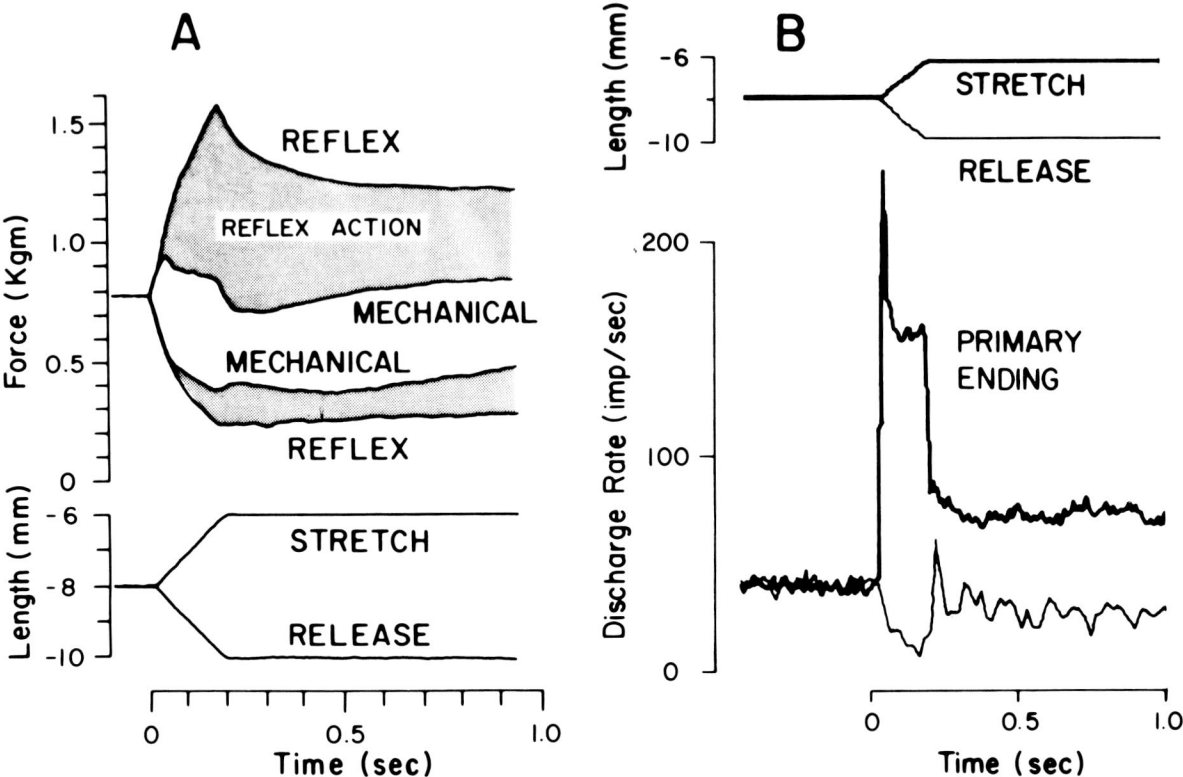

FIG. 35. Asymmetry of reflex action and its origin in primary endings. The response of soleus muscle in the decerebrate cat to stretch and release applied at 12.5 mm/s are compared in A. The responses labeled mechanical represent the changes in force that would occur if there were no reflexly generated changes in motor unit discharge or in the number of motor units recruited. Reflex action is the difference between the overall reflex and its mechanical component. *Part B* illustrates the response of primary spindle afferent, examined under closely comparable conditions. The greater reflex action associated with stretch, as contrasted with release, appears to be due mainly to the greater dynamic response of primary endings to stretch, as contrasted with release. [From Houk, Rymer, and Crago (137).]

siderable fusimotor drive (134), making them a less likely potential source of EMG asymmetry.

One should also consider the possibility that, due to nonlinearities or selective sensitivities, the tendon organ pathway operates in an asymmetric manner. Tendon organ discharge has been shown to provide an excellent sample of instantaneous total muscle force, with some dynamic sensitivity, during reflexively activated muscle contractions (133) and during locomotion (245). Tendon organ response to rising versus declining muscle force is also relatively symmetrical under both static and dynamic conditions, and there seems to be no evidence that the tendon organ is selectively responsive to the mechanical component of reflex responses (134). On present evidence, therefore, it seems unlikely that tendon organ receptors are an important source of EMG asymmetry.

While the asymmetry of the primary ending response to stretch and release is very likely to contribute to the asymmetry of the EMG, other mechanisms could also be important. For example, interneurons and motoneurons could also introduce a rectifying stage when they fall below threshold during phases of declining excitation. In those circumstances where spinal excitability is sufficient to prevent such a lower bound saturation, existing evidence indicates that spinal transmission is relatively linear (242, 287).

Compensation for Yielding

In *Stiffness Regulation*, p. 266, we described one possible scheme in which regulation of this property might arise as the result of linear feedback from receptors sensitive to length and force. This arrangement, which follows from the layout in Figure 1, is that of a linear force-length comparator, in which the values of muscle length and/or force are sensed and compared before an error signal can be computed. There are features of the transient responses, however, that are not well accounted for by the linear force-length comparator notion. One is that the magnitude of the asymmetry in reflex action discussed in the previous section is too large to be accounted for on the basis of linear feedback (226). A second discrepancy, discussed in this section, concerns the timing of the yield in relation to the latency of reflex action. It will be apparent from the data reviewed here that the compensatory signal begins too soon to be explained on the basis of an afferent detection of the onset of yield.

To consider the muscle yield first, the amplitude of stretch at which yield occurs increases with increasing stretch velocity; consequently, the time to yield does not decline simply in inverse proportion to stretch velocity. Recent measurements of the time to yield in the cat soleus (134) have shown that yield occurs at about 36 ms when stretch is applied at 10 mm/s, and it falls to about 18 ms for stretch velocities exceeding 30 mm/s. When the onset of reflex action is estimated from the point of departure between records of the reflex response and the underlying mechanical component, it is seen to be about 20 ms and to be largely independent of stretch velocity (134, 224). Under the same conditions, the onset of EMG change occurs approximatey 10 ms after stretch begins. In other words, the onset of the EMG response that appears to be responsible for yield compensation arises about 10 ms before the yield could have occurred.

The arguments concerning latency of compensatory responses become even more forceful if one attempts to allow for the times for excitation and propagation of signals from spindle receptors and tendon organs. These times were measured in the same series of experiments in which the latency of yield and of reflex action were estimated (134). Typical minimum values, estimated from onset of a rapid stretch (100 mm/s) were as follows: activation of primary endings 5 ms, secondary endings 7 ms, and tendon organs 5 ms (provided that the tendon organ in question was above threshold). The addition of afferent conduction time (2–4 ms), central (spinal) delays (1–3 ms), efferent conduction time (2–3 ms), neuromuscular transmission (1 ms), and excitation-contraction coupling (5–10 ms) means that a minimum loop delay of perhaps 20 ms must intervene before events sensed by muscle proprioceptors can result in a compensatory force change. Since reflex action can begin as early as 20 ms after stretch onset, if this compensatory signal is based on a simple force-length comparison, the yield would have had to occur at or near stretch onset. Instead, the yield is delayed by at least 18 ms.

These considerations suggest that some form of prediction is involved in yield compensation. Furthermore the mechanism cannot simply be the use of time derivative elements in the feedback pathways, since a prediction based on the rate of force or length change would be of limited value in anticipating the occurrence of an abrupt event like muscle yield. Instead one can attribute several of the predictive features of the motor servo to nonlinearities in the response properties of primary endings. Dynamic responses to stretch are large and those to release are small (i.e., the asymmetry shown in Fig. 35*B*); this is well matched to the probability that stretch will cause a failure in stiffness whereas release will not. Stretch responses rise rapidly to plateau values (differential sensitivity to small and large stretch), which insures a large, quick response that is well matched to the probability that there will soon be an abrupt failure in stiffness.

In the example shown in Figure 34 there is a close match between the time of yield and the onset of reflex action, but this it not always the case. At higher stretch velocities reflex action is delayed beyond the time of yield, whereas at lower velocities it may occur well in advance of yield (134, 226). Based on the kinematic data for cat locomotion reported by Goslow and colleagues (90), the 12.5-mm/s velocity in Figure 34 is intermediate within the physiological range. Although it is tempting to attribute this correspondence to evolutionary design, the idea is difficult to evaluate.

The latency of compensation depends on the length of the conduction pathway, which can vary appreciably between species and also between muscle groups in the same species (cf. ref. 187 for some values in humans). In contrast the latency of yield might not vary substantially if the percentage of length change associated with yield were an invariant feature (cf. *Instantaneous Stiffness and Short-Range Elasticity*, p. 272). However, one must also consider the extent to which relative stretch velocities vary with species size and with muscle group. The delay in yield associated with lower velocities in larger animals would help compensate for longer conduction times. On the other hand, more distal muscles are probably subjected to higher stretch velocities than more proximal ones, which would aggravate the problems associated with longer conduction pathways. One should not expect more than a rather rough match between time to yield and onset of reflex action. The low-pass filtering properties of the muscles and of inertial loads would tend to smooth out the deleterious effects of small discrepancies in timing.

It is apparent from the speculative nature of the previous discussion that more data comparing mechanical responses with reflex action would be helpful. What hinders this effort, particularly in experiments with intact subjects, is the difficulty in obtaining valid estimates of underlying mechanical components of response. One approach is to concentrate on force responses prior to the onset of reflex action, but even then the response is complicated by the presence of reaction forces associated with limb inertia and by onset oscillations in the stretching apparatus. The peculiar force transients at stretch onset reported previously (114, 206) undoubtedly contain inertial components, but they may also contain indications of muscle yield prior to reflex action. The force and EMG traces in Figure 36 show several phases associated with a subject using his arms to halt a free fall of his body. The subject was blindfolded and did not know when he would contact a supporting surface; thus the buildup of triceps EMG prior to contact (time zero) represents a programmed preparation of a postural

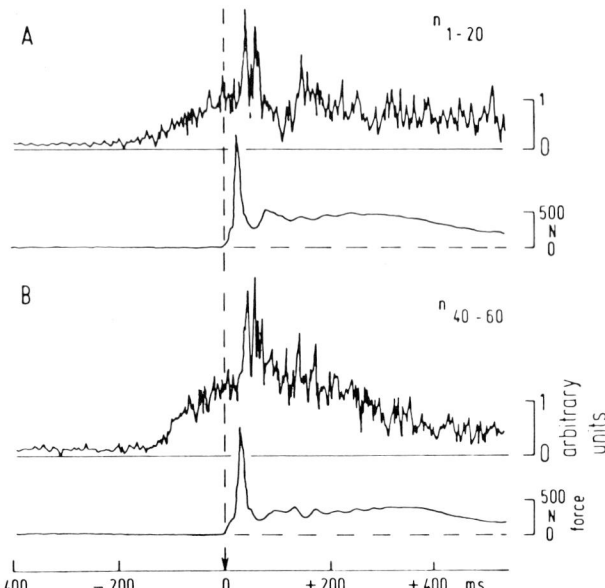

FIG. 36. EMG responses from left triceps brachii collected during a series of 60 falls, in which subject falls forward until movement is arrested by outstretched arms. Records are centered about the moment of impact. *Upper traces* in each panel are rectified EMG. *Lower traces* are of vertical force exerted against a platform. *Panel A* shows averaged responses to first 20 falls, *Panel B*, the response to the last 20 falls in the sequence. [From Dietz et al. (52).]

state. The rise in force after contact was gradual initially (finger and soft tissue contact) but became a sharp spike as the base of the hand impacted with the supporting surface. The spike undoubtedly contains an inertial reaction component, whereas the dip after this could conceiveably represent muscle yield. If so, the timing of the EMG response is appropriate to prevent the dip from continuing and to establish a plateau level of supporting force.

The previous results appear to provide a highly relevant example of yield compensation, but the complexities in the interpretation of intact subject data are also apparent. Recent efforts to separate out inertial, muscle mechanical, and reflexive components of force development and stiffness (5, 164) provide tentative support for yield compensation and also suggest that we will soon be able to make much better comparisons between the easily controlled results obtained with functionally isolated muscles and the highly practical results obtained with intact subjects.

Predictive Compensation: Feedforward vs. Nonlinear Feedback Viewpoints

The analysis provided in the previous section suggests that compensation for yielding represents the action of a predictive mechanism, since the compensatory EMG signal is generated before the time at which an error in stiffness actually occurs (i.e., in preparation for the yield). In a more conventional type of feedback regulator the compensatory signal would be produced by the error in stiffness and thus would occur only after the yield in muscle force had been detected by sensors such as tendon organs. The production of a compensatory signal in advance of the error is instead more typical of the actions of a feedforward regulator as discussed in *Feedback, Feedforward, and Adaptive Systems*, p. 260.

The reflex pathway from spindle receptors does in fact operate in a feedforward mode under the conditions imposed in most experimental studies of functionally isolated muscles. This is because muscle length is rigidly controlled by the stretching apparatus, which opens the length-feedback loop. Muscle force is not allowed to influence its own length as it normally does by its direct action on the mechanical load (Fig. 1). Thus under certain experimental conditions spindle receptors function as feedforward sensors, whereas under most natural conditions they function as feedback sensors. The predictive mechanism is likely operative in both cases. Correspondingly it seems unwise to use the feedforward nomenclature, since this would stress operation under restricted experimental conditions, rather than operation under more natural circumstances. Rather, it seems wiser to attribute the predictive aspects of motor servo performance to nonlinear feedback, resulting from the presence of nonlinear sensors (primary endings) in the length-feedback pathway. In addition, we would point out that the term predictive compensation is not wedded to either the feedforward or the feedback viewpoint.

Vibration and the Stretch Reflex

The marked sensitivity of spindle primary endings to tendon vibration has been utilized as a tool to investigate the central actions of primary and, indirectly, secondary spindle afferents. These studies depend upon two useful attributes of vibration. First, provided that vibration is of sufficient amplitude and frequency, virtually every primary ending in the muscle will be discharging at the vibration frequency. Second, vibration effectively clamps the discharge of primary endings, making them unresponsive to static length change and largely unresponsive to superimposed constant velocity stretch.

The relation between vibration frequency and Ia-afferent discharge can be used the estimate the gain of the Ia-projection. For example, Matthews (197) reported that the force output of the TVR, measured in the soleus muscle of the decerebrate cat, increased in proportion to vibration frequency over a range of about 50–300 Hz. If one presumes that all of the primary endings in the muscle were discharging at the vibration frequency, the slope of this relation between frequency and reflex force provides an estimate of net Ia effectiveness. Matthews reported slopes ranging from 1.5 to 8.5 g/Hz with a mean of 4 g/Hz. Expressed in terms of afferent discharge, these units become g· impulse^{-1}·s, measured over the total Ia-afferent population of the muscle. Broadly comparable estimates were also reported by Kanda and Rymer (1977).

These estimates can be used to calculate primary ending contributions to the stretch reflex. For example, if one assumes a mean positional sensitivity of the primary ending of 5 impulses·s^{-1}·mm^{-1} (97, 135), then the primary ending contribution to static reflex stiffness is probably no more than 20 g/mm (approximately 0.2 N/mm). The stiffnesses of the stretch reflexes were typically about 100 g/mm (measured in the same preparations). Based on these calculations and the assumption that the residual stiffness (here approximately 80 g/mm) was induced by secondary spindle afferent projections, Matthews suggests that the secondary input may be as much as four times more potent than that derived from primary endings. While there are a number of reasons why this approach may underestimate the magnitude of Ia effects [see Matthews (202) for analysis], the Ia contribution is quite unlikely to be sufficient to account for the stretch reflex.

The assumption that the mechanical response of the muscle was not a significant source of static stiffness (202) may not be entirely accurate, although it probably was not a source of large-scale error (cf. ref. 102). The problem of uncertain mechanical contribution was circumvented by Kanda and Rymer (154), who used changes in static length and vibration of one muscle (the medial gastrocnemius) to examine reflex output in a synergist (the lateral gastrocnemius). Estimates of primary and secondary effects calculated in this manner were closely comparable to those reported by Matthews (202), ranging from equal effect to five times greater secondary action.

The relative contributions of the reflex and mechanical components can also be compared readily by including an assessment of mechanical response in the analysis. Figure 37, derived from a study using the soleus muscle of the decerebrate cat (134), compares the stretch response superimposed upon an established TVR with the stretch reflex initiated from a comparable initial force. There is also included an estimate of the muscle mechanical response.

The superposition of reflex, vibration, and mechanical records highlights several important differences between the responses. Clearly the mechanical contribution to static force is negligible at the initial length used here, supporting Matthews contention that mechanical properties do not account for the (residual) stiffness previously described. Also, superimposed vibration has suppressed almost all of the initial dynamic force increase of the stretch reflex—in fact, the resulting force transient looks rather like the underlying muscle response. In spite of the rough similarity of muscle and reflex response in the initial phase, the later portion of the vibration response diverges sharply from the mechanical record and approaches the magnitude of the full stretch reflex. This latter divergence suggests that some additional source of excitation is being introduced by muscle stretch. Jack and Roberts (147) argued that such excitation may result from more secure entrainment of primary ending discharge

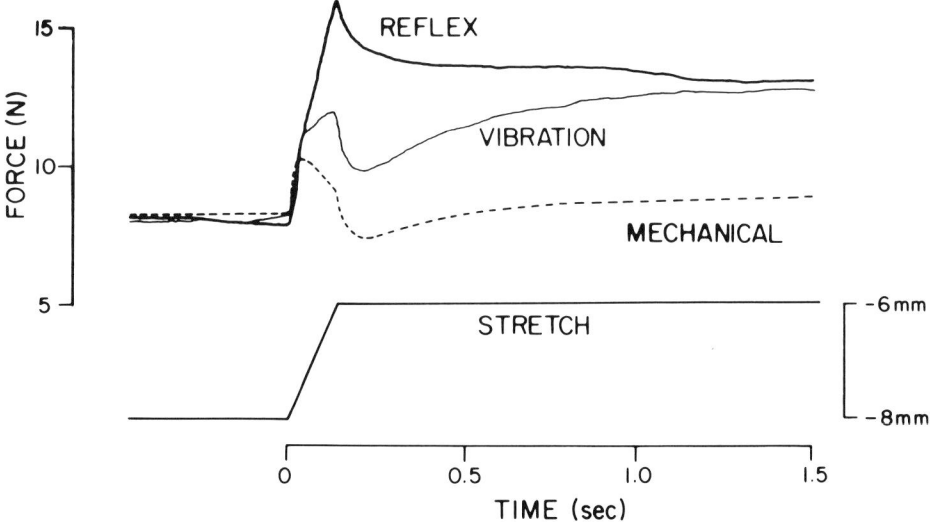

FIG. 37. Vibration of the soleus muscle in the decerebrate cat prevents reflex compensation for muscle yield. Longitudinal tendon vibration was used to block the stretch response of primary endings to demonstrate the importance of the dynamic response in the transient phase of stiffness regulation. The initial force of the normal reflex response was augmented to match that developed in the presence of vibration with a cross-extensor reflex. The difference between reflex and vibration *traces* is attributed mainly to primary endings, whereas the difference between vibration and mechanical *traces* is attributed mainly to secondary endings, although tendon organ inhibition may limit the magnitude of this component. Mechanical *trace* is an estimate, based on stretch of muscle stimulated electrically at 8 pulses/s via the ventral roots. Reflex and vibration responses are ensemble averages. [From Houk, Rymer, and Crago (137).]

at the longer muscle length; however, the relative similarity of the initial mechanical and vibration force transients indicates that practically all the primary endings were entrained at the initial length. The additional excitation induced by stretch was quite probably caused by the activation of some other stretch-sensitive receptor, such as the secondary endings. Moreover the close similarity of stretch reflex and vibration response indicates that this secondary ending contribution was probably very potent and may be largely responsible for the static stiffness. Finally, while the late increase in vibration response shown in Figure 37 was not always large in other preparations (134), it was almost always larger than the mechanical component, suggesting that a secondary contribution was uniformly present.

The experiment combining vibration and stretch also provides evidence supporting a predictive or anticipatory role for the primary ending in preventing muscle yield during stretch. Specifically Figure 37 also shows that vibration suppressed virtually all of the initial dynamic force increase in the stretch reflex leaving a residual force transient rather like the yield of the mechanical response. Recordings from spindle primary endings during vibration and stretch (134) reveal that the primary dynamic response is largely occluded by the vibration. Although the primary ending may respond with more than one impulse for each vibration cycle during large amplitude dynamic stretch (204), this effect is usually relatively modest. Vibration had virtually no effect on secondary endings, so these endings are unlikely to be involved; however, tendon organs often show variable force-dependent phase-locking of discharge (28). Augmented tendon organ discharge may have caused the reflex suppression; however, evidence cited earlier (*Loop Gain of Force Feedback*, p. 288) suggests that the central actions of Ib-afferents are modest in the decerebrate preparation. The yield in force during vibration more likely arises because the dynamic response of the primary ending has been essentially eliminated. Preservation of the dynamic response of the primary ending is associated with yield compensation, while an occlusion of the dynamic response allows yield to take place. Apparently the dynamic response is being used to compensate for yield in an anticipatory manner.

Velocity Dependence and Damping

To this point, we have emphasized the springlike behavior of the motor servo. However, given that muscles act upon substantial inertial loads, and given the existence of significant loop delays, the damping properties of motor servo action are likely to be important in preventing oscillation and instability. Oscillatory behavior in man-made mass-spring systems is often minimized by viscous damping, in which the damping element produces a restoring force proportional to movement velocity. This would require that dynamic force output of the motor servo exceed the static force and that the dynamic increase be proportional to movement velocity. With this analogy in mind, it is instructive to examine velocity sensitivity of the motor servo response.

The velocity sensitivity appears to be sharply different for small- versus large-amplitude movements. Small-amplitude responses have been examined using sinusoidal length changes, in which the frequency of the applied sinusoid can be equated broadly to the velocity of the ramp stretch. As we have described earlier in *Dynamic Features of Force Development*, p. 297, under these conditions the primary ending shows linear velocity dependence above a corner frequency of about 2 Hz; and this velocity dependence is apparently transmitted to the motor output without evident modification in frequency response. These features, which are analogous to those of a high-pass filter, are well matched to compensate for the low-pass features of muscle, resulting in a net flat frequency response relation (242). In sum, reflex force output shows essentially no dependence on velocity in the small-signal region.

For larger stretches, velocity sensitivity is most readily assessed by measuring the force produced at a particular amplitude of ramp stretch, over a wide range of stretch velocities. Figure 38, derived from a study performed on the functionally isolated soleus in the decerebrate cat (132), shows that the force increase that occurs with increasing stretch velocity is rather modest—a 100-fold increase in velocity is accompanied by less than a 2-fold increase in reflex muscle force. The force increases are largely confined to slow stretch velocities, less than 5 mm/s (226). Similar modest velocity dependence has been reported in a number of other studies on isolated animal muscles that used either constant velocity stretches (193, 270) or sinusoidal movements (150, 171, 252, 254). There is also comparable modest velocity dependence evident in the response of the human long thumb flexor to ramp stretch covering a wide range of velocities (257). In no case was the force increase simply proportional to the change in velocity.

When plotted on linear coordinates, the relation between force increment and velocity for the functionally isolated soleus is a negatively accelerating curve (226), which indicates that a power or logarithmic function might best fit the data. In a recent study of soleus reflex response to ramp stretch (136), the relation between the log of dynamic force increment and log of stretch velocity was shown to be well fitted by a straight line with a slope of 0.2. A straight-line relation on log-log coordinates implies that a power function (here with fractional exponent 0.2) would best describe the velocity dependence of motor servo output during constant velocity stretch. Similar exponent values were shown by plots of log EMG increment versus log velocity. Overall, the force increase recorded with increasing velocity is quite modest and

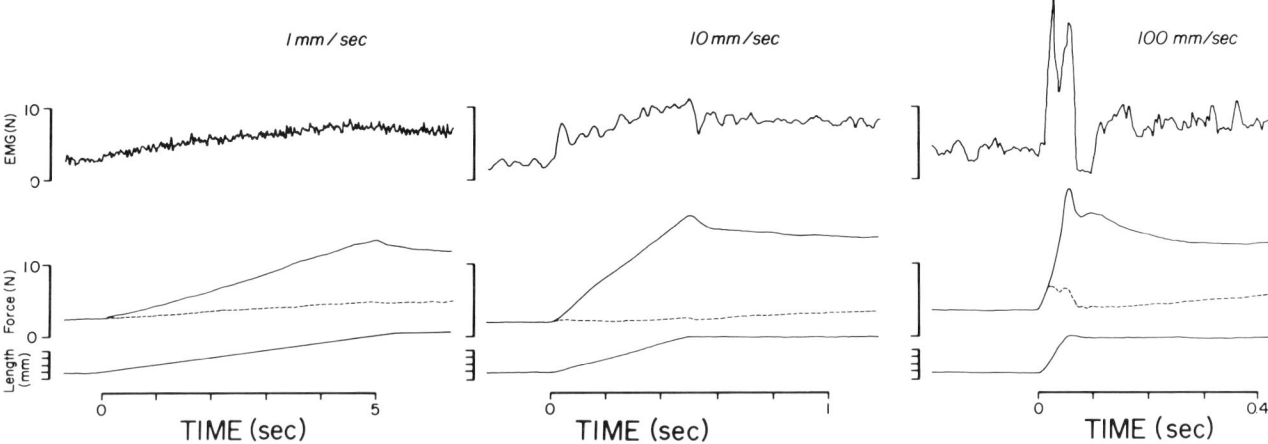

FIG. 38. Lack of dependence of EMG and force of the soleus on stretch velocity. Records show averaged response to 10 mm stretch, applied at three velocities, 1, 10, and 100 mm/s. Force output, measured at ramp end, shows approximately a 2-fold increase for a 100-fold increase in stretch velocity. EMG increment measured at the same point is slightly larger, but increase is still modest in comparison with increase in velocity. *Dashed traces* represent the mechanical responses. [From Houk (132).]

has a character quite different from that shown by a linear damping element.

There are a number of parallels between the velocity dependence of motor servo output and the velocity dependence of spindle receptors assessed during ramp stretch that suggest that spindle receptors are the major contributing mechanism. For example, when the increment in discharge of primary and secondary endings is measured at a constant stretch amplitude, over a wide range of stretch velocities, the relation between rate increment and velocity is linear on log-log coordinates, with slope of 0.2–0.4 (137, 258). In analogy with the discussion of the previous paragraph, this relation implies that the rate increment is a fractional power function of velocity. It is perhaps of further interest that the velocity exponents of primary and secondary endings are essentially comparable, which implies that either (or both) could be responsible for the velocity dependence of the motor output and that neither type of receptor, alone or in combination, would promote simple linear viscous damping.

While the lack of simple velocity dependence implies that the motor servo does not provide linear damping, there may be a tendency for damping effects to be more prevalent at low stretch velocities, where force increases more steeply with increasing velocity. This type of response is perhaps more akin to static friction than to viscosity, in that the response is sensitive to the presence of movement but not very sensitive to the particular velocity at which the movement takes place. While the functional advantage of a system showing such frictional properties remains to be determined, it would seem likely that this type of feedback would resist the onset of motion of inertial systems (when movement amplitudes and velocities are invariably small) but would be relatively unimportant for larger, more rapid movements.

Summary

Comparison of parametric dependencies of stretch reflexes with corresponding dynamic properties of areflexive muscle and muscle proprioceptors provides helpful insight concerning motor servo function. The dependence on initial force suggests that as force increases there is a progressive shift from a reflexive to a mechanical dominance. Dynamic incremental stiffness is less dependent on initial force than is the underlying muscle mechanical component, which is similar to the results for static stiffness discussed in *Dependence of Incremental Stiffness on Initial Force*, p. 287. Comparison of reflex and mechanical dependencies on amplitude demonstrates a marked improvement in linearity that results from reflex action. Nevertheless, reflexes may show 2–4 times greater stiffness for small stretches (about 1% of physiological range) than for larger ones. This difference is attributable to mechanical properties in the dynamic phase and probably to the differential sensitivity of primary endings in the static phase.

Comparison of responses to stretch versus release reveals marked asymmetry of reflex action. The greater increase in motor output during stretch (as contrasted with decrease during release) is attributable to a similar asymmetry in the dynamic responses of primary endings. Since the mechanical components show an opposite asymmetry, it appears that asymmetric reflex action serves as an important compensatory mechanism contributing to stiffness regulation. Reflex action begins too soon after stretch onset to be accounted for by a linear force-length comparator model. Instead, it is attributable to nonlinear sensor properties of primary endings. These properties result in predictive compensation, since they insure that a large reflex is initiated shortly after stretch onset. This reflex is effective in compensating for the yield in muscle mechanical force that does not occur until several milliseconds later.

The results obtained by using vibration to clamp and control primary ending discharge help to define the relative importance of primary and secondary endings. The large dynamic responses of primary endings are particularly important under dynamic conditions in maintaining motor servo stiffness during stretch. Responses of secondary endings probably are especially important in regulating static stiffness.

For small-amplitude stretches motor output shows a proportional dependence on velocity, which derives from the properties of spindle receptors and compensates for the low-pass characteristics of muscle. With intermediate to large stretch amplitudes, however, motor output and reflex force both show fractional power dependencies on velocity that derive from similar properties of spindle receptors and of areflexive muscle. This results in a frictionlike force opposing motion that may be advantageous in providing damping at low velocities without greatly slowing large and rapid movements.

IMPLEMENTATION OF MOVEMENT COMMANDS

To this point, we have concerned ourselves largely with the problem of motor servo regulation, which is to say that the reference signal for the motor servo is unchanging. Under these conditions, applied perturbations in load force or in position cause the system to traverse the characteristic force-length relations described in earlier sections. A rather different outcome arises if the reference signal is varied intentionally, in which case it is called a command signal. In this section, we describe how such variations in the reference signal give rise to changes in the locus of static and dynamic force-length curves. Depending on the characteristics of the load, these locus transitions usually induce a state of disequilibrium, which gives rise to movement.

Before we can consider precisely how variations in the command signal may give rise to movement, we must review the ways in which the motor commands are distributed to the key efferent elements—α-, β-, and γ-motoneurons. We also review the ways in which the afferent signals, especially those derived from spindle receptors, interact with and modify the discharge of motoneurons during movement.

α-γ-Relations

The efferent innervation of the muscle spindle has been described in detail in the chapter by Matthews in this *Handbook*. In this section, we focus on those aspects of the efferent innervation of extrafusal and intrafusal muscle that are most relevant to the movement control hypotheses discussed earlier (Figs. 7–9; see also *Spindle Receptors as . . . Detectors*, p. 265,

Conditional Feedback and Servo Assistance, p. 265, and *β-System and . . . Zero Sensitivity*, p. 266). Recordings from spindle receptor afferents during isometric contraction of human forearm (278–280, 282, 283) and leg muscles (29–32), from hindlimb muscle afferents during locomotion of the cat (104, 174, 246, 247, 262), and from jaw-closing muscles of the monkey (176) have shown that spindle afferent discharge rate increases with the onset of muscle activity. Simultaneous excitation of spindle receptor afferents and of muscle is also evident during slow shortening of flexor muscles in the cat hindlimb, (174, 246) and during slow shortening of human finger flexors (281). These findings have been uniformly interpreted as implying joint activation or coactivation of α- and γ-motoneurons (*Spindle Receptors as . . . Detectors*, p. 265).

In some studies coactivation has been associated with increases in spindle receptor discharge that parallel increasing force over a considerable range (32, 283). This covariation has been interpreted to imply that increases in fusimotor discharge rate and in fusimotor recruitment continue up to high levels of motor output. Moreover abrupt discontinuities in spindle afferent discharge (32), which occur over a range of force levels, have been attributed to recruitment of γ-motoneurons.

In contrast a number of studies report evidence that increased spindle afferent discharge and muscle contraction may not uniformly coexist. For example, spindle afferent discharge may decline or cease completely during shortening of cat jaw muscles (41) or of contracting hamstring muscles of the running cat preparation (174, 246). In the falling cat, spindle afferent discharge in hindlimb muscles may also decline without obvious external shortening of the active muscle (247). It has also been reported that the threshold for activation of spindle receptors in human pretibial muscles may be varied independently of changes in skeletomotor output (34).

There is also evidence that spindle receptors may be activated by efferent command in the absence of muscle excitation. For example, recordings in hindlimb muscles of the decerebrate cat (243, 260, 291) have shown that activation of muscle by the crossed extensor and other reflexes consistently gives rise to acceleration of spindle afferent discharge at stimulus intensities insufficient to activate α-motoneurons. Furthermore recordings from afferents in jaw-closing muscles of the monkey (176) and tranquilized cat (272) show that spindle afferent discharge characteristically increases before the onset of EMG activity. It follows that the lower threshold for activation of spindle afferent fibers (and therefore fusimotor neurons) may not depend upon the particular preparation, but it may simply be a consequence of differences in the experimental arrangement. Although joint excitation of spindle receptors and of muscle is common, it is not always the rule.

A number of major unresolved problems exist in relation to the control of intrafusal and extrafusal innervation. The first and perhaps the major problem concerns the complexity of the control mechanism. One proposition holds that the presence of independent innervation of α- and γ-motoneurons implies that functionally independent control mechanisms necessarily exist (34, 98) and that they are likely to be utilized in the course of movement control. This argument has been extended to include the proposition that static and dynamic fusiomotor neurons may also be subject to independent control. The alternative position is that the command signals to α- and γ-neurons are essentially coupled and that independent activation of these neuronal elements does not normally arise (cf. ref. 284). A second problem, largely unexplored at present, is that augmentation in spindle afferent discharge may not be due solely to γ-innervation—β-fibers cannot now be ignored. The role of β-fibers is addressed in the next section.

The argument for independent activation of α- and γ-motoneurons resides partly in the observation that, during some forms of movement, EMG activity may be present in a muscle from which no spindle afferent discharge is being recorded. Based on the cited examples it seems that these observations have often been made under circumstances in which the shortening velocity of the muscle was substantial and in which the effects of concurrent fusiomotor activation may have been overwhelmed by the rapid muscle shortening (244).

The other argument advanced in support of independent control of α- and γ-motoneurons depends upon the finding of spindle receptor activation in the absence of α-motoneuron activity. Here, increased spindle afferent discharge has been uniformly attributed to γ-fiber activation. While the spindle afferent recordings in humans do not show afferent rate increases without EMG activity (111, 112, 284), separate activation of muscle and spindle receptor afferents has been clearly demonstrated in animals, as described in earlier paragraphs. These findings suggest that the control of α- and γ-motoneurons may differ somewhat in human and animal subjects.

While it is conceivable that these results reflect fundamental differences in the patterns of activation of α- and γ-motoneurons, there are also differences in the experimental arrangement that may be at least partly responsible for the apparent differences in response. One difference is the magnitude of series compliance, especially that provided by the soft tissue present at the point of apposition of a limb with some measuring device. There is no comparable compliance in functionally isolated muscles, or in jaw muscle preparations, since the teeth form a noncompliant link. The practical outcome of this compliance is that during simultaneous and rapid excitation of α- and γ-motoneurons, the earlier onset of force in extrafusal muscle (which arises from more rapid conduction in skeletomotor axons) may limit the development of tension in intrafusal fibers by inducing internal muscle fiber shortening (260). This shortening will arise normally from lengthening of series elastic elements but is likely to be considerably augmented in the presence of a substantial soft tissue compliance.

It is evident that in contracting muscle the interaction between muscle and the muscle spindle is potentially quite complex. The problem of assessing fusimotor effects in spindle afferent responses recorded during muscular contraction can be circumvented by recording directly from γ-motoneurons in conscious, behaving animals. The technical difficulty of this exercise has limited the number of reported studies; however, during isometric contraction of jaw-closing muscles in monkey (176) and cat (272), the fusimotor neurons are activated without any measurable force and EMG activity. In view of these findings, the apparent similarity of threshold for activating α- and γ-motoneurons in human muscle may be related partly to the effects of series compliance and to the fact that voluntary activation of muscle in humans appears to induce a virtually simultaneous activation of α- and γ-motoneuron pools. While these factors may help explain the differing patterns of response, it is also possible that CNS control of γ-motoneurons is different in human muscles, a possibility that is supported by the rather low resting discharge rate recorded in human muscle spindle afferents.

The possibility of independent control of γ-static and γ-dynamic neurons may be questioned. While there is now strong evidence that electrical stimulation of different regions of the CNS appears to selectively excite γ-static and γ-dynamic neurons (cf. ref. 220), this finding does not automatically imply that these pathways are subject to independent control under physiologically relevant conditions. This is because many regions of the nervous system would normally be coactivated in the course of voluntary movement.

Positional Stiffness Deduced From Spindle Relations

In previous sections, the potential contribution of α- and γ-motoneuron excitation to motor output was discussed in relation to several models of motor servo action, such as the follow-up length servo arrangement of Merton (211) and the servo-assistance approach of Matthews (198). These models were derived largely without data on spindle afferent discharge or motor output in intact preparations. The availability of recordings from human nerves has provided descriptions of the quantitative relations between spindle receptor discharge rate and force in the same muscle, allowing these hypotheses to be investigated. For example, these relations have now been used to estimate the gain of a follow-up servo configuration in terms of the positional stiffness of the motor servo.

Using the finger flexors at the metacarpophalangeal

joint, Vallbo (283) estimated that the positional stiffness of a follow-up servo configuration was of the order of 0.03 Nm/deg. This stiffness calculation results in an upper bound since it is based on the assumption that the γ-motoneuron pathway is the sole source of command. Stiffness was calculated as the product of the positional sensitivity of spindle receptors (in pulses·$s^{-1}·deg^{-1}$) and the torque-rate relation (in Nm·$pulse^{-1}·s$), the latter being used as an upper bound of spindle afferent capacity to generate force. The resultant positional stiffness estimate (in Nm/deg) was deemed to be rather low, on the grounds that a modest load, such as 1 Nm applied at the finger tip would induce a 37° deflection at the metacarpophalangeal joint.

While the occurrence of an angular deflection of this magnitude might appear to indicate that positional stiffness, and thus length servo action, was inadequate, this analysis is somewhat arbitrary. A more objective assessment could depend upon a comparison of the normalized positional stiffness of the servo with that of the muscle, on the premise that an effective position servo should augment muscular stiffness by a substantial margin. The maximum torque output of the finger flexor is about 4 Nm, and the range of motion at the joint is 100°. Using the formulation from section *Normalized Stiffness*, p. 285, to estimate stiffness, the calculation provides a normalized value of 0.75, which can be compared with the 2.0 upper bound for the normalized mechanical stiffness of skeletal muscle provided in *Mechanically and Neurally Mediated Components*, p. 285. The resultant conclusion that motor servo stiffness is likely to be less than maximal muscle mechanical stiffness constitutes a strong argument against the hypothesis for length regulation.

β-Innervation of Muscle Spindles

Acceleration of spindle afferent discharge in contracting isometric muscle has usually been attributed to γ-motoneuron activity. While increases in discharge rate that arise in the absence of EMG activity are legitimately attributed to fusimotor action, increases arising above extrafusal threshold could arise equally from β-fiber action.

Skeletofusimotor or β-fibers are simply large-diameter motor axons that branch to innervate both intrafusal and extrafusal muscle fibers (see the chapter by Matthews in this *Handbook*). Their existence was first recognized in frog muscle (155) and they have since been identified in the muscles of many reptiles (64, 167, 220). Although β-fibers were also isolated in several mammalian muscles more than 15 years ago (1, 22, 23), these muscles were small (superficial and deep lumbricals), and their innervation was thought to be nonrepresentative. The importance of this innervation was also discounted on the premise that the β-innervation was simply a vestigial remnant of the form of innervation that prevails in more primitive species.

Based upon the use of more sensitive techniques (14, 15, 63, 115, 148), β-fiber innervation of muscle spindles has been reported in 30%–70% of mammalian muscles examined (63, 205) in several different species (64, 220), and it is now evident that their significance must be seriously reevaluated.

At this time, there is relatively little information available regarding possible functional contributions of β-motoneurons in physiologically activated muscles. Post, Rymer, and Hasan (243) have reported evidence derived from triceps surae muscles in the decerebrate cat, suggesting that the augmentation of spindle receptor afferent discharge that arises during reflexively induced isometric muscle contraction may be due largely to the activation of β-axons. This hypothesis was based, in turn, on the finding that the range of recruitment and rate modulation of γ-motoneurons was apparently quite limited in this preparation, so that both γ-motoneuron discharge rate and the capacity to recruit fresh γ-motoneurons was apparently saturated near the point of skeletomotor threshold. More recently, the use of ensemble averages of EMG that are synchronized to the spindle afferent spike has provided preliminary evidence that β-innervation may be detected by finding correlated unitary EMG activity prior to the spike occurrence (260). This EMG activity, which precedes the spike by some 5–10 ms, is the expected outcome if β-motoneuronal discharge was able to excite both intrafusal and extrafusal muscle. Nonneural interactions, however, arising from the mechanical effects of contraction of adjacent motor units could conceivably give rise to similar effects, and the technique requires further evaluation. In any event, it seems likely that β-motoneuron activity may serve to augment spindle receptor discharge above extrafusal threshold, while for animal models at least, γ-motoneurons may be much more influential at subthreshold levels of spinal excitation.

Analytical Approaches to Actions of α-, β-, and γ-Motoneurons

It is now instructive to reevaluate the observations of spindle afferent discharge from the various preparations in relation to the analytical models that were outlined in CONTROL THEORY CONCEPTS, p. 258, and HYPOTHESES OF MOTOR SERVO FUNCTION, p. 264, and in Figure 7. A potentially productive approach, described in these sections, is to treat the arrangement of extrafusal and intrafusal muscle as the equivalent of a model reference system, in which motor output is distributed to both the controlled system (the extrafusal muscle) and to a model of this system (the intrafusal fiber). If a command induces changes in the controlled system that are precisely comparable to the changes in the model, then no error signal will result. In the context of the motor servo, spindle afferents would produce no alteration in discharge under conditions in which length changes of the intrafusal fiber exactly match those of the extrafusal fibers. (The length under consideration here is the length of the contractile portions of the spindle poles. Since both intrafusal and extrafusal muscle fibers insert into the same common tendon, the external length of the system must be the same for both elements.) During command-induced excitation of the system, feedback is conditional, because it arises only under the conditions in which performance of the controlled system and of the model differ.

In relation to the spindle afferent recordings reported earlier, one possible objection to a model reference configuration is that γ-efferent discharge does not appear to vary in any simple relation with skeletomotor activity. Specifically, if γ-motoneuron output is not appreciably modulated in parallel with increasing α-motoneuron output, as suggested in the previous section, the nervous system might not be able to take advantage of the model reference arrangement. However, if β-fibers turn out to be an effective source of excitation to intrafusal fibers, then the β-motoneurons might extend the dynamic range of efferent innervation of the muscle spindle and allow a model reference arrangement to be implemented.

As was pointed out in HYPOTHESES OF MOTOR SERVO FUNCTION, p. 264, conditional feedback from spindle receptors does not presume absent afferent discharge; rather it requires that spindle receptor discharge, under appropriate loading conditions, be maintained at some constant discharge rate. There are relatively few reported circumstances in which spindle afferent discharge is unchanging in the face of command-induced changes in motor output. In the contraction of isometric muscle for example, there is characteristically an augmented discharge rate, which indicates that intrafusal tension typically rises more quickly than can be offset by force-related internal shortening. Similarly, during command-induced free shortening of muscle, as seen in human leg muscles (113) and in monkey (87) and cat jaw muscles (41), there is often a reduction in spindle afferent discharge. On the other hand, during very slow voluntary shortening of human finger flexors (281) or during flexion of hamstring muscles in the walking, intact cat (244) or jaw-closing muscles in the monkey (87), spindle afferent discharge may remain relatively constant. This latter situation presumably represents the null condition discussed in *Spindle Receptors as Model-Reference Error Detectors*, p. 265.

Overall, these findings indicate that in many naturally occurring circumstances, the properties of the intrafusal muscle are not consistently well matched to those of the extrafusal muscle and load. The major reason for a difference in behavior of the controlled system and of the model may be the dependence of the extrafusal system on load. While intrafusal and extrafusal muscle fibers might behave similarly under isolated conditions, the presence of a load will modify the response of extrafusal muscle to imposed command. The properties of the two systems might be well matched, for example, when the load is simply equal to the inertia of the limb.

An alternative arrangement, which is insensitive to load, was spelled out in *Control Configurations*, p. 262. This is the zero-sensitivity configuration, in which the difference between model and system response, the reference error, is fed back to the model to form a positive-feedback loop (Fig. 7A, option 2). We argued in *β-System and ... Zero Sensitivity*, p. 266, that this configuration is analogous to the β-arrangement, in which the reference error (spindle afferent discharge) is fed back onto the system model (intrafusal fiber) via an excitatory synaptic projection to β-motoneurons. Under the conditions in which the gain of the positive-feedback loop is 1, it can be shown (127) that the system performance should become independent of the properties of both extrafusal muscle and load and dependent solely upon the properties of the feedback pathway.

To our knowledge, there is no evidence that bears directly on the presence of a zero-sensitivity configuration in the motor servo; however, a number of related issues should be mentioned. It has been claimed that the action of β-fibers, as determined by their capacity to modulate spindle afferent discharge, is modest. If correct, this would imply a remote prospect of significant loop gain in the positive-feedback loop. On the other hand, β-effects have nearly always been examined in isometric muscles, in which β-dynamic effects might not be readily discernible. Moreover, the effects of β-axon stimulation have usually been examined in muscles devoid of fusimotor activity, which may have meant that the background tension of the intrafusal fiber was unusually low. Although no evidence of a positive-feedback configuration exists in the mammal, findings supporting the existence of such a loop have been reported in the frog preparation, in which spindle receptor response to stretch fell after section of the dorsal roots (144).

Equilibrium Point Control

The results just reviewed indicate that the relations between α-, β-, and γ-motoneurons are not fully understood at the present time, although considerable progress is being made. One might suppose that this lack of understanding would pose a major obstacle in attempts to understand movement control, but, in fact, considerable progress has been made. This success appears to be related to the finding discussed in *Actions of Control Signals on the Motor Servo*, p. 286, which is that the basic effect of a central motor command is a shift in the threshold of the stretch reflex, more or less independent of the α- and γ-motoneuron makeup of the command. Thus the salient properties of the motor servo are well summarized by force-length or torque-angle relations, which can be measured directly even though they derive from complex physiological mechanisms (TONIC STRETCH REFLEX IN FUNCTIONALLY ISOLATED MUSCLES, p. 283, and STATIC REGULATORY CHARACTERISTICS IN INTACT SUBJECTS, p. 290). Movement problems can then be understood on the basis of an interaction between one of these summary relations and the relevant mechanical load. This approach was introduced in *Summary Model*, p. 268 (cf. Figs. 11 and 12). It will be helpful to elaborate on a simple example given there that is relevant to a functionally isolated muscle before proceeding to more complex examples that deal with the elbow musculature as a whole.

Trajectory b in Figure 11 shows the hypothetical result of instructing a functionally isolated muscle to shorten by pulling on a spring that is attached to it. The movement begins from an initial postural state (filled circle) that lies long the solid force-length curve representing the properties of the stretch reflex at the initial value of central motor command. The command to move is assumed to be a step change in the value of the central motor command, which shifts the threshold of the stretch reflex to the left. Correspondingly the entire force-length relation is shifted to the left (dashed curve). This causes muscle force to rise, and as it rises the spring load is stretched while the muscle is shortened. Note that the new muscle force and length finally achieved depend on the spring constant of the load (the slope of trajectory b). The same command would result in less shortening, but more increase in muscle force, if the spring constant of the mechanical load were greater. In more general terms, the example illustrates why the actual movement produced by a given motor command is appreciably influenced by the mechanical load. It is equally clear that the movement is influenced by the stiffness of the stretch reflex. If motor servo stiffness were greater (steeper slope of dashed curve), the amount of shortening against a given spring load would also be greater. Figure 12 helps to emphasize this incessant loop of interaction between the stiffness property of the motor servo (ϕ) and the properties of the load (L).

The same basic approach can be used to analyze movements of the elbow using the torque-angle relations that have been measured for the elbow joint. The reader will recall from *Torque-Angle Relations*, p. 292, that the solid lines in Figure 31 represent the equivalent stretch reflexes of all the elbow flexor and extensor muscles acting in combination at each of three different levels of central motor command. The dashed curves are load lines describing the mechanical load in terms of the torque required at different elbow positions to support each of several different weights. The initial postural state of the elbow is specified by its angle together with the torque it exerts to counteract the mechanical load. Thus, any given equilibrium point in Figure 31 characterizes a postural state, and movement can be treated as a transition in equilibrium that occurs as a consequence of a shift in the torque-angle curve caused by a change in the level of central motor command. For example, if the central command is initially at level (2) and the load is at level 3, the initial posture is specified by the intersection at $\alpha_3^{(2)}$. A change in central command to level (1) would result in a transition to a new postural state specified by the intersection at $\alpha_3^{(1)}$, a movement to a more flexed position at which the musculature produces a slightly lower torque.

The previous examples suggest that the CNS controls movements by setting central motor commands to particular constant values and by then letting the particular modulations in torque required to execute the movement evolve as a natural consequence of mechanical and reflex interactions at the level of the motor servo. By this hypothesis errors in the selection of appropriate central motor commands are not corrected on any continuous basis; instead, error correction at this higher level is assumed to occur only as a result of discrete reaction-time movements, as in Figure 13.

Good evidence in support of this hypothesis has come from experiments in which unexpected load changes have been applied during occasional trials of well-rehearsed movements. Fel'dman (73), who studied human elbow flexion movements triggered by an auditory cue, suppressed corrective reaction-time movements by eliminating visual feedback and by asking his subjects not to intervene voluntarily. Bizzi, Polit, and collaborators (25, 26, 238) studied both head and elbow movements in primate subjects cued by a visual display; they suppressed corrective movements by eliminating visual (and sometimes other modalities) feedback during the movement. More recently Kelso and Holt (156) studied finger movements under conditions analogous to Fel'dman's. In all three sets of experiments it was shown that the final postural state was not affected by transient mechanical disturbances, ones that were sufficiently large to have caused a substantial somatosensory barrage of activity. Disturbances applied during the latent period prior to movement altered the initial limb position, and disturbances applied during the movement produced major changes in joint trajectory, but in both cases the joint angle and torque promptly settled to the same values as obtained during undisturbed control movements. In contrast the application of steady loads did disturb the final postural state, but, as shown by Fel'dman (72), the observed alterations in angle and torque were precisely the ones predicted from the stereotypic torque-angle curves described earlier and therefore did not involve changes in central motor command.

It has also been shown that interference with sensory feedback does not alter this basic result. Rhizotomized monkeys (26, 238) and human subjects with pressure blocks (156) still make movements to final positions that are not appreciably altered by transient mechanical disturbances. The absence of any major deterioration in performance probably derives from the gross similarity between the length-tension relations of areflexive muscle and the force-length relations of the intact motor servo as discussed earlier (*Mechanically and Neurally Mediated Components*, p. 285). In addition, the results indicated that the subjects often employed unusually high levels of cocontraction, presumably as a mechanism for stiffening the musculature in compensation for the absence of stretch reflexes. The latter findings suggest a shift in strategy following sensory deprivation, although it should be noted that intact subjects may also employ cocontraction during the execution of voluntary movements (74, 75). The major impact of these results, however, is to reinforce one's confidence in the notion that movements do not require a continual updating of central motor commands.

Neurologists have long debated whether or not it is proper to treat movement as a transition in posture (123, 192). The view of Holmes, who supported this idea, appears to be quite consistent with the concept of equilibrium point control. According to this concept, the CNS need only select new levels for the central motor commands sent to the motor servos controlling the body's musculature. The subsequent result, mediated by autogenetic reflexes and muscle mechanical properties, should be a smooth transition from one postural state to another. Although this explanation does not deal with the question of controlling how rapidly the transition is executed, the latter feature may be partly explained in terms of simple extensions of the equilibrium point concept. For example, slow movements could be produced by progressive shifts in reflex thresholds as contrasted with the stepwise shifts implied in the earlier discussion. Furthermore movements could be speeded up by producing an initial threshold shift that is larger than necessary, followed by a return to an appropriate static level. This would amount to a pulse-step command of the type known to control eye movements (253) and recently suggested for limb movements as well (81, 84, 85). It is clear that equilibrium point control should be given serious consideration since it is potentially capable of controlling quite general motor functions.

Stiffness Regulation vs. Stiffness Control

Stiffness regulation is defined as a preservation of a relative constancy of reflex stiffness, whereas stiffness control implies centrally induced changes in this property, produced to achieve some end such as the stiffening of a joint or the production of a movement. At several points throughout this chapter, evidence has been provided that the pattern of motor servo action is one that tends to reduce variations in stiffness. For example, the greater reflex action at low vs. high initial forces compensates for the proportional dependence of muscle mechanical stiffness on initial force, and the characteristic asymmetry of reflex action compensates for an opposite asymmetry of mechanical responses. While these observations provide support for the notion of stiffness regulation, there is no implication of stiffness control. In fact, it has already been pointed out that attempts to get subjects to control the stiffness of their musculature have met with only limited success (*Effect of Instructional Set*, p. 294, *Gain Variation vs. Gain Control*, p. 296). Stiffness is clearly increased when the musculature is brought from a relaxed to an active state, but once an activity pattern is set, there appears to be little additional capability for modulating gain to control stiffness, at least not in preparation for disturbances in posture. Another possibility, recently explored by Cooke (44) and by Sakitt (260a), is that stiffness control is used as a mechanism for making movement.

In Figure 39, *part A* shows tracking movements of a human subject and *part B* shows that analogous output from a model in which movements are produced by controlling stiffness, as elaborated in *part C*. The solid lines show force-length relations for an agonist muscle in the presence of three different central motor commands. The assumption was that these commands control spring stiffness (the slope of the line) and have no effect on the threshold of the stretch reflex (the intercept along the abscissa is held fixed). The force-length curves of the antagonists (dashed lines) are represented in the same way (note that agonist stretch unloads the antagonist). Under the assumption that the external load force is zero, model limb position is determined by the intersection of an appropriate pair of solid and dashed curves, a point that defines an equilibrium between equal and opposite forces. The simulated movements in *B* and *D* represent transitions from one equilibrium point to another produced by step changes in agonist stiffness.

The foregoing discussion clearly indicates that movements could be produced by changes in stiffness; however, this does not mean that movements are ordinarily produced in this manner. In fact, the evidence reviewed in *Actions of Control . . . Motor Servo*, p. 286, *Torque-Angle Relations*, p. 292, and *Equilibrium Point Control*, p. 311 is against the basic postulate that central motor commands set the slope of a force-length relation as assumed in Figure 39C. Instead, it appears that motor commands produce appreciable shifts of the intercept along the abscissa as shown in Figures 25 and 31. In spite of this deficiency, the stiffness control model may prove useful in understanding movement control after dorsal rhizotomy. The latter procedure disables the stretch reflex, in which case central motor commands would be expected to recruit select numbers of units from the motor pool, rather than to set reflex threshold. Correspondingly one would predict that the family of dashed curves in Figure 24 (length-tension curves at different levels of recruitment) would serve as a substitute for the normal family shown in Figure 25. The family of recruitment curves is more accurately characterized by alterations in stiffness than by changes in threshold. These considerations may help to explain

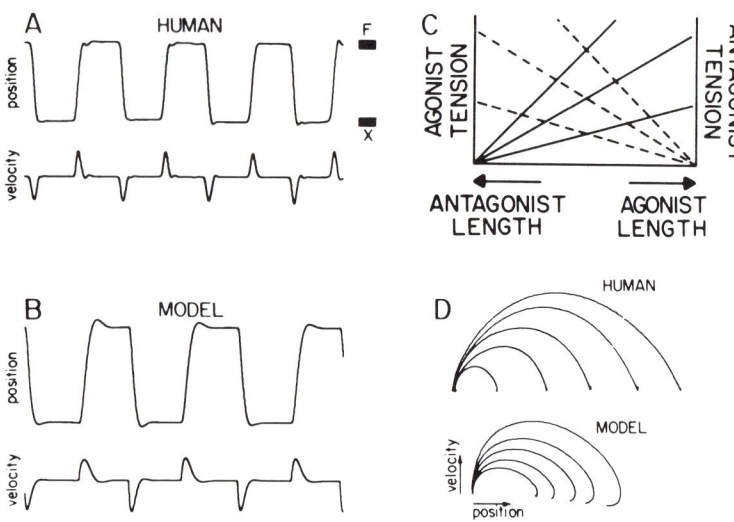

FIG. 39. Movements made by a normal human subject and by an analogue model of the limb. *A*: position and velocity records of movements made by subject during performance of visually guided step tracking task. *B*: analogous traces obtained from the model in which movements were produced by a step change in resting spring constant. *C*: a representation of a model in which the static position of a limb is treated as the point of equilibrium of opposing springs of variable stiffness. *D*: phase plane plots of movements obtained from human subject and from model. In the model, different movement amplitudes were produced by varying the size of the step in spring constant. [From Cooke (44).]

how deafferented animals are able to maintain reasonable motor control in the absence of stretch reflexes.

Perturbations During Movement

In recent years, a number of studies have examined the reflex effects of perturbations interjected in the course of ongoing movement. Such studies, which have focused largely on short-term variations in EMG response, are important in assessing possible interactions between motor servo regulation and descending commands. For example, it is conceivable that motor servo action might be augmented or reduced according to the needs of the situation, which amounts to adaptive gain control (*Adaptive Models*, p. 269). Another possibility is that reflexes would be uniformly suppressed during movement (223), or finally, descending signals and motor servo responses might simply sum in an algebraic fashion. The perturbations are here being used as probes to investigate reflex responses, but the findings are clearly relevant to life situations in which movement is frequently influenced by external environmental constraints.

The EMG response to transient perturbations during motion has been examined in human (54, 55, 91–93, 95, 165, 186, 187), monkey (25, 42), and cat preparations (244). Studies have been performed in a variety of different muscles, performing many different tasks, including visuomotor tracking (186, 187), ballistic movements (50), locomotion (53, 244), and falling (51). A number of similarities to earlier findings in stationary muscles have emerged, as well as a number of apparent differences.

The similarities are that abrupt muscle stretch induces early EMG responses, with time course and latencies comparable to those seen while stationary. In the long thumb flexors, for example, the response to abrupt interruption of voluntary flexion of the thumb may arise as early as 24 ms, a latency comparable to that seen in stationary muscle (186). Comparable medium-latency response components are also evident in shortening thumb muscles, arising at 40–55 ms after perturbation onset (186). Finally, there are also response components that may begin at medium latency but are clearly instruction dependent and appear to represent a form of reaction-time movement that can be released readily by some appropriate stimulus [(94, 255); see *Effect of Instructional Set*, p. 294].

Although the existence of these EMG responses is strong evidence that motor servo action persists in the course of movement, relatively few attempts have been made to compare directly the magnitude of the EMG responses elicited in stationary and moving limbs. One recent study (94) examined reflex transmission during movement by inserting 50-ms torque pulses prior to and early in the course of rapid plantar flexion movements of the human foot. They observed that the short-latency response to perturbation was prominent over the first 100 ms of movement but then went through a period of marked depression. This depression did not necessarily coincide with any period of EMG silence, and it was present at several different stretch velocities and amplitudes. A similar depression has been noted in the H-reflex and tendon jerk responses elicited during phasic voluntary contraction (91, 92). In contrast, Marsden and colleagues (186, 187) provide no evidence of relative inhibition when perturbations are introduced during active shortening of the long thumb flexor, although their perturbations were introduced at constant latency, well after the onset of motion, during movements performed at rather slow velocity.

In spite of the differences in EMG response, which could be dependent on the particular muscle used as well as the experimental approach, it appears that differences in EMG response to perturbation do exist in moving muscles; however, it has not yet been shown that these EMG differences result from alterations in CNS transmission or that they carry functional significance. Specifically the EMG changes simply could reflect changes in afferent input from moving limbs (see below), which would make assessment of central gain difficult. Furthermore these EMG changes may not automatically translate into comparable differences in force output, especially in light of possible nonlinearities in the dynamic EMG to force transformation in different muscles.

To pursue this problem of assessment of EMG change further, it is required that any attempt to dissect component contributions to the reflex response include appropriate estimates of the behavior of the controlled system under comparable stimulus conditions. For intact limbs, these estimates would include such things as contributions of inertial, viscous, and elastic properties of skeleton, ligaments, and muscle, excluding any reflex contributions. The only available estimate of this type in intact preparations is that of Bizzi and colleagues (25), who calculated the contributions of reflex action arising during perturbations interrupting voluntary head movement in monkeys. These authors concluded that the time course of positional change of the head was determined largely by the mechanical properties of head and neck musculoskeletal elements. Reflex action was estimated to contribute only 30% to the total force output, an increase deemed insufficient to provide effect load compensation. There was no attempt made to compare the magnitude of reflex action during movement with that observed in stationary muscles.

A number of important additional considerations are relevant to the assessment of reflex responses in moving muscle. First, regarding afferent input, the response of spindle afferents could be quite different for perturbations induced in the course of motion versus those recorded under stationary conditions. The evidence regarding changes in spindle afferent response during motion is so far incomplete; however, our recent studies derived from innervated spindles in the decerebrate cat preparation have shown that responsiveness is depressed during motion. A related issue is that afferent discharge rate during muscle shortening is determined jointly by shortening velocity and by static fusimotor bias (244). Even strong fusimotor activity may not maintain discharge when velocity of shortening exceeds 0.2 rest lengths per second (244). For lower velocities the effect of static fusimotor action becomes quite prominent. Perturbations introduced in shortening muscles may invoke little or no spindle afferent response unless velocity is less than some critical value, even in the presence of substantial fusimotor activity. Differences in afferent response may also reflect the dependence of a model reference system on load, a point addressed in an earlier section.

A final important aspect of motor servo response is that muscle properties will undoubtedly be strongly influenced by the parameters of the ongoing motion. For example, stiffness and viscosity of muscle are both changed during ongoing movement, which may influence the amplitude of response to a given load.

Compliance, Load Compensation, and Biological Design

Load compensation, length regulation, and high stiffness are essentially equivalent ways of describing what was once believed to be an important function of the motor servo. However, evidence reviewed at many points in this chapter indicates that motor servo action is not particularly effective in compensating for changes in load. The data further indicate that the stiffness of the stretch reflex is not especially high—it is not much different than the stiffness that could be achieved solely on the basis of muscle mechanical properties (assuming a fully recruited muscle). Two important functional questions that arise from these results are *1*) what possible advantages are there to regulating stiffness at a modest level? and *2*) how do we achieve load compensation when we need it?

Trajectory a in Figure 30 reviews the springlike response of the motor servo to an increase in load force. In attempting to understand potential advantages, it is helpful to emphasize the compliance of the response rather than its stiffness. Compliance is defined by the ratio of length change to force change, i.e., the inverse of stiffness and the inverse of the slope of trajectory a. While the compliance of the motor servo clearly interferes with load compensation (there is an appreciable increase in length in response to the increase in force), it may be quite beneficial in providing a suitable mechanical interface between the body and its mechanical environment (48, 127). A compliant interface would absorb the impacts of abrupt changes in load, thus attenuating their transmission to the body and head. For example, in the standing posture with knees bent, the regulation of a modest level of stiffness probably insures a good suspension system for the body. Compliance may also be advantageous for the arm musculature. If the arm should encounter an immovable obstacle in the course of a movement, it is better that the musculature yield than continue to control the position of the joint in an unchanging manner, since the latter action would require that the position of the remainder of the body change drastically in order to accommodate the commanded trajectories of joint rotations.

While compliance seems beneficial in some instances, it clearly is not when the task is to make a precise movement or to hold accurately a given limb position. The results reviewed in *Effect of Instructional Set*, p. 294, and *Gain Variation vs. Gain Control*, p. 296, suggest that rigid control of limb position is achieved mainly by the production of reaction-time movements, rather than by increasing the stiffness of the motor servo through a gain-control mechanism. Trajectory a–b in Figure 30 provides a simple hypothetical example of a load-compensated response, presumed to be mediated by an S-R processor (Fig. 13) that emits a new motor command in response to the perturbation. The manifestation of the motor command is a leftward shift in reflex threshold (dashed curve in Fig. 30). The particular response illustrated is a sequential one which characterizes the C traces in Figure 33B; the initial component is a compliant deflection mediated by the motor servo (trajectory a) followed by the response to the new motor command (trajectory b). A clean two-component sequence is not always seen (cf. Fig. 33A), due apparently to the generation of a load-compensating command prior to the completion of the motor servo response. The latter would result in a short-cut trajectory rather than the a–b sequence shown in Figure 30, although the final postural state would be no different. In the example given, load compensation is essentially perfect, since there is no net increase in muscle length even though the greater load persists.

At first thought it seems surprising that the CNS does not utilize the mechanism of adaptive gain control instead of, or in addition to, adaptive S-R processing. One likely disadvantage of the former is that the extent to which length-feedback gain can be increased is quite limited, due to myotatic time delays that promote instability and oscillation. This limitation is discussed in detail in the chapter by Rack in this *Handbook*. Another potential disadvantage is that the use of parametric gain control might unduly complicate the computation of appropriate movement commands, since the latter would have to include corrections based on the current values of stiffness. The theoretical work of Inbar (145) appears to favor the simplicity of signal adaptation (analogous to the selection of appropriate motor commands by an S-R processor) over parametric adaptation. One can also argue on the basis of evolutionary simplicity—organisms clearly require S-R processors, whereas they can get along without parametric gain control, particularly if fast reaction-time processes are available.

Finally, it is interesting to ask why there is any need for stiffness regulation, since the regulated value is not greatly different from muscle mechanical stiffness and since stiffness is not subject to any major adaptive modification. Here it is important to recall that since muscle properties are highly nonlinear, mechanical stiffness varies markedly depending on the initial conditions and on the parameters of length change. Nichols and Houk (226) argued that the improvement in linearity (equivalent to a greater constancy of stiffness) in the presence of reflex action is an important function of the motor servo. The complexity of central motor control would be increased if it were necessary to build corrective components that compensate for muscle nonlinearity into postural and movement commands.

Summary

Motor commands are distributed to α-, β-, and γ-motoneurons in combination. Most of the data suggest stereotypic patterns of activation, although the specific pattern may not be quite the same in human versus animal subjects. β-Innervation is more widespread than was formerly believed and is probably important in producing the parallel increases in spindle receptor discharge and force observed under isometric conditions. Data relevant to model reference theories of movement control is judged to be inconclusive at the present time. Regardless of the α-, β-, and γ-motoneuron makeup of movement commands, the basic outcome seems to be a simple shift in the threshold of the stretch reflex, and considerable progress in understanding movement control has been achieved on this basis.

Movements have been successfully analyzed as transitions from one postural state to another. A postural state is characterized as an equilibrium between stretch reflexes in a given musculature and the forces resulting from mechanical properties of load. Equilibrium is achieved when the muscles are sufficiently stretched to produce forces that exactly counterbalance the load. Movements are produced when a central motor command shifts the reflex thresholds of the musculature, creating a temporary disequilibrium that causes a transition to a new equilibrium state. Perturbations applied in the course of movement alter the time course of motion and provoke reflex responses, many components of which are analogous to those evoked in stationary limbs. Provided reaction-time responses are suppressed, however, the perturbations either do not alter the final postural state, or alter it in a manner predictable from the springlike properties of the motor servo. Thus the motor servo is seen as a final common processor of central motor commands.

One advantage of stiffness regulation is that it provides a springlike interface between the body and its mechanical environment. The compliance of this interface absorbs the impacts of abrupt changes in load, thus attenuating their transmission to the body and head. A disadvantage is that it provides poor load compensation and poor length regulation. Nevertheless, effective load compensation can be achieved by the superposition of appropriate reaction-time movements upon the compliant responses of the motor servo.

REFERENCES

1. ADAL, M. M., AND D. BARKER. Intramuscular branching of fusimotor fibers. *J. Physiol. London* 177: 288-299, 1965.
2. ADAM, J., C. D. MARSDEN, P. A. MERTON, AND H. B. MORTON. Proceedings: the effect of lesions in the internal capsule and the sensorimotor cortex on servo action in the human thumb. *J. Physiol. London* 254: 27P-28P, 1976.
3. ADOLPH, E. F. *Physiological Regulations*. Tempe, AZ: Cattell, 1943.
4. AHLMAN, H., S. GRILLNER, AND M. UDO. The effect of 5-HTP on the static fusimotor activity and the tonic stretch reflex of an extensor muscle. *Brain Res.* 27: 393-396, 1971.
5. ALLUM, J. H. J. Responses to load disturbance in human shoulder muscles: the hypothesis that one component is a pulse test information signal. *Exp. Brain Res.* 22: 307-326, 1975.
6. ALVORD, E. C., AND M. G. F. FUORTES. Reflex activity of extensor motor units following muscular excitation. *J. Physiol. London* 122: 302-321, 1953.
7. ARBIB, M. A. *The Metaphorical Brain: An Introduction to Cybernetics as Artificial Intelligence and Brain Theory*. New York: Interscience, 1972.
8. ASANUMA, H., K. D. LARSEN, AND H. YUMIYA. Direct sensory pathways to the motor cortex in the monkey: a basis for cortical reflexes. In: *Integration in the Nervous System*, edited by H. Asanuma and V. J. Wilson. Tokyo: Igaku Shoin, 1979, p. 223-238.
9. ASATRYAN, D. G., AND A. G. FEL'DMAN. Functional tuning of the nervous system with control of movement or maintenance of posture. I. Mechanographic analysis of the work of the joint on execution of a postural task. *Biophysics USSR* 10: 925-935, 1965.
10. ASHBY, P., C. ANDREWS, L. KNOWLES, AND J. W. LANCE. Pyramidal and extrapyramidal control of tonic mechanisms in cat. *Brain* 95: 21-30, 1972.
11. BALLIF, L., J. F. FULTON, AND E. G. T. LIDDELL. Observations on spinal and decerebrate knee jerks with special reference to their inhibition by single break shocks. *Proc. R. Soc. London Ser. B* 98: 589-607, 1925.
12. BARD, P., AND M. B. MACHT. The behavior of chronically decerebrate cats. In: *Neurological Basis of Behavior*. Boston: Little, Brown, 1958, p. 55-71. (Ciba Found. Symp.)
13. BARKER, D. The structure and distribution of muscle receptors. In: *Symposium on Muscle Receptors*, edited by D. Barker. Hong Kong: Hong Kong Univ. Press, 1962, p. 227-240.
14. BARKER, D., F. EMONET-DÉNAND, D. W. HARKER, L. JAMI, AND Y. LAPORTE. Distribution of fusimotor axons to intrafusal muscle fibers in cat tenuissimus spindles as determined by the glycogen-depletion method. *J. Physiol. London* 261: 49-70, 1976.
15. BARKER, D., F. EMONET-DÉNAND, D. W. HARKER, L. JAMI, AND Y. LAPORTE. Types of intra- and extrafusal muscle fibre innervated by dynamic skeletofusimotor axons in cat peroneus brevis and tenuissimus muscles, as determined by the glycogen depletion method. *J. Physiol. London* 266: 713-726, 1977.
16. BAWA, P., AND R. B. STEIN. Frequency response of human soleus muscle. *J. Neurophysiol.* 39: 788-793, 1976.
17. BAWA, P., AND W. G. TATTON. Motor unit response in muscles stretched by imposed displacements of the monkey wrist. *Exp. Brain Res.* 37: 417-437, 1979.
18. BELLMAN, R. E. *Adaptive Control Processes: A Guided Tour*. Princeton, NJ: Princeton Univ. Press, 1961.
19. BERNSTEIN, N. *The Coordination and Regulation of Movements*. Oxford: Pergamon, 1967.
20. BERTHOZ, A., AND S. METRAL. Behavior of a muscular group subjected to a sinusoidal and trapezoidal variation of force. *J. Appl. Physiol.* 29: 378-384, 1970.
21. BERTHOZ, A., W. J. ROBERTS, AND N. P. ROSENTHAL. Dynamic characteristics of stretch reflex using force inputs. *J. Neurophysiol.* 34: 612-619, 1971.
22. BESSOU, P., F. EMONET-DÉNAND, AND Y. LAPORTE. Occurrence of intrafusal muscle fibres innervation by branches of slow motor fibres in the cat. *Nature London* 198: 594-595, 1963.
23. BESSOU, P., F. EMONET-DÉNAND, AND Y. LAPORTE. Motor fibres innervating extrafusal and intrafusal muscle fibres in the cat. *J. Physiol. London* 180: 649-672, 1965.
24. BIANCONI, R., AND J. P. VAN DER MEULEN. The response to vibration of the end organs of mammalian muscle spindles. *J. Neurophysiol.* 26: 177-190, 1963.
25. BIZZI, E., P. DEV, P. MORASSO, AND A. POLIT. Effect of load disturbances during centrally initiated movements. *J. Neurophysiol.* 41: 542-556, 1978.
26. BIZZI, E., A. POLIT, AND P. MORASSO. Mechanisms underlying achievement of final head position. *J. Neurophysiol.* 39: 435-444, 1976.
27. BROCK, L. G., J. S. COOMBS, AND J. C. ECCLES. The recording of potentials from motoneurones with an intracellular electrode. *J. Physiol. London* 117: 431-460, 1952.
28. BROWN, M. C., I. ENGBERG, AND P. B. C. MATTHEWS. The relative sensitivity to vibration of muscle receptors in the cat. *J. Physiol. London* 192: 773-800, 1967.
29. BURKE, D., AND G. EKLUND. Muscle spindle activity in man during standing. *Acta Physiol. Scand.* 100: 187-199, 1977.
30. BURKE, D., K.-E. HAGBARTH, AND L. LOFSTEDT. Muscle spindle responses in man to changes in load during accurate position-maintenance. *J. Physiol. London* 276: 159-164, 1978.
31. BURKE, D., K.-E. HAGBARTH, AND L. LOFSTEDT. Muscle spindle activity in man during shortening and lengthening contractions. *J. Physiol. London* 277: 131-142, 1978.
32. BURKE, D., K.-E. HAGBARTH, AND N. F. SKUSE. Recruitment order of human spindle endings in isometric voluntary contractions. *J. Physiol. London* 285: 101-112, 1978.
33. BURKE, D., L. KNOWLES, C. ANDREWS, AND P. ASHBY. Spasticity, decerebrate rigidity and the clasp-knife phenomenon: an experimental study in the cat. *Brain* 95: 31-48, 1972.
34. BURKE, D., B. MCKEON, AND R. A. WESTERMAN. Induced changes in the thresholds for voluntary activation of human spindle endings. *J. Physiol. London* 302: 171-181, 1980.
35. BURKE, R. E., AND P. RUDOMÍN. Spinal neurons and synapses. In: *Handbook of Physiology. The Nervous System*, edited by E. R. Kandel. Bethesda, MD: Am. Physiol. Soc., 1977, sect. 1, vol. I, pt. 2, chapt. 24, p. 877-944.
36. BURKE, R. E., P. RUDOMÍN, AND F. E. ZAJAC. Catch property in single mammalian motor units. *Science* 168: 122-124, 1970.
37. CHAMBERS, W. W., C. N. LIU, G. P. MCCOUCH, AND E. D'AQUILI. Descending tracts and spinal shock in the cat. *Brain* 89: 377-390, 1966.
38. CHENEY, P. D., AND E. E. FETZ. Functional properties of primate cortiomotoneuronal cells (Abstract). *Society Neurosci. Abstr.* 4: 292, 1978.
39. CLAMANN, H. P., J. D. GILLIES, R. D. SKINNER, AND E. HENNEMAN. Quantitative measures of output of a motoneuron pool during monosynaptic reflexes. *J. Neurophysiol.* 37: 1328-1337, 1974.
40. CLOSE, R. I. Dynamic properties of mammalian skeletal muscles. *Physiol. Rev.* 52: 129-197, 1972.
41. CODY, F. W. J., L. M. HARRISON, AND A. TAYLOR. Analysis of activity of muscle spindles of the jaw closing muscles during normal movement in the cat. *J. Physiol. London* 253: 565-582, 1975.
42. CONRAD, B., K. MATSUNAMI, J. MEYER-LOHMANN, M. WIESENDANGER, AND V. B. BROOKS. Cortical load compensation during voluntary elbow movements. *Brain Res.* 71: 507-514, 1974.
43. COOKE, J. D. Dependence of human arm movements on limb mechanical properties. *Brain Res.* 165: 366-369, 1979.
44. COOKE, J. D. The organization of simple, skilled movements. In: *Tutorials in Motor Behaviour*, edited by G. Stelmach and J. Requin. Amsterdam: Elsevier, 1980.
45. CORDO, P. J. *Motor Unit Contributions to Reflex Regulation*

of Lengthening Muscle (Ph.D. thesis). Syracuse: State Univ. of New York, 1979.
46. CORDO, P. J., AND W. Z. RYMER. The value of unitary recruitment in reflex regulation of mechanical properties of lengthening muscles (Abstract). *Soc. Neurosci. Abstr.* 4: 294, 1978.
47. CORDO, P. J., AND W. Z. RYMER. Electromyographic contributions to reflex regulation of muscle properties in the decerebrate cat (Abstract). *Soc. Neurosci. Abstr.* 5: 366, 1979.
48. CRAGO, P. E., J. C. HOUK, AND Z. HASAN. Regulatory actions of human stretch reflex. *J. Neurophysiol.* 39: 925–35, 1976.
49. DENNY-BROWN, D. Nature of postural reflexes. *Proc. R. Soc. London Ser. B* 104: 252–301, 1929.
50. DESMEDT, J. G. R., AND E. GODAUX. Ballistic skilled movements: load compensation and patterning of motor commands. In: *Cerebral Motor Control in Man: Long Loop Mechanisms*, edited by J. E. Desmedt. Basel: Karger, 1978, p. 21–55. (Prog. Clin. Neurophysiol., vol. 4.)
51. DIETZ, V., AND J. NOTH. Pre-innervation and stretch responses of triceps bracchii in man falling with and without visual control. *Brain Res.* 142: 576–579, 1978.
52. DIETZ, V., J. NOTH, AND D. SCHMIDTBLEICHER. Interaction between pre-activity and stretch reflex in human triceps brachii during landing from forward falls. *J. Physiol. London* 311: 113–125, 1981.
53. DIETZ, V., D. SCHMIDTBLEICHER, AND J. NOTH. Neuronal mechanisms of human locomotion. *J. Neurophysiol.* 42: 1212–1222, 1979.
54. DUSFRESNE, J. R., V. S. GURFINKEL', J. F. SOECHTING, AND C. A. TERZUOLO. Response to transient disturbances during intentional forearm flexion in man. *Brain Res.* 150: 103–115, 1978.
55. DUSFRESNE, J. R., J. F. SOECHTING, AND C. A. TERZUOLO. Modulation of the myotatic reflex gain in man during intentional movements. *Brain Res.* 193: 67–84, 1980.
56. ECCLES, J. C., R. M. ECCLES, AND A. LUNDBERG. Synaptic actions on motoneurones caused by impulses in Golgi tendon organ afferents. *J. Physiol. London* 138: 227–252, 1957.
57. ECCLES, J. C., R. M. ECCLES, AND A. LUNDBERG. Types of neurone in and around the intermediate muscles of the lumbosacral cord. *J. Physiol. London* 154: 89–114, 1960.
58. ECCLES, R. M., AND A. LUNDBERG. Integrative pattern of Ia synaptic actions on motoneurones of hip and knee muscles. *J. Physiol. London* 144: 271–298, 1958.
59. ECCLES, R. M., AND A. LUNDBERG. Supraspinal control of interneurons mediating spinal reflexes. *J. Physiol. London* 147: 565–584, 1959.
60. ECCLES, R. M., AND A. LUNDBERG. Synaptic actions in motoneurones by afferents which may evoke the flexion reflex. *Arch. Ital. Biol.* 97: 199–221, 1959.
61. ELDRED, E., R. GRANIT, AND P. A. MERTON. Supraspinal control of the muscle spindle and its significance. *J. Physiol. London* 122: 498–523, 1953.
62. ELLAWAY, P. H., AND J. R. TROTT. Reflex connections from muscle stretch receptors to their own fusimotor neurons. In: *Understanding the Stretch Reflex*, edited by S. Homma. Amsterdam: Elsevier, 1976, p. 113–121.
63. EMONET-DÉNAND, F., L. JAMI, AND Y. LAPORTE. Skeleto-fusimotor axons in hind-limb muscles of the cat. *J. Physiol. London* 249: 153–166, 1975.
64. EMONET-DÉNAND, F., L. JAMI, AND Y. LAPORTE. Histophysiological observations on the skeleto-fusimotor innervation of mammalian spindles. In: *Spinal and Supraspinal Mechanisms of Voluntary Motor Control and Locomotion*, edited by J. E. Desmedt. Basel: Karger, 1980, p. 1–11. (Prog. Clin. Neurophysiol., vol. 8.)
65. ENGBERG, I., A. LUNDBERG, AND R. W. RYALL. Reticulospinal inhibition of transmission in reflex pathways. *J. Physiol. London* 194: 201–223, 1968.
66. EVANICH, M. J., AND R. V. LOURENÇO. Frequency response analysis of the diaphragm in vivo. *J. Appl. Physiol.* 40: 729–735, 1976.
67. EVARTS, E. V. Motor cortex reflexes associated with learned movements. *Science* 179: 501–503, 1973.
68. EVARTS, E. V., AND R. GRANIT. Relations of reflexes and intended movements. In: *Progress in Brain Research. Understanding the Stretch Reflex*, edited by S. Homma. Amsterdam: Elsevier, 1976, vol. 44, p. 1–14.
69. EVARTS, E. V., AND J. TANJI. Gating of motor cortex reflexes by prior instruction. *Brain Res.* 71: 479–494, 1974.
70. EVARTS, E. V., AND J. TANJI. Reflex and intended responses in motor cortex pyramidal tract neurons of monkey. *J. Neurophysiol.* 39: 1069–1080, 1976.
71. EVARTS, E. V., AND W. J. VAUGHN. Intended arm movements in response to externally produced arm displacements in man. In: *Cerebral Motor Control in Man: Long Loop Mechanisms*, edited by J. E. Desmedt. Basel: Karger, 1978, p. 178–192. (Prog. Clin. Neurophysiol., vol. 4.)
72. FEL'DMAN, A. G. Functional tuning of the nervous system control of movement or maintenance of a steady posture. II. Controllable parameters of the muscle. *Biophysics USSR* 11: 565–578, 1966.
73. FEL'DMAN, A. G. Functional tuning of the nervous system during control of movement or maintenance of a steady posture. III. Mechanographic analysis of the execution by man of the simplest motor tasks. *Biophysics USSR* 11: 766–775, 1966.
74. FEL'DMAN, A. G. Superposition of motor programs. I. Rhythmic forearm movements in man. *Neuroscience* 5: 81–90, 1980.
75. FEL'DMAN, A. G. Superposition of motor programs. II. Rapid forearm flexion in man. *Neuroscience* 5: 91–85, 1980.
76. FEL'DMAN, A. G., AND G. N. ORLOVSKY. The influence of different descending systems on the tonic stretch reflex in the cat. *Exp. Neurol.* 37: 481–494, 1972.
77. FETZ, E. E., E. JANKOWSKA, T. JOHANISSON, AND J. LIPSKI. Autogenetic inhibition of motoneurones by impulses in group Ia muscle spindle afferents. *J. Physiol. London* 293: 73–195, 1979.
78. FLITNEY, F. W., AND D. G. HIRST. Cross-bridge detachment and sarcomere 'give' during stretch of active frog's muscle. *J. Physiol. London* 276: 449–465, 1978.
79. FOCK, S., AND S. MENSE. Excitatory effects of 5-hydroxytryptamine, histamine and potassium ions on muscular group IV afferent units: a comparison with bradykinin. *Brain Res.* 105: 459–469, 1976.
80. FRANZ, M., AND S. MENSE. Muscle receptors with group IV afferent fibres responding to application of bradykinin. *Brain Res.* 92: 369–383, 1975.
81. FREUND, H. J., AND H. J. BÜDINGEN. The relationship between speed and amplitude of the fastest voluntary contractions of human arm muscles. *Exp. Brain Res.* 31: 1–12, 1978.
82. FUKUSHIMA, K., AND M. KATO. Spinal interneurones responding to group II muscle afferent fibres in the cat. *Brain Res.* 90: 307–312, 1975.
83. GHEZ, C., AND Y. SHINODA. Spinal mechanisms of the functional stretch reflex. *Brain Res.* 32: 55–68, 1978.
84. GHEZ, C., AND D. VICARIO. The control of rapid limb movement in the cat. I. Response latency. *Exp. Brain Res.* 33: 173–189, 1978.
85. GHEZ, C., AND D. VICARIO. The control of rapid limb movement in the cat. II. Scaling of isometric force adjustments. *Exp. Brain Res.* 33: 191–202, 1978.
86. GOODWIN, G. M., D. HOFFMAN, AND G. S. LUSCHEI. The strength of the reflex response to sinusoidal stretch of monkey jaw closing muscles during voluntary contraction. *J. Physiol. London* 279: 81–111, 1978.
87. GOODWIN, G. M., AND E. S. LUSCHEI. Discharge of spindle afferents from jaw-closing muscles during chewing in alert monkeys. *J. Neurophysiol.* 38: 560–571, 1975.
88. GOODWIN, G. M., G. J. MCGRATH, AND P. B. C. MATTHEWS. The tonic vibration reflex seen in the acute spinal cat after treatment with DOPA. *Brain Res.* 49: 463–466, 1973.
89. GORDON, A. M., A. F. HUXLEY, AND F. J. JULIAN. The variation

in isometric tension with sarcomere length in vertebrate muscle fibres. *J. Physiol. London* 184: 170–192, 1966.
90. GOSLOW, G. G., R. M. REINKING, AND D. G. STUART. Physiological extent, range and rate of muscle stretch for soleus, medial gastrocnemius and tibialis anterior in the cat. *Pfluegers Arch.* 341: 77–86, 1973.
91. GOTTLIEB, G. L., AND G. C. AGARWAL. Stretch and Hoffman reflexes during phasic voluntary contractions of the human soleus muscle. *Electroencephalogr. Clin. Neurophysiol.* 44: 553–561, 1978.
92. GOTTLIEB, G. L., AND G. C. AGARWAL. Response to sudden torques about ankle in man: myotatic reflex. *J. Neurophysiol.* 42: 91–106, 1979.
93. GOTTLIEB, G. L., AND G. C. AGARWAL. Response to sudden torques about ankle in man. II. Postmyotatic reaction. *J. Neurophysiol.* 43: 86–101, 1980.
94. GOTTLIEB, G. L., AND G. C. AGARWAL. Response to sudden torques about ankle in man. III. Suppression of stretch-evoked responses during phasic contraction. *J. Neurophysiol.* 44: 233–246, 1980.
95. GOTTLIEB, G. L., G. C. AGARWAL, AND L. STARK. Interactions between voluntary and postural mechanisms of the human motor system. *J. Neurophysiol.* 33: 365–381, 1970.
96. GRANIT, R. *Receptors and Sensory Perception*. New Haven: Yale Univ. Press, 1955.
97. GRANIT, R. Neuromuscular interaction is postural tone of cat's isometric soleus muscle. *J. Physiol. London* 143: 387–402, 1958.
98. GRANIT, R. *The Basis of Motor Control*. London: Academic, 1970.
99. GRANIT, R. The functional role of the muscle spindles—facts and hypotheses. *Brain* 98: 531–556, 1975.
100. GRANIT, R., J.-O. KELLERTH, AND A. J. SZUMSKI. Intracellular autogenetic effects of muscular contraction on extensor motoneurones. The silent period. *J. Physiol. London* 182: 484–503, 1966.
101. GRANIT, R, C. G. PHILLIPS, S. SKOGLUND, AND G. STEG. Differentiation of tonic from phasic alpha ventral horn cells by stretch, pinna and crossed extensor reflexes. *J. Neurophysiol.* 20: 470–481, 1957.
102. GRILLNER, S. Is the tonic stretch reflex dependent upon group II excitation? *Acta Physiol. Scand.* 78: 431–432, 1970.
103. GRILLNER, S. A role for muscle stiffness in meeting the changing postural and locomotor requirements for force development by the ankle extensors. *Acta Physiol. Scand.* 86: 92–108, 1972.
104. GRILLNER, S. Locomotion in vertebrates: central mechanisms and reflex interaction. *Physiol. Rev.* 55: 247–304, 1975.
105. GRILLNER, S., AND T. HONGO. Vestibulospinal effects on motoneurons and interneurons in the lumbosacral cord. In: *Progress in Brain Research. Basic Aspects of Central Vestibular Mechanisms*, edited by A. Brodal and O. Pompeiano. Amsterdam: Elsevier, 1972, vol. 37, p. 260–262.
106. GRILLNER, S., AND M. UDO. Is the tonic stretch reflex dependent on suppression of autogenetic inhibitory reflexes? *Acta Physiol. Scand.* 79: 13A–14A, 1970.
107. GRILLNER, S., AND M. UDO. Motor unit activity and stiffness of the contracting muscle fibres in the tonic str ch reflex. *Acta Physiol. Scand.* 81: 422–424, 1971.
108. GRILLNER, S., AND M. UDO. Recruitment in the tonic stretch reflex. *Acta Physiol. Scand.* 81: 571–573, 1971.
109. GURFINKEL', V. S., AND Y. S. LEVICK. Effects of a doublet or omission and their connection with the dynamics of the active state of human muscles. *Biofizika* 19: 925–931, 1974.
110. HAGBARTH, K.-E., AND G. EKLUND. Motor effect of vibratory stimuli in man. In: *Muscular Afferents and Motor Control. Proc. Nobel Symp. I*, edited by R. Granit. Stockholm: Almqvist & Wiksell, 1966, p. 176–186.
111. HAGBARTH, K.-E., A. HONGELL, AND B. G. WALLIN. The effect of gamma fibre block on afferent muscle nerve activity during voluntary contractions. *Acta Physiol. Scand.* 79: 27A–28A, 1970.
112. HAGBARTH, K.-E., B. G. WALLIN, D. BURKE, AND L. LOFSTEDT. Effects of the Jendrassik manoeuvre on muscle spindle activity in man. *J. Neurol. Neurosurg. Psychiatry* 38: 1143–1153, 1975.
113. HAGBARTH, K.-E., B. G. WALLIN, AND L. LOFSTEDT. Muscle spindle activity in man during voluntary fast alternating movements. *J. Neurol. Neurosurg. Psychiatry* 38: 625–635, 1975.
114. HAMMOND, P. H. An experimental study of servo action in human muscular control. In: *Proc. Int. Congr. Med. Electronics, 3rd, London, 1960*. London: IEE Conf. Publ., 1960, p. 190–199.
115. HARKER, D. W., L. JAMI, Y. LAPORTE, AND J. PETIT. Fast-conducting skeletofusimotor axons supplying intrafusal chain fibers in the cat peroneus tertius muscle. *J. Neurophysiol.* 40: 791–799, 1977.
116. HASAN, Z., AND J. C. HOUK. Analysis of response properties of deefferented mammalian spindle receptors based on frequency response. *J. Neurophysiol.* 38: 663–672, 1975.
117. HASAN, Z., AND J. C. HOUK. Transition in sensitivity of spindle receptors that occurs when the muscle is stretched more than a fraction of a millimeter. *J. Neurophysiol.* 38: 673–689, 1975.
118. HEATH, C. J., J. HORE, AND C. G. PHILLIPS. Inputs from low threshold muscle and cutaneous afferents of hand and forearm to area 3a and 3b of baboon's cerebral cortex. *J. Physiol. London* 257: 197–227, 1976.
119. HENNEMAN, E., G. SOMJEN, AND D. O. CARPENTER. Functional significance of cell size in spinal motoneurons. *J. Neurophysiol.* 28: 560–580, 1965.
120. HERTEL, H.-C., B. HOWALDT, AND S. MENSE. Responses of group IV and group III muscle afferents to thermal stimuli. *Brain Res.* 113: 201–205, 1976.
121. HILL, A. V. The heat of shortening and the dynamic constants of muscle. *Proc. R. Soc. London Ser. B* 126: 136–195, 1938.
122. HOFFER, J. A., AND S. ANDREASSEN. Regulation of soleus muscle stiffness in premammillary cats: intrinsic and reflex components. *J. Neurophysiol.* 45: 267–285, 1981.
122a. HOFFER, J. A., AND S. ANDREASSEN. Limitations in the servo regulation of soleus muscle stiffness in premammillary cats. In: *Muscle Receptors and Movement*, edited by A. Taylor and A. Prochazka. London: Macmillan. In press.
123. HOLMES, G. The clinical syptoms of cerebellar disease. *Lancet* 1: 1177–1182, 1922.
124. HOLMQVIST, B., AND A. LUNDBERG. A differential supraspinal control of synaptic actions evoked by volleys in the flexion reflex afferents in alpha motoneurones. *Acta Physiol. Scand. Suppl.* 186: 1–51, 1960.
125. HONGO, T., E. JANKOWSKA, AND A. LUNDBERG. Convergence of excitatory and inhibitory action on interneurones in the lumbosacral cord. *Exp. Brain. Res.* 1: 338–358, 1966.
126. HONGO, T., E. JANKOWSKA, AND A. LUNDBERG. The rubrospinal tract. II. Facilitation of transmission in reflex paths to motoneurons. *Exp. Brain Res.* 7: 365–391, 1969.
127. HOUK, J. C. The phylogeny of muscular control configurations. In: *Biocybernetics*, edited by H. Drischel, and P. Dettmar. Jena, E. Germany: Fischer, 1972, vol. IV, p. 125–155.
127a. HOUK, J. C. Feedback control of muscle: a synthesis of the peripheral mechanisms. In: *Medical Physiology* (13th ed.), edited by V. B. Mountcastle. St. Louis, MO: Mosby, 1974, p. 668–677.
128. HOUK, J. C. Participation of reflex mechanisms and reaction-time processes in the compensatory adjustments to mechanical disturbances. In: *Cerebral Motor Control in Man: Long Loop Mechanisms*, edited by J. E. Desmedt. Basel: Karger, 1978. (Prog. Clin. Neurophysiol., vol. 4.)
129. HOUK, J. C. A two-stage model of neural processes controlling motor output. In: *Cybernetics 1977*, edited by, G. Hauske. Munich, W. Germany: Oldenbourg, 1978, p. 35–46.
129a. HOUK, J. C. Motor control processes: new data concerning motoservo mechanisms and a tentative model for stimulus-response processing. In: *Posture and Movement: Perspective for Integrating Sensory and Motor Research on the Mammalian Nervous System*, edited by R. E. Talbott and D. R. Humphrey. New York: Raven, 1979, p. 231–241.

130. Houk, J. C. Regulation of stiffness by skeletomotor reflexes. *Annu. Rev. Physiol.* 41: 99–114, 1979.
131. Houk, J. C. Principles of system theory as applied to physiology. In: *Medical Physiology* (14th ed.), edited by V. B. Mountcastle. St. Louis, MO: Mosby, 1980, sect. 3, chapt. 7, 8, p. 227–267.
132. Houk, J. C. Afferent mechanisms mediating autogenetic reflexes. In: *Brain Mechanisms of Perceptual Awareness and Purposeful Behaviour*, edited by C. A. Marsan and O. Pompeiano. New York: Raven. In press.
133. Houk, J. C., P. E. Crago, and W. Z. Rymer. Functional properties of Golgi tendon organs. In: *Segmental Motor Control in Man*, edited by J. E. Desmedt. Basel: Karger, 1980, p. 33–43. (Prog. Clin. Neurophysiol., vol. 8.)
134. Houk, J. C., P. E. Crago, and W. Z. Rymer. Function of the spindle dynamic response in stiffness regulation—a predictive mechanism provided by nonlinear feedback. In: *Muscle Receptors and Movement*, edited by A. Taylor and A. Prochazka. London: Macmillan. In press.
135. Houk, J. C., D. A. Harris, and Z. Hasan. Non-linear behavior of spindle receptors. In: *Control of Posture and Locomotion*, edited by R. B. Stein, K. G. Pearson, R. S. Smith, and J. B. Redford. New York: Plenum, 1973. (Adv. Behav. Biol. Ser., vol. 7.)
136. Houk, J. C., W. Z. Rymer, and P. E. Crago. Complex velocity dependence of the electromyographic component of the stretch reflex (Abstract). *Proc. Int. Congr. Physiol. Sci., 27th, Paris, 1977*, vol. 13, p. 334.
137. Houk, J. C., W. Z. Rymer, and P. E. Crago. Nature of the dynamic response and its relation to the high sensitivity of muscle spindles to small changes in length. In: *Muscle Receptors and Movement*, edited by A. Taylor and A. Prochazka. London: Macmillan. In press.
138. Houk, J. C., J. J. Singer, and M. R. Goldman. An evaluation of length and force feedback to soleus muscles of decerebrate cats. *J. Neurophysiol.* 33: 784–811, 1970.
139. Hulliger, M., P. B. C. Matthews, and J. Noth. Static and dynamic fusimotor action on the response of Ia fibres to low frequency sinusoidal stretching of widely ranging amplitude. *J. Physiol. London* 267: 811–838, 1977.
140. Hultborn, H., and H. Wigström. Motor response with long latency and maintained duration evoked by activity in Ia afferents. In: *Spinal and Supraspinal Mechanisms of Voluntary Motor Control and Locomotion*, edited by J. E. Desmedt. Basel: Karger, 1980, p. 99–116. (Prog. Clin. Neurophysiol., vol. 8.)
141. Hultborn, H., H. Wigström, and B. Wangberg. Prolonged activation of soleus motoneurones following a conditioning train in soleus Ia afferents—a case for a reverberating loop? *Neurosci. Lett.* 1: 147–152, 1975.
142. Hultborn, H., H. Wigström, and B. Wangberg. Prolonged excitation in motoneurones triggered by activity in Ia afferents (Abstract). *Acta Physiol. Scand. Suppl.* 440: 62, 1976.
143. Huxley, A. F., and R. M. Simmons. Proposed mechanism of force generation in striated muscle. *Nature London* 233: 533–538, 1971.
144. Inbar, G. F., B. M. Odom, and I. H. Wagman. Muscle spindles in muscle control. I. Afferent outflow from frog muscle spindles in open and closed loop modes. *Kybernetik* 11: 119–122, 1972.
145. Inbar, G., and A. Yafe. Parameter and signal adaptation in the stretch reflex. In: *Progress in Brain Research. Understanding the Stretch Reflex*, edited by S. Homma. Amsterdam: Elsevier, 1976, vol. 44, p. 317–337.
146. Jack, J. J. B., and R. C. Roberts. Selective electrical activation of group II muscle afferent fibers. *J. Physiol. London* 241: 82–83, 1974.
147. Jack, J. J. B., and R. C. Roberts. The role of muscle spindle afferents in stretch and vibration reflexes of the soleus muscle of the decerebrate cat. *Brain Res.* 146: 366–372, 1978.
148. Jami, L., D. Lan-Couton, K. Malmgren, and J. Petit. 'Fast' and 'slow' skeleto-fusimotor innervation in cat tenuissimus spindles; a study with the glycogen depletion method. *Acta Physiol. Scand.* 103: 284–298, 1978.
149. Jankowska, E. Identification of interneurons interposed in different spinal reflex pathways. In: *Golgi Centennial Symposium: Perspectives in Neurobiology*, edited by M. Santini. New York: Raven, 1975, p. 235–246.
150. Jansen, J. K. S., and P. M. H. Rack. The reflex response to sinusoidal stretching of soleus in the decerebrate cat. *J. Physiol. London* 183: 15–36, 1966.
151. Joyce, G. C., and P. M. H. Rack. Isotonic lengthening and shortening movements of cat soleus muscle. *J. Physiol. London* 204: 475–491, 1969.
152. Joyce, G. C., P. M. H. Rack, and D. R. Westbury. The mechanical properties of cat soleus muscle during controlled lengthening and shortening movements. *J. Physiol. London* 204: 461–474, 1969.
153. Kanda, K. Contribution of polysynaptic pathways to the tonic vibration reflex. *Jpn. J. Physiol.* 22: 367–377, 1972.
154. Kanda, K., and W. Z. Rymer. An estimate of the secondary spindle receptor afferent contribution to the stretch reflex in extensor muscle of the decerebrate. *J. Physiol. London* 264: 63–87, 1977.
155. Katz, B. The efferent regulation of the muscle spindle in the frog. *J. Exp. Biol.* 26: 201–217, 1949.
156. Kelso, J. A. S., and K. G. Holt. Exploring a vibratory systems analysis of human movement production. *J. Neurophysiol.* 43: 1183–1196, 1980.
157. Kim, J. H., and L. D. Partridge. Observations on types of response to combinations of neck, vestibular, and muscle stretch signals. *J. Neurophysiol.* 32: 239–250, 1969.
158. Kirkwood, P. A., and T. A. Sears. Monosynaptic excitation of motoneurones from secondary endings of muscle spindles. *Nature London* 252: 243–244, 1974.
159. Kirkwood, P. A., and T. A. Sears. Monosynaptic excitation of motoneurones from muscle spindle secondary endings of intercostal and triceps surae muscles in the cat. *J. Physiol. London* 245: 64P–66P, 1975.
160. Kniffki, K.-D., S. Mense, and R. F. Schmidt. Chemo- and mechanosensitivity of possible metabo- and nociceptors in skeletal muscle. *Pfluegers Arch.* 362: R32, 1976.
161. Kniffki, K.-D., S. Mense, and R. F. Schmidt. Mechanisms of muscle pain: a comparison with cutaneous nociception. In: *Sensory Functions of the Skin*, edited by Y. Zotterman. New York: Pergamon, 1976, p. 463–473. (Wenner-Gren Center Int. Symp. Ser., vol. 27.)
162. Kniffki, K.-D., S. Mense, and R. F. Schmidt. Responses of group IV afferent units from skeletal muscle to stretch, contraction and chemical stimulation. *Exp. Brain Res.* 31: 511–522, 1978.
163. Kuffler, S. W., and C. C. Hunt. The mammalian small-nerve fibres; a system for efferent nervous regulation of muscle spindle discharge. *Res. Publ. Assoc. Res. Nerv. Ment. Dis.* 30: 24–47, 1952.
164. Kwan, H. C., J. T. Murphy, and M. W. Repeck. Control of stiffness by medium latency electromyographic response to limb perturbation. *Can. J. Physiol. Pharmacol.* 57: 277–285, 1980.
165. Lamarre, Y., and J. P. Lund. Load compensation in human masseter muscles. *J. Physiol. London* 253: 21–35, 1975.
166. Lang, G., and J. M. Ham. Conditional feedback systems—a new approach to feedback control. *Trans. Am. Inst. Electr. Eng., Part 2* 74: 152–161, 1955.
167. Laporte, Y., and F. Emonet-Dénand. The skeleto-fusimotor innervation of cat muscle spindle. In: *Progress in Brain Research. Understanding the Stretch Reflex*, edited by S. Homma. Amsterdam: Elsevier, 1976, vol. 44, p. 99–105.
168. Lee, R. G., and W. G. Tatton. Motor responses to sudden limb displacement in primates with specific CNS lesions and in human patients with motor system disorders. *Can. J. Neurol. Sci.* 2: 205–293, 1975.
169. Lee, R. G., and W. G. Tatton. Long loop reflexes in man:

clinical applications. In: *Cerebral Motor Control in Man: Long Loop Mechanisms*, edited by J. E. Desmedt. Basel: Karger, 1978, p. 320-333. (Prog. Clin. Neurophysiol., vol. 4.)
170. LIDDELL, E. G. T., AND C. S. SHERRINGTON. Reflexes in response to stretch (myotatic reflexes). *Proc. R. Soc. London Ser. B* 96: 212-242, 1924.
171. LIPPOLD, O. C. J. Oscillator in the stretch reflex arc and the origin of the rhythmical 8-12 C/S component of physiological tremor. *J. Physiol. London* 206: 359-382, 1970.
172. LLOYD, D. P. C. Reflex action in relation to pattern and peripheral source of afferent stimulation. *J. Physiol. London* 6: 111-210, 1943.
173. LLOYD, D. P. C. Facilitation and inhibition of spinal motoneurons. *J. Neurophysiol.* 9: 421-438, 1946.
174. LOEB, G. E., AND J. DUYSENS. Activity patterns in individual hindlimb primary and secondary muscle spindle afferents during normal movements in unrestrained cats. *J. Neurophysiol.* 42: 420-440, 1978.
175. LUCAS, M. E., AND W. D. WILLIS. Identification of muscle afferents which activate interneurons in the intermediate nucleus. *J. Neurophysiol.* 37: 282-293, 1974.
176. LUND, J. P., A. M. SMITH, B. J. SESSLE, AND T. MURAKAMI. Activity of trigeminal α- and γ-motoneurons and muscle afferents during performance of a biting task. *J. Neurophysiol.* 42: 710-725, 1979.
177. LUNDBERG, A. The supraspinal control of transmission in spinal reflex pathways. *Electroencephalogr. Clin. Neurophysiol. Suppl.* 25: 35-46, 1967.
178. LUNDBERG, A., K. MALMGREN, AND E. D. SCHOMBERG. Comments on reflex actions evoked by electrical stimulation of group II afferents. *Brain Res.* 122: 551-555, 1977.
179. LUNDBERG, A., AND G. WINSBURY. Selective activation of large afferents from muscle spindles and Golgi tendon organs. *Acta Physiol. Scand.* 49: 155-164, 1960.
180. LÜSCHER, H.-R., P. RUENZEL, E. FETZ, AND E. HENNEMAN. Postsynaptic population potentials recorded from ventral roots perfused with isotonic sucrose: connections of groups Ia and II spindle afferent fibres with large populations of motoneurons. *J. Neurophysiol.* 42: 1146-1164, 1979.
181. LÜSCHER, H.-R., P. RUENZEL, AND E. HENNEMAN. Topographic distribution of terminals of IA and group II fibers in spinal cord, as revealed by postsynaptic population potentials. *J. Neurophysiol.* 43: 968-985, 1980.
182. MACKAY, D. M., AND H. MITTELSTAEDT. Visual stability and motor control (reafference revisited). In: *Cybernetics and Bionics*, edited by W. D. Keidel, W. Handler, and M. Spreng. Munich, W. Germany: Oldenbourg, 1974, p. 71-80.
183. MACLENNAN, C. R. *Studies on the Selective Activation of Muscle Receptor Afferents* (Ph.D. thesis). Cambridge: Oxford Univ., 1971.
184. MANNARD, A., AND R. B. STEIN. Determination of the frequency response of isometric soleus muscle in the cat using random nerve stimulation. *J. Physiol. London* 229: 275-296, 1973.
185. MARSDEN, C. D., P. A. MERTON, AND H. B. MORTON. Servo action in human voluntary movement. *Nature London* 238: 140-143, 1972.
186. MARSDEN, C. D., P. A. MERTON, AND H. B. MORTON. Servo action in the human thumb. *J. Physiol. London* 257: 1-44, 1976.
187. MARSDEN, C. D., P. A. MERTON, AND H. B. MORTON. Stretch reflexes and servo actions in a variety of human muscles. *J. Physiol. London* 259: 531-560, 1976.
188. MARSDEN, C. D., P. A. MERTON, H. B. MORTON, AND J. ADAM. The effect of lesions of the dorsal columns on servo action in the human thumb. *Brain* 100: 185-200, 1977.
189. MARSDEN, C. D., P. A. MERTON, H. B. MORTON, AND J. ADAM. The effect of lesions of the sensorimotor cortex and capsular pathways on servo responses from the human long thumb flexor. *Brain* 100: 503-526, 1977.
190. MARSDEN, C. D., P. A. MERTON, H. B. MORTON, AND J. E. R. ADAM. The effect of lesions of the central nervous system on long-latency stretch reflexes in the human thumb. In: *Cerebral Motor Control in Man: Long Loop Mechanisms*, edited by J. E. Desmedt. Basel: Karger, 1978, p. 334-341. (Prog. Clin. Neurophysiol., vol. 4.)
191. MARSDEN, C. D., P. A. MERTON, H. B. MORTON, J. E. R. ADAM, AND M. HALLETT. Automatic and voluntary responses to muscle stretch in man. In: *Cerebral Motor Control in Man: Long Loop Mechanisms*, edited by J. E. Desmedt. Basel: Karger, 1978, p. 167-177. (Prog. Clin. Neurophysiol., vol. 4.)
192. MARTIN, P. J. A short essay on posture and movement. *J. Neurol. Neurosurg. Psychiatry* 40: 25-29, 1977.
193. MATTHEWS, P. B. C. The dependence of tension upon extension in the stretch reflex of the soleus muscle of the decerebrate cat. *J. Physiol. London* 147: 521-546, 1959.
194. MATTHEWS, P. B. C. A study of certain factors influencing the stretch reflex of the decerebrate cat. *J. Physiol. London* 147: 547-564, 1959.
195. MATTHEWS, P. B. C. Muscle spindles and their motor control. *Physiol. Rev.* 44: 219-288, 1964.
196. MATTHEWS, P. B. C. The reflex excitation of the soleus muscle of the decerebrate cat caused by vibration applied to its tendon. *J. Physiol. London* 184: 450-472, 1966.
197. MATTHEWS, P. B. C. Evidence that the secondary as well as the primary endings of the muscle spindles may be responsible for the tonic stretch reflex of the decerebrate cat. *J. Physiol. London* 204: 365-393, 1969.
198. MATTHEWS, P. B. C. The origin and functional significance of the stretch reflex. In: *Excitatory Synaptic Mechanisms*, edited by P. Andersen and J. K. S. Jansen. Oslo: Universitetsforlaget, 1970, p. 301-315.
199. MATTHEWS, P. B. C. *Mammalian Muscle Receptors and Their Central Actions*. Baltimore: Williams & Wilkins, 1972, p. 411-479.
200. MATTHEWS, P. B. C. The relative unimportance of the temporal pattern of the primary afferent input in determining the mean level of motor firing in the tonic vibration reflex. *J. Physiol. London* 251: 333-361, 1975.
201. MATTHEWS, P. B. C., AND G. RUSHWORTH. The selective effect of procaine on the stretch reflex and tendon jerk of soleus muscle when applied to its nerve. *J. Physiol. London* 135: 246-262, 1957.
202. MATTHEWS, P. B. C., AND R. B. STEIN. The sensitivity of muscle spindle afferents to small sinusoidal changes in length. *J. Physiol. London* 200: 723-743, 1969.
203. MCCOUCH, G. P., C. LIU, AND W. W. CHAMBERS. Descending tracts and spinal shock in the monkey. *Brain* 89: 359-376, 1966.
204. MCGRATH, G. J., AND P. B. C. MATTHEWS. Evidence from the use of vibration during procaine nerve block that the spindle group II fibres contribute excitation to the tonic stretch reflex of the decerebrate cat. *J. Physiol. London* 235: 371-408, 1973.
205. MCWILLIAM, P. N. The incidence and properties of axons to muscle spindles in the cat hind limb. *Q. J. Exp. Physiol.* 60: 25-36, 1975.
206. MELVILL-JONES, G., AND D. G. D. WATT. Muscular control of landing from unexpected falls in man. *J. Physiol. London* 219: 729-737, 1971.
207. MENDELL, L. M., AND E. HENNEMAN. Terminals of single Ia fibers: distribution within a pool of 300 homonymous motor neurons. *Science* 160: 96-98, 1968.
208. MENDELL, L. M., AND E. HENNEMAN. Terminals of single Ia fibers: location density and distribution within a pool of 300 homonymous motoneurons. *J. Neurophysiol.* 34: 171-187, 1971.
209. MENSE, S., AND R. F. SCHMIDT. Activation of group IV afferent units from muscle by algesic agents. *Brain Res.* 72: 305-310, 1974.
210. MERTON, P. A. The silent period in a muscle of the human hand. *J. Physiol. London* 114: 183-198, 1951.
211. MERTON, P. A. Speculations on the servo-control of movement. In: *The Spinal Cord*, edited by J. L. Malcolm, J. A. B. Gray,

and G. E. W. Wolstenholme. Boston: Little, Brown, 1953, p. 183–198. (Ciba Found. Symp.)
212. MILHORN, H. T., JR. *The Application of Control Theory to Physiological Systems.* Philadelphia: Saunders, 1966.
213. MILLER, A. D., AND V. B. BROOKS. Late muscular responses to torque perturbations persist during supraspinal dysfunctions in monkeys. *Exp. Brain Res.* In press.
214. MILNER-BROWN, H. S., R. B. STEIN, AND R. YEMM. Changes in firing rate of human motor units during linearly changing voluntary contraction. *J. Physiol. London* 230: 371–390, 1973.
215. MILSUM, J. H. *Biological Control Systems Analysis.* New York: McGraw-Hill, 1966.
216. MISHKIN, E., AND L. BRAUN, JR. *Adaptive Control Systems.* New York: McGraw-Hill, 1961.
217. MONSTER, A. W., AND H. CHAN. Isometric force production by motor units of extensor digitorum communis muscle in man. *J. Neurophysiol.* 40: 1432–1443, 1977.
218. MORGAN, D. L. Separation of active and passive components of short-range stiffness of muscle. *Am. J. Physiol.* 232 (*Cell Physiol.* 1): C45–C49, 1977.
219. MORGAN, D. L., U. PROSKE, AND D. WARREN. Measurements of muscle stiffness and the mechanism of elastic storage of energy in hopping kangaroos. *J. Physiol. London* 282: 253–261, 1978.
220. MURTHY, K. S. K. Vertebrate fusimotor neurones and their influences on motor behaviour. *Prog. Neurobiol. Oxford* 11: 249–307, 1978.
221. NASHNER, L. M. Adapting reflexes controlling human posture. *Exp. Brain Res.* 26: 59–72, 1976.
222. NASHNER, L. M. Fixed patterns of rapid postural responses among leg muscles during stance. *Exp. Brain Res.* 30: 13–24, 1977.
223. NAVAS, F., AND L. STARK. Sampling or intermittency in hand control system dynamics. *Biophys. J.* 8: 252–302, 1968.
224. NICHOLS, T. R. Reflex and non-reflex stiffness of soleus muscle in the cat. In: *Control of Posture and Locomotion*, edited by R. B. Stein, K. B. Pearson, R. S. Smith, and J. B. Redford. New York: Plenum, 1973, p. 407–410. (Adv. Behav. Biol., vol. 7.)
225. NICHOLS, T. R. *Soleus Muscle Stiffness and Its Reflex Control* (Ph.D. thesis). Cambridge, MA: Harvard Univ., 1974.
226. NICHOLS, T. R., AND J. C. HOUK. Improvement in linearity and regulation of stiffness that results from actions of stretch reflex. *J. Neurophysiol.* 39: 119–142, 1976.
227. NOTH, J., AND A. THILMANN. Autogenetic excitation of extensor motoneurons by group II muscle afferents in the cat. *Neurosci. Lett.* 17: 23–26, 1980.
228. PACHECO, P., AND C. GUZMAN-FLORES. Intracellular recording in extensor motoneurones of spastic cats. *Exp. Neurol.* 25: 472–481, 1969.
229. PAINTAL, A. S. Functional analysis of group III afferent fibres of mammalian muscles. *J. Physiol. London* 152: 250–270, 1960.
230. PAINTAL, A. S. Participation by pressure-pain receptors of mammalian muscles in the flexion reflex. *J. Physiol. London* 156: 498–514, 1961.
231. PARTRIDGE, L. D. Modifications of neural output signals by muscles: a frequency response study. *J. Appl. Physiol.* 20: 150–156, 1965.
232. PARTRIDGE, L. D. Signal-handling characteristics of load-moving skeletal muscle. *Am. J. Physiol.* 210: 1178–1191, 1966.
233. PARTRIDGE, L. D. Muscle properties: a problem for the motor controller physiologist. In: *Posture and Movement: Perspective for Integrating Sensory and Motor Research on the Mammalian Nervous System*, edited by R. E. Talbott and D. R. Humphrey. New York: Raven, 1979, p. 189–229.
234. PARTRIDGE, L. D., AND G. H. GLASER. Adaptation in regulation of movement and posture. A study of stretch responses in spastic animals. *J. Neurophysiol.* 23: 257–268, 1960.
235. PAVLOV, I. P. *Work of the Digestive Glands.* London: Griffin, 1910.
236. PHILLIPS, C. G. Motor apparatus of the baboon's hand. *Proc. R. Soc. London Ser. B* 173: 141–174, 1969.
237. PHILLIPS, C. G., T. P. S. POWELL, AND M. WEISENDANGER. Projection from low-threshold muscle afferents of hand and forearm to area 3a of baboon's cortex. *J. Physiol. London* 217: 419–446, 1971.
238. POLIT, A., AND E. BIZZI. Characteristics of motor programs underlying arm movements in monkeys. *J. Neurophysiol.* 42: 183–194, 1979.
239. POLLOCK, L. J., AND L. E. DAVIS. The reflex activities of a decerebrate animal. *J. Comp. Neurol.* 50: 377–411, 1930.
240. POMPEIANO, O. Alpha types of "release" studied in tension-extension diagrams from cat's forelimb triceps muscle. *Arch. Ital. Biol.* 98: 92–117, 1960.
241. POMPEIANO, O., AND P. WAND. Critical firing level of gastrocnemius soleus motoneurons showing a prolonged discharge following vibration of the homonymous muscles. *Pfluegers Arch.* 385: 263–268, 1980.
242. POPPELE, R. E., AND C. A. TERZUOLO. Myotatic reflex: its input-output relation. *Science* 159: 743–745, 1968.
243. POST, E. M., W. Z. RYMER, AND Z. HASAN. Relation between intrafusal and extrafusal activity in triceps surae muscles of the decerebrate cat: evidence for β action. *J. Neurophysiol.* 44: 383–404, 1980.
244. PROCHAZKA, A., J. A. STEPHENS, AND P. WAND. Muscle spindle discharge in normal and obstructed movements. *J. Physiol. London* 287: 57–66, 1979.
245. PROCHAZKA, A., AND P. WAND. Tendon organ discharge during voluntary movements in cats. *J. Physiol. London* 303: 385–390, 1980.
246. PROCHAZKA, A., R. A. WESTERMAN, AND S. P. ZICCONE. Discharges of single hindlimb afferents in the freely moving cat. *J. Neurophysiol.* 39: 1090–1104, 1976.
247. PROCHAZKA, A., R. A. WESTERMAN, AND S. P. ZICCONE. Ia afferent activity during a variety of voluntary movements in the cat. *J. Physiol. London* 268: 423–448, 1977.
248. RACK, P. M. H., AND D. R. WESTBURY. The effects of length and stimulus rate on tension in the isometric cat soleus muscle. *J. Physiol. London* 204: 443–460, 1969.
249. RACK, P. M. H., AND D. R. WESTBURY. The short range stiffness of active mammalian muscle and its effect on mechanical properties. *J. Physiol. London* 240: 331–350, 1974.
250. REDMAN, S. J. A quantitative approach to integrative function of dendrites. In: *Neurophysiology II*, edited by R. Porter. Baltimore: Univ. Park, 1976, p. 7–35. (Int. Rev. Physiol. Ser. Neurophysiol., vol. II.)
251. RIGGS, D. S. *Control Theory and Physiological Feedback Mechanisms.* Baltimore: Williams & Wilkins, 1970.
252. ROBERTS, T. D. M. Rhythmic excitation of a stretch reflex, revealing (a) hysteresis and (b) a difference between responses to pulling and to stretching. *Q. J. Exp. Physiol.* 48: 328–345, 1963.
253. ROBINSON, D. A. The mechanics of human saccadic eye movement. *J. Physiol. London* 174: 245–264, 1964.
254. ROSENTHAL, N. P., T. A. MCKEAN, W. J. ROBERTS, AND C. A. TERZUOLO. Frequency analysis of stretch reflex and its main subsystems in triceps surae muscles of the cat. *J. Neurophysiol.* 33: 713–749, 1970.
255. ROTHWELL, J. C., M. M. TRAUB, AND C. D. MARSDEN. Influence of voluntary intent on the human long-latency stretch reflex. *Nature London* 286: 496–498, 1980.
256. RYMER, W. Z., AND Z. HASAN. Absence of force-feedback in soleus muscle of the decerebrate cat. *Brain Res.* 184: 203–209, 1980.
257. RYMER, W. Z., Z. HASAN, AND B. CORSER. Servo-regulation of muscle contraction in man: a reevaluation. *Soc. Neurosci. Abstr.* 4: 304, 1978.
258. RYMER, W. Z., J. C. HOUK, AND P. E. CRAGO. The relation between dynamic response and velocity sensitivity for muscle spindle receptors (Abstract). *Proc. Int. Congr. Physiol. Sci., 27th, Paris, 1977,* vol. 13, p. 647.
259. RYMER, W. Z., J. C. HOUK, AND P. E. CRAGO. Mechanisms of the clasp-knife reflex studied in an animal model. *Exp. Brain Res.* 37: 93–113, 1979.

260. RYMER, W. Z., E. M. POST, AND F. R. EDWARDS. Functional roles of fusimotor and skeletofusimotor neurons studied in the decerebrate cat. In: *Muscle Receptors and Movement*, edited by A. Taylor and A. Prochazka. London: Macmillan. In press.

260a. SAKITT, B. A spring model and equivalent neural network for arm posture control. *Biol. Cybern.* 37: 227-234, 1980.

261. SCHOMBURG, E. D., AND H. B. BEHRENDS. The possibility of phase-dependent monosynaptic and polysynaptic Ia excitation to homonymous motoneurones during fictive locomotion. *Brain Res.* 143: 533-537, 1978.

262. SEVERIN, F. V. The role of the gamma-motor system in the activation of the extensor alpha-motor neurones during controlled locomotion. *Biophysics USSR* 15: 1138-1145, 1970.

263. SHERRINGTON, C. S. Decerebrate rigidity, and reflex co-ordination of movements. *J. Physiol. London* 22: 319, 1898.

264. STACEY, J. J. Free nerve endings in skeletal muscle of the cat. *J. Anat.* 105: 231-254, 1969.

265. STARK, L. *Neurological Control Systems. Studies in Bioengineering*. New York: Plenum, 1968.

266. STAUFFER, E. K., D. G. D. WATT, A. TAYLOR, R. M. REINKING, AND D. B. STUART. Analysis of muscle receptor connections by spike-triggered averaging. 2. Spindle group II afferents. *J. Neurophysiol.* 39: 1393-1402, 1976.

267. STEIN, R. B. Peripheral control of movement. *Physiol. Rev.* 54: 215-243, 1974.

268. STUART, D. G., C. G. MOSHER, R. L. GERLACK, AND R. M. REINKING. Selective activation of Ia afferents by transient muscle stretch. *Exp. Brain Res.* 10: 477-487, 1970.

269. SUGI, H. Tension changes during and after stretch in frog muscle fibers. *J. Physiol. London* 225: 237-253, 1972.

270. TAKANO, K., AND H. HENATSCH. The effect of the rate of stretch upon the development of active tension in hindlimb muscles of the decerebrate cat. *Exp. Brain Res.* 12: 422-434, 1971.

271. TATTON, W. G., S. D. FORNER, G. L. GERSTEIN, W. W. CHAMBERS, AND C. N. LIU. The effect of postcentral cortical lesions on motor responses to sudden upper limb displacement in monkeys. *Brain Res.* 96: 108-113, 1975.

272. TAYLOR, A., AND K. APPENTENG. Distinctive modes of static and dynamic fusimotor drive in jaw muscles. In: *Muscle Receptors and Movement*, edited by A. Taylor and A. Prochazka. London: Macmillan. In press.

273. TRACEY, D. J., B. WALMSLEY, AND J. BRINKMAN. "Long-loop" reflexes can be obtained in spinal monkeys. *Neurosci. Lett.* 18: 59-65, 1980.

274. TRUXAL, J. G. Control systems—some unusual design problems. In: *Adaptive Control Systems*, edited by E. Mishkin and L. Braun. New York: McGraw-Hill, 1961, chapt. 4, p. 91-118.

275. TSUKAHARA, N., AND C. OHYE. Polysynaptic activation of extensor motoneurones from group Ia fibers in the cat spinal cord. *Experientia* 20: 628-629, 1964.

276. TSYPKIN, Y. Z. Adaptive system theory today and tomorrow. In: *Sensitivity, Adaptivity, and Optimality*, edited by G. Guardabassi. Pittsburgh, PA: Int. Fed. Automatic Control, 1973, p. 47-67. (Int. Fed. Automatic Control Symp., 3rd, Ischia, Italy, 1973.)

277. TSYPKIN, Y. Z. Adaptive optimization algorithms when there is a priori uncertainty. *Autom. Remote Control USSR* 40: 857-868, 1979.

278. VALLBO, Å. B. Slowly adapting muscle receptors in man. *Acta Physiol. Scand.* 78: 315-333, 1970.

279. VALLBO, Å. B. Discharge patterns in human muscle spindle afferents during isometric voluntary contraction. *Acta Physiol. Scand.* 80: 532-566, 1970.

280. VALLBO, Å. B. Muscle spindle response at the onset of isometric voluntary contractions in man. Time difference between fusimotor and skeletomotor effects. *J. Physiol. London* 218: 405-431, 1971.

281. VALLBO, Å. B. Impulse activity from human muscle spindles during voluntary contractions. In: *Motor Control*, edited by A. A. Gydikov, N. T. Tankov, and D. S. Kosarov. New York: Plenum, 1973, p. 33-43. (Proc. 2nd Int. Symp. Mot. Control "Zlatni Pyassatsi" near Varna, Bulgaria, 1973.)

282. VALLBO, Å. B. Afferent discharge from human muscle spindles in noncontracting muscles. Steady state impulse frequency as a function of joint angle. *Acta Physiol. Scand.* 90: 303-318, 1974.

283. VALLBO, Å. B. Human muscle spindle discharge during isometric voluntary contractions. Amplitude relations between spindle frequency and torque. *Acta Physiol. Scand.* 90: 319-336, 1974.

284. VALLBO, Å. B., K.-E. HAGBARTH, H. E. TOREBJÖRK, AND B. G. WALLIN. Somatosensory, proprioceptive, and sympathetic activity in human peripheral nerves. *Physiol. Rev.* 59: 919-957, 1979.

285. VON HOLST, E., AND H. MITTELSTAEDT. Das Reafferenzprinzip (Wechselwirkugen zwischen Zentralnervensystem und Peripherie). *Naturwissenschaften* 37: 464-476, 1950.

286. WESTBURY, D. R. The response of motoneurones of the cat to sinusoidal movements of the muscles they innervate. *Brain Res.* 25: 75-86, 1971.

287. WESTBURY, D. R. A study of stretch and vibration reflexes of the cat by intracellular recording from motoneurons. *J. Physiol. London* 226: 37-56, 1972.

288. WILLIS, W. D., AND WILLIS, S. C. Properties of interneurons in the ventral spinal cord. *Arch. Ital. Biol.* 104: 354-386, 1966.

289. WILSON, D. M., AND J. L. LARIMER. The catch property of ordinary muscle. *Proc. Natl. Acad. Sci. USA* 61: 909-916, 1968.

290. WOLPAW, J. Electromagnetic muscle stretch strongly excites sensorimotor cortex neurons in behaving primates. *Science* 203: 465-467, 1979.

291. WUERKER, R. B., AND E. HENNEMAN. Reflex regulation of primary (annulospiral) stretch receptors via gamma motoneurons in the cat. *J. Neurophysiol.* 26: 539-550, 1963.

292. ZARZECKI, P., Y. SHINODA, AND H. ASANUMA. Projection from area 3a to the motor cortex by neurons activated from group I muscle afferents. *Exp. Brain Res.* 33: 269-282, 1978.

CHAPTER 9

Tremor and clonus

RICHARD B. STEIN | Department of Physiology, University of Alberta, Edmonton, Alberta, Canada

ROBERT G. LEE | Department of Medicine (Neurology), University of Calgary, Calgary, Alberta, Canada

CHAPTER CONTENTS

Types of Tremor and Clonus
  Physiological tremor
  Pathological tremors
    Resting tremor
    Postural tremor
    Intention tremor
  Anatomic relationships
  Clonus
Mechanisms of Tremor
  Mechanical oscillations
  Reflex oscillations
    Gain
    Latency
    Stability
    Interaction of mechanisms
    Resetting
  Central oscillations
    Single pacemakers
    Central feedback onto motoneurons
    Interneuronal networks
    Supraspinal oscillators
Conclusions

RHYTHMIC OSCILLATIONS are a feature of many biological activities controlled by the nervous system: e.g., respiration, locomotion, mastication. The time periods of these basic oscillations vary widely but are often several seconds, as for example in respiration. Voluntary movements of the limbs can be made at various frequencies, up to a limit of about 6 Hz (94). Frequencies near this upper limit are found in rather skilled movements such as handwriting, and it has been suggested that many of the common letters are produced by modulating a basic 6-Hz oscillation (55). The limit of 6 Hz is not absolute, and Smith et al. (111) have recently found that by using special mechanisms a cat can shake its paw at 11 Hz to remove water or other material.

In trying to maintain a steady posture or to perform a voluntary movement, almost invariably there are unwanted or involuntary oscillations that are generally referred to as tremor or clonus. Tremor cannot be defined by frequency alone, because, for example, if the oscillations generated from an outstretched limb are measured, a range of frequencies that spans the entire range of voluntary movements (45, 99) can be observed and may extend to considerably higher frequencies. Indeed, if one measures the magnitude of the different frequency components under these conditions, the largest components generally occur at low frequencies (below 5 Hz). The movements at low frequency are usually quite random, and interest has centered on higher frequency components that are often more oscillatory. If one measures the acceleration of a limb, which may be related to the forces generated as a result of neural activity, the most prominent peak is often near 10 Hz. Note that by measuring acceleration one is merely accentuating the high-frequency components, because the acceleration (in $\mu m/s^2$) of a sine wave of constant amplitude increases as the square of its frequency in cycles per second (or inversely as the square of the period in seconds).

Because of its possible correlation with neuronal activity, neurophysiologists and neurologists have tended to focus mainly on a narrow band of frequencies around 10 Hz (from 8 to 12 Hz) in studying the so-called normal physiological tremor associated with the posture or voluntary movements of a normal subject. Simply by loading a limb of a normal human subject with different masses and springs, however, Joyce and Rack (66) were able to produce substantial rhythmic oscillations at frequencies from 2 to more than 20 Hz. Similarly in a common experimental paradigm (33) in which a monkey holds a lever attached to a torque motor, the loading may be such that a tremor frequency near 6 Hz is observed, which can be changed to about one-half that frequency, e.g., by cooling the dentate nucleus [reviewed by Brooks (8)].

To summarize, tremor may be defined operationally as an involuntary movement characterized by a rhythmical oscillation about a fixed point or trajectory. In addition to the normal physiological tremor introduced above, rhythmic oscillations occur as a prominent feature of a number of different neurological diseases in animals and in the human being. Oscillations similar to these pathological tremors can be produced experimentally by placing selective lesions or applying drugs at a number of different sites within the central nervous system. The cooling of the dentate nucleus mentioned in the last paragraph is merely a reversible manner of blocking the activity of this area (see the chapter by Brooks and Thach in this *Handbook*).

The difficulty in defining the title of this chapter illustrates the kind of problem faced in writing a review of tremor and clonus. [Note that we have avoided the difficult question of what distinguishes a voluntary from an involuntary movement (27) and have not tried to distinguish those oscillations referred to as tremor from those referred to as clonus.] Therefore the nature and level of this chapter is quite different from that found in many other chapters of this *Handbook*, in which the subject matter is easily defined and presented in a detailed, didactic fashion. The rationale for including a chapter on this subject is that tremor has attracted a great deal of interest from both neurophysiologists and clinical neurologists. As a sustained rhythmical oscillation, it lends itself well to experimental investigation, and in many respects tremor provides a unique opportunity for the direct application of mathematical principles and theoretical considerations to gain a better understanding of both normal oscillatory mechanisms in intact nervous systems and abnormal oscillations that develop as a result of disease processes or experimental lesions.

This chapter is intended to be read by a wide audience and for the most part is concise and nontechnical. Rather than attempting to present a comprehensive review of the vast, diffuse, and often poorly controlled clinical literature dealing with tremor, we have chosen to present in section TYPES OF TREMOR AND CLONUS, p. 326, a brief, clinically oriented survey of the various forms of physiological and pathological tremor that occur in human subjects. For example, in dealing with tremors arising from disorders in the cerebellum or the basal ganglia, it clearly is not possible to go into the detail found in the chapters by Brooks and Thach and by DeLong and Georgopoulos in this *Handbook* devoted to these structures. Nonetheless experimental models of tremor in animals produced by surgical or pharmacological techniques are discussed briefly, and parallels are drawn between these types of tremor and spontaneously occurring tremors in the human being.

Some general properties of oscillations in mechanical systems are reviewed in section MECHANISMS OF TREMOR, p. 332, which serves as a basis for discussing specific mechanisms underlying the generation of tremor in physiological systems. To the extent that we have had to select certain aspects for treatment, rather than attempting to provide a general framework, the reader may be stimulated to fill in the many gaps still remaining in our present understanding of tremor and clonus. The reader may also wish to refer to a recently published book (28) that deals in more detail with some types of tremor. The role of feedback in normal movement, which is relevant to some aspects of tremor, is considered in more detail in the chapters by Houk and Rymer and by Rack in this *Handbook*.

TYPES OF TREMOR AND CLONUS

Physiological Tremor

From a clinical point of view, tremor that occurs in human subjects can be broadly subdivided into physiological or normal tremor and pathological tremors. Physiological tremor is a low-amplitude oscillation that, with suitable recording techniques, can be demonstrated in nearly all normal subjects. Although it is most apparent in the outstretched fingers, physiological tremor occurs in other parts of the body, including the lower extremities, the head, and even the tongue (83). As discussed above, the frequency is variable and depends on the age of the subject, the part of the body being examined, and the technique used to record the tremor. The 8- to 12-Hz component observed in the fingers of young adults (78, 83) generally occurs at lower frequencies (around 6 Hz) in young children and elderly persons (83). The tremor in proximal muscles also tends to be lower in frequency than that in distal muscles (83).

Physiological tremor is not present in the totally relaxed extremity but increases in parallel with the tonic activation of muscles to maintain a fixed posture opposing gravity or other external forces (postural tremor). Usually it persists without much change in amplitude during the execution of a voluntary movement, except insofar as the activation of the muscles (and hence the tremor) must be increased to produce a movement [but see Neilson and Lance (94)].

There are a number of factors that accentuate this type of tremor, giving rise to what is sometimes referred to as enhanced physiological tremor. These include fatigue, anxiety, excess alcohol intake, increased metabolism such as that which occurs with hyperthyroidism, and intravenous infusion of adrenaline. As a result of these observations, it has been suggested that endogenous catecholamines may play a role in the generation of physiological tremor, possibly by a direct action on β-adrenergic receptors in the muscles of the extremity [see Marsden (78)]. Although adrenergic mechanisms may be involved in enhanced physiological tremor, the mechanism of their action remains unclear.

The mechanisms responsible for various forms of tremor are considered in detail in section MECHANISMS OF TREMOR, p. 332. A short discussion of possible mechanisms underlying physiological tremor is introduced at this point, however, because it is likely that all of the mechanisms proposed for pathological tremors make some contribution to physiological tremor. The major mechanisms can be considered under three broad categories: *1*) mechanical factors, *2*) reflex oscillations, and *3*) central oscillations.

The mechanical properties of a limb can be considered as a mass-spring system that is capable of developing sustained oscillations provided there is some additional source of energy to maintain these oscillations. The natural resonant frequency depends on the mass of the system and has been calculated to be approximately 9 Hz for the human wrist, but the natural frequency is considerably lower for more proximal parts of the limb and higher for the fingers [see Marsden (78)].

One possible external source of energy that has been considered is the ballistic effect of the heartbeat (11). The ballistocardiac impulse undoubtedly makes some contribution to tremor recorded from the fingers, and oscillations occurring in time with the heartbeat can be recorded in completely denervated limbs or after paralysis with succinylcholine (78). It seems unlikely, however, that this is the major mechanism responsible for the 8- to 12-Hz tremor recorded in the outstretched fingers of normal human subjects. Marsden et al. (81) have investigated the ballistocardiac effect using cross-spectral analysis and coherence of tremor between the two hands, and have concluded that less than 10% of the tremor recorded from the outstretched fingers can be accounted for by the heartbeat.

A second driving force that may interact with the mechanical resonant properties of a limb to produce tremor is provided by the firing of motoneurons. Normally motoneurons fire in an asynchronous manner, so during voluntary activation the normal firing of motor units would not be expected to produce substantial tremor, even though the firing rates at recruitment are close to the frequency of physiological tremor. However, if there is a tendency for motor unit discharges to become grouped or synchronized, something that occurs with fatigue and isometric training (87), the possibility then exists for motor unit firing to generate oscillations in an extremity. Furthermore, if one considers that motor units firing at 8–10 Hz give rise to an unfused tetanus, then it is conceivable that during a steady maintained contraction the most recently recruited motor units, which are larger than those recruited initially (89), could give rise to rhythmical twitches of the muscle at a frequency around 10 Hz (29).

Several lines of evidence suggest that physiological tremor is at least partially due to oscillations occurring as a result of instability of the servomechanism associated with the spinal stretch reflex (45, 47, 66, 73). It is well recognized that oscillations can develop if appropriate delays are introduced into a mechanical system with positive feedback (see section MECHANISMS OF TREMOR, p. 332). Physiological tremor is absent in the disorder tabes dorsalis (46), in which the afferent part of the reflex loop is interrupted. This observation lends support to the concept that oscillations in reflex loops contribute to physiological tremor, although deafferentation clearly also affects the excitability of motoneurons. Further evidence suggesting involvement of segmental reflex mechanisms has been provided by Lippold (73), who has shown that physiological tremor can be modified or reset by perturbations applied to the outstretched fingers. Others have challenged this explanation for physiological tremor, however, pointing out that it may persist in a totally deafferented limb (79), that the frequency remains relatively constant in widely separated muscles regardless of the length of the stretch-reflex loop [(72); but see ref. 93], and that the tremor frequency is not altered by ischemia of a limb sufficient to interrupt the stretch-reflex arc (4, 72).

The possibility that physiological tremor is driven by central oscillations arising from supraspinal structures has also been considered (71). Synchronization of motor unit discharges as a possible factor contributing to tremor has already been mentioned, and it is possible that synchronization could occur in response to synchronous discharges originating at higher levels in the nervous system. Synchronization could also arise from reflex feedback, and methods that try to separate peripheral mechanisms (involving mechanical factors and reflex feedback) from those arising wholly in the central nervous system are discussed in section MECHANISMS OF TREMOR, p. 332.

The similarity in frequency between the α-rhythm of the electroencephalogram (EEG) and physiological tremor has led to speculation that some common form of central nervous system pacemaker may be giving rise to both types of oscillation [reviewed by Lippold (74)]. No firm evidence to support this hypothesis has emerged, however, and Jasper and Andrews (63) demonstrated that the tremor of limb muscles did not remain in phase with the EEG. Marsden and co-workers' observations (81) that the phase and frequency of physiological tremor in a subject's two hands are not necessarily the same also argue against this type of tremor being driven by a central oscillator.

Therefore the origin of physiological tremor remains uncertain, despite the fact that it has been the subject of numerous investigations. Probably no single mechanism can be implicated, and the available evidence suggests that tremor arises as a result of interaction between firing patterns of motor units, feedback in segmental reflex mechanisms, and mechanical properties of the extremity, with perhaps a contribution from some as yet unspecified oscillating mechanism within the central nervous system.

Pathological Tremors

Although several distinct types of pathological tremors exist, there has not been universal agreement among clinicians as to how they should be classified, and the descriptive nomenclature is confusing and sometimes inconsistent. Terms such as *static tremor* and *action tremor* have been used by various authors to describe different entities. Attempts to classify tremors on an anatomic basis by using terms such as *cerebellar tremor* and *striatal tremor* have not been entirely satisfactory, because clinically similar tremors may occur with lesions in several different locations in the central nervous system.

The most widely accepted clinical classification of pathological tremor is based on the posture or type of volitional activity during which the tremor is likely to occur (83). Some forms of tremor characteristically are present when the extremity is at rest and disappear with the initiation of voluntary movement, whereas other types are most apparent when the arms are held outstretched to maintain a fixed posture. Another form of tremor becomes most apparent during the execution of a target-directed voluntary movement. Thus, using these criteria, it is possible to subdivide pathological tremors into three major categories: *1*) resting tremor, *2*) postural tremor, and *3*) intention tremor.

In the following sections we describe each of these types of tremor in terms of the symptoms found in a single disease state in which it features prominently. It should be noted, however, that there is some overlap among these categories. Parkinsonian tremor, which is the classical example of resting tremor, may persist during voluntary movement, and cerebellar disorders may be associated with tremors that have features of both postural and intention tremor. To fully categorize pathological tremors, it is necessary to consider other criteria, including associated neurological signs, the amplitude and frequency of oscillation, and the patterns of discharge in electromyographic (EMG) activity from agonist and antagonist muscles.

RESTING TREMOR. The well-known clinical features of the resting tremor of Parkinson's disease were well described more than 150 years ago (100). This tremor is slower than physiological tremor and some other forms of pathological tremor, and it occurs at a frequency of 4–7 Hz. It is most pronounced in the distal muscles of the upper extremity, where the combination of flexion-extension and pronation-supination gives rise to the characteristic "pill-rolling" movements. At least in the early stages of the disease, the tremor of parkinsonism is a classical resting tremor that disappears when the involved muscles are activated voluntarily. Later in the disease the tremor may persist during voluntary effort and may significantly interfere with skilled movements. Some parkinsonian patients show evidence of a second, more rapid type of tremor in the 8- to 10-Hz range occurring during voluntary contraction of muscles, and it has been suggested that there may be two separate types of tremor in Parkinson's disease—the classical 4- to 7-Hz resting tremor and a more rapid tremor that is possibly an exaggeration of physiological tremor (43, 72). Recently Stiles and Pozos (117) found a continuous range of frequencies in parkinsonian tremor between 4 and 9 Hz, with the frequency varying inversely with tremor amplitude. Furthermore a virtually similar amplitude dependence was observed under conditions in which physiological tremor became greatly exaggerated in normal subjects (116). Because the frequency of physiological tremor can be affected by external factors acting through the peripheral nervous system, Stiles and Pozos (117) suggested that similar peripheral mechanisms may be operative for both normal and parkinsonian tremor (see also ref. 60).

Electromyographic recordings show that parkinsonian tremor is associated with alternating bursts of activity in antagonistic muscle groups (110). This is said to be distinct from another disease entity referred to as *essential tremor* (see POSTURAL TREMOR, p. 328), where synchronous coactivation of opposing groups of muscles can occur. Our own observations indicate, however, that alternating activation of opposing muscle groups does occur in some forms of essential tremor and that coactivation can occur in parkinsonian tremor.

Most of the symptoms of parkinsonism can be attributed to the now well-recognized abnormality in the nigrostriatal system that results in a deficiency of striatal dopamine (59). Classical resting tremor develops in less than one-half of the patients with Parkinson's disease, however (R. G. Lee, unpublished observations), and the presence of tremor tends to be uncorrelated with other features of the disease such as rigidity (91) and akinesia (lack of movement), suggesting that the tremor arises from somewhat different mechanisms than the other features of Parkinson's disease. Furthermore tremor is not a common feature of the parkinsonian syndrome that develops as a complication of treatment with psychotropic drugs (82) such as phenothiazines, which may block striatal dopamine receptors. Treatment of Parkinson's disease with L-dopa suppresses a resting tremor in many patients, but the results are less consistent and predictable than the improvement in rigidity and akinesia (85). Therefore it seems likely that factors in addition to striatal dopamine deficiency are involved in the generation of parkinsonian tremor (see the chapter by DeLong and Georgopoulos in this *Handbook*).

POSTURAL TREMOR. Among the pathological tremors, the most common example of a postural tremor is benign "essential" tremor. Clinicians tend to lump together under this term a number of different forms of tremor that may not all be related to the same mechanism. The classical form of essential tremor is not present in an extremity that is completely at rest. As in physiological tremor, it appears when the limbs are maintained in a fixed posture. Some forms of essential tremor may show features of intention tremor in that they are aggravated during an intended or voluntary movement. Although essential tremor is most apparent in the distal upper extremities, it can involve other body parts, including the head, the face, and even the muscles involved in speaking. Most cases of essential tremor develop during early adult life. There is a strong family history of a similar form of tremor, and in this situation the disorder is referred to as heredofamilial tremor. A clinically similar tremor may also develop during later life, in which case it is referred to as senile tremor.

The frequency of essential tremor is usually 8–10 Hz in young adults, but, as is the case with physiological tremor, the frequency is slower in young children and in persons of advancing age. Marshall (83) points out that the frequency of essential tremor for an individual within a certain age group is the same as the frequency of physiological tremor for that age group. The similarities in frequency and other characteristics between these two forms of tremor suggest that at least some forms of essential tremor may represent nothing more than exaggerated physiological tremor.

As the term *essential* implies, the cause of this form of tremor is unknown. No specific central nervous system lesions have been demonstrated in patients with essential tremor, and in the majority of cases there are no associated neurological abnormalities. In a large series of patients with essential tremor, however, Baxter et al. (7) have observed an increased incidence of other motor disorders, such as abnormal posturing (dystonia) and spasmodic movements of the neck (torticollis).

The question of central oscillations versus peripheral reflex mechanisms has been introduced in relation to physiological tremor and is considered in more detail in subsection INTENTION TREMOR, p. 329. It is pertinent to mention here, however, that the phase of essential tremor can be modified or reset by mechanical perturbations applied to an extremity (113). This suggests that external inputs must play at least some role in the generation of this form of tremor.

Clinicians have long been aware of the fact that ingestion of even small amounts of alcohol is remarkably effective in suppressing essential tremor, although the exact site or mode of action is unknown (83). It is also well recognized that anxiety or intravenous infusion of adrenergic substances accentuate both physiological tremor and essential tremor. Furthermore, propranolol, a β-adrenergic blocker, has been shown to be an effective form of treatment for essential tremor (124).

A number of experiments have been carried out in an attempt to determine the specific sites at which these drugs act to modify tremor. Marsden et al. (80) demonstrated that intra-arterial infusion of isoproterenol into an extremity accentuated physiological tremor only in that extremity. Furthermore this effect could be blocked locally by intra-arterial propranolol injected into the same extremity. These observations suggest that the accentuation of physiological tremor by adrenergic substances occurs as a result of their action on peripheral β-adrenergic receptors within the muscle or extremity.

With the many similarities that exist between essential tremor and physiological tremor, one might suspect that the beneficial effects of propranolol in essential tremor occur due to blockage of peripheral β-adrenergic receptors. This does not appear to be true, however. Young et al. (126) showed, in a study similar to that carried out by Marsden (80), that intra-arterial propranolol given to patients with essential tremor did not suppress the tremor in the injected extremity, suggesting that propranolol exerts its effect on essential tremor by blocking β-receptors at other sites, possibly within the central nervous system.

INTENTION TREMOR. Intention tremor, as the name implies, occurs during the execution of an intended voluntary movement. Characteristically there is little tremor at rest or during maintenance of a fixed posture. As the subject carries out a controlled target-directed movement, however, such as the finger-nose test employed by clinicians, coarse rhythmical oscillations develop around the trajectory of the intended movement. The frequency varies between 3 and 7 Hz, and the amplitude of the oscillations becomes progressively larger as the target is approached.

Intention tremor is the most common of several forms of tremor that occur in association with injuries or disease involving the cerebellum or its projections. Cerebellar tremor was studied over an extended period of time by Holmes and has been well described in his classic review papers (56, 57). Cerebellar disorders may also be associated with postural tremors, and in severe cases there may be an almost constant rhythmic oscillation of the entire body, including the trunk and the head, that occurs with any attempt to maintain a fixed posture. On the other hand, as in Parkinson's disease, tremor is not found in all cases of cerebellar damage.

Clinical pathological correlations from studies on human beings indicate that intention tremor occurs as a result of lesions involving either the deep cerebellar nuclei, particularly the dentate, or their efferent projections in the superior cerebellar peduncle (24). Animal models of cerebellar intention tremor have been produced by cerebellectomy (26), by red nucleus lesions (107), by selective stereotactic lesions involving the dentate (42), or by reversible cooling of the deep cerebellar nuclei (9, 16, 120). The normal function of these areas and their interconnections is dealt with in the chapter by Brooks and Thach in this *Handbook* (see also Fig. 1). Experimental cerebellar tremor in animals is similar to intention tremor in human beings in that it becomes more prominent as the animal reaches out to obtain food or to carry out some other form of target-directed movement.

The clinical literature contains references to another form of tremor known as *rubral tremor*, thought to be associated with lesions in or near the red nucleus (see ref. 83). Clinically, this tremor has features of both postural tremor and intention tremor. In fact, there is sufficient overlap among what has been described as rubral tremor and other forms of tremor that there would not seem to be adequate justification for identifying rubral tremor as a distinct and separate entity. Considering the fact that much of the outflow from the dentate nucleus is directed to the red nucleus, it is not surprising that lesions of either structure or of the pathways connecting them result in clinically similar tremors. Experimental lesions of the red nucleus (107) produce intention tremor similar to that developing after cerebellectomy.

Anatomic Relationships

Figure 1 illustrates schematically some of the structures and pathways believed to be involved in the generation of tremor. This figure is obviously oversimplified and is not intended to illustrate the anatomic details of these pathways. It serves as a conceptual basis for further discussion of the anatomic and physiological mechanisms underlying tremor, however, and helps integrate some of the clinical observations already discussed with the results of experimental studies.

The multiple projections among the structures shown in Figure 1 can be considered to form a series of interconnecting loops or circuits. One of these includes the inferior olive and its projections to the cerebellum, the dentatorubral pathway (from the dentate nucleus of the cerebellum to the red nucleus), and connections back from the red nucleus to the inferior olive. A second major system consists of the substantia nigra and the corpus striatum and the reciprocal connections between these structures. Superimposed on these brain stem and diencephalic circuits is a third system with projections from the corpus striatum to the globus pallidus, from the globus pallidus to the ventrolateral (VL) and ventroanterior (VA) nuclei of the thalamus, and from there to the motor cortex and then back to the corpus striatum. Note that part of the output from the dentate nucleus of the cerebellum also projects through the VL-VA nuclei of the thalamus to the motor cortex. There are many other loops such as those involving the globus pallidus and the subthalamic nucleus or the motor cortex and cerebellum that could be involved, but their role in the generation of tremor is not clear, and they are not considered further here (compare the chapters by DeLong and Georgopoulos and by Brooks and Thach).

The numbers on the illustration in Figure 1 are intended to identify the structures involved in tremor generation or sites where lesions either produce or abolish tremor. These are considered in sequence:

1. This indicates the site of lesions in the superior cerebellar peduncle that are believed to give rise to intention tremor. This is a common site for demyelinating plaques in multiple sclerosis, a disorder in which intention tremor is a common feature. As already mentioned, experimental lesions involving the origin of this pathway in the dentate nucleus in monkeys produce intention tremor with characteristics similar to those seen in disorders in human beings.

2. It is uncertain whether the inferior olive, through its connections to the cerebellum, is involved in the generation of any of the spontaneously occurring pathological tremors. Neurons in this nucleus, however, do develop abnormal bursting activity associated with the rapid 7- to 12-Hz tremor produced by the drug harmaline (70), and similarities have been drawn between experimental harmaline tremor and essential tremor in human beings (see further discussion in section MECHANISMS OF TREMOR, p. 332).

Brief mention is made here of another type of abnormal rhythmical movement, palatal myoclonus. This consists of rhythmical contractions of the soft palate and related muscles that occur at a frequency of about 120 Hz. It occurs as a result of brain stem lesions that interrupt the central tegmental tract, the major site of connections between the red nucleus and the inferior olive (49). Thus it is apparent that the olivocerebellorubral loop is involved to some extent in the generation of several forms of tremor or abnormal oscillatory activity.

3. Degeneration of dopaminergic neurons in the pars compacta of the substantia nigra is a constant feature of Parkinson's disease. Although additional factors may be involved in the generation of parkin-

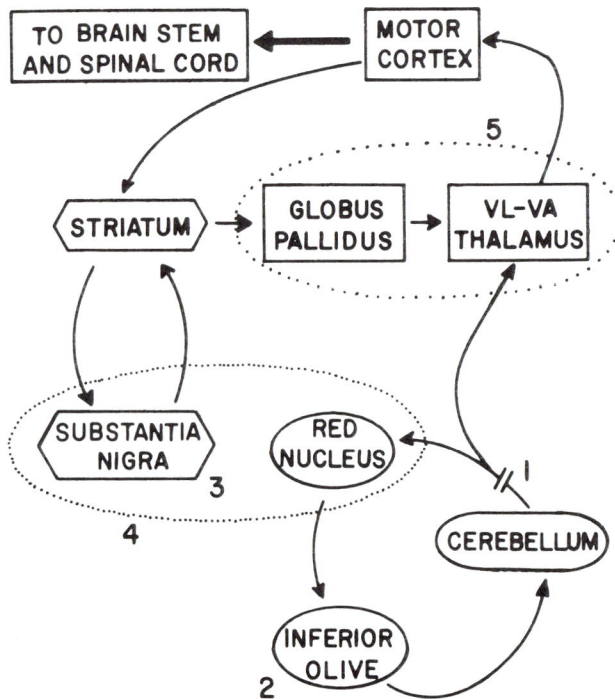

FIG. 1. Supraspinal anatomical structures involved in various types of tremor. See discussion in text. Numbers identify structures involved in tremor generation or sites where lesions either produce or abolish tremor.

sonian tremor, there is ample evidence that replacement therapy with L-dopa reduces or abolishes this form of tremor.

4. The dotted line in Figure 1 surrounding the substantia nigra and the red nucleus is intended to represent the site of ventral mesencephalic lesions that give rise to a parkinsonian tremor in monkeys. To consistently produce a tremor, these lesions must involve elements of both substantia nigra or its efferent pathways and the olivocerebellorubral system (102). Lesions of substantia nigra alone are not sufficient to produce tremor in monkeys.

5. Stereotactic lesions within the area indicated by 5 in Figure 1, involving either globus pallidus or more commonly VL thalamus, abolish parkinsonian tremor (18, 92). Similarly placed lesions may have a beneficial effect on cerebellar intention tremor and some forms of essential tremor (17). Further evidence for involvement of these structures in parkinsonian tremor is provided by several investigators who have demonstrated rhythmically discharging units in the globus pallidus that fire in association with the tremor (1, 64). Whether these units are actually driving the tremor, or whether they are merely responding to peripheral inputs from the moving extremities or to central oscillators elsewhere in the central nervous system, remains uncertain.

The points outlined above confirm the notion that the structures shown in Figure 1 are involved in some manner in the generation of tremor. It is apparent, however, that there are several missing pieces of information that must be incorporated into this scheme before a comprehensive theory to explain pathological tremors can be developed. Nevertheless, the motor system does include a number of internal feedback loops of the type shown in Figure 1 that are potentially capable of developing oscillations if modulating influences are removed. For example, oscillations in the corticopallidothalamic loop might result if the degeneration of the nigrostriatal system were to remove inhibitory influences on striatal neurons. Based on his extensive experiments on monkeys, Lamarre (68) made the interesting suggestion that there are two primary tremor-generating systems in the brain that he referred to as the thalamocortical and olivocerebellar systems.

Clonus

Although not generally considered in the same category as spontaneously occurring tremors, clonus represents another form of oscillation in a physiological system and is discussed briefly here. Clonus is a sustained rhythmical contraction, usually initiated by applying a sudden rapid stretch to a muscle, and tends to persist as long as the muscle is maintained under some degree of stretch. Generally it occurs in association with lesions involving descending motor pathways in the brain stem or spinal cord, and it is usually, but not invariably, associated with other signs of reflex hyperexcitability such as spasticity and increased tendon jerks. Clinically, clonus is most easily demonstrated in the gastrocnemius-soleus muscle group following sudden forceful dorsiflexion of the ankle, but it may also occur in other muscles such as the quadriceps or wrist flexors. The frequency of ankle clonus in human subjects varies between 5 and 8 Hz.

Clonus appears to be analogous to rhythmical oscillations that develop in stretched muscles in certain experimental preparations such as the premammillary cat (40, 93). Commonly clonus occurs in the human being following complete transection of the spinal cord. The most widely accepted explanation for clonus, based at least partially on observations on the silent period in decerebrate cats by Denny-Brown (23), is that clonus is due to "self-reexcitation" of hyperactive stretch reflexes, an example of an oscillation that is maintained entirely by reflex mechanisms (14, 15, 93) and is not dependent on central nervous system oscillations that are present in the spinal cord and brain stem (41). The brisk reflex contraction of the muscle that occurs in response to the initial stretch results in unloading the spindles. As the muscle relaxes and begins to lengthen during the silent period the spindles are again stretched, and this gives rise to another reflex contraction of the muscle. This explanation requires an assumption that the spindles are in an abnormally sensitive state and does not account for the occasional examples of clonus that occur without evidence of reflex hyperexcitability in the form of spasticity or exaggerated tendon jerks.

Some support for the sequence of events outlined above has been provided by recordings from single muscle afferents in patients with clonus (44, 118). Both of these groups have shown that the spindle discharges occur only during the relaxation or lengthening phase of the cycle and not during both contraction and relaxation phases, as is the situation with either voluntary alternating movements or parkinsonian tremor.

An alternative explanation for clonus has been proposed by Walsh (121), who observed that clonus in human beings could not be synchronized or entrained by an externally applied oscillation occurring at a frequency close to that of the clonus. Instead, the two oscillations proceeded independently, waxing and waning at a "beat" frequency. This result suggested to Walsh that clonus might be driven by an independent spinal oscillator rather than being generated by reflex mechanisms. This suggestion, however, does not automatically follow from the presence of beating, as discussed in subsection *Reflex Oscillations*, p. 334.

In summary, the various forms of tremor and clonus can be classified clinically in terms of *1*) associated disease entities (e.g., parkinsonian tremor, cerebellar tremor), *2*) the state in which they are most prominent (e.g., rest tremor, postural tremor, or intention tremor), *3*) the anatomical structures involved, and *4*) the frequency or other characteristics of the oscillations. From a physiological point of view, it would be desirable to classify tremor in terms of underlying functional mechanisms. The next section considers the extent to which such a classification is possible at the present time.

MECHANISMS OF TREMOR

Having briefly reviewed the types of tremor found physiologically and clinically, we now turn to a consideration of possible mechanisms. Some of the factors that determine the amplitude and frequency of tremor can be appreciated by considering the general properties of oscillations in a mechanical system (see the chapters by Rack and by Houk and Rymer in this *Handbook*). We therefore digress briefly to consider the mathematical properties of mechanical oscillations before returning to their role in tremor.

Mechanical Oscillations

The simplest type of oscillation is a mechanical one in which a mass M interacts with a spring of stiffness K, as shown in Figure 2A. In an ideal frictionless system, the mass would oscillate indefinitely at an amplitude A with a natural frequency f_n and a position $y(t)$ given by

$$y(t) = A \sin (2\pi f_n t) \quad (1)$$

where

$$f_n = \frac{1}{2\pi} \sqrt{K/M} \quad (2)$$

In all real systems there is some damping, as indicated by the dashpot with viscosity D in Figure 2A.

The effect of the dashpot (20) is to make the oscillation decay in response to a brief perturbation

$$y(t) = A e^{pt} \sin (2\pi f_d t) \quad (3)$$

where A is a constant depending on the magnitude of the perturbation, f_d is the damping frequency that is related to the natural frequency by

$$f_d = f_n \sqrt{1 - \zeta^2} \quad (4)$$

p is the rate constant for the exponential decay or growth of the oscillation given by

$$p = 2\pi f_n \zeta \quad (5)$$

and ζ is the damping ratio and is related to the other parameters by

$$\zeta = \frac{1}{2} \cdot \frac{D}{\sqrt{KM}} \quad (6)$$

A simple mass-spring system such as shown in Figure 2 can be described by a second-order differential equation, and is often referred to as a second-order system. Another important property of a second-order damped system is that it can be driven at a range of frequencies, even though it oscillates most easily at the frequency f_d when ζ is small. Note that the damping frequency in Equation 4 does not exist when $\zeta > 1$, because the quantity under the square root becomes negative. The ability to respond to a given frequency (called the frequency response) can be obtained by standard methods from Equation 3. Frequency-response curves for a few values of damping are shown in Figure 2B. In a second-order system, the response falls off as the second power of frequency at high frequencies (a slope of -2 on the log-log plot of Fig. 2).

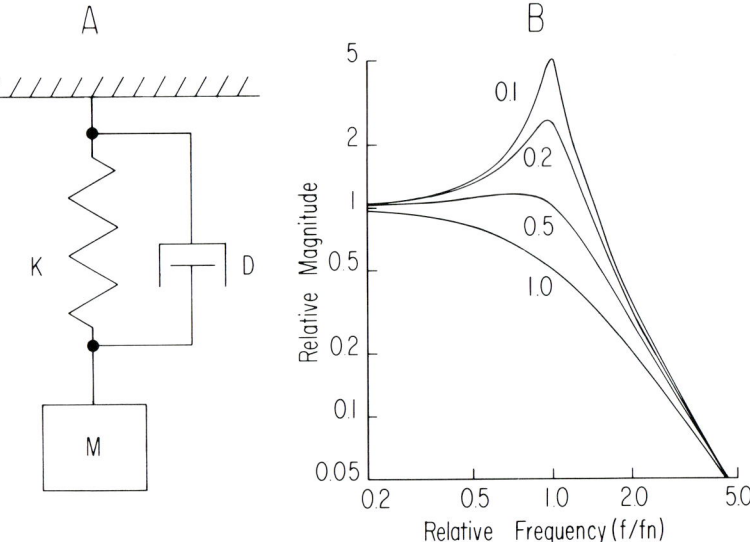

FIG. 2. *A*: schematic representation of mechanical oscillator consisting of mass, M, spring of stiffness, K, and dashpot with viscosity, D. *B*: relative magnitude of responses to forces of different frequencies (relative to the natural frequency, f_n) for several values of damping ratio (0.1–1). Note that for low damping ratios ($\zeta \ll 1$), which occur when viscosity, D, is low according to Equation 6, the response is highly peaked, with maximum when $f \sim f_n$.

Figure 3A indicates that a limb can be considered as a mass-spring system to a crude, first approximation. The mass consists of the bones and flesh being supported (in this figure the forearm) plus any external load. The muscle behaves as a nonlinear spring in that force does not increase in proportion to extension (Fig. 3B). In addition, the stiffness of a muscle fiber depends on its activity (105, 106), and some amount of active contraction is required just to maintain the limb in the position shown in Figure 3A. The slope of the classical length-tension curve of Figure 3B gives the incremental stiffness of a muscle (see also the chapter by Partridge and Benton in this *Handbook*). In the absence of active contraction, the stiffness increases with length. In the presence of a tetanic contraction, the stiffness is much greater at short lengths but changes less at longer lengths, and the change of stiffness with length even becomes negative at very long lengths (105, 106). The region of negative stiffness is often beyond the maximum physiological length, but the variations of stiffness with length and contraction do highlight the fact that tremor of a mechanical origin varies due to changes in stiffness, K, as well as mass, M.

In an intact limb, angular (rather than linear) movements occur around a joint, and we should refer to torque rather than force, inertia rather than mass and angular stiffness. Nonetheless the same form of equations applies. Proximal muscles are working against an inertia or mass (i.e., the distal part of the limb, as well as any external load) larger than the generally smaller distal muscles. The stiffness of the larger proximal muscles may also be greater, however, so it does not automatically follow that the tremor frequency is lower when the more proximal muscle is studied. In addition, muscle stiffness is further modified by reflex factors, and it has been argued (see the chapter by Houk and Rymer in this *Handbook*) that one of the major roles of reflexes is to regulate muscle stiffness.

Damping enters the neuromuscular system in several ways. There is some friction or viscosity when a muscle moves with respect to other structures in the limb. In addition there is some viscosity within the muscle that is described by the classical force-velocity curve (52). An additional source is caused by the presence of some bonds between thick and thin filaments even in the resting state. These bonds can bend a few percent of muscle length (53) and throughout the range act as short-range elasticity. Over a longer distance, however, these bonds break and reform and act as a viscosity. It is uncertain to what extent this modifies the classical picture, which described muscle (as shown in Fig. 3C) in terms of an internal elastic element K_i in series with an elastic element K_p that was in parallel with a viscous element (52). The viscous element described by Hill's force-velocity curve is also nonlinear, but a number of studies have shown that for small fluctuations about a given length, such as those that occur during physiological tremor, muscles and their loads can be modeled adequately by an equivalent linear system (5, 6, 77). The parameters of this system, however, vary for different lengths or other changes in muscle properties.

A final essential element for this simple model of muscle is an active-state element. The active state is a measure of a muscle's ability to contract, which rises rapidly and then decays roughly exponentially with time following a muscle action potential. There are

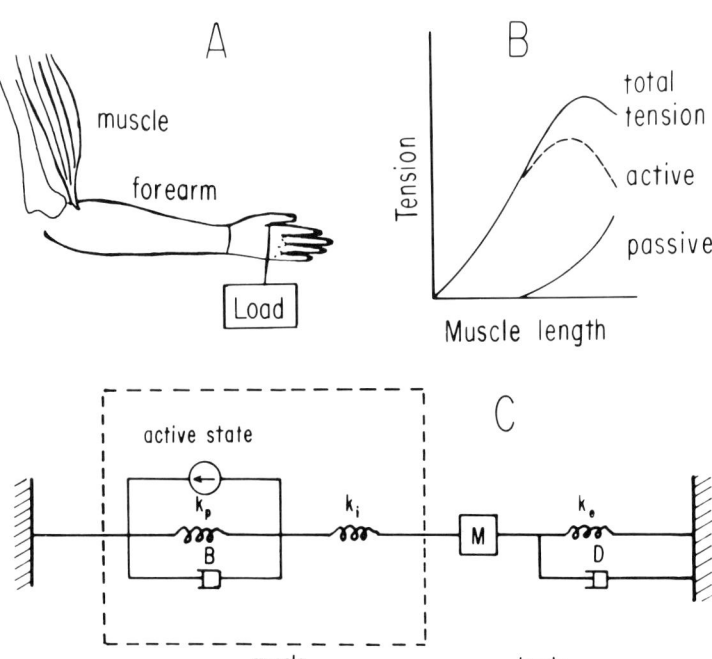

FIG. 3. *A*: schematic diagram of biceps muscle contracting against mass of forearm and its load. *B*: classic length-tension curve of muscle. Slope of this curve gives muscle stiffness, K, which depends on muscle length and state of muscle (whether it is actively contracting or is passive). *C*: more complete mechanical diagram indicating interaction between components of muscle and its load. [*C* from Oğuztöreli and Stein (96).]

thus two time constants describing the overall behavior of muscle: a viscoelastic time constant and one for the decay of the active state. Sometimes the two constants that produce a critically damped second-order system (i.e., $\zeta = 1$) are similar (77). This system responds as rapidly as possible without a tendency for undershoot or oscillations at a particular frequency (see Fig. 2B). The mass-spring system described previously represents an underdamped second-order system. When a load that can contain masses, dashpots, and springs (including the elasticity of antagonist muscles) is added to the simple model of muscle, a fourth-order system may result (114). Mathematically the resultant system shown in Figure 3C can have at most one preferred frequency of oscillation, and the response to a brief input decays with time. Thus, a mechanical oscillation requires a continuing input if it is to be maintained over a period of time.

To what extent do these properties of mechanical systems determine human tremors? At one extreme Brumlik and Yap (12) proposed a purely mechanical origin for the tremor that remains even in a normal subject at rest; i.e., in the absence of any electrical activity (EMG) in appropriate muscles. Their suggestion was that the pulses of blood entering the limb with each heartbeat were sufficient to maintain an oscillation or rest tremor indefinitely. The fact that components of tremor were observed at much higher frequencies than that of the heartbeat (e.g., 10 Hz) could be due to the tendency for the limbs to oscillate mechanically at this higher frequency. In fact, a component of tremor is observed at the frequency of the heartbeat (~1 Hz) and this can be reduced by occluding the blood supply to the limb (99). The frequencies of mechanical oscillations vary widely, from about 0.2 Hz for breathing-induced oscillations to nearly 30 Hz for mechanical perturbations to the fingers (45). Out of this greater than 100-fold range of frequencies, only a fivefold range (about 3–15 Hz) is normally considered. The mechanical resonant frequency of the human forearm varies between 4 and 8.5 Hz (66), so the tremor that remains in the absence of any EMG activity must be due to mechanical factors.

Even in the presence of neural and muscular activity, mechanical factors can play an important role. For example, even uncorrelated activity of motoneurons may maintain a mechanical oscillation. The word uncorrelated is an important one, because reflexly or centrally induced oscillations acting on a pool of motoneurons tend to synchronize the times of the motoneuronal discharges. Various methods have been used to study synchronization based on probability theory (119): cross-correlation or spectral techniques between two spike trains (29), or between a single spike train and the population of fibers producing the surface EMG (88), or the tremor recorded simultaneously (32). Reflexly or centrally generated tremors may, of course, interact with mechanical oscillations, but if there is no correlation between motor units we can largely rule out these factors. Many studies have indicated that during voluntary contractions of normal human subjects motor units are often unsynchronized in their discharge (e.g., ref. 88), although synchronization can be produced by an exercise training program (87), fatigue (90), or disease states (30).

In a sense the rhythmic discharge of motoneurons can be regarded as a centrally generated tremor, each motoneuron serving as an independent pacemaker. Rietz and Stiles (108), however, using an animal model, found that the tremor frequency was largely independent of the rate of stimulation of motoneurons. This study is the latest in a series of such experiments going back to the last century (109). In human physiological tremor, however, Allum et al. (2) have proposed that the firing rate of motoneurons (which is often about 10 impulses/s), together with the filtering properties of muscle, directly determine the frequency of physiological tremor. The evidence for this is considered further in subsection *Central Oscillations*, p. 338.

Reflex Oscillations

The simplest reflex is known as the stretch or resistance reflex, because it tends to resist perturbations. Therefore it is initially surprising to think that such reflexes produce oscillations, but in fact many feedback systems can give rise to oscillations as a result of inherent delays in such systems. The stretch reflex is tested clinically by tapping a tendon with a hammer to produce a brief, phasic stretch of the muscle. The muscle resists by contracting, but the contraction may occur after the stretch produced by the tendon tap is completed because of the reflex delays. Indeed, if the reflexes are brisk enough, the relaxation of the muscle to its original length following contraction (which represents a secondary stretch of the muscle) may be sufficient to generate further contractions, as mentioned previously. Such damped oscillations were well studied already in 1929 (23) and have been proposed as the basis for normal physiological tremor and clonus (73). Quantitative studies on the properties of muscles have also been carried out to determine their effect on oscillatory behavior. A number of conclusions can be drawn from these studies.

GAIN. The gain of a reflex pathway should be measured as a dimensionless quantity (i.e., the ratio of an output and input, both of which have the same units, such as the shortening produced against a particular load per unit of extension of a muscle). Conventionally, physiologists measure reflex gain as the force produced per unit extension of a muscle under isometric conditions. The ratio of these two quantities has the units of stiffness. Houk [(58); also see the chapter by Houk and Rymer in this *Handbook*] has argued that stiffness is a controlled variable that is not easily varied independently of overall force level [see also (54)]. Nonetheless, to the extent that reflex gain can be varied independently it mainly affects the tendency for oscillation (p in Eq. 3) rather than changing the frequency of oscillation [f in Eq. 3; see (85)]. Note that if p is positive, the oscillation tends to grow with time, whereas if p is negative the oscillation decays. The more negative the value of p, the more rapid is the decay of the oscillation. The increased gain after spinal cord section, as tested by hyperactive tendon jerks and spasticity, is often accompanied by rhythmical oscillations in the form of clonus. A tendency for damped oscillations approximately of the form given by Equation 3 can be observed even in normal subjects under some conditions during a steady voluntary contraction (73, 112), because reflex gain is increased in parallel with force during voluntary contractions (38). With increasing force, muscle stiffness also increases, so that the frequency of oscillation also tends to increase (67).

LATENCY. The latency of the reflex pathway mainly affects the frequency, f, of oscillation without as marked an influence on the tendency for oscillation, p (95). Slowing the speed of muscular contraction has a less marked influence on frequency. By cooling a limb, which slows muscular contraction (plus neuromuscular transmission and neural conduction velocity to some extent), Lippold (73) was able to lower the frequency of physiological tremor by a couple of cycles per second, which he took as evidence for the reflex basis of physiological tremor.

It has also been suggested that longer loop reflex pathways, by virtue of their greater latency, could contribute to the lower frequency oscillations found in certain disease states (114). There is as yet no supportive evidence for this suggestion, and indeed quite low frequencies of oscillation can be found in the clonus of spinal patients where these long-loop pathways are presumably interrupted. The same lesions, however, interrupt pathways that activate γ-motoneurons and in turn muscle-spindle afferents. Hagbarth et al. (44) have managed with percutaneous needle electrodes to record from single muscle spindle afferents in such patients. Their records indicate substantial delays from the time the muscle begins to lengthen to the time muscle spindles begin to discharge, which might account for the low frequency of clonus in these patients. Even in the total absence of γ-activity, muscle spindles are exceedingly sensitive to small perturbations (37) once their threshold for firing is reached. The reason that clonus is observed only when a muscle is stretched somewhat is presumably because the stretch is needed to reach the threshold of the muscle spindles.

Another interesting suggestion has been put forward by Stiles (116). It has long been known that tremor becomes more marked during fatigue and that its frequency falls under these conditions. Stiles found that tremor amplitude and frequency are linked by a power function with a negative fractional exponent. When tremor amplitude increased to the levels normally found in clonus or in parkinsonian tremor after maintaining a steady force for some minutes (117), the frequency was also similar. Although he did not relate his results quantitatively to a mechanism, Stiles felt that his results were consistent with the view that normal physiological tremor is due to a combination of mechanical and reflex mechanisms. In this view, clonus is just an exaggerated physiological tremor that results from a high-reflex gain (see also ref. 39).

STABILITY. Although reflex gain and delays affect the stability of a reflex pathway, stabilization (i.e., a reduced tendency for oscillations) primarily results from the sluggishness of muscles. Muscles are simply unable to follow high-frequency changes (115). In the study mentioned previously, Lippold (73) noted that cooling the muscle, and hence making it even more sluggish, reduced the amplitude of tremor markedly.

Matthews (84) suggested that the velocity sensitivity of muscle afferents might stabilize oscillations (see also the chapter by Matthews in this *Handbook*), because the velocity of a sinusoidal signal leads the length by 90° and therefore can cancel phase lags from other sources. Computations showed, however, that although the velocity sensitivity of muscle afferents could compensate for the phase lags of muscle and for reflex delays at low frequencies (see also ref. 104), the velocity sensitivity was such that it contributed to oscillations at higher frequencies (115). These ideas were recently confirmed experimentally by Goodwin et al. (36), who interrupted the reflex pathway to jaw muscles in the monkey. In the absence of reflexes the magnitude of tremor was reduced above 10 Hz, but the magnitude of lower frequency oscillations was markedly increased. The magnitude of the spontaneous fluctuations at lower frequencies (<3 Hz) under both conditions was much greater than the more rhythmic oscillations at higher frequencies, which we generally refer to as tremor (see also ref. 45). Thus resistance reflexes from muscle spindles serve a useful function in reducing low-frequency fluctuations, even if they increase higher frequency tremor to some extent.

Another suggestion is that the multiple reflex pathways from muscle afferents with different latencies (reviewed in ref. 27) contribute to stability of limb position (96). This theoretical suggestion has not been tested experimentally as yet, although one aspect fits well with common observations. The calculations showed an asymmetry because long-latency (e.g., supraspinal) pathways were more effective in damping out oscillations from short-latency (e.g., spinal) pathways than vice versa. Clinically it is often difficult for patients with supraspinal disorders to control tremor, even though spinal mechanisms appear intact.

INTERACTION OF MECHANISMS. Mechanical and reflex oscillations can interact in various ways. The resulting tremor can be *1)* near the frequency of the mechanical oscillation if one or the other is dominant, *2)* at an intermediate frequency if the two frequencies are not too far apart, or *3*) at more than one frequency, although generally the two components have different amplitudes and degrees of damping (96). These possibilities have all been observed experimentally. Joyce and Rack (66) loaded the forearms of normal human subjects and observed that one frequency of tremor varied with the natural frequency of the load, whereas a second frequency was independent of load and consistent with that expected from the spinal stretch reflex. Furthermore Cussons et al. (19) selectively increased the presumed reflex oscillations by vibrating a muscle at 100 Hz to produce a vibration reflex. Nichols et al. (93) have recently studied premammillary decerebrate cats in which the discharge of muscle spindle afferents, as well as motoneurons, was directly measured. In addition, all muscles in the hindlimb except the soleus were denervated, and the soleus muscle was directly connected to various inertial and elastic loads. The results fully confirm those of Rack and collaborators and the predictions of the model studies (see Fig. 3).

Interaction of peripheral and central oscillations is also possible. In Figure 4A a central oscillation at 5 Hz is considered in a model system consisting of a muscle (Fig. 3C) but no reflex connections. The muscle simply follows the 5-Hz input, although it attenuates the input somewhat. If sensory feedback of sufficient magnitude is added (Fig. 4B), the frequency approximately doubles. In the example shown, the transition occurred over a period of approximately 1 s, and the oscillation remained somewhat irregular. Such transitions (to an irregular oscillation at about twice the frequency) have often been described in parkinsonian patients (e.g., ref. 43) following the onset of voluntary activity. These calculations [(97); and R. B. Stein, unpublished observations] support the idea that these transitions result from the interaction between a central oscillator in parkinsonian patients and reflex mechanisms.

RESETTING. One property that distinguishes reflex and mechanical oscillations from purely central oscillations is their sensitivity to resetting by external stimuli. This was studied mathematically (97) in a reflex model where an oscillation was initiated by one pulse, and at a later time a second pulse was applied. The oscillation continued at the same frequency but generally with a change in phase (Fig. 4D). Figure 5A shows the change in phase of the oscillation as a function of the relative amplitude of the second pulse and the phase at which it occurred. Note that the change in phase may be either positive or negative and depends on the amplitude of the stimulus as well; i.e., the larger the stimulus, the more complete the resetting. With complete resetting the phase would be changed one degree for every degree of change in the phase of the stimulus, which would give a slope of one on a plot such as that shown in Figure 5A. Because the phase change is a continuous function of the time of the input pulse, there must be a region where the

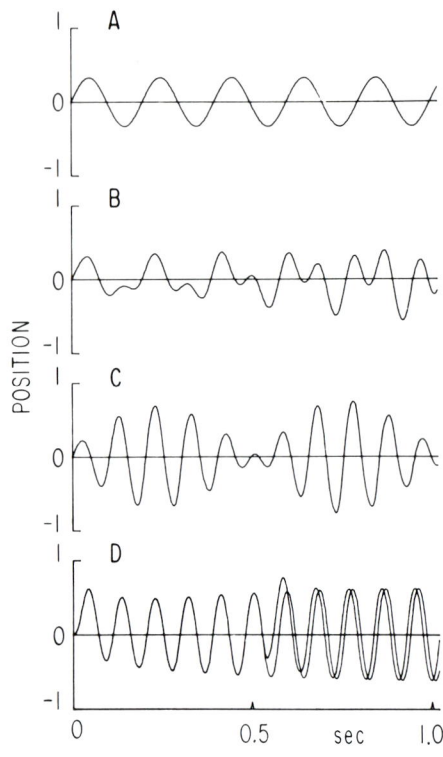

FIG. 4. *A*: in absence of sensory feedback, rhythmic input (at 5 Hz) from central nervous system produces a change in muscle length or limb position at same frequency as input, but filtered somewhat in amplitude (model calculation based on Fig. 3C). *B*: after adding sensory feedback to model, frequency approximately doubles (to nearly 11 Hz) over shown period of 1 s. See Oğuztöreli and Stein (96) for details of assumed spinal stretch reflex pathway. A saturation type of nonlinearity was included to limit or normalize range of positions to ±1 in all parts of figure. *C*: applying an external 9-Hz oscillation in limb position with same amount of sensory feedback produces clear modulation in envelope with "beat" frequency near 2 Hz. *D*: applying brief perturbation at $t = 0$ in absence of sinusoidal inputs produces slowly growing reflex oscillation. Second pulse at $t = 0.525$ s can reset oscillation without greatly modifying amplitude.

curves pass, with negative slope, back through zero phase shift. Over much of the plot, however, the calculations show an approximately linear relation, with a positive slope between the change in phase and the phase of the stimulus pulse.

This positive slope has been called a resetting index (113) and normally varies from 0 (no resetting) to 1 (complete resetting). If there is a purely central origin for a particular type of tremor (as in Fig. 4A), and sensory inputs do not affect the tremor generator, the resetting index is near 0. On the other hand, if the oscillation is generated by reflex pathways alone, adequate reflex stimulation should completely reset the tremor (index near 1). Intermediate examples can also be imagined where tremor involves interactions between reflex mechanisms and central oscillators, and intermediate values of the resetting index might be expected.

To test these ideas experimentally, torque pulses were applied to patients at various phases of an ongoing tremor that involved wrist musculature (113).

The torque pulses stretched either wrist extensors or flexors, and changes in the timing of EMG bursts from these muscles were then followed for several cycles of the tremor. Resetting indexes are shown for patients with essential tremor (Fig. 5B) and with Parkinson's disease (Fig. 5C). Note that the resetting index for the patient with essential tremor is high, indicating a strong involvement of sensory feedback. This response has consistently been observed and supports the theory that essential tremor represents an exaggerated physiological tremor that is largely dependent on reflex and mechanical factors.

Walsh (121) argued against this theory because of his finding that a beat frequency can be set up between an ongoing tremor and an applied oscillation in patients with both clonus and essential tremor. Beats arise, however, in a purely reflex model system (Fig. 4C) in which a 9-Hz input is applied to a system tending to oscillate at nearly 11 Hz from reflex feedback. A waxing and waning of the oscillation at a beat frequency of about 2 Hz is clearly seen. Thus the presence of beat frequencies is consistent with the notion that clonus and essential tremor are caused by peripheral rather than by central mechanisms.

The patients with Parkinson's disease show much less resetting, which indicates a large central component in the tremor of this disease. In fact, the results from parkinsonian patients were somewhat variable, and the mechanisms underlying parkinsonian tremor are discussed in subsection SUPRASPINAL OSCILLATORS, p. 339, after considering central oscillations in general. Walsh (122) has also observed beats when applying rhythmic forces to resting limbs of parkinsonian patients. The same qualifications, however, apply to these observations as to those for clonus that are mentioned earlier in this subsection.

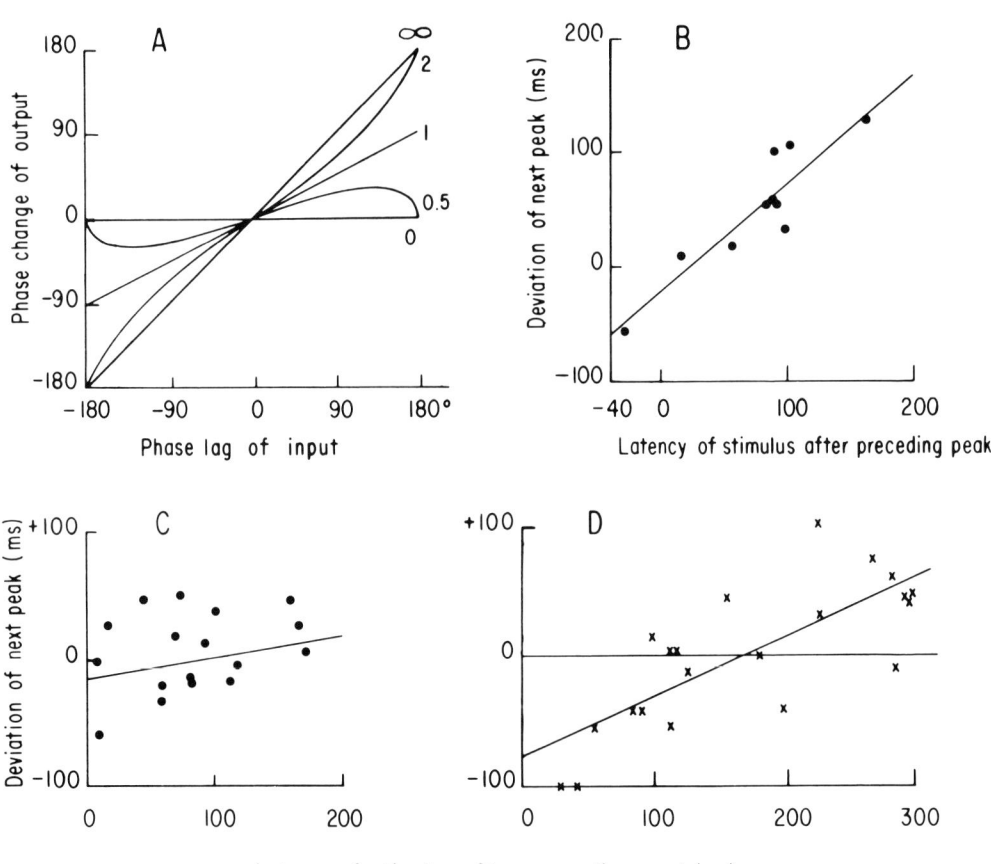

FIG. 5. *A*: effect of brief pulse at different phases of sinusoidal oscillation in resetting oscillation. Increasing amplitude of pulse (relative amplitudes are given on *right*) increases degree of resetting. This is indicated by *slope of linear portion of curve* that increases over range of 0 to 1 for linear model. [Described in detail by Oğuztöreli and Stein (97).] *B*: torque pulses applied to patient with essential tremor largely reset electromyogram (EMG) peaks associated with ongoing oscillation (slope near 1). Times are given in ms relative to 240-ms period of tremor (~4 Hz). *C*: similar pulses applied to patient with parkinsonian tremor had little effect on timing of EMG peaks (slope not significantly greater than 0). Frequency of tremor was 5 Hz. *D*: torque pulses applied to monkey with intention tremor produced by cooling cerebellar nuclei. Intermediate degree of resetting for peaks of positive velocity is observed (slope near 0.5). [*A* from Oğuztöreli and Stein (97); *B* and *C* from Stein, Lee, and Nichols (113); *D*, replotted from Villis and Hore (120).]

Central Oscillations

Abnormal functioning of central nervous structures can lead to tremor in several ways. We consider various possibilities separately before discussing the difficult question of the extent to which each mechanism takes part in the generation of particular forms of tremor.

SINGLE PACEMAKERS. The simplest form of centrally generated oscillation comes from the rhythmicity of single motoneurons (Fig. 6A). Each motor unit can then be considered as an independent pacemaker producing a partially fused and hence oscillatory contraction in its constituent muscle fibers (35). Because of the range of firing rates, the variability in the discharge properties of single motor units, and the asynchrony between the contractions of different motor units, random fluctuations might be expected with a wide range of frequency components. Allum et al. (2), however, have pointed out that there are several factors that tend to limit the peak frequency to the range of 8–12 Hz, commonly found in normal physiological tremor. First, motoneurons are recruited in an orderly fashion according to size during voluntary contractions in the human being [(48, 89); see the chapter by Henneman and Mendell in this *Handbook*]. Thus the motoneurons that are just above their threshold for recruitment at a given force threshold are the largest active units in terms of force. They also tend to fire at frequencies closest to their lower limit of steady firing (6–10 Hz), and it is at the lowest frequencies that the contractions are least fused (i.e., the oscillations in force are largest). Even though the oscillations are not sinusoidal and therefore contain harmonics of the spike repetition rate, the sluggishness of the mechanical systems means that higher harmonics are less prominent. These factors combine to produce a peak near 10 Hz in the spectrum of normal physiological tremor.

Allum et al. (2) have attempted to quantify the argument by measuring the range of frequencies produced by different motor units. They measured the size of the units and the magnitudes of the oscillations that would be produced at each frequency. If the discharge of motor units in the subjects studied was uncorrelated, this would then constitute a necessary and sufficient condition for proving that normal physiological tremor is due to the asynchronous unfused

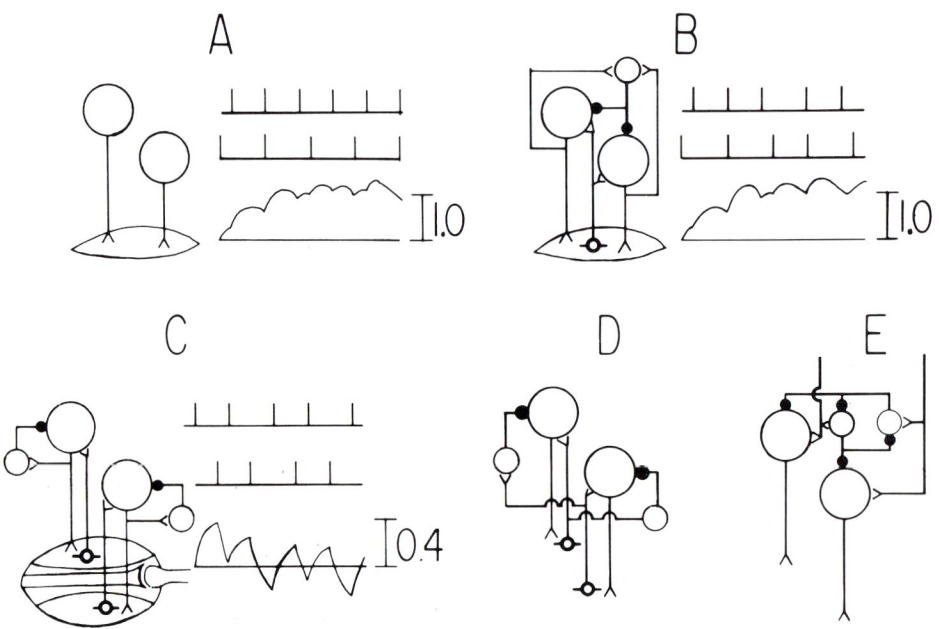

FIG. 6. *A*: independent motoneurons (indicated schematically on *left*) firing at less than tetanic rates (*upper right*) produce random fluctuations in force (*lower right*) that contain frequency components corresponding to their individual firing rates. *B*: coupling within motoneuron pool from sensory feedback (see connections from muscle spindle) or from central feedback (see connections from Renshaw cell) gradually produce more rhythmic tremor of small amplitude. *C*: coupling between antagonistic motoneuron pools involves mechanical linkage, which is sensed by muscle receptors and produces an alternating tremor. Note change in relative scale used in plotting tension. *D*: reflex connections from muscle receptors (Ia inhibitory interneurons are shown) can again increase the amplitude and rhythmicity of the tremor. Muscle not shown. *E*: central oscillators (mutually inhibitory interneurons which receive excitation from higher centers are shown) can have a similar effect and the relative importance of central and peripheral influences is often difficult to determine. The symbols used in all parts of the figure are as follow: motoneuron, ○; interneuron, ○; muscle spindle, —○—; excitatory synapse, —<; inhibitory synapse, —●. The times of motoneuronal firing in *A* to *C* could be produced by a number of simple neural models, and the resulting force fluctuations were computed using second-order model of muscle (5, 77).

contractions of constituent motor units. Under other conditions, however, motor units are synchronized, and further mechanisms must be included in the explanation of tremor.

CENTRAL FEEDBACK ONTO MOTONEURONS. Within the spinal cord there are a number of feedback pathways that could synchronize motoneurons. For example, as shown in Figure 6B, every time there is a burst of activity in a group of motoneurons, this excites Renshaw cells that inhibit the motoneurons from firing for a period of time. The motoneurons then tend to fire again as a group when the inhibition wears off. This type of central feedback is analogous in many ways to reflex feedback. It is often difficult to distinguish between the two feedbacks, particularly because Renshaw cells have rarely, if ever, been recorded in animal models of tremor, much less in tremors in the human being. Nonetheless a grouping of impulses in motoneurons with negative serial correlations (i.e., long intervals following short intervals, as shown in Fig. 6B) has been observed in normal physiological tremor (32) and in cerebellar disease (3), and the possible role of Renshaw cells in producing these patterns has been discussed. Summation of the afterhyperpolarizations following two impulses in a motoneuron also tends to produce a longer than average interval until the next impulse (see the chapter by Baldissera, Hultborn, and Illert in this *Handbook*). Thus negative serial correlations can arise from mechanisms within a motoneuron as well as from central feedback.

A combination of sensory feedback and central feedback could also produce alternation in antagonistic groups of motoneurons through mechanical linkage around a joint (Fig. 6C). Another circuit that has often been proposed to strengthen such oscillations (10, 123) is mutually inhibitory connections between antagonistic motoneuron pools. No direct connections of this type, however, have been shown for mammalian motoneurons (61). Similar effects could again be produced by reflex connections, and the well-known Ia inhibition from muscle spindles in one muscle to antagonistic motoneurons (Fig. 6D) might function to produce reciprocal activity in two motoneurons pools (86).

INTERNEURONAL NETWORKS. The central oscillators considered to this point involve motoneurons in the generation of the oscillation, and because of the many reflex connections that end on motoneurons, the rhythm should be reset to some extent by adequate reflex stimulation. As indicated, many of the centrally generated patterns could also be produced by reflexes, and experimentally the two groups are difficult to distinguish. Other types of central oscillators that involve interneuronal pacemakers or networks (Fig. 6E), however, should be less accessible to sensory input. Such central oscillators have been investigated in recent years in the spinal cord for the generation of walking [(41); and see the chapter by Grillner in this *Handbook*] and in the brain stem for breathing (125) and chewing [(21); see the chapter by Luschei and Goldberg in this *Handbook*]. In each of these natural oscillatory movements, sensory inputs that reset the rhythms or change their frequency (21, 31, 41, 125) have been described. Central networks that generate forms of tremor such as in Parkinson's disease (68) often seem remote from sensory input; we now consider such disease states in which the tremor may be due to supraspinal oscillators.

SUPRASPINAL OSCILLATORS. As shown in Figure 5, it is difficult to reset tremor in some parkinsonian patients, yet in others the tremor can be reset by sensory input (113). Different parkinsonian patients show a wide variation in symptoms. Tremor, rigidity, and bradykinesia may all be present to different degrees. Perhaps certain sensory projections to a presumed tremor generator are spared in some patients, but no correlation between symptomology, reflexology, and resetting of tremor has been obtained.

Stiles and Pozos (117) observed a striking inverse relation between tremor amplitude and frequency in 18 parkinsonian patients. Furthermore, the relation was similar to tremors of varying amplitudes induced in normal subjects, suggesting that a similar combination of reflex and mechanical factors might apply. Correlation of results, however, does not necessarily imply a common mechanism, and there is good evidence for the central generation of parkinsonian tremor. In recording with microelectrodes from peripheral nerves of parkinsonian patients (44), two bursts of activity in muscle-spindle afferents were found in each cycle of oscillation in contrast to results with patients showing clonus. The first burst occurred when the muscles were being stretched, whereas the second occurred when the muscles were actively contracting. The second burst could occur only if there were substantial inputs onto γ-motoneurons that innervate the intrafusal muscle fibers on which muscle spindle endings lie. This input is thought to come from tremor-generating centers in the brain.

In primate models of Parkinson's disease (69, 101), evidence for central generators is stronger than that in human beings. Cutting appropriate dorsal roots to abolish reflexes did not diminish, or could even increase, the parkinsonian tremor (98). Rhythmic activity at the tremor frequency could also be recorded in various areas of the central nervous system (motor cortex, thalamus, motoneurons) before and after curarizing animals to block the tremor movements and rhythmic feedback associated with them (65). Evidence for central tremor generators has also been obtained from deafferentation (34, 103) and rhythmic firing (30) in human beings, but it is weaker than in primates, and even the data for the primates can be questioned (117).

The literature on the mechanisms underlying cerebellar tremor is also mixed. Denny-Brown (25) reported that deafferentation abolished cerebellar intention tremor in monkeys. Liu and Chambers (75), however, claimed that in cerebellar-lesioned deafferented monkeys some intention tremor could be seen during goal-directed movements. Recently Villis and Hore (120) obtained strong evidence for peripheral involvement in experiments in which the cerebellar nuclei were cooled reversibly using implanted cooling probes developed by Brooks et al. (9). These workers were able to show that *1)* the tremor frequency could be increased by increasing the spring stiffness or the level of activity required of the monkey working against a lever, *2)* the frequency was decreased by the addition of masses to the lever, *3)* the frequency was not changed much but the amplitude was decreased by the addition of viscous damping, and *4)* the tremor could be reset by applying torque pulses during the period in which the position of the handle was maintained steady against a load. This last point was not quantified, but the data shown in their Figure 3 have been replotted in Figure 5D. A substantial degree of resetting is seen, although it is not as complete as in some patients with essential tremor. Studies using the same species [e.g., human beings (50)] and the same stimulus conditions are required to confirm this point. Nonetheless, there seems to be clear evidence of peripheral involvement in experimental cerebellar tremor (see also ref. 13).

The mode of action for these reflexes is unclear, but Higgins et al. (51) showed that ablating cerebellar inputs in a decerebrate cat produced a phase lag in the response to sinusoidal stretches. This suggests that the cerebellum was responsible for producing some phase advance [perhaps by activating dynamic γ-motoneurons (62)] that might enhance the stability of the system (see also the chapters by Rack and by Brooks and Thach in this *Handbook*].

Tremor can also be generated by specifically affecting the function of cerebellar and related structures. For example, the drug harmaline produces rhythmic activity in the inferior olive in phase with tremor of the limbs (22) and the rhythmic activity is not abolished even when the olive is disconnected from the rest of the nervous system (76). Thus supraspinal oscillators could play a role in cerebellar tremor, although they may not be as important as in Parkinson's disease. Further studies are clearly required, but a number of tentative conclusions can be reached.

CONCLUSIONS

1. If there is no motoneuronal activity, oscillations can occur in the limb position of a normal subject at rest due to blood pulsations interacting with the mechanical properties of the limb.

2. If, during a normal voluntary contraction to maintain a posture, the motoneurons in a pool discharge asynchronously (i.e., in a statistically uncorrelated way), fluctuations in force arise from the rhythmic discharge of motoneurons producing partially fused contractions of motor units. The partially fused contractions can, under these conditions, form the basis of normal postural (physiological) tremor.

3. Some normal subjects show synchronization of motor units due to reflex or central mechanisms. Reflex oscillations can be enhanced by appropriate loading of the limb. Increased reflex gain in certain spinal patients (who generally show spasticity) leads to prominent reflex oscillations known as clonus.

4. Essential tremor has a strong reflex involvement in that it can largely be reset by external perturbations. As indicated by the name, the underlying mechanisms remain unclear.

5. Cerebellar tremor can also be modified by peripheral factors, but tremor-like activity can also arise in the inferior olive in the absence of sensory inputs.

6. Parkinsonian tremor in different patients may or may not be reset by external inputs. It is suggested that the tremor is generated centrally, but that sensory connections to these central structures are affected to varying degrees in different patients.

7. The various types of tremor and clonus can tentatively be placed on a continuum in terms of central nervous system involvement ranging from mechanical (including muscle) mechanisms to reflex factors to central pattern generation. In this continuum, normal rest tremor < normal postural tremor < clonus < essential tremor < cerebellar tremor < parkinsonian tremor.

REFERENCES

1. ALBE-FESSARD, D., G. GUIOT, Y. LAMARRE, AND G. ARFEL. Activation of thalamocortical projections related to tremorogenic process. In: *The Thalamus*, edited by D. P. Purpura and M. D. Yahr. New York: Columbia Univ. Press, 1966, p. 237-254.
2. ALLUM, J. H. J., V. DIETZ, AND H. J. FREUND. Neuronal mechanisms underlying physiological tremor. *J. Neurophysiol.* 41: 557-571, 1978.
3. ANDREASSEN, S. *Interval Patterns of Single Motor Units* (Ph.D. thesis). Copenhagen: Tech. Univ. Denmark, 1978.
4. ANDREWS, C. J., P. D. NEILSON, AND J. W. LANCE. The comparison of tremors in normal, Parkinsonian, and athetotic man. *J. Neurol. Sci.* 19: 53-61, 1973.
5. BAWA, P., A. MANNARD, AND R. B. STEIN. Effects of elastic loads on the contractions of cat muscles. *Biol. Cybern.* 22: 129-137, 1976.
6. BAWA, P., AND R. B. STEIN. The frequency response of human soleus muscle. *J. Neurophysiol.* 39: 788-793, 1976.
7. BAXTER, D. W., S. LAL, AND M. RASMINSKY. Essential tremor and dystonic syndromes. *Can. J. Neurol. Sci.* 6: 74, 1979.
8. BROOKS, V. B. Control of intended limb movements by the lateral and intermediate cerebellum. In: *Integration in the Nervous System*, edited by H. Asanuma and V. J. Wilson. Tokyo: Igaku Shoin, 1979, p. 321-357.
9. BROOKS, V. B., I. B. KOZLOVSKAYA, A. ATKIN, F. E. HORVATH, AND M. UNO. Effects of cooling dentate nucleus on tracking-task performance in monkeys. *J. Neurophysiol.* 36: 974-995, 1973.

10. BROWN, T. G. The intrinsic factors in the act of progression in the mammal. *Proc. R. Soc. London Ser. B* 83: 308-319, 1911.
11. BRUMLIK, J. On the nature of normal tremor. *Neurology* 12: 159-179, 1962.
12. BRUMLIK, J., AND C.-B. YAP. *Normal Tremor—A Comparative Study.* Springfield, IL: Thomas, 1970.
13. CHASE, R. A., J. K. CULLEN, JR., S. A. SULLIVAN, AND A. K. OMMAYA. Modification of intention tremor in man. *Nature London* 206: 485-487, 1965.
14. CLARE, M. H., W. H. MILLS, AND G. H. BISHOP. Reflex factors in clonus and tremor. *J. Appl. Physiol.* 3: 714-731, 1951.
15. COOK, W. A., JR. Antagonistic muscles in the production of clonus in man. *Neurology* 17: 779-781, 1967.
16. COOKE, J. D., AND J. S. THOMAS. Forearm oscillation during cooling of the dentate nucleus in the monkey. *Can. J. Physiol. Pharmacol.* 54: 430-436, 1976.
17. COOPER, I. S. Neurosurgical alleviation of the intention tremor of muscle sclerosis and cerebellar disease. *N. Engl. J. Med.* 263: 441-444, 1960.
18. COOPER, I. S. Motor functions of the thalamus with recent observations concerning the role of the pulvinar. *Int. J. Neurol.* 8: 238-259, 1971.
19. CUSSONS, P. D., P. B. C. MATTHEWS, R. B. MUIR, AND J. D. G. WATSON. Enhancement of human elbow tremor by muscle vibration. *J. Physiol. London* 278: 42P-43P, 1978.
20. D'AZZO, J. J., AND C. H. HOUPIS. *Feedback Control Systems Analysis and Synthesis.* New York: McGraw-Hill, 1966.
21. DELLOW, P. G., AND J. P. LUND. Evidence for central patterning of rhythmical mastication. *J. Physiol. London* 215: 1-15, 1971.
22. DE MONTIGNY, C., AND Y. LAMARRE. Rhythmic activity induced by harmaline in the olivo-cerebello-bulbar system of the cat. *Brain Res.* 53: 81-95, 1973.
23. DENNY-BROWN, D. On the nature of postural reflexes. *Proc. R. Soc. London Ser. B* 104: 252-301, 1929.
24. DENNY-BROWN, D. *The Basal Ganglia and Their Relation to Disorders of Movement.* London: Oxford Univ. Press, 1962.
25. DENNY-BROWN, D. *The Cerebral Control of Movement.* Springfield, IL: Thomas, 1966.
26. DENNY-BROWN, D., AND S. GILMAN. Depression of gamma innervation by cerebellectomy. *Trans. Am. Neurol. Assoc.* 90: 96-101, 1965.
27. DESMEDT, J. E. (editor). *Progress in Clinical Neurophysiology, Cerebral Motor Control in Man: Long Loop Mechanisms.* Basel: Karger, 1978, vol. 4.
28. DESMEDT, J. E. (editor). *Progress in Clinical Neurophysiology, Physiological Tremor, Pathological Tremors and Clonus.* Basel: Karger, 1978, vol. 5.
29. DIETZ, V., E. BISCHOFBERGER, C. WITZ, AND H.-J. FREUND. Correlation between the discharges of two simultaneously recorded motor units and physiological tremor. *Electroencephalogr. Clin. Neurophysiol.* 40: 97-105, 1976.
30. DIETZ, V., W. HILLESHEIMER, AND H.-J. FREUND. Correlation between tremor and firing pattern of motor units in Parkinson's Disease. *J. Neurol. Neurosurg. Psychiatry* 37: 927-937, 1974.
31. DUYSENS, J. Reflex control of locomotion as revealed by stimulation of cutaneous afferents in spontaneously walking premammillary cats. *J. Neurophysiol.* 40: 737-751, 1977.
32. ELBLE, R. J., AND J. E. RANDALL. Motor-unit activity responsible for the 8- to 12-Hz component of human physiological finger tremor. *J. Neurophysiol.* 39: 370-383, 1976.
33. EVARTS, E. V., AND J. TANJI. Reflex and intended responses in motor cortex pyramidal tract neurons of monkey. *J. Neurophysiol.* 39: 1069-1080, 1976.
34. FOERSTER, O. Resection of the posterior nerve roots of spinal cord. *Lancet* 2: 76-79, 1911.
35. FREUND, H.-J., J. H. BÜDINGEN, AND V. DIETZ. Activity of single motor units from human forearm muscles during voluntary isometric contractions. *J. Neurophysiol.* 38: 933-946, 1975.
36. GOODWIN, G. M., D. HOFFMAN, AND E. S. LUSCHEI. The strength of the reflex response to sinusoidal stretch of monkey jaw closing muscles during voluntary contraction. *J. Physiol. London* 279: 81-111, 1978.
37. GOODWIN, G. M., M. HULLIGER, AND P. B. C. MATTHEWS. The effects of fusimotor stimulation during small amplitude stretching on the frequency response of the primary ending of the mammalian muscle spindle. *J. Physiol. London* 253: 175-206, 1975.
38. GOTTLIEB, G. L., AND G. C. AGARWAL. Postural adaptation. The nature of adaptive mechanisms in the human motor system. In: *Control of Posture and Locomotion,* edited by R. B. Stein, K. G. Pearson, R. S. Smith, and J. B. Redford. New York: Plenum, 1973, p. 197-210.
39. GOTTLIEB, G. L., AND G. C. AGARWAL. Physiological clonus in man. *Exp. Neurol.* 54: 616-621, 1977.
40. GRANIT, R. Observations on clonus in the cat's soleus muscle. *Anales Fac. Med. Montivideo* 44: 305-310, 1959.
41. GRILLNER, S. Locomotion in vertebrates: central mechanisms and reflex interaction. *Physiol. Rev.* 55: 247-304, 1975.
42. GROWDON, H., W. W. CHAMBERS, AND C. N. LIU. An experimental dyskinesia in the Rhesus monkey. *Brain* 90: 603-632, 1967.
43. GURFINKEL, V. S., AND S. M. OSOVETS. Mechanism of generation of oscillations in the tremor form of Parkinsonism. *Biofizika* 18: 731-738, 1973.
44. HAGBARTH, K. G., G. WALLIN, L. LOFSTETT, AND S. M. AQUILONIUS. Muscle spindle activity in alternating tremor of Parkinsonism and in clonus. *J. Neurol. Neurosurg. Psychiatry* 38: 636-641, 1975.
45. HALLIDAY, A. M., AND J. W. T. REDFEARN. An analysis of the frequency of finger tremor in healthy subjects. *J. Physiol. London* 134: 600-611, 1956.
46. HALLIDAY, A. M., AND J. W. T. REDFEARN. Finger tremor in tabetic patients and its bearing on the mechanism producing the rhythm of physiological tremor. *J. Neurol. Neurosurg. Psychiatry* 21: 101-108, 1958.
47. HENATSCH, H. D. Instability of the proprioceptive length servo: Its possible role in tremor phenomena. In: *Neurophysiological Basis of Normal and Abnormal Motor Activities,* edited by M. D. Yahr and D. P. Purpura. New York: Raven, 1967, p. 75-89.
48. HENNEMAN, E. Peripheral mechanisms involved in the control of muscle. In: *Medical Physiology* (13th ed.), edited by V. B. Mountcastle. St. Louis: Mosby, 1974, p. 617-635.
49. HERMANN, C., JR., AND J. W. BROWN. Palatal myoclonus: a reappraisal. *J. Neurol. Sci.* 5: 473-492, 1967.
50. HEWER, R. L., R. COOPER, AND M. H. MORGAN. An investigation into the value of treating intention tremor by weighting the affected limb. *Brain* 95: 549-590, 1972.
51. HIGGINS, D. C., L. D. PARTRIDGE, AND G. H. GLASER. A transient cerebellar influence on stretch responses. *J. Neurophysiol.* 25: 684-692, 1962.
52. HILL, A. V. The heat of shortening and the dynamic constants of muscle. *Proc. R. Soc. London Ser. B* 126: 136-195, 1938.
53. HILL, D. K. Tension due to interaction between sliding filaments in resting striated muscle. The effect of stimulation. *J. Physiol. London* 199: 637-684, 1968.
54. HOFFER, J. A., AND S. ANDREASSEN. Factors affecting the gain of the stretch reflex and soleus muscle stiffness in premammillary cats. *Soc. Neurosci. Abstr.* 4: 935, 1978.
55. HOLLERBACH, J. M. *A Study of Human Motor Control Through Analysis and Synthesis of Handwriting* (Ph.D. thesis). Cambridge: MIT, 1978.
56. HOLMES, G. The symptoms of acute cerebellar injuries due to gunshot injuries. *Brain* 40: 461-535, 1917.
57. HOLMES, G. The cerebellum of man. *Brain* 62: 1-30, 1939.
58. HOUK, J. C. Regulation of stiffness by skeletomotor reflexes. *Annu. Rev. Physiol.* 41: 99-114, 1979.
59. HORNYKIEWICZ, D. The mechanisms of action of L-DOPA in Parkinson's disease. *Life Sci.* 7: 1249-1260, 1974.
60. HUFSCHMIDT, H. S. Proprioceptive origin of Parkinsonian tremor. *Nature London* 200: 367-368, 1963.
61. HULTBORN, H. Convergence on interneurons in the reciprocal

Ia inhibitory pathway to motoneurones. *Acta Physiol. Scand. Suppl.* 375: 1–42, 1972.
62. JANSEN, J. K. S., AND P. B. C. MATTHEWS. The central control of the dynamic response of muscle spindle receptors. *J. Physiol. London* 161: 357–378, 1962.
63. JASPER, H. H., AND H. L. ANDREWS. Brain potentials and voluntary muscle activity in man. *J. Neurophysiol.* 1: 87–100, 1938.
64. JASPER, H. H., AND G. BERTRAND. Thalamic units involved in somatic sensation and voluntary and involuntary movements in man. In: *The Thalamus*, edited by D. P. Purpura and M. D. Yahr. New York: Columbia Univ. Press, 1966, p. 365–384.
65. JOFFROY, A. J., AND Y. LAMARRE. Rhythmic unit firing in the precentral cortex in relation with postural tremor in a deafferented limb. *Brain Res.* 27: 386–389, 1971.
66. JOYCE, G. C., AND P. M. H. RACK. The effects of load and force on tremor at the normal human elbow joint. *J. Physiol. London* 240: 375–396, 1974.
67. JOYCE, G. C., P. M. H. RACK, AND H. F. ROSS. The forces generated at the human elbow joint in response to imposed sinusoidal movements of the forearm. *J. Physiol. London* 240: 351–374, 1974.
68. LAMARRE, Y. Tremorgenic mechanisms in primates. In: *Advances in Neurology*, edited by B. Meldrum and C. D. Marsden. New York: Raven, 1975, p. 10, 23–34.
69. LAMARRE, Y., AND J. P. CORDEAU. Étude du mécanisme physiopathologique responsable, chez le singe, d'un tremblement expérimental de type parkinsonien. *Actual. Neurophysiol.* 7: 141–166, 1967.
70. LAMARRE, Y., AND M. WEISS. Harmaline-induced rhythmic activity of alpha and gamma motoneurons in the cat. *Brain Res.* 63: 430–434, 1973.
71. LANCE, J. W., AND J. G. MCLEOD. *A Physiological Approach to Clinical Neurology*. London: Butterworth, 1975.
72. LANCE, J. W., R. S. SCHWAB, AND E. A. PETERSON. Action tremor and the cogwheel phenomenon in Parkinson's disease. *Brain* 86: 95–110, 1963.
73. LIPPOLD, O. C. J. Oscillation in the stretch reflex arc and the origin of the rhythmical 8–12 c/s component of physiological tremor. *J. Physiol. London* 206: 359–382, 1970.
74. LIPPOLD, O. C. J. *The Origin of the Alpha Rhythm*. Edinburgh: Churchill Livingstone, 1973.
75. LIU, C. N., AND W. W. CHAMBERS. A study of cerebellar dyskinesia in the bilaterally deafferented forelimbs of the monkey (*Macaca mulatta* and *Macaca speciosa*). *Acta Neurobiol. Exp.* 31: 263–289, 1971.
76. LLINÁS, R., AND R. A. VOLKIND. The olivo-cerebellar system: functional properties as revealed by harmaline-induced tremor. *Exp. Brain Res.* 18: 69–87, 1973.
77. MANNARD, A., AND R. B. STEIN. Determination of the frequency response of isometric soleus muscle in the cat using random nerve stimulation. *J. Physiol. London* 229: 275–296, 1973.
78. MARSDEN, C. D. The mechanisms of physiological tremor and their significance in pathological tremors. In: *Progress in Clinical Neurophysiology. Physiological Tremor, Pathological Tremors and Clonus*, edited by J. E. Desmedt. Basel: Karger, 1978, vol. 5, p. 1–16.
79. MARSDEN, C. D., T. H. FOLEY, AND D. A. L. OWEN. Peripheral beta-adrenergic receptors concerned with tremor. *Clin. Sci.* 33: 53–65, 1967.
80. MARSDEN, C. D., J. C. MEADOWS, G. W. LANGE, AND R. S. WATSON. Effect of deafferentation on human physiological tremor. *Lancet* 2: 700–702, 1967.
81. MARSDEN, C. D., J. C. MEADOWS, G. W. LANGE, AND R. S. WATSON. The role of the ballistocardiac impulse in the genesis of physiological tremor. *Brain.* 92: 647–662, 1969.
82. MARSDEN, C. D., D. TARSY, AND R. J. BALDESSARINI. Spontaneous and drug-induced movement disorders in psychotic patients. In: *Psychiatric Aspects of Neurologic Disease*, edited by F. Benson and D. Blumer. New York: Grune & Stratton, 1975, p. 219–265.

83. MARSHALL, J. Tremor. In: *Handbook of Clinical Neurology*, edited by P. J. Vinken and G. W. Bruyn. Amsterdam: North Holland, 1970, vol. 6 p. 809–825.
84. MATTHEWS, P. B. C. Muscle spindles and their motor control. *Physiol. Rev.* 44: 219–288, 1964.
85. MCDOWELL, F. H., G. H. MARKHAM, J. E. LEE, L. J. TRECIOKAS, AND R. D. ANSEL. The clinical use of levodopa in the treatment of Parkinson's disease. In: *Recent Advances in Parkinson's Disease*, edited by F. H. McDowell and C. H. Markham. Philadelphia: Davis, 1971, p. 175–201.
86. MILLER, S., AND P. D. SCOTT. The spinal locomotor generator. *Exp. Brain Res.* 30: 387–403, 1977.
87. MILNER-BROWN, H. S., R. B. STEIN, AND R. G. LEE. Synchronization of human motor units: possible roles of exercise and supra-spinal reflexes. *Electroencephalogr. Clin. Neurophysiol.* 38: 245–254, 1974.
88. MILNER-BROWN, H. S., R. B. STEIN, AND R. YEMM. The contractile properties of human motor units during voluntary isometric contractions. *J. Physiol. London* 228: 285–306, 1973.
89. MILNER-BROWN, H. S., R. B. STEIN, AND R. YEMM. The orderly recruitment of human motor units during voluntary isometric contractions. *J. Physiol. London* 230: 359–370, 1973.
90. MORI, S. Entrainment of motor unit discharges as a neuronal mechanism of synchronization. *J. Neurophysiol.* 38: 859–870, 1975.
91. MORTIMER, J. A., AND D. D. WEBSTER. Evidence for a quantitative association between EMG stretch responses and Parkinsonian rigidity. *Brain Res.* 162: 169–173, 1979.
92. NARABAYASHI, H., AND C. OHYE. Parkinsonian tremor and nucleus ventralis intermedius (Vim) of the human thalamus. In: *Progress in Clinical Neurophysiology. Physiological Tremor, Pathological Tremors and Clonus*, edited by J. E. Desmedt. Karger: Basel, 1978, vol. 5, p. 165–182.
93. NICHOLS, T. R., R. B. STEIN, AND P. BAWA. Spinal reflexes as a basis for tremor in the premammillary cat. *Can. J. Physiol. Pharmacol.* 56: 375–383, 1978.
94. NEILSON, P. D., AND J. W. LANCE. Reflex transmission characteristics during voluntary activity in normal man and patients with movement disorders. In: *Progress in Clinical Neurophysiology. Physiological Tremor, Pathological Tremors and Clonus*, edited by J. E. Desmedt. Karger: Basel, 1978, vol. 5, p. 263–299.
95. OĞUZTÖRELI, M. N., AND R. B. STEIN. An analysis of oscillations in neuro-muscular systems. *J. Math. Biol.* 2: 87–105, 1975.
96. OĞUZTÖRELI, M. N., AND R. B. STEIN. The effects of multiple reflex pathways on the oscillations in neuro-muscular systems. *J. Math. Biol.* 3: 87–101, 1976.
97. OĞUZTÖRELI, M. N., AND R. B. STEIN. Interactions between centrally and peripherally generated neuromuscular oscillations. *J. Math. Biol.* 7: 1–30, 1979.
98. OHYE, C., R. BOUCHARD, L. LAROCHELLE, P. BÉDARD, R. BOUCHER, B. RAPHY, AND L. J. POIRIER. Effect of dorsal rhizotomy on postural tremor in the monkey. *Exp. Brain Res.* 10: 140–150, 1970.
99. PADSHA, S. M., AND R. B. STEIN. The bases of tremor during a maintained posture. In: *Control of Posture and Locomotion*, edited by R. B. Stein, K. G. Pearson, R. S. Smith, and J. B. Redford. New York: Plenum, 1973, p. 415–419.
100. PARKINSON, J. *An Essay on the Shaking Palsy*. London: Wittingham & Newland, 1817.
101. POIRIER, L. J. Experimental and histological study of midbrain dyskinesias. *J. Neurophysiol.* 23: 534–551, 1960.
102. POIRIER, L. J., G. BOUVIER, P. BÉDARD, R. BOUCHER, L. LAROCHELLE, A. OLIVIER, AND P. SINGH. Essai sur les circuits neuronaux impliqués dans le tremblement postural et l'hypokinésie. *Rev. Neurol.* 120: 15–40, 1969.
103. POLLACK, L. J., AND L. DAVIS. Muscle tone in Parkinsonian states. *Arch. Neurol. Psychiatry* 23: 303–319, 1930.
104. POPPELE, R. E., AND C. A. TERZUOLO. Myotatic reflex: Its input-output relation. *Science* 159: 743–745, 1968.
105. RACK, P. M. H., AND D. R. WESTBURY. The effects of length

and stimulus rate on tension in the isometric cat soleus muscle. *J. Physiol. London* 204: 443–460, 1969.
106. RAMSEY, R. W., AND S. F. STREET. The isometric length-tension diagram of isolated skeletal muscle fibers of the frog. *J. Cell. Comp. Physiol.* 15: 11–34, 1940.
107. RANISH, N. A., AND J. F. SOECHTING. Studies on the control of some simple motor tasks. Effects of thalamic and red nuclei lesions. *Brain Res.* 102: 334–345, 1976.
108. RIETZ, R. R., AND R. N. STILES. A viscoelastic-mass mechanism as a basis for normal postural tremor. *J. Appl. Physiol.* 37: 852–860, 1974.
109. SCHÄFER, E. A. On the rhythm of muscular response to volitional impulses in man. *J. Physiol. London* 7: 111–117, 1886.
110. SHAHANI, B. T., AND R. R. YOUNG. Action tremors: a clinical neurophysiological review. In: *Progress in Clinical Neurophysiology. Physiological Tremor, Pathological Tremors and Clonus*, edited by J. E. Desmedt. Basel: Karger, 1978, vol. 5, p. 129–137.
111. SMITH, J. L., B. BETTS, V. R. EDGERTON, AND R. F. ZERNICKE. Rapid ankle extension during paw shakes: selective recruitment of fast ankle extensors. *J. Neurophysiol.* 43: 612–620, 1980.
112. STEIN, R. B., AND P. BAWA. Reflex responses of human soleus muscle to small perturbations. *J. Neurophysiol.* 39: 1105–1116, 1976.
113. STEIN, R. B., R. G. LEE, AND T. R. NICHOLS. Modification of ongoing tremors and locomotion by sensory feedback. *Electroencephalogr. Clin. Neurophysiol. Suppl.* 34: 511–519, 1978.
114. STEIN, R. B., AND M. N. OĞUZTÖRELI. Tremor and other oscillations in neuro-muscular systems. *Biol. Cybern.* 22: 147–157, 1976.
115. STEIN, R. B., AND M. N. OĞUZTÖRELI. Does the velocity sensitivity of muscle spindles stabilize the stretch reflex? *Biol. Cybern.* 23: 219–228, 1976.
116. STILES, R. N. Frequency and displacement amplitude relations for normal hand tremor. *J. Appl. Physiol.* 40: 44–54, 1976.
117. STILES, R. B., AND R. S. POZOS. A mechanical-reflex oscillator hypothesis for Parkinsonian hand tremor. *J. Appl. Physiol.* 40: 990–998, 1976.
118. SZUMSKI, A. J., DORIS BURG, A. STRUPPLER, AND F. VELHO. Activity of muscle spindles during muscle twitch and clonus in normal and spastic human patients. *Electroencephalogr. Clin. Neurophysiol.* 37: 589–597, 1974.
119. TAYLOR, A. The significance of grouping of motor unit activity. *J. Physiol. London* 162: 259–269, 1962.
120. VILLIS, J., AND J. HORE. Effects of changes in mechanical state of limb on cerebellar intention tremor. *J. Neurophysiol.* 40: 1214–1224, 1977.
121. WALSH, E. G. Clonus: beats provoked by the application of a rhythmic force. *J. Neurol. Neurosurg. Psychiatry* 39: 266–274, 1976.
122. WALSH, E. G. Beats produced between a rhythmic applied force and the resting tremor of Parkinsonism. *J. Neurol. Neurosurg. Psychiatry* 42: 89–94, 1979.
123. WILSON, D. M., AND I. WALDRON. Models for the generation of the motor output pattern in flying locusts. *Proc. IEEE* 56: 1058–1064, 1968.
124. WINKLER, J. F., AND R. R. YOUNG. Efficacy of chronic propranolol therapy in action tremors of the familial, senile, or essential varieties. *N. Engl. J. Med.* 290: 984–988, 1974.
125. WYMAN, R. J. Neural generation of the breathing system. *Annu. Rev. Physiol.* 39: 417–448, 1977.
126. YOUNG, R. R., J. H. GROWDON, AND B. T. SHAHANI. Beta-adrenergic mechanisms in action tremor. *N. Engl. J. Med.* 293: 950–953, 1975.

CHAPTER 10

Motor units: anatomy, physiology, and functional organization

R. E. BURKE | *Laboratory of Neural Control, National Institute of Neurological and Communicative Disorders and Stroke, National Institutes of Health, Bethesda, Maryland*

CHAPTER CONTENTS

Motor Unit Types
   Muscle fiber types: histochemical profiles and
      ultrastructural correlations
      Anatomy and ultrastructure
      Neuromuscular junction specializations
   Motor unit types: physiological profiles in
      experimental animals
      A word about methodology
      Motor unit population of cat medial gastrocnemius
        muscle
      Physiological and histochemical profiles of muscle units
      Twitch-contraction times and myofibrillar ATPase
      Fatigability and metabolic profiles
   Motor units in human muscle
   Stability of motor unit types
      Alterations of demand within the physiological range
      Nonphysiological alterations
   Developmental considerations
   Skeletofusimotor units
Anatomical Considerations
   Anatomy of muscle units
      Regionalization within a muscle
      Innervation ratios and muscle unit "size"
   Anatomy of motor nuclei
      Numbers of motoneurons and motor units
   Motoneuron anatomy in relation to unit type
Physiology of α-Motoneurons and Their Synaptic Inputs in
      Relation to Motor Unit Type
   Electrophysiological properties intrinsic to motoneurons
   Organization of synaptic input
      Group Ia synaptic efficacy
      Monosynaptic supraspinal inputs
      Polysynaptic input systems
   Control of motoneuron excitability: interactive factors
      Synaptic efficacy
      Intrinsic membrane properties
Control of Muscular Action: Recruitment and Rate
      Modulation
   Motor unit recruitment
      Recruitment patterns and motor unit types
      Precision and stereotypy in recruitment process
      Are major shifts in recruitment order possible?
   Output modulation by rate and pattern of motoneuron firing
      Motoneuron firing characteristics
      Effects of firing rate and firing pattern on muscle
        unit output
   Recruitment or rate and pattern modulation?
Summary and Concluding Comments

EARLY IN THIS CENTURY, Sherrington found it useful to measure muscular action in terms of "biological" or "functional" elements in addition to conventional physical units. In a 1925 paper with Liddell (455), he defined this functional element, the motor unit, as "the motoneurone axone and its adjunct muscle-fibres ..." (p. 511) and clearly described the notion of orderly recruitment of such motor units in the control of motor output (see also ref. 631). Sherrington considered every muscular action to result from the activation of variable numbers of motor units, each corresponding to "a so-to-say quantum reaction, which forms the basis, by combinations temporal and numerical, of all grading of the muscle as effector organ ..." (p. 326 in ref. 217). This concept of the motor unit as the functional quantum of muscle action remains a cornerstone of present models of motor system organization and of the neural control of movement. It does no violence to history to include the entire motoneuron, as well as its motor axon, in the current definition of the motor unit (Fig. 1), and it is sometimes convenient to use the term muscle unit to denote the set of skeletal muscle fibers innervated by an individual motoneuron (100). The functional inseparability of motoneuron and muscle unit was emphasized by Tokizane and Shimazu (692) in their use of the term neuromuscular unit as a synonym for motor unit.

Sherrington's notion of the motor unit implicitly assumed that *1*) all fibers of the muscle unit portion are activated by each motor axon spike, thus producing the same mechanical action; and *2*) a given muscle fiber belongs to only one motor unit (i.e., that there is little or no polyneuronal innervation of muscle fibers by different motoneurons). Subsequent experimental work has shown that both assumptions are essentially correct but neither is universally true. For example, neuromuscular transmission is sufficiently powerful to cause quite reliable activation of muscle unit fibers (543), but occasional failures of fiber activation have been observed in rat diaphragm motor units studied in vitro, even with input frequencies as low as 10 Hz

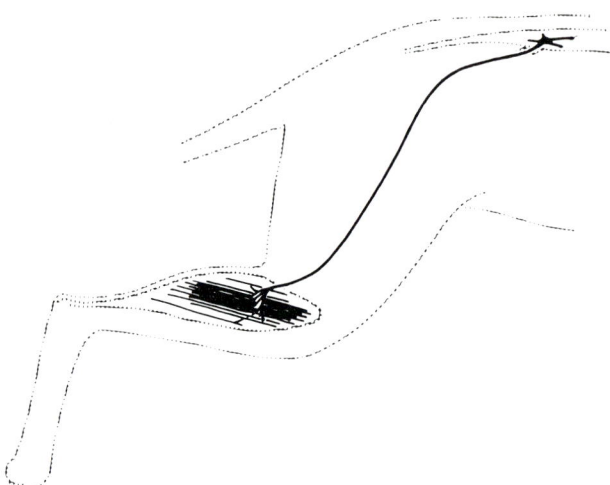

FIG. 1. Diagram of typical motor unit belonging to an ankle extensor muscle in the cat hindlimb, including the motoneuron lying in the spinal cord, its axon leaving the cord via a ventral root and peripheral nerve to reach the target muscle, where it branches profusely to innervate a set of muscle fibers (muscle unit) distributed within the anatomical confines of the muscle (see also Figs. 12, 13).

(427). Whether or not activation failure is significant under in vivo conditions remains to be clarified (see subsection FATIGUABILITY AND METABOLIC PROFILES, p. 358). As to the second point, there is little or no polyneuronal innervation of individual muscle fibers in adult muscles (35, 254, 86, 718), although persistent polyneuronal innervation can occur after reinnervation of denervated muscle (e.g., ref. 267). Polyneuronal innervation is widespread in immature limb muscles during the first few weeks of life in both rat and cat, but it disappears relatively rapidly during postnatal maturation (refs. 35, 85, 572; also see subsection *Developmental Considerations*, p. 364). Thus, the coupling between motoneuron and muscle unit can be viewed as both functionally reliable and anatomically exclusive in normal adult muscles. The neural and muscular portions form an indivisible entity, and both parts are considered together in this chapter. There is thus inevitable overlap between this discussion and some aspects of the chapters in this *Handbook* by Partridge and Benton on muscle and by Henneman and Mendell on motoneuron organization. I hope that the different points of view expressed in these chapters are complementary rather than merely repetitive.

When Sherrington defined the motor unit, he was unaware of the motor innervation of muscle spindles. We now separate two distinct classes of muscle fibers: the large skeletal (or "extrafusal") fibers that make up the main bulk of muscles, and the much smaller intrafusal fibers that are present only within the muscle spindles. We must in addition consider three classes of motoneurons: *1*) the skeletomotor motoneurons (α-motoneurons) that innervate skeletal muscle fibers exclusively; *2*) the fusimotor motoneurons (γ-motoneurons) that innervate intrafusal fibers exclusively; and *3*) the skeletofusimotor motoneurons (β-motoneu-

rons) that innervate both skeletal and intrafusal muscle fibers. Detailed discussions of these categories can be found in the chapter by Matthews in this *Handbook* and in his monograph of 1972 (480). For simplicity, this chapter uses the Greek letter designations for the motoneurons and deals only with material related to α- and β-motoneurons and their extrafusal muscle units. Unless otherwise specified, the discussion in this chapter refers only to muscle fibers (and muscle units) that are innervated by en plaque neuromuscular endings and that exhibit propagated action potentials with all-or-none twitch responses, in contrast to the "true" slow, nontwitch muscle fibers that are innervated by en grappe endings, present in some amphibian muscles (431, 446) and in mammalian extraocular muscles [(135); for reviews see refs. 366 and 544].

Finally it should be clear that movement results from the action of forces on the skeleton arising from the environment (e.g., gravity and external loads) and from active contraction of skeletal muscles. A systematic study of the control of movement by the central nervous system (CNS) must consider both classes of forces together with the anatomical design of the moving body (see the chapter by Alexander in this *Handbook*; see also ref. 6). This chapter takes a much narrower view, limiting consideration to the motor units that are the functional quanta by which the CNS grades muscle action. The first three sections deal with the characteristics of muscle units and their motoneurons to give an essentially static view of current evidence about the patterns of motor unit organization. The fourth section reviews evidence about how such organizations may function in a dynamic sense during behavioral movements.

MOTOR UNIT TYPES

If all of the motor units that make up a given muscle were similar, description of their physiological, structural, and biochemical characteristics would be relatively simple. Muscle units would then be simply scaled down versions of whole muscles and all motoneurons in a given population might be represented adequately by a single example. In fact, however, this is rarely the case; most motor unit populations so far studied display considerable ranges of properties, which suggests that significant differences exist within them. It is, of course, a subjective judgment whether the individual elements in a population under study are "similar" or "different" (e.g., ref. 640), but when the elements exhibit a wide range of interrelated characteristics, there is a natural tendency to group them into categories, if only to systematize and communicate experimental observations. Such categories are useful insofar as they allow prediction of attributes of the population that are not themselves classification criteria (e.g., refs. 104, 642). In other words, the categories assume "meaning" if they become more, rather than less, well defined as additional information is considered. Research on motor units well illustrates the advantages as well as the disadvantages of this process.

Since Ranvier's classic observations (571) over a century ago on the differences between slowly contracting "red" and rapidly contracting "white" muscles, these categories have been considered to be functionally meaningful. By inference there should be at least two equivalent categories of motor units. Histologists had long recognized that muscle fibers in many muscles are heterogeneous in appearance (e.g., refs. 94, 184, 320), but the suggestion (320) that fast-twitch white muscles might in fact contain some slowly contracting motor units was not pursued by physiologists until relatively recently, mainly because of technical limitations. The development of muscle fiber histochemistry and the resulting notion of muscle fiber "types" provided an important stimulus for systematic physiological study of individual motor units in a variety of muscle and species. Histochemical observations also provide an important link for making inferences about motor unit composition and usage patterns in human muscles, based on results from more accessible animal preparations (e.g., see subsection *Motor Unit Recruitment*, p. 386). Thus it seems useful to discuss the issue of muscle fiber types per se before dealing with the properties of motor units.

Muscle Fiber Types: Histochemical Profiles and Ultrastructural Correlations

The 1960s saw rapid development of methods for reliable histochemical study of the differences between muscle fibers, with consequent identification of a variety of muscle fiber types [(203, 532, 591, 659); see reviews in ref. 540 and chapt. 3 in ref. 202]. Most mammalian muscles, including those of humans, contain fibers with diverse histochemical characteristics and are in this sense "heterogeneous" (e.g., Fig. 2A and C; see also refs. 17, 202, 224, 228, 394, 401). In fact, histochemically homogeneous muscles such as the cat soleus (Fig. 2B, D) are quite exceptional.

Histochemical methods make it possible to visualize relatively subtle differences between muscle fibers with regard to some aspects of their structural proteins [for example, the ATPase activity of the myofibrillar material at an alkaline pH, with (AC-ATPase) or without (M-ATPase) pretreatment in acidic buffers] as well as for relative activities of a wide variety of metabolic enzyme systems, including mitochondrial oxidative enzymes such as succinic dehydrogenase (SDH) and NADH dehydrogenase (NADH-D) and enzymes related to anaerobic glycolysis, such as menadione-linked α-glycerophosphate dehydrogenase (α-GPD). The histochemical profiles of fiber types also include the relative amounts of metabolic substrates (such as glycogen and neutral fat) present in them. Because of the apparent lability of metabolic enzymes and substrates, particularly in pathological material,

many authors regard the myofibrillar ATPase reactions as the most useful determinant of fiber types (e.g., refs. 77, 78, 202, 242, 609). More recently, the application of methods that permit immunofluorescent labeling of specific varieties of myosin (20, 319), and even particular myosin subfragments (278–280), has added further refinement.

During the past 20 years a number of fiber classification schemes have been suggested along with an even greater variety of terminologies. Close (148) has attempted to reconcile some of these classifications (see also ref. 552) but a comprehensive concordance is difficult because of interspecies and intermuscle differences (see refs. 22, 52, 104, 122, 225, 434, 528, 607, 737). Table 1 shows the patterns of staining, or histochemical profiles, for the fiber types recognized in several species (guinea pig, cat, and human) together with two widely used systems of fiber nomenclature [(44, 77, 552); see also ref. 202] that are essentially interchangeable. The scheme of Brooke and Kaiser (types I, IIA, and IIB; see refs. 77, 78, 202) is based primarily on ATPase reactivity patterns, while that of Peter and co-workers (552) also considers patterns of metabolic enzymes [FG, fast twitch, glycolytic; FOG, fast twitch, oxidative and glycolytic; SO, slow twitch, oxidative]. The explicit inference of contraction speed from ATPase staining intensity alone makes this nomenclature less "neutral" than the I-IIA-IIB system; the latter is used in this chapter. The material in Table 1 is representative of findings in heterogeneous limb muscles of cat (17, 111, 112, 153, 343, 528, 621), guinea pig (44, 552), and human (202, 247, 607), where interspecies differences are relatively minor. The same fiber types are represented in the axial muscles of the cat (132, 579). The histochemical profiles of rat muscle fibers are somewhat different, particularly with respect to the ATPase reactions [see Fig. 7; (432, 433, 621, 735, 736)], and the classifications in Table 1 do not apply in all details. Furthermore the profile of the type I fibers found in the homogeneous slow-twitch soleus muscle of the cat is also different from that of the type I fibers in heterogeneous muscles in that species [compare Fig. 2A and B; (110, 122, 528, 621)]. The fiber types in the rat soleus, which is quite heterogeneous, are also not identical with any of those in the equally heterogeneous tibialis anterior (434, 621). With regard to the muscles innervated by cranial nerves, the patterns of histochemical profiles found in extraocular muscles are considerably more complex than is indicated in Table 1 (e.g., refs. 8, 483, 544), but the fiber types present in jaw muscles (677) of the cat fit reasonably well with those found in the somatic musculature. Middle ear muscles represent an interesting compromise in that they appear to contain some true slow (i.e., nontwitch) fibers (246, 257), as do extraocular muscles, but their motor units and ATPase histochemistry match the organization found in heterogeneous limb muscles (680, 681).

The intensity of reaction product deposition in his-

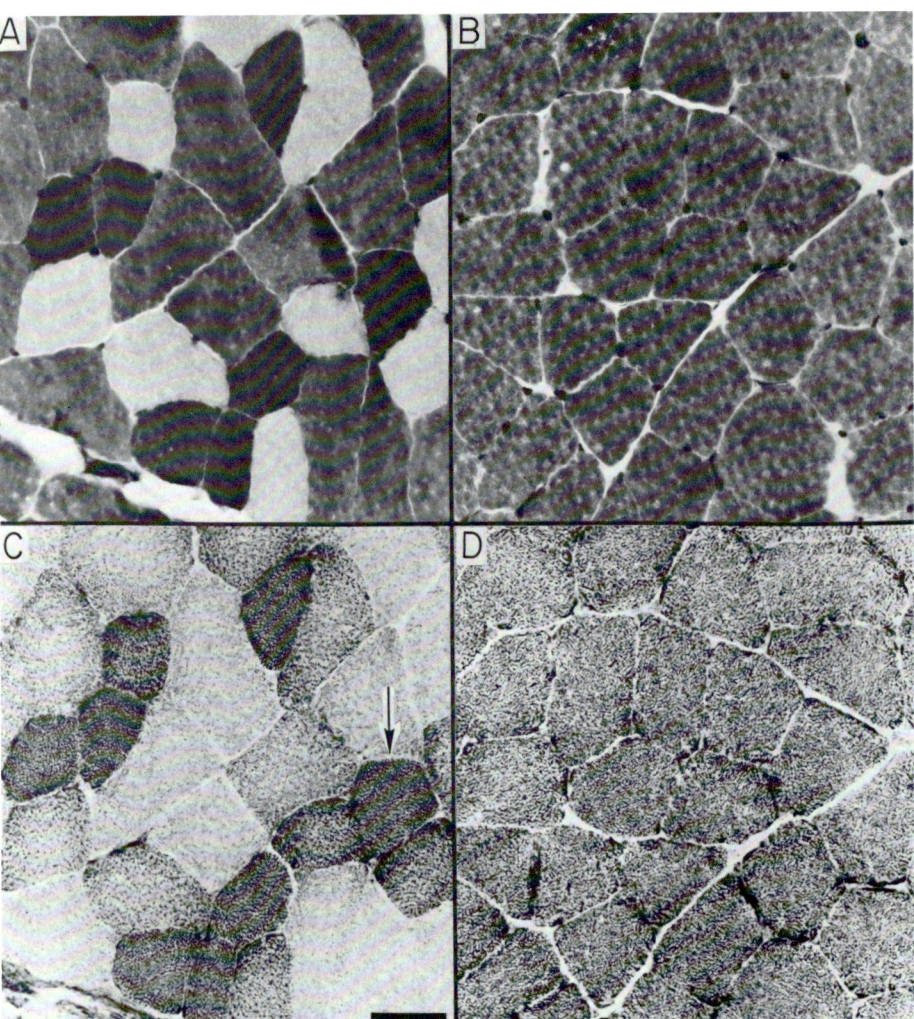

FIG. 2. Histochemical profiles of fibers in heterogeneous (A, C) and homogeneous (B, D) cat muscles. Photomicrographs of representative serial sections of heterogeneous lateral gastrocnemius (LG; panels A, C) and homogeneous soleus (SOL; panels B, D) muscles in the same cat processed as a single block of tissue and photographed under identical conditions. Panels A and B are from a section stained for myofibrillar ATPase activity after incubation in an acidic buffer at pH 4.65 (see Table 1; AC-ATPase). Panels C and D are from a serial section stained for oxidative enzyme NADH-dehydrogenase (Table 1). When comparing AC-ATPase and NADH staining patterns for individual fibers (the histochemical profile), at least 3 fiber types can be recognized in LG but only 1 in SOL. Note that appearance of an LG fiber with the profile characteristic of type S muscle units (panel C, arrow) is not identical to appearance of SOL fibers. Calibration bar in C is 100 μm. [Adapted from Burke and Tsairis (122).]

tochemical stains is usually interpreted in terms of the activity of particular enzymes or the concentration of metabolic substrates. Although such interpretations are generally consistent with biochemical assays of whole muscles with particular fiber-type predominance [see Table 1; (552)], some degree of care is nevertheless necessary in interpreting histochemical profiles (e.g., refs. 78, 202, 327; see subsections TWITCH-CONTRACTION TIMES AND MYOFIBRILLAR ATPASE, p. 355, and FATIGABILITY AND METABOLIC PROFILES, p. 358). For example, although the biochemical Ca^{2+}-activated ATPase activity of adult actomyosin fits well with ATPase histochemistry [Table 1; (552)], this is not necessarily the case with fetal or immature muscles (329, 528). Also interpretation of oxidative enzyme histochemistry is complicated by the affinity for the reaction product (e.g., in NADH-D preparations) for lipid-containing structures as well as for the mitochondrial sites of enzymatic action (e.g., chapt. 2 in ref. 202).

Despite the detailed differences between muscles and species noted above and the technical problems of interpretation, it is nevertheless fair to say that muscle fibers in adult mammals exhibit three basic histochemical and biochemical profiles [see Table 1; (22, 202, 552, 591)]. Minority subgroups with characteristics intermediate between the major groups have long been recognized (e.g., refs. 225, 591, 646), but the

TABLE 1. *Histochemical Profiles and Biochemical Features for Major Muscle Fiber Types Present in Many Cat, Guinea Pig, and Human Mixed Muscles*

Fiber Type	IIB[a],FG[b]	IIAB[a]	IIA[a],FOG[b]	I[a],SO[b]
Corresponding Motor Unit Type[c]	FF	F(int)	FR	S
Histochemical Profiles				
Myofibril ATPase, pH 9.4	High	High	High	Low
AC-ATPase, pH 4.3[d]	Low		Low	High
AC-ATPase, pH 4.6[d]	Medium	Medium	Low	High
NADH dehydrogenase[e]	Low	Medium	Medium–high	High
Succinic dehydrogenase	Low	Medium	Medium–high	High
Men.- α-GPD[f]	High		High	Low
Glycogen	High	High	High	Low
Phosphorylase	High		High	Low
Neutral fat	Low		Medium	High
Capillary supply	Sparse		Rich	Rich
Fiber diameter, cat	Large	Large–medium	Medium–small	Small
Biochemical Features[g]				
Actomyosin ATPase, $\mu mol \cdot min^{-1} \cdot mg^{-1}$, pH 9.4	0.27		0.16	0.04
Lactate dehydrogenase, $\mu mol \cdot min^{-1} \cdot g^{-1}$	449		218	105
Succinic dehydrogenase, $\mu mol \cdot min^{-1} \cdot g^{-1}$	0.72		2.49	1.95
Hexokinase, $nmol \cdot min^{-1} \cdot g^{-1}$	297		620	978
Cytochrome c, nmol/g	1.9		18	6.5
Myoglobin, mg/g	0.31		1.44	1.39

[a] Nomenclature of Brooke and Kaiser (77). [b] Nomenclature of Peter et al. (552): FG, fast twitch, glycolytic; FOG, fast twitch, oxidative, glycolytic; SO, slow twitch, oxidative. [c] Nomenclature of Burke et al. (111): FF, fast twitch, fatigable; F(int), fast twitch, intermediate; FR, fast twitch, fatigue resistant; S, slow twitch. [d] ATPase staining after preincubation with acidic buffers at indicated pH values. [e] In the NADH dehydrogenase and succinic dehydrogenase stains, the patterns of reaction product deposition are different in FOG and SO fibers (refs. 552, 659). [f] Menadione-linked α-glycerophosphate dehydrogenase. [g] Mean values for whole guinea pig muscles with indicated fiber-type predominance. [From Table 1 in ref. 552.]

distinctions between the major groups are sufficiently clear and correlative data are sufficiently compelling (see subsection PHYSIOLOGICAL AND HISTOCHEMICAL PROFILES OF MUSCLE UNITS, p. 354) that a basic tripartite division can be regarded as well established. There is one kind of fiber with relatively low myofibrillar ATPase activity at alkaline pH (type I) and at least two distinct varieties of fibers with high ATPase activity (type II fibers).

The class of type I fibers is clearly different in many respects from any of the type II varieties, both morphologically and biochemically, and type I myosin is antigenically distinct from that in type II fibers (277, 278, 280). Type I fibers have much less capacity for anaerobic glycolysis than either of the type II varieties but rather appear to depend almost exclusively on aerobic metabolism. There is less interfiber variation in metabolic enzymes among type I than among type II fibers (e.g., ref. 644). These conclusions, drawn from studies of animal muscles, have recently been confirmed in elegant biochemical studies of individual human muscle fibers that had been identified histochemically (247, 691).

The distinctions between subclasses of type II fibers are based on several factors (see Table 1). Type IIB fibers have a high evident capacity for anaerobic glycolysis (e.g., high α-GPD and considerable stored glycogen with little free lipid), but they exhibit little evident capacity for aerobic metabolism (e.g., low levels of NADH-D and SDH) and they have little myoglobin. The type IIA fibers resemble IIB in their capacity for anaerobic metabolism but, contrastingly, also have a considerable capacity for aerobic metabolism, with high activity of NADH-D, SDH, hexokinase, and cytochrome c, and high content of myoglobin. The ATPase staining intensities are different in IIA and IIB fibers when muscle sections are pretreated with acidic buffers (Table 1, AC-ATPase; see refs. 77, 78), and recent work using immunocytochemical methods suggests that IIB and IIA fibers contain different ratios of "fast" myosin light chains (279). Furthermore these two fiber types also contain different patterns of certain isoenzymes, such as those of lactate dehydrogenase (613). In light of other physiological and anatomical differences between the motor units associated with IIA or IIB muscle units (subsections MOTOR UNIT POPULATION OF CAT MEDIAL GASTROCNEMIUS MUSCLE, p. 353; INNERVATION RATIOS AND MUSCLE UNIT "SIZE," p. 369; and section PHYSIOLOGY OF α-MOTONEURONS AND THEIR SYNAPTIC INPUTS IN RELATION TO MOTOR UNIT TYPE, p. 378), it seems likely that these categories are in fact distinct. The type IIAB fibers noted in Table 1 are present in small proportions in cat limb muscles and may well represent a true "intermediate" type between IIA and IIB (see subsection PHYSIOLOGICAL AND HISTOCHEMICAL PROFILES OF MUSCLE UNITS, p. 354).

In addition to the above, there is a third category of

type II fiber, called type IIC. The type IIC fiber has been described as a "primitive" type, perhaps a relatively undifferentiated precursor of IIA and IIB (78, 79), but the interpretation of this fiber type in the organization of motor units remains unsettled at present (subsections MOTOR UNIT POPULATION OF CAT MEDIAL GASTROCNEMIUS MUSCLE, p. 353, and PHYSIOLOGICAL AND HISTOCHEMICAL PROFILES OF MUSCLE UNITS, p. 354; see also ref. 607).

ANATOMY AND ULTRASTRUCTURE. The average diameter of muscle fibers is frequently correlated with their histochemical type, at least within a given heterogeneous muscle. In many animals (e.g., cat, rat, guinea pig) there is a clear inverse relation between fiber diameter and oxidative enzyme staining (e.g., Fig. 2 in ref. 436) such that average diameters are scaled as: IIB > IIA > I (see Table 1). In general, the capillary supply (e.g., measured as numbers surrounding fibers of a given type) is directly correlated with oxidative staining [Table 1; (592)]. These two facts combine to suggest that fiber types with high oxidative capacity are presumably dependent on blood-borne oxygen and metabolites and should have relatively small diameters to maximize surface-to-volume ratios and reduce diffusion distances to a practical minimum. The price to be paid is, of course, that fewer myofibrils can be packed into a single fiber, and force output per fiber would thus diminish.

This easy generalization has a certain appeal but there are many exceptions to the size-type correlation, including many muscles in humans (e.g., ref. 202), especially in normal females (76), where type I fibers may be larger than type II on the average. The type I fibers in cat soleus muscle are about the same size as the low-oxidative type IIB fibers of the gastrocnemius (see Fig. 2), even though their metabolic patterns and fatigue resistance are very different (subsection MOTOR UNIT POPULATION OF CAT MEDIAL GASTROCNEMIUS MUSCLE, p. 353). An extreme example of disparity occurs in human masseter muscle, where the low oxidative fibers are very much smaller in average dimensions than the high-oxidative fibers, and the largest fibers by far are the type I (586). Exercise history (see subsection ALTERATIONS OF DEMAND WITHIN THE PHYSIOLOGICAL RANGE, p. 362) and other factors still to be elucidated may well play important roles in conditioning relative fiber sizes, and simple generalizations about this issue seem unwarranted.

Ultrastructural studies of muscle have demonstrated that fibers with different histochemical profiles exhibit corresponding differences in average Z line width; in the number, volume, and position of mitochondria within the fibers; and in the average volume and complexity of the T tubule and sarcoplasmic reticulum systems (230, 231, 276, 277, 463, 534, 617, 619, 619a, 694). Eisenberg and Kuda [see Fig. 3; (231)] have confirmed the general patterns found in many studies (see especially refs. 276, 277), using histochem-

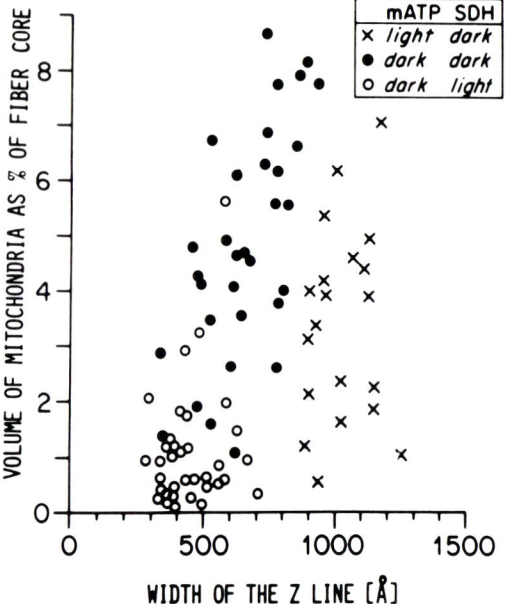

FIG. 3. Ultrastructural features of histochemically identified muscle fibers. Scatter diagram comparing Z line width (abscissa) and mitochondrial volume (ordinate, expressed as percentage of fiber core volume) measured from electron micrographs of guinea pig medial gastrocnemius muscle fibers that had been frozen, thawed, and then fixed. Serial cryostat sections of the same fibers were stained for myofibrillar ATPase at alkaline pH (mATP) and for the oxidative enzyme succinic dehydrogenase (see Table 1), permitting comparison of ultrastructural features in histochemically typed fibers. Using nomenclature of Table I, *crosses* are type I, *filled circles* are type IIA, and *open circles* are type IIB. [From Eisenberg and Kuda (231).]

ically typed fibers to show that type I fibers generally have the widest Z lines, the largest number of mitochondria (distributed rather evenly throughout the fibers, as is consistent with the fine, unbroken network of reaction product particles in oxidative histochemical reactions; e.g., Figs. 2 and 6), and the least well-developed sarcotubular systems. Fibers with the IIA profiles also have large numbers of mitochondria, with many in subsarcolemmal aggregates, consistent with the irregular oxidative reaction product deposition with subsarcolemmal accumulations in SDH or NADH-D preparations (see refs. 111, 659). Compared with type I fibers, type IIA fibers generally have somewhat narrower Z lines and rather well-developed sarcoplasmic reticulum and tubular systems. The IIB fibers exhibit the narrowest Z lines, and they have relatively few mitochondria (concomitant with their relatively weak staining for mitochondrial oxidative enzymes) but very highly developed sarcotubular systems.

NEUROMUSCULAR JUNCTION SPECIALIZATIONS. There is conflicting evidence as to whether or not the morphology of neuromuscular junctions (NMJs) is specialized in relation to postsynaptic fiber type. A direct correlation between the size of the NMJ (whether of axon terminal apparatus or of cholinesterase-stained sole plate) and the diameter of the innervated muscle fiber has been repeatedly described (e.g., refs. 14, 68, 422, 442, 527, 533), and NMJ size has a positive correlation with amount of transmitter released (442). Observations on other details of junctional morphology and fiber type interrelations, however, are less consistent.

The morphological features of NMJs found in "fast-twitch" (i.e., mixed) muscles are reported to be rather similar, at least on the average, to those found in slow-twitch muscles (usually soleus), although a wide range of dimensions and complexity have been seen in both kinds of muscles (e.g., refs. 235, 527, 611). In contrast, studies in which end plates within a given mixed muscle were compared in relation to postsynaptic fiber type [e.g., in fowl (68), in rat (422, 541), in mouse (533), and in humans (517)] indicate a considerable degree of correlated specialization (see also ref. 446). For example, the NMJs on the large-diameter "white" fibers (equivalent to the type IIB of Table 1) tend to have larger and more complex pre- and postsynaptic structures, as compared to the endings on "red" fibers (equivalent to type I fibers), as well as having larger evident stores of synaptic vesicles (517, 541). Terminals on "intermediate" fibers (probably equivalent to type IIA) exhibit an intermediate degree of complexity. The lack of clear-cut differences between soleus and mixed muscle NMJs may well indicate that the endings in the slow-twitch soleus are not typical of junctions on slow-twitch fibers in more heterogeneous muscles.

With respect to physiological differences, there are almost no direct data on neuromuscular transmission as related to fiber type within a given heterogeneous population of twitch fibers in mammalian muscle. However, McArdle and Albuquerque (484) have shown that the frequency of spontaneous miniature end-plate potentials (MEPPs) in heterogeneous slow-twitch rat muscles is about double that found in the heterogeneous fast muscle, as would be consistent with the finding of Kuno and co-workers (442) that larger end plates exhibit faster spontaneous MEPP release. There are pharmacological observations that end plates in cat soleus differ from those in predominately fast muscle with respect to blockade of transmission by competitive versus depolarizing blocking agents (397, 398) and to blockade by tetanus toxin (204).

Motor Unit Types: Physiological Profiles in Experimental Animals

A decade after Gordon's and Phillips' demonstration (298) of slow-twitch components in the fast tibialis anterior of the cat, other investigators began to find slow-twitch motor units in other nominally fast muscles, including rat tail (658) and cat intercostal (10). However, systematic description of the full range of motor unit properties in an individual muscle really began with the work of Bessou and colleagues (57) on the first deep lumbrical muscle of the cat. These authors demonstrated wide variations in twitch-contraction times, tetanic tensions, and motor axon conduction velocities in this unit population, as well as close, monotonic interrelations between these properties. These points were later confirmed (Fig. 4, filled symbols) in the same laboratory for the superficial lumbrical [(15); see also ref. 417]. In a now classic series of papers published in 1965, Henneman and colleagues described in detail the range of contraction times, tension outputs, and axonal conduction velocities for large samples of motor units in the cat medial gastrocnemius (732) and soleus muscles (491). Henneman and Olson (361) suggested that particular combinations of such properties must be related to the histochemical differences between muscle fibers, although there was no direct evidence for this at the time.

These pioneering studies revealed a number of general points that have since been repeatedly confirmed. First, within a given unit population, the motor units with the slowest twitch contraction all tend to produce rather small tensions, while the faster contracting units tend to produce a wider range of tensions, including some with quite large force outputs. This correlation is much closer and monotonic among cat lumbrical motor units (15, 57) than in the gastrocnemius population (Fig. 4, *right graph*; see also refs. 111, 732). The patterns of correlation clearly differ between these muscles, suggesting that muscle identity (and presumably functional usage) condition the organization observed (e.g., refs. 299, 662). Second, motor units found in histochemically heterogeneous lumbrical [in rat (735); in cat (J. Toop and R. E. Burke, unpublished material)] and gastrocnemius muscles (Fig. 2) exhibit much wider variation in physiological properties than those present in the homogeneous soleus (Fig. 4, *left graph*). Third, the relatively slow-twitch, small-force units tend to be innervated by relatively slowly conducting motor axons (see Figs. 20 and 21). Again force and conduction velocity are rather precisely related among lumbrical motor units [Fig. 4, *right*; (15, 57)]. In the gastrocnemius, the faster contracting units also tend to be innervated by motor axons with relatively fast conduction velocities but the correlation is very much weaker than in the lumbricals (compare open and solid-symbol distributions in Fig. 4, *right*; see also Fig. 21).

Since the mid-1960s, a large number of studies of motor unit populations have appeared. These include, in the cat, further work on the unit populations of medial gastrocnemius (100, 111, 112, 118, 345, 537, 566, 575, 662), the soleus (28, 33, 100, 110, 387, 515), the tibialis anterior and extensor digitorum longus (207, 299, 300, 387, 515), the flexor digitorum longus (31, 205, 454, 536), the peroneus brevis and longus (387), the tibialis posterior (63, 488), and the plantaris, flexor hellucis longus, and flexor digitorum brevis (301, 717a).

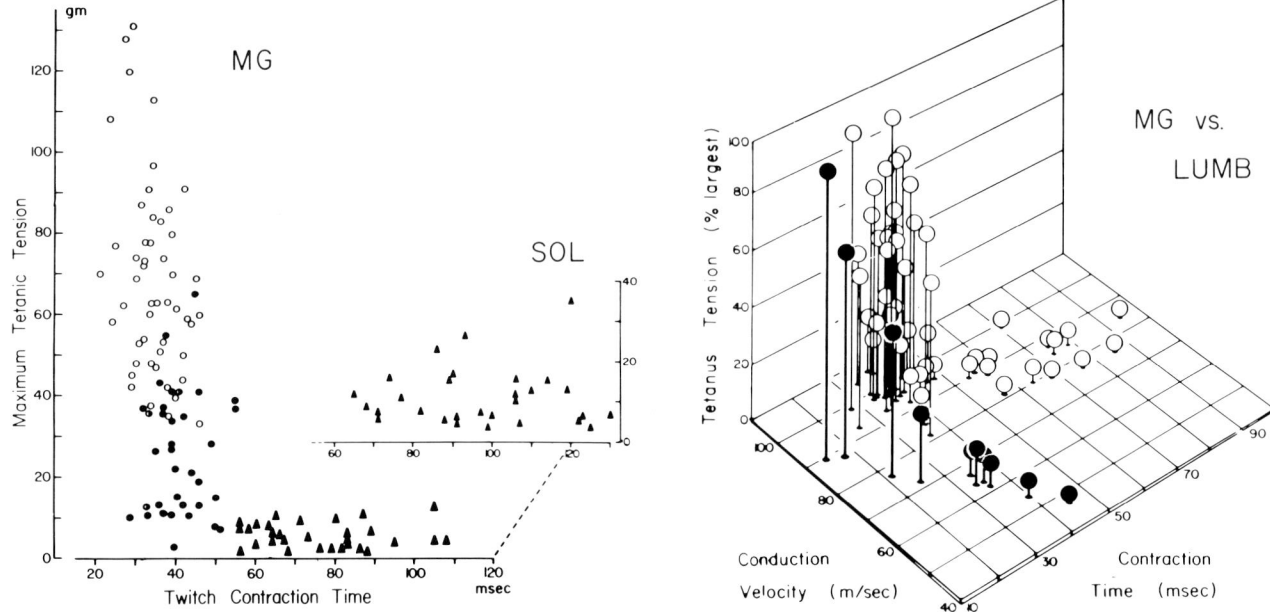

FIG. 4. Physiological profiles of motor unit samples from 3 different cat muscles. *Left*, comparison of units in medial gastrocnemius (MG) and soleus (SOL). Scatter diagrams show tetanic tension outputs (ordinate) and isometric twitch contraction times (abscissa). Note that data scatter is much greater for MG sample than for SOL. Motor unit types denoted by the following symbols: type FF units, *open circles*; type FR, *filled circles*; type S, *filled triangles*. *Right*, 3-dimensional diagram comparing physiological profiles of motor units in cat superficial lumbrical muscle (*filled circles*) with units in cat medial gastrocnemius (*open circles*). Tetanic tension output (*vertical* ordinate) is normalized as percentage of the largest unit in each sample. Note precise, monotonic relation between all 3 variables in data from lumbrical sample compared to greater scatter of points in gastrocnemius sample. The range of variation for tetanic tensions and contraction times was approximately the same in the 2 muscles (although with different absolute values), but the range of axonal conduction velocities was much wider for lumbrical than for gastrocnemius units. [*Left* from Burke and Tsairis (122). *Right*, data for lumbrical muscle from Appelberg and Emonet-Dénand (15); data for medial gastrocnemius from Burke et al. (118).]

In the rat, data are available for units in the soleus (12, 145, 432, 433), the extensor digitorum longus (12, 145), the flexor hallucis longus (462), and the tibialis anterior (227). Individual units in the extensor digitorum communis of the baboon forelimb were examined by Eccles et al. (219) and in the rabbit soleus by Bagust (29). Finally, the unit population in the medial gastrocnemius of the skunk provides an interesting contrast to its composition in the cat (701). Motor unit populations in amphibian muscles (464, 638, 639), reptile muscles (347, 348), and extraocular muscles (e.g., ref. 288) provide further comparative data that underscore the general interrelations noted above. The many differences in the details of organization between motor unit populations in various muscles and species are undoubtedly related to factors of body size, metabolic rates, movement speed, and the mechanical demands imposed by different motor habits (e.g., refs. 148, 701). Much remains to be done to clarify these potentially very important interrelations.

A WORD ABOUT METHODOLOGY. Assessment of the physiological properties of motor units requires functional isolation of individual units by *1*) dissection of fine filaments of centrally cut ventral roots so that electrical stimulation activates only one motor axon to the muscle of interest (e.g., refs. 57, 491) or *2*) penetration of the innervating motoneuron with an intracellular micropipette electrode, stimulating the cell with current pulses passed directly into it (100, 194). Most of the work cited in subsection *Motor Unit Types: Physiological Profiles in Experimental Animals* (p. 351) was done using ventral root dissection, which requires very careful attention to limit stimulation to a single motor axon to the target muscle (i.e., repeated testing to ensure that stimulation of the ventral root filament produces an all-or-none mechanical and electrical response in the muscle, and that antidromic stimulation of the muscle nerve in the periphery produces only one detectable all-or-none antidromic spike in the same ventral root filament; see ref. 667 for details). Only the peripheral portion of a motor unit can be studied by stimulating cut ventral rootlets—i.e., the distal motor axon and the muscle unit. Intracellular recording and stimulation of individual motoneurons (100, 194) provides more secure functional isolation during stimulation and, in addition, permits study of the electrophysiological (section PHYSIOLOGY

OF α-MOTONEURONS AND THEIR SYNAPTIC INPUTS IN RELATION TO MOTOR UNIT TYPE, p. 378) and morphological (subsection *Motoneuron Anatomy in Relation to Unit Type,* p. 377) characteristics of the innervating motoneuron and its synaptic inputs. Both methods are capable, under favorable conditions, of sampling a relatively large proportion of a given motor unit pool, but both may introduce some element of sampling bias in that smaller motoneurons and their finer motor axons may well be more susceptible to damage by either root dissection or intracellular penetration, with consequent underrepresentation in the final samples. The spatial density of motoneurons along the motor cell column (see subsection *Anatomy of Motor Nuclei,* p. 372) may contribute a difference between the methods in that close cell packing promotes more effective sampling with a micropipette but can hamper isolation of individual motor axons in ventral root filaments.

The conditions under which mechanical muscle unit responses are recorded can influence the reported results. Most studies have been done under nominally "isometric" conditions, although truly isometric conditions are not attainable in practice (there is always some visible deformation of the muscle during activity of single muscle units). Some work (e.g., refs. 100, 111, 112, 732) has involved setting whole muscle length and resultant passive tension to a level that gives a maximum twitch and tetanus responses for a majority of tested units. In other studies (e.g., refs. 31, 301, 566, 575), muscle length was adjusted to produce individual maximum responses, which can vary from one unit to another (454). In addition, muscle temperature and blood flow, the time history of unit activation (see subsection EFFECTS OF FIRING RATE AND FIRING PATTERN ON MUSCLE UNIT OUTPUT, p. 397), and the general condition of the experimental animal can also affect the observed mechanical unit responses. Despite such methodological variations, comparison of the data from different studies of a given muscle and animal species suggests that the choice of method does not seriously distort the general patterns of observed mechanical properties regardless of differences in details.

MOTOR UNIT POPULATION OF CAT MEDIAL GASTROCNEMIUS MUSCLE. Although each motor unit population is to some extent unique, the evidence just discussed suggests that heterogeneous motor unit populations are organized in basically similar ways. For purposes of further explication, it is useful to consider in some detail one population for which there are extensive data, not only about muscle unit characteristics but also about the innervating motoneurons and the synaptic input impinging upon them.

In their original study of the cat medial gastrocnemius (MG), Wuerker and colleagues (732) did not attempt any formal classification of motor unit types. Burke (100) later suggested that it is useful to divide MG motor units into fast-twitch (type F) and slow-twitch (type S) categories, simply on the basis of twitch-contraction time. The same author subsequently (102) noted that his type F units could be roughly divided into two groups on the basis of tetanic force output, strength of input from group Ia muscle spindle afferents, and reflex responsiveness to muscle stretch. In 1971, Olson and Swett (537) proposed a tripartite classification scheme for cat MG motor units in which unit categories were first separated by the presence or absence of repetitive muscle fiber activity following a high-frequency tetanus (termed PTRA), a phenomenon with origin at the neuromuscular junction (654, 655). The units without PTRA were then divided more loosely into two groups, one with generally large force outputs that were fatigue sensitive and another with intermediate force outputs and more resistance to fatigue. Olson and Swett opted for three unit categories largely because of the histochemical evidence for three muscle fiber types (subsection *Muscle Fiber Types: Histochemical Profiles and Ultrastructural Correlations,* p. 347). At the same time, Burke and co-workers [(112); see also ref. 111] introduced a tripartite classification scheme based on a different combination of physiological parameters, including *1*) the shape of standardized unfused tetanic responses (the "sag" property; see, e.g., Fig. 30*B*, *D*) and *2*) the relative fatigability of the unit during a standard stimulus sequence (the "fatigue index"; see Fig. 5). It is highly probable that both ways of dividing the MG unit population produce roughly equivalent motor unit groups.

The evidence available to date strongly suggests that motor units, like muscle fiber types (see Table 1), are best classified using multiple criteria (104, 111, 112, 537), or what is termed a "polythetic" classification (642). When the interrelations between four properties of muscle unit mechanical responses are considered (Fig. 5), the data points for cat MG units cluster into groups (111, 112). One group, without sag (stippled circles in Fig. 5), all had high resistance to fatigue, small tetanic tension outputs, and relatively long twitch-contraction times. These are referred to simply as slow-twitch, or type S, units, as in earlier work (100–102) and are probably equivalent to the PTRA units of Olson and Swett (537). The remaining units all exhibited sag in unfused tetani through a wide range of input frequencies (e.g., Fig. 30) and had relatively short twitch-contraction times ($<$ 55 ms); these are referred to collectively as fast-twitch, or type F, units. The F group exhibits a bimodal distribution of fatigue indices. The more fatigable group (fatigue index values $<$ 0.25) tended to produce relatively large tetanic forces; these are called type FF (or fast twitch, fatigable) and are probably equivalent to the large, fatigable units without PTRA of Olson and Swett (537). The other type F group exhibited greater resistance to fatigue (fatigue index values $>$ 0.75) but produced less tetanic force; these are called type FR (or fast twitch, fatigue resistant) units and are probably

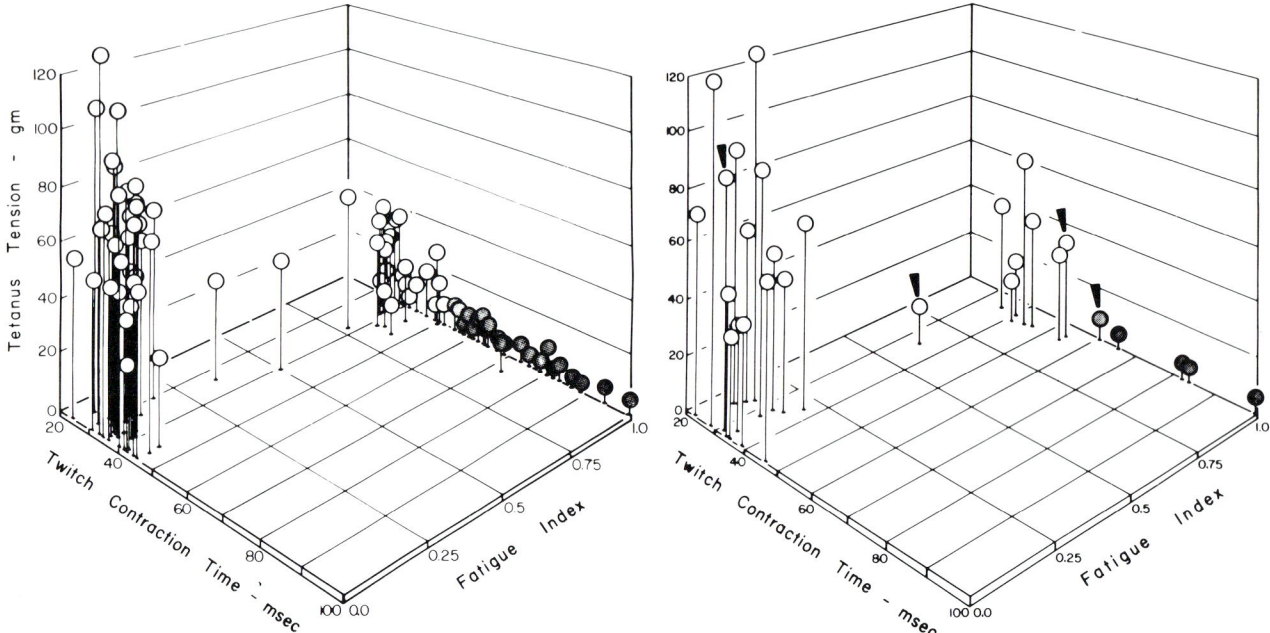

FIG. 5. Multivariate physiological profiles of motor units in cat medial gastrocnemius (MG) muscle, displayed on 3-dimensional graphs. *Left*, data from a sample of 81 MG units studied in 3 cats. *Stippled circles* denote units without "sag" in unfused tetani (type S units); *open circles* denote units with sag (type F). Type F units are divided according to fatigue index as follows: type FF, fatigue index less than 0.25; type F(int), fatigue index between 0.25 and 0.75; type FR, fatigue index greater than 0.75. Increasing values of fatigue index denote increasing resistance to fatigue during a standardized sequence of tetani. *Right*, diagram same as *left* but including data from an additional 28 MG units, each of which was also studied histochemically by the glycogen-depletion method (see text). Histochemical profiles of the 4 units denoted by *arrows* (1 of each motor unit type) are illustrated in Figure 6. [From Burke et al. (111).]

equivalent to the medium-force, fatigue-resistant units of Olson and Swett (537). A small proportion (about 5%; see also Fig. 35) of the type F population had fatigue index values between 0.25 and 0.75; these can be referred to as type F(int), or fast-twitch, intermediate units (118).

The classification criteria used for the above scheme produced clear and easily defined separation between unit groups (111, 112). Fast- and slow-twitch unit groups were identified using the sag property rather than twitch-contraction times per se because there was a continuous distribution of twitch-contraction times (Fig. 5). The presence or absence of sag provided a clear division into two categories despite the fact that this phenomenon has no current mechanistic connotation (see subsection EFFECTS OF FIRING RATE AND FIRING PATTERN ON MUSCLE UNIT OUTPUT, p. 397). It may be noted that Cooper and Eccles (164) described sag in records of unfused tetanic contractions of whole cat gastrocnemius but found it absent in the slow twitch soleus. Other studies of cat MG motor units have used this type of classification scheme with more or less comparable results (345, 566, 567, 575). The motor unit populations of the cat tibialis anterior (207), flexor digitorum longus muscles (205), flexor hallucis longus (717a), and tibialis posterior (488) can be divided into the same unit types using these criteria.

The data in Figure 5 represent an example of the advantages and difficulties introduced by a classification scheme. It is clearly advantageous to have labels for different groups of motor units, particularly when they convey some sense of physiological differences. However, it must also be recognized that the distributions of parameters such as twitch-contraction time or tetanic-force output are continuous, albeit skewed. Even within the data cluster that represents a given unit type, there is considerable variation, although certainly less than that for the population as a whole. By their very nature, classification schemes tend to emphasize differences between groups, and this can easily lead to a certain rigidity in thinking—something to be avoided in any scientific inquiry. Although this chapter is written with the explicit assumption that the muscle fiber and motor unit types discussed above are indeed meaningfully different from one another, it is important to keep this cautionary note in mind.

PHYSIOLOGICAL AND HISTOCHEMICAL PROFILES OF MUSCLE UNITS. The most direct study to date of the interrelations between the morphological, histochemical, and physiological characteristics of muscle fibers is that of Lännergren and Smith (446), who examined these features in individual fibers from the iliofibularis muscle of the toad *Xenopus* (see also ref. 244). They described three groups among the true twitch fibers:

one with relatively fast-twitch contractions (mean 29.3 ms time to peak) and little resistance to fatigue, another with somewhat longer contraction times (mean 37.2 ms) and considerably greater resistance to fatigue, and a third with the longest twitch-contraction times (mean 53.8 ms) and the greatest resistance to fatigue. Each category corresponded to a different histochemical fiber profile (oxidative enzyme and fat stains) and a distinctive morphology of the en plaque neuromuscular junctions. The same authors (639) later showed that iliofibularis motor units displayed the same distributions of physiological properties as the single fibers. This finding suggests that the observed physiological-histochemical correlations apply to whole muscle units, and it provides the best available evidence that muscle fibers belonging to a given muscle unit are identical in mechanical as well as histochemical properties.

There have been no comparable studies of single muscle fibers in mammalian muscle, although Luff and Atwood (463) have compared some mechanical and electrical properties of single fibers in mouse muscles with the ultrastructure of other fibers in the same muscles. Instead the correlation between muscle fiber histochemistry and physiology has been examined at the level of motor units, the muscle fibers of which are identified by the loss of glycogen after prolonged stimulation of individual motor axons or motoneurons. This glycogen-depletion method, suggested by Krnjevic and Miledi (428), was first used successfully by Edström and Kugelberg (227) to histochemically identify fibers belonging to individual muscle units in the rat tibialis anterior (see also refs. 74, 198, and discussion in subsection *Anatomy of Muscle Units*, p. 367). Although they were unable to deplete fibers in the most fatigue-resistant units (their type C), Edström and Kugelberg (227) concluded that there was a direct correlation between oxidative staining affinity and unit fatigue resistance but, surprisingly, found no relation with twitch-contraction times (all of their units were equally fast twitch).

Burke and colleagues (111, 112) later used the glycogen-depletion approach to label muscle units belonging to the full range of types found in the cat MG muscle (Figs. 5 and 6). All 15 type FF units studied histochemically (see Fig. 5, *right graph*) exhibited the same staining profile as the FF unit shown in Figure 6 (type IIB in Table 1). Similarly all 7 type FR units and all 5 type S units showed type-specific histochemical profiles as the FR and S units in Figure 6 (types IIA and I, respectively; see Table 1). The one F(int) unit studied histochemically (Fig. 5; referred to as an unclassified unit in Table 2 in ref. 111) exhibited the histochemical profile (Fig. 6, *second row*) of IIB fibers in ATPase staining but was like IIA in oxidative staining. Thus it is referred to as type IIAB in Table 1. The match between the physiological and histochemical profiles of muscle units is such that each set of characteristics can be used to predict the other (104, 111, 112).

In the above work, selected examples of each unit type were examined for histochemical uniformity by comparing profiles in large numbers (80–140) of glycogen-depleted unit fibers. In all cases studied, the fibers belonging to a given muscle unit were identical (111), providing strong evidence that the individual fibers making up a muscle unit are of the same histochemical type. With few exceptions (227, 432, 433), rat motor units have also been found to be histochemically uniform (74, 198). In view of the findings of Smith and Lännergren (639) previously noted, it seems reasonable to assume that fibers in a given muscle unit are also effectively identical in mechanical properties.

The main physiological differences between classes of muscle units are found in twitch-contraction times, fatigability, and average tetanic force output. Before going further, it is useful to consider the factors that may produce such differences between muscle units. Contraction time and fatigability are considered in subsections TWITCH-CONTRACTION TIMES AND MYOFIBRILLAR ATPASE, p. 355, and FATIGABILITY AND METABOLIC PROFILES, p. 358, respectively; the factors that control force output are discussed in subsection INNERVATION RATIOS AND MUSCLE UNIT "SIZE," p. 369.

TWITCH-CONTRACTION TIMES AND MYOFIBRILLAR ATPASE. The terms fast and slow are relative and no absolute twitch-contraction times can be associated with them. Muscle units in the tiny extraocular (e.g., refs. 288, 449) or middle ear muscles (680) of the cat exhibit very brief twitch-contraction times (3–13 ms) compared to units in the much larger medial gastrocnemius (20–100 ms; see Fig. 5), but the range of values within each population is similar (about four- to fivefold). The range of twitch-contraction times in the cat lumbrical is also roughly four- to fivefold [see Fig. 4; (15, 57, 417)]. These populations are in this sense heterogeneous, including fast and slow motor units, and their muscles are also heterogeneous by ATPase histochemistry (subsection *Motor Unit Types: Physiological Profiles in Experimental Animals*, p. 351). One can conclude that ATPase heterogeneity is correlated with wide ranges of twitch-contraction times.

Isometric twitch-contraction time depends on many things, including muscle fiber length and the characteristics of the series elastic element, the time course of the series of processes involved in excitation-contraction coupling (including Ca^{2+} release from the sarcoplasmic reticulum and binding to regulator proteins), the rate of cross-bridge cycling and of myofilament relaxation (including the kinetics of Ca^{2+} dissociation from regulator proteins and its reuptake into the sarcoplasmic reticulum), mechanical fiber loading, the previous history of fiber activation, fatigue effects, and possibly other factors (see discussions in refs. 144, 148, 150, 165, 403, 463, 717). The relative importance of these potentially independent factors is unsettled (e.g., ref. 403), but there is general agreement that the intrinsic speed of shortening of the myofibrils is probably a critical feature (148, 200, 321). There is, in turn,

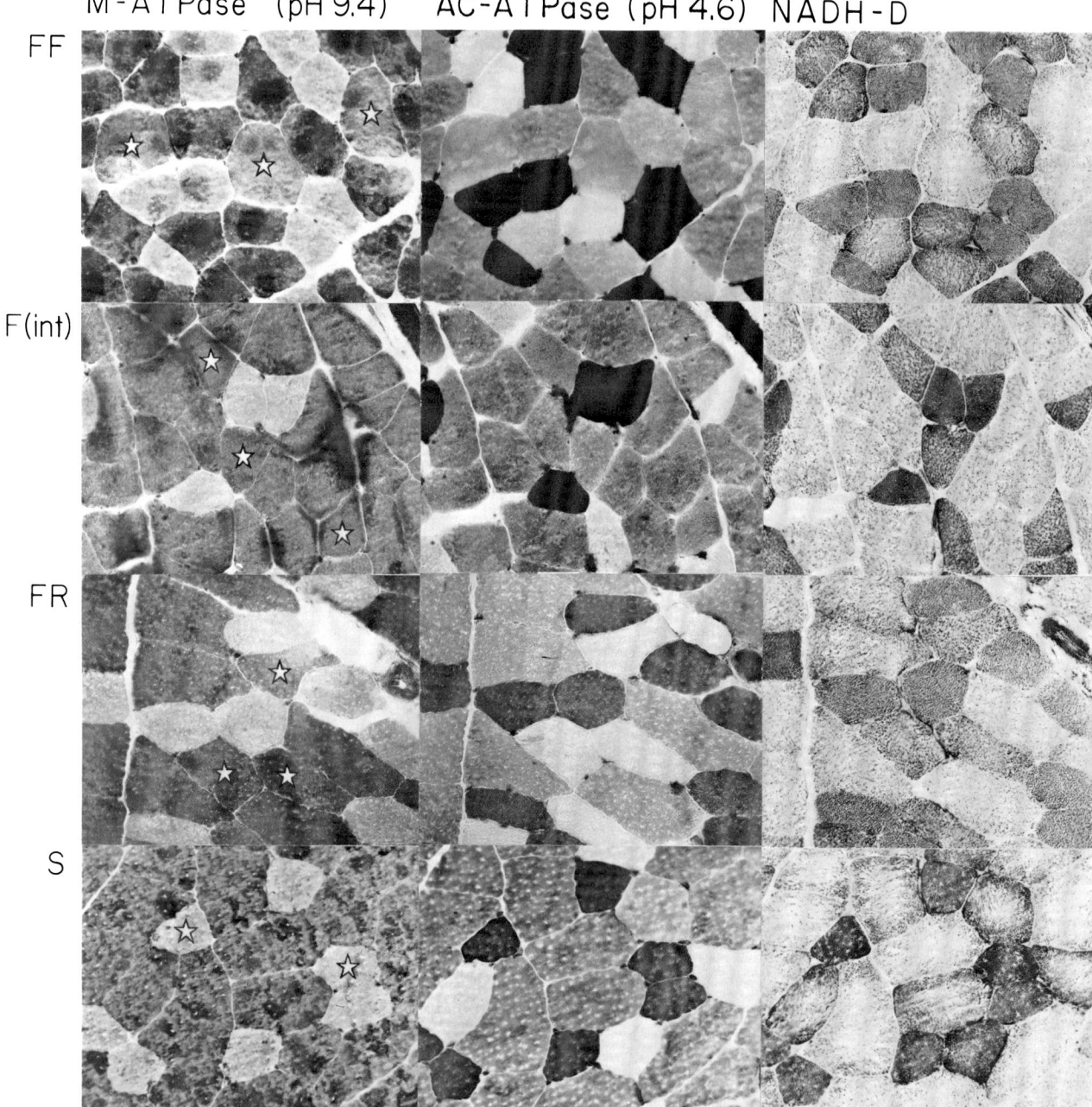

FIG. 6. Histochemical profiles of 4 physiologically identified muscle units from cat medial gastrocnemius (MG; see Fig. 5), representing each of the unit types present in that muscle. Muscle fibers belonging to the studied units were identified in each case by glycogen depletion (not illustrated, but see Fig. 12) and are indicated by *stars* in *left column* of photomicrographs. *Left column*, sections stained for myofibrillar ATPase (M-ATPase) activity at pH 9.4, in which the F units are all heavily stained (type II) and the S unit is relatively light (type I; see Table 1). Distinction between the various type II fibers can be made on the basis of ATPase activity after acidic preincubation (AC-ATPase, pH 4.6, *middle column*, in which 3 staining levels can be seen) and by relative staining for oxidative enzyme, NADH dehydrogenase (NADH-D; *right column*), for which all of the unit types except type FF display rather heavy staining. With reference to Table 1, FF unit fibers are of the IIB histochemical type, F(int) unit fibers are type IIAB, FR fibers are type IIA, and S units fibers are type I. [Unpublished photomicrographs of material from experiments described in Burke et al. (111).]

evidence that the speed of ATP hydrolysis by myosin is closely linked to intrinsic shortening velocity per sarcomere. For example, Barany showed in 1967 (39) that the biochemically measurable Mg^{2+}- and actin-activated ATPase activity of whole muscle myosin from a great variety of animals is directly correlated with the speed of muscle contraction. Table 1 shows that there is a general correlation between ATPase activity assessed by histochemical (at alkaline pH) and biochemical methods (see also refs. 328, 552). Whole mammalian muscles exhibit relatively fast sarcomere shortening when they are composed predominately of type II fibers, with high myofibrillar ATPase staining (see Table 5 in ref. 148). Although the details of the interrelation between ATP splitting and the mechanical events of contraction are by no means clarified (e.g., refs. 131, 361, 403), myosin ATPase activity can thus be regarded as an important rate-limiting factor (148, 507).

Given the above conclusion, it is useful to compare M-ATPase staining and twitch-contraction times in glycogen-depleted muscle units. With regard to cat gastrocnemius, the fibers of the nominally fast-twitch units [FF, F(int), and FR] all exhibit more intense M-ATPase staining than the fibers of the slow-twitch type S units (Fig. 6). It is also true, however, that the contraction times for fast-twitch units vary over at least a twofold range (Fig. 5), without corresponding gradations in M-ATPase staining (Fig. 6). Furthermore the range of contraction times of MG type S units documented histochemically (Fig. 5, *right*) nearly overlaps that of the type FR group despite the difference in their ATPase staining (compare Fig. 5 arrows with Fig. 6). Motor units of the histochemically homogeneous cat soleus (see Fig. 2) are, with rare exceptions [(345); R. Burke, R. Dum, and M. O'Donovan, unpublished results], all type S, but they also exhibit a twofold range in contraction times (Fig. 4; see also refs. 110, 122, 515; cf. ref. 28). Thus myofibrillar ATPase homogeneity does not necessarily guarantee muscle units with identical contraction times.

In contrast to these results in cat muscle, Kugelberg (432, 433) has described a very close correlation between the intensity of M-ATPase staining and twitch contraction times of muscle units in the heterogeneous rat soleus (Fig. 7). It is noteworthy that muscle fibers in the rat soleus exhibit a direct relation between M-ATPase staining and oxidative enzyme staining, rather than the roughly inverse relation that prevails among fibers in other heterogeneous muscles (Table 1; Fig. 6), including other muscles in the rat (e.g., ref. 331). This provides further example of the intermuscle and interspecies differences that make it difficult to arrive at a universial classification of muscle fiber and motor unit types.

The relation between M-ATPase histochemistry

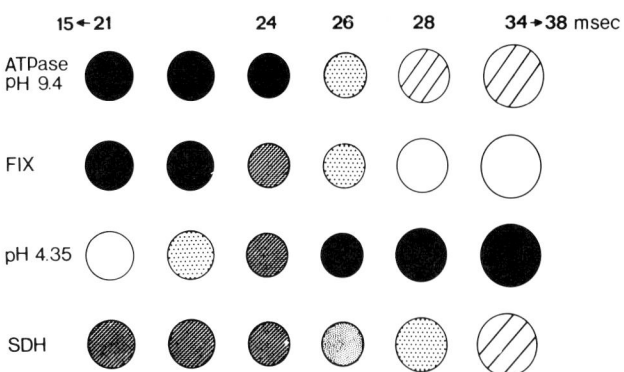

FIG. 7. Histochemical profiles (determined in glycogen-depletion experiments) representative of physiologically studied muscle units in rat soleus (SOL) muscle, separated according to their isometric twitch contraction times (in milliseconds; numbers above each column). *Shading* denotes staining intensity and size of *circles* represents relative fiber area. *Top 3 rows* represent ATPase staining under different conditions (alkaline and acid pH as in Table 1; FIX, after cold formaldehyde fixation). *Bottom row* shows staining for the oxidative enzyme, succinic dehydrogenase (SDH; see Table 1). Note parallel staining pattern between alkaline ATPase and SDH and inverse relation of both to fiber area, which is different from the pattern found in most other heterogeneous muscles (see Table 1, Fig. 6). [From Kugelberg (432).]

and contraction times of histochemically defined muscle units fits with Barany's (39) data, but clearly other factors must also be considered. With regard to limitations of methodology, there is a degree of nonspecificity to the ATPase histochemical reaction (e.g., refs. 78, 202, 327, 329), which is insensitive to the actin-activated ATPase reactivity of myofibrils (see ref. 279). Recent immunofluorescence studies of Gauthier and Lowey (279) suggest that the ratio of the A_2 and A_1 light chains of fast myosin (A_2:A_1) is greater in IIB fibers than in IIA fibers (true in both rat and cat; G. F. Gauthier, personal communication). The S_1 myosin subfragment associated with the A_2 light chain appears to have higher actin-activated ATPase activity than the A_1 subfragment, although the Mg^{2+}-dependent activity is the same (714). Whether or not such molecular-level differences can explain the subtle differences between IIA and IIB fibers in ATPase reactivity remains to be clarified. It is of interest, however, to note that, statistically, FF muscle units (with the IIB fiber type) contract slightly faster than type FR (with the IIA fiber type; e.g., Figs. 4, 5). Another factor to be considered is the possibility of mechanical errors in twitch measurements from units in large muscle masses. The latter objection seems less probable in the case of Lannergren and Smith's study (446) of individual muscle fibers of the toad, which have (among the twitch fibers) a twofold range of contraction times, without evident differences in M-ATPase staining (638, 640).

In summary there is a general but not universally

precise correlation between the rate of ATP hydrolsis by myosin and various measures of mechanical contraction speed. The rate of cross-bridge cycling (formation and breakage; see refs. 383, 403) must be important to this correlation, and this rate probably reflects both intrinsic characteristics of myosin (e.g., refs. 40, 383) as well as the kinetics of intrafiber Ca^{2+} fluxes (e.g., refs. 155, 200, 403, 717). Assays of fiber ATPase activity measure only the former, but the kinetics of Ca^{2+} release from the sarcoplasmic reticulum (SR), its binding to regulator proteins, and its reuptake into the SR also play important roles in regulating contraction speed (e.g., see ref. 270). It is interesting to note in this regard that fast- and slow-twitch muscle fibers, functionally "skinned" in vitro, exhibit different sensitivities to Ca^{2+}; fast-twitch fibers require twice the Ca^{2+} concentration for half-maximum force production compared to slow-twitch fibers (rabbit diaphragm; ref. 368).

The SR membrane from slow muscle transports Ca^{2+} much more slowly than SR from fast muscle (258), and changes in contraction time induced by chronic electrical stimulation of muscle (NONPHYSIOLOGICAL ALTERATIONS, p. 363) correlate better with SR Ca^{2+} uptake rates than with myofibrillar ATPase activity (356). Furthermore the SR system is less extensive and well developed in slowly contracting fibers than in fast ones (*Muscle Fiber Types: Histochemical Profiles and Ultrastructural Correlations*, p. 347). Jorgensen and co-workers (402) have recently used immunofluorescence histochemistry to localize two important SR proteins, the Mg^{2+}-Ca^{2+}-activated ATPase involved in Ca^{2+} pumping, and calsequestrin, which is presumably involved in local Ca^{2+} binding within the SR. Their results suggest that the ATPase protein in type I and II SR is qualitatively similar but present in much lower concentration in the SR of slow-twitch type I fibers. Calsequestrin appears to be present in about the same concentration in SR membrane of types I and II fibers, although the overall fluorescence intensity is less in type I fibers because of the more limited SR membrane system. These considerations also fit with observed differences in contraction times and suggest that histochemical M-ATPase activity alone should not be overinterpreted in terms of implied fiber contraction times (see also ref. 554).

FATIGABILITY AND METABOLIC PROFILES. For present purposes, fatigue can be regarded as a decrement in output force from a muscle unit, usually as the result of repeated activation. As with twitch-contraction time, the fatigue in indirectly activated muscle units involves a complex set of factors, some poorly understood, which can include any or all of the following: *1)* failure of neuromuscular transmission, *2)* failure of the muscle fiber action potential, *3)* failure of excitation-contraction coupling, and *4)* failure of the contractile machinery itself. The relative importance of these various factors to observed fatigue in individual motor units remains to be clarified. There is evidence [(80, 634, 663); but cf. refs. 62, 496] that failure of neuromuscular transmission can be significant even at moderate firing rates (20–50 pulses/s). Such failures can be due to depression of the end-plate potential below muscle fiber threshold (427, 684), to changes in fiber threshold itself (427), or to failure of the presynaptic action potential to invade terminal branches of the motor axon (427, 429). Fatigue effects on the muscle fiber action potential per se appear significant mainly at high firing rates (50 pulses/s or greater over periods of several seconds; see ref. 468). Both resting and action potential amplitudes in muscle fibers decrease during stimulus sequences that can lead to mechanical fatigue (55), although mechanical force output changes are predominant (210). This dissociation has led to the idea that some part of the fatigue process may be accounted for by a failure in the process coupling the action potential to activation of the contractile machinery (excitation-contraction coupling; see refs. 210, 229, 704), perhaps as a result of phosphocreatine depletion and H^+ accumulation (519). Finally, one must consider failure of the contractile machinery itself as a potential cause for decreased output force during fatigue (e.g., ref. 496). This has been attributed to failure to generate the ATP required for crossbridge cycling (180), although mechanical fatigue has been observed despite normal intrafiber ATP levels (519).

It has been known for many years that slow-twitch red muscles are more resistant to fatigue than the nominally fast-twitch white muscles. The in vivo color of whole muscles is due to multiple factors, including resting blood flow, capillary density, and myoglobin concentration [(577); see also ref. 264]. The muscle fiber types associated with gross red coloration (types I and IIA) have high concentrations of mitochondria and myoglobin compared to the type IIB fibers that predominate in white muscles, and their mitochondria display a greater intrinsic capacity for oxidative metabolism than mitochondria isolated from type IIB fibers (e.g., ref. 24). The high myoglobin content of type I and IIA fibers (Table 1) fits with high oxidative capacity, since myoglobin facilitates the entry of blood-borne oxygen into muscle fibers (729). Type I and IIA fibers are characteristically surrounded by a greater number and density of capillaries than the IIB fibers (e.g., refs. 377, 592, 607), and their often smaller diameter (see subsection *Muscle Fiber Types: Histochemical Profiles and Ultrastructural Correlations*, p. 347) suggests an optimization to ensure efficient uptake of blood-borne metabolites (e.g., ref. 706). The neutral fat content in I and IIA fibers (Table 1) suggests that they utilize fatty acids in oxidative metabolism, along with carbohydrates (see ref. 633).

The positive correlation between oxidative capacity and fatigue resistance is evident when analyzed at the level of individual muscle units (111, 227, 436). Type S and FR units (Fig. 5), associated with the high oxidative types I and IIA fibers (Fig. 6), are relatively resistant to fatigue during prolonged repetitive stimulation; FF units, composed of type IIB fibers with low oxidative capacity, are much less fatigue resistant. Experience with glycogen-depletion experiments strongly suggests that susceptibility to glycogen loss varies directly with susceptibility to mechanical fatigue (111, 227, 432–434, 436). Although mechanical fatigue can occur in vitro without substantial loss of fiber glycogen (519), exhaustive exercise in vivo clearly depletes both muscle and liver glycogen markedly (e.g., refs. 37, 261, 294, 295), and refilling of intrafiber glycogen stores is a slow process in humans, taking up to 48 h for completion (e.g., ref. 559).

The capacity to regenerate ATP by oxidative mechanisms thus appears to account for much of the observed difference between muscle units in resistance to fatigue (see ref. 180). There is something of a paradox, however, evident in Table 1; type IIA fibers (equivalent to the type FR physiological profile) have a higher absolute activity of an oxidative marker enzyme, SDH, than type I fibers (equivalent to the type S profile), even though the fatigue resistance of FR motor units is significantly less than that exhibited by type S units (111, 122). Part of this apparent discrepancy may be accounted for by the fact that slowly contracting muscle fibers may well require less ATP to generate a given force output than fast fibers in isometric contractions (e.g., refs. 27, 289, 291, 717).

The role of neuromuscular transmission failure in motor unit fatigue is difficult to assess. The experimenter cannot directly observe the mechanical action of all the individual muscle unit fibers at the same time. Rather he has only the EMG potential as an index of the completeness of muscle unit activation, and changes in the single unit EMG do not necessarily reflect neuromuscular failure (see ref. 111). Continuous stimulation can lead to rapid failure of both mechanical output and EMG amplitude in individual motor units (e.g., refs. 537, 732), which is perhaps due at least in part to neuromuscular as well as muscle fiber fatigue characteristics. In contrast intermittent stimulation usually results in greater dissociation between force output decline and EMG change (Fig. 8; see also ref. 111), which suggests that mechanical fatigue during intermittent tetanization is due mainly to processes occurring at the level of the muscle fibers themselves and not (at least in the early stages) to failure of neuromuscular transmission.

Motor Units in Human Muscle

Human muscles contain both fast- and slow-twitch fibers (209). Despite extensive electromyographic (EMG) studies of human motor units, however, information about their mechanical properties has become available only recently. Denny-Brown and Pennybacker (187) showed in 1938 that it was possible in certain patients with motoneuron disease to detect the force changes associated with the firing of an individual motor unit (see also ref. 185), but systematic

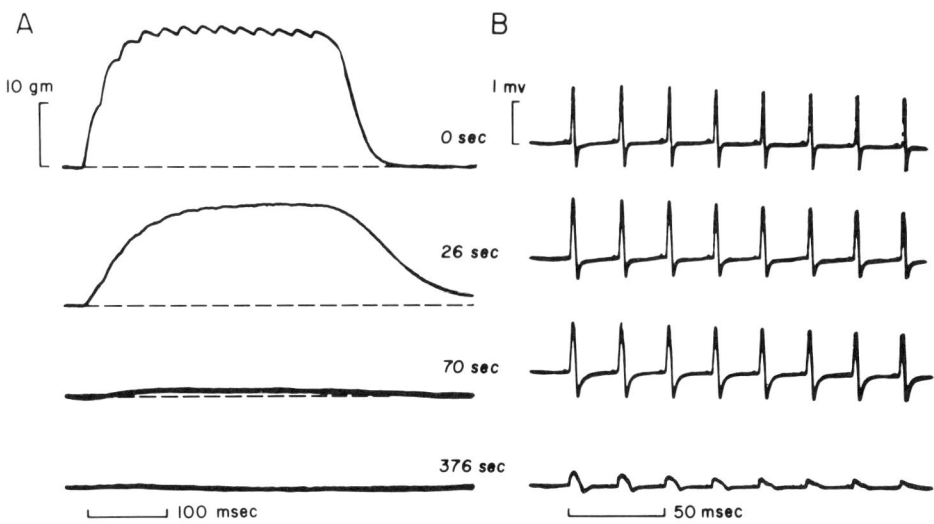

FIG. 8. A particularly clear example of dissociation of EMG decrement from mechanical fatigue during intermittent tetanization of type FF muscle unit in cat MG muscle. Mechanical (A) and electromyographic (B; note faster time base) responses during repeated tetanization (13 pulses at 40 Hz repeated every 1 s) show marked slowing of mechanical response after only 26 tetani (26-s record) and almost complete mechanical fatigue after 70 tetani (910 pulses in 70 s), when EMG responses are almost unchanged in amplitude, although individual spikes are widened. Up to this point, fatigue process appears to be primarily, if not exclusively, intrinsic to muscle fibers themselves. Markedly diminished EMG spike after 376 tetani could be due either to change in muscle fiber action potentials or to failure of neuromuscular transmission, or both (see subsection FATIGABILITY AND METABOLIC PROFILES, p. 358). (From R. Burke, D. Levine, P. Tsairis, and F. Zajac, unpublished records; see ref. 111.)

studies of mechanical properties of units in normal muscles had to await the development of appropriate technical advances, primarily the introduction of computer-averaging methods. In the last decade, computer averaging has been applied to this problem to educe the mechanical response of a single muscle unit from records of whole muscle force, synchronizing the averager either to electrical stimuli delivered to the muscle nerve or its intramuscular branches, or to the single unit EMG potential during voluntary activation (spike-triggered averaging).

In 1970, Buchthal and Schmalbruch (92) used intramuscular stimulation to produce contractions of "small bundles" of muscle fibers in a variety of human muscles, averaging the resultant force with a transducer system impaled into the tendon. They made no claim about recording from individual motor units but reported a wider range of twitch-contraction times from the bundles in some muscles (e.g., biceps brachii, 16–84 ms) than in others (e.g., triceps brachii, 16–68 ms; platysma, 30–58 ms). They noted that more slowly contracting bundles prevailed in muscles with a high proportion of mitochondria-rich, oxidative muscle fibers and showed that these slow responses tended to disappear after local circulatory arrest, implying a dependence on aerobic metabolism. Sica and McComas (632) later reported that surface stimulation of the nerve to the human extensor hallucis brevis produced all-or-none twitch responses that they ascribed to contraction of individual muscle units. They also observed a wide range of twitch-contraction times (35–98 ms) but found no correlation between contraction times and twitch forces. Both surface and intramuscular stimulation were used by D. Burke and co-workers (98) to study motor units in the human abductor digiti minimi. They found that units in this small intrinsic hand muscle exhibit a continuous Gaussian distribution of twitch-contraction times (mean about 65 ms, range 40–100 ms), with a continuous distribution of fatigue resistance as well. Taylor and Stephens [(678); see also ref. 317] have argued that the intramuscular stimulation technique can be used under some conditions to produce functional isolation of individual human muscle units. Using this method, the St. Thomas' Hospital group (275, 531) have reported that units in the human MG muscle have mechanical characteristics basically similar to those in the cat MG (Fig. 9, *bottom*). Glycogen depletion of a small sample of these units produced results analogous to those in the cat.

The spike-triggered averaging (STA) method, also introduced by Buchthal and Schmalbruch (92), was later applied systematically by Milner-Brown et al. (500, 501) to examine the properties of individual muscle units in the human first dorsal interosseous (1st DI) muscle during steady voluntary contractions. The mechanical unit "twitch" thus educed from whole muscle force can be ascribed to the action of an individual muscle unit with greater certainty than is the case with electrical stimulation methods as long as there is no statistical correlation between firings in different motor units (500). Synchronization of discharge between different motor units can occur when

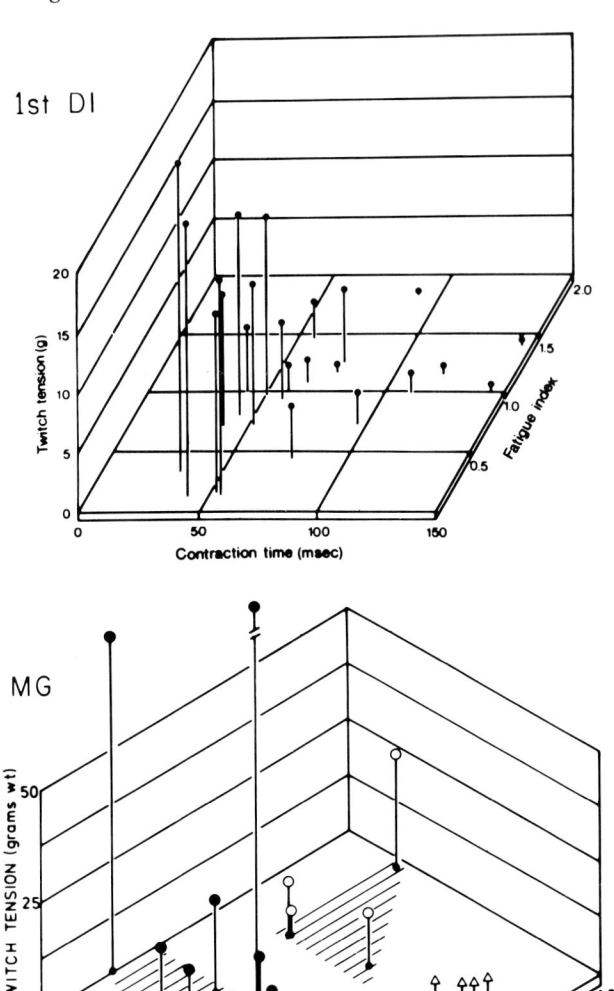

FIG. 9. Three-dimensional diagrams illustrating physiological profiles of motor units sampled from 2 different human muscles. *Upper graph*: motor units sampled by spike-triggered averaging from human 1st dorsal interosseous muscle (1st DI). *Lower graph*: motor units sampled by intramuscular stimulation from human medial gastrocnemius. *Symbols* and *shading* denote units and data regions interpreted to be equivalent to the type FF (*filled circles*), type FR (*open circles*), and type S (*triangles*) motor units described in the cat MG (see Fig. 5). Definition of fatigue index differs in the 2 studies but, as in Fig. 5, increasing values denote increasing fatigue resistance. Note that pattern of correlations between contraction time, force output, and fatigue resistance are generally similar to those found in cat muscle (compare with Fig. 5), although the data distribution in the interosseous sample seems more continuous, in keeping with the cat lumbrical muscle (see Fig. 4, *right*). [*Top graph* from data of Stephens and Usherwood (664); *bottom graph* from O'Donovan (531); see also ref. 275.]

a common input is sufficiently powerful (547), and such synchronizations are seen in some normal individuals (195), particularly after forceful contractions (396, 498).

Unfortunately even without synchronization the twitch educed by STA methods usually represents the average of components in partly fused tetanic contractions (see Fig. 30). The degree of consequent distortion depends on the frequency of unit firing relative to the actual twitch-contraction time (see subsection EFFECTS OF FIRING RATE AND FIRING PATTERN ON MUSCLE UNIT OUTPUT, p. 397); the faster the rate of firing, the less well the educed responses resemble true twitches (93, 500). The mechanical compliance of tissues (e.g., skin and tendons) interposed between the active unit and the force transducer can also introduce distortion, especially when muscle forces (and series compliances) vary during voluntary recruitment of motor units with different force thresholds (510). Monster and Chan (510) in fact suggest that all the muscle units they studied in the human extensor digitorum communis (EDC) should be regarded as fast twitch (as seems true also in the baboon; ref. 219), even though human forearm muscles contain substantial proportions of type I fibers (401). The same suggestion has been made with regard to the human abductor digiti minimi (98). It seems important to keep such methodological limitations in mind when comparing data from human and animal studies.

Using STA methods, Milner-Brown and colleagues (501) found a 3-fold range in contraction times for the twitches of 1st DI muscle units (30–90 ms; confirmed by Desmedt and Godeaux, ref. 190) and a 10-fold range in twitch forces (from 0.1 g to about 10 g). However, unlike results in animal muscle (e.g., Figs. 4 and 5), there was only a weak correlation between force and contraction time. The latter point is also evident in other STA studies of motor units in human jaw muscles (287, 738) and in the extensor digitorum communis (EDC) of the forearm (510). This difference may well result from the mechanical distortion inherent in some applications of the STA method. Stephens and Usherwood (664), however, have used the same method in human 1st DI and have found patterns of correlation between force outputs, contraction times, and fatigability that are similar to those found in animal muscle (Fig. 9, 1st DI). Overall it seems fair to conclude that the organization of motor unit populations in humans is basically the same as found in many animal muscles, and that the results from systematic studies in humans and other species are complementary rather than divergent.

Stability of Motor Unit Types

The physiological, biochemical, and structural interrelations that characterize the three basic types of muscle fibers, as discussed in subsections *Muscle Fiber Types: Histochemical Profiles and Ultrastructural Correlations* (p. 347) and *Motor Unit Types: Physiological Profiles in Experimental Animals* (p. 351), suggest the existence of trade-offs necessary to optimize particular properties at the expense of others. For example, the metabolic cost of force production seems least in slowly contracting muscle, but the price paid is limited shortening velocity (subsection TWITCH-CONTRACTION TIMES AND MYOBIFRILLAR ATPASE, p. 355), although there is evidence that efficiency during contraction at different speeds can be optimized by "fine-tuning" the myosin present in particular fiber types (see ref. 289). In addition, resistance to fatigue is often associated with relatively small fiber size and limited force production (subsection FATIGABILITY AND METABOLIC PROFILES, p. 358). These considerations in turn suggest that the interrelated characteristics recognized as "fiber types" may be relatively stable in the face of changing conditions. Assessment of whether or not muscle fiber and/or motor unit types change when challenged depends critically on how much alteration can occur before the observer can (or will) recognize "conversion" of one type to another or identify the existence of a new type. Since some notion of types is inherent to communication of observations, this problem has been (and probably will continue to be) a source of difficulty (e.g., ref. 331).

The extensive literature dealing with adaptations of muscle to challenge defies concise summary because the variety of approaches, animal species, and methods of observation have generated often conflicting results and because the complexity of the neuromuscular system is such that critical variables are, for the most part, uncontrolled and sometimes uncontrollable. Effects are inferred by comparing "treated" with "control" whole muscles, often in different subjects, introducing problems of sampling errors and comparability. A discussion of the general issue of "trophic" control of muscle characteristics is beyond the scope of this chapter (see reviews in refs. 147, 148, 199, 325, 326, 332, 333, 450, 453, 605). This discussion is limited to some aspects of differential effects on the fiber and unit types found in mammalian muscle.

It is useful to separate two kinds of manipulations or challenges that have been used to investigate the mutability of muscle fiber and unit characteristics. The first is manipulations within the physiological range of conditions encountered by intact animals. The other is those outside these limits. The physiological range includes functional demands that can be achieved without damage to, or direct interference with, the target motor unit population, such as exercise training or limb immobilization. A quite different kind of challenge results when the motor unit pool is directly damaged, as in denervation and reinnervation by the same or foreign motoneurons, or is faced with conditions not normally encountered in the intact animal, as when muscle fibers are stimulated synchronously over long periods by electrical pulses delivered either directly or via the muscle nerve. The stability of muscle fiber types (and by inference, motor unit types) appears to be quite different under these two sets of challenges.

ALTERATIONS OF DEMAND WITHIN THE PHYSIOLOGICAL RANGE. *Exercise training.* The effects produced in muscle fibers by exercise depend importantly on its nature and duration (e.g., refs. 106, 221, 371, 551, 607). To my knowledge there have been no studies of the effect of exercise on individual muscle units. Inferences thus depend on data derived from studies of whole muscles, many of which involve human subjects because of the wide interest in optimizing athletic ability. Three general classes of exercise regimes are usually recognized: *1*) highly repetitive, relatively low-resistance movements (< 70% maximum aerobic capacity) such as endurance running or swimming; *2*) movements against high resistance (> 100% aerobic capacity) with relatively low repetition rates—weight lifting is the best example; and *3*) an intermediate category of "power" movements, such as are encountered in jumping and sprinting (see ref. 221).

The major effect of endurance training on muscle per se is to cause a highly significant increase in the oxidative metabolic capacity of whole muscles, measured biochemically (e.g., refs. 45, 261, 336, 365, 370, 371, 682) or histochemically (e.g., refs. 45, 293, 336, 375). This effect also includes an increased capacity for fatty acid metabolism (371, 505, 506) and some increase in fiber cross-sectional area, which is greater in type I fibers than in type II (608). There is an associated increase in whole muscle fatigue resistance (46, 262) and in the capillary supply evident histologically (9, 473) and functionally (377). At moderate levels of exercise demand, oxidative capacity increases most dramatically in muscles composed mainly of type IIA fibers, whereas higher demand levels are necessary before the capacity increases in muscle dominated by type IIB fibers (682). This fits with the apparent usage patterns of the equivalent FR and FF motor unit types in normal movement (see subsection RECRUITMENT PATTERNS AND MOTOR UNIT TYPES, p. 386). There is less effect on anaerobic metabolic capacity (221, 607), although muscle glycogen is sometimes elevated by training (290, 336). Many of the adaptive metabolic changes in endurance-trained muscle have a glycogen-sparing effect (261, 336, 607).

Most studies in adult animals and in humans have denied any change in the proportion of type I to type II fibers after endurance training (see refs. 106, 221, 292, 375, 607, 608). Where such changes have been described (263, 334, 336, 393, 516, 656), they have been of relatively small magnitude and possibly accounted for by considerations of sampling and/or comparability of controls. Subject age and the identity of the muscle studied can be important, since Syrovy and co-workers (672) found evidence for an increased percentage of type II fibers in the soleus of exercised rats only in young animals and not in older ones, and no such change was found in the fast extensor digitorum longus at any age. The enhancement of oxidative staining with endurance exercise, discussed above, suggests that there may be some reversible (250) conversion of type IIB to IIA fibers. Although most histochemical studies of this phenomenon do not include data on the pH profile of ATPase reactions that are necessary for subtyping type II fibers, a few recent studies of endurance training in human athletes suggest that the appropriate ATPase changes do in fact occur in some fibers (9, 375, 607).

The effects of intensive dynamic exercise such as sprinting and jumping and of weight lifting have been less thoroughly studied. Sprint running produces similar but less dramatic changes in oxidative capacity (424, 656, 690) but there may be a greater relative effect on anaerobic mechanisms [(336); but cf. ref. 690]. Lipid metabolism seems unchanged (656). On the other hand, weight lifting or intermittent isometric exercise produces reversible muscle fiber hypertrophy (e.g., ref. 292) with relatively little change in histochemistry or in metabolic enzyme patterns [(221, 226, 262, 689); cf. also ref. 477].

Studies of muscle fiber populations in human athletes trained for various events suggest appropriate metabolic adaptations (see ref. 607) in that, for example, the leg muscles of distance runners tend to have a very high proportion of high oxidative (both type I and IIA) fibers (e.g., refs. 166, 392, 564, 565). An opposite trend (i.e., toward greater proportion of type IIB fibers) is suggested in biopsies from weight lifters (564). The interpretation of such results, however, is complicated by the very wide variation in fiber type proportions in human subjects irrespective of training (e.g., ref. 401) and in which a genetic influence seems strong. Komi and co-workers (421) have recently shown that the histochemical mosaic of human monozygotic twins is almost identical, whereas that of dizygotic twins varies over a much wider range, similar to that of unrelated individuals. One may thus suppose that genetically controlled differences in fiber type (and presumably motor unit type) composition of muscles may be one factor that leads to success in particular types of athletic performance.

The muscle hypertrophy that follows chronic disability of synergists (called compensatory hypertrophy; e.g., refs. 65, 186, 286, 335, 471) is sometimes considered analogous to weight-lifting exercise. The analogy may not be entirely apt, but both treatments do produce muscle fiber hypertrophy (see, e.g., refs. 292, 696). The only available study of individual motor units in chronic compensatory hypertrophy (707) indicates that the type composition of the motor unit population is essentially unchanged by this challenge (cat MG muscle), although tetanic force per unit increased significantly, especially among the fatigue-resistant unit types (S and FR). Guth and Yellin (331) have described an apparent transformation of type II into type I muscle fibers in compensatory hypertrophy in rat plantaris, but most other studies have not confirmed this finding in adult animals (see ref. 708 for references).

A converse challenge is represented by manipulations designed to decrease muscle activity (disuse), including mechanically immobilizing a limb, reducing its motor inflow by spinal section and deafferentation, and cutting the muscle's tendon. Tenotomy produces pathological effects in muscle fibers (e.g., refs. 211, 243, 490) and seems best regarded as "nonphysiological." As with other studies of this general type, the results of immobilization vary greatly with methods, muscle, animal species, and parameters observed (e.g., refs. 69, 223, 260, 474, 477, 494, 695). Of particular importance is the length at which the muscle is fixed (211, 272, 674). Motor units in chronically immobilized cat show no significant interconversions of type even after 6 mo of joint pinning (109, 482). The primary effect was marked diminution of tetanic force output per muscle unit, more marked in the fatigue-resistant S and FR units than in FF, with concomitant fiber atrophy in fibers of the associated histochemical type. The same pattern of atrophy (i.e., type I = type IIA > type IIB) has been seen in human muscle among patients with severe arthritis with joint immobilization (78), again without change in the histochemical mosaic.

In summary the existing data indicate that at least in adult fully matured muscles (see, e.g., refs. 516, 672), alterations of demand within the physiological range do not produce significant interconversions of fast-twitch and slow-twitch motor units (defined on the basis of ATPase histochemistry and fragmentary data on muscle unit physiology), implying that the characteristic features that define these types are robust and relatively stable. This is not true, however, with regard to the metabolic profiles and the associated resistance to muscle fatigue, which are very responsive to alterations in functional demand.

NONPHYSIOLOGICAL ALTERATIONS. In contrast to the previous subsection, there is considerable evidence that direct interference with the integrity of motor units (e.g., by axonal damage and regeneration) or prolonged electrical stimulation of muscle either directly or indirectly both produce alterations in muscle that involve myosin characteristics as well as metabolic profiles. Perhaps the clearest example is the self-reinnervation of a denervated heterogeneous muscle by its own motoneurons. Within 4-8 wk after neuromuscular connections are reestablished (711), the normal mosaic of histochemical fiber types (see Fig. 2A, C) is changed by the appearance of local collections of fibers with the same histochemical profile [referred to as type grouping; (408); see also ref. 734]. After the situation has stabilized, the fiber types present are the same as found in normal muscle.

Glycogen-depletion experiments have shown that after reinnervation a single motor axon often innervates contiguous groups of fibers [(74, 432, 435); see also ref. 620], as opposed to the normal, even. scattering characteristic of normal muscle units (subsection *Anatomy of Muscle Units*, p. 367). This is apparently due to the fact that regenerating axons tend to branch very locally (2, 220) much more than is apparent in normal innervation. This local "sprouting" also partially accounts for type grouping, which becomes increasingly pronounced after repeated axonal damage (see ref. 202). Histochemical fiber type differences survive denervation (e.g., ref. 407), and motor axons appear to reinnervate denervated fibers irrespective of their original type (56, 498, 716, 717a), although some late reorganization has been observed in amphibian muscle (622). The limited evidence available about individual muscle units after self-reinnervation suggests that their physiological profiles are similar to normal units, although with rather different ranges of tetanic force output [(32, 717a); R. E. Burke, R. P. Dum, and M. J. O'Donovan, unpublished observations]. These observations indicate that some denervated muscle fibers must change completely from one type to another when reinnervated by a motoneuron of a different unit type, implying that the motoneuron in some way can specify quite completely the characteristics of muscle fibers it innervates (see also ref. 379). The same conclusion has been reached in the many experiments in which motor nerves to fast-twitch and slow-twitch muscles have been interchanged (cross reinnervation; see refs. 79, 96, 146, 147, 201, 330, 462, 498, 593, 605, 715; reviewed in ref. 97). The interpretation of the results of foreign innervation are often complicated by the heterogeneous nature of the motor unit populations involved (e.g., ref. 587). This difficulty can be resolved in principle by studies of individual motor units after cross reinnervation, but, to date, such studies have not been reported in detail (see refs. 30, 105, 206).

There is now abundant evidence that electrical stimulation at low frequencies (usually 10 Hz), if delivered to a nominally fast-twitch muscle often enough (several hours per day to continuous stimulation) and long enough (over periods of weeks or months), can cause dramatic changes in metabolic enzyme patterns (mainly increases in oxidative systems; 545, 554, 555, 585, 702), increased resistance to fatigue (545, 554, 605), decreased average fiber diameter (82, 554), and increased capillarity (82) and active blood flow (378). No such effects are observed in similarly stimulated slow-twitch muscles (554). Chronically applied tonic stimulation also alters the myosin of fast-twitch fibers, reducing ATPase activity and producing the emergence of light-chain components characteristic of slow-fiber myosin (600, 605, 647), with prolongation of twitch-contraction time (545, 554, 605, 606). Changes in contraction time, however, can be found before detectable changes in myosin composition and are instead temporally correlated with decreased rates of Ca^{2+} transport in SR membrane fragments [(356); see subsection TWITCH-CONTRACTION TIMES AND MYOFIBRILLAR ATPASE, p. 355].

The effects of chronically imposed low-frequency stimulation are powerful and can, in fact, oppose the changes expected from fast-slow nerve cross union (605) or from denervation (460). It has also been suggested that stimulation in short bursts at relatively high frequency (a "phasic" pattern) can produce increased glycolytic metabolic capacity without other changes (585), but the effect is much less dramatic than those produced by sustained low-frequency activation (82). These observations clearly indicate that patterned activity, at least when externally imposed, exerts a powerful control over the characteristics of muscle fibers (and, by inference, of motor units). Whether or not this mechanism accounts for the normal maturation and maintenance of muscle fiber characteristics remains to be determined, since motoneurons of fast- and slow-twitch units do not necessarily exhibit dramatically different firing rates or firing patterns (see subsection MOTONEURON FIRING CHARACTERISTICS, p. 394).

Developmental Considerations

Muscle fibers presumably destined to be either fast twitch or slow twitch (type I or II, judged by ATPase histochemistry) are recognizable at birth in some species, including cat (344, 475, 528, 693), guinea pig (406), rat [(329); but cf. ref. 411], pig (163), monkey (51), and human (256). This suggests that fiber specification can take place in utero before maturation of motor patterns. The formation of embryonic myotubes takes place over a finite time span that may involve several discrete generations (411, 412, 728). In some species type I fibers are formed in an initial wave of myogenesis, and subsequent generations (presumably destined to become type II fibers) later form around them (23, 728). Since type I fibers tend to occur in the center of fiber fascicles (most dramatically in pig muscle; see refs. 163, 511), this biphasic pattern of myotube differentiation could partly explain the adult histochemical mosaic (411). During early development, type I fibers appear to mature earlier than type II fibers in the guinea pig (245).

It is not known whether the two waves of myotube formation noted above coincide with the arrival of axons from different sets of motoneurons, but this seems possible on the basis of studies of motor innervation in chick and rodent embryos. Bennett and Pettigrew (53) found that myotube formation in the embryonic rat diaphragm begins with the arrival of the first "pioneering" motor axons. The process then proceeds actively as motor axons continue to arrive and establish functional synapses (see also refs. 411, 413), with widespread multiple innervation that remains until after birth (see subsection INNERVATION RATIOS AND MUSCLE UNIT "SIZE", p. 369). Subsequent to establishing peripheral connections (538, 562), a significant proportion of motoneurons die, at least in the chick and toad (see refs. 341, 342, 561), but this phenomenon appears to precede most of the disappearance of polyneuronal innervation.

The importance of the motoneurons to the process of muscle fiber maturation and differentiation is suggested by several lines of evidence. The association between a particular set of motoneurons and their target whole muscle appears to be determined very early in embryonic development (see refs. 444, 445, 513). Denervation of immature muscle inhibits, albeit not completely, the maturation of normal fiber types (245, 406, 625). Myotubes in tissue culture can develop into myofibers, but they do not differentiate fiber types without neural innervation (25, 259). Full maturation and even ultimate survival of myofibers in adult regenerating muscle also require motor innervation at a critical period (130, 351, 399, 508). These observations are all consistent with the idea that motoneuron identity plays a key role in the specification of muscle fiber and unit characteristics (see also ref. 703). The mechanisms that specify motoneuron identity remain unknown, but some recent observations of human fiber histochemistry suggest a strong genetic influence. Komi and co-workers (421) have shown that the histochemical composition of human muscles in nonidentical twins varies widely for a given muscle, as it does in the general population (e.g., refs. 401, 607), but the fiber proportions found in identical (monozygotic) twins is remarkably similar.

Physiological studies of whole muscle in neonatal cats show that both fast and slow muscles initially exhibit similarly slow contraction, which speeds up over the first few weeks after birth (95, 346, 380, 477, 718). Interestingly the slow-twitch soleus (SOL) of both cat and guinea pig exhibits a significant proportion of type II fibers (344, 406, 693) in the few weeks after birth, when its twitch-contraction time is relatively fast, but these then disappear as the muscle matures to its adult, slow-twitch state (95). Denervation of soleus in adult guinea pigs causes reappearance of type II fibers (406, 407).

The normal pattern of physiological and histochemical maturation can be altered also by changing motor demands, as occurs with spinal cord section (with and without concomitant cutting of dorsal roots) or immobilization of the limb (406, 477). The histochemical mosaic of heterogeneous muscles is also more malleable during compensatory hypertrophy in immature animals [(618); see also ref. 471]. Furthermore the disappearance of polyneuronal innervation in developing rat muscles is altered by changes in activation patterns [(54, 530); but see also ref. 688]. Thus although prespecification seems to be important in the initial organization of motor unit populations, later alterations in motor demands apparently can also condition the ultimate distribution of fiber types, and by implication, of motor unit types.

The ontogeny of individual motor units has been studied in developing cats. In the first 2 wk after birth, the range of twitch-contraction times of units in soleus and a variety of heterogeneous muscles is relatively narrow, although soleus units tend to have the slower contraction times [Fig. 10; (34, 346)]. Hammarberg and Kellerth (346) have shown that the adult motor unit pattern (i.e., the presence of recognizable FF, FR, and S units) is established gradually after the second or third postnatal week and is fully established by about 6 wk of age (Fig. 10), when kittens have established their adult motor patterns (e.g., ref. 475). This temporal sequence corresponds very closely to the pattern of histochemical fiber maturation (344, 528, 693), to the loss of polyneuronal innervation (35, 718), and to the enlargement of motor axons (e.g., refs. 529) and of ventral horn neurons, presumably mostly motoneurons (476, 495, 612). Maturation occurs earlier in forelimb than in hindlimb (528, 529), and there is a corresponding rostral-to-caudal gradient in the birth (see refs. 522, 523) and cellular maturation (495, 612) of motoneurons. This period is also characterized by active remodeling of synaptic terminals on ventral horn neurons (158, 159, 594), with possible differences between motoneurons maturing into the various motor unit types (595). The differentiation of motoneurons into fast and slow groups is probably begun in utero, since motor axons of the heterogeneous flexor hallucis longus in newborn kittens (later composed primarily of fast-twitch unit types) consistently exhibit faster average axonal conduction velocities than cells innervating the slow soleus (380, 582), as they do in adult cats (subsection *Electrophysiological Properties Intrinsic to Motoneurons*, p. 379). However, the differentiation of afterhyperpolarization durations in fast and slow motoneurons does not occur until later (271, 346, 380).

The temporal correlation between all of these events in the process of motor unit pool maturation strongly suggests that they are importantly interrelated. Much remains to be done however, to clarify the mechanisms and messages that must be involved in the specification of numbers and properties of the different motor unit types in different muscles.

Skeletofusimotor Units

Motor system physiologists who work with mammals are accustomed to thinking of extrafusal and intrafusal muscle fibers as innervated by separate sets of motoneurons (α and γ, respectively). Innervation of extra- and intrafusal fibers by common (skeletofusimotor) motoneurons, as in the frog (see ref. 638), seems a primitive organization in both evolutionary and control system contexts. For more than a decade (58), however, evidence has been accumulating, mainly from the work of Laporte and colleagues (447, 448), that the skeletofusimotor, or β, pattern of innervation not only exists in mammals (mainly the cat), but may be relatively widespread. For convenience the combination of a β-motoneuron and the extra- and intrafusal muscle fibers innervated by it are referred to in this section as a β-motor unit.

Unequivocal physiological demonstration of the β-innervation pattern requires special conditions and precautions (58). The discharge of muscle spindle afferents is altered by activity of both extra- and intrafusal muscle fibers (see the chapter by Matthews in this *Handbook*). Emonet-Dénand and co-workers (237, 238), however, have clearly dermonstrated the presence of β-innervation in a variety of muscles of the cat and rabbit hindlimb (see Fig. 11), including both smaller (e.g., lumbricals, peroneus digit quinti, and tenuissimus) and larger muscles (e.g., flexor hallucis longus, peroneus brevis, tibialis anterior, and soleus). More recently Barker and colleagues (42) have used the glycogen-depletion method to study the intra- and extrafusal fiber types involved in the β-innervation pattern.

There are two clearly distinguishable types of β-motor units (see ref. 448). The first type to be identified involves motor axons with relatively slow conduction velocities [39–92 ml/s, with most <80 m/s; (237)] that innervate primarily the type of intrafusal nuclear bag fiber referred to as bag_1 (42). Almost all of these produce a dynamic modulation of primary (group Ia) spindle afferent sensitivity (237). The extrafusal fibers

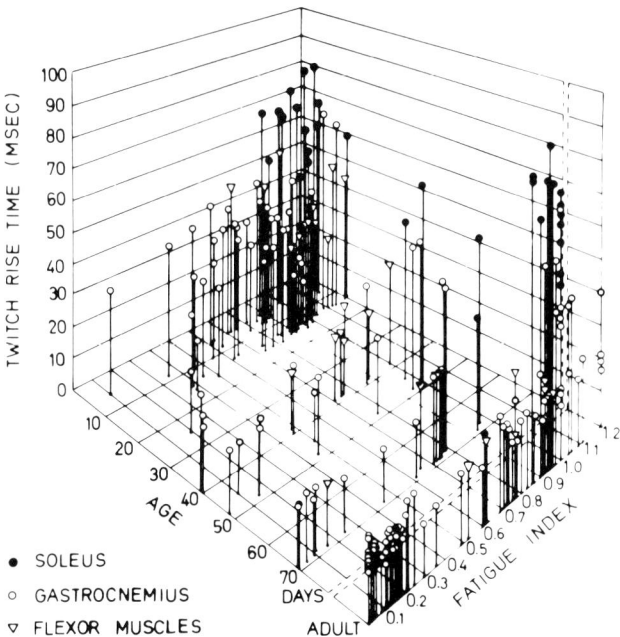

- ● SOLEUS
- ○ GASTROCNEMIUS
- ▽ FLEXOR MUSCLES

FIG. 10. Three-dimensional diagram illustrating physiological profiles (isometric-twitch–rise time and fatigue index) of motor units sampled from various hindlimb muscles (see symbol key) of cats of different postnatal age (*left* abscissa). Note that most units found during the 1st 2 postnatal wk are slowly contracting and relatively fatigue resistant, and that adult pattern becomes evident (despite small sample sizes) between 40 and 70 days after birth. [From Hammarberg and Kellerth (346).]

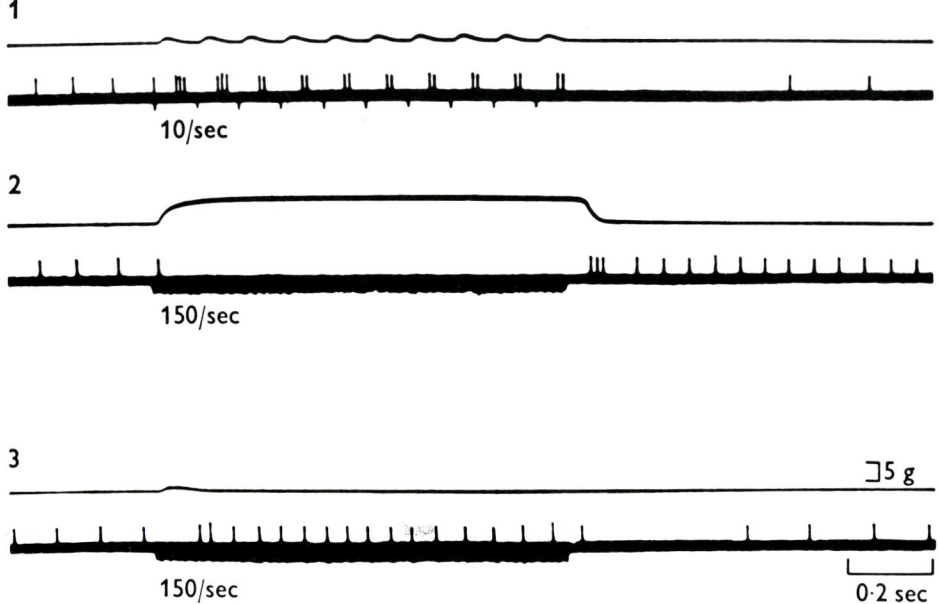

FIG. 11. Physiological evidence for innervation of extrafusal and intrafusal muscle fibers by a single skeletofusimotor (β) axon (conduction velocity 41 m/s) in rabbit lumbrical muscle. *Upper trace* in each record is isometric lumbrical force; *lower trace* is discharge of a primary (group Ia) muscle spindle afferent from the same muscle. Stimulation of the motor axon at 10/s (*record 1*) produces extrafusal twiches and brief bursts of Ia activity during each relaxation phase; tetanization at 150/s (*record 2*) produces fused mechanical response and silencing of afferent discharge, as would be expected for the α-innervation pattern. However, after partial curarization (*record 3*) sufficient to block extrafusal (note mechanical failure) but not intrafusal neuromuscular transmission, the same tetanus produces acceleration of Ia discharge, showing that motor axon must also inactivate intrafusal muscle fibers. [From Emonet-Dénand et al. (238).]

innervated by these slow or dynamic β-axons, identified by glycogen depletion (42), have all been type I fibers and are thus probably all type S muscle units physiologically (subsection PHYSIOLOGICAL AND HISTOCHEMICAL PROFILES OF MUSCLE UNITS, p. 354). Only one example of a slow β-unit has been studied both histochemically and physiologically in the cat soleus, and it proved to have unremarkable extrafusal unit characteristics (123). It is of interest to note that the bag₁ intrafusal fiber has a histochemical profile that is quite different from that of extrafusal type I fibers (see ref. 41). This fact is not a clear violation of the apparent rule that muscle fibers innervated by the same motoneuron are histochemically identical (subsection PHYSIOLOGICAL AND HISTOCHEMICAL PROFILES OF MUSCLE UNITS, p. 354), since intrafusal bag fibers are probably multiply innervated by γ-dynamic axons as well (41, 239). The neuromuscular end plates believed to represent the intrafusal terminations of β-axons (p₁ plates; see ref. 42) are morphologically similar to extrafusal end plates (41).

A second category of β-motor units has recently been demonstrated by Harker and co-workers [(352); see review in ref. 447]. They showed that some fast-conducting motor axons (conduction velocities > 85 m/s) innervating type II extrafusal muscle fibers also innervate relatively long nuclear chain fibers within some muscle spindles (cat peroneus tertius muscle).

Jami and colleagues (386) have reported additional examples of such fast β-units using glycogen-depletion methods and found that these units exert a largely static action on spindle afferents. The fast β-axons were found to innervate type IIA extrafusal fibers, associated with the FR motor unit type (subsection PHYSIOLOGICAL AND HISTOCHEMICAL PROFILES OF MUSCLE UNITS, p. 354).

Assessment of the functional significance of the existence of β-motor units depends in part on their prevalence in various muscle groups. The p₁ plate endings occur rather commonly in various muscles of cat and rat (41). In relatively small muscles like tenuissimus and abductor digiti quinti of the cat, McWilliam (492) observed that 30%–40% of spindles can have β-innervation, and some spindles in rat tail muscles appear to receive only β-axons (13). In the somewhat larger peroneus brevis of the cat, Emonet-Dénand and Laporte (239) found that almost three-fourths of the spindles received at least one β-axon, all but two conducting with slow velocity (45–75 m/s). Almost one-third of the motor axons conducting in this range innervated one or more spindles, suggesting that a substantial fraction of the type S motor unit population in peroneus brevis (see ref. 387) may in fact be β-motor units. As discussed in subsection GROUP IA SYNAPTIC EFFICACY (p. 381), type S and type FR motor units receive powerful monosynaptic excitatory input from spindle primary (group Ia) afferents, and this is almost certain to apply to those S and FR units that are in fact β-motor units (239). The existence of such positive feedback to a type S (slow) β-unit in cat soleus has been directly demonstrated (123). This point is significant, since it has been repeatedly shown that γ-motoneurons do not receive direct projections from muscle spindle afferents [(213, 308); see ref. 114]. The possible role in motor control of the unbreakable α-γ-coactivation represented by the β-innervation pattern awaits clarification (see discussion in the chapter by Houk and Rymer in this *Handbook*).

ANATOMICAL CONSIDERATIONS

Muscles can be regarded as ensembles of muscle units, usually (but not always) commingled in parallel arrangements. The internal architecture of mammalian muscles can be complex, however, with fibers originating from and inserting on large areas of bone, fascia, or aponeurosis, often at angles different from the main axis of the parent muscle and with fiber lengths that are not only shorter than the whole muscle, but that also exhibit regional variations (e.g., refs. 5, 184, 233, 273, 518, 553). Some muscles span one joint, others span two or more (e.g., the long muscles of the digits), and their functional effect (e.g., as flexor or extensor) can vary with limb position. These issues are discussed in the chapter by Alexander in this *Handbook*, where further references can be found. They are clearly important to a complete picture of functioning motor unit populations and of the differences between the populations found in various muscles.

Anatomy of Muscle Units

In general a motor axon innervates fibers limited to one anatomical muscle, although the inevitable exception has been reported in the cat's foot where a single motor axon can branch in the plantar nerve to innervate muscle fibers in adjacent lumbrical slips (240). Since muscle units include many fibers, the innervating motor axon must branch repeatedly. Most of such branching takes place within the muscle proper (254), but some branching occurs in peripheral nerves and increases in frequency as the nerve nears its entry into the muscle proper (217, 282, 669, 731).

Until relatively recently, the fibers belonging to an individual muscle unit were believed to be arranged in localized collections of contiguous fibers (motor subunits), with these in turn scattered through a more extensive motor unit territory [(89); see ref. 91 for review]. The motor subunit hypothesis was based largely on electromyographic (89) and anatomical studies of both normal and diseased human muscle (730). Earlier physiological data (428, 525) and more recent results from glycogen-depletion experiments in animals [(74, 121, 198, 227); see also subsection PHYSIOLOGICAL AND HISTOCHEMICAL PROFILES OF MUSCLE UNITS, p. 354], however, have provided strong evidence that motor subunits in fact are not present in normal muscles.

Prolonged repetitive stimulation of an individual motoneuron or its axon leads to the appearance of fibers within the target muscle that are completely devoid of their normal glycogen content [see Fig. 12; (227)], without other alterations in their histological or histochemical appearance (110, 111). Glycogen-free fibers of otherwise normal appearance are rare in normal muscle, and their presence in large numbers in this situation makes it highly probable that most, if not all, of the glycogen-depleted fibers were in fact innervated by the stimulated motoneuron (110–112, 198, 227). It does not follow, however, that every fiber belonging to the stimulated muscle unit is detectably depleted of glycogen, particularly in the fatigue-resistant type S units [(110, 121); see subsection FATIGABILITY AND METABOLIC PROFILES, p. 358]. The completeness of glycogen depletion is apparently related to the original content of and the metabolic dependence on intrafiber glycogen, both of which vary inversely with fatigue resistance (subsection FATIGABILITY AND METABOLIC PROFILES, p. 358). As an additional complication, Barker and co-workers (42) have recently shown that glycogen loss can be quite localized along the fiber length, so that unit fibers cannot be detected at some levels of sectioning. The phenomenon of regional glycogen depletion is so far unexplained but it may relate to the observation that the muscle action potential is smaller (and fiber activation perhaps less complete) in regions of the fiber distant from the neuromuscular junction (685). This problem plus the complications introduced by fiber angulation and the internal structure of pennate muscles (e.g., Fig. 13) make it difficult to rely on glycogen depletion to obtain accurate estimates of innervation ratios [(121); see subsection INNERVATION RATIOS AND MUSCLE UNIT "SIZE," p. 369].

Although the results of glycogen-depletion experiments must be interpreted with some caution, they strongly indicate that the fibers belonging to given muscle unit are scattered rather evenly through an extensive territory in both rat and cat hindlimb muscles, with occasional pairs of contiguous depleted fibers and infrequent triplets but clearly no "subunits" (Fig. 12; see refs. 74, 121, 198, 432, 433). A similar pattern seems present in normal human muscle units on the basis of recent single-fiber electromyographic (EMG) studies (232, 648, 650) and by rare observations of glycogen depletion in patients with abnormal activity of individual units (myokymia; see Fig. 3.42 in ref. 202).

A muscle unit's "territory" is usually pictured as a two-dimensional map (e.g., Fig. 12 and individual section maps in Fig. 13) but is in fact a three-dimensional volume (Fig. 13). The volume occupied by a given muscle unit can be quite extensive, perhaps as much as one-seventh of the total muscle volume in the case

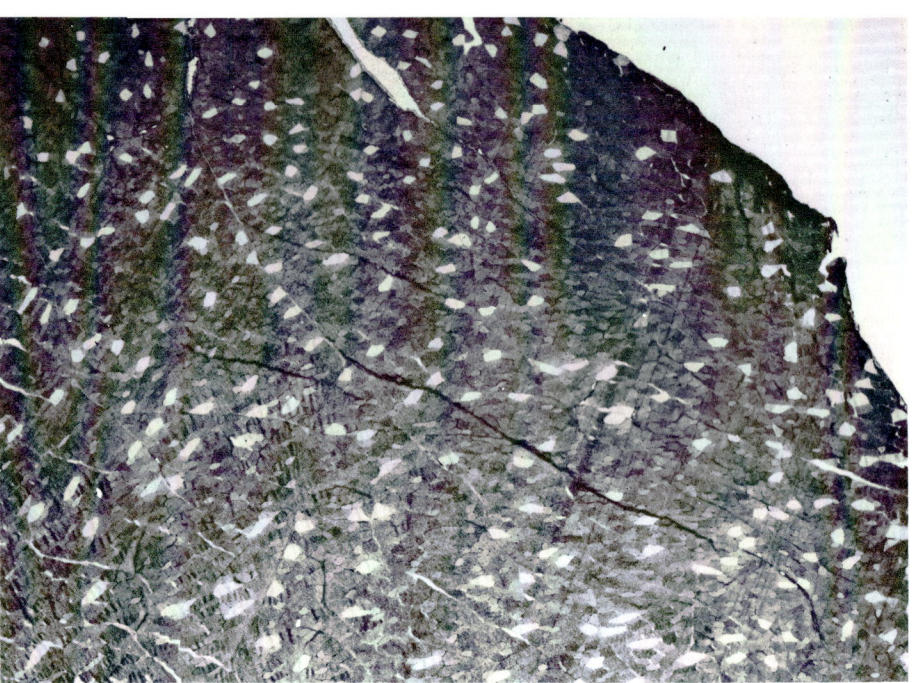

FIG. 12. Medium magnification photomicrograph of glycogen-depleted fibers belonging to a type FF muscle unit in cat medial gastrocnemius (MG), showing relatively low density of unit fibers and rather uniform scattering through the unit territory. A full reconstruction of this muscle unit is shown in Fig. 13 (Left MG). Area illustrated measures approximately 8.0 × 5.4 mm. [From material of Burke and Tsairis (121).]

of the cat MG unit illustrated in Figure 13, and units in the cat soleus appear to occupy even larger fractions of whole muscle volume [Fig. 13; (110)]. The average density of unit fibers within the muscle unit territory is 2–5 fibers per 100 for the readily depleted type FF and FR units of cat MG (121) and appears even lower in cat SOL (Fig. 13), although the latter finding may be due partly to incomplete glycogen depletion in SOL fibers (110). Thus any given region of the territorial volume must be shared by many other interdigitating muscle units [at least 20–50 in cat MG; (121)]. Results from rat muscle are comparable (198, 227, 432, 433). Electromyographic studies in large human muscles (e.g., biceps brachii) give similar estimates for average territorial density of muscle unit fibers (91) and further suggest that unit territories in limb muscles may sometimes measure up to 11 mm in diameter [(90, 91); see also refs. 409, 650], again with considerable overlapping (253). There seems to be remarkably little difference between the average territorial diameters in various human muscles, irrespective of muscle size, but within a given muscle there can be a three- to fivefold range in territorial diameter from one unit to another (90). It may be that the average density of unit fibers within the territory is relatively constant, irrespective of the innervation ratio, but this point remains to be demonstrated definitively. The density of muscle unit fibers does appear to increase with aging in human subjects, implying possible disappearance of some motoneurons with consequent reorganization of innervation (395, 653).

REGIONALIZATION WITHIN A MUSCLE. It has been recognized for many years that a given muscle can vary in color from one portion to another, with the "deeper" parts tending to have redder color (see ref. 184). Modern histochemical studies have documented this "regionalization," so that the high-oxidative fiber types (type I and sometimes IIA; see subsection *Motor Unit Types: Physiological Profiles in Experimental Animals*, p. 351) tend to predominate in parts of muscles lying toward the center of the limb, while the more superficial portions tend to contain a greater preponderance of the low-oxidative type IIB fibers (296, 579, 591, 735). In the cat MG muscle, a bandlike region along the dorsal margin contains over 75% type IIB fibers, compared to 50% for the whole muscle overall (see Figs. 9 and 10 in ref. 119). The developmental and functional meaning of regionalization of fiber types remains to be clarified. It is not self-evident that fibers in the deeper portions of muscles operate with greater mechanical advantage (296). It does seem possible, however, that the red, high-oxidative portions have a higher resting blood flow than the white parts (377), so that locating them toward the center of the limb would minimize conductive heat loss to the environment. Histochemical regionalization is certainly most dramatic in small mammals with high metabolic rates, such as the rat (735), in which heat conservation may well be a significant problem.

Regionalization of fiber types implies a corresponding difference in the proportions of different unit types from one part of the muscle to another (subsection

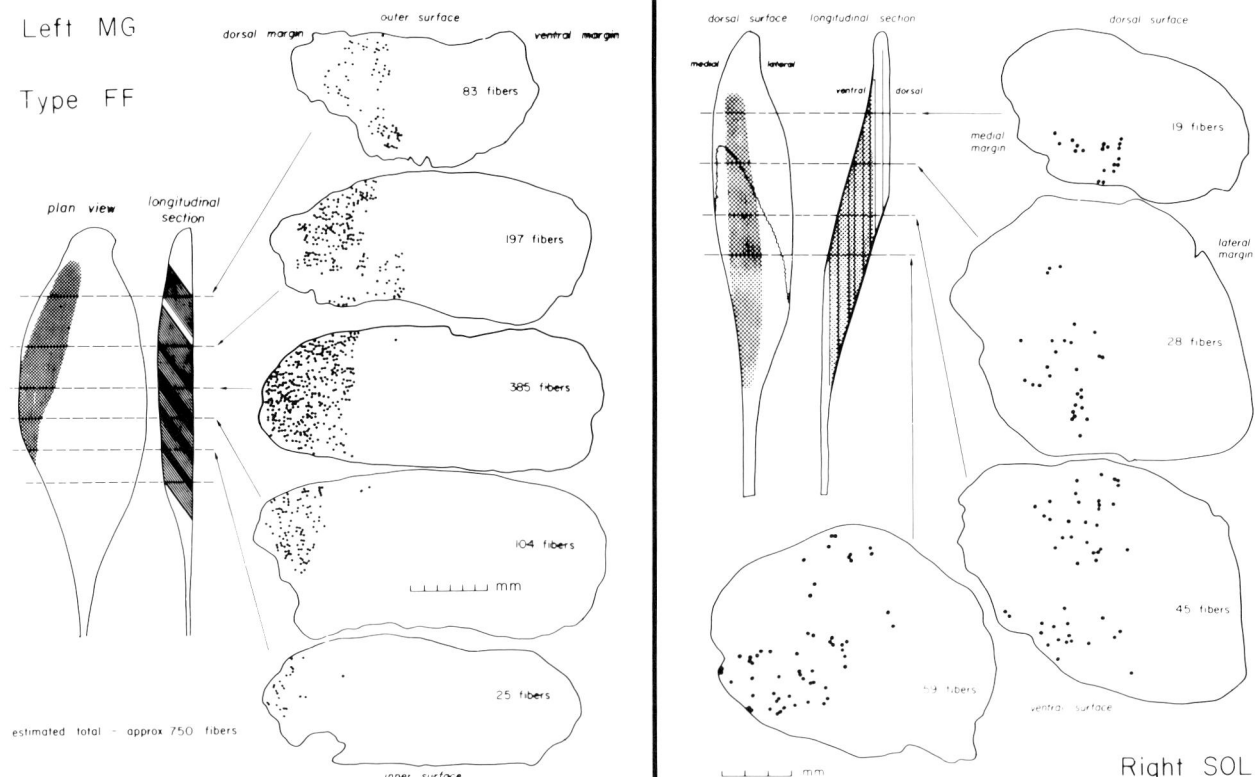

FIG. 13. Reconstructions of the territories of a type FF muscle unit in cat medial gastrocnemius (MG, *left panel*; see also Fig. 12) and of a type S unit in cat soleus (SOL; *right panel*). In each case, glycogen-depleted muscle fibers (*dots*) are plotted on outlines of cross sections taken along the muscle at different levels, as indicated on whole muscle diagrams on *right* of each *panel*. The angulation of fiber bundles within MG and SOL is shown on longitudinal section diagrams; *shading* denotes approximate extent of unit territory projected onto muscle surface in each view. Counts of glycogen-depleted fibers in each cross section are indicated on section maps. Territory of SOL unit appears to occupy a larger fraction of the whole muscle volume than does the MG unit. [*Left panel* from Burke and Tsairis (121); *right panel* from Burke et al. (110).]

PHYSIOLOGICAL AND HISTOCHEMICAL PROFILES OF MUSCLE UNITS, p. 354). Whatever the functional advantage of this inhomogeneity, there is an interesting correspondence with the spatial distribution of mucle receptor organs [(71); see also the chapters by Matthews and by Houk and Rymer in this *Handbook*]. The intramuscular distribution of muscle spindles and Golgi tendon organs is not uniform (465, 670); rather these receptors are usually distributed within those regions with local predominance of high-oxidative fiber types [(580, 735); see review in ref. 41]. Since the corresponding type S and FR motor units receive powerful excitatory feedback from primary spindle afferents (subsection GROUP Ia SYNAPTIC EFFICACY, p. 381), the proximity between spindles and high-oxidative muscle units suggests that there may be some spatial topography of reflex feedback (see refs. 64, 71, 152, 724), with perhaps some element of local mechanical interaction between spindles and nearby muscle units (725).

Golgi tendon organs are excited by mechanical force produced by the muscle fibers in series with them. Individual motor units are capable of causing significant discharge modulation in tendon organs (374, 667), and anatomical and physiological evidence indicates that all of the recognized motor unit types contribute fibers in series with tendon organs and cause their discharge (307, 388, 576). In addition all three unit types produce, on the average, roughly equivalent effects on tendon organs, but summation of the effects of simultaneously active units is often less than linear (307).

INNERVATION RATIOS AND MUSCLE UNIT "SIZE". The number of muscle fibers innervated by a given motoneuron is termed the innervation ratio for that motor unit. The overall average innervation ratio ($\overline{IR}$) for units in a particular muscle can be estimated simply by dividing the total number of muscle fibers present (M) by the total number of motoneurons (N) that innervate them (see last column in Table 2). Neither of these numbers is easily obtained, however, and estimates of both are subject to experimental error. Total muscle fiber counts are especially difficult in muscles with complex internal architecture. The numbers of innervating motoneurons have been estimated by counting the large axons that survive in a motor nerve after removal of appropriate dorsal root ganglia

TABLE 2. *Data for Muscles and Motor Unit Populations that Permit Calculation of Relative Innervation Ratios and Specific Force Outputs for Defined Motor Unit Types in Three Cat Hindlimb Muscles*

	Muscle Fiber Types			
	IIB + IIAB	IIA	I	

A. *Observed Percent Composition of Whole Muscle*

				M
MG	55.3	20.2	24.5	12,000[a]
FDL	52.8	36.9	10.3	5,000[b]
SOL			100.0[c]	25,000[d]

B. *Observed Mean Fiber Areas,* μm^{2e}

MG	4,503 (72.1)	2,370 (13.9)	1,980 (14.0)
FDL	2,628 (69.0)	1,403 (25.7)	1,023 (5.3)
SOL			3,738 (100.0)

	Properties of Equivalent Motor Unit Types			
	FF + F(int)	FR	S	

C. *Observed Percent Composition of Motor Unit Pool*[f]

				N
MG	51.8 (140)	23.0 (62)	25.2 (69)	270[g]
FDL	32.2 (42)	56.3 (73)	11.5 (15)	130[h]
SOL			100.0[c] (140)	140[g]

D. *Observed Mean Tetanic Force,* g[i]

				Total force sum
MG	71.4 (81.3)	28.7 (14.5)	7.6 (4.2)	12,292
FDL	30.0 (75.6)	5.3 (23.4)	1.1 (1.0)	1,663
SOL			10.5 (100.0)	1,470

E. *Calculated RIRs*[j]

				$M:N$
MG	1.07 (674)	0.88 (554)	0.97 (611)	630
FDL	1.64 (328)	0.66 (132)	0.90 (180)	200
SOL			1.00 (179)	179

F. *Observed Mean Axonal Conduction Velocities,* m/s

MG	98.9	99.6	83.4
FDL	99.0	98.3	84.1
SOL			72.0

G. *Calculated Specific Tensions,* kg/cm^2

MG	2.35	2.18	0.63
FDL	3.48	2.86	0.60
SOL			1.57

MG, medial gastrocnemius; FDL, flexor digitorum longus; SOL, soleus; M, estimated total number of muscle fibers; N, estimated total number of motoneurons that innervate M; RIR, relative innervation ratio. In parts A, C, and D, data for MG are from ref. 111, data for FDL are from ref. 207, and data for SOL are from ref. 110 unless otherwise noted. [a] See ref. 121. [b] Estimated from fiber length data in ref. 5 and cross-section counts from ref. 718, together with unpublished data of R. P. Dum, J. Toop, and R. E. Burke. [c] Normal cat SOL muscle contains a small (0%-5%) proportion of type II fiber and a few fast-twitch motor units (ref. 345), which are ignored here. [d] Ref. 143; see also ref. 110. [e] Numbers in parentheses are percentage of total cross-sectional area represented by each fiber type. Fiber area data for MG and SOL from refs. 110 and 111 updated from unpublished observations of R. Dum, J. Toop, R. F. Mayer, and R. E. Burke. [f] Numbers in parentheses are estimated absolute number of units of each motor unit type. [g] Compromise estimate from data in refs. 72 and 119; see also subsection *Anatomy of Motor Nuclei*. [h] Compromise estimate from data in ref. 72 together with unpublished counts of HRP-labeled FDL motoneurons of R. P. Dum and R. E. Burke. [i] Numbers in parentheses are aggregate force contributed by each unit type as percentage of total force sum obtained with unit numbers in C. [j] Numbers in parentheses are estimated absolute innervation ratios.

(see refs. 72, 217, 594) or by counting the motoneuron cell bodies labeled by retrograde transport of horseradish peroxidase after intramuscular injection (see subsection NUMBERS OF MOTONEURONS AND MOTOR UNITS, p. 376).

Using direct counts of motor axons and muscle fibers, Clark (143) estimated that an average muscle unit in the cat SOL contains 140-200 fibers (see also ref. 110). In the synergist MG, however, the average IR is estimated at between 550 and 675 fibers per unit in the cat (depending on motor unit type; part E in Table 2; see also ref 121), about 790 fibers per unit for the monkey (731), and up to 2,000 fibers per unit in the human MG [(255); see also ref. 89]. Buchthal (89) has reviewed much of the available material that permits estimates of average IRs in human muscles.

These ratios, not surprisingly, tend to be large in large limb muscles (e.g., 600–1,700 in biceps brachii and gastrocnemius), smaller in intrinsic hand muscles (100–340 in first lumbrical or dorsal interosseous; see also ref. 255), and very small in extraocular muscle (13–20 fibers per unit). Such estimates, however, provide no evidence related to possible differences in IRs in different types of motor units.

The IRs of different unit types within the same motor pool are of interest, since there is wide variation in tetanic force output [e.g., over a 100-fold range in the cat MG; subsection MOTOR UNIT POPULATION OF CAT MEDIAL GASTROCNEMIUS MUSCLE (p. 353); Fig. 6; (111)]. The simplest explanation for the variation in force output per unit is to postulate an equivalent variation in IRs, with the latter perhaps correlated with the identity and/or the size of the innervating motoneuron and motor axon. Since technical problems preclude the use of glycogen-depletion methods to attack this issue directly (see ref. 121), indirect estimates of the average IRs for different motor unit types must suffice. Such estimates assume 1) that muscle fiber histochemistry accurately reflects physiological unit type (subsection MOTOR UNIT POPULATION OF CAT MEDIAL GASTROCNEMIUS MUSCLE, p. 353); 2) that ventral root dissection or intracellular penetration provides a reasonably accurate sampling of the composition of motor unit pools; and 3) that the muscles and unit pools that yield physiological and histochemical data are in fact comparable.

The average IR for a given motor unit type ($\overline{IR}_i$) can be estimated as

$$\overline{IR}_i = (M/N) \times (p_i/q_i) \qquad (1)$$

where p_i and q_i are the respective relative frequencies of the ith fiber type and its equivalent physiological motor unit type. The ratio p_i/q_i can be termed the relative IR (or RIR) for that unit type. For example, if the percentages of histochemical fiber types and equivalent motor unit types are roughly the same, then the $\overline{IR}_i$ for each unit type would also be the same (121).

Table 2 shows how data about fiber types (parts A and B) and equivalent motor unit types (parts C and D) can be used to arrive at estimates of both relative and absolute average IRs for a given motor unit type (part E) and of the specific force output of their muscle fibers (part G). Several points emerge from the data in Table 2. The heterogeneous MG and flexor digitorum longus (FDL) muscles in the cat differ somewhat in fiber type proportions (part A) but differ more dramatically in their motor unit composition (part C). More than one-half of the FDL pool is composed of type FR motor units, and, as a consequence, the average IR calculated for FDL type FR units (IR = 132) is only about one-third (RIR = 0.66) of that estimated for FDL type FF units (IR = 328, RIR = 1.64; part E). In contrast, all of the unit types in MG have similar calculated IRs (554–674), within 12% of the overall mean IR (RIR range, 0.88–1.07, part E; see also ref. 121). When either relative or absolute IR estimates (part E) are compared with the average axonal conduction velocities for the various unit types within a given pool (part F), there is clearly no strong correlation. These data provide no support for the intuitively appealing notion that large, fast conducting motoneuron axons innervate more muscle fibers than small, slow ones (217).

There are large differences among motor units in average tetanic force per unit, both between different muscle pools and between unit types within a given muscle (see subsection *Motor Unit Types: Physiological Profiles in Experimental Animals*, p. 351), but comparisons in Table 2 between mean tetanic force data (part D) and IR estimates (part E) show only weak correlation. This is due to the fact that maximum tetanic force output (P_j) for an individual muscle unit is the product of three factors

$$P_j = IR_j \times \overline{A}_j \times S_i \qquad (2)$$

where IR_j is the unit innervation ratio, $\overline{A}_j$ is the average area of the unit's muscle fibers, and S_i is the specific tension output for the equivalent fiber type, expressed as force per unit of cross-sectional fiber area (see ref. 148). The differences between motor units in tetanic force output must be evaluated with respect to all three of the relevant factors.

Using Equation 2 and the required data from parts B, D, and E of Table 2, one can calculate the implied S_i for each fiber and motor unit group (part G). The estimates of 2.2–3.6 kg/cm^2 found for the fast-twitch unit types fits well with data from whole heterogeneous muscles of various mammals (see ref. 148), and the value obtained for the slow-twitch SOL units (1.6 kg/cm^2) is also reasonably close to accepted values (see refs. 148, 518). However, the S_i estimates for the type S units in the heterogeneous MG and FDL muscles are much lower than expected from whole muscle data (about 0.6 kg/cm^2; see ref. 121). If these low estimates are in fact correct (cf. ref. 225), the small forces produced by type S units in heterogeneous muscles would be due mainly to their relatively small fiber areas and low specific tension, and not to small IRs. An explanation for the low specific tension of the heterogeneous muscle S fibers is lacking but it could relate to intrinsic properties of the heterogeneous S unit myosin, which differs histochemically from that in SOL [see subsection *Muscle Fiber Types: Histochemical Profiles and Ultrastructural Correlations*, p. 347, and Fig. 2]. Ultrastructural data from the rat tibialis anterior shows that myofibrillar packing density is about the same in presumably fast- versus slow-twitch fibers, although the fibrils themselves are thinner in the latter [(619); see also ref. 619a]. The S_i estimates for SOL fibers suggests that low specific-force output is not necessarily characteristic of all slow-twitch muscle.

Because of the multiple factors involved (Eq. 2), it is impossible to assess the probable range of IRs for individual motor units simply on the basis of their tetanic force outputs. One also needs, at the least, information about the average cross-sectional area of the fibers belonging to the individual muscle unit under study. The three-dimensional diagram in Figure 14 illustrates this point, using data from glycogen-depleted MG motor units in which both P_j and A_j were measured (121). Fast-twitch (circles) and slow-twitch units (triangles) are plotted on different planes that represent the different estimates for S_i (Table 2, part G). These data, though limited, suggest that IRs for individual motor units can vary over at least a four- to fivefold range within a given unit type. If the assumed S_i values in fact apply to each unit, then the fivefold range of IRs can explain only that much of the observed range in P_j for all cat MG motor units (25-fold for F units and about 16-fold for S; see Fig. 6). The remainder must be accounted for by interunit variation in mean fiber areas, which can be considerable (Fig. 14). A similar analysis in the cat SOL suggests that IRs in that homogeneous unit population can vary over as much as an eightfold range (110), explaining a larger fraction of the tetanic force range than is the case in the heterogeneous MG (see also ref. 28).

The factors that control IRs in different unit types and in various motor unit populations remain to be elucidated (see subsection *Developmental Considerations*, p. 364; see also ref. 394). There is a great deal of polyneuronal innervation of individual muscle fibers at birth in both rodents (53, 85, 572, 688) and kittens (31, 718), which disappears during the first weeks of postnatal life as muscle fibers mature to their adult types (subsection *Developmental Considerations*, p. 364). Counts of ventral root axons in postnatal rats (265) suggest that the maturation process after birth does not involve significant continued motoneuron death. Thompson and co-workers (688) have suggested that the disappearance of polyneuronal innervation results from two processes: *1*) a tendency for motoneurons at a particular stage of development to restrict their peripheral field of innervation (see also ref. 687) and *2*) competitive peripheral interaction between end plates on the same muscle fiber (see refs. 53, 430). Studies of partially denervated rodent muscle suggest that a given motoneuron, when mature, can support as many as 4-5 times its normal number of motor end plates and muscle fibers (84, 687), but this capacity is less during the period of removal of polyneuronal innervation (687). What remains unknown is how the identity of the surviving innervation is determined, especially in view of the fact that there is detectable muscle fiber differentiation before, as well as during, the disappearance of polyneuronal innervation (subsection *Developmental Considerations*, p. 364).

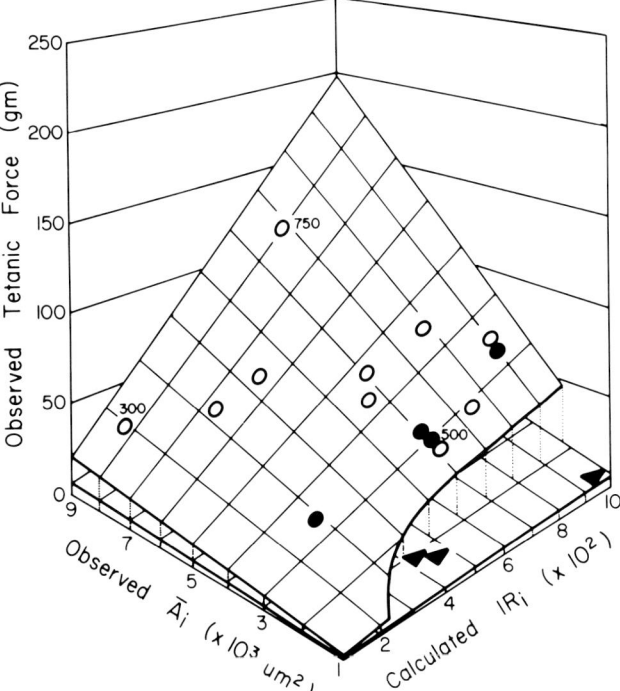

FIG. 14. Three-dimensional diagram showing dependence of isometric tetanic force from a muscle unit on unit innervation ratio, mean fiber area, and specific tension per unit fiber area. The 2 planes in the diagram represent loci for different specific tensions: 2.2 kg/cm² (the larger slope plane, for type F units) and 0.6 kg/cm² (the lower plane for type S units: see Table 2 for derivation of these estimates for cat medial gastrocnemius muscle). Innervation ratio for an individual motor unit can be estimated when its tetanic force output and average fiber area is known and a reasonable estimate of the specific force output per unit fiber area can be assumed. *Plotted points* represent different medial gastrocnemius (MG) motor units for which force and fiber area data are available (121); *open circles* denote FF units; *filled circles* are type FR units; and *filled triangles* (plotted on the 0.6 kg/cm² plane) represent type S units (see Table 2). *Numbers* next to 3 of the *points* are innervation ratio estimates from reconstructions of glycogen-depleted units (121). If the values assumed for specific tension per unit area are correct, these data suggest that innervation ratios for cat MG units vary over a 4- to 5-fold range, with little systematic difference between fast- and slow-twitch units.

Anatomy of Motor Nuclei

In all vertebrates the motoneurons lie in the ventral gray matter of the spinal cord (e.g., ref. 521), mainly in the lateral part referred to as lamina IX in the cytoarchitectonic map of Rexed (578) where they form local nuclear collections including a medial group innervating axial musculature and a lateral group innervating the limb [(234, 235); see ref. 645 for discussion and references]. The motoneurons that innervate a particular muscle (i.e., a motor nucleus) can be identified by chromatolysis after axonal injury (e.g., refs. 589, 645, 700), a relatively subtle change that affects large neurons more than small ones (589), or by retrograde transport of tracer substances such as horseradish peroxidase (426), which labels a large proportion of motoneurons without apparent regard to cell size (119,

612). One may then define a motor nucleus as a localized collection of motoneurons with axons in a particular muscle nerve that innervate muscle units within an anatomically defined muscle. Whether or not there are local subgroups within the nuclei of multifunctional muscles remains an open question.

Motor nuclei are organized into more or less definite longitudinal columns with predictable locations that emerge during embryonic development as the limb buds mature from proximal to distal (588). Maps of these columns and nuclei for limb muscles are available for a variety of species, including frog (171), chick (443), rat (75, 283, 284, 404), cat (589, 590, 665), and rhesus monkey (574, 645). Maps are also available for neck (581) and cranial nerve motor nuclei (4, 425, 438, 470). Sharrard (628) reconstructed the nuclear positions in the lumbosacral spinal cord of humans, using material from patients with poliomyelitis and showed that the human motor nuclei are organized in a pattern very similar to that found in the cat. The design of the motor cell columns is in fact quite stereotyped in mammals and birds, considering the differences between species in overall spinal cord anatomy (443).

Anatomical studies of motor nuclei with the horseradish peroxidase (HRP) method (see refs. 426, 504) have confirmed and extended earlier results with cell marking by chromatolysis. For example, the MG and SOL nuclei in the cat (119, 612) occupy the same column in the center of the ventral horn, with some rostral shift of the bulk of SOL cells (Fig. 15). According to Romanes' findings (589, 590), the cells that

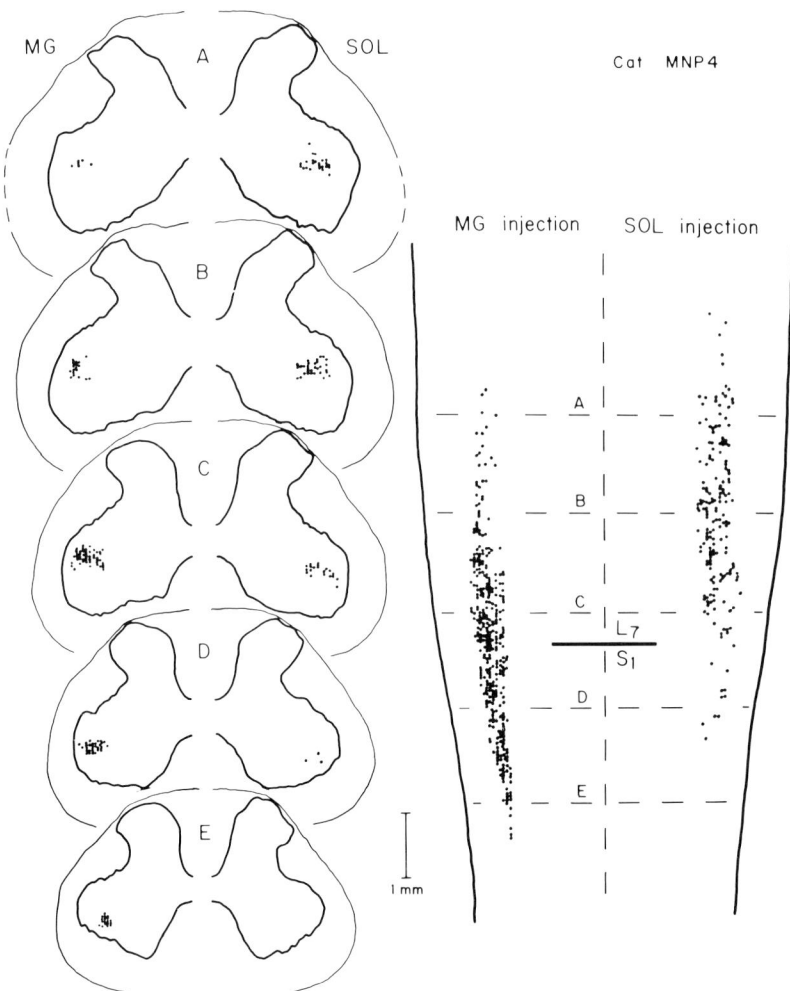

FIG. 15. Reconstructions of medial gastrocnemius (MG) and soleus (SOL) motor nuclei in a cat spinal cord, showing a dorsal view (*right*, with lateral spinal cord margins indicated by *solid lines*) and 5 levels of cross sections (*left*, levels indicated by *letters* and *dashed lines* on dorsal view diagram). Motoneurons (*dots*) were identified after retrograde transport of horseradish peroxidase injected into left MG and right SOL muscles of the same animal. Reconstructions were made from serial sagittal sections and show all labeled cells on the dorsal view. Cells indicated on cross-section reconstructions were only those within 300 μm of the selected level. The MG and SOL nuclei share the same motor cell column and are about the same overall size even though SOL contains only about one-half the number of motoneurons. [From Burke et al. (119).]

innervate the lateral gastrocnemius, popliteus and tibialis posterior muscles should also share this column, with some further rostral shift. Such anatomical associations between nuclei of muscles not strictly related in function suggest that anatomical and developmental proximity rather than strict functional synergy probably determines the identities of motor nuclei sharing a given column.

The soma diameters of labeled motoneurons in the MG and SOL nuclei (Fig. 16) show a bimodal distribution (see also ref. 700), reflecting the marked differences in average cell size between the larger α- and smaller γ-motoneurons [(119, 612, 666); see subsection *Motoneuron Anatomy in Relation to Unit Type*, p. 377]. Large and small motoneurons are randomly intermingled throughout each motor cell column (119), as is consistent with previous evidence indicating that γ-motoneurons are not spatially segregated (88, 526, 720). Furthermore there is no tendency for motoneurons within the larger versus smaller halves of the α-motoneuron size range to occur in local clusters, which is consistent with physiological evidence that motoneurons of different unit types can lie adjacent to one another (121). Local neuronal density, however, can vary along the length of both the motor cell column as a whole (683) and along an individual motor nucleus [see Fig. 15; (119)].

In the cat there is a rough somatotopic relation between the longitudinal position of an MG motoneuron in the motor cell column and the intramuscular location of its muscle unit; the most rostral motoneurons tend to innervate muscle units near the dorsal margin of the muscle, whereas the most caudal cells innervate units located near the ventral margin [(671); see also ref. 444]. This finding suggests that neighboring motoneurons innervate interdigitating muscle units (451). One may then infer that observed regionalization of muscle fiber types (subsection REGIONALIZATION WITHIN A MUSCLE, p. 368) indicates an equivalent local variation in motor unit type predominance along a nuclear column (119), even though there is almost certainly no strict anatomical segregation of motoneurons by type (121) or by relative motoneuron size (119, 140). Further verification is difficult as there seem to be no anatomical or histochemical characteristics that clearly distinguish motoneurons of different types (subsection *Motoneuron Anatomy in Relation to Unit Type*, p. 377). Despite the histochemical differences between muscle fibers (subsections *Muscle Fiber Types: Histochemical Profiles and Ultrastruc-*

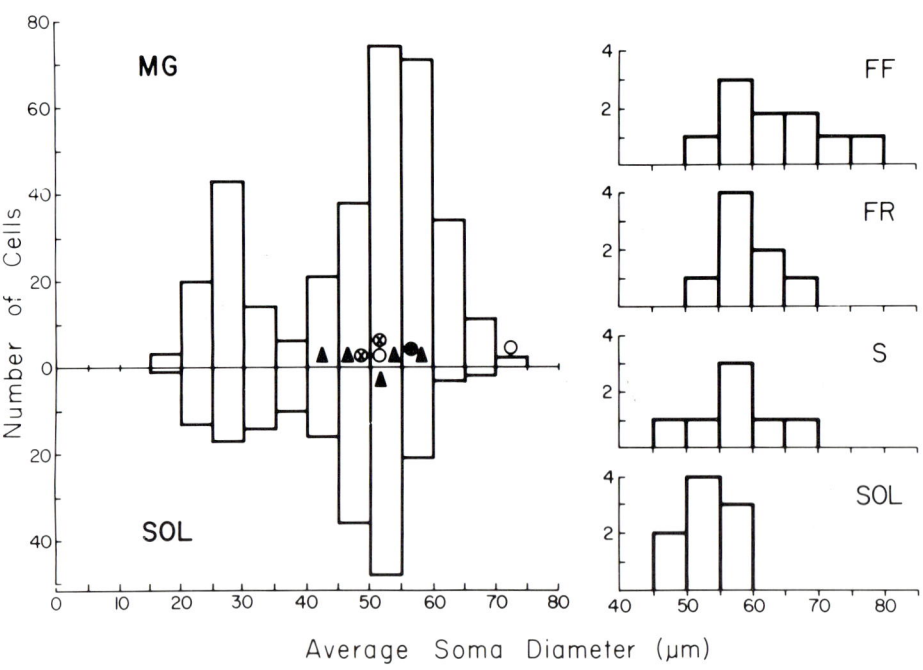

FIG. 16. Comparison of average soma sizes of cat medial gastrocnemius (MG) and soleus (SOL) motoneurons. Histogram on *left* shows average soma diameter of MG and SOL motoneurons labeled by retrograde transport of horseradish peroxidase (HRP) from same preparation as illustrated in Fig. 15. The smaller peak in this bimodal size distribution is assumed to represent γ-motoneurons. Superimposed symbols denote average soma measurements of HRP-labeled cells (9 gastrocnemius and 1 SOL) like those shown in Fig. 17, with unit type as follows (○ = FF; ⊗ = F(int); ● = FR; ▲ = S). Histograms on *right* are a more extensive set of data on type-identified, HRP-labeled triceps surae motoneurons. These data indicate that, in general, the motoneurons of type S units are somewhat smaller than those of F units, but there is considerable overlap between the groups, at least in some dimensions. [*Left* adapted from Burke et al. (119); *right* from data of S. Cullheim, J.-O. Kellerth, and B. Ulfhake, personal communication.]

tural Correlations, p. 347, and PHYSIOLOGICAL AND HISTOCHEMICAL PROFILES OF MUSCLE UNITS, p. 354), all ventral horn neurons in the α-motoneuron size range exhibit essentially identical histochemistry (high anaerobic and low oxidative enzyme capacities), while smaller cells (presumed γ-motoneurons and interneurons) have the opposite profile (128, 129).

An interesting facet of motor nucleus architecture is the existence, in some regions, of longitudinally oriented "bundles" of motoneuron dendrites (614–616, 665). These bundles are particularly prominent in the phrenic nerve nucleus and in brachial cord motor nuclei innervating proximal musculature (665). The tendency for dendrites to be longitudinally oriented varies from one part of the cord to another (181, 665). An extreme example has been found in the lumbar cord of the rat, where two large, dense collections of longitudinally oriented dendrites occur, with some desmosomelike specialization at apposing membranes [(11); see also ref. 479]. Direct intracellular staining of individual motoneurons in the cervical cord shows a predominance of longitudinal dendrites (596), but equivalent studies of hindlimb motoneurons demonstrate a much more radial dendritic spread [Fig. 17; (48, 173)]. Nevertheless horseradish peroxidase (HRP) labeling of groups of synergistic α-motoneurons (Fig. 18) suggests the existence of longitudinal dendritic associations even in radially organized trees. Whether or not the close apposition between some motoneuron dendrites can explain the small degree of apparent ephaptic electrical interaction between α-motoneurons demonstrated by Nelson (520) is not clear (479).

It seems important to stress that the major fraction of the synaptic inputs to motoneurons occurs on their dendrites, which account for more than 80% of their total membrane area (see ref. 569). When considering

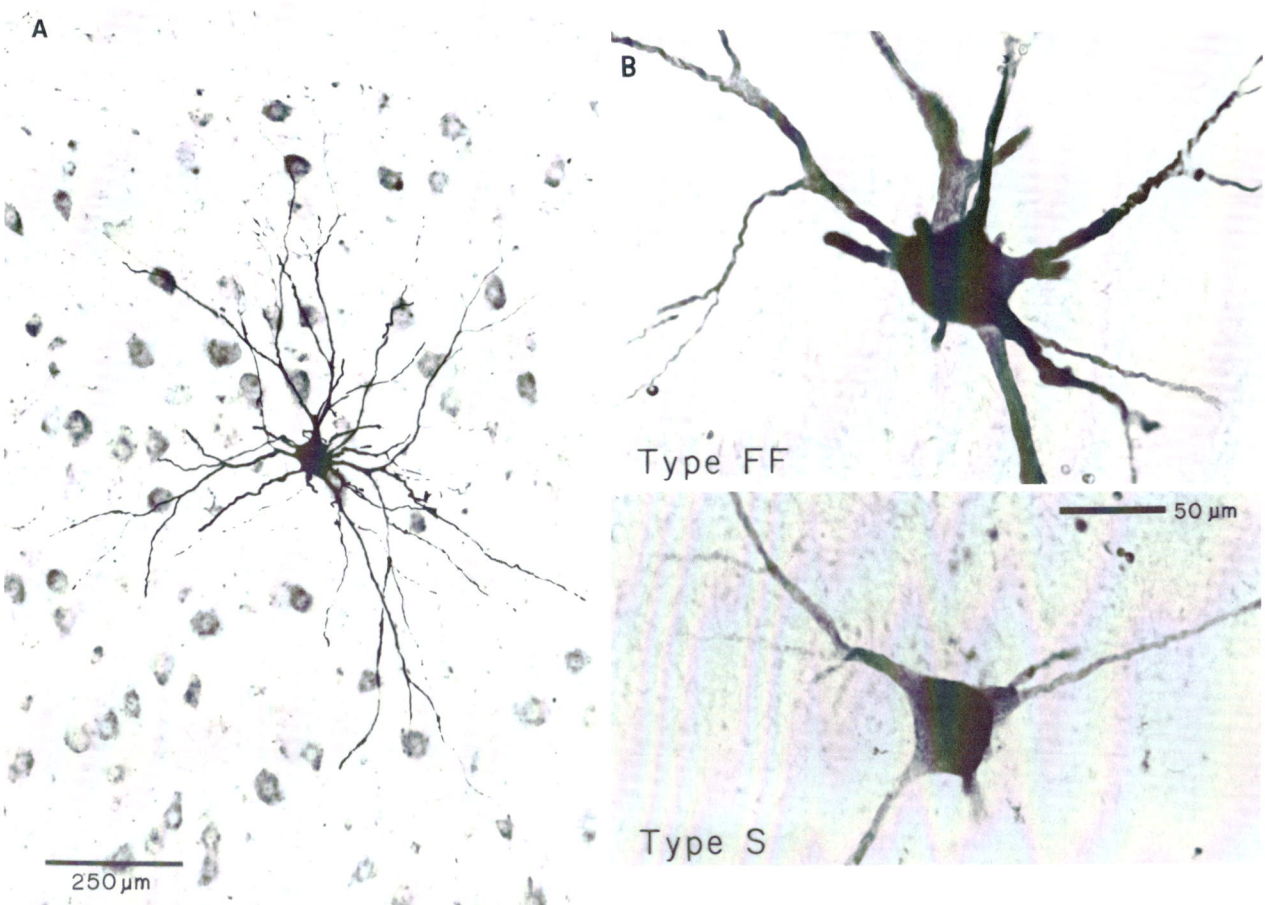

FIG. 17. Montage photomicrographs of 3 gastrocnemius motoneurons, identified as to motor unit type and labeled by intracellular iontophoresis of horseradish peroxidase (see ref. 124 for methods). *Left panel* shows, at low magnification, a type FR motoneuron in thick section, superimposed on Nissl-stained cell bodies of other ventral horn cells. The complete dendritic tree is not evident, but it is clear that dendrites extend out of the ankle extensor cell column into the columns of toe plantar flexors (dorsal) and hamstring (ventral) nuclei. *Right,* higher magnification shows, in another cat, a comparison in which type S motoneuron is clearly smaller and has fewer main stem dendrites than the FF neuron. These differences are not always so pronounced, as illustrated in Fig. 16.

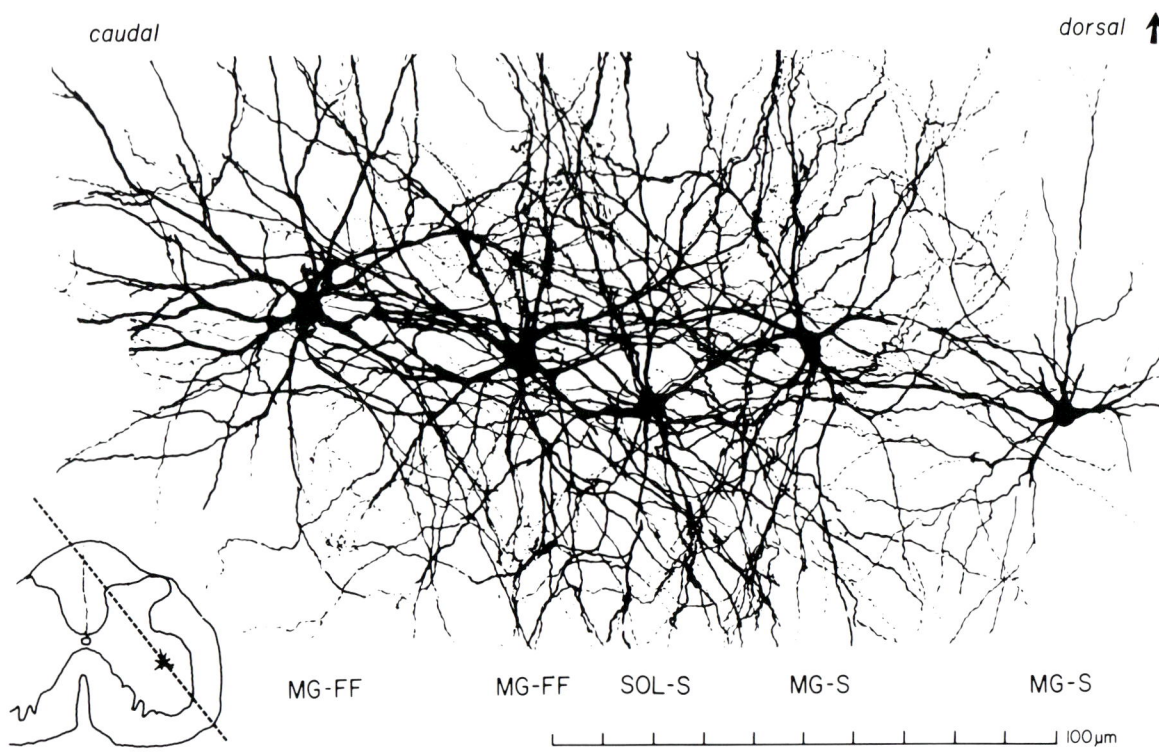

FIG. 18. Photomontage reconstruction of 5 HRP-labeled α-motoneurons: 4 medial gastrocnemius (MG) and 1 soleus (SOL), showing appearance of longitudinal dendritic associations between neighboring cell despite the basic radial arrangement of dendrites of any 1 cell. Reconstruction made by superimposing low-power photomicrographs, each enlarged onto photolithographic film, of 5 serial sections (pseudosagittal plane of sectioning shown in *inset* on *lower left*). Sections were each 75 μm thick so total reconstruction includes about 475-μm thickness. (From R. E. Burke, M. J. O'Donovan, M. J. Pinter, and A. Lev Tov, unpublished experiments; see ref. 124 for methods.)

the implications of localized motor cell columns, it should be remembered that radially oriented dendrites can project far beyond the nuclear column defined by the positions of cell somata (Figs. 15, 17), whereas the longitudinal dendrites might be expected to run within those columns. Dendritic anatomy has potentially important implications for the distribution of synaptic inputs impinging on particular species of motoneurons or even on particular sets of dendrites (e.g., ref. 616), but much remains to be done to clarify this issue.

NUMBERS OF MOTONEURONS AND MOTOR UNITS. Estimates of the total number of α-motoneurons (and therefore of motor units) in a given motor nucleus are needed for calculation of innervation ratios (see Table 2) and are directly relevant to clinical studies of neuromuscular diseases and the effects of aging in human subjects (see refs. 486, 487). Such estimates have been made by counting the larger myelinated axons in muscle nerves either after degeneration of the afferent fiber component by dorsal root ganglion removal (72, 217, 594, 731), or, in human muscles, by simply assuming a standard percentage of afferent axons (89). Data from human nerves (reviewed in ref. 89) suggest that large muscles possess more motor units than small ones, but the variation is much less than the range of muscle sizes. The bulky MG of humans appears to have about 580 motor axons (about twice the number found in the cat; Table 2), while the very much smaller first dorsal interosseous has about 119 (255; see also ref. 89). However, the nerve to the tiny external rectus oculi, which must produce very finely graded output, can contain over 1,700 motor axons (89). Thus function as well as muscle size must affect the numbers of motor units in particular muscles (see ref. 255).

Axon counts in muscle nerves consistently overestimate the actual number of motoneurons because of axonal branching that takes place in the nerve (282, 669), with a frequency that not only increases as the nerve approaches entry into the muscle (217, 731) but that varies unpredictably from one nerve to another (see ref. 594). The numbers of motoneurons directly labeled by the chromatolysis or HRP methods are consistently smaller than axon counts (e.g., refs. 119, 589). Both labeling methods may well underestimate the actual numbers of motoneurons in a given motor pool, although this error seems much less with HRP (119, 612). There is rather good agreement (within about 15%) between cell body and motor axon counts in studies of the MG and SOL nuclei in the cat, at least for the cells and axons in the α-motoneuron size range (see ref. 119). The numbers given in part *C* of

Table 2 (column N) are compromise figures based on such comparisons.

Recently, electrophysiological methods have been applied to make estimates of the number of functional motor units in certain human muscles (38, 485). Such estimates and the conclusions that have been drawn from them remain controversial, since they depend on special assumptions that may well not have wide application (e.g., refs. 87, 98, 251, 594).

Motoneuron Anatomy in Relation to Unit Type

It has long been assumed that there should be a direct correlation between the diameter of a motor axon and the size of its parent motoneuron (e.g., refs. 305, 363). Motor axon diameter is directly correlated with its conduction velocity [(382); see also ref. 712] and (under some conditions) the amplitude of its extracellular action potentials (139, 478). The fact that slow-twitch muscle units are innervated by relatively slowly conducting axons (subsection *Motor Unit Types: Physiological Profiles in Experimental Animals*, p. 351) therefore suggests that their motoneurons are correspondingly smaller than the cells that innervate the fast-twitch units (100, 216, 305, 306, 361, 439). Newer anatomical methods now permit direct tests of this relation.

Unlike axons, α-motoneurons are complex structures (e.g., ref. 3; see Fig. 17) and their "size" can refer to the diameter, surface area, or volume of the cell soma alone, which can be measured relatively easily, or to the dimensions and/or surface area of the entire neuron including soma and dendrites, which are much more difficult to estimate (e.g., ref. 48). Fortunately these measurements are correlated in motoneurons, since there is a more or less proportional scaling between somatic and dendritic dimensions [(48, 469); see also ref. 713]. Barrett and Crill (48) have shown by direct measurement of intracellularly labeled α-motoneurons (of undetermined unit type) that axonal conduction velocity is directly, but not very closely, correlated with total cell membrane area (see Fig. 2 in ref. 114), as it is also with average soma diameter (172).

This evidence suggests that some caution is necessary when equating "large" and "small" motoneurons with fast- and slow-twitch motor units. Recent direct anatomical studies of identified motoneurons amplify this need for caution. For example, Figure 16 shows that the average soma diameters of α-motoneurons (average soma diameter > 37.5 μm; see refs. 119) that innervate the homogeneous type S SOL muscle are only slightly smaller than those measured from the MG motor pool, which contains both fast- and slow-twitch units [mean values 50.1 μm versus 53.1 μm, respectively; (119, 612)]. There is thus considerable overlap between the soma size distributions in these contrasting motor nuclei (see subsection *Motor Unit Types: Physiological Profiles in Experimental Animals*, p. 351), even though type S motoneurons make up only about 25% of the MG population (Table 2).

Direct assessment of the anatomical size and complexity of motoneurons functionally identified as innervating different muscle unit types can now be done using intracellular injection of HRP (124, 156, 157, 174, 410). For example, the type S motoneuron illustrated in Figure 17 is clearly smaller in average soma diameter (43 μm) and has fewer main stem dendrites (7) than the type FF cell (54-μm diameter and 11 dendrites). The symbols plotted within the histogram bars on the left in Figure 16 show the average soma diameters measured for 10 type-identified motoneurons (R. Burke, B. Walmsley, and J. Hodgson, unpublished data). The histograms on the right illustrate a larger data sample supplied by J.-O. Kellerth, S. Cullheim, and B. Ulfhake. These direct observations confirm the view that motoneuron size (at least the dimensions of the soma) is correlated with motor unit type (see also subsection *Electrophysiological Properties Intrinsic to Motoneurons*, p. 379), but they also suggest that the differences between unit groups are surprisingly small, with many examples of overlap.

Whether or not there are anatomical differences in the dendritic trees of different motoneuron types remains to be determined, but it may be noted that Barrett and Crill (48) observed little evident correlation between soma size and the number of primary motoneuron dendrites. Observations on HRP-labeled, type-identified α-motoneurons confirm this (J. Kellerth and B. Ulfhake, personal communication) and show that α-motoneurons of the triceps surae muscles have, on average, 11–12 primary dendrites, irrespective of motor unit type (R. Burke, unpublished observations). Electrophysiological measurements (subsection *Electrophysiological Properties Intrinsic to Motoneurons*, p. 379) indicate that motoneuron dendrites are scaled roughly in proportion to somatic size, preserving relatively constant electrotonic length and dendritic:somatic conductance ratio (see also ref. 114), so that the dendrites of smaller motoneurons are probably scaled accordingly in anatomical dimensions.

The potential power of the intracellular marking methods in enlarging our knowledge of motor unit differences is illustrated in recent studies from the Karolinska group (156, 157, 175, 410). Ultrastructural studies of identified motoneurons suggest that the proportions and spatial distribution of C and M boutons differ systematically between FR and S motoneurons (157, 410). Such differences may well be related to the unit type-specific differences in synaptic organization found in electrophysiological studies (*Organization of Synaptic Input*, p. 381). The synaptic reorganization that takes place prenatally appears to involve phagocytosis of C boutons by the motoneurons themselves, in contrast to other synaptic types (595), but the origin of the C boutons remains unknown.

Using light microscopy Cullheim and Kellerth (175) have demonstrated that the extent and complexity of the recurrent motor axon collaterals differs depending on motor unit type, such that the collaterals of type S motoneurons exhibit the fewest detectable "swellings" (presumably synaptic endings), while the collaterals of type FF units have by far the largest numbers (see Fig. 19). Type FR collaterals are rather close to type S in this regard. This difference is consistent with the suggestion that the collaterals of larger motor axons provide the most powerful recurrent excitatory input to Renshaw interneurons, which in turn project most powerfully to the smaller motoneurons, producing recurrent inhibition (see subsection GROUP Ia SYNAPTIC EFFICACY, p. 381; see also ref. 86). These authors (174, 175) have also shown that the recurrent collaterals from α-motoneurons end not only in the ventromedial gray matter, where the Renshaw interneurons are known to occur (e.g., ref. 389), but also have a significant number of terminal swellings (about 20% of the total) within the motor cell column of the parent motor nucleus. These swellings make direct, monosynaptic contact with α-motoneurons, including (occasionally) the same motoneuron giving rise to the collateral system (176). These recurrent collateral systems are quite localized and their endings all occur within about 300–600 μm of the parent cell body. It is of interest that, collectively, type FF motoneurons have the fewest recurrent projections into the triceps motor nucleus as compared to the other unit types (Table 1 in ref. 175), despite the fact that they exhibit the largest total number of recurrent endings (Fig. 19).

The functional role of direct recurrent projections between motoneurons of the same nucleus is completely unknown. Presumably these endings are cholinergic and it is known that acetylcholine depolarizes the motoneuron membrane, although it does so rather unconventionally with slow time course and negligible conductance change (741). Excitatory interactions between neighboring α-motoneurons in both the frog (318, 472, 643) and cat spinal cord (285, 520) have been interpreted as ephaptic or electrotonic (see, e.g., ref. 643), possibly between closely apposed dendrites in the dendritic "bundles" (see ref. 479; see above). However, Gogan and co-workers (285) could not rule out a true synaptic projection, albeit of small magnitude and limited occurrence [14 of 97 tested cells; (285); cf. also ref. 627]. It seems possible that direct recurrent projections between local groups of α-motoneurons may have less conventional functions, perhaps allied to "trophic" influences. It would be of considerable interest, for example, if such direct intermotoneuronal connections occur preferentially between cells of the same motor unit type. Huizar and co-workers (379) have shown that partial denervation of the cat SOL muscle leads to detectable alterations in afterpotentials in the remaining, evidently undamaged SOL motoneurons. Axonal sprouting has also been observed among undamaged frog motoneurons in response to contralateral axotomy [(600); but cf. ref. 83]. These results suggest that information must somehow be transmitted from axotomized to undamaged cells and the recurrent collaterals could, at least in principle, be one route for such intercellular communication. An intraspinal route for such interactions, however, has been denied by Brown and co-workers in the mammalian cord (83), where other evidence suggests an "antidromic" message originating in the periphery [(178, 272); see also subsection *Electrophysiological Properties Intrinsic to Motoneurons*, p. 379].

PHYSIOLOGY OF α-MOTONEURONS AND THEIR SYNAPTIC INPUTS IN RELATION TO MOTOR UNIT TYPE

A review of the cellular neurophysiology of motoneurons is available in the *Handbook of Physiology, The Nervous System*, volume 1 (114), and material in this section overlaps with the chapter by Henneman and Mendell in this *Handbook*. This section deals briefly only with the physiology of motoneurons and their synaptic inputs in direct relation to motor unit type, with the latter defined on the basis of the characteristics of the innervated muscle unit (subsection

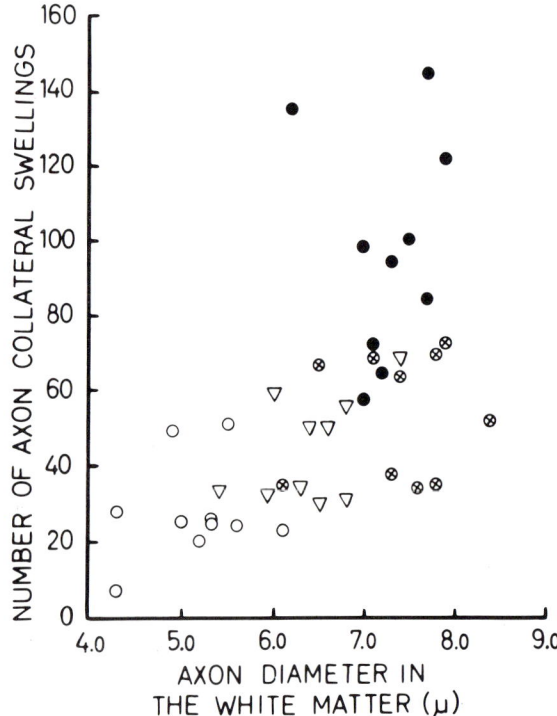

FIG. 19. Graph showing relation between diameter of intraspinal motor axon (abscissa) and number of swellings (presumably synaptic terminations) on recurrent collaterals from same axons, measured from type-identified motoneurons labeled by intracellular horseradish peroxidase iontophoresis (as in Fig. 17). ●, Gastrocnemius type FF; ⊗, gastrocnemius FR; ▽, gastrocnemius S; ○, SOL type S. Distribution of axonal diameters fits axonal conduction velocities for same unit types (see Figs. 20, 21). The FF units as a group exhibit significantly more recurrent collateral swellings than the other types that, in contrast, display a positive linear correlation between axon diameter and number of collateral swellings. [From Cullheim and Kellerth (174).]

PHYSIOLOGICAL AND HISTOCHEMICAL PROFILES OF MUSCLE UNITS, p. 354). One major point is that no combination of motoneuronal properties, whether anatomical (subsection *Motoneuron Anatomy in Relation to Unit Type*, p. 377) or electrophysiological, serves to divide the motor unit population into unambiguous classes as can be done using muscle unit characteristics (see also ref. 100).

Electrophysiological Properties Intrinsic to Motoneurons

The electrophysiological properties of a motoneuron are essentially those of its cell membrane, topologically distorted into the complex shape including soma, dendrites, and axon (see ref. 114). This viewpoint permits discussion of two distinguishable but interrelated categories of motoneuron properties: *1*) those that depend directly on the anatomical size and architecture of the neuron or its axon (i.e., the topology of the membrane) and *2*) those that do not necessarily depend on cell architecture but are intrinsic to the membrane per se.

The axonal conduction velocity (CV), whole neuron input resistance (R_N), and dendritic electrotonic length are all examples of topology-related motoneuron properties. The direct correlation between CV and several measures of motor axon and motoneuron size is discussed in subsection *Motoneuron Anatomy in Relation to Unit Type* (p. 377). Motoneuron input resistance (R_N; the resistive load presented by the cell to a constant current step passed into the soma through an intracellular pipette; e.g., refs. 160, 161, 266) varies inversely with CV [Fig. 20; (48, 415)], as well as with anatomical size (48, 469) and motor unit type [Fig. 20; (100)]. The R_N depends on both the size of the cell (in terms of its total membrane area, A_N) and the specific resistivity of the cell membrane, r_m, as well as on the equivalent electrotonic length, L, of its aggregate dendritic tree, as follows

$$R_N = r_m/A_N \, (L/\tanh L) \qquad (3)$$

This equation is rearranged from Equation 5.16 of Rall's chapter in the *Handbook of Physiology, The Nervous System*, volume 1 (569), which should be consulted for a detailed discussion. Clearly R_N reflects motoneuron size (i.e., A_N) only insofar as r_m and L are invariant in the motor unit pool.

Electrophysiological measurements indicate that L ranges between 1 and 2, with a mean value of about 1.5, in most cat α-motoneurons (see ref. 114 for references), including both F and S motoneurons of the MG pool [Table 3; (120)]. Direct comparison of electrophysiological and anatomical data in the same motoneurons (of unspecified type) indicates that r_m can vary over a twofold range from cell to cell, with mean values between 1,700 and 2,700 Ω·cm², depending on initial assumptions (48, 469). Comparable observations are not yet available for type-identified motoneurons, but it is known that the membrane time constant (t_m;

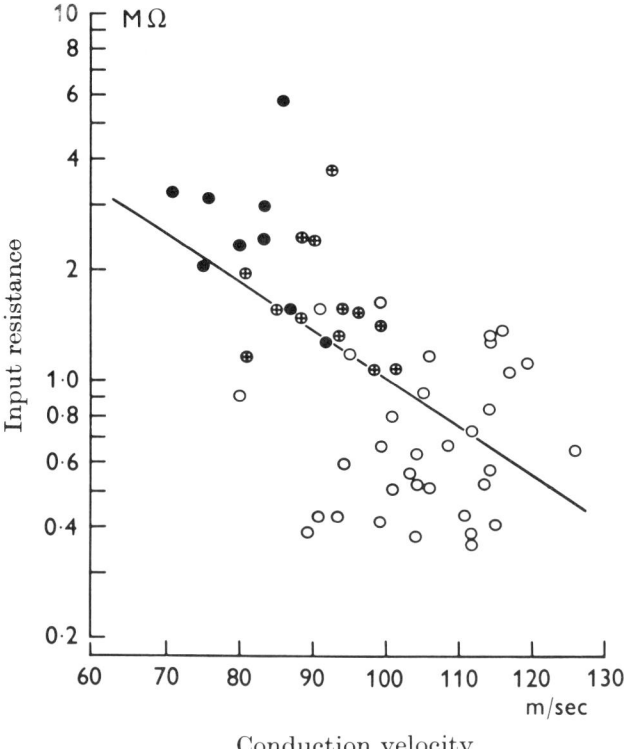

FIG. 20. Relation between axonal conduction velocity (abscissa) and motoneuron input resistance (ordinate; note logarithmic scale) in a sample of type F (*open circles*) and type S (*crossed circles*) motoneurons of cat gastrocnemius, plus a group of type S units from soleus (*filled circles*). There is a clear negative correlation despite considerable scatter. Note that input resistance values of gastrocnemius S units is, on the average, somewhat less than those of soleus, as fits with more recent anatomical data; see subsection *Motoneuron Anatomy in Relation to Unit Type*, p. 377, especially Figure 16. [From Burke (100).]

the product of r_m and the specific membrane capacitance, c_m) is, on the average, much the same in motoneurons of fast-twitch and slow-twitch units [see Table 3; (120)]. If c_m is constant, these data suggest that the differences between R_N in motoneurons of the various motor unit groups (Fig. 20; Table 3) are largely due to differences in cell size, although some systematic variation in r_m may also contribute (101). The interrelations between axonal CV, R_N, and the emerging direct anatomical data (subsection *Motoneuron Anatomy in Relation to Unit Type*, p. 377) all indicate that, on the average, motoneurons of type S units are smaller than those of type F, although there is clearly overlap between these groups (Fig. 16). Recent R_N measurements in identified type FF and FR motoneurons in the cat tibialis anterior (TA) and extensor digitorum longus (EDL) suggest further (Table 3; see also ref. 207) that the FR motoneurons may be somewhat smaller on the average than the type FF (see also Fig. 16).

Motoneuron properties that are not directly dependent on cell anatomy include *1*) the membrane time constant, τ_m; *2*) the afterhyperpolarization (AHP)

TABLE 3. *Physiological Properties of α-Motoneurons Belonging to Defined Types of Motor Units in Adult Cat Hindlimb Muscles*

Property	Muscle	FF	FR	S
Axonal conduction velocity, m/s	MG[a]	98.7 ± 1.5	99.6 ± 6.8	83.4 ± 7.7
	SOL[b]			71.5 ± 7.5
	TA + EDL[c]	97.4 ± 6.5	97.5 ± 6.4	82.6 ± 7.6
Afterhyperpolarization, ms	MG + LG[d]	110 ± 36	101 ± 26	136 ± 25
	SOL[d]			198 ± 30
Neuron input resistance, MΩ	TA + EDL[c]	0.9 ± 0.3	1.3 ± 0.5	2.0 ± 0.6
	SOL[e]			2.4 ± 1.2
		F[e]		
	MG + LG[e]	0.8 ± 0.3		1.9 ± 0.7
Membrane time constant, ms	MG + LG[e]	5.0 ± 1.7		7.0 ± 1.7
	SOL[e]			5.6 ± 1.7
Electrotonic length, λ	MG + LG[e]	1.6 ± 0.3		1.4 ± 0.2
	SOL[e]			1.6 ± 0.2

Data given as mean ± 1 SD. [a] Data from refs. 111, 118. [b] Data from ref. 110. [c] Data from ref. 207. [d] Data from ref. 346. [e] Data from refs. 100, 101, 120, in which FF and FR unit types were not distinguished. MG, medial gastrocnemius; SOL, soleus; TA, tibialis anterior; EDL, extensor digitorum longus; LG, lateral gastrocnemius.

that follows the all-or-none motoneuron action potential; and *3*) voltage-dependent membrane properties that are related to the generation of action potentials, such as accomodation and other nonlinear behaviors (see ref. 114 for general discussion and references). Note that neuronal architecture must still be kept in mind because intrinsic membrane properties can and probably do vary from one region of the cell to another (e.g., refs. 196, 197, 698; see also ref. 114).

The duration of the AHP varies with motor unit type; it is shorter on the average in FF and FR motoneurons than in type S cells, whether the latter occur in heterogeneous or homogeneous (i.e., SOL) motor pools [Table 3; (100, 345)]. Since the AHP is probably the most important mechanism that limits the steady-state firing frequency of α-motoneurons (324, 414), the direct correlation between AHP duration and twitch-contraction time (100, 416) represents an appropriate match between motoneuron and muscle unit properties (see also subsection *Output Modulation by Rate and Pattern of Motoneuron Firing*, p. 394). Because of the powerful influence of motoneuron firing frequency on muscle unit properties (subsection NONPHYSIOLOGICAL ALTERATIONS, p. 363), it has been suggested that this matching reflects a cause-and-effect relation in mature motor unit populations (271, 379), if not in early postnatal populations (380). Czeh and co-workers (178) have shown a decrease in AHP duration in SOL motoneurons after blocking axonal conduction by application of tetrodotoxin cuffs to the SOL muscle nerve, which also occurs following axotomy (440). This decrease can be prevented by chronic electrical stimulation below, but not above, the cuff. This striking finding suggests that the AHP duration may depend in part on some message delivered by retrograde transport from the periphery, implying the existence of centripetal as well as centrifugal controls in the match between motoneuron and muscle unit characteristics (cf. subsection *Stability of Motor Unit Types*, p. 361; see also ref. 452).

The process referred to as accomodation, when present, results in a progressive refractoriness (or increase in threshold) during the slowly rising or steady transmembrane depolarizations (see ref. 114 for discussion and references). Motoneurons that exhibit significant accommodation tend to fire in self-limited bursts while those without it can fire in sustained, steady trains for long periods. Demonstrable accommodation tends to be more pronounced among some fast-twitch (type F) motoneurons than among type S (113), as seems appropriate to the fatigue resistance of type S muscle units. Whether or not those type F motoneurons that exhibit little or no accommodation (113) innervate the fatigue-resistant type FR muscle units is unknown (cf. ref. 416).

With regard to other membrane properties involved in spike generation, there is rather little evidence for significant differences between motoneurons of different unit types [(439, 560); see ref. 114]. On the other hand, recent voltage clamp experiments of Schwindt and Crill (623) suggest that those α-motoneurons with relatively high R_N (presumably mainly type S cells; see Table 3) tend to exhibit a negative slope region in the subthreshold current-voltage curve. This type of net inward current (possibly carried by Ca^{2+} as in the frog; see ref. 47) is associated with pacemaker activity in invertebrate neurons (e.g., ref. 641), and it appears to promote repetitive firing (623). If the magnitude of this voltage-dependent inward current is indeed systematically high in type S motoneurons, it could represent an important membrane specialization linked to muscle unit characteristics and thus to motor unit function.

Organization of Synaptic Input

The relative responsiveness of motoneurons to graded inputs (i.e., sequential recruitment and gradations of functional threshold within a motor unit pool; subsection *Motor Unit Recruitment*, p. 386) implies corresponding quantitative or qualitative differences in the distribution of synaptic inputs to those motoneurons. It is difficult, however, to make inferences about quantitative input organization on the basis of firing patterns alone because of the multiplicity of factors that control motoneuron responses to synaptic input. Rather the relative efficacy of a given synaptic input is most directly assessed by intracellular recording under conditions that permit unambiguous measurement of postsynaptic potentials (PSPs) that are generated in type-identified (or otherwise "labeled") motoneurons by the action of functionally identified afferent inputs. Unfortunately these conditions apply strictly only to certain input systems that project to motoneurons either directly (monosynaptically) or disynaptically through a well-defined set of last-order interneurons. Quantitative estimates of synaptic efficacy require that the observed PSPs represent synchronous activity in all of the afferents in the system under study (i.e., a maximum composite PSP; see ref. 114) or in a known fraction of them, including single afferent fibers (see the chapter by Henneman and Mendell in this *Handbook*). This section focuses on the assessment of synaptic efficacy from the amplitude of composite PSPs measured in motoneurons of defined unit type. Discussions of the organization of synaptic input to α-motoneurons in general are available elsewhere (e.g., see refs. 114, 423, 466, 467, 557, 558, 626).

GROUP Ia SYNAPTIC EFFICACY. The monosynaptic excitatory connection from primary, or group Ia, muscle spindle afferents to α-motoneurons is the clearest example of an input amenable to intracellular quantitation. Despite many unresolved questions about the mechanism of Ia synaptic action (see ref. 114, 573) and its functional role in movement (see the chapters by Matthews and by Houk and Rymer in this *Handbook*), it is clear (457) that Ia-afferents project directly and powerfully to the α-motoneurons that innervate the same muscle from which they emerge (the homonymous connection) as well as to the motoneurons of functional synergists (heteronymous connections). The amplitude of the composite excitatory postsynaptic potential (EPSP) produced by electrical stimulation of the homonymous muscle nerve is generally larger than that produced by the heteronymous nerves (101, 215), due largely to differences in the connectivity patterns established by homonymous and heteronymous Ia-afferents (see the chapter by Henneman and Mendell in this *Handbook*). The efficacy or strength of this input system can be quantitated in terms of the maximum amplitude of composite Ia EPSPs since *1*) all Ia-afferents in a muscle nerve can be reliably and synchronously activated (e.g., ref. 214); *2*) their central effect is almost, if not exactly, synchronous (99, 440); and *3*) the shortest latency EPSP is monosynaptic and its peak is not contaminated by other synaptic effects, such as from group Ib-afferents (214) or the relatively weak and more delayed monosynaptic effects from group II spindle afferents (657). It is also necessary to ensure that the conditions of measurement are comparable from cell to cell (see refs. 101, 102, 118).

In 1957 Eccles and co-workers (215) showed that in the cat the amplitude of Ia EPSPs tends to be largest among motoneurons innervating red, slow-twitch muscles (SOL and anconeus). Burke (101, 102) later demonstrated in the cat MG motor nucleus that homonymous (MG) and heteronymous (LG-SOL) Ia EPSPs are larger, on the average, in cells of type S units than in type F (e.g., Fig. 23). More recent results (117, 118) demonstrate that Ia EPSP amplitudes scale rather precisely with motor unit type, in direct correlation with the fatigue resistance of the innervated muscle units and in inverse relation with their tetanic force outputs (Fig. 21). The same pattern of scaling has been found in the ankle flexors TA and EDL (208) and in the toe extensor, flexor digitorum longus (FDL; ref. 205). It is not known whether the strength of monosynaptic group II excitation (419, 657) also scales with motor unit type.

The same pattern of input efficacy (i.e., PSP amplitudes scaled with unit type as S > FR > FF) is evident for the disynaptic inhibition evoked in MG motoneurons by stimulation of group Ia-afferents from ankle flexor nerves (112, 118). The interpretation of inhibitory postsynaptic potential (IPSP) amplitudes is in this case complicated by the fact that maximum Ia IPSPs in MG motoneurons require facilitation by conditioning volleys from other inputs converging onto the Ia inhibitory interneurons (112, 118, 372). Furthermore it is well known that IPSPs are sensitive to changes in membrane potential or intracellular ionic composition (162), so that intercell comparisons require careful control of these variables.

It is of interest to mention another disynaptic inhibitory system at this point—the recurrent inhibition of motoneurons by Renshaw interneurons activated by motor axon collaterals (see ref. 114 for general details). Although there are no direct data on identified motor units, the efficacy of recurrent inhibition is generally stronger among the motoneurons to slow-twitch muscles than among the cells that innervate heterogeneous muscles (212), suggesting an organization similar to that found for Ia inputs. If confirmed for F and S motoneurons within a single motor nucleus, it makes an interesting counterpoint to the suggestion that the

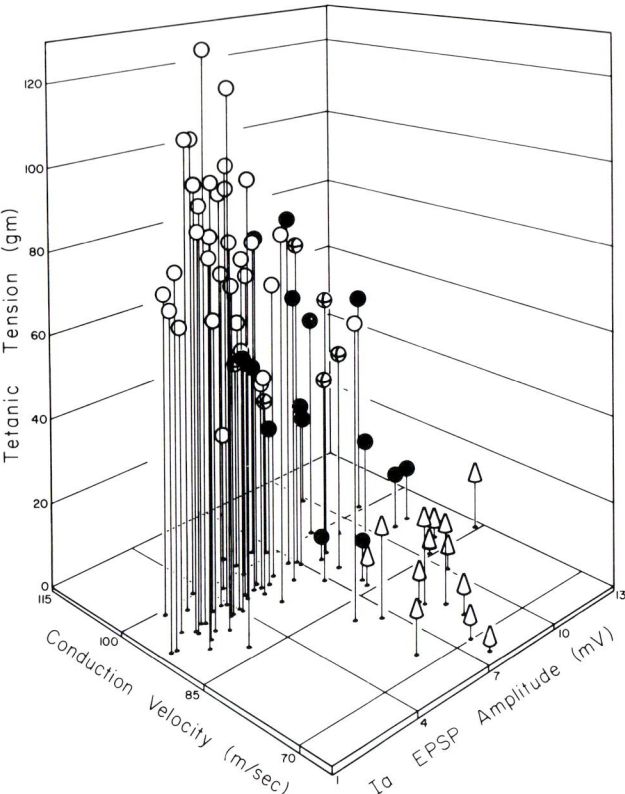

FIG. 21. Three-dimensional diagram illustrating interrelations between muscle unit tetanic-force output, motor axon conduction velocity, and amplitude of homonymous (i.e., medial gastrocnemius nerve stimulation) group Ia EPSPs in a sample of MG motor units. There is a rather good negative correlation between tetanic tensions and Ia EPSP amplitudes, but neither of these variables is well correlated with axonal conduction velocities. The type F group (denoted by *circles*) exhibits a narrow range of conduction velocities but broad ranges of both tension output and Ia EPSP size. *Open circles*, type FF; *crossed circles*, type F (int); *filled circles*, type FR; *cones*, type S. [From data of Burke et al. (118).]

recurrent collaterals of type F motoneurons may produce greater recurrent effects than type S collaterals [(174, 604); see also ref. 114], whereby activation of F motoneurons may reduce the firing probability of S call [see also subsections *Motoneuron Anatomy in Relation to Unit Type* (p. 377), and ARE MAJOR SHIFTS IN RECRUITMENT ORDER POSSIBLE? (p. 391)].

MONOSYNAPTIC SUPRASPINAL INPUTS. In the cat, two brain stem pathways project monosynaptically to α-motoneurons (see ref. 114) and quantitative data are available for the one projecting from the vestibulospinal tract (VST) to MG motoneurons (118). Surprisingly no correlation was found between the amplitude of monosynaptic VST EPSPs and motor unit type or any of the other features related to unit type. This agrees with earlier data of Grillner and co-workers (309), who found no correlation between amplitude of descending monosynaptic VST EPSPs and either Ia EPSP amplitude or the duration of the AHP.

In primates (unlike carnivores), the corticospinal tract projects directly to some α-motoneurons (see ref. 114 for references). The organization of this system with regard to unit type is of great interest but, unfortunately, there is no information available about the efficacy of corticomotoneuronal (CM) excitation in identified motor unit types. Phillips and co-workers (151) have demonstrated a rough direct relation between the average amplitudes of Ia and CM EPSPs among the various motor nuclei innervating the baboon forelimb. They found a negative correlation between the axonal conduction velocity of motoneurons and the amplitude of CM EPSPs in the extensor digitorum communis but, in contrast, a positive correlation among median nerve cells. The negative relation suggests an input organization similar to that found for group Ia-afferents in the cat MG (Fig. 21), but the positive correlation suggests the opposite. These authors concluded that the data did not permit any general formulation except that the pattern of CM excitation varies depending on the particular motor nucleus involved (p. 161 in ref. 151).

POLYSYNAPTIC INPUT SYSTEMS. It is essentially impossible to precisely quantitate the synaptic effects evoked in different motoneurons by complex and incompletely understood polysynaptic pathways, since the observed PSPs are usually mixtures of excitatory and inhibitory components with variable timing (e.g., see ref. 218). Nevertheless electrical stimulation of many hindlimb skin and muscle nerves in the anesthetized cat produces mainly IPSPs in extensor motoneurons that tend to be larger in amplitude in type F motoneurons [(112); see also ref. 218], which suggests that the scaling of synaptic systems that produce polysynaptic inhibition of extensors and excitation of flexors (i.e., the "flexor reflex afferents" or FRA; see ref. 218) is similar to that of Ia excitation (S > FR > FF; subsection GROUP Ia SYNAPTIC EFFICACY, p. 381). The recruitment patterns observed during reflex and voluntary activation of heterogeneous motor pools (see subsection RECRUITMENT PATTERNS AND MOTOR UNIT TYPES, p. 386) are such that other polysynaptic input systems may well be similarly organized. Some excitatory polysynaptic pathways, however, display a different pattern.

Denny-Brown (183) obtained early evidence for the existence of an alternative, reverse organization of synaptic input that can produce preferential excitation among motoneurons of "fast" muscles (see subsection ARE MAJOR SHIFTS IN RECRUITMENT ORDER POSSIBLE? on p. 391). Similar examples based on comparisons between synaptic potentials recorded in motoneurons of "fast" versus "slow" muscle nuclei have been reported by Preston and Whitlock (563) for corticospinal excitation in monkey hindlimb motor nuclei (MG and SOL comparisons), by Hongo and co-workers (373) for rubrospinal effects in these two nuclei in the cat, and by Illert and colleagues (384) for disynaptic excitation from the pyramidal tract to the various heads of the

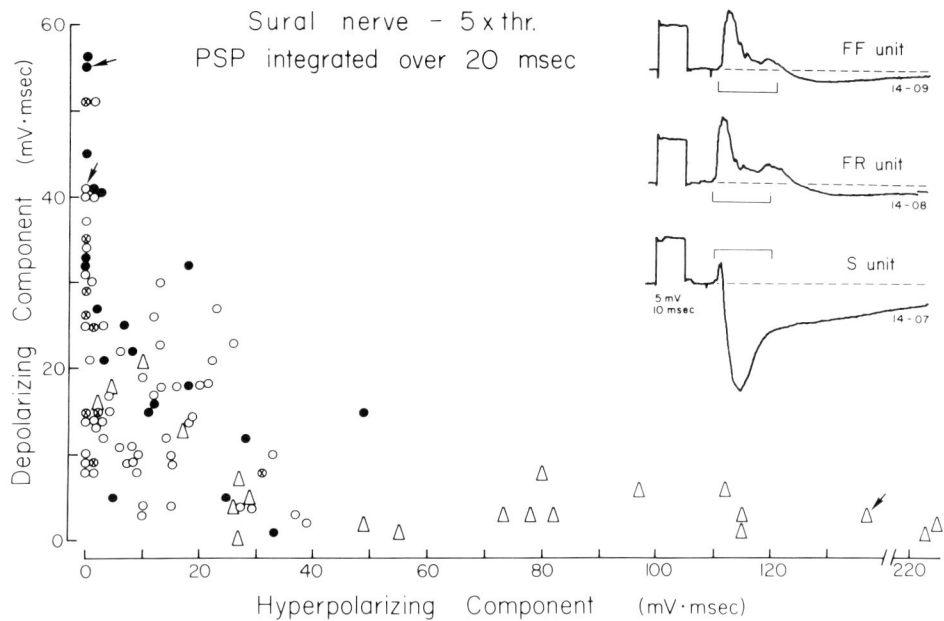

FIG. 22. Comparison of polysynaptic potentials (PSP) produced in medial gastrocnemius (MG) motoneurons by stimulating ipsilateral sural nerve at 5× threshold for the most excitable fibers. *Inset* records show computer averages (20 sweeps) of sural PSPs produced in 3 motoneurons recorded sequentially in the same cat within a 90-min period, showing marked difference in amount of early excitation between the F and S units. *Brackets* indicate 20-ms epochs over which voltage-time integrals of depolarizing and hyperpolarizing components were integrated for display in *lower graph* (data points indicated by *arrows*). Each of the 105 points in the graph came from a different MG motoneuron, with membrane potentials ranging between −60 and −75 mV. *Open circles,* type FF; *crossed circles,* type F(int); *filled circles,* type FR; *triangles,* type S. Despite some overlap in scatter, type S motoneurons have significantly smaller early polysynaptic excitation than type F units. [From Burke et al. (117).]

triceps brachii of cat. Both Megirian (493) and Rosenberg (597) found evidence that the distribution of polysynaptic excitation from cutaneous afferents was not uniform among the motoneurons in a given motor nucleus. In a similar vein, Wilson and Talbot (723) found little correlation between the effectiveness of monosynaptic versus polysynaptic excitation in flexor motor nuclei.

This kind of indirect evidence raised the possibility that different patterns of polysynaptic input exist within a single motor nucleus. Burke and co-workers (108, 117) have confirmed this suggestion directly, using type-identified motor units in the cat MG pool. They showed that in the cat the polysynaptic PSPs produced by electrical shocks to ipsilateral distal hindlimb skin nerves (the sural and, less reliably, the saphenous nerves) or to the red nucleus contain short-latency excitatory components that are much more pronounced among both FF and FR motoneurons than among type S cells, in which they are sometimes absent (Fig. 22; see also refs. 16 and 241). Despite the lack of precise quantitation, these observations suggest that certain polysynaptic excitatory pathways are organized in a pattern that is roughly the reverse of that found for Ia excitation and inhibition (see Figs. 27 and 35; see subsection ARE MAJOR SHIFTS IN RECRUITMENT ORDER POSSIBLE? on p. 391). The fact that the presence of polysynaptic excitation from cutaneous and descending sources covary within a given motor unit population (16, 108, 241) suggests that these pathways may share common interneurons.

Control of Motoneuron Excitability: Interactive Factors

Before describing the process of motor unit recruitment and its relation to motor unit type (subsection *Motor Unit Recruitment*, p. 386), it is useful to consider in a more general way the factors that control motoneuron excitability. These can be divided into two categories: *1)* those that control synaptic efficacy, all of which involve an interaction between the characteristics of presynaptic elements and the properties of postsynaptic motoneurons (mainly those related to cell anatomy) and *2)* those that are intrinsic to the motoneuron membrane, all of which are related to the process of spike generation. It is assumed that motoneuron excitability at any time reflects the balance of all of the excitatory and inhibitory synaptic effects reaching it at that moment.

SYNAPTIC EFFICACY. The factors that control synaptic efficacy (measured in terms of synaptic potential am-

TABLE 4. *Factors that Control Amplitude of Synaptic Potential in α-Motoneurons*

Presynaptic	Interaction	Postsynaptic
Number of Ia terminals per cell, N	Synaptic density, N/A	Total membrane area of cell, A
Average amount of transmitter released per terminal	Average conductance change per terminal, G_s	Receptor sensitivity
		Synaptic driving potential, $V_m - E_s$
Spatial distribution of synaptic terminals on motoneuron surface	Electrotonic attenuation and nonlinear interaction	Electrotonic architecture of motoneuron, which depends on cell anatomy and time constant, $\tau_m = r_m \times c_m$

V_m, instantaneous transmembrane potential; E_s, ionic equilibrium potential for the synaptic process; τ_m, neuronal membrane time constant; r_m, specific membrane resistivity in $\Omega \cdot cm^2$; c_m, specific membrane capacitance in $\mu F/cm^2$.

plitudes; see subsection GROUP Ia SYNAPTIC EFFICACY, p. 381) are given in Table 4. This discussion assumes that the synaptic systems under consideration are "chemical" in nature; i.e., they involve chemical transmitter substances that produce postsynaptic ionic conductance changes and consequent flow of ionic currents (see ref. 114). The "presynaptic" factors deal with the anatomy of synaptic terminations arising from a given input system (i.e., the numbers and spatial distribution of terminals on the extended motoneuron membrane) and with the characteristics of the individual terminals (i.e., the average amount of transmitter substance liberated). Not listed in Table 4 are *1*) the nature of the presynaptic transmitter and *2*) the characteristics of the associated postsynaptic receptors and transmembrane ionic balances, all of which control the polarity (i.e., excitatory or inhibitory) of the resulting PSPs.

The 10-fold range in group Ia EPSPs observed in the cat MG motor unit pool [Fig. 21; (101, 102, 118)] provides a useful example of the interaction between pre- and postsynaptic factors controlling PSP amplitude. The available evidence suggests that group Ia synapses are widely distributed over the entire receptive membrane of α-motoneurons with, perhaps, some dendritic predominance of input in those cells with the larger Ia EPSPs (Fig. 12 in ref. 101; see ref. 114 for further discussion). There is, in addition, little systematic difference between the MG motoneuron types in electrotonic architecture (subsection *Electrophysiological Properties Intrinsic to Motoneurons*, p. 379). Therefore the factors in the bottom row of Table 4 are probably not major sources of the observed range in group Ia synaptic efficacy (see also ref. 742).

The situation with Ia input sufficiently approximates the simple case of spherical neurons (see ref. 103) so that the steady-state voltage change, V, produced by a theoretical step change in conductance from Ia synapses would vary as

$$V \sim r_m \times (G_s \times N/A) \times (V_m - E_s) \qquad (5)$$

where the terms are defined in Table 4 (101, 103). There is no evidence for systematic variation in r_m or V_m in relation to motor unit type or motoneuron size (subsection *Electrophysiological Properties Intrinsic to Motoneurons*, p. 379; Table 3) and no evidence that the Ia EPSP driving potential, E_s, differs in different units. Therefore it appears likely that the variation in group Ia EPSP amplitudes in cat motoneurons can be attributed largely to equivalent variation in either the individual synaptic conductance, G_s, or in the synaptic density, N/A, of group Ia-terminals (101, 103, 124, 697, 742). In principle the role of synaptic density should be resolved by direct anatomical studies of group Ia-synaptic contacts on α-motoneurons of identified unit type (see ref. 124). Since the spatial distribution of the inhibitory terminals of group Ia inhibitory interneurons is also evidently restricted to regions on and near the motoneuron soma (107, 177), the same reasoning can be applied to explain the correlation between Ia IPSP amplitudes and motor unit type [(117, 118); subsection GROUP Ia SYNAPTIC EFFICACY, p. 381].

In view of the importance that has been attributed to motoneuron size in governing the effects of synaptic action and firing probability in motoneurons (see, e.g., refs. 179, 359, 363, 364), it seems important to note that motoneuron size (A_N) appears in Table 4 and Equation 5 as the denominator of the synaptic density term. Although there is a correlation between R_N and Ia EPSP amplitudes when the full range of motor units is considered [Fig. 23; (101, 102)], this is much weaker within either the F or S unit group alone, even though within each group there is a large variation in EPSP amplitudes. Furthermore the average amplitudes of Ia EPSPs in type S and type FR motoneurons are rather similar (see Fig. 21), although other indexes all suggest that FR motoneurons are, on the average, larger than type S (subsection *Motoneuron Anatomy in Relation to Unit Type*, p. 377, and *Electrophysiological Properties Intrinsic to Motoneurons*, p. 379). These observations emphasize the fact that the size and associated input resistance of postsynaptic motoneurons are important to synaptic efficacy only as they interact with the spatial organization, density, and conductance characteristics of the synaptic system under consideration.

INTRINSIC MEMBRANE PROPERTIES. Although it seems likely that relative synaptic efficacy is the key factor that controls functional "threshold grades" and motor unit recruitment patterns (subsection *Motor Unit Recruitment*, p. 386), some intrinsic motoneuron

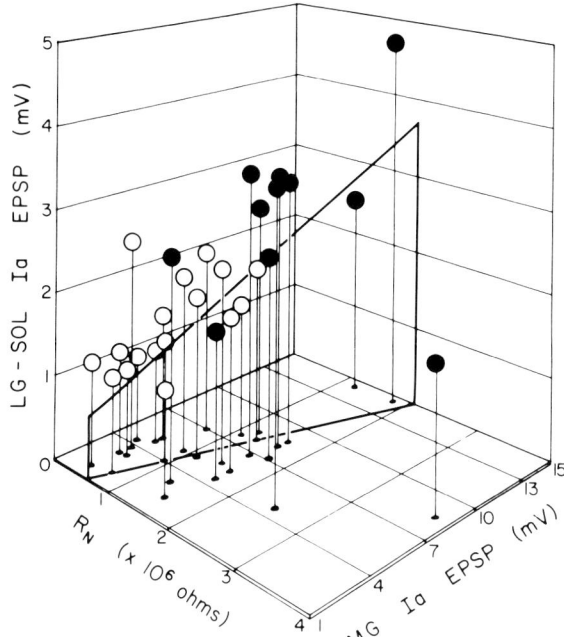

FIG. 23. Three-dimensional diagram showing interrelation between motoneuron input resistance (R_N) and maximum amplitudes of homonymous (MG) and heteronymous (LG-SOL) group Ia EPSPs in a sample of MG motoneurons. *Open circles* denote type F units; *filled circles* denote type S units. *Trapezoid* drawn through data points indicates least-squares fit to data. Although all 3 variables display positive correlations, that between MG and LG-SOL EPSP amplitudes is much stronger ($r = 0.64$) than the correlation between either set of EPSP data and R_N (0.44 and 0.40, respectively). If the F and S groups are considered separately, there is little correlation between R_N and EPSP amplitude, whereas that between the EPSP amplitudes themselves remains evident. The dissociation between EPSP size and R_N suggests that input resistance per se is not a critical factor in regulating synaptic efficacy in this system. [From data of Burke (101).]

properties not listed in Table 4 may also play a role. As noted in subsection *Electrophysiological Properties Intrinsic to Motoneurons* (p. 379), the presence of accommodation and of significant voltage-dependent inward currents are both likely to vary systematically with motor unit type. The former would tend to reduce the excitability of fast-twitch units during long-lasting excitatory input, while the latter would tend to increase it for the slow-twitch units. A quantitative assessment of the role of these factors is not possible with the data available.

Other factors may be mentioned for completeness, although there is little evidence for a systematic variation in any of them in relation to unit type or excitability profiles within motor pools. If the absolute voltage threshold required for spike initiation were systematically different among motoneurons, then the same depolarization level would produce firing in some cells and not in others. Recent data indicate that such threshold variations are not correlated with unit type or its related features (560). Graded excitability could also in principle be due to systematic variations in the true resting membrane potential i.e., the point at which synaptic effects begin their march toward the spike-threshold voltage), but there is no evidence for this among the very incomplete existing data. It is intuitively obvious that small, high-resistance neurons should require less transmembrane current to reach spike threshold than large cells. This has been demonstrated experimentally (415), but it is exactly this factor (i.e., synaptic current) that is controlled by the key interactions noted in Table 4. The weight of the evidence available at this time strongly suggests that the factors that control the excitability profile in a motor unit pool are those related to synaptic efficacy, with a relatively minor role for the intrinsic characteristics of motoneuron membranes. There is little evidence for the existence of truly distinct "tonic" and "phasic" groups of α-motoneurons (305, 306; cf. ref. 357) on the basis of intrinsic neuronal properties.

CONTROL OF MUSCULAR ACTION: RECRUITMENT AND RATE MODULATION

The level of activity in a given muscle (i.e., force and/or work output) is controlled in two ways: *1*) by varying the number and identity of motor units active at any moment (recruitment and derecruitment of motor units with particular characteristics) and *2*) by varying the rate and pattern of motoneuron firing, with resultant modulation of mechanical output from the muscle unit. The concept of recruitment was introduced by Sherrington [(455); see also p. 71 in ref. 303], and its relation to fast and slow muscle action was systematically examined by Denny-Brown (183) in Sherrington's laboratory. The role of firing-rate modulation in motor control has a similarly distinguished pedigree, having been emphasized in classic single-unit recording experiments of Adrian and Bronk (1).

The relative importance of either mechanism at low- versus high-output levels probably depends importantly on the detailed organization of the particular motor unit pool under study (see subsection *Recruitment or Rate and Pattern Modulation?* on p. 402), but the available evidence suggests that, in general, both mechanisms operate over the entire range of output control in heterogeneous motor unit pools. This discussion focuses on *1*) description of the recruitment process and its relation to motor unit type (cf. the chapter by Henneman and Mendell in this *Handbook*) and *2*) consideration of the effects of variations in the rate and pattern of motoneuron firing on muscle unit output (cf. the chapter by Partridge and Benton in this *Handbook*). The present discussion is oversimplified in terms of muscular action in behaviorally significant movements such as locomotion (e.g., see refs. 514, 679), but it is representative of the level of motor unit analysis possible with available technology. Current conceptual models of animals in motion (e.g., ref. 489) utilize different sorts of simplifications.

Motor Unit Recruitment

In a classic paper published in 1929, Denny-Brown (183) showed that motor units in the slow-twitch, red SOL muscle were more readily recruited into stretch and crossed-extension reflexes than the units in the faster, paler synergist gastrocnemii. He described (p. 294–295 in ref. 183) a hierarchy of functional "threshold grades," such that "units of lowest threshold grade are present in the red slow extensors and . . . the units of highest threshold are confined almost exclusively to the pale muscles." Denny-Brown suggested that the grading of functional thresholds is due to a corresponding scaling of excitatory and inhibitory synaptic efficacy, which is also related to muscle unit characteristics in a stable and predictable way. The term threshold grade is essentially the same as the "excitability" of a given motoneuron as measured relative to the other cells in the same motor pool under a particular set of conditions. The threshold grade reflects the level of synaptic drive required to fire the motoneuron and is thus quite different from the true voltage threshold for spike initiation discussed in subsection INTRINSIC MEMBRANE PROPERTIES, p. 384.

RECRUITMENT PATTERNS AND MOTOR UNIT TYPES. Evaluation of relative threshold grades and recruitment patterns in a given motor unit population requires some way to "label" individual units in order to recognize their activity patterns in experimental records and to establish their positions in the organizational hierarchy of the pool. Ideally one would like to be able to map the hierarchy of functional thresholds onto a multidimensional distribution of motor unit characteristics like that subsumed under the rubric of motor unit "types" (e.g., Figs. 5 and 21). This sort of complete picture has yet to be attained, but there is sufficient indirect evidence from animal and human experiments to indicate the general correlation between functional thresholds and unit types.

Studies of motor unit recruitment during voluntary activation in humans have used EMG techniques to follow the activity of single muscle units, where the amplitude and shape of the unit's EMG potential is its label. This EMG "signature" depends on a complex interplay between technical factors (electrode design, placement, and mechanical stability) and muscle unit anatomy (such as innervation ratio, fiber diameter, spatial density of unit fibers; see, e.g., refs. 91, 420, 648), which limits the interpretation of EMG potentials with respect to other muscle unit characteristics. Spike-triggered averaging of muscle unit force (STA; see subsection *Motor Units in Human Muscle*, p. 359) offers an added set of identifying labels (twitch force and contraction time; Fig. 24), but this also depends ultimately on the reliability of the EMG signature.

Recruitment studies in animals can use unit labels that refer to properties of motoneurons, including the amplitude of extracellular motor axon spike potentials (e.g., refs. 252, 305, 306, 358, 363, 364) or the axonal conduction velocity measured directly (e.g., refs. 142, 405; see also ref. 268) or indirectly (139). The interpretation of these data is hampered by variable strength in the correlations between conduction velocity and other unit characteristics (see *Motor Unit Types: Physiological Profiles in Experimental Animals*, p. 351, and *Electrophysiological Properties Intrinsic to Motoneurons*, p. 379). A few studies have attempted to examine firing patterns of individual motor units under conditions that permit direct identification of muscle unit type. These studies used recording and stimulation methods applied either to the innervating motoneuron (102) or to the motor axon in continuity (248, 249, 369). Although the intracellular method permits the most complete characterization of individual motor units (subsection A WORD ABOUT METHODOLOGY, p. 352), it has the disadvantage that even minimal damage to the motoneuron can result in altered functional threshold (e.g., ref. 138). The axon-in-continuity techniques, while technically demanding, appear most promising to provide reliable direct data about threshold-unit type relations.

As discussed in detail in the chapter by Henneman and Mendell in this *Handbook*, the overwhelming majority of systematic studies of motor unit recruitment in both human and animal muscle indicate that under many conditions the ordering of functional thresholds and consequent recruitment is more or less stereotyped and repeatable. The lowest threshold, first-recruited units tend to produce small EMG potentials (e.g., refs. 185, 187, 252, 338, 437, 524, 535, 549), with small twitch forces and slow contraction times (Fig. 24; e.g., refs. 92, 191, 317, 501, 509). Low-threshold units predominate in the deeper portions of the human biceps brachii (136), where histochemical type I muscle fibers predominate (394). The axons of the lowest threshold α-motoneurons have relatively small extracellular spike potentials (305, 358, 359) and slow conduction velocities (139, 268), and the motoneurons themselves tend to exhibit relatively high input resistance (R_N; see subsection *Electrophysiological Properties Intrinsic to Motoneurons*, p. 379) and large amplitude group Ia EPSPs [(102); see subsection GROUP Ia SYNAPTIC EFFICACY, p. 381]. These observations combine to clearly indicate that the lowest threshold motor units in heterogeneous populations are the slow-twitch type S, or their equivalent, as implied by Denny-Brown's early results (183).

Denny-Brown's conclusion (183) that the units of highest functional threshold should be those with the fastest contraction has also been confirmed by recent

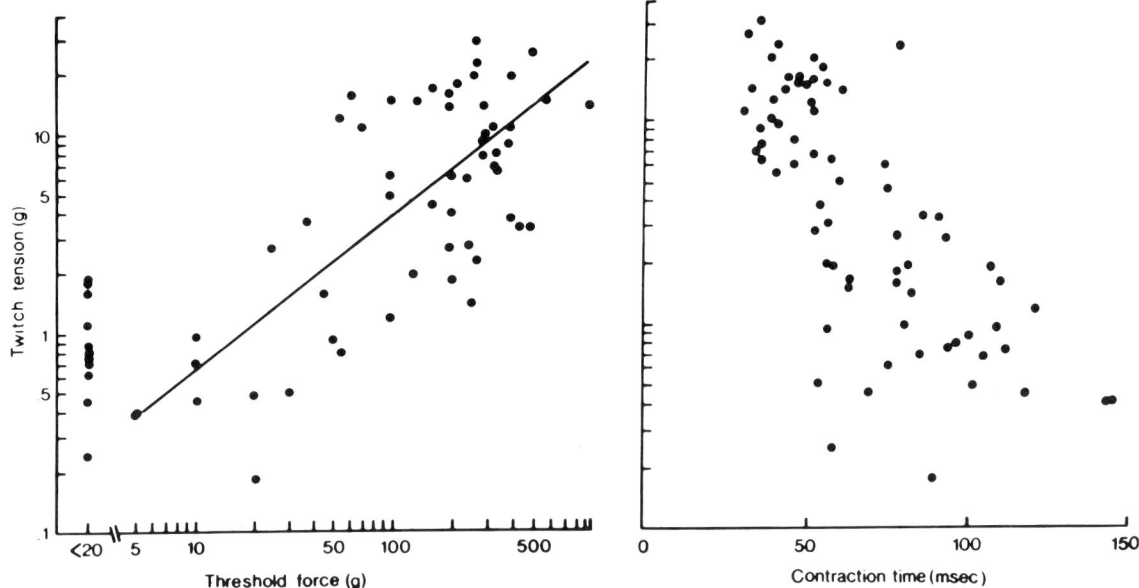

FIG. 24. Relations between muscle unit mechanical properties, obtained by spike-triggered averaging method)see subsection *Motor Units in Human Muscle*, p. 359), and functional thresholds of their motoneurons in a human hand muscle (first dorsal interosseous). The ordinate for both graphs is the "twitch" force, which is positively correlated with the voluntary threshold force required for steady firing (*left graph*) and negatively correlated with twitch contraction time (*right graph*). *Points plotted in < 20 column on left graph* all had force thresholds less than 20 g but were not more precisely characterized. Comparison of the 2 graphs indicates that motor units with lowest voluntary thresholds tend to produce small individual forces, and many have slow contraction as well. The highest threshold units all tend to have both rapid contraction and large force output. [Adapted from Stephens and Usherwood (664).]

studies using the STA method [Fig. 24; (191, 501, 664)]. In the decerebrate cat, the units with highest threshold during stretch reflexes are the type F units with relatively large force output (102), which almost certainly correspond to the type FF (fast twitch, fatigable) units found in that population (subsection MOTOR UNIT POPULATION OF CAT MEDIAL GASTROCNEMIUS MUSCLE, p. 353). The extremes of the recruitment spectrum are thus rather clearly defined regarding unit type and all that implies. The problem arises in defining the rest of the spectrum; this involves looking at the entire recruitment process in detail.

There is a rather strong direct correlation between functional threshold and mechanical force output among individual motor units in human hand and arm muscles throughout the recruitment range [Fig. 24; (190, 501, 509, 510, 644)], which remains the same in both slow and rapid movements (93, 191, 192, 323). In the decerebrate cat, relatively small force type F units with large group Ia EPSPs (most of them probably type FR; see Fig. 21) exhibit low-threshold behavior during stretch reflexes (102). Harris and Henneman (353) have recently shown that the low-threshold (up to 8% of full pool recruitment) motoneurons in the cat plantaris pool exhibit a roughly bimodal distribution of preferred firing frequencies, which is consistent with the view that both fast- (i.e., type FR) and slow- (i.e.,

type S) twitch units can have relatively low reflex thresholds.

Faden and Zajac (248, 249) have examined directly the relation between motor unit type and threshold hierarchy in the cat plantaris (PL) motor unit pool during electrically evoked and stretch-evoked monosynaptic reflexes in type-identified units. They compared reflex thresholds for pairs of PL units either directly or using critical firing level measurements (see the chapter by Henneman and Mendell in this *Handbook*) by isolating PL axons for recording and stimulation in ventral root filaments in continuity. This method permitted them to compare reflex thresholds with directly measured axonal conduction velocity and with muscle unit properties without damage to the motoneuron. When the units compared were of different types, the observed reflex thresholds were invariably (21/21 pairs) in the following sequence: S < FR < F(int) < FF. Similarly, when compared with respect to muscle unit tetanic force output, the unit with the lower functional threshold always exhibited the smaller tetanic tension (42/42 comparisons). In contrast, the correlation between reflex threshold and axonal conduction velocity was less strong, in that the unit with the lower threshold had the slower conduction velocity only in about 71% of the pairs (30/42 comparisons). With only one exception, the units with discordant scaling of thresholds versus axonal conduction velocities occurred among the fast-twitch units, which in the MG pool (e.g., Fig. 21) exhibit a narrow range of conduction velocities with complete overlap between FF and FR groups. If the interrelations between motor unit type, tetanic tension, and group Ia synaptic efficacy are similar in the PL and MG unit pools (Fig. 21), as seems likely, then the scaling of reflex thresholds among PL units would match the general scaling of Ia synaptic efficacy, as it does in the MG pool (102). This would provide additional evidence that group Ia synaptic efficacy is a major factor that determines the scaling of functional thresholds during stretch or electrically evoked group Ia reflexes, as discussed in subsection *Control of Motoneuron Excitability: Interactive Factors* (p. 383).

The evidence discussed thus far is compatible with the view that motor units in heterogeneous muscles are recruited in a sequence related to motor unit type: S → FR → FF. Additional supportive evidence comes from studies in human subjects in whom the pattern of histochemical fiber type "usage" has been inferred from the relative depletion of intrafiber glycogen during exercise of different intensities (e.g., refs. 167, 294, 295). The susceptibility to glycogen depletion varies among the different fiber types (see subsection FATIGABILITY AND METABOLIC PROFILES, p. 358), and the results of such studies must be interpreted with some caution (see ref. 106). Nevertheless low-to-moderate levels of sustained work output (< 35% of maximum, measured by mechanical output or oxygen uptake indexes) produce glycogen loss primarily in the type I muscle fibers that are ordinarily difficult to deplete, suggesting that the equivalent type S motor units are the ones primarily activated (295). This occurs even when the activity is prolonged to exhaustion (167), implying that higher threshold units are not brought into play under the tested conditions. Increasing the level of work output produces progressive glycogen loss in type II fibers, as well as in type I fibers. During isometric contractions, glycogen loss is mainly in type I fibers at force levels < 20% of maximum voluntary contraction (MVC) but almost exclusively in type II fibers after short bouts of exhausting contractions > 20% of maximum voluntary contraction (294).

The patterns of glycogen depletion in animal muscles during exhaustive running or swimming are similar (i.e., type I fibers are depleted first), and glycogen loss at moderate levels of work output begins among the type IIA fibers (equivalent to the type FR motor units) and progresses pari passu with increasing output to include increasing depletion among IIB fibers (18, 19, 37, 281, 456, 668). The IIA → IIB pattern of glycogen loss implies increasing reliance on the more anaerobic muscle units with increasing speed of locomotion (281, 668), but there are also intriguing discontinuities in the depletion pattern at points of gait transitions from run to gallop (668) that may reflect changing mechanical efficiency (133, 679). In the prosimian *Galago*, hindlimb muscle fibers exhibit greater glycogen depletion among type IIA than among type IIB fibers after treadmill running, but a reverse pattern is evident if the animals are made to hop or jump (133). Depletion in IIB fibers (equivalent to type FF units in the cat) indicates that these must certainly be activated during jumping, but this does not necessarily imply that FF units are selectively recruited. Rather such actions may simply not be sufficiently sustained to produce type I (or even IIA) depletion even though S and FR motor units also participate (see ref. 106 for discussion).

The patterns of glycogen depletion in different muscle fiber types during dynamic exercise suggests that motor units equivalent to type S are the ones first brought into play in normal voluntary movements that require small force or work outputs, but that these are closely followed by recruitment among the fatigue-resistant type FR units. The latter clearly seems to be functionally important, since running at moderate speeds can be sustained for long periods. In cat ankle extensor muscles, the peak force outputs observed during moderate speed running are such that they could be sustained by the available type S and FR motor units (708; see below). The fatigue-sensitive FF units (or their equivalents) seem to be reserved for high-force quick movements, such as jumping, that are not sustained. It should be noted that the suggested patterns of motor unit usage also fit very well with the metabolic adaptations found in the various fiber types following chronic exercise demand of various kinds (subsection ALTERATIONS OF DEMAND WITHIN THE PHYSIOLOGICAL RANGE, p. 362).

Given sufficient information about the characteristics of individual motor units in a particular pool, the functional consequences of particular recruitment sequences can be explored semiquantitatively (e.g., refs. 31, 118, 732) if one assumes some "rule of recruitment" that can specify the order in which units are activated and deactivated. The feature chosen as the ordering "rule" should ideally be causal to threshold scaling (e.g., synaptic efficacy; see subsection *Control of Motoneuron Excitability: Interactive Factors*, p. 383), or should at least covary with the causal factors (e.g., axonal conduction velocity, motor unit type, muscle unit tetanic tension; see Fig. 21). Unfortunately, the only direct test of the match between synaptic efficacy (in this case, group Ia input) and threshold scaling (firing during stretch reflexes) of necessity used intracellular recording methods (102). This study is flawed by the lack of direct, simultaneous comparisons between different units and by the possibility that intracellular penetration changed the true functional threshold (138), although the results did demonstrate that susceptibility to stretch-evoked motoneuron discharge varied directly with the amplitude of composite group Ia EPSPs. Henneman and his colleagues have argued that an ascending scale of motoneuron size, as reflected by axonal conduction velocity, is a valid recruitment rule under many conditions [(137, 361, 363, 364); see the chapter by Henneman and Mendell in this *Handbook*]. The results of Faden and Zajac (249; see above), however, suggest that motor unit type or isometric tetanic tension are perhaps more accurate predictors of reflex recruitment than is axonal conduction velocity, particularly among fast-twitch motor units.

In all motor unit populations thus far examined adequately, axonal conduction velocity, tetanic tension, motor unit type, and group Ia EPSP amplitudes all exhibit significant covariation, and thus the threshold hierarchies that would be predicted by each of these recruitment rules would all be generally similar. Recruitment sequences arranged according to unit type (i.e., S → FR → F(int) → FF), tetanic tension, or group Ia EPSP amplitude would be mutually congruent throughout the whole unit population. Recruitment strictly according to increasing axonal conduction velocity would be less well organized among the fast-twitch units, since they exhibit in some populations a narrow range in CV with complete overlap between FF, F(int), and FR groups (Fig. 21). Nevertheless the functional consequences that were suggested by Henneman and Olson (361) to emerge from the original "size principle" are entirely consistent with the S → FR → F(int) → FF sequence, as they are with its theoretical advantages as recently discussed, for example, by Hatze (355). It should be noted, however, that a sequence based strictly on motor axon conduction velocity would be very well related to force output and contraction times among cat lumbrical units (see ref. 418) because of the close correlations among these properties in this population (Fig. 4).

It is an instructive and not altogether fanciful exercise to explore the consequences of a recruitment sequence based on the scaling of synaptic input efficacy, such as that of monosynaptic excitation from group Ia muscle spindle afferents. Although it is widely accepted that this relatively powerful sensory system is important to the control of many kinds of movements, the exact nature of its influence is a matter of considerable current debate (see the chapters by Houk and Rymer and by Matthews in this *Handbook*), and group Ia excitation is certainly not the only synaptic system relevant to motor control. Its use in constructing a "recruitment model" can be defended on two grounds: *1*) it is the only excitatory input system for which sufficient quantitative data is available, and *2*) the resulting threshold hierarchies are generally consistent with other data about recruitment sequences. Since Ia excitation is not the only relevant synaptic input system, the latter fact suggests that many other synaptic systems are probably similarly organized (see subsection *Organization of Synaptic Input*, p. 381).

In Figure 25 the sequence of functional thresholds in a large sample of cat MG motoneurons is assumed to vary inversely with the amplitude of homonymous

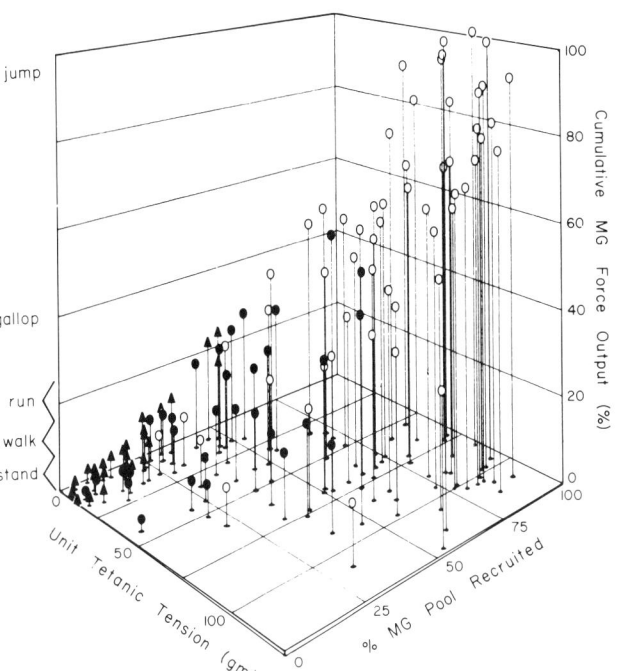

FIG. 25. A "recruitment model" for cat medial gastrocnemius (MG) motor pool using Ia EPSP amplitude as the "recruitment rule" to generate a sequential ordering of units. The MG motor units included in this 3-dimensional diagram are arrayed incrementally along the *right-hand* abscissa (% MG Pool Recruited) in strict accord with decreasing amplitude of the MG group Ia EPSP measured in each motoneuron (data from ref. 118; see also Fig. 21). The isometric tetanic force produced by each individual unit is plotted against the *left-hand* abscissa (Unit Tetanic Tension). *Vertical dimension* is cumulative isometric force that would be produced as each unit is recruited in sequence, expressed as percentage of total force (i.e., 100 %) expected from the entire MG muscle when all units are added together. *Filled symbols* indicate fatigue-resistant unit types, with types FR and F(int) indicated by *filled ovals* and type S units by *filled triangles*. Type FF units are indicated by *open ovals*. The ranges of forces actually produced by MG muscle in intact cats during standing, walking, running, and maximum vertical jumping are indicated along the *left-hand vertical* ordinate (data from ref. 707), expressed as percentage of maximum MG output during fused isometric tetani. When ordered according to Ia EPSP amplitude, the first-recruited half of the MG population consists almost entirely of fatigue-resistant units [types S, FR, and F(int)], which together produce only about 25% of the maximum force available from the MG unit population. See text for further discussion.

group Ia EPSPs. This recruitment model explores the consequences in terms of unit types, fatigue resistance, and individual unit force outputs (see also ref. 117). Motor units in the most readily activated quarter of the MG population are mostly type S, with great fatigue resistance but small individual force outputs (subsection *Motor Unit Types: Physiological Profiles in Experimental Animals*, p. 351). Since each unit adds only a small increment of force, the cumulative force generated by this most excitable 25% of the population is less than 10% of the total possible from the entire MG pool. Quadrupedal standing in the cat requires less than 10% of full isometric MG output as measured in situ in the intact animal [Fig. 25, left vertical ordinate; (707)]. Since the type S units in this easily recruited quarter of the pool should be energetically efficient in sustained quasi-isometric actions such as postural maintenance (see ref. 289), this quantitative correspondence is intuitively satisfying.

The units that would be recruited in the second quarter of the MG pool (i.e., 25%–50% recruitment) are primarily type FR, which are also relatively resistant to fatigue but produce larger individual forces than type S, so that incremental force rises more rapidly than in the first quarter (see also Fig. 1 in ref. 31). The cumulative force that would be produced by linear summation of the isometric action of the first-recruited half of the MG pool would, in this model, come to about 25% of the maximum possible MG force. In the experiments of Walmsley, Hodgson, and Burke (707), treadmill locomotion ranging from slow walk to fast running requires 10%–25% of maximum MG force (Fig. 25, left ordinate). The advantage of fatigue resistance to an activity such as locomotion is obvious, but it also appears advantageous to have it performed by fast-contracting muscle fibers, which may become energetically more efficient during relatively rapid shortening movements (26, 289, 717). Since only moderate force levels are required, it again seems to make sense to grade these by addition and subtraction of units with moderate individual force outputs [(31); see also ref. 661]. The relatively small forces involved in locomotion may seem surprising, but it should be noted that efficiency in locomotion derives from body design and the recovery of kinetic energy by stretching active muscles (see ref. 133). The results of glycogen-depletion studies in exercising human subjects are entirely consistent with the quantitative predictions of this model.

The highest threshold half of the MG pool in this model consists almost exclusively of the relatively large force type FF units that produce a steep rise in incremental force as they are recruited. Because of the fatigability of FF units, it would be expected that MG forces greater than 25%–30% of maximum should occur in infrequent bursts and, indeed, they occur only during fast gallop and vertical jumping movements (707). Such movements occur only intermittently in cats, which are relatively sedentary predators.

The available evidence (see also *Motor Unit Types: Physiological Profiles in Experimental Animals*, p. 351, and section PHYSIOLOGY OF α-MOTONEURONS AND THEIR SYNAPTIC INPUTS IN RELATION TO MOTOR UNIT TYPE, p. 378) suggests that the organization of heterogeneous motor unit populations, from synaptic input to muscle unit output, is rather precisely matched to functional demands placed on them. For example, one may suppose that roughly 75% of the isometric force-generating capacity of the cat MG muscle resides in fatigable type FF units, because this normally sedentary predator requires such output forces only infrequently during hunting or escape behaviors. In contrast, the MG muscle of the striped skunk, *Mephitis*, contains neither type FF units nor fibers with the equivalent type IIB histochemical profile (701). The motor habits of the skunk (a wide-ranging, slow-moving scavenger without need to escape from predators) differ greatly from those of the cat and the organization of its MG motor unit pool seems appropriately different (701). In the same vein, Maxwell and co-workers (481) have shown that hindlimb muscles of dogs have greater total oxidative capacity by both biochemical and histochemical criteria than homologous muscles in the cat (and lion; see ref. 18), as befits the differences between the active versus sedentary habits of these carnivores. As information accumulates from such comparative studies, we may expect clarification of the reasons behind observed differences between muscles and animal species.

Precision and Stereotypy in Recruitment Process

While the process of motor unit recruitment is basically orderly under many conditions (see also the chapter by Henneman and Mendell in this *Handbook*), it is important to discuss whether the functional threshold grade of a given motoneuron is completely invariant under a variety of different conditions and whether major restructuring of the threshold hierarchy can occur under some conditions. If functional thresholds were precisely fixed in the motor pool hierarchy, irrespective of input source, then the efficacy of all synaptic input systems would have to be scaled precisely in parallel (subsection *Control of Motoneuron Excitability: Interactive Factors*, p. 383), which is inconsistent with the available evidence (subsection *Organization of Synaptic Input*, p. 381). Invariance of threshold grade would also imply that the exact identities of units active or inactive would be completely specified simply by the level of pool output (137, 363, 364, 492). Again, however, there is evidence that the fundamental order found in the recruitment process is neither completely precise nor stable but rather varies significantly with input source and with time, as do most other biological processes.

The early results of Denny-Brown (183) suggested that the hierarchy of functional thresholds indeed varies depending on the source of input drive [see subsection ARE MAJOR SHIFTS IN RECRUITMENT ORDER POSSIBLE? (p. 391)]. In the mid-1950s, Lloyd and McIntyre (459) showed that the probability of motoneuron firing (the "firing index") can be quite different when homonymous versus heteronymous monosynaptic reflex responses are compared in individual cells, and Wilson and Talbot (723) demonstrated differences in monosynaptic versus polysynaptic firing thresholds among flexor motoneurons. More recently, Kernell and Sjöholm (418) and Clamann and Kukulka (141) have described such threshold differences when comparing motoneuron responses to supraspinal versus dorsal root inputs. All of these results are compatible with the observation that the amplitudes of homonymous and heteronymous Ia-EPSPs are not perfectly correlated [see Fig. 23; (101, 118)], and the amplitudes of vestibulospinal and Ia monosynaptic EPSPs are poorly correlated in the same set of motoneurons (subsection MONOSYNAPTIC SUPRASPINAL INPUTS, p. 382). It seems fair to conclude that the threshold hierarchy and consequent recruitment order do vary with input source. This issue is discussed in more detail in subsection ARE MAJOR SHIFTS IN RECRUITMENT ORDER POSSIBLE? (p. 391).

It is also known that the firing probability for individual motoneurons in relation to the total motor pool responsiveness fluctuates over time despite an apparently constant input. Lloyd and McIntyre (458) demonstrated such fluctuations in monosynaptic reflex responses, a phenomenon due at least in part to presynaptic mechanisms (601, 602). Rall and Hunt (570) then showed that the functional threshold ("critical excitability level") for a given motoneuron can vary in a manner quite independent of the fluctuations in total pool response, implying the existence of underlying variations in the distribution of relevant synaptic drives to different cells within the pool. More recently, Rudomin and Madrid (603) have shown that the range of threshold fluctuations can be altered by experimental conditions or by conditioning input in synaptic systems that do not directly impinge on the test motor pool (see also ref. 601). The apparent divergence between these kinds of results and reports of precisely fixed and invariant threshold hierarchies probably depends in large measure on experimental design and on the sensitivity of the test systems used.

There is a divergence of opinion about whether functional thresholds are precisely fixed in human subjects (see also the chapter by Henneman and Mendell in this *Handbook*). A number of authors have reported that there is some degree of threshold flexibility during voluntary activation of individual motor units, permitting selective activation among units with relatively low thresholds (e.g., refs. 49, 354, 636, 675, 705). Person (548) has demonstrated greater variability in recruitment and derecruitment patterns among units in the rectus femoris muscle when voluntary movements are unconstrained than when they are more stereotyped (see also refs. 185, 705). Other studies, however, report essentially no flexibility in voluntary recruitment (362, 686) and attribute earlier findings to technical factors or to study of muscles with multiple functions (686).

In summary, the weight of existing evidence indicates that the scaling of functional thresholds and consequent ordering of motor unit recruitment is not precisely the same with different input drives, nor is it entirely stable over time. The degree of variability discussed thus far, however, is relatively minor and does not negate the existence of a fundamental order in the recruitment of motor units in a heterogeneous motor pool. The evidence for a general stability of functional threshold grades under many conditions is overwhelming, and the evidence supporting the idea that recruitment is closely related to motor unit type is also extensive, if not complete (subsection RECRUITMENT PATTERNS AND MOTOR UNIT TYPES, p. 386). Whether or not individual motor units can be selectively activated under voluntary control by human subjects, particularly when their relative thresholds are even modestly different, seems inconclusive at present and demands further careful evaluation.

ARE MAJOR SHIFTS IN RECRUITMENT ORDER POSSIBLE? Although what will be called the "usual" recruitment sequence holds in a great variety of situations, there are exceptions of sufficient magnitude to be termed "major" shifts or dislocations in the threshold hierarchy. These are of interest for what they imply about the organization of motor unit control by the CNS. Examples of major dislocations include *1*) exclusive recruitment of normally high-threshold units, *2*) an interchange in recruitability between units with very different thresholds, or *3*) simultaneous excitation of some motoneurons and inhibition of others within the same motor unit population.

Sherrington (629) introduced the idea of major shifts in *The Integrative Action of the Nervous System*, in which he postulated the existence of

> two separable systems of motor innervation ... controlling two sets of musculature ... the very muscles that to the observer are most obviously under excitation by the *tonic* system are those most obviously inhibited by the *phasic* reflex system. (From p. 302 of the 1947 reprint; emphasis in the original.)

Denny-Brown (183) extended this notion with his observation that tilting the head of a decerebrate cat could generate greater tension in the fast-twitch extensor heads than in the slow-twitch synergist SOL, a pattern opposite that seen in stretch reflexes. In the 1932 monograph *Reflex Activity of the Spinal Cord*, by Sherrington and his colleagues (170), there is a description of simultaneous excitation of the fast-twitch ankle extensors and inhibition of the slow-twitch SOL (again in the decerebrate cat; see p. 73–80 and their Fig. 37). These authors (p. 78 in ref. 170) concluded that

> there are two distinct types of ipselateral [sic] excitation in the hind limb, the one minimal in degree, widely distributed in areal source and affecting the pale, rapidly contracting gastrocnemius more than soleus, the other ... powerful and exciting the slowly contracting red soleus and having an areal source restricted to proximal nerves.

The notion of differential control of red and pale muscles (or of slow- and fast-twitch motor units) has received relatively little attention in the face of repeated reports of the usual recruitment order, perhaps partly because the conditions appropriate for a clear demonstration of differential control are not easily achieved. The whole muscle experiments of the Sherrington school do not, of course, necessarily imply that major shifts in thresholds are possible within a single motor unit pool, but evidence for this has come from more recent experiments in both animals and humans.

A number of polysynaptic and descending synaptic systems in animals appear to be organized in patterns different from that expected to produce the usual hierarchy of functional thresholds (POLYSYNAPTIC INPUT SYSTEMS, p. 382). In particular, cutaneous afferents from the skin of the foot and ankle (in the territory of the sural and saphenous nerves) produce facilitation of some ankle extensor motoneurons in the cat (339, 493, 597). Burke and co-workers (108, 117) found that this polysynaptic excitation was most pronounced in motoneurons innervating fast-twitch muscle units (see POLYSYNAPTIC INPUT SYSTEMS, p. 382, and Fig. 22). With this in mind, Kanda and co-workers (405) recently showed that low-threshold MG motoneurons (tentatively identified as type S on the basis of conduction velocity and excitability profiles) in the decerebrate cat, given a background of excitation by stretch or tonic vibration reflexes, can be inhibited by stimulation of ankle skin at the same time that much higher threshold motoneurons (presumably type F) are powerfully excited (Fig. 26A).

Cutaneous inputs in humans can also alter threshold hierarchies (see ref. 337). Very recent human studies by Stephens and colleagues (660) have demonstrated

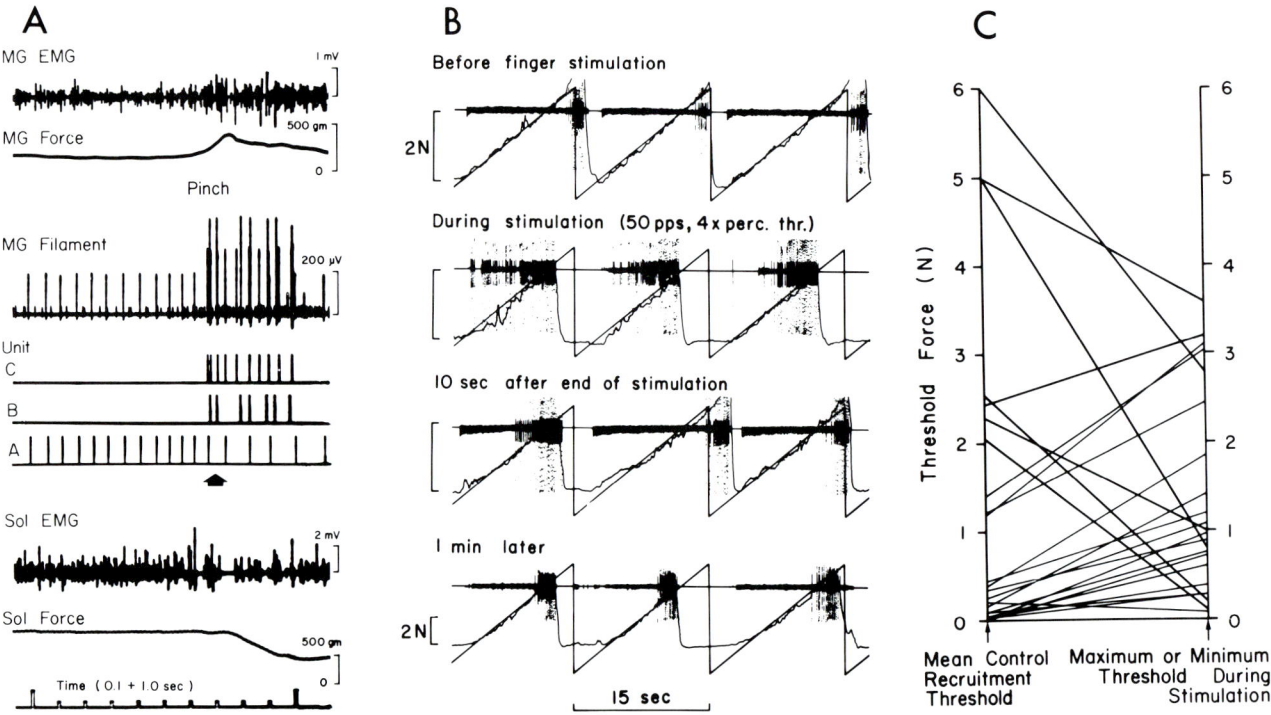

FIG. 26. Examples of differential modulation of functional thresholds of motor units within the same pool. A: motor axons recorded in a fine filament of the medial gastrocnemius (MG) muscle nerve during tonic vibration reflex (decerebrate cat). One α-motoneuron axon (unit A, conduction velocity about 73 m/s) showed low-threshold firing to stretch and vibration but was slowed (i.e., inhibited) by a light pinch to the ipsilateral ankle at the same time that 2 other MG axons with much higher functional thresholds (B and C, conduction velocities 79 and 85 m/s, respectively; both unresponsive to stretch and tendon vibration) were excited to discharge. The whole soleus (SOL) muscle (*lower traces*) was inhibited at the same time as MG unit A. B: EMG recordings of 2 motor units in human first dorsal interosseous (1st DI) muscle (*upper traces*) during isometric ramp contractions (*lower traces, irregular line*) in which subject repeatedly tracks a ramp force target (regular sawtooth). Note small EMG spike of low-threshold unit (A) and larger spike of much higher threshold unit (B) in *top set of traces*. *Second set of traces*, during delivery of continuous electrical stimuli (50 pulse/s at strength 4 times perceptible threshold) to the index finger skin, show that the force threshold for unit B decreased whereas that of A increased, so that B occasionally fired before A. After skin stimulation ended (*lower sets of traces*), relative thresholds of units A and B returned slowly to control values. Force calibration is 2 N for all records. C: graph of voluntary force thresholds for 1st DI units before (*left* ordinate, mean values) and during skin stimulation (*right* ordinate, maximum or minimum values, depending on trend of overall change), from experiments as in B. Skin stimulation raised thresholds for most low-threshold units and decreased them in high-threshold units, resulting in an overall narrowing of the threshold differences. Simultaneous enhancement of excitability in some units and depression of others within the same motor unit population can be regarded as a major change in the pattern of functional thresholds. [A from Kanda, Burke, and Walmsley (405); B and C from J. A. Stephens, unpublished data (see ref. 660).]

differential effects of local skin stimulation on the thresholds for voluntary activation among motor units in the first dorsal interosseous muscle (1st DI). Threshold forces for unit recruitment were determined without stimulation and then during continuous application of electrical stimuli to the index finger at nonnoxious intensities (Fig. 26B). In most cases studied, the force threshold for voluntary recruitment of the low-threshold units slowly increased and that for high-threshold units decreased (Fig. 26C). At least some of these threshold dislocations were clearly of a major order (J. A. Stephens, personal communication). Rather similar threshold changes (increasing for low threshold and vice versa) have recently been reported for human knee extensor motor units during the shivering response to skin cooling (478a; see also ref. 730a).

Grimby and Hannerz have published a series of papers (e.g., refs. 312–315) in which variable recruitment patterns of human motor units were found when one or another set of conditions was changed. Basmajian and co-workers (666) have reported that voluntary "isolation" of individual motor units in human muscle involves an apparent inhibition of neighboring units. Unfortunately none of these reports included data on the relative thresholds of the units being compared, so it is difficult to judge whether truly major dislocations occurred (see discussion in ref. 359). In a recent paper (316), however, Grimby and Hannerz showed rather clearly that some high-threshold motor units in the short toe extensor muscle (EDB) could be recruited in isolation, without low-threshold units, when the requested movement was a very rapid activation of a previously relaxed EDB. These high-threshold, intermittently firing units tend to have faster axonal conduction velocities than the lower threshold units that tend to fire continuously at low frequencies (70). At about the same time, Desmedt and Godaux (190, 191) denied the existence of preferential activation of high-threshold units during very rapid, or "ballistic," contractions of the human tibialis anterior (see also refs. 93, 192). These conflicting results are perhaps best reconciled by postulating that voluntary activation of human motor units is produced by synaptic systems very powerfully biased to produce the usual pattern of recruitment but that under exceptional conditions the synaptic balance is such that it permits selective activation of ordinarily high-threshold units.

In summary, the evidence available indicates that major dislocations in the ordering of threshold grades within individual motor unit pools does occur under some conditions in both animals and humans. Such reordering clearly implies corresponding differences in the organization of the relevant synaptic inputs to the pool, since major shifts would not be possible if all inputs were distributed in even approximately parallel organizations (see also subsection *Organization of Synaptic Input*, p. 381). At least two quite different patterns of input organization are necessary to produce the observed results (see ref. 405).

One possible scheme is shown in the diagram in Figure 27, which is based on data from the cat. Many input systems, including Ia excitation and other systems similarly distributed (subsection GROUP Ia SYNAPTIC EFFICACY, p. 381), appear to be scaled as indicated by the width of stippled arrows on the left in Figure 27. In contrast, the input from the polysynaptic excitatory pathway from distal skin (subsection POLYSYNAPTIC INPUT SYSTEMS, p. 382) appears to be distributed roughly as indicated by the dashed arrows on the right, at least for purposes of argument. Activation of the motor unit pool represented by the cells A through D would follow the usual order when the input drive is dominated by systems on the left to produce the orderly recruitment and derecruitment sequences diagrammed at the top of Figure 27. Input dominated by excitation distributed in the reverse

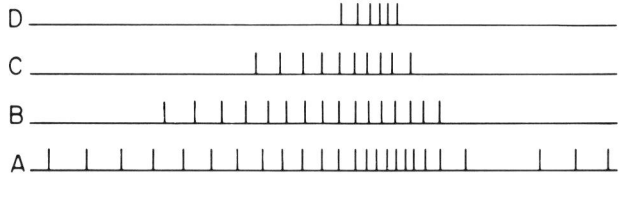

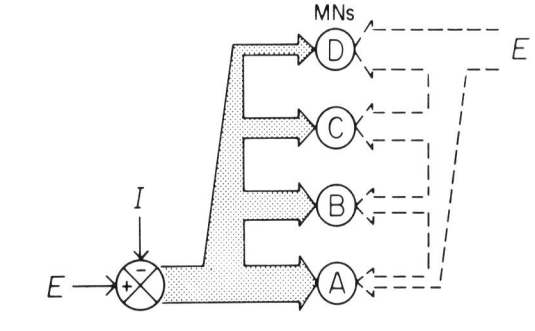

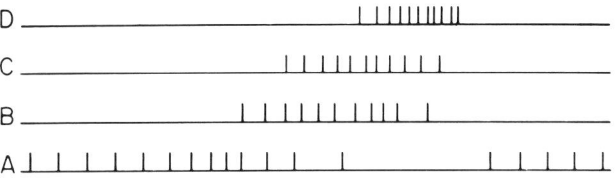

FIG. 27. Diagram of a recruitment model in which functional thresholds of motoneurons (MNs, labeled *A–D*) are controlled by the efficacy of synaptic input to them, represented by *width* of *arrows*. Synaptic input [including both excitatory (*E*) and inhibitory (*I*) effects] organized to produce the gradation of efficacy indicated by *stippled arrows* should produce recruitment and derecruitment sequences like those shown in the *upper* set of spike diagrams. Addition of an input with the reverse organization, as indicated by *dashed arrows*, could produce dislocations as shown in *lower* set of spike diagrams (as in Fig. 26). See text for further discussion. [From Kanda, Burke, and Walmsley (405).]

pattern (as on the right) could, in principle, produce preferential activation of the normally high-threshold motoneurons. Simultaneous synaptic drive distributed according to both input patterns (including some fraction of inhibition from the left) would be expected to produce complex firing patterns as diagrammed at the bottom of Figure 27, as have in fact been observed experimentally (405). In effect, simultaneous excitatory input via the opposite organizations would narrow the difference between high- and low-threshold units (Fig. 26C), perhaps to promote synchronous activation of the entire population such as must occur in maximal output actions like jumping or galloping (708). It is of interest to note that the same effect would be produced if, as discussed in subsection GROUP Ia SYNAPTIC EFFICACY, p. 381, there exists a preferential recurrent inhibition from high-threshold to low-threshold α-motoneurons. A compression of the usual threshold range might be advantageous, particularly in nonstereotyped movements requiring quick response and wide dynamic range.

To summarize this subsection, there is little evidence to support Sherrington's notion of truly separate tonic and phasic motor systems in the strict sense of those terms, since all movements include both elements. However, it is not too far from Sherrington's idea to suggest that stereotyped and rhythmic movements like locomotion may involve largely "hard-wired" motor programs (see the chapter by Grillner in this *Handbook*) that, for intuitively satisfying reasons of functional and metabolic economy (see subsections TWITCH-CONTRACTION TIMES AND MYOFIBRILLAR ATPASE, p. 355; FATIGABILITY AND METABOLIC PROFILES, p. 358; and RECRUITMENT PATTERNS AND MOTOR UNIT TYPES, p. 386), produce the usual [i.e., S → FR → F(int) → FF] recruitment sequence. Conversely, nonstereotyped "facultative" movements might well utilize other neural organizations to bypass the constraints inherent in the hard-wired networks in order to optimize mechanical effectiveness, as, for example, in rapid, forceful alternating movements, where more or less selective activation of rapidly contracting muscle units would permit fast relaxation as well as contraction (636a). Finally, as suggested above, both systems could act in concert to promote synchronous activation of the motor unit pool.

Output Modulation by Rate and Pattern of Motoneuron Firing

The classic studies of motoneuron discharge by Adrian and Bronk (1) stressed the role of firing frequency in the control of motor output, whereas Sherrington and his colleagues (subsection *Motor Unit Recruitment*, p. 386) stressed the recruitment mechanism. It is now clear, after a great deal of systematic investigation, that both mechanisms are important to the control of total muscle output and that they are interrelated. It is likely, however, that the range of modulation due to the rate and pattern of motoneuron firing varies from one motor pool to another, with narrower ranges characteristic of muscles rich in slow-twitch fibers [(192, 310, 311); see also ref. 418]. This section attempts to make several general points: *1*) the ranges of steady motoneuron firing frequencies are often (but not always) related to the properties of the innervated muscle units and to the functional nature of the parent muscle, *2*) the patterns of firing in a given motor axon (i.e., the sequence of interspike intervals making up the short-term time history of activations) have an effect on muscle unit output at least as significant as that of the average firing rate, and *3*) the long-term time history of muscle unit activation also modulates output significantly by mechanisms with persistent effects (postactivation potentiation and fatigue).

MOTONEURON FIRING CHARACTERISTICS. Virtually all studies to date agree that α-motoneurons of animals and humans tend to fire steadily at relatively slow rates (minimum rates of 6–12 pulses/s) when activated near their functional thresholds (see Fig. 28). Maximum rates during sustained firing are much more variable, depending on animal species, muscle, and experimental conditions; these rates can range from about 15 to over 50 pulses/s in steady voluntary contractions in humans, depending on the muscle (see Fig. 28; see also, e.g., refs. 61, 136, 189, 268, 338, 349, 502, 510, 524, 549, 676). Similar ranges have been found in animals for motor units firing under reflex drive (e.g., refs. 102, 183, 733) or during fictive locomotion (624, 635, 740). The firing rate of extraocular motoneurons can, in contrast, be much higher (e.g., ref. 43), in keeping with the rapid contraction characteristics of their muscle units (e.g., ref. 288).

The tendency for motoneurons to fire repetitively at low rates when activated by presumably steady, just-suprathreshold drive may well be explained by the relatively long duration of the spike afterpotentials (subsection *Electrophysiological Properties Intrinsic to Motoneurons*, p. 379) that include a late depolarizing component that increases firing probability at long intervals (see also ref. 114). Maximum firing rates are constrained mainly by the duration of the AHP, which reduces the probability of cell firing at relatively short intervals (see refs. 324, 414). The importance of the AHP mechanism to frequency control is further evident in the tendency toward a negative correlation between serial interspike intervals (549), probably produced by the negative serial dependence of AHP conductance on the immediately preceding interval (324, 385). Given this evidence, it is not surprising that motoneurons of slow-twitch units, with relatively long AHPs (subsection *Electrophysiological Properties Intrinsic to Motoneurons*, p. 379), tend to fire more slowly on the average than fast-twitch cells (e.g., refs. 102, 183, 302, 310, 311, 512). Average firing rates are considered important in the development and maintenance of fast- versus slow-twitch muscle units (sub-

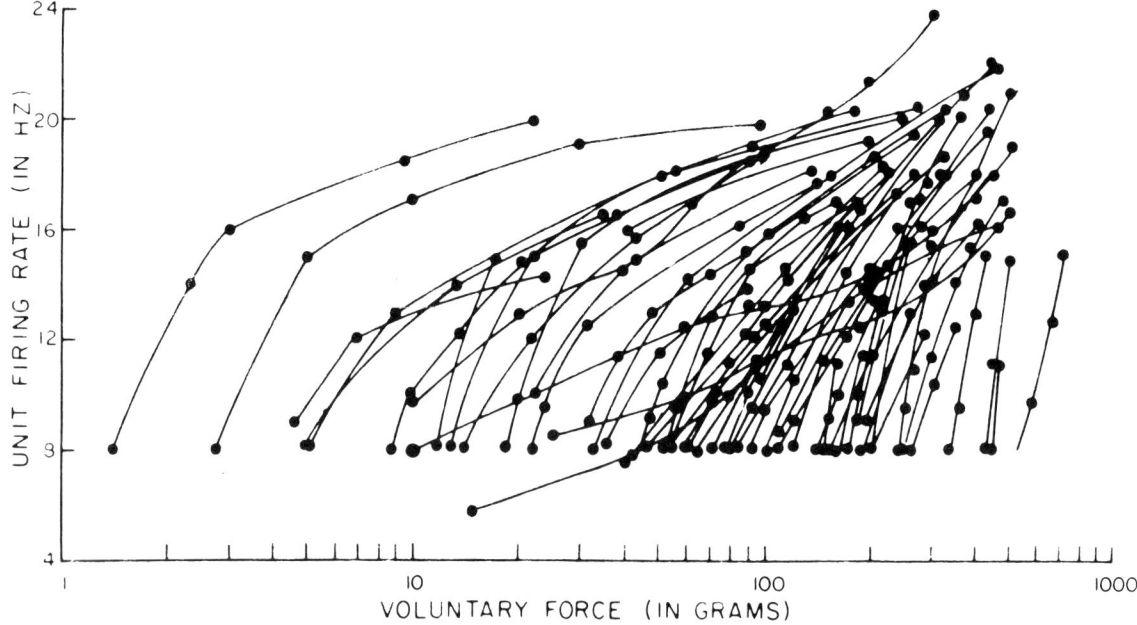

FIG. 28. Steady firing frequencies (ordinate) observed for individual motor units in human extensor digitorum communis muscle, recorded throughout a wide range of voluntary forces (abscissa). Note that virtually all units begin firing at about the same steady rate (8 Hz) and increase in rate to 16–24 Hz as total force output increases. Note also that highest threshold units display smallest range of variation but have high-force frequency slopes. [Adapted from Monster and Chan (510).]

section NONPHYSIOLOGICAL ALTERATIONS, p. 363). There is a paradox evident in studies of human muscle, however, in that the units that display the largest total range of steady firing frequencies are almost invariably the low-threshold units (presumably slow twitch; e.g., refs. 136, 268, 548), and maximum frequencies within heterogeneous unit populations are much the same in all units throughout the entire range of steady voluntary contraction [e.g., Fig. 28; (502, 510)]. However, it is true that for any given force level, the slope of the curve relating firing rate to force output is linearly related to measures of muscle unit size and threshold, such that high-threshold units display greater local changes in firing rate than low-threshold units (509).

In addition to steady motoneuron firing, many normal movements involve short trains with few spikes, such as those that occur during locomotion (e.g., refs. 624, 635, 740) or other repetitive movements (e.g., ref. 323) or at the onset of rapid movements (192, 322). Under these conditions, "instantaneous" maximum firing rates (the reciprocal of individual interspike intervals) can be very high (intervals of 8–15 ms, equivalent to rates of 66–125 pulses/s) as, for example, in human distal leg muscles when "ballistic" action is performed as rapidly as possible without attempts to track a particular force trajectory [Fig. 29; (70, 190, 316)]. One or two very short (8–15 ms) intervals are in fact commonly observed at the start of burst firing in both human and animal muscles (e.g., refs. 183, 185, 188, 192, 297, 322, 524, 740). This phenomenon of "doublet" discharge is found in both low-threshold (524) and high-threshold motoneurons (e.g., ref. 316) and occurs in motoneurons stimulated by steps of depolarizing current (e.g., refs. 36, 126, 503). Doublet firing can be ascribed to two intrinsic motoneuron properties: *1*) the tendency for the AHP conductance to summate during repetitive firing, making its depressant effect less powerful during the first interval than later in the train (324, 385) and *2*) the mechanism of "delayed depolarization," which tends to enhance the probability of discharge in the immediate wake of a preceding action potential (e.g., refs. 125, 127). The latter mechanism can in fact produce closely timed doublets at any point during a train (126, 127). For more detailed discussion of the mechanisms that control motoneuron firing, see the reviews by Burke and Rudomin in the *Handbook of Physiology, The Nervous System*, volume 1 (114) and those by Granit (304) and Gustafsson (324).

Tokizane and Shimazu (692) have argued that two distinct types of motor unit firing patterns can be identified in human subjects: *1*) a tonic (or T) pattern with relatively low firing frequencies and regular discharge intervals, characteristic of many low-threshold units and *2*) a kinetic (or K) pattern with higher frequencies and much greater tendency to irregular discharge even during apparently steady contractions, characteristic of higher threshold units (see also refs. 316, 338, 349, 710). More recently, Warmolts and Engel (710) showed that motor unit discharges during voluntary contraction tended to be easily activated and to occur in regular, low-frequency trains when re-

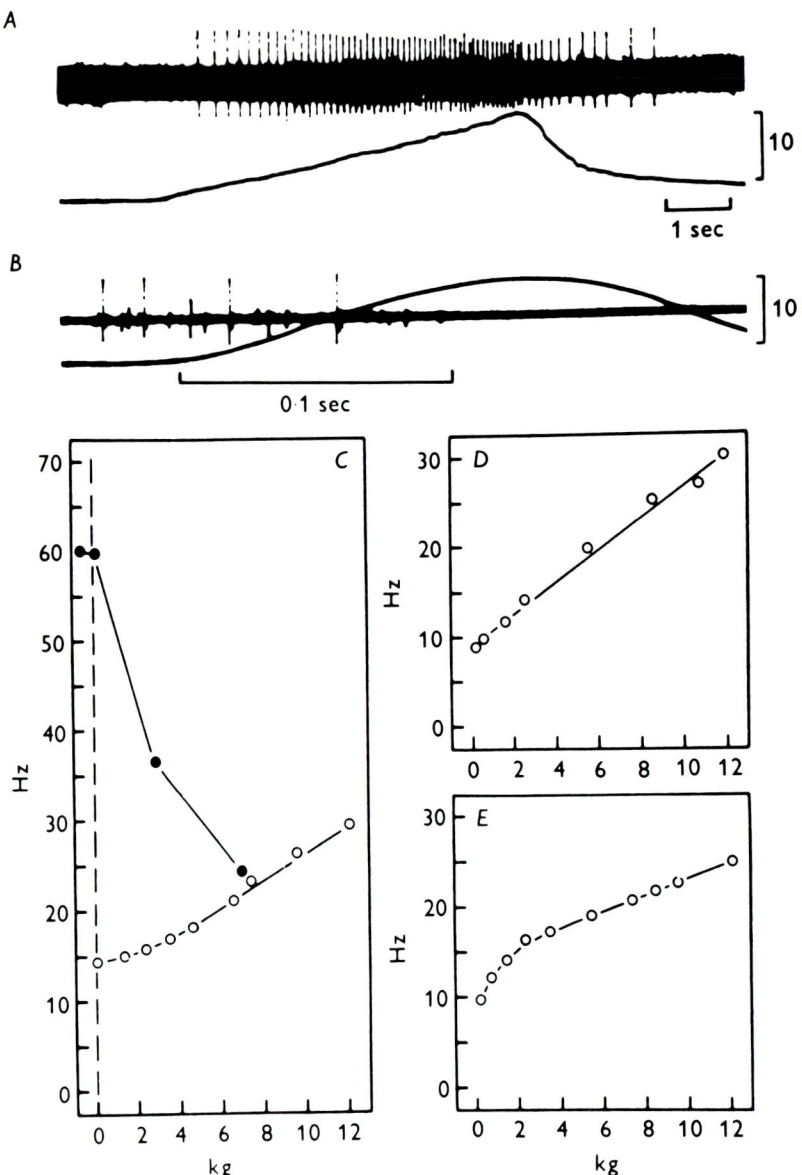

FIG. 29. Comparison of firing patterns (*upper traces* in *A, B*) from an individual motor unit in human ankle dorsiflexor, tibialis anterior, during a slow ramp contraction reaching 10 kg of force in 5 s (*record A; lower trace* is the force record) versus a ballistic contraction reaching 10 kg in 0.11 s. (*record B*; note change in time scale). The unit of interest (*large spike*) began to fire before any measurable force output in the ballistic contraction (i.e., its force "threshold" was 0), but during the slow ramp contraction its force threshold was about 2 kg. Graphs in *C, D,* and *E* illustrate the mean instantaneous frequency (ordinate; open circles) attained at the output force indicated on the abscissa during 10-kg ramp contractions lasting 1 s, 5 s, and 10 s, respectively. *Filled circles* in *C* show the mean instantaneous frequency attained during 5 ballistic contractions like that in *record B*. The firing patterns are similar in all of the ramp contractions, with gradually increasing instantaneous frequency (10–30 Hz), but the pattern is reversed in the ballistic contractions, with the highest frequency at the onset of activity (60 Hz). [From Desmedt and Godaux (190).]

corded from muscle regions dominated by type I fibers (three of four suitable cases). Regions dominated by type II fibers (one of four cases) contained only high-threshold units that tended to fire only in high-frequency bursts.

The bimodal distribution of firing patterns related to fast- versus slow-twitch unit types that is suggested by the above evidence is intuitively appealing, but most systematic studies have failed to confirm the existence of clearly distinguishable T or K groups in human EMG records (e.g., refs. 136, 182, 269, 349, 652, 676). Instead the data from relatively large samples of units suggest that the distribution of firing patterns within a given motor unit pool is effectively continuous between the extremes represented by the T and K categories, with a large proportion of "intermediate" patterns. There is little reason to doubt that the low-threshold, low-frequency, regular-interval T units are largely, if not exclusively, equivalent to type S, while the high-threshold, high-frequency, "bursty" units (e.g., refs. 70, 316) are probably equivalent to the fast-contracting, large-force, fatigable units called type FF in the cat (subsection MOTOR UNIT POPULATION OF CAT MEDIAL GASTROCNEMIUS MUSCLE, p. 353). It is not clear, however, what unit types are represented among the intermediate firing patterns (70), which could well include units of all the major types. It seems also possible that exercise training can reversibly alter the regularity (169) and synchronization (499) of motoneuron firing.

Tokizane and Shimazu (692) clearly showed that units in different muscles exhibit different ranges of steady firing rates; small distal muscles tend toward higher maximum frequencies than proximal muscles, and a similar pattern is seen comparing rostral with caudal muscles (see also refs. 73, 586, 652). The tendency to burst firing in ballistic contractions also varies from muscle to muscle; it is much less prevalent in the slowly contracting human SOL than in the faster masseter and first dorsal interosseous populations (192).

EFFECTS OF FIRING RATE AND FIRING PATTERN ON MUSCLE UNIT OUTPUT. A general discussion of the effect of activation rate and pattern on muscle fibers and whole muscles can be found in the chapter by Partridge and Benton in this *Handbook* (see also refs. 131, 367). Discussion of the mechanisms underlying excitation-contraction coupling and the production of mechanical force can be found in recent reviews (270, 383, 719). This subsection deals only with the rather limited observations on isometric contractions of individual motor units responding to stimulus trains that mimic those found in physiological usage.

The isometric-force output from an active muscle unit depends not only on its "built-in" characteristics (e.g., contraction time, tetanic-force output; subsection *Motor Unit Types: Physiological Profiles in Experimental Animals*, p. 351), but also on the time history of previous activations. Each activation appears to engage two interrelated mechanisms, one with pronounced but short-lasting effects (early enhancement and later depression, with time course measurable in tens to hundreds of milliseconds) and the other with effects that are weak for any single activation but that summate during repetitive activity and thereafter decay slowly (time course measured in minutes or even hours). The latter effects include two well-recognized phenomena: *1*) the enhancement of force output that follows high-frequency tetanization of muscle called posttetanic potentiation (PTP) and *2*) the decrement in force that can be attributed to muscle fiber fatigue (see subsection FATIGABILITY AND METABOLIC PROFILES, p. 358). The dependence of force output on activation history appears to reflect the fact that at normal temperatures the contractile machinery in mammalian skeletal muscle fibers is incompletely activated by a single impulse (i.e., the "active state" is submaximal; see refs. 148, 149, 270); it is this degree of "completeness" that can be modulated by repetitive activation.

The summation of force during unfused tetanic contractions of mammalian muscle is highly nonlinear, with significant serial dependence between successive activations (e.g., refs. 164, 598), which results in hysteresis in the relation between muscle force and activation frequency during sinusoidal input modulation (542). Examples of this serial dependence in individual muscle units are shown in Figure 30A and C. When force-time integrals for individual response components (pseudotwitches) are graphed as a function of interstimulus interval (Fig. 31), it is clear that the additions contributed by successive pulses change rapidly with small changes in pulse interval. Force-time integrals are useful to quantitate such responses, since

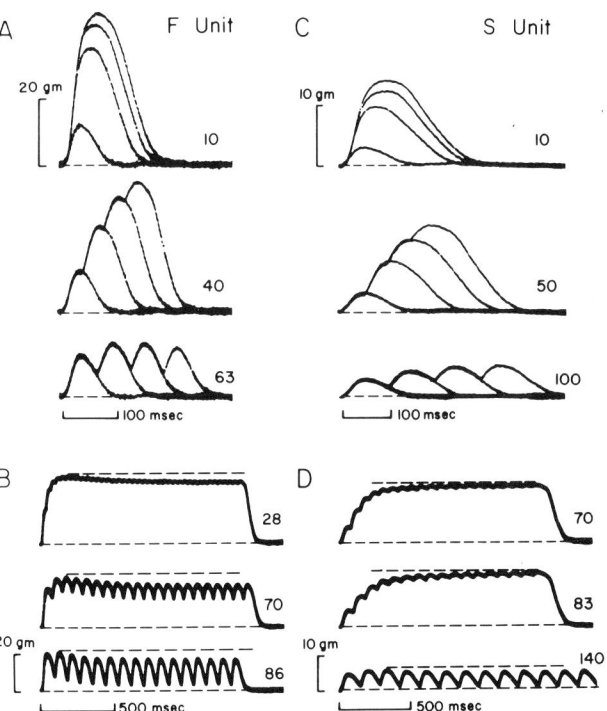

FIG. 30. Isometric force records from a type F (*A, B*) and a type S (*C, D*) motor unit showing (*A, C*) superimposed responses to 1, 2, 3, and 4 pulses at interpulse intervals noted at the end of each *record* (in ms) and (*B, D*) unfused tetanic responses to constant-frequency pulse trains, again with intervals noted at *right* of each *record*. Note presence of "sag" (see also subsection MOTOR UNIT POPULATION OF CAT MEDIAL GASTROCNEMIUS MUSCLE, p. 353) in all of the F unit tetani but only in the slowest (140-ms interval) tetanus to type S unit. *Records* in *A, C* show that at shortest stimulus interval (10 ms), the 2nd pulse in a train adds the greatest increment of force and force-time integral (see Fig. 31). [From data of Burke et al. (116).]

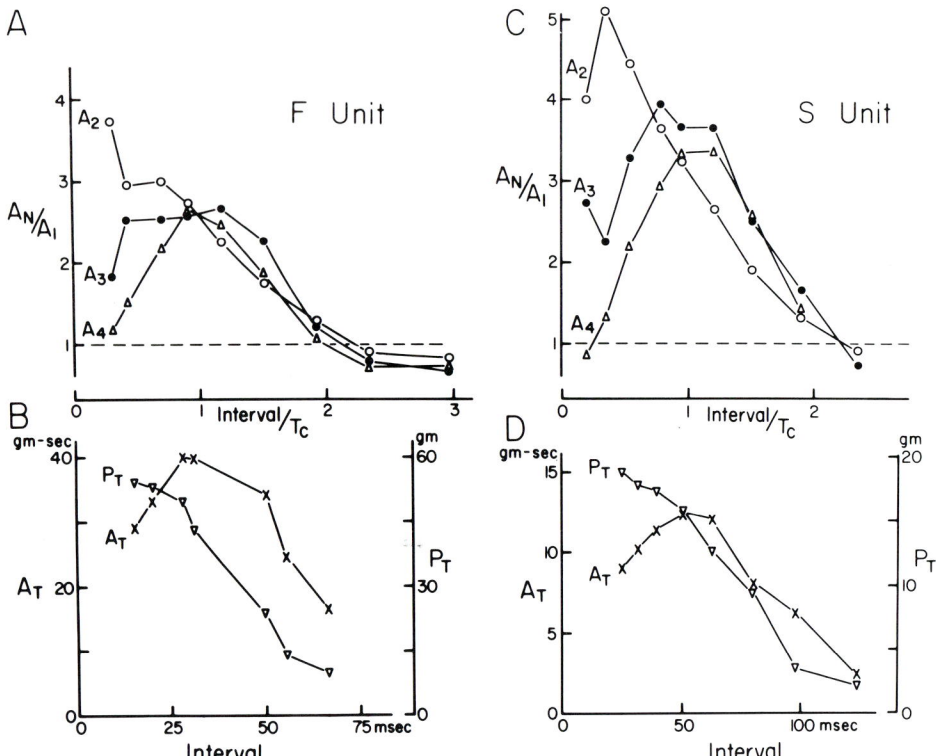

FIG. 31. Graphs showing force-time integrals (ordinates) of mechanical responses from same units illustrated in Figure 30, plotted in each case against the interval between pulses in the input trains (abscissae). *Graphs A and C* show, for the F and S units respectively (sample records in Fig. 30A, C), the force-time integral added to the already developed isometric force by the 2nd(A_2), 3rd (A_3), and 4th (A_4) pulses at the indicated intervals, with integral expressed relative to that produced by the single twitch (A_1). In general, A_2 is predominant when 2nd pulse arrives at intervals less than the isometric twitch contraction time (T_C); at longer intervals, each pulse produces about the same increment in force-time integral. *Lower graphs (B, D)* show cumulative force-time integral for 1st 15 pulses (A_T; plotted relative to *left-hand* ordinates) during different trains (sample records in Fig. 30B and D). The abscissa scale is exactly the same as in A and C but indicates absolute interpulse interval in ms. Note that shape of the A_T curves roughly match those of A_3 curves above. *Curves* labeled P_T indicate absolute isometric force attained at peak of 15th response during tetani at the various frequencies (referred to the *right-hand* ordinate in each case). Maximum slope of P_T curve occurs with intervals that produce the largest force-time integrals. [From data of Burke et al. (116).]

they are insensitive to changes in response shape and are apparently quantitatively related to ATP turnover in muscle fibers [(400); see also ref. 568].

The isometric input-output curves (Fig. 31) for individual type F and S muscle units are similar when plotted as functions of isometric-twitch contraction time (T_C). The force-time integral added by a second pulse in a train (A_2 in Fig. 31A and C) usually maximizes with the shortest interpulse intervals (8–10 ms) and decreases more or less monotonically with increasing interval, to fall below the single twitch value (A_1) at intervals greater than about twice T_C. The additions made by the third and fourth pulses (A_3 and A_4 respectively) are greatest (and usually intersect the A_2 curve) at interpulse intervals near T_C. After the fourth or fifth pulse in a given train, subsequent pulses all contribute roughly the same force-time integral, so that the input-output curves for longer tetani (curves A_T in Fig. 31B and D) have approximately the same shape as the A_4 curves (116). Equivalent observations have been made for isotonic contraction of frog muscles (546). The plateau force reached during longer trains (curves P_T in Fig. 31B, D) has a sigmoid relation to interpulse interval (164), and these curves usually rise most steeply when interpulse intervals range between 1 and 2 times T_C. In Figures 30 and 31 this would be equivalent to input frequency ranges of about 15–30 pulses/s for the F unit and about 9–18 pulses/s for the S unit, which are compatible with the respective ranges of firing frequencies observed among comparable motor units during voluntary or reflex activity (see subsection MOTONEURON FIRING CHARACTERISTICS, p. 394).

Input-output curves like those in Figure 31 for limb motor units suggest that the physiological range of firing frequencies (6–30 pulses/s) should produce very effective modulation of force output during infused tetani (i.e., curves P_T). Furthermore muscle units activated repetitively with pulse intervals near T_C should produce near maximum force-time integrals for each motoneuron spike. The integral of force over time in isometric contractions has the physical dimensions of momentum and can probably be regarded as proportional to the instantaneous work that could be done by the muscle if it became free to move (116). Furthermore Jobsis and Duffield (400) have shown that energy utilization by active muscle is proportional to the isometric force-time integral. One may conclude that both fast- and slow-twitch muscle units produce their maximum isometric output per impulse when activated at interpulse intervals near their respective T_C values, which are quite compatible with observed maximum rates during steady firing for both fast- and slow-twitch motor units (subsection MOTONEURON FIRING CHARACTERISTICS, p. 394).

Rack and Westbury (567a) have demonstrated that isometric tension output from the cat SOL muscle varies significantly with muscle length when stimulated at relatively low frequencies (5–15 pulses/s), so that output at a given frequency is maximal when the muscle is near its maximum physiological length. These authors showed in the same paper that the tension output from the whole muscle was smoothed and somewhat enhanced by asynchronous stimulation of multiple subsets of motor units. This suggests that mechanical interactions between muscle units introduce functionally useful nonlinearities into the process of tension addition during the recruitment process. Joyce and co-workers (402a, 402b) also showed that nonlinearities in muscle force output during lengthening and shortening are markedly affected by activation frequency. These complexities, which are discussed further in the chapter by Houk and Rymer in this *Handbook*, must be kept in mind when considering the link between activation frequency and mechanical action in normal movement.

Given the fact that low frequency ranges produce large modulation of muscle unit output, what then is to be gained by high firing rates (50–100 pulses/s) during short-burst firing or by the insertion of a short-interval "doublet" into a lower frequency pulse train (subsection MOTONEURON FIRING CHARACTERISTICS, p. 394)? Obviously the maximum rate of rise in force is attained only during fused tetani at high input frequencies. Such may well be required during the intense, short-duration bursts that occur in ballistic movements [e.g., Fig. 29; (191, 316)] or in high-speed galloping and jumping (see refs. 708, 637). The functional utility of doublet firing is, however, less self-evident.

Blaschko and co-workers (66), and later Wilson and Larimer (721), showed that insertion of a short, high-frequency burst into an otherwise low-frequency stimulus train can produce remarkably long-lasting enhancement of isometric force output in nontwitch arthropod muscles. Wilson and Larimer referred to this effect as a "catch property," although its mechanism is probably different from that of the catch effect seen in certain specialized molluscan muscles (699). Wilson and co-workers (722) later demonstrated the same effect in arthropod twitch muscles, and a qualitatively similar catch property has also been found in mammalian muscle units under isometric conditions (115, 116, 739). A particularly dramatic example is shown in Figure 32, in which a type S muscle unit in cat MG muscle was stimulated with three different pulse trains, each having almost identical average frequencies but differing in one or two interpulse intervals. In this example, output force was modulated primarily by the pattern and not by the average frequency of the input train.

Catch enhancement of isometric force output varies in magnitude with the frequency of the underlying steady-input train, such that it is maximum when intervals are between 1 and 2 times T_C (Fig. 5 in ref. 116), again equivalent to the preferred steady firing frequency ranges observed under physiological conditions. Although the catch effect is most dramatic in type S muscle units, it is also present to a degree in F units (Fig. 33B), but its duration is curtailed by the sag property that depresses force output from fast-twitch muscle units over a wide range of steady input frequencies [(116); see also subsection MOTOR UNIT POPULATION OF CAT MEDIAL GASTROCNEMIUS MUSCLE, p. 353). Despite its limited duration, catch enhancement could well be operative in F units during short bursts of activity.

In contrast to the serially dependent enhancements discussed above, the sag property represents a depression of force output that depends on the immediate

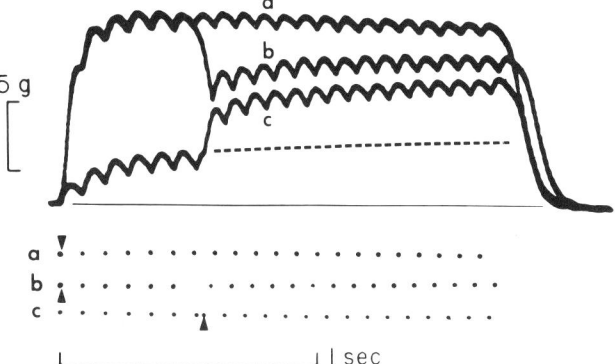

FIG. 32. The "catch" effect in a type S muscle unit from cat medial gastrocnemius (MG). Superimposed traces of 3 isometric responses to pulse trains with average frequencies of about 12.5 pulses/s but different interval structures (*diagrams a–c below*). The addition of a single extra pulse (*arrow*) within 10 ms of the 1st pulse in the basic train (*pattern a*) produced marked and persistent enhancement of force output (*record a*) even though the basic train rate is unchanged. Widening one interval slightly during this catch enhancement (*pattern b*) caused a drop in output force that was then "caught" again at a new force level (*record b*). A modest shortening of a single interval (*pattern c; arrow*) produced an equivalently modest catch enhancement (*record c*). [From Burke et al. (115). Copyright 1970 by the American Association for the Advancement of Science.]

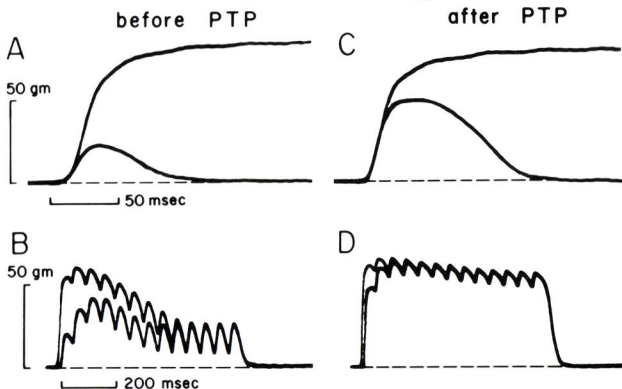

FIG. 33. Effect of posttetanic potentiation (PTP) on mechanical responses of a type F muscle unit in cat medial gastrocnemius (MG). *Top records* are superimposed traces of a single twitch and a fused tetanus before (*A*) and after (*C*) repeated high-frequency (200 Hz) tetanization. Note that there is a marked increase in twitch force and duration and more rapid rising phases of the twitch and tetanus after PTP, but that there is no change in fused-tetanus plateau force. *Lower records* illustrate unfused tetanic responses to low-frequency (approximately 20 Hz) stimulation with (larger response) and without a single extra pulse within 10 ms of the 1st (a "doublet," to illustrate the catch effect; see Fig. 32). In contrast to the S unit in Fig. 32, catch enhancement is not sustained (*record C*); instead, force output decays with a time course similar to that of the "sag" of tension in the basic tetanus. After PTP the initial doublet produces much less catch enhancement, and the tetani with and without the extra pulse converge within 200 ms. [From data of Burke et al. (116).]

history of preceding activations. At very low frequencies (interpulse intervals greater than about twice T_C), sag is present in tetanic responses of *both* F and S muscle units (e.g., Fig. 30*B, D*), and it it presumably identical with the mechanism that produces depression of the second response to paired stimuli at intervals greater than twice T_C (Fig. 31*A* and *C*). However, sag remains evident at higher input frequencies only in the F units, which is useful for distinguishing them from the type S (see subsection MOTOR UNIT POPULATION OF CAT MEDIAL GASTROCNEMIUS MUSCLE, p. 353). This difference in the shape of unfused tetanic responses in whole muscles has been noted for many years (e.g., refs. 164, 598) but remains unexplained. Burke and co-workers (116) have suggested that the sag represents a systematic decrease in the duration of the active state during the later phases of a regular, low-frequency tetanus (see Fig. 8 in ref. 116). The large difference between F and S muscle units in the expression of the sag phenomenon may be related to the differences between their myosins or to the kinetics of intrafiber Ca^{2+} fluxes, perhaps secondary to the demonstrable differences in sarcoplasmic reticulum in presumed F and S muscle fibers (see subsections *Muscle Fiber Types: Histochemical Profiles and Ultrastructural Correlations*, p. 347 and TWITCH-CONTRACTION TIMES AND MYOFIBRILLAR ATPASE, p. 355).

The serial dependencies discussed above develop and decay rather quickly (i.e., in tens or hundreds of milliseconds) and require relatively few stimuli for full expression (< 10). In contrast, muscle-force output can also be modulated by mechanisms that develop and decay over time scales measured in minutes or even hours and that require many activations (hundreds or thousands) for full expression. Force-output depression due to fiber fatigue is one of these mechanisms (see subsection FATIGABILITY AND METABOLIC PROFILES, p. 358), but the prolonged enhancement of mechanical output that follows sustained repetitive activation of muscle fibers is of particular interest here.

The phenomenon of posttetanic potentiation (PTP) of twitch force after sustained, high-frequency tetani has been known for many years (e.g., refs. 81, 149, 154, 193). The mechanism is intrinsic to muscle fibers and is not due to repetitive fiber activation (655; cf. subsection MOTOR UNIT POPULATION OF CAT MEDIAL GASTROCNEMIUS MUSCLE, p. 353) or to changes in muscle fiber action potentials (350). All of the motor unit types studied in cat heterogeneous muscles (such as MG and FDL, for example) exhibit potentiation of twitch force after repeated tetanization (111, 205), although the effect appears to decay more quickly in type S units (R. Burke, unpublished observations). The latter fact may account in part for the suggestion of Bagust and co-workers (33) that PTP occurs only in fast-twitch muscle units (in addition these authors used only rather brief, single conditioning tetani). It is clear, however, that the type S units present in the cat SOL muscle exhibit little PTP of twitch amplitude, and most, in fact, show depression of twitch force following high-frequency tetani (posttetanic depression; refs. 33, 110), as is the case with the whole SOL muscle (81). The absence of PTP in most SOL type S units represents a significant difference from the type S units found in heterogeneous muscles (see also subsections MOTOR UNIT POPULATION OF CAT MEDIAL GASTROCNEMIUS MUSCLE, p. 353 and PHYSIOLOGICAL AND HISTOCHEMICAL PROFILES OF MUSCLE UNITS, p. 354). It is of interest in this connection that Schmalbruch (619a) has recently reported that the longitudinal tubules of the SR system are less well developed in cat SOL fibers than in either the fast- or slow-twitch fibers in MG. Additional clues to the mechanism of PTP may perhaps be found in further systematic comparisons between the ultrastructure and cellular biophysics of these two varieties of slowly contracting muscle fibers (see subsection *Muscle Fiber Types: Histochemical Profiles and Ultrastructural Correlations*, p. 347).

Prolonged potentiation can also follow activity at moderate frequencies. This submaximal PTP is referred to as postactivation potentiation (116), although it is probably the same as the well-known "positive staircase" phenomenon (e.g., refs. 193, 340). Postactivation potentiation is likely to be important in normal movement, since it can occur during firing at frequencies well within the normal range (subsection MOTONEURON FIRING CHARACTERISTICS, p. 394). It may well be involved in the stretching and warming-up maneuvers of animals and humans when they prepare for movement after a period of motor inactivity.

The PTP that follows long tetanization usually results in some prolongation of the twitch contraction time, but such changes are much less dramatic than the effects on twitch force [e.g., Fig. 33A and C; Fig. 34, $T_C(1)$ and $T_C(2)$ versus $P_{tw}(1)$ and $P_{tw}(2)$; see also refs. 33, 111]. Systematic study of PTP effects in individual muscle units is difficult because the initial response observed may or may not represent a baseline state. As an extreme example, muscle units are occasionally encountered that produce virtually no detectable twitch force until tetanized several times, whereupon twitch responses grow dramatically (R. Burke, unpublished observations). In general, however, the units with relatively large twitch responses in a given type category tend to show less percentage increase after PTP than units with smaller twitches (Fig. 4 in ref. 111; see also ref. 33).

For any given muscle unit, there is a limit to twitch potentiation such that its maximum twitch:tetanus ratio can be established. For units in cat MG, the average twitch:tetanus ratios (using maximally potentiated twitch responses) differ for the various unit types; they are largest (0.58) for type FF, somewhat smaller (0.43) for type FR, and smallest (0.31) for type S [(111); see also refs. 33, 662]. Twitch:tetanus ratios are of interest in that they give some indication of the degree of contractile machinery activation possible in a single response relative to the maximum level of the active state produced in fused tetanic contractions. The differences between unit type groups suggest that more complete activation is possible in type FF than in type FR and S units after a single input pulse.

Posttetanic, or more generally, postactivation potentiation modifies the input-output characteristics of muscle units in significant ways. For example, the unfused tetani of the F unit shown in Figure 33 are obviously changed by prior tetanization, both in shape and force output, and the catch effect is much diminished in the potentiated response. This is also true for the more sustained catch effects in type S units (Fig. 6 in ref. 116). The graph in Figure 34 illustrates the changes produced in the input-output curves of unfused tetani (as in Fig. 31B and D) in the initial and maximally potentiated state. The fused tetanic force (P_o) is unchanged by PTP, but the muscle unit generates larger plateau forces [compare curves $P_T(1)$ with $P_T(2)$] and much greater force-time integrals [curves $A_T(1)$ versus $A_T(2)$] during unfused tetani throughout the input interval range. Different levels of postactivation potentiation would be expected to produce families of curves between those illustrated, so that the isometric-force output of a given muscle unit would be predictable only with knowledge of the long-term as well as short-term time history of the input pulses to it (116).

It is beyond the scope of this chapter to discuss possible mechanisms for the pulse-history effects described in this section, and indeed there is rather little experimental evidence bearing on this problem. However, it is striking that both the rapidly decaying and slowly decaying enhancements of force output appear to occlude one another, suggesting some commonality of mechanism. Studies of intrafiber Ca^{2+} release during twitch and tetanic responses in frog muscle indicate that the free Ca^{2+} concentration does not correlate at all well with force output (67), making it appear unlikely that the serial dependence of force output on input pattern is explainable simply on the basis of the concentration of free activator Ca^{2+} available at any moment. However, Winegrad (726, 727) has shown that Ca^{2+} is released from the terminal cisternae of the sarcoplasmic reticulum, but it is taken up again all along the longitudinal tubules, with significant (tens of seconds) delays in the complete cycle. This agrees with recent immunohistochemical evidence that the Ca^{2+}-Mg^{2+}-activated ATPase protein associated with reuptake is distributed uniformly along the SR tubules, while the Ca^{2+}-binding protein, calsequestrin,

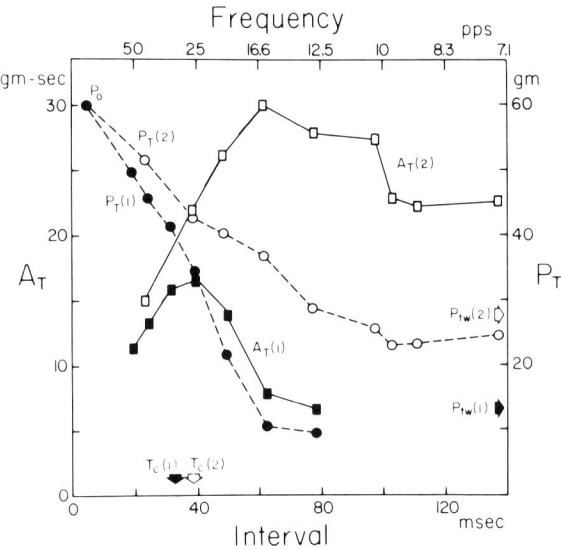

FIG. 34. Input-output graph (as in Fig. 31B and D) for a type F muscle unit in cat medial gastrocnemius (MG), showing the effect of posttetanic potentiation (PTP) on mechanical output during short tetani at various frequencies. *Continuous lines* denote force-time integrals under 1st 14 responses (A_T) in tetani under initial conditions [i.e., before repeated tetanization to produce maximal PTP; curve $A_T(1)$, *filled squares*] and after tetanization [i.e., during PTP; curve $A_T(2)$, *open squares*]. Plateau force reached by the 14th response during the same tetani (P_T; *dashed curves*) is shown for initial conditions [$P_T(1)$; *filled circles*] and during maximum PTP ($P_T(2)$; *open circles*). Both *curves* converge to the same maximum force in fused tetani (P_o), but the potentiated tetani generate more peak force at all lower frequencies (see also Fig. 33). The PTP produces a greater increase in twitch force (*arrows* labeled P_{tw}, referred to *right-hand* ordinate) than in twitch contraction time (*arrows* labeled T_C, referred to *lower* abscissa). The PTP has the effect of lowering and broadening the range of input frequencies over which muscle unit output is most effectively modulated by input rate (compare with Fig. 31 and attendant discussion). [From Burke et al. (116).]

appears to be localized to the terminal cisternae (402). The dissociation of activator Ca^{2+} from the regulatory proteins of the myofilaments is also relatively slow (see ref. 60) and is partly dependent on developed force (see ref. 270). If the removal of Ca^{2+} is indeed a relatively slow process, then some part of the serial dependence in input-output relations could be due to the kinetics of intrafiber Ca^{2+} movements (155). Similarly, if cross-bridge formation involves cooperative binding of more than one Ca^{2+} (e.g., ref. 21; see also ref. 270), a nonlinear threshold effect might result. For example, a single-input pulse could result in partial activation of some fraction of the regulatory proteins without contractile element activation (51, 134). More complete contractile element activation could then be accomplished by relatively small amounts of additional Ca^{2+} released by subsequent pulses with the proper timing (67). Both the short-term effects of pulse patterns and the slowly decaying effects of postactivation potentiation may thus result from the still incompletely understood movements and bindings of activator Ca^{2+} within muscle fibers (see refs. 270 and 719 for further discussion).

Recruitment or Rate and Pattern Modulation?

Given the existence of recruitment versus rate and pattern modulation as alternative mechanisms, it is important to attempt to define their relative importance in the control of total muscle force. There is some disagreement in the literature on this issue. For example, Grillner and Udo (311) have reported that recruitment of cat SOL motor units occurred in stretch reflexes primarily when active tension was less than 50% of its final value and that few, if any, additional units became active even though active reflex force increased above that level. The same authors (310) also reported a remarkably narrow range (6–10 pulses/s) of firing frequencies for SOL motor units in stretch reflexes, suggesting that rate modulation is very limited at any level of output in this motor pool. In a similar vein, Severin and colleagues (624) have suggested that recruitment rather than rate modulation is the main mechanism grading motor output (presumably much below maximum levels) during fictive locomotion in the decerebrate cat preparation, although their records do show interesting variations in pulse patterns (including doublets) that could well be important in modulating mechanical output (subsection EFFECTS OF FIRING RATE AND FIRING PATTERN ON MUSCLE UNIT OUTPUT, p. 397). As a contrasting example, Monster and Chan [see Fig. 28; (510)] have shown that both recruitment of new units and significant changes in steady motoneuron firing rate occur throughout the entire range of voluntary force output in the human extensor digitorum communis.

Milner-Brown and colleagues (502) have discussed this issue in some detail and used their data on motor units in the human first dorsal interosseous muscle (see subsection *Motor Units in Human Muscle*, p. 359) to estimate the relative importance of recruitment versus rate modulation in voluntary contraction. They concluded that recruitment is the major mechanism at low levels of force output but that rate modulation becomes more and more important as force output increases, so that it is the dominant factor at high-force outputs. The same conclusion was reached by Monster and Chan (510) using data from the extensor digitorum communis of humans. Although both sets of authors used linear equations (and linear assumptions) to model the highly nonlinear output of muscle units, their formulations are the most complete available that include data about the mechanical properties of muscle units and the firing rates of the parent motoneurons as they relate to steady force production. The positive correlation between functional threshold and motor unit force (e.g., Fig. 25) ensures that a recruitment mechanism will predominate at low levels of total force output.

During fast tracking movements and in ballistic contractions (as rapid as possible without tracking), the threshold for recruitment is related to the future force produced during the contraction and not to the force level at the moment of recruitment [see Fig. 29; (93, 190, 192)]. In such movements, firing pattern is probably more important than firing rate per se.

In summary it seems clear that both recruitment and rate and pattern modulation are important to the control of total muscle force. One or the other mechanism may dominate depending on the nature of the muscle or the nature and speed of the action under study.

SUMMARY AND CONCLUDING COMMENTS

This chapter attempts to review currently available material on the properties of individual motor units and their organization into populations (motor unit pools) with a common function. A motor unit consists of a motoneuron and the extrafusal muscle fibers innervated by it (the muscle unit portion); they are the quanta into which all muscular activity (and resultant movements) can be decomposed. From a functional viewpoint, muscles are simply collections of muscle units mechanically coupled together (subsection *Anatomy of Muscle Units*, p. 367) and innervated by motoneurons in a contiguous motor nucleus (subsection *Anatomy of Motor Nuclei*, p. 372).

Motor units can be divided into definable types on the basis of the mechanical properties of the muscle unit portion (subsection MOTOR UNIT POPULATION OF CAT MEDIAL GASTROCNEMIUS MUSCLE, p. 353), and the resultant groupings correspond (subsection PHYSIOLOGICAL AND HISTOCHEMICAL PROFILES OF MUSCLE UNITS, p. 354) to the various types of muscle fibers recognized on the basis of histochemical and morphological characteristics (subsection *Muscle Fiber Types*:

Histochemical Profiles and Ultrastructural Correlations, p. 347). Most muscles in animals from amphibians to humans contain heterogeneous mixtures of various unit types; homogeneous motor pools made up entirely of a single unit type are exceptional. Furthermore some motor units include intrafusal as well as extrafusal muscle fibers in their peripheral muscle units (skeletofusimotor or β-motor units; subsection *Skeletofusimotor Units*, p. 365). This diversity suggests that the different groups of motor units are specialized for particular roles during movement.

Comprehensive models of motor control must take into account the diversity within motor unit pools, but the complications introduced by this diversity are mitigated when motor units are considered according to type (which carries information about multiple interrelated characteristics) rather than by any single characteristic. There are only a few clearly defined types, and there is considerable commonality of features within a type (subsection *Motor Unit Types: Physiological Profiles in Experimental Animals*, p. 351). The diagram in Figure 35 illustrates the interrelatedness among the characteristics of motor units in a given population (in this case, the MG pool of the cat hindlimb), including properties of motoneurons and synaptic inputs as well as of muscle units. Identi-

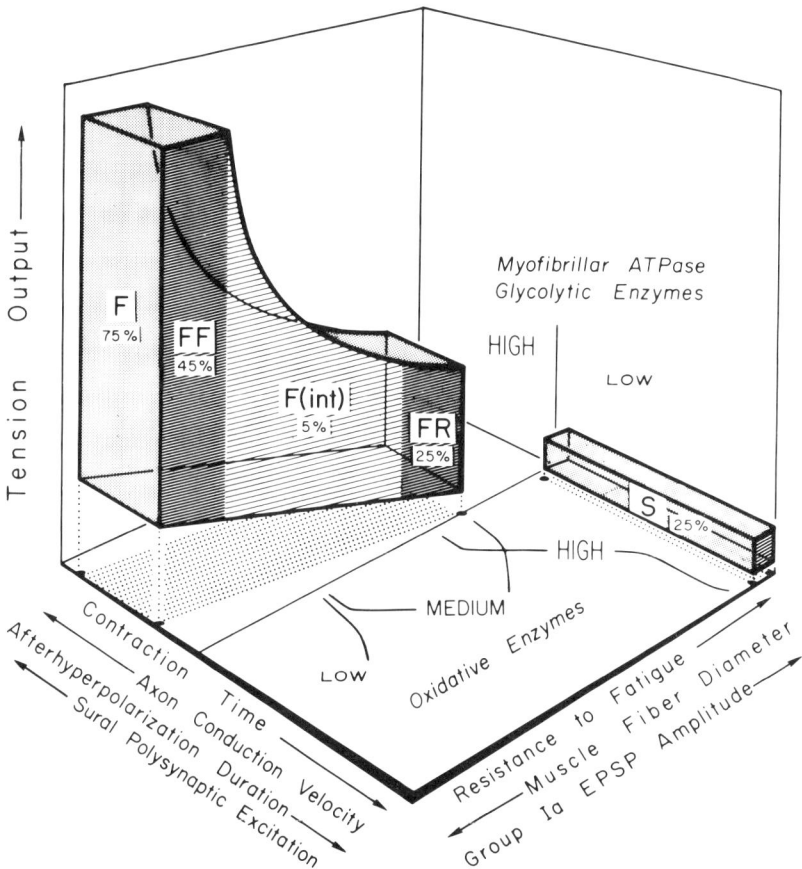

FIG. 35. Three-dimensional diagram summarizing the interrelations between a variety of features of the physiological, morphological, and histochemical profiles of motor units found in the cat medial gastrocnemius (MG) population. Muscle unit properties include tetanic force output, twitch contraction time, resistance to fatigue, myofibrillar ATPase staining at alkaline pH, metabolic enzyme patterns (anaerobic and oxidative), and average muscle fiber diameter. Motoneuron properties included are axonal conduction velocity and duration of the afterhyperpolarization. Contrasting patterns of synaptic organization are represented by amplitude of monosynaptic group Ia EPSP (*right* abscissa) and by the apparent strength of polysynaptic excitatory input from distal hindlimb skin (sural nerve; *left* abscissa). The diagram is based on displays such as in Figs. 2 and 5 and on material like that in Tables 1–3. It should be clear that this summary somewhat distorts reality in that the various features specified are not all distributed in exactly the way displayed, but the general trends are as illustrated. The diagram is not intended to be all inclusive (other characteristics could be added to one or another axis) but rather emphasizes the fact that a great many properties of motoneurons and their muscle units display correlated variation, which can be communicated by the notion of motor unit "types." The types identified in the cat MG, along with their percentages in that population, are indicated on the *shaded boxes*, which denote the approximate loci of the clusters of data points seen in the actual data displays, such as in Figure 5. [Adapted from Burke (104). In: *The Nervous System. The Basic Neurosciences*, edited by R. O. Brady. Copyright 1975 by Raven Press, New York.]

fication of clusters, or types, of units provides a useful and even necessary step in attempts to understand the organization behind the diversity. The correlations among physiological, histochemical, and morphological characteristics appear to reflect specializations designed to optimize particular properties of muscle (subsections TWITCH-CONTRACTION TIMES AND MYOFIBRILLAR ATPASE, p. 355; FATIGABILITY AND METABOLIC PROFILES, p. 358; and *Anatomy of Muscle Units*, p. 367) and the distinctions between unit and fiber types are robust in that they remain relatively stable in the face of changing demand within the physiological range (subsection ALTERATIONS OF DEMAND WITHIN THE PHYSIOLOGICAL RANGE, p. 362).

The distinctions between fiber and unit types are apparently controlled by the activity patterns or the cellular identities (or, more likely, some combination of both) of the innervating motoneurons (subsections NONPHYSIOLOGICAL ALTERATIONS, p. 363, and *Developmental Considerations*, p. 364), although the electrophysiological (subsection *Electrophysiological Properties Intrinsic to Motoneurons*, p. 379) and morphological (subsection *Motoneuron Anatomy in Relation to Unit Type*, p. 377) characteristics of motoneurons themselves do not permit unambiguous identification of motor unit types. The centrifugal trophic control of muscle units by motoneurons is well documented although the mechanisms involved remain obscure. There is growing indication, however, that a reverse communication (i.e., from muscle unit to motoneuron; subsection NONPHYSIOLOGICAL ALTERATIONS, p. 363) may also play a role in maintaining the normal pattern of interrelations that we recognize as motor unit types.

The relatively small amount of data so far available strongly suggest that the organization of synaptic inputs to motoneurons in a given motor pool is rather precisely matched with motor unit type (subsection *Organization of Synaptic Input*, p. 381). At least two different patterns have been demonstrated to exist in the cat lumbosacral spinal cord, one in which synaptic efficacy is directly related to fatigue resistance and inversely related to unit force output, of which group Ia excitation is the best-documented example (subsection GROUP Ia SYNAPTIC EFFICACY, p. 381) and the other in which excitatory input is stronger among the fast-twitch units than in the slow-twitch units, a pattern found for a particular set of cutaneous afferents from distal hindlimb skin (subsection POLYSYNAPTIC INPUT SYSTEMS, p. 382). Indirect evidence strongly suggests that many synaptic systems are organized in parallel with the group Ia input pattern (subsection RECRUITMENT PATTERNS AND MOTOR UNIT TYPES, p. 386). Synaptic efficacy appears to be the key factor in the complex of interactions that control the hierarchy of functional thresholds within a motor pool (subsection *Control of Motoneuron Excitability: Interactive Factors*, p. 383).

The control of muscle force by the central nervous system during normal movement involves two basic mechanisms: *1*) the recruitment of motor units in an orderly fashion so that total output reflects both the numbers and the individual properties of the units active at any level of output and *2*) the modulation of force output from individual units by the frequency and pattern of motoneuron firing (section CONTROL OF MUSCULAR ACTION: RECRUITMENT AND RATE MODULATION, p. 385). A great deal of evidence from both animals and humans (subsection RECRUITMENT PATTERNS AND MOTOR UNIT TYPES, p. 386) indicates that under many conditions small-force, fatigue-resistant, slow-twitch units are activated at the lowest output levels, such as occur in (but are not confined to) postural maintenance. Somewhat greater force levels, such as those that occur in locomotion, require activation of moderate-force, fast-twitch, fatigue-resistant units. High-force outputs that may be required only infrequently in many animals appear to involve the large-force, fast-twitch, but fatigable, units that can make up the bulk of some unit populations. This recruitment pattern is consistent with the organization of input systems typified by the group Ia input from muscle spindles (subsection GROUP Ia SYNAPTIC EFFICACY, p. 381). Under specialized conditions, major dislocations in the expected sequence of functional thresholds have been observed (subsection ARE MAJOR SHIFTS IN RECRUITMENT ORDER POSSIBLE? on p. 391), suggesting that alternative synaptic organization patterns (subsection POLYSYNAPTIC INPUT SYSTEMS, p. 382) may have physiological importance in some movement strategies.

Although it remains for future work to document directly the usage patterns of the different motor unit types in normal movements, the existing indirect evidence (subsection *Motor Unit Recruitment*, p. 386) strongly suggests that the interrelations observed from synaptic input to muscle fiber biochemistry, here subsumed under the rubric of motor unit types, represent functional specializations by which the motor unit pool of any muscle is precisely tailored to the functional demands ordinarily encountered by it. Further evidence to support this conclusion should come from comparisons of motor unit populations in various animals and in different muscles as they relate to motor habits and mechanical demands. However, direct documentation of this intuitively satisfying picture must await the development of technical methods that permit unambiguous type-identification of individual motor units as they are used for normal, behaviorally significant movements.

There are many exciting questions about the neurobiology of motor units that concern the mechanisms by which the normal interrelations are maintained (i.e., the trophic interaction between muscle and motoneuron); there is also the developmental question of how the system arrives at its mature state. With respect to the maintenance of motor unit characteristics, there is good evidence that activity pattern is an important, although probably not exclusive, trophic factor (subsection *Stability of Motor Unit Types*, p. 361). However, the role of activity patterns per se during development is more problematic. The functional thresholds and consequent activity patterns of motoneurons depend on a complex interaction between presynaptic organization and postsynaptic properties (subsection *Control of Motoneuron Excitability: Interactive Factors*, p. 383), in which no single factor seems predominant. A random distribution of synaptic efficacy within a motor pool (due to differences in synaptic density, for example) might seem tenable as an organizing factor if only one input system were critical, but this model is difficult to reconcile with the fact that the organization of many input systems are found correlated with unit type (subsection *Organization of Synaptic Input*, p. 381). There appears to an early, strong, genetically related specification of motor unit types and of the type composition of a given motor pool that is difficult to reconcile with random selection (subsection *Developmental Considerations*, p. 364). There is considerable current interest in this fascinating question and, hopefully, the next edition of this *Handbook* will report more complete answers.

REFERENCES

1. ADRIAN, E. D., AND D. W. BRONK. The discharge of impulses in motor nerve fibres. Part II. The frequency of discharge in reflex and voluntary contractions. *J. Physiol. London* 67: 119-151, 1929.
2. AITKEN, J. T. Growth of nerve implants in voluntary muscle. *J. Anat.* 84: 38-49, 1950.
3. AITKEN, J. T., AND J. E. BRIDGER. Neuron size and neuron population density in the lumbosacral region of the cat's spinal cord. *J. Anat.* 95: 38-53, 1962.
4. AKAGI, Y. The localization of the motor neurons innervating the extraocular muscles in the oculomotor nuclei of the cat and rabbit, using horseradish peroxidase. *J. Comp. Neurol.* 181: 745-762, 1978.
5. AL-AMOOD, W. S., AND R. POPE. A comparison of the structural features of muscle fibres from a fast- and slow-twitch muscle of the pelvic limb of the cat. *J. Anat.* 113: 49-60, 1972.
6. ALEXANDER, R. McN. The mechanics of jumping by a dog (*Canis familiaris*). *J. Zool.* 173: 549-573, 1974.
8. ALVARADO, J., AND C. VAN HORN. Muscle cell types of the cat inferior oblique. In: *Basic Mechanisms of Ocular Motility and Their Clinical Implications*, edited by G. Lennerstrand and P. Bach-y-Rita. Oxford: Pergamon, 1975, p. 15-45.
9. ANDERSEN, P., AND J. HENRIKSSON. Training induced changes in the subgroups of human type II skeletal muscle fibres. *Acta Physiol. Scand.* 99: 123-125, 1977.
10. ANDERSEN, P., AND T. A. SEARS. The mechanical properties and innervation of fast and slow motor units in the intercostal muscles of the cat. *J. Physiol. London* 173: 114-129, 1964.
11. ANDERSON, W. J., M. W. STROMBERG, AND E. J. HINSMAN. Morphological characteristics of dendrite bundles in the lumbar spinal cord of the rat. *Brain Res.* 110: 215-227, 1976.
12. ANDREW, B. L., AND N. J. PART. Properties of fast and slow motor units in hind limb and tail muscles of the rat. *Q. J. Exp. Physiol.* 57: 213-225, 1972.
13. ANDREW, B. L., N. J. PART, AND F. WAIT. Muscle spindles without γ-efferents. *J. Physiol. London* 219: 28P-29P, 1971.
14. ANZENBACHER, H., AND W. ZENKER. Über die Grössenbeziehung der Muskelfasern zu ihren motorischen Endplatten und Nerven. *Z. Zellforsch. Mikrosk. Anat.* 60: 860-871, 1963.
15. APPELBERG, B., AND F. EMONET-DÉNAND. Motor units of the first superficial lumbrical muscle of the cat. *J. Neurophysiol.* 30: 154-160, 1967.
16. ARAKI, T., K. ENDO, Y. KAWAI, K. ITO, AND Y. SHIGENAGA. Supraspinal control of slow and fast spinal motoneurons of the cat. In: *Progress in Brain Research. Understanding the Stretch Reflex*, edited by S. Homma. Amsterdam: Elsevier, 1976, vol. 44, p. 413-432.
17. ARIANO, M. A., R. B. ARMSTRONG, AND V. R. EDGERTON. Hindlimb muscle fiber populations of five mammals. *J. Histochem. Cytochem.* 21: 51-55, 1973.
18. ARMSTRONG, R. B., P. MARUM, C. W. SAUBERT, H. J. SEEHERMAN, AND C. R. TAYLOR. Muscle fiber activity as a function of speed and gait. *J. Appl. Physiol.: Respirat. Environ. Exercise Physiol.* 43: 672-677, 1977.
19. ARMSTRONG, R. B., C. W. SAUBERT, R. E. SEMBROWICH, R. E. SHEPHERD, AND P. D. GOLLNICK. Glycogen depletion in rat skeletal muscle fibers at different intensities and durations of exercise. *Pfluegers Arch.* 352: 243-256, 1974.
20. ARNDT, T., AND F. A. PEPE. Antigenic specificity of red and white muscle myosin. *J. Histochem. Cytochem.* 23: 159-168, 1975.
21. ASHLEY, C. C., AND D. G. MOISESCU. Model for the action of calcium in muscle. *Nature London New Biol.* 237: 208-211, 1972.
22. ASHMORE, C. R., AND L. DOERR. Comparative aspects of muscle fiber types in different species. *Exp. Neurol.* 31: 408-418, 1971.
23. ASHMORE, C. R., D. W. ROBINSON, P. RATTRAY, AND L. DOERR. Biphasic development of muscle fibers in the fetal lamb. *Exp. Neurol.* 37: 241-255, 1972.
24. ASHMORE, C. R., G. TOMPKINS, AND L. DOERR. Comparative aspects of mitochondria isolated from αW, αR, and βR muscle fibers of the chick. *Exp. Neurol.* 35: 413-420, 1972.
25. ASKANAS, V., S. A. SHAFIQ, AND A. T. MILHORAT. Histochemistry of cultured aneural chick muscle. Morphological maturation without differentiation of fiber types. *Exp. Neurol.* 37: 218-230, 1972.
26. AWAN, M. Z., AND G. GOLDSPINK. Energy utilization by mammalian fast and slow muscle in doing external work. *Biochim. Biophys. Acta* 216: 229-230, 1970.
27. AWAN, M. Z., AND G. GOLDSPINK. Energetics of the development and maintenance of isometric tension by mammalian fast and slow muscles. *J. Mechanochem. Cell Motil.* 1: 97-108, 1972.
28. BAGUST, J. Relationship between motor nerve conduction velocities and motor unit contraction characteristics in a slow-twitch muscle of the cat. *J. Physiol. London* 238: 269-278, 1974.
29. BAGUST, J. The effects of tenotomy upon the contraction characteristics of motor units in rabbit soleus muscle. *J. Physiol. London* 290: 1-10, 1979.
30. BAGUST, J., H. J. FINOL, D. M. LEWIS, S. WEBB, AND R. A. WESTERMAN. Motor units of cross-reinnervated fast and slow twitch muscles. *J. Physiol. London* 239: 45P-46P, 1974.
31. BAGUST, J., S. KNOTT, D. M. LEWIS, J. C. LUCK, AND R. A. WESTERMAN. Isometric contractions of motor units in a fast twitch muscle of the cat. *J. Physiol. London* 231: 87-104, 1973.
32. BAGUST, J., AND D. M. LEWIS. Isometric contractions of motor units in self-reinnervated fast and slow twitch muscles of the cat. *J. Physiol. London* 237: 91-102, 1974.
33. BAGUST, J., D. M. LEWIS, AND J. C. LUCK. Post-tetanic effects in motor units of fast and slow twitch muscle of the cat. *J. Physiol. London* 237: 115-121, 1974.
34. BAGUST, J., D. M. LEWIS, AND R. A. WESTERMAN. The prop-

erties of motor units in a fast and slow twitch muscle during post-natal development in the kitten. *J. Physiol. London* 237: 75-90, 1972.
35. BAGUST, J., D. M. LEWIS AND R. A. WESTERMAN. Polyneuronal innervation of kitten skeletal muscle. *J. Physiol. London* 229: 241-255, 1973.
36. BALDISSERA, F., AND B. GUSTAFSSON. Firing behaviour of a neurone model based on the afterhyperpolarization conductance time course. First interval firing. *Acta Physiol. Scand.* 91: 528-544, 1974.
37. BALDWIN, K. M., J. S. REITMAN, R. L. TERJUNG, W. W. WINDER, AND J. O. HOLLOSZY. Substrate depletion in different types of muscle and in liver during prolonged running. *Am. J. Physiol.* 225: 1045-1050, 1973.
38. BALLANTYNE, J. P., AND S. HANSEN. A new method for the estimation of the number of motor units in a muscle. I. Control subjects and patients with myasthenia gravis. *J. Neurol. Neurosurg. Psychiatry* 37: 907-915, 1974.
39. BÁRÁNY, M. ATPase activity of myosin correlated with speed of muscle shortening. *J. Gen. Physiol.* 50: 197-216, 1967.
40. BÁRÁNY, M., AND K. BÁRÁNY. A proposal for the mechanism of contraction in intact frog muscle. In: *The Mechanism of Muscle Contraction.* Cold Spring Harbor: Cold Spring Harbor Lab., 1973, p. 635-646. (Cold Spring Harbor Symp. Quant. Biol., 1973, vol. 37.)
41. BARKER, D. The morphology of muscle receptors. In: *Handbook of Sensory Physiology. Muscle Receptors*, edited by C. C. Hunt. Berlin: Springer-Verlag, 1974, vol. 3, pt. 2, p. 1-190.
42. BARKER, D., F. EMONET-DÉNAND, D. W. HARKER, L. JAMI, AND Y. LAPORTE. Types of intra- and extrafusal muscle fibre innervated by dynamic skeletofusimotor axons in cat peroneus brevis and tenuissimus muscles as determined by the glycogen depletion method. *J. Physiol. London* 266: 713-726, 1977.
43. BARMACK, N. H. Recruitment and suprathreshold frequency modulation of single extraocular muscle fibers in the rabbit. *J. Neurophysiol.* 40: 779-790, 1977.
44. BARNARD, R. J., V. R. EDGERTON, T. FURUKAWA, AND J. B. PETER. Histochemical, biochemical and contractile properties of red, white and intermediate fibers. *Am. J. Physiol.* 220: 410-414, 1971.
45. BARNARD, R. J., V. R. EDGERTON, AND J. B. PETER. Effect of exercise on skeletal muscle. I. Biochemical and histochemical properties. *J. Appl. Physiol.* 28: 762-766, 1970.
46. BARNARD, R. J., V. R. EDGERTON, AND J. B. PETER. Effect of exercise on skeletal muscle. II. Contractile properties. *J. Appl. Physiol.* 28: 767-770, 1970.
47. BARRETT, E. F., AND J. N. BARRETT. Separation of two voltage-sensitive potassium currents, and demonstration on a tetrodotoxin-resistant calcium current in frog motoneurons. *J. Physiol. London* 255: 737-744, 1976.
48. BARRETT, J. N., AND W. E. CRILL. Specific membrane properties of cat motoneurones. *J. Physiol. London* 239: 301-324, 1974.
49. BASMAJIAN, J. V. Control and training of individual motor units. *Science* 141: 440-441, 1963.
50. BAWA, P., AND W. G. TATTON. Motor unit responses in muscles stretched by imposed displacements of the monkey wrist. *Exp. Brain Res.* 37: 417-437, 1979.
51. BEATTY, C. H., G. M. BASINGER, AND R. M. BOELK. Differentiation of red and white fibers in muscle from fetal, neonatal and infant rhesus monkeys. *J. Histochem. Cytochem.* 15: 93-103, 1967.
52. BEATTY, C. H., G. M. BASINGER, C. C. DULLY, AND R. M. BOELK. Comparison of red and white voluntary skeletal muscles of several species of primates. *J. Histochem. Cytochem.* 14: 590-600, 1966.
53. BENNETT, M. R., AND G. PETTIGREW. The formation of synapses in striated muscle during development. *J. Physiol. London* 241: 515-545, 1974.
54. BENOIT, P., AND J. P. CHANGEUX. Consequences of tenotomy on the evolution of multi-innervation on developing rat soleus muscle. *Brain Res.* 99: 354-358, 1975.

55. BERGMANS, J., AND G. MARECHAL. Rapport entre potentiel d'action et tension du muscle strié. *Arch. Int. Physiol. Biochim.* 68: 377-379, 1960.
56. BERNSTEIN, J. J., AND L. GUTH. Nonselectivity in establishment of neuromuscular connections following nerve regeneration in the rat. *Exp. Neurol.* 4: 262-275, 1961.
57. BESSOU, P., F. EMONET-DÉNAND, AND Y. LAPORTE. Relation entre la vitesse de conduction des fibres nerveuses motrices et le tempe de contraction de leurs unites motrices. *C. R. Acad. Sci. Ser. D* 256: 5625-5627, 1963.
58. BESSOU, P., F. EMONET-DÉNAND, AND Y. LAPORTE. Motor fibres innervating extrafusal and intrafusal muscle fibres in the cat. *J. Physiol. London* 180: 649-672, 1965.
59. BETZ, W. J., J. H. CALDWELL, AND R. R. RIBCHESTER. The size of motor units during post-natal development of rat lumbrical muscle. *J. Physiol. London* 297: 463-478, 1980.
60. BEZANILLA, F., AND P. HOROWICZ. Fluorescence intensity changes associated with contractile activation in frog muscle stained with Nile Blue A. *J. Physiol. London* 246: 709-735, 1975.
61. BIGLAND, B., AND O. LIPPOLD. Motor unit activity in the voluntary contraction of human muscle. *J. Physiol. London* 125: 322-335, 1954.
62. BIGLAND-RITCHIE, B., D. A. JONES, AND J. J. WOODS. Excitation frequency and muscle fatigue: electrical responses during human voluntary and stimulated contractions. *Exp. Neurol.* 64: 414-427, 1979.
63. BINDER, M. D., W. E. CAMERON, AND D. G. STUART. Speed-force relations in the motor units of cat tibialis posterior. *Am. J. Phys. Med.* 57: 57-65, 1978.
64. BINDER, M. D., J. S. KROIN, G. P. MOORE, E. K. STAUFFER, AND D. G. STUART. Correlation analysis of muscle spindle responses to single motor unit contractions. *J. Physiol. London* 257: 325-336, 1976.
65. BINKHORST, R. A., AND M. A. VAN'T HOF. Force-velocity relationship and contraction trace of the rat fast plantaris muscle due to compensatory hypertrophy. *Pfluegers Arch.* 342: 145-158, 1973.
66. BLASCHKO, H., M. CATTELL, AND J. L. KAHN. On the nature of the two types of response in the neuromuscular system of the crustacean claw. *J. Physiol. London* 73: 25-35, 1931.
67. BLINKS, J. R., R. RUDEL, AND S. R. TAYLOR. Calcium transients in isolated amphibian skeletal muscle fibres: detection with Aequorin. *J. Physiol. London* 277: 291-323, 1978.
68. BOESIGER, B. Comparaison morphologique, biometrique et histochimique des fibres musculaires et de leurs terminaisons nerveuses motrices de differents muscles de la caille japonaise, *Coturnix coturnix japonica. Acta Anat.* 71: 274-310, 1968.
69. BOOTH, F. W., AND J. R. KELSO. Effect of hind-limb immobilization on contractile and histochemical properties of skeletal muscle. *Pfluegers Arch.* 342: 231-238, 1973.
70. BORG, J., L. GRIMBY, AND J. HANNERZ. Axonal conduction velocity and voluntary discharge properties of individual short toe extensor motor units in man. *J. Physiol. London* 277: 143-152, 1978.
71. BOTTERMAN, B. R., M. D. BINDER, AND D. G. STUART. Functional anatomy of the association between motor units and muscle receptors. *Am. Zool.* 18: 135-152, 1978.
72. BOYD, I. A., AND M. R. DAVEY. *Composition of Peripheral Nerves.* Edinburgh: Livingstone, 1968.
73. BRACCHI, F., M. DECANDIA, AND T. GUALTIEROTTI. Frequency stabilization in the motor centers of spinal cord and caudal brain stem. *Am. J. Physiol.* 210: 1170-1177, 1966.
74. BRANDSTATER, M. E., AND E. H. LAMBERT. Motor unit anatomy: type and spatial arrangement of muscle fibers. In: *New Developments in Electromyography and Clinical Neurophysiology*, edited by J. E. Desmedt. Basel: Karger, 1973, vol. 1, p. 14-22.
75. BRINK, E. E., J. I. MORRELL, AND D. W. PFAFF. Localization of lumbar epaxial motoneurons in the rat. *Brain Res.* 170: 23-41, 1979.
76. BROOKE, M. H., AND W. K. ENGEL. The histographic analysis

of human muscle biopsies with regard to fiber types. *Neurology* 19: 221-233, 1969.
77. BROOKE, M. H., AND K. K. KAISER. Muscle fibre types: how many and what kind? *Arch. Neurol. Chicago* 23: 369-379, 1970.
78. BROOKE, M. H., AND K. K. KAISER. The use and abuse of muscle histochemistry. *Ann. NY Acad. Sci.* 228: 121-144, 1974.
79. BROOKE, M. H., E. WILLIAMSON, AND K. K. KAISER. The behaviour of four fiber types in developing and reinnervated muscle. *Arch. Neurol. Chicago* 25: 360-366, 1971.
80. BROWN, G. L., AND B. D. BURNS. Fatigue and neuromuscular block in mammalian skeletal muscle. *Proc. R. Soc. London Ser. B* 136: 182-195, 1949.
81. BROWN, G. L., AND U. S. VON EULER. The after effects of a tetanus on mammalian muscle. *J. Physiol. London* 93: 39-60, 1938.
82. BROWN, M. C., M. A. COTTER, O. HUDLICKA, AND G. VRBOVA. The effects of different patterns of muscle activity on capillary density, mechanical properties and structure of slow and fast rabbit muscles. *Pfluegers Arch.* 361: 241-250, 1976.
83. BROWN, M. C., R. L. HOLLAND, AND R. IRONTON. Evidence against an intraspinal signal for motoneurone sprouting in mice. *J. Physiol. London* 291: 35P-36P, 1979.
84. BROWN, M. C., AND R. IRONTON. Sprouting and regression of neuromuscular synapses in partially denervated mammalian muscles. *J. Physiol. London* 278: 325-348, 1978.
85. BROWN, M. C., J. K. S. JANSEN, AND D. VAN ESSEN. Polyneuronal innervation of skeletal muscle in new-born rats and its elimination during maturation. *J. Physiol. London* 261: 387-422, 1976.
86. BROWN, M. C., AND P. B. C. MATTHEWS. An investigation into the possible existence of polyneuronal innervation of individual skeletal muscle fibres in certain hind-limb muscles of the cat. *J. Physiol. London* 151: 436-457, 1960.
87. BROWN, W. F., AND H. S. MILNER-BROWN. Some electrical properties of motor units and their effects on the methods of estimating motor unit numbers. *J. Neurol. Neurosurg. Psychiatry* 39: 249-257, 1976.
88. BRYAN, R. N., D. L. TREVINO, AND W. D. WILLIS. Evidence for a common location of alpha and gamma motoneurons. *Brain Res.* 38: 193-196, 1972.
89. BUCHTHAL, F. The general concept of the motor unit. *Res. Publ. Assoc. Res. Nerv. Ment. Dis.* 38: 3-30, 1961.
90. BUCHTHAL, F., F. ERMINIO, AND P. ROSENFALCK. Motor unit territory in different human muscles. *Acta Physiol. Scand.* 45: 72-87, 1959.
91. BUCHTHAL, F., AND P. ROSENFALCK. On the structure of motor units. In: *New Developmens in Electromyography and Clinical Neurophysiology*, edited by J. E. Desmedt. Basel: Karger, 1973, vol. 1, p. 71-85.
92. BUCHTHAL, F., AND H. SCHMALBRUCH. Contraction times and fibre types in intact human muscle. *Acta Physiol. Scand.* 79: 435-452, 1970.
93. BÜDINGEN, H. J., AND H. J. FREUND. The relationship between the rate of rise of isometric tension and motor unit recruitment in a human forearm muscle. *Pfluegers Arch.* 362: 61-67, 1976.
94. BULLARD, H. H. Histological as related to physiological and chemical differences in certain muscles of the cat. *Johns Hopkins Hosp. Rep.* 18: 323, 1919.
95. BULLER, A. J., J. C. ECCLES, AND R. M. ECCLES. Differentiation of fast and slow muscles in the cat hind limb. *J. Physiol. London* 150: 339-416, 1960.
96. BULLER, A. J., J. C. ECCLES, AND R. M. ECCLES. Interactions between motoneurons and muscles in respect of the characteristic speeds of their responses. *J. Physiol. London* 150: 417-439, 1960.
97. BULLER, A. J., AND R. POPE. Plasticity in mammalian skeletal muscle. *Philos. Trans. R. Soc. London Ser. B* 278: 295-305, 1977.
98. BURKE, D., W. F. SKUSE, AND A. K. LETHLEAN. Isometric contraction of the abductor digiti minimi muscle in man. *J. Neurol. Neurosurg. Psychiatry* 37: 825-834, 1974.
99. BURKE, R. E. Composite nature of the monosynaptic excitatory post synaptic potential. *J. Neurophysiol.* 30: 1114-1136, 1967.
100. BURKE, R. E. Motor unit types of cat triceps surae muscle. *J. Physiol. London* 193: 141-160, 1967.
101. BURKE, R. E. Group Ia synaptic input to fast and slow twitch motor units of cat triceps surae. *J. Physiol. London* 196: 605-630, 1968.
102. BURKE, R. E. Firing patterns of gastrocnemius motor units in the decerebrate cat. *J. Physiol. London* 196: 631-654, 1968.
103. BURKE, R. E. On the central nervous system control of fast and slow twitch motor units. In: *New Developments in Electromyography and Clinical Neurophysiology*, edited by J. E. Desmedt. Basel: Karger, 1973, vol. 1, p. 69-94.
104. BURKE, R. E. A comment on the existence of motor unit "types." In: *The Nervous System. The Basic Neurosciences*, edited by R. O. Brady. NY: Raven, 1975, vol. 1, p. 611-619.
105. BURKE, R. E., R. P. DUM, M. J. O'DONOVAN, J. TOOP, AND P. TSAIRIS. Properties of soleus muscle and of individual soleus muscle units after cross-reinnervation by FDL motoneurons. *Neurosci. Abstr.* 5: 765, 1979.
106. BURKE, R. E., AND V. R. EDGERTON. Motor unit properties and selective involvement in movement. In: *Exercise and Sport Sciences Reviews*, edited by J. H. Wilmore and J. F. Keogh. New York: Academic, 1975, vol. 3, p. 31-81.
107. BURKE, R. E., L. FEDINA, AND A. LUNDBERG. Spatial synaptic distribution of recurrent and group Ia inhibitory systems in cat spinal motoneurones. *J. Physiol. London* 214: 305-326, 1971.
108. BURKE, R. E., E. JANKOWSKA, AND G. TEN BRUGGENCATE. A comparison of peripheral and rubrospinal synaptic input to slow and fast twitch motor units of triceps surae. *J. Physiol. London* 207: 709-732, 1970.
109. BURKE, R. E., K. KANDA, AND R. F. MAYER. The effect of chronic immobilization on defined types of motor units in cat medial gastrocnemius. *Neurosci. Abstr.* 1: 763, 1975.
110. BURKE, R. E., D. N. LEVINE, M. SALCMAN, AND P. TSAIRIS. Motor units in cat soleus muscle: physiological, histochemical and morphological characteristics. *J. Physiol. London* 238: 503-514, 1974.
111. BURKE, R. E., D. N. LEVINE, P. TSAIRIS, AND F. E. ZAJAC. Physiological types and histochemical profiles in motor units of the cat gastrocnemius. *J. Physiol. London* 234: 723-748, 1973.
112. BURKE, R. E., D. N. LEVINE, F. E. ZAJAC, P. TSAIRIS, AND W. K. ENGEL. Mammalian motor units: physiological-histochemical correlation in three types in cat gastrocnemius. *Science* 174: 709-712, 1971.
113. BURKE, R. E., AND P. G. NELSON. Accommodation to current ramps in motoneurons of fast and slow twitch motor units. *Int. J. Neurosci.* 1: 347-356, 1971.
114. BURKE, R. E., AND P. RUDOMIN. Spinal nervous and synapses. In: *Handbook of Physiology. The Nervous System. Cellular Biology of Neurons*, edited by E. R. Kandel. Bethesda, MD: Am. Physiol. Soc., sect. 1, vol. 1, pt. 2, chapt. 24, p. 877-944.
115. BURKE, R. E., P. RUDOMIN, AND F. E. ZAJAC. Catch property in single mammalian motor units. *Science* 168: 122-124, 1970.
116. BURKE, R. E., P. RUDOMIN, AND F. E. ZAJAC. The effect of activation history on tension production by individual muscle units. *Brain Res.* 109: 515-529, 1976.
117. BURKE, R. E., W. Z. RYMER, AND J. V. WALSH. Functional specialization in the motor unit population of cat medial gastrocnemius muscle. In: *Control of Posture and Locomotion*, edited by R. B. Stein, K. G. Pearson, R. S. Smith, and J. B. Redford. New York: Plenum, 1973, p. 29-44.
118. BURKE, R. E., W. Z. RYMER, AND J. V. WALSH, JR. Relative strength of synaptic input from short-latency pathways to motor units of defined type in cat medial gastrocnemius. *J. Neurophysiol.* 39: 447-458, 1976.
119. BURKE, R. E., P. L. STRICK, K. KANDA, C. C. KIM, AND B. WALMSLEY. Anatomy of medial gastrocnemius and soleus motor nuclei in cat spinal cord. *J. Neurophysiol.* 40: 667-680, 1977.
120. BURKE, R. E., AND G. TEN BRUGGENCATE. Electrotronic characteristics of alpha motoneurones of varying size. *J. Physiol. London* 234: 749-765, 1973.

121. BURKE, R. E., AND P. TSAIRIS. Anatomy and innervation ratios in motor units of cat gastrocnemius. *J. Physiol. London* 234: 749-765, 1973.
122. BURKE, R. E., AND P. TSAIRIS. The correlation of physiological properties with histochemical characteristics in single muscle units. *Ann. NY Acad. Sci.* 228: 145-159, 1974.
123. BURKE, R. E., AND P. TSAIRIS. Histochemical and physiological profile of a skeletofusimotor (β) unit in cat soleus muscle. *Brain Res.* 129: 341-345, 1977.
124. BURKE, R. E., B. WALMSLEY, AND J. A. HODGSON. HRP anatomy of group Ia afferent contacts on alpha motoneurons. *Brain Res.* 160: 347-352, 1979.
125. CALVIN, W. H. A third mode of repetitive firing: self-regenerative firing due to large delayed depolarizations. In: *Control of Posture and Locomotion*, edited by R. O. Stein, K. G. Pearson, R. S. Smith, and J. B. Redford. New York: Raven, 1973, p. 173-177.
126. CALVIN, W. H. Three modes of repetitive firing and the role of threshold time course between spikes. *Brain Res.* 69: 341-346, 1974.
127. CALVIN, W. H., AND P. C. SCHWINDT. Steps in production of motoneuron spikes during rhythmic firing. *J. Neurophysiol.* 35: 297-310, 1972.
128. CAMPA, J. F., AND W. K. ENGEL. Histochemistry of motor neurones and interneurons of the cat lumbar spinal cord. *Neurology* 20: 559-568, 1970.
129. CAMPA, J. F., AND W. K. ENGEL. Histochemical and functional correlations in anterior horn neurons of the cat spinal cord. *Science* 171: 198-199, 1971.
130. CARLSON, B. M., AND E. GUTMANN. Contractile and histochemical properties of sliced muscle grafts regenerating in normal and denervated rat limbs. *Exp. Neurol.* 50: 319-329, 1976.
131. CARLSON, F. D., AND D. R. WILKIE. *Muscle Physiology.* Englewood Cliffs, NJ: Prentice-Hall, 1974.
132. CARLSON, H. Histochemical fiber composition of lumbar back muscles in the cat. *Acta Physiol. Scand.* 103: 198-209, 1978.
133. CAVAGNA, G. A., N. C. HEGLUND, AND C. R. TAYLOR. Mechanical work in terrestrial locomotion: two basic mechanisms for minimizing energy expediture. *Am. J. Physiol.* 233 (*Regulatory Integrative Comp. Physiol.* 2): R243-R261, 1977.
134. CECCHI, G., F. COLOMO, AND V. LOMBARDI. Force-velocity relation in normal and nitrate-treated frog single muscle fibres during rise of tension in an isometric tetanus. *J. Physiol. London* 285: 257-273, 1978.
135. CHIARIANDINI, D. J., AND E. STEFANI. Electrophysiological identification of two types of fibres in rat extraocular muscles. *J. Physiol. London* 290: 453-465, 1979.
136. CLAMANN, H. P. Activity of single motor units during isometric tension. *Neurology* 20: 256-260, 1970.
137. CLAMANN, H. P., J. D. GILLIES, AND E. HENNEMAN. Effects of inhibitory inputs on critical firing level and rank order of motoneurons. *J. Neurophysiol.* 37: 1350-1360, 1974.
138. CLAMANN, H. P., AND S. J. GOLDBERG. Uncertainty of recruitment order when tested with intracellular techniques. *Neurosci. Abstr.* 1: 167, 1975.
139. CLAMANN, H. P., AND E. HENNEMAN. Electrical measurement of axon diameter and its use in relating motoneuron size to critical firing level. *J. Neurophysiol.* 39: 844-851, 1976.
140. CLAMANN, H. P., AND C. G. KUKULKA. The relation between size of motoneurons and their position in the cat spinal cord. *J. Morphol.* 153: 461-466, 1977.
141. CLAMANN, H. P., AND C. G. KUKULKA. Reversals of recruitment order in medial gastrocnemius produced by stimulation of Deiters nucleus. *Neurosci. Abstr.* 3: 269, 1977.
142. CLAMANN, H. P., AND A. C. NGAI. Recruitment order in three different reflex responses elicited in a hindlimb flexor muscle in the cat. *Neurosci. Abstr.* 4: 293, 1978.
143. CLARK, D. A. Muscle counts of motor units: a study in innervation ratios. *Am. J. Physiol.* 96: 296-304, 1931.
144. CLOSE, R. The relation between intrinsic speed of shortening and duration of the active state of muscle. *J. Physiol. London* 180: 542-559, 1965.
145. CLOSE, R. Properties of motor units in fast and slow skeletal muscles of the rat. *J. Physiol. London* 193: 45-55, 1967.
146. CLOSE, R. Dynamic properties of fast and slow skeletal muscles of the rat after nerve cross-union. *J. Physiol. London* 204: 331-346, 1969.
147. CLOSE, R. Neural influences on physiological properties of fast and slow limb muscles. In: *Contractility of Muscle Cells and Related Processes*, edited by R. J. Podolsky. Englewood Cliffs, NJ: Prentice-Hall, 1971, p. 175-188.
148. CLOSE, R. Dynamic properties of mammalian skeletal muscles. *Physiol. Rev.* 52: 129-197, 1972.
149. CLOSE, R., AND J. F. Y. HOH. The after-effects of repetitive stimulation on the isometric twitch contraction of rat fast skeletal muscle. *J. Physiol. London* 197: 461-477, 1968.
150. CLOSE, R. I., AND A. R. LUFF. Dynamic properties of inferior rectus muscle of the rat. *J. Physiol. London* 236: 259-270, 1974.
151. CLOUGH, J. F., D. KERNELL, AND C. G. PHILLIPS. The distribution of monosynaptic excitation from the pyramidal tract and from primary spindle afferents to motoneurones of the baboon's hand and forearm. *J. Physiol. London* 198: 145-166, 1968.
152. COHEN, L. A. Localization of the stretch reflex. *J. Neurophysiol.* 16: 272-285, 1954.
153. COLLATOS, T. C., V. R. EDGERTON, J. L. SMITH, AND B. R. BOTTERMAN. Contractile properties and fiber type compositions of flexors and extensors of elbow joint in cat: implications for motor control. *J. Neurophysiol.* 40: 1292-1300, 1977.
154. COLOMO, F., AND P. ROCCHI. Staircase effect and post-tetanic potentiation in frog nerve-single muscle fiber preparation. *Arch. Fisiol.* 64: 189-266, 1965.
155. CONNOLLY, R., W. GOUGH, AND S. WINEGRAD. Characteristics of the isometric twitch of skeletal muscle immediately after a tetanus. A study of the influence of the distribution of calcium within the sarcoplasmic reticulum on the twitch. *J. Gen. Physiol.* 57: 697-709, 1971.
156. CONRADI, S., J.-O. KELLERTH, AND C.-H. BERTHOLD. Electron microscopic studies of cat spinal α-motoneurons. II. A method for the description of neuronal architecture and synaptology from serial sections through the cell body and proximal dendritic segments. *J. Comp. Neurol.* 184: 741-754, 1979.
157. CONRADI, S., J.-O. KELLERTH, C.-H. BERTHOLD, AND C. HAMMARBERG. Electron microscopic studies of cat spinal α-motoneurons. IV. Motoneurons innervating slow twitch (type S) units of the soleus muscle. *J. Comp. Neurol.* 184: 769-782, 1979.
158. CONRADI, S., AND L.-O. RONNEVI. Spontaneous elimination of synapses on cat spinal motoneurons after birth: do half of the synapses on the cell bodies disappear? *Brain Res.* 92: 505-510, 1975.
159. CONRADI, S., AND L.-O. RONNEVI. Ultrastructure and synaptology of the initial axon segment of cat spinal motoneurons during early postnatal development. *J. Neurocytol.* 6: 195-210, 1977.
160. COOMBS, J. S., D. R. CURTIS, AND J. C. ECCLES. The electrical constants of the motoneurone membrane. *J. Physiol. London* 145: 505-528, 1959.
161. COOMBS, J. S., J. C. ECCLES, AND P. FATT. The electrical properties of the motoneurone membrane. *J. Physiol. London* 130: 291-325, 1955.
162. COOMBS, J. S., J. C. ECCLES, AND P. FATT. The specific ionic conductances and the ionic movements across the motonerone membrane that produce the inhibitory post-synaptic potential. *J. Physiol. London* 130: 326-373, 1955.
163. COOPER, C. C., R. G. CARSENS, L. L. KASTENSCHMIDT, AND E. J. BRISKEY. Histochemical characterization of muscle differentiation. *Dev. Biol.* 23: 169-184, 1970.
164. COOPER, S., AND J. C. ECCLES. The isometric responses of mammalian muscles. *J. Physiol. London* 69: 377-385, 1930.
165. COSTANTIN, L. L. Activation in striated muscle. In: *Handbook of Physiology. The Nervous System. Cellular Biology of Neurons*, edited by E. R. Kandel. Bethesda, MD: Am. Physiol. Soc., 1977, sect. 1, vol. I, pt. 1, chapt. 7, p. 215-259.
166. COSTILL, D. L., W. J. FINK, AND M. L. POLLOCK. Muscle fiber composition and enzyme activities of elite distance runners.

Med. Sci. Sports 8: 96–100, 1976.
167. COSTILL, D. L., P. D. GOLLNICK, E. D. JANSSON, B. SALTIN, AND E. M. STEIN. Glycogen depletion pattern in human muscle fibres during distance running. *Acta Physiol. Scand.* 89: 374–383, 1973.
169. CRACROFT, J. D., AND J. H. PETAJAN. Effect of muscle training on the pattern of firing of single motor units. *Am. J. Phys. Med.* 56: 183–194, 1977.
170. CREED, R. S., D. DENNEY-BROWN, J. D. ECCLES, E. G. T. LIDDELL, AND C. S. SHERRINGTON. *Reflex Activity of the Spinal Cord*. London: Oxford Univ. Press, 1932.
171. CRUCE, W. L. R. The anatomical organization of hindlimb motoneurons in the spinal cord of the frog, *R. catesbiana*. *J. Comp. Neurol.* 153: 59–76, 1974.
172. CULLHEIM, S. Relations between cell body size, axon diameter and axon conduction velocity of cat sciatic α-motoneurons stained with horseradish peroxidase. *Neurosci. Lett.* 8: 17–20, 1978.
173. CULLHEIM, S., AND J.-O. KELLERTH. Combined light and electron microscopic tracing of neurons, including axons and synaptic terminals, after intracellular injection of horseradish peroxidase. *Neurosci. Lett.* 2: 307–313, 1976.
174. CULLHEIM, S., AND J.-O. KELLERTH. A morphological study of the axons and recurrent axon collaterals of cat α-motoneurones supplying different functional types of muscle unit. *J. Physiol. London* 281: 301–313, 1978.
175. CULLHEIM, S., AND J.-O. KELLERTH. A morphological study of the axons and recurrent axon collaterals of cat sciatic α-motoneurons after intracellular staining with horseradish peroxidase. *J. Comp. Neurol.* 178: 537–558, 1978.
176. CULLHEIM, S., J.-O. KELLERTH, AND S. CONRADI. Evidence for direct synaptic interconnections between cap spinal α-motoneurons via the recurrent axon collaterals: a morphological study using intracellular injection of horseradish peroxidase. *Brain Res.* 132: 1–10, 1977.
177. CURTIS, D. R., AND J. C. ECCLES. The time courses of excitatory and inhibitory synaptic actions. *J. Physiol. London* 145: 529–546, 1959.
178. CZEH, G., R. GALLEGO, N. KUDO, AND M. KUNO. Evidence for the maintenance of motoneurone properties by muscle activity. *J. Physiol. London* 281: 239–252, 1978.
179. DAVIS, W. J. Functional significance of motoneuron size and soma position in swimmeret system of the lobster. *J. Neurophysiol.* 34: 274–288, 1971.
180. DAWSON, M. J., D. G. GADIAN, AND D. R. WILKIE. Muscular fatigue investigated by phosphorus nuclear magnetic resonance. *Nature London* 274: 861–866, 1978.
181. DEKKER, J. J., D. G. LAWRENCE, AND H. G. J. M. KUYPERS. The location of longitudinally running dendrites in the ventral horn of the cat spinal cord. *Brain Res.* 51: 319–325, 1973.
182. DELUCA, C. J., AND W. J. FORREST. Probability distribution function of the inter-pulse intervals of single motor unit action potentials during isometric contractions. In: *New Developments in Electromyography and Clinical Neurophysiology*, edited by J. E. Desmedt. Basel: Karger, 1973, vol. 1, p. 638–647.
183. DENNY-BROWN, D. On the nature of postural reflexes. *Proc. R. Soc. London Ser B* 104: 252–301, 1929.
184. DENNY-BROWN, D. The histological feature of striped muscle in relation to its functional activity. *Proc. R. Soc. London Ser. B* 104: 371, 1929.
185. DENNY-BROWN, D. Interpretation of the electromyogram. *Arch. Neurol. Psychiatry* 61: 99–128, 1949.
186. DENNY-BROWN, D. Experimental studies pertaining to hypertrophy, regeneration and degeneration. *Res. Publ. Assoc. Res. Nerv. Ment. Dis.* 38: 147–196, 1960.
187. DENNY-BROWN, D., AND J. B. PENNYBACKER. Fibrillation and fasciculation in voluntary muscle. *Brain* 61: 311–344, 1938.
188. DENSLOW, J. S. Double discharges in human motor units. *J. Neurophysiol.* 11: 209–215, 1948.
189. DERFLER, B., AND L. J. GOLDBERG. Spike train characteristics of single motor units in the human masseter muscle. *Exp. Neurol.* 61: 592–608, 1978.
190. DESMEDT, J. E., AND E. GODAUX. Ballistic contractions in man: characteristic recruitment pattern of single motor units of the tibialis anterior muscle. *J. Physiol. London* 264: 673–694, 1977.
191. DESMEDT, J. E., AND E. GODAUX. Fast motor units are not preferentially activated in rapid voluntary contractions in man. *Nature London* 267: 717–719, 1977.
192. DESMEDT, J. E., AND E. GODAUX. Ballistic contractions in fast or slow human muscles: discharge patterns of single motor units. *J. Physiol. London* 285: 185–196, 1978.
193. DESMEDT, J. E., AND K. HAINAUT. Kinetics of myofilament activation in potentiated contraction: staircase phenomenon in human skeletal muscle. *Nature London* 217: 529–532, 1968.
194. DEVANANDAN, M. S., R. M. ECCLES, AND R. A. WESTERMAN. Single motor units of mammalian muscles. *J. Physiol. London* 178: 359–367, 1965.
195. DIETZ, V., E. BISCHOFBERGER, C. WITA, AND H.-J. FREUND. Correlation between the discharges of two simultaneously recorded motor units an physiological tremor. *Electroencephalogr. Clin. Neurophysiol.* 40: 97–105, 1976.
196. DODGE, F. A. The nonuniform excitability of central neurons as exemplified by a model of the spinal motoneuron. In: *The Neurosciences: Fourth Study Program*, edited by F. O. Schmitt. Boston: MIT Press, 1979, p. 439–455.
197. DODGE, F. A., AND J. W. COOLEY. Action potential of the motoneuron. *IBM J. Res. Dev.* 17: 219–229, 1973.
198. DOYLE, A. M., AND R. F. MAYER. Studies of the motor unit in the cat. *Bull. Sch. Med. MD.* 54: 11–17, 1969.
199. DRACHMAN, D. B. Trophic interactions between nerves and muscles: the role of cholinergic transmission (including usage) and other factors. In: *Biology of Cholinergic Function*, edited by A. M. Goldberg and I. Hanin. New York: Raven, 1976, p. 161–186.
200. DRACHMAN, D. B., AND D. M. JOHNSTON. Development of a mammalian fast muscle: dynamic and biochemical properties correlated. *J. Physiol. London* 234: 29–42, 1973.
201. DUBOWITZ, V. Cross-innervated mammalian skeletal muscle: histochemical, physiological and biochemical observations. *J. Physiol. London* 193: 481–496, 1967.
202. DUBOWITZ, V., AND M. H. BROOKE. *Muscle Biopsy: A Modern Approach*. London: Saunders, 1973.
203. DUBOWITZ, V., AND A. G. E. PEARSE. A comparative histochemical study of oxidative enzyme and phosphorylase activity in skeletal muscle. *Histochemie* 2: 105–117, 1960.
204. DUCHEN, L. W., AND D. A. TONGE. The effects of tetanus toxin on neuromuscular transmission and on the morphology of motor end-plates in slow and fast skeletal muscle of the mouse. *J. Physiol. London* 228: 157–172, 1973.
205. DUM, R. P., R. E. BURKE, AND J. A. HODGSON. Analysis of the motor unit population in cat flexor digitorum longus (FDL) muscle. *Neurosci. Abstr.* 4: 294, 1978.
206. DUM, R. P., R. E. BURKE, M. J. O'DONOVAN, AND J. TOOP. The properties of whole FDL muscle and of individual FDL muscle units after cross-reinnervation by soleus motoneurons in cat. *Neurosci. Abstr.* 5: 766, 1979.
207. DUM, R. P., AND T. T. KENNEDY. Physiological and histochemical characteristics of motor units in cat tibialis anterior and extensor digitorum longus muscles. *J. Neurophysiol.* 43: 1615–1630, 1980.
208. DUM, R. P., AND T. T. KENNEDY. Synaptic organization of defined motor-unit types in cat tibialis anterior. *J. Neurophysiol.* 43: 1631–1644, 1980.
209. EBERSTEIN, A., AND J. GOODGOLD. Slow and fast twitch fibers in human skeletal muscle. *Am. J. Physiol.* 215: 535–541, 1968.
210. EBERSTEIN, A., AND A. SANDOW. Fatigue mechanisms in muscle fibers. In: *Effect of Use and Disuse on Neuromuscular Function*, edited by E. Gutmann and P. Hnik. Prague: Czech. Acad. Sci., 1963, p. 515–526.
211. ECCLES, J. C. Investigations on muscle atrophies arising from disuse and tenotomy. *J. Physiol. London* 103: 253–266, 1944.
212. ECCLES, J. C., R. M. ECCLES, A. IGGO, AND M. ITO. Distribution of recurrent inhibition among motoneurones. *J. Physiol. Lon-*

don 159: 479-499, 1961.
213. ECCLES, J. C., R. M. ECCLES, A. IGGO, AND A. LUNDBERG. Electrophysiological studies on gamma motoneurones. *Acta Physiol. Scand.* 50: 32-40, 1960.
214. ECCLES, J. C., R. M. ECCLES, AND A. LUNDBERG. Synaptic actions on motoneurons in relation to the two components of the group Ia muscle afferent volley. *J. Physiol London* 136: 527-546, 1957.
215. ECCLES, J. C., R. M. ECCLES, AND A. LUNDBERG. The convergence of monosynaptic excitatory afferents on to many different species of alpha motoneurones. *J. Physiol. London* 137: 22-50, 1957.
216. ECCLES, J. C., R. M. ECCLES, AND A. LUNDBERG. The action potentials of the alpha motoneurones supplying fast and slow muscles. *J. Physiol. London* 142: 275-291, 1958.
217. ECCLES, J. C., AND C. S. SHERRINGTON. Numbers and contraction values of individual motor units examined in some muscles of the limb. *Proc. R. Soc. London Ser. B* 106: 326-357, 1930.
218. ECCLES, R. M., AND A. LUNDBERG. Synaptic actions in motoneurons by afferents which may evoke the flexion reflex. *Arch. Ital. Biol.* 97: 199-221, 1959.
219. ECCLES, R. M., C. G. PHILLIPS, AND C. P. WU. Motor innervation, motor unit organization and afferent innervation of M. extensor digitorum communis of the baboon's forearm. *J. Physiol. London* 198: 179-192, 1968.
220. EDDS, M. V. Collateral regeneration of residual motor axons in partially denervated muscles. *J. Exp. Zool.* 113: 507-552, 1950.
221. EDGERTON, V. R. Mammalian muscle fiber types and their adaptability. *Am. Zool.* 18: 113-125, 1978.
222. EDGERTON, V. R., R. J. BARNARD, J. B. PETER, C. A. GILLESPIE, AND D. R. SIMPSON. Overloaded skeletal muscles of a nonhuman primate (*Galago senegalensis*). *Exp. Neurol.* 37: 322-339, 1972.
223. EDGERTON, V. R., R. J. BARNARD, J. B. PETER, A. MAIER, AND D. R. SIMPSON. Properties of immobilized hind-limb muscles of the *Galago senegalensis*. *Exp. Neurol.* 46: 115-131, 1975.
224. EDGERTON, V. R., J. L. SMITH, AND D. R. SIMPSON. Muscle fiber type populations in human leg muscles. *Histochem. J.* 7: 259-266, 1975.
225. EDJTEHADI, G. D., AND D. M. LEWIS. Histochemical reactions of fibres in a fast twitch muscle of the cat. *J. Physiol. London* 287: 439-453, 1979.
226. EDSTRÖM, L., AND B. EKBLOM. Differences in sizes of red and white muscle fibres in vastus lateralis of musculus quadriceps femoris of normal individuals and athletes. Relation to physical performance. *J. Clin. Lab. Invest.* 30: 175-181, 1972.
227. EDSTRÖM, L., AND E. KUGELBERG. Histochemical composition, distribution of fibres and fatiguability of single motor units. Anterior tibial muscle of the rat. *J. Neurol. Neurosurg. Psychiatry* 31: 424-433, 1968.
228. EDSTRÖM, L., AND B. NYSTRÖM. Histochemical types and sizes of fibres in normal human muscles. A biopsy study. *Acta Neurol. Scand.* 45: 257-269, 1969.
229. EDWARDS, R. H. T., D. K. HILL, D. A. JONES, AND P. A. MERTON. Fatigue of long duration in human skeletal muscle after exercise. *J. Physiol. London* 272: 769-778, 1977.
230. EISENBERG, B. R., AND A. M. KUDA. Discrimination between fiber populations in mammalian skeletal muscle by using ultrastructural parameters. *J. Ultrastruct. Res.* 54: 76-88, 1976.
231. EISENBERG, B. R., AND A. M. KUDA. Retrieval of cryostat sections for comparison of histochemistry and quantitative electron microscopy in a muscle fiber. *J. Histochem. Cytochem.* 25: 1169-1177, 1977.
232. EKSTEDT, J. Human single muscle fiber action potentials. *Acta Physiol. Scand. Suppl.* 226: 1-96, 1964.
233. ELFTMAN, H. Biomechanics of muscle. *J. Bone Jt. Surg.* 48A: 363-377, 1966.
234. ELLIOTT, H. C. Studies on the motor cells of the spinal cord. I. Distribution in the normal human cord. *Am. J. Anat.* 70: 95-117, 1942.
235. ELLIOTT, H. C. Studies on the motor cells of the spinal cord. II. Distribution in the normal human foetal cord. *Am. J. Anat.* 72: 29-38, 1943.
236. ELLISMAN, M. H., J. RASH, L. A. STRAEHELIN, AND K. R. PORTER. Studies of excitable membranes. II. A comparison of specializations at neuromuscular junctions and un-junctional sarcolemmas of mammalian fast and slow twitch muscle fibres. *J. Cell Biol.* 68: 752-774, 1976.
237. EMONET-DÉNAND, F., L. JAMI, AND Y. LAPORTE. Skeletofusimotor axons in hind-limb muscles of the cat. *J. Physiol. London* 249: 153-166, 1975.
238. EMONET-DÉNAND, F., E. JANKOWSKA, AND Y. LAPORTE. Skeletofusimotor fibres in the rabbit. *J. Physiol. London* 210: 669-680, 1970.
239. EMONET-DÉNAND, F., AND Y. LAPORTE. Proportion of muscle spindles supplied by skeletofusimotor axons (β-axons) in peroneus brevis muscle of the cat. *J. Neurophysiol.* 38: 1390-1394, 1975.
240. EMONET-DÉNAND, F., Y. LAPORTE, AND U. PROSKE. Contraction of muscle fibers in two adjacent muscles innervated by branches of the same motor axon. *J. Neurophysiol.* 34: 132-138, 1971.
241. ENDO, K., T. ARAKI, AND Y. KAWAI. Contra- and ipsilateral cortical and rubral effects on fast and slow spinal motoneurone of the cat. *Brain Res.* 88: 91-98, 1975.
242. ENGEL, W. K. Fiber-type nomenclature of human skeletal muscle for histochemical purposes. *Neurology* 24: 344-348, 1974.
243. ENGEL, W. K., M. H. BROOKE, AND P. G. NELSON. Histochemical studies of denervated or tenotomized cat muscle: illustrating difficulties in relating experimental animal conditions to human neuromuscular diseases. *Ann. NY Acad. Sci.* 138: 160-185, 1966.
244. ENGEL, W. K., AND R. L. IRWIN. A histochemical-physiological correlation of frog skeletal muscle fibers. *Am. J. Physiol.* 213: 511-518, 1967.
245. ENGEL, W. K., AND G. KARPATI. Impaired skeletal muscle maturatiion following neonatal neurectomy. *Dev. Biol.* 17: 713-723, 1968b.
246. ERULKAR, S. D., M. L. SHELANSKI, B. L. WHITSEL, AND P. OGLE. Studies of muscle fibers of the tensor of the cat. *Anat. Rec.* 149: 279-289, 1964.
247. ESSEN, B., E. JANSSON, J. HENRIKSSON, A. W. TAYLOR, AND B. SALTIN. Metabolic characteristics of fibre types in human skeletal muscle. *Acta Physiol. Scand.* 95: 153-165, 1975.
248. FADEN, J. S. *Recruitment Order and Its Relationship to the Neural and Muscular Properties of Motor Units in the Cat* (Ph.D. dissertation). College Park, MD: Univ. of Maryland, 1978.
249. FADEN, J. S., AND F. E. ZAJAC. Direct comparison of recruitment order with neural and muscular properties of motor axons. *Neurosci. Abstr.* 3: 271, 1977.
250. FAULKNER, J. A., L. C. MAXWELL, AND D. A. LIEBERMAN. Histochemical characteristics of muscle fibers from trained and detrained guinea pigs. *Am. J. Physiol.* 222: 836-840, 1972.
251. FEASBY, T. E., AND W. F. BROWN. Variation of motor unit size in the human extensor digitorum brevis and thenar muscles. *J. Neurol. Neurosurg. Psychiatry* 37: 916-926, 1974.
252. FEDDE, M. R., P. D. DE WET, AND R. L. KITCHELL. Motor unit recruitment pattern and tonic activity in respiratory muscles of *Gallus domesticus*. *J. Neurophysiol.* 32: 995-1004, 1969.
253. FEINDEL, W. Anatomical overlap of motor units. *J. Comp. Neurol.* 101: 1-14, 1954.
254. FEINDEL, W., J. R. HINSHAW, AND G. WENDELL. The pattern of motor innervation in mammalian striated muscle. *J. Anat.* 86: 35-48, 1952.
255. FEINSTEIN, B., B. LINDEGARD, E. NYMAN, AND G. WOHLFART. Morphological studies of motor units in normal human muscles. *Acta Anat.* 23: 127-142, 1955.
256. FENICHEL, G. A histochemical study of developing human skeletal muscle. *Neurology* 16: 741-745, 1966.
257. FERNAND, V. S. V., AND A. HESS. The occurrence, structure

and innervation of slow and twitch muscle fibres in the tensor tympani and stapedius of the cat. *J. Physiol. London* 200: 547–554, 1969.
258. FIEHN, W., AND J. B. PETER. Properties of the fragmented sarcoplasmic reticulum from fast-twitch and slow-twitch muscles. *J. Clin. Invest.* 50: 570–573, 1971.
259. FISCHBACH, G. D., AND P. G. NELSON. Cell culture in neurobiology. In: *Handbook of Physiology. The Nervous System. Cellular Biology of Neurons*, edited by E. R. Kandel. Bethesda, MD: Am. Physiol. Soc., 1977, sect. 1, vol. I, pt. 2, chapt. 20, p. 719–774.
260. FISCHBACH, G. D., AND N. ROBBINS. Changes in contractile properties of disused soleus muscles. *J. Physiol. London* 201: 305–320, 1969.
261. FITTS, R. H., F. W. BOOTH, W. W. WINDER, AND J. O. HOLLOSZY. Skeletal muscle respiratory capacity, endurance, and glycogen utilization. *Am. J. Physiol.* 228: 1029–1033, 1975.
262. FITTS, R., D. CAMPION, F. NAGLE, AND R. CASSENS. Contractile properties of skeletal muscle from trained miniature pig. *Pfluegers Arch.* 343: 133–141, 1973.
263. FITTS, R. H., AND J. O. HOLLOSZY. Contractile properties of rat soleus muscle: effects of training and fatigue. *Am. J. Physiol.* 233 (*Cell Physiol.* 2): C86–C91, 1977.
264. FOLKOW, B., AND H. D. HALICKA. A comparison between 'red' and 'white' muscle with respect to blood supply, capillary surface area and oxygen uptake during rest and exercise. *Microvas. Res.* 1: 1–14, 1968.
265. FRAHER, J. P. A numerical study of cervical and thoracic ventral roots. *J. Anat.* 118: 127–142, 1974.
266. FRANK, K., AND M. G. F. FUORTES. Stimulation of spinal motoneurones with intracellular electrodes. *J. Physiol. London* 134: 451–470, 1956.
267. FRANK, E., J. K. S. JANSEN, T. LØMO, AND R. H. WESTGAARD. The interaction between foreign and original motor nerves innervating the soleus muscle of rats. *J. Physiol. London* 247: 725–743, 1975.
268. FREUND, H.-J., H. J. BÜDINGEN, AND V. DIETZ. Activity of single motor units from human forearm muscles during voluntary isometric contractions. *J. Neurophysiol.* 38: 933–946, 1975.
269. FREUND, H.-J., V. DIETZ, C. W. WITA, AND H. KAPP. Discharge characteristics of single motor units in normal subjects and patients with supraspinal motor disturbances. In: *New Developments in Electromyography and Clinical Neurophysiology*, edited by J. E. Desmedt. Basel: Karger, 1973, vol. 3, p. 242–250.
270. FUCHS, F. Striated muscle. *Ann. Rev. Physiol.* 36: 461–502, 1974.
271. GALLEGO, R., P. HUIZAR, N. KUDO, AND M. KUNO. Disparity of motoneurone and muscle differentiation following spinal transection in the kitten. *J. Physiol. London* 281: 253–265, 1978.
272. GALLEGO, R., M. KUNO, R. NUÑEZ, AND W. D. SNIDER. Dependence of motoneurone properties on the length of immobilized muscle. *J. Physiol. London* 291: 179–189, 1979.
273. GANS, C., AND W. J. BOCK. The functional significance of muscle architecture—a theoretical analysis. *Ergeb. Anat. Entwicklungsgesch.* 38: 116–141, 1965.
274. GARNETT, R. A. F., M. J. O'DONOVAN, J. A. STEPHENS, AND A. TAYLOR. Evidence for the existence of three motor unit types in normal human gastrocnemius. *J. Physiol. London* 280: 65P, 1978.
275. GARNETT, R. A. F., M. J. O'DONOVAN, J. A. STEPHENS, AND A. TAYLOR. Motor unit organization of human medial gastrocnemius. *J. Physiol. London* 287: 33–43, 1979.
276. GAUTHIER, G. F. On the relationship of ultrastructural and cytochemical features to color in mammalian skeletal muscle. *Z. Zellforsch. Mikrosk. Anat.* 95: 462–482, 1969.
277. GAUTHIER, G. F. Ultrastructural identification of muscle fiber types by immunocytochemistry. *J. Cell Biol.* 82: 391–400, 1979.
278. GAUTHIER, G.F., AND S. LOWEY. Polymorphism of myosin among skeletal muscle fiber types. *J. Cell Biol.* 74: 760–779, 1977.
279. GAUTHIER, G. F., AND S. LOWEY. Distribution of myosin isoenzymes among skeletal muscle fiber types. *J. Cell Biol.* 81: 10–25, 1979.
280. GAUTHIER, G. F., S. LOWEY, AND A. W. HOBBS. Fast and slow myosin in developing muscle fibres. *Nature London* 274: 25–29, 1978.
281. GILLESPIE, C. A., D. R. SIMPSON, AND V. R. EDGERTON. Motor unit recruitment as reflected by muscle fiber glycogen loss in a prosimian (Bushbaby) after running and jumping. *J. Neurol. Neurosurg. Psychiatry* 37: 817–824, 1974.
282. GILLIATT, R. W. Axon branching in motor nerves. In: *Control and Innervation of Skeletal Muscle*, edted by B. L. Andrew. Edinburgh: Livingstone, 1966, p. 53–60.
283. GLATT, H. R., AND C. G. HONEGGER. Retrograde axonal transport for cartography of neurones. *Experientia* 29: 1515–1517, 1973.
284. GOERING, J. H. An experimental analysis of the motor-cell columns in the cervical enlargement of the spinal cord in the albino rat. *J. Comp. Neurol.* 46: 125–151, 1928.
285. GOGAN, P., J. P. GUERITAUD, G. HORCHELLE-BOSSAVIT, AND S. TYC-DUMONT. Direct excitatory interactions between spinal motoneurones of the cat. *J. Physiol. London* 272: 755–767, 1977.
286. GOLDBERG, A. L., C. JABLECKI, AND J. B. LI. Effects of use and disuse on amino acid transport and protein turnover in muscle. *Ann. NY Acad. Sci.* 228: 190–201, 1974.
287. GOLDBERG, L. J., AND B. DERFLER. Relationship among recruitment order, spike amplitude, and twitch tension of single motor units in human masseter muscle. *J. Neurophysiol.* 40: 879–890, 1977.
288. GOLDBERG, S. J., G. LENNERSTRAND, AND C. D. HULL. Motor unit responses in the lateral rectus muscle of the cat: intracellular current injection of abducens nucleus neurons. *Acta Physiol. Scand.* 96: 58–63, 1976.
289. GOLDSPINK, G. Energy turnover during contraction of different types of muscle. In: *Biomechanics VI-A*, edited by E. Asmussen and K. Jorgensen. Baltimore: Univ. Park Press, 1978, vol. 2A, p. 27–39. (Int. Ser. Biomech.)
290. GOLDSPINK, G., AND K. F. HOWELLS. Work-induced hypertrophy in exercised normal muscles of different ages and the reversibility of hypertrophy after cessation of exercise. *J. Physiol. London* 239: 179–193, 1974.
291. GOLDSPINK, G., R. E. LARSON, AND R. E. DAVIES. The immediate supply and cost of maintenance of isometric tension for different muscles in the hamster. *Z. Vgl. Physiol.* 66: 389–397, 1970.
292. GOLLNICK, P. D., R. B. ARMSTRONG, B. SALTIN, C. W. SAUBERT, W. L. SEMBROWITCH, AND R. E. SHEPHERD. Effect of training on enzyme activity and fiber composition of human skeletal muscle. *J. Appl. Physiol.* 34: 107–111, 1973.
293. GOLLNICK, P. D., R. B. ARMSTRONG, C. W. SAUBERT, K. PIEHL, AND B. SALTIN. Enzyme activity and fiber composition in skeletal muscle of untrained and trained men. *J. Appl. Physiol.* 33: 312–319, 1972.
294. GOLLNICK, P. D., J. KARLSSEN, K. PIEHL, AND B. SALTIN. Selective glycogen depletion in skeletal muscle fibres of man following sustained contractions. *J. Physiol. London* 241: 59–67, 1974.
295. GOLLNICK, P. D., K. PIEHL, AND B. SALTIN. Selective glycogen depletion pattern in human muscle fibres after exercise of varying intensity and at varying pedalling rates. *J. Physiol. London* 241: 45–57, 1974.
296. GONYEA, W. J., AND G. C. ERICSON. Morphological and histochemical organization of the flexor carpi radialis muscle in the cat. *Am. J. Anat.* 148: 329–344, 1977.
297. GORDON, G., AND A. HOLBOURN. The mechanical activity of single motor units in reflex contraction of skeletal muscles. *J. Physiol. London* 110: 26–35, 1949.
298. GORDON, G., AND C. G. PHILLIPS. Slow and rapid components

in a flexor muscle. *Q. J. Exp. Physiol.* 38: 35–45, 1953.
299. GOSLOW, G. E., W. E. CAMERON, AND D. G. STUART. The fast twitch motor units of cat ankle flexors. 1. Tripartite classification on basis of fatigability. *Brain Res.* 134: 35–46, 1977.
300. GOSLOW, G. E., W. E. CAMERON, AND D. G. STUART. The fast twitch motor units of cat ankle flexors. 2. Speed-force relations and recruitment order. *Brain Res.* 134: 47–57, 1977.
301. GOSLOW, G. E., E. K. STAUFFER, W. C. NEMETH, AND D. G. STUART. Digit flexor muscles in the cat: their action and motor units. *J. Morphol.* 137: 335–352, 1972.
302. GRANIT, R. Neuromuscular interaction in postural tone of the cat's soleus muscle. *J. Physiol. London* 143: 387–402, 1958.
303. GRANIT, R. *Charles Scott Sherrington: An Appraisal.* London: Nelson, 1966.
304. GRANIT, R. *Mechanisms Regulating the Discharge of Motoneurons.* Liverpool: Liverpool Univ. Press, 1972.
305. GRANIT, R., H.-D. HENATSCH, AND G. STEG. Tonic and phasic ventral horn cells differentiated by post-tetanic potentiation in cat extensors. *Acta Physiol. Scand.* 37: 114–126, 1956.
306. GRANIT, R., C. G. PHILLIPS, S. SKOGLUND, AND G. STEG. Differentiation of tonic from phasic alpha ventral horn cells by stretch, pinna and crossed extensor reflexes. *J. Neurophysiol.* 20: 470–481, 1957.
307. GREGORY, J. E., AND U. PROSKE. The responses of Golgi tendon organs to stimulation of different combinations of motor units. *J. Physiol. London* 295: 251–262, 1979.
308. GRILLNER, S., T. HONGO, AND S. LUND. Descending monosynaptic and reflex control of γ-motoneurones. *Acta Physiol. Scand.* 75: 592–613, 1969.
309. GRILLNER, S., T. HONGO, AND S. LUND. The vestibulospinal tract. Effects on alpha-motoneurones in the lumbosacral spinal cord in the cat. *Exp. Brain Res.* 10: 94–120, 1970.
310. GRILLNER, S., AND M. UDO. Motor unit activity and stiffness of the contracting muscle fibers in the tonic stretch reflex. *Acta Physiol. Scand.* 81: 422–424, 1971.
311. GRILLNER, S., AND M. UDO. Recruitment in the tonic stretch reflex. *Acta Physiol. Scand.* 81: 571–573, 1971.
312. GRIMBY, L., AND J. HANNERZ. Recruitment order of motor units on voluntary contraction: changes induced by proprioceptive afferent activity. *J. Neurol. Neurosurg. Psychiatry* 31: 565–573, 1968.
313. GRIMBY, L., AND J. HANNERZ. Differences in recruitment order of motor units in phasic and tonic flexion reflex in 'spinal man.' *J. Neurol. Neurosurg. Psychiatry* 33: 562–570, 1970.
314. GRIMBY, L., AND J. HANNERZ. Differences in recruitment order and discharge pattern of motor units in the early and late flexion reflex components in man. *Acta Physiol. Scand.* 90: 555–564, 1974.
315. GRIMBY, L., AND J. HANNERZ. Disturbances in voluntary recruitment order of low and high frequency motor units on blockade of proprioceptive afferent activity. *Acta Physiol. Scand.* 96: 207–216, 1976.
316. GRIMBY, L., AND J. HANNERZ. Firing rate and recruitment order of toe extensor motor units in different modes of voluntary contraction. *J. Physiol. London* 264: 865–879, 1977.
317. GRIMBY, L., J. HANNERZ, AND B. HEDMAN. Contraction time and voluntary discharge properties of individual short toe extensor motor units in man. *J. Physiol. London* 289: 191–201, 1979.
318. GRINNELL, A. D. A study of the interaction between motoneurones in the frog spinal cord. *J. Physiol. London* 182: 612–648, 1966.
319. GRÖSCHEL-STEWART, U., K. MESCHEDE, AND I. LAHR. Histochemical and immunochemical studies on mammalian striated muscle fibres. *Histochemie* 33: 79–85, 1973.
320. GRÜTZNER, P. Zur Anatomie und Physiologie der quergestreiften Muskeln. *Recl. Zool. Suisse* 1: 665–684, 1884.
321. GULATI, J. Force-velocity characteristics for calcium-activated mammalian slow-twitch and fast-twitch skeletal fibers from the guinea pig. *Proc. Natl. Acad. Sci. USA* 73: 4693–4697, 1976.
322. GURFINKEL, V. S., M. L. MIRSKII, A. M. TARKO, AND T. D. SURGULADZE. Function of human motor units on initiation of muscle tension. *Biofizika* 17: 303–310, 1972.
323. GURFINKEL, V. S., T. D. SURGULADZE, M. L. MIRSKII, AND A. M. TARKO. Activity of human motor units during rhythmic movements. *Biofizika* 15: 1090–1095, 1970.
324. GUSTAFSSON, B. After hyperpolarization and the control of repetitive firing in spinal neurones of the cat. *Acta Physiol. Scand. Suppl.* 416: 1–47, 1974.
325. GUTH, L. "Trophic" influences of nerve on muscle. *Physiol. Rev.* 48: 645–687, 1968.
326. GUTH, L. A review of the evidence for the neural regulation of gene expression in muscle. In: *Contractility of Muscle Cells and Related Processes*, edited by R. J. Podolsky. Englewood Cliffs, NJ: Prentice-Hall, 1971, p. 189–201.
327. GUTH, L. Fact and artifact in the histochemical procedure for myofibrillar ATPase. *Exp. Neurol.* 41: 440–450, 1973.
328. GUTH, L., AND F. J. SAMAHA. Qualitative differences between actomyosin ATPase of slow and fast mammalian muscle. *Exp. Neurol.* 25: 138–152, 1969.
329. GUTH, L., AND F. J. SAMAHA. Erroneous interpretations which may result from application of the "myofibrillar ATPase" histochemical procedure to developing muscle. *Exp. Neurol.* 34: 465–475, 1972.
330. GUTH, L., P. K. WATSON, AND W. C. BROWN. Effects of cross-reinnervation on some chemical properties of red and white muscles of rat and cat. *Exp. Neurol.* 20: 52–69, 1968.
331. GUTH, L., AND H. YELLIN. The dynamic nature of the so-called "fiber types" of mammalian skeletal muscle. *Exp. Neurol.* 31: 277–300, 1971.
332. GUTMANN, E. Neurotrophic relations. *Annu. Rev. Physiol.* 38: 177–216, 1976.
333. GUTMANN, E. Problems in differentiating trophic relationships between nerve and muscle cells. In: *Motor Innervation of Muscle*, edited by S. Thesleff. New York: Academic, 1976, p. 323–343.
334. GUTMANN, E., AND I. HAJEK. Differential reaction of muscle to excessive use in compensatory hypertrophy and increased phasic activity. *Physiol. Bohemoslov.* 20: 205–212, 1971.
335. GUTMANN, E., S. SCHIAFFINO, AND V. HANZLIKOVA. Mechanism of compensatory hypertrophy in skeletal muscle of the rat. *Exp. Neurol.* 31: 451–464, 1971.
336. GUY, P. S., AND D. H. SNOW. The effect of training and detraining on muscle composition in the horse. *J. Physiol. London* 269: 33–51, 1977.
337. GYDIKOV, A. A. Pattern of discharge of different types of alpha motoneurones and motor units during voluntary and reflex activities under normal physiological conditions. In: *Biomechanics V*, edited by P. V. Komi. Baltimore: Univ. Park Press, 1975, vol. A, p. 45–57. (Int. Ser. Biomech.)
338. GYDIKOV, A., AND D. KOSAROV. Some features of different motor units in human biceps brachii. *Pfluegers Arch. Gesamte Physiol. Menschen Tiere* 347: 75–88, 1974.
339. HAGBARTH, K.-E. Excitatory and inhibitory skin areas for flexor and extensor motoneurones. *Acta Physiol. Scand. Suppl.* 94: 1–58, 1952.
340. HAJDU, S. Mechanism of the Woodworth staircase phenomenon in heart and skeletal muscle. *Am. J. Physiol.* 216: 206–214, 1969.
341. HAMBURGER, V. Cell death in the development of the lateral motor column of the chick embryo. *J. Comp. Neurol.* 160: 535–546, 1975.
342. HAMBURGER, V. The developmental history of the motor neuron. *Neurosci. Res. Program Bull.* 15: (Suppl. April) 1–37, 1977.
343. HAMMARBERG, C. Histochemical staining patterns of muscle fibres in the gastrocnemius, soleus and anterior tibial muscles of the adult cat, as viewed in serial sections stained for lipids and succinic dehydrogenase. *Acta Neurol. Scand.* 50: 272–284, 1974.
344. HAMMARBERG, C. The histochemical appearance of developing muscle fibres in the gastrocnemius, soleus and anterior tibial

muscles of the kitten, as viewed in serial sections stained for lipids and succinic dehydrogenase. *Acta Neurol. Scand.* 50: 285-301, 1974.

345. HAMMARBERG, C., AND J.-O. KELLERTH. Studies of some twitch and fatigue properties of different motor unit types in the ankle muscles of the adult cat. *Acta Physiol. Scand.* 95: 231-242, 1975.

346. HAMMARBERG, C., AND J.-O. KELLERTH. The postnatal development of some twitch and fatigue properties of single motor units in the ankle muscles of the kitten. *Acta Physiol. Scand.* 95: 243-257, 1975.

347. HAMMOND, G. R., AND R. M. A. P. RIDGE. Properties of twitch motor units in snake costocutaneous muscle. *J. Physiol. London* 276: 525-533, 1978.

348. HAMMOND, G. R., AND R. M. A. P. RIDGE. Post-tetanic potentiation of twitch motor units in snake costocutaneous muscle. *J. Physiol. London* 276: 535-554, 1978.

349. HANNERZ, J. Discharge properties of motor units in relation to recruitment order in voluntary contraction. *Acta Physiol. Scand.* 91: 374-384, 1974.

350. HANSON, J., AND A. PERSSON. Changes in the action potential and contraction of isolated frog muscle after repetitive stimulation. *Acta Physiol. Scand.* 81: 340-348, 1971.

351. HANZLIKOVA, V., AND S. SCHIAFFINO. Studies on the effect of denervation in developing muscle. III. Diversification of myofibrillar structure and origin of heterogeneity of muscle fibre types. *Z. Zellforsch. Mikrosk. Anat.* 147: 75-85, 1973.

352. HARKER, D. W., L. JAMI, Y. LAPORTE, AND J. PETIT. Fast-conducting skeletofusimotor axons supplying intrafusal chain fibers in the cat peroneus tertius muscle. *J. Neurophysiol.* 40: 791-799, 1977.

353. HARRIS, D. A., AND E. HENNEMAN. Identification of two species of alpha motoneurons in cat's plantaris pool. *J. Neurophysiol.* 40: 16-25, 1977.

354. HARRISON, V. F., AND O.A. MORTENSEN. Identification and voluntary control of single motor unit activity in the tibialis anterior muscle. *Anat. Rec.* 144: 109-116, 1962.

355. HATZE, H. A teleological explanation of Weber's law and the motor unit size law. *Bull. Math. Biol.* 41: 407-425, 1979.

356. HEILMANN, C., AND D. PETTE. Molecular transformations in sarcoplasmic reticulum of fast-twitch muscle by electro-stimulation. *Eur. J. Biochem.* 93: 437-446, 1979.

357. HENATSCH, H.-D., F. J. SCHULTE, AND G. BUSCH. Wandelbarkeit des tonisch-phäsischen Reaktionstype einzelner Extensor-Motoneurone bei Variation ihrer Antriebe. *Pfluegers Arch. Gesamte Physiol. Menschen Tiere* 270: 161-173, 1959.

358. HENNEMAN, E. Relations between size of neurons and their susceptibility to discharge. *Science* 126: 1345-1346, 1957.

359. HENNEMAN, E., H. P. CLAMANN, J. D. GILLIES, AND R. D. SKINNER. Rank order of motoneurons within a pool: law of combination. *J. Neurophysiol.* 37: 1338-1349, 1974.

361. HENNEMAN, E., AND C. B. OLSON. Relations between structure and function in the design of skeletal muscles. *J. Neurophysiol.* 28: 581-598, 1965.

362. HENNEMAN, E., B. T. SHAHANI, AND R. R. YOUNG. Voluntary control of human motor units. In: *The Motor System: Neurophysiology and Muscle Mechanisms*, edited by M. Shahani. Amsterdam: Elsevier, 1976, p. 73-78.

363. HENNEMAN, E., G. SOMJEN, AND D. O. CARPENTER. Functional significance of cell size in spinal motoneurons. *J. Neurophysiol.* 28: 560-580, 1965.

364. HENNEMAN, E., G. SOMJEN, AND D. O. CARPENTER. Excitability and inhibitibility of motoneurons of different sizes. *J. Neurophysiol.* 28: 599-620, 1965.

365. HENRIKSSON, J., AND J. S. REITMAN. Quantitative measures of enzyme activities in type I and type II muscle fibres of man after training. *Acta Physiol. Scand.* 97: 392-397, 1976.

366. HESS, A. Vertebrate slow muscle fibers. *Physiol. Rev.* 50: 40-62, 1970.

367. HILL, A. V. *First and Last Experiments in Muscle Mechanics*. Cambridge: Cambridge Univ. Press, 1970.

368. HOAR, P. E., AND W. G. L. KERRICK. Rabbit diaphragm: two types of fibres determined by calcium-strontium activation and protein content. *J. Physiol. London* 295: 345-352, 1979.

369. HOFFER, J. A., M. J. O'DONOVAN, AND G. E. LOEB. A method for recording and identifying single motor units in intact cats during walking. *Neurosci. Abstr.* 5: 374, 1979.

370. HOLLOSZY, J. O. Biochemical adaptations in muscle: effects of exercise on mitochondrial oxygen uptake and respiratory enzyme activity in skeletal muscle. *J. Biol. Chem.* 242: 2278-2282, 1967.

371. HOLLOSZY, J. O., AND F. W. BOOTH. Biochemical adaptations to endurance exercise in muscle. *Annu. Rev. Physiol.* 38: 273-291, 1976.

372. HONGO, T., E. JANKOWSKA, AND A. LUNDBERG. The rubrospinal tract. I. Effects on alpha-motoneurones innervating hindlimb muscles in cats. *Exp. Brain Res.* 7: 344-364, 1969.

373. HONGO, T., E. JANKOWSKA, AND A. LUNDBERG. The rubrospinal tract. II. Facilitation of interneuronal transmission in reflex paths to motoneurones. *Exp. Brain Res.* 7: 365-391, 1969.

374. HOUK, J. C., AND E. HENNEMAN. Responses of Golgi tendon organs to active contractions of the soleus muscle. *J. Neurophysiol.* 30: 466-481, 1967.

375. HOUSTON, M. E. The use of histochemistry in muscle adaptation: a critical assessment. *Can. J. Appl. Sport Sci.* 3: 109-118, 1978.

377. HUDLICKA, O. Effect of training on macro- and microcirculatory changes in exercise. In: *Exercise and Sport Science Reviews*, edited by R. S. Hutton. New York: Academic, 1977, vol. 5, p. 181-230.

378. HUDLICKA, O., M. BROWN, M. COTTER, M. SMITH, AND G. VRBOVA. The effect of long-term stimulation of fast muscles on their bloodflow, metabolism and ability to withstand fatigue. *Pfluegers Arch.* 369: 141-149, 1977.

379. HUIZAR, P., M. KUNO, N. KUDO, AND Y. MIYATA. Reaction of intact spinal motoneurones to partial denervation of the muscle. *J. Physiol. London* 265: 175-191, 1977.

380. HUIZAR, P., M. KUNO, AND Y. MIYATA. Differentiation of motoneurones and skeletal muscles in kittens. *J. Physiol. London* 252: 465-479, 1975.

381. HULTBORN, H., E. PIERROT-DESEILLIGNY, AND H. WIGSTRÖM. Recurrent inhibition and after hyperpolarization following motoneuronal discharge in the cat. *J. Physiol. London* 297: 253-266, 1979.

382. HURSH, J. B. Conduction velocity and diameter of nerve fibers. *Am. J. Physiol.* 127: 131-139, 1939.

383. HUXLEY, A. F. Muscular contraction. *J. Physiol. London.* 243: 1-43, 1974.

384. ILLERT, M., A. LUNDBERG, AND R. TANAKA. Integration in descending motor pathways controlling the forelimb in the cat. I. Pyramidal effects on motoneurones. *Exp. Brain Res.* 26: 509-519, 1976.

385. ITO, M., AND T. OSHIMA. Temporal summation of after hyperpolarization following a motoneurone spike. *Nature London* 195: 910-911, 1962.

386. JAMI, L., D. LAN-COUTON, K. MALMGREN, AND J. PETIT. Histophysiological observations on fast skeleto-fusimotor axons. *Brain Res.* 164: 53-59, 1979.

387. JAMI, L., AND J. PETIT. Correlation between axonal conduction velocity and tetanic tension of motor units in four muscles of the cat hind limb. *Brain Res.* 96: 114-118, 1975.

388. JAMI, L., AND J. PETIT. Heterogeneity of motor units activating single Golgi tendon organs in cat leg muscles. *Exp. Brain Res.* 24: 485-493, 1976.

389. JANKOWSKA, E., AND S. LINDSTRÖM. Morphological identification of Renshaw cells. *Acta Physiol. Scand.* 81: 428-430, 1971.

390. JANKOWSKA, E., J. RASTAD, AND J. WESTMAN. Intracellular application of horseradish peroxidase and its light and electron microscopical appearance in spinocervical tract cells. *Brain Res.* 105: 557-562, 1976.

391. JANSEN, J. K., W. THOMPSON, AND D. P. KUFFLER. The formation and maintenance of synaptic connections as illustrated by studies of the neuromuscular junction. In: *Progress in Brain Research. Maturation of the Nervous System*, edited by M. A. Corner, R. E. Baker, N. E. Van De Poll, D. F. Swaab, and H. B. M. Uylings. Amsterdam: Elsevier, 1977, vol. 48, p. 3-18.

392. JANSSON, E., AND L. KAIJSER. Muscle adaptation to extreme endurance training in man. *Acta Physiol. Scand.* 100: 315-324, 1977.

393. JANSSON, E., B. SJÖDIN, AND P. TESCH. Changes in muscle fibre type distribution in man after physical training. *Acta Physiol. Scand.* 104: 235-237, 1978.

394. JENNEKENS, F. G. I., B. E. TOMLINSON, AND J. N. WALTON. Data on the distribution of fibre types in five human limb muscles. *J. Neurol. Sci.* 14: 245-257, 1971.

395. JENNEKENS, F. G. I., B. E. TOMLINSON, AND J. N. WALTON. The extensor digitorum brevis: histological and histochemical aspects. *J. Neurol. Neurosurg. Psychiatry* 35: 124-132, 1972.

396. JESSOP, J., AND O. C. J. LIPPOLD. Altered synchronization of motor unit firing as a mechanism for long-lasting increases in the tremor of human hand muscles following brief, strong effort. *J. Physiol. London* 269: 29P-30P, 1977.

397. JEWELL, P. A., AND E. J. ZAIMIS. A differentiation between red and white muscle fibres in the cat based on responses to neuromuscular blocking agents. *J. Physiol. London* 124: 417-428, 1954.

398. JEWELL, P. A., AND E. J. ZAIMIS. Changes at the neuromuscular junction of red and white muscle fibres in the cat induced by disuse atrophy and by hypertrophy. *J. Physiol. London* 124: 429-442, 1954.

399. JIRMANOVA, I., AND S. THESLEFF. Ultrastructural study of experimental muscle degeneration and regeneration in the adult rat. *Z. Zellforsch. Mikrosk. Anat.* 131: 77-97, 1972.

400. JÖBSIS, F. F., AND J. C. DUFFIELD. Force, shortening and work in muscular contractions: relative contributions to overall energy utilization. *Science* 156: 1388-1392, 1967.

401. JOHNSON, M. A., J. POLGAR, D. WEIGHTMAN, AND D. APPLETON. Data on the distribution of fibre types in thirty-six human muscles. An autopsy study. *J. Neurol. Sci.* 18: 111-129, 1973.

402. JORGENSEN, A. O., V. KALNINS, AND D. H. MACLENNAN. Localization of sarcoplasmic reticulum proteins in rat skeletal muscle by immunofluorescence. *J. Cell Biol.* 80: 372-384, 1979.

402a. JOYCE, G. C., P. M. H. RACK, AND D. R. WESTBURY. The mechanical properties of cat soleus muscle during controlled lengthening and shortening movements. *J. Physiol. London* 204: 461-475, 1969.

402b. JOYCE, G. C. AND P. M. H. RACK. Isotonic lengthening and shortening movements of cat soleus muscle. *J. Physiol. London* 204: 475-491, 1969.

403. JULIAN, F. J., AND M. R. SOLLINS. Regulation of force and speed of shortening in muscle contraction. In: *The Mechanism of Muscle Contraction*. Cold Spring Harbor: Cold Spring Harbor Lab, 1973, p. 635-646. (Cold Spring Harbor Symp. Quant. Biol., 1973, vol. 37.)

404. KAIZAWA, J., AND I. TAKAHASHI. Motor cell columns in rat lumbar spinal cord. *Tohoku J. Exp. Med.* 101: 25-34, 1970.

405. KANDA, K., R. E. BURKE, AND B. WALMSLEY. Differential control of fast and slow twitch motor units in the decerebrate cat. *Exp. Brain Res.* 29: 57-74, 1977.

406. KARPATI, G., AND W. K. ENGEL. Correlative histochemical study of skeletal muscle after suprasegmental denervation, peripheral nerve section, and skeletal fixation. *Neurology* 18: 681-692, 1968.

407. KARPATI, G., AND W. K. ENGEL. Histochemical investigation of fiber type ratios with the myofibrillar ATP-ase reaction in normal and denervated skeletal muscles of guinea pig. *Am. J. Anat.* 122: 145-156, 1968.

408. KARPATI, G., AND W. K. ENGEL. 'Type grouping' in skeletal muscles after experimental reinnervation. *Neurology* 18: 447-455, 1968.

409. KATO, M., AND J. TANJI. Volitionally controlled single motor units in human finger muscles. *Brain Res.* 40: 345-357, 1972.

410. KELLERTH, J.-O., C.-H. BERTHOLD, AND S. CONRADI. Electron microscopic studies of serially sectioned cat spinal α-motoneurons. III. Motoneurons innervating fast-twitch (type FR) units of the gastrocnemius muscle. *J. Comp. Neurol.* 184: 755-767, 1979.

411. KELLY, A. M., AND D. L. SCHOTLAND. The evolution of the 'checkerboard' in a rat muscle. In: *Research in Muscle Development and the Muscle Spindle*, edited by B. O. Banker, R. J. Poszybylski, J. P. Van Der Menlen, and M. Victor. Amsterdam: Excerpta Medica, 1972, p. 32-48.

412. KELLY, A. M., AND S. I. ZACKS. The histogenesis of rat intercostal muscle. *J. Cell Biol.* 42: 135-153, 1969.

413. KELLY, A. M., AND S. I. ZACKS. The fine structure of motor endplate morphogenesis. *J. Cell Biol.* 41: 154-169, 1969.

414. KERNELL, D. The limits of firing frequency in cat lumbosacral motoneurones possessing different time course of afterhyperpolarization. *Acta Physiol. Scand.* 65: 87-100, 1965.

415. KERNELL, D. Input resistance, electrical excitability, and size of ventral horn cells in cat spinal cord. *Science* 152: 1637-1640, 1966.

416. KERNELL, D. Rhythmic properties of motoneurones innervating muscle fibres of different speed in m. gastrocnemius medialis of the cat. *Brain Res.* 160: 159-162, 1979.

417. KERNELL, D., A. DUCATI, AND H. SJÖHOLM. Properties of motor units in the first deep lumbrical muscle of the cat's foot. *Brain Res.* 98: 37-55, 1975.

418. KERNELL, D., AND H. SJÖHOLM. Recruitment and firing rate modulation of motor unit tension in a small muscle of the cat's foot. *Brain Res.* 98: 57-72, 1975.

419. KIRKWOOD, P. A., AND T. A. SEARS. Monosynaptic excitation of motoneurones from muscle spindle secondary endings of intercostal and triceps surae muscles in the cat. *J. Physiol. London* 245: 64-66P, 1975.

420. KNOTT, S., D. M. LEWIS, AND J. C. LUCK. Motor unit areas in a cat limb muscle. *Exp. Neurol.* 30: 475-483, 1973.

421. KOMI, P. V., J. H. T. VIITASALO, M. HAVU, A. THORSTENSSON, B. SJÖDEN, AND J. KARLSSON. Skeletal muscle fibres and muscle enzyme activities in monozygous and dizygous twins of both sexes. *Acta Physiol. Scand.* 100: 385-392, 1977.

422. KORNELIUSSEN, H., AND O. WAERHAUG. Three morphological types of motor nerve terminals in the rat diaphragm, and their possible innervation of different muscle fiber types. *Z. Anat. Entwicklungsgesch.* 140: 73-89, 1973.

423. KOSTYUK, P. G. Supraspinal mechanisms on a spinal level. In: *The Motor System: Neurophysiology and Muscle Mechanisms*, edited by M. Shahani. Amsterdam: Elsevier, 1976, p. 211-235.

424. KOWALSKI, K., E. E. GORDON, A. MARTINEZ, AND J. ADAMEK. Changes in enzyme activities of various muscle fiber types in rat induced by different exercises. *J. Histochem. Cytochem.* 17: 601-607, 1969.

425. KRAMMER, E. B., T. RATH, AND M. F. LISCHKA. Somatotopic organization of the hypoglossal nucleus: a HRP study in the rat. *Brain Res.* 170: 533-537, 1979.

426. KRISTENSSON, K., Y. OLSSON, AND J. SJÖSTRAND. Axonal uptake and retrograde transport of exogenous protein in the hypoglossal nerve. *Brain Res.* 32: 399-406, 1971.

427. KRNJEVIC, K., AND R. MILEDI. Failure of neuromuscular propagation in rats. *J. Physiol. London* 140: 440-461, 1958.

428. KRNJEVIC, K., AND R. MILEDI. Motor units in the rat diaphragm. *J. Physiol. London* 140: 427-439, 1958.

429. KRNJEVIC, K., AND R. MILEDI. Presynaptic failure of neuromuscular propagation in rats. *J. Physiol. London* 149: 1-22, 1959.

430. KUFFLER, D., W. THOMPSON, AND J. K. S. JANSEN. The elimination of synapses in multiply-innervated skeletal muscle fibres of the rat: dependence on distance between end-plates. *Brain Res.* 138: 353-358, 1977.

431. KUFFLER, S. W., AND E. M. VAUGHAN-WILLIAMS. Small-nerve junction potentials, the distribution of small motor nerves to frog skeletal muscle, and the membrane characteristics of the

fibres they innervate. *J. Physiol. London* 121: 289–317, 1953.
432. KUGELBERG, E. Histochemical composition, contraction speed and fatiguability of rat soleus motor units. *J. Neurol. Sci.* 20: 177–198, 1973.
433. KUGELBERG, E. Adaptive transformation of rat soleus motor units during growth. Histochemistry and contraction speed. *J. Neurol. Sci.* 27: 269–289, 1976.
434. KUGELBERG, E., AND L. EDSTRÖM. Differential histochemical effects of muscle contractions on phosphorylase and glycogen in various types of fibres: relation to fatigue. *J. Neurol. Neurosurg. Psychiatry* 31: 415–423, 1968.
435. KUGELBERG, E., L. EDSTRÖM, AND M. ABBRUZZESE. Mapping of motor units in experimentally innervated rat muscle. *J. Neurol. Neurosurg. Psychiatry* 33: 319–329, 1970.
436. KUGELBERG, E., AND B. LINDEGREN. Transmission and contraction fatigue of rat motor units in relation to succinate dehydrogenase activity of motor unit fibres. *J. Physiol. London* 288: 285–300, 1979.
437. KUGELBERG, E., AND C. R. SKOGLUND. Natural and artificial activation of motor units—a comparison. *J. Neurophysiol.* 9: 399–412, 1946.
438. KUME, M., AND M. UEMURA, K. MATSUDA, R. MATSUSHIMA, AND N. MIZUNO. Topographical representation of peripheral branches of the facial nerve within the facial nucleus: a HRP study in the cat. *Neurosci. Lett.* 8: 5–8, 1978.
439. KUNO, M. Excitability following antidromic activation in spinal motoneurones supplying red muscles. *J. Physiol. London* 149: 374–393, 1959.
440. KUNO, M. Quantal components of excitatory synaptic potentials in spinal motoneurones. *J. Physiol. London* 175: 81–99, 1964.
442. KUNO, M., S. A. TURKANIS, AND J. N. WEAKLY. Correlation between nerve terminal size and transmitter release at the neuromuscular junction of the frog. *J. Physiol. London* 213: 545–556, 1971.
443. LANDMESSER, L. The distribution of motoneurones supplying chick hind limb muscles. *J. Physiol. London* 284: 371–389, 1978.
444. LANDMESSER, L. The development of motor projection patterns in the chick hind limb. *J. Physiol. London* 284: 391–414, 1978.
445. LANDMESSER, L., AND D. G. MORRIS. The development of functional innervation in the hind limb of the chick embryo. *J. Physiol. London* 249: 301–326, 1975.
446. LÄNNERGREN, J., AND R. S. SMITH. Types of muscle fibres in toad skeletal muscle. *Acta Physiol. Scand.* 68: 263–274, 1966.
447. LAPORTE, Y. Innervation of cat muscle spindles by fast conducting skeletofusimotor axons. In: *Integration in the Nervous System*, edited by H. Asanuma and V. J. Wilson. Tokyo: Igaku-Shoin, 1979, p. 3–10.
448. LAPORTE, Y., AND F. EMONET-DÉNAND. The skeleto-fusimotor innervation of cat muscle spindle. In: *Progress in Brain Research. Understanding the Stretch Reflex*, edited by S. Homma. Amsterdam: Elsevier, 1976, vol. 44, p. 99–105.
449. LENNERSTRAND, G. Mechanical studies on the retractor bulbi muscle and its motor units in the cat. *J. Physiol. London* 236: 43–55, 1974.
450. LENTZ, T. L. Neurotrophic regulation at the neuromuscular junction. *Ann. NY Acad. Sci.* 228: 323–337, 1974.
451. LETBETTER, W. D. Influence of intramuscular nerve branching on motor unit organization in medial gastrocnemius muscle. *Anat. Rec.* 178: 402, 1974.
452. LEWIS, D. M., J. BAGUST, S. M. WEBB, R. A. WESTERMAN, AND H. FINOL. Axon conduction velocity modified by re-innervation of mammalian muscle. *Nature London* 270: 745–746, 1977.
453. LEWIS, D. M., C. J. C. KEAN, AND J. D. MCGARRICK. Dynamic properties of slow and fast muscle and their trophic regulation. *Ann. NY Acad. Sci.* 228: 105–120, 1974.
454. LEWIS, D. M., J. C. LUCK, AND S. KNOTT. A comparison of isometric contractions of the whole muscle with those of motor units in a fast-twitch muscle of the cat. *Exp. Neurol.* 37: 68–85, 1972.
455. LIDDELL, E. G. T., AND C. S. SHERRINGTON. Recruitment and some other factors of reflex inhibition. *Proc. R. Soc. London Ser. B* 97: 488–518, 1925.
456. LINDHOLM, A., H. BJERNELD, AND B. SALTIN. Glycogen depletion pattern in muscle fibers of trotting horses. *Acta Physiol. Scand.* 90: 475–484, 1974.
457. LLOYD, D. P. C. Reflex action in relation to pattern and peripheral source of afferent stimulation. *J. Neurophysiol.* 6: 111–120, 1943.
458. LLOYD, D. P. C., AND A. K. MCINTYRE. Monosynaptic reflex responses of individual motoneurons. *J. Gen. Physiol.* 38: 771–787, 1955.
459. LLOYD, D. P. C., AND A. K. MCINTYRE. Transmitter potentiality of homonymous and heteronymous monosynaptic reflex connections of individual motoneurons. *J. Gen. Physiol.* 38: 789–799, 1955.
460. LØMO, T. The role of activity in the control of membrane and contractile properties of skeletal muscle. In: *Motor Innervation of Muscle*, edited by S. Thesleff. New York: Academic, 1976, p. 289–321.
461. LØMO, T., R. H. WESTGAARD, AND H. A. DAHL. Contractile properties of muscle: control by pattern of muscle activity in the rat. *Proc. R. Soc. London Ser. B* 187: 99–103, 1974.
462. LUFF, A. R. Dynamic properties of fast and slow skeletal muscles in the cat and rat following cross-innervation. *J. Physiol. London* 248: 83–96, 1975.
463. LUFF, A. R., AND H. L. ATWOOD. Membrane properties and contraction of single muscle fibers in the mouse. *Am. J. Physiol.* 222: 1435–1440, 1972.
464. LUFF, A. R., AND U. PROSKE. Properties and motor units of the frog sartorius muscle. *J. Physiol. London* 258: 673–685, 1976.
465. LUND, J. P., F. J. R. RICHMOND, C. TOULOREMIS, Y. PATRY, AND Y. LAMARRE. The distribution of Golgi tendon organs and muscle spindles in masseter and temporalis muscles of the cat. *Neuroscience* 3: 259–270, 1978.
466. LUNDBERG, A. Convergence of excitatory and inhibitory action on interneurones in the spinal cord. In: *The Interneuron*, edited by M.A.B. Brazier. Univ. Calif. Press, 1969, p. 231–265. (UCLA Forum Med. Sci.)
467. LUNDBERG, A. Multisensory control of spinal reflex pathways. In: *Progress in Brain Research. Reflex Control of Posture and Movement*, edited by R. Granit and O. Pompeiano. Amsterdam: Elsevier, 1979, vol. 50, p. 11–28.
468. LÜTTGAU, H. C. The effect of metabolic inhibitors on the fatigue of the action potential in single muscle fibres. *J. Physiol. London* 178: 45–67, 1965.
469. LUX, H. D., P. SCHUBERT, AND G. W. KREUTZBERG. Direct matching of morphological and electrophysiological data in cat spinal motoneurones. In: *Excitatory Synaptic Mechanisms*, edited by P. Andersen and J. K. S. Jansen. Oslo: Universitetsforlaget, 1970, p. 189–198.
470. LYON, M. J. The central location of motor neurons to the stapedius muscle in the cat. *Brain Res.* 143: 437–444, 1978.
471. MACKOVA, E., AND P. HNIK. Time course of compensatory hypertrophy of slow and fast rat muscles in relation to age. *Physiol. Bohemoslov.* 21: 9–17, 1972.
472. MAGHERINI, P. C., W. PRECHT, AND P. C. SCHWINDT. Evidence for electrotonic coupling between frog motoneurons in the in situ spinal cord. *J. Neurophysiol.* 39: 474–483, 1976.
473. MAI, J. V., V. R. EDGERTON, AND R. J. BERNARD. Capillarity of red, white and intermediate muscle fibers in trained and untrained guinea pigs. *Experientia* 26: 1222–1223, 1970.
474. MAIER, A., J. L. CROCKETT, D. R. SIMPSON, C. W. SAUBERT, AND V. R. EDGERTON. Properties of immobilized guinea pig hindlimb muscles. *Am. J. Physiol.* 231: 1520–1526, 1976.
475. MAIER, A., AND E. ELDRED. Postnatal growth of the extra- and intrafusal fibers in the soleus and medial gastrocnemius muscles of the cat. *Am. J. Anat.* 141: 161–178, 1974.
476. MANABU, S., M. NOBORU, AND K. AKIRA. Postnatal differentiation of cell body volumes of spinal motoneurons innervating

slow-twitch and fast-twitch muscles. *J. Comp. Neurol.* 175: 27-36, 1977.
477. MANN, W. S., AND B. SALAFSKY. Enzymic and physiological studies of normal and disused developing fast and slow cat muscles. *J. Physiol. London* 208: 33-47, 1970.
478. MARKS, W. B., AND G. E. LOEB. Action currents, intermodal potentials, and extracellular records of myelinated mammalian nerve fibers derived from node potentials. *Biophys. J.* 16: 655-668, 1976.
478a. MASUDA, M., H. KURATA, AND S. MORIMOTO. Functional differentiation of single human motor units produced by external cooling during voluntary muscle contraction. *Jikeikai Med. J.* 26: 221-230, 1979.
479. MATTHEWS, M. A., W. D. WILLIS, AND V. WILLIAMS. Dendrite bundles in lamina IX of cat spinal cord: a possible source for electrical interaction between motoneurons? *Anat. Rec.* 171: 313-327, 1971.
480. MATTHEWS, P. B. C. *Mammalian Muscle Receptors and Their Central Actions.* Baltimore: Williams & Wilkins, 1972.
481. MAXWELL, L. C., J. K. BARCLAY, D. E. MOHRMAN, AND J. A. FAULKNER. Physiological characteristics of skeletal muscles of dogs and cats. *Am. J. Physiol.* 233 (*Cell Physiol.* 2): C14-C18, 1977.
482. MAYER, R. F., R. E. BURKE, AND K. KANDA. Immobilization and muscle atrophy. *Trans. Am. Neurol. Assoc.* 101: 145-150, 1976.
483. MAYR, R. Structure and distribution of fibre types in the external eye muscles of the rat. *Tissue Cell* 3: 433-462, 1971.
484. MCARDLE, J. J., AND E. X. ALBUQUERQUE. A study of the reinnervation of fast and slow mammalian muscles. *J. Gen Physiol.* 61: 1-23, 1973.
485. MCCOMAS, A. J., P. R. W. FAWCETT, M. J. CAMPBELL, AND R. E. P. SICA. Electrophysiological estimation of the numbers of motor units within a human muscle. *J. Neurol. Neurosurg. Psychiatry* 34: 121-131, 1971.
486. MCCOMAS, A. J., R. E. P. SICA, AND M. J. CAMPBELL. Numbers and sizes of human motor units in health and disease. In: *New Developments in Electromyography and Clinical Neurophysiology*, edited by J. E. Desmedt. Basel: Karger, 1973, vol. 1, p. 55-63.
487. MCCOMAS, A. J., R. E. P. SICA, A. R. M. UPTON, AND F. PETITO. Sick motoneurons and muscle disease. *Ann. NY Acad. Sci.* 228: 261-279, 1974.
488. MCDONAGH, J. C. *The Muscle Units of Cat Tibialis Posterior: Classification Based on Unit Neuromechanical Properties and Whole Muscle Histochemistry* (Ph.D. dissertation). Tucson: Univ. of Arizona, 1979.
489. MCMAHON, T. A. Using body size to understand the structural design of animals: quadrupedal locomotion. *J. Appl. Physiol.* 39: 619-627, 1975.
490. MCMINN, R. M. H., AND G. VRBOVA. Motoneurone activity as a cause of degeneration in the soleus muscle of the rabbit. *Q. J. Exp. Physiol.* 52: 411-415, 1967.
491. MCPHEDRAN, A. M., R. B. WUERKER, AND E. HENNEMAN. Properties of motor units in a homogeneous red muscle (soleus) of the cat. *J. Neurophysiol.* 28: 71-84, 1965.
492. MCWILLIAM, P. N. The incidence and properties of β axons to muscle spindles in the cat hindlimb. *Q. J. Expt. Physiol.* 60: 25-36, 1975.
493. MEGIRIAN, D. Bilateral facilitatory and inhibitory skin areas of spinal motoneurones of cat. *J. Neurophysiol.* 25: 127-137, 1962.
494. MELICHNA, J., AND E. GUTMANN. Stimulation and immobilization effects on contractile and histochemical properties of denervated muscle. *Pfluegers Arch.* 352: 165-178, 1974.
495. MELLSTRÖM, A., AND S. SKOGLUND. Quantitative morphological changes in some spinal cord segments during postnatal development. *Acta Physiol. Scand. Suppl.* 81: 331, 1969.
496. MERTON, P. A. Voluntary strength and fatigue. *J. Physiol. London* 123: 553-564, 1954.
498. MILEDI, R., AND E. STEFANI. Non-selective reinnervation of slow and fast muscle fibers in the rat. *Nature London* 222: 569-571, 1969.
499. MILNER-BROWN, H. S., R. B. STEIN, AND R. G. LEE. Synchronization of human motor units: possible roles of exercise and supraspinal reflexes. *Electroencephalogr. Clin. Neurophysiol.* 38: 245-254, 1975.
500. MILNER-BROWN, H. S., R. B. STEIN, AND R. YEMM. The contractile properties of human motor units during voluntary isometric contractions. *J. Physiol. London* 228: 285-306, 1973.
501. MILNER-BROWN, H. S., R. B. STEIN, AND R. YEMM. The orderly recruitment of human motor units during voluntary isometric contractions. *J. Physiol. London* 230: 359-370, 1973.
502. MILNER-BROWN, H. S., R. B. STEIN, AND R. YEMM. Changes in firing rate of human motor units during linearly changing voluntary contractions. *J. Physiol. London* 230: 371-390, 1973.
503. MISCHELEVICH, D. J. Repetitive firing to current in cat motoneurons as a function of muscle unit twitch type. *Exp. Neurol.* 25: 401-409, 1969.
504. MIZUNO, N., A. KONISHI, AND M. SATO. Localization of masticatory motoneurons in the cat and rat by means of retrograde axonal transport of horseradish peroxidase. *J. Comp. Neurol.* 164: 105-116, 1975.
505. MOLÉ, P. A., AND J. O. HOLLOSZY. Exercise-induced increase in the capacity of skeletal muscle to oxidize palmitate. *Proc. Soc. Exp. Biol. Med.* 134: 789-792, 1970.
506. MOLÉ, P. A., L. B. OSCAI, AND J. O. HOLLOSZY. Adaptation of muscle to exercise: increase in levels of palmitoyl CoA synthetase, carnitine palmityltransferase, and palmityl CoA dehydrogenase, and in the capacity to oxidize fatty acids. *J. Clin. Invest.* 50: 2323-2330, 1971.
507. MOMMAERTS, W. F. H. M. Energetics of muscular contraction. *Physiol. Rev.* 49: 427-508, 1969.
508. MONG, F. S. F. Histological and histochemical studies on the nervous influence on minced muscle regeneration of triceps surae of the rat. *J. Morphol.* 151: 451-462, 1977.
509. MONSTER, A. W. Firing rate behavior of human motor units during isometric voluntary contraction: relation to unit size. *Brain Res.* 171: 349-354, 1979.
510. MONSTER, A. W., AND H. CHAN. Isometric force production by motor units of extensor digitorum communis muscle in man. *J. Neurophysiol.* 40: 1432-1443, 1977.
511. MOODY, W. G., AND R. G. CASSENS. Histochemical differentiation of red and white muscle fibres. *J. Anim. Sci.* 27: 961-968, 1968.
512. MORI, S. Discharge patterns of soleus motor units with associated changes in force exerted by foot during quiet stance in man. *J. Neurophysiol.* 36: 458-471, 1973.
513. MORRIS, D. G. Development of functional motor innervation in supernumerary hindlimbs of the chick embryo. *J. Neurophysiol.* 41: 1450-1465, 1978.
514. MORRISON, J. B. The mechanics of muscle function in locomotion. *J. Biomech.* 3: 432-451, 1970.
515. MOSHER, C. G., R. L. GERLACH, AND D. G. STUART. Soleus and anterior tibial motor units of the cat. *Brain Res.* 44: 1-11, 1972.
516. MÜLLER, W. Temporal progress of muscle adaptation to endurance training in hindlimb muscles of young rats. *Cell Tissue Res.* 156: 61-88, 1974.
517. MURATA, F., AND T. OGATA. The ultrastructure of neuromuscular junction of human red, white and intermediate muscle fibers. *Tohoku J. Exp. Med.* 99: 289-301, 1969.
518. MURPHY, R. A., AND A. C. BEARDSLEY. Mechanical properties of the cat soleus muscle in situ. *Am. J. Physiol.* 227: 1008-1013, 1974.
519. NASSAR-GENTINA, V., J. V. PASSONEAU, S. I. RAPOPORT, AND J. L. VERGARA. Metabolic correlates of fatigue and of recovery from fatigue in single frog muscle fibers. *J. Gen. Physiol.* 72: 593-606, 1978.
520. NELSON, P. G. Interaction between spinal motoneurons of the cat. *J. Neurophysiol.* 29: 275-287, 1966.
521. NIEUWENHUIS, R. Comparative anatomy of the spinal cord.

In: *Progress in Brain Research. Organization of the Spinal Cord*, edited by J. C. Eccles and J. P. Schadé. Amsterdam: Elsevier, 1964, vol. 11, p. 1-55.

522. NORNES, H. O., AND M. CARRY. Neurogenesis in spinal cord of mouse: an autoradiographic analysis. *Brain Res.* 159: 1-16, 1978.

523. NORNES, H. O., AND G. D. DAS. Temporal pattern of neurogenesis in spinal cord of rat. I. An autoradiographic study—time and sites of origin and migration and settling patterns of neuroblasts. *Brain Res.* 73: 121-138, 1974.

524. NORRIS, F. H., AND E. L. GASTEIGER. Action potentials of single motor units in normal muscle. *Electroencephalogr. Clin. Neurophysiol.* 7: 115-126, 1955.

525. NORRIS, F. H., AND R. L. IRWIN. Motor unit area in a rat muscle. *Am. J. Physiol.* 200: 944-946, 1961.

526. NYBERG-HANSEN, R. Anatomical demonstration of γ-motoneurons in the cat's spinal cord. *Exp. Neurol.* 13: 71-81, 1965.

527. NYSTRÖM, B. Fibre diameter increase in nerves to "slow-red" and "fast-white" cat muscles during postnatal development. *Acta Neurol. Scand.* 44: 265-294, 1968.

528. NYSTRÖM, B. Postnatal development of motor nerve terminals in "slow-red" and "fast-white" cat muscles. *Acta Neurol. Scand.* 44: 363-383, 1968.

529. NYSTRÖM, B. Histochemistry of developing cat muscles. *Acta Neurol. Scand.* 44: 405-439, 1968.

530. O'BRIEN, R. A. D., A. J. C. OSTBERG, AND G. VRBOVA. Observations on the elimination of polyneuronal innervation in developing mammalian skeletal muscle. *J. Physiol. London* 282: 571-582, 1978.

531. O'DONOVAN, M. J. *Physiological and Histochemical Correlations in Human Muscle*. London: Univ. of London (St. Thomas' Hospital Medical School), 1978. Dissertation.

532. OGATA, T. A histochemical study of the red and white muscle fibres. *Acta Med. Okayama* 12: 216-239, 1958.

533. OGATA, T. A histochemical study on the structural differences of motor endplate in the red, white and intermediate muscle fibers of mouse limb muscle. *Acta Med. Okayama* 19: 149-153, 1965.

534. OGATA, T., AND F. MURATA. Cytological features of three fiber types in human skeletal muscle. *Tohoku J. Exp. Med.* 99: 225-245, 1969a.

535. OLSON, C. B., D. O. CARPENTER, AND E. HENNEMAN. Orderly recruitment of muscle action potentials. *Arch. Neurol.* 19: 591-597, 1968.

536. OLSON, C. B., AND C. P. SWETT. A functional and histochemical characterization of motor units in a heterogeneous muscle (flexor digitorum longus) of the cat. *J. Comp. Neurol.* 128: 475-498, 1966.

537. OLSON, C. B., AND C. P. SWETT. Effect of prior activity on properties of different types of motor units. *J. Neurophysiol.* 34: 1-16, 1971.

538. OPPENHEIM, R. W., AND I.-W. CHU-WANG. Spontaneous cell death of spinal motoneurons following peripheral innervation in the chick embryo. *Brain Res.* 125: 154-160, 1977.

539. OPPENHEIM, R. W., I. W. CHU-WANG, AND J. L. MADERDRUT. Cell death of motoneurons in the chick embryo spinal cord. III. The differentiation of motoneurons prior to their induced degeneration following limb-bud removal. *J. Comp. Neurol.* 177: 87-112, 1978.

540. PADYKULA, H. A., AND G. F. GAUTHIER. Morphological and cytochemical characteristics of fiber types in normal mammalian skeletal muscle. In: *Exploratory Concepts in Muscular Dystrophy and Related Disorders*, edited by A. T. Milhorat. Amsterdam: Excerpta Med., 1967, p. 117-128.

541. PADYKULA, H. A., AND G. F. GAUTHIER. The ultrastructure of the neuromuscular junctions of mammalian red, white and intermediate skeletal muscle fibers. *J. Cell Biol.* 46: 27-41, 1970.

542. PARTRIDGE, L. D. Signal-handling characteristics of load-moving skeletal muscle. *Am. J. Physiol.* 210: 1178-1191, 1966.

543. PATON, W. D. M., AND D. R. WAUD. The margin of safety of neuromuscular transmission. *J. Physiol. London* 191: 59-90, 1967.

544. PEACHEY, L. D. The structure of the extraocular muscle fibers of mammals. In: *The Control of Eye Movements*, edited by P. Bach-y-Rita, C. C. Collins, and J. E. Hyde. New York: Academic, 1971, p. 47-66.

545. PECKHAM, P. H., J. T. MORTIMER, AND J. P. VAN DER MEULEN. Physiologic and metabolic changes in white muscle of cat following induced exercise. *Brain Res.* 50: 424-429, 1973.

546. PENNYQUICK, C. J. Response of fast muscle to series of impulses. *J. Exp. Biol.* 41: 291-298, 1964.

547. PERKEL, D. H., G. L. GERSTEIN, AND G. P. MOORE. Neuronal spike trains and stochastic joint processes. II. Simultaneous spike trains. *Biophys. J.* 7: 419-440, 1967.

548. PERSON, R. S. Rhythmic activity of a group of human motoneurones during voluntary contraction of a muscle. *Electroencephalogr. Clin. Neurophysiol.* 36: 585-595, 1974.

549. PERSON, R. S., AND L. P. KUDINA. Discharge frequency and discharge pattern of human motor units during voluntary contraction of muscle. *Electroencephalogr. Clin. Neurophysiol.* 32: 471-483, 1972.

550. PETAJAN, J. H., AND B. A. PHILIP. Frequency control of motor unit action potentials. *Electroencephalogr. Clin. Neurophysiol.* 27: 66-72, 1969.

551. PETER, J. B. Histochemical, biochemical, and physiological studies of skeletal muscle and its adaptation to exercise. In: *Contractility of Muscle Cells and Related Processes*, edited by R. J. Podolsky. Englewood Cliffs, NJ: Prentice-Hall, 1971, p. 151-173.

552. PETER, J. B., R. J. BARNARD, V. R. EDGERTON, C. A. GILLESPIE, AND K. E. STEMPEL. Metabolic profiles of three fiber types of skeletal muscle in guinea pigs and rabbits. *Biochemistry* 11: 2627-2633, 1972.

553. PETERS, S. E., AND C. RICK. The actions of three hamstring muscles of the cat: a mechanical analysis. *J. Morphol.* 152: 315-328, 1978.

554. PETTE, D., B. U. RAMIREZ, W. MÜLLER, R. SIMON, G. U. EXNER, AND R. HILDEBRAND. Influence of intermittent long-term stimulation on contractile, histochemical and metabolic properties of fibre populations in fast and slow rabbit muscles. *Pfluegers Arch.* 361: 1-7, 1975.

555. PETTE, D., M. E. SMITH, H. W. STAUDTE, AND G. VRBOVA. Effects of long-term electrical stimulation on some contractile and metabolic characteristics of fast rabbit muscles. *Pfluegers Arch.* 338: 257-272, 1973.

556. PEYRONNARD, J.-M., AND Y. LAMARRE. Electrophysiological and anatomical estimation of the number of motor units in the monkey extensor digitorum brevis muscle. *J. Neurol. Neurosurg. Psychiatry* 40: 756-764, 1977.

557. PHILLIPS, C. G. The Ferrier lecture, 1968. Motor apparatus of the baboon's hand. *Proc. R. Soc. London Ser. B* 173: 141-174, 1969.

558. PHILLIPS, C. G. Pyramidal apparatus for control of the baboon's hand. In: *New Developments in Electromyography and Clinical Neurophysiology*, edited by J. E. Desmedt. Basel: Karger, 1973, vol. 3, p. 136-144.

559. PIEHL, K. Time course for refilling of glycogen stores in human muscle fibres following exercise induced glycogen depletion. *Acta Physiol. Scand.* 90: 297-302, 1974.

560. PINTER, M. J., R. L. CURTIS, AND M. J. HOSKO. On the relationships between selected parameters of motoneuron—motor unit "type" and the absolute voltage threshold of the motoneuron. *Neurosci. Abstr.* 4: 302, 1978.

561. PRESTIGE, M. C. Differentiation, degeneration, and the role of the periphery: quantitative considerations. In: *The Neurosciences. Second Study Program*, edited by F. O. Schmitt. New York: Rockefeller Univ. Press, 1970, p. 73-82.

562. PRESTIGE, M. C. Evidence that at least some of the motor nerve cells that die during development have first made peripheral connections. *J. Comp. Neurol.* 170: 123-134, 1976.

563. PRESTON, J. B., AND D. G. WHITLOCK. A comparison of motor

cortex effects on slow and fast muscle innervations in the monkey. *Exp. Neurol.* 7: 327–341, 1963.
564. PRINCE, F. P., R. HIKIDA, AND F. C. HAGERMAN. Human fiber types in power lifters, distance runners and untrained subjects. *Pfluegers Arch.* 363: 19–26, 1976.
565. PRINCE, F. P., R. S. HIKEDA, AND F. C. HAGERMAN. Muscle fiber types in women athletes and non-athletes. *Pfluegers Arch.* 371: 161–165, 1977.
566. PROSKE, U., AND P. M. E. WAITE. Properties of types of motor units in the medial gastrocnemius muscle of the cat. *Brain Res.* 67: 89–102, 1974.
567. PROSKE, U., AND P. M. E. WAITE. The relation between tension and axonal conduction velocity for motor units in the medial gastrocnemius muscle of the cat. *Exp. Brain Res.* 26: 325–328, 1976.
567a. RACK, P. M. H., AND D. R. WESTBURY. The effects of length and stimulus rate on tension in the isometric cat soleus muscle. *J. Physiol. London* 204: 443–460, 1969.
568. RALL, J. A. Dependence of energy output on force generation during muscle contraction. *Am. J. Physiol.* 235 (*Cell Physiol.* 4): C20–24, 1978.
569. RALL, W. Core conductor theory and cable properties of neurons. In: *Handbook of Physiology. The Nervous System. Cellular Biology of Neurons*, edited by E. R. Kandel. Bethesda, MD: Am. Physiol. Soc., 1977, sect. 1, vol. 1, pt. 1, chapt. 3, p. 39–97.
570. RALL, W., AND C. C. HUNT. Analysis of reflex variability in terms of partially correlated excitability fluctuations in a population of motoneurons. *J. Gen. Physiol.* 39: 397–422, 1956.
571. RANVIER, L. De quelgues faits relatifs à l'histologie et à la physiologie des muscles striés. *Arch. Physiol. Norm. Pathol.* 1: 5–18, 1874.
572. REDFERN, P. A. Neuromuscular transmission in new-born rats. *J. Physiol. London* 209: 701–709, 1970.
573. REDMAN, S. Junctional mechanisms at group Ia synapses. *Prog. Neurobiol.* 12: 33–83, 1979.
574. REED, A. F. The nuclear masses in the cervical spinal cord of *Macaca mulatta*. *J. Comp. Neurol.* 72: 187–206, 1940.
575. REINKING, R. M., J. A. STEPHENS, AND D. G. STUART. The motor units of cat medial gastrocnemius: problem of their categorisation on the basis of mechanical properties. *Exp. Brain Res.* 23: 301–313, 1975.
576. REINKING, R. M., J. A. STEPHENS, AND D. G. STUART. The tendon organs of cat medial gastrocnemius: significance of motor unit type and size for the activation of Ib afferents. *J. Physiol. London* 250: 491–512, 1975.
577. REIS, D. J., AND G. F. WOOTEN. The relationship of blood flow to myoglobin, capillary density, and twitch characteristics in red and white skeletal muscle in cat. *J. Physiol. London* 210: 121–135, 1970.
578. REXED, B. The cytoarchitectonic organization of the spinal cord in the cat. *J. Comp. Neurol.* 96: 415–496, 1952.
579. RICHMOND, F. J. R., AND V. C. ABRAHAMS. Morphology and enzyme histochemistry of dorsal muscles of the cat neck. *J. Neurophysiol.* 38: 1312–1321, 1975.
580. RICHMOND, F. J. R., AND V. C. ABRAHAMS. Morphology and distribution of muscle spindles in dorsal muscles of the cat neck. *J. Neurophysiol.* 38: 1322–1339, 1975.
581. RICHMOND, F. J. R., D. A. SCOTT, AND V. C. ABRAHAMS. Distribution of motoneurons to neck muscles, biocater cervicis, oplenius and complexus in the cat. *J. Comp. Neurol.* 181: 451–464, 1978.
582. RIDGE, R. M. A. P. The differentiation of conduction velocities of slow twitch and fast twitch muscle motor innervations in kittens and cats. *Q. J. Exp. Physiol.* 52: 294–304, 1967.
583. RILEY, D. A. Histochemical changes in ATPase activity during regeneration of skeletal muscle fibers. *Exp. Neurol.* 41: 690–704, 1973.
584. RILEY, D. A. Tenotomy delays the postnatal development of the motor innervation of the rat soleus. *Brain Res.* 143: 162–167, 1978.
585. RILEY, D. A., AND E. F. ALLIN. The effects of inactivity, programmed stimulation, and denervation on the histochemistry of skeletal muscle fiber types. *Exp. Neurol.* 40: 391–413, 1973.
586. RINGQVIST, M. Histochemical enzyme profiles of fibres in human masseter muscles with special regard to fibres with intermediate myofibrillar ATPase reaction. *J. Neurol. Sci.* 18: 133–141, 1973.
587. ROBBINS, N., G. KARPATI, AND W. K. ENGEL. Histochemical and contractile properties of the cross-innervated guinea pig soleus muscle. *Arch. Neurol.* 20: 318–329, 1969.
588. ROMANES, G. J. The development and significance of the cell columns in the ventral horn of the cervical and upper thoracic spinal cord of the rabbit. *J. Anat.* 76: 112–130, 1941.
589. ROMANES, G. J. The motor cell columns of the lumbo-sacral spinal cord of the cat. *J. Comp. Neurol.* 94: 313–363, 1951.
590. ROMANES, G. J. The motor pools of the spinal cord. In: *Progress in Brain Research. Organization of the Spinal Cord*, edited by J. C. Eccles and J. P. Schadé. Amsterdam: Elsevier, 1964, vol. 11, p. 93–119.
591. ROMANUL, F. C. A. Enzymes in muscle. I. Histochemical studies of enzymes in individual muscle fibers. *Arch. Neurol.* 11: 355–368, 1964.
592. ROMANUL, F. C. A. Capillary supply and metabolism of muscle fibers. *Arch. Neurol.* 12: 497–509, 1965.
593. ROMANUL, F. C. A., AND J. P. VAN DER MEULEN. Slow and fast muscles after cross innervation. *Arch. Neurol.* 17: 387–402, 1967.
594. RONNEVI, L.-O. Spontaneous phagocytosis of boutons on spinal motoneurons during early postnatal development. An electron microscopical study in the cat. *J. Neurocytol.* 6: 487–504, 1977.
595. RONNEVI, L.-O. Spontaneous phagocytosis of C-type synaptic terminals by spinal α-motoneurons in newborn kittens. An electron microscopic study. *Brain Res.* 162: 189–199, 1979.
596. ROSE, P. K., AND F. J. R. RICHMOND. A morphological description of motoneurons in the upper cervical spinal cord of the adult cat. *Neurosci. Abstr.* 3: 278, 1977.
597. ROSENBERG, M. E. Synaptic connexions of alpha extensor motoneurones with ipsilateral and contralateral cutaneous nerves. *J. Physiol. London* 207: 231–255, 1970.
598. ROSENBLUETH, A., AND R. RUBIO. Tetanic summation in isotonic and isometric responses. *Arch. Int. Physiol. Biochim.* 68: 165–180, 1960.
599. ROTSHENKER, S. Sprouting of intact motoneurons induced by neuronal lesion in the absence of denervated muscle fibers and degenerating axons. *Brain Res.* 155: 354–356, 1978.
600. RUBINSTEIN, N., K. MABUCHI, F. PEPE, S. SALMONS, J. GERGELY, AND F. SRETER. Use of type-specific antimyosins to demonstrate the transformation of individual fibers in chronically stimulated rabbit fast muscles. *J. Cell Biol.* 79: 252–261, 1978.
601. RUDOMIN, P., R. E. BURKE, R. NÚÑEX, J. MADRID, AND H. DUTTON. Control by presynaptic correlation: a mechanism affecting information transmission from Ia fibers to motoneurons. *J. Neurophysiol.* 38: 267–284, 1975.
602. RUDOMIN, P., AND H. DUTTON. Effects of conditioning afferent volleys on variability of monosynaptic responses of extensor motoneurons. *J. Neurophysiol.* 32: 140–157, 1969.
603. RUDOMIN, P., AND J. MADRID. Changes in correlation between monosynaptic responses of single motoneurons and in information transmission produced by conditioning volleys to cutaneous nerves. *J. Neurophysiol.* 35: 44–64, 1972.
604. RYALL, R. W., M. F. PIERCEY, C. POLOSA, AND J. GOLDFARB. Excitation of Renshaw cells in relation to orthodromic and antidromic excitation of motoneurons. *J. Neurophysiol.* 35: 137–148, 1972.
605. SALMONS, S., AND F. A. SRETER. Significance of impulse activity in the transformation of skeletal muscle type. *Nature London* 263: 30–34, 1976.
606. SALMONS, S., AND G. VRBOVA. The influence of activity on some contractile characteristics of mammalian fast and slow

muscles. *J. Physiol. London* 201: 535–549, 1969.

607. SALTIN, B., J. HENRIKSSON, E. NYGAARD, P. ANDERSEN, AND E. JANSSON. Fiber types and metabolic potentials of skeletal muscles in sedentary man and endurance runners. *Ann. NY Acad. Sci.* 301: 3–29, 1977.

608. SALTIN, B., K. NAZAR, D. L. COSTILL, E. STEIN, E. JANSSON, B. ESSEN, AND P. D. GOLLNICK. The nature of the training response: peripheral and central adaptations to one-legged exercise. *Acta Physiol. Scand.* 96: 289–305, 1976.

609. SAMAHA, F. J., L. GUTH, AND R. W. ALBERS. Phenotypic differences between the actomyosin ATPase of the three fiber types of mammalian skeletal muscle. *Exp. Neurol.* 26: 120–125, 1970.

610. SANES, J. R., L. M. MARSHALL, AND V. J. MCMAHON. Reinnervation of muscle fiber basal lamina after removal of myofibers. *J. Cell Biol.* 78: 176–198, 1978.

611. SANTA, T., AND A. G. ENGEL. Histometric analysis of neuromuscular junction ultrastructure in rat red, white and intermediate muscle fibres. In: *New Developments in Electromyography and Clinical Neurophysiology,* edited by J. E. Desmedt. Basel: Karger, 1973, vol. 1, p. 41–54.

612. SATO, M., N. MIZUNO, AND Z. KONISHI. Postnatal differentiation of cell body volumes of spinal motoneurons innervating slow-twitch and fast-twitch muscles. *J. Comp. Neurol.* 175: 27–36, 1977.

613. SAWAKI, S., AND J. B. PETER. Occurrence and distribution of isoenzymes in different types of skeletal muscle fibers. *Exp. Neurol.* 35: 421–430, 1972.

614. SCHEIBEL, M. E., AND A. B. SCHEIBEL. Spinal motoneurons, interneurons and Renshaw cells. A Golgi study. *Arch. Ital. Biol.* 104: 328–353, 1966.

615. SCHEIBEL, M. E., AND A. B. SCHEIBEL. Organization of spinal motoneuron dendrites in bundles. *Exp. Neurol.* 28: 106–112, 1970.

616. SCHEIBEL, M. E., AND A. B. SCHEIBEL. Developmental relationship between spinal motoneuron dendrite bundles and patterned activity in the forelimb of cats. *Exp. Neurol.* 30: 367–373, 1971.

617. SCHIAFFINO, S., V. HANZLIKOVA, AND S. PIEROBON. Relations between structure and function in rat skeletal muscle fibers. *J. Cell Biol.* 47: 107–119, 1970.

618. SCHIAFFINO, S., AND S. PIEROBON-BORMIOLI. Adaptive changes in developing rat skeletal muscle in response to functional overload. *Exp. Neurol.* 40: 126–137, 1973.

619. SCHMALBRUCH, H. "Rote" Muskelfasern. *Z. Zellforsch. Mikrosk. Anat.* 119: 120–146, 1971.

619a. SCHMALBRUCH, H. The membrane systems in different fibre types of the triceps surae muscle of cat. *Cell Tissue Res.* 204: 187–200, 1979.

620. SCHMALBRUCH, H., AND Z. KAMIENIECKA. Histochemical fiber typing and staining intensity in cat and rat muscles. *J. Histochem. Cytochem.* 23: 395–401, 1975.

621. SCHMIDT, H., AND E. STEFANI. Re-innervation of twitch and slow muscle fibres of the frog after crushing the motor nerves. *J. Physiol. London* 258: 99–123, 1976.

622. SCHWARTZ, M. S., E. STÅLBERG, H. H. SCHILLER, AND B. THIELE. The reinnervated motor unit in man. A single fibre EMG multielectrode investigation. *J. Neurol. Sci.* 27: 303–312, 1976.

623. SCHWINDT, P., AND W. E. CRILL. A persistent negative resistance in cat lumbar motoneurons. *Brain Res.* 120: 173–178, 1977.

624. SEVERIN, F. V., M. L. SHIK, AND G. N. ORLOVSKII. Work of muscles and single motor units during controlled locomotion. *Biophysics* 12: 762–772, 1967.

625. SHAFIQ, S. A., S. A. ASIEDRE, AND A. T. MILHORAT. Effect of neonatal neurectomy on differentiation of fiber types in rat skeletal muscle. *Exp. Neurol.* 35: 529–540, 1972.

626. SHAPOVALOV, A. I. Extrapyramidal control of primate motoneurons. In: *New Developments in Electromyography and Clinical Neurophysiology,* edited by J. E. Desmedt. Basel: Karger, 1973, vol. 3, p. 145–158.

627. SHAPOVALOV, A. I., AND B. I. SHIRIAEV. Two types of electrotonic EPSP evoked in amphibian motoneurons by ventral root stimulation. *Exp. Brain Res.* 33: 313–323, 1978.

628. SHARRARD, W. J. W. The distribution of the permanent paralysis in the lower limb in poliomyelitis. *J. Bone Jt. Surg.* 37: 540–558, 1955.

629. SHERRINGTON, C. S. *The Integrative Action of the Nervous System.* New Haven: Yale Univ. Press, 1906. (Reprinted 1947.)

630. SHERRINGTON, C. S. Remarks on some aspects of reflex inhibition. *Proc. R. Soc. London Ser. B* 97: 519–545, 1925.

631. SHERRINGTON, C. S. Ferrier Lecture—some functional problems attaching to convergence. *Proc. R. Soc. London Ser. B* 105: 332–362, 1929.

632. SICA, R. E. P., AND A. J. MCCOMAS. Fast and slow twitch units in a human muscle. *J. Neurol. Neurosurg. Psychiatry* 34: 113–120, 1971.

633. SIMONSON, E. Depletion of energy yielding substances. In: *Physiology of Work Capacity and Fatigue,* edited by E. Simonson. Springfield, IL: Thomas, 1971, p. 31–49.

634. SIMONSON, E. Transmission fatigue. In: *Physiology of Work Capacity and Fatigue,* edited by E. Simonson. Springfield, IL: Thomas, 1971, p. 211–237.

635. SJÖSTROM, A., AND P. ZANGGER. Muscle spindle control during locomotor movements generated by the deafferented spinal cord. *Acta Physiol. Scand.* 97: 281–291, 1976.

636. SMITH, H. M., JR., J. V. BASMAJIAN, AND S. F. VANDERSTOEP. Inhibition of neighboring motoneurons in conscious control of single spinal motoneurons. *Science* 183: 975–976, 1974.

636a. SMITH, J. L., B. BETTS, V. R. EDGERTON, AND R. F. ZERNICKE. Rapid ankle extension during paw shakes: selective recruitment of fast ankle extensors. *J. Neurophysiol.* 43: 612–620, 1980.

637. SMITH, J. L., V. R. EDGERTON, B. BETTS, AND T. C. COLLATOS. EMG of slow and fast ankle extensors of cat during posture, locomotion, and jumping. *J. Neurophysiol.* 40: 503–513, 1977.

638. SMITH, R. S., G. BLINSTON, AND W. K. OVALLE. Skeletomotor and fusimotor organization in amphibians. In: *Control of Posture and Locomotion,* edited by R. B. Stein, K. G. Pearson, R. S. Smith, and J. B. Redford. New York: Plenum, 1973, p. 105–117.

639. SMITH, R. S., AND J. LÄNNERGREN. Types of motor units in the skeletal muscle of *Xenopus laevis. Nature London* 217: 281–283, 1968.

640. SMITH, R. S., AND W. K. OVALLE. Varieties of fast and slow extrafusal muscle fibres in amphibian hind limb muscles. *J. Anat.* 116: 1–24, 1973.

641. SMITH, T. G., JR., J. L. BARKER, AND H. GAINER. Requirements for bursting pacemaker potential activity in molluscan neurons. *Nature London* 253: 450–452, 1975.

642. SOKAL, R. R. Classification: purposes, principles, progress, prospects. *Science* 185: 1115–1123, 1974.

643. SONNHOF, U., D. W. RICHTER, AND R. TAUGNER. Electrotonic coupling between frog spinal motoneurons. An electrophysiological and morphological study. *Brain Res.* 138: 197–215, 1977.

644. SPAMER, C., AND D. PETTE. Activities of malate dehydrogenase, 3-hydroxyacyl-CoA dehydrogenase and fructose-1,6-diphosphatase with regard to metabolic subpopulations of fast- and slow-twitch fibres in rabbit muscles. *Histochemistry* 60: 9–19, 1979.

645. SPRAGUE, J. M. A study of motor cell localization in the spinal cord of the rhesus monkey. *Am. J Anat.* 82: 1–26, 1948.

646. SPURWAY, N. C. Cluster analysis and the typing of muscle fibres. *J. Physiol. London* 280: 39P–40P, 1978.

647. SRETER, F. A., J. GERGELY, S. SALMONS, AND F. ROMANNE. Synthesis by fast muscle of myosin light chains characteristic of slow muscle in response to long-term stimulation. *Nature New Biol.* 241: 17–19, 1973.

648. STÅLBERG, E., AND J. EKSTEDT. Single fibre EMG and microphysiology of the motor unit in normal and diseased human muscle. In: *New Developments in Electromyography and Clin-*

ical Neurophysiology, edited by J. F. Desmedt. Basel: Karger, 1973, vol. 1, p. 113-129.
649. STÅLBERG, E., J. EKSTEDT, AND A. BROMAN. The electromyographic filter in normal human muscles. *Electroencephalogr. Clin. Neurophysiol.* 31: 429-438, 1971.
650. STÅLBERG, E., M. S. SCHWARTZ, B. THIELE, AND H. H. SCHILLER. The normal motor unit in man—a single fibre EMG multielectrode investigation. *J. Neurol. Sci.* 27: 291-301, 1976.
651. STÅLBERG, E., AND B. THIELE. Transmission block in terminal nerve twigs. A single fiber electromyographic finding in man. *J. Neurol. Neurosurg. Psychiatry* 35: 52-59, 1972.
652. STÅLBERG, E., AND B. THIELE. Discharge patterns of motoneurones in humans. A single fiber EMG study. In: *New Developments in Electromyography and Clinical Neurophysiology*, edited by J. E. Desmedt. Basel: Karger, 1973, p. 234-241.
653. STÅLBERG, E., AND B. THIELE. Motor unit fibre density in the extensor digitorum communis muscle. *J. Neurol. Neurosurg. Psychiatry* 38: 874-880, 1975.
654. STANDAERT, F. G. Post-tetanic repetitive activity in the cat soleus nerve. Its origin, course, and mechanism of generation. *J. Gen. Physiol.* 47: 53-70, 1963.
655. STANDAERT, F. G. The mechanisms of post-tetanic potentiation in cat soleus and gastrocnemius muscles. *J. Gen. Physiol.* 47: 987-1001, 1964.
656. STAUDTE, H. W., G. U. EXNER, AND D. PETTE. Effects of short-term, high intensity (sprint) training on some contractile and mechanical characteristics of fast and slow muscles of the rat. *Pfluegers Arch.* 344: 159-168, 1973.
657. STAUFFER, E. K., D. G. D. WATT, A. TAYLOR, R. M. REINKING, AND D. G. STUART. Analysis of muscle receptor connections by spike-triggered averaging. 2. Spindle group II afferents. *J. Neurophysiol.* 39: 1393-1402, 1976.
658. STEG, G. Efferent muscle innervation and rigidity. *Acta Physiol. Scand.* 61: (Suppl. 225), p. 1-53, 1964.
659. STEIN, J. M., AND H. A. PADYKULA. Histochemical classification of individual skeletal muscle fibers of the rat. *Am. J. Anat.* 110: 103-116, 1962.
660. STEPHENS, J. A., R. GARNETT, AND N. P. BULLER. Reversal of recruitment order of single motor units produced by cutaneous stimulation during voluntary muscle contraction in man. *Nature London* 272: 362-364, 1978.
661. STEPHENS, J. A., AND D. G. STUART. The motor units of cat medial gastrocnemius: speed-size relations and their significance for the recruitment order of motor units. *Brain Res.* 91: 177-195, 1975.
662. STEPHENS, J. A., AND D. G. STUART. The motor units of cat medial gastrocnemius. Twitch potentiation and twitch-tetanus ratio. *Pfluegers Arch.* 356: 359-372, 1975.
663. STEPHENS, J. A., AND A. TAYLOR. Fatigue of maintained voluntary muscle contraction in man. *J. Physiol. London* 220: 1-18, 1972.
664. STEPHENS, J. A., AND T. P. USHERWOOD. The mechanical properties of human motor units with special reference to their fatiguability and recruitment threshold. *Brain Res.* 125: 91-97, 1977.
665. STERLING, P., AND H. G. J. M. KUYPERS. Anatomical organization of the brachial spinal cord of the cat. II. The motoneuron plexus. *Brain Res.* 4: 16-32, 1967.
666. STRICK, P. L., R. E. BURKE, K. KANDA, C. C. KIM, AND B. WALMSLEY. Differences between alpha and gamma motoneurons labeled with horseradish peroxidase by retrograde transport. *Brain Res.* 113: 582-588, 1976.
667. STUART, D. G., C. G. MOSHER, R. L. GERLACH, AND R. M. REINKING. Mechanical arrangement and transducing properties of Golgi tendon organs. *Exp. Brain Res.* 14: 274-292, 1972.
668. SULLIVAN, T. E., AND R. B. ARMSTRONG. Rat locomotory muscle fiber activity during trotting and galloping. *J. Appl. Physiol: Respirat. Environ. Exercise Physiol.* 44: 358-363, 1978.
669. SUNDERLAND, S., AND J. O. LAVARACK. The branching of nerve fibres. *Acta Anat.* 17: 46-61, 1953.
670. SWETT, J. E., AND E. ELDRED. Distribution and numbers of stretch receptors in medial gastrocnemius and soleus muscles of the cat. *Anat. Rec.* 137: 453-460, 1960.
671. SWETT, J., E. ELDRED, AND J. S. BUCHWALD. Somatotopic cord-to-muscle relations in efferent innervation of cat gastrocnemius. *Am. J. Physiol.* 219: 762-766, 1970.
672. SYROVY, I., E. GUTMANN, AND J. MELICHNA. Effect of exercise on skeletal muscle myosin ATPase activity. *Physiol. Bohemoslov.* 21: 633-638, 1972.
673. SYSKA, H., S. V. PERRY, AND I. P. TRAYER. A new method of preparation of troponin I (inhibitory protein) using affinity chromatography. Evidence for three different forms of troponin I in striated muscle. *FEBS Lett.* 40: 253-257, 1974.
674. TABARY, J. C., C. TABARY, C. TARDIEU, G. TARDIEU, AND G. GOLDSPINK. Physiological and structural changes in the cat's soleus muscle due to immobilization at different lengths by plaster casts. *J. Physiol. London* 224: 231-244, 1972.
675. TANJI, J., AND M. KATO. Recruitment of motor units in voluntary contraction of a finger muscle in man. *Exp. Neurol.* 40: 759-770, 1973.
676. TANJI, J., AND M. KATO. Firing rate of individual motor units in voluntary contraction of abductor digiti minimi muscle in man. *Exp. Neurol.* 40: 771-783, 1973.
677. TAYLOR, A., F. W. J. CODY, AND M. A. BOSLEY. Histochemical and mechanical properties of the jaw muscles of the cat. *Exp. Neurol.* 38: 999-109, 1973.
678. TAYLOR, A., AND J. A. STEPHENS. Study of human motor unit contractions by controlled intramuscular microstimulation. *Brain Res.* 117: 331-335, 1976.
679. TAYLOR, C. R. Why change gaits? Recruitment of muscles and muscles fibers as a function of speed and gait. *Am. Zool.* 18: 153-161, 1978.
680. TEIG, E. Tension and contraction time of motor units of the middle ear muscles in the cat. *Acta Physiol. Scand.* 84: 11-21, 1972.
681. TEIG, E., AND H. A. DAHL. Actomyosin ATPase activity of middle ear muscles in the cat. *Histochemie* 29: 1-7, 1972.
682. TERJUNG R. Muscle fiber involvement during training of different intensities and durations. *Am. J. Physiol.* 230: 946-950, 1976.
683. TESTA, C. Functional implications of the morphology of spinal ventral horn neurons of the cat. *J. Comp. Neurol.* 123: 425-443, 1964.
684. THESLEFF, S. Motor end plate densitization by repetitive nerve stimuli. *J. Physiol. London* 148: 659-664, 1959.
685. THESLEFF, S., F. VYSKOCIL AND M. R. WARD. The action potential in end-plate and extrajunctional regions of rat skeletal muscle. *Acta Physiol. Scand.* 91: 196-202, 1974.
686. THOMAS, J. S., E. M. SCHMIDT, AND F. T. HAMBRECHT. Facility of motor unit control during tasks defined directly in terms of unit behaviors. *Exp. Neurol.* 59: 384-395, 1978.
687. THOMPSON, W., AND J. K. S. JANSEN. The extent of sprouting of remaining motor units in partly denervated immature and adult rat soleus muscle. *Neuroscience* 2: 523-535, 1977.
688. THOMPSON, W., D. P. KUFFLER, AND J. K. S. JANSEN. The effect of prolonged, reversible block of nerve impulses on the elimination of polyneuronal innervation of new-born rat skeletal muscle fibres. *Neuroscience* 4: 271-281, 1979.
689. THORSTENSSON, A., B. HULTEN, W. VAN DOBELN, AND J. KARLSSON. Effect of strength training on enzyme activities and fibre characteristics in human skeletal muscle. *Acta Physiol. Scand.* 96: 392-398, 1976.
690. THORSTENSSON, A., B. SJÖDIN, AND J. KARLSSON. Enzyme activities and muscle strength after "sprint training" in man. *Acta Physiol. Scand.* 94: 313-318, 1975.
691. THORSTENSSON, A., B. SJÖDIN, P. TESCH, AND J. KARLSSON. Actomyosin ATPase, myokinase, CPK and LDH in human fast and slow twitch muscle fibres. *Acta Physiol. Scand.* 99: 225-229, 1977.
692. TOKIZANE, T., AND H. SHIMAZU. *Functional Differentiation of Human Skeletal Muscle. Corticalization and Spinalization of Movements.* Springfield, IL: Thomas, 1964, p. 60.

693. TOMANEK, R. A histochemical study of postnatal differentiation of skeletal muscle with reference to functional overload. *Dev. Biol.* 42: 305-314, 1975.
694. TOMANEK, R. J., C. R. ASMUNDSON, R. R. COOPER, AND R. J. BARNARD. Fine structure of fast-twitch and slow-twitch guinea pig muscle fibers. *J. Morphol.* 139: 47-65, 1973.
695. TOMANEK, R. J., AND D. D. LUND. Degeneration of different types of skeletal muscle fibres. II. Immobilization. *J. Anat.* 118: 531-541, 1974.
696. TOMANEK, R. J., AND Y. K. WOO. Compensatory hypertrophy of the plantaris muscle in relation to age. *J. Gerontol.* 25: 23-29, 1970.
697. TRAUB, R. D. A model of a human neuromuscular system for small isometric tensions. *Biol. Cybernetics* 26: 159-167, 1977.
698. TRAUB, R. D., AND R. LLINAS. The spatial distribution of ionic conductances in normal and axotomized motoneurons. *Neuroscience* 2: 829-849, 1977.
699. TWAROG, B. M. Factors influencing contraction and catch in *Mytilus* smooth muscle. *J. Physiol. London* 191: 847-856, 1967.
700. VAN BUREN, H. M., AND K. FRANK. Correlation between the morphology and potential field of a spinal motor nucleus in the cat. *Electroencephalogr. Clin. Neurophysiol.* 19: 112-126, 1965.
701. VAN DE GRAAFF, K. M., E. C. FREDERICK, R. G. WILLIAMSON, AND G. E. GOSLOW, JR. Motor units and fiber types of primary ankle extensors of the skunk (*Mephitis mephitis*). *J. Neurophysiol.* 40: 1424-1431, 1977.
702. VAN DER MEULEN, J. P., P. H. PECKHAM, AND J. T. MORTIMER. Use and disuse of muscle. *Ann. NY Acad. Sci.* 228: 177-189, 1974.
703. VÉLEZ, S. J., AND R. J. WYMAN. Synaptic connectivity in a crayfish neuromuscular system. II. Nerve-muscle matching and nerve branching patterns. *J. Neurophysiol.* 41: 85-96, 1978.
704. VERGARA, J. L., S. I. RAPOPORT, AND V. NASSAR-GENTINA. Fatigue and posttetanic potentiation in single muscle fibers of the frog. *Am. J. Physiol.* 232 (*Cell Physiol.* 1): C185-C190, 1977.
705. WAGMAN, I. H., D. S. PIERCE, AND R. E. BURGER. Proprioceptive influences in volitional control of individual motor units. *Nature London* 207: 957-958, 1965.
706. WAHREN, J., G. AHLBORG, P. FELIG, AND L. JORFELDT. Glucose metabolism during exercise in man. In: *Muscle Metabolism During Exercise*, edited by B. Pernow and B. Saltin. New York: Plenum, 1971, p. 189-203.
707. WALMSLEY, B., J. A. HODGSON, AND R. E. BURKE. Forces produced by medial gastrocnemius and soleus muscles during locomotion in freely moving cats. *J. Neurophysiol.* 41: 1203-1216, 1978.
708. WALSH, J. V., R. E. BURKE, W. Z. RYMER, AND P. TSAIRIS. Effect of compensatory hypertrophy studied in individual motor units in medial gastrocnemius muscle of the cat. *J. Neurophysiol.* 41: 496-508, 1978.
709. WAND, P. AND O. POMPEIANO. Contribution of different size motoneurons to Renshaw cell discharge during stretch and vibration reflexes. In: *Progress in Brain Research, Reflex Control of Posture and Movement*. Amsterdam: Elsevier, 1979, vol. 50, p. 45-60.
710. WARMOLTS, J. R., AND W. K. ENGEL. Open biopsy electromyography. I. Correlation of motor unit behavior with histochemical muscle fiber type in human limb muscle. *Arch. Neurol. Psychiatry* 27: 512-517, 1972.
711. WARSZAWSKI, M., N. TELERMAN-TOPPET, J., DURDU, G. L. GRAFF, AND C. COERS. The early stages of neuromuscular regeneration after crushing the sciatic nerve in the rat. Electrophysiological and histological study. *J. Neurol. Sci.* 24: 21-32, 1975.
712. WAXMAN, S. G., AND M. V. L. BENNETT. Relative conduction velocities of small myelinated and non-myelinated fibres in the central nervous system. *Nature New Biol.* 238: 217-219, 1972.
713. WEBBER, C. L., AND K. PLESCHKA. Structural and functional characteristics of individual phrenic motoneurons. *Pfluegers Arch.* 364: 113-121, 1976.
714. WEEDS, A. G., AND R. S. TAYLOR. Separation of subfragment-1 isoenzymes from rabbit skeletal muscle myosin. *Nature London* 257: 54-56, 1975.
715. WEEDS, A. G., D. R. TRENTHAM, C. J. C. KEAN, AND A. J. BULLER. Myosin from cross-innervated cat muscles. *Nature London* 247: 135-139, 1974.
716. WEISS, P., AND A. HOAG. Competitive reinnervation of rat muscles by their own and foreign nerves. *J. Neurophysiol.* 9: 413-418, 1946.
717. WENDT, I. R., AND C. L. GIBBS. Energy production of mammalian fast- and slow-twitch muscles during development. *Am. J. Physiol.* 226: 642-647, 1974.
717a. WESTERMAN, R. A., H. S. CHAN, S. P. ZICCONE, D. SRIRATANA, X. DENNETT, AND K. A. TATE. Plasticity of motor reinnervation in the kitten. In: *Neural Growth and Differentiation*, edited by E. Meisami and M. A. B. Brazier. New York, Raven Press, 1979, pp. 397-432.
718. WESTERMAN, R. A., D. M. LEWIS, J. BAGUST, G. EDJTEHADI, AND D. PALLOT. Communication between nerves and muscles: postnatal development in kitten hindlimb fast and slow twitch muscle. In: *Memory and Transfer of Information*, edited by H. Zippel. Plenum, 1973, p. 255-291.
719. WHITE, D. C. S., AND J. THORSON. The kinetics of muscle contraction. *Prog. Biophys.* 27: 173-255, 1973.
720. WILLIS, W. D., R. D. SKINNER, AND M. A. WEIR. Field potentials of alpha and gamma motoneurons and Renshaw cells in response to activation of motor axons. *Exp. Neurol.* 25: 57-69, 1969.
721. WILSON, D. M., AND J. L. LARIMER. The catch property of ordinary muscle. *Proc. Natl. Acad. Sci. USA* 61: 909-916, 1968.
722. WILSON, D. M., D. O. SMITH, AND P. DEMPSTER. Length and tension hysteresis during sinusoidal and step function stimulation of arthropod muscle. *Am. J. Physiol.* 218: 916-922, 1970.
723. WILSON, V. J., AND W. H. TALBOT. Pattern of discharge of flexor motoneurons. *J. Neurophysiol.* 27: 451-463, 1964.
724. WINDHORST, U. Considerations on mechanisms of focused signal transmission in the multi-channel muscle stretch system. *Biol. Cybernetics* 31: 81-90, 1978.
725. WINDHORST, U., AND J. MEYER-LOHMANN. The influence of extrafusal muscle activity on the discharge patterns of primary muscle spindle endings. *Pfluegers Arch.* 372: 131-138, 1977.
726. WINEGRAD, S. Intracellular calcium movements of frog skeletal muscle during recovery from tetanus. *J. Gen. Physiol.* 51: 65-83, 1968.
727. WINEGRAD, S. The intracellular site of calcium activation of contraction in frog skeletal muscle. *J. Gen. Physiol.* 55: 77-88, 1970.
728. WIRSEN, C., AND K. W. LARSSON. Histochemical differentiation of skeletal muscle in foetal and newborn mice. *J. Embryol. Exp. Morphol.* 12: 759-767, 1964.
729. WITTENBERG, J. B. Myoglobin-facilitated oxygen diffusion: role of myoglobin in oxygen entry into muscle. *Physiol. Rev.* 50: 559-636, 1970.
730. WOHLFART, G. Muscular atrophy in diseases of the lower motor neurones. Contribution to the anatomy of motor units. *Arch. Neurol. Psychiatry* 61: 599-620, 1949.
730a. WOLF, S. L., AND W. D. LETBETTER. Effect of skin cooling on spontaneous EMG activity in triceps surae of the decerebrate cat. *Brain Res.* 91: 151-155, 1975.
731. WRAY, S. H. Innervation ratios for large and small limb muscles in the baboon. *J. Comp. Neurol.* 137: 227-250, 1969.
732. WUERKER, R. B., A. M. MCPHEDRAN, AND E. HENNEMAN. Properties of motor units in a heterogeneous pale muscle (m. gastrocnemius) of the cat. *J. Neurophysiol.* 28: 85-99, 1965.
733. WYMAN, R. J., I. WALDRON, AND G. M. WACHTEL. Lack of fixed order of recruitment in cat motoneuron pools. *Exp. Brain Res.* 20: 101-114, 1974.
734. YELLIN, H. Neural regulation of enzymes in muscle fibers of red and white muscle. *Exp. Neurol.* 19: 92-103, 1967.
735. YELLIN, H. A histochemical study of muscle spindles and their relationship to extrafusal fiber types in the rat. *Am. J. Anat.* 125: 31-46, 1969.

736. YELLIN, H. Differences in histochemical attributes between diaphragm and hindleg muscles of the rat. *Anat. Rec.* 173: 333–339, 1972.
737. YELLIN, H., AND L. GUTH. The histochemical classification of muscle fibers. *Exp. Neurol.* 26: 424–432, 1970.
738. YEMM, R. The orderly recruitment of motor units of the masseter and temporal muscles during voluntary isometric contraction in man. *J. Physiol. London* 265: 163–174, 1977.
739. ZAJAC, F. E. Recruitment and rate modulation of motor units during locomotion. In: *Progress in Clinical Neurophysiology. Recruitment Patterns of Motor Units and the Gradation of Muscle Force*, edited by J. E. Desmedt. Basel: Karger, 1978, vol. 9.
740. ZAJAC, F. E., AND J. L. YOUNG. Discharge patterns of motor units during cat locomotion and their relation to muscle performance. In: *Neural Control of Locomotion*, edited by R. M. Herman, S. Grillner, P. S. G. Stein, and D. G. Stuart. New York: Plenum, 1976, p. 789–793.
741. ZIEGLGÄNSBERGER, W., AND C. REITER. A cholinergic mechanism in the spinal cord. *Neuropharmacology* 13: 519–527, 1974.
742. ZUCKER, R. S. Theoretical implications of the size principle of motoneurone recruitment. *J. Theoret. Biol.* 38: 587–596, 1973.

CHAPTER 11

Functional organization of motoneuron pool and its inputs

ELWOOD HENNEMAN | Department of Physiology, Harvard Medical School, Boston, Massachusetts

LORNE M. MENDELL | Department of Physiology, Duke University Medical Center, Durham, North Carolina

CHAPTER CONTENTS

Morphological Considerations
  Columnar arrangement of motoneuron pool
  Dimensions of α-motoneurons and distribution of cell size
  Scaling of motoneurons
  Initial segment of α-motor axons
  Axon collaterals of α-motoneurons
  Recurrent inhibitory feedback from motoneurons
  Direct synaptic interconnections between spinal motoneurons
  Species of motoneurons
  Terminals of motoneurons in muscle
  Morphology of neuromuscular junctions
  Matching the properties of motoneurons and the muscle fibers they supply
  Concluding comments
Firing Patterns of Individual Motoneurons and Motor Units
  Functional significance of size of motoneurons
  Measurement of total output of motoneuron pools
  Critical firing levels of motoneurons
  Relation of critical firing level to axon diameter and motoneuron size
  Effects of inhibitory inputs on critical firing level and rank order during repetitive firing
  Recruitment of motor units in humans
  Evidence regarding alternative patterns of recruitment
  Evidence regarding voluntary selective control of motor units
  Size principle in other species
  Modulation of firing rate
Organization of Input to Motoneuron Pools
  Anatomical studies
    The motoneuron
    Anatomy of Ia-branches to motoneurons
    Ia-synapses on motoneurons
  Techniques used to study EPSPs elicited by impulses in single afferent fibers
    EPSPs recorded from single motoneurons
    EPSPs recorded from populations of motoneurons
  Amplitudes of EPSPs elicited by impulses in single fibers
    Variability of EPSP amplitudes
    Factors responsible for variability in EPSP amplitudes
  Boutons of Ia-fibers on motoneurons
    Physiological analysis of location of boutons
    Efficacy of synapses on different parts of motoneuron
  Physiology of Ia-terminals
  Distribution of Ia excitation to motoneuron pools
    Percentage of motoneurons receiving terminals from single Ia-fibers
    Factors influencing percentage of motoneurons receiving homonymous projections
  Comparison of projections to homonymous and heteronymous motoneurons
  Correlations between morphology and function
  Latency of EPSPs
  Other examples of divergence in inputs to motoneurons
  Ia-projections to motoneurons controlling other parts of the body
  Group II input from secondary endings in muscle spindles
  Inhibitory inputs to motoneurons
    Ia inhibitory interneurons
    Renshaw cells
  Group Ib input from Golgi tendon organs
  Monosynaptic input from descending pathways
  Topographic factors governing development of connections of Ia-fibers to motoneurons
  Concluding comments
Nonuniformity of Motoneurons
  Early classification of tonic and phasic types of motoneurons
  Significance of nonuniformity of muscle fibers
  Motoneuron properties independent of size
  Differential responses of motoneurons to injected currents
  Influence of muscle on developing and mature motoneurons
  Evidence from human disease
  Concluding comments
How Size of Motoneurons Determines Their Susceptibility to Discharge
  Properties of motoneurons that influence susceptibility to discharge
  Role of input in determining susceptibility to discharge
Some Principles Underlying Organization of Motoneuron Pools
  How sensitivity in gradation of tension is achieved
  Basis for relation between motoneuron size and the force its motor unit develops
  Actual sensitivity in grading muscular tension
  Mathematical derivation of a "principle of maximum grading sensitivity"
  Recruitment order and minimum energy principle
  Collective action of motoneuron pool: role of input
  The size principle in Ia and group II sensory fibers
  How does the central nervous system use the motoneuron pool?

ALL OF THE activity in the nervous system that influences movement converges ultimately on motoneurons. For this reason, Sherrington called motoneurons the "final common path" to muscle. The cells and axons that compose this common path are by no means uniform in their properties. They differ systematically from each other in size and other properties and form a functional ensemble whose collective properties are far more extensive than those of any single motoneuron. The organization of this population of cells derives from the intrinsic properties of the motoneurons and from the inputs they receive.

In order to discuss this organization in a logical manner, this review is divided into six sections.

1. An anatomical description of the motoneuron pool and certain aspects of the morphology of individual motoneurons is given. This account is limited to information that seems relevant to a discussion of functional organization.

2. The role of a motoneuron pool is to translate a large, heterogeneous inflow of signals from certain peripheral structures and from many parts of the nervous system into a much smaller and simpler output that will produce precisely controlled tensions in a particular muscle. The characteristics of this output, as judged by the firing patterns of individual motoneurons and motor units, are described. From the body of information available from studies on animals and humans a set of simple rules is derived that governs the behavior of the motoneuron pool as a whole and the muscle it supplies.

3. Physiological studies on afferent systems that send impulses directly or indirectly to the motoneuron pool are described and an attempt is made to infer some general principles that govern the organization of such inputs.

4. The fourth section reviews evidence regarding the nonuniformity of motoneurons. The chief purpose is to determine whether the differences between motoneurons in a single pool are sufficiently basic to classify them into different types or species. Other information essential to a proper appreciation of pool organization is also included.

5. Some of the factors underlying the differences in the susceptibility of motoneurons to discharge are discussed. A new hypothesis regarding the role of terminal arborizations of afferent fibers on motoneurons is advanced to explain the size principle of recruitment. Recent experimental evidence supporting this hypothesis is presented.

6. Lastly, some theoretical and mathematical treatments of principles underlying the functional organization of the motoneuron pool are called to the reader's attention, although space does not permit extensive discussion of them.

The field with which this chapter deals is changing rapidly. We wish to emphasize that this account does not provide a comprehensive review of the world literature in this area. It is selective and attempts to impart understanding rather than a mere accumulation of facts.

MORPHOLOGICAL CONSIDERATIONS

The purpose of this section is to provide a morphological basis for the physiological findings that are described in later parts of this chapter. Particular emphasis is placed on the dimensions of motoneurons, the uniform scaling of the different parts of the neuron, the distribution of cell sizes, and the functional implications of these factors.

Columnar Arrangement of Motoneuron Pool

The population of motoneurons innervating a particular muscle is called a "pool" (78). The members of a pool are not readily identifiable with ordinary staining techniques, because they appear to be intermingled with other motoneurons in the gray matter of the ventral horn. By sectioning muscle nerves Romanes (302) showed that the chromatolyzed motoneurons supplying hindlimb muscles in the cat were disposed in longitudinal columns within lamina IX. A recently developed technique (230) has made it possible to label the motoneurons supplying a particular muscle more clearly than with chromatolysis, so that they stand out distinctly from other cells. When the enzyme horseradish peroxidase (HRP) is injected into a muscle, it is taken up by the motor axons in the muscle and carried rapidly by retrograde axoplasmic flow back to their cell bodies, where it appears, after an appropriate chemical reaction, as brown, intracytoplasmic granules. If the intramuscular injection of HRP is well dispersed, so that all the motor terminals are exposed to it, a high percentage of the motoneurons is found to contain the HRP reaction product. Intracellular transport of the enzyme makes it possible to define all the dendritic and axonal projections of motoneurons in some cases.

Figure 1 illustrates the locations of labeled cells in an experiment (47) in which HRP was injected into the left medial gastrocnemius (MG) and the right soleus (SOL) muscles of a cat. After reconstruction of the histological material, it was apparent that the motoneurons innervating each of these muscles formed a column of cells parallel with the long axis of the spinal cord in the lateral part of the ventral horn. Throughout most of their courses the two pools overlap to some extent. This arrangement permits close apposition of pools supplying related muscles, which may facilitate the organization of input common to them and of interconnections between them. Both α-motoneurons, which innervate the ordinary, large extrafusal muscle fibers, and γ-motoneurons, which supply the small intrafusal muscle fibers, were labeled with HRP. The latter cells (originally called "small" motoneurons) were distributed randomly throughout both cell columns. Since they provide the motor innervation for spindles located in the muscle supplied by the α-motoneurons, they should be regarded as special components of the same pool. A third type of cell, the β-motoneuron, which innervates both extra- and intrafusal fibers, has recently been described by Emonet-Dénand et al. (108).

Dimensions of α-Motoneurons and Distribution of Cell Size

Physiological studies reveal that the functions of motoneurons are highly correlated with their size. In particular, the relations between the size of a motoneuron and *1)* its susceptibility to discharge by excitatory inputs, *2)* the suppression of its firing by inhibitory inputs, and *3)* the properties of the motor units it supplies prompted Henneman et al. (159) to conclude that there was a "size principle" underlying these correlations.

The α-motoneurons are large cells with soma diameters ranging from about 30 to 70 μm (339) and a mean diameter of 48 μm, assuming they are spheres (121). The distribution of their cell volumes (soma and dendrites) in the rhesus monkey is shown by the histogram in Figure 2, a rescaled version of one constructed from measurements of all of the motoneurons in the seventh cervical segment (161). This highly skewed distribution, with a preponderance of cells at the smaller end of the scale, is characteristic of motoneuron pools supplying large and small muscles in all species.

Using electrophysiological techniques, Clamann and Kukulka (62) found no evidence that motoneurons are distributed spatially according to size within the pools supplying the medial gastrocnemius or plantaris muscles as Wyman (355) had suggested. Their study indicates that any sufficiently large sample of motoneurons obtained in a restricted region of the motoneuron pool or in the ventral root filaments issuing from it contains a wide range of sizes.

Differences in the sizes of motoneurons allow for considerable variation in the number of boutons on their surfaces. A summary of some early estimates of synaptic density was compiled by Illis (179). Conradi (71) made an extensive electron microscope examination of cat motoneurons and Barrett and Crill (14) carried out a detailed study of the soma and dendritic trees of several motoneurons that had been injected with Procion dye. Combining the results of these two studies, Barrett (12) estimated the total number of synaptic endings at 20,000–50,000 per cell, depending on its size.

The great differences in the surface area of motoneurons, and possibly in their geometry, may be the major cause for the wide range of input resistances they exhibit (0.3–6.0 MΩ). The functional significance of input resistance in determining excitability and inhibitability is discussed in later parts of this chapter.

Scaling of Motoneurons

Early anatomists were intrigued by the wide range of sizes and by the geometry of the neurons they found in the nervous system. Deiters (86) was apparently the first to recognize that the diameter of an axon is proportional to the size of its cell body. Cajal (291) also showed that the size of a neuron is related to the diameter of its axis cylinder and, further, to the number and thickness of its collaterals and terminals. As examples of large cells with thick axons he cited spinal motoneurons, giant corpuscles of the torpedo, Golgi cells of the cerebellum, horizontal cells of the retina, and, as a case of special interest, the Mauthner cell. In contrast, he pointed out that small neurons, such as the granular cells of the cerebellum and fascia dentata, and the bipolar cells of the retina, all have thin axons, which give off few collaterals. In his chapter dealing with dorsal root ganglia, Cajal points out that ganglion cells of large volume have thick axons and those of small volume have thin axons (Figs. 157–159 in ref. 291). Many other examples could be noted. The giant cells that have been described in various species invariably have large axons; small cells never do. In the mammalian nervous system, there seem to be no striking exceptions to this general rule.

The dimensions and proportions of spinal motoneurons have recently been scrutinized in more detail and with a greater variety of techniques than those of other types of neurons because of the body of information that clearly relates their functional characteristics to their size. After studying motoneurons physiologically with intracellular electrodes that were filled with a dye to mark them, Barrett and Crill (13) then examined the labeled cells histologically. Using the conduction velocity of the axons as a measure of their diameter (174), they found that axonal diameter correlated closely with the size of the cell body and the extent of its dendritic tree. By injecting horseradish peroxidase intracellularly (324) it is now possible to perform dimensional analyses of physiologically characterized neurons more precisely than ever before. With this technique, Cullheim (80) has confirmed and extended Barrett and Crill's findings by purely morphological methods. The mean diameters of the cell bodies of sciatic motoneurons injected with HRP ranged from 44 to 71 μm, which is in good agreement with the results of electron microscope studies (71). In Figure 3 the diameters of α-motor axons at the initial segment and in the white matter are plotted against the sizes of the parent cell bodies. In spite of the scatter, due largely to representing cell size by the mean diameters in just one plane, significant ($P < 0.001$) positive correlations are present in both cases. In Figure 4 the axon conduction velocities are plotted against cell body sizes, initial segment diameters, and mean axon diameters in the white matter, with significant positive correlations in all three cases.

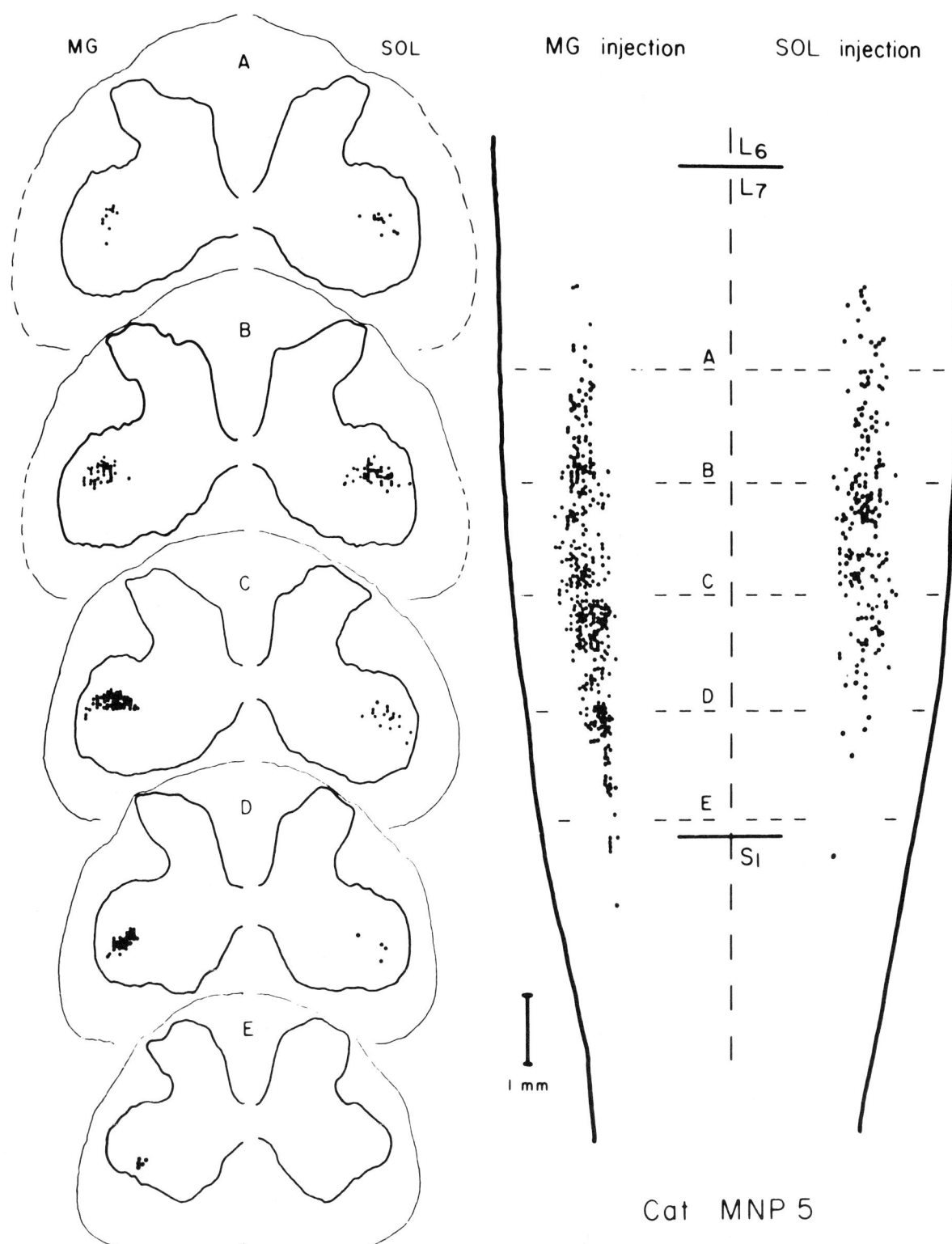

Initial Segment of α-Motor Axons

Physiological studies indicate that impulses are normally generated in the initial segment (IS) of a motoneuron's axon (75, 118). If other factors are equal, a given depolarization of the soma should cause a larger flow of transmembrane current in a thin IS than in a thick one. Thin initial segments may, therefore, have lower thresholds than thick ones (183). Cullheim and Kellerth (82) have used intracellular injections of horseradish peroxidase to delineate the intramedullary parts of the axons of sciatic α-motoneurons in the adult cat. The IS was invariably the narrowest part of the motor axon. Its diameters ranged from 2.3 to 4.9 µm (mean = 3.5 µm) and its lengths varied from 20 to 35 µm (mean = 26 µm). No correlation was found between its diameter and length. When the diameters of the IS were plotted against those of the same axon in the white matter, a significant ($P < 0.001$) positive correlation was found, as illustrated in Figure 5. In view of these considerations, the dimensions and membrane properties of the initial segment may play a role in determining the relative excitability of motoneurons. Their importance, relative to that of other factors, is, however, difficult to assess without further information.

Axon Collaterals of α-Motoneurons

The number and total extent of the axon collaterals of a motoneuron are related to the size of the cell and its functional properties. Cajal (291) found that a correlation existed between the diameter of central axons and the size of their collateral trees. Cullheim and Kellerth's study (82) with horseradish peroxidase shows that this finding applies to α-motoneurons. This suggests that stronger physiological effects may be exerted by recurrent collateral systems from large motor axons than from small ones. The number of first-order collaterals given off by a single axon ranged from 0 to 6. Most first-order collaterals give off 2–5 branches of about equal size. The number of collateral end branches originating from one first-order collateral varied from 1 to 39 and the total number of such branches from a single motor axon ranged from 0 to 69. A significant positive correlation exists between the diameter of the first-order collateral and the number of its end branches. This is another example of the scaling principle in motoneurons.

Cullheim and Kellerth (81) have also used horseradish peroxidase to examine the axon collaterals of different types of motor units as classified by Burke et al. (40, 41). In this study, they were concerned chiefly with "axon collateral swellings," discrete out-bulgings that usually are identifiable as synaptic boutons under the electron microscope. All motor units with fewer than 30 axon collateral swellings were found to be of the slowly contracting, slowly fatiguing (S) type or the soleus-S (SOL-S) type (see the chapter by Burke in this *Handbook*), while those with more than 80 swell-

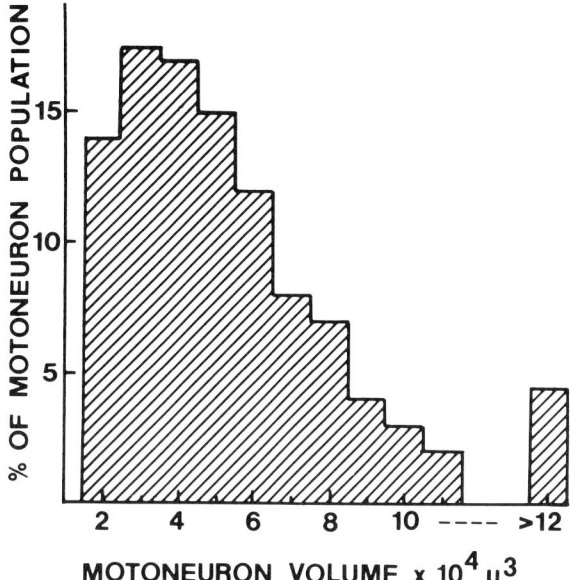

FIG. 2. Distribution of motoneuron sizes in the 7th cervical segment of 6 normal rhesus monkeys. [Adapted from Hodes et al. (161).]

FIG. 1. Reconstructions of medial gastrocnemius (MG) and soleus (SOL) nuclei from serial sagittal sections in cat. *Right*, dorsal view of spinal cord outline (white matter–pia boundary in *heavy lines*) on which are superimposed positions (*dots*) of MG (left hemicord) and SOL motoneuron cell bodies (right hemicord). Boundaries between L_6, L_7, and S_1 segments (identified by dorsal root entry zones), are indicated by *horizontal heavy lines*; midline denoted by *vertical dashed line*. *Dashed lines* across the cord denote levels (labeled A–E) at which reconstructions of cross sections were made. *Left*, reconstructions of cross sections at levels A–E showing white matter–pia boundary in *light lines* and gray-white matter boundary in *heavy lines*. *Dashed lines* at most lateral parts of cross sections indicate estimated outline; the most lateral parts were lost in sectioning. All diagrams drawn on same scale. Neurons indicated on each cross-section diagram are cells located within 300 µm rostral and caudal to that level. [From Burke et al. (47).]

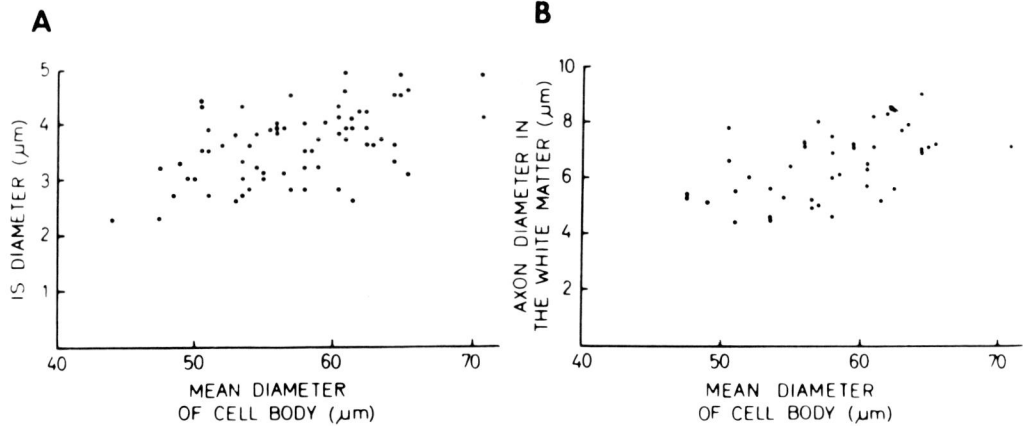

FIG. 3. *A*: diameters of sciatic α-motor axons of cat at initial segment (IS) are plotted against mean diameters of their parent cell bodies ($n = 68$). Linear correlation coefficient $(r) = +0.522$ ($P < 0.001$). *B*: mean diameters of sciatic α-motor axons in white matter are plotted against mean diameters of their parent cell bodies ($n = 42$). Linear correlation coefficient $(r) = +0.516$ ($P < 0.001$). [From Cullheim (80).]

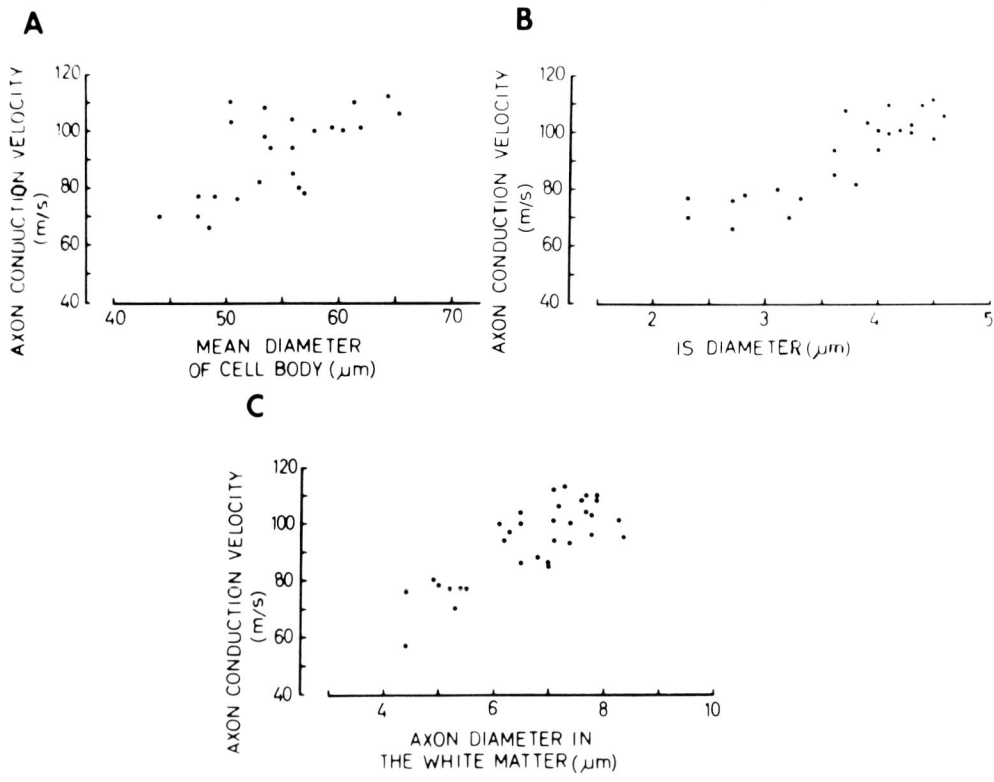

FIG. 4. Axon conduction velocities in cat are plotted in *A* against size of parent cell bodies ($n = 24$), in *B* against axon diameters at initial segment IS ($n = 24$), and in *C* against axon diameters in white matter ($n = 33$). In *A* the linear correlation coefficient $(r) = +0.673$ ($P < 0.001$); in *B*, $r = +0.869$ ($P < 0.001$); and in *C*, $r = +0.804$ ($P < 0.001$). [From Cullheim (80).]

ings were exclusively of the fast, fatiguing type. The mean number of swellings found were as follows: FF = 98.1 ± 29.6; FR = 53.8 ± 16.5; S = 44.4 ± 14.1; SOL-S = 27.8 ± 13.1 (FF is fast, fatiguing; FR is fast, fatigue resistant). These differences were statistically significant. The axon collateral systems of the FF and FR motor units showed considerable differences, adding morphological support to the physiological classification of these two types. The authors believe that the large variations in the axon collateral trees are at least partly correlated with differences in the types of motor units they supply. Since different types of motor units vary in the size of their motoneurons, it is difficult to judge whether motoneuron size or motor-unit type correlates more closely with the morphology of axon collateral trees.

Recurrent Inhibitory Feedback from Motoneurons

Control of a muscle demands various types of coordinated activity of its motoneurons. Much of this coordination is produced by inputs that are shared by a large percentage of the motoneuron pool, as described in section ORGANIZATION OF INPUT TO MOTONEURON POOLS, p. 460. Another type of coordination, still poorly understood, results from short-latency feedback mechanisms. Renshaw (297, 298) demonstrated that each time a motoneuron discharged an impulse a recurrent collateral of that axon transmitted a corresponding signal that excited a special group of interneurons located mainly in the ventral portion of lamina VII near the motoneuron pool. These interneurons, called Renshaw cells, send their axons back to motoneurons in the pool of origin, where they exert inhibitory effects. This inhibitory feedback is modulated by activity in dorsal root fibers and descending systems. Its function, however, is not at all clear. Consistent with other findings that large motoneurons exert greater effects than small ones, Ryall et al. (307) reported that Renshaw cells are more strongly excited by collaterals of large motoneurons than of small ones.

Direct Synaptic Interconnections Between Spinal Motoneurons

The possibility of even more direct interactions between motoneurons via recurrent collaterals was recognized many years ago. Cajal (291) reported that some collaterals arborize extensively in the region of their motoneurons and suggested that they made synaptic contacts with them. Later, collaterals terminating not only in the Renshaw cell area but also among motoneurons were described by the Scheibels (309, 310). No wholly convincing demonstration of direct synaptic transmission from one motoneuron to another has been made to date in mammals. Cullheim et al. (83), however, recently provided the best morphological evidence that direct interconnections exist. By injecting horseradish peroxidase into motoneurons of the cat's triceps surae he and his colleagues were able to trace some motor axons and recurrent collaterals to their terminations with both the light and electron microscope. In addition to the expected projection to the Renshaw cell area, axon collaterals were frequently found terminating within the motor nuclei, where at least some of them made direct contact with triceps motoneurons. The presence of a synaptic complex at these junctions "satisfied the morphological criteria needed for postulating a genuine synaptic connection." (83).

Several reports of physiological interactions between motoneurons have appeared. Short-latency facilitation of motoneurons by antidromic excitation of adjacent motoneurons was described by Nelson (267). Recurrent excitation of frog motoneurons by antidromic volleys was also reported by Grinnell (140),

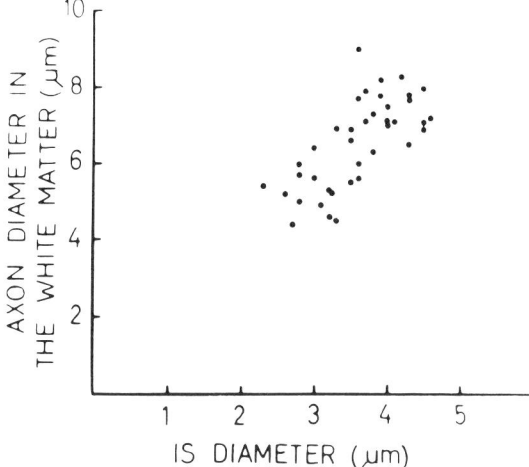

FIG. 5. Relation between axonal diameters in spinal cord white matter and diameters of initial segments (IS) for 39 sciatic α-motor axons in cat. Linear correlation coefficient $(r) = +0.698$ $(P < 0.0001)$. [From Cullheim and Kellerth (82).]

and evidence that this is transmitted electrically between the somadendritic regions of the motoneuron membranes was recently advanced by Magherini et al. (248). Excitatory interactions between cat motoneurons that could be mediated by recurrent collaterals have been described by Gogan et al. (124). However, an unequivocal demonstration of the physiological effect of activity in these collaterals has not yet been made.

Species of Motoneurons

For some time it was assumed that the motoneurons supplying a muscle were a homogenous population of cells differing only in size and in certain size-dependent properties. Recent physiological studies (145, 146), however, indicate that there may be two or more species of α-motoneurons in a pool, differing in characteristics that are independent of size. Just as there are distinct types of muscle fibers in a single mammalian muscle, there may be different species of motoneurons that innervate them and are responsible for their contractile properties. However, no morphological basis for distinguishing different types of cells within a pool, except by their size, has been discovered to date. Studies on the distribution of enzyme activity in anterior horn cells have been carried out by Penny and colleagues (279) in the hope of identifying different species of motoneurons histochemically. Cytophotometric measurements of the activities of five oxidative enzymes (succinate, malate, lactate, NAD^+-linked isocitrate, and NADH dehydrogenases) have been made in the spinal cord of rabbits. The findings indicate a unimodal distribution of the activities of all of these enzymes. Although the results do not offer a means of identifying different species of motoneurons, they are consistent with the "constant proportion" hypothesis of Pette and co-workers (281) with regard to oxidative enzyme activity. This was based on the finding that in a number of tissues, including the brain, the activities of mitochondrial enzymes were always in constant ratio to each other, although the absolute activities varied from tissue to tissue. It should be emphasized that although there was a unimodal distribution of the activities of all the enzymes studied, there was a very wide range of activities among anterior horn cells.

For the present, therefore, the only evidence indicating that there are different species of motoneurons in a pool comes from physiological studies that are described in section FIRING PATTERNS OF INDIVIDUAL MOTONEURONS AND MOTOR UNITS, p. 435. Whether the motoneurons innervating different types of muscles, such as the extraocular muscles, constitute different species is a question requiring information that is not yet available.

Terminals of Motoneurons in Muscle

Cajal (291) recognized that the number of terminals a motor axon gave off was proportional to the diameter of its axon and, thus, to the size of its cell body. Eccles and Sherrington (102) devoted considerable attention to the branching of motor fibers and proposed that "the larger fiber prepares early to form an extensive motor unit," since division of large fibers begins far proximal to the muscle. Thus the size of a motoneuron is an important element in determining the capacity of its motor unit to produce tension. However, other factors such as the type of muscle fibers it supplies also play a role.

The average "size" of a motor unit is determined by dividing the number of fibers in a muscle by the number of α-motor axons in the nerve supplying it. The extrinsic eye muscles contain as few as 3–6 fibers per motor unit. In the soleus of the cat, Clark (64) found an innervation ratio of 120:1. The mean innervation ratios vary widely in different muscles and may reach 1,000:1 or more in some large limb muscles. Innervation ratio is usually correlated with delicacy of movement.

What is important for this discussion is the fact that innervation ratios vary widely within a single muscle as a direct function of the conduction velocity and diameter of the motor axon. This became apparent in the 1960s when a technique was developed that made it possible to activate a single motor unit in an otherwise quiescent muscle and to study its properties in isolation (20, 352). The axon of a single motor unit was separated from others supplying the same muscle by repeatedly subdividing ventral root filaments until a thin strand was found that contained only one axon supplying the muscle under investigation. The conduction velocity of this axon was obtained from measurements of conduction time and distance. When single motor units were stimulated at various rates there were striking differences in the maximal tetanic tensions they produced. In the soleus muscle, the maximal tetanic tensions varied from about 3 to 40 g (253); in the medial gastrocnemius they ranged from about 0.5 to 120 g, a more than 200-fold difference. A definite relation between axonal conduction velocity (proportial to diameter) and maximal tetanic tension was found in the deep and superficial lumbrical muscle of the cat (6, 20) and in the soleus muscle of the cat (253). As illustrated by the three examples in Figure 6 a linear relationship between conduction velocity and maximum tetanic tension was found in all 10 experiments on the soleus muscle. For other large limb muscles the evidence has been controversial (11, 262, 273, 283, 353). A recent paper emphasized the importance of sample size in such studies (10). Jami and Petit (185), therefore, investigated four leg muscles (peroneus brevis, peroneus longus, soleus, and tibialis anterior), examining 25%–50% of the motor unit population in each muscle. As Figure 7 illustrates, these large samples showed unequivocally that there is a demonstrable relation between the logarithm of the tetanic tensions developed by motor units and the conduction velocities of their motor axons. A total of 453 units was studied to construct Figure 7. Axonal conduction velocities were grouped in classes of

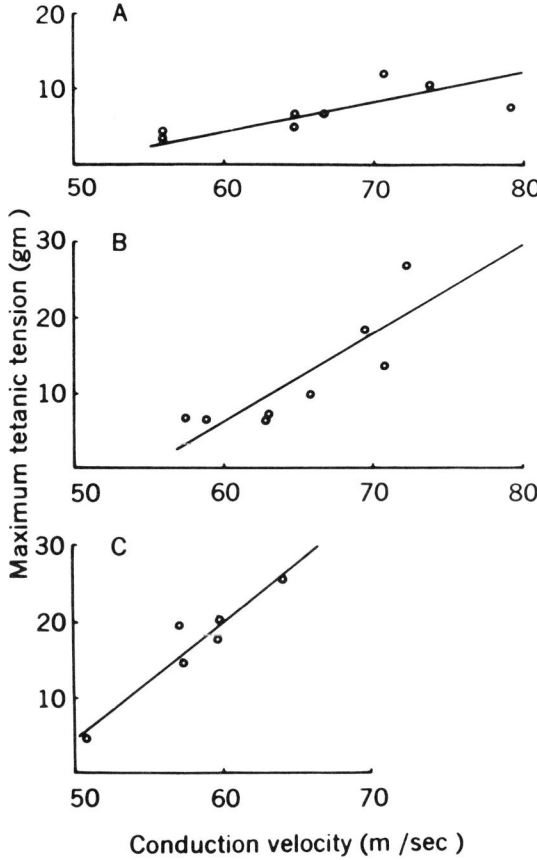

FIG. 6. Relation between maximum tetanic tension of individual motor units in cat soleus muscle and conduction velocity of their axons in 3 different experiments. [From McPhedran, Wuerker, and Henneman (253).]

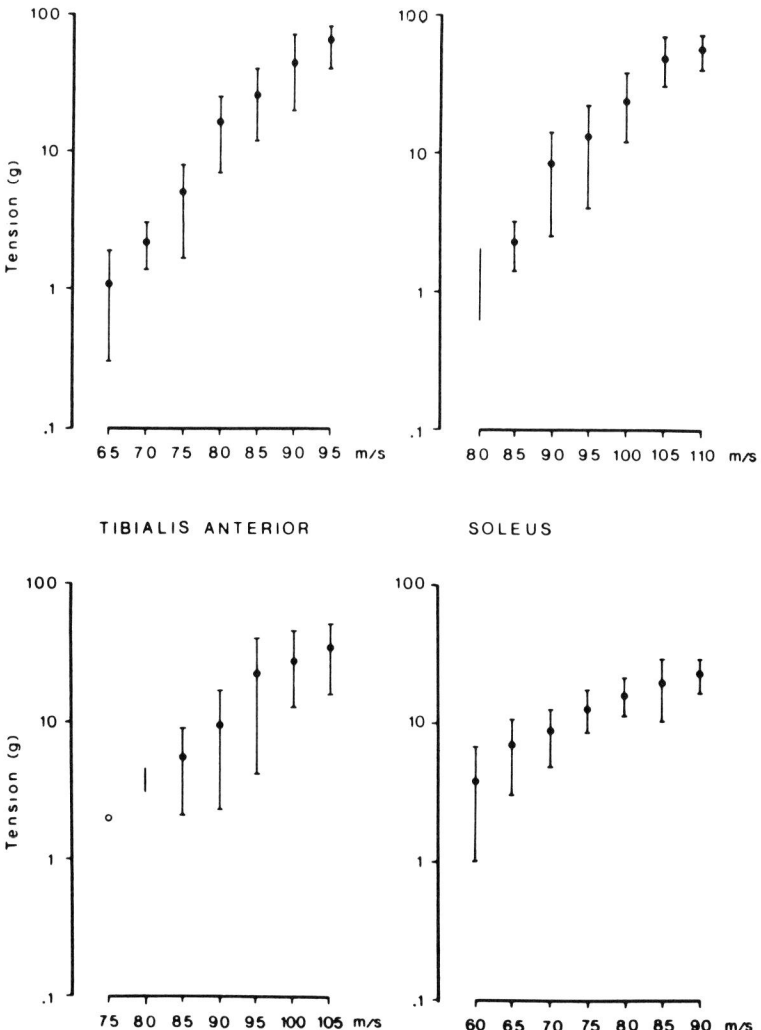

FIG. 7. Relation between logarithm of tetanic tensions developed by motor units and the conduction velocities of their motor axons in 4 leg muscles of the cat. *Heavy dots* on *vertical bars* indicate mean value of tension ± SD. For peroneus longus and tibialis anterior, intervals corresponding to conduction velocities under 85 m/s contained too few motor units to allow valid calculation of mean tension. Range of tensions developed by these motor units are represented by a *vertical bar*. *Open circle* represents tension of a single unit. For soleus, 4 motor units innervated by axons, either faster than 90 m/s or slower than 60 m/s. are not represented. [From Jami and Petit (185).]

5 m/s intervals. This study provides a firm basis for the conclusion that axonal conduction velocity and tetanic tension are correlated in large limb muscles. It does not, however, explain whether the number or type of muscle fibers, or both, are responsible for the correlation. It seems likely that within each type of motor unit there are units with numbers of muscle fibers that vary systematically with the conduction velocity of the axon.

The distributions of maximal tetanic tensions for soleus and medial gastrocnemius muscles in the cat are plotted in Figure 8. In both histograms the largest number of motor units occurs in the 0–10-g range. In general there is a progressive decrease in the number of motor units in each higher decade. In a study of the flexor digitorum longus, Olson and Swett (273) grouped the 83 units developing less than 10 g each on an expanded scale, with intervals of 1 g. Even within this restricted range, there was a clear tendency for the number of units in each 1-g interval to decrease in number as their tensions increased. These histograms are typical of all muscles that have been studied in this way, including such specialized muscles as the tensor tympani (336) and those that move the eye. The functional significance of this distribution pattern is discussed later in this section (*Matching the Properties of Motoneurons and the Muscle Fibers They Supply*, p. 433). It is sufficient now to point out that the abundance of small units makes possible precise, finely graded control of muscle tension in the lower

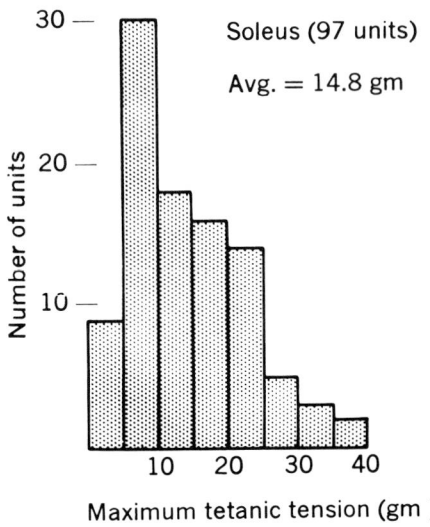

FIG. 8. Distribution of maximal tetanic tensions of motor units of cat's soleus (A) and medial gastrocnemius (B). [A, from Mc-Phedran, Wuerker, and Henneman (253); B from Wuerker, Mc-Phedran, and Henneman (353).]

ranges, whereas the presence of very large units provides for the addition of large increments of tension during maximal efforts.

Clark (64) found an innervation ratio of 120:1 for the soleus muscle. Correcting his estimate for the small γ-fibers to muscle spindles, which constitute about 33% of the total motor outflow in muscle nerves, an average innervation ratio of 180:1 is obtained. This applies to the average motor unit which develops 14.8 g of tetanic tension. By extrapolation the smallest motor unit (3.2 g) and the largest unit (40.4 g) in this sample consist of 39 and 491 muscle fibers, respectively. Since the cat's soleus is homogenous throughout, consisting entirely of β-fibers whose diameters and histochemical appearance are extremely uniform (157), these estimates should be reasonably accurate.

This type of analysis cannot be applied to the gastrocnemius muscle, because it has three types of fibers differing in size and contractile properties.

Only one study has been carried out on the anatomy and innervation ratios of identified types of motor units (49). Direct morphological determination of innervation ratios required complete reconstruction of the three-dimensional distribution of each motor unit's fibers within the whole medial gastrocnemius muscle. Technical difficulties limited satisfactory reconstructions to two type FF units. The results indicated that the muscle unit territories extend through a large fraction of the whole muscle volume, and within this territory the density of fibers belonging to a single unit is relatively low. At least 40–50 motor units probably share any one region within the medial gastrocnemius. Burke and Tsairis (49) conclude that "an average muscle unit in the cat medial gastrocnemius contains between 400 and 800 muscle fibers irrespective of physiological type." Unfortunately the number of motor units satisfactorily reconstructed was too small to provide a direct morphological test of the physiological findings described above; i.e., muscle units that produce small tensions contain fewer fibers than larger tension units. This conclusion was particularly compelling in the case of the homogenous soleus muscle of the cat. In harmony with this conclusion are the results of Knott and colleagues (210), who showed in studies of single motor units that there was a clear correlation between the surface area from which an EMG could be recorded, and the EMG amplitude and the maximum tension the unit produced. This correlation seems to indicate that strong motor units contain more muscle fibers that are more widely dispersed in the muscle than weaker units.

Morphology of Neuromuscular Junctions

This description of motoneurons would be incomplete without including information on the junctions they form with muscle fibers. Only certain aspects of this topic that are germane to the subject of this chapter are described. Three types of neuromuscular junctions can be distinguished ultrastructurally (274). The most obvious differences between them are the total sizes of the junctions and the amounts of surface area they present for the discharge and reception of transmitter. The axonal terminals on red fibers are small and elliptical. The areas of contact they make on a single fiber are relatively discrete and separate. The junctional folds, which the sarcoplasmic membrane of the muscle forms, are relatively shallow, sparse, and irregular in their arrangement. Axoplasmic vesicles are moderate in number and sarcoplasmic vesicles are rare. Axonal terminals on white fibers are longer and flatter and have a much greater area for release of acetylcholine. The postjunctional surface formed by the branching, closely spaced junctional folds provides a vast receptive area for the transmitter. At adjacent contacts on the same muscle fiber the junctional folds may merge with one another, so that synaptic contiguity is more continuous and widespread. Axoplasmic and sarcoplasmic vesicles are numerous. Intermediate fibers receive relatively large axonal terminals. Their junctional folds are the most widely spaced and deepest of the three types. They are relatively straight and unbranched. Axoplasmic vesicles are less numerous than in white fibers. Sarcoplasmic vesicles are conspicuous near the deeper portions of the junctional folds. According to Padykula and Gauthier (274), junctions on intermediate fibers are not just a gradation between the types on red and white fibers but are a distinct third type.

On the presynaptic side of the myoneural junction the dimensions and form of the axonal terminals are correlated with the caliber of the parent axon (271). On the postsynaptic side there is a positive correlation between the size of the end plate and the muscle fiber diameter in mammals (5, 66, 69, 144, 271). Moreover, the distinctive features of the three types of junctions are correlated with the diameters of their muscle fibers (274). The larger a muscle fiber, the smaller its input resistance (198) and the greater the amount of transmitter required to depolarize it to its firing threshold. Therefore, large white fibers require extensive synaptic surfaces. Kuno and colleagues (223) showed a positive correlation between the end-plate area and the diameter of muscle fibers. They also demonstrated that the number of quanta of transmitter released by a presynaptic impulse was positively correlated with the size of the end plate. The greater number of synaptic vesicles in the axonal terminals on white fibers is presumably associated with release of more acetylcholine over a wider area. The resulting end-plate potential is sufficient in amplitude and extent to set up a propagated impulse in the large, low-resistance muscle fiber. Smaller junctions with fewer vesicles are adequate to ensure transmission to the more easily excited red fibers.

The pre- and postsynaptic differences in neuromuscular junctions that are associated with the three types of muscle fibers are perhaps another indication that there may be three species of motoneurons supplying heterogeneous muscles. There is convincing evidence that the activity pattern that motoneurons impress on the muscle fibers they supply determines many of the morphological, chemical, and functional properties of the muscle fibers (308). It is quite possible that these activity patterns also determine the structural and functional characteristics of neuromuscular junctions. Although this has not been demonstrated, it seems likely because prolonged stimulation of a muscle nerve can transform the muscle fibers it innervates from one type to another (308). It is probable that the neuromuscular junctions transmitting these impulse patterns are also transformed, since they must be adapted to the types of muscle fibers they supply.

Matching the Properties of Motoneurons and the Muscle Fibers They Supply

In the preceding sections it was pointed out that the dendrites, the axon, and the axonal terminals of motoneurons are all scaled in proportion to the size of the cell body. As a consequence of this scaling principle, the postsynaptic effects a motoneuron produces at its various axonal terminals are also proportional to the size of the cell. The most obvious of these size-related effects is the capacity to produce tension. The influence of a motoneuron on its muscle fibers, however, goes far beyond tension production. The pattern of contractile activity it induces in them causes them to develop a distinctive set of morphological, chemical, and functional properties (308). Since the firing patterns and mean daily activity of motoneurons vary systematically with cell size (and perhaps cell species) throughout a pool, the characteristics induced in their muscle units vary correspondingly. The basic mechanisms by which contractile activity in a muscle induces changes in its own properties are not understood, but they clearly enable the muscle to adapt to the amount and pattern of usage it experiences. The result of this adaptation is that the contractile properties of motor units are well matched to the activity patterns of their motoneurons.

Figure 9 illustrates the distribution of some of the properties of motor units that have been studied in typical limb muscles. The histogram is a smoothed version of the one shown in Figure 8 in which the maximal tetanic tensions of gastrocnemius motor units are plotted against the number of units in each 10-g tension range. As noted in subsection *Dimensions of α-Motoneurons and Distribution of Cell Size*, p. 425, this skewed distribution, with a preponderance of units producing small tensions, resembles the distribution of cell volumes in Figure 2. The large number of units at the left end of the histogram have axons of small diameter and, thus, are innervated by a correspondingly large population of small motoneurons. The few motor units generating large tensions have thick axons and are supplied by a small number of large motoneurons.

The largest motoneurons, which typically discharge in brief, high-frequency bursts, supply motor units with large, pale type A muscle fibers that contract rapidly and, therefore, require the fast rates of activation they receive from their motoneurons to produce fused tetanic contractions. These motor units fatigue quickly, sometimes in a few seconds, a characteristic that matches the brief duration of firing in their motoneurons. Their susceptibility to fatigue may be related to lack of an abundant blood supply and to insufficient mitochondria that contain the enzymes necessary for aerobic metabolism. Instead, these pale fibers utilize glycogen, which is capable of supplying energy anaerobically at a rapid rate, but only for a brief time. The glycogen is quickly depleted, and after

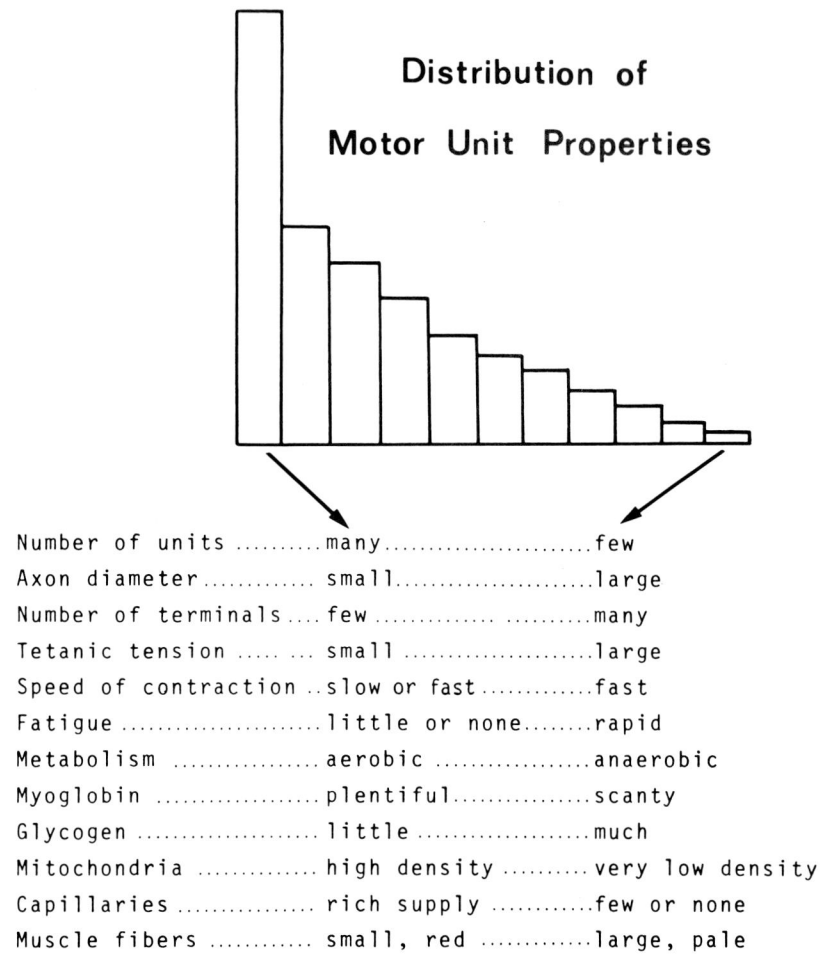

FIG. 9. Smoothed version of histogram in Figure 8B, illustrating distribution of some of the properties of motor units in typical limb muscles. Height of columns indicates relative numbers of motor units with the properties listed below. [From Henneman (154). Skeletal muscle: the servant of the nervous system. In: *Medical Physiology* (14th ed.), edited by V. B. Mountcastle. St. Louis, MO: The C. V. Mosby Co., 1980.]

a short period of maximal activity the tension output drops to a low level and may take a long time to recover. In contrast, the units that produce the smallest tensions consist of thin, red fibers that are least susceptible to fatigue. These units can maintain their maximal tensions almost indefinitely, as is often necessary in postural activities. They are dependent on oxidative metabolism for contractile energy. Their muscle fibers are richly supplied with capillaries and mitochondria. Their small diameters serve to reduce the distance over which oxygen and other metabolites must be transported from capillaries to mitochondria. All of these characteristics are well matched to the high level of daily activity in their motoneurons. As these examples illustrate, the distribution of firing patterns in a motoneuron pool has its counterpart in muscle where there is a matching distribution of contractile properties in the corresponding motor units (37, 45, 50).

The adaptive mechanisms that determine what properties develop in a motor unit are probably all responding to the same influence, i.e., the activity pattern of their motoneuron. It is perhaps not surprising, therefore, that the contractile properties in a motor unit are found in only certain combinations. The occurrence within one motor unit of a certain capacity for producing tension, a particular contraction speed, a characteristic range of firing rates, a specific susceptibility to neuromuscular and contractile fatigue, a distinctive histochemical profile, and well-defined morphological properties probably represents a set of correlated adaptations. The particular combination of properties occurring in a unit undoubtedly is the one with the greatest functional utility, because all of the properties were determined by the same activity pattern. The advantages of combining certain properties will become clearer in section FIRING PATTERNS OF INDIVIDUAL MOTONEURONS AND MOTOR UNITS, p. 435, when the actual discharge patterns of individual motoneurons are described and the operations of the pool as a whole are defined.

Concluding Comments

The morphological studies summarized in this section indicate that motoneurons differ widely in size and that all of their parts (dendrites, soma, initial segment, axon, collaterals, intramuscular terminals, and neuromuscular end plates) are scaled in proportion to each other. Taken as a whole, the observations make an impressive array of evidence, providing an anatomical basis for a size principle.

Although the morphological observations suggest that in some respects large motoneurons are simply expanded versions of small ones, the physiological findings of Harris and Henneman (145, 146) and others to be described later in section NONUNIFORMITY OF MOTONEURONS, p. 485, indicate that motoneurons may also differ in ways not related to their size. Cullheim and Kellerth (81) report that the number of recurrent collateral outbulgings (interpreted as synaptic terminals) of a motoneuron correlate as well or better with the type of muscle fibers innervated as with the axonal diameter. In view of the anatomical evidence already described and further physiological findings to be presented in the next section, it is probable that the functional properties of motoneurons correlate not only with their size but also with the neuromuscular junctions they form and the types of muscle fibers they supply.

FIRING PATTERNS OF INDIVIDUAL MOTONEURONS AND MOTOR UNITS

Functional Significance of Size of Motoneurons

Present concepts of the organization of the motoneuron pool can be traced to the interest of early histologists in the significance of neuronal size and shape. Ramón y Cajal (291) disposed of many of the conjectures of his day by demonstrating that the diameter of a nerve fiber is related directly to the size of its cell body and by giving numerous examples of this relation throughout the nervous system. His findings have been repeatedly confirmed, in particular for motoneurons, by electrical and anatomical studies. Functional relations between the diameters of axons and their electrical properties did not become apparent until the introduction of the oscilloscope and the studies of Erlanger and Gasser in *Electrical Signs of Nervous Activity* (109). In particular, Gasser (120) showed that the amplitude of a nerve impulse recorded externally from a peripheral nerve is related directly to the diameter of the fiber in which it is conducted. Thus, when impulses of different amplitudes are recorded from the same nerve, the largest signal signifies the firing of the largest fiber in the nerve and the discharge of the biggest cell body. Smaller signals indicate firing in correspondingly smaller fibers and cells. Electrical and anatomical criteria were used to classify nerve fibers into three main types (A, B, C) differing in size, and the first tentative attempts to correlate fiber types with their functions were made.

The voltages required to excite axons with external electrodes increase as the diameters of axons decrease (109). It does not follow, however, that large neurons can be more easily discharged synaptically than small ones. The situation, in fact, appears to be just the reverse, as Henneman (153) demonstrated in studies on motoneurons. Reflexes were elicited in lumbar ventral roots by electrical stimulation of dorsal roots or large nerve trunks. When shocks of sufficient strength were used, the response consisted of two phases (Fig. 10). The first phase was a brief, relatively synchronous

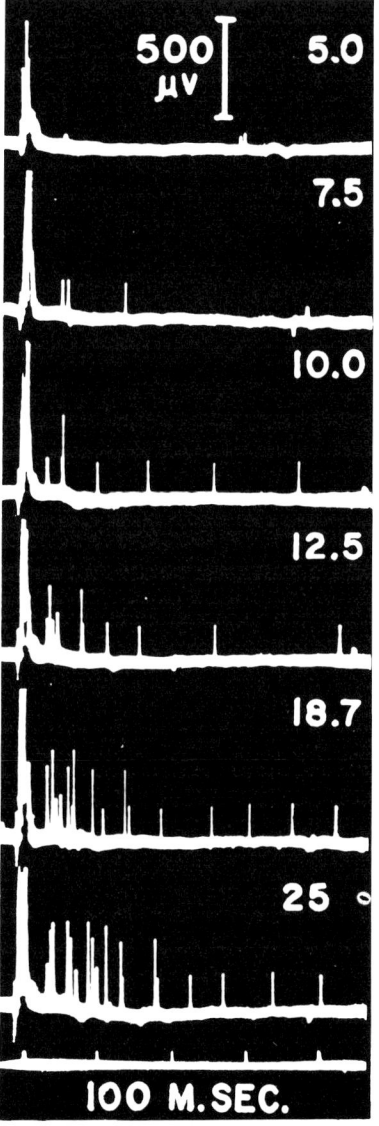

FIG. 10. Reflex discharges recorded from a filament of 7th lumbar ventral root in response to stimulation of ipsilateral sciatic nerve of cat. Numbers at right of each tracing indicate relative intensity of stimulation. Initial deflection on *left* of each tracing is the early discharge referred to in text. [From Henneman (153).]

discharge of short latency, followed by rhythmic firing sometimes lasting one second or more (the late phase of the well-known flexor reflex). To analyze the second phase of the reflex in detail, monophasic recordings were taken from fine filaments of ventral roots dissected under a low-power microscope. Individual impulses of single motor fibers that discharged repetitively could readily be distinguished in these records by their amplitudes. As the stimulus applied to the ipsilateral sciatic nerve was increased, progressive changes in the late response occurred. The top record in Figure 10 shows that the stimuli reaching the motoneurons were well above threshold for the early reflex but were insufficient to evoke a late discharge. The three small spikes shown in this trace were probably impulses in γ-motoneurons. Increase in the stimulus strength then caused a single α-motoneuron to discharge three times. Further increases in stimulus intensity caused progressively longer trains of impulses in this fiber. At a higher stimulus intensity a second unit, with spikes about twice the amplitude of the first, made its appearance, thereafter discharging two, four, and five times in response to stronger shocks. A third and still larger unit appeared with stronger shocks, firing twice at this intensity and four times at higher intensity. Recruitment of progressively larger motoneurons with increase in stimulus intensity was observed regularly. Discharges of slightly smaller motoneurons with stronger shocks were occasionally observed in single tracings, but not as a regular occurrence. In general, units that differed most in spike amplitude also varied most in the strength of stimulation required to discharge them. Even small gradations in the spike amplitude of motoneurons, however, were associated with measureable differences in their reflex threshold.

From these observations it appeared that motoneurons may be graded according to their susceptibility to synaptic discharge in a flexor reflex. At the upper end of the scale are the largest cells, requiring the most intense stimulation. Smaller cells require correspondingly less intense stimulation. At the lower end of the scale are the γ-motoneurons. In most recordings from ventral root filaments these cells can be seen firing steadily without externally applied stimulation. The tendency to be continuously active is perhaps an indication that these small cells are so susceptible to excitation that the spontaneous activity of the spinal cord is sufficient to keep them firing.

Although the discharge patterns recorded from different ventral root filaments varied, certain features were regularly observed. The most notable were *1)* recruitment of larger units and lengthening of discharge trains with stronger shocks; *2)* regularity in the rhythm of discharges of each motoneuron, with progressive decrease in their rate of firing with increasing train length; and *3)* an inverse relation between spike height and train length. These characteristics suggest that the excitatory process responsible for the observed discharges of motoneurons was a prolonged firing of internuncial cells, reaching an early peak of intensity from which it declined smoothly to a resting level. At its maximum the internuncial input was apparently sufficient to cause repetitive firing in a wide range of cell sizes. As the excitatory activity subsided, it fell below the levels necessary to fire the larger cells but remained adequate to discharge smaller cells. Hence the patterns in Figure 10: short trains of large spikes and longer trains of smaller impulses.

It should be emphasized that the relationship between motoneuron size and susceptibility to discharge in these experiments was observed in recordings from ventral root filaments where axons from several pools of flexor motoneurons were intermingled. Undoubtedly, the observed firing originated in different pools of flexor motoneurons (322). Nevertheless, the relationships between input intensity and the size of output signals held with few exceptions. This suggests that several pools of flexor motoneurons, whose activity is closely related during withdrawal reflexes, may function like one large, common pool in response to certain inputs. In 1926 Creed and Sherrington (79) studied the concurrent contractions of flexor muscles in the "flexion" reflex and concluded:

> From the point of view of the afferent nerve the muscular entity executing the [flexor] reflex movement is . . . not this or that muscle but a composite aggregate of motor units scattered through and forming parts of a number of separate and even distant muscles. This composite collection is given functional solidarity and homogeneity by the likeness of threshold and latency obtaining among its units in regard to the afferent nerve bringing them into action. An increment in stimulus does not break this homogeneity but merely brings to it a certain addition again composed of units mutually similar in threshold and latency although made up from muscles anatomically separate.

These studies suggested that orderly recruitment of motoneurons according to their size might be a general phenomenon, not limited to flexor reflexes. To investigate this possibility a more comprehensive series of experiments was carried out using a variety of inputs. A convenient means of evoking a reflex discharge of motoneurons is to stretch an extensor (antigravity) muscle in a decerebrate cat. In such preparations the normal response to stretch is exaggerated and the slightest elongation of the muscle results in the discharge of motoneurons and the development of reflex tension (233). The reflex is highly specific, the response being limited to the motoneurons of the muscle that is stretched or its closest synergists.

Figure 11 illustrates the results of stretching the triceps surae muscle and recording from a filament of the seventh lumbar ventral root. The tension applied to the tendon of the muscle is measured by the separation of the upper beams and the ventral root discharge appears in the lowest tracings. With the muscle completely relaxed the only activity usually recorded

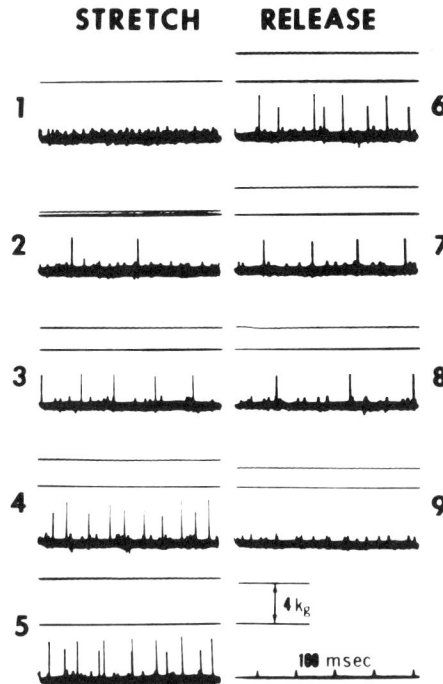

FIG. 11. Stretch-evoked responses of 2 α-motoneurons recorded from a filament of 7th lumbar ventral root of cat. Amount of tension applied and developed reflexly is indicated by separation of 2 top beams in each frame. Several seconds elapsed between successive frames while muscle was stretched (1–5) and released (6–9). [From Henneman et al. (159).]

was a continuous series of impulses of very low amplitude (not seen in this tracing). This activity was derived from the axons of γ-motoneurons, which are of smaller diameter than the α-fibers.

In Figure 12 a series of single sweeps is reproduced to illustrate recruitment in a filament containing the axons of five triceps motoneurons. With increasing stretch progressively larger impulses appeared, which are numbered from 1 to 5. The recruitment order was 1, 2, 3, 4, 5; the order of dropout was 5, 4, 3, 2, 1.

Figure 13 illustrates the distribution of stretch thresholds for 208 motoneurons. The tensions required to elicit maintained rhythmic firing ranged from less than 0.4 kg to more than 8 kg.

These observations (159), together with those already described, suggested that orderly recruitment must depend on differences in the excitabilities of the motoneurons themselves, on some systematic difference in the input they received that was correlated with their sizes, or on a combination of these factors. To distinguish between these possibilities, recruitment was examined, using a number of different inputs. A variety of spinal reflexes was elicited to discharge flexor or extensor motoneurons (160). Responses of pairs of units to the same, simultaneously delivered stimuli were compared. In general, the smaller of any two responding units was discharged at a lower intensity of stimulation regardless of whether the stimuli arose ipsilaterally or contralaterally, physiologically or electrically, whether the responses were elicited monosynaptically or polysynaptically, or whether the motoneurons were flexor or extensor. In a further series of experiments (325) trains of electrical stimuli were also applied to brain stem motor areas, cerebellum, basal ganglia, and motor cortex of the cat. Regardless of the site of stimulation, motoneurons whose axons yielded the smallest impulses in ventral root filaments were discharged at the lowest thresholds and other units were recruited in order of increasing size. By comparing each responsive unit with all of the others in the same filament, a total of 396 pairs of motoneurons was examined. In 86% of comparisons the smaller unit had the lower threshold, in 4% the thresholds were indistinguishable, and in 10% the larger unit had the lower threshold. The use of electrical stimulation with widely spaced electrodes must have resulted in discharges from several pools of motoneurons. The low incidence of exceptions to orderly recruitment suggests that most of the descending activity reaches motoneuron pools through a few penultimate internuncial circuits (243) that transform this activity into highly ordered patterns of input. In conjunction with previous findings, the results suggested that the susceptibility of a motoneuron to discharge is strongly correlated with its size regardless of the source of the excitation and the neural circuits that transmit it to the motoneurons. Input is not excluded as an important factor in this correlation, but it is difficult to understand how each of the various inputs in these experiments could supply more excitatory fibers to small cells than to large ones, as some authors (36, 192) suggest.

Susceptibility to inhibition is also correlated with cell size, as illustrated in Figure 14. The upper portion of the figure shows orderly recruitment of three triceps motoneurons with increasing stretch. After the normal pattern of recruitment had been established a 4-kg stretch, sufficient to elicit tonic firing of all three motoneurons, was applied by elongating the triceps to a fixed length. This stretch was maintained while the effects of inhibition, shown below, were recorded. Weak inhibition silenced the largest unit. Inhibition of moderate intensity suppressed firing of the unit of intermediate size as well, leaving the smallest unit discharging until a still stronger inhibition eliminated all responses to stretch. During each of the brief periods after inhibition there was a partial but incomplete recovery of the original pattern of response. Results of this kind were obtained in a variety of experiments. In general, the larger the unit, the more readily it was silenced by inhibition. Regardless of the existing level of excitatory drive, regardless of whether the motoneurons were responding rhythmically to stretch or monosynaptically to synchronous volleys, and regardless of whether the inhibition was direct, internuncially mediated, autogenetic, or recurrent, the susceptibility of each cell to inhibition appeared to be closely correlated with its size. It was concluded that

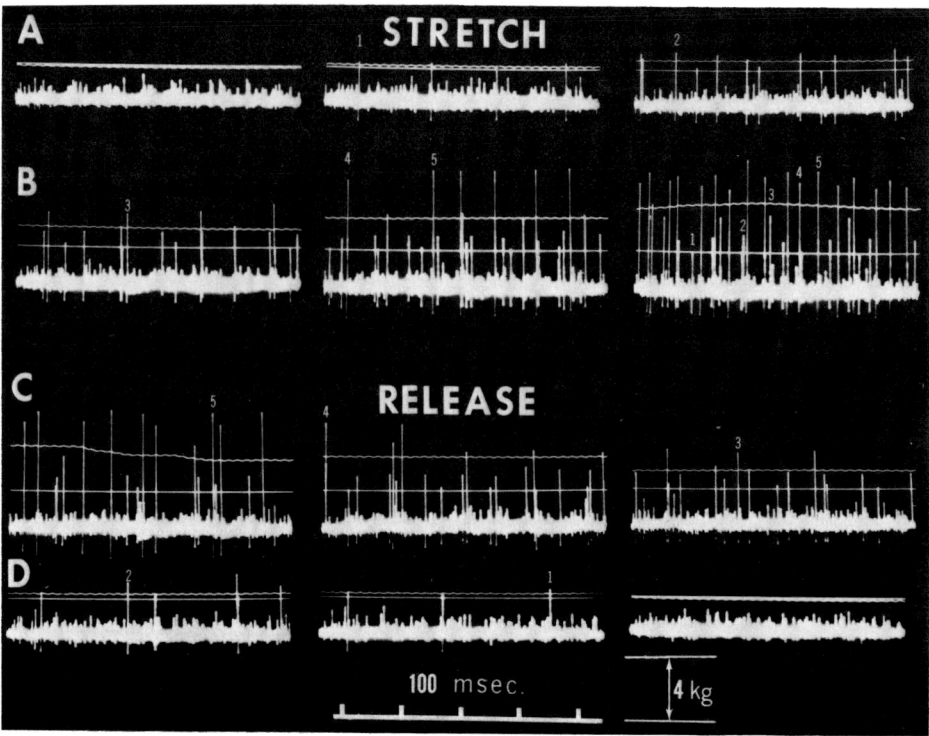

FIG. 12. Stretch-evoked responses of 5 α-motoneurons recorded from a filament of the 1st sacral ventral root of cat. Numbers above action potentials indicate rank of units according to size. [From Henneman et al. (159).]

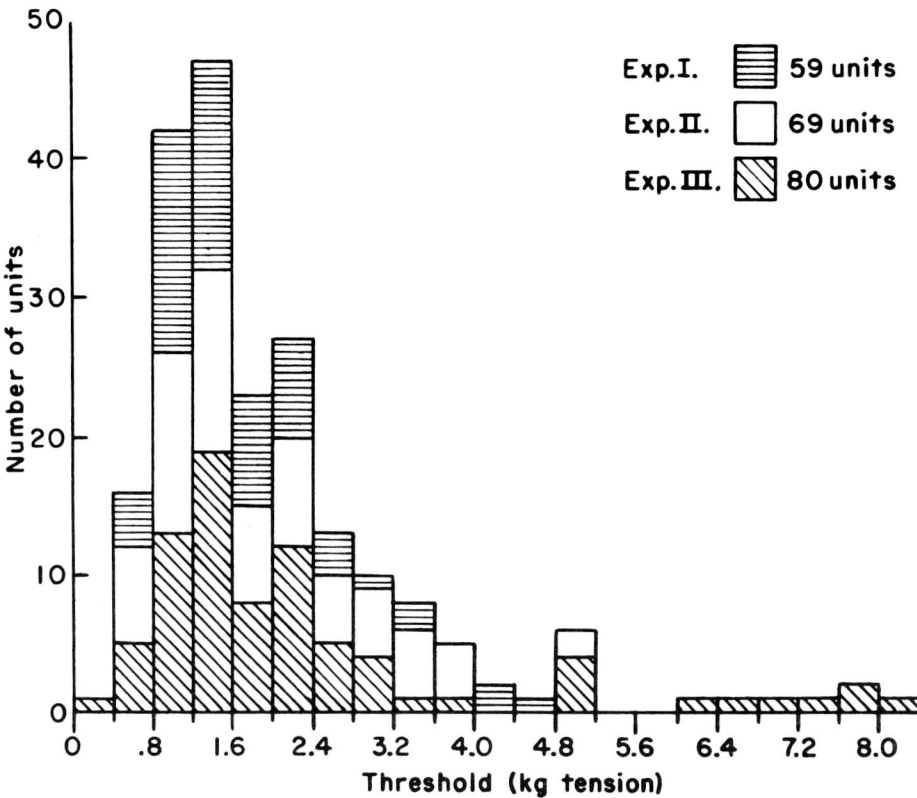

FIG. 13. Frequency distribution of thresholds of tonic responses to stretch in 3 experiments on cats. Abscissa, threshold tension of deefferented triceps muscle. Ordinate, number of units whose thresholds fell between values indicated on abscissa. [From Henneman et al. (159).]

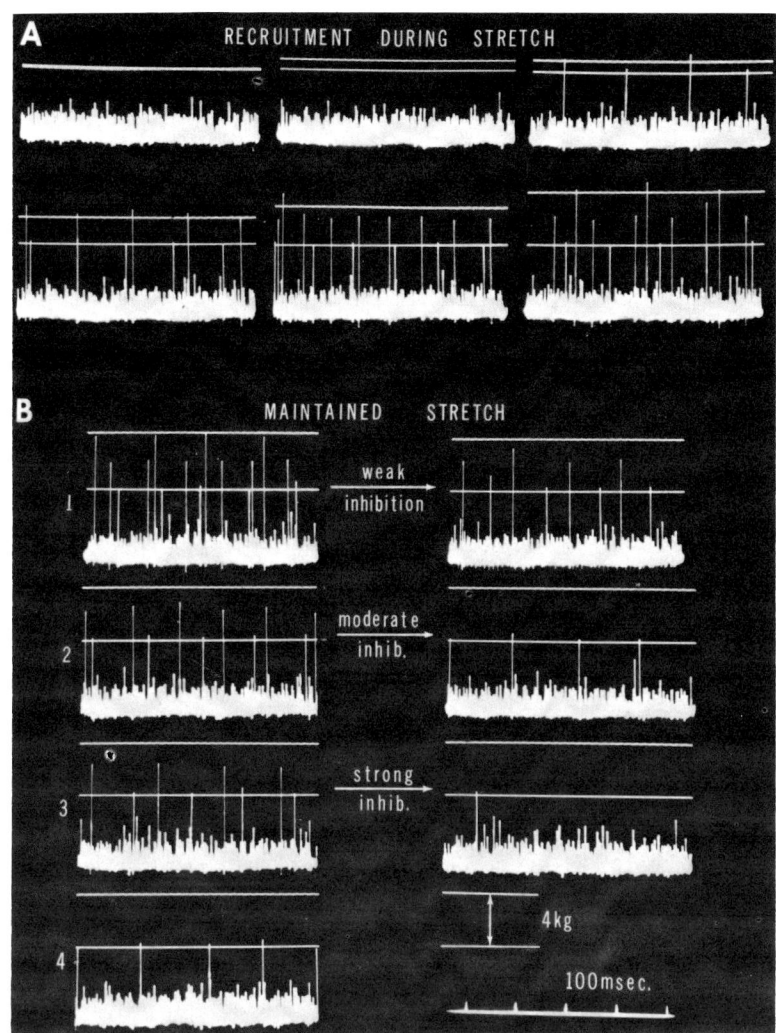

FIG. 14. A: orderly recruitment in cat of 3 triceps motoneurons of different sizes in response to increasing degrees of stretch. Tension produced by stretch of triceps muscle indicated by separation of top *traces* in each frame. B: orderly inhibition of same 3 units during a constant stretch of 4 kg. Records *1–4* on *left* show control responses of stretch before, between and after 3 inhibitory stimulations. Records on *right* were obtained during 100/s stimulation of ipsilateral deep peroneal nerve at 3 intensities. Largest unit was silenced first (*line 1*), intermediate unit next (*line 2*), and smallest unit last (*line 3*). Note lasting effects produced by brief inhibitions, i.e., failure to recover to previous levels in *lines 2* and *4*. [From Henneman et al. (160).]

whereas the excitability of motoneurons (including the role of input) is an inverse function of cell size, their inhibitability is a direct function of cell size.

The net effects of cell size, excitatory input, and inhibition on the responses of three different motoneurons are represented quantitatively by means of three-dimensional graphs in Figure 15. The responses of the smallest and most excitable unit, which was spontaneously active with the muscle relaxed, are plotted in Figure 15A. The stretch threshold of the intermediate unit (Fig. 15B) was between 0 and 5 mm extension and that of the largest and least excitable unit was between 5 and 10 mm. At all levels of stretch the intensity of inhibitory stimulation required to silence a unit was always the greatest for the most excitable cell (Fig. 15A). In Figure 15D the responses of all the motor units are combined in the contractile response of the whole muscle.

In summary, by 1966 it had been shown that the neural energy required to discharge a motoneuron, the energy it transmits and releases in its muscle, its excitability and inhibitability, its mean rate of firing, and even its rate of protein synthesis (280) are all correlated with its size. This set of correlations was referred to as the "size principle" (159, 160).

Measurement of Total Output of Motoneuron Pools

By 1965 it had been shown that there was a striking degree of orderliness in both the neural and contractile properties of motor units. From the outset, however, apparent exceptions in recruitment order had been noted. It was difficult to ascertain whether these were due to *1*) decreased amplitude of impulses in injured fibers; *2*) recording of impulses from separate but synergistic pools, due to mixture of their axons in ventral root filaments; or *3*) true departures from the general principle that cell size is highly correlated with susceptibility to discharge. There was clearly a need for defining the operations of the motoneuron pool in quantitative terms so that the activity of each cell could be related to that of the entire pool. A technique was devised for measuring the simultaneous discharge of all the cells in a pool, and, from this, the percentage of output during any monosynaptic reflex (59). The method is illustrated in Figure 16. The combined nerves to the medial gastrocnemius muscle (MG) and the lateral gastrocnemius and soleus muscles (LG-S), which together make up the triceps surae muscle, were stimulated with brief shocks (1 shock/s) that set up antidromic volleys in all of the α-motor fibers of these nerves and dromic volleys in all of the group Ia-fibers. The antidromic volley was recorded in the distal half of the seventh lumbar or first sacral ventral root (L_7VR or S_1VR) and displayed on one trace of a two-beam oscilloscope. The dromic volley elicited a monosynaptic reflex in the proximal half of the same ventral root, which was displayed on the other trace. The base lines of these two traces are superimposed in Figure 17. The left potential in each pair of responses is the antidromic volley. It is a measure of the discharge of all of the MG and LG-S motor fibers in this ventral root. The right potential in each pair is the monosynaptic reflex. Its size is determined by the number of MG and LG-S motoneurons discharged during the reflex and the sizes of their action potentials. Before a 12-s conditioning tetanus to the muscle nerves at 500 shocks/s, the amplitude of the reflex was less than one-half that of the antidromic volley (top row of responses in Fig. 17). After the tetanus the reflex increased in amplitude due to posttetanic potentiation (PTP) (237) and reached temporary equality with the antidromic volley (left side of second row). Thereafter, the reflex response gradually declined back to its original amplitude. At the peak of PTP all of the MG and LG-S motoneurons were evidently discharged reflexly, as nearly as could be determined by comparison of amplitudes. A more accurate measure of a compound action potential can be obtained by integrating it electronically. This was done in the experiments described below. The time integrals had an absolute accuracy of 1%–2% and varied by less than 0.2% on repeated trials. Thus, any monosynaptic reflex could be described quantitatively, using a scale of output running from 0 to 100%.

Critical Firing Levels of Motoneurons

With the technique just described the monosynaptic reflexes of a large population of triceps motoneurons were recorded in decerebrate cats (155). Simultaneously the monosynaptic reflexes of one triceps motoneuron were recorded from a thin filament of ventral root. The vertical lines in the top tracing of Figure 18 are the time integrals of successive population reflexes recorded at a rate of 1/s. The height of each line varies with the number of motoneurons discharged and their sizes. Just before this series was recorded the combined MG and LG-S nerves were tetanized. The responses in Figure 18 were recorded during the decline in the resulting PTP. As long as the responses of the triceps population exceeded a certain level, the triceps unit below discharged in every reflex. When the population response declined below this level, the unit ceased to respond. The first failure of the unit to discharge was followed by two successive responses before the unit ceased to fire completely. Careful examination of the record reveals that the first failure was associated with a smaller population response than were the next two unit responses. The "critical firing level" (CFL) of this unit was, thus, between the levels associated with the first failure and the smaller of the next two population responses. The difference between these levels was less than 1% of the maximal output of the triceps pool in this experiment.

The records in Figure 18 suggest that CFL is very sharply defined. When the PTP was repeated several times and sufficient observations were available within the critical range, however, it was usually apparent that there was a slight degree of uncertainty in the firing of the motoneuron; i.e., there was a narrow range of population responses within which a unit might or might not respond monosynaptically. This is evident in Figure 19, which reproduces the responses of three typical triceps units with relatively sharp "thresholds." The plateau at the beginning of the top trace on the left indicates the 100% level of the population response at the peak of potentiation. During the decline in potentiation each of the three units abruptly stopped responding at a different level and did not discharge again in that series. Close inspection revealed, however, that the unit that ceased firing at approximately the 60% level actually discharged once at 58.6% and failed to respond several times just above the 60% level. The range over which the unit's response was unpredictable was called the uncertain range. The

FIG. 15. Graphic representation of discharge frequency of 3 motoneurons of different sizes (A–C) in triceps surae of cat, and of contractile tension developed by the muscle itself (D) in response to varying degrees of excitation and inhibition: x-axis, intensity of inhibitory stimulation applied to ipsilateral deep peroneal nerve; y-axis, frequency of discharge in A–C and contractile tension in D; z-axis, stretch of triceps surae, in millimeters. Data for all 4 graphs obtained simultaneously. Cells were subjected simultaneously to various mixtures of excitatory (z-axis) and inhibitory (x-axis) stimuli. Each plotted point represents mean of 2 successive determinations. Inhibitory stimuli were 100/s shocks applied for 0.9-s periods at 4-s intervals. Note that unit A (smallest) fired spontaneously without stretch, unit B began to discharge between 0 and 5 mm of stretch, and unit C (the largest) between 5 and 10 mm. [From Henneman et al. (160).]

CHAPTER 11: ORGANIZATION OF MOTONEURON POOL 441

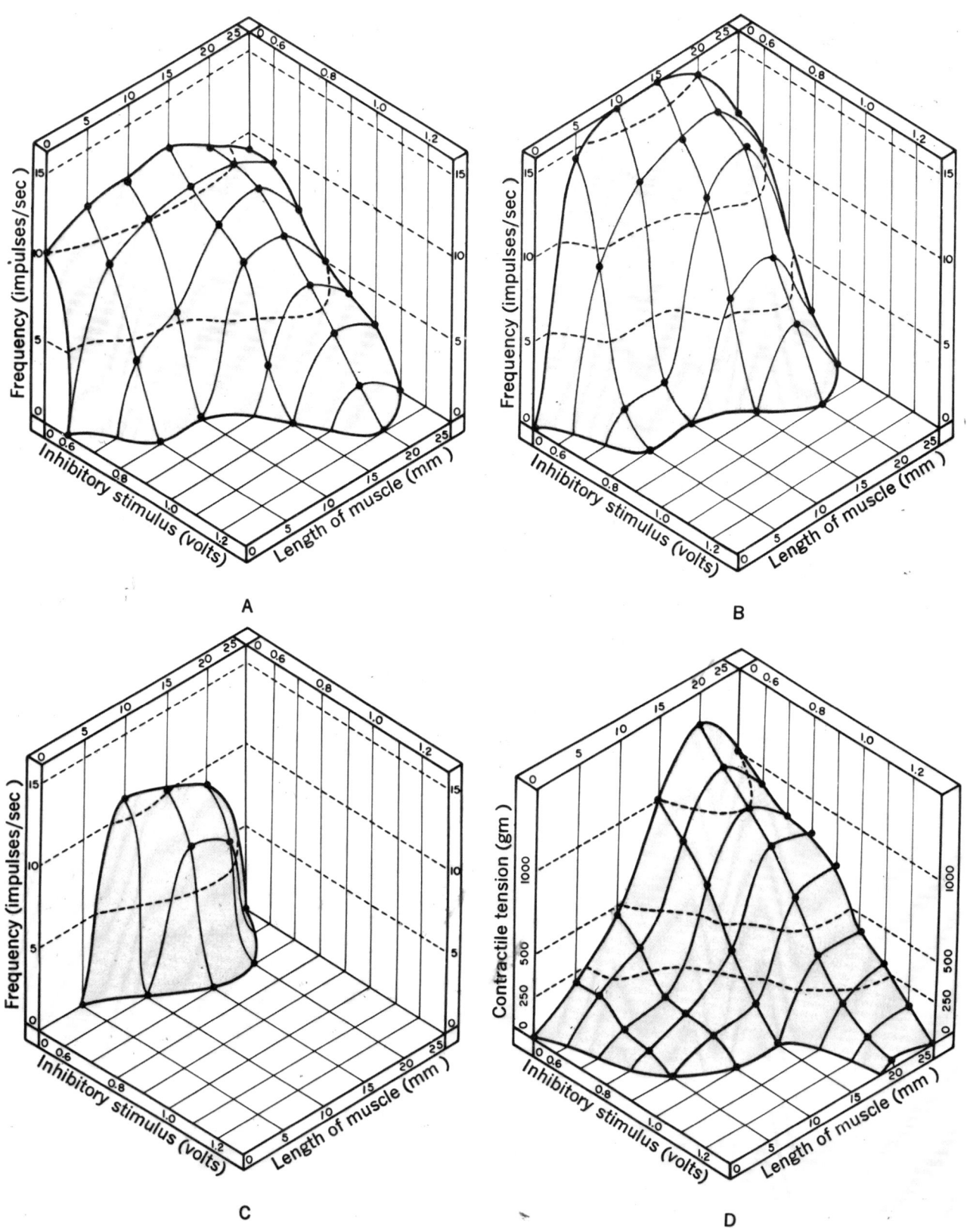

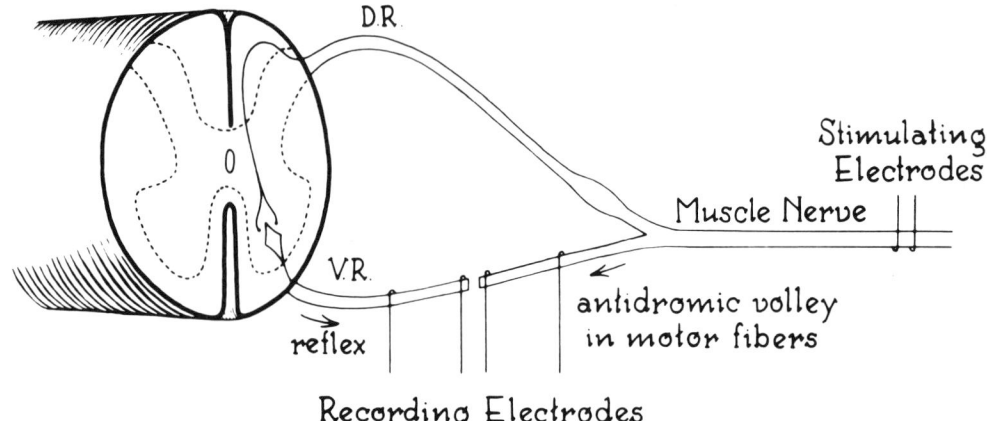

FIG. 16. Scheme of experiment used to measure maximal monosynaptic discharge of a motoneuron pool. DR, dorsal root; VR, ventral root. [From Clamann, Henneman, et al. (59).]

critical firing level was defined as the arithmetic mean of the uncertain range. In this series of experiments 203 triceps units were examined. Their CFLs ranged from 0 to 98.7%. The mean uncertain range for the entire group (2.1%) did not vary systematically with the CFL.

No technique was available for measuring critical firing levels directly during repetitive firing; instead, it was possible to make use of the order of recruitment in pairs of motoneurons as a measure of their susceptibility to repetitive discharge and to compare this order with the critical firing levels established in monosynaptic tests. Two examples of this approach are shown in Figure 20. Recordings were taken from two different pairs of plantaris motoneurons in the same experiment. As the intensity was first increased and then decreased manually, the two units commenced and ceased their firing at different intensities of stimulation, thus signaling their different thresholds to repetitive discharge. In both pairs of units the motoneuron with the lower CFL (shown at the ends of traces b and c) began to discharge sooner during the increase in stimulation intensity and ceased firing later during the decrease. In the lower pair of units, differing in CFL by 3.1%, the onsets of firing were farther apart, and the last discharges were more separated in time than in the upper pair of units, which differed by only 1.7%.

Sixty-two pairs of motoneurons were compared as illustrated in Figures 20 and 21. In 57 of these pairs the unit with the lower CFL in monosynaptic tests was invariably the more susceptible to repetitive firing. In 5 pairs, which differed in CFLs by only 1.7%, 1.1%, 2.0%, 2.1%, and 5.0%, the unit with the lower CFL was slightly less susceptible to repetitive firing. The minor disagreements between the two methods of ranking motoneurons were probably due to obtaining insufficient data in estimating the CFL monosynaptically. They tended to disappear when a longer series of monosynaptic reflexes was recorded for this purpose. The repetitive stimulation used in these experiments

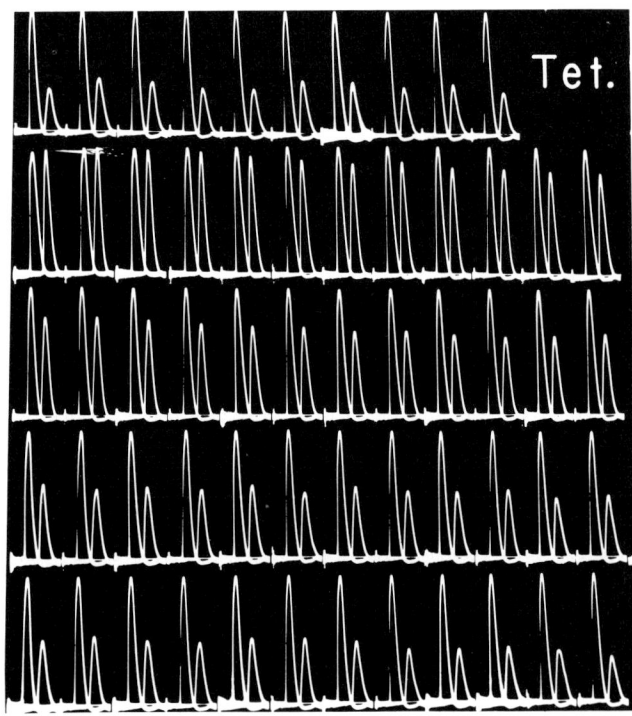

FIG. 17. Pairs of responses in cat recorded as in Figure 16 from proximal and distal halves of 1st sacral ventral root in response to single-shock stimulation of combined nerves to medial and lateral gastrocnemius (MG and LG). Left and right deflections of each pair are antidromic and reflex responses, respectively, displayed on superimposed traces of a 2-beam oscilloscope. First 10 pairs in *top row* recorded before 12-s tetanus (500 shocks/s) to MG and LG nerves. Subsequent pairs recorded at 2-s intervals after tetanus. [From Clamann, Henneman, et al. (59).]

activated several afferent systems in addition to the group Ia-fibers and presumably elicited descending activity from higher centers as well as recurrent inhibition from the motoneuron discharges. The results, therefore, have considerable generality. They apply to mixtures of inputs that might occur under normal conditions, not merely to group Ia inputs.

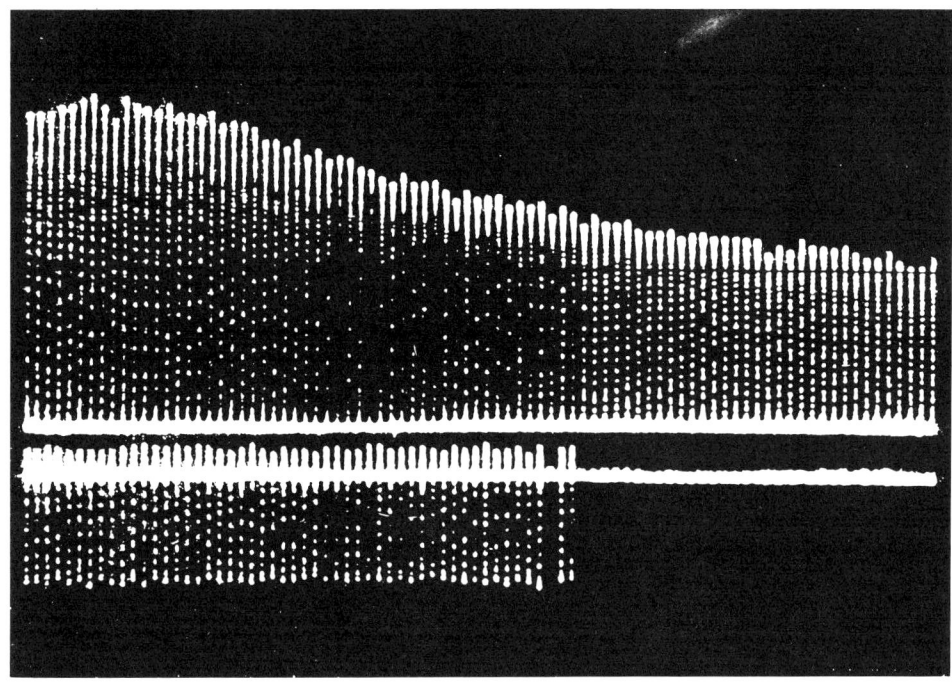

FIG. 18. Simultaneous recordings in cat of a series of monosynaptic reflexes of triceps surae pool (*top*) and a single triceps motoneuron (*bottom*) showing critical firing level of the latter. *Top trace*, time integrals of monosynaptic reflexes recorded at 1/s from proximal half of 1st sacral ventral root. Height of each vertical line measures size of population response. *Bottom trace*, monosynaptic reflexes of a single triceps motoneuron recorded from a small filament of 7th lumbar ventral root. Records were made during decline in posttetanic potentiation following a brief train of conditioning shocks that were applied to the combined medial gastrocnemius and lateral gastrocnemius and soleus nerves at 500/s. [From Henneman et al. (155).]

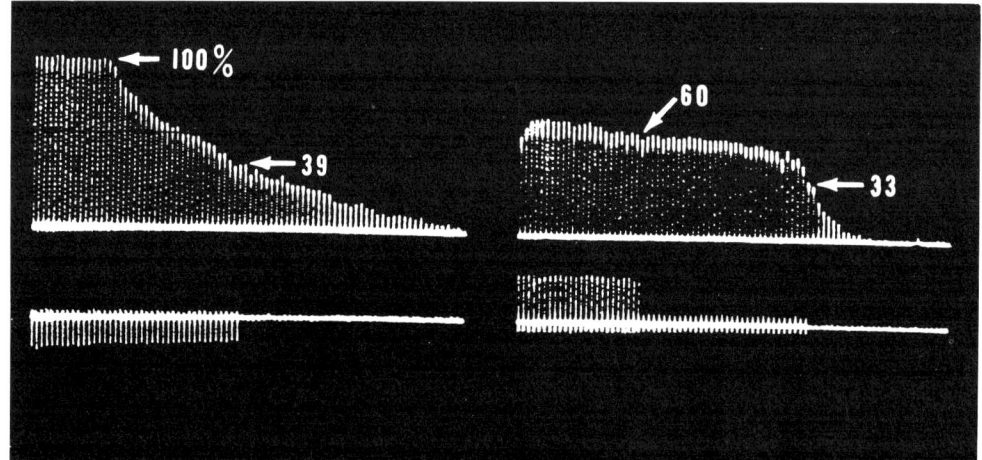

FIG. 19. Critical firing levels of 3 triceps motoneurons in cat. Single unit in *bottom left* had a sharp threshold at 39%. The 2 units in *bottom right* tracing had thresholds of 60% and 33%. Plateau in *top left* record indicates 100% discharge level of triceps pool. [From Henneman et al. (155).]

Relation of Critical Firing Level to Axon Diameter and Motoneuron Size

Defining the CFL and relating it to rank order in repetitive firing made it important to correlate CFL with axonal diameter and motoneuron size by direct quantitative methods. A technique was devised to do this, which is fully described in reference 60. It involved three separate procedures. *1*) Monosynaptic reflexes of single motor fibers were recorded monophasically from ventral root filaments. A resistor was placed in shunt across the recording electrodes and its value was varied until the action potentials were reduced by one-half. The resistance of the nerve filament

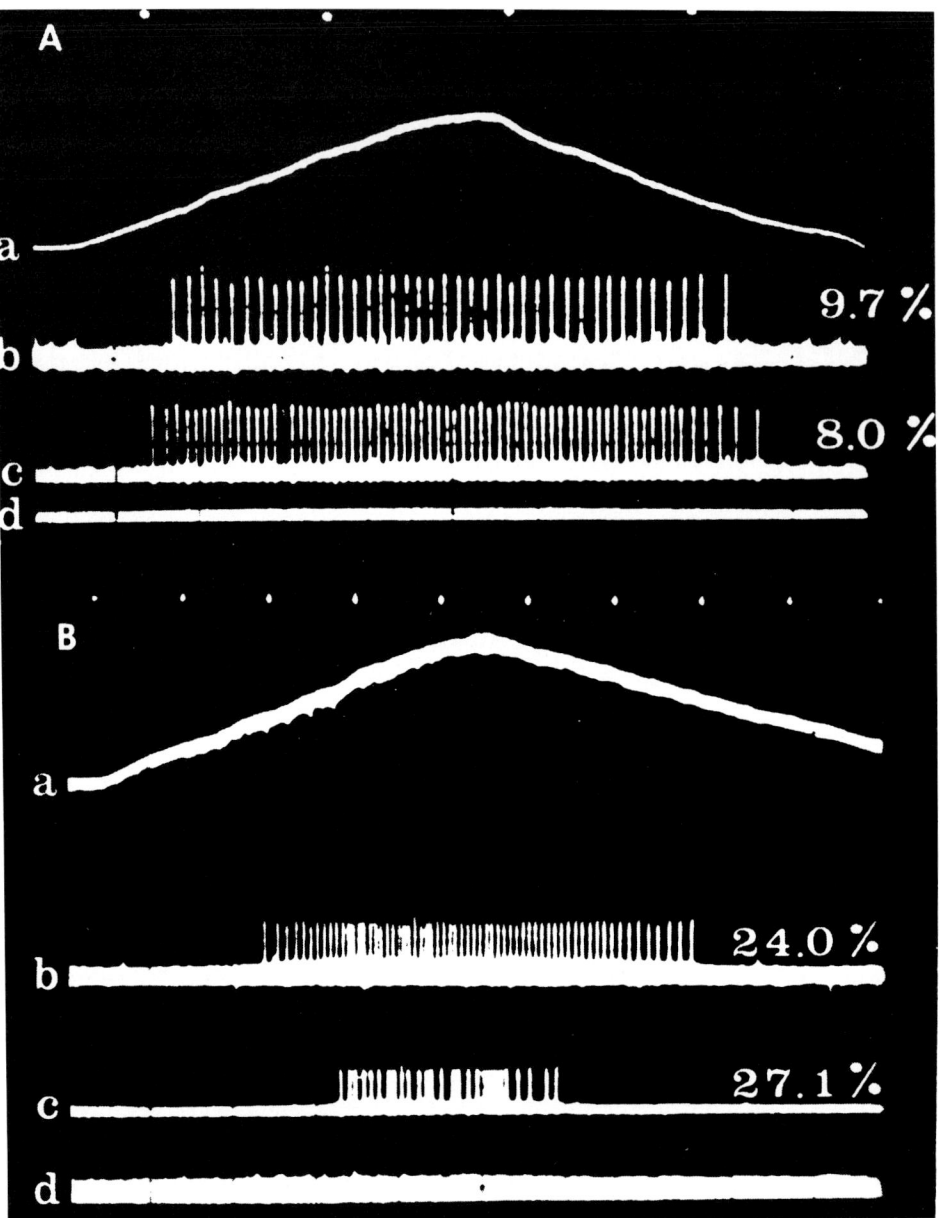

FIG. 20. Susceptibilities of 2 pairs of cat plantaris motoneurons with known critical firing levels (CFLs) to repetitive discharge in cat. Electrical stimulation of plantaris nerve at 300 stimuli/s in both cases. Stimulus intensity (i.e., voltage) indicated by level of *trace a* with reference to *base line d*. Responses of plantaris units recorded on *traces b* and *c*. CFLs indicated at right end of these traces. Time marks at 1-s intervals for both *top* and *bottom* records. [From Henneman et al. (155).]

was then equal to that of the shunt. Dividing the voltage of the action potentials by the resistance of the filament gave the axonal action current. *2)* In experiments in which impulses were conducted antidromically over long distances to yield accurate measurements of conduction velocity, it was shown that the axonal current of an impulse varied as the square of its conduction velocity. *3)* After the sizes of the impulses had been normalized in accordance with the resistances of their ventral root filaments, a direct correlation was found between impulse size and CFL.

Since both CFL and axon diameter were related to impulse size, they were related to each other, as illustrated in Figure 22.

The linearity of the data points in Figure 22 suggests that CFL is a function of a single continuous variable, which is probably cell size. If CFL is precisely and linearly related to cell size, it must be concluded that the distribution of input to the pool and any other factors that contribute to the relationship are also correlated with cell size. It is appropriate, therefore, to ask whether the scatter in the data points of Figure

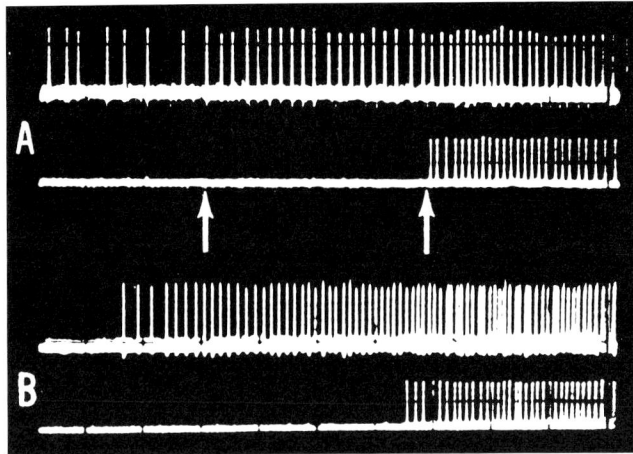

FIG. 21. Differences in susceptibility to repetitive firing of 2 cat plantaris motoneurons whose critical firing levels were 12.0% (*top*) and 15.5% (*bottom*). *A*: shocks applied to plantaris nerve were supramaximal for all group Ia-fibers. Frequency was switched from 20 shocks/s initially to 30 shocks/s at 1st *arrow*, and to 40 shocks/s at 2nd *arrow*. *B*: frequency of stimulation was 500 shocks/s throughout and intensity was increased gradually as trace moved from left to right. [From Henneman et al. (155).]

22 indicates a degree of variability or nonlinearity in this relationship. When the experimental observations were repeated several times, variations were noted that were sufficient to account for all of the scatter. Technical limitations, therefore, account for the observed scatter. Barrett and Crill (14) have demonstrated close relationships between input impedance and conduction velocity and between soma size and conduction velocity. Their observations are consistent with the conclusion that CFL is a function of a single continuous variable such as cell size, but, of course, they do not provide direct proof of the relationship.

Effects of Inhibitory Inputs on Critical Firing Level and Rank Order During Repetitive Firing

Although the motoneuron pool in the preceding experiments was subjected to a variety of excitatory and inhibitory influences, the specific inputs used to elicit monosynaptic reflexes and repetitive firing were predominantly excitatory to the pool. An important question to be answered was whether the critical firing levels and rank orders obtained in such experiments would be affected by the deliberate application of various types of inhibition.

The oscillographic record reproduced in Figure 23 illustrates the effects of a potent inhibitory input from the lateral popliteal nerve on the monosynaptic reflexes of a pool of plantaris motoneurons and a single unit from the same population. The top trace records the time integrals of the monosynaptic reflexes of the plantaris population elicited at 2-s intervals during the declining phase of a posttetanic potentiation. The lower trace, recorded simultaneously, shows the re-

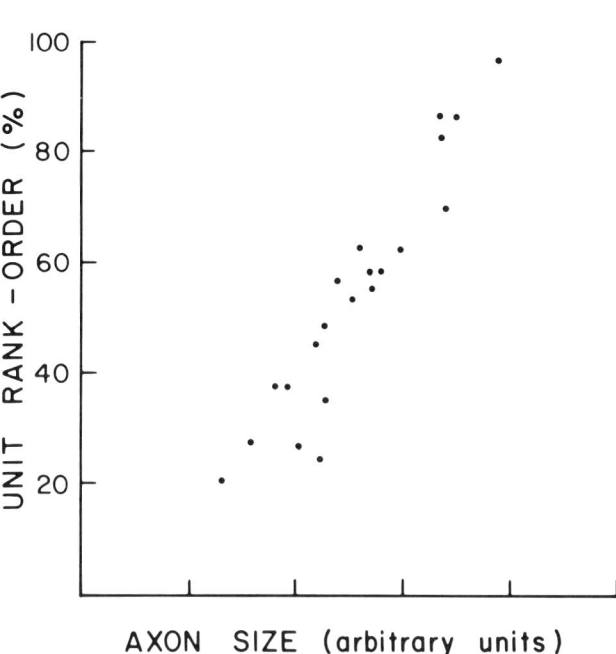

FIG. 22. Relation between axon size and critical firing level (rank order) of 21 cat plantaris motoneurons isolated in a single experiment. [From Clamann and Henneman (60).]

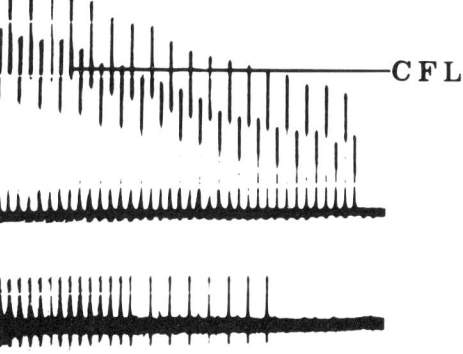

FIG. 23. Critical firing level (CFL) of a cat plantaris motoneuron with and without inhibitory input from lateral popliteal nerve. *Top*, time integrals of monosynaptic reflexes of plantaris population elicited at 2-s intervals during declining phase of posttetanic potentiation. *Bottom*, simultaneous responses of a plantaris unit with a critical firing level of 61%. Alternate reflexes preceded by a 200-ms train of pulses to lateral popliteal nerve. *Horizontal line* indicating critical firing level drawn as described in text. [From Clamann, Gillies, and Henneman (58).]

sponses of a single plantaris unit with a CFL of 61%. Alternate reflexes of the plantaris pool were preceded by a 200-ms train of pulses applied to the lateral popliteal nerve. The parameters of this pulse train were adjusted to cause a 20% average inhibition of the maximum monosynaptic reflex of the plantaris pool. As the monosynaptic reflexes declined from their peak, the absolute amount of inhibition resulting from the peroneal input remained approximately constant. The single unit in the lower tracing discharged without exception as long as the corresponding population responses reached the level indicated by the horizontal line labeled CFL. This line was drawn at a level equal to the size of the smallest uninhibited population response that was accompanied by a unit discharge, and just above the largest inhibited response without a unit discharge. The CFL of this unit was, thus, unchanged by the addition of a potent inhibitory input. The effects of inhibition on 32 triceps surae units with CFLs ranging from 3% to 87% were examined as above by stimulating antagonistic nerves in the same hindlimb or inhibitory sites in the medial reticular formation. The general conclusion was that inhibition had no significant effect on CFL in these experiments.

Experiments were also carried out to study the effects of inhibition on the repetitive firing of motoneurons. As a rule, when any two motoneurons belonging to the same pool were compared directly for susceptibility to inhibition, the results could be predicted from prior measurements of their critical firing levels. This was always the case when the CFLs differed by more than 2.5% and was usually true when they were closer together. The records reproduced in Figure 24 illustrate this point. They show the effects of recurrent inhibition and lateral popliteal inhibition on the monosynaptic reflexes and the repetitive firing of a pair of plantaris motoneurons. In each of the four comparisons shown in this figure the upper unit had a slightly higher CFL (18.6% in traces 1 and 3 and 18.4% in traces 2 and 4). Each of the underlined monosynaptic reflexes shown in A1 and A2 was preceded and accompanied by a 100-ms train of shocks (100/s) applied to the proximal portion of the seventh lumbar ventral root. The antidromic volleys set up by this stimulation resulted in recurrent inhibition mediated by Renshaw cells. Although 9 of the 18 reflexes in trace 1 were inhibited by this input, only 1 of those in trace 2 was silenced. In the absence of recurrent inhibition, both units responded every time. In A3 and A4 the same pair of units is seen responding rhythmically to repetitive stimulation of the plantaris nerve. When continuous recurrent inhibition was begun, as indicated by the thicker base line in A4, the upper unit ceased firing and the lower unit slowed to about one-half its original rate of discharge. In Figure 24B, the same pair of units was subjected to an inhibitory input elicited by stimulating the lateral popliteal nerve at

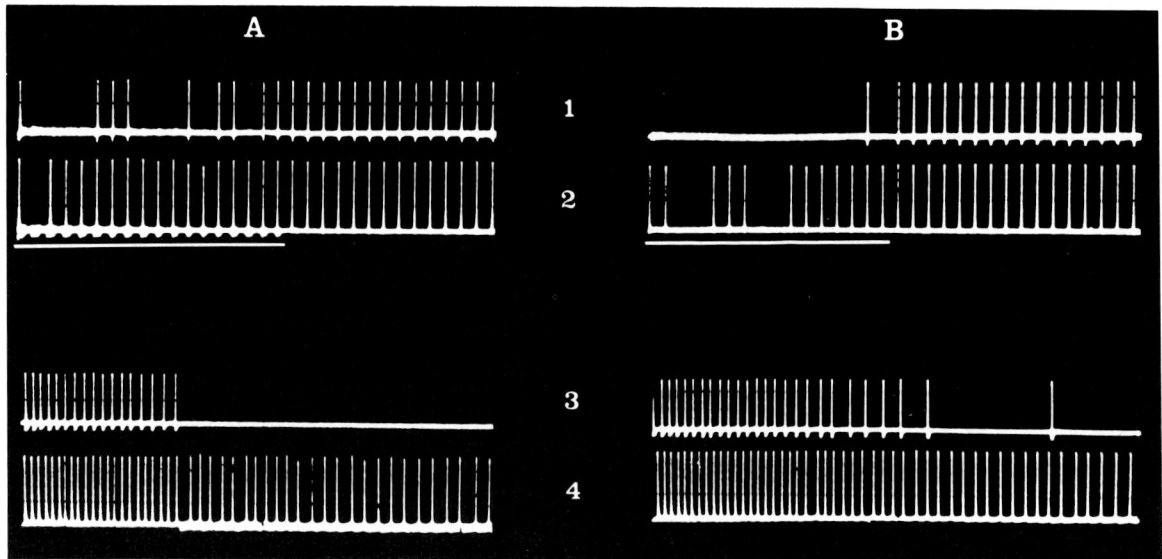

FIG. 24. Effects of recurrent inhibition (A) and lateral popliteal inhibition (B) in cat on monosynaptic reflexes (*traces 1, 2*) and repetitive firing (*traces 3, 4*) of a pair of plantaris motoneurons with critical firing levels of 18.6% (*top*) and 18.4% (*bottom*). A: in *traces 1, 2* the underlined reflexes were preceded and accompanied by a 100-ms train of shocks (100/s) to proximal portion of 7th lumbar ventral root. Antidromic volleys set up by stimulation in A1, A2 resulted in recurrent inhibition mediated by Renshaw cells. Of the 18 reflexes in *trace 1*, 9 were inhibited by this input; in *trace 2* only 1 reflex was silenced. In A3, A4 the same pair of units is seen responding rhythmically to repetitive stimulation of the plantaris nerve. When continuous recurrent inhibition was begun, indicated by *thick base line* in A4, *top unit* ceased firing and *bottom unit* slowed to about one-half original rate of discharge. B: same pair of units was subjected to inhibitory input elicited by stimulating lateral popliteal nerve at 100/s. In B1, B2 the underlined monosynaptic reflexes were somewhat more susceptible to this inhibition than to the recurrent inhibition. Of the 16 reflexes receiving this inhibition, 15 in *trace 1* and 4 in *trace 2* were silenced. In B3, B4 the same pair of units firing rhythmically in response to 100/s stimulation of the plantaris nerve was subjected to an inhibitory input whose intensity was gradually increased as the traces moved across the oscilloscope. The *top unit* was finally suppressed by this input whereas the *bottom unit* was only slowed in rate. [Clamann, Gillies, and Henneman (58).]

100/s. The underlined monosynaptic reflexes in B1 and B2 were somewhat more susceptible to this inhibition than to the recurrent inhibition. Of the 16 reflexes receiving this inhibition, 15 in trace 1 and 4 in trace 2 were silenced. In B3 and B4 the same pair of units firing rhythmically in response to 100/s stimulation of the plantaris nerve was subjected to an inhibitory input whose intensity was gradually increased as the traces moved across the oscilloscope. The upper unit was finally suppressed by this input, whereas the lower one was only slowed in rate. All four comparisons in Figure 24 reveal that the unit with a slightly lower CFL was the more resistant to inhibition regardless of the mode of firing or the type of inhibition.

In a wide variety of experimental conditions the activity of individual motoneurons is determined by the relative magnitudes of the excitatory and inhibitory inputs. The quantitative relations between the two types of input and their effects were examined more closely by measuring the intensities of the stimuli used to produce the inputs. The record reproduced in Figure 25 is an example of the experimental data obtained. Two plantaris units, whose CFLs had been measured previously, were set into rhythmic discharge by 100/s stimulation of the plantaris nerve. A sample of the excitatory stimuli was led to the oscilloscope. The stimulus strength of this input was constant during each test period but varied in different tests. The lateral popliteal nerve was stimulated at 100/s to produce a competing inhibition. The stimulus strength of this input was gradually increased manually as the beam moved across the screen. The intensity of the inhibition required to silence each of the plantaris units was determined by measuring the level of the trace at the time of their last discharge. Similar measurements were made at six different levels of excitatory input. The results are graphed in Figure 26. The data for the lower unit, with a critical firing level of 12.7%, are plotted with filled circles and a solid-line curve; those for the upper unit, with a critical firing level of 18.8%, are represented by open circles and a dashed curve. The plot shows that every increase in the excitatory stimuli required a proportionate increase in the inhibitory stimuli required to silence the two plantaris units. For each of the six excitatory inputs, the corresponding inhibitory input was greater for the unit with the lower critical firing level. Furthermore, the difference between the two inhibitory inputs was approximately the same at all levels of excitation. It must be emphasized that the stimulus intensities plotted in Figure 26 do not necessarily correspond to the magnitudes of the neural inputs that result from the stimulations. Until the actual neural inputs can be measured directly (no technique is currently available for this purpose) the quantitative validity of these results remains to be verified. Still, the findings provide evidence for the tentative conclusion that inhibition often produced effects that are similar to a simple reduction in excitation. They also suggest that the competition between excitation and inhibition in these experiments is a simple algebraic process.

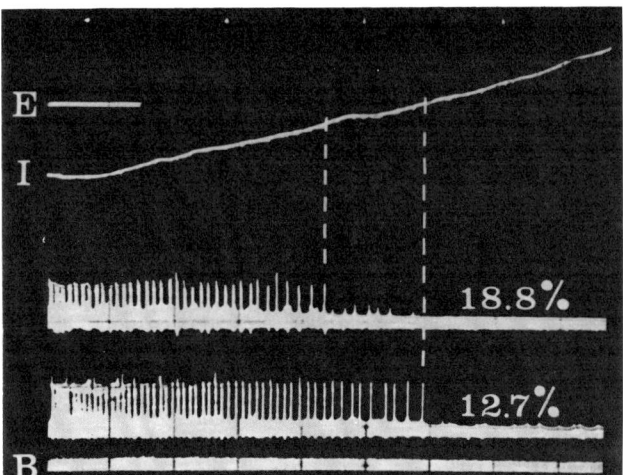

FIG. 25. Records illustrating quantitative relationships between intensity of excitatory stimulus causing 2 cat motoneurons with critical firing levels of 18.8% and 12.7% to discharge repetitively and intensity of inhibitory stimulus required to silence them. Stimulus strength of excitatory input (100/s stimulation of a plantaris nerve), indicated by level of *line E* with reference to *base line B*, was constant during each test but varied in different tests. Stimulus strength of inhibitory input (100/s stimulation of lateral popliteal nerve), indicated by *line I*, was increased as trace moved across screen. Intensity of inhibition required to silence each unit was measured at time of their last discharges, indicated by *dashed lines*. Time signals at top of record represent 1-s intervals. [From Clamann, Gillies, and Henneman (58).]

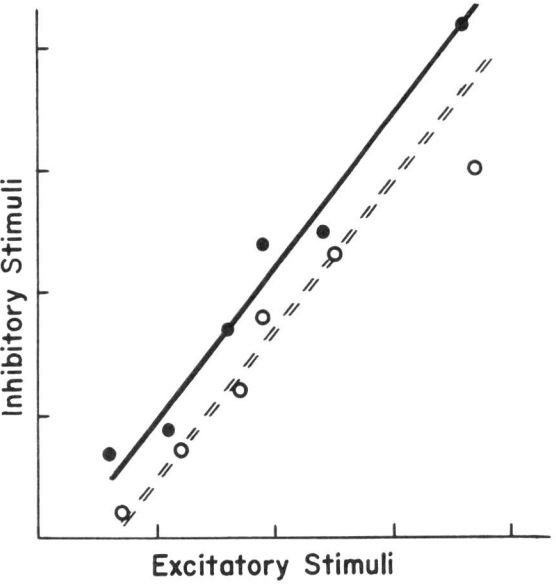

FIG. 26. Graph showing linear relation between strength of excitatory stimuli causing each of 2 cat motoneurons to discharge repetitively and strength of inhibitory stimuli required to silence them. Data obtained as illustrated in Figure 25. Data for *lower unit*, with critical firing level of 12.7%, are plotted with *filled circles* and *solid line*; data for *upper unit*, with a critical firing level of 18.8%, are represented by *open circles* and *dashed line*. [From Clamann, Gillies, and Henneman (58).]

The effects of inhibition on 133 pairs of plantaris motoneurons are compiled in Table 1. In 123 pairs (92%) the rank order for repetitive discharge was the same as for monosynaptic reflexes. The differences in the CFLs for this group of units ranged from 0.2% to 72.1% and the mean difference was 15.9%. In the 10 remaining pairs with differences in CFLs from 0.4% to 9.9% and a mean difference of 3.2%, the rank order was reversed for repetitive firing. In three monosynaptic comparisons, i.e., 1.8%, inhibition reversed the original rank order. In two of them the differences in CFLs were 1.0% and 0.4%. In four comparisons, i.e., 2%, inhibition reversed the rank order established for repetitive discharge. The mean difference in CFLs in these four pairs of units was 0.8%.

The six inputs used in these experiments were selected to provide contrasting types of inhibition for testing: postsynaptic and presynaptic, spinal and supraspinal, unilateral and contralateral, recurrent and nonrecurrent, cutaneous and muscular, and mixed and pure. Although these inhibitory systems and the effect they exert differ from one another in many respects, their effects on the rank order of motoneurons in both monosynaptic and repetitive tests were indistinguishable. As Table 1 indicates, none of the inputs caused a significant number of reversals. The small percentages of reversals in Table 1 all occurred in pairs that were nearly equal in CFL.

Recruitment of Motor Units in Humans

Despite the human and technical limitations involved, studies on motor units in humans have added greatly to the information gained from animal experiments and facilitated its interpretation. Human subjects can voluntarily make delicately graded contractions, hold a desired tension, produce rapid or slow contractions on demand, and, by monitoring their performance on an oscilloscope, attempt to alter the order of recruitment. Actions that are difficult or impossible to study in animals can often be carried out quite simply by a cooperative subject. Furthermore, the results are not open to the criticisms that they are due to limited or unphysiological inputs, to the effects of anesthesia, or to abnormal preparations such as decerebrates. In humans, recordings are usually taken from muscles instead of nerves. Hence artifacts due to shifting of the position of the electrodes relative to the active muscle fibers must be minimized. This movement has been a serious problem in some studies, leading to apparent reversals in recruitment order, and it requires constant vigilance from experimenters. In a study by Olson, Carpenter, and Henneman (272), orderly recruitment of muscle action potentials of increasing amplitude was demonstrated on several cat muscles. Some of the factors influencing the recorded size of motor unit potentials and the apparent order of recruitment were discussed. They included the distance of the active fibers from the electrodes, differences in the diameters of muscle fibers, and possible variations in the density of the fibers of a single motor unit. It is noteworthy that orderly recruitment was readily observed in the cat soleus, a homogeneous muscle in which differences in histochemical fiber types and diameters were not significant factors.

Milner-Brown et al. (258) used the action potentials of single motor units in the first dorsal interosseous muscle of human subjects to trigger an averager that recorded the twitch contractions of motor units in that muscle. Those contractions that were time locked with the trigger signals from a particular unit were extracted by an averaging process from the other contractile activity in the muscle. The twitch tension of each unit was related to the total force produced by the whole muscle at the instant of recruitment. Figure 27 shows the number of motor units plotted on a linear scale and on a logarithmic scale, with the tensions indicated. As in experiments on motor units in cats (253, 273, 353), there was an approximately exponential relation between the numbers of motor units isolated in each size range and the tensions they produced (many units developing small tensions, few units generating large forces). The three-dimensional figure of Burke et al. (41) illustrating a tripartite classification of motor units unintentionally gives the impression that large motor units are much more numerous than small ones. Milner-Brown et al. (258) concluded that motor units in human muscles are recruited in orderly progression according to the amount of tension they develop. The larger motor units, which were recruited at higher threshold forces, tended to have shorter contraction times than the smaller units, as is commonly found in animal studies (35, 253, 353). Milner-Brown et al. (258) added in their discussion that

> these findings strongly confirmed the "size principle" expounded by Henneman.... Indeed, the degree of ordering... is remarkably high (linear correlation coefficients > 0.8 for all three subjects) when one considers that the recordings were made in experiments over a

TABLE 1. *Effects of Inhibition on Pairs of Motoneurons*

Source of Inhibitory Input	Monosynaptic Reflexes		Repetitive Discharge	
	No. of tests	No. of reversals of rank order	No. of tests	No. of reversals of rank order
Lateral peroneal nerve	36	0	38	1
Posterior biceps semi-tendinosus nerve	36	1	37	0
Sural nerve	7	0	8	0
L_7 ventral root	29	1	49	0
Contralateral S_1 dorsal root	32	1	34	2
Brain stem	30	0	30	1
Totals	170	3	196	4

Adapted from Clamann, Gillies, and Henneman (58).

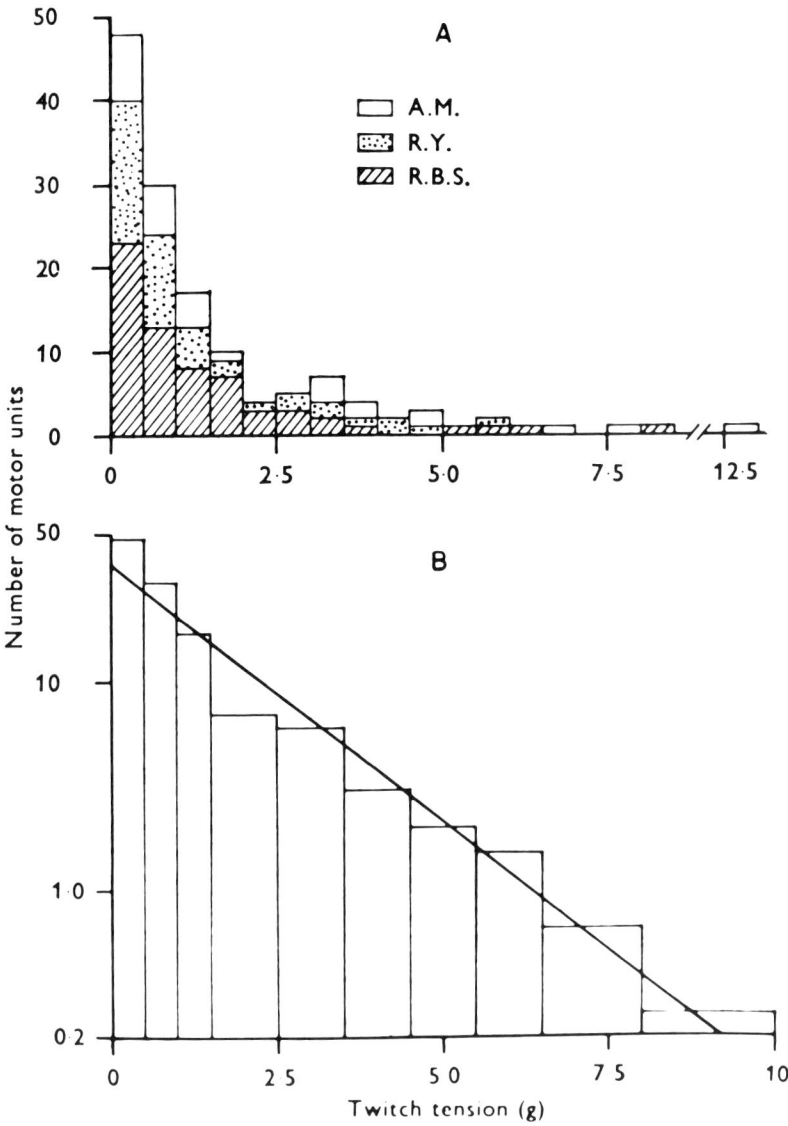

FIG. 27. Number of human motor units having the twitch tensions indicated. A: linear scale. B: logarithmic scale. Distributions are similar for all 3 subjects. The computed best-fitting line on the semilog plot (B) indicates an approximately exponential relation between number of motor units and twitch tension. [From Milner-Brown et al. (258).]

period of several months, and that there are inevitably many uncontrolled variables in human experiments. Since the size of a unit recruited (ΔF) is proportional to the mean force level (F) over such a wide range, the fractional increments in force ($\Delta F/F$) produced by recruiting each unit will be constant.... This result is reminiscent of the constant Weber functions ($\Delta S/S$) sometimes obtained when just-noticeable differences (ΔS) are measured at various stimulus intensities (S) in sensory experiments...

See Henneman and Olson (157) for a fuller discussion of this analogy. Using the same averaging technique, Yemm (359) also found a nearly linear relationship between recruitment force and twitch tension in the more powerful masseter and temporal muscles for the 0-6-kg force range. Subsequently, Goldberg and Derfler (125) demonstrated strong positive correlations between threshold force of recruitment, EMG spike amplitude, and twitch tension in the masseter over longer and greater ranges of force (10-s plateaus varying from 1 to 47 kg).

The relation between the tension a motor unit develops and the conduction velocity (i.e., diameter) of its axon has also been well documented in humans. Freund et al. (115) reported that the total muscle forces at which motor units were recruited were a direct function of their axonal conduction velocities (CVs). Recently Grimby and Hannerz (139) and Borg et al. (23) published studies on the discharge properties of short toe extensor motor units activated voluntarily. Certain motor units could be driven continuously by voluntary effort at frequencies of 10/s or less. These units gradually accelerated their firing with increases in contraction strength, and had maximum rates below 30/s during a sustained contraction but above 60/s in twitch contractions. This group of units was found to have CVs between 30 and 45 m/s. In contrast, larger units with CVs between 40 and 54 m/s could not be driven continuously, did not fire repeatedly at rates below 20/s, accelerated rapidly with increasing effort, and attained maximal firing rates above 100/s. Units that were intermediate between these two groups had intermediate CVs. In a prolonged contraction of constant strength only continuously firing units were active. In brief rapid contractions both types of units participated. Thus, a clear relationship was established between the voluntary discharge properties of a unit and its axonal CV, as one would expect from animal studies. The authors (23, 139) point out that the axonal CV of a motor unit is directly related to the histochemistry of its muscle fibers, to their twitch time, and to twitch amplitude, and inversely related to the input resistance and afterhyperpolarization of its motoneuron. Since the voluntary discharge properties are related to CV, they should also be related to the other characteristics noted above. Accordingly, the voluntary discharge properties may be a valuable index to the other parameters of a motor unit that are difficult to study in humans. It is clear from this summary that the voluntary discharge properties of human motor units do not differ significantly from the characteristics of motor units in animals responding involuntarily to various experimental inputs.

One function of the motoneuron pool that has received little attention so far is its control of the precise timing of the mechanical events in single motor units relative to each other and to the development of tension in the entire muscle. In an important study Büdingen and Freund (30) analyzed the mechanical aspects of recruitment as they relate to the motoneuronal events. Single motor units from the human extensor indicis muscle were investigated during voluntary isometric contractions of equal amplitude carried out at different speeds, as illustrated in Figure 28A. As Tanji and Kato (335) had shown, the threshold force of recruitment for all motor units apparently decreased as the speed of contraction was increased. Plots of the threshold forces versus the rates of increase in tension had approximately the same slopes in seven different units of the same muscle (Fig. 28C). This monotonic decrease in threshold was consistently observed in all units tested. No evidence was found to indicate that high-threshold units were preferentially activated in fast, phasic (2,000 g/s) contractions.

Due to the general decrease in all force thresholds with faster contractions, the total time between the recruitment of low- and high-threshold units diminished considerably. This is apparent in Figure 28B, which plots the rate of rise of tension against the time elapsing between the beginning of the voluntary muscle contraction and the onset of firing in three of its motor units. Both scales are logarithmic. With rapid contraction (300–3,000 g/s) recruitment was greatly compressed in time. The delay in the onset of firing in low- and high-threshold units decreased from about 2,500 ms in the slowest contractions to less than 100 ms in the fastest. The parallel curves indicate again that although the high-threshold units started firing much sooner in rapid contractions than in slow ones, they were not preferentially activated.

The relation of the first twitch contraction of a unit to the total muscle force is the mechanical counterpart of electrical recruitment. By measuring the contraction time of a unit, the change in total muscle force that occurs within that time during a rising contraction can be calculated. In Figure 28D the increase in total muscle force that occurs within the mean contraction time of the muscle is plotted on the ordinate against the rate of rise of tension. The average decrease of the threshold force of recruitment of 12 units of this muscle with increasing rates of rise of tension is plotted for comparison. The two slopes are almost equal but of opposite direction. Hence, the sum of these two variables is approximately constant over the range examined in these experiments. The decrease in the threshold force of recruitment with increasing rate of rise of tension almost exactly cancels the increase of force in the whole muscle during the contraction time. As a result, the authors (30) conclude that the mechanical recruitment of a motor unit occurs at approximately the same force level regardless of the rate of rise of tension.

This analysis provides new insights into the organization of the motoneuron pool. Since the order of recruitment does not change with the rate of rise of tension, Büdingen and Freund argue that "... the proportion between the force generated by recruitment and by firing rate modulation of the units activated prior to a particular unit remains unchanged. This demonstrates how precise the tuning is between the recruitment of units and the activity of those already recruited." The findings demonstrate that the activation of the motoneurons in a pool is organized to achieve precise mechanical effects, i.e., stable relations between the force output of the individual motor units at the time of their mechanical recruitment and the corresponding force outputs of the whole muscle. These observations help to explain why the size and excitability of a motor unit are necessarily related to its contraction time, rate of firing, and recruitment order.

As described above, recruitment is orderly in contractions of up to 2,500 g/s. Desmedt and Godaux (90) have developed a technique for investigating even faster "ballistic" contractions that are completed in too short a time to be controlled by sensory feedback signals from the activated muscles. The commands in ballistic movements are presumably preprogrammed and must be dispatched to the segmental circuits and

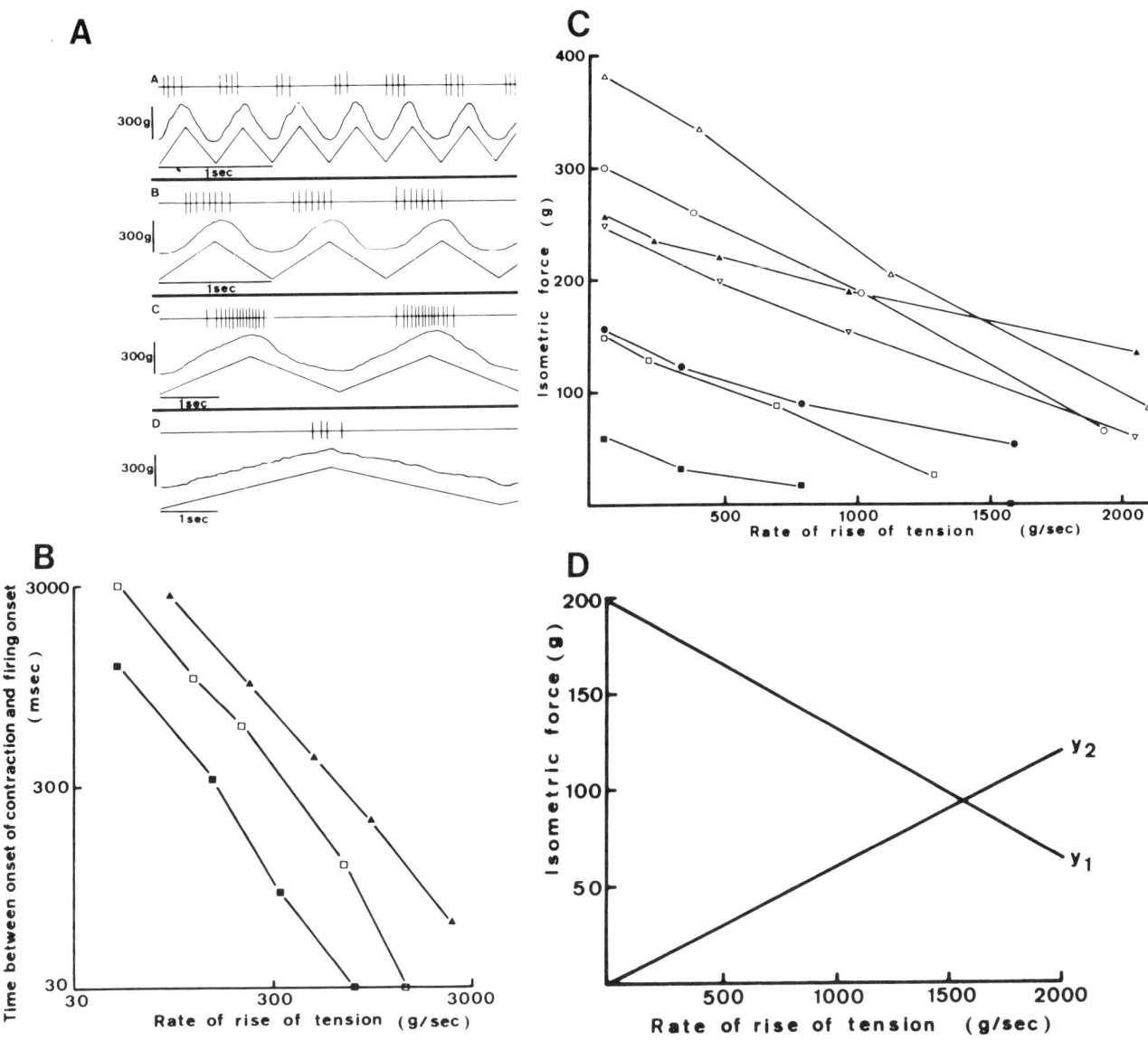

FIG. 28. *A*: firing pattern of a high-threshold unit recorded from human extensor indicis during isometric contractions with different rates of rise of tension (A–D). Each registration shows (*top to bottom*) the spike record, isometric force, and tracking signal which was visually displayed to the subject. Time scale in *bottom 2 records* is one-half that of *top 2 records*. During increasingly faster contractions, unit starts firing at successively lower force levels. *B*: dependence of time between beginning of muscle contraction and firing onset of 3 motor units on rate of rise of tension. Double logarithmic scale. Faster contraction causes earlier recruitment. *C*: change of threshold force of recruitment (ordinate) associated with variation of rate of rise of isometric tension. Recordings from 7 motor units of extensor indicis of 3 subjects (■, ▲, ●). *D*: regression line of change of threshold force of recruitment on rate of rise of isometric tension ($y_1 = -0.067x + 198.66$) calculated from 12 motor units of extensor indicis. The increase of muscle force that occurs within the mean contraction time of the muscle is shown for comparison ($y_2 = 0.060x$). [From Büdingen and Freund (30).]

motoneurons before the contraction begins. For study of these movements, subjects were asked to make 50 or more ballistic contractions of tibialis anterior muscle at intervals of several seconds. Peak forces ranging from 0.05 to 12.0 kg were produced in less than 0.15 s each. During each contraction the action potentials of the discharging unit at the recording site were recorded along with the total contractile force. The 50 or more contractions were then ranked in order of increasing peak force and the corresponding activity of each unit was compiled as in Table 2. Unit 1 fired in all 52 trials; units 2–5 failed to respond below certain peak forces, but discharged with increasing probability in the progressively stronger contractions listed in the table. The lower part of Table 2 gives the thresholds of the same 5 units for ballistic and slow ramp con-

TABLE 2. *Motor Unit Threshold Data*

Trial	Force, kg	Unit 1	Unit 2	Unit 3	Unit 4	Unit 5	Trial	Force, kg	Unit 1	Unit 2	Unit 3	Unit 4	Unit 5
1	0.07	+	−	−	−	−	27	2.27	+	+	+	−	−
2	0.08	+	−	−	−	−	28	2.42	+	+	+	−	−
3	0.15	+	−	−	−	−	29	2.72	+	+	+	+	−
4	0.30	+	−	−	−	−	30	2.75	+	+	+	−	−
5	0.30	+	−	−	−	−	31	3.18	+	+	+	+	−
6	0.31	+	−	−	−	−	32	3.20	+	+	+	−	−
7	0.31	+	−	−	−	−	33	3.33	+	+	+	+	−
8	0.37	+	−	−	−	−	34	3.48	+	+	+	+	−
9	0.38	+	−	−	−	−	35	3.51	+	+	+	+	−
10	0.45	+	+	−	−	−	36	3.78	+	+	+	+	−
11	0.46	+	+	−	−	−	37	4.54	+	+	+	+	+
12	0.53	+	−	−	−	−	38	4.84	+	+	+	+	+
13	0.75	+	+	−	−	−	39	4.99	+	+	+	+	+
14	0.90	+	+	−	−	−	40	5.15	+	+	+	+	+
15	0.90	+	+	−	−	−	41	5.30	+	+	+	+	+
16	0.91	+	+	−	−	−	42	5.45	+	+	+	+	+
17	1.06	+	+	−	−	−	43	5.75	+	+	+	+	+
18	1.06	+	+	−	−	−	44	6.96	+	+	+	+	+
19	1.06	+	+	−	−	−	45	8.03	+	+	+	+	+
20	1.14	+	+	+	−	−	46	8.10	+	+	+	+	+
21	1.21	+	+	+	−	−	47	8.18	+	+	+	+	+
22	1.36	+	+	−	−	−	48	8.63	+	+	+	+	+
23	1.38	+	+	+	−	−	49	9.54	+	+	+	+	+
24	1.51	+	+	−	−	−	50	9.69	+	+	+	+	+
25	1.81	+	+	+	−	−	51	10.90	+	+	+	+	+
26	1.82	+	+	+	−	−	52	12.70	+	+	+	+	+

Unit	Ballistic force threshold, kg — Range	Mean	Ramp force threshold, kg — Range	Mean ± SD
1	0–0.07	0.035	0.14–0.48	0.34 ± 0.15
2	0.38–0.75	0.56	3.50–4.10	3.70 ± 0.28
3	1.06–1.81	1.43	3.60–4.40	4.14 ± 0.36
4	2.72–3.33	3.02	11.98–13.15	12.66 ± 0.57
5	3.78–4.54	4.16	13.73–16.41	15.46 ± 0.93

+, Motor unit discharge; −, no discharge. Ballistic threshold was estimated by taking mean between maximum peak force for which a unit never discharged and minimum force for which it always fired. Ramp threshold estimated from data of 10 separate ramp contractions producing 12 kg in 8 s.   [Adapted from Desmedt and Godaux (90).]

tractions. The two sets of thresholds were compared by the rank correlation method, which yielded a very high correlation coefficient (0.95). Four other muscles (masseter, first dorsal interosseous, tibialis, and soleus) were later studied by the same investigators (91) with similar results. Since the pyramidal tract is strongly involved in ballistic movements, it was suggested that pyramidal signals impinge on the motoneuron pool in a pattern similar to that of the group Ia and II spindle afferent fibers from the muscle itself.

Further evidence was provided by Desmedt and Godaux (92), who studied motor units in the first dorsal interosseous muscle with the spike-triggered averaging technique, which allows the investigator to extract the tension myogram of individual twitch contractions. It was clear with this approach that the more rapidly contracting units were not preferentially recruited in ballistic contractions. In fact, the fast motor units were recruited after the slow motor units even in fast contractions (94). This part of the study also showed that the motor units recruited at the initial stage of a small ballistic movement produced smaller forces than the higher threshold units.

Finally, evidence was presented (93, 95) that vibration-induced inhibition of motor units silences them in exactly the reverse order from that in which they were recruited, as originally described in animal experiments (58, 159).

Thus, many of the findings described in the early part of this chapter have been confirmed in experiments on human subjects, so that anesthesia, decerebration, and other procedures, such as extensive denervation and prolonged immobilization, could not influence the results. In addition, studies on humans have added important new findings that provide further insight into the organization of the motoneuron pool.

Evidence Regarding Alternative Patterns of Recruitment

As the preceding sections have indicated, there is abundant evidence from animal and human studies that motoneurons in a pool are usually recruited in a stereotyped and repeatable order according to their size. However, exceptions to this usual order have been noted since the first investigations were reported and interest in their possible functional significance has increased. The early studies (159, 160) in which discharges of motoneurons were recorded from ventral root filaments showed apparent reversals of recruitment order in 11%–13% of comparisons. The extent to which these reversals were due to minor injuries to fibers in dissected ventral root filaments or to the possible mixture of axons from closely related but different pools was not known. With later, more quantitative techniques (155) reversals were seldom observed in comparisons of units that differed by more than 2.5% in CFL (but see ref. 61). This led to the belief that recruitment order was relatively, but not absolutely, fixed. Departures from the standard order of recruitment have been reported by several authors (136, 137, 138, 335, 356, 206). Some of these studies have suffered from lack of information about the relative thresholds of different units, difficulty in repeating observations, and various technical limitations. Any deviation from the standard order of recruitment deserves special attention, however, because it indicates that there are deficiencies in our knowledge of the mechanisms underlying recruitment and may provide useful clues regarding these mechanisms. This section reviews evidence concerning variations in the order of recruitment in animals and human subjects.

The best examples of variations in the order of recruitment are those illustrated in a study of Kernell and Sjöholm (206), who produced maintained contractions of the first deep lumbrical muscle of the cat's foot either by electrical stimulation of the contralateral motor cortex or by pinching the foot pad, which elicits a toe extensor reflex. The small size of this lumbrical muscle permitted the investigators to record the discharges of all the motor units of the muscle electromyographically as well as the tensions they produced. Cortical stimulation as well as pad pinching customarily recruited small units before large ones. The order of recruitment caused by pad pinching often differed, however, from that caused by cortical stimulation. The most complete analyses of recruitment were made in lumbricals containing five motor units or less. Data from only six such muscles were compiled in Table 3, but the results were confirmed in muscles with large numbers of units. A difference in recruitment order between two units in the table indicates that one of them could be silent while the other one was discharging repetitively for at least 0.5 s. Table 3 shows pooled data from 23 motor units, analyzed in a manner similar to that used by Henneman et al. (159). The recruitment threshold for each unit was compared to that for every other unit in the muscle. Thirty-four pairwise comparisons were possible. In a clear majority of pairs the smaller unit had the lower threshold. Exceptions were not rare, however. Unfortunately, they varied in an unpredictable manner from cat to cat and sometimes in the same preparation. Motor-unit pairs exhibiting some kind of sequence exception in response to cortical stimulation generally showed

TABLE 3. *Recruitment Order and Amplitude of Motor Unit Spikes in Contractions Elicited by Cortical Stimulation and by Pinching the Foot Pad*

Motor Unit	Cortex	Pad	Cortex = Pad
All pairs			
Small always before large	27	24	20
Tie	1	1	0
Large may precede small	6 (3)	9 (5)	2
Pairs of nonsimilar units			
Small always before large	23	20	17
Tie	1	1	0
Large may precede small	4 (1)	7 (3)	1

Data for all 23 motor units of 6 small muscles (1st deep lumbricals of cat's foot). Recruitment threshold of each motor unit was compared to that of each other unit in same muscle. Total of 34 pairwise comparisons were made. Peak-to-peak amplitudes of motor unit spikes were measured. Cortex, recruitment patterns in response to cortical stimulation; Pad, recruitment patterns in response to pad pinching; Cortex = Pad, same recruitment pattern for both kinds of stimuli. Numbers in parentheses indicate number of pairs where large unit consistently preceded small. Nonsimilar unit refers to pairs where spike size and twitch amplitude in one unit were at least 30% larger than in the other. [From Kernell and Sjöholm (206).]

an ascending size order of recruitment in response to pad pinching and vice versa. Hence, the exceptions were not the result of some difference in excitability between the various motoneurons, but were probably due to differences in the distribution of input. In six cats cortical stimulation was compared before and after section of dorsal roots L_5–S_3. No obvious effect was produced by this procedure. In view of observations of Thomas et al. (337), it would be valuable to know whether the first deep lumbrical muscle in the cat is uni- or multifunctional, since only the latter type showed reversals in their experiments.

In a study of a larger pool of motoneurons, Kanda et al. (192) used bipolar hook electrodes on small natural filaments of the MG muscle nerve or fine bipolar EMG electrodes to record electromyographically from motor units. Stretch or vibration of the MG or SOL muscles was used to elicit reflex discharges of motoneurons. Prompted by early reports (78) that certain peripheral inputs could facilitate muscle tension in the fast gastrocnemius while simultaneously inhibiting tension in the closely related, slow soleus, Kanda and colleagues (192) used electrical or natural stimulation of sural nerve afferents to alter the discharge patterns of MG motoneurons. The results were variable in different preparations. Some low-threshold units responding to stretch or vibration of the MG muscle exhibited brief slowing or cessation of firing at about the same time that higher threshold units, not responsive to stretch or vibration, were powerfully recruited by stimulation of sural afferents. As Figure 29 illustrates, the durations of the reversals produced by sural stimulation were measured in tenths of seconds. Activity in the lowest threshold unit (unit A) slowed and then ceased during the brief period when the higher threshold units (B–E) were recruited. Units

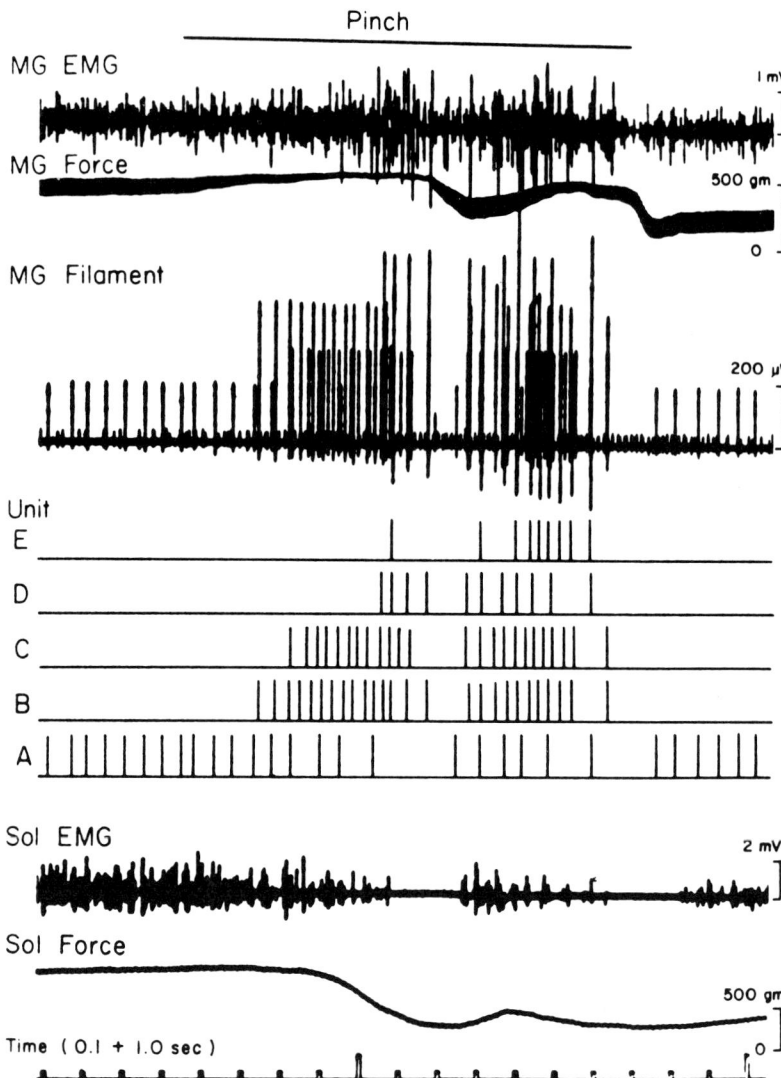

FIG. 29. Records of EMG activity and force outputs of medial gastrocnemius (*top 2 traces*) and soleus (*bottom 2 traces*) muscles of cat, together with simultaneous record of activity of a small number of medial gastrocnemius (MG) motor axons in a natural filament of MG muscle nerve (*3rd trace*). During MG vibration (160 Hz, 90 μm) activity in whole MG increased and that in soleus (SOL) showed a smaller increase. Pinching the skin over the lateral ankle with toothed forceps produced 2 bursts of MG activity, with recruitment of large amplitude motor axons in the MG filament, but caused quite complete suppression of SOL activity. Isolated activity of 5 identifiable MG motoneuron axons is shown in A–E. Note slowing of unit A discharge during each burst of activity in the higher threshold units B–E. [From Kanda et al. (192).]

D and E began to fire only during a 0.2-s pause in the activity of unit A. While the firing behavior of unit A was similar to the activity pattern in the whole soleus muscle in Figure 29, the spike patterns in the higher threshold units (B–E) were unlike those of SOL motoneurons or unit A. The authors interpret these records "as a clear and unambiguous example of differential control of alpha motoneurons within a single motor unit pool." It should be noted that units B–E were recruited in the order of their conduction velocities as Table 4 indicates. The authors point out that the findings in no way suggest that recruitment order is at times chaotic, but rather may be intrinsically orderly within different subgroups of a population. They add that "differential control is unusual and hard to demonstrate." As previously noted, Clamann, Gillies, and Henneman (58) found no evidence that inhibitory inputs in general or sural inputs in particular caused such differential effects. This study leaves the impression that differential control plays minor roles of brief duration. At present, the findings have the greatest value "as clues for further investigation of synaptic input" (192).

The CFL of motoneurons may also be altered differentially by certain inputs. The CFL was defined (subsection *Critical Firing Levels of Motoneurons*,

TABLE 4. *Axonal Conduction Velocities of Motor Units*

Unit	Conduction Distances, mm		
	22	24	37.2
E	88		
D	88	80	97
C	85	86	
B	79	80	89
A	73	70	81
Gamma		28	

Velocities, in m/s, measured at 3 different conduction distances in experiment shown in Figure 29. Distal electrodes fixed on muscle nerve near entry to muscle; position of proximal pair varied. [Adapted from Kanda et al. (192).]

p. 440) for monosynaptic responses to homonymous inputs. Since it correlates closely with motoneuron size (60), with recruitment order in mechanically or electrically elicited stretch reflexes, and with response to various inhibitory inputs, it is regarded as a good index of the rank order of a motoneuron with respect to all other cells in the pool. Clamann and Kukulka (61) have shown that more than two-thirds of MG motoneurons showed a different CFL in response to $L_7 + S_1DR$ stimulation than to stimulation of one dorsal root (DR) alone. The same authors (63) have demonstrated that CFLs obtained by stimulating $L_7 + S_1DR$ are altered by electrical stimulation of Deiter's nucleus. This stimulation lowered the CFLs of motoneurons with axonal conduction velocities greater than 100 m/s and raised CFLs of those with conduction velocities below 85 m/s. The effects may be due to inhibition of small motoneurons or facilitation of large cells. There is some evidence that both effects occur. The significance of results achieved with artificial inputs that are far removed from natural ones is uncertain. The inability of human subjects to control rank order voluntarily (subsection *Evidence Regarding Voluntary Selective Control of Motor Units*, p. 457) suggests that the inputs used in these experiments are not under voluntary differential control.

The most substantial group of studies on recruitment in human subjects are those of Grimby and Hannerz and their collaborators. They used EMG recording techniques in a variety of muscles, reflexes, and voluntary movements. Various examples of reversals in recruitment order were described in normal subjects and neurological patients. One of their most recent papers (139) is summarized here, because it seems to represent the culmination of skills, experience, and conclusions that 10 years of experimentation have developed. References to their earlier studies are found in this paper and in a more recent one by Borg et al. (23). In these two publications, the firing rates and recruitment orders of motor units in the short toe extensors of normal human subjects were investigated in great detail. Two distinct types of motor units and a large group of intermediate units could be distinguished by their firing patterns. About one-half of all the motor units could be driven continuously by voluntary efforts, increased slowly in firing rate with greater contraction strength, and discharged for long periods of time. Some of these "continuously firing long-interval units" (c.l.m.u.s.) discharged regularly at 8–10/s, while others did not attain regularity until frequencies at 10–15/s. During sustained maximum efforts c.l.m.u.s. fired at 30–50/s and even more rapidly in brief twitches of maximum rapidity and strength.

About 10% of the motor units could not be driven continuously, but only for brief intervals. These "intermittently firing short interval motor units" (i.s.m.u.s.) could not be driven voluntarily by weak or moderate sustained contractions of constant strength and did not fire at rates below 20/s. With strong efforts they discharged intermittently during steady contractions or in brief high-frequency bursts reaching 100/s during rapid increases in contraction strength. Nearly one-half of the motor units had discharge properties somewhere between those of c.l.m.u.s. and i.s.m.u.s. These "intermediate" units had various degrees of so-called endurance, according to Grimby and Hannerz. Certain motor units could be driven continuously in the initial stage of an experiment but gradually lost this capacity after repeated contractions. The lack of endurance noted by Grimby and Hannerz resembles the rapid cessation of firing in large motoneurons of cats whose muscle nerves are being stimulated repetitively at high frequencies, as noted earlier in this section. This phenomenon is not understood, but it may be due to a decrease in the effectiveness of the high-frequency input. It could hardly be due to failure of contractile mechanisms, since the EMG does not measure these.

One c.l.m.u. and one i.s.m.u. were studied simultaneously under many conditions. In sustained isometric contractions the c.l.m.u. was recruited before the i.s.m.u. In a prolonged isometric contraction of constant strength or even during prolonged maximum effort only the c.l.m.u. fired. On acceleration the i.s.m.u. was not recruited before the c.l.m.u. had attained firing intervals as short as 30–40 ms, i.e., not before the c.l.m.u. had discharged near its maximum sustained frequency. On rapid acceleration the i.s.m.u. was recruited earlier. In twitch contractions selective activation of the i.s.m.u. occurred if the muscle was relaxed before the twitch and minimum duration of the twitch was intended. Some training was necessary before the subject was capable of adjusting his contraction so that only the i.s.m.u. was activated. Even after intense training, however, the subject could not activate the i.s.m.u. selectively on each trial. The authors (139) concluded that "under the experimental conditions used, the subjects were not capable of systematic activation of only i.s.m.u.s." In a subsequent paper (23) it was shown that c.l.m.u.s. had conduction velocities between 30 and 45 m/s; i.s.m.u.s. conducted at 40–54 m/s and intermediate units had intermediate conduction velocities. Thus, a relationship was established between voluntary discharge properties and axonal conduction velocity (cell size). This finding indicates how closely these studies on human motor units resemble those on animals previously described.

As this summary indicates, there appear to be some differences in the results of Grimby and Hannerz (139) and those of Desmedt and Godaux (90-92) previously described. These may only be due to differences in experimental conditions. Grimby and Hannerz believe that in the rapid ballistic contractions of Desmedt and Godaux isometric contractions were studied rather than isotonic, as their paper states, and that this accounts for the difference in their results.

As mentioned earlier, both c.l.m.u.s. and i.s.m.u.s. participate in ballistic isotonic contractions if the contractions are not made in any special way. If the muscle is relaxed before a ballistic contraction and both maximum speed and minimum duration of contraction are intended, i.s.m.u.s. can be recruited briefly in isolation, i.e., according to the authors, "the order of recruitment can be reversed."

If, however, the muscle is slightly contracted or stretched before a ballistic contraction and lower force and a longer duration of contraction is intended, c.l.m.u.s. can be recruited without i.s.m.u.s. According to Grimby and Hannerz, "a pre-existing contraction or stretch of the muscle is necessary for studies of isometric twitch contraction and this explains the absence of recruitment order flexibility..." in the studies of Milner-Brown et al. (258) and Desmedt and Godaux (90). Figure 30 (139) illustrates the basis for their conclusions. One c.l.m.u. and one i.s.m.u. were recruited. In sustained contraction, the c.l.m.u. was recorded before the i.s.m.u. (A). On prolonged maximum effort, only the c.l.m.u. responded (B). When sudden, rapid, and short contractions were intended, selective or predominant action of the i.s.m.u. occurred (C and D).

Comparison of the latter condition with the 100-ms time mark indicates that these reversals were of very brief duration, and the authors point out that their occurrence was "unpredictable." Whether the mechanisms for reversal of recruitment order can be used systematically, and have real functional utility, remains to be demonstrated.

The recent experiments of Stephens and colleagues (330) have added a fascinating new observation to the study of recruitment in humans. Motor units in the first dorsal interosseous muscle (1DI) were recorded along with the force produced by abduction of the index finger. During normal voluntary abduction, motor units were recruited into activity in a fixed order, according to their size, as contraction was increased. Subjects were unable to contract their 1DI in such a way that the unit with the normally higher threshold of a pair discharged first or alone. Continuous stimulation of the digital nerves of the index finger at 50/s through ring electrodes around the finger, however, changed the order of recruitment in many cases. As stimulation was continued for 2-4 min the unit that normally had the lowest threshold (1) gradually decreased in firing rate until unit 2 was discharging alone. When unit 1 stopped firing, the subject was able to keep unit 2 active alone at a contraction strength lower than the recruitment threshold for this unit in control conditions. Unit 1 could be made to fire, but only if the force of contraction was greater than that

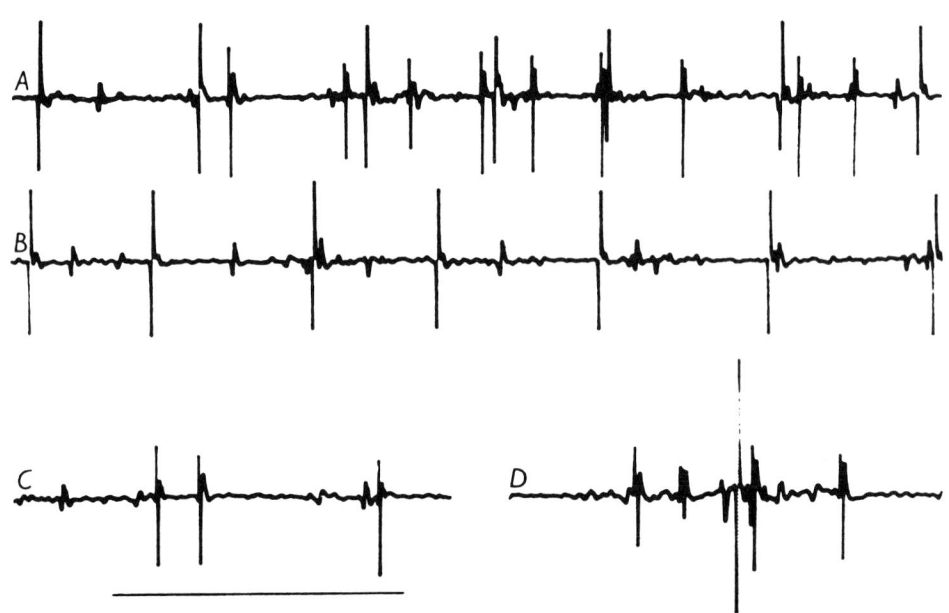

FIG. 30. Simultaneous recording of one continuously firing long-interval motor unit and one intermittently firing short-interval motor unit in human. A: increasing contraction. B: prolonged maximum effort. C, D: rapid twitches. Time bar, 100 ms. [From Grimby and Hannerz (139).]

at which unit *2* fired alone. The recruitment order was thus reversed. According to the authors, the subject was quite unable to contract the muscle so that the previously low-threshold unit (*1*) fired alone. After stimulation was discontinued, several minutes were required for the control pattern to return. As the effect of the stimulus wore off, unit *1* increased its firing rate, although the force exerted by the subject was decreasing. Unit *2* could no longer be fired alone at this time.

In further studies on the 1DI by Garnett and Stevens (119) each subject was asked to track a moving target on an oscilloscope by moving the index finger. During each contraction, the recruitment threshold was defined as that level of force at which the unit first fired continuously. During subsequent trackings, the index finger was stimulated via the ring electrode. In general, units recruited at less than 150 g (6% max force) had their thresholds raised by the skin stimulation. Units with thresholds above 150 g had their thresholds lowered. As in the previous experiments, 2–4 min of stimulation was required to produce these changes and 1–2 min passed before they had completely subsided.

The long delay in the onset of these effects, their duration, and their slow subsidence are difficult to explain. The results indicate that prolonged stimulation of cutaneous nerves may result in nonhomogeneous distribution of inputs to a motoneuron pool. At present, it is hard to put these findings in appropriate perspective; it is even difficult to judge whether they are physiologically normal. The first dorsal interosseous muscle is used in manipulative tasks, giving rise to cutaneous input of various types. However, brief stimulation of the digital nerves, such as might occur normally, had little effect on recruitment in these experiments. A number of intriguing questions are, therefore, raised by these findings.

The foregoing review of evidence relating to alternative orders of recruitment indicates that this topic is not ready for any definitive conclusions. Differences in recruitment order have been demonstrated under circumstances that usually leave their significance uncertain. In general, they have been of short duration, unpredictable in occurrence, and not under voluntary control. The unpredictability of departures from the usual order contrasts with the predictability of the standard order, as Grimby and Hannerz' studies emphasize. Further experimentation rather than speculation is needed to clarify these problems.

Evidence Regarding Voluntary Selective Control of Motor Units

To understand the significance of deviations from the usual recruitment order or of variability within it, it was important to establish the degree of selective control that the central nervous system could exercise voluntarily or even unconsciously over individual motor units.

After an initial report of selective activation of single motor units in humans by Harrison and Mortenson (147), Basmajian (17–19) has repeatedly claimed that when human volunteers are provided with visual and auditory feedback from their active motor units, they easily learn within 10–15 min to control the activity of any single unit within a given muscle. Since these reports disagreed with the majority of observations on animals and humans showing a relatively fixed order of recruitment, an attempt was made to determine whether human subjects could indeed learn to exercise selective control over their motor units. Subjects were asked to discharge motor units in the extensor indicis proprius muscle by dorsiflexing the index finger. After establishing the usual order of recruitment for two motor units that were clearly distinguishable on the oscilloscope, subjects were instructed either to reverse the usual order or to silence the activity of unit *1* without silencing unit *2*. These were considered to be simple but crucial tests of the claims for selective control (158). All nine subjects were able, without difficulty, to cause discharges of a single motor unit on the oscilloscope and to control its rate of firing from most recording sites. Slight voluntary increases in muscle contraction usually resulted in an increase in the firing rate of the first motor unit and the recruitment of a second somewhat larger action potential that followed the same pattern as the first. When the subject was asked to reduce tension in the muscle, the second unit was silenced before the first and there was a progressive decrease in the firing rate of the first; the latter finally stopped when the muscle was at complete rest. This pattern of recruitment could easily be reproduced in all subjects without special training.

In six of the nine subjects no changes in recruitment order were observed despite two hours of training and the help of audiovisual feedback. In each experiment recordings were made from many sites, and the subject was encouraged to explore maneuvers that might lead to alteration in recruitment. At each new site at least 20–30 minutes was spent attempting to alter the normal order. In not a single instance, out of hundreds of trials, was any one of these six subjects able to recruit two units in their usual small-to-large order and then turn off unit *1* without silencing unit *2*. It should be emphasized that even under almost isotonic conditions the most minimal movements of the index finger, scarcely visible to observers, were associated with activity in both units. The CFLs of these pairs of motoneurons probably differed only slightly, yet no reversals in recruitment order occurred.

The results at almost all recording sites in the three remaining subjects were similar to those just described. In each of these subjects, however, there was one site at which some variability in recruitment order was observed. Although one unit was recruited first and dropped out last in the majority of tests, the unit that was usually recruited second was occasionally the first to respond and could then be activated repetitively for some seconds without any activity in the first unit. These changes in recruitment order seemed to occur randomly. None of the subjects could, on demand, activate unit 2 at will or alternate the activity of the two units in sequence.

These studies agree with numerous reports that human subjects can easily isolate single active units and control their frequency by simply changing the contractile force voluntarily. This isolation is apparent rather than real, however, and selective control could only be demonstrated for the lowest threshold unit within recording range. There was no evidence of true voluntary or conscious control over the order of recruitment. These results demonstrate that the pattern of recruitment in human subjects is relatively but not absolutely fixed in the sense that it is not subject to voluntary control.

In contrast to the results just described, a number of studies have been published (9, 18, 194, 341) suggesting that human subjects can activate motor units selectively, provided they are given visual or auditory cues signaling the occurrence of firing. To investigate these claims Thomas et al. (337) recently studied three different muscles. In two, the abductor pollicis brevis and the extensor digitorum brevis, they were able to demonstrate a significant number of reversals of recruitment order. These are both muscles with more than one action. The reversals observed occurred only between units with thresholds that differed by less than 50 g and were accomplished by using the muscle for movements in different directions. Reversals between units with perceptibly different thresholds, when activated along the same axis of contraction, were spontaneously reported to be "impossible" by all subjects. In the first dorsal interosseous muscle, which has only one action, no reversals could be demonstrated. "Thus, it appears," the authors conclude, "that recruitment order reversals are possible to a limited extent in multi-functional muscles, but not in single function muscles" (337).

Size Principle in Other Species

Recruitment of motoneurons in order of increasing size by excitatory inputs of progressive intensity is not limited to mammals. It has been observed in a wide variety of animals as phylogenetically distinct as cats (160) and lobsters (85). Since its first description in the cat (153), it has been reported in the natural motor output to crab leg muscles (52) and eyestalk muscles (165), as well as in cockroaches (277, 278), locusts (168), dragonflies (257), mantids (301), water bugs (342), newts (333), fish (169), chickens (113), skunks (340), and humans (115).

Davis (85) has made a comprehensive study of the functional significance of motor neuron size in the swimmeret system of the lobster. The advantages of the invertebrate preparation enabled him to measure soma diameter directly, as well as conduction velocity and extracellular spike amplitude in motor neurons which could be identified from animal to animal. He found that these indices of motor neuron size were strongly correlated with each other and also with numerous functional properties of the motor neurons, including adaptation to intracellular depolarization and neuromuscular effect, as well as recruitment sequence and discharge pattern during natural motor output.

Lobster motor neurons are driven in rhythmic bursts of impulses by an "oscillator" in the corresponding abdominal ganglion. Coordinated movements of the four pairs of swimmeret appendages are brought about by interactions between these oscillators. The oscillators, in turn, are controlled by identified excitatory and inhibitory "command" interneurons. Stimulation of an excitatory command fiber in an isolated nervous system elicits the rhythmic pattern of motor output that normally causes swimmeret beating. The underlying neuronal mechanisms are, therefore, unusually amenable to analysis.

The diameters of the somata were measured with an ocular micrometer. They ranged from 25 to 125 μm. Large cells invariably had rapid axonal conduction velocities and large extracellular impulses as illustrated in Figure 31. In neurons supplying a given muscle, the relation between conduction velocity and

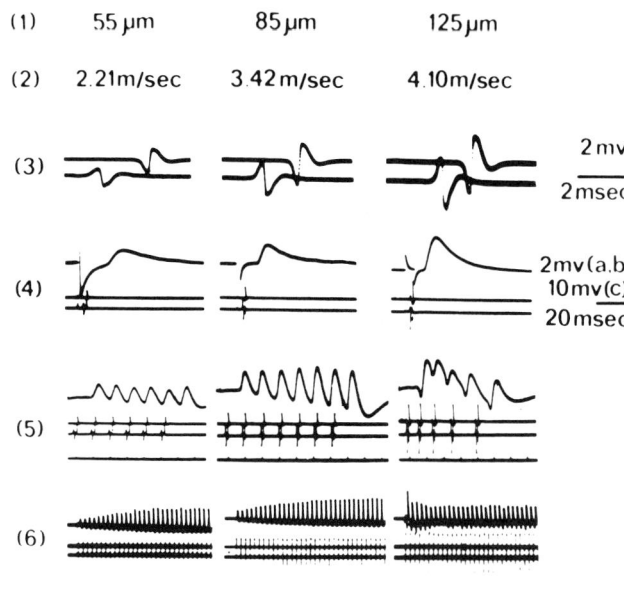

FIG. 31. Properties of a small (A), medium (B), and large (C) motor neuron of lobster innervating the main power stroke muscle. 1, Soma diameters; 2, axonal conduction velocities; 3, amplitudes of action potentials recorded with 2 extracellular electrodes at different positions on the motor nerve; 4, amplitudes of excitatory junctional potentials (EJPs) recorded from a single muscle fiber (*top trace* in each record); 5, adaptation to a maintained intracellular depolarizing current; and 6, facilitation properties of extracellular EJPs (*top trace* in each record) during 50-Hz stimulation. Note antifacilitation produced by the largest motoneuron. Time marks in *row 5 (lowest trace)*, 0.1 ms. [From Davis (85).]

soma diameter was approximately linear. Since conduction velocity is positively correlated with axon diameter, soma and axon diameter were positively correlated as well. These indices of motor neuron size were measured in dozens of experiments and found to correlate well with several functional properties of the motor neuron.

A long-duration pulse of depolarizing current injected into a soma caused a series of action potentials in the motor axon. Small motor neurons typically responded with a train of evenly spaced impulses; in large motor neurons the interspike intervals became progressively longer during the train. Accommodation at the site of spike initiation was presumably the cause of this adaptation. Smaller motor neurons could also be driven at higher maximum frequencies, an indication that their refractory periods were probably shorter. It was regularly observed that the relative increase in stimulus current needed to cause a given increase in discharge frequency was related to motor neuron size. That is, pacemaker sensitivity was apparently inversely related to size.

The size of a motor neuron was also correlated with its effect on the muscle fibers it supplied. The smallest cells evoked the smallest excitatory junctional potentials (EJPs), which on repetition displayed the most neuromuscular facilitation (Fig. 31, line 4). The EJPs of the largest motor neurons, in fact, nearly always showed antifacilitation (Fig. 31, line 6). These results indicate that small and large motor neurons supplying swimmerets have functional properties usually attributed to slow and fast crustacean motor neurons (33).

Increases in the frequency of stimulation of single command interneurons caused a greater frequency of rhythmic bursts and also resulted in recruitment of additional motor neurons. This recruitment proceeded in the order of increasing motor neuron size. The thresholds of these motor neurons to natural synaptic inputs, therefore, increased with their size as in vertebrates. When electrodes were placed so that the activity of all of the motor neurons could be monitored at the same time, it was apparent that with regard to the recruitment sequence, at least, the size principle governs the entire population of swimmeret motor neurons, rather than simply the smaller groups of cells innervating single muscles. Recruitment of motor neurons in order of increasing size occurred before and after abolishing all sensory feedback from proprioceptors and other sense organs. Thus, the size principle in the swimmeret system does not depend on intact reflexes, but results instead from central properties. Davis (85) also showed that the temporal structure of bursts of motor neuron impulses depends strongly on the size of the motor neuron. He had pointed out also that a number of other properties are correlated with the dimensions of cells, adding further support to the use of the more inclusive term size principle to describe the many implications of motor neuron size.

The widespread distribution of the size principle suggests that some rules governing the output of neuronal networks are common to both simple and complex nervous systems (85). There is, moreover, suggestive evidence that the size principle may apply not only to motor neurons but to other neural cells as well. Orderly recruitment of interneurons is apparent in acridid auditory interneurons (304); the sensitivity of pacemaker cells is said to be inversely related to their size (33), and the size of sensory neurons in general may play a role in determining their excitability (32, 357).

Modulation of Firing Rate

In 1929, Adrian and Bronk (3) noted that the force of a voluntary contraction could be increased by two mechanisms. The number of actively contracting motor units could be increased ("recruitment") or the rates of the units already discharging could be accelerated ("frequency coding," "rate coding," "rate modulation"). Adrian and Bronk gave a major role to rate modulation. Recently recruitment has been emphasized more because several investigators found little increase in firing rate except near threshold (24, 128, 135). Moreover, the firing rate appeared to be stable over a wide range of voluntary forces in humans (21, 57, 191).

Using the first dorsal interosseous muscle (1DI) of humans, Milner-Brown et al. (259) averaged the steady discharge rate of single motor units at just above the threshold required to recruit them. During voluntary contractions over a wide range of forces, the relative importance of recruitment and rate coding were compared. Subjects were asked to generate linearly increasing or decreasing forces by moving the index finger laterally and tracking a triangular wave form on an oscilloscope. Single motor units began firing at 8.4 ± 1.3 impulses/s and increased their rates by 1.4 ± 0.6 impulses/s for each 100-g increment of force. The mean firing rate did not depend on the threshold for recruitment, although a relationship has been noted in other muscles (21, 57). At intermediate rates of increasing and decreasing force, firing varied linearly with force over the entire range examined. During slow increases in force, firing rate tended to reach a plateau; during rapid increases an initial train of impulses at a nearly constant rate occurred.

At each level the percentage of extra force due to recruitment and that due to increased firing rate could be computed for the population of units recorded. Recruitment accounts for the majority of the increase at low levels. Although larger motor units were recruited at higher levels, they were relatively few compared to the number of units already active, so that the higher firing rate in the previously active units produced most of the extra force. Over the range considered, increased rate produced about two-thirds and recruitment only about one-third of the total force accounted for.

Wani and Guha (343) have proposed a mathematical model based on these findings of Milner-Brown et al. (259) and on the contractile characteristics of motor units in animals (253, 353) and in humans (29, 57). The model finds the twitch tension, firing frequency, and tension of any motor unit in the muscle at any instant during the gradation process. Expressions are also derived for finding total tension, tension due to recruitment, and tension due to rate coding after the recruitment of any motor unit in the muscle. The model quantifies the interplay between recruitment and rate coding. The characteristics of the motor units of the 1DI, evaluated with the model, closely resemble those obtained experimentally by Milner-Brown et al. (259).

In another very small muscle (the first deep lumbrical of the cat) similar observations have been made (206). The tension produced by lumbrical motor units may easily be more than doubled by synaptically induced changes in firing rate. Kernell and Sjölholm (206) go through a brief formal argument showing that if the motor units of a muscle behave like lumbrical motor units, the importance of rate modulation would remain valid regardless of the number of motor units in the muscle.

It may be assumed that these findings apply to large muscles, though with some modifications. In the lumbrical muscle of the cat rate modulation is important before all motor units are recruited. During a stretch reflex in the cat soleus muscle, however, a gradual recruitment may apparently occur without much modulation of firing rates (89, 128, 135). Even a modest amount of rate modulation, in the range of 5-10 impulses/s, would have a significant influence on the strength of a tonic reflex in the muscle, as Kernell (204) points out.

The widespread distribution of Ia-terminals to practically all homonymous motoneurons (255) is an important factor in rate modulation. Mendell and colleagues (269, 270) have shown that this is common in limb muscles (see section ORGANIZATION OF INPUT TO MOTONEURON POOLS, this page). Any increase in synaptic excitation to the pool would, thus, occur simultaneously in all motoneurons, including those already firing. In a discharging motoneuron this would tend to cause an increase in firing rate. Therefore, an increase in the number of recruited motoneurons would commonly be expected to be accompanied by some increase in firing rate among all the discharging members of the pool. This is what has been observed.

In a contracting soleus muscle, as Kernell (204) points out, a given length change tends to produce a greater relative change in tension at low stimulus rates than at higher ones (132, 249, 284). Thus, according to Grillner (132) the stiffness $\Delta F/\Delta L$ (where F = force and L = length) of a soleus contraction would, in theory, be greater if it were caused by many units firing at slower rates than if it were produced by fewer units discharging at higher rates. The close relationship between recruitment and firing rates seen in all recordings, however, makes it unlikely that the soleus pool has these alternatives. For questions of motor control, it is important to understand which mechanisms may be responsible for the amount of rate modulation that occurs in parallel with recruitment.

Kernell (204) has been analyzing this problem with models containing only five motoneurons. The factors that influence the relation between recruitment and rate modulation are treated theoretically. They include the slope of the frequency-current relation of the motoneurons, the distribution of recruitment thresholds, the effects of recurrent inhibition, and other factors. If appropriately distributed, for example, a strong recurrent inhibition may have a very marked effect on the rate-recruitment relation.

More recently Hatze (149) has made a theoretical study of the contributions of recruitment and rate coding under static conditions. An "activation sensitivity index" is derived from an "excitation variable," and it is stated that this index is a "precise indicator of the relative importance of the two control mechanisms for any mode of contraction." The index is applied to both experimental and stimulation results. The author reports that the index "confirms earlier and more intuitively based conclusions that recruitment is the major mechanism responsible for the grading of the force output at low levels (up to about 30% of the maximum tetanic force), while at intermediate and high force levels rate coding is the dominant factor." Thus, experiments, models, and mathematical studies seem to be in general agreement.

ORGANIZATION OF INPUT TO MOTONEURON POOLS

The firing patterns of motoneurons and motor units described in the previous section are determined by the intrinsic properties of the motoneurons and by the distribution of input to them. Each motoneuron receives thousands of terminal boutons from primary sensory fibers, spinal interneurons, and supraspinal fibers. In spite of the great diversity of input, both excitatory and inhibitory, that they receive, motoneurons innervating the same muscle function as collective entities. The activity of each cell in a pool is closely correlated with the activity of all the other cells in the pool.

The purpose of this section is to review and evaluate recent studies detailing how inputs are distributed to motoneurons. There is little emphasis on synaptic mechanisms, which are well covered in recent reviews by Burke and Rudomin (44) and Redman (295).

Many of our present ideas concerning convergence and divergence in the nervous system, particularly in the spinal cord, derive from the work of Cajal, Sherrington, and Lloyd. Cajal (291) provided evidence that single sensory fibers branch and send terminals to several motoneurons. From physiological studies,

Sherrington and colleagues (78, 321) inferred that many inputs converge on the motoneuron pool supplying a given muscle. Simultaneous activation of different converging inputs could evoke responses that were larger than the sum of the separately evoked reflexes. This summation was interpreted as the result of subliminal activation of some motoneurons by each input alone. Additive effects in motoneurons, due to "overlap" of "subliminal fringes," were believed to bring additional motoneurons to threshold.

A convenient way to begin this discussion of input to motoneurons is to describe recent findings on group Ia-fibers that transmit impulses directly to motoneurons. The inference of monosynaptic contact first became possible after Lorente de Nó (239) had shown that the synaptic delay at the motoneurons in the third cranial nucleus varied from 0.5–0.6 to 0.8–0.9 ms. Renshaw (296) demonstrated that there were spinal reflex arcs consisting of only two neurons (one synaptic delay). Lloyd (235) went on to show that Ia-fibers from spindles were the only primary sensory fibers to make monosynaptic contacts with motoneurons. These early conclusions have been amended since recent studies revealed the existence of monosynaptic connections from group II fibers supplying secondary receptors in spindles, as described in subsection *Group II Input From Secondary Endings in Muscle Spindles*, p. 479.

The introduction of intracellular recording by Eccles and collaborators (25) permitted direct access to the excitatory and inhibitory events occurring in motoneurons. Intracellular recording revealed that the excitatory event was a depolarizing potential, an excitatory postsynaptic potential (EPSP). When a muscle nerve was stimulated, the amplitude of the EPSP was determined in part by the number of Ia-fibers conducting impulses to the motoneuron (99). This subject and corresponding findings for inhibitory postsynaptic potentials (IPSPs) are discussed extensively from an electrophysiological point of view in the first volume of this *Handbook* section on the nervous system (44) and are not treated here.

The early intracellular investigations of synaptic input used electrical stimulation of peripheral nerves. They allowed estimates of the number and potency of Ia inputs from various sources to different motoneuron pools (99, 103). The extent to which Ia action is focused upon particular motoneurons began to become apparent. To understand how individual motoneurons function as parts of an ensemble, however, it must be known how the terminals of afferent fibers are distributed to the members of the pool. It was necessary, therefore, to study the effects of impulses in single Ia-fibers on individual motoneurons and to determine the distribution of these effects.

Anatomical Studies

In this subsection recent anatomical findings are surveyed with special emphasis on features that are important to the problem of distribution of Ia-fiber connections to motoneurons. The discussion of this subsection is qualitative; a more quantitative treatment is given in subsection *Correlations Between Morphology and Function*, p. 476, where physiological and anatomical results are correlated.

THE MOTONEURON. Motoneurons are large cells in the ventral horn whose axons exit the spinal cord via the ventral roots and run in peripheral nerves to supply muscle fibers. They include both α-motoneurons, which innervate extrafusal muscle fibers responsible for muscular force, and γ-motoneurons, which supply intrafusal muscle fibers of the muscle spindle. The Ia-fibers project monosynaptically to α-motoneurons but not to γ-motoneurons (98). This account is therefore restricted to α-motoneurons and synapses upon them.

An important feature of the motoneuron is its very large surface area, which has been estimated in dye-filled neurons as ranging from 79,000 to 250,000 μm^2 (14). According to these authors 80%–90% of this surface area is dendritic.

Motoneurons have 5–20 dendrites, each of which divides frequently, with daughter branches tending to be smaller in diameter than the parents. The details of this branching have become important in the development of mathematical models of dendritic function (see ref. 288 for review). Dendrites are oriented predominantly in the rostrocaudal direction. These branches often extend more than 1 mm in either direction from the cell body (87, 311, 332). Dendrites from different cells are often arranged in bundles (251, 311, 312). The functional significance of this bundling is unknown.

All dendritic regions as well as the soma receive synaptic connections; there are no regions devoid of synapses (122, 354). Some order has been found in the termination of various presynaptic systems on motoneurons (218); however, motoneurons do not receive a highly topographic, layered series of connections from various sources as do cerebellar Purkinje cells, for example.

ANATOMY OF Ia-BRANCHES TO MOTONEURONS. The Ia-fiber has a very extensive series of central connections, including cells of Clarke's column, spinal cord interneurons, and α-motoneurons (44). Only those branches terminating on α-motoneurons are of concern here. Early studies at the level of the light microscope (180, 327, 331, 334) gave confusing results, perhaps because the transverse sections used failed to provide a sufficiently comprehensive view of the dominant rostrocaudal polarity of the motoneuron. Similarly, the Ia-fiber, which also has an important rostrocaudal component, could not be viewed in its proper perspective in transverse sections.

Scheibel and Scheibel (310), using Golgi techniques and sagittal sections in kitten spinal cords, however, were able to reconstruct the entire intraspinal course of Ia-fibers. They described how afferent fibers bifurcate upon entering the spinal cord from the dorsal root and run in both the rostral and caudal directions in the dorsal columns. Several branches are given off from the dorsal column and drop ventrally through the medial part of the dorsal horn and into the ventral horn (Fig. 32), where their collaterals are organized primarily in a mediolateral plane. Each collateral provides terminal branches to the deeper layers of the dorsal horn and also to motoneurons in the ventral horn. It has since been learned that group II fibers also project into the ventral horn (117) and make monosynaptic contact with motoneurons (subsection *Group II Input From Secondary Endings in Muscle Spindles*, p. 479); Ia-fibers, therefore, cannot be identified simply by the presence of a projection into the ventral horn.

The anatomy of single Ia-fibers has recently been examined in much more detail by staining single identified cells with HRP (26, 51, 163). Reconstructions from either cross sections (26, 163) or sagittal sections (51) reveal a picture (Fig. 32) that is qualitatively similar to the Scheibels' description. Several collaterals from each Ia-fiber leave the dorsal columns and drop down into the ventral horn to make contact with motoneurons. Rostrocaudal spread of individual collaterals within the ventral horn was limited (Fig. 32). The terminal fields of individual collaterals did not overlap. A more quantitative discussion of these findings is deferred until subsection *Correlations Between Morphology and Function*, p. 476, where both physiological and anatomical results can be evaluated together. However, a reasonable conclusion at this point is that the morphology of Ia-fibers allows each of them access to large numbers of motoneurons.

Ia-SYNAPSES ON MOTONEURONS. This system contributes only a small proportion (fewer than 5%) of the total number of boutons on these cells (71, 72, 252; see subsection *Correlations Between Morphology and Function*, p. 476). This has complicated the analysis, particularly from the point of view of statistical reliability (for review see ref. 73 and also ref. 212). Conradi (71), using ultrastructural methods, has described the bouton population on motoneurons and estimated which types are contributed by group Ia-fibers. Only type M and larger type S boutons, which are 3-7 μm in diameter and contain clear spherical vesicles, become fewer in number following dorsal rhizotomy; degenerating boutons were not found sufficiently often in this study to warrant quantitative analysis (but see ref. 222). Most boutons (e.g., types T, P, C, and smaller type S) survive this procedure, indicating that their axons have not been injured and, therefore, are not derived from sensory fibers. Conradi (71) found that type M and S boutons of sensory origin were localized primarily on the proximal dendrites, where they were estimated to make up about 0.5% of the total (see also ref. 212). In a similar study, McLaughlin (252) found only type M boutons, which also were most concentrated on proximal dendrites of motoneurons. An additional factor that may further decrease the total number of boutons on distal dendrites is the diminished surface area per unit of length in distal regions of the motoneuron (14). These regional ultrastructural studies are extremely difficult, due to the widespread dendritic tree and the heterogeneous inputs, only a small portion of which arise from the afferent system of interest.

Studies on the identity of group Ia-boutons and the

FIG. 32. Morphology of Ia-collaterals to motoneurons and arrangements of boutons on dendrites. *A*: sagittal section through lumbosacral cord of 40-day-old kitten (section shown at *right*). Primary fibers in dorsal columns (a) send ventrally directed branches to ventral horn (b) to terminate in region of motoneurons (c and d) that have sagitally running dendrites. Primary afferent branches also give off branches to dorsal horn and intermediate zone; these are described in more detail in the original illustration of Scheibel and Scheibel (310) from which this figure is modified. *B*: scale drawing illustrating morphology of collaterals of a single triceps surae Ia-fiber as revealed by horseradish peroxidase (HRP) filling. This 3-dimensional representation provides both a cross-sectional (transverse) and sagittal perspective. The Ia-fiber in the dorsal columns is drawn as a *thick black line* along with the dorsal root ganglion cell and dorsal root portion of the cell. Four collaterals emanating from the dorsal column region are illustrated, each one coursing through the dorsal horn (in a ventrolateral and rostral direction) to terminate in the cylindrical motoneuron region (lamina IX). Other terminals are given off by the same fiber in laminae VI and VII. *C*: morphology of a single soleus Ia-fiber in the dorsal columns with 9 branches given off to ventral horn; HRP technique. Two motoneurons—soleus (SOL), which innervates type S motor unit, and lateral gastrocnemius (LG), which innervates a type F, fatigue-resistant motor unit (R)—were also filled with HRP. *Circles* and *stippling* denote somata and maximum dendritic extents of these neurons. Note that at most only 2 of 9 Ia-fiber branches have access to each of these motoneurons. Also ventrally directed collaterals of this fiber do not exhibit rostral component shown by Brown and Fyffe (Fig. 32*B*). *Top* and *bottom solid lines* denote dorsal and ventral borders of cord. *Dotted lines* represent dorsal and ventral limits of ventral horn. *D*: origins of primary collaterals of MG, LG-S, and posterior tibial (PT) Ia-fibers. *E*: schematic drawing of disposition of Ia-fiber boutons on α-motoneurons. In each case, both Ia-fiber and motoneuron filled with HRP. Note in SOL motoneuron that bouton A is on proximal dendrites in contrast to B-F, which are on distal dendrites. Terminals on LG-type FR motoneuron are of en passant variety (triplet) and of terminal variety. [*A*, adapted from Scheibel and Scheibel (310); *B* and *D*, from Brown and Fyffe (26); *C* and *E*, from Burke et al. (51).]

CHAPTER 11: ORGANIZATION OF MOTONEURON POOL 463

distribution of this population on the motoneuron surface are fundamental to our understanding of Ia-motoneuron synaptic transmission. To further analyze the mechanisms by which input can lead to highly organized output behavior, however, we must also be able to describe where the boutons from single Ia-fibers terminate on single motoneurons. For example, different types of motoneurons might have systematically different locations for Ia inputs, which would contribute to the order in which they are recruited. In order to study the termination of single Ia-fibers on motoneurons it is necessary to label them with some

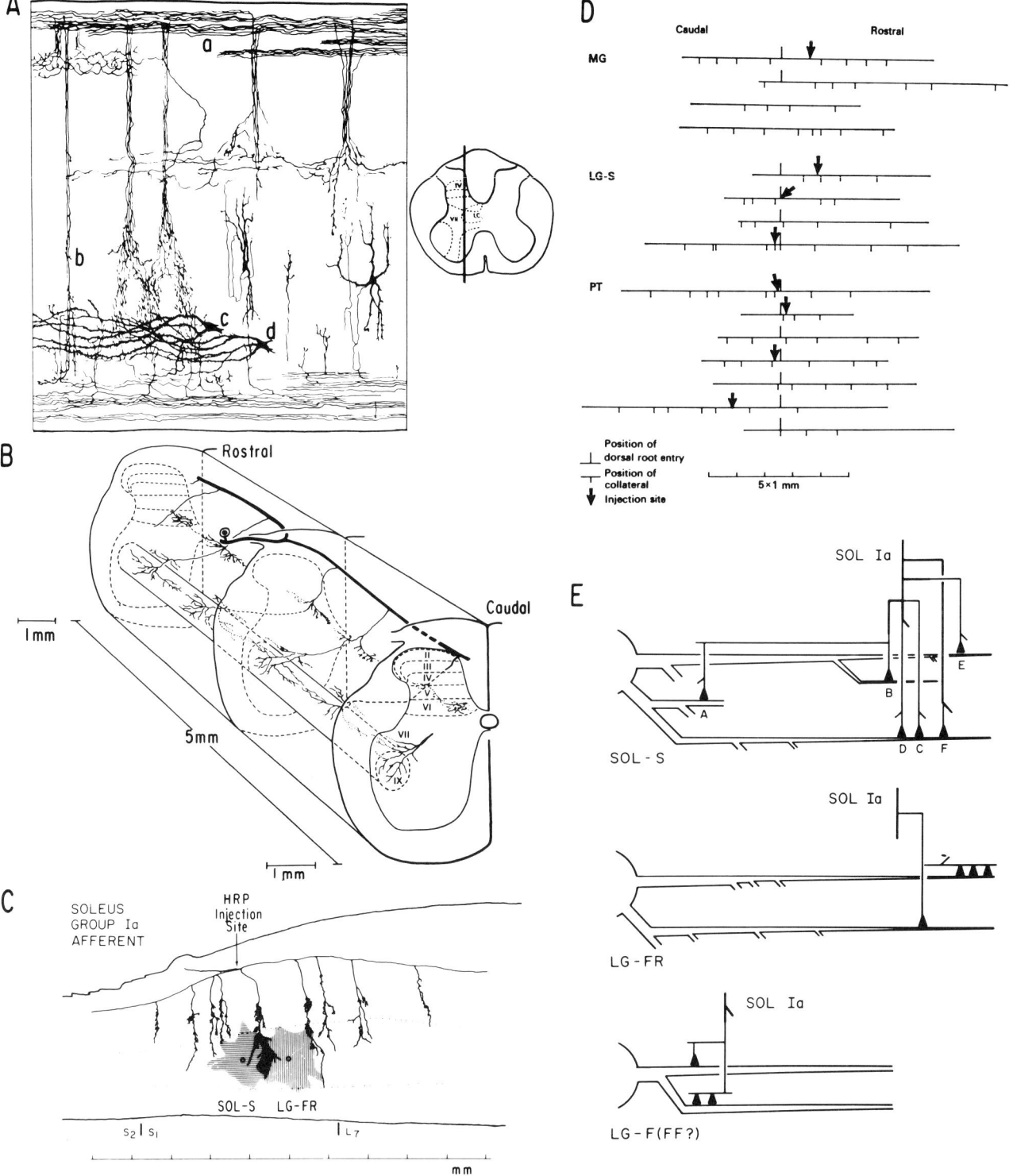

marker, so that their boutons can be identified. A particularly thorny problem in such an analysis is the relatively extensive dendritic tree of the motoneuron, which makes it difficult to sample the entire postsynaptic surface available to the Ia-fiber. Iles (177) labeled small groups of dorsal root fibers with cobalt and studied the terminals given off by single Co^{2+}-filled fibers to single motoneurons. These studies were necessarily limited to regions near the soma, since the motoneurons were only lightly stained and dendrites could not easily be followed. The boutons tended to be clustered, although this impression may have been biased by the relative difficulty in seeing boutons other than juxtasomatic ones.

An important advance in this analysis has been recently published by Burke et al. (51). Horseradish peroxidase was injected into a physiologically characterized Ia-fiber. Similar techniques were used to inject HRP into identified motoneurons (homonymous or heteronymous in relation to the Ia-fiber) at a different time during the same experiment. The sagitally sectioned spinal cord was then processed to identify the HRP reaction product, which is easily visible. Both Ia-fiber terminals and motoneuron dendrites fill very extensively, perhaps completely. Since synaptic connections occur between Ia-fibers and a high proportion of homonymous and heteronymous motoneurons (subsection PERCENTAGE OF MOTONEURONS RECEIVING TERMINALS FROM SINGLE Ia-FIBERS, p. 473), this technique has a high yield even though no physiological evidence is obtained for connectivity between the filled afferent and motoneuron. The results were quite dramatic: a single Ia-fiber sends several collaterals into the ventral horn, only one making contact with the single motoneuron whose dendrites are easily visible. Most boutons are localized close to one another but in one such case (of three reported), the Ia-collateral was observed to terminate with several boutons on different closely related dendritic branches and also to send a process terminating in a single bouton close to the soma (Fig. 32). These results are presently limited to light microscope observations where synaptic contact can only be inferred. Furthermore, no correlative information is yet available on the shape of the EPSPs produced by Ia-fibers whose bouton numbers and locations are known (subsection PHYSIOLOGICAL ANALYSIS OF LOCATION OF BOUTONS, p. 468).

Despite the exciting progress of these anatomical studies, much of the current knowledge concerning the details of Ia-fiber connections to motoneurons comes from physiological studies.

Techniques Used to Study EPSPs Elicited by Impulses in Single Afferent Fibers

EPSPS RECORDED FROM SINGLE MOTONEURONS. Kuno (215) was the first to study EPSPs that were elicited in motoneurons by impulses in single afferent fibers. This was done by electrical stimulation of a fine strand of a muscle nerve dissected until it apparently contained a single Ia-fiber. Burke and Nelson (42) investigated rhythmic EPSPs recorded intracellularly during stretch of the homonymous muscle. These EPSPs exhibited characteristics indicating that they were evoked directly or indirectly by impulses in single Ia-fibers (i.e., silence during muscle contraction, increased firing rate as a function of stretch, regular discharge), but they could be detected in only 10% of the motoneurons that were penetrated. Letbetter et al. (232) recorded EPSPs evoked by intracellular stimulation of Ia-cell bodies in dorsal root ganglia. Several investigators have stimulated peripheral nerves and have severed dorsal roots progressively to achieve single fiber inputs. Others have worked with filaments containing a small number of Ia-fibers and adjusted the peripheral shock to stimulate only a single fiber (176, 182). In order to resolve these small EPSPs clearly from other synaptic noise, averaging techniques have been used.

One of the most useful methods is to trigger an averaging computer with single Ia impulses recorded from a dorsal root filament. Only EPSPs that are time locked with these impulses are resolved; all other intracellular activity is averaged out (Fig. 33). This technique does not require a dorsal root filament with only one active Ia-fiber. In fact, the presence of two active Ia-fibers in a filament allows the investigator to trigger first off one afferent and later the other and, thus, to study the EPSPs produced by two different Ia-fibers in the same motoneuron (256, 315). This technique, first used by Mendell and Henneman (254, 255), is called spike-triggered averaging (STA). Watt et al. (345) and Nelson and Mendell (269) have devised techniques to ensure before beginning intracellular recording that fibers have not been damaged central to the recording point during dissection.

EPSPS RECORDED FROM POPULATIONS OF MOTONEURONS. The limitations of studying EPSPs in single motoneurons have recently been removed by a new technique introduced by Lüscher, Henneman, et al. (244), which permits recording of EPSPs from large populations of cells. By infiltrating a ventral root with isotonic sucrose solution so that its extracellular resistance is extremely high, the interiors of its axons can be used as wick electrodes to record voltage changes in all the motoneurons of that spinal segment. With an averaging computer triggered by the action potentials from a functionally isolated, but intact afferent, the synaptic effect of a Ia impulse upon a large population of motoneurons can be extracted from the physiological and electrical noise in the recording system. Some of the early results of studying input with this technique are described in subsection FACTORS RESPONSIBLE FOR VARIABILITY IN EPSP AMPLITUDES, p. 466.

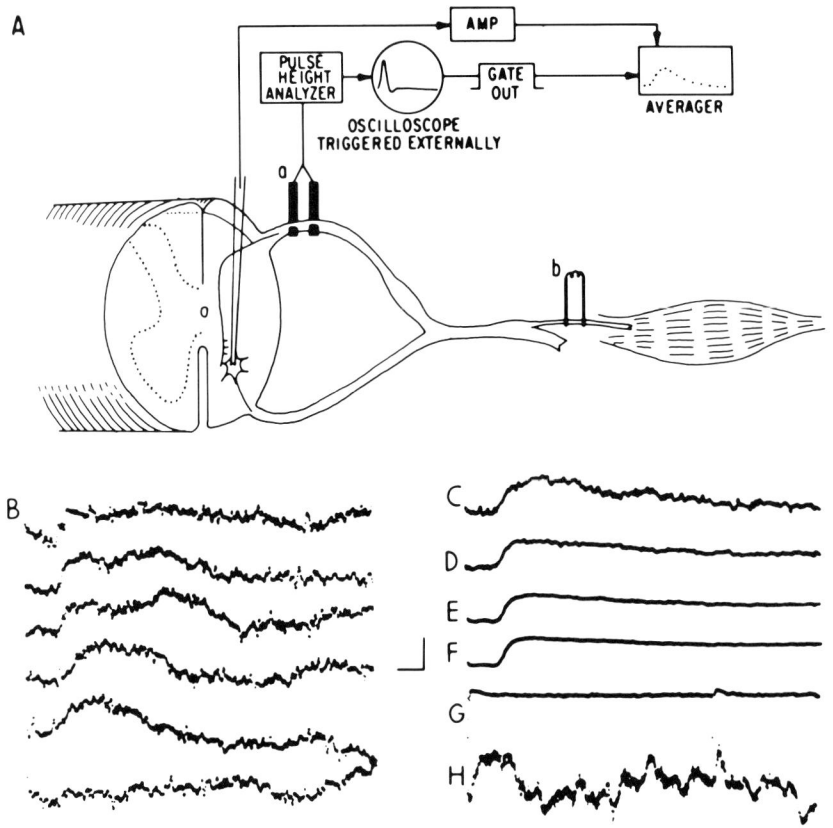

FIG. 33. *A*: arrangement for spike-triggered averaging. Muscle-stretch activated group Ia impulse recorded from dorsal rootlet (a) is used to trigger an averaging computer, using a pulse-height analyzer to select impulses of constant height produced by a single fiber. Each trigger pulse causes averager to process the next several milliseconds of signal recorded from the microelectrode impaling the motoneuron. Motoneuron is identified by antidromic invasion following muscle nerve stimulation (b). If Ia-fiber acting as source of trigger signal sends terminals to motoneuron, then an EPSP is averaged. *B*: examples of single 20-ms records (sweeps) from a medial gastrocnemius (MG) motoneuron triggered by an MG group Ia impulse. The EPSP is seen at start of sweep superimposed on highly variable synaptic activity. Note variability in amplitude of Ia-evoked EPSP. *C–F*: 4, 16, 64, and 256 sweeps are averaged, respectively. Note improvement in resolution of EPSP as number of sweeps averaged is increased. Only potentials synchronized with the MG afferent are preserved. Others are asynchronous with respect to the trigger signal and so are averaged out. *G, H*: dorsal root recording (*G*) and simultaneous intracellular recording from motoneuron (*H*) at slower sweep speed. Note 2 Ia impulses in *G* and synaptic noise in *H*. Calibration, 500 μV for *B–F*, and *H*; 0.7 ms for *B–F*; 5 ms for *H*. [*A*, adapted from Mendell and Henneman (255).]

Amplitudes of EPSPs Elicited by Impulses in Single Fibers

VARIABILITY OF EPSP AMPLITUDES. Consideration of the results in studies performed in different laboratories with the various methods described above, indicates that the average size of EPSPs elicited by impulses in single fibers depends on the techniques used to measure them. It is important to recognize that the EPSP at any synapse does not have a fixed amplitude but varies in size from stimulus to stimulus (42, 215, 256). Whether this variability is due to differences in transmitter release from terminals (34, 215, 256), intermittent conduction in presynaptic terminals (106), or the superposition of synaptic noise on a constant EPSP (105) is not yet clear (see ref. 44 and subsection *Physiology of Ia-Terminals*, p. 472). The extent of this variability is itself subject to some control (305). Whatever its cause, reliable comparisons can only be made between averaged EPSPs.

The EPSPs obtained by electrical stimulation methods (176, 182, 219) are much larger on the average than those obtained using spike-triggered averaging (254–256, 266, 269, 315, 345). Examination of typical amplitude distributions for each technique (Fig. 34) reveals important differences at both ends of the spectrum; spike-triggered averaging yields no EPSPs larger than 800 μV, with more than one-half of them being smaller than 100 μV. In contrast, very few EPSPs evoked by electrical stimulation are smaller than 100 μV and they range in amplitude up to and beyond 2 mV.

Differences between the EPSPs obtained by spike-triggered averaging and electrical stimulation might

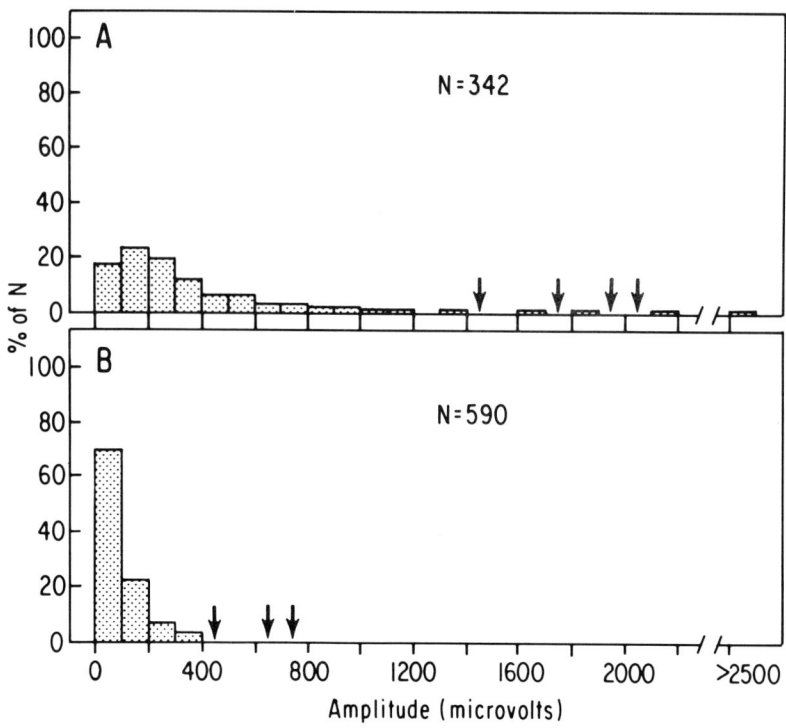

FIG. 34. Amplitude histograms of single-fiber EPSPs in homonymous and heteronymous motoneurons. *A*: histogram obtained using electrical stimulation method. *B*: histogram with spike-triggered averaging method. *Arrows* represent values of less than 1% of N. Afferents and motoneurons are mainly from triceps surae and semitendinosus muscle groups in *A* and exclusively so in *B*. [*A*, from Jack et al. (82); *B*, from data of Mendell and Henneman (255), Nelson and Mendell (269, 270), Scott and Mendell (315).]

be explained by a number of factors. For example, a criterion used in the studies with electrical stimulation, namely that the EPSP exhibit a single time course with no discontinuities, might fail occasionally, so that the EPSP would be elicited by impulses in more than a single fiber. This would account for the few relatively large EPSPs, but unless this were a common occurrence it would not explain why so few averaged EPSPs of less than 100 µV were recorded under these conditions. However, this method selects Ia-fibers with the lowest electrical threshold and impulses in fast conducting fibers have been shown in other experiments (255) to evoke the largest EPSPs (see the next subsection). Furthermore, it seems possible that motoneurons would receive less interneuronal and afferent input under these conditions than during spike-triggered averaging, when the muscle is stretched and a large fraction of the dorsal rootlets are still intact. The synaptic potentials produced by these other inputs might tend to act as a shunt, thereby reducing the amplitude of EPSPs evoked by the Ia-fiber under study (15, 38).

The rhythmic EPSPs recorded by Burke and Nelson (42) had mean amplitudes ranging from 680 µV to 1,570 µV. These may have been the largest EPSPs evoked by Ia-fibers, perhaps the only ones large enough to be detected in single sweeps. They were detected in only about 10% of the motoneurons from which recordings were made. It is also possible that these EPSPs were elicited by an interneuron that was driven rhythmically by Ia impulses.

The wide range of mean EPSP amplitudes described above may be due to the use of different techniques. It is worth reemphasizing that the spike-triggered averaging technique provides the most complete assurance that only a single fiber is generating the EPSP and that it is a Ia-fiber. This technique has consistently yielded EPSPs smaller than 800 µV in animals with intact spinal cords. Larger EPSPs in such preparations have only been obtained using the other techniques. Despite these differences there is general agreement that most EPSPs are 200–300 µV or less. Their small size indicates that a considerable Ia convergence is required to discharge motoneurons. However, under normal conditions the motoneuron membrane potential might hover close enough to threshold so that input from a few Ia-fibers would be sufficient to discharge it.

FACTORS RESPONSIBLE FOR VARIABILITY IN EPSP AMPLITUDES. Even when variability introduced by the use of different techniques is eliminated, a wide range of EPSP amplitudes is observed. Certain factors influencing EPSP amplitude have been identified. Mendell and Henneman (255) reported that the mean EPSP amplitude evoked in experiments in which large afferent fibers (measured by conduction velocity) were stimulated, was larger than in experiments when small afferents were stimulated. This finding has been extended by Henneman and colleagues (244), who have recorded the electrotonic potential from an entire ventral root that had been perfused with isotonic sucrose (subsection *Techniques Used to Study EPSPs Elicited by Impulses in Single Afferent Fibers*, p. 464). The root was held under constant conditions, during which the projections of many Ia-afferent fibers were studied using the spike-triggered averaging technique. The size of the response, which reflects both the number of motoneurons activated as well as the amplitudes of their individual EPSPs, was found to be systematically greater for large Ia-fibers than for small ones within a given experiment (Fig. 35). These results suggest that larger sensory fibers exert more potent synaptic actions, perhaps by giving off more terminal branches. A further example of the capacity of different afferent fibers to evoke EPSPs of different amplitudes is provided by lateral gastrocnemius Ia-afferents, which evoke larger EPSPs on the average than medial gastrocnemius, soleus (315), or semitendinosus Ia-afferent fibers (269) despite similar conduction velocities.

Mendell and Henneman (255) also found that when experiments were performed in high spinal, unanesthetized preparations, the EPSPs were on the average about twice as large as in intact, unanesthetized preparations. This was attributed to the lack of anesthetic; however, recent experiments (268) suggest that acute transection of the spinal cord in the anesthetized preparation can also lead to considerably larger EPSPs via mechanisms which are still obscure. These results underscore the importance of the experimental conditions in determining EPSP amplitude.

The existence of pre- and postsynaptic sites at which EPSPs evoked by Ia-fibers can be influenced is now well accepted. Stimulation of various segmental (101, 216) and supraspinal areas (53, 54) results in depolarization of Ia-terminals and depression of EPSPs without any change in their time course. This is probably due to presynaptic inhibition (314). Whether there is diminished release of transmitter due to presynaptic depolarization (195) or prevention of impulse propagation at terminal branch points by cathodal block (167), or both, is not known. The EPSP amplitude might also be diminished by shunting if it were evoked during an afferent barrage in other fibers converging on the same motoneuron (15, 38). These mechanisms are discussed in more detail in Burke and Rudomin's review (44). For the present, it is sufficient to note that alterations on either side of the synapse can affect the amplitude of the EPSP and that differences in descending, segmental, or propriospinal activity determined by the type of experimental preparation might cause variations in EPSPs.

Another source of systematic variability in EPSP amplitude is the input resistance of the motoneuron

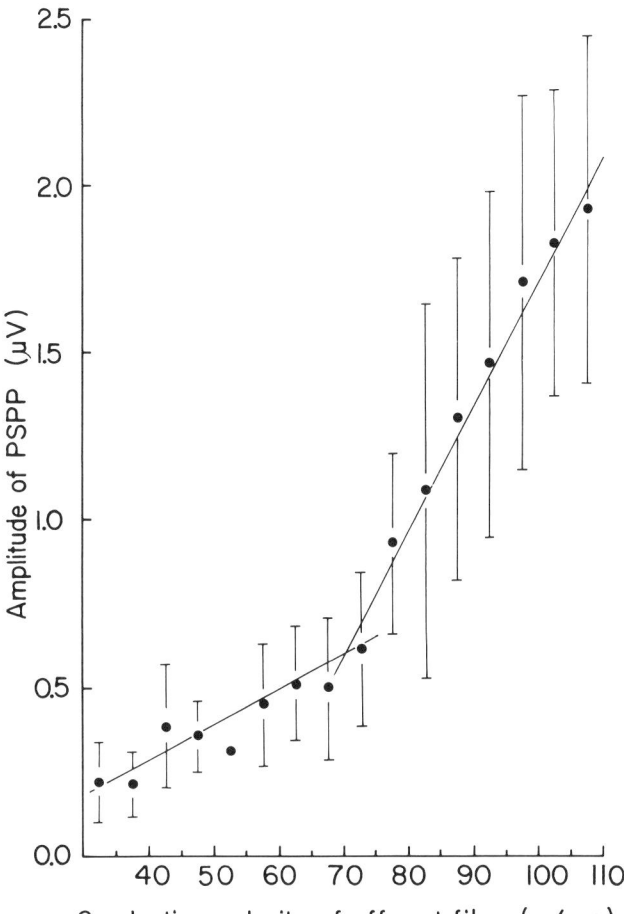

FIG. 35. Plot of mean amplitudes of postsynaptic population potentials (PSPPs) elicited by afferent impulses with mean condition velocities shown on abscissa. The PSPPs were evoked by impulses in single group Ia and II fibers of cat medial gastrocnemius muscle, using spike-triggered averaging. Responses recorded from 1st sacral ventral root and lower part of 7th lumbar ventral root. The 153 data points were grouped in pentads of conduction velocity and mean and standard deviations of PSPPs for each group are shown. Mean data points fell into 2 groups, each of which was fitted with a straight line by method of least squares, using point at 72.5 m/s for both calculations. [From Lüscher, Henneman, et al. (244).]

(203). Several investigators (36, 220, 255) have observed that EPSPs are larger on the average in small motoneurons that have larger input resistances than in large ones with small input resistances (Fig. 36).

Further evidence for the role of cell size is that individual EPSPs are larger in soleus than in medial or lateral gastrocnemius motoneurons (315). This factor undoubtedly contributes to the greater reflex excitability of small motoneurons than large ones (see section HOW SIZE OF MOTONEURONS DETERMINES THEIR SUSCEPTIBILITY TO DISCHARGE, p. 491).

The use of axonal conduction velocity to assess variations in EPSP properties in motoneurons of different sizes is justified by the substantial evidence that recruitment order is a function of motor axon diameter, which is proportional to axonal conduction veloc-

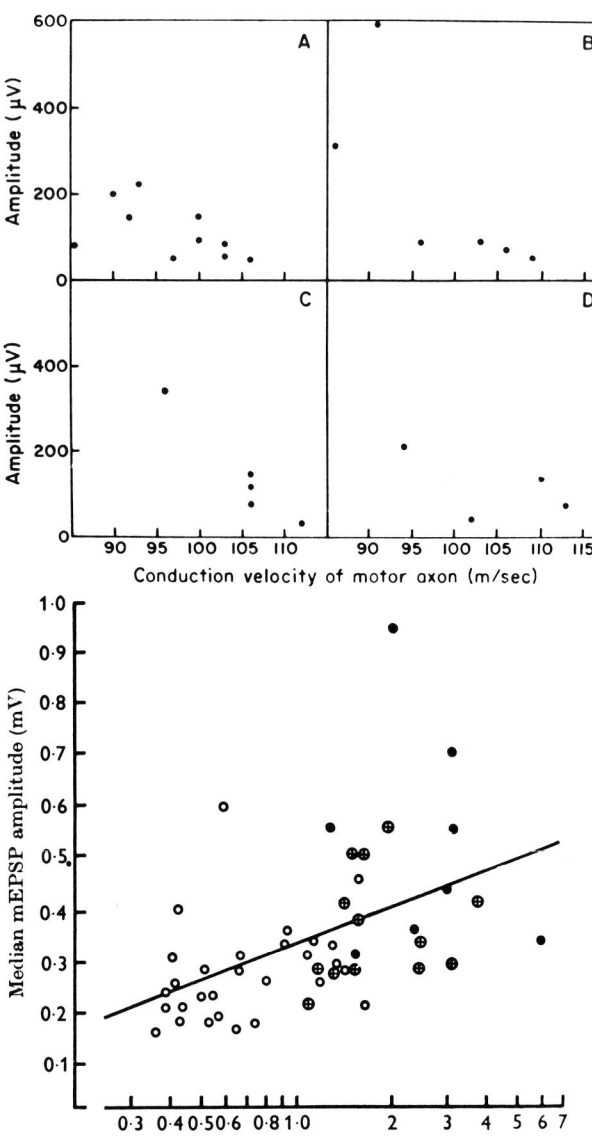

FIG. 36. Dependence of amplitude of single-fiber EPSPs on size of motoneuron in cat. *Top,* relationship between EPSP amplitude (obtained by spike-triggered averaging) and motor axon conduction velocity determined for 4 separate group Ia afferent fibers. Axonal conduction velocity determined by antidromic stimulation. Medial gastrocnemius (MG) Ia-fibers and motoneurons in each case. Note inverse relationship. *Bottom,* each point represents median value of amplitude distribution of a presumed single-fiber EPSP evoked in a motoneuron during stretch of triceps surae. The EPSPs are not restricted to those generated by Ia-fibers. Many of these EPSPs are probably produced by interneurons. It is assumed that variation of these EPSPs with motoneuron input resistance as shown would also occur in the subpopulation of Ia-evoked EPSPs. Small cells with large input resistance (203) generate larger EPSPs. ○, Gastrocnemius motoneurons supplying type F (rapidly contracting) motor units; ⊕, MG motoneurons supplying type S (slowly contracting) motor units; and ●, soleus motoneurons. [*Top* from Mendell and Henneman (255); *bottom* from Burke (36).]

ity (see sections FIRING PATTERNS OF INDIVIDUAL MOTONEURONS AND MOTOR UNITS, p. 435, and NON-UNIFORMITY OF MOTONEURONS, p. 485). However, these studies may provide an incomplete picture.

Burke et al. (46) have demonstrated that motoneurons supplying muscle units of various types generate aggregate EPSPs whose amplitudes appear to depend more on motor unit type (obtained from intracellular stimulation of the motoneuron and measurement of the resultant muscle contraction) than on axonal conduction velocity. Although motoneurons in type FF (fast, fatiguing) motor units have conduction velocities similar to those supplying type FR units (fast, fatigue resistant), the aggregate EPSPs are apparently smaller in the former. This subject is discussed in greater detail in the chapter by Burke in this *Handbook.*

Boutons of Ia-Fibers on Motoneurons

PHYSIOLOGICAL ANALYSIS OF LOCATION OF BOUTONS. The time course of individual EPSPs is a good indication of the location of the active boutons on motoneurons. Analysis of aggregate EPSPs (36) is complicated by asynchrony in the arrival of the afferent impulses as well as by differences in the location of the active synapses. In order to use EPSP time course to infer synaptic location precisely, certain information concerning the electrical properties of the cell soma and its dendrites as well as the time course of the synaptic current must be known. These topics have been treated at length in reviews by Rall (288) and by Burke and Rudomin (44) in the first volume of this *Handbook* section on the nervous system and also in a recent review by Redman (294); they are discussed only briefly here.

Rall (286–288) has developed an electrical model of the motoneuron in which the dendrites are represented as cylinders divided into compartments of equal electrotonic length. The EPSPs produced by activation of single compartments and also by simultaneous or sequential activation of several compartments have been computed (286). The EPSPs generated by the action of boutons located on distal dendrites would, in general, be expected to have slower time courses than those elicited by somatic boutons (Fig. 37A). An additional variable, which may affect the shape of an EPSP, is the time course of the synaptic current. Indirect evidence suggests that this may vary from synapse to synapse (176) perhaps as a result of conduction-time differences in the presynaptic terminal systems (141, 177, 275). A relatively slow EPSP might result from a fast-current transient acting on distal dendrites or from a slow-current transient acting on the proximal dendrites or soma. A very fast EPSP is likely to result from a brief-current transient acting proximally. Factors that may also influence the time course of an EPSP include the time constant of the postsynaptic cell (τ; $3 < \tau < 12$ ms) and the ratio of dendritic to somatic conductance (ρ; $3 < \rho < 25$).

The influence of the distance between synapse and recording point on the time course of synaptic potentials was first demonstrated experimentally by Fatt and Katz (112) at the neuromuscular junction (Fig. 37B). As the recording microelectrode was moved

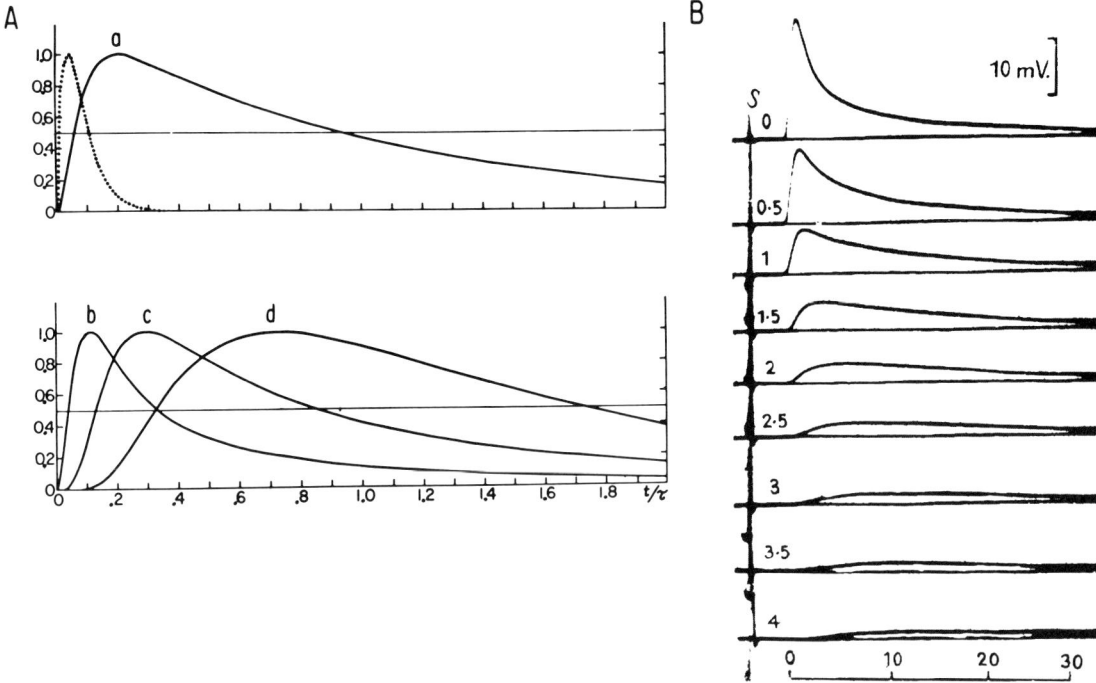

FIG. 37. *A*: EPSP shapes computed for input restricted to specific regions of the dendritic tree of cat. All EPSPs assumed to be recorded from compartment 1 (the soma) of a 10-compartment motoneuron. Compartments 2–10 represent dendritic regions of equal electrotonic length but increasing distance from the soma. *Top*, time course of the conductance transient generating EPSPs is given by *dotted line*; a is EPSP expected for a transient delivered to all compartments simultaneously. *Bottom*, b–d are EPSPs expected for transients delivered to compartments 1, 4, and 8, respectively. Ordinate is in arbitrary units; to produce EPSPs with equal peak amplitudes as shown, intensity of conductance changes for d > c > b > a. Note differences in time course of EPSPs, and for b–d, note differences in time of their onset. *B*: end plate potentials at different locations in same muscle fiber (frog sartorius in vitro). Microelectrode was inserted sequentially into curarized fiber and end plate potential in response to motor nerve stimulation was measured. Numbers at *left* of each trace represent distance in millimeters from end plate focus. S is the stimulus artifact. Time is in ms. [*A*, from Rall (287); *B*, from Fatt and Katz (112).]

progressively farther from the synapse, the end plate potentials (EPPs) became slower and smaller (see next subsection). This is in qualitative agreement with the predictions of the Rall model (Fig. 37). Individual EPSPs in motoneurons show similar variations (176, 182, 255, 263, 269, 289, 315) suggesting the basic correctness of the Rall analysis. Moreover, half-width (duration at half amplitude) and rise time (time to peak) are positively correlated (176, 182, 255, 263, 269, 289, 315) as predicted by the theory (287). Impulses in a single Ia-fiber produce EPSPs of very different time courses in different motoneurons (Fig. 38*A*). Conversely, impulses in two Ia-fibers can elicit slow and fast EPSPs in the same motoneuron (Fig. 38*B*). The time course of an individual EPSP is not an intrinsic property of either the Ia-fiber or the motoneuron alone; other factors that vary from synapse to synapse also influence the time course.

Some individual EPSPs have half-widths that are too long for the rise time (based on Rall's calculations for input localized to a single compartment and a simple synaptic current time course). Occasionally, such EPSPs appear to consist of two well-defined components (Fig. 38*C*), but this is exceptional. These observations indicate either a compound time course for synaptic current or more than one location for the synaptic boutons from a single afferent fiber, or both. Rall et al. (289) concluded that some synapses were probably distributed to more than one compartment. A similar conclusion was reached by Mendell and Weiner (256), who compared EPSPs produced by two Ia-fibers in the same motoneuron (see anatomical evidence in support of this in subsection *Anatomical Studies*, p. 461).

Methods of calculating the distance from synapses to soma from EPSP time course have been described by Jack et al. (182). Use of these techniques (176, 182) has revealed that the majority of Ia-EPSPs are generated by terminals located on the proximal half of the dendritic tree. Synapses on the soma and distal dendrites occur relatively infrequently. This distribution agrees with the anatomical findings of Conradi and McLaughlin (71, 72, 252) as described in subsection *Anatomical Studies*, p. 461. Studies have been limited to EPSPs with simple time courses. The electrical stimulation methods used by these investigators prob-

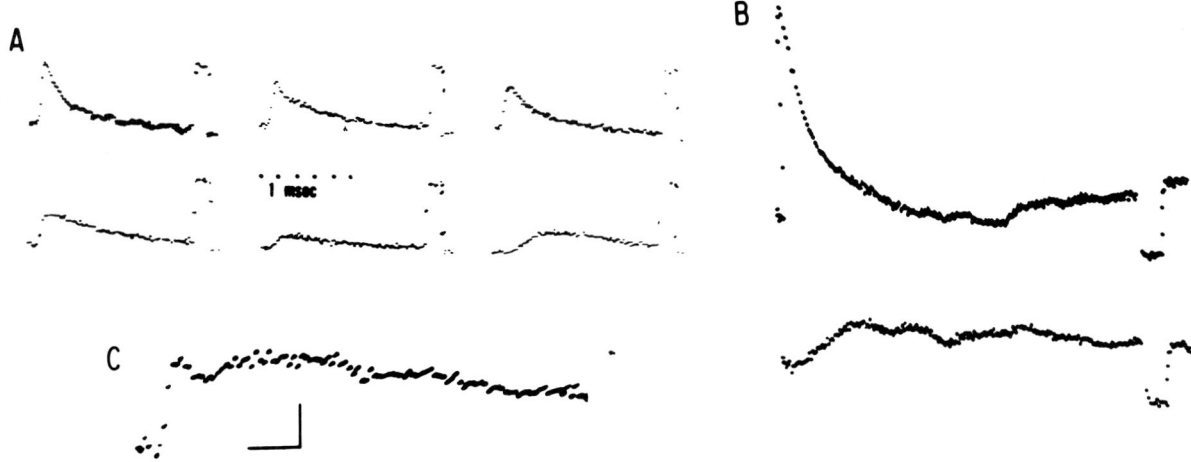

FIG. 38. *A*: single-fiber excitatory postsynaptic potentials (EPSPs) obtained using spike-triggered averaging produced by the same medial gastrocnemius (MG) Ia-afferent fiber in 6 different MG motoneurons in cat. Note different shapes of the 6 EPSPs. Calibration pulse at the end of each sweep is 200 μV. *B*: single-fiber EPSPs (by spike-triggered averaging) produced in the same LG motoneuron by an LG Ia-fiber (*top*) and a soleus Ia-fiber (*bottom*). Calibration pulse is 100 μV, 1 ms. Note differences in shape of these EPSPs. *C*: example of a single fiber EPSP (MG Ia-fiber and MG motoneuron) with compound shape (spike-triggered averaging). Calibration is 1 ms, 50 μV. [*A*, from Mendell and Henneman (255); *B*, from Scott and Mendell (315); *C*, from Mendell and Henneman (255).]

ably activated the largest Ia-afferent fibers. These indirect estimates of the location of synaptic terminals may, therefore, be biased.

The rise times of individual EPSPs are longer in small than in large motoneurons (315). A similar conclusion was reached by Burke (36) from analysis of composite EPSPs. These data alone cannot be used to infer that synaptic terminals are located more distally in small motoneurons because the longer time constants of small motoneurons (48) would tend to prolong EPSPs irrespective of the location of the terminals. However, Jack et al. (181) have taken the time-constant factor into account and have shown a tendency for Ia-terminals on small motoneurons to be located more distally than those on large cells. In experiments on individual motoneurons, they found no evidence that Ia-fibers with different peripheral conduction velocities terminate on different parts of the somadendritic tree. Conduction velocity of Ia-afferent fibers central to the dorsal root ganglion is considerably less than in the periphery (238).

EFFICACY OF SYNAPSES ON DIFFERENT PARTS OF MOTONEURON. Rall's analysis has been instructive in evaluating the effects exerted by boutons located on different regions of the motoneuron surface. Rinzel and Rall (300) have calculated that an input transient (current source) delivered to a single dendritic branch generates a much smaller EPSP at the soma (by factors of up to 235) than the same input at the soma itself. Several factors enter into the analysis, including nonlinear summation in the dendrites, the attenuation introduced by the dendritic cable, the number of neighboring branches activated (288), and the properties of the current, e.g., steady vs. transient (15, 290).

Data on individual EPSPs suggest less attenuation of distally generated EPSPs than predicted by Rall's theoretical studies. A negative correlation between EPSP amplitude and rise time would be expected, but this is actually weak as shown in Figure 39A (see also refs. 22, 34, 217, 255, 256). Rise time may not be an accurate indication of synaptic location because of the variations in synaptic-current time course (α) as well as motoneuron time constant (τ). However, the findings of Iansek and Redman (176) indicate that dendritic EPSPs recorded at the soma are about the same amplitude as those generated at the soma where synaptic distance is estimated taking ρ and τ into account (Fig. 39B). The correlation between amplitude and half-width is unexpectedly positive (see ref. 256 for discussion).

The small differences between amplitudes of EPSPs produced by dendritic and somatic synapses do not necessarily argue against the Rall motoneuron model. The prediction that dendritic synapses should evoke smaller EPSPs than somatic ones requires assumptions concerning the uniformity of synaptic input, postsynaptic receptors, and motoneuron properties at those parts of the motoneuron. Differences in these properties have been postulated to explain the similarity in amplitudes of distally and proximally generated EPSPs. These include increased receptor sensitivity at dendritic synapses (176, 256), enhanced resistivity of dendritic membrane compared to the soma (111, 175, 196), a greater number or size of boutons at dendritic synapses (294), and a regional membrane specialization with reversal potentials that are more positive for dendritic synapses, with a resultant decrease in nonlinear summation (294). At present, none of these explanations has decisive experimental sup-

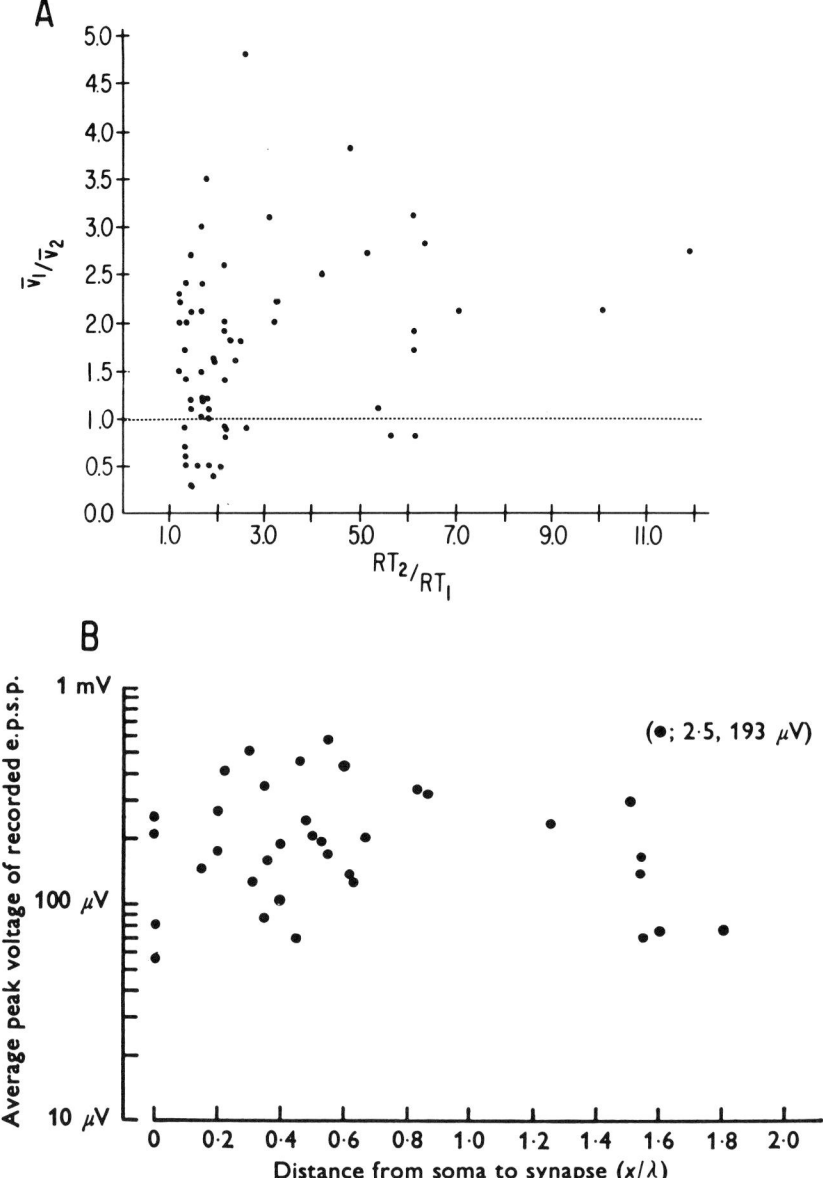

FIG. 39. *A*: plot of ratio of excitatory postsynaptic potential (EPSP) amplitudes ($\bar{V}_1/\bar{V}_2$) against ratio of their rise times (RT_2/RT_1). Each *point* was obtained by consideration of 2 averaged single-fiber EPSPs (spike-triggered averaging) evoked by different Ia-fibers in the same motoneuron. Medial gastrocnemius (MG) Ia-fibers and MG motoneurons throughout. By definition $RT_1 < RT_2$ so that $RT_2/RT_1 > 1$. Furthermore $\bar{V}_1/\bar{V}_2$, the ratio of the amplitudes, is defined so that amplitude of faster rising EPSP is in numerator. Majority of points have $\bar{V}_1/\bar{V}_2 > 1$ suggesting a tendency for faster rising EPSPs to be larger than slower rising ones. Correlation between $\bar{V}_1/\bar{V}_2$ and RT_2/RT_1 is very weak. *B*: plot of single-fiber EPSP amplitude (obtained by electrical stimulation) against distance (in units of space constant λ) between the terminals and the electrode (assumed to be in soma). The EPSPs are chiefly from hamstring and triceps surae motoneurons with both homonymous and heteronymous combinations. [*A*, from Mendell and Weiner (256); *B*, from Iansek and Redman (176).]

port; in fact, anatomical studies suggest that Ia-boutons on dendrites are not greater in size (222) or density (72) than those on more proximal regions.

Nonlinear summation of synaptic potentials would be expected if the EPSPs approached the equilibrium potential and/or if appreciable shunting of one by the other took place. Kuno and Miyahara (219) concluded that substantial nonlinear summation could occur among the unit EPSPs produced by impulses in a single Ia-fiber because the observed amplitude histogram was narrower than expected from the quantal analysis (i.e., fewer large potentials). However, Burke (34) demonstrated that aggregate EPSPs evoked by volleys in different muscle nerves sum linearly in the majority of cases. The maximum deviation from perfect linearity was 17% (i.e., 83% of the expected value calculated from adding the separately evoked EPSPs). Since the terminals of a single fiber are more likely to be clustered than those from two muscle nerves, this difference in summation is not surprising. Furthermore, it is likely (219) that this effect would be greatest for dendritic terminals where the EPSPs would be expected to be largest due to locally high input resistance. The occurrence of very large synaptic potentials at dendritic terminals has been confirmed by Iansek and Redman (176).

The inference of nonlinear summation was also made (269, 315) to explain the finding that the expected aggregate EPSP amplitude, calculated from individual EPSP amplitudes, was usually larger than the experimentally determined value (99, 103). The Ia-terminals from a single muscle nerve may be in much closer proximity on the motoneuron than those from different muscle nerves. This could account for the smaller amount of nonlinear summation in the results of Burke (34). It would be important to learn whether certain combinations of inputs or types of motoneurons exhibit more nonlinear summation than others.

Many authors have tended to equate the amplitude of the synaptic potential recorded at the soma with its effectiveness in causing action potentials. However, since the ultimate effect of EPSPs is to cause depolarization of the initial segment, and since summation of EPSPs is necessary to reach threshold, the duration of the EPSP is an important variable. Barrett and Crill (15) have suggested that the time integral of an EPSP is perhaps a better measure of an EPSP's effectiveness. Rall (285) has made the interesting suggestion that dendritically generated EPSPs, which are usually slower (measured at the soma) than somatically generated ones, might act to regulate excitability. More proximally placed inputs would be apt to cause specific impulse patterns. Lüscher, Henneman, et al. (244) have provided experimental support for these suggestions. Theoretical work indicating the importance of the first derivative of EPSP time course in raising the probability of firing (209, 211) is also consistent with these ideas.

Physiology of Ia-Terminals

It is not feasible at present to make satisfactory intracellular or extracellular recordings from identified regions of Ia-terminals. The recording of individual EPSPs in a motoneuron, however, may provide some indirect evidence regarding Ia-terminals, permitting inferences to be made concerning their function.

Kuno (215) suggested that fluctuations in EPSP amplitude at a particular synapse were the result of a variable release of transmitter. He plotted the distribution of amplitudes resulting from stimulation of single Ia-fibers or small numbers of them. These amplitude histograms were found to have multiple peaks that satisfied Poisson statistics or, in some cases, binomial statistics. Quantal content was generally less than 5 with occasional synapses exhibiting values up to 20–25 (215, 219, 220). Similar findings were made by Burke and Nelson (42) and Mendell and Weiner (256). These results suggested that transmitter release mechanisms at the Ia-motoneuron synapse were qualitatively similar to those at the neuromuscular junction (88). The number of units released by a single impulse at the neuromuscular junction, however, is about 2–3 orders of magnitude greater than at the Ia-motoneuron synapse.

Edwards et al. (105) analyzed similar data but applied different calculation procedures. Charge transfer (time integral of the voltage) rather than peak amplitude of the EPSP was used for analysis. Furthermore, they took account of variability introduced by the synaptic noise. The distributions of EPSP plus noise and noise alone were calculated. They solved for the signal distribution, which, when convolved with the observed noise distribution, gives the EPSP plus noise distribution. In over one-third of the individual EPSPs only a single peak was obtained for the EPSP charge distribution, and in about another one-third, two peaks were found whose amplitudes did not have a simple integral relationship as in a quantized process. Peaks corresponding to failures, which were quite common in the earlier analyses, were seen only rarely. These results suggested neither a Poisson nor a binomial process.

These two approaches lead to very different conclusions: individual EPSPs in single sweeps are very small and are accompanied by considerable synaptic noise from other inputs, making direct analysis difficult. Fitting the observed distribution with a Poisson process (256) or calculating a peak charge distribution (105) requires statistical verification (e.g., χ^2 analysis) and this has been obtained in both cases. The major difficulty is that there is no unique solution to this problem and statistical methods cannot determine that one solution is significantly better than another.

Edwards et al. (106) used their convolution technique to analyze two individual EPSPs whose compound shapes made it very unlikely that the responsible terminals were located on a single compartment of the motoneuron. Calculation of the charge histograms revealed that each EPSP consisted of two peaks. The EPSP associated with each peak was found to have a different shape and the probability of occurrence of these peaks was different. These results were interpreted as indicating two sets of terminals from a Ia-fiber located on different compartments of the motoneuron with different probabilities of activation. This suggested intermittent conduction in the presynaptic terminals. The alternate possibility, namely that these intermittent events reflected a stochastic release process, was rejected because the charge histograms did not satisfy binomial or Poisson statistics.

An important common thread in these two groups of results is that stochastic or probabilistic processes probably occur at some locus along the path of the presynaptic Ia-fiber. At present, it is not clear if this is in the terminals and consists, for example, of a quantized release process obeying Poisson or binomial statistics, or if it is located at points of fiber branching, which can be regions of low safety factor (141, 275). At issue is the nature of the unit or smallest EPSP produced by a single fiber. (See refs. 44, 51 for further discussion.) In a more general context, attempts to deal fully with the relationship between the anatomy of the Ia-fiber distribution to motoneurons and the resultant functional action must await resolution of these problems.

Distribution of Ia Excitation to Motoneuron Pools

PERCENTAGE OF MOTONEURONS RECEIVING TERMINALS FROM SINGLE Ia-FIBERS. In studying EPSPs produced by impulses in single Ia-fibers, the opportunity arises to determine the percentage of motoneurons in an identified pool to which a given Ia-fiber projects. Both Ia-fibers and motoneurons are identified by their responses to electrical stimulation of muscle nerves. The spike-triggered averaging technique is particularly suited to this type of study because impulses can be recorded from a single Ia-afferent in an intact dorsal rootlet for many hours, and the responses of many motoneurons can be studied. Mendell and Henneman (254, 255) demonstrated that activation of single MG Ia-fibers evoked EPSPs in virtually all (94%) MG motoneurons. They inferred that each of the approximately 60 Ia-fibers (56) from MG projected to each of the 300 α-motoneurons (102) innervating this muscle. Kuno and Miyahara (220) performed a similar experiment but found a much lower percentage (44%). They ascribed this difference to their inability to resolve very small EPSPs, since, rather than averaging, they examined single sweeps. This illustrates an obvious but important technical problem in such studies, namely that failure to detect small EPSPs can lead to an underestimate of the total Ia projection. The presence of a tonic inhibitory process (pre- or postsynaptic) could cause the same problem. Recent evidence indicates the existence of such processes in preparations with intact spinal cords (see next subsection) and suggests that they play an important role in determining the percentage of functioning synapses.

Scott and Mendell (315) investigated the projection of all three types of triceps surae efferents (MG, LG, SOL) to their homonymous motoneurons in the intact preparation (Table 5). Although the majority of Ia impulses from MG elicited EPSPs in virtually all homonymous motoneurons, a significant minority evoked EPSPs in only 65% or less of the homonymous pool. The average percentage for all MG Ia-afferent fibers in these experiments was 78%. This decrease from 94% reported by Mendell and Henneman (255)

TABLE 5. *Percentage of Triceps Surae Motoneurons Receiving Homonymous or Heteronymous Projections From Ia-Fibers of Triceps Surae Muscles as Indicated by Spike-Triggered Averaging*

Afferent	Motoneuron		
	MG	LG	SOL
MG	78	54	63
	(89)	(69)	(24)
LG	49	71	68
	(49)	(84)	(19)
SOL	42	74	100
	(46)	(61)	(18)

MG, medial gastrocnemius; LG, lateral gastrocnemius; SOL, soleus. Values represent percentage of motoneurons that develop excitatory postsynaptic potentials. Numbers in parentheses represent total number of observations. [From Scott and Mendell (315).]

was attributed to the finding of these more narrowly projecting afferents. Similar Ia-fibers were found to arise from the LG muscle. Soleus Ia-fibers projected to all (100%) of the SOL motoneurons, but the sample size for this study was relatively small, and this result may be less reliable than for MG and LG afferents. Fibers projecting to less than 65% of homonymous motoneurons have been called type Y. They have conduction velocities similar to fibers projecting to more than 80% of motoneurons, called type X fibers. These are arbitrary classifications, and fibers with intermediate projection percentages exist. Type Y fibers tend to produce smaller EPSPs than type X fibers. It is possible that the smaller projections of type Y fibers result from inability to detect the smaller EPSPs they produce. More recent studies in preparations with spinal cord transection indicate that connectivity has been underestimated in intact preparations and that the error is particularly severe for type Y fibers (see next subsection). Similar connectivity has been reported by Watt et al. (345) for triceps surae afferents and by Nelson and Mendell (269) for semitendinosus afferent fibers. In the latter case a mixture of type Y and type X afferent fibers was seen in about the same proportion as observed for triceps afferent fibers.

FACTORS INFLUENCING PERCENTAGE OF MOTONEURONS RECEIVING HOMONYMOUS PROJECTIONS. Estimates of the projections of single MG Ia-fibers to MG motoneurons in preparations anesthetized with pentobarbital and with intact spinal cords have ranged from 78% to 94% (255, 315). This variation reflects at least in part the proportion of type Y afferent fibers in the sample (269, 315) and the sizes (conduction velocity) of the afferent fibers (Table 6). In anesthetized preparations with spinal cord transections at T_{13} or L_5, single Ia impulses elicit EPSPs in 98% of the homonymous motoneuron pool and no type Y fibers are ever encountered (268). Since these changes occur soon after transection (subject to time required to record from enough motoneurons and also to sampling error), growth of new terminals is an unlikely explanation. It seems more probable that these "new" connections already existed in the intact cord but were inactive. This increase in functioning connections can occur in preparations exhibiting normal EPSP amplitudes (268, 270), so it seems unlikely that an improvement in resolution of small EPSPs is the major factor responsible for the higher percentage of projections observed.

Since the changes after transection occur in a monosynaptic pathway, their locus must be restricted to the presynaptic terminal arborizations or to the synapse itself. It is known that descending impulses can cause presynaptic depolarization of Ia-terminals (53, 54), which might diminish or eliminate conduction through terminal branches (167) and reduce release of transmitter (198, 234). Interruption of this descending input following spinal cord transection might increase the number of motoneurons to which presynaptic impulses have access by a process of presynaptic disinhibition. Under these conditions the distinction between type X and type Y afferent fibers would disappear, since each afferent could evoke EPSPs in each homonymous motoneuron. It follows that these differences observed in preparations with intact spinal cords may reflect functional (e.g., effects of presynaptic inhibition) rather than anatomical factors (i.e., number of motoneurons to which terminals are sent).

In conclusion, it appears that projections to motoneurons can be underestimated in experiments on the intact spinal cord because of inhibitory effects exerted on terminals by systems desending from more rostral regions. The findings as a whole suggest that each Ia-fiber sends terminals to all of its homonymous motoneurons.

Comparison of Projections to Homonymous and Heteronymous Motoneurons

As early as Sherrington's observations (233) it was clear that input to heteronymous motoneurons was weaker than that to homonymous motoneurons. The studies carried out by Lloyd (235) using ventral root discharges, and subsequently by Eccles and collaborators (99, 103) using intracellular recording, confirmed the existence of a weaker monosynaptic excitatory input from Ia-fibers to heteronymous than homonymous motoneurons.

In the context of the previous analysis of Ia-evoked EPSPs, the smaller aggregate EPSPs in heteronymous motoneurons might have resulted from fewer projections to heteronymous motoneurons, smaller EPSPs in the motoneurons, or both. There is agreement among several groups that single Ia-fibers project more widely to homonymous than to heteronymous motoneurons (220, 255, 269, 315, 345). This remains true even after spinal cord transection (268). In early studies (255, 345) individual EPSPs in homonymous motoneurons (MG) were found to be only slightly larger on the average than in heteronymous motoneurons (LG plus SOL). It was concluded that the larger aggregate EPSPs in homonymous motoneurons were due to the projection of more Ia-fibers to homonymous than to heteronymous motoneurons.

This issue was subsequently reexamined by Scott and Mendell (315), who made a special effort to distinguish the projections to LG and SOL motoneurons (whose axons run in the same peripheral nerve), since EPSPs would be expected to be larger in SOL cells due to their smaller size (subsection FACTORS RESPONSIBLE FOR VARIABILITY IN EPSP AMPLITUDES, p. 466). In these studies motoneurons were first classified by antidromic stimulation as either MG or LG-SOL. If they were LG or SOL, the motoneuron was stimulated intracellularly to localize the muscle in which the contraction occurred. The projections from LG and SOL Ia-afferent fibers to these three types of motoneurons were also examined. The results (Table 7) were subjected to a two-way analysis of variance, which showed conclusively that, on the average, individual EPSPs from any of the three afferents were larger in homonymous than in heteronymous moto-

TABLE 6. *Relationship of Axonal Conduction Velocity of Ia-Afferent Fibers and α-Motoneurons to Percent of Homonymous Projections Linking Them*

Conduction Velocity Range, m/s	Projection Frequency From Afferent Fibers	Projection Frequency to Motoneurons
70–80	50% (16)	89% (45)
80–90	81% (80)	78% (131)
90–100	77% (103)	76% (114)
100–110	87% (87)	83% (95)
110–120	96% (25)	82% (17)

Data derived from studies on homonymous projections, including medial and lateral gastrocnemius, soleus and semitendinosus. Numbers in parentheses represent total number of observations. Ia-afferent conduction velocity was often not available. Values in left column refer to conduction velocities of Ia-fibers (middle column) and to conduction velocities of motoneurons (right column). [From data of Mendell and Henneman (255); Nelson, Mendell, et al. (268); and Scott and Mendell (315).]

TABLE 7. *Mean Amplitude of Excitatory Postsynaptic Potentials Elicited by Homonymous and Heteronymous Inputs*

Afferent	Motoneuron		
	MG	LG	SOL
MG	95 (69)	59 (37)	79 (15)
LG	76 (24)	14 (60)	84 (13)
SOL	50 (19)	65 (45)	143 (18)

Excitatory postsynaptic potentials (EPSPs) in triceps surae motoneurons produced by impulses in triceps surae group Ia-afferent fibers. EPSPs obtained by spike-triggered averaging. Values are in microvolts. Values in parentheses are number of observations making up each mean value. Note that largest values are on diagonal representing homonymous combinations. [From Scott and Mendell (315).]

neurons, excluding other factors such as the tendency for EPSPs to be larger in SOL motoneurons because of their small size. The largest EPSPs (greater than 150 μV) occurred almost exclusively in homonymous motoneurons; small EPSPs occurred in both types. In several cases, the EPSPs evoked in the same motoneuron by impulses in one homonymous afferent and one heteronymous afferent were compared (Fig. 38B). Under these more controlled experimental conditions where motoneuron properties were identical for each comparison, the homonymous EPSP was found to be significantly larger on the average than the heteronymous one.

A possible explanation for larger EPSPs in homonymous motoneurons might be a tendency for Ia-fibers to terminate in a preferred location (173, 236), e.g., closer to the soma of these cells (but see subsection EFFICACY OF SYNAPSES ON DIFFERENT PARTS OF MOTONEURON, p. 470). Jack and Porter (184) did, in fact, find a tendency for aggregate EPSPs in homonymous motoneurons to have slightly briefer rise times than in heteronymous ones (but see ref. 220). Scott and Mendell (315) confirmed this finding (see also ref. 263) although the differences in mean rise time, which were very small, could hardly account for the differences in amplitude, given the very weak relationship between amplitude and rise time (see subsection EFFICACY OF SYNAPSES ON DIFFERENT PARTS OF MOTONEURON, p. 470). Thus, it seems likely that factors other than location of terminals on the somadendritic tree account for larger EPSPs in homonymous motoneurons.

Similar studies have been carried out on the projections of Ia-fibers from the semitendinosus muscle to homonymous and heteronymous (posterior biceps, semimembranosus) motoneurons (269). The results confirmed the findings obtained from analysis of triceps surae connections, namely, that homonymous Ia-fibers project to a higher percentage of motoneurons and elicit larger EPSPs than heteronymous fibers.

Attempts to account for differences in projections to homonymous and heteronymous motoneurons can only be speculative at this time. It is important to emphasize that the higher percentage of homonymous projections might be due to the larger individual EPSPs they elicit. The EPSPs too small to be resolved would undoubtedly be more common in heteronymous motoneurons and would therefore reduce the projection frequency to motoneurons in this pool more than to the homonymous pool. However, if resolution were improved, it seems likely that additional small EPSPs would be found more frequently in heteronymous motoneurons. Since the mean EPSP amplitude is calculated taking into account only nonzero values, the differences in mean EPSP amplitude between homonymous and heteronymous motoneurons might be even larger than those found with the present level of resolution.

Since large EPSPs cannot be accounted for by a more proximal location of the active boutons on the soma-dendritic membrane, other factors must be responsible. Kuno (215) proposed that EPSP amplitude was related to the mean quantal content of the EPSP, which was verified for individual EPSPs by Mendell and Weiner (256). A more general conclusion, in view of the discussion in subsection *Physiology of Ia-Terminals*, p. 472, is that larger EPSPs are produced by the action of a greater number of functional presynaptic "units."

A specific proposal (269) that could account for these observations is that afferent fibers give off more boutons on the average to homonymous than to heteronymous motoneurons (Fig. 40). This would result in a larger mean EPSP in homonymous motoneurons. If, in addition, the number of boutons exhibited variability about these means, one would expect *1*) a smaller number of Ia-projections to heteronymous motoneurons, since a greater portion of this distribution of bouton numbers would be truncated at 0 (no boutons; therefore no projection); and *2*) restriction of the largest EPSPs to homonymous motoneurons (315), since only homonymous projections would include the largest number of boutons. It is possible that

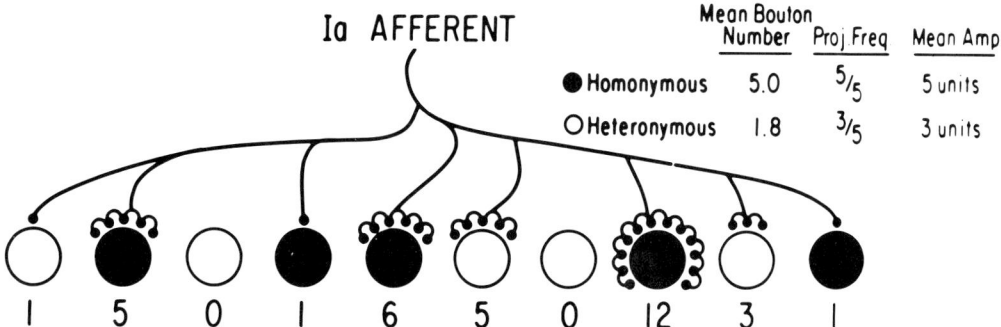

FIG. 40. Model of projection of single Ia-fiber to homonymous and heteronymous motoneurons (*circles*). Systematic differences in mean number of boutons provided by single Ia-fibers to homonymous and heteronymous motoneurons would lead to differences in projection frequency and excitatory postsynaptic potential (EPSP) amplitude in these 2 types of projections. Mean bouton number was chosen using estimates of Iles (177) as a guide. *Numbers* below each *circle* represent number of boutons provided by single Ia-fiber to each motoneuron.

motoneurons have a fixed number of receptor sites for each type of afferent fiber, with more reserved for homonymous than heteronymous Ia-fibers. This hypothesis implies a variable number of boutons per Ia-fiber (51, 177). In its simplest form, it requires that the boutons be identical, so that their number is the decisive variable. The evidence for this is by no means clear. Some investigators (222, 252) have reported that all Ia-boutons are similar, whereas Conradi (72) has described two types, M and S (subsection *Anatomical Studies*, p. 461). It is conceivable that the boutons on homonymous motoneurons may be qualitatively different from those on heteronymous cells, e.g., the larger type M boutons may be restricted to homonymous motoneurons. Another variable of possible significance is bouton size. At the neuromuscular junction the number of quanta released is directly correlated with the size of the nerve terminals (223). Current evidence suggests that there is a fivefold variation in the length of bouton contacts on motoneurons (222), which may account for differences in synaptic efficacy. Variations in the areas of synaptic contact may explain the differences in the amplitude of EPSPs, which occur upon stimulation of small and large Ia-fibers (subsection VARIABILITY OF EPSP AMPLITUDES, p. 465). The optimal technique for resolving these issues may involve filling single afferents and motoneurons with HRP, followed by ultrastructural analysis of the synapse—a difficult task.

Correlations Between Morphology and Function

In a Golgi study on kittens Scheibel and Scheibel (310) provided anatomical evidence that may explain some of the physiological findings that have been described. It is now generally agreed that the soma and dendrites of motoneurons are disposed in a predominantly longitudinal column running for a considerable distance in the rostrocaudal axis of the spinal cord (309, 332). According to Scheibel and Scheibel, each primary Ia-fiber in the dorsal column of the kitten gives off a series of primary afferent collaterals at intervals of 100–200 μm (Fig. 32). These collaterals leave the dorsal column "at right angles and drop ventrally with almost plumb-line precision" (310). Several collaterals run together, forming a "microbundle", which passes perpendicularly through the dendritic field of the motoneurons. Each primary afferent collateral gives off terminals that ramify almost entirely in the mediolateral plane with little rostrocaudal extension. Thus, the terminal field of each collateral is virtually two-dimensional and makes contact with a very limited extent of the longitudinally running motoneurons. The thickness of these two-dimensional fields varies from 10 to 50 μm, with a mean of about 25 μm.

The primary afferent collaterals projecting into the ventral horn at different rostrocaudal levels allow each single Ia-fiber to make contact with virtually all motoneurons in the homonymous pool despite the extent of the pool (up to 8 mm) along the rostrocaudal axis (47, 302). Scheibel and Scheibel (310) suggested that a single Ia-fiber might project to 90–900 α-motoneurons. Physiological studies indicate that a Ia-fiber from MG makes contact with virtually all of the 300 MG motoneurons and at least 60% of the 600 heteronymous cells belonging to the LG and SOL pools.

An important difference between the results of Golgi studies on kittens and more recent studies with horseradish peroxidase (26, 51, 163) is in the number and spacing of the ventrally directed Ia-collaterals. Scheibel and Scheibel (310) reported that 10–100 collaterals were given off at intervals of 100–200 μm. Studies with HRP indicate that only 5–11 collaterals are given off at intervals of about 1 mm. Depending upon which set of figures is used, each collateral could contact as many as 50–60 motoneurons (26) or as few as about 10 (177, 310).

These differences between the number and spacing of collaterals are not easily resolved at this time. It does not seem likely that some branches of Ia-fibers have failed to be filled with HRP, since recent physiological mapping of these collaterals using spike-triggered averaging of the presynaptic spike (see next subsection) indicated that the number of collaterals has not been underestimated (265). A more intriguing possibility is that since the Golgi studies were performed in kittens whereas adult cats were used for the HRP and electrophysiological work, the collateral pattern may undergo changes during maturation. How such reorganization occurs is not known, and no descriptions of degenerating branches are available. However, a substantial loss of boutons from certain regions of the motoneuron occurs in the period immediately after birth (74, 303), and this remodeling process may be related in some manner to reorganization of the Ia-projection.

Many individual EPSPs have time courses indicating that the active Ia-terminals are located in close proximity to each other (e.g., on a single compartment of the motoneuron). In commenting upon this fact, Mendell and Henneman (255) used the then available evidence on spacing between collaterals, i.e., 100–200 μm (310), to conclude that although many collaterals from the same Ia-fiber might have access to any motoneuron whose dendritic tree has a rostrocaudal extent of 1–2 mm (332), the time courses of the EPSPs indicated that only one of these collaterals might actually synapse on the motoneuron. This suggested an interesting possibility, namely, that after one set of endings from a particular Ia-fiber is established on a motoneuron, no others from different collaterals of the same fiber can develop, even on other dendrites of that motoneuron. With the more recent information indicating a spacing of 1 mm between collaterals, it now seems unlikely that more than a single collateral of a Ia-fiber has access to a given motoneuron. However, it remains to be seen whether individual EPSPs in the kitten have a more complex time course than in the adult, suggesting early functional Ia-motoneuron connections that are later eliminated, as has been observed at the neuromuscular junction (28, 293).

Latency of EPSPs

Early studies with aggregate EPSPs elicited by volleys in Ia-fibers fixed their synaptic delay at about 0.5 ms (25). When individual EPSPs were investigated, however, it became apparent that synaptic delay varied considerably from synapse to synapse. Variability was first seen when the interval between the arrival of the dorsal root impulse and the onset of the EPSP was measured (255). Intracellular recording from the motoneuron with spike-triggered averaging often reveals a small brief wave that precedes the onset of the EPSP; this has been interpreted as the arrival of the afferent impulse in the terminal region (189, 345). Munson and Sypert (263) demonstrated that the latency between this presynaptic spike and EPSP onset also fluctuates, thereby localizing the variability to the synapse itself.

A major factor underlying differences in synaptic delay is probably the time required for electrotonic conduction in motoneuron dendrites. This was analyzed by Rall (287) and Iles (178), who showed that EPSPs generated in the distal dendrites of a model motoneuron should exhibit longer delays than those produced in the soma or proximal dendrites. This prediction was confirmed in experiments showing (Fig. 41) that the latencies of EPSPs increased with their rise times (255, 263). Differences in the synaptic delays of homonymous and heteronymous EPSPs were also observed that were consistent with the differences in their rise times [Fig. 41; (263)].

In addition to these differences from synapse to synapse, variability in delay has also been observed in single sweeps at a given synapse (34, 70, 215, 218, 266, 295). This phenomenon is similar to that described previously at the neuromuscular junction (16, 197). The variability in delays at motoneurons has been localized to the synaptic region by the finding that the latency of the presynaptic spike is constant, unlike the fluctuations in latency observed in the subsequent EPSPs (70). These delays can vary by as much as 300–400 μs but most of them are within a 100-μs range and the distribution of latencies is unimodal. The EPSPs with the shorter latencies have the same time courses

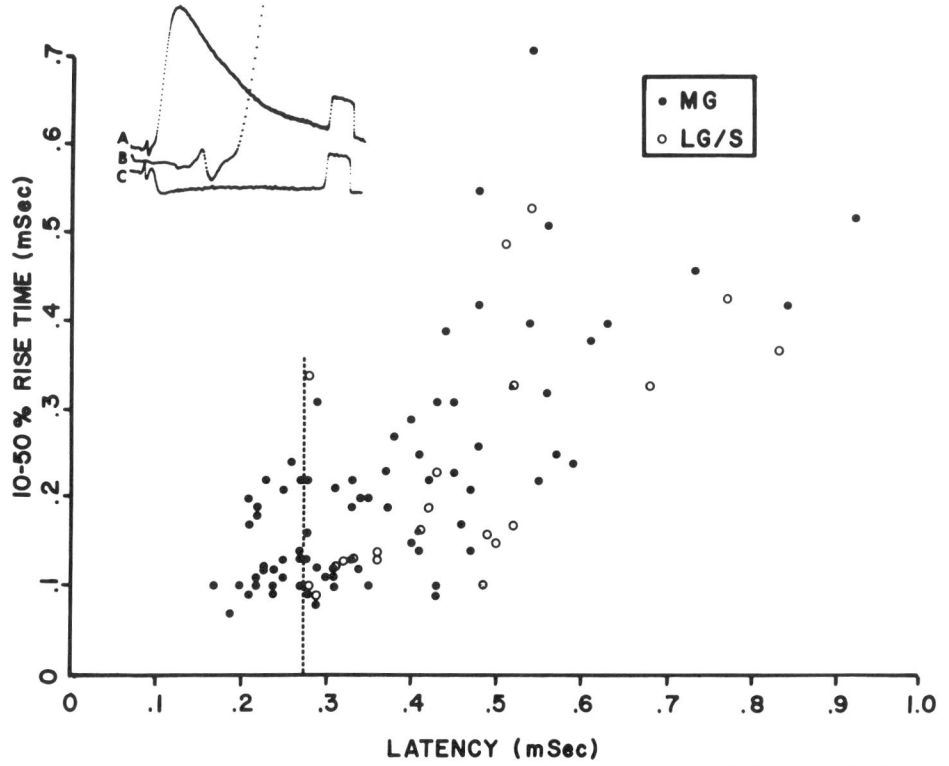

FIG. 41. Scatter diagram of relationship between rise time and latency for single-fiber excitatory postsynaptic potentials (EPSPs) in 78 medial gastrocnemius (MG) and 23 lateral gastrocnemius and soleus (LG-SOL) motoneurons. MG Ia-afferent fibers throughout. *Dashed vertical line* at 0.27 ms denotes minimum latency recorded in heteronymous LG-SOL motoneurons. *Inset* shows intracellular (A), extracellular (C) records from a motoneuron with spike-triggered averaging. Note reversal of EPSP, but not diphasic prespike following withdrawal of electrode. Calibration pulses 50 μV, 1 ms. B is same as A with both scales expanded by 4. Latency was measured from negative (downward going) peak of prespike to onset of EPSP. [From Munson and Sypert (263).]

(rise time, half-width) as those with the longer latencies, which suggests that they are generated by the same terminals and that the latency fluctuations are a property of the release process (70).

These findings are consistent with the idea that the Ia-motoneuron synapse is chemical rather than electrical (266). This issue is currently controversial and further discussion is beyond the scope of this chapter (see review in ref. 295).

One consequence of these fluctuations in latency is that temporal parameters (e.g., rise time) of averaged individual EPSPs are composite values. Any attempt to estimate location of synaptic terminals based on EPSP time course (subsection PHYSIOLOGICAL ANALYSIS OF LOCATION OF BOUTONS, p. 468) is affected by this process, since measured values are somewhat larger than the actual ones.

Other Examples of Divergence in Inputs to Motoneurons

Less direct methods of studying the inputs to motoneurons also indicate considerable divergence of afferent terminals to a motoneuron pool, resulting in a significant degree of correlated firing in the cells of the pool. Working in the respiratory system, Sears and Stagg (317) have used spike-triggered averaging to show, by means of pre- and poststimulus time histograms, that the discharge of motor axons is highly correlated with the firing of other motor axons. This result was perhaps predictable in view of previous findings that impulses in single Ia-fibers excite all the members of a pool at approximately the same time. Use of the EMG rather than recordings from motor nerves makes the Sears and Stagg technique suitable for human studies, which is an important advantage.

The preceding study led to the hypothesis that the joint occurrence of EPSPs elicited in motoneurons by impulses in branches of common stem presynaptic fibers causes a transient depolarization in one respiratory motoneuron at the time of discharge in another motoneuron of the same pool. The hypothesis was tested by averaging the synaptic noise of inspiratory motoneurons (209). A depolarization centered around the time of the trigger spikes was consistently observed and was designated the average common excitation (a.c.e.) potential. The a.c.e. potentials had a mean amplitude of 32 μV when the trigger signals came from a filament in the same segment, but only 19 μV when the filament was two segments rostral to the motoneuron. The a.c.e. potentials were recorded when either α- or γ-discharges served as triggers. This was regarded as evidence for α-γ-coactivation by common presynaptic axons. The authors have developed a theory that accounts for the main features of the a.c.e. potential.

Another indication that impulses in branches of common stem presynaptic fibers are an important mechanism for correlating the activity of members of a motoneuron pool was noted by Rudomin and colleagues (see review in ref. 44). They report that fluctuations in the amplitudes of Ia-evoked EPSPs are correlated to a significant degree in different motoneurons in a pool from which intracellular recordings are made simultaneously (305). Primary-afferent depolarization, which may affect many related Ia-terminals synchronously, may account for some of the correlations in motoneuron discharge. Whether widespread depolarization occurs via the action of interneurons, which branch to terminate on many Ia-terminals, or because of correlated firing among large pools of interneurons having relatively narrow projections, is not known. Whatever the mechanism, the findings suggest that modifications in synaptic input may be exerted in such a way as not to disturb the relative strengths of inputs to motoneurons in a pool, and thus preserve recruitment order.

Ia-Projections to Motoneurons Controlling Other Parts of the Body

The previous discussions have centered on reflex connections involving the hindlimb of the cat. In this subsection functional aspects of Ia-motoneuron connections for muscles controlling other regions of the body are briefly discussed.

Forelimb muscles in the baboon have a substantial complement of spindles. Afferent fibers from them project to both homonymous and heteronymous motoneurons (65). Projections to heteronymous motoneurons are generally, although not always, weaker than those to homonymous motoneurons as measured by their mean aggregate EPSP. The differences, however, do not appear to be as great as for motoneurons supplying cat hindlimb muscles.

The spike-triggered averaging technique has been used to examine the monosynaptic connections made by afferents from jaw elevator muscle spindles to masseter and temporalis motoneurons (7). Intracellular recording revealed monosynaptic projections in only 14 of 91 instances and a mean amplitude of only 18 μV. These connections were studied further by using the spike-triggered averaging procedure to measure the extracellular fields produced by impulses in single Ia-fibers. These fields were found to be highly localized within the motor nucleus and were found to be somewhat larger in response to input from dynamic spindles than from static ones, again confirming the smaller monosynaptic action from the slower conducting fibers of smaller diameter discussed in subsection FACTORS RESPONSIBLE FOR VARIABILITY IN EPSP AMPLITUDES, p. 466. The authors explained this very limited projection as possibly resulting from the compound structure of these muscles, which have multiple insertion points, unlike limb muscles with single insertions. Spindles from a given part of the muscle might therefore project to only certain functionally related motoneurons.

Considerable effort has been devoted to the study

of reflexes in respiratory muscles, where it is known that a powerful monosynaptic reflex exists from large-diameter fibers (316) and a weaker one from group II fibers (207, 208). The details of the distribution of Ia-fibers from external and internal intercostal muscles in various segments to the motoneurons innervating these muscles are not known. Since prevention of spindle unloading by tracheal occlusion during inspiration causes increased inspiratory motoneuron discharge (76), it would appear that Ia excitation is directed toward homonymous motoneurons, as in limb muscle reflexes.

Neck muscles are well supplied with spindles that send fibers to make monosynaptic connections with motoneurons innervating these muscles. Recent experiments indicate that these connections are quite selective (4), with splenius group Ia-fibers sending few terminals to biventer cervicis and complexus motoneurons, and spindles of the latter muscles sending Ia-terminals to their own motoneurons rather than to those supplying splenius. This organization is similar to that seen for limb muscles with respect to projections to homonymous and heteronymous motoneurons. Functional studies indicate that splenius and the biventer cervicis–complexus group have different actions (299). Despite the existence of these well-defined monosynaptic connections as revealed by recording aggregate EPSPs, monosynaptic reflexes to these muscles may be hard to demonstrate under some experimental conditions (1).

These examples indicate that the widespread projections of Ia-fibers from hindlimb muscles in the cat are not necessarily present in all Ia-motoneuron systems. One must be careful in extrapolating findings from this well-studied system to all others.

Group II Input From Secondary Endings in Muscle Spindles

In the past few years it has become apparent that group II fibers from muscle spindles must send some of their terminals directly to homonymous motoneurons (207, 208, 244, 328). Early studies using electrical stimulation of group II fibers in muscle nerves with unavoidable activation of their Ia- and Ib-fibers had revealed central synaptic effects, similar to those elicited by impulses in cutaneous fibers, that were inhibitory to extensor motoneurons (104, 229). The different synaptic effects of impulses in group II and group Ia fibers were always puzzling because of the similarity in location and adequate stimulus of their receptors. The use of the spike-triggered averaging technique to study the connections of group II spindle fibers has demonstrated the existence of a monosynaptic excitatory projection to homonymous extensor motoneurons (Fig. 42) and the probable existence of polysynaptic projections to motoneurons from the same fibers. Although the conduction time in the central processes of group II fibers was slower than that of Ia-fibers, synaptic delay, as measured from the prespike to the onset of the EPSP, was identical to that of EPSPs elicited by Ia impulses (328), as illustrated in Figure 42.

Stauffer et al. (328) found that impulses in group II fibers from MG spindles evoked EPSPs in 52% of MG motoneurons and in 26% of LG-S cells, compared to 87% and 61%, respectively, for impulses in Ia-fibers under similar experimental conditions (345). The mean amplitudes of the group II EPSPs were 38 μV and 12 μV compared with 67 μV and 54 μV for Ia-EPSPs. These findings suggest that group II fibers give off fewer terminals to motoneurons than Ia-fibers. This is consistent with the conclusion reached in examining EPSPs elicited by impulses in Ia-fibers of different diameters (Table 1). The smaller EPSPs evoked by impulses in group II fibers probably represent an extension of the relationship between Ia-fiber diameter and individual EPSP size. Lüscher, Henneman, et al. (244) found that the amplitudes of the postsynaptic population potentials (PSPPs) recorded from an entire ventral root were directly related to the conduction velocities of the Ia or group II impulses that evoked the PSPPs. Of course, factors other than afferent fiber diameter probably influence the size of PSPPs. For example, if the number of terminals given off by an afferent fiber is a function of the diameter of that fiber, the relationship between conduction velocity of afferent fiber and amplitude of EPSP should be the same for both group Ia and group II afferents. However, Lüscher, Henneman, et al. found different slopes relating these variables, which indicates that factors other than the number of terminals alone influence the size of a PSPP.

Lüscher, Henneman, et al. (244) have also found that the rise times of PSPPs evoked by group II impulses are slower than those of PSPPs elicited by Ia impulses. This indicates that the synaptic terminals given off by group II fibers may be located, on the average, more distally on the dendritic tree than terminals from Ia-fibers. These results suggest a possible distinction between dendritic and somatic activity. The more dendritically located synapses, generating slower EPSPs (measured at the soma) might be chiefly responsible for the maintenance and regulation of the general excitatory state of the motoneuron pool. They would be well suited to process input from secondary endings, which are most sensitive to the static length of the muscle. In contrast, the more proximally located input would be apt to cause rapid triggering of reflex discharge. This would be an appropriate response to input from primary receptors, which are most sensitive to rapid changes in muscle length. The sustained synaptic activity in the dendrites, produced by input from secondary endings may, therefore, modify the effectiveness of the input from primary endings. This functional distinction in the central processing of signals from primary and secondary endings may shed some light on how inputs from different peripheral

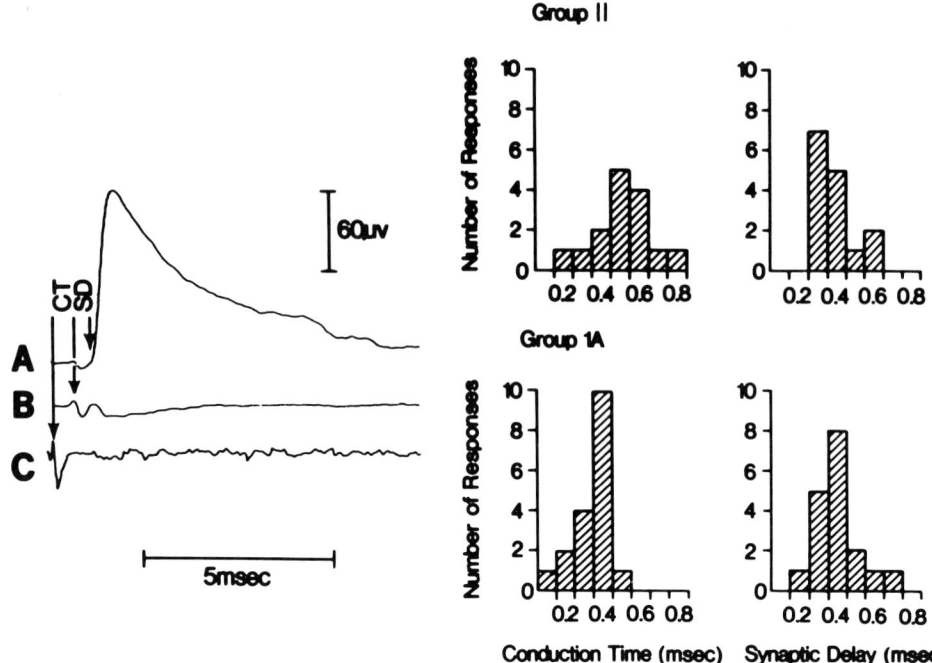

FIG. 42. Comparison of synaptic delay associated with single-fiber excitatory postsynaptic potentials (EPSPs) produced by group Ia and group II fibers in cat. *Left*, trace A represents potential recorded inside a medial gastrocnemius (MG) motoneuron with spike-triggered averaging from a group II afferent fiber. The large upward potential is EPSP, which is preceded by a brief diphasic potential considered to arise from activity in presynaptic terminals of group II fiber. *Trace B* is record obtained by spike-triggered averaging from a position just outside motoneuron. The early potential is not inverted, indicating that it is produced outside motoneuron and unlike EPSP, which reverses, showing that it is generated across the membrane. *Trace C* is averaged record recorded from group II fiber in dorsal rootlet. Interval from dorsal root spike to presynaptic spike is conduction time (CT) and remaining time to EPSP onset is synaptic delay (SD). *Right*, histograms of conduction time and synaptic delay for group II fibers (*top*) and group Ia-fibers (*bottom*). Note similarities in synaptic delay for both types of fiber and trend for shorter conduction time in (the larger) group-Ia fibers. [From Stauffer et al. (328).]

receptors can act together at the level of the motoneurons.

Inhibitory Inputs to Motoneurons

Motoneurons also receive inhibitory inputs which play an important role in determining their discharge properties. Recruitment and critical firing level studies have shown that inhibitory inputs from many sources affect motoneurons according to their size, with large motoneurons being more easily silenced. This is opposite to the situation with excitatory inputs where large motoneurons are the least susceptible to discharge (section FIRING PATTERNS OF INDIVIDUAL MOTONEURONS AND MOTOR UNITS, p. 435). The organization of inhibitory inputs to motoneurons is, unfortunately, more difficult to characterize because the projections from the periphery are not monosynaptic.

Burke et al. (46) have obtained evidence that the amplitude of aggregate disynaptic IPSPs in antagonist motoneurons is directly correlated with the amplitude of their monosynaptic EPSPs, the largest IPSPs being found in small cells. Since the small cells in a pool are the last to be silenced by inhibition, additional factors must be involved in determining susceptibility to inhibition, e.g., the amount of excess excitation (section FIRING PATTERNS OF INDIVIDUAL MOTONEURONS AND MOTOR UNITS, p. 435). The mechanism by which an orderly distribution of inhibitory input is achieved without interfering with recruitment order is not known. It apparently does not involve widely diverging projections at each synaptic level (see next subsection).

IA INHIBITORY INTERNEURONS. The only interneuronal input studied systematically at the level of individual IPSPs is the projection from interneurons mediating disynaptic Ia inhibition (188, 189). The appropriate interneurons were identified from their pattern of responses to peripheral muscle nerve stimulation and by their projection into the motoneuron pool. Their synapses on antagonistic motoneurons were studied by a modified version of the spike-triggered averaging described in subsection *Techniques Used to Study EPSPs Elicited by Impulses in Single Afferent Fibers*, p. 464 (Fig. 43). Instead of natural activation of the interneuron, it was made to fire by iontophoresis of glutamate. The interneuronal spikes triggered the

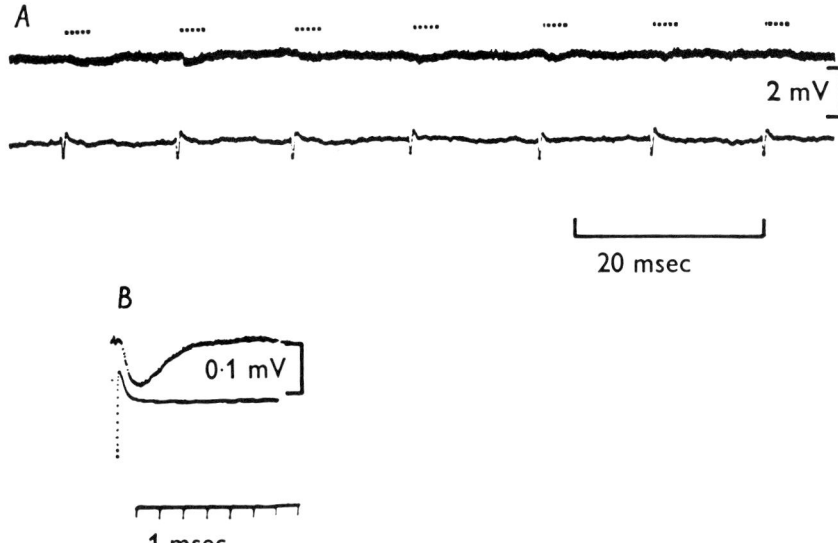

FIG. 43. Inhibitory postsynaptic potential (IPSP) in a cat motoneuron analyzed by spike-triggered averaging. A: *top trace* is intracellular record from a posterior biceps or semitendinosus motoneuron. *Bottom trace* is extracellular spike activity from an interneuron satisfying the criteria required for a Ia-interneuron. Interneuron is excited by iontophoretically applied glutamate and discharges rhythmically. Each spike is associated with an IPSP (overlaid by row of *dots*). B: averages of 512 sweeps triggered by interneuronal spike from motoneuron (*above*) and interneuron (*below*). Trigger level was set so that averaging began at beginning of interneuronal spike. [From Jankowska and Roberts (189).]

computer, which averaged the intracellular postsynaptic potential in the motoneuron. The IPSPs were also examined in single sweeps without averaging.

The projection of 12 quadriceps-activated interneurons (Q) was examined in 43 posterior biceps–semitendinosus motoneurons (PBST) that were within 100 μm of the interneuronal terminals. A projection from a Q interneuron to this subset of PBST motoneurons was found in 38 of 43 instances (88%). Since single Q interneurons were found to project to about 50% of the length of the PBST motor pool, giving off terminals to about 40% of this region and innervating about 90% of the neurons within this restricted region, it was estimated that single Q interneurons terminate on about 20% of the entire PBST motor pool. The PBST interneurons were found to innervate a somewhat smaller proportion of Q motoneurons. It was suggested that a divergence of single Ia-fibers to supply a large proportion of the interneurons, as is the case with the monosynaptic Ia–motoneuron projection (subsection PERCENTAGE OF MOTONEURONS RECEIVING TERMINALS FROM SINGLE Ia-FIBERS, p. 473), could result in a widespread effect from single Ia-fibers to motoneurons over this disynaptic inhibitory pathway.

The mean amplitude of these individual IPSPs was 52 μV. The distribution of amplitudes in repeated trials indicates a quantal release mechanism (224). Comparison with the mean aggregate IPSP (3.6 mV) suggested that about 70 interneurons converge on each PBST motoneuron.

Shape-index plots (half-width vs. rise time) indicate that these interneuronal terminals are located on the proximal dendrites or soma, since the rise times and half-widths were always quite brief. Individual Ia-EPSPs exhibit a much wider range of rise times and half-widths, which overlaps the values observed for these IPSPs. Reversal of individual IPSPs by intracellular chloride injection was always seen, also suggesting that the boutons from a single interneuron were grouped on the soma of the motoneuron. Complex nonuniform reversals were often seen in the case of aggregate IPSPs.

In many cases, averaged individual IPSPs were preceded by a small spike similar to that occurring prior to individual EPSPs (subsection *Latency of EPSPs*, p. 477). The latency between presynaptic spike and IPSP onset ranged from 0.28 to 0.42 ms, which is consistent with a monosynaptic connection.

The distribution of disynaptic inhibition from MG Ia-fibers to motoneurons has been studied with the spike-triggered averaging technique (345). Although the amplitude of the recorded IPSP is a poor measure of this disynaptic projection, because the interposed interneuron does not allow the motoneuron to respond in one-to-one fashion, a useful estimate of the divergence of single Ia-fibers to target cells connected via interneurons can be obtained. The IPSPs with latencies consistent with a disynaptic pathway (1.2–2.4 ms) were found primarily in tibialis anterior and extensor digitorum longus motoneurons, ankle flexors which one would expect to show disynaptic IPSPs in response to MG Ia impulses. Longer latency IPSPs suggestive of trisynaptic action were also observed, again mostly in ankle flexors.

RENSHAW CELLS. Another well-defined inhibitory input to α-motoneurons is provided by Renshaw cells. These cells are situated in the ventral horn medial to α-motoneurons (186). They are activated by the recurrent axon collaterals of motoneurons and respond to ventral root stimulation with a characteristic high-frequency repetitive discharge (97, 348). The output of these cells is directed toward α- and γ-motoneurons (97), other Renshaw cells (306), and interneurons mediating Ia inhibition to motoneurons (172). In each case, their action is inhibitory. A more complete review of these topics is given by Burke and Rudomin (44).

Antidromic stimulation studies have revealed that Renshaw cell axons can project to sites up to 12 mm apart along the spinal cord (190). These fibers are not restricted to the gray matter, but run in the ventral funiculi. Terminals to the motor nuclei appear to be limited to within 4 mm of the Renshaw cell. More distant terminals apparently go to Ia inhibitory interneurons (190). There is no direct evidence concerning the degree of convergence of Renshaw cells on motoneurons; in particular, the amplitudes of their individual IPSPs are not known, so that comparison with their aggregate IPSP is not feasible. Although the recurrent IPSP is finely graded upon ventral root stimulation suggesting substantial convergence from these cells (97, 348), Renshaw cells discharge more rapidly in response to increasing strength of stimulation. The increase in IPSP amplitude could, therefore, represent temporal summation as well as spatial summation. The finding that a single Renshaw cell gives off terminals to motoneurons only within 4 mm of its cell body suggests that divergence of single cells cannot include an entire motoneuron pool whose cells can extend over as much as 10 mm (302). Although the number of motoneurons contacted by a single Renshaw cell is not known (313), the distribution of recurrent inhibitory action seems to be restricted to the motor pool whose nerve is stimulated and to its synergists (97). In addition, motoneurons receiving this inhibitory action tend to be located in close proximity to the antidromically activated ones, which is not surprising in view of the short-range projection of Renshaw cells to motoneurons (190).

There is evidence that activation of large motor axons produces a much larger excitatory effect on Renshaw cell firing than activation of small motor axons (193, 307). The notion that large motor axons provide a more powerful input to Renshaw cells is further supported (307) by evidence that small reflex ventral root volleys (in small fibers) elicit much smaller Renshaw effects than similarly sized antidromic volleys (in large fibers). These observations are further examples of the size principle; larger motoneurons exert larger synaptic effects than small cells. Since studies with electrical stimulation suggest that Renshaw inhibition is most potent in small cells (97, 131, 214), it has been suggested that during some phasic movements large motoneurons might be able to selectively inhibit small cells. However, the evidence discussed in section FIRING PATTERNS OF INDIVIDUAL MOTONEURONS AND MOTOR UNITS, p. 435, indicates that recruitment occurs according to the size principle for both fast ballistic movements as well as for slow ramp movements and that deliberate application of Renshaw cell inhibition does not silence firing in small motoneurons before that in larger cells (see Fig. 24).

Analysis of the effects exerted by Ia-interneurons and Renshaw cells on motoneurons requires consideration of the other inputs that drive these interneurons as well as the synaptic relationship between them. Such a discussion is beyond the scope of this chapter, but the reader is referred to recent articles and reviews on this subject (e.g., refs. 116, 171, and the chapter by Baldissera, Hultborn, and Illert in this *Handbook*).

Group Ib Input From Golgi Tendon Organs

Tendon organs respond primarily to tension produced by the active contraction of motor units directly in series with the receptor (166). Previous studies (100, 229) indicated that activity in this projection to motoneurons was mediated by a circuit with one interneuron, i.e., a disynaptic afferent pathway, and was inhibitory to homonymous motoneurons. The Ib-fibers do not send terminals directly into the ventral horn. Many of their terminals end in lamina VI (27, 163, 347) where they synapse with a well-localized group of interneurons (240). The complete projection of these interneurons is not known, but many of their axons go directly to motoneurons. In addition, such interneurons receive extensive convergence from other segmental and descending pathways (242).

The distribution of Ib effects to motoneurons of various species has been studied by means of spike-triggered averaging (345). In numerous homonymous and heteronymous motoneurons IPSPs were seen after prolonged averaging (400–16,000 sweeps). The responses were somewhat jagged and irregular despite this extensive averaging, an indication that only occasional Ib impulses triggered the discharge of the inhibitory interneuron that elicited the IPSP. Nevertheless, these potentials were more clearly defined than similarly evoked EPSPs found chiefly in the motoneurons of direct and indirect antagonist muscles. The IPSP latencies ranged from 0.6 to 6.0 ms, suggesting the existence of di- and trisynaptic linkages from Ib-fibers to motoneurons. The amplitudes of these responses were small (5.2 ± 3.5 μV), as would be expected in averaging over pathways involving more than one synapse. These results, obtained with physiological excitation of receptors, confirm earlier, less direct methods in showing that impulses from Golgi tendon organs exert disynaptic inhibitory effects on both homonymous and heteronymous motoneurons. They also confirm the existence of excitatory connections to motoneurons of antagonists. These studies suggest that the projection from individual Ib-fibers is not sufficiently focused on the interneurons to fire them reliably, judging from the relative infrequency of responses in motoneurons. Recent HRP studies (163) on single Ib-fibers demonstrate that they distribute collaterals at several rostrocaudal levels to interneurons, much as Ia-fibers do.

Monosynaptic Input From Descending Pathways

A number of descending systems project monosynaptically to motoneurons. In particular, evidence exists for direct projections from vestibulospinal, reticulospinal, rubrospinal, and corticospinal systems. However, these projections differ substantially from one another. In some cases, the nature of a given projection varies with the species of animal. This general subject has recently been reviewed by Burke and Rudomin (44).

The vestibulospinal tract is well organized in all mammalian species. Two uncrossed descending systems exist: the lateral vestibulospinal tract originating from the cells of the lateral vestibular (Deiters') nucleus and the medial vestibulospinal pathway, which originates from the medial vestibular nucleus. The lateral system has a strong excitatory projection to neck motoneurons and to hindlimb extensor motoneurons, particularly those of the knee and ankle (133, 349) but not to motoneurons supplying forelimb muscles (349). One descending fiber may influence neurons in both cervical and lumbar segments (2). Monosynaptic vestibular effects on motoneurons are quite weak, with maximal composite EPSPs generally smaller than 2 mV (133, 241). Spike-triggered averaging studies have revealed a limited divergence from descending fibers to motoneurons with relatively small individual EPSPs (less than 40 μV). The time course of these individual EPSPs as well as of aggregate EPSPs (292) suggests more proximal locations of vestibular terminals than of Ia-terminals generally.

The medial vestibulospinal tract terminates exclusively in rostral spinal cord segments. An unusual feature is the generation of monosynaptic IPSPs in neck motoneurons (349). This pathway has been studied with the spike-triggered averaging technique and it was found that the IPSPs were generally smaller than 80 μV. Their reversibility with somatic hyperpolarizing currents as well as their brief times to peak (292) indicate that these IPSPs are generated at proximal boutons. Single fibers in this tract project to less than 50% of the motoneurons in a pool.

Two descending systems with relatively little direct input to motoneurons are the rubrospinal and reticulospinal tracts. In the cat only a small monosynaptic rubrospinal projection to α-motoneurons exists (164) although this crossed pathway provides terminals to all levels of the spinal cord. A small monosynaptic projection to motoneurons supplying distal muscles exists in the monkey. Comparison of the spontaneous EPSPs, ranging from 0.2 to 0.6 mV in amplitude (319), with the aggregate EPSPs (less than 1.2 mV) suggests a restricted convergence of different fibers from the red nucleus on single α-motoneurons. Effects of membrane polarization indicate that terminals of rubrospinal fibers are located at similar distances from the soma as Ia-terminals (320). The reticulospinal pathway is uncrossed and projects both in cat and monkey to hindlimb flexors (134, 241), forelimb flexors and extensors (349), and neck and back motoneurons (350). The small size of aggregate EPSPs again indicates relatively limited convergence from this source on α-motoneurons (318).

The corticospinal pathway is largely crossed and makes monosynaptic connections with flexor and extensor motoneurons, supplying forelimbs and hindlimbs in the monkey, but not in the cat. In the cat, individual fibers may send terminals to both cervical and lumbar cord (323). The aggregate EPSPs are in general large compared to those produced by volleys in reticulospinal and rubrospinal pathways. A much stronger projection is directed to motoneurons controlling distal than proximal muscles (65, 187, 282). Injection of intracellular currents (320) indicates that the active terminals are more proximal than those from Ia-fibers. The smoothly graded nature of the aggregate EPSP indicates that there is considerable convergence from corticospinal axons onto α-motoneurons (187, 282).

In primates some descending systems are reported to terminate selectively on large α-motoneurons. Rubrospinal (8, 39) and large corticospinal (8) axons send excitatory terminals to large motoneurons. Small cells in the same pool are apparently unaffected or, in some cases, are inhibited. Corticospinal axons of smaller diameter distribute their terminals more uniformly to motoneurons of all sizes. In cats these systems do not project directly to motoneurons, but in humans there is apparently a larger direct projection. Detailed physiological studies of these descending projections similar to those on single Ia-fibers have not been carried out. Other direct projections that are involved in movement, such as the vestibulospinal (8), exert excitatory actions on both small and large motoneurons in the same pool. At present there is little evidence that higher centers and their projections are used in isolation to achieve special patterns of recruitment within a pool.

Topographic Factors Governing Development of Connections of Ia-Fibers to Motoneurons

One of the most important questions facing neuroscientists is how the neurons in the brain establish their specific patterns of connections. The projections of primary sensory neurons to motoneurons provide a specific example of this connectivity that has obvious advantages for study. Since motoneurons to different muscles are often adjacent to one another and slightly intermingled in the spinal cord (44, 302), ingrowing afferent fibers must have some way of establishing the necessary orderly connectivity. Various hypotheses have been advanced to explain the precision of such connections. The chemoaffinity hypothesis formulated by Sperry (326) proposes that neurons become chemically differentiated during development depending on the positions they occupy. This enables the axons of neurons to recognize matching or complementary labels on target neurons. Eccles (96) proposed that the surface properties of motoneurons are the basis for recognition by afferent fibers. The finding that the mean size of an aggregate EPSP is larger in homonymous than heteronymous motoneurons (99) led Eccles to postulate that Ia-fibers establish connections with motoneurons by a process of "species recognition." The foregoing parts of this section provide considerable new evidence consistent with the hypothesis of species specificity (see also refs. 225–228 for evidence concerning inherent species specificity of motoneurons).

Others have challenged the notion of a unique role for species specificity, suggesting "that there is a certain stage in the development of most neural centers during which they become topographically polarized in such a way that the constituent neurons acquire some determining characteristic that establishes the spatial organization of the projection as a whole" (77). Basing their arguments on genetic considerations and analogies with sensory systems, Wyman et al. (355, 356) have suggested that topographic factors may account for connectivity in the spinal cord without specification of connections by neuronal species. A recent study with a new electrophysiological technique (156) provides considerable new evidence regarding the importance of such topographic factors.

Postsynaptic population potentials (PSPPs), evoked in large numbers of motoneurons by impulses in single Ia-fibers or spindle group II fibers, were recorded simultaneously from two adjacent ventral roots perfused with isotonic sucrose. By comparing the amplitudes of these PSPPs with the entry points of the afferent fibers, the distribution of their terminals was inferred. The Ia impulses entering a spinal segment evoked larger PSPPs in its motoneurons than in those of the adjacent segment. The size of the PSPP was correlated with the exact entry level of the afferent fiber, indicating that Ia-fibers give off more endings to motoneurons located near the entry point. Figure 44 reproduces records from a typical experiment that illustrate how the cord entry points of three afferent fibers influenced the amplitudes of the PSPPs their impulses evoked. The conduction velocity, entry point, and muscle of origin of each of the three afferent fibers are shown schematically in Figure 44A–C. The PSPPs recorded simultaneously from the lower part of L_7VR and from S_1VR are reproduced. In each pair of records the larger PSPP was recorded from the spinal segment that the afferent fiber entered. The entry points of these gastrocnemius fibers were extremely important in determining the size of the PSPPs they evoked. These general findings indicate that a Ia-fiber gives off more terminals to motoneurons in the regions near its entry point. Connectivity is not determined entirely by species specificity as some early findings may suggest.

To demonstrate the effect of the precise level of entry on the amplitude of a PSPP, data from individual experiments were utilized. Figure 45 illustrates how the amplitudes of PSPPs depend on both the conduction velocities and entry points of the afferent impulses eliciting them. The conduction velocity and the entry level of the afferent fibers are plotted on the horizontal plane. The amplitude of the corresponding PSPPs are plotted on the vertical scale. Data from 11 out of 22 afferent units in this experiment were selected for display according to the following criteria. First, six units with the same entry level (2.0 ± 0.2 mm) were chosen to illustrate the effects of their different conduction velocities. Second, seven units with the same conduction velocities (84 ± 1.0 m/s) were selected to show the effects of their different levels of entry. The illustration shows how the amplitude of PSPPs increases with the conduction velocity of the impulses evoking them. A clear maximum of PSPP amplitude can be seen for units entering the caudal part of S_1DR (illustrating that PSPPs are largest when entry level and recording level coincide). The PSPP size decreases for units entering the cord either more cranially or more caudally. The decrease in amplitude with distance is, however, not symmetrical in both directions. These findings suggest that somatotopic factors are more important than previously believed in the development of these monosynaptic connections. The somatotopic distribution of terminals described here provides a possible explanation for the topographically localized stretch reflexes within a single muscle originally described by Cohen (67, 68) and the focusing of signal transmission in the multichannel muscle stretch system postulated by Windhorst (351).

Concluding Comments

The action of a motor pool is determined to a large extent by the distribution of afferent input to its individual members of motoneurons. The best studied afferent input to spinal α-motoneurons is provided by group Ia-fibers. The most striking result is that each single Ia-fiber distributes the excitatory action to all homonymous motoneurons even though these can number in the hundreds. In general the amount of excitatory action (EPSP amplitude) is greatest in small motoneurons. Consideration of the details of transmission at this synapse reveals a number of factors that might influence EPSP amplitude; these include presynaptic processes such as terminal invasion

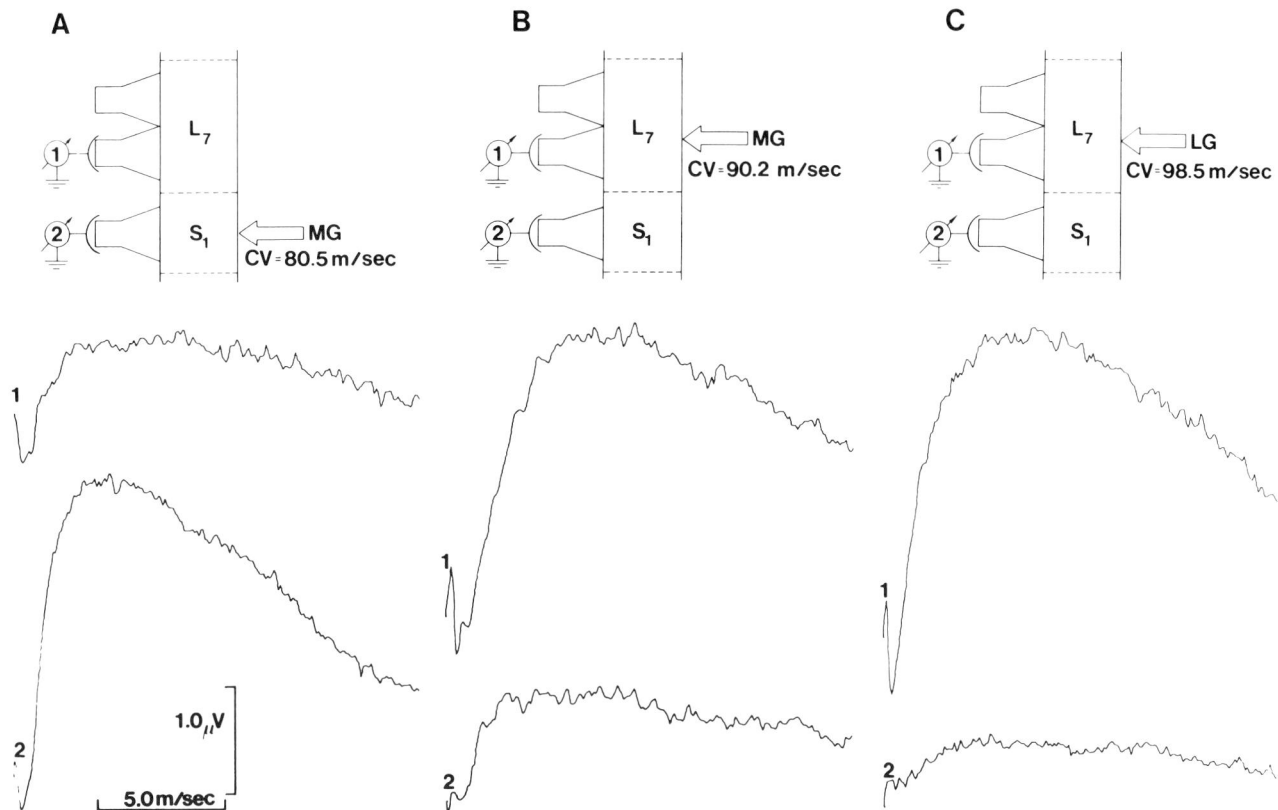

FIG. 44. Influence of entry level of Ia-fiber of cat on amplitude of postsynaptic population potentials (PSPPs) its impulses elicit. Data are from a single experiment. Schematic drawings in *top* of figure illustrate recording arrangements on ventral roots (VR); CV represents conduction velocity. *Arrow* points at spinal segment that the afferent fiber enters. The PSPPs recorded from caudal part of 7th lumbar ventral root (L_7VR) and 1st sacral ventral root (1) and 1st sacral (S_1VR) (2) are reproduced below. *A*: Ia-fiber arising in medial gastrocnemius (MG) enters through S_1 dorsal root. *B*: Ia-fiber from MG enters spinal segment L_7. *C*: Ia-fiber from lateral gastrocnemius (LG) enters spinal segment L_7. Each PSPP was averaged 4,096 sweeps. [From Lüscher, Ruenzel, and Henneman (246).]

and release from boutons, both of which may be subject to external control. Postsynaptic factors include location of synapses on the somadendritic tree as well as motoneuron properties such as resistance. A discussion of the possible mechanism generating the inverse relation between EPSP amplitude and motoneuron size is deferred to section HOW SIZE OF MOTONEURONS DETERMINES THEIR SUSCEPTIBILITY TO DISCHARGE, p. 491.

The global projection of Ia input to homonymous α-motoneurons stands in marked contrast to the organization of all other segmental (heteronymous Ia, interneuronal) and descending systems where single fibers appear to have a much more restricted projection to α-motoneurons. At present it is not known whether these act to fractionate the motor pool, in effect preventing its collective action, or whether these systems are themselves activated in a manner that ensures the stereotyped action of the pool expected from the group Ia-fiber input. Information presented in section FIRING PATTERNS OF INDIVIDUAL MOTONEURONS AND MOTOR UNITS, p. 435, suggests that at least under most experimental conditions, the motor pool behaves in a uniform manner, indicating that the organization of these motoneuronal inputs is extremely important.

NONUNIFORMITY OF MOTONEURONS

Motoneurons differ in their shape, size, connections, and electrical properties. Whether these differences are sufficiently basic to classify motoneurons into different types or species is a major issue in this field. The facts that the contractile properties of muscle fibers are so strongly influenced by the discharge patterns of their motoneurons and that muscle fibers are classified into at least three types, have led investigators to look for corresponding types of motoneurons. To date there is no clear basis, however, in their histochemistry or ultrastructure for making sharp distinctions between motoneurons.

The differences described below are essential for a proper appreciation of the organization of the motoneuron pool. They are also of practical importance for an understanding of certain neuromuscular disease processes, as is noted below.

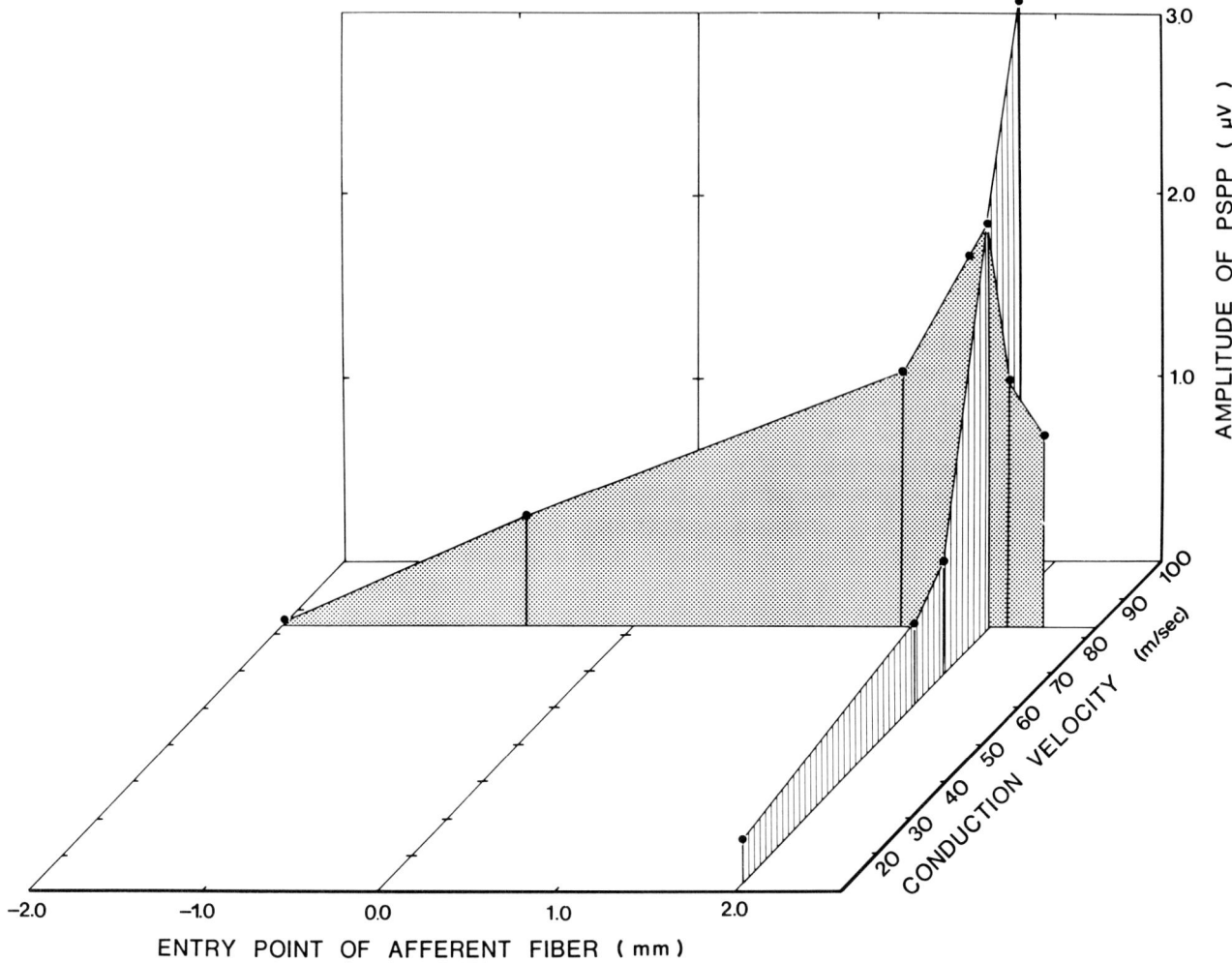

FIG. 45. Three-dimensional graph illustrating relationship between amplitude of postsynaptic population potentials (PSPPs) and conduction velocity and spinal entry point of afferent impulses evoking them. Amplitudes were averaged over 4,096 sweeps and were recorded from 1st sacral ventral root. Data were derived from a single experiment. All afferent fibers had origin in medial gastrocnemius muscle. [From Lüscher, Ruenzel, and Henneman (246).]

Early Classification of Tonic and Phasic Types of Motoneurons

As a result of earlier studies, Granit believed that there were probably two types of motoneurons, those that subserve long-lasting "tonic" or postural motor functions and those that initiate brief "phasic" responses. To determine whether these tonic and phasic motoneurons were basically different types of cells, Granit and colleagues (129) devised tests to accentuate the differences between them. Recordings were made from axons of ankle extensor motoneurons in ventral root filaments of decerebrate cats. After the response of each unit had been recorded during three control stretches, the muscle nerve was stimulated electrically at 500 impulses/s for 10 s with the myograph disconnected. Beginning 20 s after the tetanus, the response of each unit was reexamined every 10 s. In the posttetanic or potentiated state the responses to a constant 10-mm stretch fell into two main categories: 1) a tonic discharge that went on for a long time, and 2) a phasic discharge, consisting of only one or two impulses during the rising phase of the stretch. Intermediate units were seen but were given little attention. The phasic units generated larger spikes in general than the tonic ones in the ventral root recordings.

Following this work, the terms tonic and phasic came into common use to distinguish two types of motoneurons and their responses to stretch. In an early paper Henneman (153) also noted that some units tended to fire tonically whereas others responded phasically, and that these firing patterns were correlated with motoneuron size. Later, Henneman and colleagues (159) demonstrated, however, that motoneurons should not be divided into fixed tonic and phasic types, because, depending on the relation between their size and the existing level of excitatory and inhibitory input, they may change from one category to the other or behave in either mode.

Tonic and phasic are, therefore, appropriate terms

to characterize a given response, but not a particular motoneuron.

Significance of Nonuniformity of Muscle Fibers

Since the widespread use of histochemical techniques, it has been apparent that most mammalian muscles are composed of fibers differing widely in diameter, mitochondrial density and distribution, capillarity, myoglobin concentration, enzymatic content, and background staining. Furthermore, when activated individually, the motor units in these muscles show major differences in contractile tension and speed, susceptibility to fatigue, and recruitment order.

There is considerable evidence that many of these differences in muscle fibers and motor units are determined by the properties of the motoneurons that supply them. Cross-innervation studies, initiated by Buller et al. (31) and repeatedly substantiated by others, indicate that motoneurons play a dominant role in determining the contractile properties of the muscle fibers they innervate. The extent of this influence is revealed strikingly by the appearance of new types of muscle fibers in the previously homogeneous soleus of the cat after reinnervation of the muscle by the nerve to a mixed muscle (358).

In conjunction, these findings suggest that the histochemical and physiological characteristics, which have led to the identification of three types of muscle fibers and motor units, may be due in part to differences in the types of motoneurons supplying them. In the past ten years Henneman and colleagues (159, 160, 253, 352) have demonstrated that many of the properties of motor units and motoneurons are highly correlated with the size of the neural soma. Size-dependent differences in motoneurons, however, would presumably lead to a continuous gradation in the histological appearance of muscle fibers rather than to three distinct types. Gradations are apparent in the appearance and properties of muscle fibers, but recognition of different fiber types indicates that factors independent of cell size may also affect the differentiation process.

Motoneuron Properties Independent of Size

Harris and Henneman (145) analyzed this problem by isolating single motor axons of the plantaris pool in ventral root filaments of decerebrate cats, measuring their cortical firing levels (CFLs), and comparing their firing rates (FRs) during repetitive stimulation of the plantaris nerve. Units in the 0%–8% range of CFLs (thus varying little in size) were found to differ either very little or quite widely in maximal FR, as illustrated in Figure 46. Apparently these units were sampled randomly from two populations, one firing rapidly, the other slowly. The ratio between the two rates remained approximately constant regardless of the intensity or rate of input the units received, as long as

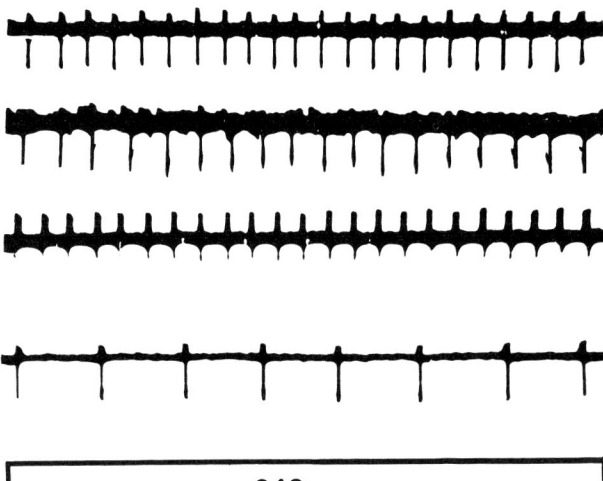

FIG. 46. Maximal firing rates of 4 plantaris motoneurons of cat with approximately equal critical firing levels recorded simultaneously during first 940 ms of their response to electrical stimulation of plantaris nerve. Stimulus parameters adjusted to produce maximal firing rates. *Bottom unit* fires significantly slower than *top 3 units*, giving impression of having been sampled from a different population than the others. [From Harris and Henneman (145).]

both of them discharged rhythmically (Fig. 47). In single experiments 10–15 of the smallest units in the pool (all with CFLs in the 0%–8% range) were isolated and compared. Statistical analyses and visual inspection of these small samples again suggested the existence of two populations of motoneurons. Analysis also indicated that the FRs of units in single experiments were not sampled from any one of a variety of parametric, single-modal distributions. This implies that the data were sampled from a distribution having more than one mode, which indicates the existence of separate populations of motoneurons among the small units of the pool. Pooling of the normalized data from different experiments revealed a bimodal histogram, reinforcing the conclusion that there are two types of small α-motoneurons in the plantaris pool. It is possible that inputs to the motoneuron pool other than the group Ia volleys used in the determination of CFLs, i.e., inputs that might be effective only during repetitive stimulation of the muscle nerve, could result in more synaptic drive on one cell than another. In a recent study (58) six different sources of inhibitory input did not alter the CFL of motoneurons or their relative rank order during repetitive firing. This argues against the possibility that certain motoneurons in a pool have completely different sets of inputs than others, but it does not entirely dispose of input as an explanation for differences in FR. Any systematic difference in input to cells of similar size that was sufficient to account for fast- and slow-firing populations of motoneurons might be considered an adequate basis for defining different types of cells based on their connectivity. There is, however, reason to be doubtful about drawing this conclusion. Chapple (55) has shown that pairs of bilaterally homologous motoneurons in

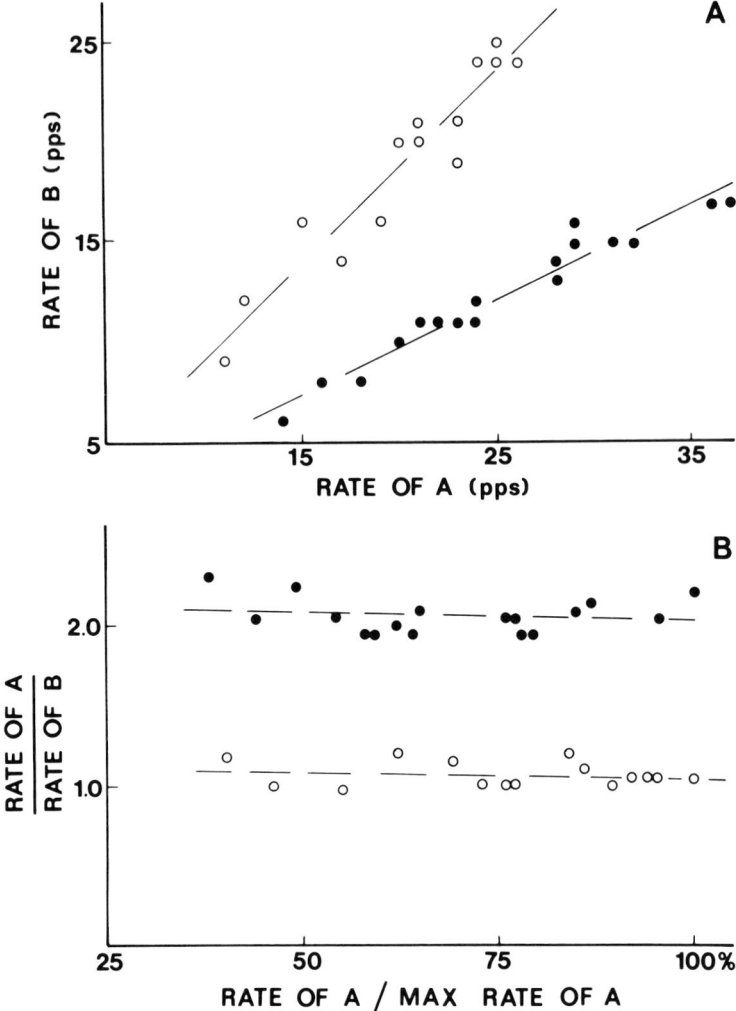

FIG. 47. Firing rates (averaged over first second) of 2 pairs of units of cat with similar critical firing levels, compared simultaneously. Data obtained by applying a wide range of stimulus intensities and frequencies to plantaris nerve. *A*: for each pair of units firing rate (FR) of 1 unit is plotted versus FR of other unit. *Dashed lines* indicate linear regression. *B*: ratio of FRs of each pair plotted as a function of the rate of 1 of the units expressed as a percentage of its maximum rate. *Bottom pair (open circles)* had very similar FRs (ratio ≃ 1.0); *top pair (closed circles)* had widely differing FRs (ratio > 2.0). Linear regression lines with slopes near zero indicate ratio of FRs remained constant for all these inputs. [From Harris and Henneman (145).]

the hermit crab are physiologically asymmetrical in their tonic frequencies. Those on the left side fire at higher frequencies than those on the right. The conduction velocities of the motoneurons on the two sides did not differ appreciably and no significant differences in the axon or soma diameters of motoneurons injected with cobalt were apparent on the two sides. Chapple concluded that the source of the symmetry was not in the motoneurons themselves but arose centrally in the absence of any major peripheral asymmetry.

Further evidence regarding differences in the properties of motoneurons that are not dependent on size has recently been obtained by Harris and Henneman (146). Motoneurons of similar size were compared in FR during repetitive stimulation of the plantaris nerve to establish control values and also during added stimulation of various inhibitory nerves. Criteria were developed whereby pairs of units, previously classified by their FRs, could be independently classified according to their responses to inhibitory inputs. The ability to distinguish motoneurons consistently by more than one set of criteria reinforces the evidence summarized above, that physiologically different populations of cells exist within a single motoneuron pool. The findings indicate that cells that respond unequally to inhibition either receive different amounts of input from certain inhibitory sources or react differentially to the same amounts of these inputs.

Another indication that the motoneurons innervating different types of motor units may vary in their essential properties appears in a recent study by Burke and his colleagues (46). The maximum amplitudes of aggregate EPSPs produced in MG motoneurons were found to be related to the type of muscle fibers they supplied. On the average, EPSPs were the largest in motoneurons of type S units, somewhat smaller in type FR units, and smallest in type FF units. Group Ia EPSPs were also correlated inversely with motor unit tension production and directly with resistance to fatigue.

If different types of motoneurons are present in the same pool and the sizes of their aggregate EPSPs are correlated with the types of muscle fibers they supply, the order of recruitment should perhaps correlate more closely with motor unit type than motoneuron size. Faden and Zajac (110) investigated recruitment order in motor units of known type by dissecting out small, unsevered ventral root filaments. Axonal conduction velocity was measured for each unit and the tension and EMG they produced when stimulated were recorded. After identification of motor unit type according to the criteria of Burke et al. (41) the intact filaments were cut and recruitment order was examined by direct comparisons of firing in different filaments. A variety of reflex maneuvers was used in these comparisons, including tendon taps, muscle stretches, repetitive shocks to the muscle nerve, and single shocks after posttetanic potentiation. In all of the 11 pairs of units studied in these difficult experiments, the unit producing the largest tension, fatiguing most rapidly, and having the highest conduction velocity was recruited last. The unit with the higher conduction velocity had the larger tetanic tension in 60 out of 76 comparisons, with the reverse in 4 cases. There were 12 "ties."

The authors conclude that "these results are consistent with the hypothesis that recruitment order is solely based on motoneuron size, which, in turn, is highly correlated with the size and fatigability of the innervated motor unit." Units defined as FF, FR, and S were included in the study.

Differential Responses of Motoneurons to Injected Currents

The responses of motoneurons to current injected through an intracellular electrode have been studied by a number of investigators (114, 130, 200–202, 276). Although injected current is not a natural input, it is a useful means of studying the membrane properties of motoneurons. None of the papers cited above attempted to relate the firing patterns of the motoneurons to the properties of the muscle fibers they supplied. Mishelevich (260) has investigated this problem. Motoneurons of the LG, MG, SOL, and plantaris (PL) were designated as fast units if their motor unit twitch times were 30 ms or less; they were classified as slow if their twitch times were 40 ms or more. Slightly more than one-half of the motoneurons supplying fast-twitch muscle fibers and all those innervating slow fibers fired repetitively (i.e., more than once) to an intracellular current step. All but two of the repetitively firing cells continued discharging for the duration of the current pulse (usually 1 s). The average current applied to produce rhythmic firing was only about 30% above rheobase for a single spike. Currents of up to 175% above rheobase for a single spike were used in testing motoneurons that did not respond repetitively.

All the motoneurons examined had resting membrane potentials of 50 mV or greater. When the motoneurons were grouped according to the amplitude of their antidromic action potentials, those between 57 and 78 mV had many more nonrepetitive cells than those between 79 and 96 mV, indicating that injury due to penetration correlates with nonrepetitive firing. Nevertheless, all the motoneurons supplying slow-twitch units fired repetitively whereas only one-half to two-thirds of the fast units did, depending on the minimum amplitude chosen.

These groups could also be differentiated on the basis of their rheobase. Cells with antidromic action potentials greater than 72 mV had rheobasic values as follows: fast, nonrepetitive units, 19.0 ± 9.3 nA; fast, repetitive units, 7.9 ± 6.6 nA; slow, repetitive units, 3.7 ± 2.9 nA.

Mishelevich's results are consistent with the general lack of accommodation in motoneurons supplying slow-twitch fibers and with the various degrees of accommodation found in cells innervating fast-twitch fibers.

Kernell (200–202) concluded that most cat motoneurons in good condition will respond repetitively to current injection. The currents he used, however, often far exceeded those that may occur normally. With the more stringent criteria used in Mishelevich's study, distinctions in repetitive response can apparently be made between motoneurons innervating different types of muscle fibers. These distinctions are not correlated with any known differences in synaptic input to motoneurons; they presumably depend on the membrane properties of the motoneurons.

Influence of Muscle on Developing and Mature Motoneurons

It has been known for some time that muscles exert an important influence on the motoneurons that innervate them. The full extent of this influence has not been determined but is under active investigation.

Many motoneurons die during early stages of development. This probably occurs because they fail to form adequate connections with muscle (see ref. 143). If the limb bud of an embryo is removed before motor innervation is established, all the corresponding motoneurons degenerate (142). If an additional limb bud is grafted onto the embryo, enlarging the peripheral target organ (162), fewer motoneurons degenerate than normally. Development of motoneurons apparently requires the presence of, or connections with, skeletal muscle. The mechanisms underlying these developmental effects are obscure.

Partial denervation of the soleus muscle in adult cats alters the electrical properties of the soleus motoneurons whose axons are intact as well as those whose axons are severed (170). Section of lumbosacral dorsal roots does not produce these effects, hence they are not mediated by sensory impulses (221). Czéh et al. (84) pursued this problem by showing that transection of the thoracic cord resulted in a significant decrease in the duration of the afterhyperpolarization (AHP) following action potentials. This change, which occurred within 8 days, was prevented by daily stimulation of the sciatic nerve. The AHP of soleus motoneurons was also shortened appreciably within 8 days after blocking conduction in the soleus nerve with a tetrodotoxin cuff. This change was prevented by chronic stimulation of the soleus nerve peripheral to but not central to the cuff. It was concluded that motoneuron properties in an adult probably depend partly upon some factors associated with activity of the innervated muscle and that such factors are carried in the motor axons by retrograde axoplasmic flow rather than by nerve impulses. In line with this reasoning is the finding that disuse atrophy of muscle, which occurred after cord section in these experiments, has been shown to be associated with a decrease in the rate of protein synthesis and an increase in its rate of degradation (126, 127). Other mechanisms, however, are also considered in the authors' discussions.

To date there is no evidence indicating whether different muscle fibers exert type-specific retrograde effects on their motoneurons. The results of cross-innervation experiments, in which motor nerves originally supplying fast muscles cause the development of three types of muscle fibers in the homogenous soleus muscle, suggest that the influence of motoneurons on muscles may be more powerful than the retrograde effects of the muscle on the motoneuron. The latter, however, may simply be more subtle influences that appear less potent.

Evidence From Human Disease

When an abnormal pattern of recruitment is recorded from a muscle, biopsy is almost certain to reveal pathology. Electromyography (EMG) of the most superficial parts of the muscle followed by an open biopsy of 2-5 mm of muscle around the tip of the electrodes may lead to a diagnosis of long-standing myopathy even in muscles that appear grossly normal. In a survey of 110 selected patients, Warmoltz and Engel (344) discovered a small group of patients with the following characteristics: *1*) initial activation on minimal to mild voluntary contraction; *2*) well-maintained rhythmic firing with little effort at frequencies of 6-10 s; *3*) sustained discharge through all ranges from mild to maximal forces; *4*) acceleration of firing rates with stronger contractions to a maximum of 18-20/s. In this group of cases open biopsy disclosed that 95%-99% of the muscle fibers of these normally heterogeneous muscles (biceps brachii or quadriceps femoris) were small and red.

Motor units from another group of patients had completely different characteristics: *1*) sudden or vigorous contraction required for activation; *2*) either discharge of brief bursts lasting 0.5-5.0 s with no capacity to sustain them longer (during this time they fired steadily at 10-25/s or sputtered irregularly) or discharge only once or twice; *3*) peak firing frequencies reaching 16-50/s at the height of bursts accompanying maximal contractions; *4*) more rapid initial and peak discharge frequencies with increasingly vigorous contraction. Biopsies from these patients contained 96%-100% pale (type A) fibers. In brief, the normal recruitment pattern, with its wide range of potential sizes and frequencies, was lacking in both these groups.

It is a reasonable, but unproven, inference that the motoneurons supplying one type of muscle fiber in these cases were susceptible to a disease process to which the motoneurons supplying the other type of muscle fibers were resistant. The muscle fibers supplied by the susceptible motoneurons were denervated as a result. The motoneurons innervating the healthy muscle fibers apparently remained relatively intact. These cells presumably put out axonal collaterals that supplied the denervated muscle fibers and in time converted them to the type characteristic of their own activity pattern, as in cross-innervation experiments.

There are puzzling features in these studies. The findings suggest that the motoneurons supplying heterogeneous muscles may differ significantly in their susceptibility to disease. The extreme uniformity of the muscle population that eventually results is surprising and difficult to explain. It is unlikely that the motoneurons themselves are as homogeneous as the appearance of the muscle fibers suggests. The converted muscle fibers appear to be normal as judged by their electrical properties. In five cases showing selective, widespread, moderately severe atrophy of large, pale fibers, and in four cases with milder involvement, the amplitude and duration of the low-threshold unitary potentials appeared normal, suggesting that they were derived from normal red fibers not then involved in a disease process. In seven of these nine cases the only recognizable EMG abnormality was failure to achieve a full "interference pattern" of large and small spikes with maximal effort. These studies seem to require the existence of at least two types of motoneurons. Variations in motoneuron properties or in the properties of the muscle fibers they innervate may account for the differences in susceptibility to disease that apparently exist. However, the recent work already described on motoneurons with similar critical firing levels but widely differing firing rates suggests that there are at least two populations of motoneurons with size-independent properties sufficiently different to account for different susceptibility to disease.

Concluding Comments

The various types of evidence described in this section clearly indicate that the motoneurons in a pool are not uniform in their basic properties. Tentatively, one may conclude that there are at least three types of motoneurons in a pool. Differences in their firing characteristics presumably account for the widely differing properties of the muscle fibers they supply. Until clear distinctions between the histochemistry, ultrastructure, or membrane properties of motoneurons can be demonstrated, however, it seems premature to classify motoneurons into specific types as has been done for muscle fibers. This is an area with important clinical implications, as indicated in subsection *Evidence From Human Disease*, p. 490.

HOW SIZE OF MOTONEURONS DETERMINES THEIR SUSCEPTIBILITY TO DISCHARGE

Analysis of the firing patterns of motoneurons leaves little doubt that susceptibility to discharge is highly correlated with motoneuron size. This conclusion poses a difficult question. Why are small motoneurons fired more readily than large ones by almost all types of excitatory inputs, and why are they more resistant to silencing by inhibition?

Kuno (214) has shown that the resting membrane potentials of small and large motoneurons do not differ and that approximately the same degree of depolarization is required to discharge them. If their firing thresholds are not significantly different, then the properties of the motoneurons themselves, the input to them, or both of these factors in combination must somehow result in larger depolarizations (EPSPs) in small cells than in large ones. A simple experiment illustrates that this inference is correct, at least under special experimental conditions. If a muscle nerve is stimulated so that a synchronous volley is conducted centrally in all of its Ia-fibers, the effect of this standard input can be examined by recording the "composite" or "aggregate" EPSP it produces in motoneurons of the homonymous pool. These aggregate EPSPs vary inversely in amplitude with the size of the motoneuron from which they are recorded (36, 99). An explanation for this particular correlation has recently been found (245), which also accounts for the more general relationship between the size of motoneurons and their susceptibility to discharge. This is described in the subsection entitled *Role of Input in Determining Susceptibility to Discharge*, p. 493.

According to Ohm's Law ($E = IR$), the aggregate EPSP (E) is the product of the total synaptic current (I) produced by all of the active Ia-endings on a motoneuron and the resistance (R), which the membrane of the soma and dendrites offers to this current.

$$\text{aggregate EPSP} = \text{synaptic current} \times \text{input resistance of cell} \quad (1)$$

In the next subsection some of the properties of motoneurons that influence Equation 1 are described.

Properties of Motoneurons That Influence Susceptibility to Discharge

As Equation 1 suggests, the input resistance of the motoneuron is an important factor in determining the size of its aggregate EPSPs and its susceptibility to discharge. This resistance varies inversely with the surface area of the cell's membrane, directly with its specific resistance per unit area and to some extent perhaps with the density of the synaptic boutons that partly cover the surface. According to Conradi (72) the boutons may cover more than 50% of the motoneuron surface.

The importance of input resistance in determining the size of synaptic potentials was demonstrated by Katz and Thesleff (199). When miniature endplate potentials (MEPPs) were recorded from different frog muscle fibers, their mean amplitudes varied by factors of more than 10 to 1, although the mean quantum of acetylcholine eliciting the MEPPs was approximately constant. By determining the input resistances of the individual muscle fibers, which are a function of their diameters, Katz and Thesleff found that the greater the resistance, the larger the MEPP.

This result was important to subsequent considerations of the relationship between cell size and susceptibility to discharge. The application of this finding to the motoneuron, however, has been difficult, because the surface area, which determines the input resistance, also determines the number of boutons on the cell (122) and, thus, influences the total synaptic current generated under various conditions.

Although the input resistance of the motoneuron does not per se account for its susceptibility to discharge, it has been shown to be a good index to its size. Kernell (203) showed experimentally that the input resistance of a cell is inversely related to its axonal conduction velocity and, thus, to its dimensions. Barrett and Crill (13) and Cullheim (80) extended Cajal's original findings by demonstrating specifically in motoneurons the close relationship between axon diameter in the white matter and at the initial segment, and between axonal conduction velocity and cell size. Barrett and Crill (13) and Lux et al. (247) also confirmed Kernell's (203) finding that axonal conduction velocity and input resistance are inversely correlated by carrying out electrical measurements on impaled motoneurons before filling them with a dye and later examining them morphologically.

In view of the preceding observations, it is not surprising that several investigators have shown that the aggregate EPSP of a motoneuron is directly proportional to its input resistance. Eccles et al. (99) were the first to note that small motoneurons have larger aggregate EPSPs than bigger ones. The five tables in which their observations are compiled summarize a great deal of data concerning the size of aggregate EPSPs for many different species of motoneurons.

Kernell (203) reasoned that with synapses of similar size and location the current generated by a given conductance change should alter the soma membrane potential more in a cell with a high than in one with a low input resistance, as Katz and Thesleff's (199) findings predicted. Thus, he argued, less current (for example, a smaller number of active synapses) would presumably be needed for eliciting a repetitive discharge in a cell with a high input resistance. Using four different methods of measuring input resistance, he found that cells with slowly conducting axons had higher resistances than those with rapidly conducting axons.

Accepting "the notion that there is a relation between motoneuron size, cell input impedance and amplitude of synaptic potentials," Burke (36) set out to examine the basis for these relationships by studying the characteristics of group Ia synaptic input to triceps surae motoneurons. A significant positive correlation was found between the maximum amplitudes of homonymous aggregate EPSPs evoked electrically and the input resistance values across the entire population of units studied. A similar correlation, though somewhat less strong, was found for heteronymous EPSPs. The amplitudes of "unitary miniature EPSPs (mEPSPs) of presumed group Ia origin," elicited by small static stretches were also examined. A significant positive correlation was found between the median amplitudes of the mEPSP distributions and the input resistance values. Positive correlations were also noted between the amplitudes of the median mEPSPs and the maximum homonymous aggregate EPSPs in the cells for which both data points were available. The duration of the aggregate EPSPs in high-resistance (type S) cells tended to be significantly longer than in lower resistance (type F) cells. This observation could not be entirely accounted for by the relatively small difference in the mean time constants of the two types of cells. For these reasons and because of a theoretical analysis he carried out, Burke concluded that "the density of Ia synaptic terminals tends to be higher on type S motoneurons than on type F cells." This valuable set of data and the theoretical analysis accompanying it led Burke to the conclusion that small motoneurons with a high input resistance are more susceptible to discharge because they receive a higher density of Ia-endings than large cells, although additional factors were believed to be important as well (36).

Despite the generally agreed facts that input resistance is a function of motoneuron size and surface area and, as Equation 1 indicates, is an important factor governing the size of EPSPs and susceptibility to discharge, its role vis-à-vis other factors is difficult to define precisely. This is because the surface area, which determines the input resistance, also determines the number of boutons on a cell. The additional number of boutons on large cells may exactly compensate for the decrease in input resistance, as Zucker's (360) calculations indicate. Barrett and Crill (13) have demonstrated that small motoneurons have a slightly higher specific resistance than large ones. This suggests that input resistance is disproportionately higher in small cells and might explain their larger EPSPs.

Other systematic differences between large and small motoneurons might also help to explain the observed relationship between EPSP amplitude and cell size. For example, if small motoneurons had a shorter total electrotonic length (L), Ia-synapses might be closer on the average to the soma, thereby causing larger EPSPs. Burke and ten Bruggencate (48) have shown, however, that there is no systematic relationship between cell size and L and it has already been noted that Ia-terminals on small cells are not closer to the soma (subsection PHYSIOLOGICAL ANALYSIS OF LOCATION OF BOUTONS, p. 468).

Before concluding this section, it should be noted that there is strong experimental support (see review in ref. 44) for the concept that the all-or-none action potential of a motoneuron is generated in the initial segment of the axon (axon hillock plus nonmedullated segment). According to Eccles et al. (99), the aggregate EPSP "will be virtually identical with the depolarization produced in the initial segment." This belief was consistent with the observation that "homonymous and heteronymous EPSPs are indistinguishable with respect to the level of depolarization at which they initiate the discharge of impulses" (99). It is possible that the threshold of the initial segment may influence the susceptibility of a motoneuron to discharge, but Kuno's (214) finding that the same degree of depolarization is required to fire large and small cells does not support this notion.

Although differences in the amplitudes of aggregate EPSPs of small and large cells are undoubtedly useful in explaining susceptibility to discharge, it is also important to keep in mind that motoneuron threshold is sometimes considered to be that level of membrane potential at which the cell begins to discharge repetitively. A property of motoneurons that may be crucial in allowing them to fire repetitively in response to steady current is the slow potassium conductance that is turned on following an impulse (205). Using computer modeling techniques, Traub (338) has shown that the time constant governing the decay of this slow potassium conductance may be smaller in large cells than in small ones. This postulate is apparently necessary to obtain the correct impulse frequency vs. injected current relationships in small and large cells. It emphasizes the importance of inherent membrane properties in addition to geometrical considerations and organization of synaptic input in determining how susceptibility to discharge is established. Burke and Nelson (43) have demonstrated that large motoneurons have a tendency to exhibit greater accommodation than small ones, another example of a size-related property that may contribute to the functioning of the size principle. Although motoneuron size is not the only variable influencing recruitment order, it appears that other important factors are also functions of cell size.

Finally, in attempting to evaluate the general significance of input resistance, it is pertinent to consider whether it bears the same relationship to inhibitory as to excitatory inputs. The data needed to answer this question are less numerous and not as easy to interpret for inhibitory as for excitatory inputs, because inhibitory inputs are not as precisely controlled, the responses are harder to measure, and the afferent circuits are generally at least disynaptic. Nevertheless, it has been found in a number of experimental circumstances that IPSPs are larger in smaller motoneurons (46, 131, 152, 214). In the study by Burke et al. (46) the same motoneurons that yielded large aggregate EPSPs also exhibited large disynaptic IPSPs. Hence it is likely that input resistance or cell size influences the responses to all inputs, both excitatory and inhibitory.

Role of Input in Determining Susceptibility to Discharge

A number of theoretical analyses have been made to explain the size-dependent susceptibility of motoneurons to discharge by Ia volleys (36, 329, 338, 360). These formulations relied on the experimental data that were available, but they also depended on a number of stated and unstated assumptions that were of uncertain validity. It was apparent that until these theories could be tested experimentally they had to be regarded chiefly as speculative exercises.

Recently, however, a hypothesis was developed that could be tested experimentally (245). The essential features of this hypothesis are as follows. Since motoneurons of different sizes reportedly have equal densities of synaptic boutons (122), those with large surface areas must have proportionally more boutons. In particular, if large motoneurons supplying the medial gastrocnemius have more endings from Ia-fibers coming from that muscle, this is due not to receiving projections from more Ia-fibers, but to more extensive arborization of individual Ia-fibers on these cells, because each motoneuron receives terminals from essentially all Ia-fibers coming from its muscle (255). The more numerous branch points, terminal boutons, and boutons en passant in extensive arborizations presumably lower the safety factor for propagation (177). Experimental evidence indicates that an impulse in a motor axon may fail to invade all of its branches (213) and that transmission failures may occur in Ia-synapses on motoneurons (105–107). It follows that the larger the motoneuron, the more extensive are the terminal arborizations on it and the greater is the possibility that impulses in them will die out at certain points and the smaller will be the percentage of Ia-endings that are activated by maximal volleys in its Ia-fibers. Anything than facilitates invasion of Ia-terminals and activation of synaptic endings should lead to larger aggregate EPSPs, and this tendency should be greater in large than in small motoneurons.

To test this hypothesis, intracellular recordings were made from motoneurons of anesthetized cats. First, the input resistance (IR) of each motoneuron was measured, which provided a reliable estimate of its size (13, 203). Then the medial gastrocnemius nerve was stimulated with brief shocks (1/s) that set up afferent volleys in all of its Ia-fibers. The monosynaptic EPSPs evoked by the volleys were recorded and a series of 16 responses was averaged electronically and written out on an x-y plotter. The muscle nerve was then tetanized at 500 impulses/s for 10 s and a posttetanic series of EPSPs was recorded and averaged. Lloyd (237) showed that conditioning tetani of this frequency and duration caused hyperpolarization of the Ia-fibers and a dramatic increase in the amplitude of the monosynaptic reflexes elicited by volleys in them. This "posttetanic potentiation" (PTP) gradually declined back to control levels in 2–3 min.

Figure 48 illustrates typical effects of PTP on the EPSPs of three motoneurons of different sizes. The lower traces in the three pairs of records illustrate that the average size of the aggregate EPSPs before potentiation varied directly with the input resistance of the motoneuron. This confirmed previous observations (36). The upper traces are the averages of 16 EPSPs following the tetanus. The percent potentiations in *A*, *B*, and *C* were 123, 92, and 11, respectively.

Figure 49*A* plots the relationship between input resistance and amplitude of control EPSPs in data pooled from nine experiments. Figure 49*B* illustrates how percent potentiation was related to input resistance in the same experiment. As the hypothesis predicts, the greatest potentiation occurred in motoneurons with the lowest *IR*, i.e., in the largest cells. The least potentiation and the largest control EPSPs were found in motoneurons with the highest *IR*s. Less branching would be expected in Ia-fibers approaching these small cells, and few inactive endings should be available to increase synaptic input during PTP. It has generally been assumed that PTP is due to release of more transmitter from a fixed number of active endings. This assumption, however, predicts that the effect of PTP is independent of cell size, so it is no longer tenable.

If the hypothesis is correct, PTP might be expected to cause small increases in the conduction time required for Ia volleys to invade additional terminals and to activate more synaptic knobs. The flow of synaptic currents at the various endings might be less synchronous, i.e., more prolonged due to these delays (177), but it is difficult to predict the effects of PTP on the time course of EPSPs without precise infor-

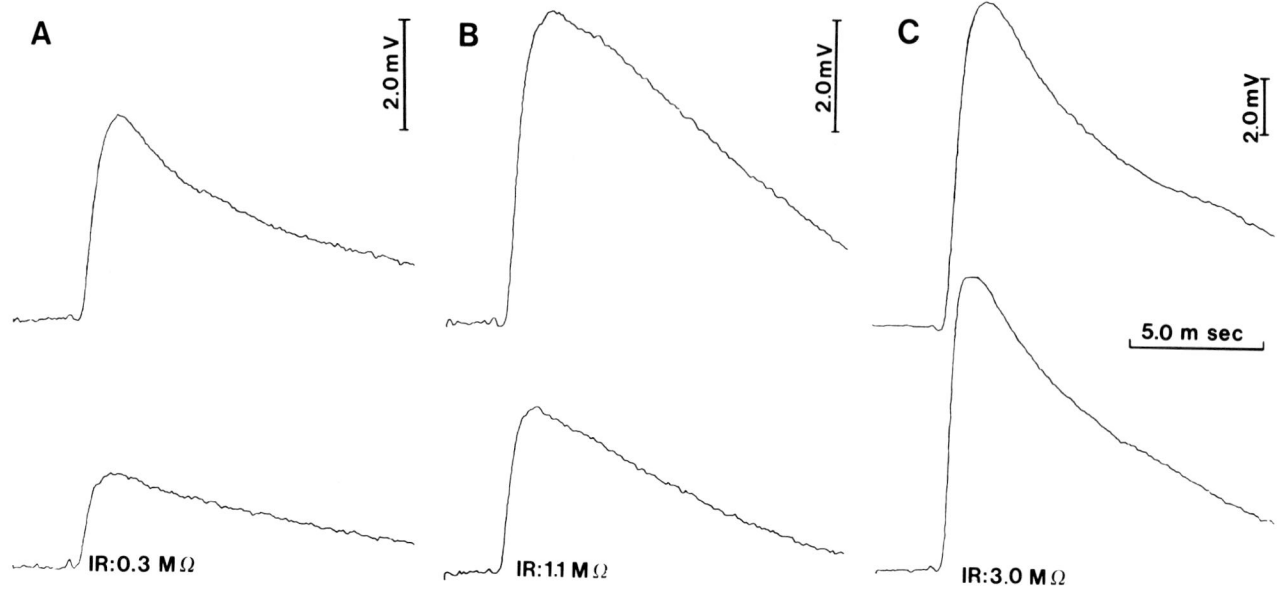

FIG. 48. Examples of aggregate excitatory postsynaptic potentials (EPSPs) recorded from 3 medial gastrocnemius motoneurons of cat to illustrate effects of posttetanic potentiation on cells of different input resistance (IR) and size. *Bottom traces* illustrate that average size of aggregate EPSPs before potentiation varied directly with IR of motoneuron. *Top traces* are averages of 16 EPSPs following tetanus. Percent potentiations in *A–C* were 123, 92, and 11, respectively. [From Lüscher, Ruenzel, and Henneman (245).]

mation about the geometry of the terminal arborization of Ia-fibers. Figure 50 is a plot of the changes in rise time in EPSPs versus the changes in their half-widths. With a few exceptions PTP increased both rise time and half-width, but the magnitudes of these changes do not seem to be related.

These experimental findings are consistent in all respects with the hypothesis that has been proposed. They suggest that invasion of Ia-terminals is a graded process that is generally more complete in the terminal arborizations on small cells because they have fewer branch points. The percentage of Ia-boutons that are activated by afferent impulses depends on this process. The surface area that a motoneuron presents to approaching Ia-fibers may influence their tendency to branch and, thus, indirectly it may determine its own susceptibility to discharge.

SOME PRINCIPLES UNDERLYING ORGANIZATION OF MOTONEURON POOLS

Although this chapter has been devoted primarily to the organization of the motoneuron pool, it should be apparent that the properties of motoneurons and of the muscle fibers they supply are so interdependent that neither can be understood in isolation from the other. In the course of evolution all of the features of the combined neuromuscular system have been subjected to selection pressures. Some capacities that survival might tend to optimize, however, are mutually exclusive. The control system that has evolved, therefore, represents compromises between conflicting needs. Its characteristics suggest that four requirements took precedence and played major roles in determining the final organization. Survival, with its emphasis on speed, endurance, and agility of movement, apparently placed a premium on *1*) maximal sensitivity in the control of muscular tension and *2*) maximal economy in expenditure of contractile energy. Less obvious, but increasingly essential as the complexity of the central nervous system increased, was the need for a mechanism that provided *3*) collective action from a large population of neurons and *4*) as nearly automatic operation as possible at the final output stage. These aspects of the neuromuscular system are discussed briefly in the concluding sections of this chapter in order to provide further insight into the organization of the motoneuron pool.

How Sensitivity in Gradation of Tension is Achieved

The experimental results in section FIRING PATTERNS OF INDIVIDUAL MOTONEUTRONS AND MOTOR UNITS, p. 435, reveal the basic principle involved in the grading of muscular tension. The first step in the grading process is that the motoneuron pool functions incrementally by adding progressively larger units to its total neural output as the net excitatory input increases. As excitation decreases or inhibition increases, the pool operates decrementally by subtracting progressively smaller units from its output. These operations depend on the distribution of cell sizes in

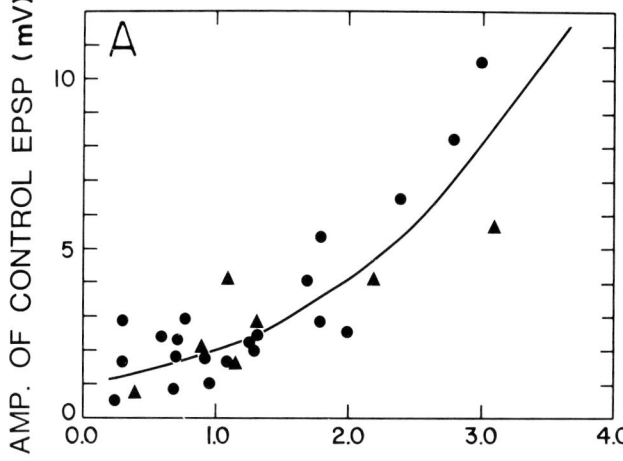

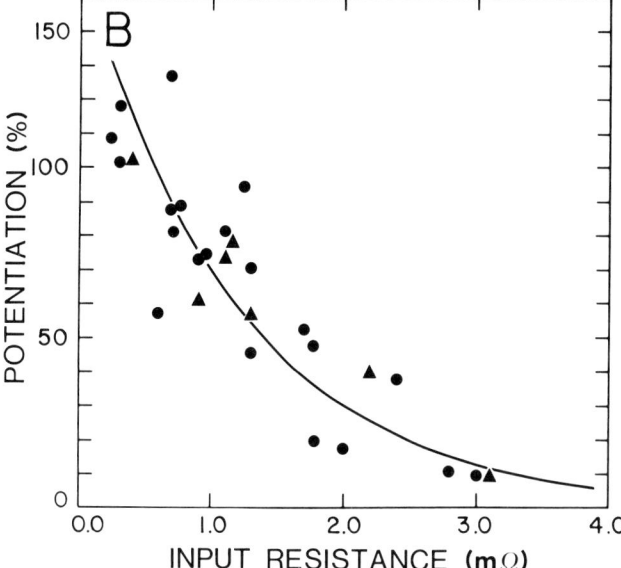

FIG. 49. Relation between input resistance and amplitude of aggregate excitatory postsynaptic potentials (EPSPs) before (A) and during (B) posttetanic potentiation in cat. *Circles*, medial gastrocnemius motoneurons; *triangles*, semitendinosus motoneurons. [From Lüscher, Ruenzel, and Henneman (245).]

the pool and certain correlates of cell size that determine susceptibility to discharge. The pool is organized as a graded hierarchy. Rank order in this hierarchy is defined in terms of susceptibility to discharge by physiological inputs. The lowest ranking cell requires the smallest net excitatory input to be fired; the highest ranking cell requires the largest. Experimental analysis has shown that whenever a particular motoneuron responds monosynaptically, all the lower ranking cells in the pool discharge with it. Thus, all the monosynaptic reflex outputs (O) have the form

$$O_T = O_1 + O_2 + O_3 \ldots O_X \qquad (2)$$

where O_T is the total monosynaptic output and O_X is the highest ranking cell discharged by a particular input.

Equation 2 is a concise formulation of a basic law of combination that specifies how the activities of motoneurons are combined in monosynaptic reflexes. The same law applies when the monosynaptic reflex is conditioned by various mixtures of excitation and inhibition. Figure 51 illustrates some of the features of pool organization schematically. Each vertical line in the figure represents a motoneuron whose relative size is indicated by its amplitude. Small motoneurons, which are most numerous, are finely graded in size and highly susceptible to discharge. Large cells are far less numerous, differ more widely in size, and require much larger inputs to be fired. Resistance to inhibition is distributed in the same general pattern, but in the reverse order, the largest motoneurons being most readily silenced by inhibitory inputs. Figure 51 should be regarded as a simplified illustrative scheme rather than as an accurate quantitative representation of experimental findings.

As described in section FIRING PATTERNS OF INDIVIDUAL MOTONEURONS AND MOTOR UNITS, p. 435, recruitment follows the same order during repetitive firing as it does in monosynaptic reflexes. Since rate of firing is a function of size and other factors, a more general form of Equation 2 is required to represent the output of a pool during repetitive activity

$$O_T = f_1 O_1 + f_2 O_2 + f_3 O_3 + \ldots f_X O_X \qquad (3)$$

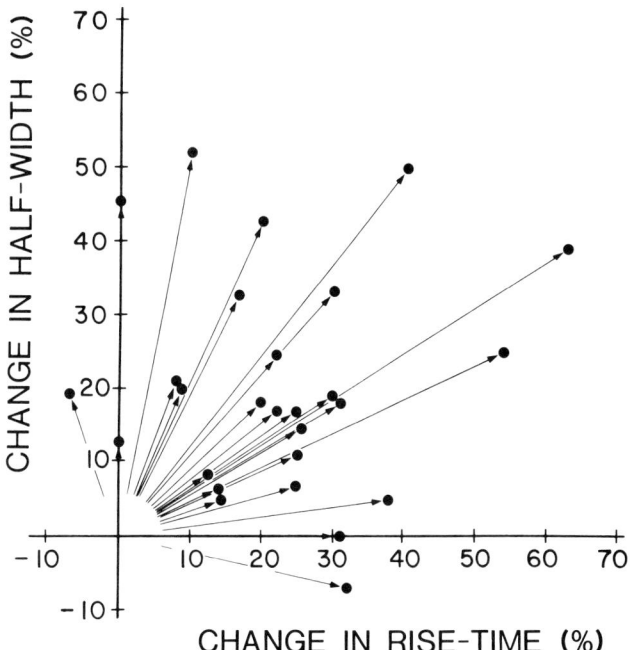

FIG. 50. Plot of changes in rise times of excitatory postsynaptic potentials (EPSPs) versus changes in their half-widths following a tetanus to cat muscle nerve at 500/s for 10 s. *Arrows* indicate directions of change. [From Lüscher, Ruenzel, and Henneman (245).]

where f_1-f_X represent firing rates determined by input to the pool and the size and other properties of the motoneurons. In general, the firing rate of a motoneuron at recruitment and its maximal rate of discharge increase with its size. Monster and Chan (261) recorded the firing rates of pairs of motor units in the extensor digitorum muscle of humans during voluntary isometric contractions with values of force up to 500 g. The simultaneously recorded values were plotted against one another, as illustrated in Figure 52.

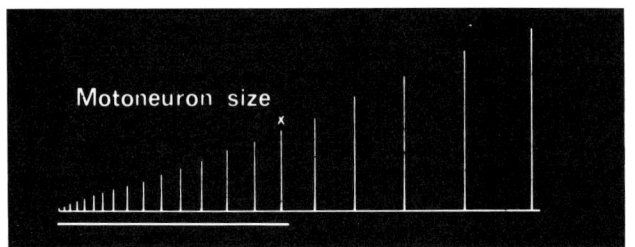

FIG. 51. Some features of a motoneuron pool. Heights of *vertical lines* represent sizes of motoneurons. Their spacing indicates relative numbers of cells of different sizes. *Horizontal line* below base line shows combination of motoneurons firing in response to a given input. Largest cell discharged denoted by X. [From Henneman (154a). Organization of the motoneuron pool: the size principle. In: *Medical Physiology* (14th ed.), edited by V. B. Mountcastle. St. Louis, MO: The C. V. Mosby Co., 1980.]

The small spread of the data points of each pair (8 pairs are shown) reveals that firing rate variations among the units of each pair were highly correlated and maintained an orderly pattern. The dashed straight lines, indicating the relative rates of change in the firing rates of the units in each pair, had linear regression coefficients of > 0.9 in 80% of the pairs. Nonlinearities were observed in several pairs involving very low threshold units. Analysis of the slopes of the dashed lines showed that the higher threshold (i.e., larger) unit of a pair generally increased its firing rate more rapidly than the lower threshold unit, as the results of animal experiments had also revealed. The slopes of the regression lines were found to depend on the threshold differences between members of a pair. Rate modulation occurs systematically throughout the pool, enhancing the sensitivity of the gradation process.

Basis for Relation Between Motoneuron Size and the Force Its Motor Unit Develops

Recruitment of motoneurons results in the activation of motor units developing progressively larger twitch and tetanic tensions. The total force produced by the muscle grows in direct proportion to the output of the motoneuron pool. Two factors account for the

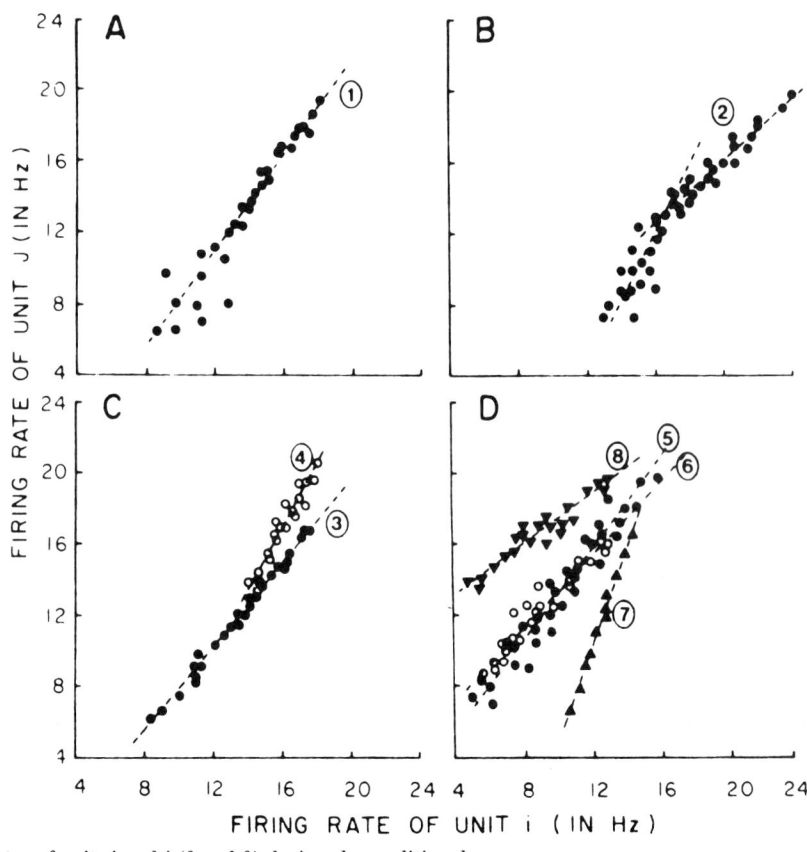

FIG. 52. Concomitant changes in mean firing rates of units i and j (f_i and f_j) during slow volitional changes in an isometric contraction in human. The f_i-f_j relationship of each pair is approximated by 1 or 2 straight (*dashed*) lines. The same i unit was used in pairs 5-8. [From Monster and Chan (261).]

correspondence between neural and contractile output. *1)* The scaling principle, described in MORPHOLOGICAL CONSIDERATIONS, p. 424, implies that larger motoneurons have larger axons that give off more terminals and innervate more muscle fibers. All of the muscle fibers of a motor unit in mammals normally participate in its activities. This purely dimensional aspect of the size principle probably explains the linear relationship between the size of a motoneuron and the tension capacity of its motor unit in the cat's soleus (Fig. 6). In this "homogeneous" red muscle all of the muscle fibers have approximately the same cross-sectional areas. Judging from their uniform histochemical reactions and fine structure, each fiber presumably has the same capacity for developing tension. The maximal force produced by a motor unit, therefore, depends on the number of fibers it comprises, although other factors are not excluded. *2)* In heterogeneous muscles the types of muscle fibers, with their various sizes and contractile properties, are related to the sizes of their motoneurons. In these muscles force also increases monotonically with neural output. The slope of the relationship between these variables, however, becomes steeper as larger motoneurons are recruited. The presence of different types of fibers endows muscles with a much wider range of contractile properties, making them more versatile servants of the motoneuron pool.

Actual Sensitivity in Grading Muscular Tension

It is instructive to consider how much sensitivity over control of muscular tension would be afforded by recruitment alone without considering the contribution of rate modulation. Henneman and Olson (157) made such calculations, based on data obtained from the medial gastrocnemius muscle of the cat (Table 8). It is obvious that a large number of small motor units, varying only slightly in size, could provide extremely fine control at the low end of the tension scale. What happens to fine control at the other end of the scale where the largest units recruited may contribute up to 120 g to the total tension? To answer this question, the relation of the various possible increments of tetanic tension to the total tension already developed prior to each new addition must be calculated. To do this, all of the maximal tetanic tensions of MG motor units measured experimentally were grouped in decades. Line 1 in Table 8 gives the sums of the unit tensions in each decade. Line 2 contains the total cumulative tensions, i.e., the sum of all the unit tensions in each column, plus the totals of all columns to the left. The percent of tension contributed by new units to the tensions already developed by all units of smaller size is shown in line 3. For example, 6.4% in the left-hand column was obtained by dividing 10 g (the smallest unit in the next column) by 156.3 g (the cumulative total of all units below 10 g). If all increments of tension are viewed as percentages of the preexisting total tension in this manner, there is no loss of fine control as the total tension approaches a maximum.

This treatment of the data is intended only as an example of a basic principle in the control of muscle tension. A number of factors combine to make the actual control much finer and more precise than the data in the table indicate. There are about three times as many motor units in an average MG muscle as there were in the experimental sample used to construct Table 8. Hence, each addition to the total tension is an even smaller percentage of the total tensions. With more units the spectrum of sizes is more nearly continuous and the thresholds of the motoneurons at the low end of the scale are much closer together than at the high end. Finally and most importantly, units are actually recruited in overlapping fashion. New units are added to the total discharge well before the last recruits reach their maximal tension levels. Rate modulation adds enormously to the fineness of the grading process. The result is a smooth crescendo of total tension.

Mathematical Derivation of a "Principle of Maximum Grading Sensitivity"

Henneman et al. (159) pointed out that the grading of output in a muscle is somewhat analogous to the

TABLE 8. *Percent Contribution of Single Motor Units to Tension Developed by All Smaller Motor Units of Medial Gastrocnemius*

Grouping of Units	<10 g	10.0–19.9	20.0–29.9	30.0–39.9	40.0–49.9	50.0–59.9	60.0–69.9	70.0–79.9	80.0–89.9	90.0–99.9	100.0–109.9	110.0–120.0
1. Total tensions, g	156	152	387	252	358	323	443	519	587	278	107	345
2. Cumulative totals, g	156	308	695	947	1,305	1,628	2,071	2,590	3,177	3,455	3,562	3,907
3. Percent contribution of 1 unit to cumulative tensions of samples	6.4	6.5	4.3	4.2	3.8	3.7	3.4	3.1	2.8	2.9	3.1	3.1
4. Percent contribution of 1 unit to cumulative tensions, estimated for whole muscle	2.1	2.2	1.4	1.4	1.3	1.2	1.1	1.0	0.9	1.0	1.0	1.0

Adapted from Henneman and Olson (157).

grading of sensation. The smallest increment that can be added to the force exerted by a muscle becomes greater as the total force increases, just as the smallest increment of sensory stimulation required to produce a "just noticeable difference" in sensation becomes larger as the sensation itself increases in intensity.

Starting with the experimental results of Milner-Brown et al. (258), Hatze (149) has derived mathematically a "motor unit size law" that is synonymous with the size principle of recruitment. From this he has also derived an expression relating the proportion of active muscle mass to the sequential order number of a newly recruited unit. He concludes that his motor unit size law is a consequence of the minimum entropy principle and "since a minimization of the fluctuations in the recruitment sequence implies a maximization of the grading sensitivity of the muscle's force output, it appears more appropriate to speak of a principle of maximum grading sensitivity" (150).

Recruitment Order and Minimum Energy Principle

Hatze and Buys (151) have shown mathematically that the sequential order of motor unit recruitment found experimentally coincides with the order predicted when the total energy expenditure of the muscle is minimized at all levels of force output. If the sequence of recruitment is determined by the size principle, as discussed in the previous subsection, but the same sequence can independently be predicted from a minimum energy hypothesis, then it follows that the rate of energy expenditure per unit of muscle mass must be a monotonically increasing function of the relative motor unit size (as Fig. 4 in ref. 151 illustrates). Studies of heat production in contracting muscle (123, 346) tend to support this conclusion, but detailed analysis of the relative energy cost of tension production in motor units of different size and type is lacking.

Collective Action of Motoneuron Pool: Role of Input

One of the properties of a motoneuron pool that enables it to perform its complex functions is its capacity to operate as a collective entity. What organizational principle enables the individual motoneurons to work together smoothly as an ensemble? Unquestionably, the arrangement of the afferent fibers to the pool provides this cohesion. The distribution of the terminals of single Ia-fibers to all the homonymous motoneurons is an example of how this is accomplished in the case of one afferent system. As a result, the signals in a single Ia-fiber affect every cell in the pool at approximately the same time. Although the 60 Ia-fibers from the cat's MG muscle usually fire asynchronously, the 300 motoneurons in the MG pool receive the same combinations of Ia inputs from the MG in approximately the same temporal sequences. Thus, the total Ia input waxes and wanes in near synchrony throughout the pool. This arrangement provides some insight into the organizational principle underlying the collective action of the pool. The extent to which this model applies to other inputs remains to be seen.

The Size Principle in Ia and Group II Sensory Fibers

The organization of the motoneuron pool depends heavily on its input. Recently the size principle has been shown (244) to apply, at least in part, to sensory fibers that impinge directly on motoneurons. The larger the Ia or group II fiber, the greater are the excitatory effects on its impulses on motoneurons. Some indication of how the size of afferent fibers governs the amplitude of synaptic effects presynaptically as well as postsynaptically is emerging. The size of a sensory neuron not only determines the magnitude of the effect its impulses produce, but also influences the locations where these effects are exerted postsynaptically.

The size of a primary stretch afferent from muscle is also correlated with its responsiveness to stretch. Differences in the dynamic properties of primary and secondary endings have been reported by several investigators (148, 231, 250). Furthermore, Matthews (250) showed that the dynamic responses of primary and secondary endings were related to the conduction velocities of the afferent fibers, and that sensitivity to velocity of stretch increased with fiber size.

The evidence that the synapses from group II and Ia afferents are located on different parts of the somatodendritic membrane, in conjunction with a suggestion of Rall (285), indicates a functional distinction between dendritic and somatic activity. Dendritic synapses would be more appropriate for the regulation of the general excitatory state of the motoneuron pool. They would be well suited to process input from secondary endings, which are most sensitive to static changes in muscle length. More proximally located input would be more apt to cause rapid triggering of reflex discharge, an appropriate response to input from primary endings that are most sensitive to rapid changes in muscle lengths. Thus, both ends of these sensory fibers follow the size principle and enable the motoneuron pool to respond to the various types of changes occurring within its muscle.

How Does the Central Nervous System Use the Motoneuron Pool?

No definite answer to this question can be given at present, but it is surely pertinent to ask "what are the functional implications of the precise and nearly invariant rank order that has been demonstrated for the higher centers where commands originate?" To consider this question in broad perspective, imagine that no rank order exists. The central nervous system has at its disposal motor units with a wide range of contractile properties. How should it select those it needs for a particular task, and how should it combine them to produce the muscle tension it desires? It is conceivable that the central nervous system might use the 300 motoneurons in the cat's medial gastrocnemius pool like the keys of a large adding machine, picking any combination of cells to yield the proper total. This notion is implicit in suggestions that motoneurons can be activated in a selective manner. However, this proposition would require 300 separately activable inputs, so that each of the 300 motoneurons could be fired selectively, a very demanding requirement. It would also necessitate circuits to do something much more difficult, namely to calculate what combinations of active units would produce the correct total tensions. This would require formidable circuitry and considerable neural delay. Consider the number (n) of possible combinations that might occur. For a pool consisting of 300 cells, such as the MG pool, n is calculated as follows

$$n = \sum_{k=1}^{300} \frac{300!}{k!\,(300-k)!}$$

In this example $n > 10^{90}$.

Feedback signals from muscle could not replace circuits to precalculate the total tension. They would be too slow and, in any case, they would be needed to determine the size of the feedback correction. The solution that has evolved is the rank-ordered pool, which relieves the central nervous system of the necessity for selective activation of motoneurons and provides a simple rule for their combination.

REFERENCES

1. ABRAHAMS, V. C., R. RICHMOND, AND P. K. ROSE. Absence of monosynaptic reflex in dorsal neck muscles of the cat. *Brain Res.* 92: 130–131, 1975.
2. ABZUG, C., M. MAEDA, B. W. PETERSON, AND V. J. WILSON. Branching of individual lateral vestibulospinal axons at different spinal cord levels. *Brain Res.* 56: 327–330, 1973.
3. ADRIAN, E. D., AND D. W. BRONK. The discharge of impulses in motor nerve fibers. II. The frequency of discharge in reflex and voluntary contractions. *J. Physiol. London* 67: 119–151, 1929.
4. ANDERSON, M. E. Segmental reflex inputs to motoneurons innervating dorsal neck musculature in the cat. *Exp. Brain Res.* 28: 175–187, 1977.
5. ANZENBACHER, H., AND W. ZENKER. Über die Grössenbeziehung der Muskelfasern zu ihren motorischen Endplatten und Nerven. *Z. Zellforsch. Mikrosk. Anat.* 60: 860–871, 1963.
6. APPELBERG, B., AND F. EMONET-DÉNAND. Motor units of the first superficial lumbrical muscle of the cat. *J. Neurophysiol.* 30: 154–160, 1967.
7. APPENTENG, K., M. J. O'DONOVAN, G. SOMJEN, J. A. STEPHENS, AND A. TAYLOR. The projection of jaw elevator muscle spindle afferents to fifth nerve motoneurons in the cat. *J. Physiol. London* 279: 409–423, 1978.
8. ARAKI, T., K. ENDO, Y. KAWAI, K. ITO, AND Y. SHIGENAGA. Supraspinal control of slow and fast spinal motoneurons of the cat. In: *Progress in Brain Research. Understanding the Stretch Reflex*, edited by S. Homma. Amsterdam: Elsevier, 1976, vol. 44, p. 413–432.
9. BAGINSKY, R. G. Voluntary control of motor unit activity by visual and aural feed-back. *Electroencephalogr. Clin. Neurophysiol.* 27: 724–725, 1969.
10. BAGUST, J. Relationships between motor nerve conduction velocities and motor unit contraction characteristics in a slow twitch muscle of the cat. *J. Physiol. London* 238: 269–278, 1974.
11. BAGUST, J., S. KNOTT, D. M. LEWIS, J. C. LUCK, AND R. A. WESTERMAN. Isometric contractions of motor units in a fast twitch muscle of the cat. *J. Physiol. London* 231: 87–104, 1973.
12. BARRETT, J. N. Motoneuron dendrites: role in synaptic integration. *Federation Proc.* 34: 1398–1407, 1975.
13. BARRETT, J. N., AND W. E. CRILL. Specific membrane resistivity of dye-injected cat motoneuron. *Brain Res.* 28: 556–561, 1971.
14. BARRETT, J. N., AND W. E. CRILL. Specific membrane properties of cat motoneurons. *J. Physiol. London* 239: 301–324, 1974.
15. BARRETT, J. N., AND W. E. CRILL. Influence of dendritic location and membrane properties on the effectiveness of synapses in cat motoneurons. *J. Physiol. London* 239: 325–345, 1974.
16. BARRETT, E. F., AND C. F. STEVENS. Quantal independence and uniformity of presynaptic release kinetics at the frog neuromuscular junction. *J. Physiol. London* 227: 665–689, 1972.
17. BASMAJIAN, J. V. Control and training of individual motor units. *Science* 141: 440, 1963.
18. BASMAJIAN, J. V. Control of individual motor units. *Am. J. Phys. Med.* 46: 480, 1967.
19. BASMAJIAN, J. V. Electromyography comes of age. *Science* 176: 603, 1972.
20. BESSOU, P., F. EMONET-DÉNAND, AND Y. LAPORTE. Relation entre la vitesse de conduction des fibres nerveuses motrices et le temps de contraction de leurs unités motrices. *C. R. Acad. Sci.* 256: 5625–5627, 1963.
21. BIGLAND, B., AND O. C. J. LIPPOLD. Motor unit activity in the voluntary contraction of human muscle. *J. Physiol. London* 125: 322–335, 1954.
22. BLANKENSHIP, J. E., AND M. KUNO. Analysis of spontaneous subthreshold activity in spinal motoneurons of the cat. *J. Neurophysiol.* 31: 195–209, 1968.
23. BORG, J., L. GRIMBY, AND J. HANNERZ. Axonal conduction velocity and voluntary discharge properties of individual short toe extensor motor units in man. *J. Physiol. London* 277: 143–152, 1978.
24. BRACCHI, F., M. DECANDIA, AND T. GUALTIEROTTI. Frequency stabilization in the motor centers of spinal cord and caudal brain stem. *Am. J. Physiol.* 210: 1170–1177, 1966.
25. BROCK, L. G., J. S. COOMBS, AND J. C. ECCLES. The recording of potentials from motoneurons with an intracellular electrode. *J. Physiol. London* 117: 431–460, 1952.
26. BROWN, A. G., AND R. E. W. FYFFE. The morphology of group Ia afferent fiber collaterals in the spinal cord of the cat. *J. Physiol. London* 274: 111–127, 1978.
27. BROWN, A. G., AND R. E. W. FYFFE. The morphology of Group Ib muscle afferent fiber collaterals. *J. Physiol. London* 277: 44–45, 1978.
28. BROWN, M. C., J. K. S. JANSEN, AND D. VAN ESSEN. Polyneuronal innervation of skeletal muscle in newborn rats and its elimination during maturation. *J. Physiol. London* 261: 387–422, 1976.
29. BUCHTHAL, F., AND H. SCHMALBRUCH. Contraction times and fibre types in intact human muscle. *Acta Physiol. Scand.* 79: 435–452, 1970.
30. BÜDINGEN, H. J., AND H. J. FREUND. The relationship between the rate of rise of isometric tension and motor unit recruitment in a human forearm muscle. *Pfluegers Arch.* 362: 61–67, 1976.

31. BULLER, A. J., J. C. ECCLES, AND R. M. ECCLES. Interactions between motoneurons and muscles in respect of the characteristic speeds of their responses. *J. Physiol. London* 150: 417-439, 1960.
32. BULLOCK, T. H. Comparative aspects of some biological transducers. *Federation Proc.* 12: 666-672, 1953.
33. BULLOCK, T. H., AND G. A. HORRIDGE. *Structure and Function in the Nervous Systems of Invertebrates.* San Francisco: Freeman, 1965.
34. BURKE, R. E. Composite nature of the monosynaptic excitatory postsynaptic potential. *J. Neurophysiol.* 30: 1114-1137, 1967.
35. BURKE, R. E. Motor unit types of cat triceps surae muscle. *J. Physiol. London* 193: 141-160, 1967.
36. BURKE, R. E. Group Ia synaptic input to fast and slow twitch motor units of cat triceps surae. *J. Physiol. London* 196: 605-630, 1968.
37. BURKE, R. E. On the central nervous control of fast and slow twitch motor units. In: *New Developments in Electromyography and Clinical Neurophysiology. Human Reflexes, Pathophysiology of Motor Systems, Methodology of Human Reflexes,* edited by J. E. Desmedt. Basel: Karger, 1973, vol. 3, p. 69-94.
38. BURKE, R. E., L. FEDINA, AND A. LUNDBERG. Spatial synaptic distribution of recurrent and group Ia inhibitory systems in cat spinal motoneurons. *J. Physiol. London* 214: 305-326, 1971.
39. BURKE, R. E., E. JANKOWSKA, AND G. TEN BRUGGENCATE. A comparison of peripheral and rubrospinal synaptic input to slow and fast twitch motor units of triceps surae. *J. Physiol. London* 207: 709-732, 1970.
40. BURKE, R. E., D. N. LEVINE, M. SALCMAN, AND P. TSAIRIS. Motor units in cat soleus muscle: physiological, histochemical and morphological characteristics. *J. Physiol. London* 238: 503-514, 1974.
41. BURKE, R. E., D. N. LEVINE, P. TSAIRIS, AND F. E. ZAJAC III. Physiological types and histochemical profiles in motor units of the cat gastrocnemius. *J. Physiol. London* 234: 723-748, 1973.
42. BURKE, R. E., AND P. G. NELSON. Synaptic activity in motoneurons during natural stimulation of muscle spindles. *Science* 151: 1088-1091, 1966.
43. BURKE, R. E., AND P. G. NELSON. Accommodation to current ramps in motoneurons of fast and slow twitch motor units. *Int. J. Neurosci.* 1: 347-356, 1971.
44. BURKE, R. E., AND P. RUDOMIN. Spinal neurons and synapses. In: *Handbook of Physiology. The Nervous System. Cellular Biology of Neurons,* edited by E. Kandel. Bethesda, MD: Am. Physiol. Soc., 1977, sect. 1, vol. I, pt. 2, chapt. 24, p. 877-944.
45. BURKE, R. E., W. Z. RYMER, AND J. V. WALSH, JR. Functional specialization in the motor unit population of cat medial gastrocnemius muscle. In: *Control of Posture and Locomotion,* edited by R. B. Stein, K. B. Pearson, R. S. Smith, and J. B. Redford. New York: Plenum, 1974. (Adv. Behav. Biol. Ser., vol. 7.)
46. BURKE, R. E., W. Z. RYMER, AND J. V. WALSH, JR. Relative strength of synaptic input from short-latency pathways to motor units of defined type in cat medial gastrocnemius. *J. Neurophysiol.* 39: 447-458, 1976.
47. BURKE, R. E., P. L. STRICK, K. KANDA, C. C. KIM, AND B. WALMSLEY. Anatomy of medial gastrocnemius and soleus motor nuclei in cat spinal cord. *J. Neurophysiol.* 40: 667-680, 1977.
48. BURKE, R. E., AND G. TEN BRUGGENCATE. Electrotonic characteristics of alpha motoneurons of varying size. *J. Physiol. London* 212: 1-20, 1971.
49. BURKE, R. E., AND P. TSAIRIS. Anatomy and innervation ratios in motor units of cat gastrocnemius. *J. Physiol. London* 234: 749-765, 1973.
50. BURKE, R. E., AND P. TSAIRIS. The correlation of physiological properties with histochemical characteristics in single muscle units. *Ann. NY Acad. Sci.* 228: 145-159, 1974.
51. BURKE, R. E., B. WALMSLEY, AND J. A. HODGSON. Structural-functional relations in monosynaptic action on spinal motoneurons. In: *Integration in the Nervous System,* edited by H. Asanuma and V. J. Wilson. Toyko: Igaku-Shoin, 1979, p. 27-45.
52. BUSH, B. M. H. Proprioceptive reflexes in the legs of *Carcinus maenas* (L.). *J. Exp. Biol.* 39: 89, 1962.
53. CANGIANO, E., W. A. COOK, AND O. POMPEIANO. Primary afferent depolarization in the lumbar cord evoked from the fastigial nucleus. *Arch. Ital. Biol.* 107: 321-340, 1969.
54. CARPENTER, D., I. ENGBERG, AND A. LUNDBERG. Primary afferent depolarization evoked from the brain stem and the cerebellum. *Arch. Ital. Biol.* 104: 73-85, 1966.
55. CHAPPLE, W. D. Motoneurons innervating the dorsal superficial muscles of the hermit crab, *Pagurus pollicarus,* and their reflex asymmetry. *J. Comp. Physiol.* 121: 413-431, 1977.
56. CHIN, N. K., M. COPE, AND M. PANG. Number and distribution of spindle capsules in seven hindlimb muscles of the cat. In: *Symposium on Muscle Receptors,* edited by D. Barker. Hong Kong: Hong Kong Univ. Press, 1962, p. 241-248.
57. CLAMANN, H. P. Activity of single motor units during isometric tension. *Neurology* 20: 254-260, 1970.
58. CLAMANN, H. P., J. D. GILLIES, AND E. HENNEMAN. Effects of inhibitory inputs on critical firing level and rank order of motoneurons. *J. Neurophysiol.* 37: 1350-1360, 1974.
59. CLAMANN, H. P., J. D. GILLIES, R. D. SKINNER, AND E. HENNEMAN. Quantitative measures of output of a motoneuron pool during monosynaptic reflexes. *J. Neurophysiol.* 37: 1328-1337, 1974.
60. CLAMANN, H. P., AND E. HENNEMAN. Electrical measurement of axon diameter and its use in relating motoneuron size to critical firing level. *J. Neurophysiol.* 39: 844-851, 1976.
61. CLAMANN, H. P., AND C. G. KUKULKA. Evidence for selective inputs to a motoneuron pool. *Neurosci. Abst.* 2: 539, 1976.
62. CLAMANN, H. P., AND C. G. KUKULKA. The relation between size of motoneurons and their position in the cat spinal cord. *J. Morphol.* 153: 461-466, 1977.
63. CLAMANN, H. P., AND C. G. KUKULKA. Reversals of recruitment order in medial gastrocnemius produced by stimulation of Deiters' nucleus. *Neurosci. Abst.* 3: 269, 1977.
64. CLARK, D. A. Muscle counts of motor units: a study in innervation ratios. *Am. J. Physiol.* 96: 296-304, 1931.
65. CLOUGH, J. F. M., D. KERNELL AND C. G. PHILLIPS. The distribution of monosynaptic excitation from the pyramidal tract and from primary spindle afferents to motoneurons of the baboon's hand and forearm. *J. Physiol. London* 198: 145-166, 1968.
66. COËRS, C. Les variations structurelles normales et pathologiques de la jonction neuromusculaire. *Acta Neurol. Psychiatr. Belg.* 55: 741-866, 1955.
67. COHEN, L. A. Localization of stretch reflex. *J. Neurophysiol.* 16: 272-285, 1953.
68. COHEN, L. A. Organization of stretch reflex into two types of direct spinal arcs. *J. Neurophysiol.* 17: 443-453, 1954.
69. COLE, W. V. Structural variations of nerve endings in the striated muscle of rat. *J. Comp. Neurol.* 108: 445-464, 1957.
70. COLLATOS, T. C., A. NIECHAJ, S. J. NELSON, AND L. M. MENDELL. Fluctuations in time of onset of Ia-motoneuron EPSPs in the cat. *Brain Res.* 160: 514-518, 1979.
71. CONRADI, S. Ultrastructure and distribution of neuronal and glial elements on the motoneuron surface in the lumbosacral spinal cord of the adult cat. *Acta Physiol. Scand. Suppl.* 332: 5-48, 1969.
72. CONRADI, S. Ultrastructure of dorsal root boutons on lumbosacral motoneurons of the adult cat. *Acta Physiol. Scand. Suppl.* 332: 85-115, 1969.
73. CONRADI, S. Functional anatomy of the anterior horn motor neuron. In: *The Peripheral Nerve,* edited by D. H. Landon. London: Chapman Hall, 1976, p. 279-329.
74. CONRADI, S., AND L. O. RONNEVI. Spontaneous elimination of synapses on cat spinal motoneurons after birth: do half of the synapses on the cell bodies disappear? *Brain Res.* 92: 505-510, 1975.

75. COOMBS, J. S., D. R. CURTIS, AND J. C. ECCLES. The generation of impulses in motoneurons. *J. Physiol. London* 139: 232–249, 1957.
76. CORDA, M., G. EKLUND, AND C. V. EULER. External intercostal and phrenic alpha motor responses to changes in respiratory load. *Acta Physiol. Scand.* 63: 391–400, 1965.
77. COWAN, W. M. The development of the brain. *Sci. Am.* 241: 113–133, 1979.
78. CREED, R. S., D. DENNY-BROWN, J. C. ECCLES, E. G. T. LIDDELL, AND C. S. SHERRINGTON. *Reflex Activity of the Spinal Cord*. London: Oxford Univ. Press, 1932.
79. CREED, R. S., AND C. SHERRINGTON. Observations on concurrent contraction of flexor muscles in the flexion reflex. *Proc. R. Soc. London Ser. B* 100: 258–267, 1926.
80. CULLHEIM, S. Relations between cell body size, axon diameter and axon conduction velocity of cat sciatic alpha-motoneurons stained with horseradish peroxidase. *Neurosci. Letters* 8: 17–20, 1978.
81. CULLHEIM, S., AND J. O. KELLERTH. A morphological study of the axons and recurrent axon collaterals of cat alpha-motoneurons supplying different functional types of muscle unit. *J. Physiol. London* 281: 301–313, 1978.
82. CULLHEIM, S., AND J. O. KELLERTH. A morphological study of the axons and recurrent axon collaterals of cat sciatic α-motoneurons after intracellular staining with horseradish peroxidase. *J. Comp. Neurol.* 178: 537–558, 1978.
83. CULLHEIM, S., J. O. KELLERTH, AND S. CONRADI. Evidence for direct synaptic interconnections between cat spinal α-motoneurons via the recurrent axon collaterals: a morphological study using intracellular injection of horseradish peroxidase. *Brain Res.* 132: 1–10, 1977.
84. CZÉH, G., R. GALLEGO, N. KUDO, AND M. KUNO. Evidence for the maintenance of motoneuron properties by muscle activity. *J. Physiol. London* 281: 239–252, 1978.
85. DAVIS, W. J. Functional significance of motoneuron size and soma position in swimmeret system of the lobster. *J. Neurophysiol.* 34: 274–288, 1971.
86. DEITERS, O. *Untersuchung über Gehirn and Rückenmark des Menschen und der Säugethiere*. Braunschweig, 1865.
87. DEKKER, J. J., D. G. LAWRENCE, AND H. G. J. M. KUYPERS. The location of longitudinally running dendrites in the ventral horn of the cat spinal cord. *Brain Res.* 51: 319–325, 1973.
88. DEL CASTILLO, J., AND B. KATZ. Quantal components of the end plate potential. *J. Physiol. London* 124: 560–573, 1954.
89. DENNY-BROWN, D. Nature of postural reflexes, *Proc. R. Soc. London Ser. B* 104: 252–301, 1929.
90. DESMEDT, J. E., AND E. GODAUX. Ballistic contractions in man: characteristic recruitment pattern of single motor units of the tibialis anterior muscle. *J. Physiol. London* 264: 673–693, 1977.
91. DESMEDT, J. E., AND E. GODAUX. Critical evaluation of the size principle of human motoneuron recruitment in ballistic movements and in vibration-induced inhibition or potentiation. *Trans. Am. Neurol. Assoc.* 102: 104–108, 1977.
92. DESMEDT, J. E., AND E. GODAUX. Fast motor units are not preferentially activated in rapid voluntary contractions in man. *Nature London* 267: 717–719, 1977.
93. DESMEDT, J. E., AND E. GODAUX. Ballistic skilled movements: load compensation and patterning of the motor commands. In: *Progress in Clinical Neurophysiology. Cerebral Motor Control in Man: Long Loop Mechanisms*, edited by J. E. Desmedt. Basel: Karger, 1978, vol. 4, p. 21–55.
94. DESMEDT, J. E., AND E. GODAUX. Ballistic contractions in fast or slow human muscles: discharge patterns of single motor units. *J. Physiol. London* 285: 185–196, 1978.
95. DESMEDT, J. E., AND E. GODAUX. Mechanism of the vibration paradox: excitatory and inhibitory effects of tendon vibration on single soleus muscle motor units in man. *J. Physiol. London* 285: 197–207, 1978.
96. ECCLES, J. C. *The Physiology of Synapses*. New York: Academic, 1964.
97. ECCLES, J. C., R. M. ECCLES, A. IGGO, AND M. ITO. Distribution of recurrent inhibition among motoneurons. *J. Physiol. London* 159: 479–499, 1961.
98. ECCLES, J. C., R. M. ECCLES, A. IGGO, AND A. LUNDBERG. Electrophysiological studies on gamma motoneurons. *Acta Physiol. Scand.* 50: 32–40, 1960.
99. ECCLES, J. C., R. M. ECCLES, AND A. LUNDBERG. The convergence of monosynaptic excitatory afferents onto many different species of alpha motoneurons. *J. Physiol. London* 137: 22–50, 1957.
100. ECCLES, J. C., R. M. ECCLES, AND A. LUNDBERG. Synaptic actions on motoneurons caused by impulses in Golgi tendon organ afferents. *J. Physiol. London* 138: 227–252, 1957.
101. ECCLES, J. C., R. M. ECCLES, AND F. MAGNI. Central inhibitory action attributable to presynaptic depolarization produced by muscle afferent volleys. *J. Physiol. London* 159: 147–166, 1961.
102. ECCLES, J. C., AND C. S. SHERRINGTON. Numbers and contraction values of individual motor-units examined in some muscles of the limb. *Proc. R. Soc. Lond. Ser. B* 106: 326, 1939.
103. ECCLES, R. M., AND A. LUNDBERG. Integrative pattern of Ia synaptic actions of motoneurons of hip and knee muscles. *J. Physiol. London* 144: 271–298, 1958.
104. ECCLES, R. M., AND A. LUNDBERG. Synaptic actions in motoneurons by afferents which may evoke the flexion reflex. *Arch. Ital. Biol.* 97: 199–221, 1959.
105. EDWARDS, F. R., S. J. REDMAN, AND B. WALMSLEY. Statistical fluctuations in charge transfer at Ia synapses on spinal motoneurons. *J. Physiol. London* 259: 665–688, 1976.
106. EDWARDS, F. R., S. J. REDMAN, AND B. WALMSLEY. Nonquantal fluctuations and transmission failures in charge transfer at Ia synapses on spinal motoneurons. *J. Physiol. London* 259: 689–704, 1976.
107. EDWARDS, F. R., S. J. REDMAN, AND B. WALMSLEY. The effect of polarizing currents on unitary Ia excitatory postsynaptic potentials evoked in spinal motoneurons. *J. Physiol. London* 259: 705–723, 1976.
108. EMONET-DÉNAND, F., L. JAMI, AND Y. LAPORTE. Skeleto-fusimotor axons in hind-limb muscles of the cat. *J. Physiol. London* 249: 153–166, 1975.
109. ERLANGER, J., AND H. S. GASSER. *Electrical Signs of Nervous Activity*. Philadelphia: Univ. Pennsylvania Press, 1937.
110. FADEN, J. S., AND F. F. ZAJAC. Direct comparison of recruitment order with neural and muscular properties of motor units. *Soc. Neurosci. Abstr.* 3: 271, 1977.
111. FATT, P. Sequence of events in synaptic activation of a motoneurone. *J. Neurophysiol.* 20: 61–80, 1957.
112. FATT, P., AND B. KATZ. An analysis of the end-plate potential recorded with an intracellular electrode. *J. Physiol. London* 115: 320–370, 1951.
113. FEDDE, M. R., P. D. DE WET, AND R. L. KITCHELL. Motor unit recruitment pattern and tonic activity in respiratory muscles of *Gallus domesticus*. *J. Neurophysiol.* 32: 995–1004, 1969.
114. FRANK, K., AND M. G. F. FUORTES. Accommodation of spinal motoneurons of cats. *Arch. Ital. Biol.* 98: 165–170, 1960.
115. FREUND, H.-J., H. J. BÜDINGEN, AND V. DIETZ. Activity of single motor units from human forearm muscles during voluntary isometric contractions. *J. Neurophysiol.* 38: 933–946, 1975.
116. FU, T. C., H. HULTBORN, R. LARSSON, AND A. LUNDBERG. Reciprocal inhibition during the tonic stretch reflex in the decerebrate cat. *J. Physiol. London* 284: 345–369, 1978.
117. FU, T. C., AND E. D. SCHOMBURG. Electrophysiological investigation of the projection of secondary muscle spindle afferents in the cat spinal cord. *Acta Physiol. Scand.* 91: 314–329, 1974.
118. FUORTES, M. G. F., K. FRANK, AND M. C. BECKER. Steps in the production of motoneuron spikes. *J. Gen. Physiol.* 40: 732–752, 1957.
119. GARNETT, R., AND J. A. STEPHENS. Changes in the recruitment threshold of motor units in human first dorsal interosseous muscle produced by skin stimulation. *J. Physiol. London* 282: 13–14, 1978.

120. GASSER, H. The classification of nerve fibers. *Ohio J. Sci.* 41: 145, 1941.
121. GELFAN, S. Neuron and synapse populations in the spinal cord: indication of role in total integration. *Nature London* 198: 162, 1963.
122. GELFAN, S., AND A. G. RAPISARDA. Synaptic density on spinal neurons of normal dogs and dogs with experimental hindlimb rigidity. *J. Comp. Neurol.* 123: 73-95, 1964.
123. GIBBS, C. L., AND W. R. GIBSON. Energy production of rat soleus muscle. *Am. J. Physiol.* 223: 864-871, 1972.
124. GOGAN, P., J. P. GEURITAUD, G. HORCHELLE-BOSSAVIT, AND S. TYC-DUMONT. Direct excitatory interactions between spinal motoneurons of the cat. *J. Physiol. London* 272: 755-767, 1977.
125. GOLDBERG, L. J., AND B. DERFLER. Relationship among recruitment order, spike amplitude, and twitch tension of single motor units in human masseter muscle. *J. Neurophysiol.* 40: 879-890, 1977.
126. GOLDSPINK, D. F. The influence of immobilization and stretch on protein turnover of rat skeletal muscle. *J. Physiol. London* 264: 267-282, 1977.
127. GOLDSPINK, D. F. The influence of activity on muscle size and protein turnover. *J. Physiol. London* 264: 283-296, 1977.
128. GRANIT, R. Neuromuscular interaction in postural tone of the cat's isometric soleus muscle. *J. Physiol. London* 143: 387-402, 1958.
129. GRANIT, R., H. D. HENATSCH, AND G. STEG. Tonic and phasic ventral horn cells differentiated by post-tetanic potentiation in cat extensors. *Acta Physiol. Scand.* 37: 114-126, 1956.
130. GRANIT, R., D. KERNELL, AND G. K. SHORTESS. Quantitative aspects of repetitive firing of mammalian motoneurons, caused by injected currents. *J. Physiol. London* 168: 911-931, 1963.
131. GRANIT, R., J. E. PASCOE, AND G. STEG. The behaviour of tonic alpha and gamma motoneurons during stimulation of recurrent collaterals. *J. Physiol. London* 138: 381-400, 1957.
132. GRILLNER, S. Muscle stiffness and motor control—forces in the ankle during locomotion and standing. In: *Motor Control*, edited by A. A. Gydikov, N. T. Tankov, and D. S. Kosarov. New York: Plenum, 1973, p. 195-215. (Proc. Int. Symp. Motor Control "Zlatni Pyassatsi," 2nd, near Varni, Bulgaria, 1973.)
133. GRILLNER, S., T. HONGO, AND S. LUND. The vestibulospinal tract. Effects on alpha-motoneurons in the lumbosacral spinal cord in the cat. *Exp. Brain Res.* 10: 94-120, 1970.
134. GRILLNER, S., T. HONGO, AND S. LUND. Convergent effects on alpha motoneurons from the vestibulospinal tract and a pathway descending in the medial longitudinal fasciculus. *Exp. Brain Res.* 12: 457-479, 1971.
135. GRILLNER, S., AND M. UDO. Recruitment in the tonic stretch reflex. *Acta Physiol. Scand.* 81: 571-573, 1971.
136. GRIMBY, L., AND J. HANNERZ. Recruitment order of motor units in voluntary contraction: changes induced by proprioceptive afferent activity. *J. Neurol. Neurosurg. Psychiatry* 31: 565-573, 1968.
137. GRIMBY, L., AND J. HANNERZ. Differences in recruitment order and discharge pattern of motor units in the early and late flexion reflex components in man. *Acta Physiol. Scand.* 90: 555-564, 1974.
138. GRIMBY, L., AND J. HANNERZ. Disturbances in voluntary recruitment order of low and high frequency motor units on blockade of proprioceptive afferent activity. *Acta Physiol. Scand.* 96: 207-216, 1976.
139. GRIMBY, L., AND J. HANNERZ. Firing rate and recruitment order of toe extensor motor units in different modes of voluntary contraction. *J. Physiol. London* 264: 865-879, 1977.
140. GRINELL, A. D. A study of the interaction between motoneurons in the frog spinal cord. *J. Physiol. London* 182: 612-648, 1966.
141. GROSSMAN, Y., M. E. SPRIA, AND I. PARNAS. Differential flow of information into branches of a single axon. *Brain Res.* 64: 379-386, 1973.
142. HAMBURGER, V. Regression vs. peripheral control of differentiation in motor hypoplasia. *Am. J. Anat.* 102: 365-410, 1958.
143. HAMBURGER, V. Cell death in the development of the lateral motor column of the chick embryo. *J. Comp. Neurol.* 160: 535-546, 1975.
144. HARRIS, C. The morphology of the myoneural junction as influenced by neurotoxic drugs. *Am. J. Pathol.* 30: 501-519, 1954.
145. HARRIS, D. A., AND E. HENNEMAN. Identification of two species of alpha motoneurons in cat's plantaris pool. *J. Neurophysiol.* 40: 16-25, 1977.
146. HARRIS, D. A., AND E. HENNEMAN. Different species of alpha motoneurons in same pool: further evidence from effects of inhibition on their firing rates. *J. Neurophysiol.* 42: 927-935, 1979.
147. HARRISON, V. F., AND O. A. MORTENSON. Identification and voluntary control of single motor unit activity in the tibialis anterior muscle. *Anat. Rec.* 144: 109, 1962.
148. HARVEY, R. J., AND P. B. C. MATTHEWS. The response of deefferented muscle spindle endings in the cat's soleus to slow extension of the muscle. *J. Physiol. London* 157: 370-392, 1961.
149. HATZE, H. The relative contribution of motor unit recruitment and rate coding to the production of static isometric muscle force. *Biol. Cybernetics* 27: 21-25, 1977.
150. HATZE, H. A teleological explanation of Weber's Law and the motor unit size law. *Bull. Math. Biol.* 41: 407-425, 1979.
151. HATZE, H., AND J. D. BUYS. Energy-optimal controls in the mammalian neuromuscular system. *Biol. Cybernetics* 27: 9-20, 1977.
152. HENATSCH, H. D., AND F. J. SCHULTE. Reflexerregung und Eigenhemmung tonischer und phossicher Alpha-motoneurone wahrend chemischer Dauererregung der Muskelspindeln. *Pfluegers Arch.* 268: 134-147, 1958.
153. HENNEMAN, E. Relation between size of neurons and their susceptibility to discharge. *Science* 126: 1345-1347, 1957.
154. HENNEMAN, E. Skeletal muscle: the servant of the nervous system. In: *Medical Physiology* (14th ed.), edited by V. B. Mountcastle. St. Louis: Mosby, 1980, p. 674-702.
154a. HENNEMAN, E. Organization of the motoneuron pool: the size principle. In: *Medical Physiology* (14th ed.), edited by V. B. Mountcastle. St. Louis: Mosby, 1980, p. 718-741.
155. HENNEMAN, E., H. P. CLAMANN, J. D. GILLIES, AND R. D. SKINNER. Rank-order of motoneurons within a pool: law of combination. *J. Neurophysiol.* 37: 1338, 1974.
156. HENNEMAN, E., H.-R. LÜSCHER, AND P. RUENZEL. Terminal distribution of Ia and group II spindle afferent fibers in the spinal cord as revealed by postsynaptic population potentials recorded from two adjacent spinal segments. *Neurosci. Abstr.* 5: 724, 1979.
157. HENNEMAN, E., AND C. B. OLSON. Relations between structure and function in the design of skeletal muscles. *J. Neurophysiol.* 28: 581-598, 1965.
158. HENNEMAN, E., B. T. SHAHANI, AND R. R. YOUNG. Voluntary control of human motor units. In: *The Motor System: Neurophysiology and Muscle Mechanisms*, edited by M. Shahani. Amsterdam: Elsevier, 1976, p. 73-78.
159. HENNEMAN, E., G. SOMJEN, AND D. O. CARPENTER. Functional significance of cell size in spinal motoneurons. *J. Neurophysiol.* 28: 560-580, 1965.
160. HENNEMAN, E., G. SOMJEN, AND D. O. CARPENTER. Excitability and inhibitibility of motoneurons of different sizes. *J. Neurophysiol.* 28: 599-620, 1965.
161. HODES, R., S. M. PEACOCK, JR., AND D. BODIAN. Selective destruction of large motoneurons by poliomyelitis virus. II. Size of motoneurons in the spinal cord of rhesus monkeys. *J. Neuropathol. Exp. Neurol.* 8: 400-410, 1949.
162. HOLLYDAY, M., AND V. HAMBURGER. Reduction of the naturally occurring motor neuron loss by enlargement of the periphery. *J. Comp. Neurol.* 170: 311-320, 1976.
163. HONGO, T., N. ISHIZUKA, H. MANNEN, AND S. SASAKI. Axonal trajectory of single group Ia and Ib fibers in the cat spinal cord. *Neurosci. Letters* 8: 321-328, 1978.
164. HONGO, T., E. JANKOWSKA, AND A. LUNDBERG. The rubrospinal tract. I. Effects on alpha motoneurons innervating hind-

limb muscles in cats. *Exp. Brain Res.* 7: 344-364, 1969.
165. HORRIDGE, G. A., AND M. BURROWS. Tonic and phasic systems in parallel in the eyecup responses of the crab *Carcinus*. *J. Exp. Biol.* 49: 269, 1968.
166. HOUK, J., AND E. HENNEMAN. Responses of Golgi tendon organs to active contractions of the soleus muscle of the cat. *J. Neurophysiol.* 30: 466-481, 1967.
167. HOWLAND, B., J. Y. LETTVIN, W. S. MCCULLOCH, W. PITTS, AND P. D. WALL. Reflex inhibition by dorsal root interaction. *J. Neurophysiol.* 18: 1-17, 1955.
168. HOYLE, G. Exploration of neuronal mechanisms underlying behaviour in insects. In: *Neural Theory and Modeling: Proceedings*, edited by R. F. Reiss. Stanford, CA: Stanford Univ. Press, 1964, p. 346-376. (Ojai Symp., 1962.)
169. HUGHES, G. M., AND C. M. BALLINTIJN. Electromyography of the respiratory muscles and gill water flow in the dragonet. *J. Exp. Biol.* 49: 583, 1968.
170. HUIZAR, P., N. KUDO, M. KUNO, AND Y. MIYATA. Reaction of intact spinal motoneurons to partial denervation of the muscle. *J. Physiol. London* 265: 175-191, 1977.
171. HULTBORN, H. Transmission in the pathway of reciprocal Ia inhibition to motoneurons and its control during the tonic stretch reflex. In: *Progress in Brain Research. Understanding the Stretch Reflex*, edited by S. Homma. Amsterdam: Elsevier, 1976, vol. 44, p. 235-255.
172. HULTBORN, H., E. JANKOWSKA, AND S. LINDSTROM. Recurrent inhibition from motor axon collaterals of transmission in the Ia inhibitory pathway to motoneurons. *J. Physiol. London* 215: 591-612, 1971.
173. HUNT, C. C. Monosynaptic reflex response of spinal motoneurons to graded afferent stimulation. *J. Gen. Physiol.* 38: 813-832, 1955.
174. HURSH, J. B. Conduction velocity and diameter of nerve fibers. *Am. J. Physiol.* 127: 131-139, 1939.
175. IANSEK, R., AND S. J. REDMAN. An analysis of the cable properties of spinal motoneurons using a brief intracellular current pulse. *J. Physiol. London* 234: 613-636, 1973.
176. IANSEK, R., AND S. J. REDMAN. The amplitude, time course and charge of unitary excitatory post-synaptic potentials evoked in spinal motoneuron dendrites. *J. Physiol. London* 234: 665-688, 1973.
177. ILES, J. F. Central terminations of muscle afferents on motoneurons in the cat spinal cord. *J. Physiol. London* 262: 91-117, 1976.
178. ILES, J. F. The speed of passive dendritic conduction of synaptic potentials in a model motoneuron. *Proc. R. Soc. London Ser. B* 197: 225-229, 1977.
179. ILLIS, L. Spinal cord synapses in the cat: the normal appearances by the light microscope. *Brain* 87: 543-554, 1964.
180. ILLIS, L. The relative densities of monosynaptic pathways to the cell bodies and dendrites of the cat ventral horn. *J. Neurol. Sci.* 4: 259-270, 1967.
181. JACK, J. J. B., S. MILLER, R. PORTER, AND S. J. REDMAN. The distribution of group Ia synapses on lumbosacral motoneurons in the cat. In: *Excitatory Synaptic Mechanisms*, edited by P. Anderson and J. K. S. Jansen. Oslo: Universitetsforlaget, 1970, p. 199-205.
182. JACK, J. J. B., S. MILLER, R. PORTER, AND S. J. REDMAN. The time course of minimal excitatory post-synaptic potentials evoked in spinal motoneuron by group Ia afferent fibers. *J. Physiol. London* 215: 353-380, 1971.
183. JACK, J. J. B., D. NOBLE, AND R. W. TSIEN. *Electric Current Flow in Excitable Cells*. Oxford: Clarendon, 1975, p. 502.
184. JACK, J. B., AND R. PORTER. Rapidly and slowly rising components of monosynaptic excitatory postsynaptic potentials in spinal motoneurons. *J. Physiol. London* 186: 106-107, 1966.
185. JAMI, L., AND J. PETIT. Correlation between axonal conduction velocity and tetanic tension of motor units in four muscles of the cat hind limb. *Brain Res.* 96: 114-118, 1975.
186. JANKOWSKA, E., AND S. LINDSTROM. Morphological identification of Renshaw cells. *Acta Physiol. Scand.* 81: 428-430, 1971.
187. JANKOWSKA, E., Y. PADEL, AND R. TANAKA. Projections of pyramidal tract cells to alpha motoneurons innervating hind limb muscles in the monkey. *J. Physiol. London* 249: 637-667, 1975.
188. JANKOWSKA, E., AND W. J. ROBERTS. An electrophysiological demonstration of the axonal projections of single spinal interneurons in the cat. *J. Physiol. London* 222: 597-622, 1972.
189. JANKOWSKA, E., AND W. J. ROBERTS. Synaptic actions of single interneurons mediating reciprocal Ia inhibition of motoneurons. *J. Physiol. London* 222: 623-642, 1972.
190. JANKOWSKA, E., AND D. O. SMITH. Antidromic activation of Renshaw cells and their axonal projections. *Acta Physiol. Scand.* 88: 198-214, 1973.
191. KAISER, E. I., AND I. PETERSEN. Muscle action potentials studied by frequency analysis and duration measurements. *Acta Neurol. Scand.* 41: (Suppl. 13) 213-236, 1965.
192. KANDA, K., R. E. BURKE, AND B. WALMSLEY. Differential control of fast and slow twitch motor units in the decerebrate cat. *Exp. Brain Res.* 29: 57-74, 1977.
193. KATO, M., AND K. FUKUSHIMA. Effect of differential blocking of motor axons on antidromic activation of Renshaw cells. *Exp. Brain Res.* 20: 135-143, 1974.
194. KATO, M., AND J. TANJI. Volitionally controlled single motor units in human finger muscles. *Brain Res.* 40: 345-357, 1972.
195. KATZ, B. The transmission of impulses from nerve to muscle, and the subcellular unit of synaptic action. *Proc. R. Soc. London Ser. B* 155: 455-477, 1962.
196. KATZ, B., AND R. MILEDI. A study of spontaneous miniature potentials in spinal motoneurons. *J. Physiol. London* 168: 389-422, 1963.
197. KATZ, B., AND R. MILEDI. The measurement of synaptic delay and the time course of acetylcholine released at the neuromuscular junction. *Proc. R. Soc. London Ser. B* 161: 483-495, 1965.
198. KATZ, B., AND R. MILEDI. A study of synaptic transmission in the absence of nerve impulses. *J. Physiol. London* 192: 407-436, 1967.
199. KATZ, B., AND S. THESLEFF. On the factors which determine the amplitude of the miniature end plate potential. *J. Physiol. London* 137: 267-278, 1957.
200. KERNELL, D. The adaptation and the relation between discharge frequency and current strength of cat lumbosacral motoneurons stimulated by long-lasting injected currents. *Acta Physiol. Scand.* 65: 65-73, 1965.
201. KERNELL, D. High-frequency repetitive firing of cat lumbosacral motoneurons stimulated by long-lasting injected currents. *Acta Physiol. Scand.* 65: 74-86, 1965.
202. KERNELL, D. The limits of firing frequency in cat lumbosacral motoneurons possessing different time course of afterhyperpolarization. *Acta Physiol. Scand.* 65: 87-100, 1965.
203. KERNELL, D. Input resistance, electrical excitability, and size of ventral horn cells in cat spinal cord. *Science* 152: 1637-1640, 1966.
204. KERNELL, D. Recruitment, rate modulation and the tonic strength reflex. *Progress in Brain Research. Understanding the Stretch Reflex*, edited by S. Homma. Amsterdam: Elsevier, 1976, vol. 44, p. 257-266.
205. KERNELL, D., AND H. SJOHOLM. Repetitive impulse firing: comparisons between neuron models based on "voltage clamp equations" and spinal motoneurons. *Acta Physiol. Scand.* 87: 40-56, 1973.
206. KERNELL, D., AND H. SJÖHOLM. Recruitment and firing rate modulation of motor unit tension in a small muscle of the cat's foot. *Brain Res.* 98: 57-72, 1975.
207. KIRKWOOD, P. A., AND T. A. SEARS. Monosynaptic excitation of motoneurons from secondary endings of muscle spindles. *Nature London* 252: 243-244, 1974.
208. KIRKWOOD, P. A., AND T. A. SEARS. Monosynaptic excitation of motoneurons from muscle spindle secondary endings of intercostal and triceps surae muscles in the cat. *J. Physiol. London* 245: 64-66, 1975.

209. KIRKWOOD, P. A., AND T. A. SEARS. The synaptic connexions to intercostal motoneurons as revealed by the average common excitation potential. *J. Physiol. London* 275: 103-134, 1978.
210. KNOTT, S., D. M. LEROIS, AND J. C. LUCK. Motor unit area in a cat limb muscle. *Exp. Neurol.* 30: 475-483, 1971.
211. KNOX, C. K. Cross-correlation functions for a neuronal model. *Biophys. J.* 14: 567-582, 1974.
212. KOZIOL, J. A., AND H. C. TUCKWELL. Analysis and estimation of synaptic densities and their spatial variation on the motoneuron surface. *Brain Res.* 150: 617-624, 1978.
213. KRNJEVIĆ, K., AND R. J. MILEDI. Failure of neuromuscular propagation in rats. *J. Physiol. London* 140: 440-461, 1958.
214. KUNO, M. Excitability following antidromic activation in spinal motoneurons supplying red muscles. *J. Physiol. London* 149: 374-393, 1959.
215. KUNO, M. Quantal components of excitatory synaptic potentials in spinal motoneurons. *J. Physiol. London* 175: 81-99, 1964.
216. KUNO, M. Mechanism of facilitation and depression of the excitatory synaptic potential in spinal motoneurons. *J. Physiol. London* 175: 100-112, 1964.
217. KUNO, M. Quantum aspects of central and ganglionic synaptic transmission in vertebrates. *Physiol. Rev.* 51: 647-678, 1971.
218. KUNO, M., AND R. LLINAS. Enhancement of synaptic transmission by dendritic potentials in chromatolyzed motoneurons of the cat. *J. Physiol. London* 210: 807-821, 1970.
219. KUNO, M., AND J. T. MIYAHARA. Non-linear summation of unit synaptic potentials in spinal motoneurons of the cat. *J. Physiol. London* 201: 465-477, 1969.
220. KUNO, M., AND J. T. MIYAHARA. Analysis of synaptic efficacy in spinal motoneurons from "quantum" aspects. *J. Physiol. London* 201: 479-493, 1969.
221. KUNO, M., Y. MIYATA, AND E. J. MUÑOZ-MARTINEZ. Differential reactions of fast and slow alpha motoneurons to axotomy. *J. Physiol. London* 240: 725-739, 1974.
222. KUNO, M., E. J. MUÑOZ-MARTINEZ, AND M. RANDIC. Synaptic action in Clarke's column neurons in relation to afferent terminal size. *J. Physiol. London* 228: 343-360, 1973.
223. KUNO, M., S. A. TURKANIS, AND J. N. WEAKLY. Correlation between nerve terminal size and transmitter release at the neuromuscular junction of the frog. *J. Physiol. London* 213: 545-566, 1971.
224. KUNO, M., AND J. N. WEAKLY. Quantal components of the inhibitory synaptic potential in spinal motoneurons of the cat. *J. Physiol. London* 224: 287-303, 1972.
225. LAMB, A. The projection patterns of the ventral horn to the hind limb during development. *Dev. Biol.* 54: 82-99, 1976.
226. LAMB, A. H. Neuronal death in the development of the somatotopic projections of the ventral horn in *Xenopus*. *Brain Res.* 134: 145-150, 1977.
227. LANDMESSER, L. The development of motor projection patterns in the chick hind limb. *J. Physiol. London* 284: 391-414, 1978.
228. LANDMESSER, L., AND D. G. MORRIS. The development of functional innervation in the hind limb of the chick embryo. *J. Physiol. London* 249: 301-326, 1975.
229. LAPORTE, Y., AND D. LLOYD. Nature and significance of the reflex connections established by large afferent fibers of muscular origin. *Am. J. Physiol.* 169: 609-621, 1952.
230. LAVAIL, J. H., AND M. M. LAVAIL. The retrograde intra-axonal transport of horseradish peroxidase in the chick visual system: a light and electron microscopic study. *J. Comp. Neurol.* 157: 303-358, 1974.
231. LENNERSTRAND, G. Position and velocity sensitivity of muscle spindles in the cat. I. Primary and secondary endings deprived of fusimotor activation. *Acta Physiol. Scand.* 73: 281-299, 1968.
232. LETBETTER, W. D., W. D. WILLIS, AND W. M. THOMPSON. Monosynaptic excitation of motoneurons by single dorsal root ganglion cells. *Federation Proc.* 27: 749, 1968.
233. LIDDELL, E. G. T., AND C. S. SHERRINGTON. Reflexes in response to stretch (myotatic reflexes). *Proc. R. Soc. London Ser. B* 96: 212-242, 1924.
234. LILEY, A. W. The effects of presynaptic polarization on the spontaneous activity of the mammalian neuromuscular junction. *J. Physiol. London* 134: 427-443, 1956.
235. LLOYD, D. P. C. Reflex action in relation to pattern and peripheral source of afferent stimulation. *J. Neurophysiol.* 6: 111-119, 1943.
236. LLOYD, D. P. C. Integrative pattern of excitation and inhibition in two-neuron reflex arcs. *J. Neurophysiol.* 9: 439-444, 1946.
237. LLOYD, D. P. C. Post-tetanic potentiation of response in monosynaptic reflex pathways of the spinal cord. *J. Gen. Physiol.* 33: 147-170, 1949.
238. LOEB, G. Decreased conduction velocity in the proximal projections of myelinated dorsal root ganglion cells in the cat. *Brain Res.* 103: 381-385, 1976.
239. LORENTE DE NÓ, R. Limits of variation of the synaptic delay of motoneurons. *J. Neurophysiol.* 1: 187-194, 1938.
240. LUCAS, M. E., AND W. D. WILLIS. Identification of muscle afferents which activate interneurons in the intermediate nucleus. *J. Neurophysiol.* 37: 282-293, 1974.
241. LUND, S., AND O. POMPEIANO. Monosynaptic excitation of alpha motoneurons from supraspinal structures in the cat. *Acta Physiol. Scand.* 73: 1-21, 1968.
242. LUNDBERG, A., K. MALMGREN, AND E. D. SCHOMBURG. Role of joint afferents in motor control exemplified by effects on reflex pathways from Ib afferents. *J. Physiol. London* 284: 327-343, 1978.
243. LUNDBERG, A., U. NORSELL, AND P. VOORHOEVE. Pyramidal effects on lumbo-sacral interneurons activated by somatic afferents. *Acta Physiol. Scand.* 56: 220-229, 1962.
244. LÜSCHER, H.-R., P. RUENZEL, E. FETZ, AND E. HENNEMAN. Postsynaptic population potentials recorded from ventral roots perfused with isotonic sucrose: connections of groups Ia and II spindle afferent fibers with large populations of motoneurons. *J. Neurophysiol.* 42: 1146-1164, 1979.
245. LÜSCHER, H.-R., P. RUENZEL, AND E. HENNEMAN. How the size of motoneurons determines their susceptibility to discharge. *Nature London* 282: 859-861, 1979.
246. LÜSCHER, H.-R., P. RUENZEL, AND E. HENNEMAN. Topographic distribution of terminals Ia and Group II fibers in the spinal cord, as revealed by post-synaptic population potentials. *J. Neurophysiol.* 43: 968-985, 1980.
247. LUX, H. D., P. SCHUBERT, AND G. W. KREUTZBERG. Direct matching of morphological and electrophysiological data in cat spinal motoneurons. In: *Excitatory Synaptic Mechanisms*, edited by P. Anderson and J. K. S. Jansen. Oslo: Universitetsforlaget, 1970, p. 189-198.
248. MAGHERINI, P. C., W. PRECHT, AND P. C. SCHWINDT. Evidence for electrotonic coupling between frog motoneurons in the in situ spinal cord. *J. Neurophysiol.* 39: 474-483, 1976.
249. MATTHEWS, P. B. C. The dependence of tension upon extension in the stretch reflex of the soleus muscle of the decerebrate cat. *J. Physiol. London* 147: 521-546, 1959.
250. MATTHEWS, P. B. C. The response of de-efferented muscle spindle receptors to stretching at different velocities. *J. Physiol. London* 168: 660-678, 1963.
251. MATTHEWS, M. A., W. D. WILLIS, AND V. WILLIAMS. Dendrite bundles in lamina IX of cat spinal cord: a possible source for electrical interaction between motoneurons. *Anat. Rec.* 171: 313-328, 1971.
252. MCLAUGHLIN, B. J. Dorsal root projections to the motor nuclei in the cat spinal cord. *J. Comp. Neurol.* 144: 461-474, 1972.
253. MCPHEDRAN, A. M., R. B. WUERKER, AND E. HENNEMAN. Properties of motor units in a homogeneous red muscle (soleus) of the cat. *J. Neurophysiol.* 28: 71-84, 1965.
254. MENDELL, L. M., AND E. HENNEMAN. Terminals of single Ia fibers: distribution within a pool of 300 homonymous motor neurons. *Science* 160: 96-98, 1968.
255. MENDELL, L. M., AND E. HENNEMAN. Terminals of single Ia fibers: location, density, and distribution within a pool of 300 homonymous motoneurons. *J. Neurophysiol.* 34: 171-187, 1971.
256. MENDELL, L. M., AND R. WEINER. Analysis of pairs of individ-

ual Ia-EPSPs in single motoneurons. *J. Physiol. London* 255: 81–104, 1976.
257. MILL, P. J. Neural patterns associated with ventilatory movements in dragonfly larvae. *J. Exp. Biol.* 52: 67, 1970.
258. MILNER-BROWN, H. S., R. B. STEIN, AND R. YEMM. The orderly recruitment of human motor units during voluntary isometric contractions. *J. Physiol. London* 230: 359–370, 1973.
259. MILNER-BROWN, H. S., R. B. STEIN, AND R. YEMM. Changes in firing rate of human motor units during linearly changing voluntary contractions. *J. Physiol. London* 230: 371–390, 1973.
260. MISHELEVICH, D. J. Repetitive firing to current in cat motoneurons as a function of muscle unit twitch type. *Exp. Neurol.* 25: 401–409, 1969.
261. MONSTER, A. W., AND H. CHAN. Isometric force production by motor units of extensor digitorum communis muscle in man. *J. Neurophysiol.* 40: 1432–1443, 1977.
262. MOSHER, C. G., R. L. GERLACH, AND D. G. STUART. Soleus and anterior tibial motor units of the cat. *Brain Res.* 44: 1–11, 1972.
263. MUNSON, J. B., AND G. W. SYPERT. Latency-rise time relationship in unitary postsynaptic potentials. *Brain Res.* 151: 404–408, 1978.
264. MUNSON, J. B., AND G. W. SYPERT. Properties of central Ia afferent fibers projecting to motoneurons. *Neurosci. Abstr.* 4: 569, 1978.
265. MUNSON, J. B., AND G. W. SYPERT. Properties of single central Ia fibers projection to motoneurons. *J. Physiol. London* 296: 315–328, 1979.
266. MUNSON, J. B., AND G. W. SYPERT. Properties of single fiber excitatory post-synaptic potentials in triceps surae motoneurons. *J. Physiol. London* 296: 329–342, 1979.
267. NELSON, P. G. Interaction between spinal motoneurons of the cat. *J. Neurophysiol.* 29: 275–287, 1966.
268. NELSON, S. G., T. C. COLLATOS, A. NIECHAJ, AND L. M. MENDELL. Immediate increase in Ia-motoneuron synaptic transmission caudal to spinal cord transection. *J. Neurophysiol.* 42: 655–664, 1979.
269. NELSON, S. G., AND L. M. MENDELL. Projection of single knee flexor Ia fibers to homonymous and heteronymous motoneurons. *J. Neurophysiol.* 41: 778–787, 1978.
270. NELSON, S. G., AND L. M. MENDELL. Enhancement in Ia-motoneuron synaptic transmission caudal to chronic spinal cord transection. *J. Neurophysiol.* 42: 642–654, 1979.
271. NYSTROM, B. Postnatal development of motor nerve terminals in "slow-red" and "fast-white" cat muscles. *Acta Neurol. Scand.* 44: 363–383, 1968.
272. OLSON, C. B., D. O. CARPENTER, AND E. HENNEMAN. Orderly recruitment of muscle action potentials: motor unit threshold and EMG amplitude. *Arch. Neurol. Chicago* 19: 591–597, 1968.
273. OLSON, C. B., AND C. P. SWETT, JR. A functional and histochemical characterization of motor units in a heterogeneous muscle (flexor digitorum longus) of the cat. *J. Comp. Neurol.* 128: 475–498, 1966.
274. PADYKULA, H. A., AND G. F. GAUTHIER. The ultrastructure of the neuromuscular junctions of mammalian red, white and intermediate skeletal muscle fibers. *J. Cell Biol.* 46: 27–41, 1970.
275. PARNAS, I. Differential block at high frequency of branches of a single axon innervating two muscles. *J. Neurophysiol.* 35: 903–914, 1972.
276. PASCOE, J. E. The responses of anterior horn cells to applied currents. *Acta Physiol. Scand.* 42: (Suppl. 145) 112–113, 1957.
277. PEARSON, K. G., AND J. F. ILES. Discharge patterns of coxal levator and depressor motoneurons of the cockroach, *Periplaneta americana*. *J. Exp. Biol.* 52: 139, 1970.
278. PEARSON, K. G., R. B. STEIN, AND S. K. MALHOTRA. Properties of action potentials from insect motor nerve fibers. *J. Exp. Biol.* 53: 299–316, 1970.
279. PENNY, J. E., J. R. KUKUMS, M. J. EADIE, AND J. H. TYRER. Quantitative oxidative enzyme histochemistry of the spinal cord. Part 1. Distribution of enzyme activity in anterior horn cells. *J. Neurol. Sci.* 26: 179–185, 1975.

280. PETERSON, R. P. Cell size and rate of protein synthesis in ventral horn neurons. *Science* 153: 1413–1414, 1966.
281. PETTE, D., M. KLINGENSBERG, AND TH. BÜCHER. Comparable and specific proportions in the mitochondrial enzyme activity pattern. *Biochem. Biophys. Res. Commun.* 7: 425–429, 1962.
282. PORTER, R., AND J. HORE. Time course of minimal corticomotoneuronal excitatory postsynaptic potentials in lumbar motoneurons of the monkey. *J. Neurophysiol.* 32: 443–451, 1969.
283. PROSKE, U., AND P. M. E. WAITE. Properties of types of motor units in the medial gastrocnemius muscle of the cat. *Brain Res.* 67: 89–101, 1974.
284. RACK, P. M. H., AND D. R. WESTBURY. The effects of length and stimulus rate on tension in the isometric cat soleus muscle. *J. Physiol. London* 204: 443–460, 1969.
285. RALL, W. Branching dendritic trees and motoneuron membrane resistivity. *Exp. Neurol.* 1: 491–527, 1959.
286. RALL, W. Theoretical significance of dendrites for neuronal input-output relations. In: *Neuronal Theory and Modeling: Proceedings*, edited by R. Reiss. Stanford, CA: Stanford Univ. Press, 1964, p. 73–97. (Ojai Symp., 1962.)
287. RALL, W. Distinguishing theoretical synaptic potentials computed for different soma-dendritic distributions of synaptic input. *J. Neurophysiol.* 30: 1138–1168, 1967.
288. RALL, W. Core conductor theory and cable properties of neurons. In: *Handbook of Physiology. The Nervous System. Cellular Biology of Neurons*, edited by E. Kandel. Bethesda, MD: Am. Physiol. Soc., 1977, sect. 1, vol. I, pt. 1, chapt. 3, p. 39–97.
289. RALL, W., R. E. BURKE, T. G. SMITH, P. G. NELSON, AND K. FRANK. Dendritic location of synapses and possible mechanisms for the monosynaptic EPSP in motoneurons. *J. Neurophysiol.* 30: 1169–1193, 1967.
290. RALL, W., AND J. RINZEL. Branch input resistance and steady attenuation for input to one branch of a dendritic neuron model. *Biophys. J.* 13: 648–688, 1973.
291. RAMÓN Y CAJAL, S. *Histologie du Système de l'Homme et des Vertèbres*. Paris: Maloine, 1909.
292. RAPAPORT, S., A. SUSSWEIN, Y. UCHINO, AND V. J. WILSON. Synaptic actions of individual vertibular neurons on cat neck motoneurons. *J. Physiol. London* 272: 367–382, 1977.
293. REDFERN, P. A. Neuromuscular transmission in newborn rats. *J. Physiol. London* 209: 701–709, 1970.
294. REDMAN, S. J. A quantitative approach to the integrative function of dendrites. In: *International Review of Physiology: Neurophysiology II*, edited by R. Porter. Baltimore: Univ. Park, 1976, vol. 10, p. 1–36.
295. REDMAN, S. J. Junctional mechanisms at group Ia synapses. *Prog. Neurobiol. NY* 12: 33–83, 1979.
296. RENSHAW, B. Activity in the simplest spinal reflex pathways. *J. Neurophysiol.* 3: 373–387, 1940.
297. RENSHAW, B. Influence of discharge of motoneurons upon excitation of neighboring motoneurons. *J. Neurophysiol.* 4: 167–183, 1941.
298. RENSHAW, B. Central effects of centripetal impulses in axons of spinal ventral roots. *J. Neurophysiol.* 9: 191–204, 1946.
299. RICHMOND, F. J. R., AND V. C. ABRAHAMS. Morphology and enzyme histochemistry of dorsal muscles of the cat neck. *J. Neurophysiol.* 38: 1312–1321, 1975.
300. RINZEL, J., AND W. RALL. Transient response in a dendritic neuron model for current injected at one branch. *Biophys. J.* 14: 759–790, 1974.
301. ROEDER, K. D., L. TOZIAN, AND E. A. WEIANT. Endogenous nerve activity and behavior in the mantis and cockroach. *J. Insect Physiol.* 4: 45, 1960.
302. ROMANES, G. J. The motor cell columns of the lumbo-sacral spinal cord of the cat. *J. Comp. Neurol.* 94: 313–363, 1951.
303. RONNEVI, L. O., AND S. CONRADI. Ultrastructural evidence for spontaneous elimination of synaptic terminals on spinal motor neurons in the kitten. *Brain Res.* 80: 335–339, 1974.
304. ROWELL, C. H. F., AND J.M. MCKAY. An acridid auditory interneuron. I. Functional connexions and response to single sounds. *J. Exp. Biol.* 51: 231, 1969.

305. Rudomín, P., R. E. Burke, R. Núñez, J. Madrid, and H. Dutton. Control by presynaptic correlation: a mechanism affecting information transmission from Ia fibers to motoneurons. *J. Neurophysiol.* 38: 267-284, 1975.
306. Ryall, R. W. Renshaw cell mediated inhibition of Renshaw cells: patterns of excitation and inhibition from impulses in motor axon collaterals. *J. Neurophysiol.* 33: 257-270, 1970.
307. Ryall, R. W., M. F. Piercey, C. Polosa, and J. Goldfarb. Excitation of Renshaw cells in relation to orthodromic and antidromic excitation of motoneurons. *J. Neurophysiol.* 35: 137-148, 1972.
308. Salmons, S., and F. A. Sreter. Significance of impulse activity in the transformation of skeletal muscle type. *Nature London* 263: 30-34, 1976.
309. Scheibel, M. E., and A. B. Scheibel. Spinal motoneurons, interneurons and Renshaw cells. A Golgi study. *Arch. Ital. Biol.* 104: 328-353, 1966.
310. Scheibel, M. E., and A. B. Scheibel. Terminal patterns in cat spinal cord. III. Primary afferent collaterals. *Brain Res.* 13: 417-443, 1969.
311. Scheibel, M. E., and A. B. Scheibel. Organization of spinal motoneuron dendrites in bundles. *Exp. Neurol.* 28: 106-112, 1970.
312. Scheibel, M. E., and A. B. Scheibel. Developmental relationship between spinal motor neuron dendrite bundles and patterned activity in the forelimb of cats. *Exp. Neurol.* 30: 367-373, 1971.
313. Scheibel, M. E., and A. B. Scheibel. Inhibition and the Renshaw cell: a structural critique. *Brain Behav. Evol.* 4: 53-93, 1971.
314. Schmidt, R. F. Presynaptic inhibition in the vertebrate nervous system. *Ergeb. Physiol. Biol. Chem. Exp. Pharmakol.* 63: 20-101, 1971.
315. Scott, J. G., and L. M. Mendell. Individual EPSPs produced by single triceps surae Ia afferent fibers in homonymous and heteronymous motoneurons. *J. Neurophysiol.* 39: 679-692, 1976.
316. Sears, T. A. Some properties and reflex connections of respiratory motoneurons of the cat's thoracic spinal cord. *J. Physiol. London* 175: 386-403, 1964.
317. Sears, T. A., and D. Stagg. Short-term synchronization of intercostal motoneuron activity. *J. Physiol. London* 263: 357-381, 1976.
318. Shapovalov, A. I., and N. R. Gurevich. Monosynaptic and disynaptic reticulospinal actions on lumbar motoneurons of the cat. *Brain Res.* 21: 249-263, 1970.
319. Shapovalov, A. I., O. A. Karamyan, G. G. Kurchavyi, and Z. A. Repina. Synaptic actions evoked from the red nucleus on the spinal alpha-motoneurons in the Rhesus monkey. *Brain Res.* 32: 325-348, 1971.
320. Shapovalov, A. I., and G. G. Kurchavyi. Effects of transmembrane polarization and TEA injection on monosynaptic actions from motor cortex, red nucleus and group Ia afferents on lumbar motoneurons in the monkey. *Brain Res.* 82: 49-67, 1974.
321. Sherrington, C. S. *The Integrative Action of the Nervous System.* New Haven, CT: Yale Univ. Press, 1906.
322. Sherrington, C. S. Flexion-reflex of the limb, crossed extension-reflex and reflex stepping and standing. *J. Physiol. London* 40: 28-121, 1910.
323. Shinoda, Y., A. P. Arnold, and H. Asanuma. Spinal branching of corticospinal axons in the cat. *Exp. Brain Res.* 26: 215-234, 1976.
324. Snow, P. J., P. K. Rose, and A. G. Brown. Tracing axons and axon collaterals of spinal neurons using intracellular injection of horseradish peroxidase. *Science* 191: 312-313, 1976.
325. Somjen, G., D. O. Carpenter, and E. Henneman. Responses of motoneurons of different sizes to graded stimulation of supraspinal centers of the brain. *J. Neurophysiol.* 28: 958-965, 1965.
326. Sperry, R. W. Chemoaffinity in the orderly growth of nerve fiber patterns and connections. *Proc. Natl. Acad. Sci. USA.* 50: 703-710, 1951.
327. Sprague, J. M. The distribution of dorsal root fibers on motor cells in lumbosacral spinal cord of the cat and the site of excitatory and inhibitory terminals in monosynaptic pathways. *Proc. R. Soc. London Ser. B* 149: 534-556, 1958.
328. Stauffer, E. K., D. G. D. Watt, A. Taylor, R. M. Reinking, and D. G. Stuart. Analysis of muscle receptor connections by spike triggered averaging. 2. Spindle group II afferents. *J. Neurophysiol.* 39: 1393-1402, 1976.
329. Stein, R. B., and R. Bertoldi. The size principle: a synthesis of neurophysiological data. In: *Progress in Clinical Neurophysiology. Recruitment Patterns of Motor Units and the Gradation of Muscle Force,* edited by J. E. Desmedt. Basel: Karger, In press.
330. Stephens, J. A., R. Garnett, and N. P. Buller. Reversal of recruitment order of single motor units produced by cutaneous stimulation during voluntary muscle contraction in man. *Nature London* 272: 362-364, 1978.
331. Sterling, P., and H. G. J. M. Kuypers. Simultaneous demonstration of normal boutons and degenerating nerve fibers and their terminals in the spinal cord. *J. Anat.* 100: 723-732, 1966.
332. Sterling, P., and H. G. J. M. Kuypers. Anatomical organization of the brachial spinal cord of the cat. II. The motoneuron plexus. *Brain Res.* 4: 16-32, 1967.
333. Szekely, G., G. Czeh, and G. Voros. The activity pattern of limb muscles in freely moving normal and deafferented newts. *Exp. Brain Res.* 9: 53, 1969.
334. Szentagothai, J. The anatomical basis of synaptic transmission of excitation and inhibition of motoneurons. *Acta Morphol. Acad. Sci. Hung.* 8: 287-309, 1958.
335. Tanji, J., and M. Kato. Recruitment of motor units in voluntary contraction of a finger muscle in man. *Exp. Neurol.* 40: 759-770, 1973.
336. Teig, E. Tension and contraction times of motor units of the middle ear muscles in the cat. *Acta Physiol. Scand.* 84: 11-21, 1972.
337. Thomas, J. S., E. M. Schmidt, and F. T. Hambrecht. Facility of motor unit control during tasks defined directly in terms of unit behaviors. *Exp. Neurol.* 59: 384-395, 1978.
338. Traub, R. D. Motoneurons of different geometry and the size principle. *Biol. Cybernetics* 25: 163-176, 1977.
339. Van Buren, J. M., and K. Frank. Correlation between the morphology and potential field of a spinal motor nucleus in the cat. *Electroencephalogr. Clin. Neurophysiol.* 19: 112-126, 1965.
340. Van de Graaff, K. M., E. C. Frederick, R. G. Williamson, and G. E. Goslow, Jr. Motor units and fiber types of primary ankle extensors of the skunk (*Mephitis mephitis*). *J. Neurophysiol.* 40: 1424-1431, 1977.
341. Wagman, I. H., D. S. Pierce, and R. E. Burges. Proprioceptive influence in volitional control of individual motor units. *Nature London* 207: 957-958, 1965.
342. Walcott, B., and M. Burrows. The ultrastructure and physiology of the abdominal airguide retractor muscles in the giant water bug, *Lethocerus. J. Insect Physiol.* 15: 1865, 1969.
343. Wani, A. M., and S. K. Guha. A model for gradation of tension-recruitment and rate coding. *Med. Biol. Eng.* 13: 870-874, 1975.
344. Warmoltz, J. R., and W. K. Engel. Open-biopsy electromyography. I. Correlation of motor unit behavior with histochemical muscle fiber type in human limb muscle. *Arch. Neurol.* 27: 512-517, 1972.
345. Watt, D. G. D., E. K. Stauffer, A. Taylor, R. M. Reinking, and D. G. Stuart. Analysis of muscle receptor connections by spike-triggered averaging. 1. Spindle primary and tendon organ afferents. *J. Neurophysiol.* 39: 1375-1392, 1976.
346. Wendt, I. R., and C. L. Gibbs. Energy production of rat extensor digitorum longus muscle. *Am. J. Physiol.* 224: 1081-1086, 1973.

347. WILLIS, W. D., R. NÚÑEZ, AND P. RUDOMÍN. Excitability changes of terminal arborizations of single Ia and Ib afferent fibers produced by muscle and cutaneous conditioning volleys. *J. Neurophysiol.* 39: 1150-1159, 1976.

348. WILLIS, W. D., AND J. C. WILLIS. Properties of interneurons in the ventral spinal cord. *Arch. Ital. Biol.* 104: 354-386, 1966.

349. WILSON, V. J., AND M. YOSHIDA. Comparison of effects of stimulation of Deiters' nucleus and medial longitudinal fasciculus on neck, forelimb, and hindlimb motoneurons. *J. Neurophysiol.* 32: 743-758, 1969.

350. WILSON, V. J., AND M. YOSHIDA. Monosynaptic inhibition of neck motoneurons by the medial vestibular nucleus. *Exp. Brain Res.* 9: 365-380, 1969.

351. WINDHORST, V. Cross correlations between discharge patterns of primary muscle spindle endings in active triceps-surae muscles of the cat. *Neurosci. Lett.* 5: 63-67, 1977.

352. WUERKER, R. B., AND E. HENNEMAN. Reflex regulation of primary (annulospiral) stretch receptors via gamma motoneurons in the cat. *J. Neurophysiol.* 26: 539-550, 1963.

353. WUERKER, R. B., A. M. MCPHEDRAN, AND E. HENNEMAN. Properties of motor units in a heterogeneous pale muscle (M. gastrocnemius) of the cat. *J. Neurophysiol.* 28: 85-99, 1965.

354. WYCKOFF, R. W. G., AND J. Z. YOUNG. The motor neuron surface. *Proc. R. Soc. London Ser. B* 144: 440-450, 1955.

355. WYMAN, R. J. Somatotopic connectivity or species recognition connectivity? In: *Control of Posture and Locomotion*, edited by R. B. Stein, K. B. Pearson, R. S. Smith, and J. B. Redford. New York: Plenum, 1974, p. 45-53. (Adv. Behav. Biol. Ser., vol. 7.)

356. WYMAN, R. J., I. WALDRON, AND G. W. WACHTEL. Lack of fixed order of recruitment in cat motoneuron pools. *Exp. Brain Res.* 20: 101-114, 1974.

357. YATSUKI, Y., S. YOSHINO, AND J. CHEN. Action current of the single lateral line nerve of the fish. II. On the discharge due to stimulation. *Jpn. J. Physiol.* 1: 179-194, 1951.

358. YELLIN, H. Neural regulation of enzymes in muscle fibers of red and white muscle. *Exp. Neurol.* 19: 92-103, 1967.

359. YEMM, R. The orderly recruitment of motor units of the masseter and temporal muscles during voluntary isometric contraction in man. *J. Physiol. London* 265: 163-174, 1977.

360. ZUCKER, R. S. Theoretical implications of the size principle of motoneuron recruitment. *J. Theor. Biol.* 38: 587-596, 1973.

CHAPTER 12

Integration in spinal neuronal systems

FAUSTO BALDISSERA | *Laboratorio di Fisiologia dei Centri Nervosi, Consiglio Nazionale delle Ricerche, Milan, Italy*

HANS HULTBORN | *Department of Physiology, University of Göteborg, Göteborg, Sweden*

MICHAEL ILLERT | *Physiologisches Institut der Universität München, Munich, Germany*

CHAPTER CONTENTS

Methodological Considerations
　Selective stimulation of primary afferents
　Stimulation of central motor systems
　Methods for investigation of convergence at interneuronal level
Spinal Neuronal Circuits Used in Common by Segmental
　　　Afferents and Supraspinal Motor Centers
　Recurrent inhibition
　　Convergence onto Renshaw cells
　　Actions of Renshaw cells on spinal neurons
　　Functional considerations
　Pathways from Ia-afferents and their control by γ-motoneurons
　　Reflex pathways from group Ia muscle spindle afferents
　　Segmental and supraspinal control of γ-motoneurons
　　Functional consequences of α-γ-linkage
　Reflex pathways from Ib tendon organ afferents
　　Pattern of Ib actions in α-motoneurons
　　Convergence in Ib pathways
　　Interneurons interposed in Ib pathways to α-motoneurons (Ib-interneurons)
　　Functional considerations
　Reflex pathways from cutaneous and joint afferents and from
　　　groups II and III muscle afferents
　　Cutaneous afferents
　　Joint afferents
　　Secondary spindle afferents
　　Reflex pathways from the "flexor reflex afferents"
　Propriospinal neurons
　　Propriospinal pathways relaying descending motor commands
　　Propriospinal neurons for interlimb coordination
　　Other propriospinal systems
　Presynaptic inhibition of transmission from primary afferents
　　Effects from primary afferents to primary afferent terminals
　　Segmental control of pathways to primary afferents
　　Effects from supraspinal centers to primary afferent terminals
　　Primary afferent hyperpolarization
　　Functional considerations
Reticulospinal Inhibition of Segmental Reflex Transmission
　Dorsal reticulospinal system
　Ventral reticulospinal pathways
　Monoaminergic reticulospinal pathways
　Decerebrate preparation
Direct Projections of Descending Pathways to α-Motoneurons
Ascending Pathways That Monitor Segmental Interneuronal
　　　Activity
　　Evidence that ascending FRA pathways monitor activity in
　　　interneurons of reflex pathways
　　Information via ascending collaterals of interneurons
　　Ventral flexor reflex tracts
　　Ventral spinocerebellar tract
General Summary and Epilogue
　General summary
　Epilogue

IN THE INTRODUCTION to one of the first reviews of the spinal cord physiology, Foster (186) wrote that "reflex action may be said *par excellence* the function of the spinal cord" but he also added that "the cord contains a number of more or less complicated mechanisms capable of producing, as reflex result, co-ordinated movement altogether similar to those which are called forth by will. Now it must be an economy to the body that the will should make use of these mechanisms already present, by acting directly on their centers, rather than it should have recourse to a special apparatus of its own of a similar kind." This idea that spinal mechanisms should be used by higher centers in the generation of motor activities has until recently not developed beyond the Sherringtonian concept of a number of spinal common paths versus the final common path (550). In the meantime spinal reflexes and descending motor activities were as a rule considered to be separate entities that share the "final common path" (i.e., the motoneurons) as output but are otherwise independent in their organization [cf. chapters on motor control of the preceding edition of this *Handbook* (123, 155, 395, 476)]. This analytical approach was partly due to the compelling need for neurophysiologists to isolate from the overwhelming complexity of the nervous system simple subsystems that could be submitted to an experimental analysis. It has now been firmly established, however, that only a limited number of descending and reflex pathways maintain their individuality up to the contact with the motoneurons and that most of them share common interneurons or propriospinal neurons with other pathways. Therefore the integration of supraspinal influences with afferent signals from the periphery to a great extent occurs already at a premotoneuronal level.

A detailed knowledge of the organization of the internuncial apparatus of the spinal cord is still lacking, but a few groups of interneurons have already been systematically analyzed with regard to their synaptic input as well as to their projections to other neurons. This has been achieved partly by recording from the interneurons themselves, but in most cases our information on interneurons interposed in various pathways is still based on indirect evidence obtained by recording their effects on motoneurons. Taken together, the results of various studies have disclosed a number of neuronal networks that at this stage may be described as "functional units" of the spinal cord (550) in the sense that they are connected to a certain afferent input and exert a given action onto motoneurons. This chapter is primarily devoted to a description of such functional units and to how the brain can utilize them in its control of the final common pathway. The fact that most of the descending control of the final common pathway is integrated with afferent activity at an interneuronal level raises the need for a feedback mechanism that will allow the brain to assess the end result of this convergence. One section of this chapter therefore deals with ascending pathways that appear to monitor activity of interneurons in these functional units. Emphasis on interneuronal integration in this chapter is not intended to shadow the existence and relevance of the direct connections from supraspinal centers to motoneurons; their special significance is considered in DIRECT PROJECTIONS OF DESCENDING PATHWAYS TO α-MOTONEURONS, p. 567.

METHODOLOGICAL CONSIDERATIONS

Progress in research on interneuronal integration has been tightly linked to the development of techniques that permit selective activation of primary afferents and of specific nuclei or tracts in the central nervous system as well as recording of synaptic responses in motoneurons and other neurons in the spinal cord. The aim of this methodological section is limited to a description of some problems that are of immediate relevance for the interpretation of the experimental results discussed in the following sections.

Selective Stimulation of Primary Afferents

Electrical stimulation of peripheral nerves has been widely used to investigate reflex actions from primary afferents (cf. ref. 444). This is explained by the easy control of an electrical stimulus and by the possibility to estimate central latencies from the synchronous arrival of the afferent volley to the spinal cord. Differences in the axon diameters of afferents from different receptors and the consequent differences in excitability to electrical stimuli allowed relatively selective stimulation of at least some identifiable groups of afferents. This approach proved particularly valuable in the case of muscle afferents (68, 134, 136, 148, 368), even though the degree of threshold separation varies with the muscle and is never complete (106, 316, 317, 570).

In many cases activation of the receptors rather than their afferents proved more selective. When the nerve is left in continuity with the receptor-bearing muscle, selective activation of primary muscle spindle (group Ia) afferents can be achieved, at least for some muscles, by brief stretches or sinusoidal vibration of small amplitude (70, 179, 429, 569). Activation of afferents from Golgi tendon organs can be elicited during extrafusal contraction brought about by stimulation of α-efferents in ventral roots (304), but central actions by such a stimulus are difficult to interpret because of the concomitant changes in discharge of other receptors (282, 515). A synchronous and selective activation of Ib tendon organ afferents can, however, be obtained by electrical stimulation of nerves after increasing the thresholds for excitation of Ia-afferents (to a level above the threshold for Ib-afferents) by prolonged muscle vibration (105).

Isolated activation of secondary muscle spindle afferents is more difficult to achieve. Electrical stimulation of muscle nerves with a special waveform of the stimulating current (brief rise time, slow decay), together with a "reversed" polarity of the electrodes (anode proximal), seems to block conduction in group I but not in group II afferents (316, 318). This method, of course, does not exclude activation of group II afferents of non–spindle origin that are present to some extent in different muscle nerves (66). A more selective adequate activation of group II spindle afferents can be obtained in the cases when a synchronous activation is not requested. Spindle secondary endings increase their firing frequency both to an increase in muscle length and to static γ-efferent stimulation. If the primary endings are continuously activated by a low-amplitude–high-frequency vibration, an additional increase in muscle length (or stimulation of static γ-efferents) would then cause a selective increase in the firing of secondary afferents against the background of a constant high-frequency firing of the Ia-afferents (344, 442, 605). As demonstrated by Jack and Roberts (316, 319), it is indispensible to control that the Ia fibers indeed follow the vibration (one to one) at both muscle lengths in order to interpret the reflex effects of such input fractionation.

In the case of cutaneous fibers, only low-threshold mechanoreceptors are represented in the Aα-fiber size range, but there is a great overlap in conduction velocity for afferents from receptors of different submodalities (76, 307). Low-threshold mechanoreceptors, thermoreceptors, and nociceptors are all represented among the thinner afferents [Aδ- and C-fibers; (76, 307)]. Graded electrical stimulation of cutaneous nerves therefore cannot be used for selective activation of afferents mediating specific modalities; for that purpose it is necessary to resort to adequate receptor stimulation (cf. refs. 83, 321).

Stimulation of Central Motor Systems

In comparison with the abundant literature dealing with selective activation of different types of primary afferents, there has been surprisingly little interest in the difficulties of interpreting effects produced by electrical stimulation of motor centers in the brain. Problems connected with stimulation of a "motor center" have been considered in some detail in a series of papers regarding the rubrospinal tract (37, 38, 274–277) as well as elsewhere (e.g., ref. 32).

For some distinct groups of cells such as the red nucleus and Deiters' nucleus, it is possible to record field potentials evoked by antidromic stimulation of their axons in the spinal cord. The thresholds for descending effects can then be compared with the distribution of antidromic field potentials for different electrode positions in and around the nucleus. With stimulation at a particular site within a nucleus, it is also possible to determine whether a given effect disappears after transection of the appropriate descending tract in the spinal cord or remains after lesions severing other descending fiber systems. When activation of a large fraction of the neurons in a particular nucleus is attempted, coactivation of other fiber systems or cell groups is virtually unavoidable. For example, near-maximal stimulation of neurons in the red nucleus activates at least two extrarubral systems with effects on the spinal cord (37). In this special case the problem was solved by choosing a stimulus site ventral to the red nucleus, where the interpositorubral fiber bundle can be activated at low stimulus strength. This activation is then followed by an indirect, synaptically evoked synchronous discharge of all rubrospinal neurons (38). In other situations interpretation requires excluding the possibility of antidromic activation of fiber systems projecting to a nucleus via their axon collaterals (i.e., pyramidal tract fibers in case of the red nucleus and reticulospinal fibers in Deiters' nucleus).

It is possible to record the summed activity in descending fibers from dissected spinal cord fascicles or from the surface of the intact spinal cord (triphasic recording) following electrical stimulation of supraspinal centers. When such descending volleys are monitored at the segmental level, they can be used to judge the synaptic linkage of actions in spinal neurons from the fastest conducting descending fibers in the same way as for afferent incoming volleys following peripheral nerve stimulation. In the case of descending volleys one must take into account that even weak electrical stimuli in the brain coactivate neurons with different fiber diameter. Therefore, it is usually only possible to judge the synaptic linkage of short-latency effects related to the fastest conducting fibers. A long segmental delay from the earliest component of the descending volley may reflect monosynaptic connections from slower fibers; polysynaptic effects from the fastest fibers are only indicated when there is pronounced temporal facilitation and/or spatial facilitation or inhibition from segmental inputs.

Effects evoked by electrical stimulation of the reticular formation are particularly difficult to interpret. The cells with descending projections are widely distributed and collaterals from other motor centers are abundant. Furthermore ascending fibers from the spinal cord terminate in the reticular formation; if these ascending neurons have collaterals in the spinal cord, stimulating them antidromically may give synaptic actions that could be misinterpreted as evoked by reticulospinal neurons (cf. ASCENDING PATHWAYS THAT MONITOR SEGMENTAL INTERNEURONAL ACTIVITY, p. 569). In view of these difficulties it is worthwhile to note that selective methods are available for investigation of effects exerted from the monoaminergic reticulospinal pathways (cf. *Monoaminergic Reticulospinal Pathways*, p. 562).

Methods for Investigation of Convergence at Interneuronal Level

The introduction of monosynaptic test reflexes to assess motoneuronal excitability (387, 393, 501) opened the way for studies on excitatory and inhibitory convergence onto motoneurons. By systematically varying the intervals between the conditioning and test stimuli, it was even possible to study the time course of the synaptic actions brought about by the conditioning volleys. These studies were followed by intracellular recording of synaptic potentials in motoneurons (128). Information regarding convergence onto interneurons interposed in reflex pathways to the recorded motoneurons could then be obtained, in a corresponding way, by studying how the synaptic potentials evoked from primary afferents are influenced from other neuronal systems (407, 412), as illustrated diagrammatically in Figure 1. In Figure 1A activation of either primary afferents or descending systems has no effect on the motoneuron, since the stimulation strength has been adjusted to be subliminal for activation of the interposed interneurons. If combined stimulation of both systems elicits a postsynaptic potential (PSP) in the motoneuron, it should be due to spatial summation of subliminal excitatory actions from systems I and II on common interneurons. The appearance of a motoneuronal PSP depends on the level of excitability within the interneuronal pool, and it is often more convenient to use test and conditioning

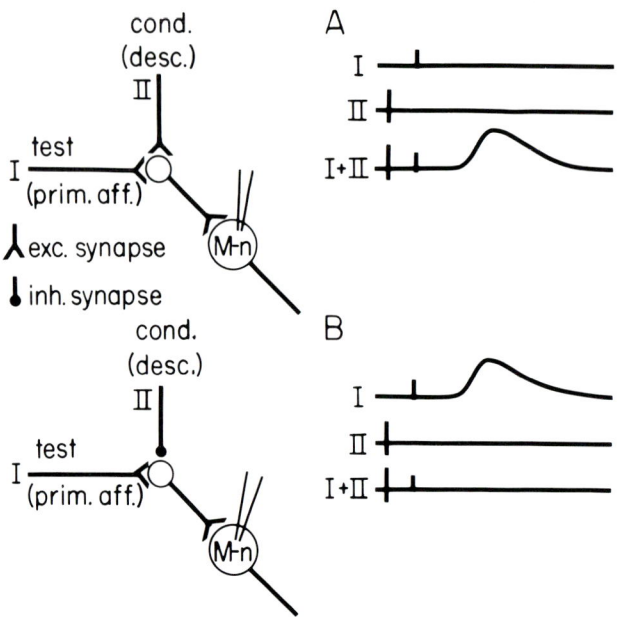

FIG. 1. Indirect technique used to investigate convergence in interneurons of reflex pathways. Diagram exemplifies convergence from primary afferents (I, prim. aff.) and descending pathways (II, desc.) on common excitatory interneurons projecting to motoneurons. Neuronal circuits are illustrated on *left*. *A*: example of excitatory convergence from both sources. *B*: example of convergence of excitation from prim. aff. and inhibition from desc. pathways. Interneurons represent a population of interneurons with identical convergence. *Traces* on *right* give idealized intracellular records from a single motoneuron after the test stimulus (I, prim. aff.), the conditioning (cond.) stimulus (II, desc.), and combined stimulation (I+II). This example refers to convergence from descending fibers and primary afferents, but the technique can be used for convergence from any source. See text for explanation. [Adapted from Lundberg (412) in *The Nervous System. The Basic Neurosciences.* ©1975, Raven Press, N. Y.]

stimuli that individually excite some interneurons (see, e.g., Figs. 12 and 18). Excitatory convergence onto common interneurons is then inferred when the PSP from combined stimulation of both systems is larger than the algebraic sum of the PSPs evoked by separate stimuli. A modification of this technique allows one to establish convergence of excitation and inhibition on common interneurons (Fig. 1*B*). Assume that activation of system I evokes a test PSP and that conditioning stimulation of system II is without effect in the motoneurons. A decrease or abolishment of the test PSP after combined stimulation suggests then that the conditioning volley (II) has an inhibitory effect on the interneurons, provided that it neither changes the membrane conductance in the motoneurons nor gives presynaptic inhibition of transmission from the primary afferents of system I. In Figure 1*B* inhibition is indicated as postsynaptic on the soma of the interneurons, and the decrease of the PSP in motoneurons is due to a corresponding decrease in the number of fired interneurons. By varying the conditioning-test interval it is possible to deduce the latency and time course of the PSP evoked in interneurons by conditioning stimuli. Although this method is rather simple, it allows several important conclusions to be made, and it has in fact provided most of the present information regarding convergence on interneurons.

When the effects of descending conditioning volleys on a disynaptic test PSP from primary afferents are investigated, it is easy to interpret the results because there is only one interneuron in the tested pathway. When the test PSP is mediated by a chain of interneurons, however, it is usually not possible to decide at what level the descending action is exerted. In such cases it is sometimes an advantage to reverse the order of test and conditioning stimuli and use a disynaptic descending PSP as a test. Effects produced on the descending PSP by conditioning volleys in polysynaptic reflex pathways then give a measure of convergence on last-order interneurons projecting directly to motoneurons (cf. Fig. 15*I–K*).

A more direct approach to studying interneuronal integration is to record directly from the interneurons. It is often difficult, however, to draw conclusions from such results because the projections of the analyzed interneurons are usually unknown and therefore the interneurons may be only tentatively identified as belonging to a given reflex pathway. With accumulating knowledge on convergence from the "indirect" approach of recording from motoneurons, high probability candidates may, nevertheless, be recognized. To provide a final proof, one may analyze the unitary action of single interneurons on the assumed target motoneurons by simultaneously recording from both of them. This was first achieved in invertebrates by Kandel et al. (345) with a spike-triggered averaging technique. The method was then successfully used for studies of a spinal interneuronal system by Jankowska and Roberts [(335, 336); *Pathways From Ia-Afferents and Their Control by γ-Motoneurons*, p. 519] and for a vestibular system by Rapoport et al. (498) and Hikosaka et al. (262). When interneurons have been identified as belonging to a particular reflex pathway, direct recording may greatly expand the knowledge on the segmental and descending convergence onto them.

SPINAL NEURONAL CIRCUITS USED IN COMMON BY SEGMENTAL AFFERENTS AND SUPRASPINAL MOTOR CENTERS

In this section we describe a number of neuronal networks—spinal functional units—that are involved in various segmental reflexes. Throughout this presentation evidence is presented on how the available functional units in the spinal cord interact with each other and how the brain uses them to control the final common pathway, the α-motoneurons. We begin with the circuitry of the recurrent inhibition through Renshaw cells, not only because it appears to be the simplest example, but also because of its unique feature of being activated by the final motor output rather than by a special afferent input. The following subsections deal with reflex pathways from different peripheral receptor systems. The particular attention given to reflex pathways from Ia-afferents does not imply that they are more important than others but rather reflects the fact that the Ia pathways are currently the most completely characterized of the many spinal functional units, with detailed morphological and functional identification of all their constituents including the receptor control by γ-motoneurons. Other subsections are devoted to propriospinal systems and to pathways transmitting primary afferent depolarization.

Recurrent Inhibition

Renshaw (501) demonstrated that antidromic impulses in motor axons reduce the excitability of α-motoneurons projecting to the same or synergic muscles. This phenomenon, which became known as "recurrent inhibition," is due to activation by motor axon collaterals of a group of interneurons that in turn inhibit motoneurons [cf. refs. 130, 253, 607; see the chapter by Burke and Rudomin in the first volume of this *Handbook* section on the nervous system (82)]. These interneurons have been called Renshaw cells (139) and are located in the ventral horn medial to the motor nuclei (326, 328, 590, 591, 607). In addition to their well-known projection to α-motoneurons, Renshaw cells also connect with γ-motoneurons, interneurons mediating reciprocal group Ia inhibition of motoneurons (Ia inhibitory interneurons), other Renshaw cells, and cells of origin of the ventral spinocerebellar tract (VSCT neurons). Besides their excitation from motor axon collaterals, Renshaw cells also receive excitatory and inhibitory synaptic inputs from many other sources. The existence of a complex convergence from a number of segmental reflex pathways and descending tracts suggests that the local feedback regulation provided by the recurrent pathway is not stereotyped but might be used in a versatile manner.

Before the pathway of recurrent inhibition is discussed, brief reference should be made to the recent morphological finding that axon collaterals of α-motoneurons can establish direct contacts with homonymous α-motoneurons without any intercalated interneurons [(110–112); see also the chapter by Burke in this *Handbook*]. This connection reveals an interesting possibility for mutual motoneuronal interaction and might prove important for the concerted activity within a motor nucleus.

CONVERGENCE ONTO RENSHAW CELLS. *Motor axon collaterals*. Recurrent collaterals show terminal branching with the highest density of swellings (synaptic boutons) where the Renshaw cells are located (110, 111). It has been known for a long time that not all motor axons give off recurrent collaterals (87, 516, 517, 493), and it has recently been shown that the presence of the initial collaterals is correlated with the motoneuron species (110): collaterals were always given off by motoneurons innervating long muscles at the ankle or knee but were absent in the case of motoneurons of short plantar muscles of the foot. This observation might indicate that the Renshaw system is primarily concerned with control of the proximal muscles (limb position) rather than of the distal ones (movements of the digits).

Each individual Renshaw cell is excited by axon collaterals of many motoneurons, as evidenced both by their smoothly growing responses to increasing intensity of stimulation of individual nerves and by excitation evoked from several nerves (133, 139, 399, 510). The convergence onto Renshaw cells is not organized at random but appears to follow a rather specific pattern. Motor axon collaterals distribute only within a distance of less than 1 mm from their parent cell bodies [(110, 111); see, however, refs. 516 and 517 for immature kittens]; consequently excitation can be obtained only from motor nuclei located in the immediate neighborhood of a given Renshaw cell (133, 513). In fact only part of a motor nucleus may project to a given Renshaw cell, since some nuclei are 8–9 mm long in the cat spinal cord (84, 504). Since Renshaw cells are excited mainly by motoneurons of synergic muscles but not by those of strict antagonists (133, 511), convergence onto individual cells is restricted further by factors other than proximity.

The pool of motoneurons innervating a muscle is not homogeneous. In addition to the division into α- and γ-motoneurons, the α-motoneurons may be further subdivided into different types depending on the properties of the neurons themselves and the muscle fibers they innervate—fast, fatiguing (FF); fast, fatigue resistant (FR); and slow (S) units (see the chapter by Burke in this *Handbook*). Although activation of both γ- and α-motor axons has no greater effect on Renshaw cells than activation of α-motor axons alone (139, 224), a selective blockade of α-motor axons disclosed that antidromic volleys in γ-motor axons may cause a liminal excitation of at least some Renshaw cells (346). Since the α-motoneurons seem to be recruited in a specific order during motor performance (see the chapters by Henneman and Mendell and by Burke in this *Handbook*), knowledge of the relative contribution of the various subgroups of α-motoneurons is indeed important for a functional evaluation of the Renshaw system. A specialized convergence pattern onto Renshaw cells might result in a preferential mobilization of them in some types of movements and not in others. Anatomical investigations by Cullheim and Kellerth (111) have now shown that the number of synaptic contacts of recurrent collaterals of a motoneuron is correlated with the motor unit type. In the case of motoneurons of triceps surae, collaterals are much more numerous for FF units than for FR or S units, and are particularly sparse for S units of the soleus. These findings are compatible with the view that the Renshaw cells are activated more effectively by large α-motoneurons than by small ones (see discussion in refs. 131, 224), but the degree of collateralization does not allow final predictions about the synaptic linkage and potency. The electrophysiological evidence is both more conflicting and less direct. The conventional view holds that Renshaw cells are only excited by a relatively large monosynaptic reflex discharge (139, 502, 514), which has led to the conclusion that the smallest motoneurons, which are recruited first in a monosynaptic reflex, are rather inefficient in producing recurrent inhibition. Although the relation between the size of monosynaptic reflex and Renshaw cell discharge varies from one Renshaw cell to another [(297); see also ref. 346], this input-output relation is linear when the summed activity in a pool of Renshaw cells is considered (297, 346, 505). Unfortunately this is not easily interpreted in terms of excitation contributed by the size spectrum of motor units for two reasons. First, the size of the monosynaptic reflex recorded in ventral roots is not linearly related to the number of recruited motor units, since larger motor axons contribute more to the size of the monosynaptic reflex than smaller ones. Second, the number of spikes evoked in a Renshaw cell burst is not linearly related to the excitatory input because of a saturation of Renshaw cell firing in the case of large responses. The contribution of small motoneurons to Renshaw cell excitation is consequently overestimated. The observed linear relation might indeed be taken to indicate that large motoneurons contribute more than small ones. The importance of this issue requires additional quantitative experimental evidence.

It is generally assumed that axon collaterals have strong synaptic linkage with Renshaw cells, a view that has been based mainly on the finding that single antidromic motor axon volleys cause a burst of spikes at a very high frequency (502). This view is now supported by the effects of intracellular stimulation of individual motoneurons on simultaneously recorded Renshaw cells (506, 507, 592); in some cases (see Fig.

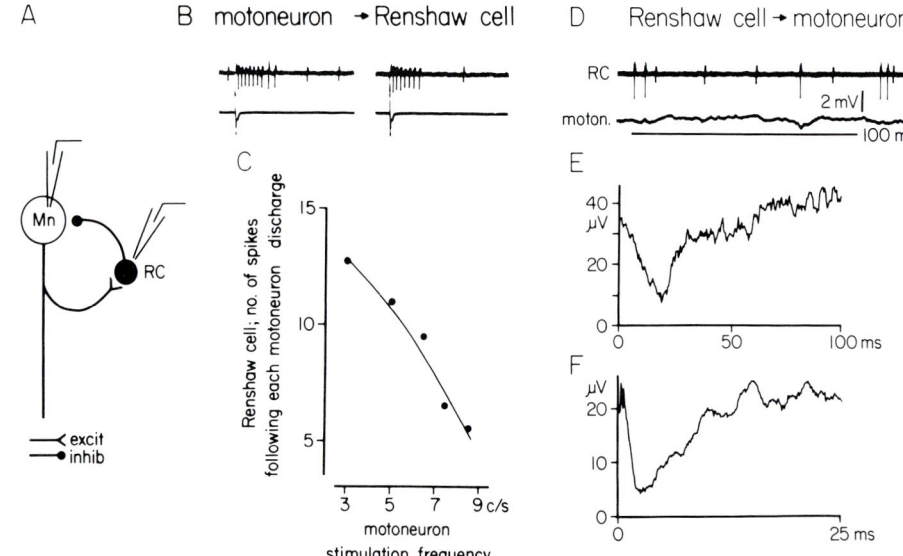

FIG. 2. Relations between individual motoneurons and individual Renshaw cells. *A*: illustration of experimental arrangement and neuronal circuit. Excitatory effect on Renshaw cells (RC) by single impulses in motoneurons (Mn) and inhibitory effect of individual Renshaw cells onto individual motoneurons were investigated with the aid of 2 microelectrodes: 1 used for intracellular stimulation of and recording from motoneurons, and 1 used for extracellular recording from Renshaw cells. The 2nd electrode was filled with 3 M sodium glutamate, which allowed electrophoretic application of glutamate to induce repetitive firing of the recorded Renshaw cells. *B*: 2 samples of burst firing in a Renshaw cell (*upper traces, large spikes*) following single action potentials in the motoneuron (timing shown by *lower trace*). Stimulation frequency of motoneuron was 8.5 impulses/s. Time calibration in *D* applies also to records in *B*. *C*: graph showing rapid decrease of number of spikes in Renshaw cell burst firing following each motoneuronal spike with increasing stimulation frequency. *Dots* represent mean value of several trials (cf. records in *B*) at different stimulation frequencies. This example shows the most powerful excitatory coupling of 21 tested cases. *D*: slow repetitive firing of Renshaw cell (*upper trace, large spike*) with simultaneous recording of membrane potential of motoneuron (*lower trace*; voltage calibration applies to intracellular recording). Same motoneuron and Renshaw cell that was illustrated in *B, C*. *E*: averaged record of membrane potential in motoneuron following single discharges of the Renshaw cell (the Renshaw cell firing with "doublets" or "triplets" are excluded). Same motoneuron and Renshaw cell that was illustrated in *B-D*. Note remarkably long time course of this unitary IPSP. *F*: a more typical time course of a presumed unitary IPSP from a Renshaw cell in a different motoneuron. Pretriggered averaging was used in both *E* and *F*; zero on abscissa refers to a time 1 ms before occurrence of spike of Renshaw cell. (From L. Van Keulen, unpublished material. See ref. 592.)

2) a repetitive discharge of a single motoneuron produced firing of the analyzed Renshaw cell at a much higher frequency (507, 592).

Segmental afferents. Activity in segmental afferents may influence Renshaw cells apart from the indirect excitation that is produced by motoneuronal reflex discharge. Polysynaptic excitation has been described after stimulation of *1*) dorsal roots (113, 114, 485, 512); *2*) ipsilateral group II and III muscle afferents; *3*) cutaneous afferents (114, 485, 512); and *4*) contralateral high-threshold afferents (614). In all cases there was evidence showing that indirect excitation via discharging motoneurons was not—or was only partly—responsible for the observed Renshaw cell activation. In addition to excitatory input, Renshaw cells receive polysynaptic inhibition from both ipsi- and contralateral segmental afferents (114, 189, 485, 512, 612, 614). They receive inhibition also during the late long-lasting flexor reflex revealed after injection of dopa (51). The latter effect may be of special interest in view of the relation of these late reflexes to the generation of locomotion (REFLEX PATHWAYS FROM THE "FLEXOR REFLEX AFFERENTS," p. 541). Studies on Renshaw cell activity during "fictive" (and partly also actual) locomotion are, however, still conflicting. The reports by Severin et al. (537) and by Feldman and Orlovsky (175) suggest that the ability of a train of antidromic volleys in the motor axons to inhibit α-motoneurons and Ia inhibitory interneurons is reduced during treadmill locomotion. These authors therefore inferred that Renshaw cells are inhibited during locomotion. McCrea and Jordan (444a), however, could not reveal a generalized depression in the recurrent pathway with direct recording of Renshaw cell firing during fictive locomotion (cf. also ref. 492).

Supraspinal systems. There is ample evidence that Renshaw cell activity may also be affected from supraspinal levels. Inhibitory and excitatory effects have been evoked by electrical stimulation of the cerebral cortex (261, 430), the capsula interna (351), the red nucleus (620), the cerebellum (49, 220, 254, 255), the reticular formation (254, 255, 430), and the thalamus (430). It has further been shown that recurrent inhibition of α-motoneurons is more potent in the decerebrate than in the spinal state (267) and that transmission in the recurrent pathways is enhanced by activation of bulbospinal noradrenergic pathways (15). It is difficult to ignore the possibility that these effects are partly secondary to alterations in motoneuronal activity, but there is usually evidence suggesting that at least part of the descending action is mediated via separate channels to the Renshaw cells. The descending pathways and the segmental linkages mediating their effects are not yet established.

Virtually nothing is known about the type of motor activity in which the descending control of Renshaw cells is involved. Recent studies in humans, however, seem to offer a promising approach to this problem, since it is now possible to estimate recurrent inhibition by a specially designed method of paired Hoffmann's reflexes (86). This method has been used to study the excitability of Renshaw cells during voluntary movements of the ankle joint [(294, 487); R. Katz and E. Pierrot-Deseilligny, personal communication]. During weak contractions of triceps surae, the excitability of Renshaw cells inhibiting soleus motoneurons increased more than could be explained by the input from motor axon collaterals. On the other hand, during stronger contractions the excitability decreased. These observations indicated an excitatory and inhibitory control of these Renshaw cells during weak and strong movements, respectively (see FUNCTIONAL CONSIDERATIONS, p. 518).

ACTIONS OF RENSHAW CELLS ON SPINAL NEURONS. Direct morphological and electrophysiological investigations of single Renshaw cells disproved the early suggestions (see refs. 516, 517) that they are Golgi type II neurons. Renshaw cells are in fact funicular cells with axons that enter the spinal white matter to project over distances of more than 12 mm rostrally or caudally (326, 328, 337, 513, 591). In limb segments there is no evidence for contralateral projections of Renshaw cells (139, 266, 609), although crossed recurrent inhibition has been found in motoneurons of tail muscles in lower sacral segments (334).

α-Motoneurons. Following activation of the motoneurons to a particular muscle, recurrent inhibition is evoked in a number of motor nuclei. The largest recurrent inhibitory postsynaptic potentials (IPSPs) are evoked in motoneurons of the same motor nucleus, but many other motoneurons are also strongly inhibited (131, 139, 292, 579). In a search for some rules behind the distribution of recurrent inhibition, it was first noticed that the size of the recurrent IPSPs in motoneurons was correlated to the distance between these recipient neurons and the nuclei from which the Renshaw cells were activated (131, 139, 501, 579, 613). It was therefore suggested that distribution of recurrent inhibition depends primarily on the distance between motoneurons (the proximity hypothesis), thus cutting across all functional classifications (131). The subsequent observation that motoneurons innervating synergic muscles are linked by strong mutual recurrent inhibition suggested, however, that its distribution rather depends on functional factors (131, 292, 613). In fact the positive correlation between the pattern of distribution of the recurrent inhibition from a given muscle nerve and of the monosynaptic excitation from the Ia-afferents in the same nerve (summarized in Fig. 3) proved independent of the location of the motor nuclei. In the gracilis motoneuron of Figure 4 large recurrent IPSPs were evoked from the Ia synergists semitendinosus and posterior biceps (see *Pathways From Ia Afferents and Their Control by γ-Motoneurons,* p. 519, for distribution of Ia effects) whose motor nuclei are located some segments away. On the other hand, recurrent inhibition was never found be-

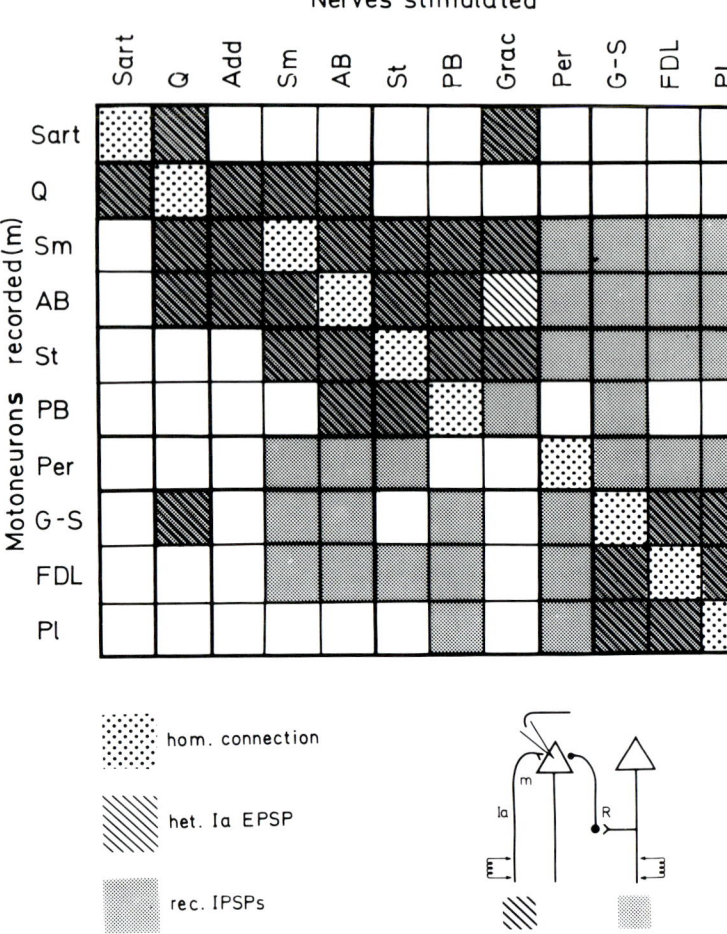

FIG. 3. Comparison of patterns of monosynaptic excitation from muscle spindle Ia-afferents and recurrent inhibition via motor axon collaterals in motor nuclei supplying various hindlimb muscles in cat. Experimental arrangement and neuronal circuits as illustrated in the scheme. Motor nuclei recorded from are listed to *left* of diagram and nerves whose orthodromic and antidromic effects were compared are indicated *above*. Homonymous connections, always with both Ia excitation and recurrent inhibition, are indicated by *dotted areas*. Heteronymous Ia excitation and recurrent inhibition are indicated by *hatched* and *shaded areas*, respectively. Diagram is constructed from data obtained in the cat. It indicates a complete overlap of Ia excitation and recurrent inhibition, but with recurrent inhibition more widely distributed than Ia excitation. Sart, sartorius; Q, quadriceps; Sm, semimembranosus; AB, anterior biceps; St, semitendinosus; PB, posterior biceps; Per, peroneus; G-S, gastrocnemius-soleus; FDL, flexor digitorum longus; Pl, plantaris; Add, adductor femoris and longus; Grac, gracilis. [Data for Ia pathways from Eccles et al. (135) and Eccles and Lundberg (147); data for recurrent inhibition from Hultborn et al. (292), Eccles et al. (131), and Wilson et al. (613).]

tween motor nuclei of strict antagonists at the same joint, not even in cases when the nuclei have a similar segmental location. The striking overlap between distribution of Renshaw inhibition and Ia excitation, however, should not conceal the fact that recurrent inhibition is more extensively distributed than Ia excitation (see Fig. 3). It has been suggested (292) that the additional recurrent connections may link muscles that act in some "functional synergisms" in movements and postures not reflected by the Ia input.

Knowledge of the distribution of recurrent inhibition within the motor nucleus is still incomplete. If the Renshaw circuit mainly subserves a negative feedback of motoneurons, one would expect the activity of a given group of motoneurons to act either selectively on themselves or diffusely on all motoneurons innervating the same muscle. Intracellular records from triceps surae motoneurons suggest that there is a more or less linear relation between the amount of recurrent inhibition and the size of the monosynaptic reflex in both "small" and "large" motoneurons (296), as would be expected in the case of a diffuse distribution. A quantitatively more powerful effect of recurrent inhibition on slow motor units has been postulated, since maximal recurrent IPSPs are generally larger in small motoneurons than in large ones (131, 362). The more effective suppression of discharges of "tonic" than of "phasic" motoneurons during stimulation of ventral

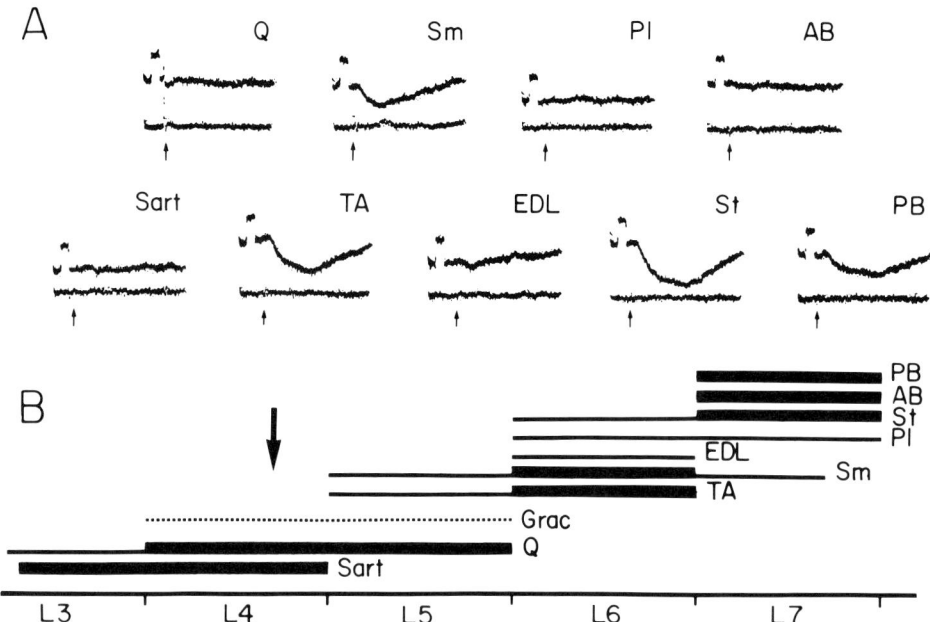

FIG. 4. Convergence of recurrent inhibition in a primate (baboon) gracilis (Grac) motoneuron with correlation to location of motor nuclei whose efferent axons have been stimulated. *A*: *upper traces* are intracellular averaged records (calibration pulse 1 mV, 4 ms) from the gracilis motoneuron. *Lower traces* are simultaneous records from the cord dorsum. Dorsal roots have been cut and nerves indicated have been stimulated at supramaximal strength for α-fibers (arrival of volleys at spinal cord indicated by *arrows*). *B*: segmental location of motor nuclei tested in *A* (at the end of each experiment the rostrocaudal distribution of motor nuclei were tested by stimulation of individual ventral roots with simultaneous recording from peripheral muscle nerves). Position of recorded gracilis motoneuron is indicated by *arrow*. Results suggest that recurrent inhibition is not organized according to proximity principle. Note large recurrent IPSPs from semitendinosus and posterior biceps whose motor nuclei are among the most caudal ones, but no effect at all from quadriceps despite a similar rostrocaudal location of quadriceps and gracilis motor nuclei. Q, quadriceps; Sm, semimembranosus; Pl, plantaris; AB, anterior biceps; Sart, sartorius; TA, tibialis anterior; EDL, extensor digitorum longus; St, semitendinosus; PB, posterior biceps. (From H. Hultborn, E. Jankowska, and S. Lindström, unpublished material. Cited in ref. 292.)

roots also supports that notion (224). However, such results do not necessarily indicate a preferential projection of Renshaw cells on small motoneurons; they can at least partly be explained by the differences in input resistance of small tonic and large phasic motoneurons (see the chapter by Burke in this *Handbook*). Recent work (H. Hultborn, R. Katz, and R. Mackel, unpublished data) indeed suggests that there is no difference in the synaptic conductance underlying a maximal autogenetic recurrent IPSP in small and large triceps surae motoneurons, respectively.

γ-Motoneurons. Recurrent inhibition of γ-motoneurons has long been denied (132, 224, 308). However, later studies firmly established its presence (71, 159, 160, 231) and showed that it may be evoked at threshold for activation of α-motor axons (160). Recurrent inhibition was found in both dynamic and static γ-motoneurons (160, 231), but it appeared not to be evenly distributed: some motoneurons are not inhibited at all, and others are affected to a variable extent (160).

Ia inhibitory interneurons. Antidromic volleys in ventral roots or peripheral nerves effectively depress transmission in the Ia inhibitory pathways to α-motoneurons (see REFLEX PATHWAYS FROM GROUP Ia MUSCLE SPINDLE AFFERENTS, p. 519, examples are given in Fig. 10). The depression is caused by postsynaptic inhibition of the interposed interneurons (the Ia inhibitory interneurons) by Renshaw cells (circuit in Fig. 10*D*). To reveal the organization of the recurrent inhibition of these interneurons, its origin was compared with the origin of the Ia IPSP evoked in the same motoneurons (292). It was found that the recurrent depression of Ia IPSPs were invariably produced by motor axons in the same muscle nerves whose Ia-afferents evoked them. Thus, for example, the Ia IPSPs from quadriceps in posterior biceps motoneurons were effectively depressed by stimulation of motor fibers to the quadriceps muscle. The depression of Ia IPSPs from other nerves, if found, was always much weaker than that evoked from the nerves with afferents eliciting the Ia IPSPs.

Since sets of α-motoneurons and Ia inhibitory interneurons that receive the same Ia connections may often act together ("corresponding neurons", see RE-FLEX PATHWAYS FROM GROUP Ia MUSCLE SPINDLE

AFFERENTS, p. 519), it was of interest to compare the origin of the recurrent inhibition of these two groups of neurons. It turned out that the distribution of recurrent effects are very similar, with "corresponding neurons" always inhibited from the same efferent motor fibers (292). This parallelism appeared even more striking when these actions were quantitatively analyzed. Large recurrent IPSPs in motoneurons were matched by strong inhibition of the corresponding Ia inhibitory interneurons and smaller IPSPs in the α-motoneurons with weaker effects on the Ia inhibitory interneurons (see Table 6 in ref. 292). It was therefore proposed that α-motoneurons and "corresponding" Ia inhibitory interneurons are inhibited by the same Renshaw cells. That implies that recurrent effects on both target neurons are subject to the same influences from segmental and supraspinal systems and that the functions of these projections probably are inseparable (see further in FUNCTIONAL CONSIDERATIONS, this page).

Renshaw cells. Although first reported by Renshaw (502), mutual inhibition between Renshaw cells was often doubted (139, 614) until convincing evidence for its existence was obtained more recently by Ryall and co-workers (510, 513). Relatively little is known about the distribution of this inhibition, but apparently a given Renshaw cell most strongly inhibits functionally related Renshaw cells, i.e., those that are activated from the same motor axon collaterals (510). If so, the mutual inhibition between Renshaw cells could serve to focus "recurrent inhibition of motoneurons into particular channels" and might also "shorten the duration of recurrent inhibition" (510).

FUNCTIONAL CONSIDERATIONS. Recurrent inhibition of α-motoneurons has mostly been described in terms of a "stabilizing" and "limiting" feedback that would reduce the sensitivity of neurons to changes in their excitatory drive (stabilization) and decrease the frequency of their discharge to a given input when compared to a system without a recurrent feedback (limitation). These ideas, which are self-obvious for any system of recurrent inhibition, have been developed in connection with experiments showing a low steady firing of triceps surae motoneurons during the stretch reflex (see ref. 253). It was later proposed that recurrent inhibition not only stabilizes motor output but also changes its spatial pattern and possibly enhances motor contrast, just as sensory contrast is sharpened by recurrent inhibition in the *Limulus* eye (500). This proposal received some support when it was demonstrated that recurrent inhibition is more effective on monosynaptic reflexes to synergistic than to homonymous muscles [(69); cf. ref. 610]. With additional knowledge about the distribution of recurrent depression of reciprocal Ia inhibition and the extensive supraspinal control of Renshaw cells (ACTIONS OF RENSHAW CELLS ON SPINAL NEURONS, p. 515), it became possible to formulate the hypothesis of a recurrent control of the spatial pattern of motor activity in more specific terms (292). It was suggested that inhibition of Renshaw cells (suppressing recurrent inhibition of both motoneurons and Ia inhibitory interneurons) would permit expression of the full pattern of Ia actions, including heteronymous excitation and reciprocal inhibition. In contrast facilitation of Renshaw cells (enhancing recurrent inhibition) would instead tend to restrict spatially the effect of Ia activity to excitation of homonymous motoneurons, providing optimal conditions for the control of individual muscles via the γ-loop. It is not yet proved, however, that the relative effectiveness of the recurrent inhibition of homonymous and heteronymous α-motoneurons and of the corresponding Ia inhibitory interneurons is actually distributed as required by this hypothesis.

It has also been suggested that recurrent inhibition may affect the temporal pattern of motoneuronal activity. Gelfand and co-workers (201, 202) thus suggested that it might serve to prevent the synchronized firing that might otherwise be evoked by strong common excitatory inputs to many motoneurons in a nucleus (cf. refs. 350, 534). Some experimental support for this idea has been given recently (3, 619).

According to another hypothesis (293), the Renshaw system would primarily serve as a variable gain regulator at the motoneuronal level rather than to modify the pattern of motor activity. The hypothesis is based on the assumption that the relation between synaptic depolarization of motoneurons by a central command and the muscular force generated by the ensuing motoneuronal activity depends on the amount of the negative feedback given by Renshaw cells as illustrated in Figure 5. The hypothetical diagram (Fig. 5B) relates the excitatory synaptic current (input) to the activity of a pool of motoneurons (output) during inhibitory or excitatory control of Renshaw cells. The very weakest motoneuronal activity would result in a negligible recurrent inhibition, but with the increasing activity more recurrent inhibition will be progressively added. The amount of added recurrent inhibition should be larger when the Renshaw cells are facilitated and smaller when they are inhibited (cf. ref. 295), with the resulting different slopes (gain) of the input-output relations under these two conditions. It was pointed out (293) that a "low gain" condition (facilitation of Renshaw cells) would allow supraspinal force-generating circuits to play over a considerable part of their working range and yet cause only small changes in muscular force, whereas a "high gain" state (inhibition of Renshaw cells) would allow the central command to generate larger forces for a given drive. Such a variable gain control at motoneuronal level may thus optimize the resolution of the motor output during weak as well as strong contractions. Recent experiments in humans (ACTIONS OF RENSHAW CELLS ON SPINAL NEURONS, p. 515) indeed suggest that weak contractions of triceps surae are accompanied by facilitation of Renshaw cells and strong contractions are associated with their inhibition.

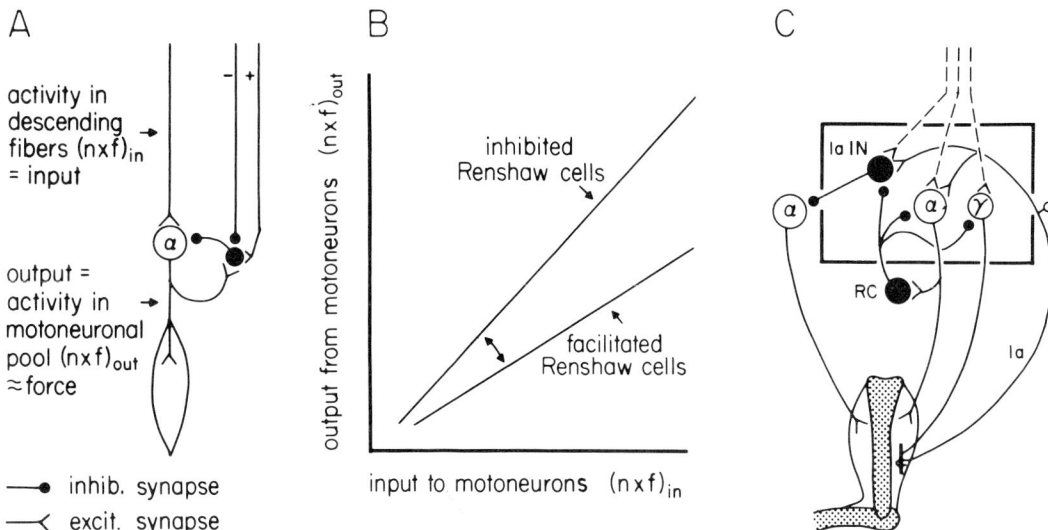

FIG. 5. Diagrams illustrating the hypothesis that Renshaw system serves as a variable gain regulator at motoneuronal level. *A*: input and output connections of α-motoneurons and Renshaw cells. *B*: simplified diagram of input-output relations of a motoneuronal pool during inhibition and facilitation of transmission in recurrent pathway. *C*: concept of motor output stage. Neurons constituting output are framed by *thick lines*. *Hatched lines* indicate parallel connections to α- and γ-motoneurons and corresponding Ia inhibitory interneurons. α, α-Motoneurons; γ, γ-motoneurons; RC, Renshaw cells; Ia IN, Ia inhibitory interneurons. [Adapted from Hultborn et al. (293).]

Voluntary muscle contractions probably involve parallel and balanced excitation of α- and γ-motoneurons of a muscle as well as of the interneurons inhibiting its antagonists (see subsection FUNCTIONAL CONSEQUENCES OF α-γ-LINKAGE, p. 529). Therefore all three groups of neurons can be considered together as forming an "output stage" of the motor system [Fig. 5C; (293)]. Since recurrent inhibition of motoneurons and Ia inhibitory interneurons that build up such an output stage is apparently mediated by the same pool of Renshaw cells (see ACTIONS OF RENSHAW CELLS ON SPINAL NEURONS, p. 515) the gain control will be exerted in parallel on all the three types of neurons, leaving the required balance between them undisturbed.

Pathways From Ia-Afferents and Their Control by γ-Motoneurons

Two main reasons for the continuing interest in the reflex actions from the primary endings of the muscle spindles (Ia-afferents) are the existence of a separate efferent innervation of the intrafusal fibers (γ-innervation) that modulate their sensitivity and the possibility of the use of such modulation in generating movements. In 1953 Merton (449) proposed that the brain may control the muscle length by a fusimotor discharge: the resulting intrafusal contraction with concomitant acceleration of Ia firing frequency was thought to produce an excess of α-motor discharge until the muscle had shortened sufficiently to reduce the Ia firing toward its original value. This "follow-up length servo" concept (259, 449) was later modified (217, 441) with the proposal that muscle Ia spindle afferents, rather than act as primary drive, provide a "servo assistance" (443, 444) during movements. Central to the servo-assistance concept is the idea that intra- and extrafusal fibers should shorten in parallel during muscle contractions due to coactivation of α- and γ-motoneurons. If extrafusal shortening is prevented, an increased discharge of the Ia-afferents (an error signal) will augment α-motoneuronal firing and thereby add force to the extrafusal contraction. Both servo concepts reflect the intimate functional relation between the γ-motoneurons and primary spindle afferents and require that they are regarded as parts of one and the same "functional unit." Consequently Ia-afferents and γ-motoneurons are treated together in this section. The central effects of muscle spindle secondary endings are discussed separately in subsection *Reflex Pathways From Cutaneous and Joint Afferents and From Groups II and III Muscle Afferents*, p. 535, since, with present knowledge, they seem to be more related to other reflex effects than those associated with Ia-afferents.

REFLEX PATHWAYS FROM GROUP Ia MUSCLE SPINDLE AFFERENTS. *Pathways to agonist α-motoneurons. Monosynaptic pathways.* Lloyd (390–392) demonstrated that α-motoneurons are excited monosynaptically by the most rapidly conducting (group I) muscle afferents. Indirect evidence suggested that Ia-afferents were responsible for this effect, as was ultimately proved with adequate activation of muscle spindles and intracellular recording from α-motoneurons [(429); cf. ref. 444]. Whereas early studies emphasized

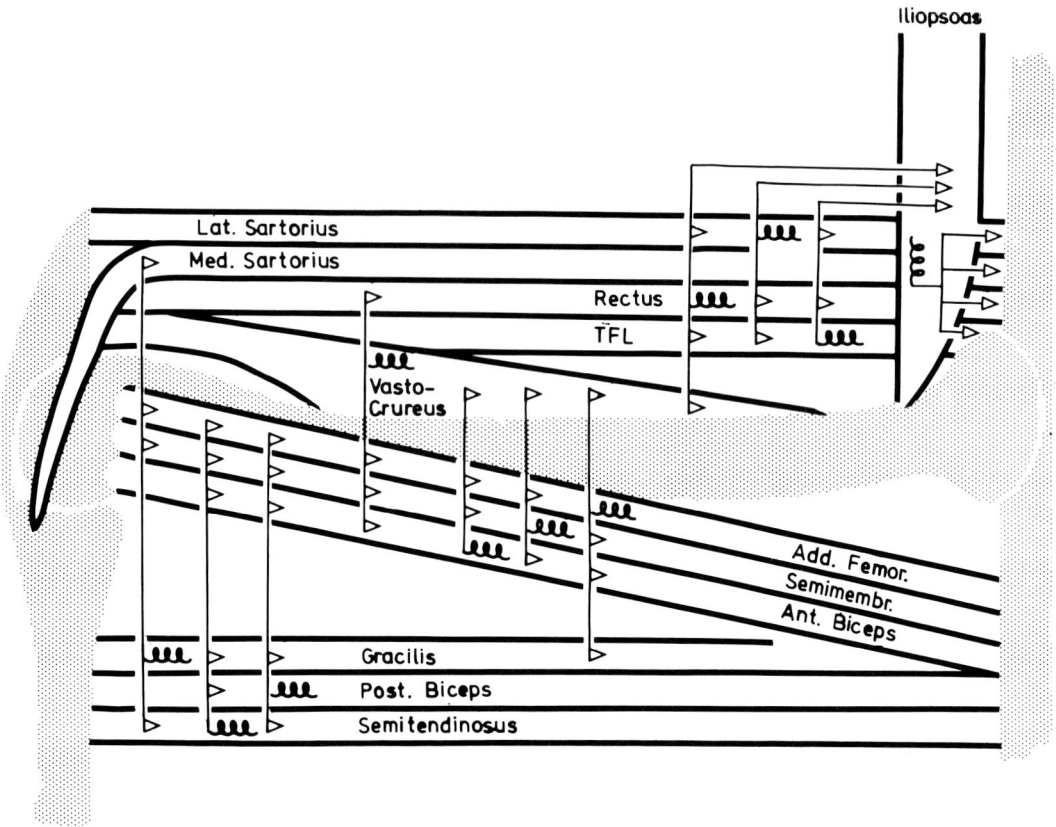

FIG. 6. Distribution of heteronymous monosynaptic excitation evoked by impulses in muscle spindle Ia-afferents from proximal hindlimb muscles in cat. Ia-afferents of an individual muscle (indicated by *coils*) evoke excitatory effects via monosynaptic pathways in α-motoneurons of muscles (marked by *open triangles*). TFL, musculus tensor fasciae latae. [Adapted from Eccles and Lundberg (147).]

the localized (homonymous) origin of monosynaptic Ia excitation (101, 102, 378, 503), the technique of facilitating monosynaptic test reflexes revealed effects from synergic (heteronymous) muscles acting at the same joint as well (369, 393, 394). These findings led to the concept of the "myotatic unit," which includes those muscles operating together at a given joint (excited together by Ia-afferents) and muscles with antagonistic function at the same joint (inhibited by the same Ia-afferents) [(394); see further in subsection SEGMENTAL AND SUPRASPINAL CONTROL OF γ-MOTONEURONS, p. 527]. A much wider distribution of Ia excitation to motoneurons was revealed with intracellular recording techniques (99, 135, 147, 188, 520, 608).

Figure 6 summarizes the main monosynaptic Ia connections to motoneurons of proximal muscles of the hindlimb of the cat and provides several examples that are not in accordance with the original idea of the myotatic unit: an individual nucleus may draw its Ia excitation from a wide receptive field and, vice versa, afferents from one muscle may supply Ia excitation to many motor nuclei. Muscles interconnected by Ia pathways are often denoted as "Ia synergists," although they may not act in strict mechanical synergy. Correspondingly, wide Ia connections were found in the baboon hindlimb though with some interesting differences (T. Hongo, A. Lundberg, and C. G. Phillips, unpublished observations).[1] For example, in the cat the slow soleus motoneurons receive substantial heteronymous Ia excitation from medial and lateral gastrocnemius, while medial gastrocnemius motoneurons are much more isolated with only small heteronymous effects from soleus (135). In the baboon the situation is reversed with large heteronymous Ia effects to medial gastrocnemius and small actions to soleus motoneurons. This different organization in cats and primates suggests that the widespread Ia connections in higher animals are not vestigial but have been subject to phylogenetic adaptation. In view of the ability of cats to perform precise skilled forelimb movements, it is interesting to note that widespread Ia connections are a characteristic feature also of their forelimbs (188, 608). Even more interesting are the similar wide Ia connections between muscles of the baboon's forearm and hand (99); in some of these motor nuclei (e.g., of flexor digitorum communis) the heteronymous Ia ex-

---

[1] Tables of Ia connections are available on request from Prof. A. Lundberg, Dept. of Physiology, University of Göteborg, Göteborg, Sweden.

citatory postsynaptic potentials (EPSPs) are considerably larger than the homonymous ones.

The effects caused by the wide distribution of Ia excitation must be considered in relation to reflex adjustments accompanying the classic myotatic reflex. Stretch of the quadriceps, for example, will generate monosynaptic excitation of motoneurons of the knee extensors themselves, of hip extensors and, interestingly, of the ankle extensor soleus, and thus will contribute to readjust the position of the limb (135). Furthermore, the motoneurons of the slow muscles receive a larger aggregate of EPSPs than do the motoneurons of the fast ones, which suggests that Ia excitation may be especially important in postural reflexes [(135); see the chapters by Henneman and Mendell; Burke; Matthews; and Houk and Rymer in this *Handbook*].

For an adequate contribution to the motor output in movements where Ia-afferent discharge is maintained by a fusimotor drive, the excitation from Ia-afferents should be restricted to α-motoneurons of muscles participating in the centrally initiated movement. The simplifying assumption is often made that γ-initiated Ia activity reaches only homonymous motoneurons, but it obviously tends to facilitate all Ia synergists. The Ia pathways might therefore be of special importance in movements that involve a co-contraction of muscle groups linked in Ia synergism. It has thus been suggested that the Ia pattern has evolved to assist locomotion in the (cat) hindlimb (166, 408) and the grasp reflex in the primate forelimb (99). It is, however, generally assumed that γ-operated Ia effects contribute also to movements that do not involve all Ia synergists. If servo assistance (cf. subsection FUNCTIONAL CONSEQUENCES OF α-γ-LINKAGE, p. 529) is given by Ia pathways in these cases, the activation of the α-motoneurons must depend on additional background excitation from other sources. It certainly seems unlikely that motoneurons could be mobilized by Ia activity from heteronymous muscles if they themselves do not receive direct depolarization by the central motor command.

Polysynaptic excitatory Ia pathways. It has been postulated repeatedly that, in addition to their monosynaptic projection, Ia-afferents may have more complex polysynaptic excitatory pathways to α-motoneurons (7, 225, 271, 343, 582), but it is only recently that such circuits have been clearly demonstrated (301, 302, 525). Hultborn et al. (302) demonstrated that selective activation of Ia-afferents in the decerebrate cat may lead to a long-lasting (up to several minutes) increase in excitability of α-motoneurons to homonymous and synergistic muscles in addition to the monosynaptic reflex response. This is illustrated in Figure 7B, C where a long-lasting depolarization of a triceps surae motoneuron follows a short train of Ia impulses. The latency of this response was in the order of 60–70 ms. The original excitability level could be restored at any time by a train of impulses in skin afferents. Such a long-lasting activity indicates that the neuronal network underlying this response includes some kind of positive feedback mechanisms (such as closed interneuronal circuits that can support a reverberating activity). This mechanism would be localized within the central nervous system, since the increase in excitability could be obtained after section of the ventral roots and/or after section of the muscle nerves, which excludes involvement of a peripheral loop (cf. refs. 191, 581).

A similar long-latency and long-lasting response has recently been recorded in acute spinal cats (Fig. 7D, E). It appeared, however, only after intravenous (i.v.) injection of the serotonin precursor 5-hydroxytryptophan (see subsection *Monoaminergic Reticulospinal Pathways*, p. 562), which suggests that the responsible segmental circuits depend on facilitation by descending serotonergic pathways.

The polysynaptic network(s) activated from Ia-afferents probably has a function different from that (those) of the monosynaptic Ia-motoneuron connections described above. It should allow interactions between Ia-afferents and other segmental and supraspinal systems, as evidenced in the spinal cat for skin afferents and descending serotonergic pathways (see Fig. 7). It also has the peculiar capacity to integrate the effect of Ia activity reaching the spinal cord during a prolonged period. A continuous or interrupted train of Ia impulses leads to a steady augmenting autogenetic excitation (301) that is reminiscent of the tonic vibration reflex in humans (120, 154, 257, 365) or animals (343). Furthermore since the long-latency Ia excitation is easily elicited in the unanesthetized decerebrate cat, it is likely to contribute to the maintenance of the rigidity and the enhanced stretch reflexes seen in that preparation. The long-latency Ia excitation must further be considered with regard to the finding that the most important part of the load compensation reflex during voluntary contractions occurs at latencies too long to be explained by monosynaptic Ia excitation (258, 259). It has been suggested that these later components are partly mediated via "long loops" (or transcortical pathways) [(434, 435, 445); see the chapter by Porter in this *Handbook*], but the long-latency segmental polysynaptic Ia excitation may obviously contribute.

Pathways to antagonist α-motoneurons. Reciprocal Ia inhibition is mediated by a disynaptic pathway (30, 140), and the convergence onto the interposed interneurons is the main object of the following paragraphs.

Pattern of reciprocal Ia inhibition of α-motoneurons. Lloyd (394) considered the reciprocal inhibition as a counterpart of excitation in a myotatic unit and thus thought it to be limited to the motoneurons of strict antagonists at the same joint. Again intracellular recording revealed a more extensive distribution [Fig. 8; (147)]. Thus a given motor nucleus draws its Ia inhibition not only from its strict mechanical antagonists but usually also from other muscles connected

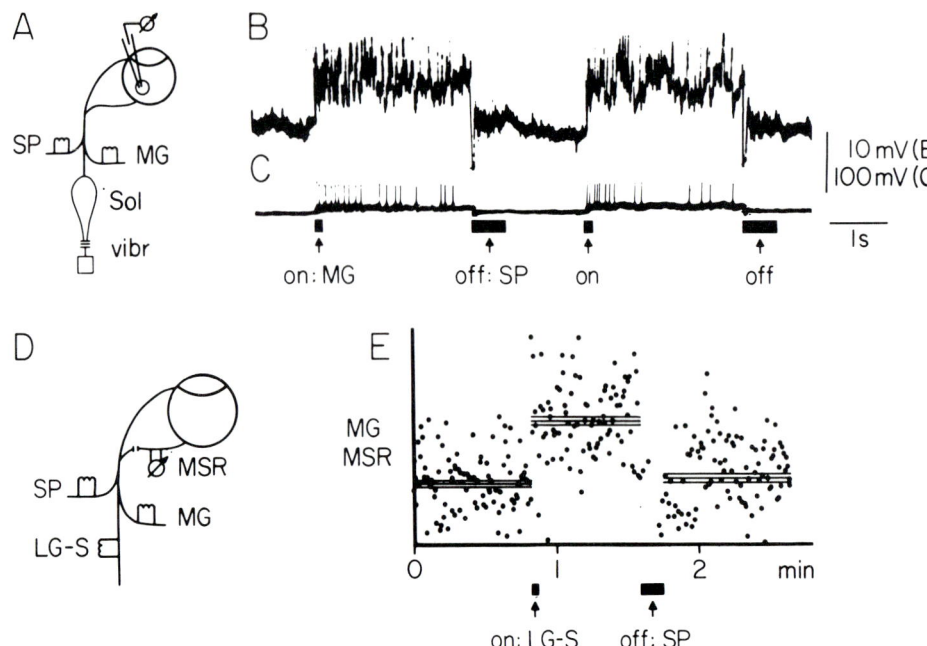

FIG. 7. Long-lasting excitability increase of α-motoneurons induced via polysynaptic Ia pathways. B, C: simultaneous intracellular records at different gains from a triceps surae motoneuron in a decerebrate, decerebellate cat (experimental arrangement in A). Ventral roots were intact, but γ-loop was opened by relaxation with gallamine triethiodide (Flaxedil). Short stimulus trains to medial gastrocnemius nerve (on: MG) caused a depolarizing shift of membrane potential and a firing of motoneuron. This effect was reversed by a short stimulus train to superficial peroneal nerve (off: SP). D, E: monosynaptic reflexes (MSR) evoked by stimulation of nerve from medial gastrocnemius and recorded from central end of cut S_1–L_7 ventral roots (γ-loop open) in a spinal unanesthetized cat after injection of 5-hydroxytryptophan (50 mg/kg; experimental arrangement in D). E: integrated amplitude of MSR (arbitrary units, *horizontal lines* give mean ± SEM) is plotted against time. Stimulation of lateral gastrocnemius-soleus nerve (on: LG-S) increased amplitude of MSR while a short stimulus train to the SP nerve (off: SP) brought it back to control value. Values obtained during LG-S or SP stimulation are not included in the calculation. [A–C adapted from Hultborn and Wigström (301); D, E from H. Hultborn and H. Wigström, unpublished observations.]

with them in Ia synergism (147, 315). Reciprocal Ia inhibition, however, is not found between adductors and abductors (147).

In the cases when Ia-afferents from several muscles evoke disynaptic inhibition in one motor nucleus, it might be relayed either by independent lines or via common interneurons. The different Ia signals would be integrated in the motoneurons themselves in the former case, and, at the level of the inhibitory interneurons, in the latter (147). Application of the spatial facilitation technique demonstrated that whenever activity in Ia-afferents from several muscles evoked inhibition in a motor nucleus, convergence of Ia-afferents occurred onto common interneurons [Fig. 9; (299)]. In addition the pattern of convergence on the interneurons appeared to be identical with that found on α-motoneurons.

Parallel input to α-motoneurons and to interneurons mediating reciprocal Ia inhibition to antagonists. The finding of a similar origin of monosynaptic Ia excitation to α-motoneurons and to the interneurons interposed in the pathway of reciprocal Ia inhibition (usually referred to as Ia inhibitory interneurons) was the first of a series of observations showing that these two groups of cells are as a rule influenced in parallel. This appeared to be true for their input from both supraspinal and segmental systems (275, 286, 409) and is further illustrated in the following sections. Because of this parallelism, α-motoneurons and Ia inhibitory interneurons with the same monosynaptic input from Ia-afferents have been denoted as "corresponding neurons." It might be pointed out that the parallel distribution of effects to the corresponding motoneurons and interneurons reflects the most intimate relation between the Ia synergists and their antagonists and ensures the control by the same fiber systems of both excitation (contraction) of agonists and reciprocal inhibition (relaxation) of antagonists (FUNCTIONAL CONSEQUENCES OF α-γ-LINKAGE, p. 529).

Recurrent inhibition of Ia inhibitory interneurons. Inhibition of Ia inhibitory interneurons by volleys in motor axon collaterals is one example of parallel inhibitory actions on α-motoneurons and on the interneurons mediating Ia inhibition of the antagonistic muscles. The Ia IPSPs in motoneurons are consider-

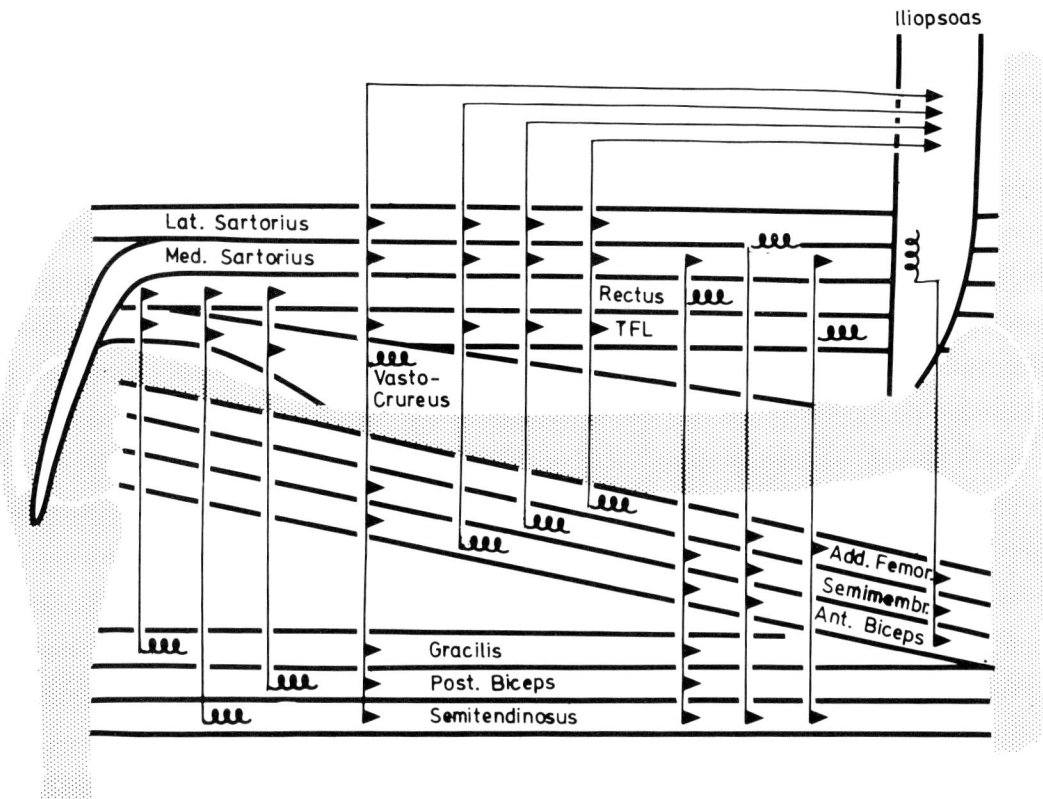

FIG. 8. Distribution of disynaptic inhibition evoked by impulses in muscle spindle Ia-afferents from proximal hindlimb muscles in cat. Ia-afferents of an individual muscle (indicated by *coils*) evoke inhibitory actions via disynaptic pathways in α-motoneurons of muscles (marked by *closed triangles*). TFL, musculus tensor fasciae latae. [Adapted from Eccles and Lundberg (147).]

ably decreased when they are preceded by stimulation of ventral roots [Fig. 10; (290)]. This depression was attributed to postsynaptic inhibition of the interposed Ia inhibitory interneurons, since it occurs without a concomitant presynaptic depolarization of Ia-afferents and without change in conductance of the motoneuronal membrane (290). The depression is evoked from efferent motor fibers to the muscles whose Ia-afferents produce the IPSPs (292). For example, Ia IPSPs evoked from the knee extensor quadriceps in motoneurons innervating the knee flexors, posterior biceps, and semitendinosus are depressed by antidromic volleys in the quadriceps nerve (Fig. 10). The same antidromic volleys would thus inhibit quadriceps motoneurons and corresponding Ia inhibitory interneurons (see subsection *Recurrent Inhibition*, p. 513). Intracellular records of subsequently identified Ia inhibitory interneurons allowed direct visualization of their recurrent inhibition [see Fig. 10; (287, 291)]. It should be added that recurrent inhibition of interneurons in afferent and descending pathways to motoneurons seems to be limited to those mediating reciprocal Ia inhibition (172, 173, 285, 300). Recurrent depression of IPSPs in motoneurons therefore indicates that they are mediated by the Ia inhibitory interneurons.

Identification of the Ia inhibitory interneurons.
With the criterion of convergence of monosynaptic excitation from Ia afferents and disynaptic inhibition from the appropriate motor axon collaterals, the interneurons mediating reciprocal Ia inhibition to α-motoneurons were searched for systematically in the spinal gray matter (291). Neurons with the required convergence were found in lamina VII, in a region dorsal and dorsomedial to the motor nuclei (Fig. 10). The recurrent IPSPs recorded in them were evoked with a disynaptic latency and had the same time course as in α-motoneurons. Figure 10E–G shows records from a lamina VII interneuron with monosynaptic excitation from quadriceps Ia-afferents and disynaptic inhibition from the ventral roots of the fifth and sixth lumbar segments (L_5–L_6 ventral roots), indicating that it should have mediated Ia inhibition to motoneurons of knee flexors. To obtain direct evidence that such neurons are indeed inhibitory and project to α-motoneurons, their axonal projections and synaptic actions on motoneurons of knee flexors were investigated (335, 336). Figure 10I–K shows simultaneous records of extracellular spike activity, evoked by ejection of glutamate from the recording electrode, of a lamina VII interneuron with monosynaptic input from quadriceps, together with postsynaptic potentials in a motoneuron of posterior biceps or semitendinosus. This

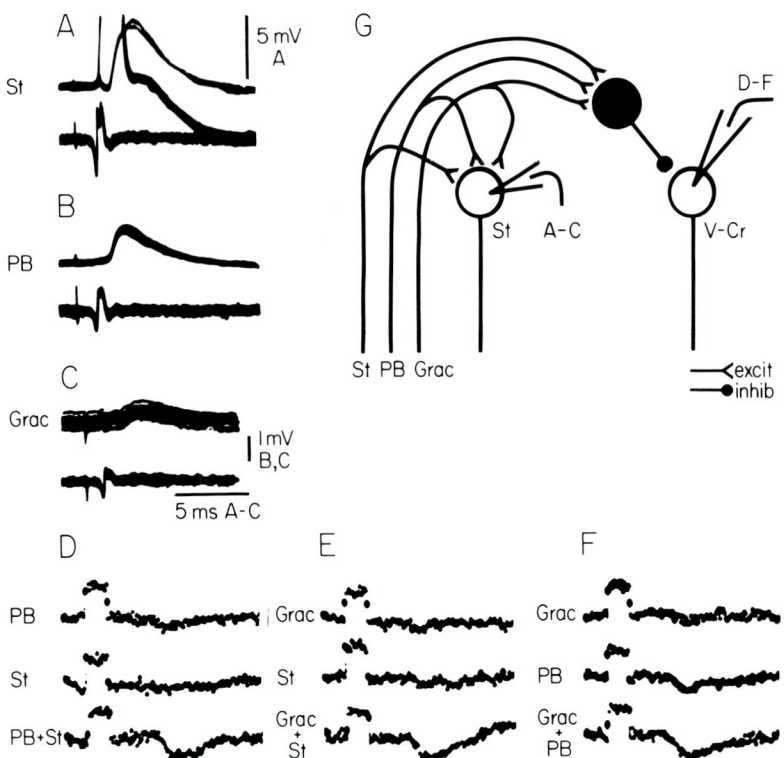

FIG. 9. Convergence of Ia-afferents on α-motoneurons and interneurons that mediate disynaptic Ia inhibition to motoneurons of antagonists (Ia inhibitory interneurons). Scheme in G illustrates experimental arrangement and neuronal circuits. A–C: upper traces are intracellular records from a semitendinosus (St) motoneuron (identified by antidromic invasion in A). Lower traces are records from L$_7$ dorsal root entry zone. Voltage calibrations apply to intracellular records. Activation of Ia-afferents from St, posterior biceps (PB), and gracilis (Grac) muscles evokes monosynaptic EPSPs. D–F: intracellular (averaged) records from a vastocrureus (V-Cr) motoneuron (direct antagonist to St). Calibration pulse: 2 ms, 0.5 mV. Stimulation strength (in times threshold of lowest threshold afferent fibers): D) PB, 1.2; St, 1.1; E) Grac, 1.3; St, 1.05; F) Grac, 1.3; PB, 1.2. Appearance of disynaptic IPSPs in motoneuron (bottom traces in D–F) upon conjoint stimulation of PB and St (D), Grac and St (E), and Grac and PB (F) demonstrates convergence of monosynaptic excitation from respective Ia-afferents on common inhibitory interneurons that thus receive same excitatory convergence as the St motoneurons. [A–C adapted from Eccles et al. (135); D–F adapted from Hultborn and Udo (299).]

and similar examples constitute the final proof that these ventral horn interneurons really mediate the reciprocal Ia inhibition.

Ia inhibitory interneurons, identified by synaptic convergence pattern, have also been studied morphologically (327). Intracellular staining with procion yellow established the location of a number of neurons, their axonal projections, and various morphological characteristics and corroborated the conclusion based on electrophysiological studies (335) that Ia inhibitory interneurons are funicular cells.

Input to Ia inhibitory interneurons from primary afferents and segmental pathways. Group Ia-afferents. Direct records from Ia inhibitory interneurons confirmed convergence of Ia-afferents from synergists (287, 291) as was postulated from motoneuronal recordings. They also revealed a disynaptic inhibition by Ia-afferents from antagonists [Fig. 11; (287)]. This inhibition is depressed by conditioning stimulation of motor axons (Fig. 11B–E) and should therefore be relayed by other Ia inhibitory interneurons, referred to as "opposite" Ia inhibitory interneurons (Fig. 11L). The mutual inhibition of Ia inhibitory interneurons may be favorable in γ-assisted contractions of a given agonist muscle that would otherwise be inhibited disynaptically by antagonist Ia afferents activated by the resulting passive stretch (287, 536).

Flexor reflex afferents [(FRA); see subsection *Reflex Pathways From Cutaneous and Joint Afferents and From Groups II and III Muscle Afferents*, p. 535]. Transmission in the pathway mediating reciprocal Ia inhibition of α-motoneurons is influenced via both short- and long-latency FRA pathways. The short-latency pathways facilitate transmission of Ia inhibition to both flexor and extensor motoneurons (72, 172, 173) by exciting Ia inhibitory interneurons (288). In addition to excitation, Ia inhibitory interneurons are also inhibited from the FRAs (288). This inhibition is partly secondary to FRA excitation of opposite Ia inhibitory interneurons and partly medi-

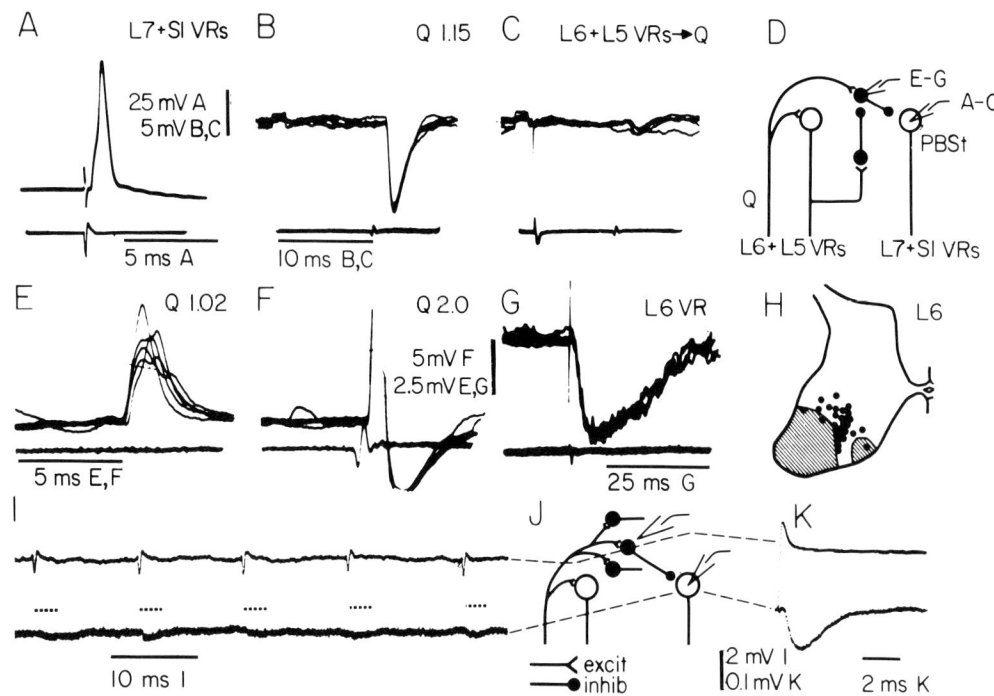

FIG. 10. Identification of interneurons mediating disynaptic Ia inhibition (Ia inhibitory interneurons) from quadriceps (Q) afferents to posterior biceps and semitendinosus (PBSt) motoneurons. Experimental arrangement and neuronal circuits are illustrated in *D* (for records *A–G*) and *J* (for records *I*, *K*). *Upper traces* in *A–G* are intracellular records from a PBSt motoneuron (*A–C*) and a lamina VII interneuron (*E–G*). *Lower traces* are records from L₅ dorsal root entry zone. *Upper trace* in *I* is an extracellular record from a lamina VII interneuron that is excited by electrophoretic ejection of glutamate from the recording electrode. *Lower trace* is a simultaneous intracellular record from a PBSt motoneuron. *K* shows averaged intracellular response from *I* (*lower trace*) triggered by extracellular interneuronal spike (*upper trace*). Voltage calibrations refer to intracellular records. Stimulation strength of Q nerve is given in times threshold of lowest threshold afferent fibers; stimulation of ventral roots (VRs) was supramaximal for α-fibers. *A–C*: disynaptic Ia IPSPs from Q afferents in a PBSt motoneuron (*A*, *B*) and its depression by conditioning stimulation of L₅ + L₆ VRs (*C*). *E–G*: lamina VII interneuron with convergence required for mediation of effects recorded in PBSt motoneuron of *A–C*, i.e., monosynaptic activation from Q Ia-afferents (*E*, *F*) and recurrent inhibition from L₆ VR (*G*). *H*: summarizing diagram giving location in L₆ of a number of interneurons with convergence illustrated in *E–G*. *I–K*: synaptic action in a PBSt motoneuron by an interneuron with convergence shown in *E–G* and location shown in *H*. Monosynaptic unitary IPSP evoked by interneuronal activity proves that interneuron with monosynaptic Ia excitation and disynaptic inhibition from motor axons mediates reciprocal Ia inhibition. [*A–C* from H. Hultborn, E. Jankowska, and S. Lindström, unpublished records; *E–G* adapted from Hultborn et al. (287); *H* adapted from Hultborn et al. (291); *I–K* adapted from Jankowska and Roberts (336).]

ated through pathways not shared with Ia-afferents. The distribution of FRA effects to flexor- and extensor-coupled Ia inhibitory interneurons (288) resembles that found in flexor and extensor α-motoneurons, respectively (148, 266, 268, 611). The long-latency FRA pathways also activate Ia inhibitory interneurons (193); the ipsilateral pathways excite interneurons mediating Ia inhibition to extensors, and the contralateral pathways excite those to flexors.

In addition to their effects via common FRA pathways, low-threshold cutaneous afferents may activate Ia inhibitory interneurons via separate "private" pathways (172, 288). Inhibition or mixed effects from these afferents can also be seen but it has not been established if these actions are relayed through private pathways or through channels belonging to the FRA.

Input to Ia inhibitory interneurons from supraspinal systems. It was first established for the corticospinal tract (425), and later for other descending systems, that supraspinal motor centers may facilitate transmission of reciprocal Ia inhibition to α-motoneurons by either mono- or polysynaptic excitation of the interposed interneurons.

Vestibulospinal tract. The ipsilateral vestibulospinal tract is so far the only descending pathway in the cat known to project directly to Ia inhibitory interneurons. The monosynaptic connection was shown first by the time course of facilitation of reciprocal Ia inhibition of motoneurons to knee, hip, and some ankle flexors and hip extensors [Fig. 11*A–C*; (236, 237, 298)] and later by direct recording from the interneurons themselves [Fig. 11*I–L*; (289)]. Note that the monosynaptic cou-

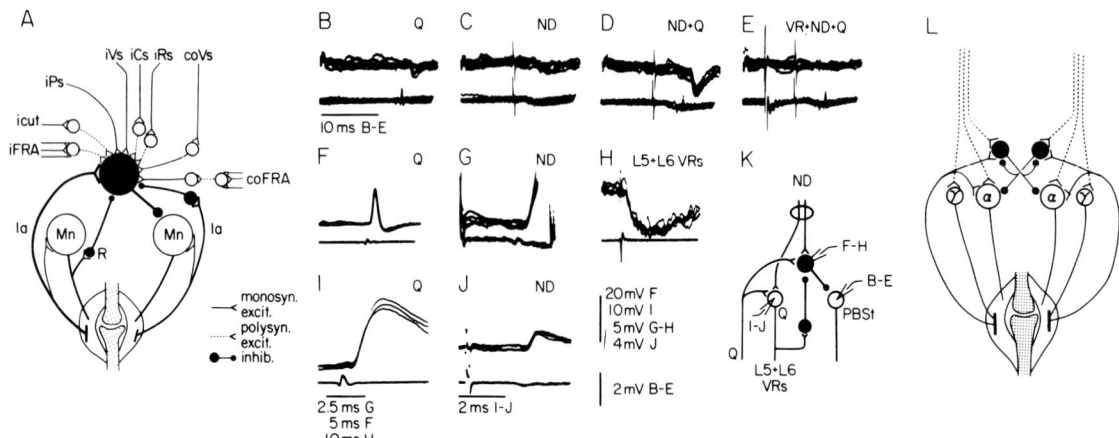

FIG. 11. Connections to interneuron in reciprocal Ia inhibitory pathway. *A*: circuit diagram of some connections to interneuron in reciprocal Ia inhibitory pathway. i, Ipsilateral; co, contralateral; Vs, vestibulospinal tract; Cs, corticospinal tract; Rs, rubrospinal tract; Ps, propriospinal tract; cut, cutaneous afferents; FRA, flexor reflex afferents; Mn, motoneurons; R, Renshaw cells. *B–K*: parallel projection from nucleus vestibularis lateralis (ND) onto α-motoneurons and corresponding Ia inhibitory interneurons. Experimental arrangement and neuronal circuits as illustrated in *K*. *Upper traces* are intracellular records from a posterior biceps–semitendinosus motoneuron (PBSt; *B–E*), a quadriceps (Q) motoneuron (*I, J*), and a Ia inhibitory interneuron (*F–H*) presumably intercalated in the Ia inhibitory pathway from Q to PBSt. *Lower traces* are records from dorsal root entry zone in L$_7$ (*B–E*) or L$_5$ (*F–J*). Voltage calibrations refer to intracellular records. Ipsilateral ND stimulated with 80 μA in *C–E* and 200 μA in *G*. Q nerve (*B–E, F*) stimulated with 1.1 times threshold of the lowest threshold afferent fibers. Ventral roots (VR) were stimulated with single stimuli, supramaximal for α-fibers. *B–E*: facilitation of the Q Ia IPSP in a PBSt motoneuron from vestibulospinal tract (*B–D*) and depression of facilitated IPSP from L$_5$ + L$_6$ VRs (*E*). Results indicate convergence of vestibulospinal excitation and inhibition from motor axon collaterals on common Ia inhibitory interneurons projecting to PBSt motoneurons. *F–H*: monosynaptic excitation from the ND (*G*) of a Q-activated Ia inhibitory interneuron (*F*) and its disynaptic inhibition from L$_5$ + L$_6$ VRs (*H*). Note that these direct recordings from interneuron (*F–H*) correspond to convergent actions from the ND and the VR on the Ia IPSP recorded in the PBSt motoneuron (*B–E*). *I, J*: monosynaptic activation of a Q motoneuron (*I*, homonymous EPSP) from lateral vestibulospinal tract (*J*). *L*: schematic drawing of parallel projections (*broken lines*) onto α- and γ-motoneurons innervating a muscle and the Ia inhibitory interneuron inhibiting the motoneurons of its antagonist. Notice also the mutual inhibition between opposite Ia inhibitory interneurons. Further description in the text. [*B–E* adapted from Hultborn and Udo (298); *F–H* adapted from Hultborn et al. (289); *I, J* adapted from Grillner et al. (240); *L* adapted from Hultborn et al. (287).]

pling between the vestibulospinal tract and the interneurons inhibiting flexor motoneurons parallels the monosynaptic vestibulospinal projection to extensor motoneurons [Fig. 11*G, H*; (240)]. The disynaptic vestibulospinal inhibition of knee flexor motoneurons (236, 240) is depressed by volleys in motor axons, as would be required if the Ia inhibitory interneurons relay this inhibition [Fig. 11*E, F*; (300)]. A corresponding vestibulospinal inhibition of Ia inhibitory interneurons to extensors seems to be mediated by the same Ia inhibitory interneurons that inhibit flexor motoneurons, i.e., the mutual inhibitory connection described above (289). A similar parallel control of motoneurons and Ia inhibitory interneurons is exerted also from the contralateral vestibulospinal tract (278).

Corticospinal tract. In cat hindlimb segments conditioning stimulation of the corticospinal tract facilitates transmission in Ia inhibitory pathways to both extensor and flexor α-motoneurons by a polysynaptic excitation of the interposed interneurons (425). The polysynaptic corticospinal inhibition of motoneurons is strongly affected by Renshaw cells and therefore appears to be mediated to a great extent by Ia inhibitory interneurons (300). Intracellular records from Ia inhibitory interneurons that project to hindlimb motoneurons disclose polysynaptic corticospinal excitation and, in addition, polysynaptic inhibition (289). The inhibition was considerably depressed by conditioning ventral root stimulation. It should therefore be at least partly mediated by opposite Ia inhibitory interneurons, since recurrent inhibition of interneurons in afferent and descending pathways seems to be limited to those mediating reciprocal Ia inhibition.

A more direct coupling between corticospinal tract fibers and Ia inhibitory interneurons has been found in the forelimb segments of the cat [disynaptic; (315)] and in the hindlimb segments of primates [monosynaptic; (333)]. In both cases the corticospinal inhibition of motoneurons turned out to be largely, if not exclusively, mediated by Ia inhibitory interneurons.

Rubrospinal tract. Volleys in the rubrospinal tract facilitate Ia inhibition of cat hindlimb flexor and extensor motoneurons via polysynaptic pathways (275, 298), and direct recording from Ia inhibitory interneurons revealed di- and polysynaptic rubrospinal EPSPs (289). Either di- or trisynaptic inhibition of Ia inhibitory interneurons was also regularly found. Trisynaptic inhibition was partly relayed by opposite Ia inhibitory interneurons; disynaptic IPSPs seemed to be mediated by interneurons of private cutaneous pathways and FRA pathways (300).

Propriospinal systems. In their projection to spinal neurons, descending pathways may utilize propriospinal systems (see subsection *Propriospinal Neurons*, p. 549). Up to now at least two propriospinal systems have been found to act on Ia inhibitory interneurons; one system consists of short-axoned neurons with somata in the third and fourth cervical segments (C_3–C_4) and projecting mainly to the forelimb segments (314); the other system consists of intermediate and long-axoned neurons originating between the fourth cervical and third thoracic segments (C_4–T_3) and projecting to the hindlimb segments (332). In both cases intracellular records revealed that IPSPs evoked in α-motoneurons from these propriospinal systems are mediated by Ia inhibitory interneurons (315, 332). Since the respective propriospinal neurons can be activated monosynaptically from descending tracts, the supraspinal motor centers can act directly on Ia inhibitory interneurons without mediation by other segmental reflex pathways. This type of descending control is similar to certain actions on α-motoneurons that are relayed by propriospinal neurons (cf. *Propriospinal Neurons*, p. 549).

Organization of pathways acting in parallel on motoneurons and Ia inhibitory interneurons. As described in the preceding paragraphs the distribution of effects from primary afferents and descending pathways are very similar for α-motoneurons and their corresponding Ia inhibitory interneurons. This raises the question of to what extent transmission in various pathways projecting to Ia inhibitory interneurons are also facilitated from the segmental and descending systems that modulate transmission in corresponding pathways to α-motoneurons (287–289). This has been most extensively investigated for the rubrospinal tract, but similar results have been obtained for other systems as well. It emerged that the organization of corresponding pathways to both sets of neurons is virtually identical. For example, disynaptic rubrospinal EPSPs and IPSPs in α-motoneurons and corresponding Ia inhibitory interneurons are both facilitated by activation of cutaneous pathways and FRA pathways (35, 289). Such findings could most easily be explained by collateral projections of individual descending tract fibers and segmental interneurons onto α-motoneurons and their corresponding Ia inhibitory neurons. An alternative possibility would be that separate but similar subsystems project to either of these two types of neurons. The latter possibility would more readily allow for a flexible control of pairs of antagonist muscle groups (cf. discussion in subsection FUNCTIONAL CONSEQUENCES OF α-γ-LINKAGE, p. 529). These alternatives are not mutually exclusive, and neither can be ruled out on the basis of available data.

SEGMENTAL AND SUPRASPINAL CONTROL OF γ-MOTONEURONS. The length-servo hypothesis (449) stimulated considerable interest in the central control of γ-motoneurons. When it was recognized (440) that there are two subgroups of γ-motoneurons that have preferential actions on the dynamic or static sensitivity of the muscle spindle afferents (see the chapter by Matthews in this *Handbook*), the possibility of their independent control also became important. In the analysis of fusimotor control it must be kept in mind that intrafusal muscle fibers are innervated both by γ-motoneurons and by collaterals of motor fibers that innervate extrafusal muscle fibers (cf. ref. 367 and the chapters by Burke and by Matthews in this *Handbook*). The parallel skeletofusimotor innervation is the rule in amphibians [see review by Barker (43)] and was found some time ago in the cat (61), but its common occurrence in felines became clear only recently (164). The skeletofusimotor fibers are denoted β-fibers although their conduction velocity is in the α-range; indeed no difference has so far been found between motoneurons that innervate only extrafusal muscle fibers and those that also innervate intrafusal fibers (see ref. 85). Although it is not known how β- and γ-innervation interact in the control of the muscle spindle, the preservation of the combined skeletofusimotor fibers in mammals will obviously tend to secure a parallel contraction of intrafusal and extrafusal fibers, which is independent of the γ-route.

In reviewing the central control of γ-activity we have chosen to emphasize the parallelism of actions of various neuronal systems on α- and γ-motoneurons that innervate the same muscle. The actions on γ-motoneurons can be inferred indirectly from changes in the responses of muscle spindle afferents or observed directly by recording from γ-motoneurons. A differentiation between the control of either static or dynamic γ-motoneurons requires afferent recording; direct recording is necessary when studying the segmental organization of the pathways controlling γ-motoneurons. The two methods are thus complementary. It shall be noted, however, that the presence of skeletofusimotor fibers complicates the interpretation of central effects on γ-motoneurons inferred from observing changes in the discharges of muscle spindle afferents.

Afferent control of γ-motoneurons. Group I afferents. There is no indication of monosynaptic Ia excitation of γ-motoneurons (132, 163, 239, 303, 308, 602), which is a notable exception from the general rule of parallel actions on α- and γ-motoneurons. Excitation from Ia-afferents may, however, reach dynamic γ-motoneurons via a polysynaptic spinal pathway, and it has been suggested that this might reinforce α-motoneuronal discharge to maintain a constant muscle length during postural activity (162, 163, 191, 581).

Inhibition of γ-motoneurons by group I afferents from homonymous and synergic muscles has been repeatedly reported (157, 163, 191, 239, 303), but its Ia or Ib origin has not yet been established. In the few γ-motoneurons investigated intracellularly, the origin of the inhibition evoked by electrical stimulation of nerves (239) resembled that of Ib inhibition of α-motoneurons (subsection *Reflex Pathways From Ib Tendon Organ Afferents*, p. 530). On the other hand, adequate activation of muscle receptors suggests that both Ia- and Ib-fibers may contribute to it (162, 163, 191). It has furthermore been postulated that some inhibition of γ-motoneurons by impulses in Ia-afferents may in fact be evoked indirectly via Renshaw cells that are activated secondary to Ia excitation of α-motoneurons (163, 191, 239). Whatever pathway is used, group I inhibition is more effective in static than in dynamic neurons (190, 191, 239). This may explain why it was not found in acute spinal cats (308), a preparation in which most static fusimotor neurons are silent (5, 53, 231).

Group II afferents. In general secondary muscle spindle afferents have effects on γ-motoneurons similar to the action of other flexor reflex afferents (see subsection *Reflex Pathways From Cutaneous and Joint Afferents and From Groups II and III Muscle Afferents*, p. 535). They excite γ-motoneurons (both dynamic and static) that project to flexors and evoke a mixture of inhibitory and excitatory effects in those that project to extensors (53, 231, 602). Whereas most of these actions seem to be relayed in the common FRA pathways, there are also indications of some separate lines. Thus Appelberg et al. (28) described an autogenetic disynaptic excitation of dynamic γ-motoneurons from secondary endings. They proposed that this pathway could provide a positive feedback for the adjustment of the dynamic sensitivity of muscle spindles when a muscle meets an increasing load during contraction. Disynaptic group II EPSPs were likewise found in α-motoneurons (416), and these group II actions thus provide another possible example of parallel effects onto α- and γ-motoneurons.

Flexor reflex afferents. As in α-motoneurons, the FRAs activate γ-motoneurons through short- and long-latency pathways. The short-latency effects most often follow the pattern of ipsilateral flexor and crossed extensor reflexes in α-motoneurons (303), but mixed or reversed effects are also common (cf. ref. 232) with some differences in effects to dynamic and static γ-motoneurons. In spinal preparations the FRAs more effectively activate dynamic than static γ-motoneurons to flexors (53); in the same preparations dynamic γ-motoneurons are spontaneously active whereas static ones are not. After injection of dopa (cf. subsection *Monoaminergic Reticulospinal Pathways*, p. 562) short-latency FRA activation is depressed in dynamic and increased in static γ-motoneurons, and the spontaneous discharge of these neurons is subject to similar changes; firing of dynamic γ-motoneurons is depressed but appears in static γ-motoneurons. It is not known whether these changes in FRA responses are due to a general change in the excitability of the γ-motoneurons or to a specific effect on the short-latency interneuronal pathways. The latter possibility has been discussed by Bergmans and Grillner (53) who suggested that the opposite responses of flexor γ-motoneurons after dopa injection might reflect interactive inhibitory relations between the pathways to dynamic and static γ-motoneurons. No such opposite FRA effects have been found in γ-motoneurons to extensors. Although in the spinal state only the dynamic γ-motoneurons are spontaneously active (5, 231), their activity is enhanced after injection of dopa in parallel with the appearance of resting activity of static γ-motoneurons (231). Short-latency FRA effects are evoked in all extensor γ-motoneurons. Inhibition is mainly present in dynamic motoneurons; excitation occurs in both dynamic and static motoneurons (28, 231).

In addition to the short-latency effects described above, flexor and extensor γ-motoneurons are subject to long-latency FRA effects after injection of dopa [cf. subsection *Reflex Pathways From Cutaneous and Joint Afferents and From Groups II and III Muscle Afferents*, p. 535; (53, 231, 242)]. They are excited from ipsi- and contralateral FRAs, respectively. The excitation reaches both dynamic and static γ-motoneurons in parallel to the long-latency effects on α-motoneurons. It has therefore been suggested that the long-latency synaptic actions on α- and γ-motoneurons are mediated by common pathways (53).

Descending control of γ-motoneurons. There have been many studies on the supraspinal control of γ-motoneurons. In the 1950s [(156, 223); see also ref. 157] it was found that stimulation almost anywhere in the reticular formation of the brain stem is effective in activating γ-motoneurons. There are short-latency effects that are reciprocal for flexor and extensor γ-motoneurons, and there are also long-latency, long-lasting actions that are similar on both extensor and flexor γ-motoneurons (221, 560). The latter are greatly dependent on the level of the anesthesia (598), and can be mobilized by a "pinna twist" (222, 522, 523, 527). They have been viewed as part of a general arousal response (218, 219), but it is unknown to what extent they are coupled to the corresponding widespread facilitation of α-motoneurons.

Monosynaptic actions from the brain stem on γ-motoneurons appear, on the other hand, to be closely linked to the actions of the same systems on α-motoneurons (DIRECT PROJECTIONS OF DESCENDING PATHWAYS TO α-MOTONEURONS, p. 567). Thus monosynaptic excitation is evoked in extensor α- and γ-motoneurons from the lateral vestibular nucleus and in flexor α- and γ-motoneurons from fibers descending in the medial longitudinal fasciculus (239). In both cases it seems that the excitation is selectively exerted on the static γ-motoneurons [(52, 231); see also ref. 90]. These monosynaptic projections represent the most clearcut examples of parallel control of α- and γ-motoneurons from descending systems, and they could provide a substrate for tightly coupled α-γ-coactivation.

The γ-motoneurons are also controlled from the mesencephalon. Spontaneously discharging neurons nearly always change their frequency during rubral stimulation (27), and there is evidence that the rubrospinal influence on fusimotor neurons (27) closely parallels that to α-motoneurons with respect to both the sign of the action and its minimal synaptic linkage (274). Dynamic and static γ-motoneurons to flexors are excited, whereas those to extensors receive mainly inhibition (dynamic neurons) or mixed rubrospinal effects (static neurons). Stimulation within the region dorsal to the red nucleus selectively increases the dynamic sensitivity of muscle spindles (25, 26, 29). The efferent pathway transmitting this effect descends ipsilaterally to the inferior olive and, after being relayed in the lower brain stem, reaches the contralateral dorsolateral funiculus of the spinal cord (25, 339, 340).

Stimulation of the motor cortex or the corticospinal tract evokes pronounced excitatory and inhibitory actions in γ-motoneurons projecting to flexors and extensors, respectively, with the effects distributed to both static and dynamic cells (180, 599, 622). In all these studies fusimotor effects were obtained before the effects of central stimulation were noticeable in α-motoneurons. This could be relevant to the question of whether or not there exist separate and independent cortical projections to α- and γ-motoneurons (352, 353). The minimal synaptic linkage of the corticospinal excitation of γ-motoneurons is monosynaptic in the monkey (100, 230) and disynaptic in the cat (180), similar to the corticospinal projection to α-motoneurons in both species [cf. section DIRECT PROJECTIONS OF DESCENDING PATHWAYS TO α-MOTONEURONS, p. 567; (60, 312)].

FUNCTIONAL CONSEQUENCES OF α-γ-LINKAGE. In his hypothesis of the follow-up length servo, Merton (449) postulated that in "ordinary movements" the γ-loop constitutes an independent route for motor control but is less important in "urgent movements," which were thought to be produced by direct activation of α-motoneurons. The results of systematic investigations in decerebrate cats strongly suggest, however, that the gain of the γ-operated stretch reflex is too low to allow the operation of an unaided follow-up servo (see ref. 444). Meanwhile it had been postulated that movements depend on coactivation of α- and γ-motoneurons (217). A neuronal system acting in α-γ-linkage would exert synaptic depolarization of α-motoneurons both directly (α-route) and indirectly (γ-route), and the discharge of α-motoneurons would accordingly depend on spatial facilitation of the two effects. With this organization the γ-loop would provide servo assistance to movements (444). It is important for the coordination of movements that reciprocal inhibition of antagonists be coupled to excitation of agonist muscles. The hypothesis of "α-γ-linkage in reciprocal inhibition" postulates that neuronal systems acting in α-γ-linked movements excite in parallel not only α- and γ-motoneurons to agonists but also Ia inhibitory interneurons to antagonists (275, 409). As discussed above (subsection REFLEX PATHWAYS FROM GROUP Ia MUSCLE SPINDLE AFFERENTS, p. 519), corresponding α-motoneurons and Ia inhibitory interneurons have identical input from most segmental and descending systems. The servo assistance given by the γ-loop should therefore support not only the contraction of agonists but also the relaxation of antagonists.

Although parallel connections exist to α- and γ-motoneurons and to corresponding Ia inhibitory interneurons, other evidence is needed to prove that the central nervous system really operates these pathways in accordance with the above hypothesis. Such confirmation has now been obtained for *1)* α-γ-coactivation for respiratory movements (cat), jaw movements (cat and monkey), stepping (cat), and voluntary movements in humans; and *2)* coactivation of α-motoneurons and corresponding Ia inhibitory interneurons for stepping (cat) and voluntary movements (humans).

Coactivation of α- and γ-motoneurons under physiological conditions was first demonstrated with recordings from spindle afferents of respiratory muscles [(153, 171); see also refs. 532, 533 for recording of efferent fibers]. The afferent discharge increased when the muscles shortened during contraction and decreased during passive lengthening in the relaxation phase. This pattern reversed after a selective blockade of γ-fibers and was therefore attributed to the efferent activation of the muscle spindles in parallel with the extrafusal shortening. Similar observations have been made for jaw movements [(401, 578); see, however, refs. 207, 577] and during locomotion in decorticated and decerebrated cats (481, 535, 536). Simultaneous recording from α- and γ-efferents during "fictive" locomotion (see the chapter by Grillner in this *Handbook*) in spinal cats revealed that the coactivation can also be produced by the spinal circuitry that generates locomotor alternations (562). Recordings from primary muscle spindle afferents in the intact freely moving cat demonstrated the existence of α-γ-coactivation also in this preparation, but with an unexpected degree of independence (397, 398, 494–496), in contrast to a rather rigid coactivation in reactions that asked for isometric contraction against an imposed load. These findings suggest therefore that the degree of central coupling between the inputs to both sets of motoneurons may depend on the intended movement.

Coactivation of α- and γ-motoneurons has also been found in humans (583–585, 588). During voluntary isometric contractions of wrist and finger muscles, the discharge patterns of single spindle afferents indicate a very tight coupling between α- and γ-motoneurons. The linkage appears to be remarkably rigid in three basic aspects. First, the fusimotor outflow is spatially restricted to the contracting muscle and does not even reach synergists (584). Second, the timing of the Ia firing at the beginning of a contraction suggests that the activity in α- and γ-efferents leaves the spinal cord simultaneously (585), which implies a tight temporal linkage. Finally, there is a close relation between the firing frequency of spindle afferents and the strength of the isometric contractions (588). Acceleration of spindle afferent firing can be seen also during attempted voluntary contractions when conduction in α-fibers (and thus extrafusal contraction) is prevented by a pressure block of the nerve (78). It can therefore be concluded that parallel contraction of extra- and intrafusal fibers during isometric voluntary contraction in humans depends on a tight α-γ-coactivation, although the extent to which skeletofusimotor (β) fibers may contribute is still unknown.

Vallbo et al. (589) made a provisional assessment of the quantitative importance in humans of the excitatory drive to α-motoneurons that is supplied by the enhanced spindle inflow during voluntary muscle contraction. In spite of the close α-γ-coupling described above, they concluded that the contribution of muscle spindle afferents to α-activation is quite small. Vallbo (588) further stated that the muscle spindles and their central connections "do not constitute a very powerful mechanism to hold muscle length constant when the load varies." On the other hand, the primary endings may respond very distinctly to small irregularities of active movements (77, 586, 587), and Vallbo (586) therefore suggested that their role might be to reduce variations in speed of movements caused by small variations in load or frictional resistance or by an irregular skeletomotor outflow. These experiments in humans [as well as the inconsistent spindle driving in freely moving cats; (494–496)] shift the balance of evidence away from the idea of a servo assistance (cf. ref. 444) and back toward the early suggestion by Kuffler and Hunt (361) that the chief function of the fusimotor fibers is "to maintain the afferent flow from spindles in spite of a certain amount of muscle shortening," so that their information input could be preserved at all times.

The function of the γ-system must, however, be considered separately for the two subgroups of γ-motoneurons that govern different parameters of muscle spindle sensitivity (see the chapter by Matthews in this *Handbook*). The dynamic γ-motoneurons control the sensitivity of the primary endings to stretches of small amplitudes, and they may therefore have special significance in situations in which the spindles should react to small perturbations and irregularities. Only static fibers are able to increase the firing of primary (and secondary) endings during muscle shortening (374). Consequently if the γ-loop and muscle spindles contribute to the excitation of α-motoneurons during extrafusal shortening, the central command has to include the static γ-motoneurons. It may be, however, that the most important aspect of the coactivation of static γ-motoneurons with α-motoneurons is to ensure that the muscle spindle afferents are ready to respond to small perturbations added on a large active muscle shortening in line with the suggestion by Kuffler and Hunt (361). On the basis of such general considerations, the central nervous system might be expected to use the available possibility for separate control of static and dynamic γ-motoneurons. The current experiments on freely moving animals and on voluntary movements in humans seem to offer promising possibilities to answer these questions.

Coactivation of α-motoneurons and of corresponding Ia inhibitory interneurons has been demonstrated in natural movements, as required by the hypothesis of "α-γ-linkage in reciprocal inhibition." The directly recorded activity of Ia inhibitory interneurons was enhanced in locomotion of the mesencephalic cat when the muscles that supply Ia excitation contracted (175). Their rhythmic activation persisted after interruption of the γ-loop by deafferentation, showing that the Ia inhibitory interneurons are at least in part driven by the central locomotor command. Compatible results have been obtained for voluntary movements in humans (575, 576). Tanaka (575, 576) found that group I volleys from the pretibial flexors were not effective in inhibiting monosynaptic test reflexes (Hoffmann's reflex) of the antagonist triceps surae muscle at rest, although they did so during voluntary ankle flexion. This finding suggests that the central motor command for ankle flexion includes excitation of Ia inhibitory interneurons projecting to triceps surae motoneurons.

It remains to be established how rigid is the coactivation of α- and γ-motoneurons and corresponding Ia inhibitory interneurons. A flexible control from central motor areas seems necessary for an optimal operation of the γ-system in various types of movements (see above and refs. 397, 398, 494–496). The coupling would be rather rigid if collaterals of the same central neurons reached all target cells; parallel but separate projections to each subgroup of target cells would provide the possibility for a selective control. Such an independent control has actually been demonstrated in several experimental situations in which the coupling between α- and γ-motoneurons was analyzed (107, 221, 352, 353), but no corresponding evidence has yet been found for α-motoneurons and corresponding Ia inhibitory interneurons.

Reflex Pathways From Group Ib Tendon Organ Afferents

The early demonstration of the clasp-knife phenomenon [(553); see ref. 444] revealed that receptors in a given muscle not only supply reflex excitation but also can produce reflex inhibition of its own motoneurons. Subsequently the Ib tendon organ afferents were shown to be a main source of this autogenetic inhibition. The Ib inhibition was for a long time regarded mainly as a protective reflex against muscle overloading [see review by Haase et al. (253)] because of the high threshold of the receptors to passive stretch (306, 439). This view became untenable with the demonstration that active contraction of only a few motor units (or even a single unit) may activate tendon organs (281, 338, 566). It is furthermore well established that the Ib actions in α-motoneurons are not limited to autogenetic effects and that interneuronal transmission in both excitatory and inhibitory Ib reflex pathways is controlled from higher centers (cf. ref. 412). The latter findings and the low-receptor threshold during active force generation suggest rather that Ib pathways are engaged in the continuous control of motoneuronal excitability (404, 413). Experiments on the convergence within the Ib pathways to α-motoneurons have stimulated interest in the Ib projection onto the interposed interneurons. The available evidence suggests that such interneurons are shared by many segmental and supraspinal systems and that their activity may only partially relate to activity of Ib-afferents.

PATTERN OF Ib ACTIONS IN α-MOTONEURONS. Laporte and Lloyd (369) tested conditioning effects of graded electrical stimulation of various hindlimb muscle nerves on monosynaptic test reflexes. They ascribed reflex actions, which were additional to the facilitation and inhibition from Ia-afferents, to activation of Ib-fibers. They observed two main effects, both of which involve muscles operating at the same joint: *1*) inhibition of motoneurons projecting to synergists (an effect that was assumed to be evoked in homonymous motoneurons as well); and *2*) excitation of motoneurons to antagonists. Since these actions were opposite the pattern of the myotatic reflex, they were referred to as the inverse myotatic reflex (369). Sometimes inhibitory actions were found between muscles not belonging to the same myotatic unit. The conclusion on Ib origin of these actions received strong support from experiments in which effects of adequate stimulation of muscle spindles and tendon organs were compared (215, 216, 304).

With intracellular recording from motoneurons in the low spinal cat and electrical stimulation of muscle afferents [using the slight threshold difference of Ia- and Ib-fibers to differentiate Ia and Ib actions (68)], the pattern of the inverse myotatic reflex was confirmed [(134, 136); see also ref. 415], but both excitatory and inhibitory effects were shown to be more widely distributed than was apparent in experiments with monosynaptic test reflexes. The effects were mainly evoked from extensors. The Ib reflex actions revealed during conditioning stimulation of the red nucleus were even more widely distributed, and new projections linking together muscles that operate one or several joints apart were described (275). Hongo et al. (275) demonstrated the presence of inhibitory pathways from extensors to flexor nuclei and from flexors to extensor nuclei for muscles acting at neighboring joints. For muscles operating further apart, inhibitory pathways from flexors to flexor nuclei and excitatory paths from flexors to extensor nuclei were also revealed. These experiments demonstrated that information from tendon organ afferents of an individual muscle may reach nearly all motor nuclei of a limb and cut across even the functional division of the muscles into flexors and extensors.

Perl (478, 479) and Holmqvist (266) have shown that electrical stimulation of group I afferents from flexor or extensor muscles produces a mixture of excitatory or inhibitory effects in contralateral flexor and extensor motoneurons, but it was not possible to separate Ia and Ib effects. Selective stimulation of Ib-afferents (105) from the soleus muscle revealed that they excite contralateral flexor and extensor muscles crossing the ankle (47). However, with the present knowledge of Ia contribution to Ib inhibition in motoneurons, the very low threshold at which electrical stimulation evoked effects in chronic spinal animals (266) is suggestive of Ia participation as well. It thus emerges that the contribution of Ib-afferents to such a classical crossed-reflex response as the "Philippson's reflex" [contraction of contralateral knee extensors, by flexion of the knee; (483, 552, 553)] is still unclear.

CONVERGENCE IN Ib PATHWAYS. Both the excitatory and the inhibitory Ib actions on ipsilateral α-motoneurons are relayed in pathways with di- or trisynaptic linkages (136, 369). Using the spatial facilitation technique, it has been shown that afferents from different muscles that contribute to these actions converge at the intercalated interneurons (415). The paragraphs that follow describe additional convergence from segmental and descending pathways.

Ia-afferents. It was assumed for a long time that autogenetic and synergic inhibition of motoneurons from group I muscle afferents was exclusively evoked from tendon organs. Recent experiments have shown, however, that Ia-afferents also may contribute to such inhibition. Both di- and trisynaptic IPSPs are evoked in homonymous and synergic motoneurons by adequate activation of Ia-afferents from ankle and toe extensors (179). They are smaller than the maximal IPSPs evoked either by electrical stimulation of all group I fibers or by selective electrical stimulation of Ib-fibers after the electrical threshold of Ia-axons had been raised by long-lasting, high-frequency vibration of the muscles (105). Spatial facilitation between inhibitory effects of Ia- and Ib-afferents indicates that inhibition is mediated by neurons common to both pathways [(417); E. E. Fetz, E. Jankowska, and J. Lipski, unpublished observations; see also ref. 322]. This finding of Ia-Ib convergence in segmental interneurons suggests that reflex actions from muscle spindle and tendon organ afferents are linked, at least so far as autogenetic and synergic inhibition are concerned. It remains to be established if Ia-afferents similarly contribute to ipsilateral Ib excitation of motoneurons or to other inhibitory effects from Ib-afferents.

Cutaneous and joint afferents. The Ib effects seen in the low spinal animal (136) are effectively facilitated from low-threshold cutaneous and joint afferents [Fig. 12; (417, 419)]. This has been found for both excitatory and inhibitory Ib actions, and the time course indicates a disynaptic linkage from cutaneous and joint afferents to the interneurons of the common pathways. Because of the different organization of the cutaneous pathways in fore- and hindlimb segments (see *Reflex Pathways From Cutaneous and Joint Afferents and From Groups II and III Muscle Afferents*, p. 535), it is interesting to note that cutaneous facilitation is more marked for Ib effects among different forelimb muscles than for Ib effects among different hindlimb muscles (313).

Cortico- and rubrospinal tracts. Stimulation of the cortico- and rubrospinal tracts facilitates transmission in excitatory and inhibitory pathways from Ib-afferents to α-motoneurons by excitatory action on the interposed interneurons (275, 313, 425). Both descending tracts act with such a short segmental delay that a monosynaptic linkage from the tract fibers to the interneurons was postulated. In the lumbar cord this direct coupling was demonstrated for the rubrospinal tract [Fig. 12; (275)] and in the cervical cord for both the rubro- and corticospinal tracts (313).

Reticulospinal systems. Ipsilateral Ib pathways are subject to an inhibitory control from the brain stem. This was first evidenced with the demonstration that reflex transmission in both excitatory and inhibitory pathways is tonically inhibited in the decerebrate state (see subsection *Decerebrate Preparation*, p. 564). Further analysis of this descending control disclosed at least two descending inhibitory systems controlling transmission in Ib reflex pathways. Stimulation of the medullary reticular formation effectively depressed excitatory and inhibitory Ib actions in α-motoneurons at strengths that neither changed their membrane conductance nor evoked any primary afferent depolarization (167). This effect is mediated by the dorsal reticulospinal system with axons descending in the dorsal quadrant of the lateral funiculus (see subsection *Dorsal Reticulospinal System*, p. 560). Inhibition of Ib transmission to motoneurons can also be evoked by activity in noradrenergic reticulospinal pathways, as

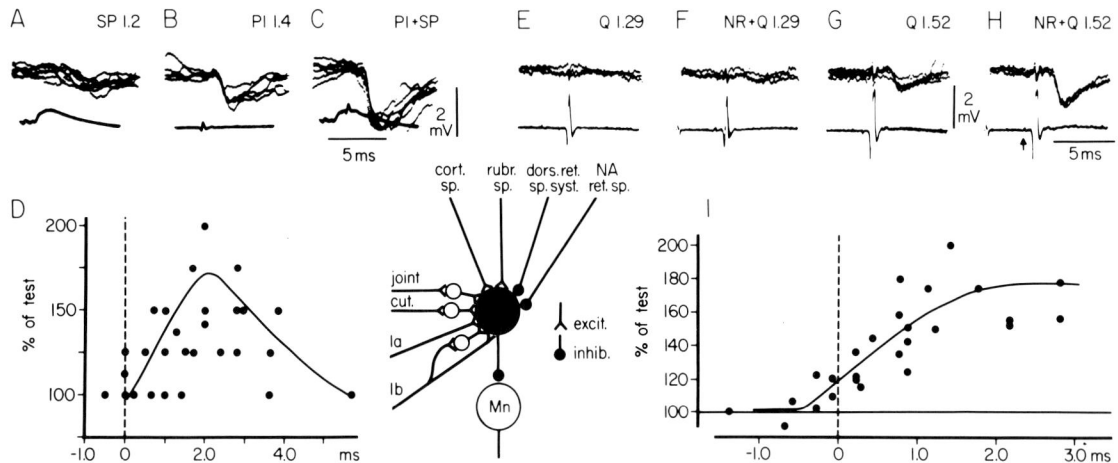

FIG. 12. Convergence on interneurons in Ib inhibitory pathway to motoneurons. *Upper traces,* intracellular recordings from motoneurons to gastrocnemius-soleus (*A–C*) and to flexor digitorum longus (*E–H*). *Lower traces,* incoming volleys recorded from L$_7$ dorsal root entry zone. Voltage calibrations refer to intracellular records. Stimulus strengths of peripheral nerves are given in multiples of thresholds for lowest threshold afferents. *A–C*: facilitatory interaction in inhibitory transmission to motoneurons from Ib muscle afferents from plantaris (Pl) and cutaneous afferents in superficial peroneal nerve (SP). *E–H*: facilitatory interaction between a single descending volley in rubrospinal tract (stimulation of red nucleus, NR) and a Ib volley in quadriceps nerve (Q); *G*, *H* compare the lack of facilitation with weaker nerve stimulation that mainly activates Ia-afferents in *E*, *F*. Arrow below records in *H* indicates time of arrival of the fastest descending volleys in rubrospinal tract to the L$_6$ level. Corresponding *graphs* in *D* and *I* show time course of facilitation obtained by varying conditioning-testing interval. Zero on abscissa indicates simultaneous arrival at segmental level of both conditioning and testing volleys. Delay of facilitation by a cutaneous volley (*D*) suggests a disynaptic linkage to Ib inhibitory interneurons. Facilitatory action at simultaneous arrival (and even with the conditioning volley arriving slightly after the test) in the case of rubrospinal volley (*I*) strongly indicates a monosynaptic linkage from rubrospinal tract. Circuit diagram summarizes most of the neuronal connections to Ib inhibitory interneurons. [*A–C* adapted from Lundberg et al. (417); *E–H* adapted from Hongo et al. (275).]

evidenced in the acute spinal cat by the depression of Ib actions after i.v. injection of dopa (see *Monoaminergic Reticulospinal Pathways*, p. 562).

INTERNEURONS INTERPOSED IN Ib PATHWAYS TO α-MOTONEURONS (Ib-INTERNEURONS). Identification of the interneurons interposed in reflex pathways from Ib tendon organ afferents to α-motoneurons (the Ib-interneurons) has not yet advanced as far as the identification of Ia inhibitory interneurons (*Pathways From Ia-Afferents and Their Control by γ-Motoneurons*, p. 519). However, high probability candidates exist among the group I–activated interneurons in the intermediate nucleus in laminae V and VI (115, 116, 132, 168, 273, 277, 323, 400, 407, 420), where large monosynaptic focal potentials are evoked by volleys in group I muscle afferents (141). Many of the mono- or disynaptically excited group I interneurons in this area also receive input from both descending pathways and segmental systems, as is required for interneurons that mediate Ib effects to α-motoneurons (from the indirect method of recording in motoneurons; summarized in Fig. 12). For example, disynaptic excitation from cutaneous afferents (273) and excitation from corticospinal fibers (420) were found in a substantial number of interneurons, and they often received monosynaptic excitation from the rubrospinal tract (277). Inhibition from the dorsal reticulospinal system was also recorded in some of the interneurons located in the intermediate nucleus (168).

Many of the laminae V and VI interneurons are monosynaptically excited by both Ia- and Ib-afferents (Fig. 13). Existence of two different populations of group I–excited interneurons, with input from either Ia- or Ib-afferents, was postulated in initial studies (137), but later investigations suggested that convergence onto individual cells from the two afferent systems is very common (117, 273, 277, 323). Most of these group I–excited interneurons were, in addition, monosynaptically excited by descending fibers, possibly rubro- and corticospinal (Fig. 13C), and disynaptically excited from cutaneous afferents [Fig. 13B; (323)]. Since Ia- and Ib-afferents should converge onto common interneurons in the Ib reflex pathways (according to indirect evidence from motoneuronal recording), these laminae V and VI interneurons seem suitable candidates for Ib-interneurons. Intracellular staining with horseradish peroxidase demonstrated that several of them indeed project to the motor nuclei (115, 116, 323), as was also the case for the neuron shown in Figure 13. Of course these findings do not exclude the possibility that Ib excited interneurons

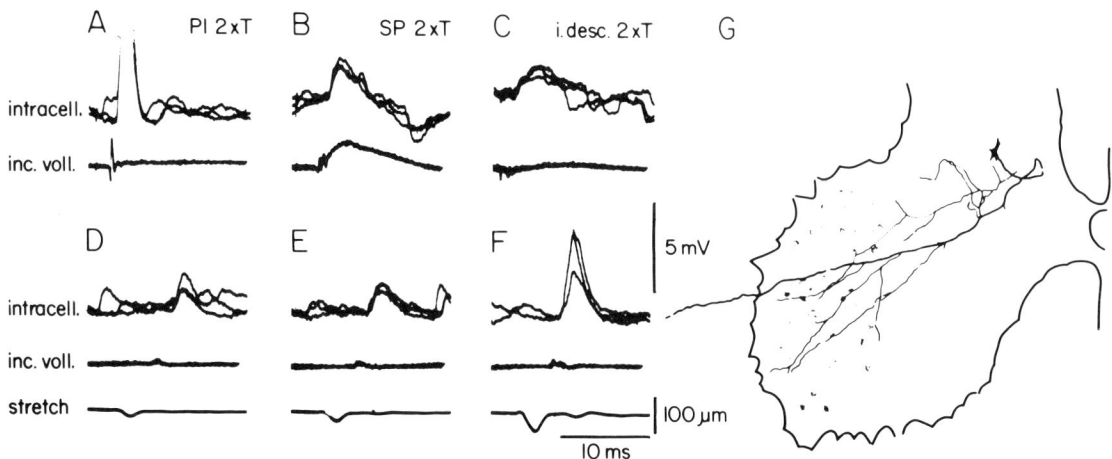

FIG. 13. Convergence onto a lamina V and VI interneuron possibly interposed in Ib reflex pathways to motoneurons. *Upper traces (A–F)*, intracellular records from a lamina V and VI interneuron; *lower traces (A–C)* and *middle traces (D–F)*, records of afferent volleys from L₇ dorsal root entry zone; *lower traces (D–F)*, records of changes in muscle length (increase in length downward). *A–C*: convergence of monosynaptic excitation from group I afferents in nerve from plantaris (Pl), of disynaptic excitation from cutaneous afferents in superficial peroneal nerve (SP) and of monosynaptic excitation from ipsilateral descending fibers (i. desc.). Stimulus strength is given in times threshold for lowest threshold fibers. *D–F*: analysis by graded brief stretches of plantaris muscle of contribution from muscle spindle Ia-afferents and Golgi tendon organ Ib-afferents to the group I excitation illustrated in *A*. Small stretch in *D* (cf. calibration to right of *F*) selectively activates muscle spindle Ia-afferents, the larger muscle stretches in *E* and *F* are near maximal for Ia-afferents and above threshold for Ib-afferents, respectively. This series of records thus strongly indicates that both Ia- and Ib-afferents contribute monosynaptic excitation. *G*: reconstruction of soma and part of the axonal projections of interneuron whose excitatory input is illustrated in *A–F*. Interneuron was stained by ejecting horseradish peroxidase from the microelectrode after the recording. Notice the axonal projection into region of motoneurons (large neurons, probably motoneurons, are indicated by *hatched areas*). (From E. Jankowska, T. Johannisson, and J. Lipski, unpublished observations.)

without Ia convergence also take part in reflex transmission to motoneurons (cf. ref. 179), especially since there is little information on whether the group I pathways that mediate autogenetic and synergic inhibition to motoneurons are homogeneous or whether there exist parallel interneuronal lines with different patterns of input convergence.

The laminae V and VI interneurons are further characterized by an indirect inhibitory control from group I muscle afferents from wide receptive fields (117, 273, 277, 323). The significance of this control is difficult to evaluate, but it should be noted that the rubrospinal tract can select among alternative Ib reflex pathways, perhaps by interactive inhibition between the different segmental systems (275, 277).

FUNCTIONAL CONSIDERATIONS. With particular reference to the inhibitory autogenetic Ib effects, Houk and Henneman (280) developed the idea of a tension feedback that would help keep the force constant for any level of motoneuronal activity despite variations caused by factors such as muscle fatigue and velocity of shortening (force-velocity relation). Realizing the inherent contradiction between a length servo (from muscle spindles) and a tension servo (from Golgi tendon organs), Houk et al. (282) also discussed the possibility that "during certain motor tasks length feedback is inhibited and force feedback is facilitated so as to provide a system controlling muscular force rather than length." They pointed out that the descending control of the mediating interneurons probably could provide for this change and that a pure force feedback might be advantageous, for example, during exploratory movements. A flexible balance between the stretch reflex and autogenetic inhibition has also been discussed by Newsom Davis and Sears (458) for the respiratory musculature during breathing and vocalization, and by Bergmans et al. (50) for the hindlimb in different phases of gait. However, in later discussions Nichols and Houk (459) and Crago et al. (108) looked on the conjoint effects provided by the feedback from muscle spindle and Golgi tendon organs as more rigidly coupled and argued that together they regulate muscle stiffness in a way that compensates for the highly asymmetrical mechanical properties of contracting muscles during lengthening and shortening (see also the chapter by Houk and Rymer in this *Handbook*). They reached the tentative conclusion that the main function of these proprioceptive reflexes was to compensate for inherent nonlinearities in muscle properties rather than to compensate for perturbations in force and length that occur in the interaction with the external world during motor behavior.

Although the servo concept provided a valuable impetus for discussions on the Ib actions on motoneurons, it nevertheless seems too limited to incorporate all essential elements in our present knowledge. First of all it must be kept in mind that only a minor part of the Ib inhibitory action is autogenetic and that supraspinal centers seem able to choose from the available patterns of Ib effects (in addition to their quantitative control of transmittability). These aspects are certainly difficult to reconcile with a function specifically linked to the biophysical properties of the contracting homonymous muscle or even with any simple form of force servo that refers to individual muscles. Under all circumstances it must be remembered that the regulated object is not the activity of the individual homonymous muscle but rather the action of virtually all the limb muscles in a flexible pattern. The extensive convergence on the Ib-interneurons from peripheral receptors of different modalities indeed raises the question of whether the pathway is primarily related to the Golgi tendon organs or if the excitation of the interneurons would be more adequately discussed in terms of conjoint action from muscle, skin, and joint afferents (419). For the time being it seems easier to handle the former concept, i.e., to regard the convergence from Ia-, skin, and joint afferents as a control of transmission from Ib-afferents. This line of reasoning is illustrated by the following example of the possible significance of the convergence from joint afferents (419).

The majority of joint receptors, at least from the knee (23, 75, 97, 176, 177, 227, 228, 563), are most effectively activated at either end position and this should facilitate Ib inhibition at the end of an active limb extension and contribute to the decrease of extensor activity in the terminal phase of the movement. Since this phase is usually influenced by dynamic forces, e.g., during locomotion (166), it may be important to have a segmental mechanism to control the relaxation rather than to depend solely on a centrally programmed timing [(419); see further in subsection JOINT AFFERENTS, p. 538)]. Within the framework of this example, a role may also be given to reciprocal Ib excitation, which may assist in braking the movement by activating antagonists. The same line of reasoning has been applied also for the facilitation of Ib inhibition from cutaneous afferents (417), with the assumption that the facilitation of the inhibitory Ib pathway in an exploratory movement is drawn from a skin field activated when the moving limb meets an obstacle. Active touch could under some conditions produce a decrease of agonist activity so as not to apply force to objects. The view reflected in these examples is not necessarily contradictory to the force-servo theory. The role of a servo is to keep some parameter constant in spite of external disturbances. The supraspinal control of Ib-interneurons would set the gain of the servo and/or the desired level of force toward which the servo aims. It may be questioned, however, how purposeful this servo concept is when the gain of the servo may also continuously change with the changing activity in converging afferent systems (Ia-, joint, and skin afferents; cf. ref. 417).

Before closing the discussion on the reflex actions from Ib-afferents, special mention should be made of the excitatory Ib effects. It has been tacitly assumed that the main reflex action from Ib-afferents is the inhibitory one and the excitatory Ib pathways have therefore received little attention. Transmission in them is characterized by the same facilitatory support from descending and segmental systems as the inhibitory pathways, and the distribution of the excitatory effects is to some extent reciprocal to the inhibitory ones. The Ib excitation has therefore been viewed mainly as subsidiary to the inhibition (411, 412), as in the example discussed above on the facilitation of inhibitory and excitatory Ib pathways from joint afferents (419). Lundberg (411), however, proposed that Ib excitation may have a more independent function under some conditions. He suggested that a descending command may activate motoneurons via excitatory Ib-interneurons. The wide convergence onto the interneurons of Ib-afferents from many muscles would then cause an additional excitation of them when Golgi tendon organs fired during the active movement (411), and that, in turn, would reinforce the movement. Such positive feedback could have a powerful load compensating effect, but would differ from the Ia load compensation in that it would not operate primarily on the homonymous muscles but on the limb movement as a whole.

Reflex Pathways From Cutaneous and Joint Afferents and From Groups II and III Muscle Afferents

Electrical stimulation of cutaneous and joint afferents and of groups II and III muscle afferents, evokes very powerful synaptic actions in motoneurons, but knowledge of the pathways by which these effects are mediated is nevertheless very incomplete. Eccles and Lundberg (148) suggested that a common reflex pathway from these afferents existed and the afferents contributing to it were considered together as the flexor reflex afferents (FRA). It was emphasized from the beginning that the same afferents may have other separate reflex connections as well that do not belong to the common reflex pathway referred to above (268). Nevertheless the simplistic idea that an individual afferent system contributes to only one reflex has tended to survive (cf. ref. 565). The FRA concept implied that a reflex pathway should be defined by the convergence on its interneurons rather than by individual afferent systems, since each of them may contribute to several reflex pathways of diverse functions. In accordance with this view it was found by Hongo et al. (273) that convergence from several afferent systems is very common among spinal interneurons, and the preceding subsections show that there is now increasing evidence for such convergence on interneurons in several well-defined reflex pathways.

In a recent review on the interneuronal organization in reflex feedback systems, it was pointed out by Lundberg (413) that

... all active movements lead to activation of receptors in muscles, joints and skin. If so, why should a feedback system controlling a movement utilize only a single afferent system to control the movement. From a teleological point of view it seems much more sensible that different receptors which might give useful information combine in this regulation, and this is best achieved if their afferents converge on the same interneurones so that they form a common reflex pathway.

The first step toward understanding such reflex systems, however, is knowledge of the actions evoked by the individual afferent systems. At the present stage it still seems necessary to consider in isolation effects from cutaneous, joint, and muscle spindle secondary afferents. We begin with a brief description of reflexes from cutaneous afferents, among which are examples of specialized reflexes, which perhaps are mediated by "private" interneuronal paths (i.e., pathways other than the common FRA pathways).

CUTANEOUS AFFERENTS. Although spinal reflex studies began with the flexor reflexes evoked from skin, it soon appeared that cutaneous stimuli could also give other reflex responses. Limb extension may be evoked in response to genitocrural stimulation (554), and light pressure on the plantar surface elicits the extensor thrust (549). The pathways mediating these reflexes have not been analyzed electrophysiologically, but more information is available regarding another specialized reflex evoked from the foot.

Gentle pressure on the central plantar cushion in the cat hindlimb activates muscles that plantar-flex (i.e., extend) the toes, with the strongest effects in the flexor digitorum brevis and weaker effects in the synergic toe extensors, flexor digitorum longus, and plantaris [(165); cf. also ref. 260]. Excitation is also evoked in motoneurons to other intrinsic plantar muscles, e.g., the lumbricals and the interossei, but not to the extensors of the ankle, knee, and hip. There was no evidence for a significant reciprocal inhibition to the antagonist toe flexor muscles that give dorsiflexion of the toes. Stronger mechanical stimulation of the plantar cushion instead facilitated monosynaptic test reflexes in these flexor muscles and also inhibited test reflexes to ankle, knee, and hip extensors, but these effects have been interpreted as part of a general flexor reflex. The toe extensor reflex is an interesting example of a highly specialized reflex that acts selectively on a limited number of functionally related muscles and is evoked from a very distinct skin region. The toe pads and hairy skin of the toes do not contribute, and gentle manipulation of the toes is also ineffective, suggesting that proprioceptors do not contribute. Experiments with the spatial facilitation technique (Fig. 14) have shown that the interneurons that mediate the toe extensor reflex from the plantar cushion are also ex-

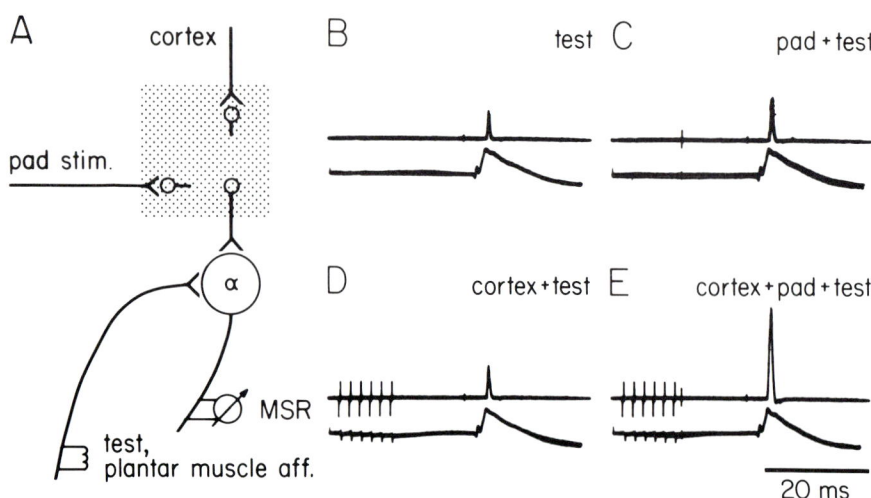

FIG. 14. Facilitation from corticospinal tract of a cutaneous reflex originating from plantar cushion. Scheme in *A* illustrates experimental arrangement and the involved neuronal circuits. *Stippled area* symbolizes a pool of interneurons and emphasizes that the actions from both systems are relayed in polysynaptic pathways. Actual site of interaction is not known. *Upper traces* in *B–E* are records from ventral root; *lower traces* are simultaneous recordings from dorsal root entry zone. Monosynaptic test reflex of plantar muscles (*B*) is moderately facilitated by a weak (conditioning) electrical stimulus to the pad (*C*). Stimulation of cortex (*D*) had no detectable effect on test reflex, but combined action from the 2 conditioning systems resulted in a large spatial facilitation (*E*). [Adapted from Engberg (165).]

cited from the corticospinal tract (165). Engberg (165) proposed that the toe extensor reflex may stabilize the foot during standing and during the stance phase of the step. It may also contribute to the downward extension of the toes that is needed for the completion of the stance phase of the step as the foot pushes off.

There is evidence also for other specialized cutaneous reflexes. For example, Hagbarth (256) has described reflex activation of extensors from restricted skin areas (generally the area that covers the muscle). During locomotion in spinal cats impulses in low-threshold mechanoreceptors in the skin of the hindlimb and the belly evoke short-latency reflexes (22, 183, 524). Hair stimulation of the dorsum of the foot during the swing phase of the step cycle elicits a response that resembles the tactile placing reaction (42, 497).[2] Transmission of these reflexes is subject to a cyclic modulation during locomotion, which is described in the chapter by Grillner in this *Handbook*.

The information available regarding interneuronal reflex paths from the skin is largely based on experiments with electrical stimulation of skin nerves in which it is particularly difficult to decide if an action is evoked by a specialized reflex path from skin or mediated by common FRA pathways (there is also the possibility of actions via reflex paths from Ia- and Ib-afferents; cf. subsections *Pathways From Ia-Afferents and Their Control by γ-Motoneurons*, p. 519, and

[2] The classic tactile placing reaction is often interpreted as a cortical reflex, since it is abolished by lesions in the sensorimotor cortex (8, 42). The relation between that reaction and the response seen during locomotion in spinal animals is discussed in the chapter by Grillner in this *Handbook*.

Reflex Pathways From Ib Tendon Organ Afferents, p. 530). A differentiation is sometimes possible, as when the FRAs evoke inhibition in fast motor units to triceps surae while volleys in some skin nerves produce excitatory PSPs in the same motoneurons (80). As illustrated in Figure 15 both corticospinal (314, 425) and rubrospinal volleys (275, 314) cause a facilitation of transmission in excitatory and inhibitory pathways activated by electrical stimulation of skin nerves. Descending action on specialized reflex pathways from skin has been inferred because facilitation of cutaneous PSPs is sometimes produced without concomitant effects on PSPs from high-threshold muscle afferents (275). In hindlimb segments of the cat, the minimum linkage in reflex pathways from cutaneous pathways is trisynaptic (see ref. 412). Since conditioning volleys in cutaneous afferents facilitate transmission in disynaptic excitatory and inhibitory (Fig. 15*I*–*K*) pathways from the red nucleus, it appears that rubrospinal fibers impinge on the last-order interneurons in these reflex arcs (35). Interneurons excited disynaptically from cutaneous afferents and monosynaptically from rubrospinal fibers have been found, as required, in layers VI and VII (277). More dorsally located interneurons that are monosynaptically activated from cutaneous afferents do not have this rubrospinal projection but may receive monosynaptic excitation from corticospinal fibers (178, 420). The differential termination of the cortico- and rubrospinal tracts in the spinal gray matter has also been determined by mapping their monosynaptic focal potentials [Fig. 15*L*; (277)]. It thus seems possible that the cortico- and rubrospinal fibers control the same reflex

CHAPTER 12: INTEGRATION IN SPINAL NEURONAL SYSTEMS 537

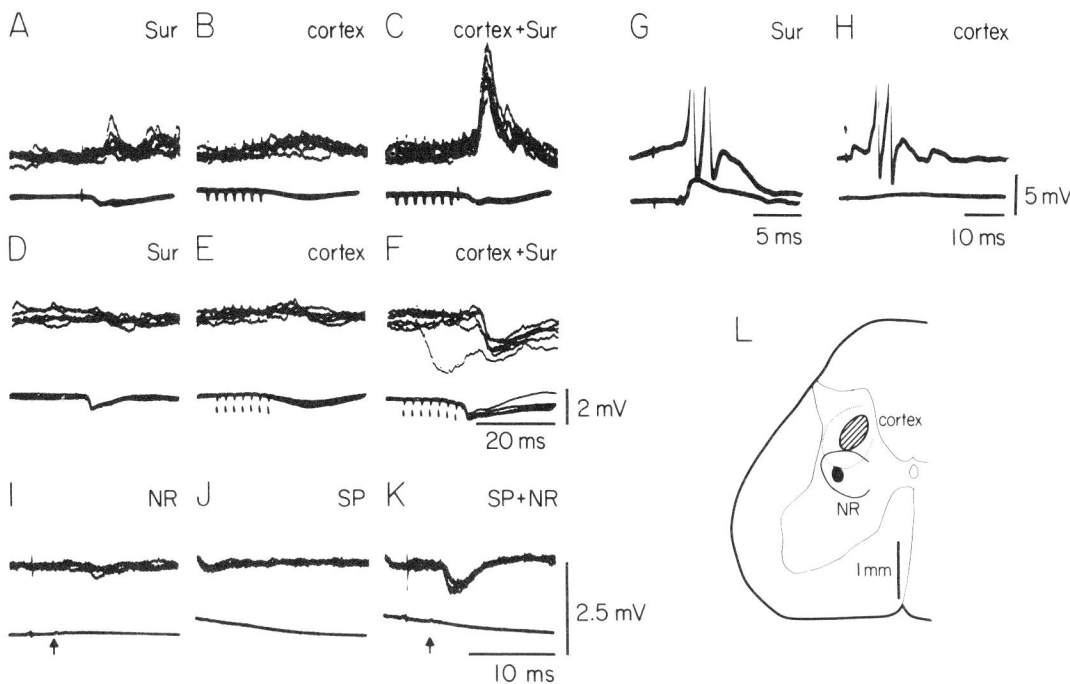

FIG. 15. Interaction of cortico- and rubrospinal tracts with lumbar cutaneous reflex pathways. *Upper traces* in *A–K* are intracellular records from different α-motoneurons and interneurons. *A–C*: posterior biceps–semitendinosus motoneuron. *D–F*: gastrocnemius-soleus motoneuron. *I–K*: pretibial flexor motoneuron supplied by deep peroneal nerve. *G, H*: L_7 dorsal horn interneuron. *Lower traces* are records from dorsal root entry zone at the respective segmental levels. Voltage calibrations refer to intracellular records. *A–F*: facilitation of cutaneous actions from cortex. Liminal synaptic actions evoked from sural nerve (Sur; stimulated alone in *A* and *D*) were conditioned by preceding stimulation of cortex (*C* and *F*). Cortex was stimulated alone in *B* and *E*. The ensuing increase of the polysynaptic potentials indicates excitatory convergence by corticospinal volleys and cutaneous afferent volleys on interneurons in excitatory and inhibitory cutaneous reflex pathways. *G, H*: monosynaptic activation of a lumbar dorsal horn interneuron from cutaneous (Sur) afferents (*G*) and short-latency (probably monosynaptic) activation from the cortex (*H*). This pattern suggests that, in the action illustrated in *A–F*, the corticospinal tract may project monosynaptically onto first-order interneurons in lumbar cutaneous pathways. *I–K*: monosynaptic excitation from rubrospinal tract of last order interneurons in a cutaneous reflex pathway. *I* shows a liminal IPSP evoked from red nucleus (NR) with a single shock of 200 μA (*arrows* below surface records in *I* and *K* mark arrival at segmental level of descending volley in rubrospinal tract). Conditioning stimulation of superficial peroneal nerve (SP) at 1.4 times threshold of the lowest threshold afferents increased the disynaptic rubrospinal IPSP (*K*; SP alone in *J*). *L*: comparison of location in cat lumbar cord of focal potentials evoked from rubrospinal and corticospinal tracts. Transverse section shows areas in which field potentials were evoked from indicated sites with an amplitude above 80% (*black* and *hatched area*) and 50% (*continuous* and *interrupted lines*) of their maximal amplitudes. Dorsal location of field from cortex and ventral location of NR field would be compatible with hypothesis that corticospinal fibers interact with first--order interneurons (cf. *A–F, G, H*) and rubrospinal fibers interact with last-order interneurons (cf. *I–K*) in trisynaptic cutaneous reflex pathways in the lumbar spinal cord. [*A–F* from Lundberg and Voorhoeve (425); *G, H* adapted from Lundberg et al. (420); *I–K* adapted from Baldissera et al. (35); *L* adapted from Hongo et al. (277).]

path but act at different stages in the interneuronal chain (277, 412).

Mention should be made of the recent finding that the organization of cutaneous reflex pathways of the forelimb of the cat seems to differ from that of the hindlimb. In the case of the forelimb the shortest latencies indicate a disynaptic pathway between cutaneous afferents and motoneurons, and further analysis strongly suggests that both the cortico- and rubrospinal tract monosynaptically excite the interposed neurons (314).

Lundberg (412) has suggested that the descending and primary afferent convergence on common interneurons allows cutaneous afferent impulses to reinforce a descending command mediated by these interneurons. Thus if a descending command for plantar flexion of the toes is mediated by interneurons of the toe extensor reflex, the contact with the ground may then reinforce that movement. Similar mechanisms may operate in the control of the grip of the hand in primates. For example, Marsden et al. (433, 434) have shown that a load compensating servo control of thumb flexion in humans is abolished when the skin of the thumb is anesthetized (although these authors suggested that this cutaneous effect is due to an interaction in the sensorimotor cortex—long-loop reflex—rather than at spinal segmental levels). A large fraction of single afferent units from the glabrous skin of the human hand are activated during voluntary finger movements even without skin contact with external objects (284). A cutaneous feedback may therefore play a role in shaping the motor output even when there is no contact with an object.

The above discussion has emphasized the conjoint activation of interneurons from descending fibers and cutaneous fibers. In other cases the "primary" event may be the reflex action, and the descending effect may then more suitably be described as facilitation of a reflex. For example, if tactile placing is regarded as a purposeful reflex reaction that depends on spinal circuitry, its disappearance after cortical lesions (42) may be explained as due to a removal of a descending facilitatory support (185).

JOINT AFFERENTS. Adequate activation of joint receptors can evoke reflex responses in motoneurons (152, 229). For example, manipulation of the knee joint, including inflation of the capsule, which effectively activates Ruffini endings (23), characteristically produces flexor facilitation and extensor inhibition (152). It is not known whether such effects are due to the contribution from joint afferents to the FRA pathways or whether they are mediated by other pathways specific to joint receptors. It was originally reported that the FRA effect occurred at a strength 2.5 times electrical threshold for the joint nerve (148), and Matthews (444) thus assumed that nociceptivelike afferents were responsible. However, activation of the FRA pathways requires considerable summation, and such results therefore cannot exclude the contribution of lower threshold afferents. Recently, positive evidence was obtained by Lundberg et al. (419), showing that FRA effects from the joint nerves may be evoked at a strength less than twice threshold. Since large effects were produced in a threshold range, activating fibers containing very few afferents that respond to noxious stimuli (75), they postulated that specific joint mechanoreceptors do in fact contribute to the FRA (419).

There is also evidence for reflex responses evoked by low-threshold joint afferents, which presumably are not mediated by the FRA pathways. Such effects were first observed during rubrospinal facilitation (275) but recently have also been observed in spinal cats (419). Also, apart from their contribution to FRA paths, joint afferents may have their main actions by operating in conjunction with other receptor systems in the limb. The possible role of the convergence of Ib-afferents and joint afferents on common interneurons was discussed in a preceding section (subsection *Reflex Pathways From Ib Tendon Organ Afferents*, p. 530). The finding that reflex transmission from cutaneous afferents can depend on limb position [(245); see also ref. 184; cf. subsection *Reflex Pathways From Cutaneous and Joint Afferents and From Groups II and III Muscle Afferents*, p. 535; and see the chapter by Grillner in this *Handbook*] is now being analyzed with respect to the possible contribution of joint receptors to this control. Rossignol and Gauthier (508) reported that the reversal of late reflexes from the FRA (cf. subsection *Reflex Pathways From Cutaneous and Joint Afferents and From Groups II and III Muscle Afferents*, p. 535) persists after deafferentation of the hip joint, which opens the possibility that this control depends on muscle as well as joint afferents. Further investigation of the effect of joint afferents on spinal interneurons is highly desirable, particularly with regard to the inhibitory actions they may exert on interneuronal paths activated from primary afferents and/or descending fibers. At present there is only scanty indirect evidence for such inhibition (419).

SECONDARY SPINDLE AFFERENTS. The detailed knowledge of the receptor function of the secondary spindle afferents and their control from static γ-motoneurons (see the chapter by Matthews in this *Handbook*) can be contrasted with the uncertainty regarding their role in reflex actions. From a teleological point of view, Matthews (444) argued for the existence of actions other than those found with electrical stimulation of group II muscle afferents (148, 369, 391). He appeared to have obtained indication for one such action by demonstrating that muscle stretch, superimposed on vibration designed to saturate Ia-afferent input, can give a large increase of the stretch reflex in extensor muscles of decerebrate cats [(442); see also ref. 344]. Matthews (442) postulated that this additional activation was from spindle secondaries. This hypothesis was functionally attractive, but no reflex pathway was known that could mediate this action in the decerebrate state. However, Matthews' hypothesis received support when experiments with spike-triggered averaging showed that impulses in secondaries evoke monosynaptic EPSPs in motoneurons (349, 565). The monosynaptic effects were overlooked in earlier experiments with electrical stimulation of muscle nerves but have since been confirmed both for extensors and flexors (418). The available evidence suggests that this monosynaptic connection is weak compared with that from Ia-afferents, but further investigation of the relative potency of the monosynaptic pathways from the two systems of spindle afferents is desirable. Meanwhile Jack and Roberts (319) have reported findings that may at least partly explain Matthews' results. They found that vibratory stimuli are not always able to drive the primaries during the stretch reflex contraction that they evoke, but that vibration gives "full driving" during a superimposed stretch of the tendon, with the result that Ia excitation and the consequent stretch reflex increases. Jack and Roberts (319) postulated "as the most economical interpretation" that the only major excitatory effect is from Ia-afferents. Accordingly it seems that Matthews' results cannot be taken to indicate the existence of potent autogenetic excitatory reflex from secondaries in the decerebrate cat. It is therefore necessary to return to interneuronal reflex pathways that are known to exist.

Studies of conditioning effects on monosynaptic test reflexes showed that volleys in group II muscle afferents excite flexors and inhibit extensors; these effects were evoked both from extensor and flexor nerves (369, 391). These results were later confirmed with intracellular recording (148). Hunt (305) showed that secondary spindle afferents account for virtually all group II afferents in the nerve to medial gastrocnemius and soleus (cf. also ref. 66 and in particular ref. 316). The same appears to hold true for flexor digitorum longus (66), while a substantial number of non–spindle afferents exist among group II afferents from the pretibial flexors (66, 316). Accordingly, although the effects from extensors and flexors are very similar, it is uncertain whether the effects from flexors are entirely from spindle afferents. The following discussion refers to effects from gastrocnemius-soleus or flexor digitorum and hallucis longus.

From measurements of central latencies of interneuronally mediated group II PSPs, it has been postulated that the minimal linkage is disynaptic in the excitatory pathway to flexors and trisynaptic in the inhibitory pathway to extensors (148, 416). Other polysynaptic actions may also be evoked from group II afferents. In the decerebrate state (cf. *Decerebrate Preparation*, p. 564) reflex transmission from group II afferents may be completely inhibited at an interneuronal level (149). However, after a low pontine lesion there is a partial release from this descending inhibitory control, and group II volleys may then evoke inhibition of flexors instead of the excitation that is found after a spinal transection (268). On the basis of these findings, it was suggested that secondary spindle afferents have alternative excitatory and inhibitory pathways to flexor motoneurons. The existence of an alternative excitatory pathway to extensor motoneurons is indicated by the finding that, in some spinal cats, group II volleys evoke EPSPs in extensors instead of the usual IPSPs (Fig. 16). The latency of these EPSPs suggests a disynaptic linkage (416).

When attempting to investigate convergence on the interneurons mediating group II EPSPs, little or no spatial facilitation was found even between muscles such as triceps surae and flexor digitorum longus (416). There was, however, a high degree of occlusion between group II EPSPs from these nerves, which is most easily explained by convergence on common interneurons. Lack of significant temporal facilitation in transmission of the group II EPSPs, indicating a

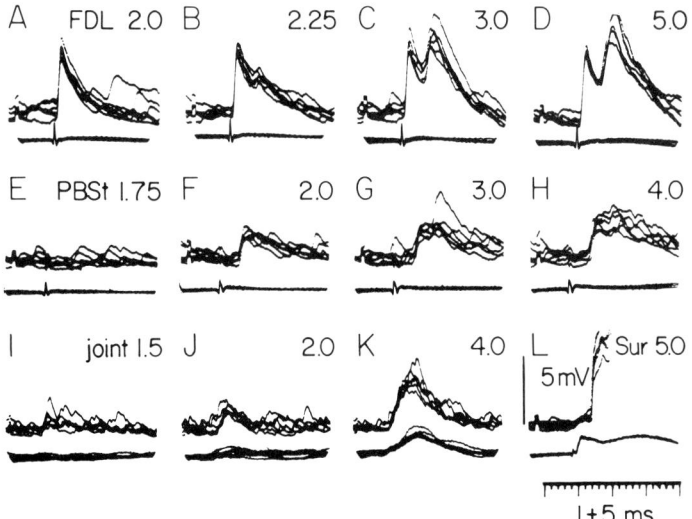

FIG. 16. EPSPs from group II muscle afferents, joint afferents, and cutaneous afferents in a motoneuron to flexor digitorum longus. *Upper traces*, intracellular records; *lower traces*, incoming volleys recorded from dorsal root entry zone in L_7. Stimulus strengths are given in multiples of threshold for each nerve. Voltage calibration applies to intracellular records. *A–D*: graded stimulation of nerve from flexor digitorum longus (FDL; maximal homonymous Ia EPSP at 2 times threshold in *A*). *E–H*: graded stimulation of nerves from posterior biceps and semitendinosus (PBSt). *I–K*: graded stimulation of posterior knee joint nerve. *L*: stimulation of cutaneous afferents in sural nerve (Sur). To estimate the central latency of group II effects, it is necessary to relate them to arrival of the group II volley to the spinal cord. The group II incoming volley was therefore recorded at end of experiment from transected dorsal root. Minimum linkage for group II EPSP in extensor motoneurons seems to be disynaptic. Notice similarity of group II actions from FDL and PBSt as well as from joint and skin afferents. (From A. Lundberg, K. Malmgren, and E. Schomburg, unpublished observations; see ref. 416.)

small subliminal fringe, was taken to suggest that these interneurons were fired from one or a few group II afferents. Some spatial facilitation was, however, evoked from cutaneous afferents (A. Lundberg, K. Malmgren, and E. D. Schomburg, unpublished observations), suggesting more graded cutaneous excitatory action on interneurons intercalated in the disynaptic group II pathways to motoneurons. Because of the peculiar characteristics of this disynaptic group II pathway, it has not been feasible to use the indirect spatial facilitation technique for extensive studies of convergence patterns, and it is not known if afferents other than cutaneous afferents converge onto these interneurons.

It is noteworthy that independent of whether the synaptic group II PSPs were inhibitory or excitatory in flexor and extensor motoneurons the polysynaptic PSPs produced by these afferents and by group III muscle afferents, joint afferents, and cutaneous afferents usually are qualitatively similar (cf. Fig. 16). It was for this reason that group II afferents were originally classified among the FRA (148, 268). Appelberg et al. (28) have found that volleys in group II muscle afferents often evoke EPSPs in dynamic γ-motoneurons to extensors although group III volleys give IPSPs in the same neurons, and they therefore suggested the existence of a separate pathway from group II afferents. A similar dissociation of group II and group III effects may be observed in extensor α-motoneurons (Fig. 9 in ref. 148), but they are less frequently encountered than the concordant effects referred to above (A. Lundberg, personal communication). Taken together these observations seem to suggest that there are several reflex pathways from secondary afferents with different convergence on their interneurons.

The termination of group II afferents in the spinal cord has been investigated with the recording of focal potentials and with antidromic activation of individual afferents. Monosynaptic focal potentials were found in the dorsal horn and more ventrally in the lateral part of layer VII (195). Antidromic activation of identified secondaries was likewise obtained from the two regions (196). The antidromic activation from the ventral region occurred after relatively long latencies, suggesting slow conduction in terminal branches.

A preliminary investigation revealed that some interneurons in the ventral terminal area are monosynaptically activated by group II afferents (A. Lundberg, K. Malmgren, and E. D. Schomburg, personal communication; Fig. 17). Fine gradation of stimulus strength in a few cells showed that the EPSPs were made up of a very limited number of unitary EPSPs, as was suggested for interneurons of the disynaptic excitatory reflex pathway (416). More graded excit-

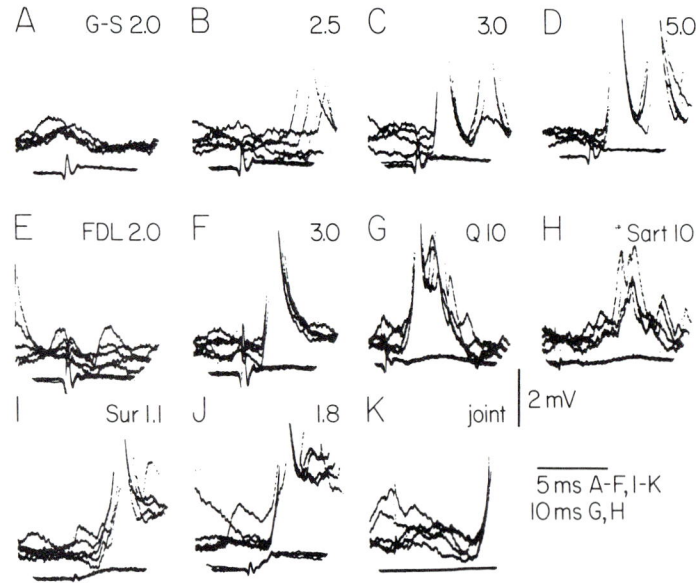

FIG. 17. EPSPs from group II muscle afferents, cutaneous afferents, and joint afferents in a lamina VII interneuron. *Upper traces,* intracellular records; *lower traces,* incoming volleys recorded from dorsal root entry zone in L$_7$. Stimulus strengths are given in multiples of threshold for each nerve. Voltage calibration applies to intracellular records. *A–D*: graded stimulation of nerve from gastrocnemius-soleus (G-S). *E, F*: graded stimulation of nerve from flexor digitorum longus (FDL). *G, H*: stimulation of quadriceps (Q) and sartorius (Sart) nerves. *I, J*: stimulation of sural nerve (Sur). *K*: stimulation of posterior knee joint nerve (joint). Central latency from arrival of group II incoming volley to spinal cord (as judged from recording from transected dorsal roots at end of experiment) of the group II effects from G-S (*C, D*) and from FDL (*G*) indicates a monosynaptic linkage from group II afferents. Note additional convergence of polysynaptic EPSPs from group II afferents (*C, D, H*) and from cutaneous and joint afferents. This type of interneuron has a pattern of convergence that makes it a likely candidate for transmitting the type of reflex actions illustrated in Fig. 16. (From A. Lundberg, K. Malmgren, and E. Schomburg, unpublished observations.)

atory action was evoked from cutaneous afferents. Excitation by volleys in group III muscle afferents and joint afferents and monosynaptic EPSPs from group I afferents were evoked in some of these neurons. Monosynaptic rubrospinal excitation was also encountered. These interneurons need to be investigated in much more detail to find out if they belong to disynaptic excitatory pathways to motoneurons from secondary afferents.

Concerning the function of the interneuronal reflex pathways to which secondaries contribute, it seems impossible to go beyond the general suggestion that they may add to or subtract from the fusimotor-controlled Ia effects, depending on the selection of excitatory or inhibitory paths by higher centers.

REFLEX PATHWAYS FROM THE "FLEXOR REFLEX AFFERENTS." In spinal cats electrical stimulation of groups II and III muscle afferents, joint afferents, and cutaneous afferents evokes polysynaptic actions according to the pattern of the ipsilateral flexion reflex and the crossed extension reflex, with appropriate reciprocal synaptic action on antagonist motoneurons (148). These afferent systems were therefore characterized as the flexor reflex afferents (FRA). The collective designation FRA serves primarily to emphasize the common central action of these different afferent species, which would be most easily understood if they converged on common interneurons in the reflex pathways. Results obtained with the spatial facilitation technique show that cutaneous, joint, and high-threshold muscle afferents do indeed converge on interneurons in reflex pathways to motoneurons (Fig. 6 in ref. 413), although there is no such evidence in the case of group II afferents. The original reason for grouping all these afferents (including group II) together was not only related to their common reflex actions on motoneurons, but also to the finding that they act together on ascending spinal pathways and that in all cases the actions were drawn from large receptive fields including muscle afferents from both flexors and extensors (269). Lundberg (404) suggested long ago that these ascending neurons signaled activity in the interneurons of the reflex pathways from the FRA and pointed out that many spinocerebellar neurons appeared to signal such information. It is now known that FRA information is in fact signaled by a large number of neurons belonging to different ascending pathways (see ASCENDING PATHWAYS THAT MONITOR SEGMENTAL INTERNEURONAL ACTIVITY, p. 569). These findings suggest that the reflex pathways from the FRA might have a role in motor control not related to the nociceptive flexor reflex. This hypothesis was supported by evidence that interneurons in the FRA pathways are excited from various supraspinal motor centers and thus may mediate excitation from the brain to motoneurons. Participation of the FRA pathways in motor control necessitates the assumption that these afferent species include not only nociceptive afferents but also afferents that are activated during an active limb movement (411, 413). There is actually experimental evidence to show that muscle contraction secondary to stimulation of α-efferents activates afferents that contribute to the FRA system [J. Bergmans, S. Grillner, and A. Lundberg, unpublished observations; illustrated and quoted by Lundberg (413)].

In the following subsections we consider separately the short-latency FRA pathways and the long-latency pathways that are released by administration of dopa (cf. subsection *Monoaminergic Reticulospinal Pathways*, p. 562).

Short-latency FRA pathways. In the acute spinal animal, volleys in the ipsilateral FRA evoke polysynaptic (central latencies of a few milliseconds) EPSPs in flexor motoneurons and IPSPs in extensor motoneurons, but even in this preparation other actions may occur, indicating the existence of alternative reflex pathways from the FRA (148). More direct evidence for such pathways was obtained in conjunction with studies of the inhibitory control of reflex pathways from supraspinal centers. Powerful tonic inhibition is exerted on transmission in all reflex pathways from the FRA in the decerebrate cat (subsection *Decerebrate Preparation*, p. 564). As we mentioned in connection with reflex pathways from secondary spindle afferents (subsection SECONDARY SPINDLE AFFERENTS, p. 538), it is possible to obtain a partial release from this tonic control by a transverse medial lesion in the lower pons (268). After such a lesion IPSPs are evoked in flexor motoneurons not only from group II muscle afferents but also by volleys in cutaneous, joint, and group III muscle afferents. The low pontine lesion also gives release of transmission in the inhibitory pathway from the FRA to extensor motoneurons so that the low pontine state is characterized by a generalized inhibition from the FRA. Release of transmission in the excitatory pathway to flexor motoneurons from the FRA, which mediates the dominating action in the spinal state, occurs only after a more caudal medullary lesion. These findings strongly suggest the existence of alternative reflex pathways from the FRA to flexor motoneurons. The possibility that the pathways giving opposite synaptic actions are supplied by afferents of different receptors was rejected by Holmqvist and Lundberg (268) on the grounds that it would require "two sets of receptor systems from skin, muscle and joint with afferents in the same diameter ranges, and both of them supplying actions to flexor motoneurones from the same extensive fields" (268). These authors furthermore concluded that "the pathways conveying the reciprocal actions of excitation to flexor and inhibition to extensor motoneurones from the FRA are controlled from the brain by separate neuronal systems and that these reciprocal actions can be differentially controlled" (268). The results thus question the general validity of Sherrington's view that the inhibitory process in the flexion reflex "is part and parcel of the reflex reaction so that inhibition goes on side by side with excitation of other muscles opposed to those which are inhibited" [(550), p. 90 in the 1947 edition].

By the same criteria there are also alternative pathways from the FRA to extensor motoneurons. Mobilization of the alternative pathway conveying excitation to extensor motoneurons could never be achieved by experimental manipulation, and the existence of such a pathway can thus be appreciated only when it opens spontaneously (148, 268, 611).

Contralateral FRA also activate common interneuronal mechanisms (266). In the spinal preparation contralateral FRA usually excite extensor motoneurons and inhibit flexor motoneurons, giving the pattern of the crossed extensor reflex (210, 554). However, crossed effects from FRA may often—more often than the ipsilateral ones—spontaneously turn into either the inverse pattern or parallel effects, i.e., excitatory or inhibitory, to both flexors and extensors (266). This finding may be correlated to previously described changes in these reflex responses [(109, 212, 341, 488); see, however, ref. 65]. There is also evidence for another excitatory FRA pathway to extensor and/or flexor motoneurons in which the interneurons are activated from FRA of both hindlimbs (332).

On the basis of these observations it can be concluded that each functional group of motoneurons (flexors and extensors) is reached by alternative (excitatory and inhibitory) pathways from both ipsilateral and contralateral FRA. In many cases transmission in these alternative pathways seems to be mutually exclusive (148, 268, 332) as if they were linked by inhibitory connections.

Several higher motor centers are known to excite interneurons of ipsilateral and crossed reflex pathways from the FRA. The evidence is largely based on experiments with the indirect technique of spatial facilitation, but some supporting evidence has also been obtained with direct recording from interneurons. For example, weak conditioning stimulation of the corticospinal tract facilitates transmission from the FRA to both flexor and extensor motoneurons [Fig. 18A–I; (425)], while stronger cortical stimulation evokes synaptic actions that resemble those from the FRA. This finding was taken to suggest that an important part of the corticospinal action in motoneurons is mediated by interneurons common to the reflex pathways from the FRA. Rubrospinal volleys evoke a similar facilitation of transmission in reflex pathways from the FRA. In some cases, however, a depression was observed that was interpreted to be evoked by activation of another FRA pathway, inhibitory to the one tested (275). The vestibulospinal tract has been found to have connections with interneurons of only some reflex pathways from the FRA and to facilitate transmission primarily in the excitatory pathways to contralateral extensor motoneurons and in the inhibitory pathways to contralateral flexor motoneurons [both via Ia inhibitory interneurons (cf. subsection *Pathways From Ia-Afferents and Their Control by γ-Motoneurons*, p. 519) and via another pathway not shared with Ia-afferents; (72)].

In several cases it has been demonstrated that the descending projection is to the last-order interneurons of the FRA paths. To show this, the conditioning effect of FRA volleys was tested on descending disynaptic PSPs (Fig. 18J–L). With this technique it was shown that rubrospinal and vestibulospinal fibers have connections with last-order interneurons in ipsilateral and crossed-reflex pathways, respectively (35, 72). The last-order interneurons in crossed-reflex pathways from the FRA presumably contribute to the disynaptic excitation that is the dominant action from the vestibulospinal tract in extensor motoneurons (72, 240, 403). It has also been demonstrated that axons of long propriospinal neurons excite last-order interneurons of a special excitatory reflex pathway to extensors that are activated from the FRA in both hindlimbs (332). There is no corresponding information concerning at which stage in the interneuronal chain the corticospinal tract acts but, since its fibers terminate more dorsally and directly excite dorsal horn interneurons, it is not unlikely that their effect is exerted at an earlier stage in the polysynaptic chain from the FRA to motoneurons (as discussed for reflex paths from cutaneous afferents; see CUTANEOUS AFFERENTS, p. 535, and Fig. 15).

Direct recordings from spinal interneurons have shown that a large number of them are activated from the FRA, and convergent descending excitation also appears to be common. This was first indicated by the actions evoked by stimulation of fiber systems in the spinal cord (137) and later for specific tracts from higher motor centers such as the corticospinal and rubrospinal tracts (277, 420), but it remains to be investigated for the vestibulospinal tract and long propriospinal fiber systems. In view of the many alternative pathways from the FRA, it is clearly difficult to identify interneurons activated from these afferents as belonging to a specific neuronal pathway. It is nevertheless important to continue the investigation of these interneurons, especially since the descending effects evoked in them may corroborate the conclusions inferred from the indirect spatial facilitation technique. Furthermore, interneuronal recordings give a clue to inhibitory effects that might be exerted from the FRA on transmission in different neuronal spinal pathways. Inhibition from FRA is indeed very common and is evoked not only in interneurons activated from other afferents but also in interneurons that are activated from the FRA (cf. Fig. 10 in ref. 273). At first it may seem strange that the same afferents can evoke opposite effects in the same interneurons, but this finding may be explained by the hypothesis of inhibitory interaction between alternative reflex pathways from the FRA discussed in the following subsections. On the other hand, the FRA inhibition of interneurons

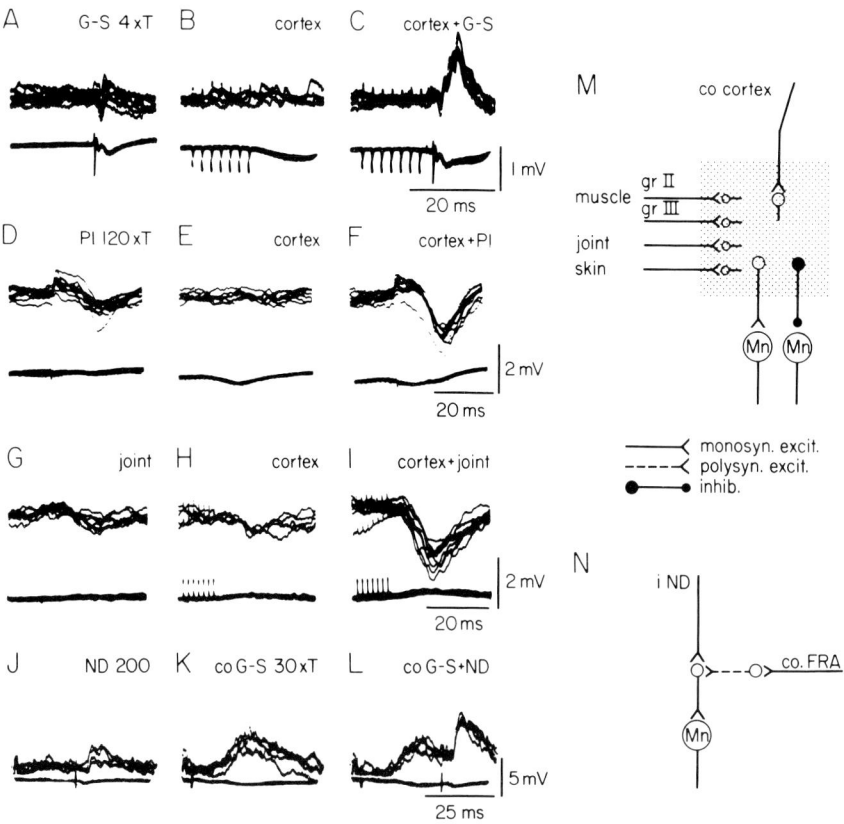

FIG. 18. Interaction of descending tracts with flexor reflex afferent (FRA) pathways. *Upper traces* show intracellular records from a posterior biceps–semitendinosus motoneuron (*A–C*), 2 gastrocnemius-soleus motoneurons (*D–F* and *G–I*), and a tibial motoneuron (*J–L*). *Lower traces* are records from dorsal root entry zone. Voltage calibrations apply to intracellular records. Stimulation strengths of gastrocnemius-soleus (G-S) in *A–C* and *J–L* and plantaris (Pl) in *D–F* are indicated in times threshold (×T) of lowest threshold afferents. Stimulation of posterior knee joint nerve (joint) in *G–I* activated high-threshold joint afferents. Stimulation strength of ipsilateral Deiters' nucleus (ND) is given in μA. *A–I*: facilitation of excitatory (*A–C*) and inhibitory (*D–I*) FRA actions from cortex (postsigmoid gyrus). *A, D, G* show responses to nerve stimulation alone. *B, E, H* show responses to stimulation of cortex alone. *C, F, I* show effects of combined stimulation. Initial negative potential in *A* and *C* is a Ia field potential (same shape at an extracellular position), the short-latency EPSP in *D* and *F* is a heteronymous Ia EPSP. The EPSP facilitated in *C* is due to activation of group II fibers. The IPSP in *F* is due to activation of relatively high-threshold group II afferents and group III afferents (stimulation of Pl with 11 ×T was without effect). *J–L*: facilitation of a disynaptic vestibulospinal EPSP from contralateral (co) FRA. *J* illustrates disynaptic vestibulospinal EPSP that is markedly increased by preceding stimulation of the coG-S (*L*; G-S alone in *K*). *M*: diagram summarizing neuronal connections revealed by records in *A–I*. Stippled area symbolizes a pool of interneurons and emphasizes that the actions from both cortex and peripheral afferents are relayed by polysynaptic pathways. Actual site of convergence is not known. Records in *A–C, D–F, G–I* do not show whether all the afferent systems are relayed via common interneurons or through separate channels. The first alternative is the most likely, however, since spatial facilitation among all these afferent systems (including cutaneous afferents) have been described in other investigations [T.-C. Fu, E. Jankowska, and A. Lundberg, unpublished observations, quoted and illustrated in Lundberg (413)], and since many interneurons in the intermediate region display the required convergence, including corticospinal excitation (420). As indicated, the same convergence applies for interneurons in excitatory (*A–C*) and inhibitory (*D–F, G–I*) pathways to motoneurons. *N*: diagram summarizing neuronal connections revealed by records in *J–L*. Interneurons mediating disynaptic vestibulospinal excitation are also last-order interneurons in the cross-extensor reflex. [*A–I* adapted from Lundberg and Voorhoeve (425); *J–L* adapted from Bruggencate and Lundberg (72).]

activated from other afferents suggests that a reflex pathway from the FRA may inhibit reflex pathways from other afferents (273). It is also worth noting that the FRA (as well as group I muscle afferents) can evoke pure inhibition in interneurons that receive excitation from descending fibers but not from primary afferents (273). If such interneurons are intercalated in pathways to motoneurons, there is the possibility that in these cases the main function of primary afferents may be to inhibit transmission from descending pathways. The most clear example of inhibitory effects from the FRA on descending transmission refers to actions on primary afferent terminals (Fig. 7 in ref. 427).

Long-latency FRA pathways. In addition to the short-latency effects discussed above, FRA volleys may also evoke synaptic effects in motoneurons (in spinal cats) with a very much longer latency and duration. Such effects are more often encountered contralateral than ipsilateral to the input (65). In extensor motoneurons the short-latency EPSP of the crossed extensor reflex is usually followed by a second EPSP with a latency of 30–50 ms and a duration of 200–300 ms (65). In "slow" motoneurons the late effect is much larger than the early one and may give a reflex discharge. Similar late long-lasting reflexes can be selectively evoked from the FRA after intravenous injection of the monoamine precursors dopa (3,4-dihydroxyphenylalanine) and 5-HTP (5-hydroxytryptophan) in spinal cats. These drugs produce dramatic changes in transmission from the FRA to *1*) motoneurons (14, 15); *2*) primary afferents (subsection *Presynaptic Inhibition of Transmission From Primary Afferents*, p. 554); and *3*) ascending tract neurons (section ASCENDING PATHWAYS THAT MONITOR SEGMENTAL INTERNEURONAL ACTIVITY, p. 569), presumably as a result of liberating monoaminergic transmitters from segmental terminals of descending fibers (subsection *Monoaminergic Reticulospinal Pathways*, p. 562). As illustrated in Figure 19, transmission in the path-

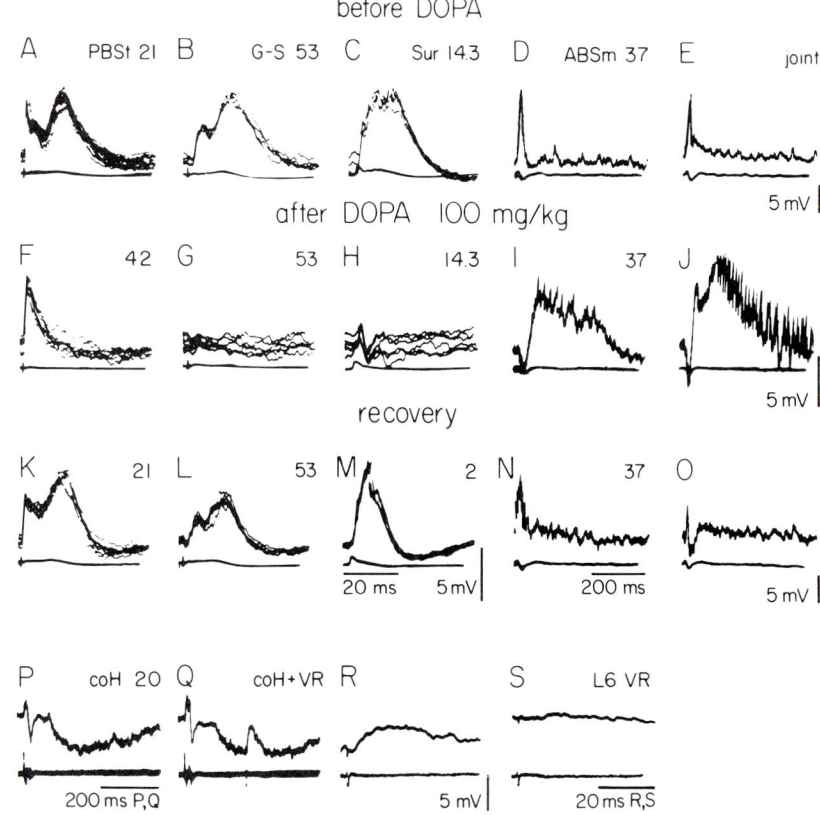

FIG. 19. Actions of flexor-reflex afferents (FRA) in α-motoneurons before and after activation of reticulospinal noradrenergic pathways by intravenous injection of L-hydroxyphenylalanine (dopa). *Upper traces* are intracellular records from 4 different posterior biceps–semitendinosus motoneurons (*A–E; F–J; K–O; P–S*). *Lower traces* are records from L_7 dorsal root entry zone. Voltage calibrations refer to intracellular records. Stimulation strength of afferent nerves is indicated in times threshold of the lowest threshold afferent fibers. Stimulation of L_6 ventral roots (VR; *Q–S*) was supramaximal for α-fibers. In *A–O* the *left 3 columns* show effect of single stimuli at fast sweep speed (calibration below *M*), the *right 2 columns* show effect of short trains of stimuli at slow time base (calibration below *N*). All records were obtained in spinal unanesthetized cats. PBSt, posterior biceps–semitendinosus; G-S, gastrocnemius and soleus; Sur, suralis; ABSm, anterior biceps and semimembranosus; joint, posterior knee joint nerve; coH, contralateral hamstring. *A–E*: polysynaptic short-latency EPSPs from FRA without dopa. *F–J*: depression of short-latency effects after injection of dopa and appearance of long-latency excitation (compare *I, J* and *D, E*). Depolarization remaining in *F* is homonymous monosynaptic Ia EPSP in the motoneuron. *K–O*: reappearance of short-latency FRA actions about 2 h after dopa and parallel disappearance of long-latency excitation. *P–S*: reciprocal inhibition of long latency obtained in a flexor motoneuron by stimulation of contralateral (co) FRA after injection of dopa. Depression of IPSP by stimulation of L_6 VR (*Q*, expanded in *R*) indicates its mediation by Ia inhibitory interneurons (L_6 VR alone in *S*). [*A–O* adapted from Jankowska et al. (324); *P–S* adapted from Fu et al. (193).]

ways of the short-latency flexor and crossed extensor reflexes is profoundly depressed after i.v. injection of dopa (about 100 mg/kg), as evidenced by the disappearance of the respective EPSPs and IPSPs (15, 324). Transmission of short-latency effects from FRA to primary afferent terminals and to ascending tract neurons is similarly inhibited (*Presynaptic Inhibition of Transmission From Primary Afferents*, p. 554, and ASCENDING PATHWAYS THAT MONITOR SEGMENTAL INTERNEURONAL ACTIVITY, p. 569).

The depression of transmission from FRA after dopa injection is surprising in view of the original observation that dopa enhances the flexion reflex in the acute spinal animal (92). However, aside from the inhibition of the early FRA effects, dopa favors the appearance of a new response consisting of a sustained discharge in ipsilateral flexors and contralateral extensors evoked after a delay of 100–200 ms and with a duration of 400–1,000 ms (15). Intracellular recording from motoneurons revealed the expected late, long-lasting EPSPs and also IPSPs in antagonist motoneurons (193, 324). Late effects evoked from FRA after administration of dopa have the same distribution to ipsi- and contralateral motoneurons as the usual flexor reflex in the untreated spinal animal. This might suggest that the two reflexes are transmitted by a single pathway, the functional properties of which are different before and after dopa. There are, however, strong indications supporting the view that the short- and long-latency effects to motoneurons are transmitted by two different although interacting pathways.

The various pieces of evidence for the latter conclusion should be mentioned here because of its importance for the later discussion on the role played by the FRA in motor control. *1)* Existence of separate pathways for the short- and long-latency effects is best evidenced for FRA actions onto primary afferent terminals. Before dopa, volleys in the FRA evoke a primary afferent depolarization (PAD) in their own terminals but not in the terminals of Ia-afferents. After dopa, however, transmission in this FRA to FRA pathway is inhibited and FRA volleys instead evoke a late PAD in terminals of Ia-afferents (subsection *Presynaptic Inhibition of Transmission From Primary Afferents*, p. 554). Thus two different FRA pathways appear to transmit PAD; one before and another after the drug injection. *2)* Some interneurons that respond as expected for cells intercalated in the pathway transmitting the late excitation to flexor motoneurons after dopa were recorded from also before dopa administration and did not then respond to volleys in the FRA (325). *3)* Prolonging the train of FRA volleys delays the onset of the long-latency responses [Fig. 21; (16, 324, 325)]. This has been interpreted as a sign of an inhibitory interaction from the short-latency FRA pathway on transmission through the long-latency path, as drawn schematically in Figure 21*I*.

The most interesting feature of the reflex pathways transmitting the late effects from the FRA is the very effective mutual inhibition between the interneuronal pathways transmitting excitation to flexor and extensor motoneurons (Fig. 20*A–L*). Transmission of the late EPSPs to ipsilateral flexor motoneurons is strongly inhibited by activation of the pathway that conveys excitation to extensor motoneurons from the contralateral FRA [Fig. 20*A–C*; (324)]. In a similar manner activation of the excitatory pathway to flexor motoneurons from the ipsilateral FRA effectively inhibits the pathway transmitting the late reflex actions to extensor motoneurons from the contralateral FRA (Fig. 20*G–I*). Since the possibility that this inhibition was exerted at motoneuronal or at primary afferent level could be excluded, it was concluded that it occurred at an interneuronal level (324). Corroborating evidence was obtained by recording from interneurons in the lumbar segments, which behaved as expected for interneurons intercalated in the long-latency FRA paths. These cells were located in the dorsolateral part of Rexed's lamina VII, dorsal to motoneurons (325). Some interneurons were excited from the ipsilateral FRA, exhibiting a late, long-lasting discharge that was strongly depressed by conditioning volleys in the contralateral FRA (Fig. 20*D–F*). These interneurons may belong to the late reflex pathway from the FRA to ipsilateral flexor motoneurons. Other neurons displayed the behavior of interneurons transmitting excitation to extensor motoneurons (Fig. 20*J–L*); a late, long-lasting discharge was evoked from the contralateral FRA, and this discharge was strongly inhibited by a conditioning volley in the ipsilateral FRA.

The FRA may also evoke late long-lasting IPSPs after dopa (Fig. 19*P–S*). Since conditioning stimulation of the appropriate ventral root gave a virtually complete removal of these IPSPs (193), it was concluded that they are mediated by the Ia inhibitory interneurons (recurrent inhibition of interneurons in afferent and descending pathways to motoneurons appears to be limited to the Ia inhibitory interneurons; see subsection REFLEX PATHWAYS FROM GROUP Ia MUSCLE SPINDLE AFFERENTS, p. 519). In keeping with these observations it was found that some of the interneurons with a late, long-lasting discharge from the FRA also are monosynaptically activated from Ia-afferents; these interneurons have subsequently been identified as Ia inhibitory interneurons (193). It can thus be concluded that the long-latency FRA pathway provides another example of a neuronal system projecting in parallel to α- and γ-motoneurons as well as to corresponding Ia inhibitory interneurons (subsection SEGMENTAL AND SUPRASPINAL CONTROL OF γ-MOTONEURONS, p. 527; Fig. 11*L*).

Half-centers and stepping. Mutual inhibition between antagonist spinal motor centers was first postulated by Graham Brown (209) to explain the finding that stepping in spinal animals may persist after deafferentation of the limb. Graham Brown (211) distinguished between "primary half-centers" (antagonist motoneurons) and "interposed half-centers" (interneuron groups projecting to motor nuclei). He developed particularly the idea of mutual inhibitory inter-

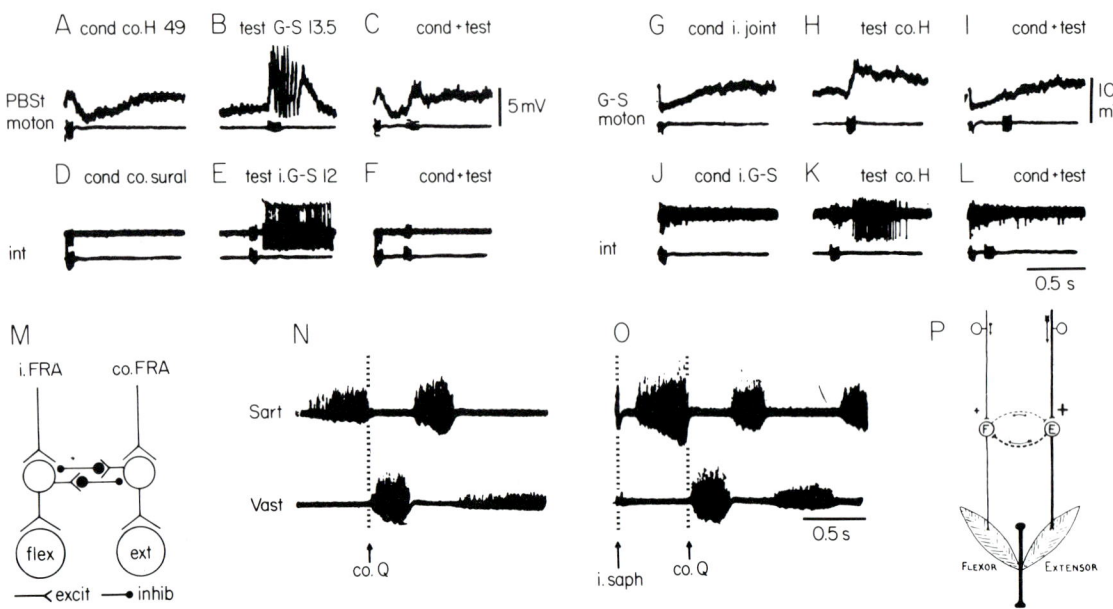

FIG. 20. Organization of a spinal network giving reciprocal activation of flexor and extensor muscles. *Upper traces* in A–C and G–I are intracellular records from 2 α-motoneurons to posterior biceps–semitendinosus muscles (PBSt) and gastrocnemius-soleus muscles (G-S) in D–F and J–L *upper traces* are extracellular records from interneurons. *Lower traces* are from dorsal root entry zone. Voltage calibrations refer to intracellular records. Stimulation strength of afferent nerves is given in times threshold of lowest threshold afferent fibers. N–O are simultaneous records from efferent nerves to a flexor and an extensor muscle. All records were obtained in spinal unanesthetized cats after injection of dopa (100 mg/kg). A–L: half-center organization of interneuronal network released after dopa. In flexor motoneuron (A–C) a train of volleys in high-threshold muscle afferents evoked the characteristic long-latency EPSP (B), which was effectively inhibited (C) by a preceding (cond) train of volleys in contralateral high-threshold muscle afferents (contralateral hamstring nerve, co.H). In the extensor motoneuron (G–I) long-latency EPSP was evoked from contralateral high-threshold muscle afferents (H) and inhibited from the ipsilateral posterior nerve to the knee joint (joint, I). D–F and J–L are corresponding records from interneurons that were located in a region dorsal to motor nuclei. Neuron in D–F was excited from high-threshold afferents in G-S (E) and inhibited from contralateral high-threshold cutaneous afferents (co. sural nerve, co.Sur; F). Neuron of J–L was excited from co.H (K) and completely inhibited from high-threshold afferents in the i.G-S (L). M: tentative diagram showing principle organization of an interneuronal network that could account for results illustrated in A–L, N,O. Inhibition could be exerted by pre- or postsynaptic actions. A single interneuron in the diagram represents a chain of neurons. N,O: alternating discharges in flexor and extensor efferents triggered by short trains of impulses in ipsilateral and contralateral FRA. Acute spinal cat pretreated with nialamide (10 mg/kg) before administration of 100 mg/kg dopa. Records from nerves to a flexor (medial sartorius, Sart) and to an extensor (medial vastus of quadriceps, Vast). N: stimulation of high-threshold afferents in contralateral quadriceps nerve (co.Q; timing of stimulus train marked by *arrow* and the *vertical interrupted line*) during a spontaneous discharge in flexor efferents is followed by a pause in flexor nerve and a discharge in extensor nerve. Activity in flexor nerve is resumed after cessation of extensor discharge, and a 2nd extensor discharge then occurs after this flexor burst. O: stimulation of ipsilateral saphenous nerve (i.saph) evokes a long-latency discharge in the flexor nerve that, after additional stimulation of co.Q, is followed by a series of alternating bursts in the efferent nerves. P: original hypothesis of organization of spinal "primary half-centers" projecting to flexor and extensor muscles with reciprocal inhibition acting between them [Graham Brown (209, 211).] As described in text, Graham Brown (214) later proposed the existence of "interposed half-centers" to describe interneurons (intercalated between primary afferents and motoneurons) with mutual inhibition as in the diagram in M. [A–C, G–I, and N from Jankowska et al. (324); D–F and J–L from Jankowska et al. (325); M adapted from Jankowska et al. (324); O from Jankowska et al. (324) illustrated in Lundberg (413); P from Graham Brown (213).]

actions between the primary half-centers [Fig. 20P; (213, 214)] and considered a possible inhibitory role of recurrent motor axon collaterals (211), but he also admitted that "for certain phenomena of rhythmic activity it is useful to presume that the interposed half-centers should mutually inhibit each other and also inhibit the antagonist 'primary half-center.'" The interneuronal network transmitting the long-latency FRA action clearly possesses the characteristics required of the interposed half-centers and is the first identified interneuronal network in the vertebrate central nervous system that may give alternating activation of flexors and extensors (Fig. 20M). The property of this network to transform peripheral inputs into rhythmic alternating activity of flexors and extensors became apparent when dopa was given after pretreatment with nialamide, an amine oxidase inhibitor (see subsection *Monoaminergic Reticulospinal Pathways*, p. 562). As illustrated in Figure 20N, O, short trains of volleys in the FRA may then evoke a series of alternating discharges in flexors and extensors (231, 324, 600). Maintained alternating activity in efferent nerves may also develop spontaneously or during continuous bilateral stimulation of the central ends of sectioned dorsal roots [fictive locomotion (249, 250)], and sequences of excitatory and inhibitory PSPs can then be recorded in motoneurons (150). After injection of dopa or of norepinephrine-mimetic substances (clonidine), locomotor movements are elicited in the acute spinal cat (intact dorsal roots) with limbs placed on the moving belt of a treadmill (73, 74, 182), which suggests a driving of the half-centers by afferent activity evoked by passive and active limb movements. Involvement of the FRA-excited "half-centers" in the circuitry generating stepping is also suggested by the finding that electrical stimulation of the locomotor region in the mesencephalon (559) at intensities just subthreshold for locomotion evokes changes in spinal cord reactivity that resemble those produced by dopa injection, i.e., depression of short-latency FRA pathways and appearance of late reflexes from the FRA (247).

Mutual inhibitory interactions between the half-centers do not by themselves explain the oscillatory behavior of the network that generates stepping. Graham Brown (211) considered that switching between them was due to a "depreciation" (fatigue) that would depend on accumulating refractoriness in the active half-center and its inhibitory pathway to the antagonist half-center. However, even if an FRA drive of the half-centers from the two hindlimbs could produce alternating activation with the help of some sort of fatigue, it does not explain how the walking movements can become well adapted to any chosen speed of a treadmill belt as is actually found after dopa (74, 182). Since the original series of studies on the organization of the pathways mediating late reflexes from the FRA, there has been one interesting development that may explain how the switching between extensor and flexor activity can be so well adapted to the belt movement. It was found (233, 245) that the late FRA reflexes do not consist of a fixed pattern of ipsilateral flexion and contralateral extension but that the destination of the reflex response depends on hip position. Grillner (233) found a switch from ipsilateral flexor to extensor activation when the hip was placed in flexion, and Grillner and Rossignol (245) found a similar reflex reversal governed by the hip position for the crossed responses. Accordingly, if the FRA activity plays a role in locomotion, switching between the half-centers might normally be governed from hip receptors (cf. ref. 246) instead of depending on some undefined fatigue, as discussed above. However, since alternating activity still can occur in fictive locomotion without afferent feedback, additional controlling factors must be present.

Interaction between short- and long-latency FRA pathways. Early evidence for the functional connections of the long-latency FRA pathways with other spinal mechanisms came from the observations that if FRA stimulation is prolonged in the dopa-treated preparation, then the late reflex response only appears when the stimulation is discontinued [Fig. 21; (16, 324, 325, 329)]. It was suggested that the same afferents that provide the excitation also inhibit transmission to the half-center network. Accordingly it was postulated that the activation of interneurons of the short-latency path would inhibit transmission in the late reflex pathways. The action of dopa would be to inhibit interneuronal transmission in the short-latency pathway, thereby releasing late reflex transmission through the half-center network. In this model (Fig. 21*I*) the short-latency paths occupy a central position, being both the receiver of the noradrenergic inhibition and the controller of the late discharge mechanism.

A possible functional correlate of this inhibition from FRA on the late reflexes is the prompt interruption of locomotor activity that occurs in all phases of stepping after activation of high-threshold cutaneous afferents (181, 601). However, the fact that volleys in the same FRA both excite and inhibit transmission to the half-center network should be considered in relation to the role of the FRA in fictive locomotion because the driving action from the FRA might be disturbed by the inhibitory action produced by the same afferents. The possibility has been considered (but not tested) that there is mutual inhibitory interaction between short-latency and long-latency pathways from the FRA so that once the latter are activated to give alternating activation, an inhibitory effect is exerted on transmission in the short-latency pathway (413). Modulation of transmission in short-latency FRA pathways during fictive locomotion has in fact been reported recently (526).

Many recent reports deal with the effect of primary afferent activity on the locomotor system (234, 235, 477, 480) and on the cyclic modulation of reflex transmission during locomotion (22, 181, 183, 524–526, 531). These results are discussed in the chapter by Grillner in this *Handbook*.

A possible role of FRA activity. The extreme complexity of reflex pathways from the FRA to motoneurons and the manyfold actions from these afferents on other neuronal systems are bewildering. There is clearly a need for some unifying hypothesis that incorporates the existence of alternative pathways and the descending excitation of the interneurons in the pathways from the FRA to motoneurons. It may be argued that higher motor centers can utilize these interneuronal pathways to transmit action to motoneurons relatively independently of primary afferent activity, if transmission from the periphery is pre-

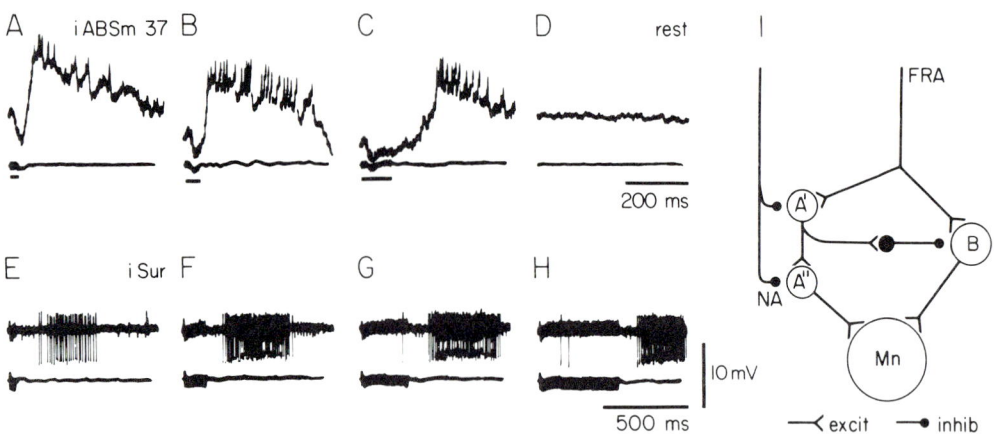

FIG. 21. Inhibitory action from short-latency flexor-reflex afferent (FRA) pathways on transmission in long-latency FRA pathways. *Upper traces* in *A–D* are intracellular records from a motoneuron innervating posterior biceps–semitendinosus muscles (PBSt); in *E–H* they are extracellular records from a lumbar interneuron located dorsal to the motor nuclei. *Lower traces* are records from dorsal root entry zone. Voltage calibration applies to intracellular records. Both neurons were recorded in unanesthetized acute spinal cats after injection of dopa (100 mg/kg). *A–D*: recording from PBSt motoneuron shows EPSPs of long latency and duration following stimulation of ipsilateral FRA (ipsilateral nerve to anterior biceps–semimembranosus muscle, iABSm; stimulation strength is 37 times threshold of lowest threshold afferent fibers). *Bars* below *A–D* indicate duration of repetitive stimulation. Notice that prolongation of repetitive stimulation of FRA delays onset of EPSP. *E–H*: stimulation of ipsilateral sural nerve (iSur) elicits long-latency and long-lasting activation of interneuron that is typical after dopa. Notice that response is delayed with prolongation of repetitive stimulation (thickening of base lines is due to stimulation artifacts). *I*: tentative diagram of neuronal connections that could explain illustrated effects. A single interneuron in the diagram represents a chain of interneurons. Inhibition of short-latency pathway A (A′ and A″) from descending noradrenergic systems (NA) releases transmission in long-latency pathway B (records *A–H* were obtained in this condition). The prolongation in onset of late discharge found in motoneurons and interneurons of B (the interneuron in *E–H* should belong to this population) illustrates inhibitory interaction from short-latency on long-latency FRA pathways. The short-latency pathway A is subdivided into A′ and A″ to accomodate the finding that the noradrenergic system may block the short-latency reflex action onto motoneurons when there is still an inhibitory action on transmission through the long-latency pathway B. Mn, motoneuron. [*A–D, I* adapted from Jankowska et al. (324); *E–H* adapted from Jankowska et al. (325).]

vented by descending inhibition (cf. section RETICULOSPINAL INHIBITION OF SEGMENTAL REFLEX TRANSMISSION, p. 560). However, it may seem more likely that the control of interneurons somehow depends on a conjoint action from descending fibers and primary afferents. The significance of the FRA activity in motor control that follows from such a standpoint would also make sense of all the ascending FRA information, which is conveyed in particular to cerebellum (section ASCENDING PATHWAYS THAT MONITOR SEGMENTAL INTERNEURONAL ACTIVITY, p. 569). Lundberg (411–413) has suggested that the role of activity in the FRA is to support descending motor commands that are mediated via interneurons in FRA pathways to motoneurons (Fig. 22). More specifically the hypothesis suggests that the descending command signal activates interneurons in one of the several alternative reflex pathways from the FRA (for example, B in Fig. 22). Through interactive inhibitory connections (demonstrated for some of them as described above) there is inhibition of transmission in the other pathways from FRA (A and C in Fig. 22). The movement that is caused by activation of the motoneurons activates different types of receptors in the active muscles, related joints, and surrounding skin, some of which

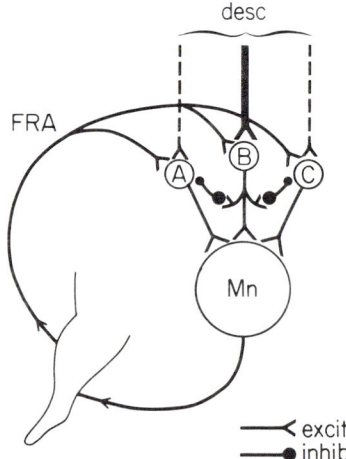

FIG. 22. Diagram showing alternative reflex pathways from flexor reflex afferents (FRA) with descending (desc) excitatory connections to interneurons of these pathways and its inhibitory interactive connections with the other reflex pathways from the FRA. Mn, motoneuron. [Adapted from Lundberg (411).]

seem to belong to the FRA. The movement thus gives rise to an impulse flow in the FRA and this activity is channeled back into the reflex path already activated from the brain, because transmission in the other alternative FRA pathways is already inhibited. A diffuse feedback system with a multisensory input from muscle, joint, and skin from a very large receptive field may thus give a selective positive reinforcement of the activity in the interneuronal path selected by the command from the brain (411–413).

Propriospinal Neurons

Investigation of propriospinal neurons was pioneered by classic anatomical studies (64, 87, 556) that described various types of spinal neurons with axonal projections restricted to the spinal cord. To differentiate them from motoneurons and long ascending tract cells, they were called "propriospinal" neurons. This definition covered neurons with axonal projections over a few or many segments as well as local interneurons. From a functional point of view a distinction between propriospinal neurons and interneurons seems important, but not on the basis of their axonal length. Neurons intercalated in reflex pathways of limb segments are referred to as "interneurons," even if many are in fact funicular cells projecting over a few segments (335–337). The neurons with cell bodies located outside the limb segments but projecting into them are the "propriospinal neurons" (314).

Many electrophysiological investigations of propriospinal connections have been directed toward an analysis of mechanisms coordinating fore- and hindlimb segments. Anatomical investigations have further indicated that propriospinal systems may also take part in transmission of supraspinal motor information to α-motoneurons (571), a role that is the main topic of this chapter (cf. refs. 354, 386, 414).

PROPRIOSPINAL PATHWAYS RELAYING DESCENDING MOTOR COMMANDS. The analysis of propriospinal systems that transmit descending motor information to α-motoneurons was initiated with the finding that activity in bulbospinal pathways activates short-axoned neurons in upper lumbar segments that then excite hindlimb α-motoneurons monosynaptically (386). Spatial facilitation was observed when activation of these neurones was combined with stimulation of the motor cortex, which indicates convergence of corticospinal fibers on these relay cells (386).

Short-axoned propriospinal neurons. Lateral cervical neurons. With lesions of descending pathways at different levels in the spinal cord (cf. ref. 568), Illert et al. (312, 313) identified a propriospinal system that is characterized by monosynaptic convergence from various supraspinal motor centers and primary cervical afferents. Disynaptic EPSPs evoked in forelimb α-motoneurons from the contralateral pyramid and the red nucleus (312, 313) remained after complete transection of the cortico- and rubrospinal tracts in the rostral part of the fifth cervical segment (C_5) but were abolished after similar lesions in the caudal C_2 segment [Fig. 23; (314)]. The combination of these results suggests that both descending tracts give off collaterals below the C_2 level that then activate a short propriospinal system with cell bodies in the C_3 and C_4 segments. These propriospinal neurons, which have axons located outside the dorsolateral funiculus in C_5, mediate disynaptic cortico- and rubrospinal excitation to forelimb motoneurons. They serve in addition as relay neurons in a trisynaptic inhibitory pathway from corticospinal fibers to forelimb motoneurons; the last-order neurons in this case are identical with segmental Ia inhibitory interneurons (315).

Further analysis with the spatial facilitation technique (see Fig. 24) revealed that the C_3–C_4 propriospinal system receives additional monosynaptic excitatory convergence from bulbospinal fibers (54), from the tectospinal tract, and from low-threshold cutaneous and group I muscle afferents from the ipsilateral forelimb (314). The primary afferents from the forelimb ascend to the propriospinal neurons in the dorsal columns.

Propriospinal neurons with the required convergence have been recorded from in the C_3 and C_4 segments (311). Their cell bodies are located mainly in the lateral part of lamina VII and their axons descend in the ventral part of the lateral funiculus; many of them terminate within the forelimb segments. Retrograde transport of horseradish peroxidase (after local injection into forelimb motor nuclei) to neurons in lamina VII of the C_3 and C_4 segments has confirmed this projection (226, 451). Extensive monosynaptic convergence from the various descending tracts is common in the great majority of these propriospinal neurons (Fig. 25). Monosynaptic excitation from forelimb afferents (Fig. 25) is less regular and rather weak when compared with the combined effects from the descending pathways. It is therefore likely that the main function of the C_3–C_4 propriospinal relay is to transmit and integrate activity from higher centers and that the convergent action of the forelimb afferents may primarily have a regulatory role on the transmission of descending activity (311, 414).

Direct records from C_3–C_4 propriospinal neurons also demonstrate intricate inhibitory projections onto them (310, 412, 414), for which the indirect evidence is scanty (314). The organization of these inhibitory pathways is not yet fully understood, but apparently different mechanisms contribute. All of the input systems that supply monosynaptic excitation to the propriospinal neurons also inhibit them via a disynaptic pathway (310, 412). Convergence of different systems on common interneurons, which probably are located in the C_3 and C_4 segments, has been demonstrated with spatial facilitation (cf. discussion in ref. 414). Since the inhibition is not necessarily coupled to monosynaptic excitation, it was suggested to be the feedforward type (310). This would give the brain the possibility, when activating a given population of propriospinal neurons required for a certain movement, to inhibit other groups projecting to different muscles in order to provide spatial selectivity. It was further discussed that the inhibitory projection from forelimb

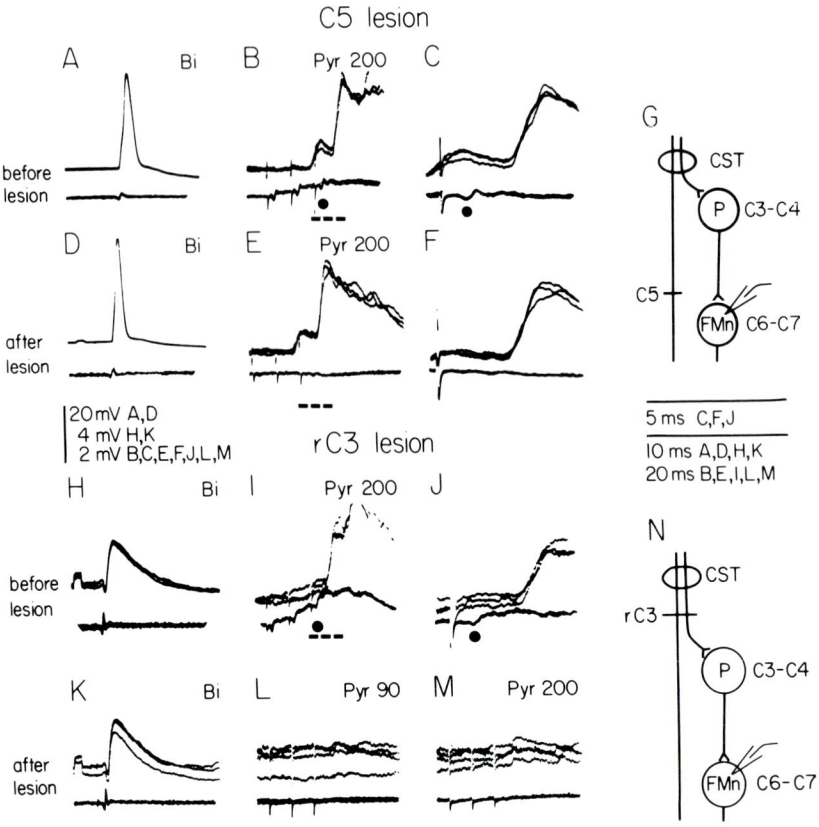

FIG. 23. Definition of propriospinal relay neurons in C_3–C_4 segments. Experimental arrangement and neuronal circuits as illustrated in G (for records A-F) and in N (for records H-M). *Upper traces,* intracellular records from 2 biceps (Bi) motoneurons (A-F; H-M); *lower traces,* records from C_6 dorsal root entry zone. Voltage calibration refers to intracellular records. Stimulation strength of contralateral pyramid (Pyr) is given in μA. Dots below surface records in B, C, I, J indicate arrival of 3rd pyramidal volley. *Dashed lines* below records B, E, I mark sections that are shown at an expanded time scale in C, F, J. A-F: disynaptic (1.5 ms) Pyr EPSP before (A-C) and after (D-F) transection of corticospinal tract (CST) in C_5. Comparison of antidromic spike potentials in A and D suggests that recording conditions before and after lesion were similar. Results indicate presence of propriospinal neurons (P) above the C_5 lesion that transmit disynaptic corticospinal excitation to forelimb motoneurons (FMn). H-M: near disappearance of disynaptic Pyr EPSP after CST transection at rostral (r) C_3. Grading of the Pyr stimulation strength in L and M suggests that the very small disynaptic EPSP that remained after lesion was a unitary response. These results indicate that the most rostral location of the propriospinal neurons intercalated in disynaptic corticomotoneuronal pathway is in caudal C_2 or rostral C_3. [Adapted from Illert et al. (314).]

afferents may not only assist supraspinal motor centers in producing feedforward inhibition but could also act as a feedback mechanism allowing signals from the forelimb to adjust propriospinal transmission during movements (414).

Stimulation of the lateral funiculus at C_6–C_8 produces monosynaptic IPSPs in C_3–C_4 propriospinal neurons (310, 412, 414) to which both descending and ascending systems contribute. Stimulation in the medullary brain stem produced IPSPs that are probably of reticulospinal origin (54). Very large IPSPs are also evoked from the lateral reticular nucleus (309, 414), and it has been tentatively suggested that these were due to antidromic activation of inhibitory axons ascending to the lateral reticular nucleus (151).

Integration in the C_3–C_4 propriospinal system has been considered in relation to the more general problem of how activity in a variety of motor pathways is coordinated (cf. discussion in ref. 314, 414). There can be little doubt that such a coordination occurs between motor centers in the brain as well as in the spinal cord. Regarding coordination in the brain, it seems likely that the cerebellar loops allow commands in different supraspinal motor centers to be shaped with due consideration to the activity in others. Another interesting possibility for cerebral and cerebellar interaction is suggested by the findings on the C_3–C_4 propriospinal system. Transmission in the fastest corticomotoneuronal pathway to the cat forelimb may be continuously controlled from the cerebellum through rubrospinal and bulbospinal systems converging onto the propriospinal neurons. Since such a regulation would involve little time lag, it would be rather favorable in rapid forelimb movements. In fact, behavioral experiments

CHAPTER 12: INTEGRATION IN SPINAL NEURONAL SYSTEMS 551

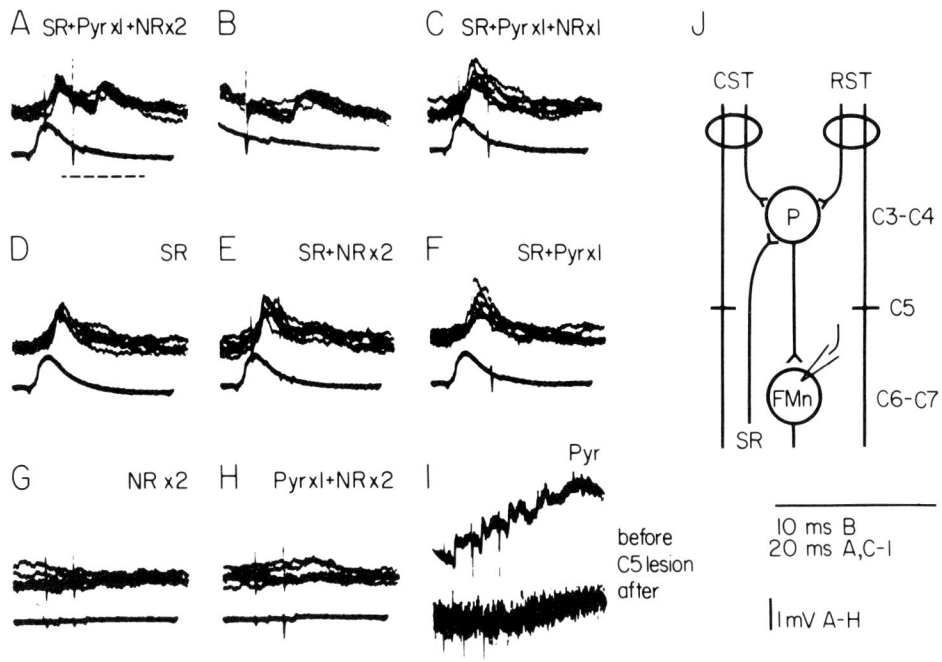

FIG. 24. Convergence on C_3–C_4 propriospinal neurons (P) from corticospinal (CST) and rubrospinal (RST) tracts and from forelimb cutaneous afferents (superficial radial nerve, SR). Experimental arrangement and neuronal circuits as illustrated in J. Convergence was judged indirectly from intracellular recording from a forelimb motoneuron (FMn; *upper traces* in A–H) with CST transected completely in C_5 (compare in I records from lateral funiculus in C_6 before, *upper trace*, and after, *lower trace*, the C_5 lesion). The same lesion transected the RST only partially. *Lower traces* in A–H are records from C_6 dorsal root entry zone. Voltage calibration applies to intracellular records. Stimulation strengths: SR, 1.5 times threshold of lowest threshold fibers; red nucleus (NR), 65 μA; pyramid (Pyr), 200 μA. Note that disynaptic EPSP appears only in A, B when 2 rubral stimuli and 1 pyramidal stimulus are given together with the cutaneous SR volley that indicates excitation of common propriospinal neurons (P). All other possible combinations were ineffective (C–H). *Dashed line* below A indicates the part of the traces that is expanded in B. [Adapted from Illert et al. (314).]

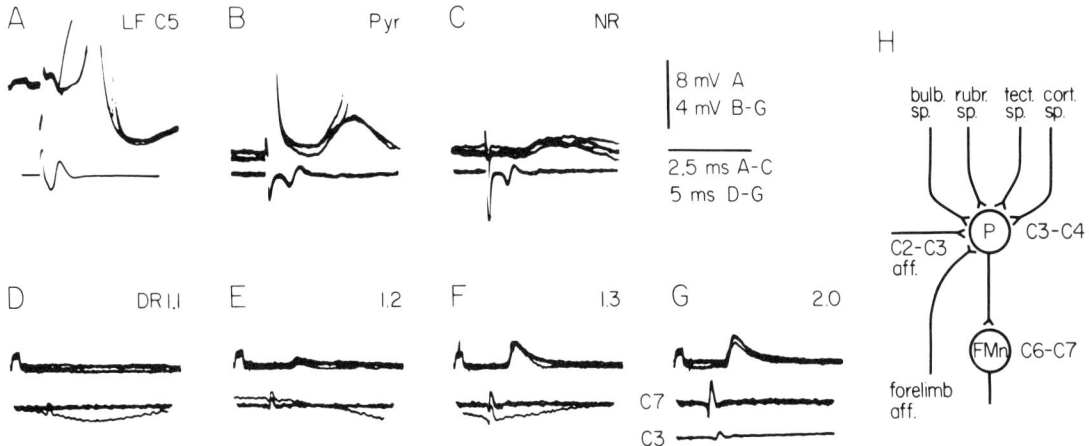

FIG. 25. Convergence on C_3–C_4 propriospinal neurons (P). Scheme in H summarizes monosynaptic excitatory convergence onto them as well as their direct projection to forelimb motoneurons (FMn). Intracellular records in A–G (*upper traces*) illustrate a propriospinal neuron (identified from the lateral funiculus in C_5 in A) with monosynaptic excitation from forelimb group I muscle afferents (D–G: deep radial nerve, DR; stimulation strength in times threshold of the lowest threshold fibers), from corticospinal tract (B: stimulation of contralateral pyramid, Pyr, with 100 μA), and from rubrospinal tract (C: stimulation of contralateral red nucleus, NR, with 100 μA). *Lower traces* are records from dorsal root entry zone in C_7 (in G also from C_3). Voltage calibration refers to intracellular records. [A–G adapted from Illert et al. (311); H from data in refs. 54, 226, 310, 311, 314.]

with differential lesions of the propriospinal axons and of the cortico- and rubrospinal tracts cranial or caudal to the C_3-C_4 propriospinal relay support this hypothesis (6, 414). They indicate that the C_3-C_4 propriospinal system is mainly used in precise rapid movements of the whole forelimb, whereas pronation-supination of the foot and manipulatory toe movements should mainly be exerted via interneuronal systems located within the forelimb segments (6).

In view of the hypothesis of a complex integration in the C_3-C_4 propriospinal relay, the observation of a collateral projection from C_3-C_4 propriospinal neurons to the lateral reticular nucleus [Fig. 26; (309)] was a most important discovery. This would supply the cerebellum with parallel information about the activity reaching the forelimb motoneurons via this system and would allow a cerebellar feedback control with minimal delay (see ASCENDING PATHWAYS THAT MONITOR SEGMENTAL INTERNEURONAL ACTIVITY, p. 569).

Lateral lumbar neurons. The cell bodies of the short-axoned propriospinal system to lumbosacral segments are located in the L_3-L_5 segments in the lateral half of laminae V-VII in the external basilar nucleus, and their axons project caudally in the dorsal part of the lateral funiculus (9, 594, 597). These neurons receive short-latency excitation from the cortico-, rubro-, and reticulospinal tracts, with a monosynaptic linkage from the latter system. In some cells the latency of rubro- and corticospinal excitation is sometimes brief enough to suggest a monosynaptic linkage, but polysynaptically relayed effects appear to be more common (597). Primary afferents from the hindlimb were reported to have no short-latency effects (594, 597) that would correspond to the absence of degenerating preterminals in this region after dorsal root section (489). However, absence of short-latency segmental effects seems to have been used as a criterion to differentiate external basilar neurons from those located in the internal basilar nucleus (cf. ref. 597). Preterminals of degenerating dorsal root fibers have been demonstrated in the latter region (489), and convergence from the corticospinal tract and segmental afferents onto common neurons of the internal basilar nucleus has also been described (355).

It has been postulated that the lateral propriospinal neurons are specialized for transmission of descending motor commands independent of primary afferent activity from the hindlimb and also that they project directly to hindlimb motoneurons and thus might mediate disynaptic rubro- and/or corticomotoneuronal excitation. Although there is some anatomical support for this hypothesis (571, 572), it was based mainly on the observation that after degeneration of long fiber systems (following hemisection of the thoracic cord), stimulation of the dorsal part of the lateral funiculus in the L_4-L_5 segments elicits monosynaptic EPSPs and IPSPs in hindlimb motoneurons (356, 357). The PSPs were suggested to be evoked by stimulation of the axons of the lateral L_3-L_5 propriospinal neurons. This is perhaps the most likely explanation but, since the L_4-L_5 segments are included in the reflex apparatus supplying the hindlimb, it seems possible that

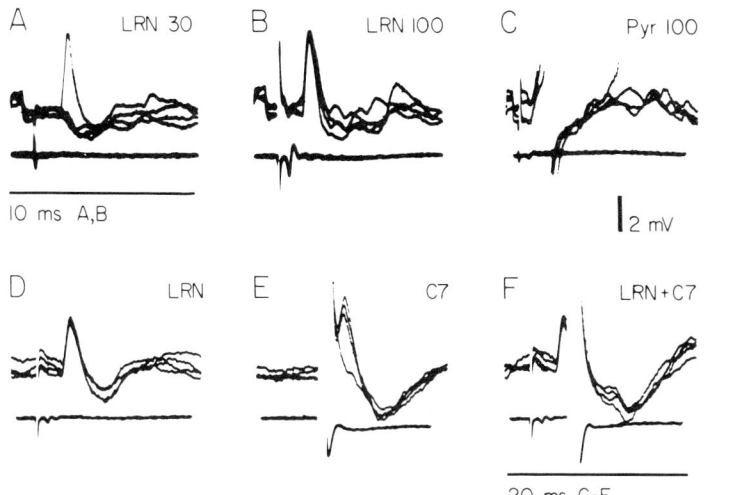

FIG. 26. Collateral projection of C_3-C_4 propriospinal neurons (P) to forelimb segments and to lateral reticular nucleus (LRN). Scheme in *G* illustrates experimental arrangement and neuronal circuits. *A-F*: upper traces, intracellular records from a propriospinal neuron in C_3 (antidromic activation from the C_7 segment in *E*); lower traces, records from C_3 dorsal root entry zone. Voltage calibration applies to intracellular records. *A, B* show antidromic activation of propriospinal neuron from LRN (stimulation strength in μA); note monosynaptic IPSP from LRN in *A* (see Fig. 39). *C* illustrates monosynaptic EPSP from contralateral pyramid (Pyr, 100 μA). *D-F*: collision of antidromic spike (*F*) evoked in propriospinal neuron from C_7 (*E*) by preceding LRN stimulation (*D*). [*A-F* adapted from Illert and Lundberg (309); *G*, data for descending projection from Illert et al. (311, 314); data for direct projection to forelimb motoneurons (FMn) from Illert et al. (314) and Grant et al. (226).]

interneurons of reflex pathways were stimulated. It is also difficult to exclude the possibility that axons of ascending neurons may have collaterals to motoneurons (cf. section ASCENDING PATHWAYS THAT MONITOR SEGMENTAL INTERNEURONAL ACTIVITY, p. 569). Accordingly, further analysis of the projection of the lateral lumbar propriospinal neurons seems desirable.

Medial lumbar neurons. Short-axoned propriospinal neurons located in L_4 and L_5 in the ventromedial part of lamina VII (453, 567, 571) have also been investigated electrophysiologically (359, 360, 545, 593, 595, 596). In most of these neurons, short-latency excitation was found from reticulospinal and vestibulospinal pathways, and convergence of monosynaptic reticulospinal and disynaptic vestibulospinal excitation was also common. This pattern was complemented in the monkey by monosynaptic excitation from the corticospinal tract (359). These medial propriospinal neurons give rise to axons that descend in the ventral funiculus (595), and stimulation experiments similar to those described above for the lateral propriospinal cells have led to the conclusion that the medial neurons act on hindlimb motoneurons by mono- and disynaptic pathways (358, 593). Hence it has been postulated that they constitute a propriospinal relay system mediating di- and polysynaptic reticulo- and vestibulospinal actions to lumbosacral motor nuclei (595, 596). These indirect conclusions have been supported by extracellular stimulation in the region of the L_4 and L_5 propriospinal neurons and by simultaneous recording of monosynaptic EPSPs or IPSPs in hindlimb motoneurons (360, 545).

Observations on the effects from primary afferents in these medial propriospinal neurons are somewhat conflicting. Vasilenko and Kostyukov (595) found little evidence for actions from the hindlimb or the dorsal root, but Kozhanov and Shapovalov (359) observed effects in many cells. In some cells synaptic actions were exclusively evoked from high-threshold afferents with polysynaptic latencies, but other cells received monosynaptic input from the periphery (359), suggesting that many of the medial propriospinal neurons integrate activity from higher centers and primary afferents. It is likely that the effects investigated by Lloyd (386) were mediated by this propriospinal system. If so, the large relayed volley recorded by Lloyd from the surface of the spinal cord indicates that this system comprises a considerable number of neurons.

Long-axoned propriospinal neurons. Long propriospinal systems that project from cervical segments to the lumbar enlargement course in the ventral and ventrolateral funiculi (206, 452, 556). Some have been investigated electrophysiologically with respect to their projection on lumbar neurons (331, 593). Neurons with somata located between the third cervical and eleventh thoracic segments (C_3 and T_{11}) and with axons in the lateral funiculus project to α-motoneurons and to interneurons of the hindlimb reflex apparatus (331, 332). Monosynaptic EPSPs and di- or polysynaptic EPSPs and IPSPs were recorded in motoneurons, disynaptic IPSPs were relayed by segmental Ia inhibitory interneurons and disynaptic EPSPs by last-order interneurons of a segmental bilateral flexion reflex pathway [(332); see subsection *Reflex Pathways From Cutaneous and Joint Afferents and From Groups II and III Muscle Afferents*, p. 535]. Long propriospinal neurons with somata between C_4 and T_7 and with axons descending in the ventral funiculus evoke disynaptic EPSPs or IPSPs in hindlimb motoneurons (593). The observation that this system seems to be more effective in influencing proximal hindlimb motoneurons than distal ones has been taken as indirect evidence that it is especially related to the regulation of postural reactions (593).

PROPRIOSPINAL NEURONS FOR INTERLIMB COORDINATION. Sherrington and Laslett (556) were the first to demonstrate the existence of long propriospinal connections between the cervical and the lumbosacral cord (cf. the chapter by Kuypers in this *Handbook*). It has always been assumed that these pathways coordinate activity between the limb enlargements, and it is therefore not surprising that transmission in them is controlled from supraspinal levels.

Descending systems. Electrical stimulation of medium- to high-threshold forelimb afferents evokes a sequence of excitation and inhibition in hindlimb motoneurons with a slight preponderance for excitation in extensor motoneurons (24, 396, 529). A special short-latency inhibitory pathway was found to α-motoneurons innervating flexor digitorum longus (24, 396, 528, 530). This early inhibition is relayed by ipsilateral pathways (cf. ref. 389) and mainly evoked from low-threshold cutaneous and mixed nerves in the ipsilateral forelimb (530). In the cat it might prevent claw protrusion (24, 396) or plantar flexion of the toes during walking (528). The same inhibition has been observed in the dog, which does not have any active claw protrusion (530). However, during normal locomotion plantar flexion of the terminal phalanges of the dog could be prevented.

Transmission in these descending propriospinal systems is modulated during fictive locomotion induced by dopa (530, 531). The short-latency IPSPs in motoneurons of flexor digitorum longus are predominantly transmitted during the active phase of this muscle, i.e., during extension and less during flexion.

Ascending systems. Propriospinal pathways ascending from the lumbar enlargements to brachial motoneurons can mediate strong excitatory and inhibitory effects on reflexes to different groups of forelimb muslcles (55, 203, 204, 450). Stimulation of groups II and III muscle afferents and group II cutaneous afferents of the hindlimb affects mainly shoulder girdle muscles and muscles innervated by the dorsal interosseus nerve. Those muscles supplied by the ulnar or median nerves are much less affected (55, 450). The ascending propriospinal pathways are influenced bilaterally from the hindlimb and mediate effects to both ipsilateral and contralateral forelimb reflex systems. The ipsilateral projections are dominant, and it has been suggested that they represent intrinsic links between the hindlimb and forelimb motor centers and may contribute facilitation to the flexors of the forelimb once the ipsilateral hindlimb has begun the first extension leading to its placing on the ground (450). One of the most striking features of this system is that it is greatly affected by an injection of dopa [(55); early discharges are facilitated and late discharges appear, cf. subsection *Reflex Pathways From Cutaneous and Joint Afferents and From Groups II and III Muscle Afferents*, p. 535]. This indicates that activation of reticulospinal monoaminergic pathways, which mobilizes the spinal locomotor generator, also influences transmission in long ascending pathways.

OTHER PROPRIOSPINAL SYSTEMS. Experiments with stimulation of the spinal cord suggest the existence of rather strong excitatory and inhibitory monosynaptic connections to trunk muscle motoneurons by short- and medium-length propriospinal neurons (37). Although the afferent and descending input to these neurons are unknown, it seems probable that such connections are important for the functional unity of the axial musculature.

Activation of neck afferents facilitates monosynaptic test reflexes to flexor and extensor muscles of the hindlimb (2) and evokes polysynaptic EPSPs in hindlimb motoneurons (347). There are apparently two propriospinal systems available for transmission of these effects. Effects from neck muscle afferents have a rather long latency (2) in comparison to effects from the forelimb, and the former are very effectively controlled from the brain (1). On the other hand, stimulation of C_1–C_3 spinal ganglia, which in addition activates afferents from intervertebral joint receptors and from short intervertebral muscles, evokes EPSPs in hindlimb motoneurons with latencies as short as those from forelimb afferents (347, 531).

Neck as well as thoracic afferents are important for the generation of the scratch reflex that is organized within the spinal cord and utilizes long propriospinal neurons (551, 555, 556). Recent experiments have considerably deepened our understanding of the mechanisms behind this behavioral reaction (56–58, 121), particularly by showing that neurons in L_4 and L_5 segments may be involved in the generation of the rhythmic oscillations (56, 57). In paralyzed preparations in which "movements" were monitored as the efferent nerve activity ("fictitious scratching") it has been shown that neurons within layer VII of these segments were modulated in their activity in relation to the scratch cycle. The basic mechanism generating the rhythm and temporal pattern is thus assumed to be located in lumbosacral segments. Propriospinal neurons from more rostral segments with axons located laterally in the lateral funiculus mediate the excitatory inflow to the rhythm generator (56, 551). For example, C_1 and C_2 propriospinal neurons with a projection to lumbar levels respond to peripheral stimuli and are tonically active during fictitious scratching (58). Thorndike (580) showed that cats can be conditioned to use hindlimb scratching to release themselves from a cage. This suggests that intraspinal mechanisms for scratching (and similar reactions) can be readily utilized by higher centers. It was later demonstrated that the corticospinal tract is essential for their mobilization (208).

Presynaptic Inhibition of Transmission From Primary Afferents

The intraspinal terminals of primary afferents are the first central sites where incoming information can be modulated. Long-lasting depolarization in primary afferents (dorsal root potentials; DRPs) was described long ago (46), but the physiological significance of this phenomenon was only generally recognized when it became conceptually associated with a depression of synaptic transmission (138, 187). The hypothesis was forwarded that primary afferent depolarization (PAD) is evoked by axoaxonal synapses and that this depolarization produces presynaptic inhibition by reducing transmitter release (129, 518).

During the 1960s detailed studies were made on the source of PAD in different categories of primary afferents. In the interpretation of these results it was generally assumed that the PAD in all cases caused presynaptic inhibition, although strong evidence for this relation exists only for the monosynaptic connection from Ia-afferents to motoneurons. Each category of primary afferents often contributes to several reflex pathways to motoneurons, primary afferents, and ascending neurons. It is not known if PAD affects transmission from primary afferents to all their target neurons in a similar way, although that seems to have been tacitly assumed in most cases. Even if these assumptions may introduce unjustifiable oversimplifications, we adhere to them in this chapter. We also disregard the possibility that the PAD evoked by discrete groups of afferents is a more unspecific effect of extracellular K^+ accumulation (cf. ref. 82) and thus, with other reviewers in this field (82, 518), view PAD as the effect of the activity in a specific neuronal pathway whose last-order interneurons have axoaxonal synapses. With these assumptions, the pathways to primary afferent terminals can be regarded as equivalent to other neuronal pathways in the spinal cord. Their functional organization, interaction, and control from higher centers can then be discussed in the same terms as the reflex pathways to motoneurons.

EFFECTS FROM PRIMARY AFFERENTS TO PRIMARY AFFERENT TERMINALS. The pattern of effects on particular species of primary afferents has been investigated either with excitability measurements using the method of Wall (603) or with intra-axonal recording. The functional organization of effects mediated by pathways to primary afferent terminals has been discussed in detail elsewhere (518); therefore only a brief summary of the main effects in the acute spinal cat is given here (Fig. 27). We refrain entirely from a discussion on the interneurons mediating PADs to various afferents because of the very scanty and indirect evidence in that field (cf. ref. 518).

Ia-terminals. Terminals of Ia-afferents from both extensors and flexors are depolarized by volleys in Ia- and Ib-afferents from ipsilateral flexor muscles as well as from the knee extensor quadriceps (144). The PAD can be evoked either by short trains of volleys in the nerves to these muscles or by muscle stretch or vibration (44, 124, 125). A short train of volleys in group I afferents from other extensors, such as triceps surae, fails to evoke PAD in Ia-terminals of other muscles but has been claimed to produce a selective action on its own terminals (119). The latter results have not been confirmed in a recent reinvestigation at normal temperature (192). Nevertheless the possibility of some selective presynaptic action on homonymous Ia-terminals cannot be discarded because Barnes and Pompeiano (45) found that relatively long-lasting vibration of triceps surae gave PAD in homonymous Ia-afferents and a corresponding long-lasting depression of the monosynaptic test reflex. It remains to be determined whether this effect is mediated by a selective pathway giving strict negative feedback or represents a marginal activation of the pathway giving more widespread action on Ia-afferents (cf. ref. 192). It should be noted in this context that there is also indirect evidence from experiments in humans for a possible presynaptic inhibition of the soleus monosynaptic test reflex (Hoffmann's reflex) induced by vibration or passive stretch of triceps surae (122).

Before we conclude this subsection a brief mention should be made of the experiments on reciprocal inhibition by Liddell and Sherrington (379). They used the stretch reflex in the quadriceps muscle to monitor the degree of reciprocal inhibition evoked by weak pulling of the hamstring muscles. A powerful inhibition was produced, but it proved to be quite resistant to strychnine. From our present knowledge that Ia IPSPs are effectively blocked by strychnine (67), it is likely that most of the inhibition seen by Liddell and Sherrington was of presynaptic origin.

Ib-terminals. There is no apparent difference in receptiveness of PAD between Ib-afferents from flexors and extensors. In either case the main input source is from Ib-afferents of both flexors and extensors without any evidence for a "local sign" (145). Weaker effects can also be evoked from contralateral Ib-afferents (126). Electrical stimulation of FRA from both hindlimbs causes a depolarization of Ib-afferents that may be considerable in unanesthetized preparations. The PAD has also been evoked by noxious radiant heat applied to the skin of the plantar pad (83).

Cutaneous afferents. Single volleys in cutaneous nerves evoke very large DRPs, which consist of two different components (93). The early component has a very restricted segmental distribution and is largely or entirely due to PAD in cutaneous afferents (93, 146). The later second component distributes over several segments and is part of a wider FRA response that also evokes PAD in cutaneous afferents. These two components are also differentiated by the fact

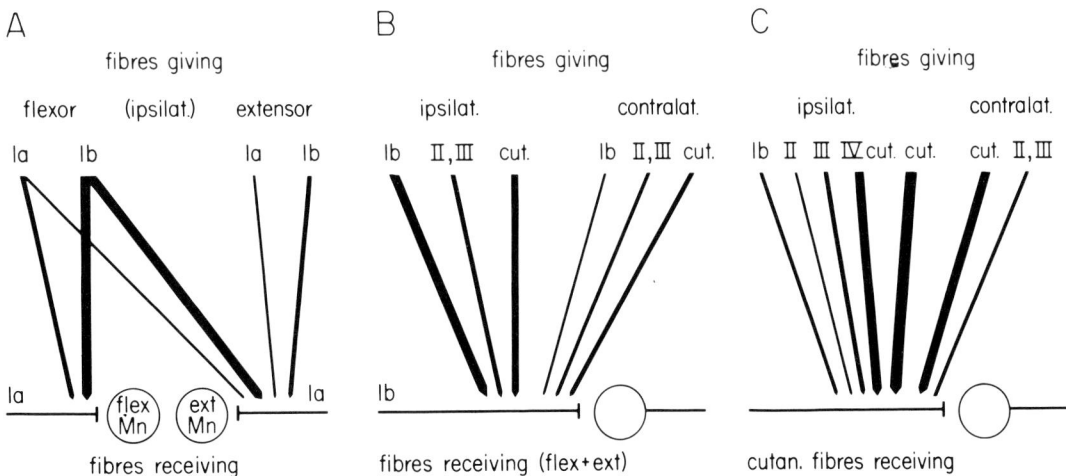

FIG. 27. Segmental afferent input depolarizing terminals of muscle spindle Ia-afferents (*A*), Golgi tendon organ Ib-afferents (*B*), and cutaneous afferents (*C*). Approximate relative amount of depolarization contributed by each input has been estimated from results quoted in text and is indicated by width of *arrows*. Mn, motoneurons; Ia, Ib, II, and III are the respective muscle afferents; Cut, myelinated cutaneous fibers. *A*: ipsilateral inputs depolarizing Ia-fibers of flexor (*left*) and extensor (*right*) muscles. *B*: ipsi- and contralateral inputs depolarizing Ib-fibers. *C*: ipsi- and contralateral inputs depolarizing cutaneous afferent fibers. Note that this pattern of effects is partly changed after administration of dopa to acute spinal cat (described in the text). [From Schmidt (518).]

that transmission in the pathway mediating the first component is unaffected in the decerebrate state; that of the second component is subject to a very effective tonic inhibition (93).

Investigations on single cutaneous afferents of known modality have revealed a great specificity in the distribution of PADs among them (320, 321). It was found that PAD is generated by two separate systems, one from rapidly adapting low-threshold receptors and the other from slowly adapting receptors. Both systems were of negative feedback character producing PAD mainly in their own terminals. Furthermore there was a spatial specificity, since the PAD was mainly evoked from the neighborhood of the receptor whose afferent was recorded (321, 519). In addition to these specific actions PAD in large cutaneous afferents is also evoked by electrical stimulation of the FRA (corresponding to the second component of the DRP) and by radiant heat applied to the skin (83). They are also depolarized by Ib volleys from ipsilateral flexors and extensors (146). Terminals of small myelinated skin nociceptor fibers appear to receive their main depolarization by damaging mechanical skin stimuli (606).

The FRA. Eccles et al. (143) suggested that the afferents belonging to the FRA act together on pathways to primary afferent terminals, as they seem to do on other reflex pathways, and that their main action is to depolarize their own terminals in a negative feedback fashion. This hypothesis was based on the finding of a long-lasting inhibitory interaction—presumed to be at least partly presynaptic—between high-threshold muscle afferents and cutaneous afferents in depressing transmission to motoneurons and in producing DRPs. The evidence that the afferents belonging to the FRA act together on primary afferent terminals is strong (93). It is also highly likely that the hypothesis of a negative feedback is a correct one, although direct evidence for it is meager. Terminals of cutaneous afferents and group II muscle afferents are depolarized from the FRA (93, 145, 146, 402), but no direct evidence is available for terminals of group III muscle afferents and of joint afferents. The effects evoked from the FRA are indeed widespread. Apart from the presumed action on their own terminals, they also act on Ib-afferents, cutaneous afferents (some of which may not be part of the FRA), and under some conditions also on Ia-afferents. The FRA also act by inhibiting transmission in some pathways to primary afferent terminals (see next subsection).

SEGMENTAL CONTROL OF PATHWAYS TO PRIMARY AFFERENTS. In some respect modulation of transmission in the pathways to primary afferents is easier to investigate than in those to motoneurons. Detailed information regarding inhibitory interactions in the internuncial apparatus of the spinal cord was first obtained for pathways to primary afferent terminals. For example, the effective depression from the FRA of the DRPs evoked by Ia volleys suggested an inhibition of transmission in the pathway to Ia-afferent terminals [Fig. 28; (402)]; this conclusion rests on the knowledge that only Ia-afferents are depolarized by Ia volleys and that FRA volleys do not depolarize Ia-terminals (see EFFECTS FROM PRIMARY AFFERENTS TO PRIMARY AFFERENT TERMINALS, p. 554). The FRA inhibition of interneuronal transmission in the pathway from Ia-afferents to Ia-afferent terminals was finally proved with the demonstration that FRA volleys blocked the increase of excitability of Ia-terminals (Fig. 28*E–H*) as well as the PAD in them. The finding that this inhibition has the same prolonged time course as the FRA-evoked PAD in other terminals strongly suggests that the FRA inhibition is caused by presynaptic inhibition—not of primary afferent terminals but of the terminals of interposed interneurons (Fig. 28*M*). The brief onset of the inhibition makes it likely that postsynaptic inhibition of interneurons also contributes (273, 402). The expected removal of presynaptic inhibition of Ia EPSPs in motoneurons has also been demonstrated (see Fig. 28*A–D*). The function of this mechanism may be to ensure that the γ-loop contributes effectively during movements depending on activation of interneuronal pathways from the FRA.

An interaction between different segmental FRA pathways to primary afferent terminals was revealed by a comparison of effects before and after activation of the noradrenergic reticulospinal pathway with dopa in acute spinal cats [(16, 50); cf. subsection *Monoaminergic Reticulospinal Pathways*, p. 562]. Without dopa, volleys in the FRA evoke PAD largely in their own terminals but not in Ia-afferents (see above). After dopa, however, the former effect is curtailed, but a late long-lasting PAD in Ia-afferents appears instead (Fig. 29); no corresponding late PAD was found in Ib- and cutaneous afferents, but some observations suggest that terminals from secondary spindle afferents also may be depolarized (50). Similar late effects are evoked in Ia-afferents from the contralateral FRA (329). As found for the late postsynaptic effects from FRA in motoneurons after dopa (Fig. 21), the onset of the late DRPs is also delayed by prolongation of stimulation. This shows that the FRA pathway mediating the late DRP also can be inhibited from the FRA (16). It was postulated that this inhibitory action is produced by activity in short-latency pathways from the FRA and that the release of transmission in the pathway giving late PAD in Ia-afferents is due to noradrenergic inhibition of these short-latency FRA pathways (Fig. 29*H*). This hypothesis was supported by the observation that the late PAD in Ia-afferents may be preceded by a primary afferent hyperpolarization (PAH) in the same afferents, presumably due to a removal of a tonic PAD in them by inhibition in the group I pathway to their terminals (16). Occasionally, particularly if dopa is given after inhibition of amine oxidase with nialamide, a large PAH may be the only effect evoked from the FRA. In this case it is

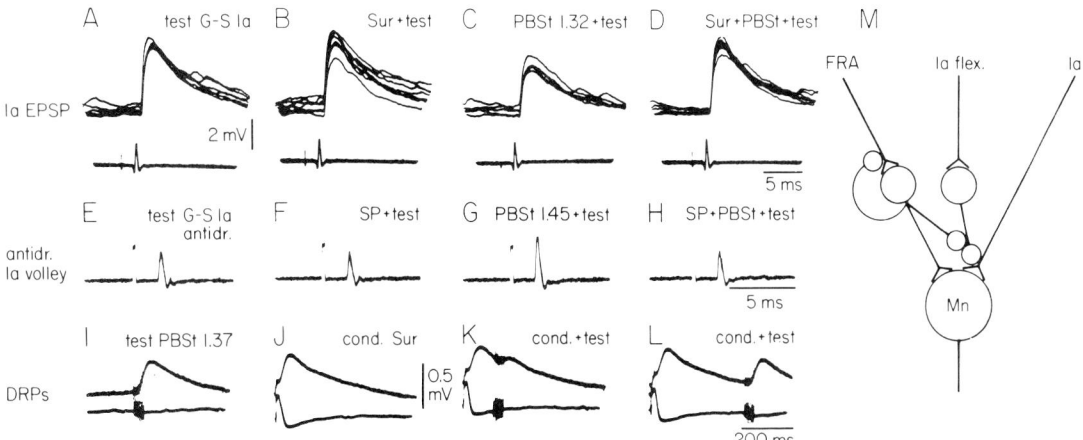

FIG. 28. Inhibitory action from flexor reflex afferents (FRA) on transmission to Ia-afferents illustrated by recording Ia EPSPs in motoneurons (A–D), by the antidromic discharge of Ia-afferents following stimulation of their terminals in the spinal cord (E–H), and by recording dorsal root potentials (I–L). A–D: upper traces, intracellular records from a gastrocnemius-soleus motoneuron (G-S); lower traces, from L₇ dorsal root entry zone. Voltage calibration refers to intracellular records. Stimulus strengths are given in multiples of threshold for lowest threshold fibers. Homonymous test Ia EPSP is shown in A. In B there is no effect by a conditioning volley in the sural (Sur) nerve. Depression in C is evoked by a short train of maximal Ia volleys in nerve from posterior biceps–semitendinosus (PBSt). With combined conditioning with sural and PBSt nerves there is a removal of the depression (D). E–H: intraspinal excitability measurements of Ia-afferent terminals in gastrocnemius-soleus (G-S) motor nucleus. Test response (E) was recorded in G-S nerve. Conditioning stimulation of superficial peroneal nerve (SP; cutaneous afferents only) does not change excitability (F). The facilitation (G, reflecting an excitability increase) is evoked by a train of PBSt Ia volleys. Record in H shows that a volley in SP can remove facilitatory action from PBSt Ia volleys. I–L: upper traces are dorsal root potentials (DRPs) recorded from the most caudal dorsal rootlet in L₆. Lower traces are recorded from L₇ dorsal root entry zone. I shows test DRP evoked from a train of maximal Ia volleys from PBSt. J shows response to stimulation of the sural nerve. In K and L there is combined stimulation of sural and PBSt nerves (cond. + test). Note pronounced depression of DRP from PBSt Ia-afferents (K) as well as the long duration of this effect (L). M: tentative diagram showing connections through which volleys in FRA depress transmission from Ia to Ia-terminals. Terminals with 2 branches are excitatory. Circles indicate presynaptic terminals making synaptic contacts with presynaptic terminals. In the diagram a single interneuron may represent a chain of interneurons. [A–L from Lund et al. (402); diagram in M from Lundberg (406).]

assumed that the spontaneous activity in the pathway to the Ia-terminals already gave maximal depolarization and that the initial PAH remained as the sole effect from the FRA.

EFFECTS FROM SUPRASPINAL CENTERS TO PRIMARY AFFERENT TERMINALS. A few years after the recognition of presynaptic inhibition as a segmental regulatory mechanism, it was found that large DRPs could also be evoked from the sensorimotor cortex and from the somatosensory area II (19, 96). At moderate strength of stimulation this DRP is mediated by corticospinal fibers (96), but extrapyramidal pathways can also contribute (272). A comparison of cortical regions from which PAD was evoked in forelimb and hindlimb segments revealed a somatotopic organization similar to that for motoneuronal activation (19).

The effects on primary afferent terminals from the sensorimotor cortex might be involved in either sensory or motor regulation. The demonstration of similar presynaptic effects from cortex in the dorsal column nuclei [(17, 18); cf. ref. 518] tended to focus the interest on regulation of sensory transmission. In this context it is of interest to mention the effects from the rubrospinal tract, which seem less likely to be related primarily to sensory transmission (Fig. 30). Generally the motor effects mediated by corticospinal and rubrospinal fibers are very similar (cf. section SPINAL NEURONAL CIRCUITS USED IN COMMON BY SEGMENTAL AFFERENTS AND SUPRASPINAL MOTOR CENTERS, p. 512), and this holds true also for the effects to primary afferent terminals. Both descending systems evoke considerable PAD in terminals of Ib- and cutaneous afferents (96, 276). There is also considerable spatial facilitation between descending cortico- or rubrospinal volleys and primary afferents both for the production of DRPs (Fig. 30) and intra-axonally recorded PAD (96, 276). The facilitation of the DRP evoked from high-threshold muscle afferents and of the second component of the cutaneous DRP indicates that cortico- and rubrospinal volleys excite interneurons in the pathway mediating PAD from the FRA, including the one giving negative feedback on FRA terminals. Cortical stimuli do not, on the other hand, depolarize Ia-fibers (19, 96). Instead they evoke inhibition in pathways from Ia-afferents to Ia-afferent

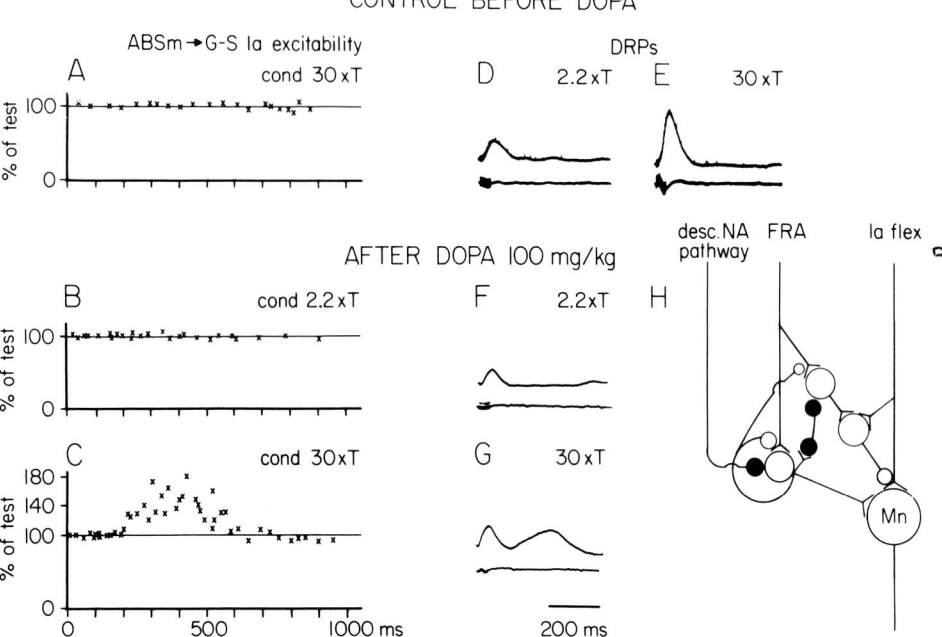

FIG. 29. Long-latency depolarization evoked from flexor reflex afferents (FRA) in Ia-terminals after dopa administration. Unanesthetized decorticate acute spinal cat. Graphs in A-C give excitability measurements of Ia-afferent terminals from gastrocnemius-soleus nerve (G-S) before (A) and after (B, C) injection of dopa. Intraspinal stimulation of G-S afferent terminals with a microelectrode (test) was conditioned (cond) with a short train of stimuli to anterior biceps–semimembranosus (ABSm) nerve (stimulation strength is indicated in times threshold, ×T, of lowest threshold afferent fibers). Abscissa gives interval between 1st conditioning volley and test stimulus to G-S terminals. Ordinate gives amplitude of conditioned response in percent of unconditioned test response. Comparison of A and C shows that after dopa FRA stimulation causes an increased excitability of Ia-fibers of long latency (conditioning group I stimulation is without effect, B). D–G illustrate simultaneous recordings of dorsal root potentials (DRPs) evoked from ABSm nerve. Comparison of E and G shows that parallel to excitability increase in Ia-terminals following stimulation of FRA there is also a long-latency DRP. H: tentative diagram of connections from FRA to Ia-afferents. *Filled circles*, connections exerting either pre- or postsynaptic inhibition; *open circles*, termination on presynaptic terminals. Excitatory synaptic terminals are indicated by two branches. Each symbol represents a chain of interneurons. It is assumed that activity in short-latency FRA pathway (*left*) inhibits long-latency pathway to Ia-afferent terminals. Inhibition from a descending noradrenergic (NA) pathway of short-latency FRA system releases transmission in long-latency path from FRA to Ia-terminals. [A–G adapted from Andén et al. (16); H from Lundberg (406).]

terminals in the same way as volleys in the FRA do and, accordingly, very effectively remove presynaptic inhibition of Ia transmission to motoneurons (402, 426). It has been postulated (402) that this corticospinal action is exerted by activation of interneurons in the FRA pathway that blocks transmission from Ia-fibers to Ia-terminals (cf. Fig. 28M). The possibility was discussed (276) that this inhibitory action from the cortex could conceal an excitatory corticospinal action on the pathway from group I afferents to Ia-terminals, a possibility further suggested by the rubral effects on Ia-afferents. Rubrospinal volleys are as effective as corticospinal ones in inhibiting transmission from Ia-afferents to Ia-terminals (276). Nevertheless it was found that weak rubral stimuli enhance the DRP produced by flexor Ia-afferents and can also give a small PAD in Ia-afferents. It remains to be learned whether a large PAD can be evoked in Ia-afferents from the red nucleus—and possibly from the sensorimotor cortex—if the competing inhibitory action can be avoided.

A large PAD is evoked in Ia-afferents from the medial longitudinal fasciculus (MLF), the ventral part of the ipsilateral medial vestibular nucleus (95, 103), the descending vestibular nucleus, the contralateral fastigial nucleus, and the vestibular nerve (88, 103). The same stimuli also give PAD in cutaneous afferents and in Ib-afferents. The two latter groups of afferents (but not Ia-afferents) are also depolarized from the intermediate zone in the anterior cerebellar cortex (89, 95) and from wide regions in the medullary reticular formation (95). It is possible that reticulospinal depolarization of primary afferent terminals contributes to the depression of reflex transmission that can be evoked from Magoun's inhibitory center (95).

There is no specific hypothesis on how the depolarization of Ia-afferent terminals (or other terminals for that matter) from the vestibular complex contributes

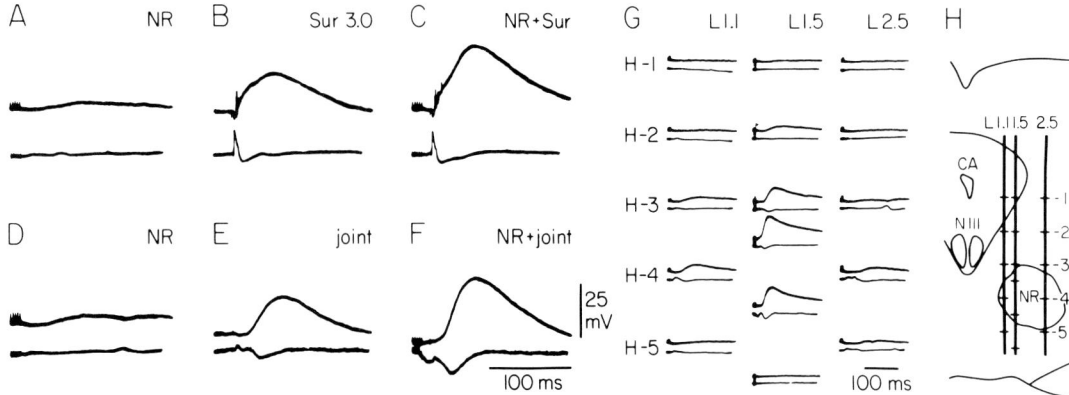

FIG. 30. Rubrospinal facilitation of segmental transmission to primary afferents. *A–G: upper traces*, dorsal root potentials (DRPs) recorded from the most caudal filament of the L$_6$ dorsal root; *lower traces*, records from cord dorsum at L$_7$. Voltage calibration beside F applies to DRPs of A–F. *A–F:* facilitation from red nucleus (NR) of DRPs evoked from cutaneous (*B, C*: sural nerve, Sur, stimulation at 3 times threshold of lowest threshold afferent fibers) and joint afferents (*E, F*: high-threshold afferents in posterior knee joint nerve). Increased amplitude of DRP in C is due to facilitation of 2nd component of cutaneous DRP that is mediated by an FRA pathway. *G, H:* origin of DRPs evoked by tegmental stimulation. The DRPs of G were evoked with 100-μA stimulation at sites marked in H in a drawing of a correspnding transverse section of brain stem. The DRPs are evoked from a rather restricted area within the NR. CA, central aqueduct; NIII, oculomotor nucleus; L, lateral and H, horizontal Horsley-Clarke coordinates. [Adapted from Hongo et al. (276).]

to regulation of posture or movements. However, some physiological role of the presynaptic inhibition of Ia transmission is suggested by the presence of PAD evoked in Ia-terminals during phasic periods of desynchronized sleep, when it probably contributes to the transient inhibition of monosynaptic reflexes that occurs during these periods (33, 36, 454, 455).

PRIMARY AFFERENT HYPERPOLARIZATION. There are by now numerous reports on positive DRPs (89, 265, 375, 446, 448) or PAH (276, 402, 427, 447, 509). It is generally assumed that PAH represents a removal of a tonic PAD and thus is caused by inhibition in the pathways to primary afferent terminals. It is therefore of special interest to consider those cases for which an inhibitory action on transmission to primary afferent terminals already has been demonstrated (subsection SEGMENTAL CONTROL OF PATHWAYS TO PRIMARY AFFERENTS, p. 556). Whenever the receiving fibers have been identified experimentally, PAH was evoked selectively in Ia-afferent terminals (as in the examples given in the preceding subsection). However, in the well-known report by Mendell and Wall (448), it was postulated that stimulation of small skin afferents produces PAH in large cutaneous afferents. Mendell (446) later concluded that the positive DRP evoked by stimulation of small fibers represents a PAH in large muscle afferents "rather than cutaneous fibers." It is noteworthy that this was already suggested during a discussion (A. Lundberg, discussion in ref. 604) when the proposition was first forwarded by Wall (604).

FUNCTIONAL CONSIDERATIONS. Schmidt (518) has wisely stated that "the evaluation of the functional role of presynaptic inhibition in the vertebral central nervous system is just as impossible a task as that of describing the functional role of postsynaptic inhibition." Nevertheless there are some distinguishing features that may serve as basis for discussion. The negative feedback character of the segmental PAD has been pointed out repeatedly (129, 518); in the case of Ib-afferents, cutaneous afferents, and the FRA the producing and the receiving fibers are identical. However, this striking organization must not overshadow the fact that these afferents may also act on terminals of other afferents. For example, Ib-afferents also act on different categories of cutaneous afferents, as do the FRA on Ib-afferents and on cutaneous afferents that may not belong to FRA. Since the FRA also act on Ia-afferents after dopa injection (subsection SEGMENTAL CONTROL OF PATHWAYS TO PRIMARY AFFERENTS, p. 556), they appear to provide an example of an afferent system that can depolarize all categories of fibers so far investigated.

The negative feedback character of presynaptic inhibition has been discussed both in relation to sensory transmission and to motor control. In connection with the facilitatory effect from the sensorimotor cortex and the red nucleus, it has been suggested that the negative feedback subserved reflex transmission to motoneurons and that when a reflex pathway to motoneurons is mobilized from these centers (EFFECTS FROM SUPRASPINAL CENTERS TO PRIMARY AFFERENT TERMINALS, p. 557), there appears to be a concomitant mobilization of the negative feedback for the afferents subserving that reflex (96, 276). This negative feedback may have a spatial focusing function, giving a local sign to the reflexes by limiting a stray excitation, as originally suggested by Eccles et al. (143). Such an action can by no means be excluded, but another possible role for the negative feedback has been emphasized by Lundberg more recently (411, 413). In subsections CUTANEOUS AFFERENTS, p. 535, and REFLEX PATHWAYS FROM THE "FLEXOR REFLEX AFFERENTS," p. 541, it was pointed out that the functional significance of the convergent excitatory action from primary afferents and higher centers on interneurons in reflex pathways to motoneurons might be that motoneurons are activated from higher centers via these interneurons and that primary afferent activity evoked by the ensuing movements might reinforce activation of motoneurons by adding to the excitation of the same interneurons. Such a positive feedback could perhaps get out of hand without a mechanism to control it. The depolarizing effect from the FRA onto their own terminals may serve as negative feedback with gain regulated from the brain by facilitation or inhibition of interneuronal transmission. It is noteworthy that the pathways from the FRA to motoneurons and primary afferents are controlled in a similar fashion from the brain not only in case of facilitation (from cortico- and rubrospinal pathways) but also with descending inhibition. Thus the dorsal reticulospinal system and the two monoaminergic reticulospinal systems act in parallel to suppress transmission in both pathways, and some of these descending pathways are responsible for the suppression in the decerebrate state (section RETICULOSPINAL INHIBITION OF SEGMENTAL REFLEX TRANSMISSION, this page). The release of transmission to primary afferent terminals from tonic descending inhibition following transverse lesions in the brain stem occurs in parallel with the release of the excitatory pathways to motoneurons (section RETICULOSPINAL INHIBITION OF SEGMENTAL REFLEX TRANSMISSION), which suggests a linkage to excitatory transmission to motoneurons, as is required by the feedback hypothesis considered above.

Despite all the attention given to the organization of the pathway from Ia- and Ib-afferents of flexor muscles to Ia-afferent terminals, there is no hypothesis that specifies its role in motor control. A hypothesis has, however, been forwarded for the function of the PAD in Ia-afferents from the FRA after dopa injection (50). This action was regarded as subsidiary to the release of the interneuronal network, which functions as spinal locomotor center (subsection *Half-centers and stepping*, p. 545). During locomotion this interneuronal network is supposed to be driven partly by activity in the FRA. It is assumed that activity in the FRA increases with the speed of locomotion and thereby enhances the presynaptic inhibition of transmission. Assuming that the stretch reflex may give servo assistance during locomotion (*Pathways From Ia-Afferents and Their Control by γ-Motoneurons*, p. 519), presynaptic inhibition seems to provide a segmental mechanism to adjust the relation of direct motoneuron excitation ("α-route") and the indirect Ia excitation mediated by the γ-loop; the demand on the γ-operated stretch reflex may be very different during slow walking and high-speed gallop. Recent work has suggested that γ-operated Ia discharge during active contraction is weak in fast locomotion; most of the Ia firing instead occurs during the very rapid muscle lengthening in the passive phase (subsection *Pathways From Ia-Afferents and Their Control by γ-Motoneurons*, p. 519). As an alternative to the previous proposition, it may be suggested that the presynaptic inhibition from FRA to Ia-terminals serves to diminish adverse effects of a "nonphysiological" Ia discharge during passive lengthening.

RETICULOSPINAL INHIBITION OF SEGMENTAL REFLEX TRANSMISSION

By generalizing the observations discussed in section SPINAL NEURONAL CIRCUITS USED IN COMMON BY SEGMENTAL AFFERENTS AND SUPRASPINAL MOTOR CENTERS, p. 512, it may be said that the principal task of the cortico-, rubro-, and vestibulospinal descending systems is to mobilize spinal functional units by their excitatory action on segmental reflex pathways and propriospinal systems. Although activity in these descending pathways often evokes inhibition in segmental interneurons, this may reflect inhibitory interactions between different segmental systems rather than a primary inhibitory function of these pathways. In contrast the main action of several reticulospinal pathways seems to be an inhibitory control of reflex transmission. Due to the complex organization of these reticulospinal systems, it seemed preferable to deal with all of them together rather than in relation to individual segmental systems. In doing so we do not follow the historical development in this field that began with the analysis of the tonic inhibition of transmission in some segmental reflex pathways in the intercollicular decerebrate cat (149, 267, 268). Instead, we first review more recent work on four reticulospinal pathways and their actions on the segmental reflex apparatus. Then follows a description of the tonic decerebrate control of reflex transmission and a discussion on which reticulospinal pathways mediate these effects.

Dorsal Reticulospinal System

Engberg et al. (167, 168) studied the effects of the dorsal reticulospinal system by electrically stimulating the ventromedial brain stem. Guided by the earlier knowledge that tonic decerebrate inhibition of reflex transmission is conveyed by pathways in the dorsolateral fasciculi [(267); see *Decerebrate Preparation*, p. 564], these experiments were performed in animals with extensive spinal cord lesions (cf. Fig. 31A) to avoid concomitant effects from ventral reticulospinal pathways and the cortico- and rubrospinal tracts. The axons of the dorsal reticulospinal system are distributed in the dorsal part of the lateral funiculus and

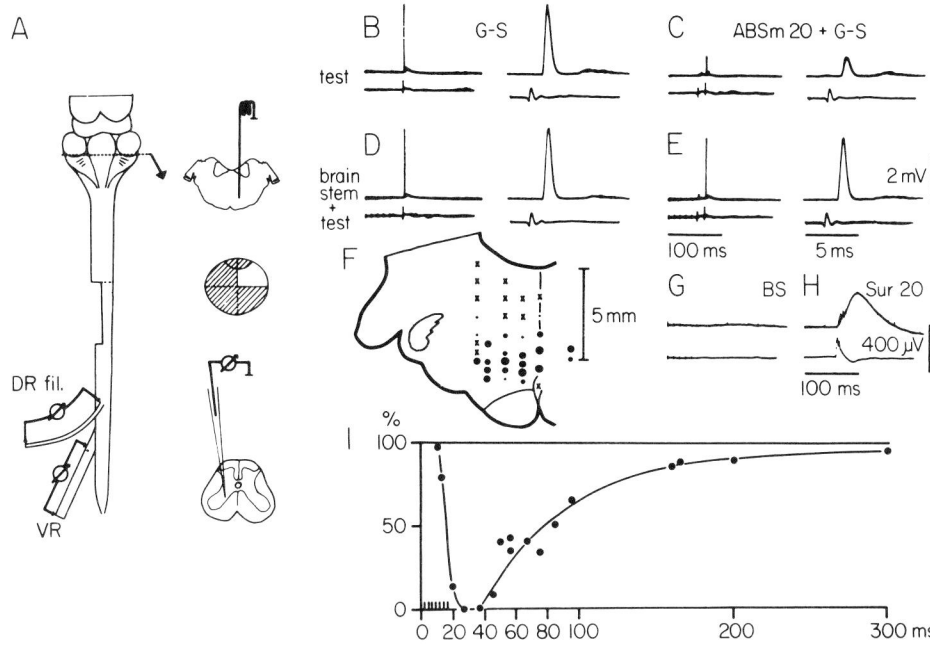

FIG. 31. Depression by dorsal reticulospinal system of flexor reflex afferent (FRA) inhibition in gastrocnemius-soleus (G-S) motor nucleus. *A*: schematic drawing of experimental arrangements. *Right*, 3 transverse sections: from brain stem (about 6 mm rostral of obex) showing the stimulation; from lower thoracic cord, *hatched area* indicating transection of whole cord except the right dorsolateral fascicle; from lumbar cord with microelectrode recording in left ventral horn. Left ventral quadrant and dorsolateral fascicle are mounted on electrodes for recording ascending discharges. Ventral root (VR) discharges are recorded from S_1 and L_7 segments, and dorsal root potentials are recorded in a caudal filament of the L_6 dorsal root (DR fil.), both on *left*. *B–E*: *upper traces*, monosynaptic reflexes recorded from ventral root; *lower traces*, incoming volleys at the dorsal root entry zone. Recording was done with 2 sweep speeds simultaneously and records therefore consist of double sets (*left traces* at slow and *right traces* at fast sweep speeds; see calibrations below *E*). *B*: monosynaptic reflex from group Ia-afferents in G-S nerve. *C*: same reflex inhibited by a preceding volley in high-threshold afferents (20 times threshold for lowest threshold fibers) from anterior biceps and semimembranosus (ABSm). *D, E*: same as *B* and *C* respectively but conditioned by a train of 5 stimuli in brain stem that removes most of FRA inhibition (compare *C* and *E*), without any effect on monosynaptic test reflex itself (compare *B* and *D*). *F*: diagram of a transverse brain stem section about 6 mm above obex. *Filled circles* of different size indicate points of stimulation and magnitude of effect on FRA inhibitory actions; × indicates points stimulated without effect on transmission from FRA. *G, H*: dorsal root records (*upper traces*) showing that no dorsal root potential (DRP) is evoked by the same brain stem (BS) stimulation that was used in *D, E*, whereas there is a large DRP with the same amplification from a single volley in the sural nerve (Sur) at 20 times threshold for the lowest threshold fibers. *I*: time course of brain stem action illustrated in *C* and *E*. Inhibition of monosynaptic reflex by the ABSm volley (100% refers to inhibition seen without preceding brain stem stimulation) is plotted against time interval between onset of brain stem stimulation and arrival of ABSm volley at the cord. [Adapted from Engberg et al. (167).]

have conduction velocities of at least 20 m/s. Since the supraspinal origin and course of this system have not been identified with any anatomically established descending tract, it has been referred to as the "dorsal reticulospinal system."

The basic finding by Engberg et al. (167) that a train of brain stem stimuli effectively depresses transmission of excitatory and inhibitory FRA effects to motoneurons is illustrated in Figure 31. It was concluded that the system acts at an interneuronal level, since FRA transmission to motoneurons could be inhibited without concomitant primary afferent depolarization or postsynaptic effects in motoneurons (Fig. 31). The example given above refers to the ordinary short-latency FRA pathways (REFLEX PATHWAYS FROM THE "FLEXOR REFLEX AFFERENTS," p. 541). Late long-lasting FRA actions sometimes developed spontaneously and resembled those obtained after injection of monoamine precursors in acute spinal preparations (subsections REFLEX PATHWAYS FROM THE "FLEXOR REFLEX AFFERENTS," p. 541, and *Monoaminergic Reticulospinal Pathways*, p. 562). These late responses are also effectively depressed by the dorsal reticulospinal system. In addition excitatory and inhibitory Ib effects are depressed; disynaptic reciprocal Ia inhibition and recurrent inhibition both are unaffected.

The action on transmission to primary afferents was also studied by Engberg et al. (167). They found that group I DRPs and the first component in the cutaneous DRPs (which is not an FRA response) are unaffected by brain stem stimuli. The DRPs evoked by FRA stimuli (including the second component in the cutaneous DRP) are, on the other hand, effectively depressed. This applied both to ordinary short-latency DRPs and to occasional late long-lasting ones. Transmission from the FRA (but not from Ia- and Ib-afferents) to ascending spinal pathways (section ASCENDING PATHWAYS THAT MONITOR SEGMENTAL INTERNEURONAL ACTIVITY, p. 569), is similarly inhibited.

The EPSPs and IPSPs evoked in lumbar interneurons by FRA stimulation are also very effectively depressed by the dorsal reticulospinal system [Fig. 32; (168)]. Since the brain stem stimulation never evoked EPSPs in interneurons, it was proposed that axons of the dorsal reticulospinal system are primarily inhibitory. In keeping with this, some interneurons displayed IPSPs with such a short latency that a monosynaptic linkage from the descending tract seemed possible (Fig. 32). It is important to note that all these interneurons with reticulospinal IPSPs were monosynaptically excited from primary afferents. If such interneurons are in fact first-order interneurons in polysynaptic FRA pathways, then it would suggest that this descending system does not inhibit reflex transmission through widespread postsynaptic effects in interneuronal chains but rather at a few selected stations early in the FRA reflex pathways (168, 407).

Ventral Reticulospinal Pathways

Stimulation in the ventromedial region of the medullary reticular formation causes a collapse of decerebrate rigidity and suppression of stretch reflexes (432). The main mechanism of this general relaxation seems to be a postsynaptic inhibition of flexor and extensor α-motoneurons (330, 384, 385) mediated by pathways in the ventral quadrants in the spinal cord. Although these strong postsynaptic effects in motoneurons made it difficult to study simultaneous effects on reflex transmission in detail, the available evidence (330) nevertheless suggests that ventral reticulospinal pathways inhibit, at an interneuronal level, transmission in pathways from cutaneous and high-threshold muscle afferents to motoneurons. Many DRPs evoked by Ia-, Ib-, and flexor reflex afferent volleys are effectively depressed by brain stem stimuli that by themselves do not evoke any PAD (427). These results suggest the existence of reticulospinal inhibition of transmission from these afferent systems to primary afferents. It should be noted that the effects on transmission to primary afferents from the ventral reticulospinal pathways differ from those effects mediated by the dorsal reticulospinal system in that transmission from Ia- and Ib-afferents is depressed only by the ventral pathways.

Monoaminergic Reticulospinal Pathways

Extensive experimental studies (13, 91, 118) suggest that virtually all monoaminergic terminals containing

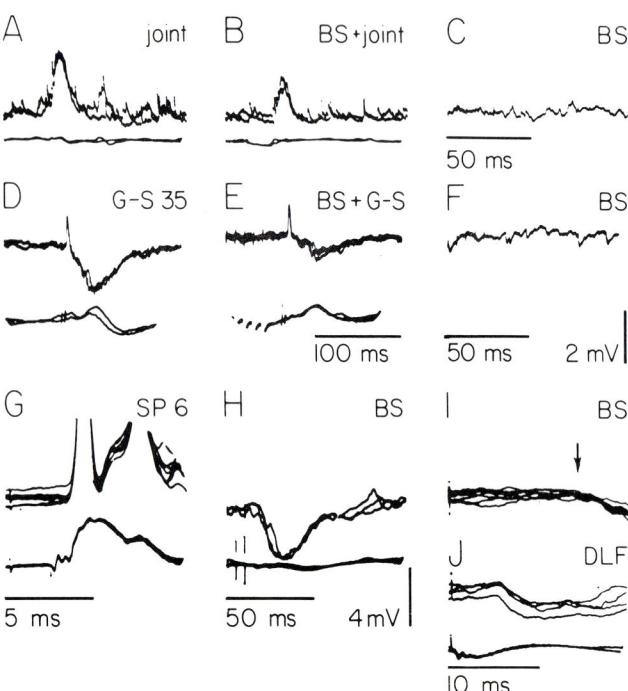

FIG. 32. Action of dorsal reticulospinal system in lumbar interneurons. *Upper traces* in *A–J* are records from 3 different interneurons (*A–C; D–F; G–J*) located at 1.8 mm–2.0 mm depth from cord dorsum. *Lower traces* are records from dorsal root entry zone (not present in *C, F, I*). Voltage calibrations refer to intracellular records. Stimulation strength for nerves is indicated in times threshold of lowest threshold afferent fibers. Experimental arrangement is shown in Fig. 31 *A*. *A–F*: excitation from high-threshold fibers of posterior knee joint nerve (*A*: joint) and inhibition from high-threshold muscle afferents of gastrocnemius-soleus nerve (*D*; G-S) were both depressed by conditioning stimulation of brain stem (*B, E*; BS). BS stimulation alone evoked neither postsynaptic potentials in interneurons (*C, F*) nor dorsal root potentials (not illustrated), which indicates inhibition from BS in FRA pathways to interneurons from which recording was done. *G–J*: interneuron with synaptic inhibition from BS. *G*: monosynaptic activation from superficial peroneal nerve (SP; stimulation at 6 times threshold for lowest threshold fibers). *H*: inhibitory postsynaptic potential (IPSP) evoked by 3 stimuli in BS. *I*: onset of IPSP evoked by a single shock (beginning of 1st deflection is marked by *arrow*). *J*: IPSP evoked by a single stimulus of contralateral dorsolateral funiculus (DLF) just rostral to spinal cord lesion. A comparison of the latencies to onset of inhibition in *I* and *J* suggests that responsible descending fibers have a conduction velocity of 25 m/s. [Adapted from Engberg et al. (168).]

norepinephrine (NA) or serotonin [5-hydroxytryptamine (5-HT)] that are present in the spinal cord have a supraspinal origin. These monoaminergic systems originate in the medulla oblongata and the lower pons (118, 200, 462), and their fibers descend widely distributed in the lateral and ventral funiculi. Very recently evidence has been obtained for a dopaminergic projection from diencephalon to the spinal cord (62, 63). It is not yet known whether this pathway extends beyond the thoracic segments, but there are at least no pharmacological results in favor of a dopaminergic action in the cat lumbar spinal cord.

Since intravenous injection of dopa (3,4-dihydroxyphenylalanine) and 5-hydroxytryptophan (5-HTP), precursors of NA and 5-HT, respectively, enhances the fluorescence in NA and 5-HT terminals (198, 199), it has been assumed that injection of dopa or of 5-HTP would force synthesis and release of monoamines from presynaptic terminals of the respective reticulospinal fibers and reproduce, in the acute spinal cat, the physiological effects that would follow selective activation of the two descending monoaminergic systems (12). The validity of this hypothesis was supported by the finding that drugs that interact with biosynthesis, liberation, and degradation of NA and 5-HT also interfere in a predictable way with actions of dopa and 5-HTP on the isolated spinal cord. A brief summary of this work is given in the following paragraphs to illustrate both the strength and remaining weak points of these arguments.

The mechanism of action of dopa on the spinal cord has been deduced from pharmacological experiments. The effect of dopa is completely antagonized by the adrenergic α-receptor blocker phenoxybenzamine and shows a 10-fold potentiation after inhibition of amine oxidase which inactivates NA (13, 15). Furthermore dopa has no effect after inhibition of aromatic-L-amino-acid decarboxylase (responsible for the synthesis of dopamine from dopa), which shows that dopa does not act directly but through catecholamine formation (13). It seems, however, that dopa does not act by a fast synthesis of NA, but rather by formation of dopamine that displaces NA from its stores and causes NA liberation from the terminals [(342); cf. however, ref. 11]. This conclusion was based on the finding that inhibition of dopamine-β-monooxygenase (which converts dopamine to NA) does not influence the effect of a single injection of dopa, while a subsequent dopa injection is rendered completely ineffective, as would be expected if the terminals were depleted of NA following the first dopa injection and were unable to form new NA from dopamine during inhibition of dopamine-β-monooxygenase (342). The effects of dopa are also reduced by pretreatment with reserpine (13), which empties NA stores and prevents synthesis of NA from dopamine.

Substances that induce a selective release from noradrenergic presynaptic terminals [such as 4,α-dimethyl-meta-tyramine; (174)] or stimulate NA receptors [e.g., clonidine; (10, 182)], replicate the actions of dopa in the acute spinal preparation (cf., however, ref. 21). Additional evidence has emerged from experiments in which a selective and reversible degeneration of the descending noradrenergic pathways was produced by injection of 6-hydroxydopamine into the cerebrospinal fluid (461). After such pretreatment with 6-hydroxydopamine, the effects of dopa on reflex transmission in the acute spinal rat are lost in parallel with the disappearance of NA terminals in the cord. At the same time, NA-mimetic drugs become more active than in the normal animal, which is interpreted as due to sensitization of NA receptors.

In apparent contradiction to the idea that dopa normally acts by release of NA exclusively from descending noradrenergic fibers, it has been demonstrated that the effects of dopa and the NA liberator 4,α-dimethyl-meta-tyramine are partially preserved in chronic spinal cats (13, 174). The cause of these effects is not yet clear but there seem to be several possibilities. For example, the spinal segments below the section may undergo profound changes after degeneration of the descending pathways, and the possibility cannot be excluded that the neurons deprived of their noradrenergic innervation develop enhanced sensitivity to dopa (or to dopamine that can be synthetized by extraneuronal decarboxylase) and to the NA liberator itself. It would also be plausible that enzymes from the degenerating terminals are taken up by neighboring glia cells that may then synthetize and release NA to act on nearby postsynaptic receptors.

The evidence on pharmacological interaction with 5-HT biosynthesis, liberation, and degradation is less detailed, but it has been demonstrated that the actions of 5-HTP are *1*) prevented by decarboxylase blockers (12, 161); *2*) increased by pretreatment with reserpine, because synthetized 5-HT is prevented from entering empty storage vesicles (573); and *3*) partly reversed by blockers of 5-HT receptors [methysergide and bromlysergic acid; (169, 170); see also ref. 205]. The effects of 5-HTP are largely retained in chronic spinal animals (20, 460, 558), and this has been explained by a possible decarboxylation at extraneuronal sites. The fact that the time course of the 5-HTP effects is very different in acute and chronic spinal cats (558) is taken to suggest that decarboxylation nevertheless may occur in the descending serotonergic terminals in the acute preparation. Strong evidence that the inhibitory effect by 5-HTP on transmission from the FRA is caused by transmitter liberation from 5-HT terminals was obtained when reserpine was given to acute spinal cats pretreated with nialamide (169). Reserpine is known to liberate monoamines from the presynaptic terminals and the large amounts liberated after amine oxidase inhibition may produce considerable synaptic effects. Since the effective depression of transmission from the FRA evoked by reserpine is not at all antagonized by the adrenergic α-receptor blocker phenoxybenzamine, but is partially antagonized by 5-HT blockers, it appears to be due to liberation of 5-HT. This conclusion was supported by the finding that reserpine has no effect on transmission from the FRA in chronic spinal cats.

As described in *Reflex Pathways From Cutaneous and Joint Afferents and From Groups II and III Muscle Afferents*, p. 535, injection of dopa or 5-HTP causes an effective depression of reflex transmission in short-latency FRA pathways to motoneurons, primary afferents, and ascending tract cells. In the case of dopa there is likewise an inhibition of transmission in Ib pathways to motoneurons. Figure 33 exemplifies the abolition of excitation from the FRA in motoneurons after dopa injection and the subsequent release caused by the α-receptor blocker phenoxybenzamine. The depression of short-latency transmission in Ib and

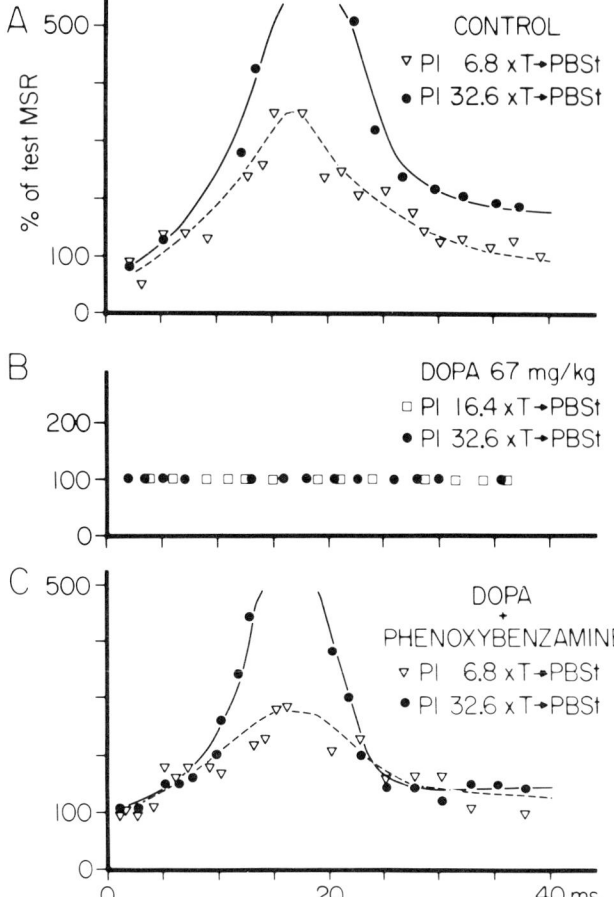

FIG. 33. Effect of dopa on transmission from high-threshold muscle afferents in motoneurons and reversal of effects by the α-receptor blocker phenoxybenzamine. Graphs show effect of single conditioning volleys on monosynaptic test reflex (MSR) from flexor posterior biceps-semitendinosus nerve (PBSt). Ordinate gives amplitude of MSR in percent of unconditioned MSR. Abscissa gives interval between arrival at spinal cord of conditioning and testing group I volleys. Strength of conditioning stimulation of plantaris nerve (Pl) is indicated in times threshold (×T) of lowest threshold afferent fibers. *A* was evoked before injection of dopa; *B* evoked 10 min after injection of dopa; and *C* evoked 25 min after dopa and 15 min after injection of phenoxybenzamine. The FRA facilitation of the flexor MSR (*A*) is abolished after dopa (*B*), which indicates inhibition of transmission in short-latency flexor reflex afferent (FRA) pathways. Reversal of inhibition by phenoxybenzamine indicates that effect of injected dopa is mediated by α-receptors. [Adapted from Andén et al. (15).]

FRA pathways after injection of monoamine precursors resembles the effects mediated by the dorsal reticulospinal system (subsection *Dorsal Reticulospinal System*, p. 560), but it is evident that these pathways are not identical because of the partial diversity of their actions on the cord. For instance, when the early FRA reflex pathways are inhibited by administration of dopa and 5-HTP, transmission through the long-latency FRA pathways is released (12, 15, 16, 324); these late responses do not appear when the short-latency pathways are inhibited by stimulation of the dorsal reticulospinal system (167). Independence of the dorsal reticulospinal system and the monoaminergic pathways is also suggested by the conduction velocity of about 20-30 m/s for the former system, whereas the unmyelinated monoaminergic reticulospinal axons, with a diameter of about 0.1-1 µm (118) should have a much lower conduction velocity.

The action of the monoaminergic precursors dopa and 5-HTP is not restricted to an inhibition of reflex transmission. In acute spinal animals they also cause an increase in the discharge of static γ-motoneurons and, in parallel, enhanced stretch reflexes [(4, 161, 0231); cf. subsection *Pathways From Ia-Afferents and Their Control by γ-Motoneurons*, p. 519]. A direct action on the central mechanisms controlling static γ-motoneurons by these drugs is probably of great importance. This seems well established for dopa, which does not directly affect the excitability of α-motoneurons (15), but in the case of 5-HTP additional factors may be important. An increased excitability of α-motoneurons is observed after injection of 5-HTP even with an open γ-loop (161, 405). The occurrence of tonic stretch reflexes should also be promoted by autogenetic excitation from a polysynaptic Ia pathway that is mobilized by 5-HTP administration [(301); subsection *Pathways From Ia-Afferents and Their Control by γ-Motoneurons*, p. 519].

The descending monoaminergic pathways originate from several regions of the brain stem (118, 200, 462), and it would therefore be expected that the consequent subgroups subserve different functions at the segmental level. From this point of view it is indeed surprising that even the noradrenergic and serotonergic systems seem to have so many effects in common. The problem of functional subgroups within these two systems is of course not readily approached by administration of transmittor precursors that simultaneously act on all terminals.

Decerebrate Preparation

Sherrington (548) studied the motor behavior in a variety of species following a transection of the brain stem in the region of the corpora quadrigemina. These preparations were characterized by a peculiar rigidity, predominantly in extensors, but sometimes also in flexors (48). The excessive muscular tone was paralleled by enhanced stretch reflexes (378). Decerebrate rigidity is the most conspicuous feature of this preparation, perhaps explaining why another aspect of this state, the depression of a variety of spinal polysynaptic reflex actions, initially drew less attention. It was later realized that the threshold for various polysynaptic excitatory and inhibitory reflexes decreased after a subsequent spinal transection (41, 376, 377, 554, 557), and this release of reflex actions was thought to be caused by disappearance of a tonic inhibitory action on the interneurons mediating the reflexes (197, 341). A detailed description of all aspects of the decerebrate state is outside the scope of this chapter; the reader is referred to Matthews' monograph (444) for a full discussion. The main emphasis here is given to the organization of the tonic inhibitory control of segmental reflex transmission that is typical for this preparation.

A very effective tonic inhibition of transmission in polysynaptic pathways from some primary afferent systems to motoneurons was demonstrated in the decerebrate state as compared with the spinal preparation, both with conditioning of monosynaptic test reflexes and with intracellular recording (149, 363). This was established for both excitatory and inhibitory pathways from flexor reflex and Ib-afferents; no corresponding depression was seen of reciprocal Ia inhibition or recurrent inhibition (149, 267). In subsequent work on decerebrate control of transmission to primary afferents (93), it was shown that transmission from FRA (but not from Ia- and Ib-afferents) was inhibited. Partial spinal cord lesions (Fig. 34) demonstrated that the supraspinal control of Ib and FRA pathways is maintained by fibers descending within the dorsal half of the lateral funiculus (267). The effect is bilateral so that the tonic inhibition persists as long as the dorsal half of the lateral funiculus on either side is intact. Section of the ventral cord quadrants does not affect transmission in Ib and FRA pathways, but decerebrate rigidity is then abolished (127), most probably due to interruption of the vestibulospinal tract.

The brain stem centers responsible for the tonic inhibition appear to be controlled from more rostral levels, since the tonic inhibitory control is less intense in the intact lightly anesthetized animal than after a subsequent decerebration (267, 269). The location of these brain stem centers is not known, but lesion experiments (93, 94, 266, 268) indicate that the centers that control the excitatory and those that control the inhibitory spinal reflex pathways from FRA have different rostrocaudal locations in the medulla and the pons (Fig. 35). Thus a medial lesion at a low pontine level causes a selective release of transmission in the inhibitory FRA pathways to α-motoneurons, Ia inhib-

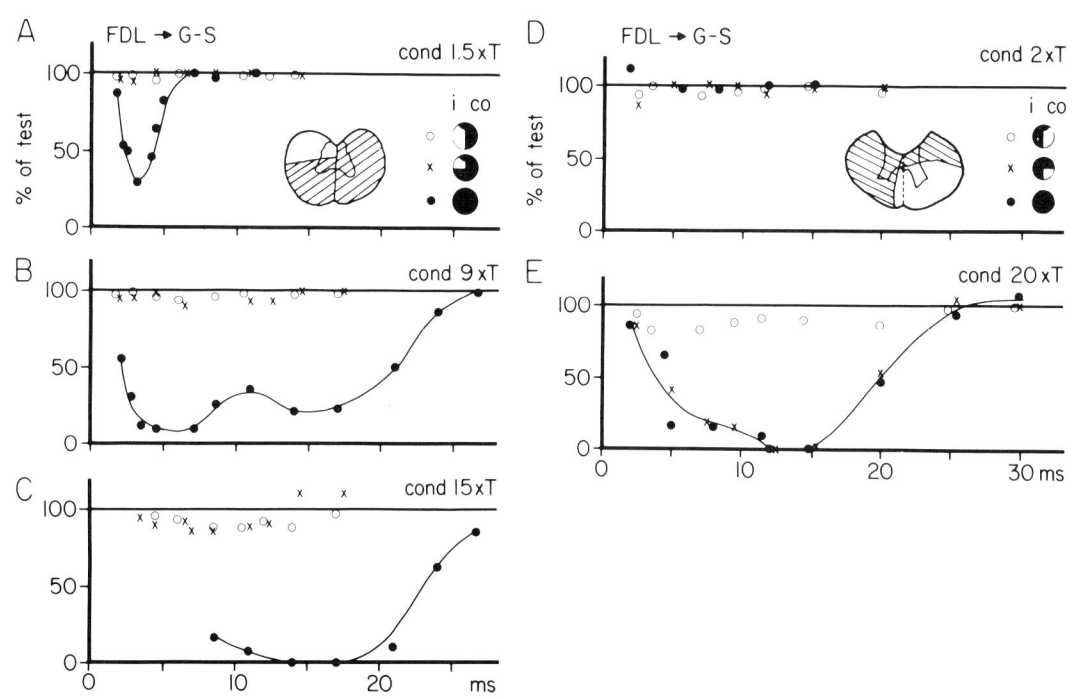

FIG. 34. Release of Ib- and flexor reflex afferent (FRA) actions after bilateral lesions of dorsolateral funiculi. Graphs show effect of single conditioning volleys in nerve to flexor digitorum longus (FDL) on monosynaptic test reflexes evoked from gastrocnemius-soleus (G-S). Ordinate gives amplitude of reflexes in percent of unconditioned test reflex. Abscissa gives interval between arrival at spinal cord of conditioning and testing group I volleys. Strength of conditioning stimulation (cond) is indicated in times threshold (×T) of lowest threshold afferent fibers. It was chosen to activate group I fibers in A and D, groups I and II fibers in B, and groups I, II, and III fibers in C and E. At each conditioning strength the curves were obtained after the ipsilateral (i) and contralateral (co) lesions indicated schematically in A (for A–C) and in D (for D, E). Transverse spinal cord drawings in A show symbols used in A–C to illustrate effects of sequential lesions; the initial lesion of the dorsal column and dorsolateral on the contralateral side, and ventral funiculi (○), the additional transection of ipsilateral ventral funiculus (×, cf. histological reconstruction to *left*), and the complete spinal transection (●). Drawings in D similarly show initial lesion of dorsal column and dorsolateral on the ipsilateral side, and ventral quadrants (○), the additional lesion of the contralateral dorsal funiculus (×, cf. histological reconstruction to *left*), and complete spinal transection (●). [Adapted from Holmqvist and Lundberg (267).]

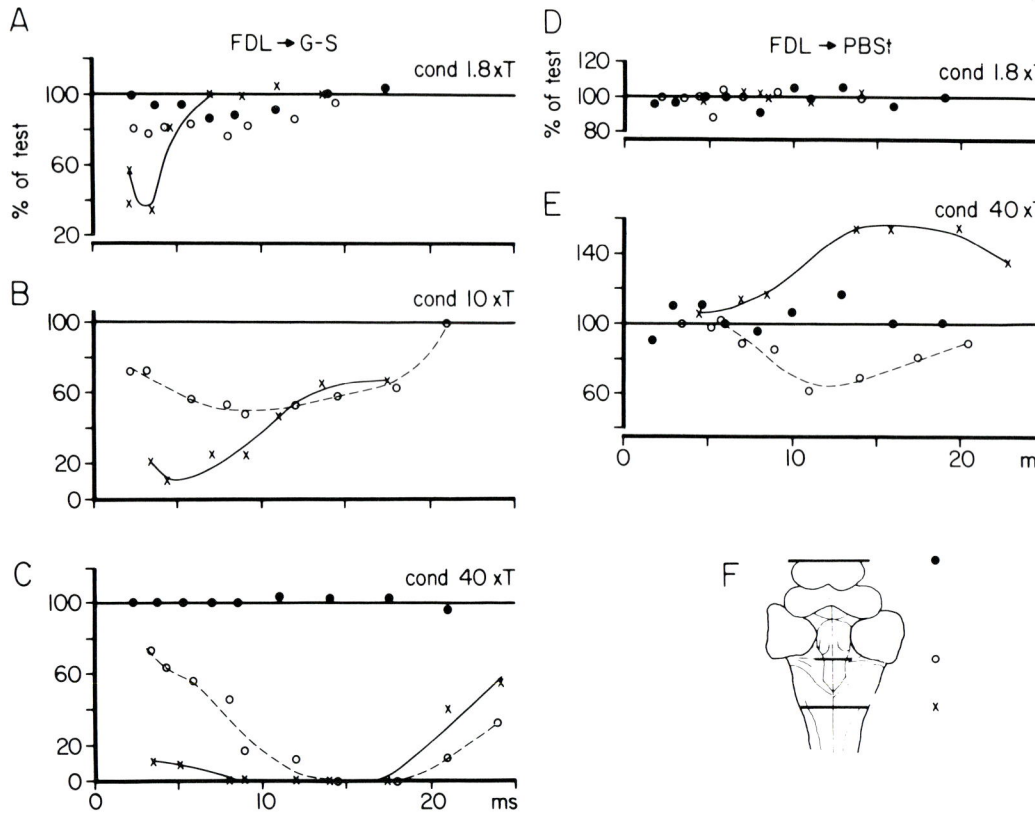

FIG. 35. Differential release of transmission in excitatory and inhibitory flexor reflex afferent pathways by brain stem lesions. Graphs show effect of single conditioning volleys in nerve to flexor digitorum longus (FDL) on monosynaptic test reflexes evoked from gastrocnemius-soleus (G-S, A–C) or from posterior biceps–semitendinosus (PBSt, D, E). Ordinate gives amplitude of reflexes in percent of unconditioned test reflexes. Abscissa gives interval between arrival at spinal cord of conditioning and testing group I volleys. Strength of conditioning stimulation (cond) is indicated in times threshold (×T) of lowest threshold afferent fibers. It was chosen to activate group I fibers in A and D, groups I and II fibers in B, and groups I, II, and III fibers in C and E. At each conditoning strength the curves were obtained after brain stem lesions indicated in F. [Adapted from Holmqvist and Lundberg (268).]

itory interneurons, and some ascending tract cells, whereas the excitatory FRA pathways to the same neurons remain blocked. Transmission in excitatory FRA pathways is restored only after medial section at the level of the obex. These results, however, do not imply that the reticulospinal cells have a different rostrocaudal distribution; it may apply only to their controlling centers. The FRA pathways to primary afferents are only released after lesions at the level of the obex (93), i.e., together with the excitatory pathways to motoneurons, Ia inhibitory interneurons, and ascending tract cells. The release, following the brain stem lesions described above, always occurs in parallel for pathways from ipsi- and contralateral FRA (266).

The decerebrate control of Ib pathways is presumably independent of the tonic inhibition of FRA pathways discussed above. In fact, the low pontine lesions that release inhibitory FRA pathways do not affect Ib pathways (268), showing that the latter are controlled from caudal brain stem areas. Furthermore a differential release of inhibitory and excitatory pathways, as found for the FRA, was not observed for pathways activated from Ib-afferents (268). The existence of two independent central control mechanisms is also suggested by spontaneous fluctuations of the decerebrate control, which may lead in the same preparation to a release of Ib transmission, while FRA pathways remain blocked or vice versa (267).

The tonic inhibitory control of segmental reflex transmission in the decerebrate state certainly includes a number of effects similar to those that can be evoked by electrical or pharmacological activation of the various reticulospinal systems described above. The question that then arises is to what extent these various systems contribute to the tonic decerebrate control. The ventral reticulospinal pathways may be excluded, since section of the ventral quadrants does not affect the decerebrate control. The descending NA system is probably not involved either, since administration of α-blockers does not cause a release from the decerebrate control (170). Administration of 5-HT antagonists, on the other hand, results in a partial release of transmission in FRA reflex pathways (and injection of amine oxidase inhibitors correspondingly increases the effectiveness of decerebrate control); therefore the decerebrate inhibition may be maintained at least partly by tonic activity in 5-HT neurons (170). However, the 5-HT pathways are probably not the only ones to contribute for at least two reasons. First, lesions of the raphe nuclei that destroy the bulk of the brain stem 5-HT cells decrease but do not abolish decerebrate inhibition (170). Furthermore administration of 5-HTP causes a release of late long-lasting FRA effects that is not a common feature of the decerebrate state. The dorsal reticulospinal system may also contribute to maintain the tonic inhibition of reflex transmission in the decerebrate state. This system not only exerts all the actions on spinal reflex transmission that are required but also descends in the dorsolateral funiculi, which are necessary to decerebrate control. Thus the available evidence makes it highly likely that both the dorsal reticulospinal system and the descending 5-HT pathways participate importantly in the tonic decerebrate control of spinal reflex pathways.

Although this section is primarily concerned with the inhibitory control of reflex transmission, some comments should be made on the relation between this tonic control in the decerebrate state and the appearance of stretch reflexes. Downman and Hussain (127) have suggested that the decerebrate inhibition of reflex transmission could be removed by selective spinal lesions without affecting muscle tone, but more recent investigations have shown that interruption of the dorsolateral funiculi has important consequences for tonic stretch reflexes. In the triceps surae, for example, the gain of the reflex (change in active tension with a given extension) is decreased after such a lesion without variations in the reflex threshold (248). The quadriceps muscle has also been reported (79) to respond with a stretch reflex only when close to its minimal physiological length (knee extended). Its contraction appeared to melt and the muscle to give way, as in the classic clasp-knife phenomenon when its length increased. These results clearly indicate that lesions of the dorsal reticulospinal system can release autogenetic inhibitory processes, which decrease the gain of the stretch reflex and disclose instead the clasp-knife phenomenon (79, 515).

DIRECT PROJECTIONS OF DESCENDING
PATHWAYS TO α-MOTONEURONS

On their way to motoneurons, both the descending supraspinal and peripheral afferent fiber systems project to a much larger extent on spinal segmental interneurons than on the motoneurons themselves. Therefore most of this chapter has been devoted to the significance of the integration at the interneuronal level. The motoneurons are, however, reached by some supraspinal systems and this section briefly summarizes these direct connections (extensive reports are given in the chapters by Kuypers, by Wilson and Peterson, and by Asanuma in this *Handbook*) to give a background for a discussion on the significance of the monosynaptic projections as compared with the polysynaptic ones.

Four main descending excitatory systems with direct projection to motoneurons have appeared in the course of the phylogenetic development, three from the brain stem (reticulo-, vestibulo-, and rubrospinal) and one from the motor cortex [(540, 542); see also the chapter by Kuypers in this *Handbook*]. The most ancient of the pathways is the reticulospinal tract, which is present in cyclostomes, teleosts, amphibians, reptiles, and mammals, including primates. In the cat, stimulation of fast-conducting reticulospinal axons evokes monosynatic EPSPs in hindlimb (238, 241, 243, 244, 543, 616), forelimb (616), trunk (37, 616), and neck (482, 616) motoneurons. In addition there is now evidence for monosynaptic reticulospinal inhibition of neck motoneurons (482). The cell bodies of reticulospinal axons with direct connections to motoneurons seem to be located in nucleus reticularis gigantocellularis (482, 542), nucleus reticularis pontis caudalis (244, 482), and nucleus reticularis ventralis (482). In the cat, their main effects are distributed to motoneurons of knee, ankle, and toe flexors of the hindlimb, but motoneurons of hip and toe extensors also receive some direct excitation (241, 616). In the monkey (546) the monosynaptic reticulospinal projection to lumbar motoneurons is preferentially onto those that innervate proximal muscles (541).

It is not known whether the ipsilateral vestibulospinal projection, present in reptiles and amphibians, has direct connections with motoneurons in these inframmalian species (cf. ref. 542). Such a connection is lacking in the rat (348), but in carnivores such as the cat, stimulation of Deiters' nucleus or of the lateral vestibulospinal tract produces monosynaptic EPSPs in lumbar motoneurons, particularly in those innervating hindlimb extensor muscles (236, 240, 241, 403, 547, 616), as well as in neck (616) and back extensor motoneurons (618). The direct vestibulospinal projections seem, on the other hand, to be absent in cat forelimb motoneurons (616). Monosynaptic vestibulospinal EPSPs are also present in primates, where they have been recorded from hindlimb extensor motoneurons (546). On the other hand, axons of the medial vestibulospinal tract can give rise to monosynaptic inhibition of neck motoneurons (617) and of back motoneurons (618) but not of limb motoneurons (616).

Monosynaptic connections between the rubrospinal tract and spinal motoneurons have been systematically found only in primates, where the motoneurons of distal limb muscles are their main target (544). Monosynaptic EPSPs are only sporadically recorded in the cat lumbar motoneurons (274, 538). In addition to these main descending tracts from the brain stem, it has been found that activation of fastigiospinal fibers produces monosynaptic excitation in neck motoneurons (615).

Direct connections between the corticospinal fibers and motoneurons have developed mainly in primates (59, 60, 484, 574), although they are also reported for the rat (158) and the raccoon (621). In primates, corticospinal fibers are reported to be preferentially distributed to the motoneurons of distal limb muscles (99, 574). In these motoneurons convergence of rubrospinal and corticospinal monosynaptic EPSPs is frequently found [Fig. 36; (539, 544)].

It is interesting to note that, whereas the direct corticomotoneuronal connections in primates develop with a general phylogenetic growth of the pyramidal system, the monosynaptic rubromotoneuronal connections appear in primates without a parallel development of the rubrospinal projection in these species [actually there is apparent diminished anatomical importance of the rubrospinal tract in higher primates; (436, 521)]. The parallel development of cortico- and rubrospinal projections to motoneurons further underlines the intimate relationship between these two tracts, which was discussed above in relation to the control of the segmental reflex transmission and of one of the propriospinal systems (SPINAL NEURONAL CIRCUITS USED IN COMMON BY SEGMENTAL AFFERENTS AND SUPRASPINAL MOTOR CENTERS, p. 512).

The main difference between monosynaptic and polysynaptic effects of descending systems onto motoneurons is that signals conveyed by the direct route bypass the integration with peripheral afferent information and intrinsic spinal activities before they reach the motoneurons. The pattern of descending commands reaching various motor nuclei is thus predetermined by the higher centers. It has therefore been suggested that the direct corticomotoneuronal connections constitute a substrate for the most refined and fractionated movements of the primate hand [(372, 373); see also the chapter by Evarts in this *Handbook*].

The functional importance of the more ancient monosynaptic projections from the reticulospinal and vestibulospinal tracts is more difficult to interpret. The finding (240) that the monosynaptic vestibulospinal excitation of cat hindlimb motoneurons is relatively weak (even lacking) in some cats raises the question of to what extent that projection might be vestigial in higher mammals, especially in view of the fact that the disynaptic vestibulospinal effects are always much larger than the monosynaptic ones.

One remarkable feature of all the monosynaptic EPSPs, which are evoked in spinal motoneurons by activity in the descending systems, is their relatively small amplitude (around 2 mV or below). This suggests that none of these systems can discharge the motoneurons when acting alone. However, this suggestion may not be valid for the highest primates, chimpanzee, and humans, since in these species anatomical evidence indicates that the corticospinal termination among the motor nuclei is much denser than that occurring in the baboon and the rhesus monkey (364, 521). In the case of the corticomotoneuronal connections, the early suggestion of a tremendous increase in amplitude of EPSPs evoked by successive impulses in

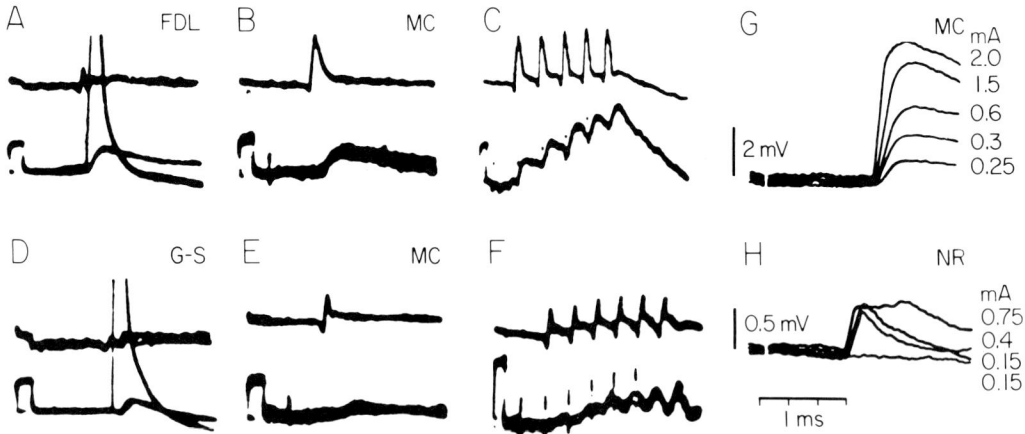

FIG. 36. Monosynaptic connections to α-motoneurons from corticospinal and rubrospinal tracts in primate (rhesus monkey). *Lower traces* in A-F are intracellular records from 2 motoneurons. *Upper traces* are cord dorsum potentials monitoring afferent incoming volleys and corticospinal volleys. All traces in G, H are intracellular records. A-F: frequency potentiation of monosynaptic excitatory postsynaptic potential (EPSP) evoked from motor cortex (MC) in a motoneuron to flexor digitorum longus (FDL, in A-C) and to gastrocnemius-soleus (G-S, in D-F). Antidromic invasion from FDL and G-S nerves in A and D, respectively. Monosynaptic EPSPs following a single shock stimulation of motor cortex are shown in B, E. Growth of monosynaptic EPSPs with repetitive stimuli shown in C, F; same stimulus strengths as in B, E, respectively. Notice the greater potentiation in F than in C. Calibration pulse 1 ms, 5 mV in A, D; 1 ms, 2 mV in B, C, E, F. G, H: convergence of monosynaptic EPSPs from motor cortex (MC) and red nucleus (NR) in an FDL motoneuron. Superimposed *traces* of monosynaptic EPSPs evoked by stimulation of MC (G) and NR (H) of different intensities given to *right* of each *trace*. Note differences in amplitude and time course from MC and NR. [A-F from Tamarova et al. (574); G, H from Shapovalov (539).]

a train (Fig. 21 in ref. 484) also must be taken into consideration. Other investigations have confirmed the occurrence of such temporal potentiation of effects from pyramidal tract fibers [Fig. 36; (366, 456, 491, 574); see also ref. 457] although a contamination of monosynaptic EPSPs by disynaptic responses in all likelihood added to the originally described effects on motoneurons. It seems therefore that even if the monosynaptic EPSPs (from cortex and red nucleus) are important for the pattern of excitation in skilled fractionated movements, they have to operate on a background excitation to be effective. The fine gradation of muscle force must then depend on a proper control of the level of the background excitation of the motoneurons. It may be envisaged that polysynaptic descending effects, the strength of which depends on the segmental afferent input and their integration at interneuronal level, may be particularly important for this aspect of motor control.

ASCENDING PATHWAYS THAT MONITOR SEGMENTAL INTERNEURONAL ACTIVITY

Systematic analysis of single-unit activity readily showed that many neurons of ascending spinal systems are activated from both skin and muscle afferents with very large receptive fields (370). Some of these neurons, subsequently shown to belong to the dorsal spinocerebellar tract (422) or to the spinocervical tract (423), also receive modality-specific monosynaptic excitation from small receptive fields; neurons belonging to other ascending tracts appear to receive only the wide-field excitation (424, 467). Many neurons, particularly those belonging to the ventral spinocerebellar tract, are also inhibited from such wide fields and diverse receptor systems (466). Lundberg (404) recognized that the skin, muscle, and joint afferents contributing to this large-field excitation or inhibition correspond to those evoking the flexor reflex actions in the acute spinal cat (i.e., the flexor reflex afferents; cf. subsection REFLEX PATHWAYS FROM THE "FLEXOR REFLEX AFFERENTS," p. 541). He postulated (404) that ascending neurons with input from the FRA do not signal peripheral events per se but rather monitor the activity of interneurons of reflex pathways. The discovery of the descending excitation of interneurons belonging to reflex pathways from the FRA (*Reflex Pathways From Cutaneous and Joint Afferents and From Groups II and III Muscle Afferents*, p. 535) made it easier to understand why higher centers need feedback information regarding this activity. The ultimate proof that ascending pathways can in fact monitor intrinsic spinal processes was given by the demonstration that ventral spinocerebellar tract cells (VSCT; subsection *Ventral Spinocerebellar Tract*, p. 573) are rhythmically activated in phase with the step cycle even after complete deafferentation of lumbar segments (31).

The hypothesis that ascending pathways monitor activity in spinal interneurons required that transmission to ascending neurons and transmission in reflex pathways to motoneurons respond identically to descending control. The analysis of those ascending pathways that could signal interneuronal activity has thus been intimately linked with studies of the supraspinal control of reflex pathways (SPINAL NEURONAL CIRCUITS USED IN COMMON BY SEGMENTAL AFFERENTS AND SUPRASPINAL MOTOR CENTERS, p. 512).

This section does not describe systematically all of the ascending pathways or subsystems that may signal information regarding intrinsic events in the spinal cord but rather concentrates on the evidence for the existence of such a function. The two principal ways in which ascending neurons may monitor interneuronal activity are shown in Figure 37. The simplest and most direct way is by an ascending collateral whereby the segmental "interneuron" would also function as an ascending tract cell. The other way is by collateral projection from the interneuron to a separate ascending neuron. There is, in fact, evidence for both of these organizations.

Evidence That Ascending FRA Pathways Monitor Activity in Interneurons of Reflex Pathways

Transmission in reflex pathways from the FRA to motoneurons and to primary afferent terminals is subject to inhibitory control from four different reticulospinal pathways (section RETICULOSPINAL INHIBITION OF SEGMENTAL REFLEX TRANSMISSION, p. 560). Three of them, the dorsal reticulospinal system, the noradrenergic, and the serotonergic reticulospinal pathways, have also been tested with regard to modulation of

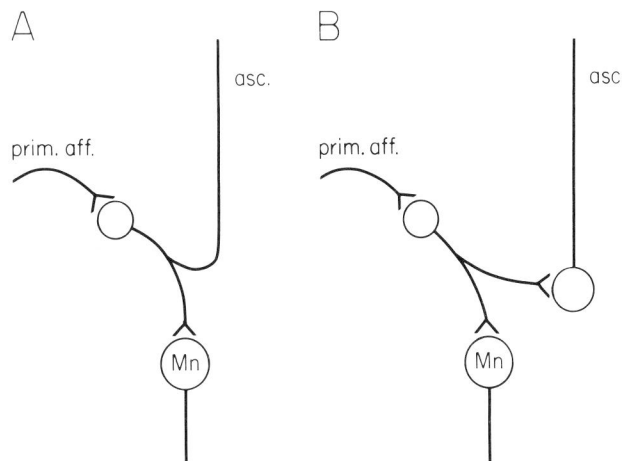

FIG. 37. Diagram illustrating 2 different ways in which ascending neurons may monitor interneuronal activity. *A*: by ascending collaterals from interneurons interposed in segmental reflex pathways. *B*: by separate ascending neurons that receive collateral projections from interneurons interposed in segmental reflex pathways. Mn, motoneuron; asc., ascending neuron; prim. aff., primary afferent.

ascending transmission from the FRA by recording the mass discharge in ventral spinobulbar pathways that are polysynaptically activated from the FRA (12, 15, 167). All three systems inhibit transmission from the FRA to ascending pathways in a way very similar to that seen in motoneurons (cf. section RETICULOSPINAL INHIBITION OF SEGMENTAL REFLEX TRANSMISSION, p. 560). The tonic inhibition of segmental reflexes in the decerebrate state (*Decerebrate Preparation*, p. 564) is also mirrored by a corresponding depression of ascending transmission (269). Figure 38 shows an example of the reversible release of crossed ascending transmission from the FRA, recorded in the ventral quadrant, obtained with a cold block of conduction in descending axons in the dorsal half of the spinal cord (note also the characteristic release of resting activity). In the decerebrate state there is also a similar tonic depression of inhibitory transmission from the FRA to VSCT neurons (269, 468). The differential release of transmission in inhibitory and excitatory pathways from the FRA to motoneurons following brain stem lesions at different levels is found also for the corresponding effects to ascending pathways (94).

Well-defined descending systems such as the corticospinal tract facilitate transmission from the FRA to motoneurons (REFLEX PATHWAYS FROM THE "FLEXOR REFLEX AFFERENTS," p. 541) and likewise facilitate FRA action on ascending tract neurons (279, 421, 431).

Volleys in this tract also evoke a discharge in those spinoreticular neurons that are excited from the FRA, and they inhibit the VSCT neurons that are inhibited from the FRA. In the latter case it was shown that corticospinal inhibition is mediated by the same interneurons that transmit inhibition from the FRA (194, 431).

Rubrospinal volleys have very similar effects. Intracellular recording from spinoreticular neurons excited from FRA also reveal rubral EPSPs, and a convergent action on common interneurons was shown by the rubral facilitation of transmission from the FRA (F. Baldissera, H. Hultborn, and A. Lundberg, unpublished findings). A similar facilitatory interaction was also found for the inhibitory FRA pathway to VSCT cells (34), and because the "reversed-conditioning technique" was used (METHODOLOGICAL CONSIDERATIONS, p. 510), it could be concluded that rubrospinal impulses monosynaptically excite last-order inhibitory interneurons to VSCT neurons just as is the case with the inhibitory reflex paths to motoneurons. Similar results have been obtained with regard to effects from the vestibulospinal tract (40). All these results provide strong indirect evidence that the synaptic effects from the FRA on ascending tract neurons reflect the activity in segmental interneurons that belong to reflex pathways to motoneurons (subsection *Reflex Pathways From Cutaneous and Joint Afferents and From Groups II and III Muscle Afferents*, p. 535).

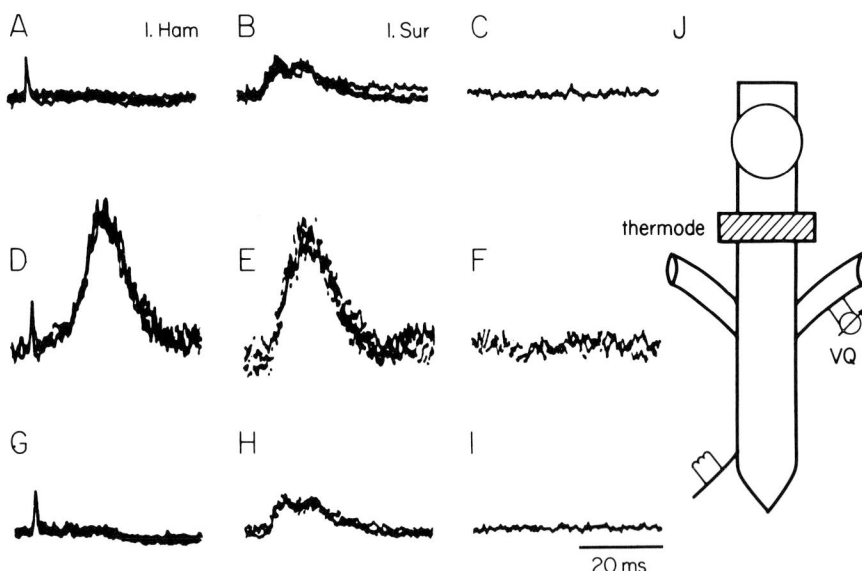

FIG. 38. Decerebrate control of transmission to ascending ventral pathways activated from flexor reflex afferents (FRA). Diagram in *J* illustrates experimental arrangement with a bilateral section of ventral quadrants (VQ) and recording from right VQ of ascending discharge evoked from high-threshold afferents in left hamstring nerve (l. Ham; *A, D, G*) and left sural nerve (l. Sur; *B, E, H*). *C, F, I* show background activity in VQ without stimulation. Comparison of records obtained before (*A–C*), during (*D–F*), and after (*G–I*) cooling of dorsal part of spinal cord (the dorsal column removed) with a thermode illustrates effective blockade of transmission from FRA to ascending tracts in decerebrate state with conducting dorsolateral funiculi (*A–C; G–I*), and release in the spinal state, i.e., during blockade of impulse transmission in dorsal part of the spinal cord (*D–F*). [Adapted from Holmqvist et al. (269).]

Information Via Ascending Collaterals of Interneurons

It is now known that many ascending neurons have collaterals in the spinal cord (252, 383, 437, 499, 564). When such collaterals are given off close to the cell body and are locally distributed, they may make synaptic contacts with interneurons that are part of a segmental motor mechanism and/or regulate ascending activity. Recently it has been shown that some ascending neurons have long collaterals that traverse several segments (264). Such long collaterals are given off by spinocerebellar neurons that are localized in C_7–T_1 segments and that receive polysynaptic inhibition from forelimb flexor-reflex afferents (263). Stimulation at different levels of the spinal cord showed that many of them could be activated antidromically not only from the cerebellar cortex but also from the lower thoracic segments (264). Accordingly these spinocerebellar neurons also function as long propriospinal neurons although their action in the lumbar spinal cord is not known. A similar double function can be ascribed to spinoreticular neurons (activated from the FRA in both hindlimbs; cf. below), which originate in the L_3–L_4 segments and terminate in the lateral reticular nucleus (G. Andersson and K.-E. Ekerot, unpublished observations). Many of them also have descending collaterals to lower lumbar segments but again with unknown action in these segments.

There is another example in the cervical spinal cord of double projecting neurons where the targets of both the ascending and descending branches are known (Figs. 26, 39). The C_3–C_4 propriospinal neurons, which serve as a relay station from higher motor centers to forelimb motoneurons (subsection PROPRIOSPINAL PATHWAYS RELAYING DESCENDING MOTOR COMMANDS, p. 549), can be antidromically activated both from the lateral reticular nucleus (LRN) and from the lateral funicle in the brachial segments (309). Stimulation in the LRN does evoke monosynaptic EPSPs in forelimb neurons, as would be expected from this double projection (Fig. 39A). The LRN and cerebellum thus appear to receive information via the ascending collaterals that mirrors the activity reaching forelimb motoneurons. Complex integration taking place in this propriospinal system, controlled by various higher centers as well as by forelimb afferents, may thus be subject to cerebellar feedback control. If the integration results in an inappropriate activity in the propriospinal neurons, the cerebellum might take corrective measures with a minimal delay so that adjustments are made before the execution of the movement (414).

Another example of an ascending collateral projec-

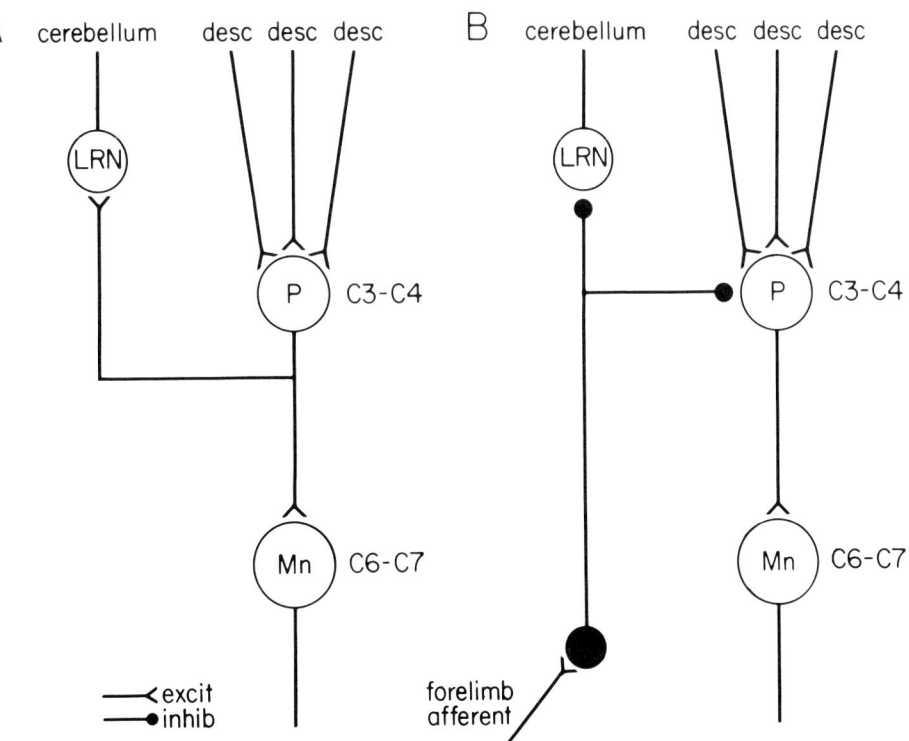

FIG. 39. Wiring diagrams illustrating 2 examples of ascending information from collaterals of neurons interposed in spinal neuronal circuits. *A*: ascending collaterals from propriospinal neurons in C_3–C_4 (P) to lateral reticular nucleus (LRN). Mn, motoneuron. This connection is illustrated in Fig. 26. *B*: ascending collaterals to LRN from inhibitory interneurons (with monosynaptic excitation from forelimb afferents) projecting to propriospinal neurons in C_3–C_4. [*A* from data of Illert and Lundberg (309); *B* from unpublished results of B. Alstermark, M. Illert, and A. Lundberg (see ref. 413).]

tion is shown in Figure 39B. It is known that long ascending inhibitory neurons terminate in the LRN (151), and some of them belong to a pathway activated from the ipsilateral forelimb afferents. This pathway is of interest in relation to the finding that stimulation in the LRN evokes monosynaptic IPSPs in the C_3–C_4 propriospinal neurons, which can be ascribed to antidromic activation of a collateral from long inhibitory neurons originating in the forelimb segments and projecting to the C_3–C_4 propriospinal neurons (414). Apparently the cerebellum (via LRN) takes interest in the activity not only of the propriospinal neurons themselves (cf. Fig. 39A) but also of a subsystem controlling them (Fig. 39B).

Ventral Flexor Reflex Tracts

It was found in the early 1960s that many ascending neurons were activated from FRA of both hindlimbs; these were classified as the bilateral ventral flexor reflex tract, or bVFRT (424, 471). Other ascending neurons were activated only from FRA of one hindlimb and were called the contralateral ventral flexor reflex tract, or coVFRT (contralateral refers to the location of the axon in the spinal cord). The further systematic analysis revealed many subsystems of the VFRT neurons. Some belong to spinoolivocerebellar pathways (371, 469, 470, 475), and others terminate in the LRN and are part of the spinoreticulocerebellar pathways (98). Furthermore the existence of additional subcategories of the VFRT neurons is indicated by their different patterns of terminations in the cerebellar cortex (472, 473). These ascending spinocerebellar systems are described in the chapter by Bloedel and Courville in this *Handbook* and here we only consider their possible functional relationship with reflex pathways from the FRA.

In this connection it should be mentioned that the bilateral receptive field from which the bVFRT is excited originally was puzzling, since it seemed to be at variance with the organization of reflex pathways to motoneurons in the acute spinal cat in which flexion reflex actions dominate ipsilaterally and extension reflex actions dominate contralaterally (cf. *Reflex Pathways From Cutaneous and Joint Afferents and From Groups II and III Muscle Afferents*, p. 535). Therefore ascending neurons that signal information from the interneuronal pathways mediating these reflexes would be expected to draw their excitation from one limb only. However, it was subsequently found that the FRA have alternative reflex pathways to motoneurons and that some are bilaterally supplied with convergence from the two limbs occurring at an interneuronal level (*Reflex Pathways From Cutaneous and Joint Afferents and From Groups II and III Muscle Afferents*, p. 535). The last-order interneurons of these bilateral reflex pathways are monosynaptically excited by volleys in both long propriospinal neurons and the vestibulospinal tract [(332); G. ten Bruggencate and A. Lundberg, unpublished observations; see ref. 413]. The bVFRT neurons are also monosynaptically excited from neurons originating in the lower brain stem (270). Further experiments revealed that bVFRT neurons are indeed monosynaptically excited from vestibulospinal neurons and that they are also monosynaptically excited by volleys in long propriospinal neurons (238).

The similarity in the convergence onto bVFRT neurons that project to LRN and onto the last-order neurons of reflex pathways bilaterally excited from the FRA certainly indicates a functional relationship. The simplest explanation would be a common origin of the two projections, as indicated in Figure 39A, with a collateral projection to LRN from the last-order neurons (identical to bVFRT cells) in the reflex pathway to motoneurons. However, in that case antidromic activation of bVFRT axons in the LRN should evoke monosynaptic EPSPs in hindlimb motoneurons. No such monosynaptic effect has so far been recorded in lumbar motoneurons innervating knee, ankle, and toe extensors or in knee flexors (B. Alstermark, A. Lundberg, and E. Sybirska, unpublished observations). It remains to be learned whether a projection exists to other motor nuclei or whether the functional organization is in fact of the type shown in Figure 37B. In the latter case, it is difficult to understand the functional significance of a parallel monosynaptic projection from vestibulospinal and long propriospinal axons onto both the ascending bVFRT neurons and the last-order neurons of the segmental reflex pathways (cf., however, subsection *Ventral Spinocerebellar Tract*, p. 573, for the interpretation of the information forwarded by the ventral spinocerebellar tract cells).

Intracellular recording from reticulocerebellar neurons in the LRN has revealed that many of the long ascending neurons projecting to the LRN, including those of bVFRT type, are inhibitory (151). Ekerot and Oscarsson (151) postulated that they carried information regarding activity in inhibitory spinal pathways. Such a function would be explicable if inhibitory neurons had an ascending collateral, as in the example illustrated in Figure 37A. However, the inhibitory bVFRT cells are probably not last-order interneurons in reflex pathways to motoneurons because, again, stimulation of the LRN on either side does not evoke monosynaptic IPSPs in hindlimb motoneurons (B. Alstermark, A. Lundberg, and E. Sybirska, unpublished observations). In relation to the discussion on inhibitory interactions between reflex pathways from the FRA (REFLEX PATHWAYS FROM THE "FLEXOR REFLEX AFFERENTS," p. 541; cf. Fig. 22), the possibility should be considered that the bVFRT forwards information on activity in an inhibitory pathway from the FRA onto another neuronal pathway to motoneurons.

In connection with the bilateral receptive fields of bVFRT, it should be recalled that both hindlimbs contribute to the PAD evoked from FRA. This holds true both for the PAD evoked in the acute spinal cat and the late PAD evoked after administration of dopa (*Presynaptic Inhibition of Transmission From Primary Afferents*, p. 554). On the basis of differences in the inhibitory effects of dopa and of the NA-mimetic drug clonidine on transmission from the FRA to motoneurons and to primary afferent terminals, Anderson and Sjölund (21) suggested that one of the channels of the ventral spinoolivocerebellar system is functionally related to pathways from the FRA to primary afferent terminals and signals information regarding transmission in these pathways. Their findings also support the hypothesis that presynaptic inhibition from the FRA has a definite function in motor control (cf. *Presynaptic Inhibition of Transmission From Primary Afferents*, p. 554). The inhibitory pathways to the LRN may also be considered in relation to the FRA inhibition of transmission to primary afferent terminals (subsection *Presynaptic Inhibition of Transmission From Primary Afferents*, p. 554). Other channels of the ventral spinoolivocerebellar system are influenced by clonidine and dopa in a way expected if they signal information regarding interneuronal activity in reflex pathways to motoneurons (561). It is noteworthy that the FRA excitation in the latter case is not of bilateral origin but is supplied from one limb, as would be expected for ascending pathways signaling information from the traditional reflex pathways from the FRA to motoneurons.

Ventral Spinocerebellar Tract

Analysis of ascending activity in the spinal cord revealed that VSCT neurons are monosynaptically excited from Ib-afferents contralateral to the ascending axons (465). The inhibitory effects from the FRA discussed above were disclosed when this monosynaptic discharge was used to test the effect of conditioning volleys in the FRA (466). This inhibitory action was confirmed with intracellular recording from VSCT neurons with cell bodies mainly in Rexed's layers VI and VII (142, 283). Another subsystem of VSCT, which takes origin from the spinal border cells of Cooper and Sherrington (104, 438), has many neurons monosynaptically excited from Ia-afferents (81, 328, 428). In addition some VSCT neurons are monosynaptically activated from both Ia- and Ib-afferents, and another subgroup is characterized by absence of monosynaptic connections from any set of primary afferents (142, 382, 428).

Intracellular analysis has also revealed that many VSCT neurons, like motoneurons, are disynaptically inhibited by volleys in group I muscle afferents (142, 382, 428). Disynaptic Ia IPSPs are common in the spinal border cells, and in one subgroup of these VSCT cells the same Ia volleys evoked both monosynaptic EPSPs and disynaptic IPSPs (251, 428). To explain these findings it was postulated that the Ia IPSP in VSCT cells was a collateral action from the inhibitory interneurons intercalated in the reciprocal Ia inhibitory pathway to motoneurons [Fig. 40A; (410)]. The VSCT cells would then carry ascending information regarding the activity in the reciprocal Ia inhibitory pathway, provided there is sufficient background excitation, which seems ensured by the parallel Ia monosynaptic excitation (Fig. 40). Lundberg (410) also suggested that the descending monosynaptic excitation of VSCT cells is in a corresponding way collateral to the descending input to interneurons of inhibitory reflex paths to motoneurons (Fig. 40B). The general input-output comparator hypothesis, based on a number of such observations, implies that inhibitory output from a set of interneurons is measured against the excitatory input to the same last-order inhibitory interneurons (410).

The detailed information available regarding the convergence onto the Ia inhibitory interneurons (subsection *Pathways From Ia-Afferents and Their Control by γ-Motoneurons*, p. 519) presents an excellent possibility to test the hypothesis of a double projection from interneurons onto motoneurons and ascending neurons (Fig. 40). The inhibitory action from recurrent motor axon collaterals provided a critical test, since it operates selectively on Ia inhibitory interneurons (subsection *Recurrent Inhibition*, p. 513). Gustafsson and Lindström (251) found that Ia IPSPs are as effectively depressed in VSCT cells as in motoneurons (Fig. 41) and also that the time course of the recurrent depression is the same in both cases. The depression was found for Ia IPSPs from flexors or extensors and was exerted whether or not a monosynaptic Ia EPSP was evoked from the same nerve. Other experiments revealed facilitation of Ia IPSP in VSCT cells from the same primary afferents (251) and the same supraspinal centers that facilitate Ia IPSPs in motoneurons (34, 40, 194). The vestibulospinal facilitation was monosynaptic (to the Ia-interneurons) and the rubrospinal was disynaptic, as for the reciprocal Ia inhibitory pathway to motoneurons (Fig. 42). The evidence from these findings, although indirect, appears to be so strong that a double projection from the Ia inhibitory interneurons is virtually proved.

In connection with the input-output comparator hypothesis it should be noted that volleys in all descending tracts that excite Ia inhibitory interneurons also may excite VSCT cells (34, 39, 194). The input-output comparator hypothesis does not imply that each VSCT cell signaling Ia inhibition receives collateral action from all the excitatory systems converging on the Ia inhibitory interneurons. Fractional sampling instead seems to be the rule. For example, some VSCT cells with collateral action from Ia inhibitory interneurons do not receive monosynaptic excitation from Ia-afferents. Such cells may signal inhibition against excitation from the vestibulo-, rubro-, and corticospinal tracts, all of which also supply excitation to the Ia inhibitory interneurons [subsection *Pathways From Ia-Afferents and Their Control by γ-Motoneurons*, p. 519; (34, 39, 194)]. It seems likely that the cerebellum,

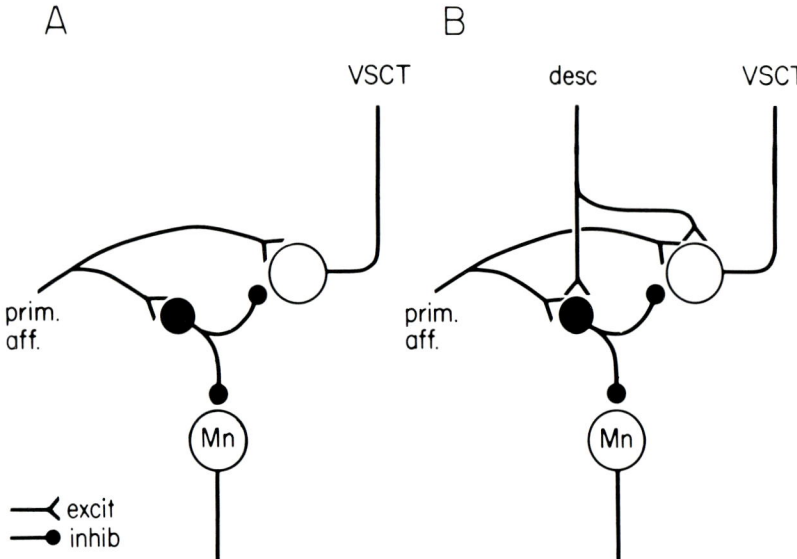

FIG. 40. Wiring diagrams illustrating hypothesis that information transferred by ventral spinocerebellar tract (VSCT) neurons reflects relation between input to and output from inhibitory segmental interneurons. *A*: diagram illustrating convergence on a VSCT neuron of monosynaptic excitation from primary afferents (prim. aff.) and disynaptic inhibition evoked from the same primary afferents. Disynaptic inhibition of VSCT neuron is due to a collateral projection from interneurons transmitting disynaptic inhibitory postsynaptic potentials to motoneurons (Mn). In this case the VSCT neuron would compare excitatory input to interneurons from primary afferents and the resulting activity of the inhibitory interneuron. *B*: in addition to connections in *A* there is also a descending motor pathway (desc) giving monosynaptic excitation and disynaptic inhibition of VSCT neuron. The descending monosynaptic excitation is collateral to excitation of interneurons, and the disynaptic inhibition is again due to collateral projection from interneuron. Such a VSCT neuron thus compares excitatory input to interneurons from primary afferents and the descending pathway with the resulting activation of the interneuron.

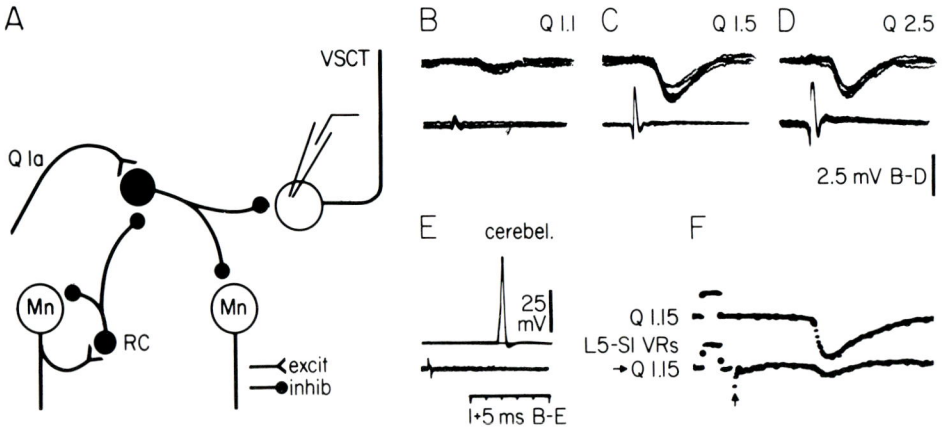

FIG. 41. Recurrent depression of a Ia inhibitory postsynaptic potential (IPSP) in a ventral spinocerebellar tract (VSCT) neuron. Experimental arrangement and relevant neuronal circuits are illustrated in *A*. Mn, motoneuron; RC, Renshaw cell; Q, quadriceps. *Upper traces* in *B–E* are intracellular records from a VSCT neuron (identification from ipsilateral anterior lobe of cerebellum in *E*). *Lower traces* are records from L_5 dorsal root entry zone. Voltage calibrations refer to intracellular records. *B–D*: disynaptic Ia IPSPs from Q nerve. Stimulation strength is indicated in times threshold of lowest threshold afferent fibers. *F*: averaged records of submaximal Ia IPSPs from Q (*upper trace*) combined with conditioning stimulation of L_5–S_1 ventral roots (VRs; *lower trace*). *Arrow* below *lower trace* indicates arrival of the VR volley to the spinal cord (calibration pulse 1 mV, 2 ms). [Adapted from Gustafsson and Lindström (251).]

to regulate reciprocal Ia inhibition, requires quantitative information regarding the contribution from each of the systems controlling the Ia inhibitory interneurons. This fractionation hypothesis implies that individual VSCT cells carry only part of the total information relating to the Ia inhibitory pathway. This concept may also help to explain why volleys in Ia-afferents evoke monosynaptic EPSPs in some VSCT

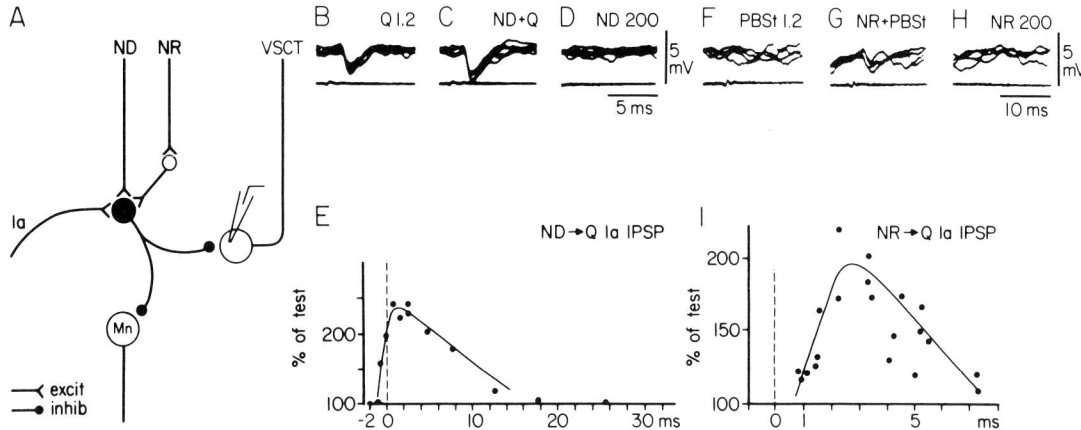

FIG. 42. Facilitation of Ia inhibitory postsynaptic potentials (IPSPs) in ventral spinocerebellar tract (VSCT) neurons from vestibulospinal and rubrospinal tracts. *A* shows experimental arrangement and relevant neuronal circuits. Mn, motoneurons; ND, Deiters' nucleus; NR, red nucleus. *Upper traces* in *B–D* and *F–H* are intracellular records from 2 different VSCT neurons. *Lower traces* are from dorsal root entry zone. Voltage calibrations refer to intracellular records. Strength of stimulation in ND and NR is indicated in μA, stimulation of nerves in times threshold of lowest threshold afferent fibers. *B–E*: facilitation of a quadriceps-evoked (Q) Ia IPSP from the ND. Graph in *E* gives amplitude of IPSP in percent of unconditioned test (ordinate) in relation to time interval between arrival of descending volley from ND (zero ms on abscissa) and incoming Q volley (*interrupted line* indicates synchronous arrival). Facilitation started with Q volley arriving slightly before ND volley, which indicates monosynaptic coupling of descending fibers with interneuron mediating the Ia IPSP. *F–I*: facilitation from NR of IPSPs evoked from posterior biceps–semitendinosus nerve (PBSt). Records in *F–H* show a facilitation of a Ia IPSP from PBSt. Graph in *I* shows time course of facilitation of a Ia IPSP from Q in another VSCT neuron. Amplitude of IPSP is given in percent of unconditioned test (ordinate) in relation to time interval in arrival of 1st rubrospinal volley (zero ms on abscissa) and the incoming Q volley (*interrupted line* indicates synchronous arrival). [*B–E* adapted from Baldissera and Roberts (40); *F–I* adapted from Baldissera and Bruggencate (34).]

cells but not disynaptic IPSPs, as implied in Figure 40 (380, 410). Clearly such cells cannot compare directly the input and output of the Ia inhibitory interneurons, but they may have the function of providing an excitatory reference to the information provided by the comparing cells. The cerebellum could obtain a measure of the transmission through the Ia inhibitory interneurons by subtracting the firing of the input-output cells from that of the reference cells.

Lundberg (410) has pointed out that some inhibitory actions on VSCT cells may be collateral not to inhibition of motoneurons but to an inhibitory input to the interneurons whose function is signaled. The monosynaptic descending IPSP elicited in some VSCT cells by stimulation of the MLF could thus be collateral to an action on segmental interneurons (39). There are two examples of inhibitory actions on VSCT neurons that may relate to reciprocal Ia inhibition. A small fraction of VSCT cells receives recurrent IPSPs from motor axon collaterals (381) indicating that VSCT cells receive collaterals from Renshaw cells, which also terminate on Ia inhibitory interneurons and α-motoneurons (subsection *Recurrent Inhibition*, p. 513). The same VSCT cells also received Ia EPSPs. Lindström and Schomburg (381) write "By comparing the output of Ia comparator VSCT cells with the output from the other type of Ia excited VSCT cells, with and without recurrent inhibition, the cerebellum can determine to which extent the output from the Ia inhibitory interneurones is determined by Ia excitation and by the recurrent inhibition respectively." Another example may be provided by the VSCT cells in which reciprocal Ia actions are evoked, e.g., monosynaptic EPSPs from knee flexor and disynaptic IPSPs from knee extensors (251, 428). As an explanation for this convergence it was suggested that such VSCT cells may "compare collateral effects from excitatory and inhibitory pathways converging on motoneurones" (410). However, this pattern may also reflect the input convergence onto the Ia inhibitory interneurons, since it has later been shown that mutual inhibitory connections exist between "opposite" Ia inhibitory interneurons [Fig. 11; (287)]. The reciprocal Ia IPSPs in these VSCT cells may thus represent the input from the opposite Ia inhibitory interneurons to those whose Ia input gives the collateral excitation (380). However, since in all likelihood "corresponding" α-motoneurons and Ia inhibitory interneurons receive collaterals from the same Ia-afferents, Ia inhibitory interneurons, and Renshaw cells (subsection *Pathways From Ia-Afferents and Their Control by γ-Motoneurons*, p. 519), it may be impossible to decide whether this VSCT information relates to synaptic effects onto Ia inhibitory interneurons or to α-motoneurons, or indeed to both of them. This problem has also been discussed in relation to the mono- and disynaptic EPSPs evoked in VSCT cells by volleys in the vestibulospinal tract (39).

It has been suggested that the VSCT signal information from other segmental reflex pathways as well. Disynaptic and/or trisynaptic IPSPs from Ib- (or possibly Ia- and Ib-) afferents are fairly common in VSCT cells (142, 382, 428). The suggestion that these IPSPs are mediated by collaterals from corresponding inhibitory pathways to motoneurons is supported by the finding that transmission to VSCT cells is facilitated by volleys in the cortico- and rubrospinal tracts (34, 194), as found for transmission in the corresponding pathway to motoneurons (subsection *Reflex Pathways From Ib Tendon Organ Afferents*, p. 530). Similarly the corresponding rubrospinal action is in both cases monosynaptically exerted on the intercalated neurons [same subsection, p. 530; (34)]. Some of the monosynaptic excitation of VSCT cells from Ib muscle afferents and from Ia- and Ib-afferents may also be collateral to the input to Ib reflex pathways to motoneurons (same subsection, p. 530). In some VSCT cells there is evidence for convergence of monosynaptic EPSPs and disynaptic IPSPs from the same Ib-afferents, as required for input-output comparing cells (382), but it is also common to find IPSPs evoked from Ia- or Ib-afferents of other nerves (382, 428). One group of VSCT cells that is characterized by a special pattern of monosynaptic group I excitation receives Ia IPSPs that are not depressed from recurrent motor axon collaterals and thus cannot be mediated by collaterals of Ia inhibitory interneurons (382). It has been suggested that these IPSPs are mediated by the Ia excited interneurons in the intermediate nucleus and that these interneurons might be inhibitory onto the Ib reflex pathway to motoneurons (277, 322, 380, 410). Further investigation of the hypothesis that VSCT carries information regarding transmission in Ib inhibitory reflex pathways to motoneurons may become possible with advancing knowledge regarding the functional organization of these reflex pathways (same subsection, p. 530). For example, to assess the finding that many VSCT cells receive large monosynaptic Ib EPSPs from hip extensors and knee flexors (142, 382, 466), it would be desirable to obtain information regarding the functional organization of reflex pathways from these muscles to motoneurons.

Monosynaptic input to VSCT from the periphery appears to exist only from Ia- and Ib-afferents, which are also the only afferents known to supply disynaptic inhibitory pathways to hindlimb motoneurons. Spinocerebellar neurons of the forelimb segments, which probably are equivalent to VSCT (263, 474), also receive monosynaptic EPSPs from cutaneous afferents. Correspondingly it has been recently shown that a disynaptic inhibitory pathway exists from cutaneous afferents to forelimb motoneurons (313); in hindlimb segments the minimal linkage appears to be trisynaptic (subsection *Reflex Pathways From Cutaneous and Joint Afferents and From Groups II and III Muscle Afferents*, p. 535). The inhibition from the FRA referred to in the beginning of this section is one of the most characteristic features in VSCT cells. These IPSPs may be mediated at least partly (410) by collaterals of last-order interneurons of the private inhibitory reflex pathways from the FRA (i.e., not shared with Ia-afferents), and VSCT cells may thus convey information from those reflex pathways whose function was discussed in subsection REFLEX PATHWAYS FROM THE "FLEXOR-REFLEX AFFERENTS," p. 541.

It must be emphasized that the available evidence suggests that individual VSCT cells may convey information on transmission through different inhibitory reflex pathways to motoneurons [the multiplicity hypothesis; (410)]. This suggests a mixture of information that might represent an integrated message regarding different inhibitory reflexes acting together in a given movement (410). This multiplicity makes it somewhat difficult to assess the significance of some descending excitatory actions on VSCT cells. For example, when rubrospinal volleys evoke monosynaptic EPSPs in a VSCT cell that receives IPSPs from Ib-afferents and the FRA (34), then the monosynaptic EPSPs may be collateral to the rubral action in the last-order inhibitory interneurons in the reflex pathway from Ib-afferents and/or the FRA, both of which are monosynaptically excited by impulses in rubrospinal fibers (subsections *Reflex Pathways From Ib Tendon Organ Afferents*, p. 530, and *Reflex Pathways from Cutaneous and Joint Afferents and From Groups II and III Muscle Afferents*, p. 535). Nevertheless the effects produced by descending volleys on VSCT cells can be well described as reflecting the actions on interneurons belonging to various reflex pathways to motoneurons and are thus in general keeping with the hypothesis that VSCT monitors transmission in these pathways.

GENERAL SUMMARY AND EPILOGUE

The main part of the experimental results that have been discussed in this chapter refer to the analysis of functional subsystems in the spinal cord, as characterized by the organization of connections to interneurons in different reflex pathways. By the indirect technique of recording synaptic responses in motoneurons as well as direct recording from interneurons, it has been shown that descending pathways connect with interneurons interposed in various segmental reflex pathways and also that activity in one reflex pathway may influence interneurons mediating other reflex actions. This approach has provided detailed knowledge of how activity in descending pathways from supraspinal motor centers interacts with the segmental neuronal circuits in the way broadly envisaged already by Foster and Sherrington (186, 550). In this closing section we first summarize the main results and their conceptual framework and then consider the possibilities to investigate how the functional subsystems are utilized during movements in animals and humans.

General Summary

The description of the spinal functional units began with an account of the recurrent inhibition that is evoked via motor axon collaterals and Renshaw cells (subsection *Recurrent Inhibition*, p. 513). This circuitry differs from all others in the sense that it is not directly linked to any specific afferent input but rather to the motor output. The negative feedback character of this pathway has long been emphasized, but more elaborate hypotheses had to await further experimental analysis. The projection of Renshaw cells to γ-motoneurons, interneurons mediating reciprocal Ia inhibition and Renshaw cells in addition to their connections with α-motoneurons, showed that recurrent inhibition from motor axon collaterals contributes to the regulation of several types of neurons that are involved in the final stage in motor control (the output stage). The pattern of distribution from different motor nuclei further shows that this regulation is mainly confined to neurons controlling synergists and antagonists of the same joint. The fact that Renshaw cells are subject to excitatory and inhibitory control from both segmental reflex pathways and descending tracts suggests that the feedback regulation provided by the recurrent pathway can be used in a versatile way during different types of movements, rather than in a stereotyped manner depending only on the input from firing motoneurons. The hypotheses on the functional role of the recurrent inhibition have focused on three possible aspects. It has thus been proposed that it may help to shape either the spatial or temporal pattern of the motor output. According to the third theory, the main effect would be to control the gain of transmission across the neurons that receive the recurrent inhibition. According to the latter hypothesis, the supraspinal facilitation and inhibition of Renshaw cells allows recurrent inhibition to serve as a variable gain regulator at the motoneuronal level in order to obtain an optimal resolution in the force generation during weak as well as strong contractions.

The following subsections were devoted to the proprioceptive reflexes from muscle spindles and Golgi tendon organs. Since the activity of muscle spindle afferents is intimately related to that of γ-motoneurons, they are regarded as parts of one and the same functional unit. The reflex action from the muscle spindle Ia-afferents and the central control of fusimotor neurons were therefore discussed together (subsection *Pathways From Ia-Afferents and Their Control by γ-Motoneurons*, p. 519). The experimental material may preferably be considered in the light either of Merton's hypothesis on a follow-up length servo of extrafusal contraction by a central activation of γ-motoneurons or of the later idea of a servo assistance due to a coactivation of α- and γ-motoneurons. In many discussions of these ideas the simplifying assumption is often made that γ-initiated Ia activity reaches only homonymous motoneurons. There is, on the contrary, a wide distribution of monosynaptic Ia excitation not only to motoneurons of close synergists at the same joint but often also of muscles acting at neighboring joints. This was first shown for the cat hindlimb but was later demonstrated also for the forelimb in the cat and the forearm and hand in the baboon. This wide distribution of Ia effects thus does not prevent the performance of discrete movements and indeed suggests that the selection of which muscles shall contract must rely on a central control of α-motoneurons rather than by excitation via the γ-loop.

In parallel with the monosynaptic excitation of motoneurons, activity in Ia-fibers also causes a reciprocal inhibition of motoneurons innervating antagonists. The reciprocal Ia inhibition is disynaptic and the interposed interneurons (Ia inhibitory interneurons) have been identified. The extensive analysis of these interneurons revealed an enormous convergence onto them from segmental as well as descending pathways. It turned out that α-motoneurons and Ia inhibitory interneurons with the same excitatory Ia input display a strikingly similar convergence, which led to the general conclusion that α-motoneurons and "corresponding" Ia inhibitory interneurons are controlled in parallel by supraspinal motor centers as well as from segmental afferent systems. This parallelism reflects the need for coordination between contraction of agonists and relaxation of antagonists in many movements.

The control of γ-motoneurons can be judged either by direct recording of their activity or indirectly from the firing of corresponding muscle spindle afferents. The latter method has the advantages of allowing separation of activity in dynamic and static γ-motoneurons and of being applicable for experiments on humans and on freely moving animals. Stimulation of segmental afferents and of various motor centers in the brain has revealed numerous examples of parallel effects onto corresponding α- and γ-motoneurons (static and/or dynamic). There is also evidence, however, for an additional separate control of γ-motoneurons that could allow for considerable flexibility in the α-γ-linkage. The analysis of activity in muscle spindle afferents from respiratory muscles during respiration in anesthetized cats and from hindlimb muscles in decerebrate cats walking a treadmill suggested a tightly linked coactivation of α- and γ-motoneurons. Recent results obtained during isometric voluntary contractions in humans also revealed a rigid coupling. In contrast recording from limb muscle afferents of freely walking cats and from jaw muscle afferents in cat and monkey now suggests a greater flexibility in the coactivation.

It now seems established that the activity in muscle spindle Ia-afferents cannot by itself produce an excitation of α-motoneurons strong enough to subserve a follow-up-length servo as envisaged by Merton. Moreover the importance of the monosynaptic Ia excitation for servo assistance, which would result in compensatory contraction during increasing loads on the muscle, has been questioned in the last years. The load compensation that actually occurs has been ascribed instead to long-loop circuits via the brain stem and the motor cortex. It has also been established recently that activity in Ia-afferents can excite homonymous motoneurons by complex polysynaptic spinal pathways. The understanding of the contribution by the γ-loop to the motor performance is thus presently less clear than it may have seemed a few years ago.

The second main proprioceptive system originates from the Golgi tendon organs (subsection *Reflex Pathways From Ib Tendon Organ Afferents*, p. 530). Their low threshold during muscle contraction suggests that this system is involved in the normal control of muscle force. The finding that activation of Ib-afferents leads to an autogenetic inhibition of α-motoneurons then led to the idea that the tendon organs and their central pathways might provide for a "force-servo" system as contrasted to an alleged "length-servo" system from muscle spindles. There are many experimental findings, however, that are not easily fitted into such an hypothesis. The distribution of inhibitory and excitatory Ib actions is very wide and the autogenetic inhibition represents only a minor part of the effects; the regulated objects are not individual muscles but virtually all the limb muscles. Moreover descending activity seems able to control the Ib actions not only quantitatively but also qualitatively by selecting the pattern of distribution. The interneurons mediating the Ib actions are also subject to a very large convergence. Besides facilitatory and inhibitory control from descending tracts, there is an extensive convergence from segmental pathways with monosynaptic excitation from muscle spindle Ia-afferents and disynaptic excitation from cutaneous and joint afferents. All this segmental convergence raises the question of whether this pathway is primarily concerned with Golgi tendon organs (with facilitation from many other sources) or if it should be considered as a pathway used in common by muscle (Ia- and Ib-), skin, and joint afferents. In any case it provides an example of a reflex whose primary effect is inhibition, which in a negative feedback fashion controls muscle tension during active movements. The supraspinal control of the interposed interneurons would adjust the gain to allow regulation over a wide range of forces commanded by the brain.

The reflex pathways from cutaneous and joint afferents and from high-threshold muscle afferents were reviewed in subsection *Reflex Pathways From Cutaneous and Joint Afferents and From Groups II and III Muscle Afferents*, p. 535. Some examples of discrete reflexes from individual afferent systems, such as the toe extensor reflex evoked from the plantar cushion, were discussed. In addition to such specific reflexes stimulation of these afferents evokes common reflex actions that in the spinal cat have the pattern of the flexion reflex, i.e., excitation of motoneurons to ipsilateral flexors and contralateral extensors with appropriate reciprocal inhibition of antagonists. Volleys in cutaneous nerves supplying very different skin areas produce qualitatively similar effects as does activity in high-threshold muscle afferents from either flexor or extensor muscles. This pattern of synaptic effects is therefore largely devoid of spatial and modality specificity. Because of their common central action these afferent systems were collectively referred to as the "flexor reflex afferents" or FRA. It was suggested that these afferents converge onto common interneurons that then project to motoneurons. This hypothesis was supported by several observations. First, many interneurons receive an excitatory convergence from all these sources. Second, spatial facilitation in motoneurons between responses evoked by different afferents within the FRA system has confirmed that some of these interneurons are indeed interposed in reflex pathways to motoneurons. Furthermore, conditioning supraspinal volleys affect transmission from all the afferents within the FRA system in a similar way. Activation of these afferents also produces conjoint actions in many ascending tract cells (either excitation or inhibition). It has been suggested that these effects in ascending tract cells are due to collateral innervation from interneurons mediating the segmental reflex actions. Such ascending pathways would thus monitor the activity in the segmental FRA pathways. Such observations make it highly likely that all of the afferents classified together in the FRA system do indeed converge upon common interneurons in reflex pathways to motoneurons. It is important to stress that such a conclusion does not refute the possibility that the same afferents in parallel support separate reflex pathways in which their spatial and modality specificity is preserved. It should also be recalled that many afferents that are part of the FRA system are not nociceptors, but are low-threshold mechanoreceptors that are activated during all types of normal movements, a fact that may be overlooked because of the term "flexor reflex afferents."

From the beginning of the analysis of the FRA pathways it became evident that the pattern of effects was not always the same; i.e., sometimes motoneurons of ipsilateral extensors were excited or those of flexors were inhibited. Various brain stem lesions in the decerebrate cat made it possible to obtain a selective control of the inhibitory and excitatory FRA pathways. In acute spinal cats, intravenous administration of the noradrenergic precursor dopa abolishes the ordinary short-latency FRA actions (both excitation and inhibition) and reveals a new long-lasting response of long latency. These observations lead to the conclusion that there are a number of alternative FRA pathways to each motor nucleus. Further analysis of these pathways suggests that activation of one of them may preclude simultaneous transmission through the other ones depending on mutually inhibitory interactions. It is likely that descending activity may mobilize any of the alternative pathways, which in turn would mediate the supraspinal action onto the selected motoneurons. It has been assumed that transmission along any particular FRA path prevents transmission through the other alternative pathways. When the motoneurons are activated through one of these paths and the movement starts, the barrage of impulses in afferents belonging to the FRA system would support transmission along the already selected path. According to this view the FRA system would then provide a positive feedback that could reinforce and prolong the descending activation. Such a positive support appears purposeful since it may relieve the descending supraspinal pathways from being solely responsible for the entire excitatory drive of the motoneurons during active movement and yet leave control with the supraspinal motor centers.

The long-latency FRA responses that are revealed in acute spinal cats after dopa administration were described in some detail. The half-center organization of the interneuronal network mediating these reflexes was discussed in relation to spinal generation of alternating activity in flexors and extensors during locomotion.

As is clear from the preceding description, the interneurons interposed in segmental reflex pathways are characterized by a great convergence from both segmental afferents and descending pathways. A similar convergence is found also in other intrinsic spinal neurons localized outside the limb segments into which they are projecting. They are referred to as propriospinal neurons (subsection *Propriospinal Neurons*, p. 549). Some propriospinal systems seem to play an important role in mediating effects from higher centers to motoneurons and interneurons of the segmental reflex apparatus. These propriospinal neurons are characterized by convergent excitatory effects from many supraspinal motor centers, but in some cases segmental afferents may contribute as well. Several short-axoned systems of this type have been described with their cell bodies localized a few segments rostral to the limb segments they innervate. Long propriospinal neurons serve to coordinate the activity in the forelimb and hindlimb segments. There are both descending and ascending propriospinal systems of this type and their neurons have an efficient input from segmental afferents though descending effects may also contribute.

The neuronal organization of the spinal cord allows for a flexible pattern of reflex action not only by interactive mechanisms at the interneuronal level but also by a presynaptic control of transmission from primary afferents (subsection *Presynaptic Inhibition of Transmission From Primary Afferents*, p. 554). In some cases the distribution of presynaptic inhibition has the general feature of a negative feedback. For example, primary afferent depolarization in cutaneous fibers is produced from other cutaneous fibers, particularly from those of the same submodality. However, the entire distribution of presynaptic inhibition between primary afferents cannot be contained within the simplifying concept of a negative feedback. Usually several classes of afferents contribute to the primary afferent depolarization in any given group of afferents and the FRA in particular seem to have access to virtually all groups of afferents.

The segmental pathways mediating primary afferent depolarization are polysynaptic, which allows for interactions at an interneuronal level. Such interaction occurs both between different segmental systems and between descending projections and segmental inputs. Stimulation of various motor centers in the brain evokes primary afferent depolarization—not indiscriminately in all types of afferents, but according to specific patterns. Such stimulation usually facilitates transmission in segmental reflex pathways to primary afferents, which are operative also in the acute spinal state. In other cases descending activity may open up segmental pathways in which transmission is normally inhibited.

The parallel effect from higher centers on the interneuronal pathways to primary afferent terminals and to motoneurons suggests that presynaptic inhibition has a regulatory function when reflex pathways to motoneurons are utilized by higher centers. It is an open question whether the presynaptic inhibition primarily serves to control the gain of the afferent transmission or has a spatial function, giving a local sign to the reflexes by limiting stray excitation.

The idea of Foster and Sherrington that higher centers use complex spinal mechanisms in their control of motor activity is now supported by the findings that activity in the cortico-, rubro-, and vestibulospinal tracts indeed utilize segmental reflex pathways by excitatory action on the interposed interneurons. In section RETICULOSPINAL INHIBITION OF SEGMENTAL REFLEX TRANSMISSION, p. 560, a number of reticulospinal pathways were described whose primary function is to inhibit interneuronal transmission in segmental pathways. There are four groups of pathways of this kind, but with partly different actions; the dorsal reticulospinal system, the ventral reticulospinal pathways, and two monoaminergic (noradrenergic and serotonergic) systems. The reticulospinal inhibition of segmental transmission is not limited to reflex pathways to motoneurons but also acts on transmission to primary afferents and ascending tract cells.

The decerebrate preparation is characterized by both a high excitability of motoneurons and the appearance of exaggerated stretch reflexes. Many years ago the importance of a release of descending excitatory action to α- and γ-motoneurons for the development of tonic stretch reflexes was stressed. However, a reticulospinal inhibition of transmission in pathways mediating autogenetic inhibition from the stretched muscles now seems to be of equal importance. The evidence suggests that the dorsal reticulospinal system and serotonergic pathways are responsible, since both of them are tonically active in the decerebrate state. Furthermore activation of the serotonergic system in the acute spinal cat causes several effects that have a strong resemblance to the decerebrate state, as for example, the reappearance of tonic stretch reflexes.

The emphasis in this chapter has been placed on integration at an interneuronal level because the effects in motoneurons from descending supraspinal and peripheral afferent fiber systems to a large extent are mediated via common interneurons. There are, however, several descending systems that also project directly onto the motoneurons (section DIRECT PROJECTIONS OF DESCENDING PATHWAYS TO α-MOTONEURONS, p. 567). In primates monosynaptic excitation of α-motoneurons has thus been described from the reticulo-, vestibulo-, rubro-, and corticospinal tracts. Signals that are conveyed by such direct routes escape the integration with peripheral afferents and intrinsic spinal activity before they reach the motoneurons. It has been suggested that, for example, the refined and fractionated movements of the primate hand are related to the development of direct corticomotoneuronal connections. The size of the monosynaptic excitation from descending pathways is quite small, and it therefore seems likely that the gradation of force must depend on a proper level of background excitation mediated by polysynaptic pathways, while the fine spatial pattern of motor activity may depend on the direct projections, especially in the case of the rubro- and corticospinal tracts.

A large number of ascending pathways seem not to convey classic sensory information but instead to monitor segmental interneuronal activity. The analysis of the latter type of ascending pathways is closely linked to parallel work on the segmental reflex circuitry, the activity of which they are assumed to monitor. Section ASCENDING PATHWAYS THAT MONITOR SEGMENTAL INTERNEURONAL ACTIVITY, p. 569, summarized the evidence for this type of ascending pathway as well as its principal organization. The first clues to suggest that many ascending pathways monitor segmental reflex activity came with the observation that many of them were affected by the same afferents that contribute to the flexor reflex actions in the acute spinal cat. It was later noticed that transmission from FRA was depressed in parallel to motoneurons and to these ascending tract cells in the decerebrate state. Stimulation of motor centers that facilitates transmission from the FRA to motoneurons (and to primary afferents) also does so for these ascending neurons. The idea that such ascending pathways are concerned with intrinsic spinal activity rather than afferent activity per se was later demonstrated by the observations of rhythmic activity in some of these cells in phase with centrally triggered movements even after deafferentation.

It has now been shown that the ascending information monitoring segmental activity may be conveyed either by separate ascending neurons that receive collateral effects from segmental interneurons or by ascending collaterals from neurons that themselves mediate synaptic actions to motoneurons. At the present stage it is not always possible to decide to which of these categories a certain ascending system belongs.

The similarity between convergence in various FRA pathways and on different subsystems of the ventral flexor reflex tract (VFRT) was discussed in some detail. The VFRT consists of many separate subsystems that are excited from the FRA and ascend in the ventral quadrants of the spinal cord. Some belong to spinoolivocerebellar pathways; others terminate in the lateral reticular nucleus and are part of spinoreticulocerebellar pathways. It was suggested that they inform the cerebellum of the activity in the different segmental interneuronal centers that are activated from the FRA.

Many ventral spinocerebellar tract neurons (VSCT) receive monosynaptic excitation from Ia- and/or Ib-afferents. The monosynaptic excitation is often followed by a disynaptic inhibition from the same nerve. It was suggested that the disynaptic inhibition is due to collateral connections from inhibitory interneurons (that otherwise project to motoneurons) and that the monosynaptic excitation reflects collateral connections from the primary afferents that activate the inhibitory interneurons. It was therefore suggested that the VSCT may carry information about the output from inhibitory interneurons, as measured against their excitatory input. This input-output comparator hypothesis has been particularly well elucidated in relation to transmission in the Ia inhibitory pathway because the convergence onto the Ia inhibitory interneurons is so well known (subsection *Pathways From Ia-Afferents and Their Control by γ-Motoneurons*, p. 519). It was found that all descending pathways known to facilitate Ia inhibition in motoneurons also did so in VSCT neurons, as would be expected with a collateral projection from Ia inhibitory interneurons. All these motor centers could also supply excitation to the VSCT cells as needed for a comparison of the input-output relation for these interneurons. Different subpopulations of the VSCT are probably concerned with similar information for other inhibitory pathways to motoneurons.

Epilogue

We hope that this review has made clear the enormous complexity of the circuitry in the spinal cord. It is certainly of a magnitude that a complete "wiring diagram" remains beyond reach. How then can the ever more detailed information contribute to a better understanding of motor control? At the moment the main returns consist of various examples that reveal features of general significance. A multitude of experimental findings on different spinal circuits have often been brought together into a few coherent ideas on their possible operation and significance during motor performance. Such synthesizing hypotheses were discussed in this chapter for several circuits such as the recurrent inhibition via motor axon collaterals (subsection *Recurrent Inhibition*, p. 513), the γ-loop, and the inhibition mediated by the Ia inhibitory interneurons (*Pathways From Ia-Afferents and Their Control by γ-Motoneurons*, p. 519), the feedback provided by the FRA system (REFLEX PATHWAYS FROM THE "FLEXOR REFLEX AFFERENTS," p. 541), and the control of forelimb movements from the brain via short propriospinal neurons (subsection *Propriospinal Neurons*, p. 549). Although a thorough analysis of the neuronal connectivity forms the necessary base for such attempts of synthesis, forthcoming hypotheses must be tested when the animal—or human—actually performs a movement in which the neuronal circuits are supposed to participate. It is therefore important that techniques have been developed that allow recording of neuronal activity and of reflex transmission during actual motor behavior. The first models related to stereotyped rhythmic movements such as breathing in the anesthetized cat or locomotion in the high decerebrate cat (cf. the chapter by Grillner in this *Handbook*). Technical developments now allow the recording of activity in single afferent fibers during voluntary movements in humans (cf. ref. 589) and during unrestrained locomotion or other movements in the cat (cf. refs. 398, 494–496). With indirect techniques it is now also possible to follow changes in transmission in various reflex pathways during voluntary movement in humans (294, 486, 576). All these methods, which were only recently introduced, will certainly be of decisive importance in the evaluation of the hypotheses that were developed on the basis of neuronal convergence.

The spinal functional units that were described in section SPINAL NEURONAL CIRCUITS USED IN COMMON BY SEGMENTAL AFFERENTS AND SUPRASPINAL MOTOR CENTERS, p. 512, can hardly be thought to operate independently of each other. The manner in which their activities are linked in meaningful cooperation will indeed be one of the major problems for future research. It can be seen, for example, how the typical features of the classic decerebrate preparation depend on the activity in specific bulbospinal pathways that cause both a suppression of transmission in some segmental pathways and a concomitant facilitation in others (RETICULOSPINAL INHIBITION OF SEGMENTAL REFLEX TRANSMISSION, p. 560). Corresponding conjoint alterations in several spinal functional units have also been studied when the animal passes from quiet wakefulness to synchronized sleep to desynchronized REM sleep (see ref. 490). Studies on locomotion in the high decerebrate cat have shown that the activity in the great majority of rubrospinal and vestibulospinal neurons is modulated in phase with the step cycle during walking on a treadmill (463, 464). With the present knowledge on the widespread segmental effects by these descending systems, it can be inferred that virtually all functional units are subject to a concerted regulation even in such a stereotyped movement. Progress in this field requires further studies during different types of normal purposeful motor behavior. The increasing possibility of recording segmental reflex activity under such conditions opens new promising perspectives.

Present address of Hans Hultborn: Department of Neurophysiology, University of Göteborg, Göteborg, Sweden.

REFERENCES

1. ABRAHAMS, V. C. Cervico-lumbar reflex interactions involving a proprioceptive receiving area of the cerebral cortex. *J. Physiol. London* 209: 45–56, 1970.
2. ABRAHAMS, V. C., AND S. FALCHETTO. Hind leg ataxia of cervical origin and cervico-lumbar spinal interactions with a supratentorial pathway. *J. Physiol. London* 203: 435–447, 1969.
3. ADAM, D., U. WINDHORST, AND G. F. INBAR. The effects of recurrent inhibition on the cross-correlated firing patterns of motoneurones (and their relation to signal transmission in the spinal cord-muscle channel). *Biol. Cybernetics* 29: 229–235, 1978.
4. AHLMAN, H., S. GRILLNER, AND M. UDO. The effect of 5-HTP on the static fusimotor activity and the tonic stretch reflex of an extensor muscle. *Brain Res.* 27: 393–396, 1971.
5. ALNAES, E., J. K. S. JANSEN, AND T. RUDJORD. Fusimotor activity in the spinal cat. *Acta Physiol. Scand.* 63: 197–212, 1965.
6. ALSTERMARK, B., A. LUNDBERG, U. NORRSELL, AND E. SYBIRSKA. Role of C3–C4 propriospinal neurones in forelimb movements in the cat. *Acta Physiol. Scand.* 105: 24A–25A, 1979.
7. ALVORD, E. C., JR., AND M. G. F. FUORTES. Reflex activity of extensor motor units following muscular afferent excitation. *J. Physiol. London* 122: 302–321, 1953.
8. AMASSIAN, V. E., H. WEINER, AND M. ROSENBLUM. Neural systems subserving the tactile placing reaction: a model for the study of higher level control of movement. *Brain Res.* 40: 171–178, 1972.
9. ANASTASIEVIC, R., D. A. VASILENKO, A. I. KOSTYUKOV, AND N. N. PREOBRAZHENSKII. Reticulofugal influences of interneurones in the lateral region of gray matter of the cat spinal cord. *Neurophysiology USSR* 5: 525–536, 1973.
10. ANDÉN, N.-E., H. CORRODI, K. FUXE, B. HÖKFELT, T. HÖKFELT, C. RYDIN, AND T. SVENSSON. Evidence for a central noradrenaline receptor stimulation by clonidine. *Life Sci.* 9: 513–523, 1970.
11. ANDÉN, N.-E., J. ENGEL, AND A. RUBENSON. Mode of action of L-DOPA on central noradrenaline mechanisms. *Naunyn-Schmiedebergs Arch. Pharmacol.* 273: 1–10, 1972.
12. ANDÉN, N.-E., M. G. M. JUKES, AND A. LUNDBERG. Spinal reflexes and monoamine liberation. *Nature London* 202: 1222–1223, 1964.
13. ANDÉN, N.-E., M. G. M. JUKES, AND A. LUNDBERG. The effect of DOPA on the spinal cord. 2. A pharmacological analysis. *Acta Physiol. Scand.* 67: 387–397, 1966.
14. ANDÉN, N.-E., M. G. M. JUKES, A. LUNDBERG, AND L. VYKLICKÝ. A new spinal flexor reflex. *Nature London* 202: 1344–1345, 1964.
15. ANDÉN, N.-E., M. G. M. JUKES, A. LUNDBERG, AND L. VYKLICKÝ. The effect of DOPA on the spinal cord. 1. Influence on transmission from primary afferents. *Acta Physiol. Scand.* 67: 373–386, 1966.
16. ANDÉN, N.-E., M. G. M. JUKES, A. LUNDBERG, AND L. VYK-

LICKÝ. The effect of DOPA on the spinal cord. 3. Depolarization evoked in the central terminals of ipsilateral Ia afferents by volleys in the flexor reflex afferents. *Acta Physiol. Scand.* 68: 322–336, 1966.

17. ANDERSEN, P., J. C. ECCLES, R. F. SCHMIDT, AND T. YOKOTA. Slow potential waves produced in the cuneate nucleus by cutaneous volleys and by cortical stimulation. *J. Neurophysiol.* 27: 78–91, 1964.

18. ANDERSEN, P., J. C. ECCLES, R. F. SCHMIDT, AND T. YOKOTA. Depolarization of presynaptic fibers in the cuneate nucleus. *J. Neurophysiol.* 27: 92–106, 1964.

19. ANDERSEN, P., J. C. ECCLES, AND T. A. SEARS. Cortically evoked depolarization of primary afferent fibers in the spinal cord. *J. Neurophysiol.* 27: 63–77, 1964.

20. ANDERSON, E. G. Bulbospinal serotonin-containing neurons and motor control. *Federation Proc.* 31: 107–112, 1972.

21. ANDERSON, G., AND B. SJÖLUND. The ventral spino-olivocerebellar system in the cat. IV. Spinal transmission after administration of clonidine and L-Dopa. *Exp. Brain Res.* 33: 227–240, 1978.

22. ANDERSSON, O., H. FORSSBERG, S. GRILLNER, AND M. LINDQUIST. Phasic gain control of the transmission in cutaneous reflex pathways to motoneurones during "fictive" locomotion. *Brain Res.* 149: 503–507, 1978.

23. ANDREW, B. L., AND E. DODT. The deployment of sensory nerve endings at the knee joint of the cat. *Acta Physiol. Scand.* 28: 287–296, 1953.

24. AOKI, M., AND A. K. MCINTYRE. Cortical and long spinal actions on lumbosacral motoneurones in the cat. *J. Physiol. London* 251: 569–587, 1975.

25. APPELBERG, B. A rubro-olivary pathway. II. Simultaneous action on dynamic fusimotor neurones and the activity of the posterior lobe of the cerebellar cortex. *Exp. Brain Res.* 3: 382–390, 1967.

26. APPELBERG, B., AND T. JENESKOG. Mesencephalic fusimotor control. *Exp. Brain Res.* 15: 97–112, 1972.

27. APPELBERG, B., T. JENESKOG, AND H. JOHANSSON. Rubrospinal control of static and dynamic fusimotor neurones. *Acta Physiol. Scand.* 95: 431–440, 1975.

28. APPELBERG, B., H. JOHANSSON, AND G. KALISTRATOV. The influence of group II muscle afferents and low threshold skin afferents on dynamic fusimotor neurones to the triceps surae of the cat. *Brain Res.* 132: 153–158, 1977.

29. APPELBERG, B., AND C. MOLANDER. A rubro-olivary pathway. I. Identification of a descending system for control of the dynamic sensitivity of muscle spindles. *Exp. Brain Res.* 3: 372–381, 1967.

30. ARAKI, T., J. C. ECCLES, AND M. ITO. Correlation of the inhibitory postsynaptic potential of motoneurones with the latency and time course of inhibition of monosynaptic reflexes. *J. Physiol. London* 154: 354–377, 1960.

31. ARSHAVSKY, YU., M. B. BERKINBLIT, O. I. FUKSON, I. M. GELFAND, AND G. N. ORLOVSKY. Origin of modulation in neurones of the ventral spinocerebellar tract during locomotion. *Brain Res.* 43: 276–279, 1972.

32. ASANUMA, H., AND I. ROSÉN. Spread of mono- and polysynaptic connections within cat's motor cortex. *Exp. Brain Res.* 16: 507–520, 1973.

33. BALDISSERA, F., AND G. BROGGI. An analysis of potential changes in the spinal cord during desynchronized sleep. *Brain Res.* 6: 706–715, 1967.

34. BALDISSERA, F., AND G. TEN BRUGGENCATE. Rubrospinal effects on ventral spinocerebellar tract neurones. *Acta Physiol. Scand.* 96: 233–249, 1976.

35. BALDISSERA, F., G. TEN BRUGGENCATE, AND A. LUNDBERG. Rubrospinal monosynaptic connexion with last-order interneurones of polysynaptic reflex paths. *Brain Res.* 27: 390–392, 1971.

36. BALDISSERA, F., M. G. CESA-BIANCHI, AND M. MANCIA. Phasic events indicating presynaptic inhibition of primary afferents to the spinal cord during desynchronized sleep. *J. Neurophysiol.* 29: 871–887, 1966.

37. BALDISSERA, F., A. LUNDBERG, AND M. UDO. Activity evoked from the mesencephalic tegmentum in descending pathways other than the rubrospinal tract. *Exp. Brain Res.* 15: 133–150, 1972.

38. BALDISSERA, F., A. LUNDBERG, AND M. UDO. Stimulation of pre- and postsynaptic elements in the red nucleus. *Exp. Brain Res.* 15: 151–167, 1972.

39. BALDISSERA, F., AND W. J. ROBERTS. Effects on the ventral spinocerebellar tract neurones from Deiters' nucleus and the medial longitudinal fascicle in the cat. *Acta Physiol. Scand.* 93: 228–249, 1975.

40. BALDISSERA, F., AND W. J. ROBERTS. Effects from the vestibulospinal tract on transmission from primary afferents to ventral spino-cerebellar tract neurones. *Acta Physiol. Scand.* 96: 217–232, 1976.

41. BALLIF, L., J. F. FULTON, AND E. G. T. LIDDELL. Observations on spinal and decerebrate knee-jerks with special reference to their inhibition by single break-shocks. *Proc. R. Soc. London Ser. B* 98: 586–607, 1925.

42. BARD, P. Studies on the cerebral cortex. 1. Localized control of placing and hopping reactions in the cat and their normal management by small cortical remnants. *Arch. Neurol. Psychiatry* 30: 40–74, 1933.

43. BARKER, D. The morphology of muscle receptors. In: *Handbook of Sensory Physiology. Muscle Receptors*, edited by C. C. Hunt. Berlin: Springer-Verlag, 1974, vol. 3, pt. 2, p. 1–190.

44. BARNES, C. D., AND O. POMPEIANO. Inhibition of monosynaptic extensor reflex attributable to presynaptic depolarization of the group Ia afferent fibers produced by vibration of flexor muscle. *Arch. Ital. Biol.* 108: 233–258, 1970.

45. BARNES, C. D., AND O. POMPEIANO. Presynaptic and postsynaptic effects in the monosynaptic reflex pathway to extensor motoneurons following vibration of synergic muscles. *Arch. Ital. Biol.* 108: 259–294, 1970.

46. BARRON, D. H., AND B. H. C. MATTHEWS. The interpretation of potential changes in the spinal cord. *J. Physiol. London* 92: 276–321, 1938.

47. BAXENDALE, R. H., AND J. R. ROSENBERG. Crossed reflexes evoked by selective activation of tendon organ afferent axons in the decerebrate cat. *Brain Res.* 127: 323–326, 1977.

48. BAZETT, H. C., AND W. G. PENFIELD. A study of the Sherrington decerebrate animal in the chronic as well as the acute condition. Original articles and clinical cases. *Brain* 65: 185–265, 1922.

49. BENECKE, R., J. MEYER-LOHMANN, AND J. GUNTAU. Inverse changes in the excitability of Renshaw cells and α-motoneurones induced by interpositus stimulation. *Pfluegers Arch.* 365: R40, 1976.

50. BERGMANS, J., R. BURKE, L. FEDINA, AND A. LUNDBERG. The effect of DOPA on the spinal cord. 8. Presynaptic and "remote" inhibition of transmission from Ia afferents to alpha motoneurones. *Acta Physiol. Scand.* 90: 618–639, 1974.

51. BERGMANS, J., R. BURKE, AND A. LUNDBERG. Inhibition of transmission in the recurrent inhibitory pathway to motoneurones. *Brain Res.* 13: 600–602, 1969.

52. BERGMANS, J., AND S. GRILLNER. Changes in dynamic sensitivity of primary endings of muscle spindle afferents induced by DOPA. *Acta Physiol. Scand.* 74: 629–636, 1968.

53. BERGMANS, J., AND S. GRILLNER. Reciprocal control of spontaneous activity and reflex effects in static and dynamic flexor γ-motoneurones revealed by an injection of DOPA. *Acta Physiol. Scand.* 77: 106–124, 1969.

54. BERGMANS, J., M. ILLERT, E. JANKOWSKA, AND A. LUNDBERG. Reticulospinal control of propriospinal neurones mediating disynaptic corticomotoneurones excitation in the cat (Abstract). *Acta Physiol. Scand.* 96: 5A, 1976.

55. BERGMANS, J., S. MILLER, AND D. J. REITSMA. Influence of L-DOPA on transmission in long ascending propriospinal pathways in the cat. *Brain Res.* 62: 155–167, 1973.

56. BERKINBLIT, M. B., T. G. DELIAGINA, A. G. FELDMAN, I. M. GELFAND, AND G. N. ORLOVSKY. Generation of scratching. I. Activity of spinal interneurons during scratching. *J. Neuro-

physiol. 41: 1040-1057, 1978.
57. BERKINBLIT, M. B., T. G. DELIAGINA, A. G. FELDMAN, I. M. GELFAND, AND G. N. ORLOVSKY. Generation of scratching. II. Nonregular regimes of generation. *J. Neurophysiol.* 41: 1058-1069, 1978.
58. BERKINBLIT, M. B., T. G. DELIAGINA, G. N. ORLOVKSY, AND A. G. FELDMAN. Activity of propriospinal neurons during scratch reflex in the cat. *Neirofiziologiia* 9: 504-511, 1977.
59. BERNHARD, C. G., AND E. BOHM. Monosynaptic corticospinal activation of fore limb motoneurones in monkeys (*Macaca mulatta*). *Acta Physiol. Scand.* 31: 104-112, 1954.
60. BERNHARD, C. G., E. BOHM, AND I. PETERSÉN. Investigations on the organization of the corticospinal system in monkeys (*Macaca mulatta*). *Acta Physiol. Scand.* 29: (Suppl. 106) 79-105, 1953.
61. BESSOU, P., F. EMONET-DÉNAND, AND Y. LAPORTE. Motor fibres innervating extrafusal and intrafusal muscle fibres in the cat. *J. Physiol. London* 180: 649-672, 1965.
62. BJÖRKLUND, A., AND G. SKAGERBERG. Evidence for a major spinal cord projection from the diencephalic A11 dopamine cell group in the rat using transmitter-specific fluorescent retrograde tracing. *Brain Res.* 177: 170-175, 1979.
63. BLESSING, W. W., AND J. P. CHALMERS. Direct projection of catecholamine (presumably dopamine)-containing neurons from hypothalamus to spinal cord. *Neurosci. Lett.* 11: 35-40, 1979.
64. BOK, S. T. Das Rückenmark. In: *Handbuch der Mikroskopischen Anatomie des Menschen. Vierter Band: Nervensystem*, edited by W. von Möllendorff. Berlin: Springer-Verlag, 1928, p. 478-578.
65. BOSEMARK, B. Some aspects on the crossed extensor reflex in relation to mononeurones supplying fast and slow contracting muscles. In: *Muscular Afferents and Motor Control, Nobel Symposium I*, edited by R. Granit. Stockholm: Almqvist & Wiksell, 1966, p. 261-268.
66. BOYD, I. A., AND M. R. DAVEY. *Composition of Peripheral Nerves.* Edinburgh: Livingstone, 1968.
67. BRADLEY, K., D. M. EASTON, AND J. C. ECCLES. An investigation of primary or direct inhibition. *J. Physiol. London* 122: 474-488, 1953.
68. BRADLEY, K., AND J. C. ECCLES. Analysis of the fast afferent impulses from thigh muscles. *J. Physiol. London* 122: 462-473, 1953.
69. BROOKS, V. B., AND V. J. WILSON. Recurrent inhibition in the cat's spinal cord. *J. Physiol. London* 146: 380-391, 1959.
70. BROWN, M. C., I. ENGBERG, AND P. B. C. MATTHEWS. The relative sensitivity to vibration of muscle receptors of the cat. *J. Physiol. London* 192: 773-800, 1967.
71. BROWN, M. C., D. G. LAWRENCE, AND P. B. C. MATTHEWS. Antidromic inhibition of presumed fusimotor neurones by repetitive stimulation of the ventral root in the decerebrate cat. *Experientia* 24: 1210-1211, 1968.
72. BRUGGENCATE, G. TEN, AND A. LUNDBERG. Facilitatory interaction in transmission to motoneurones from vestibulospinal fibres and contralateral primary afferents. *Exp. Brain Res.* 19: 248-270, 1974.
73. BUDAKOVA, N. N. Stepping movements evoked by a rhythmic stimulation of a dorsal root in mesencephalic cat [in Russian] *Fiziol. Zh. SSSR. im I. M. Sechenova* 57: 1632-1640, 1971. [Engl. transl. *Neurosci. Behav. Physiol.* 5: 355-363, 1972.]
74. BUDAKOVA, N. N. Stepping movements in the spinal cat due to DOPA administration [in Russian]. *Fiziol. Zh. SSSR im I. M. Sechenova* 59: 1190-1198, 1973.
75. BURGESS, P. R., AND F. J. CLARK. Characteristics of knee joint receptors in the cat. *J. Physiol. London* 203: 317-335, 1969.
76. BURGESS, P. R., AND E. R. PERL. Cutaneous mechanoreceptors and nociceptors. In: *Handbook of Sensory Physiology. Somatosensory System*, edited by A. Iggo. Berlin: Springer-Verlag, 1973, vol. II, p. 29-78.
77. BURKE, D., K.-E. HAGBARTH, AND L. LÖFSTEDT. Muscle spindle responses in man to changes in load during accurate position maintenance. *J. Physiol. London* 276: 159-164, 1978.

78. BURKE, D., K.-E. HAGBARTH, AND N. F. SKUSE. Voluntary activation of spindle endings in human muscles temporarily paralysed by nerve pressure. *J. Physiol. London* 287: 329-336, 1979.
79. BURKE, D., L. KNOWLES, C. ANDREWS, AND P. ASHBY. Spasticity, decerebrate rigidity and the clasp-knife phenomenon: an experimental study in the cat. *Brain* 95: 31-48, 1972.
80. BURKE, R. E., E. JANKOWSKA, AND G. TEN BRUGGENCATE. A comparison of peripheral and rubrospinal synaptic input to slow and fast twitch motor units of triceps surae. *J. Physiol. London* 207: 709-732, 1970.
81. BURKE, R., A. LUNDBERG, AND F. WEIGHT. Spinal border cell origin of the ventral spinocerebellar tract. *Exp. Brain Res.* 12: 283-294, 1971.
82. BURKE, R. E., AND P. RUDOMIN. Spinal neurons and synapses. In: *Handbook of Physiology. The Nervous System*, edited by J. M. Brookhart and V. B. Mountcastle. Bethesda, MD: Am. Physiol. Soc., 1977, sect. 1, vol. I, pt. 2, chapt. 24, p. 877-944.
83. BURKE, R. E., P. RUDOMIN, L. VYKLICKÝ, AND F. E. ZAJAC III. Primary afferent depolarization and flexion reflexes produced by radiant heat stimulation of the skin. *J. Physiol. London* 213: 185-214, 1971.
84. BURKE, R. E., P. L. STRICK, K. KANDA, C. C. KIM, AND B. WALMSLEY. Anatomy of medial gastrocnemius and soleus motor nuclei in cat spinal cord. *J. Neurophysiol.* 40: 667-680, 1977.
85. BURKE, R. E., AND P. TSAIRIS. Histochemical and physiological profile of a skeletofusimotor (β) unit in cat soleus muscle. *Brain Res.* 129: 341-345, 1977.
86. BUSSEL, B., AND E. PIERROT-DESEILLIGNY. Inhibition of human motoneurones, probably of Renshaw origin, elicited by an orthodromic motor discharge. *J. Physiol. London* 269: 319-339, 1977.
87. CAJAL, S. RAMÓN Y. *Histologie du Système Nerveux de L'Homme et des Vertébrés.* Paris: Maloine, 1909, vol. 1.
88. CANGIANO, A., W. A. COOK, JR., AND O. POMPEIANO. Primary afferent depolarization in the lumbar cord evoked from the fastigial nucleus. *Arch. Ital. Biol.* 107: 321-340, 1969.
89. CANGIANO, A., W. A. COOK, JR., AND O. POMPEIANO. Cerebellar inhibitory control of the vestibular reflex pathways to primary afferents. *Arch. Ital. Biol.* 107: 341-364, 1969.
90. CARLI, G., K. DIETE-SPIFF, AND O. POMPEIANO. Responses of the muscle spindles and of the extrafusal fibres in an extensor muscle to stimulation of the lateral vestibular nucleus in the cat. *Arch. Ital. Biol.* 105: 209-242, 1967.
91. CARLSSON, A., B. FALCK, K. FUXE, AND N.-Å. HILLARP. Cellular localization of monoamines in the spinal cord. *Acta Physiol. Scand.* 60: 112-119, 1964.
92. CARLSSON, A., T. MAGNUSSON, AND E. ROSENGREN. 5-Hydroxytryptamine of the spinal cord normally and after transection. *Experientia* 19: 359, 1963.
93. CARPENTER, D., I. ENGBERG, H. FUNKENSTEIN, AND A. LUNDBERG. Decerebrate control of reflexes to primary afferents. *Acta Physiol. Scand.* 59: 424-437, 1963.
94. CARPENTER, D., I. ENGBERG, AND A. LUNDBERG. Differential supraspinal control of inhibitory and excitatory actions from the FRA to ascending spinal pathways. *Acta Physiol. Scand.* 63: 103-110, 1965.
95. CARPENTER, D., I. ENGBERG, AND A. LUNDBERG. Primary afferent depolarization evoked from the brain stem and the cerebellum. *Arch. Ital. Biol.* 104: 73-85, 1966.
96. CARPENTER, D., A. LUNDBERG, AND U. NORRSELL. Primary afferent depolarization evoked from the sensorimotor cortex. *Acta Physiol. Scand.* 59: 126-142, 1963.
97. CLARK, F. J., AND P. R. BURGESS. Slowly adapting receptors in cat knee joint: can they signal joint angle? *J. Neurophysiol.* 38: 1448-1463, 1975.
98. CLENDENIN, M., C.-F. EKEROT, O. OSCARSSON, AND I. ROSÉN. The lateral reticular nucleus in the cat. II. Organization of component activated from bilateral ventral flexor reflex tract (bVFRT). *Exp. Brain Res.* 21: 487-500, 1974.
99. CLOUGH, J. F. M., D. KERNELL, AND C. G. PHILLIPS. The distribution of monosynaptic excitation from the pyramidal

tract and from primary spindle afferents to motoneurones of the baboon's hand and forearm. *J. Physiol. London* 198: 145-166, 1968.
100. CLOUGH, J. F. M., C. G. PHILLIPS, AND J. D. SHERIDAN. The short-latency projection from the baboon's motor cortex to fusimotor neurones of the forearm and hand. *J. Physiol. London* 216: 257-279, 1971.
101. COHEN, L. A. Localization of stretch reflex. *J. Neurophysiol.* 16: 272-285, 1953.
102. COHEN, L. A. Organization of stretch reflex into two types of direct spinal arcs. *J. Neurophysiol.* 17: 443-453, 1954.
103. COOK, W. A., JR., A. CANGIANO, AND O. POMPEIANO. Vestibular control of transmission in primary afferents to the lumbar spinal cord. *Arch. Ital. Biol.* 107: 296-320, 1969.
104. COOPER, S., AND C. S. SHERRINGTON. Gower's tract and spinal border cells. *Brain* 63: 123-134, 1940.
105. COPPIN, C. M. L., J. J. B. JACK, AND C. R. MACLENNAN. A method for the selective electrical activation of tendon organ afferent fibres from the cat soleus muscle. *J. Physiol. London* 210: 18P-20P, 1970.
106. COPPIN, C. M. L., J. J. B. JACK, AND A. K. MCINTYRE. Properties of group I afferent fibres from semitendinosus muscle in the cat. *J. Physiol. London* 203: 45P-46P, 1969.
107. CORDA, M., C. VON EULER, AND G. LENNERSTRAND. Reflex and cerebellar influences on α and on "rhythmic" and "tonic" γ activity in the intercostal muscle. *J. Physiol. London* 184: 898-923, 1966.
108. CRAGO, P. E., J. C. HOUK, AND Z. HASAN. Regulatory actions of human stretch reflex. *J. Neurophysiol.* 39: 925-935, 1976.
109. CREED, R. S., D. DENNY-BROWN, J. C. ECCLES, E. G. T. LIDDELL, AND C. S. SHERRINGTON. *Reflex Activity of the Spinal Cord.* London: Oxford Univ. Press, 1932.
110. CULLHEIM, S., AND J.-O. KELLERTH. A morphological study of the axons and recurrent axon collaterals of cat α-motoneurones supplying different hind-limb muscles. *J. Physiol. London* 281: 285-299, 1978.
111. CULLHEIM, S., AND J.-O. KELLERTH. A morphological study of the axons and recurrent axon collaterals of cat α-motoneurones supplying different functional types of muscle unit. *J. Physiol. London* 281: 301-313, 1978.
112. CULLHEIM, S., J.-O. KELLERTH, AND S. CONRADI. Evidence for direct synaptic interconnections between cat spinal α-motoneurons via the recurrent axon collaterals: a morphological study using intracellular injection of horseradish peroxidase. *Brain Res.* 132: 1-10, 1977.
113. CURTIS, D. R., J. W. PHILLIS, AND J. C. WATKINS. Cholinergic and non-cholinergic transmission in the mammalian spinal cord. *J. Physiol. London.* 158: 296-323, 1961.
114. CURTIS, D. R., AND R. W. RYALL. The synaptic excitation of Renshaw cells. *Exp. Brain Res.* 2: 81-96, 1966.
115. CZARKOWSKA, J., E. JANKOWSKA, AND E. SYBIRSKA. Axonal projections of spinal interneurones excited by group I afferents in the cat, revealed by intracellular staining with horseradish peroxidase. *Brain Res.* 118: 115-118, 1976.
116. CZARKOWSKA, J., E. JANKOWSKA, AND E. SYBIRSKA. Diameter and internodal length of axons of spinal interneurones excited by group I afferents in the cat. *Brain Res.* 118: 119-122, 1976.
117. CZARKOWSKA, J., E. JANKOWSKA, AND E. SYBIRSKA. Common interneurones in reflex pathways from group Ia and Ib afferents of knee flexors and extensors. *J. Physiol. London.* In press.
118. DAHLSTRÖM, A., AND K. FUXE. Evidence for the existence of monoamine neurons in the central nervous system. II. Experimentally induced changes in the intraneuronal amine levels of bulbospinal neuron systems. *Acta Physiol. Scand.* 64:(Suppl. 247) 1-36, 1965.
119. DECANDIA, M., L. PROVINI, AND H. TÁBOŘÍKOVÁ. Presynaptic inhibition of the monosynaptic reflex following the stimulation of nerves to extensor muscles of the ankle. *Exp. Brain Res.* 4: 34-42, 1967.
120. DEGAIL, P., J. W. LANCE, AND P. D. NEILSON. Differential effects on tonic and phasic reflex mechanisms produced by vibration of muscles in man. *J. Neurol. Neurosurg. Psychiatry* 29: 1-11, 1966.
121. DELIAGINA, T. G., A. G. FELDMAN, I. M. GELFAND, AND G. N. ORLOVSKY. On the role of central program and afferent inflow in the control of scratching movements in the cat. *Brain Res.* 100: 297-313, 1975.
122. DELWAIDE, P. J. Human monosynaptic reflexes and presynaptic inhibition. In: *New Developments in Electromyography and Clinical Neurophysiology*, edited by J. E. Desmedt. Basel: Karger, 1973, vol. 3, p. 508-522.
123. DENNY-BROWN, D. Motor mechanisms—introduction: the general principles of motor integration. In: *Handbook of Physiology. Neurophysiology*, edited by J. Field, H. W. Magoun and V. E. Hall. Washington, DC: Am. Physiol. Soc., 1960, sect. 1, vol. II, p. 781-796.
124. DEVANANDAN, M. S., R. M. ECCLES, AND T. YOKOTA. Depolarization of afferent terminals evoked by muscle stretch. *J. Physiol. London* 179: 417-429, 1965.
125. DEVANANDAN, M. S., R. M. ECCLES, AND T. YOKOTA. Muscle stretch and the presynaptic inhibition of the group Ia pathway to motoneurones. *J. Physiol. London.* 179: 430-441, 1965.
126. DEVANANDAN, M. S., B. HOLMQVIST, AND T. YOKOTA. Presynaptic depolarization of group I muscle afferents by contralateral afferent volleys. *Acta Physiol. Scand.* 63: 46-54, 1965.
127. DOWNMAN, C. B. B., AND A. HUSSAIN. Spinal tracts and supraspinal centres influencing visceromotor and allied reflexes in cats. *J. Physiol. London* 141: 489-499, 1958.
128. ECCLES, J. C. *The Neurophysiological Basis of Mind: The Principles of Neurophysiology.* Oxford: Clarendon, 1953.
129. ECCLES, J. C. Presynaptic inhibition in the spinal cord. In: *Progress in Brain Research. Physiology of Spinal Neurons*, edited by J. C. Eccles and J. P. Schadé. Amsterdam: Elsevier, 1964, vol. 12, p. 65-91.
130. ECCLES, J. C. *The Inhibitory Pathways of the Central Nervous System. The Sherrington Lectures IX.* Liverpool: Liverpool Univ. Press, 1969.
131. ECCLES, J. C., R. M. ECCLES, A. IGGO, AND M. ITO. Distribution of recurrent inhibition among motoneurones. *J. Physiol. London* 159: 479-499, 1961.
132. ECCLES, J. C., R. M. ECCLES, A. IGGO, AND A. LUNDBERG. Electrophysiological studies on gamma motoneurones. *Acta Physiol. Scand.* 50: 32-40, 1960.
133. ECCLES, J. C., R. M. ECCLES, A. IGGO, AND A. LUNDBERG. Electrophysiological investigations of Renshaw cells. *J. Physiol. London* 159: 461-478, 1961.
134. ECCLES, J. C., R. M. ECCLES, AND A. LUNDBERG. Synaptic actions on motoneurones in relation to the two components of the group I muscle afferent volley. *J. Physiol. London* 136: 527-546, 1957.
135. ECCLES, J. C., R. M. ECCLES, AND A. LUNDBERG. The convergence of monosynaptic excitatory afferents on to many different species of alpha motoneurones. *J. Physiol. London* 137: 22-50, 1957.
136. ECCLES, J. C., R. M. ECCLES, AND A. LUNDBERG. Synaptic actions on motoneurones caused by impulses in Golgi tendon organ afferents. *J. Physiol. London* 138: 227-252, 1957.
137. ECCLES, J. C., R. M. ECCLES, AND A. LUNDBERG. Types of neurone in and around the intermediate nucleus of the lumbosacral cord. *J. Physiol. London* 154: 89-114, 1960.
138. ECCLES, J. C., R. M. ECCLES, AND F. MAGNI. Central inhibitory action attributable to presynaptic depolarization produced by muscle afferent volleys. *J. Physiol. London* 159: 147-166, 1961.
139. ECCLES, J. C., P. FATT, AND K. KOKETSU. Cholinergic and inhibitory synapses in a pathway from motor-axon collaterals to motoneurones. *J. Physiol. London* 126: 524-562, 1954.
140. ECCLES, J. C., P. FATT, AND S. LANDGREN. Central pathway for direct inhibitory action of impulses in largest afferent nerve fibres to muscle. *J. Neurophysiol.* 19: 75-98, 1956.
141. ECCLES, J. C., P. FATT, S. LANDGREN, AND G. J. WINSBURY. Spinal cord potentials generated by volleys in the large muscle afferents. *J. Physiol. London* 125: 590-606, 1954.

142. ECCLES, J. C., J. I. HUBBARD, AND O. OSCARSSON. Intracellular recording from cells of the ventral spinocerebellar tract. *J. Physiol. London* 158: 486–516, 1961.
143. ECCLES, J. C., P. G. KOSTYUK, AND R. F. SCHMIDT. Presynaptic inhibition of the central actions of flexor reflex afferents. *J. Physiol. London* 161: 258–281, 1962.
144. ECCLES, J. C., F. MAGNI, AND W. D. WILLIS. Depolarization of central terminals of group I afferent fibres from muscle. *J. Physiol. London* 160: 62–93, 1962.
145. ECCLES, J. C., R. F. SCHMIDT, AND W. D. WILLIS. Depolarization of central terminals of group Ib afferent fibers of muscle. *J. Neurophysiol.* 26: 1–27, 1963.
146. ECCLES, J. C., R. F. SCHMIDT, AND W. D. WILLIS. Depolarization of the central terminals of cutaneous afferent fibers. *J. Neurophysiol.* 26: 646–661, 1963.
147. ECCLES, R. M., AND A. LUNDBERG. Integrative pattern of Ia synaptic actions on motoneurones of hip and knee muscles. *J. Physiol. London* 144: 271–298, 1958.
148. ECCLES, R. M., AND A. LUNDBERG. Synaptic actions in motoneurones by afferents which may evoke the flexion reflex. *Arch. Ital. Biol.* 97: 199–221, 1959.
149. ECCLES, R. M., AND A. LUNDBERG. Supraspinal control of interneurones mediating spinal reflexes. *J. Physiol. London* 147: 565–584, 1959.
150. EDGERTON, V. R., S. GRILLNER, A. SJÖSTRÖM, AND P. ZANGGER. Central generation of locomotion in vertebrates. In: *Neural Control of Locomotion, Advances in Behavioral Biology*, edited by R. M. Herman, S. Grillner, P. S. G. Stein and D. G. Stuart. New York: Plenum, 1976, vol. 18, p. 439–464.
151. EKEROT, C.-F., AND O. OSCARSSON. Inhibitory spinal paths to the lateral reticular nucleus. *Brain Res.* 99: 157–161, 1975.
152. EKHOLM, J., G. EKLUND, AND S. SKOGLUND. On the reflex effects from the knee joint of the cat. *Acta Physiol. Scand.* 50: 167–174, 1960.
153. EKLUND, G., C. VON EULER, AND S. RUTKOWSKI. Spontaneous and reflex activity of intercostal gamma motoneurones. *J. Physiol. London* 171: 139–163, 1964.
154. EKLUND, G., AND K.-E. HAGBARTH. Normal variability of tonic vibration reflexes in man. *Exp. Neurol.* 16: 80–92, 1966.
155. ELDRED, E. Posture and locomotion. In: *Handbook of Physiology. Neurophysiology*, edited by J. Field, H. W. Magoun, and V. E. Hall. Washington, DC: Am. Physiol. Soc., 1960, sect. 1, vol. II, p. 1067–1088.
156. ELDRED, E., AND B. FUJIMORI. Relations of the reticular formation to muscle spindle activation. In: *Reticular Formation of the Brain*, edited by H. H. Jasper, L. D. Proctor, R. S. Knighton, W. C. Noshay and R. T. Costello. Boston: Little, Brown, 1958, p. 275–283.
157. ELDRED, E., R. GRANIT, AND P. A. MERTON. Supraspinal control of the muscle spindles and its significance. *J. Physiol. London* 122: 498–523, 1953.
158. ELGER, C. E., E.-J. SPECKMANN, H. CASPERS, AND R. W. C. JANZEN. Cortico-spinal connections in the rat. I. Monosynaptic and polysynaptic responses of cervical motoneurons to epicortical stimulation. *Exp. Brain Res.* 28: 385–404, 1977.
159. ELLAWAY, P. H. Antidromic inhibition of fusimotor neurones. *J. Physiol. London* 198: 39P–40P, 1968.
160. ELLAWAY, P. H. Recurrent inhibition of fusimotor neurones exhibiting background discharges in the decerebrate and the spinal cat. *J. Physiol. London* 216: 419–439, 1971.
161. ELLAWAY, P. H., AND J. R. TROTT. The mode of action of 5-hydroxytryptophan in facilitating a stretch reflex in the spinal cat. *Exp. Brain Res.* 22: 145–162, 1975.
162. ELLAWAY, P. H., AND J. R. TROTT. Reflex connections from muscle stretch receptors to their own fusimotor neurones. In: *Progress in Brain Research. Understanding the Stretch Reflex*, edited by S. Homma. Amsterdam: Elsevier, 1976, vol. 44, p. 113–122.
163. ELLAWAY, P. H., AND J. R. TROTT. Autogenetic reflex action on to gamma motoneurones by stretch of triceps surae in the decerebrated cat. *J. Physiol. London* 276: 49–66, 1978.

164. EMONET-DÉNAND, F., L. JAMI, AND Y. LAPORTE. Skeleto-fusimotor axons in hind-limb muscles of the cat. *J. Physiol. London* 249: 153–166, 1975.
165. ENGBERG, I. Reflexes to foot muscles in the cat. *Acta Physiol. Scand.* 62: (Suppl. 235) 1–64, 1964.
166. ENGBERG, I., AND A. LUNDBERG. An electromyographic analysis of muscular activity in the hindlimb of the cat during unrestrained locomotion. *Acta Physiol. Scand.* 75: 614–630, 1969.
167. ENGBERG, I., A. LUNDBERG, AND R. W. RYALL. Reticulospinal inhibition of transmission in reflex pathways. *J. Physiol. London* 194: 201–223, 1968.
168. ENGBERG, I., A. LUNDBERG, AND R. W. RYALL. Reticulospinal inhibition of interneurones. *J. Physiol. London* 194: 225–236, 1968.
169. ENGBERG, I., A. LUNDBERG, AND R. W. RYALL. The effect of reserpine on transmission in the spinal cord. *Acta Physiol. Scand.* 72: 115–122, 1968.
170. ENGBERG, I., A. LUNDBERG, AND R. W. RYALL. Is the tonic decerebrate inhibition of reflex paths mediated by monoaminergic pathways. *Acta Physiol. Scand.* 72: 123–133, 1968.
171. EULER, C. VON. The control of respiratory movement. In: *Breathlessness*, edited by J. B. L. Howell and E. J. M. Campbell. Oxford: Blackwell, 1966, p. 19–32.
172. FEDINA, L., AND H. HULTBORN. Facilitation from ipsilateral primary afferents of interneuronal transmission in the Ia inhibitory pathway to motoneurones. *Acta Physiol. Scand.* 86: 59–81, 1972.
173. FEDINA, L., H. HULTBORN, AND M. ILLERT. Facilitation from contralateral primary afferents of interneuronal transmission in the Ia inhibitory pathway to motoneurones. *Acta Physiol. Scand.* 94: 198–221, 1975.
174. FEDINA, L., A. LUNDBERG, AND L. VYKLICKÝ. The effect of a noradrenaline liberator (4,alpha-dimethyl-meta-tyramine) on reflex transmission in spinal cats. *Acta Physiol. Scand.* 83: 495–504, 1971.
175. FELDMAN, A. G., AND G. N. ORLOVSKY. Activity of interneurons mediating reciprocal Ia inhibition during locomotion. *Brain Res.* 84: 181–194, 1975.
176. FERRELL, W. R. *Slowly Adapting Receptors in the Cat Knee Joint and Their Role in Position Sense* (Dissertation). Glasgow: Univ. of Glasgow Library, 1977.
177. FERRELL, W. R. The discharge of mechanoreceptors in the cat knee joint at intermediate angles. *J. Physiol. London* 268: 23P–24P, 1977.
178. FETZ, E. E. Pyramidal tract effects on interneurons in the cat lumbar dorsal horn. *J. Neurophysiol.* 31: 69–80, 1968.
179. FETZ, E. E., E. JANKOWSKA, T. JOHANNISSON, AND J. LIPSKI. Autogenetic inhibition of motoneurones by impulses in group Ia muscle spindle afferents. *J. Physiol. London* 293: 173–195, 1979.
180. FIDONE, S. J., AND J. B. PRESTON. Patterns of motor cortex control of flexor and extensor cat fusimotor neurons. *J. Neurophysiol.* 32: 103–115, 1969.
181. FORSSBERG, H. Stumbling corrective reaction: A phase-dependent compensatory reaction during locomotion. *J. Neurophysiol.* 42: 936–953, 1979.
182. FORSSBERG, H., AND S. GRILLNER. The locomotion of the acute spinal cat injected with clonidine i.v. *Brain Res.* 50: 184–186, 1973.
183. FORSSBERG, H., S. GRILLNER, AND S. ROSSIGNOL. Phasic gain control of reflexes from the dorsum of the paw during spinal locomotion. *Brain Res.* 132: 121–139, 1977.
184. FORSSBERG, H., S. GRILLNER, S. ROSSIGNOL, AND P. WALLÉN. Phasic control of reflexes during locomotion in vertebrates. In: *Neural Control of Locomotion. Advances in Behavioral Biology*, edited by R. M. Herman, S. Grillner, P. S. G. Stein and D. G. Stuart. New York: Plenum, 1976, vol. 18, p. 647–674.
185. FORSSBERG, H., S. GRILLNER, AND A. SJÖSTRÖM. Tactile placing reactions in chronic spinal kittens. *Acta Physiol. Scand.* 92: 114–120, 1974.

186. FOSTER, M. *A Textbook of Physiology.* London, 1879. [Cited by E. G. T. Liddell: *The Discovery of Reflexes.* Oxford: Clarendon, 1960, p. 101.]
187. FRANK, K., AND M. G. F. FUORTES. Presynaptic and postsynaptic inhibition of monosynaptic reflexes (Abstract). *Federation Proc.* 16: 39–40, 1957.
188. FRITZ, N., M. ILLERT, AND P. SAGGAU. Monosynaptic convergence of group I muscle afferents from the forelimb onto dorsal interosseus motoneurones. *Neurosci. Lett.:* (Suppl. 1) S95, 1978.
189. FROMM, C., J. HAASE, AND E. WOLF. Depression of the recurrent inhibition of extensor motoneurons by the action of group II afferents. *Brain Res.* 120: 459–468, 1977.
190. FROMM, C., AND J. NOTH. Autogenetic inhibition of γ-motoneurones in the spinal cat uncovered by Dopa injection. *Pfluegers Arch.* 349: 247–256, 1974.
191. FROMM, C., AND J. NOTH. Reflex responses of gamma motoneurones to vibration of the muscle they innervate. *J. Physiol. London* 256: 117–136, 1976.
192. FU, T.-C., H. HULTBORN, R. LARSSON, AND A. LUNDBERG. Reciprocal inhibition during the tonic stretch reflex in the decerebrate cat. *J. Physiol. London* 284: 345–369, 1978.
193. FU, T.-C., E. JANKOWSKA, AND A. LUNDBERG. Reciprocal Ia inhibition during the late reflexes evoked from the flexor reflex afferents after DOPA. *Brain Res.* 85: 99–102, 1975.
194. FU, T.-C., E. JANKOWSKA, AND R. TANAKA. Effects of volleys in cortico-spinal tract fibres on ventral spino-cerebellar tract cells in the cat. *Acta Physiol. Scand* 100: 1–13, 1977.
195. FU, T.-C., M. SANTINI, AND E. D. SCHOMBURG. Characteristics and distribution of spinal focal synaptic potentials generated by group II muscle afferents. *Acta Physiol. Scand.* 91: 298–313, 1974.
196. FU, T.-C., AND E. D. SCHOMBURG. Electrophysiological investigation of the projection of secondary muscle spindle afferents in the cat spinal cord. *Acta Physiol. Scand.* 91: 314–329, 1974.
197. FULTON, J. F. *Muscular Contraction and the Reflex Control of Movement.* Baltimore: Williams & Wilkins, 1926, p. 1–644.
198. FUXE, K. Evidence for the existence of monoamine neurons in the central nervous system. III. The monoamine nerve terminal. *Z. Zellforsch. Mikrosk. Anat.* 65: 573–596, 1965.
199. FUXE, K. Evidence for the existence of monoamine neurons in the central nervous system. IV. The distribution of monoamine terminals in the central nervous system. *Acta Physiol. Scand.* 64: (Suppl. 247) 39–85, 1965.
200. FUXE, K., AND G. JONSSON. Further mapping of central 5-hydroxytryptamine neurons: studies with the neurotoxic dihydroxytryptamines. In: *Advances in Biochemical Psychopharmacology. Serotonin: New Vistas. Histochemistry and Pharmacology,* edited by E. Costa, G. L. Gessa, and M. Sandler. New York: Raven, 1974, vol. 10, p. 1–12.
201. GELFAND, I. M., V. S. GURFINKEL, Y. M. KOTS, V. I. KRINSKII, M. L. TSETLIN, AND M. L. SHIK. Investigations of postural activity. *Biofizika* 9: 710–717, 1964.
202. GELFAND, I. M., V. S. GURFINKEL, Y. M. KOTS, M. L. TSETLIN, AND M. L. SHIK. Synchronization of motor units and associated model concepts. *Biofizika* 8: 475–486, 1963.
203. GERNANDT, B. E., AND D. MEGIRIAN. Ascending propriospinal mechanisms. *J. Neurophysiol.* 24: 364–376, 1961.
204. GERNANDT, B. E., AND M. SHIMAMURA. Mechanisms of interlimb reflexes in cat. *J. Neurophysiol.* 24: 665–676, 1961.
205. GERSHON, M. D. Biochemistry and physiology of serotonergic transmission. In: *Handbook of Physiology. The Nervous System,* edited by J. M. Brookhart and V. B. Mountcastle. Bethesda, MD: Am. Physiol. Soc. 1977, sect. 1, vol. I, pt. 1, chapt. 16, p. 573–623.
206. GIOVANELLI BARILARI, M., AND H. G. J. M. KUYPERS. Propriospinal fibers interconnecting the spinal enlargements in the cat. *Brain Res.* 14: 321–330, 1969.
207. GOODWIN, G. M., AND E. S. LUSCHEI. Discharge of spindle afferents from jaw-closing muscles during chewing in alert monkeys. *J. Neurophysiol.* 38: 560–571, 1975.
208. GÓRSKA, T., E. JANKOWSKA, AND M. MOSSAKOWSKI. Effects of pyramidotomy on instrumental conditioned reflexes in cats. II. Reflexes derived from unconditioned reactions. *Acta Biol. Exp. Warsaw* 26: 451–462, 1966.
209. GRAHAM BROWN, T. The intrinsic factors in the act of progression in the mammal. *Proc. R. Soc. London Ser. B* 84: 308–319, 1911.
210. GRAHAM BROWN, T. Studies in the physiology of the nervous system. IX. Reflex terminal phenomena-rebound-rhythmic rebound and movements of progression. *Q. J. Exp. Physiol.* 4: 331–397, 1911.
211. GRAHAM BROWN, T. The factors in rhythmic activity of the nervous system. *Proc. R. Soc. London Ser. B* 85: 278–289, 1912.
212. GRAHAM BROWN, T. Studies in the physiology of the nervous system. XI. Immediate reflex phenomena in the simple reflex. *Q. J. Exp. Physiol.* 5: 237–307, 1912.
213. GRAHAM BROWN, T. *Die Reflexfunktionen des Zentralnervensystems mit besonderer Berücksichtigung der rhythmischen Tätigkeiten beim Säugetier.* Wiesbaden: Bergmann, 1916, vol. II, p. 480–790.
214. GRAHAM BROWN, T. Studies in the physiology of the nervous system. XXVIII. Absence of algebraic equality between the magnitudes of central excitation and effective central inhibition given in the reflex centre of a single limb by the same reflex stimulus. *Q. J. Exp. Physiol.* 14: 1–23, 1924.
215. GRANIT, R. Reflex self-regulation of muscle contraction and autogenetic inhibition. *J. Neurophysiol.* 13: 351–372, 1950.
216. GRANIT, R. Reflexes to stretch and contraction of antagonists around ankle joint. *J. Neurophysiol.* 15: 269–279, 1952.
217. GRANIT, R. *Receptors and Sensory Perception.* New Haven, CT: Yale Univ. Press, 1955.
218. GRANIT, R. *The Basis of Motor Control.* London: Academic, 1970.
219. GRANIT, R. The functional role of the muscle spindles—facts and hypotheses. *Brain* 98: 531–556, 1975.
220. GRANIT, R., J. HAASE, AND L. T. RUTLEDGE. Recurrent inhibition in relation to frequency of firing and limitation of discharge rate of extensor motoneurons. *J. Physiol. London* 154: 308–328, 1960.
221. GRANIT, R., B. HOLMGREN, AND P. A. MERTON. The two routes for excitation of muscle and their subservience to the cerebellum. *J. Physiol. London* 130: 213–224, 1955.
222. GRANIT, R., C. JOB, AND B. R. KAADA. Activation of muscle spindles in pinna reflex. *Acta Physiol. Scand.* 27: 161–168, 1952.
223. GRANIT, R., AND B. R. KAADA. Influence of stimulation of central nervous structures on muscle spindles in cat. *Acta Physiol. Scand.* 27: 130–160, 1952.
224. GRANIT, R., J. E. PASCOE, AND G. STEG. The behaviour of tonic α and γ motoneurones during stimulation of recurrent collaterals. *J. Physiol. London* 138: 381–400, 1957.
225. GRANIT, R., C. G. PHILLIPS, S. SKOGLUND, AND G. STEG. Differentiation of tonic from phasic alpha ventral horn cells by stretch, pinna and crossed extensor reflexes. *J. Neurophysiol.* 20: 470–481, 1957.
226. GRANT, G., M. ILLERT, AND R. TANAKA. Integration in descending motor pathways controlling the forelimb in the cat. 6. Anatomical evidence consistent with the existence of C_3–C_4 propriospinal neurones projecting to forelimb motornuclei. *Exp. Brain Res.* 38: 87–93, 1980.
227. GRIGG, P. Mechanical factors influencing response of joint afferent neurons from cat knee. *J. Neurophysiol.* 38: 1473–1484, 1975.
228. GRIGG, P., AND B. J. GREENSPAN. Response of primate joint afferent neurons to mechanical stimulation of knee joint. *J. Neurophysiol.* 40: 1–8, 1977.
229. GRIGG, P., E. P. HARRIGAN, AND K. E. FOGARTY. Segmental reflexes mediated by joint afferent neurons in cat knee. *J. Neurophysiol.* 41: 9–14, 1978.
230. GRIGG, P., AND J. B. PRESTON. Baboon flexor and extensor fusimotor neurons and their modulation by motor cortex. *J. Neurophysiol.* 34: 428–436, 1971.
231. GRILLNER, S. The influence of DOPA on the static and the

dynamic fusimotor activity to the triceps surae of the spinal cat. *Acta Physiol. Scand.* 77: 490-509, 1969.
232. GRILLNER, S. Supraspinal and segmental control of static and dynamic γ-motoneurones in the cat. *Acta Physiol. Scand.:* (Suppl. 327) 1-34, 1969.
233. GRILLNER, S. Locomotion in the spinal cat. In: *Advances in Behavioral Biology. Control of Posture and Locomotion,* edited by R. B. Stein, K. B. Pearson, R. S. Smith and J. B. Redford. New York: Plenum, 1973, vol. 7, p. 515-535.
234. GRILLNER, S. Locomotion in vertebrates: central mechanisms and reflex interaction. *Physiol. Rev.* 55: 247-304, 1975.
235. GRILLNER, S. On the neural control of movement—a comparison of different basic rhythmic behaviors. In: *Function and Formation of Neural Systems,* edited by G. S. Stent. Berlin: Dahlem Konferenzen, 1977, p. 197-224.
236. GRILLNER, S., AND T. HONGO. Vestibulospinal effects on motoneurones and interneurones in the lumbosacral cord. In: *Progress in Brain Research. Basic Aspects of Central Vestibular Mechanisms,* edited by A. Brodal and O. Pompeiano. Amsterdam: Elsevier, 1972, vol. 37, p. 243-262.
237. GRILLNER, S., T. HONGO, AND S. LUND. Interaction between the inhibitory pathways from the Deiters' nucleus and Ia afferents to flexor motoneurones. *Acta Physiol. Scand.* 68: (Suppl. 277) 61, 1966.
238. GRILLNER, S., T. HONGO, AND S. LUND. The origin of descending fibres monosynaptically activating spinoreticular neurones. *Brain Res.* 10: 259-262, 1968.
239. GRILLNER, S., T. HONGO, AND S. LUND. Descending monosynaptic and reflex control of γ-motoneurones. *Acta Physiol. Scand.* 75: 592-613, 1969.
240. GRILLNER, S., T. HONGO, AND S. LUND. The vestibulospinal tract. Effects on alpha-motoneurones in the lumbosacral spinal cord in the cat. *Exp. Brain Res.* 10: 94-120, 1970.
241. GRILLNER, S., T. HONGO, AND S. LUND. Convergent effects on alpha motoneurones from the vestibulospinal tract and a pathway descending in the medial longitudinal fasciculus. *Exp. Brain Res.* 12: 457-479, 1971.
242. GRILLNER, S., T. HONGO, AND A. LUNDBERG. The effect of DOPA on the spinal cord. 7. Reflex activation of static γ-motoneurones from the flexor reflex afferents. *Acta Physiol. Scand.* 70: 403-411, 1967.
243. GRILLNER, S., AND S. LUND. A descending pathway with monosynaptic action on flexor motoneurones. *Experientia* 22: 390, 1966.
244. GRILLNER, S., AND S. LUND. The origin of a descending pathway with monosynaptic action on flexor motoneurones. *Acta Physiol. Scand.* 74: 274-284, 1968.
245. GRILLNER, S., AND S. ROSSIGNOL. Contralateral reflex reversal controlled by limb position in the acute spinal cat injected with clonidine i.v. *Brain Res.* 144: 411-414, 1978.
246. GRILLNER, S., AND S. ROSSIGNOL. On the initiation of the swing phase of locomotion in chronic spinal cats. *Brain Res.* 146: 269-277, 1978.
247. GRILLNER, S., AND M. L. SHIK. On the descending control of the lumbosacral spinal cord from the "mesencephalic locomotor region." *Acta Physiol. Scand.* 87: 320-330, 1973.
248. GRILLNER, S., AND M. UDO. Is the tonic stretch reflex dependent on suppression of autogenetic inhibitory reflexes? *Acta Physiol. Scand.* 79: 13A-14A, 1970.
249. GRILLNER, S., AND P. ZANGGER. Locomotor movements generated by the deafferented spinal cord. *Acta Physiol. Scand.* 91: 38A-39A, 1974.
250. GRILLNER, S., AND P. ZANGGER. On the central generation of locomotion in the low spinal cat. *Exp. Brain Res.* 34: 241-261, 1979.
251. GUSTAFSSON, B., AND S. LINDSTRÖM. Recurrent control from motor axon collaterals of Ia inhibitory pathways to ventral spinocerebellar tract neurones. *Acta Physiol. Scand.* 89: 457-481, 1973.
252. HA, H., AND C.-N. LIU. Cell origin of the ventral spinocerebellar tract. *J. Comp. Neurol.* 133: 185-206, 1968.
253. HAASE, J., S. CLEVELAND, AND H.-G. ROSS. Problems of postsynaptic autogenous and recurrent inhibition in the mammalian spinal cord. *Rev. Physiol. Biochem. Pharmacol.* 73: 74-129, 1975.
254. HAASE, J., AND J. P. VAN DER MEULEN. Effects of supraspinal stimulation on Renshaw cells belonging to extensor motoneurones. *J. Neurophysiol.* 24: 510-520, 1961.
255. HAASE, J., AND B. VOGEL. Die Erregung der Renshaw-Zellen durch reflektorische Entladungen der α-Motoneurone. *Pfluegers Arch.* 325: 14-27, 1971.
256. HAGBARTH, K.-E. Excitatory and inhibitory skin areas for flexor and extensor motoneurones. *Acta Physiol. Scand.* 26: (Suppl. 94) 1-58, 1952.
257. HAGBARTH, K.-E., AND G. EKLUND. Motor effects of vibratory stimuli in man. In: *Muscular Afferents and Motor Control. Nobel Symposium 1,* edited by R. Granit. Stockholm: Almqvist & Wiksell, 1966, p. 177-186.
258. HAMMOND, P. H. An experimental study of servo action in human muscular control. *IEE Conf. Publ. London* 3: 190-199, 1960.
259. HAMMOND, P. H., P. A. MERTON, AND G. G. SUTTON. Nervous gradation of muscular contraction. *Brit. Med. Bull.* 12: 214-218, 1956.
260. HARRIS, A. S. Mammalian plantar reflexes in terms of afferent fibers. *Am. J. Physiol.* 124: 117-125, 1938.
261. HENATSCH, H.-D., H.-J. KAESE, D. LANGREHR, AND J. MEYER-LOHMANN. Einflüsse des motorischen Cortex der Katze auf die Renshaw-Rückkoppelungshemmung der Motoneurone. *Pfluegers Arch.* 274: 51-52, 1961.
262. HIKOSAKA, O., Y. IGUSA, S. NAKAO, AND H. SHIMAZU. Direct inhibitory synaptic linkage of pontomedullary reticular burst neurons with abducens motoneurons in the cat. *Exp. Brain Res.* 33: 337-352, 1978.
263. HIRAI, N., T. HONGO, N. KUDO, AND T. YAMAGUCHI. Heterogenous composition of the spinocerebellar tract originating from the cervical enlargement in the cat. *Brain Res.* 109: 387-391, 1976.
264. HIRAI, N., T. HONGO, AND T. YAMAGUCHI. Spinocerebellar tract neurones with long descending axon collaterals. *Brain Res.* 142: 147-151, 1978.
265. HODGE, C. J., JR. Potential changes inside central afferent terminals secondary to stimulation of large- and small-diameter peripheral nerve fibers. *J. Neurophysiol.* 35: 30-43, 1972.
266. HOLMQVIST, B. Crossed spinal reflex actions evoked by volleys in somatic afferents. *Acta Physiol. Scand.* 52: (Suppl. 181) 1-67, 1961.
267. HOLMQVIST, B., AND A. LUNDBERG. On the organization of the supraspinal inhibitory control of interneurones of various spinal reflex arcs. *Arch. Ital. Biol.* 97: 340-356, 1959.
268. HOLMQVIST, B., AND A. LUNDBERG. Differential supraspinal control of synaptic actions evoked by volleys in the flexion reflex afferents in alpha motoneurons. *Acta Physiol. Scand.* 54: (Suppl. 186) 1-51, 1961.
269. HOLMQVIST, B., A. LUNDBERG, AND O. OSCARSSON. Supraspinal inhibitory control of transmission to three ascending spinal pathways influenced by the flexion reflex afferents. *Arch. Ital. Biol.* 98: 60-80, 1960.
270. HOLMQVIST, B., A. LUNDBERG, AND O. OSCARSSON. A supraspinal control system monosynaptically connected with an ascending spinal pathway. *Arch. Ital. Biol.* 98: 402-422, 1960.
271. HOMMA, S., M. MIZOTE, AND S. WATANABE. Participation of mono- and polysynaptic transmission during tonic activation of the stretch reflex arcs. *Jpn. J. Physiol.* 25: 135-146, 1975.
272. HONGO, T., AND E. JANKOWSKA. Effects from the sensorimotor cortex on the spinal cord in cats with transected pyramids. *Exp. Brain Res.* 3: 117-134, 1967.
273. HONGO, T., E. JANKOWSKA, AND A. LUNDBERG. Convergence of excitatory and inhibitory action on interneurones in the lumbosacral cord. *Exp. Brain Res.* 1: 338-358, 1966.
274. HONGO, T., E. JANKOWSKA, AND A. LUNDBERG. The rubrospinal tract. I. Effects on alpha-motoneurones innervating hindlimb muscles in cats. *Exp. Brain Res.* 7: 344-364, 1969.
275. HONGO, T., E. JANKOWSKA, AND A. LUNDBERG. The rubro-

spinal tract. II. Facilitation of interneuronal transmission in reflex paths to motoneurones. *Exp. Brain Res.* 7: 365-391, 1969.
276. HONGO, T., E. JANKOWSKA, AND A. LUNDBERG. The rubrospinal tract. III. Effects on primary afferent terminals. *Exp. Brain Res.* 15: 39-53, 1972.
277. HONGO, T., E. JANKOWSKA, AND A. LUNDBERG. The rubrospinal tract. IV. Effects on interneurones. *Exp. Brain Res.* 15: 54-78, 1972.
278. HONGO, T., N. KUDO, AND R. TANAKA. The vestibulospinal tract: crossed and uncrossed effects on hindlimb motoneurones in the cat. *Exp. Brain Res.* 24: 37-55, 1975.
279. HONGO, T., AND Y. OKADA. Cortically evoked pre- and postsynaptic inhibition of impulse transmission to the dorsal spinocerebellar tract. *Exp. Brain Res.* 3: 163-177, 1967.
280. HOUK, J., AND E. HENNEMAN. Feedback control of skeletal muscles. *Brain Res.* 5: 433-451, 1967.
281. HOUK, J., AND E. HENNEMAN. Responses of Golgi tendon organs to active contractions of the soleus muscle of the cat. *J. Neurophysiol.* 30: 466-481, 1967.
282. HOUK, J. C., J. J. SINGER, AND M. R. GOLDMAN. An evaluation of length and force feedback to soleus muscles of decerebrate cats. *J. Neurophysiol.* 33: 784-811, 1970.
283. HUBBARD, J. I., AND O. OSCARSSON. Localization of the cell bodies of the ventral spino-cerebellar tract in lumbar segments of the cat. *J. Comp. Neurol.* 118: 199-204, 1962.
284. HULLIGER, M., E. NORDH, A.-E. THELIN, AND Å. B. VALLBO. The responses of afferent fibres from glabrous skin of the hand during voluntary finger movements in man. *J. Physiol. London* 291: 233-249, 1979.
285. HULTBORN, H. Convergence on interneurones in the reciprocal Ia inhibitory pathway to motoneurones. *Acta Physiol. Scand.* 85: (Suppl. 375) 1-42, 1972.
286. HULTBORN, H. Transmission in the pathway of reciprocal Ia inhibition to motoneurones and its control during the tonic stretch reflex. In: *Progress in Brain Research. Understanding the Stretch Reflex*, edited by S. Homma. Amsterdam: Elsevier, 1976, vol. 44, p. 235-255.
287. HULTBORN, H., M. ILLERT, AND M. SANTINI. Convergence on interneurones mediating the reciprocal Ia inhibition of motoneurones. I. Disynaptic Ia inhibition of Ia inhibitory interneurones. *Acta Physiol. Scand.* 96: 193-201, 1976.
288. HULTBORN, H., M. ILLERT, AND M. SANTINI. Convergence on interneurones mediating the reciprocal Ia inhibition of motoneurones. II. Effects from segmental flexor reflex pathways. *Acta Physiol. Scand.* 96: 351-367, 1976.
289. HULTBORN, H., M. ILLERT, AND M. SANTINI. Convergence on interneurones mediating the reciprocal Ia inhibition of motoneurones. III. Effects from supraspinal pathways. *Acta Physiol. Scand.* 96: 368-391, 1976.
290. HULTBORN, H., E. JANKOWSKA, AND S. LINDSTRÖM. Recurrent inhibition from motor axon collaterals of transmission in the Ia inhibitory pathway to motoneurones. *J. Physiol. London* 215: 591-612, 1971.
291. HULTBORN, H., E. JANKOWSKA, AND S. LINDSTRÖM. Recurrent inhibition of interneurones monosynaptically activated from group Ia afferents. *J. Physiol. London* 215: 613-636, 1971.
292. HULTBORN, H., E. JANKOWSKA, AND S. LINDSTRÖM. Relative contribution from different nerves to recurrent depression of Ia IPSPs in motoneurones. *J. Physiol. London* 215: 637-664, 1971.
293. HULTBORN, H., S. LINDSTRÖM, AND H. WIGSTRÖM. On the function of recurrent inhibition in the spinal cord. *Exp. Brain Res.* 37: 399-403, 1979.
294. HULTBORN, H., AND E. PIERROT-DESEILLIGNY. Changes in recurrent inhibition during voluntary soleus contractions in man studied by an H-reflex technique. *J. Physiol. London* 297: 229-251, 1979.
295. HULTBORN, H., AND E. PIERROT-DESEILLIGNY. Input-output relations in the pathway of recurrent inhibition to motoneurones in the cat. *J. Physiol. London* 297: 267-287, 1979.
296. HULTBORN, H., E. PIERROT-DESEILLIGNY, AND H. WIGSTRÖM. Distribution of recurrent inhibition within a motor nucleus. *Neurosci. Lett.*: (Suppl. 1) S97, 1978.
297. HULTBORN, H., E. PIERROT-DESEILLIGNY, AND H. WIGSTRÖM. Recurrent inhibition and afterhyperpolarization following motoneuronal discharge in the cat. *J. Physiol. London* 297: 253-266, 1979.
298. HULTBORN, H., AND M. UDO. Convergence in the reciprocal Ia inhibitory pathway of excitation from descending pathways and inhibition from motor axon collaterals. *Acta Physiol. Scand.* 84: 95-108, 1972.
299. HULTBORN, H., AND M. UDO. Convergence of large muscle spindle (Ia) afferents at interneuronal level in the reciprocal Ia inhibitory pathway to motoneurones. *Acta Physiol. Scand.* 84: 493-499, 1972.
300. HULTBORN, H., AND M. UDO. Recurrent depression from motor axon collaterals of supraspinal inhibition in motoneurones. *Acta Physiol. Scand.* 85: 44-57, 1972.
301. HULTBORN, H., AND H. WIGSTRÖM. Motor response with long latency and maintained duration evoked by activity in Ia afferents. In: *Progress in Clinical Neurophysiology, Spinal and Supraspinal Mechanisms of Voluntary Motor Control and Locomotion*, edited by J. E. Desmedt. Basel: Karger, 1980, vol. 8, p. 99-115.
302. HULTBORN, H., H. WIGSTRÖM, AND B. WÄNGBERG. Prolonged activation of soleus motoneurones following a conditioning train in soleus Ia afferents — a case for a reverberating loop? *Neurosci. Lett.* 1: 147-152, 1975.
303. HUNT, C. C. The reflex activity of mammalian small-nerve fibres. *J. Physiol. London* 115: 456-469, 1951.
304. HUNT, C. C. The effect of stretch receptors from muscle on the discharge of motoneurones. *J. Physiol. London* 117: 359-379, 1952.
305. HUNT, C. C. Relation of function to diameter in afferent fibers of muscle nerves. *J. Gen. Physiol.* 38: 117-131, 1954.
306. HUNT, C. C., AND S. W. KUFFLER. Stretch receptor discharges during muscle contraction. *J. Physiol. London* 113: 298-315, 1951.
307. HUNT, C. C., AND A. K. MCINTYRE. Characteristics of responses from receptors from the flexor longus digitorum muscle and the adjoining interosseous region of the cat. *J. Physiol. London* 153: 74-87, 1960.
308. HUNT, C. C., AND A. S. PAINTAL. Spinal reflex regulation of fusimotor neurones. *J. Physiol. London* 143: 195-212, 1958.
309. ILLERT, M., AND A. LUNDBERG. Collateral connections to the lateral reticular nucleus from cervical propriospinal neurones projecting to forelimb motoneurones in the cat. *Neurosci. Lett.* 7: 167-172, 1978.
310. ILLERT, M., A. LUNDBERG, Y. PADEL, AND R. TANAKA. Convergence on propriospinal neurones which may mediate disynaptic corticospinal excitation to forelimb motoneurones in the cat. *Brain Res.* 93: 530-534, 1975.
311. ILLERT, M., A. LUNDBERG, Y. PADEL, AND R. TANAKA. Integration in descending motor pathways controlling the forelimb in the cat. 5. Properties of and monosynaptic excitatory convergence on C3-C4 propriospinal neurones. *Exp. Brain Res.* 33: 101-130, 1978.
312. ILLERT, M., A. LUNDBERG, AND R. TANAKA. Integration in descending motor pathways controlling the forelimb in the cat. 1. Pyramidal effects on motoneurones. *Exp. Brain Res.* 26: 509-519, 1976.
313. ILLERT, M., A. LUNDBERG, AND R. TANAKA. Integration in descending motor pathways controlling the forelimb in the cat. 2. Convergence on neurones mediating disynaptic cortico-motoneuronal excitation. *Exp. Brain Res.* 26: 521-540, 1976.
314. ILLERT, M., A. LUNDBERG, AND R. TANAKA. Integration in descending motor pathways controlling the forelimb in the cat. 3. Convergence on propriospinal neurones transmitting disynaptic excitation from the corticospinal tract and other descending tracts. *Exp. Brain Res.* 29: 323-346, 1977.
315. ILLERT, M., AND R. TANAKA. Integration in descending motor

pathways controlling the forelimb in the cat. 4. Corticospinal inhibition of forelimb motoneurones mediated by short propriospinal neurones. *Exp. Brain Res.* 31: 131-141, 1978.

316. JACK, J. J. B. Some methods for selective activation of muscle afferent fibres. In: *Studies in Neurophysiology. Essays in Honour of Professor A. K. McIntyre.* Cambridge: Cambridge Univ. Press, 1978.

317. JACK, J. J. B., AND C. R. MACLENNAN. The lack of an electrical threshold discrimination between group Ia and group Ib fibres in the nerve to the cat peroneus longus muscle. *J. Physiol. London* 212: 35P-36P, 1971.

318. JACK, J. J. B., AND R. C. ROBERTS. Selective electrical activation of group II muscle afferent fibres. *J. Physiol. London* 241: 82P-84P, 1974.

319. JACK, J. J. B., AND R. C. ROBERTS. The role of muscle spindle afferents in stretch and vibration reflexes of the soleus muscle of the decerebrate cat. *Brain Res.* 146: 366-372, 1978.

320. JÄNIG, W., R. F. SCHMIDT, AND M. ZIMMERMAN. Single unit responses and the total afferent outflow from the cat's foot pad upon mechanical stimulation. *Exp. Brain Res.* 6: 100-115, 1968.

321. JÄNIG, W., R. F. SCHMIDT, AND M. ZIMMERMAN. Two specific feedback pathways to the central afferent terminals of phasic and tonic mechanoreceptors. *Exp. Brain Res.* 6: 116-129, 1968.

322. JANKOWSKA, E. New observations on neuronal organization of reflexes from tendon organ afferents and their relation to reflexes evoked from muscle spindle afferents. In: *Progress in Brain Research. Reflex Control of Posture and Movement,* edited by R. Granit and O. Pompeiano. Amsterdam: Elsevier, 1979, vol. 50, p. 29-36.

323. JANKOWSKA, E., T. JOHANNISSON, AND J. LIPSKI. Common interneurones in reflex pathways from group Ia and Ib afferents of ankle extensors in the cat. *J. Physiol. London.* In press.

324. JANKOWSKA, E., M. G. M. JUKES, S. LUND, AND A. LUNDBERG. The effect of DOPA on the spinal cord. 5. Reciprocal organization of pathways transmitting excitatory action to alpha motoneurones of flexors and extensors. *Acta Physiol. Scand.* 70: 369-388, 1967.

325. JANKOWSKA, E., M. G. M. JUKES, S. LUND, AND A. LUNDBERG. The effect of DOPA on the spinal cord. 6. Half-centre organization of interneurones transmitting effects from the flexor reflex afferents. *Acta Physiol. Scand.* 70: 389-402, 1967.

326. JANKOWSKA, E., AND S. LINDSTRÖM. Morphological identification of Renshaw cells. *Acta Physiol. Scand.* 81: 428-430, 1971.

327. JANKOWSKA, E., AND S. LINDSTRÖM. Morphology of interneurones mediating Ia reciprocal inhibition of motoneurones in the spinal cord of the cat. *J. Physiol. London* 226: 805-823, 1972.

328. JANKOWSKA, E., AND S. LINDSTRÖM. Procion yellow staining of functionally identified interneurones in the spinal cord of the cat. In: *Intracellular Staining in Neurobiology,* edited by S. B. Kater and C. Nicholson. New York: Springer-Verlag, 1973, p. 199-209.

329. JANKOWSKA, E., S. LUND, AND A. LUNDBERG. The effect of DOPA on the spinal cord. 4. Depolarization evoked in the central terminals of contralateral Ia afferent terminals by volleys in the flexor reflex afferents. *Acta Physiol. Scand.* 68: 337-341, 1966.

330. JANKOWSKA, E., S. LUND, A. LUNDBERG, AND O. POMPEIANO. Inhibitory effects evoked through ventral reticulospinal pathways. *Arch. Ital. Biol.* 106: 124-140, 1968.

331. JANKOWSKA, E., A. LUNDBERG, W. J. ROBERTS, AND D. STUART. A long propriospinal system with direct effect on motoneurones and on interneurones in the cat lumbosacral cord. *Exp. Brain Res.* 21: 169-194, 1974.

332. JANKOWSKA, E., A. LUNDBERG, AND D. STUART. Propriospinal control of last order interneurones of spinal reflex pathways in the cat. *Brain Res.* 53: 227-231, 1973.

333. JANKOWSKA, E., Y. PADEL, AND R. TANAKA. Disynaptic inhibition of spinal motoneurones from the motor cortex in the monkey. *J. Physiol. London* 258: 467-487, 1976.

334. JANKOWSKA, E., Y. PADEL, AND P. ZARZECKI. Crossed disynaptic inhibition of sacral motoneurones. *J. Physiol. London* 285: 425-444, 1978.

335. JANKOWSKA, E., AND W. J. ROBERTS. An electrophysiological demonstration of the axonal projections of single spinal interneurones in the cat. *J. Physiol. London* 222: 597-622, 1972.

336. JANKOWSKA, E., AND W. J. ROBERTS. Synaptic actions of single interneurones mediating reciprocal Ia inhibition of motoneurones. *J. Physiol. London* 222: 623-642, 1972.

337. JANKOWSKA, E., AND D. O. SMITH. Antidromic activation of Renshaw cells and their axonal projections. *Acta Physiol. Scand.* 88: 198-214, 1973.

338. JANSEN, J. K. S., AND T. RUDJORD. On the silent period and Golgi tendon organs of the soleus muscle of the cat. *Acta Physiol. Scand.* 62: 364-379, 1964.

339. JENESKOG, T. Parallel activation of dynamic fusimotor neurones and a climbing fibre system from the cat brain stem. I. Effects from the rubral region. *Acta Physiol. Scand.* 91: 223-242, 1974.

340. JENESKOG, T. Parallel activation of dynamic fusimotor neurones and a climbing fibre system from the cat brain stem. II. Effects from the inferior olivary region. *Acta Physiol. Scand.* 92: 66-83, 1974.

341. JOB, C. Über autogene Inhibition und Reflexumkehr bei spinalisierten und decerebrierten Katzen. *Pfluegers Arch.* 256: 406-418, 1953.

342. JURNA, I., AND A. LUNDBERG. The influence of an inhibitor of dopamine-beta-hydroxylase on the effect of DOPA on transmission in the spinal cord. In: *Structure and Functions of Inhibitory Neuronal Mechanisms.* Oxford: Pergamon, 1968, p. 469-472. (Fourth Int. Meeting Neurobiol., Stockholm, September 1966.)

343. KANDA, K. Contribution of polysynaptic pathways to the tonic vibration reflex. *Jpn. J. Physiol.* 22: 367-377, 1972.

344. KANDA, R., AND W. Z. RYMER. An estimate of the secondary spindle receptor afferent contribution to the stretch reflex in extensor muscles of the decerebrate cat. *J. Physiol. London* 264: 63-87, 1977.

345. KANDEL, E. R., W. T. FRAZIER, R. WAZIRI, AND R. E. COGGESHALL. Direct and common connections among identified neurons in *Aplysia. J. Neurophysiol.* 30: 1352-1376, 1967.

346. KATO, M., AND K. FUKUSHIMA. Effect of differential blocking of motor axons on antidromic activation of Renshaw cells in the cat. *Exp. Brain Res.* 20: 135-143, 1974.

347. KENINS, P., H. KIKILLUS, AND E. D. SCHOMBURG. Short- and long-latency reflex pathways from neck afferents to hindlimb motoneurones in the cat. *Brain Res.* 149: 235-238, 1978.

348. KIBAKINA, T. V., AND A. I. SHAPOVALOV. Functional organization of reticulo- and vestibulo-spinal synaptic projections to rat lumbar motoneurons [in Russian]. *Fiziol. Zh. SSSR im I. M. Sechenov* 64: 435-442, 1978.

349. KIRKWOOD, P. A., AND T. A. SEARS. Monosynaptic excitation of motoneurones from muscle spindle secondary endings of intercostal and triceps surae muscles in the cat. *J. Physiol. London* 245: 64P-66P, 1975.

350. KIRKWOOD, P. A., AND T. A. SEARS. The synaptic connexions to intercostal motoneurones as revealed by the average common excitation potential. *J. Physiol. London* 275: 103-134, 1978.

351. KOEHLER, W., U. WINDHORST, J. SCHMIDT, J. MEYER-LOHMANN, AND H.-D. HENATSCH. Diverging influences on Renshaw cell responses and monosynaptic reflexes from stimulation of capsula interna. *Neurosci. Lett.* 8: 35-39, 1978.

352. KOEZE, T. H. The independence of corticomotoneuronal and fusimotor pathways in the production of muscle contraction by motor cortex stimulation. *J. Physiol. London* 197: 87-105, 1968.

353. KOEZE, T. H., C. G. PHILLIPS, AND J. D. SHERIDAN. Thresholds of cortical activation of muscle spindles and α motoneurones of the baboon's hand. *J. Physiol. London* 195: 419-449, 1968.

354. KOSTYUK, P. G. Interneuronal mechanisms of interaction be-

tween descending and afferent signals in the spinal cord. In: *Golgi Centennial Symposium. Proceedings*, edited by M. Santini. New York: Raven, 1975, p. 247-259.
355. KOSTYUK, P. G., AND D. A. VASILENKO. Transformation of cortical motor signals in spinal cord. *Proc. IEEE* 56: 1049-1058, 1968.
356. KOSTYUK, P. G., D. A. VASILENKO, AND E. LANG. Propriospinal pathways in the dorsolateral funiculus and their effects on lumbosacral motoneuronal pools. *Brain Res.* 28: 233-249, 1971.
357. KOSTYUK, P. G., D. A. VASILENKO, AND A. G. ZADOROZHNY. Reactions of lumbar motoneurons produced by actions of propriospinal pathways. *Neurophysiology USSR* 1: 5-14, 1969.
358. KOZHANOV, V. M. The propriospinal monosynaptic effects of the ventral descending pathways on the cat lumbar motoneurones. *Fiziol. Zh. SSSR im I. M. Sechenov* 60: 171-178, 1974.
359. KOZHANOV, V. M., AND A. I. SHAPOVALOV. Synaptic organization of the supraspinal control of propriospinal ventral horn interneurons in cat and monkey spinal cord. *Neurophysiology USSR* 9: 177-184, 1977.
360. KOZHANOV, V. M., AND A. I. SHAPOVALOV. Synaptic actions evoked in motoneurons by stimulation of individual propriospinal neurons. *Neurophysiology USSR* 9: 300-306, 1977.
361. KUFFLER, S. W., AND C. C. HUNT. The mammalian small-nerve fibers: a system for efferent nervous regulation of muscle spindle discharge. In: *Patterns of Organization in the Central Nervous System*, edited by P. Bard. Baltimore: Williams & Wilkins, 1952, p. 24-47.
362. KUNO, M. Excitability following antidromic activation in spinal motoneurones supplying red muscles. *J. Physiol. London* 149: 374-393, 1959.
363. KUNO, M., AND E. R. PERL. Alternation of spinal reflexes by interaction with suprasegmental and dorsal root activity. *J. Physiol. London* 151: 103-122, 1960.
364. KUYPERS, H. Pericentral cortical projections to motor and sensory nuclei. *Science* 128: 662-663, 1958.
365. LANCE, J. W., P. DE GAIL, AND P. D. NEILSON. Tonic and phasic spinal cord mechanisms in man. *J. Neurol. Neurosurg. Psychiatry* 29: 535-544, 1966.
366. LANDGREN, S., C. G. PHILLIPS, AND R. PORTER. Minimal synaptic actions of pyramidal impulses on some alpha motoneurones of the baboon's hand and forearm. *J. Physiol. London* 161: 91-111, 1962.
367. LAPORTE, Y. The motor innervation of the mammalian muscle spindle. In: *Studies in Neurophysiology. Essays in Honour of Professor A. K. McIntyre*, edited by R. Porter. Cambridge: Cambridge Univ., 1978, p. 45-59.
368. LAPORTE, Y., AND P. BESSOU. Étude des sous-groupes lent et rapide du groupe I (fibres afférentes d'origine musculaire de grand diamètre) chez le chat. *J. Physiol. Paris* 49: 1025-1037, 1957.
369. LAPORTE, Y., AND D. P. C. LLOYD. Nature and significance of the reflex connections established by large afferent fibers of muscular origin. *Am. J. Physiol.* 169: 609-621, 1952.
370. LAPORTE, Y., A. LUNDBERG, AND O. OSCARSSON. Functional organization of the dorsal spinocerebellar tract in the cat. II. Single fibre recording in Flechsig's fasciculus on electrical stimulation of various peripheral nerves. *Acta Physiol. Scand.* 36: 188-203, 1956.
371. LARSSON, B., S. MILLER, AND O. OSCARSSON. A spinocerebellar climbing fibre path activated by the flexor reflex afferents from all four limbs. *J. Physiol. London* 203: 641-649, 1969.
372. LAWRENCE, D. G., AND D. A. HOPKINS. The development of motor control in the rhesus monkey: evidence concerning the role of corticomotoneuronal connections. *Brain* 99: 235-254, 1976.
373. LAWRENCE, D. G., AND H. G. J. M. KUYPERS. The functional organization of the motor system in the monkey. II. The effects of lesions of the descending brain-stem pathways. *Brain* 91: 15-36, 1968.
374. LENNERSTRAND, G., AND U. THODEN. Muscle spindle responses to concomitant variations in length and in fusimotor activation. *Acta Physiol. Scand.* 74: 153-165, 1968.
375. LEVY, R. A., AND E. G. ANDERSON. The role of γ-aminobutyric acid as a mediator of positive dorsal root potentials. *Brain Res.* 76: 71-82, 1974.
376. LIDDELL, E. G. T. Spinal shock and some features in isolation-alteration of the spinal cord in cats. *Brain* 57: 386-400, 1934.
377. LIDDELL, E. G. T. The influence of experimental lesions of the spinal cord upon the knee-jerk. II. Chronic lesions. With an appendix 'a note on the "spinal" and "decerebrate" type of knee-jerk in the cat'. *Brain* 59: 160-174, 1936.
378. LIDDELL, E. G. T., AND C. S. SHERRINGTON. Reflexes in response to stretch (myotatic reflexes). *Proc. R. Soc. London Ser. B* 96: 212-242, 1924.
379. LIDDELL, E. G. T., AND C. S. SHERRINGTON. Further observations on myotatic reflexes. *Proc. R. Soc. London Ser. B* 97: 267-283, 1925.
380. LINDSTRÖM, S. Recurrent control from motor axon collaterals of Ia inhibitory pathways in the spinal cord of the cat. *Acta Physiol. Scand. (Suppl. 392)*: 1-43, 1973.
381. LINDSTRÖM, S., AND E. D. SCHOMBURG. Recurrent inhibition from motor axon collaterals of ventral spinocerebellar tract neurones. *Acta Physiol. Scand.* 88: 505-515, 1973.
382. LINDSTRÖM, S., AND E. D. SCHOMBURG. Group I inhibition in Ib excited ventral spinocerebellar tract neurones. *Acta Physiol. Scand.* 90: 166-185, 1974.
383. LIU, C.-N. Fate of cells of Clarke's nucleus following axon section in cat, with evidence of spinal collaterals from dorsal spinocerebellar tract. *Anat. Record.* 115: 342-343, 1953.
384. LLINAS, R., AND C. A. TERZUOLO. Mechanisms of supraspinal actions upon spinal cord activities. Reticular inhibitory mechanisms on alpha-extensor motoneurones. *J. Neurophysiol.* 27: 579-591, 1964.
385. LLINAS, R., AND C. A. TERZUOLO. Mechanisms of supraspinal actions upon spinal cord activities. Reticular inhibitory mechanisms upon flexor motoneurones. *J. Neurophysiol.* 28: 413-422, 1965.
386. LLOYD, D. P. C. Activity in neurons of the bulbospinal correlation system. *J. Neurophysiol.* 4: 115-134, 1941.
387. LLOYD, D. P. C. A direct central inhibitory action of dromically conducted impulses. *J. Neurophysiol.* 4: 184-190, 1941.
388. LLOYD, D. P. C. The spinal mechanism of the pyramidal system in cats. *J. Neurophysiol.* 4: 525-546, 1941.
389. LLOYD, D. P. C. Mediation of descending long spinal reflex activity. *J. Neurophysiol.* 5: 435-458, 1942.
390. LLOYD, D. P. C. Reflex action in relation to pattern and peripheral source of afferent stimulation. *J. Neurophysiol.* 6: 111-119, 1943.
391. LLOYD, D. P. C. Neuron patterns controlling transmission of ipsilateral hind limb reflexes in cat. *J. Neurophysiol.* 6: 293-315, 1943.
392. LLOYD, D. P. C. Conduction and synaptic transmission of the reflex response to stretch in spinal cats. *J. Neurophysiol.* 6: 317-326, 1943.
393. LLOYD, D. P. C. Facilitation and inhibition of spinal motoneurons. *J. Neurophysiol.* 9: 421-438, 1946.
394. LLOYD, D. P. C. Integrative pattern of excitation and inhibition in two-neuron reflex arcs. *J. Neurophysiol.* 9: 439-444, 1946.
395. LLOYD, D. P. C. Spinal mechanisms involved in somatic activities. In: *Handbook of Physiology. Neurophysiology*, edited by J. Field, H. W. Magoun, and V. E. Hall. Washington, DC: Am. Physiol. Soc., 1960, sect. 1, vol. II, chapt. 36, p. 929-949.
396. LLOYD, D. P. C., AND A. K. McINTYRE. Analysis of forelimb-hindlimb reflex activity in acutely decapitate cats. *J. Neurophysiol.* 11: 455-470, 1948.
397. LOEB, G. E., M. J. BAK, AND J. DUYSENS. Long-term unit recording from somatosensory neurons in the spinal ganglia of the freely walking cat. *Science* 197: 1192-1194, 1977.
398. LOEB, G. E., AND J. DUYSENS. Activity patterns in individual hindlimb primary and secondary muscle spindle afferents during normal movements in unrestrained cats. *J. Neurophysiol.* 42: 420-440, 1979.
399. LONGO, V. G., W. R. MARTIN, AND K. R. UNNA. A pharmacological study on the Renshaw cell. *J. Pharmacol. Exp. Ther.* 129: 61-68, 1960.
400. LUCAS, M. E., AND W. D. WILLIS. Identification of muscle

afferents which activate interneurons in the intermediate nucleus. *J. Neurophysiol.* 37: 282-293, 1974.

401. LUND, J. P., A. M. SMITH, B. J. SESSLE, AND T. MURAKAMI. Activity of trigeminal α- and γ-motoneurons and muscle afferents during performance of a biting task. *J. Neurophysiol.* 42: 710-725, 1979.

402. LUND, S., A. LUNDBERG, AND L. VYKLICKÝ. Inhibitory action from the flexor reflex afferents on transmission to Ia afferents. *Acta Physiol. Scand.* 64: 345-355, 1965.

403. LUND, S., AND O. POMPEIANO. Monosynaptic excitation of alpha motoneurones from supraspinal structures in the cat. *Acta Physiol. Scand.* 73: 1-21, 1968.

404. LUNDBERG, A. Integrative significance of patterns of connections made by muscle afferents in the spinal cord. In: *Congr. Int. Cienc. Fisiol., XXI, Buenos Aires, 1959*, p. 100-105.

405. LUNDBERG, A. Monoamines and spinal reflexes. In: *Studies in Physiology*. Berlin: Springer-Verlag, 1965, p. 186-190.

406. LUNDBERG, A. Integration in the reflex pathway. In: *Muscular Afferents and Motor Control. Nobel Symposium I*, edited by R. Granit. Stockholm: Almqvist & Wiksell, 1966, p. 275-305.

407. LUNDBERG, A. Convergence of excitatory and inhibitory action on interneurones in the spinal cord. In: *The Interneuron*, edited by M. A. B. Brazier. Los Angeles: University of California Press, 1969, p. 231-265. (UCLA Forum Med. Sci. No. 11.)

408. LUNDBERG, A. Reflex control of stepping. *The Nansen Memorial Lecture V*. Oslo: Universitetsforlaget, 1969, p. 5-42.

409. LUNDBERG, A. The excitatory control of the Ia inhibitory pathway. In: *Excitatory Synaptic Mechanisms*, edited by P. Andersen and J. K. S. Jansen. Oslo: Universitetsforlaget, 1970, p. 333-340.

410. LUNDBERG, A. Function of the ventral spinocerebellar tract. A new hypothesis. *Exp. Brain Res.* 12: 317-330, 1971.

411. LUNDBERG, A. The significance of segmental spinal mechanisms in motor control. In: *Symp. Int. Biophys. Congr., 4th, Moscow, 1972*. Moscow: Pushchino, 1973, p. 1-23.

412. LUNDBERG, A. Control of spinal mechanisms from the brain. In: *The Nervous System. The Basic Neurosciences*, edited by D. B. Tower. New York: Raven, 1975, vol. I, p. 253-265.

413. LUNDBERG, A. Multisensory control of spinal reflex pathways. *Progress in Brain Research. Reflex Control of Posture and Movement*, edited by R. Granit and O. Pompeiano. Amsterdam: Elsevier, 1979, vol. 50, p. 11-28.

414. LUNDBERG, A. Integration in a propriospinal motor centre controlling the forelimb in the cat. In: *Integration in the Nervous System*, edited by H. Asanuma and V. J. Wilson. Tokyo: Igaku shoin, 1979, p. 47-64.

415. LUNDBERG, A., K. MALMGREN AND E. D. SCHOMBURG. Convergence from Ib, cutaneous and joint afferents in reflex pathways to motoneurones. *Brain Res.* 87: 81-84, 1975.

416. LUNDBERG, A., K. MALMGREN AND E. D. SCHOMBURG. Characteristics of the excitatory pathway from group II muscle afferents to alpha motoneurones. *Brain Res.* 88: 538-542, 1975.

417. LUNDBERG, A., K. MALMGREN AND E. D. SCHOMBURG. Cutaneous facilitation of transmission in reflex pathways from Ib afferents to motoneurones. *J. Physiol. London* 265: 763-780, 1977.

418. LUNDBERG, A., K. MALMGREN AND E. D. SCHOMBURG. Comments on reflex actions evoked by electrical stimulation of group II muscle afferents. *Brain Res.* 122: 551-555, 1977.

419. LUNDBERG, A., K. MALMGREN, AND E. D. SCHOMBURG. Role of joint afferents in motor control exemplified by effects on reflex pathways from Ib afferents. *J. Physiol. London* 284: 327-343, 1978.

420. LUNDBERG, A., U. NORRSELL, AND P. VOORHOEVE. Pyramidal effects on lumbo-sacral interneurones activated by somatic afferents. *Acta Physiol. Scand.* 56: 220-229, 1962.

421. LUNDBERG, A., U. NORRSELL, AND P. VOORHOEVE. Effects from the sensorimotor cortex on ascending spinal pathways. *Acta Physiol. Scand.* 59: 462-473, 1963.

422. LUNDBERG, A., AND O. OSCARSSON. Functional organization of the dorsal spino-cerebellar tract in the cat. VII. Identification of units by antidromic activation from the cerebellar cortex with recognition of five functional subdivisions. *Acta Physiol. Scand.* 50: 356-374, 1960.

423. LUNDBERG, A., AND O. OSCARSSON. Three ascending spinal pathways in the dorsal part of the lateral funiculus. *Acta Physiol. Scand.* 51: 1-16, 1961.

424. LUNDBERG, A., AND O. OSCARSSON. Two ascending spinal pathways in the ventral part of the cord. *Acta Physiol. Scand.* 54: 270-286, 1962.

425. LUNDBERG, A., AND P. VOORHOEVE. Effects from the pyramidal tract on spinal reflex arcs. *Acta Physiol. Scand.* 56: 201-219, 1962.

426. LUNDBERG, A., AND L. VYKLICKÝ. Inhibitory interaction between spinal reflexes to primary afferents. *Experientia* 19: 247-248, 1963.

427. LUNDBERG, A., AND L. VYKLICKÝ. Inhibition of transmission to primary afferents by electrical stimulation of the brain stem. *Arch. Ital. Biol.* 104: 86-97, 1966.

428. LUNDBERG, A., AND F. WEIGHT. Functional organization of connexions to the ventral spinocerebellar tract. *Exp. Brain Res.* 12: 295-316, 1971.

429. LUNDBERG, A., AND G. WINSBURY. Selective adequate activation of large afferents from muscle spindles and Golgi tendon organs. *Acta Physiol. Scand.* 49: 155-164, 1960.

430. MACLEAN, J. B., AND H. LEFFMAN. Supraspinal control of Renshaw cells. *Exp. Neurol.* 18: 94-104, 1967.

431. MAGNI, F., AND O. OSCARSSON. Cerebral control of transmission to the ventral spino-cerebellar tract. *Arch. Ital. Biol.* 99: 369-396, 1961.

432. MAGOUN, H. W., AND R. RHINES. An inhibitory mechanism in the bulbar reticular formation. *J. Neurophysiol.* 9: 165-171, 1946.

433. MARSDEN, C. D., P. A. MERTON, AND H. B. MORTON. Servo action in human voluntary movement. *Nature London* 238: 140-143, 1972.

434. MARSDEN, C. D., P. A. MERTON, AND H. B. MORTON. Is the human stretch reflex cortical rather than spinal. *Lancet* 1: 759-761, 1973.

435. MARSDEN, C. D., P. A. MERTON, AND H. B. MORTON. Stretch reflex and servo action in a variety of human muscles. *J. Physiol. London* 259: 531-560, 1976.

436. MASSION, J. The mammalian red nucleus. *Physiol. Rev.* 47: 383-436, 1967.

437. MATSUSHITA, M. Some aspects of the interneuronal connections in cat's spinal gray matter. *J. Comp. Neurol.* 136: 57-79, 1969.

438. MATSUSHITA, M., AND Y. HOSOYA. Cells of origin of the spinocerebellar tract in the rat, studied with the method of retrograde transport of horseradish peroxidase. *Brain Res.* 173: 185-200, 1979.

439. MATTHEWS, B. H. C. Nerve endings in mammalian muscle. *J. Physiol. London* 78: 1-53, 1933.

440. MATTHEWS, P. B. C. The differentiation of two types of fusimotor fibre by their effects on the dynamic response of muscle spindle primary endings. *Q. J. Exp. Physiol.* 47: 324-333, 1962.

441. MATTHEWS, P. B. C. Muscle spindles and their motor control. *Physiol. Rev.* 44: 219-288, 1964.

442. MATTHEWS, P. B. C. Evidence that the secondary as well as the primary endings of the muscle spindles may be responsible for the tonic stretch reflex of the decerebrate cat. *J. Physiol. London* 204: 365-393, 1969.

443. MATTHEWS, P. B. C. The origin and functional significance of the stretch reflex. In: *Excitatory Synaptic Mechanism*, edited by P. Andersen and J. K. S. Jansen. Olso: Universitetsforlaget, 1970, p. 301-315.

444. MATTHEWS, P. B. C. *Mammalian Muscle Receptors and Their Central Actions*. London: Arnold, 1972.

444a. MCCREA, D. A., C. A. PRATT, AND L. M. JORDAN. Renshaw cell activity and recurrent effects on motoneurons during fictive locomotion. *J. Neurophysiol.* 44: 475-488, 1980.

445. MELVILL-JONES, G., AND D. G. D. WATT. Observations on the control of stepping and hopping movements in man. *J. Physiol. London* 219: 709-727, 1971.

446. MENDELL, L. Positive dorsal root potentials produced by stimulation of small diameter muscle afferents. *Brain Res.* 18: 375-379, 1970.
447. MENDELL, L. Properties and distribution of peripherally evoked presynaptic hyperpolarization in cat lumbar spinal cord. *J. Physiol. London* 226: 769-792, 1972.
448. MENDELL, L. M., AND P. D. WALL. Presynaptic hyperpolarization: a role for fine afferent fibers. *J. Physiol. London* 172: 274-294, 1964.
449. MERTON, P. A. Speculations on the servo-control of movement. In: *The Spinal Cord*, edited by G. E. W. Wolstenholme. London: Churchill, 1953, p. 247-255.
450. MILLER, S., D. J. REITSMA, AND F. G. A. VAN DER MECHÉ. Functional organization of long ascending propriospinal pathways linking lumbo-sacral and cervical segments in the cat. *Brain Res.* 62: 169-188, 1973.
451. MOLENAAR, I. The distribution of propriospinal neurons projecting to different motoneuronal cell groups in the cat's brachial cord. *Brain Res.* 158: 203-206, 1978.
452. MOLENAAR, I., AND H. G. J. M. KUYPERS. Cells of origin of propriospinal fibers and of fibers ascending to supraspinal levels. A HRP study in cat and rhesus monkey. *Brain Res.* 152: 429-450, 1978.
453. MOLENAAR, I., A. RUSTIONI, AND H. G. J. M. KUYPERS. The location of cells of origin of the fibers in the ventral and the lateral funiculus of the cat's lumbo-sacral cord. *Brain Res.* 78: 239-254, 1974.
454. MORRISON, A. R., AND O. POMPEIANO. Central depolarization of group Ia afferent fibers during desynchronized sleep. *Arch. Ital. Biol.* 103: 517-537, 1965.
455. MORRISON, A. R., AND O. POMPEIANO. Depolarization of central terminals of group Ia muscle afferent fibres during desynchronized sleep. *Nature London* 210: 201-202, 1966.
456. MUIR, R. B., AND R. PORTER. The effect of a preceding stimulus on temporal facilitation at corticomotoneuronal synapses. *J. Physiol. London* 228: 749-763, 1973.
457. MURAKAMI, F., N. TSUKAHARA, AND Y. FUJITO. Properties of the synaptic transmission of the newly formed cortico-rubral synapses after lesion of the nucleus interpositus of the cerebellum. *Exp. Brain Res.* 30: 245-258, 1977.
458. NEWSOM DAVIS, J., AND T. A. SEARS. The proprioceptive reflex control of the intercostal muscles during their voluntary activation. *J. Physiol. London* 209: 711-738, 1970.
459. NICHOLS, T. R., AND J. C. HOUK. Improvement in linearity and regulation of stiffness that results from actions of stretch reflex. *J. Neurophysiol.* 39: 119-142, 1976.
460. NYGREN, L.-G., K. FUXE, G. JONSSON, AND L. OLSON. Functional regeneration of 5-hydroxytryptamine nerve terminals in the rat spinal cord following 5,6-dihydroxytryptamine induced degeneration. *Brain Res.* 78: 377-394, 1974.
461. NYGREN, L.-G., AND L. OLSON. On spinal noradrenaline receptor supersensitivity: Correlation between nerve terminal densities and flexor reflexes various times after intracisternal 6-hydroxydopamine. *Brain Res.* 116: 455-470, 1976.
462. NYGREN, L.-G., AND L. OLSON. A new major projection from locus coeruleus: the main source of noradrenergic nerve terminals in the ventral and dorsal columns of the spinal cord. *Brain Res.* 132: 85-93, 1977.
463. ORLOVSKY, G. N. Activity of vestibulospinal neurons during locomotion. *Brain Res.* 46: 85-98, 1972.
464. ORLOVSKY, G. N. Activity of rubrospinal neurons during locomotion. *Brain Res.* 46: 99-112, 1972.
465. OSCARSSON, O. Functional organization of the ventral spinocerebellar tract in the cat. I. Electrophysiological identification of the tract. *Acta Physiol. Scand.* 38: 145-165, 1956.
466. OSCARSSON, O. Functional organization of the ventral spinocerebellar tract in the cat. II. Connections with muscle, joint, and skin nerve afferents and effects on adequate stimulation of various receptors. *Acta Physiol. Scand.* 42: (Suppl. 146) 1-107, 1957.
467. OSCARSSON, O. Further observations on ascending spinal tracts activated from muscle, joint, and skin nerves. *Arch. Ital. Biol.* 96: 199-215, 1958.
468. OSCARSSON, O. Functional organization of the ventral spino cerebellar tract in the cat. III. Supraspinal control of VSCT units of I-type. *Acta Physiol. Scand.* 49: 171-183, 1960.
469. OSCARSSON, O. Termination and functional organization of the ventral spino-olivocerebellar path. *J. Physiol. London* 196: 453-478, 1968.
470. OSCARSSON, O. Termination and functional organization of the dorsal spino-olivocerebellar path. *J. Physiol. London* 200: 129-149, 1969.
471. OSCARSSON, O. Functional organization of spinocerebellar paths. In: *Handbook of Sensory Physiology. Somatosensory System*, edited by A. Iggo. Berlin: Springer-Verlag, 1973, vol. II, p. 339-380.
472. OSCARSSON, O. Spatial distribution of climbing and mossy fibre inputs into the cerebellar cortex. In: *Afferent and Intrinsic Organization of Laminated Structures in the Brain*, edited by O. Creutzfeldt. *Exp. Brain Res.* Suppl. 1. Berlin: Springer-Verlag, 1976, p. 36-42.
473. OSCARSSON, O., AND B. SJÖLUND. The ventral spino-olivocerebellar system in the cat. I. Identification of five paths and their termination in the cerebellar anterior lobe. *Exp. Brain Res.* 28: 469-486, 1977.
474. OSCARSSON, O., AND N. UDDENBERG. Identification of a spinocerebellar tract activated from forelimb afferents in the cat. *Acta Physiol. Scand.* 62: 125-136, 1964.
475. OSCARSSON, O., AND N. UDDENBERG. Somatotopic termination of spino-olivocerebellar path. *Brain Res.* 3: 204-207, 1966.
476. PATTON, H. D., AND V. E. AMASSIAN. The pyramidal tract: its excitation and functions. In: *Handbook of Physiology. Neurophysiology*, edited by J. Field, H. W. Magoun and V. E. Hall. Washington, DC: Am. Physiol. Soc., 1960, sect. 1, vol. II, chapt. 34, p. 837-861.
477. PEARSON, K. G., AND J. DUYSENS. Function of segmental reflexes in the control of stepping in cockroaches and cats. In: *Neural Control of Locomotion. Advances in Behavioral Biology*, edited by R. M. Herman, S. Grillner, P. G. S. Stein and D. G. Stuart. New York: Plenum, 1976, vol. 18, p. 519-537.
478. PERL, E. R. Crossed reflex effects evoked by activity in myelinated afferent fibers of muscle. *J. Neurophysiol.* 21: 101-112, 1958.
479. PERL, E. R. Effects of muscle stretch on excitability of contralateral motoneurones. *J. Physiol. London* 145: 193-203, 1959.
480. PERRET, C. Neural control of locomotion in the decorticate cat. In: *Neural Control of Locomotion. Advances in Behavioral Biology*, edited by R. M. Herman, S. Grillner, P. S. G. Stein and D. G. Stuart. New York: Plenum, 1976, vol. 18, p. 587-615.
481. PERRET, C., AND A. BERTHOZ. Evidence of static and dynamic fusimotor actions on the spindle response to sinusoidal stretch during locomotor activity in the cat. *Exp. Brain Res.* 18: 178-188, 1973.
482. PETERSON, B. W., N. G. PITTS, K. FUKUSHIMA, AND R. MACKEL. Reticulospinal excitation and inhibition of neck motoneurons. *Exp. Brain Res.* 32: 471-489, 1978.
483. PHILIPPSON, M. L'autonomie et la centralisation dans le système nerveux des animaux. *Trav. Lab. Physiol. Inst. Solvay Bruxelles.* 7: 1-208, 1905.
484. PHILLIPS, C. G., AND R. PORTER. The pyramidal projection to motoneurones of some muscle groups of the baboon's forelimb. In: *Progress in Brain Research. Physiology of Spinal Neurons*, edited by J. C. Eccles and J. P. Schadé. Amsterdam: Elsevier, 1964, vol. 12, p. 222-245.
485. PIERCEY, M. F., AND J. GOLDFARB. Discharge patterns of Renshaw cells evoked by volleys in ipsilateral cutaneous and high-threshold muscle afferents and their relationship to reflexes recorded in ventral roots. *J. Neurophysiol.* 37: 294-302, 1974.
486. PIERROT-DESEILLIGNY, E., R. KATZ, AND C. MORIN. Evidence for Ib inhibition in human subjects. *Brain Res.* 166: 176-179, 1979.
487. PIERROT-DESEILLIGNY, E., C. MORIN, R. KATZ, AND B. BUSSEL. Influence of posture and voluntary movement on recurrent inhibition in human subjects. *Brain Res.* 124: 427-436, 1977.

488. PI-SUÑER, J., AND J. F. FULTON. The influence of proprioceptive system upon the crossed extensor reflex. *Am. J. Physiol.* 88: 453–467, 1929.
489. POGORELAYA, N. KH. Experimental-morphological study of primary afferent terminals in the base of dorsal horn of the cat spinal cord. *Neurophysiology USSR* 5: 406–414, 1973.
490. POMPEIANO, O. Mechanisms of sensorimotor integration during sleep. In: *Progress in Physiological Psychology*, edited by E. Stellar and J. M. Sprague. New York: Academic, 1970, vol. 3, p. 1–179.
491. PORTER, R. Early facilitation at corticomotoneuronal synapses. *J. Physiol. London* 207: 733–745, 1970.
492. PRATT, C. A., AND L. M. JORDAN. Recurrent inhibition of motoneurons in decerebrate cats during controlled treadmill locomotion. *J. Neurophysiol.* 44: 489–500, 1980.
493. PRESTIGE, M. C. Initial collaterals of motor axons within the spinal cord of the cat. *J. Comp. Neurol.* 126: 123–136, 1966.
494. PROCHAZKA, A., J. A. STEPHENS, AND P. WAND. Muscle spindle discharge in normal and obstructed movements. *J. Physiol. London* 287: 57–66, 1979.
495. PROCHAZKA, A., R. A. WESTERMAN, AND S. P. ZICCONE. Discharges of single hindlimb afferents in the freely moving cat. *J. Neurophysiol.* 39: 1090–1104, 1976.
496. PROCHAZKA, A., R. A. WESTERMAN, AND S. P. ZICCONE. Ia afferent activity during a variety of voluntary movements in the cat. *J. Physiol. London* 268: 423–448, 1977.
497. RADEMAKER, G. G. S. *Das Stehen*. Berlin: Springer-Verlag, 1931.
498. RAPOPORT, S., A. SUSSWEIN, Y. UCHINO, AND V. J. WILSON. Synaptic actions of individual vestibular neurones on cat neck motoneurones. *J. Physiol. London* 272: 367–382, 1977.
499. RASTAD, J., E. JANKOWSKA, AND J. WESTMAN. Arborization of initial axon collaterals of spinocervical tract cells stained intracellularly with horseradish peroxidase. *Brain Res.* 135: 1–10, 1977.
500. RATLIFF, F., H. H. HARTLINE, AND W. H. MILLER. Spatial and temporal aspects of retinal inhibitory interaction. *J. Opt. Soc. Am.* 53: 110–120, 1963.
501. RENSHAW, B. Influence of discharge of motoneurons upon excitation of neighboring motoneurons. *J. Neurophysiol.* 4: 167–183, 1941.
502. RENSHAW, B. Central effects of centripetal impulses in axons of spinal ventral roots. *J. Neurophysiol.* 9: 191–204, 1946.
503. ROBERTS, T. D. M. Reflex interaction of synergic extensor muscles of the cat hind limb. *J. Physiol. London* 117: 5P–6P, 1952.
504. ROMANES, G. J. The motor cell columns of the lumbo-sacral spinal cord of the cat. *J. Comp. Neurol.* 94: 313–363, 1951.
505. ROSS, H.-G., S. CLEVELAND, AND J. HAASE. Quantitative relation of Renshaw cell discharges to monosynaptic reflex height. *Pfluegers Arch.* 332: 73–79, 1972.
506. ROSS, H.-G., S. CLEVELAND, AND J. HAASE. Contribution of single motoneurons to Renshaw cell activity. *Neurosci. Lett.* 1: 105–108, 1975.
507. ROSS, H.-G., S. CLEVELAND, AND J. HAASE. Quantitative relation between discharge frequencies of a Renshaw cell and an intracellularly depolarized motoneuron. *Neurosci. Lett.* 3: 129–132, 1976.
508. ROSSIGNOL, S., AND L. GAUTHIER. Reversal of contralateral limb reflexes. *Proc. Int. Un. Physiol. Sci.* 13: 639, 1977.
509. RUDOMIN, P., R. NUÑEZ, J. MADRID, AND R. E. BURKE. Primary afferent hyperpolarization and presynaptic facilitation of Ia afferent terminals induced by large cutaneous fibers. *J. Neurophysiol.* 37: 413–429, 1974.
510. RYALL, R. W. Renshaw cell mediated inhibition of Renshaw cells: Patterns of excitation and inhibition from impulses in motor axon collaterals. *J. Neurophysiol.* 33: 257–270, 1970.
511. RYALL, R. W. Excitatory convergence on Renshaw cells. *J. Physiol. London* 226: 69P–70P, 1972.
512. RYALL, R. W., AND M. F. PIERCEY. Excitation and inhibition of Renshaw cells by impulses in peripheral afferent nerve fibers. *J. Neurophysiol.* 34: 242–251, 1971.
513. RYALL, R. W., M. F. PIERCEY, AND C. POLOSA. Intersegmental and intrasegmental distribution of mutual inhibition of Renshaw cells. *J. Neurophysiol.* 34: 700–707, 1971.
514. RYALL, R. W., M. F. PIERCEY, C. POLOSA, AND J. GOLDFARB. Excitation of Renshaw cells in relation to orthodromic and antidromic excitation of motoneurons. *J. Neurophysiol.* 35: 137–148, 1972.
515. RYMER, W. Z., J. C. HOUK, AND P. E. CRAGO. Mechanisms of the clasp-knife reflex studied in an animal model. *Exp. Brain Res.* 37: 93–113, 1979.
516. SCHEIBEL, M. E., AND A. B. SCHEIBEL. Spinal motoneurons, interneurons, and Renshaw cells. A Golgi study. *Arch. Ital. Biol.* 104: 328–353, 1966.
517. SCHEIBEL, M. E., AND A. B. SCHEIBEL. Inhibition and the Renshaw cell. A structural critique. *Brain Behav. Evol.* 4: 53–93, 1971.
518. SCHMIDT, R. F. Presynaptic inhibition in the vertebrate central nervous system. *Ergeb. Physiol. Biol. Exp. Pharmacol.* 63: 20–101, 1971.
519. SCHMIDT, R. F., J. SENGES, AND M. ZIMMERMANN. Presynaptic depolarization of cutaneous mechanoreceptor afferents after mechanical skin stimulation. *Exp. Brain Res.* 3: 234–247, 1967.
520. SCHMIDT, R. F., AND W. D. WILLIS. Intracellular recording from motoneurons of the cervical spinal cord of the cat. *J. Neurophysiol.* 26: 28–43, 1963.
521. SCHOEN, J. H. R. Comparative aspects of the descending fibre systems in the spinal cord. In: *Progress in Brain Research. Organization of the Spinal Cord*, edited by J. C. Eccles and J. P. Schadé. Amsterdam: Elsevier, 1964, vol. 11, p. 203–222.
522. SCHOMBURG, E. D. Fusimotorische Förderung und Hemmung bei Pinna-Reizung in Abhängigkeit vom zentralnervösen Zustand. *Pfluegers Arch.* 304: 164–182, 1968.
523. SCHOMBURG, E. D. Supraspinal interactions of anesthetic, neuroleptic and analeptic drugs on the fusimotor effects of pinna stimulation in the cat. *Exp. Brain Res.* 10: 182–196, 1970.
524. SCHOMBURG, E. D., AND H. B. BEHRENDS. Phasic control of the transmission in the excitatory and inhibitory reflex pathways from cutaneous afferents to α-motoneurones during fictive locomotion in cats. *Neurosci. Lett.* 8: 277–282, 1978.
525. SCHOMBURG, E. D., AND H. B. BEHRENDS. The possibility of phase-dependent monosynaptic and polysynaptic Ia excitation to homonymous motoneurones during fictive locomotion. *Brain Res.* 143: 533–537, 1978.
526. SCHOMBURG, E. D., H. B. BEHRENDS, AND H. STEFFENS. Alteration of transmission in segmental pathways from flexor reflex afferents (FRA) to α-motoneurones during spinal locomotor activity. *Neurosci. Lett.*: (Suppl. 1), S103, 1978.
527. SCHOMBURG, E. D., AND H. D. HENATSCH. Aktivierung lumbaler Extensor-Fusimotoneurone durch mechanische und elektrische Pinna-Reizung an decerebrierten Katzen. *Pfluegers Arch.* 304: 152–163, 1968.
528. SCHOMBURG, E. D., H.-M. MEINCK, AND J. HAUSTEIN. A fast propriospinal inhibitory pathway from forelimb afferents to motoneurones of hindlimb flexor digitorum longus. *Neurosci. Lett.* 1: 311–314, 1975.
529. SCHOMBURG, E. D., H.-M. MEINCK, J. HAUSTEIN, AND J. ROESLER. Functional organization of the spinal reflex pathways from forelimb afferents to hindlimb motoneurones in the cat. *Brain Res.* 139: 21–33, 1978.
530. SCHOMBURG, E. D., J. ROESLER, AND P. KENINS. On the function of the fast long spinal inhibitory pathway from forelimb afferents to flexor digitorum longus motoneurones in cats and dogs. *Neurosci. Lett.* 7: 55–59, 1978.
531. SCHOMBURG, E. D., J. ROESLER, AND H.-M. MEINCK. Phase-dependent transmission in the excitatory propriospinal reflex pathway from forelimb afferents to lumbar motoneurones during fictive locomotion. *Neurosci. Lett.* 4: 249–252, 1977.
532. SEARS, T. A. Investigations on respiratory motoneurones of the thoracic spinal cord. In: *Progress in Brain Research. Physiology of Spinal Neurons*, edited by J. C. Eccles and J. P. Schadé. Amsterdam: Elsevier, 1964, vol. 12, p. 259–273.
533. SEARS, T. A. Efferent discharges in alpha and fusimotor fibres of intercostal nerves of the cat. *J. Physiol. London* 174: 295–315, 1964.

534. SEARS, T. A., AND D. STAGG. Short-term synchronization of intercostal motoneurone activity. *J. Physiol. London* 263: 357–381, 1976.
535. SEVERIN, F. V. On the role of γ-motor system for extensor α-motoneurone activation during controlled locomotion [in Russian]. *Biofizika* 15: 1096–1102, 1970.
536. SEVERIN, F. V., G. N. ORLOVSKY, AND M. L. SHIK. Work of the muscle receptors during controlled locomotion. *Biophysics* 12: 575–586, 1967. [Engl. transl. 12: 502–511, 1967.]
537. SEVERIN, F. V., G. N. ORLOVSKY, AND M. L. SHIK. Recurrent inhibitory effects on single motoneurones during an electrically evoked locomotion. *Bull Exp. Biol. Med. USSR* 66: 3–9, 1968.
538. SHAPOVALOV, A. I. Excitation and inhibition of spinal neurones during supraspinal stimulation. In: *Muscular Afferents and Motor Control. Nobel Symp. I*, edited by R. Granit. Stockholm: Almqvist & Wiksell, 1966, p. 331–348.
539. SHAPOVALOV, A. I. Extrapyramidal monosynaptic and disynaptic control of mammalian alpha motoneurons. *Brain Res.* 40: 105–115, 1972.
540. SHAPOVALOV, A. I. Evolution of neuronal systems of supraspinal motor control. *Neurophysiology USSR* 4: 453–470, 1972.
541. SHAPOVALOV, A. I. Extrapyramidal control of primate motoneurons. In: *New Developments in Electromyography and Clinical Neurophysiology*, edited by J. E. Desmedt. Basel: Karger, 1973, vol. 3, p. 145–158.
542. SHAPOVALOV, A. I. Neuronal organization and synaptic mechanisms of supraspinal motor control in vertebrates. *Rev. Physiol. Biochem. Pharmacol.* 72: 1–54, 1975.
543. SHAPOVALOV, A. I., A. A. GRANTYN, AND G. G. KURCHAVYI. Short-latency reticulospinal projections to alpha-motoneurons. *Bull. Exp. Biol. Med. USSR* 64: 3–15, 1967.
544. SHAPOVALOV, A. I., O. A. KARAMJAN, G. G. KURCHAVYI, AND Z. A. REPINA. Synaptic actions evoked from the red nucleus on the spinal alpha-motoneurons in the rhesus monkey. *Brain Res.* 32: 325–348, 1971.
545. SHAPOVALOV, A. I., AND V. M. KOZHANOV. Disynaptic brainstem-propriospinal projections to mammalian motoneurones. *Neuroscience* 3: 105–108, 1978.
546. SHAPOVALOV, A. I., G. G. KURCHAVYI, O. A. KARAMJAN, AND Z. A. REPINA. Extrapyramidal pathways with monosynaptic effects upon primate α-motoneurons. *Experientia* 27: 522–524, 1971.
547. SHAPOVALOV, A. I., G. G. KURCHAVYI, AND M. P. STROGONOVA. Synaptic mechanisms of vestibulo-spinal influences on alpha-motoneurons. *Sechenov J. Physiol. USSR* 52: 1401–1409, 1966.
548. SHERRINGTON, C. S. Decerebrate rigidity, and reflex coordination of movements. *J. Physiol. London* 22: 319–332, 1898.
549. SHERRINGTON, C. S. On innervation of antagonistic muscles. Sixth Note. *Proc. R. Soc. London Ser. B* 66: 66–67, 1900.
550. SHERRINGTON, C. *The Integrative Action of the Nervous System*. New Haven: Yale Univ. Press, 1906.
551. SHERRINGTON, C. S. Observations on the scratch-reflex in the spinal dog. *J. Physiol. London* 34: 1–50, 1906.
552. SHERRINGTON, C. S. On reciprocal innervation of antagonistic muscles. Twelfth note. Proprioceptive reflexes. *Proc. R. Soc. London Ser. B* 80: 552–564, 1908.
553. SHERRINGTON, C. S. On plastic tonus and proprioceptive reflexes. *Q. J. Exp. Physiol.* 2: 109–156, 1909.
554. SHERRINGTON, C. S. Flexion-reflex of the limb, crossed extension reflex, and reflex stepping and standing. *J. Physiol. London* 40: 28–121, 1910.
555. SHERRINGTON, C. S. Notes on the scratch-reflex of the cat. *Q. J. Exp. Physiol.* 3: 213–220, 1910.
556. SHERRINGTON, C. S., AND E. E. LASLETT. Observations on some spinal reflexes and the interconnection of spinal segments. *J. Physiol. London* 29: 58–96, 1903.
557. SHERRINGTON, C. S., AND S. C. M. SOWTON. Observations on reflex responses to single break-shocks. *J. Physiol. London* 49: 331–348, 1915.
558. SHIBUYA, T., AND E. G. ANDERSON. The influence of chronic cord transection on the effects of 5-hydroxytryptophan, l-tryptophan and pargyline on spinal neuronal activity. *J. Pharmacol. Exp. Ther.* 164: 185–190, 1968.
559. SHIK, M. L., F. V. SEVERIN, AND G. N. ORLOVSKY. Control of walking and running by means of electrical stimulation of the mid-brain. *Biofizika* 11: 659–666, 1966. [Engl. transl. 11: 756–765, 1966.]
560. SHIMAZU, H., T. HONGO, AND K. KUBOTA. Two types of central influences on gamma motor system. *J. Neurophysiol.* 25: 309–323, 1962.
561. SJÖLUND, B. The ventral spino-olivocerebellar system in the cat. V. Supraspinal control of spinal transmission. *Exp. Brain Res.* 33: 509–522, 1978.
562. SJÖSTRÖM, A., AND P. ZANGGER. Muscle spindle control during locomotor movements generated by the deafferented spinal cord. *Acta Physiol. Scand.* 97: 281–291, 1976.
563. SKOGLUND, S. Anatomical and physiological studies of knee joint innervation in the cat. *Acta Physiol. Scand.* 36: (Suppl. 124) 1–101, 1956.
564. SNOW, P. J., P. K. ROSE, AND A. G. BROWN. Tracing axons and axon collaterals of spinal neurons using intracellular injection of horseradish peroxidase. *Science* 191: 312–313, 1976.
565. STAUFFER, E. K., D. G. D. WATT, A. TAYLOR, R. M. REINKING, AND D. G. STUART. Analysis of muscle receptor connections by spike-triggered averaging. 2. Spindle group II afferents. *J. Neurophysiol.* 39: 1393–1402, 1976.
566. STEPHENS, J. A., R. M. REINKING, AND D. G. STUART. Tendon organs of cat medial gastrocnemius: responses to active and passive forces as a function of muscle length. *J. Neurophysiol.* 38: 1217–1231, 1975.
567. STERLING, P., AND H. G. J. M. KUYPERS. Anatomical organization of the brachial spinal cord of the cat. II. The motoneuron plexus. *Brain Res.* 4: 16–32, 1967.
568. STEWART, D. H., J. B. PRESTON, AND D. G. WHITLOCK. Spinal pathways mediating motor cortex evoked excitability changes in segmental motoneurons in pyramidal cats. *J. Neurophysiol.* 31: 928–937, 1968.
569. STUART, D. G., C. G. MOSHER, R. L. GERLACH, AND R. M. REINKING. Selective activation of Ia afferents by transient muscle stretch. *Exp. Brain Res.* 10: 477–487, 1970.
570. SUMNER, A. J. Properties of Ia and Ib afferent fibres serving stretch receptors of the cat's medial gastrocnemius muscle. *Proc. Univ. Otago Med. School* 39: 3–5, 1961.
571. SZENTÁGOTHAI, J. Short propriospinal neurons and intrinsic connections of the spinal gray matter. *Acta Morphol. Acad. Sci. Hung.* 1: 81–94, 1951.
572. SZENTÁGOTHAI, J. Propriospinal pathways and their synapses. In: *Progress in Brain Research. Organization of the Spinal Cord*, edited by J. C. Eccles and J. P. Schadé. Amsterdam: Elsevier, 1964, vol. 11, p. 155–177.
573. TABER, C. p-Chlorophenylalanine blockade of the effect of 5-hydroxytryptophan on spinal synaptic activity (Abstract). *Federation Proc.* 30: 317, 1971.
574. TAMAROVA, Z. A., A. I. SHAPOVALOV, O. A. KARAMYAN, AND G. G. KURCHAVYI. Cortico-pyramidal and cortico-extrapyramidal synaptic effects on the monkey lumbar motoneurons. *Neirofiziologiia* 4: 587–596, 1972.
575. TANAKA, R. Reciprocal Ia inhibition during voluntary movements in man. *Exp. Brain Res.* 21: 529–540, 1974.
576. TANAKA, R. Reciprocal Ia inhibition and voluntary movements in man. In: *Progress in Brain Research. Understanding the Stretch Reflex*, edited by S. Homma. Amsterdam: Elsevier, 1976, vol. 44, p. 291–302.
577. TAYLOR, A., AND F. W. J. CODY. Jaw muscle spindle activity in the cat during normal movements of eating and drinking. *Brain Res.* 71: 523–530, 1974.
578. TAYLOR, A., AND M. R. DAVEY. Behaviour of jaw muscle stretch receptors during active and passive movements in the cat. *Nature London* 220: 301–302, 1968.
579. THOMAS, R. C., AND V. J. WILSON. Recurrent interactions between motoneurons of known location in the cervical cord of the cat. *J. Neurophysiol.* 30: 661–674, 1967.
580. THORNDIKE, E. L. Animal intelligence: an experimental study of the associative processes in animals. *Psychol. Monogr.* 2: 1–109, 1898. No. 8.

581. TROTT, J. R. The effect of low amplitude muscle vibration on the discharge of fusimotor neurones in the decerebrate cat. *J. Physiol. London* 255: 635-649, 1976.
582. TSUKAHARA, N., AND C. OHYE. Polysynaptic activation of extensor motoneurones from group Ia fibres in the cat spinal cord. *Experientia* 20: 628-629, 1964.
583. VALLBO, Å. B. Slowly adapting muscle receptors in man. *Acta Physiol. Scand.* 78: 315-333, 1970.
584. VALLBO, Å. B. Discharge patterns in human muscle spindle afferents during isometric voluntary contractions. *Acta Physiol. Scand.* 80: 552-566, 1970.
585. VALLBO, Å. B. Muscle spindle response at the onset of isometric voluntary contractions in man. Time difference between fusimotor and skeletomotor effects. *J. Physiol. London* 218: 405-431, 1971.
586. VALLBO, Å. B. Muscle spindle afferent discharge from resting and contracting muscles in normal human subjects. In: *New Developments in Electromyography and Clinical Neurophysiology,* edited by J. E. Desmedt. Basel: Karger, 1973, vol. 3, p. 251-262.
587. VALLBO, Å. B. The significance of intramuscular receptors in load compensation during voluntary contractions in man. In: *Control of Posture and Locomotion. Advances in Behavioral Biology,* edited by R. B. Stein, K. B. Pearson, R. S. Smith and J. B. Redford. New York: Plenum, 1973, vol. 7, p. 211-226.
588. VALLBO, Å. B. Human muscle spindle discharge during isometric voluntary contractions. Amplitude relations between spindle frequency and torque. *Acta Physiol. Scand.* 90: 319-336, 1974.
589. VALLBO, Å. B., K.-E. HAGBARTH, H. E. TOREBJÖRK, AND B. G WALLIN. Somatosensory, proprioceptive and sympathetic activity in human peripheral nerves. *Physiol. Rev.* 59: 919-957, 1979.
590. VAN KEULEN, L. C. M. Identification de cellules de Renshaw par l'injection intracellulaire, de la substance fluorescente "procion yellow." *J. Physiol. Paris* 63: 131A, 1971.
591. VAN KEULEN, L. C. M. Axon trajectories of Renshaw cells in the lumbar spinal cord of the cat, as reconstructed after intracellular staining with horseradish peroxidase. *Brain Res.* 167: 157-162, 1979.
592. VAN KEULEN, L. Relations between individual motoneurones and individual Renshaw cells. *Neurosci. Lett.:* (Suppl. 3), S 313, 1979.
593. VASILENKO, D. A. Propriospinal pathways in the ventral funicles of the cat spinal cord: their effects on lumbosacral motoneurones. *Brain Res.* 93: 502-506, 1975.
594. VASILENKO, D. A., AND P. G. KOSTYUK. Functional properties of interneurons activated monosynaptically by the pyramidal tract. *Zh. Vyssh. Nervn. Deyat. im I. P. Pavlova* 16: 1046, 1966. [*Neurosci. Transl.* 1: 66-72, 1967/68.]
595. VASILENKO, D. A., AND A. I. KOSTYUKOV. Brain stem and primary afferent projections to the ventromedial group of propriospinal neurones in the cat. *Brain Res.* 117: 141-146, 1976.
596. VASILENKO, D. A., AND A. I. KOSTYUKOV. Transmission of reticulofugal activity via the ventromedial group of propriospinal neurons in cat. *Neurophysiology USSR* 9: 205-209, 1977.
597. VASILENKO, D. A., A. I. KOSTYUKOV, AND A. I. PILYAVSKY. Cortico- and rubrofugal activation of propriospinal interneurons sending axons into the dorsolateral funiculus of the cat spinal cord. *Neurophysiology USSR* 4: 489-500, 1972.
598. VEDEL, J. P., AND J. MOUILLAC-BAUDEVIN. Contrôle de l'activité des fibres fusimotrices dynamiques et statiques par la formation réticulée mésencéphalique chez le chat. *Exp. Brain Res.* 9: 307-324, 1969.
599. VEDEL, J. P., AND J. MOUILLAC-BAUDEVIN. Contrôle pyramidal de l'activité des fibres fusimotrices dynamiques et statiques chez le chat. *Exp. Brain Res.* 10: 39-63, 1970.
600. VIALA, D., AND P. BUSER. Modalités d'obtention de rythmes locomoteurs chez le lapin spinal par traitements pharmacologiques (DOPA, 5-HTP, D-amphétamine). *Brain Res.* 35: 151-165, 1971.
601. VIALA, G., D. ORSAL, AND P. BUSER. Cutaneous fiber groups involved in the inhibition of fictive locomotion in the rabbit. *Exp. Brain Res.* 33: 257-267, 1978.
602. VOORHOEVE, P. E., AND R. W. VAN KANTEN. Reflex behaviour of fusimotor neurones of the cat upon electrical stimulation of various afferent fibers. *Acta Physiol. Pharmacol. Neerl.* 10: 391-407, 1962.
603. WALL, P. D. Excitability changes in afferent fibre terminations and their relation to slow potentials. *J. Physiol. London* 142: 1-21, 1958.
604. WALL, P. D. Presynaptic control of impulses at the first central synapse in the cutaneous pathway. In: *Progress in Brain Research. Physiology of Spinal Neurons,* edited by J. C. Eccles and J. P. Schade. Amsterdam: Elsevier, 1964, vol. 12, p. 92-118.
605. WESTBURY, D. R. A study of stretch and vibration reflexes of the cat by intracellular recording from motoneurones. *J. Physiol. London* 226: 37-56, 1972.
606. WHITEHORN, D., AND P. R. BURGESS. Changes in polarization of central branches of myelinated mechanoreceptor and nociceptor fibers during noxious and innocuous stimulation of the skin. *J. Neurophysiol.* 36: 226-237, 1973.
607. WILLIS, W. D. The case for the Renshaw cell. *Brain Behav. Evol.* 4: 5-52, 1971.
608. WILLIS, W. D., G. W. TATE, R. D. ASHWORTH, AND J. C. WILLIS. Monosynaptic excitation of motoneurons of individual forelimb muscles. *J. Neurophysiol.* 29: 410-424, 1966.
609. WILLIS, W. D., AND J. C. WILLIS. Properties of interneurons in the ventral spinal cord. *Arch. Ital. Biol.* 104: 354-386, 1966.
610. WILSON, V. J. Regulation and function of Renshaw cell discharge. In: *Muscular Afferents and Motor Control, Nobel Symposium I,* edited by R. Granit. Stockholm: Almqvist & Wiksell 1966, p. 317-329.
611. WILSON, V. J., AND M. KATO. Excitation of extensor motoneurons by group II afferent fibers in ipsilateral muscle nerves. *J. Neurophysiol.* 28: 545-554, 1965.
612. WILSON, V. J., AND W. H. TALBOT. Integration at an inhibitory interneurone: Inhibition of Renshaw cells. *Nature London* 200: 1325-1327, 1963.
613. WILSON, V. J., W. H. TALBOT, AND F. P. J. DIECKE. Distribution of recurrent facilitation and inhibition in cat spinal cord. *J. Neurophysiol.* 23: 144-153, 1960.
614. WILSON, V. J., W. H. TALBOT, AND M. KATO. Inhibitory convergence upon Renshaw cells. *J. Neurophysiol.* 27: 1063-1079, 1964.
615. WILSON, V. J., Y. UCHINO, R. A. MAUNZ, A. SUSSWEIN, AND K. FUKUSHIMA. Properties and connections of cat fastigiospinal neurons. *Exp. Brain. Res.* 32: 1-17, 1978.
616. WILSON, V. J., AND M. YOSHIDA. Comparison of effects of stimulation of Deiters' nucleus and medial longitudinal fasciculus on neck, forelimb, and hindlimb motoneurons. *J. Neurophysiol.* 32: 743-758, 1969.
617. WILSON, V. J., AND M. YOSHIDA. Monosynaptic inhibition of neck motoneurons by the medial vestibular nucleus. *Exp. Brain Res.* 9: 365-380, 1969.
618. WILSON, V. J., M. YOSHIDA, AND R. H. SCHOR. Supraspinal monosynaptic excitation and inhibition of thoracic back motoneurons. *Exp. Brain Res.* 11: 282-295, 1970.
619. WINDHORST, U., D. ADAM, AND G. F. INBAR. The effects of recurrent inhibitory feedback in shaping discharge patterns of motoneurones excited by phasic muscle stretches. *Biol. Cybernetics* 29: 221-227, 1978.
620. WINDHORST, U., M. PTOK, J. MEYER-LOHMANN, AND J. SCHMIDT. Effects of conditioning stimulation of the contralateral n. ruber on antidromic Renshaw cell responses and monosynaptic reflexes. *Pfluegers Arch.* 373: R 70, 1978.
621. WIRTH, F. P., J. L. O'LEARY, J. M. SMITH, AND A. B. JENNY. Monosynaptic corticospinal-motoneuron path in the raccoon. *Brain Res.* 77: 344-348, 1974.
622. YOKOTA, T., AND P. E. VOORHOEVE. Pyramidal control of fusimotor neurons supplying extensor muscles in the cat's forelimb. *Exp. Brain Res.* 9: 96-115, 1969.

CHAPTER 13

Anatomy of the descending pathways

H.G.J.M. KUYPERS | *Department of Anatomy, Erasmus University Medical School, Rotterdam, The Netherlands*

CHAPTER CONTENTS

Anatomical Techniques
   Visualization of neurons and their processes
      Light microscopy
      Electron microscopy
   Tracing of axons and identification of their terminals by techniques of anterograde labeling
      Anterograde degeneration labeling
      Anterograde transport labeling
      Orthodromic electrical stimulation
   Identification of cells of origin of fiber systems by retrograde labeling
      Retrograde degeneration labeling
      Retrograde transport labeling
      Antidromic electrical stimulation
   Identification of neurons and tracing of their axons
      Histofluorescence
      Immunohistochemistry
Anatomy of Spinal Cord and Brain Stem
   Spinal cord
      Dorsal horn
      Somatic motoneuronal cell groups
      Autonomic preganglionic motoneuronal cell groups
      Intermediate zone
   Brain stem
      Lower brain stem
      Mesencephalon
      Monoaminergic neurons
Descending Pathways
   Descending brain stem pathways
      Cells of origin
      Trajectory and terminal distribution
   Descending cortical pathways
      Corticospinal and corticobulbar pathways
      Cortical projections to cell groups of descending brain stem pathways
      Laminar distribution of cortical neurons projecting to subcortical and spinal structures
Synthesis
   Grouping of descending pathways on the basis of their terminal distribution
   Descending brain stem pathways
   Corticobulbar and corticospinal pathways
   Functional epilogue
   Conclusion

THE ANATOMY of the descending pathways of the brain is difficult to summarize at this moment because the accumulation of new data obtained by means of many recently developed techniques has resulted in rapid changes in our knowledge of this area. Moreover, these data do not all show a perfect fit, since each technique has its own astigmatism. In this chapter, therefore, reference is always made to the technique by means of which the data have been obtained.

Many of the descending brain pathways occur in a variety of vertebrates, yet for practical purposes the present survey deals only with those in mammals, especially in the common laboratory species of rat, cat, and macaque. When reliable data are available in other mammals, including human beings and their near relatives the apes, these data are also reported.

In discussing the descending pathways it has been customary to deal mainly with those distributing to the spinal cord, because this portion of the neuraxis is generally treated as being distinctly different from the supraspinal structures. However, spinal cord and lower brain stem (medulla oblongata and pons) in many respects form a unit. They possess a common architectural plan, and the descending pathways from the upper brain stem and the cerebral cortex generally are distributed to corresponding cell groups in these two portions of the neuraxis. In this chapter lower brain stem and spinal cord are therefore treated as much as possible as a unit, and the descending pathways are discussed from this vantage point.

A discussion of the anatomy of the descending pathways is bound to deal with their spatial characteristics, i.e., the location and the morphology of their cells of origin, the descending trajectories of their fibers, and the location of the cells upon which they terminate. This implies that an understanding of the anatomy of the descending pathways requires some understanding of the anatomy of brain stem and spinal cord, which therefore is also dealt with.

ANATOMICAL TECHNIQUES

Visualization of Neurons and Their Processes

The central nervous system consists of a complex network of interconnected neurons. These neurons possess a cell body with dendrites, which together carry the bulk of the receptive surface of the neuron and also give rise to an axon that may give off several collaterals. The axon and its collaterals generally carry a myelin sheath and are fitted with terminal boutons that make synaptic contacts with other neurons.

LIGHT MICROSCOPY. The descending pathways are composed of axons that are derived from neurons in cerebral cortex and brain stem and descend over varying distances into lower brain stem and spinal cord. Evidence concerning the descending pathways has been accumulated since the early 1800s when Gall and Spurzheim (208) recognized the pyramidal tract as a decussating fiber bundle extending from cerebral cortex to spinal cord.

Initially the evidence regarding the descending fiber systems in the brain was mainly obtained by light microscopic studies of normal brain material (i.e., without lesions) both in its adult form and at different stages of development. In such material the neuronal cell bodies may be demonstrated by means of the Nissl stain, which stains the nucleus and its nucleolus, as well as the so-called Nissl bodies in the cell body and the proximal parts of the dendrites. The configuration of the dendritic tree may be revealed by applying either the Golgi Cox technique (578), which mainly impregnates cell body and dendrites, or the original rapid Golgi technique and its modifications (597), which also impregnate axons and their collaterals. The usefulness of these techniques is especially derived from their visualization of only a few neurons, which, however, seem to be almost completely impregnated. Much of the axonal network as it exists in the brain may be visualized by applying the reduced silver impregnation techniques of Cajal (597), Bielschowsky (597), and Bodian (64); some of the terminal boutons are also impregnated by use of these techniques. The boutons can be visualized selectively by applying reduced silver impregnation techniques to prechromated material (21, 582). In such material the neuronal cell bodies and dendrites are then visualized indirectly by virtue of their being studded with impregnated terminals. In small pieces of tissue the terminals may also be visualized by applying the Malais zinc iodide method (4), which mainly stains synaptic vesicles.

The trajectory of the various bundles of axons can be studied indirectly by staining their myelin sheaths by means of either the original Weigert technique (597) or the Klüver Barrera technique (348), or by the Häggqvist modification (254) of the Alzheimer-Mann technique. This latter modification stains the axon and its myelin sheath with different colors and is particularly suitable for examining the fiber diameters of the different pathways (93, 138).

ELECTRON MICROSCOPY. The ultrastructure of neurons and their appendages can be studied with the aid of the electron microscope [see Palay and Chan-Palay (538)]. Thus in electron-microscopic studies the nerve terminals are shown to contain synaptic vesicles and mitochondria and to establish specialized synaptic contacts with dendrites (axodendritic contacts) and cell bodies (axosomatic contacts) as well as other fibers or terminals (axoaxonal contacts). Synaptic contacts may also be established between dendrites (dendrodendritic contacts). Interestingly enough the activity of nerve terminals may be reflected in the affinity of synaptic vesicles for the above-mentioned Malais zinc iodide stain (610). In several parts of the brain functionally different types of terminals contain different types of synaptic vesicles and may establish differently structured synaptic contacts [see discussion of synapses in Palay and Chan-Palay (538)].

To define the descending pathways it is necessary: *1*) to trace their fibers throughout the neuraxis and to identify their synaptic terminals among the many other terminals in the neuropil; *2*) to recognize their cells of origin. For these purposes techniques of "anterograde" and "retrograde" labeling have been developed.

Tracing of Axons and Identification of Their Terminals by Techniques of Anterograde Labeling

ANTEROGRADE DEGENERATION LABELING. When a neuronal cell body is destroyed or its axon is interrupted, the axon distal to the interruption, together with its myelin sheath, undergoes the so-called anterograde Wallerian degeneration (747) and ultimately disappears. This degeneration, anterograde labeling, can be used to determine the trajectory and the terminal distribution of the fibers of the descending pathways.

The degeneration of the myelin sheath can be demonstrated, either positively by the blackening of the degenerating myelin with osmium tetroxide according to the Marchi technique (669), or negatively by showing the absence of myelin in myelin-stained sections.

With the advent of the Rasdolsky technique (580) the terminal distribution of the degenerating fibers could be established. This technique, which consists of fuchsin B and light green staining of material fixed with formalin and osmic acid, stains degenerating axons and terminals with a different color than normal ones. Later it was found that degenerating axons and terminals could be visualized more effectively by applying reduced silver impregnation techniques (217, 288, 678) and especially the Nauta technique (510) and its modifications (157, 193, 773), which selectively impregnate degenerating axons and many of their terminals. Unless stated otherwise, the light-microscopic (LM) anterograde degeneration findings, referred to in the following description, have been obtained by means of the silver impregnation techniques and especially the Nauta technique and its modifications.

Gray and Hamlyn (233) showed that the anterograde degeneration technique could also be used in electron-microscopic (EM) studies because degenerating terminals show characteristic changes in their ultrastructure, starting with enlargement of the synaptic vesicles (336). In this respect it is important to realize that the EM technique is the only truly reliable means of demonstrating the terminal distribution area of a degenerating fiber system, since degenerating terminals are sometimes difficult to distinguish from axonal debris in silver-impregnated material viewed with the light microscope.

In EM studies three types of terminal degeneration may occur: i.e., *1*) the electron-dense type, in which the terminal shrinks and the ground substance as well as the mitochondria become electron dense (124); *2*) the hypertrophic type, in which a hypertrophy of the neuronal filaments occurs (233); and *3*) the electron-lucent type, in which the terminal becomes swollen and empty except for aggregates of synaptic vesicles (159). The latter two types may ultimately develop into the electron-dense type (123). After interruption of a given fiber system its terminals may degenerate at different times (576). Moreover, those in advanced stages of degeneration may no longer be recognized as terminals with certainty. To maximize the harvest of degenerating terminals the optimal survival time for the fiber system under study should therefore be established.

ANTEROGRADE TRANSPORT LABELING. Tritiated amino acids, such as [^{3}H]leucine, when injected into the brain are taken up by local cell bodies and are then incorporated into proteins. This process forms the basis for a recently developed anterograde labeling technique. Subsequently the radioactivity is transported from the cell body down the axon to the terminals, as can be demonstrated by means of autoradiography (169, 391, 686). This transport occurs in several phases, e.g., a rapid phase that carries a certain amount of radioactivity directly to the terminals (230–300 mm/day) and a slow phase that distributes radioactivity throughout the length of the axon (1–5 mm/day). (See two-component hypotheses of axonal transport discussed by Grafstein in ref. 230.) When radioactive amino acids are injected in a bundle of axons, however, the radioactivity is not transported anterogradely (137). Moreover, except for proline (363) the radioactive amino acids are also not taken up by terminals and transported retrogradely in detectable quantities to the cell body (31, 137). Yet in the anterograde transport studies the type of amino acid that is used is significant because some amino acids are not taken up by all cells (367).

The anterograde amino acid transport technique has the advantage over the degeneration technique in that it allows the tracing of the axons of neurons that are embedded in fiber bundles, because the amino acids are only taken up by and transported from cell bodies. Furthermore, by utilizing the rapid transport phase (short survival times) the termination area of a fiber system can be defined more reliably than by means of the anterograde LM degeneration technique. The anterograde amino acid transport technique also has the advantage that it can be used to trace fibers that are difficult to demonstrate by means of silver impregnation (240). Nevertheless, the technique also has some drawbacks. For example, the population of neurons that has taken up and transported the radioactivity is difficult to delineate accurately, because the size of the blackened area in autoradiographs is in part a function of the autoradiographic exposure time (236, 295). A further drawback results because fibers and terminals can only be labeled by way of their parent cell bodies. As a consequence a given bundle of axons, the cells of origin of which are not entirely known, is difficult to label. For this limited purpose the anterograde degeneration technique is therefore still the method of choice. Finally, when using the standard survival time of two weeks, cortical and brain stem descending fibers generally can only be demonstrated clearly in the cervical and thoracic segments. Longer survival times are necessary (292) for tracing them into the lumbosacral and coccygeal segments.

The anterograde amino acid transport technique can also be used in EM studies because the radioactivity can be demonstrated by means of EM autoradiography (152, 275, 276, 627). This method carries additional advantages: the ultrastructural morphology of the labeled terminals remains unaltered, and when using relatively long autoradiographic exposure times a much larger number of terminals can be labeled than by means of the anterograde EM degeneration technique (152).

Axons and terminals can also be labeled anterogradely by means of the enzyme horseradish peroxidase (HRP), which may be taken up by neurons and distributed through their axons to the terminals (424, 425). According to Graham and Karnovsky (232) the enzyme can be demonstrated histochemically in LM as well as in EM material (see RETROGRADE TRANSPORT LABELING, p. 600). Individual neurons, including cell body, dendrites, axon collaterals, and terminal, can also be visualized by injecting HRP intracellularly (142, 325, 649). Unfortunately, however, the enzyme does not proceed through axons over very large distances.

ORTHODROMIC ELECTRICAL STIMULATION. Anatomical data concerning the termination area of the various fiber systems may be complemented by electroanatomical data that are obtained by orthodromic stimulation of the fiber system under study and recording of the postsynaptic potentials of the neurons in the termination area. On the basis of the conduction velocity of the fibers and the delay between the application of the stimulus and occurrence of the postsynaptic potentials, the existence of direct connections from the fiber systems to given neurons may be inferred (89). In addition, the rise time of the excitatory postsynaptic potentials (EPSPs) may give information concerning the location of the terminals on the receptive surface of the neuron [see discussion of postsynaptic potential shape index loci by Rall (577), and of spatial distribution of Ia-terminals on motoneuronal surface by Burke and Rudomin (89)]. These data fill in a blind spot in the anatomy, because in LM as well as in EM studies synaptic contacts between fibers and the distal dendrites of a given group of neurons cannot be established. This is because in LM material the dendritic tree cannot be visualized together with the degenerating or otherwise-labeled afferent terminals, whereas in EM material the parent cell body of a postsynaptic distal dendritic element is frequently difficult to identify.

Identification of Cells of Origin of Fiber Systems by Retrograde Labeling

RETROGRADE DEGENERATION LABELING. Originally the retrograde labeling of the cells of origin of a given fiber system was achieved by utilizing the chromatolytic changes that occur in neuronal cell bodies after transection of their axons. The acute, chromatolytic changes consist of dustlike appearance of the Nissl substance, eccentricity of the nucleus, accumulation of chromatinic material along the nuclear border (71), and changes in the position of the sex chromatin, as well as changes in the enzyme activity, e.g., cholinesterase (196). These changes may lead to shrinkage of the neuron or may progress to such a degree that the neuron disappears altogether (71). The chromatolytic changes, however, may be difficult to detect in neurons with little Nissl substance. The use of young animals has therefore been advocated (69), since in such animals retrograde changes tend to be relatively more pronounced than in adult animals. Nonetheless, the method is not very sensitive, because the retrograde changes become progressively less pronounced (491) after axotomy at increasing distances from the cell body. Axons can therefore be traced over much greater distances by means of the anterograde than by means of the retrograde degeneration technique.

RETROGRADE TRANSPORT LABELING. Kristensson and Olsson (358, 360), Malmgren et al. (438), and the La Vails (397) demonstrated that the enzyme HRP is taken up by nerve terminals as well as by damaged axons and is then transported retrogradely to the parent cell body, where it can be demonstrated histochemically (232). This technique and its recent modifications (158, 241, 260, 261, 277, 437, 477, 661, 715) may be used to label retrogradely the neuronal cell bodies of fiber systems in the brain (397). It has the advantage over the retrograde degeneration technique in that HRP is transported over very large distances (381). Moreover, when some of the histochemical techniques are used, the HRP reaction products are electron opaque and therefore can also be detected with EM (85, 162, 219, 316, 359). Other substances, such as tritiated proteins (273, 659), tritiated amino acids (363), iron-dextran complex (112, 531), and several fluorescent substances (40, 375, 377) may also be transported retrogradely. These fluorescent substances may be used in combination to demonstrate the existence of divergent axon collaterals on the basis of double labeling (41, 720). This may also be achieved by combining HRP with enzymatically inactive but tritiated HRP (273).

ANTIDROMIC ELECTRICAL STIMULATION. The cells of origin of fiber systems may also be identified by means of electrical stimulation of the axons. The action potentials set up in this way in each axon travel both orthodromically toward the terminals and antidromically toward the parent cell body. Antidromic potentials invading the parent cell body can be detected by means of macroelectrode recordings (777), and recently microelectrode recordings have been used in combination with the collision technique (148). This technique makes it also possible to demonstrate the existence of axon collaterals and to determine their distribution (1).

Identification of Neurons and Tracing of Their Axons

HISTOFLUORESCENCE. In the 1960s a technique (183) was developed by means of which neurons containing certain transmitters can be recognized on the basis of their fluorescence characteristics. This technique and its recent glyoxylic acid modifications (25, 57) are based on the fact that, when treated with paraformaldehyde, serotonin and the catecholamines dopamine, norepinephrine, and epinephrine form green and yellow fluorescent compounds, respectively, which can be visualized microscopically. The cells of origin of the different groups of fluorescent fibers and their trajectories as well as their terminal distributions can be determined to some degree by means of the degeneration technique (146, 714), which is derived from the following relationship: after fiber transection the fluorescence in the distal part of the axon and its terminals decreases, while the fluorescence in the proximal part of the axon as well as in the parent cell body increases. The findings obtained with the degeneration technique may be complemented by combining histofluorescence with retrograde neuronal labeling by means of fluorescent tracers (59). The degeneration technique may also be used for histochemically demonstrating fiber pathways that contain cholinesterase (251). The cell bodies of noradrenergic neurons can also be identified histochemically on the basis of the presence of, for example, monoamine oxidase (615), an enzyme that can be demonstrated together with HRP in the same neuron (615). The same is true for acetylcholinesterase, which can also be demonstrated together with HRP in the same neuron (478).

IMMUNOHISTOCHEMISTRY. Different fluorescent systems sometimes cannot be distinguished from one another when using the above histofluorescence techniques—e.g., adrenergic and noradrenergic neurons (289). This difficulty can be overcome by using immunohistofluorescence techniques (266, 289) to demonstrate the presence of certain enzymes involved in the metabolism of a specific transmitter. When applying the indirect immunohistofluorescence technique the purified enzyme is used as an antigen to elicit antibodies against it in a species different from that to be studied. The histological material of the animal to be examined is then treated with these antibodies, which presumably become attached to the enzyme wherever it is present. This antibody-antigen complex in turn may be demonstrated by treating the sections with fluorescent or peroxidase-labeled antibodies against the antibodies of the first species, a procedure that results in the labeling of neurons and axons containing the specific enzyme. This technique (212, 721) promises to widen the horizon of neuroanatomy and ultimately may help to provide an insight into the transmitter architecture of the descending pathways.

ANATOMY OF SPINAL CORD AND BRAIN STEM

Spinal Cord

The spinal cord consists of peripherally located white matter that contains mainly axons, and centrally located gray matter that contains neuronal cell bodies. The white matter is subdivided into the ventral funiculus, which is located between the spinal ventral fissure and the ventral roots; the lateral funiculus, located between the ventral and the dorsal roots; and the dorsal funiculus, located between the dorsal roots and the midline. The lateral funiculus is subdivided into ventrolateral and dorsolateral funiculi. The gray matter may be subdivided into the dorsal horn, the motoneuronal cell groups of the ventral horn, and the intermediate zone, which in the present description thus also comprises the nonmotoneuronal cell groups in the medial and central parts of the ventral horn. According to Rexed (590, 591) the spinal gray consists of 10 horizontal laminae (numbered from I to X). This laminar arrangement is especially striking in longitudinal sections parallel to the sagittal plane (590). In transfer sections it is only truly obvious in the dorsal horn, which comprises laminae I to IV as well as the medial parts of laminae V and VI. The intermediate zone comprises the lateral parts of laminae V and VI as well as laminae VII and VIII; the motoneuronal cell groups correspond to lamina IX. Some of these laminae, however, do not necessarily represent anatomical entities with respect to their efferents and afferents. In the present description Rexed's laminae therefore are mainly used as convenient landmarks.

DORSAL HORN. The dorsal horn is regarded as the main sensory relay of the spinal gray because it contains the bulk of the neurons that distribute their fibers to supraspinal levels, including the diencephalon (6, 7, 103, 166, 706–708). These neurons are located in lamina I, in the nucleus proprius of the dorsal horn (lamina IV), in the medial parts of laminae V and VI, and in the most lateral reticulated parts of these laminae, which protrude into the dorsolateral funiculus. Strikingly enough, this entire area, which will be referred to as the dorsal horn, differs histochemically from the remainder of the spinal gray because of a high concentration of glutamate decarboxylase (470).

SOMATIC MOTONEURONAL CELL GROUPS. Somatic motoneuronal cell groups of the ventral horn, which distribute their axons to the striated muscles of body and limbs, represent a key element in motor control. This population of motoneurons displays a detailed spatial organization that has been studied most thoroughly in the ventral horn of the cat (596). The arrangement in this animal is therefore used as a model in this chapter (Fig. 1).

The basic building block of the motoneuronal population seems to be represented by a longitudinal column of motoneurons that innervate a given muscle (588, 596, 656) and in which the α- and γ-motoneurons tend to be intermixed (82, 662). The various columns innervating the different muscles are grouped into two

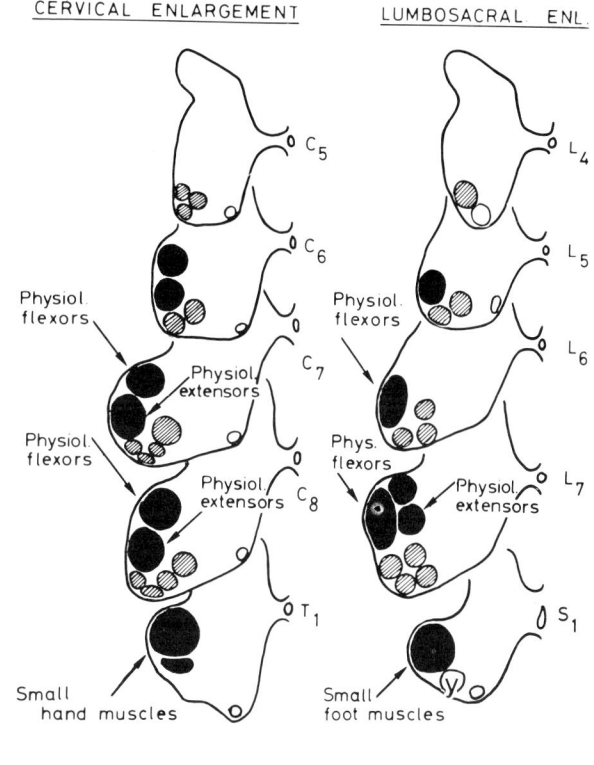

FIG. 1. Distribution of the different motoneuronal cells columns in the cervical and lumbosacral enlargements that innervate the various groups of limb muscles in cat. Note that motoneuronal cell groups innervating proximal muscles are distributed throughout the major portion of the enlargements. Cell group y in the S_1 segment distributes its fibers by way of pudendal nerve to muscles of pelvic diaphragm and vesical and rectal sphincters. [From Kuypers (373a), by permission of S. Karger AG, Basel.]

major longitudinal motoneuronal aggregates, medial and lateral, which in cross section constitute the medial and lateral motoneuronal cell groups of the ventral horn.

The motoneurons of the medial longitudinal aggregate distribute their fibers by way of the dorsal primary ramus of the spinal nerves to the axial muscles along the vertebral column, whereas the motoneurons of the lateral aggregate distribute their fibers by way of the ventral primary ramus to the remainder of the muscles of body and limbs (650). The lateral longitudinal aggregate seems to be interrupted at the caudal end of the enlargements. In the thoracic and the low sacral and coccygeal segments the lateral and the medial motoneuronal aggregates fuse to one, in which, however, the dorsal ramus motoneurons are still located ventromedial to the ventral ramus motoneurons (650). In the brachial cord (C_5–T_1, Fig. 1) and the lumbosacral cord (L_4–S_2, Fig. 1) the lateral motoneuronal aggregate enlarges in a dorsolateral direction because of the addition of several longitudinal groups of motoneuronal columns that innervate the muscles intrinsic to the extremities.

The medial longitudinal motoneuronal aggregate in the upper five cervical segments, according to retrograde degeneration (441) and HRP transport findings (592), contains the motoneuronal cell columns that innervate the neck muscles, including the sternocleidomastoid muscle (579). Some of the motoneurons innervating the splenius muscle and those innervating the muscles between scapula and vertebral column, e.g., trapezius and rhomboid muscles, are, however, located more laterally (579). Farther caudally this latter group of motoneuronal cell columns, which may be regarded as the upper portion of the lateral motoneuronal aggregate, is continuous with the motoneuronal columns in the ventromedial part of the lateral motoneuronal cell group of the brachial cord (Fig. 1); the last-mentioned columns innervate girdle muscles, i.e., the scapular muscles, the latissimus dorsi, and the pectoral and deltoid muscles (441, 588, 656). Dorsolateral to these columns, in the lateral motoneuronal aggregate of the brachial cord, two additional longitudinal groups of columns are present, one located dorsomedial to the other. According to retrograde degeneration studies (588, 656) these two groups innervate the muscles intrinsic to the upper extremity. The ventrolaterally located group contains the motoneurons that innervate the (extensor) muscles on the dorsal aspect of the arm, while the dorsomedially located group contains the motoneurons that innervate the (flexor) muscles on the ventral aspect of the arm, including the small hand muscles. Furthermore, in these two groups of columns not only a dorsoventral but also a rostrocaudal arrangement exists such that their rostral portions (C_5–C_7, Fig. 1) contain motoneurons that innervate the muscles of the upper parts of the arm, while their caudal portions (C_7–T_1, Fig. 1) contain motoneurons that innervate the muscles of the forearm and the small hand muscles. In cross section the motoneurons in the lateral motoneuronal cell group are therefore arranged from medial to dorsolateral in the following sequence: motoneurons of girdle muscles, motoneurons of extensor muscles, motoneurons of flexor muscles, and in C_8 and T_1 (Fig. 1) the motoneurons of small hand muscles.

The organization of the motoneurons in the lumbosacral cord (441, 596) is somewhat similar to that of the brachial cord. Thus the medial motoneuronal aggregate innervates the axial muscles (68), while the lateral motoneuronal aggregate innervates the muscles of the lower extremity. This latter aggregate in L_4 and L_5 (Fig. 1) contains motoneuronal cell columns that innervate lower extremity muscles attached to the pelvis, e.g., sartorius and the rectus femoris muscles (the motoneuronal columns of which are located rather ventrally) as well as the adductor magnus, the gracilis, and the vasti muscles (the motoneuronal columns of which are located more dorsally). Farther caudally these columns are aligned with groups of columns in the ventromedial part of the lateral motoneuronal cell group of the lumbosacral cord (L_6 to S_2, Fig. 1), which innervate other proximal leg muscles, e.g., the glutei and the quadratus femoris muscles (the motoneurons of which are located ventrally) and the hamstring muscles (the motoneurons of which are located in a more dorsal position). From L_6 to S_2 (Fig. 1) these columns are adjoined dorsally by three longitudinal groups of motoneuronal columns that innervate the muscles intrinsic to the leg and the foot. Two of these longitudinal groups are located side by side. The lateral group contains the motoneuronal columns that innervate muscles of the anterior aspect of the leg, e.g., the anterior tibial muscle, peroneal muscle, and extensor digitorum longus and brevis muscles that bring about dorsiflexion of the foot (physiological flexion) and of the toes. The medial group contains the motoneuronal columns that innervate muscles on the posterior aspect of the leg, e.g., gastrocnemius, soleus, and posterior tibial muscles (90) that bring about plantar flexion (physiological extension) of the foot. The third group of motoneuronal columns is located dorsal to the medial group and contains the motoneuronal columns of the long plantar flexor muscles of the toes. This group in turn overlaps caudally with a large group of motoneurons in the extreme dorsal part of the ventral horn that extends into S_1 and S_2 (Fig. 1) and innervates the small foot muscles. Thus, when proceeding in a cross section from ventromedial to dorsolateral through the L_7 lateral motoneuronal cell groups, a proximodistal arrangement is encountered whereby motoneurons innervating progressively more distal muscles are located progressively more dorsally, just as in the brachial cord. This anatomical arrangement is difficult to translate into physiological terms. It can be stated, however, that in both the lumbosacral and brachial cord the motoneurons innervating the physiological flexors intrinsic to the extremity are located relatively close to the dorsolateral funiculus.

Two other longitudinal motoneuronal aggregates are present in the spinal cord; they are rather short and are located between the medial and the lateral aggregates. One of these two, the phrenic nucleus, is located in the brachial cord in C_5 and C_6 (Fig. 1) and innervates the diaphragm (171, 656, 713, 751, 754), while the other, named the nucleus of Onuf (533, 534) or group y (596) or group x (533), is located in the lumbosacral cord in S_1 and S_2. This aggregate distributes its fibers through the pudendal nerve (596) to striated muscles of the perineal region, including the vesical and rectal sphincters (385, 613, 781).

The motoneuronal cell columns, and in particular the phrenic nucleus and Onuf's nucleus, are characterized by the presence of bundles of longitudinal dendrites (15, 153, 350, 466, 599, 621, 656), which is in keeping with horseradish peroxidase (HRP) transport findings (592, 598). The predominantly longitudinal arrangement of the motoneuronal dendrites is in contrast to the arrangement in the intermediate zone, where the dendrites are oriented mainly transversely [(657); see also Fig. 1 in Burke and Rudomin (89)]. Motoneurons, however, also possess transversely oriented dendrites, some of which radiate into the ventral and lateral funiculi and into the intermediate zone (97, 408, 592, 652). The transverse dendrites of the motoneuronal cell columns that innervate distal extremity muscles radiate mainly into the lateral parts of the intermediate zone because of their position in the ventral horn, whereas those of the motoneuronal columns that innervate more proximal muscles extend for the same reason mainly into the ventral part of the intermediate zone (592, 652).

AUTONOMIC PREGANGLIONIC MOTONEURONAL CELL GROUPS. Autonomic preganglionic motoneuronal cell groups innervate smooth muscles and glands by way of peripheral ganglia; they are concentrated in the thoracic, upper lumbar, and sacral segments. Retrograde degeneration findings in monkey (182, 556) and retrograde HRP transport findings in cat (117, 118, 163), dog (557), and guinea pig (147) indicate that many of these neurons are located in the sympathetic intermediolateral nucleus (lateral horn) from C_8 to L_3 (Fig. 1). In cross section this nucleus is adjoined medially by transverse strands of preganglionic neurons extending toward the central canal and is adjoined laterally by scattered preganglionic neurons in the lateral funiculus (cf. also ref. 564). A similar group of parasympathetic preganglionic motoneurons occurs in the sacral cord (S_1 to C_1) (150, 259, 496, 503, 556, 613, 781). Throughout the spinal cord the nucleus intermediomedialis is located close to the central canal (66, 556). It receives primarily afferent fibers from the dorsal roots (556, 652, 655) and probably contains propriospinal neurons that in the thoracic and sacral cord presumably distribute fibers to the preganglionic autonomic motoneurons (66).

INTERMEDIATE ZONE. The intermediate zone is regarded as comprising the lateral parts of laminae V and VI (the medial parts being regarded as a portion of the dorsal horn), as well as lamina VII and lamina VIII, the latter of which is located in the medial part of the ventral horn.

The neurons in the intermediate zone possess long radiating dendrites (97) that are mainly oriented transversely (622, 656), i.e., perpendicular to the bulk of the motoneuronal dendrites. The great majority of the neurons are propriospinal in nature and distribute their fibers within the spinal cord. Some of the neurons in the intermediate zone, however, also project to supraspinal levels (461, 490). The distribution of the propriospinal fibers and their collaterals is difficult to study, even in Golgi material (440), because they all enter the funiculi and after ascending and descending close to the gray matter (11, 703) reenter the gray matter to terminate in the motoneuronal cell groups and the intermediate zone (97, 144, 326, 459, 460, 463, 465, 620, 675, 676, 691). Contrary to what has frequently been assumed, short-axon neurons that distribute their fibers only through the gray matter to motoneurons apparently do not exist. Such connections do exist, but they are established by collaterals that are given off by the main propriospinal axons while passing through the gray matter on their way to the funiculi (459, 675, 676).

Direct anatomical evidence regarding the distribution of the fibers of the various propriospinal neurons is sparse; evidence that has been gathered by means of the anterograde degeneration, retrograde degeneration, and the retrograde HRP transport techniques has so far been mainly indirect.

The lengths of the various propriospinal fibers differ. Based on retrograde transport findings after HRP injections at different spinal levels (464, 490), the propriospinal neurons (Fig. 2) may be subdivided according to the length of their fibers into *long*, *intermediate*, and *short* propriospinal neurons. The long propriospinal neurons distribute their fibers throughout the length of the spinal cord, mainly by way of the ventral and ventrolateral funiculi. They are concentrated in lamina VIII and the dorsally adjoining part of lamina VII (464, 490, 645). In the upper cervical segments, however, they occupy a more lateral position in the ventral horn. The fibers from the long propriospinal neurons in the cervical cord descend bilaterally, but those from the corresponding neurons in the lumbosacral cord ascend mainly contralaterally (490). The ascending fibers from some of the neurons in lamina VIII and lamina VII are, however, distributed to supraspinal levels where they terminate, e.g., in bulbar medial tegmental field (7, 467), the inferior olive (20), and the cerebellum (462). A portion of these ascending fibers reaches as far rostrally as the meso-

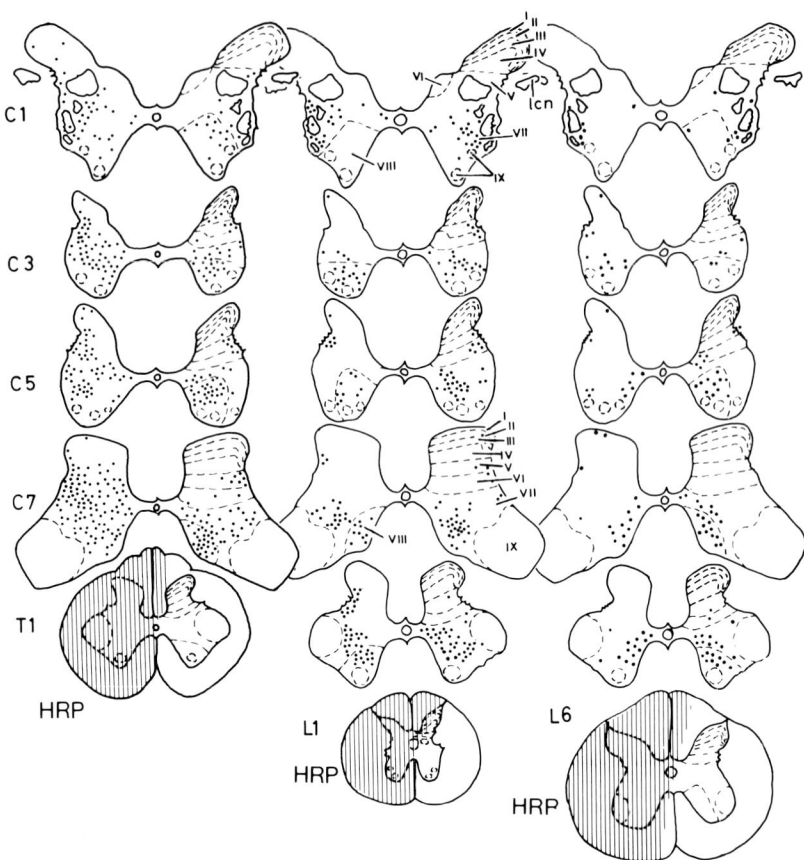

FIG. 2. Distribution of retrogradely HRP-labeled neurons in cat cervical cord after HRP injections at different spinal levels. Note that after L_6 injections the labeled long propriospinal neurons are concentrated in lamina VIII and adjoining parts of lamina VII, whereas after T_1 injections short propriospinal neurons in the dorsal and lateral part of laminae V and VII are also labeled. [Adapted from Molenaar and Kuypers (490).]

diencephalic junction and beyond (706–708). The intermediate propriospinal neurons distribute their fibers over shorter distances, e.g., from C_7 (Fig. 2) to the upper lumbar cord but not to the sacral cord. They are located in the central and medial parts of lamina VII, which, however, also contain short propriospinal neurons. The fibers from this population of intermediate propriospinal neurons are distributed bilaterally, with a dominance of the ipsilateral distribution. The short propriospinal neurons that distribute their fibers over a distance of only six to eight segments are the main occupants of the lateral parts of laminae V to VII; they distribute their fibers primarily ipsilaterally through the lateral funiculus. These conclusions, which are based on retrograde HRP transport findings, are in keeping with Golgi (622) and silver impregnation findings (460) and with retrograde as well as anterograde degeneration findings (216, 352, 491, 657, 674). Moreover, this organization of the propriospinal neurons not only applies to cat and monkey but also exists in lower vertebrates (690).

With respect to the terminal distribution of the propriospinal fibers, anterograde degeneration findings (216, 463, 465, 606, 657) indicate that the contingents of propriospinal fibers that travel in the ventral and lateral funiculi are distributed to both motoneuronal cell groups and intermediate zone (Fig. 3). In anterograde degeneration experiments with funicular lesions the distribution of the ascending propriospinal fibers can be easily determined, but that of the descending propriospinal fibers to the intermediate zone is less easy to study because it is somewhat masked by the distribution of the fibers of the descending supraspinal pathways. In cat, however, the ascending as well as the descending propriospinal fibers to the motoneuronal cell groups can be studied in detail because in this animal transection of the descending pathways does not produce heavy anterograde degeneration in the motoneuronal cell groups (522, 553). As a consequence heavy fiber degeneration observed in cat's motoneuronal cell groups after transection of the ventral and lateral funiculi must be derived almost exclusively from propriospinal fibers.

The propriospinal fibers to the cat's motoneuronal cell groups, as demonstrated by means of anterograde degeneration, are relatively short (352, 469, 606, 657), and the descending fibers are more numerous than the ascending ones (606, 657). Thus the bulk of the pro-

CHAPTER 13: ANATOMY OF DESCENDING PATHWAYS 605

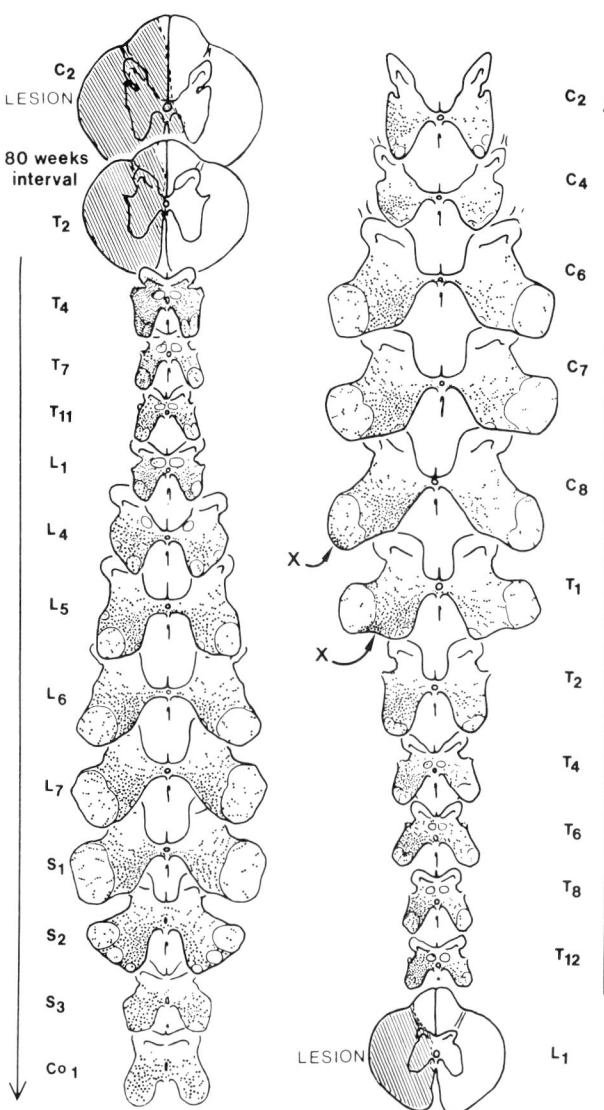

FIG. 3. Distribution of ascending and descending propriospinal fibers in cat, based on silver-impregnated anterograde fiber degeneration. Distribution of descending fibers has been obtained by hemisecting the cord at T_1–T_2 in animals in which cord had previously been hemisected at C_2 on that same side 80 wk earlier. After such a survival time the descending degeneration resulting from the C_2 hemisection can no longer be demonstrated. [From Giovanelli-Barilari and Kuypers (216).]

priospinal fibers to the motoneuronal cell groups in the brachial cord, which innervate the muscles intrinsic to the foreleg, comes from cervical segments caudal to C_2, and the bulk of the fibers to the corresponding motoneuronal cell groups in lumbosacral cord comes from lumbosacral segments caudal to L_2 and L_3. According to anterograde degeneration and electrophysiological findings (216, 465, 482, 483, 657), however, some low cervical motoneurons that innervate proximal muscles do receive a pronounced distribution of ascending propriospinal fibers from distant segments (Fig. 3), i.e., from the lower portion of the thoracic cord and the lumbar cord. The existence of this pro-

nounced distant projection may be related to the fact that some of the muscles in question (e.g., latissimus dorsi) are very large and may receive part of their sensory innervation from low thoracic dorsal roots. (For a quantitative analysis of the various types of boutons in motoneurons see ref. 127.)

The rostrocaudal distribution of the propriospinal fibers from a given group of segments to the intermediate zone extends beyond the distribution to the motoneuronal cell groups and occurs throughout the spinal cord (Fig. 3). According to anterograde degeneration findings (216, 606), however, the propriospinal fibers from a given set of segments are distributed in relatively nearby segments to all parts of the intermediate zone, whereas in distant segments their terminal distribution is largely restricted to lamina VIII and the adjoining parts of lamina VII in the ventromedial part of the intermediate zone. This is in keeping with orthodromic electrical stimulation findings (411). Other electrophysiological findings (323), however, indicate that relatively long propriospinal fibers also terminate on motoneurons. This is not necessarily at variance with the anterograde degeneration findings, because in the latter studies a few descending degenerating propriospinal fibers from the cervical cord were found to be distributed to the lumbosacral motoneuronal cell groups [Fig. 3; (216)]. Moreover, as pointed out in ANATOMICAL TECHNIQUES, p. 597, anterograde degeneration data always refer to the distribution of degenerating fibers in the motoneuronal cell groups, and neither LM nor EM degeneration data can provide information regarding synaptic contacts between long propriospinal fibers and the transverse motoneuronal dendrites that extend into the intermediate zone (652).

Anterograde degeneration findings in cat (352, 606, 657) indicate that the propriospinal fibers in the different parts of the ventral and lateral funiculi are distributed preferentially to different parts of the spinal gray, which comprise both the intermediate zone and the motoneuronal cell groups (Fig. 4).

1. In both the brachial and the lumbosacral cord, the propriospinal fibers in the dorsolateral funiculus and in the dorsal part of the ventrolateral funiculus are distributed primarily to the dorsal and lateral parts of the intermediate zone and to motoneurons in the dorsal and lateral parts of the lateral motoneuronal cell group, which innervate muscles intrinsic to the extremities (cf. ref. 355). Thus the fibers in the L_5 dorsolateral funiculus terminate only to a very limited extent in the L_5 lateral motoneuronal cell group, which mainly contains motoneurons of leg muscles attached to the pelvis; after descending caudally they terminate densely in the lateral parts of the lateral motoneuronal cell group at L_6 and especially at L_7 and S_1, which contain motoneurons of muscles intrinsic to the limb. This pattern suggests that these propriospinal fibers are distributed specifically to motoneurons of intrinsic extremity muscles.

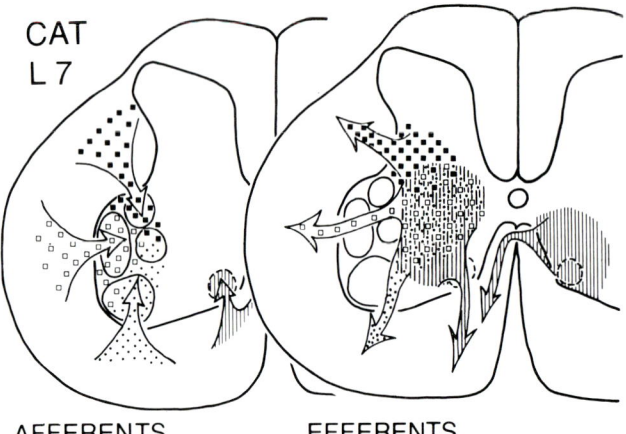

FIG. 4. *Left*: distribution of propriospinal fibers from different portions of lateral and ventral funiculi to the various motoneuronal cell groups in cat L_7 ventral horn. *Right*: distribution of neurons in different parts of intermediate zone that distribute their fibers to the various portions of lateral and ventral funiculi in cat. Data based on findings obtained by means of silver-impregnated anterograde axon degeneration and by means of retrograde cell degeneration. [Adapted from Molenaar, Rustioni, and Kuypers (491).]

2. The propriospinal fibers in the ventral part of the ventrolateral funiculus display the opposite distribution pattern. They are mainly distributed to the central and medial parts of lamina VII and to motoneurons in the ventromedial parts of the lateral motoneuronal cell group, which innervate proximal extremity and girdle muscles. Thus the fibers in the L_7 ventrolateral funiculus terminate densely in the ventromedial part of the lateral motoneuronal cell group at L_6, L_7, and upper S_1, but they are distributed to only a very limited extent to the lateral motoneuronal cell groups at low S_1, which mainly contain motoneurons of the very distal small foot muscles (596).

3. The propriospinal fibers in the ventral funiculus are distributed mainly to the ventromedial part of the intermediate zone, which characteristically contains long propriospinal neurons, and to motoneurons innervating axial and girdle muscles.

The anatomical findings concerning the differential distribution of those propriospinal fibers located in the dorsal and ventral parts of the lateral funiculus find their counterpart in recent physiological findings in cat (8), which show that, after transection of the dorsal and ventral parts of the C_5 lateral funiculus, different motor defects occur; thus transection of the dorsal part, which contains propriospinal fibers that extend to distal motoneurons, affects primarily the movement of the digits, whereas transection of the ventral part, which contains propriospinal fibers that extend to motoneurons of more proximal muscles, affects mainly movements of the limb as a whole, and these movements by their very nature also involve contraction of proximal muscles.

Retrograde degeneration findings (352, 491, 657) indicate that in the enlargements the cells of origin of the propriospinal fibers in the different funiculi are located in different parts of the intermediate zone (Fig. 4). Thus, for example, in L_7 the propriospinal fibers in the ventral funiculus and the ventral part of the lateral funiculus are mainly derived from neurons in lamina VIII and the medial and central parts of lamina VII, while the propriospinal fibers in the dorsolateral funiculus are mainly derived from neurons in the lateral parts of laminae V to VII. These findings, combined with the anterograde degeneration findings described, suggest that in the enlargements neurons in the medial and central parts of lamina VII and in the adjoining parts of lamina VIII establish widespread connections with ipsilateral motoneurons of axial, girdle, and proximal limb muscles, but to a lesser extent with motoneurons of distal limb muscles. In contrast the neurons in the dorsolateral part of lamina VII and in the lateral parts of laminae VI and V appear to represent the main source of the propriospinal fibers to the motoneurons of distal extremity muscles (Fig. 4). These anatomical inferences, which are supported by retrograde HRP transport findings (489), are reminiscent of earlier electrophysiological findings (22), especially those of Bernhard and Rexed (49), which suggest that the interneurons to the lumbosacral peroneal motoneurons are located laterally in the intermediate zone (cf. also the results in ref. 352). They are also reminiscent of the electrophysiological findings of Vasilenko (724), which show that those propriospinal fibers in the lumbar funiculus descending from above T_7 preferentially influence motoneurons of proximal muscles.

In light of this mediolateral organization of the interneuronal motoneuronal complex it would appear that the intermediate zone and the motoneuronal cell groups of the slender spinal gray in the upper cervical, the thoracic, and the upper lumbar segments correspond to the medial portions of the intermediate zone and the motoneuronal cell groups in the enlargements. This would imply that in the enlargements both the population of propriospinal neurons and that of motoneurons have expanded laterally. The distribution of the descending pathways as demonstrated by anterograde degeneration supports this conclusion (Fig. 5) and shows that, for example, those pathways terminating in the medial part of the ventral gray of the enlargements terminate throughout the width of the ventral gray at thoracic and upper lumbar levels.

The detailed electrophysiological and morphological studies of Hultborn and of Jankowska and Lindström (307, 321, 322) show that in addition to the mediolateral differential organization in the intermediate zone just described, a dorsoventral organization exists such that inhibitory interneurons (i.e., the Ia inhibitory neurons) and the Renshaw cells are characteristically concentrated in the ventral parts of the intermediate zone, that is, close to the motoneuronal cell groups, whereas they are largely lacking in the dorsal part.

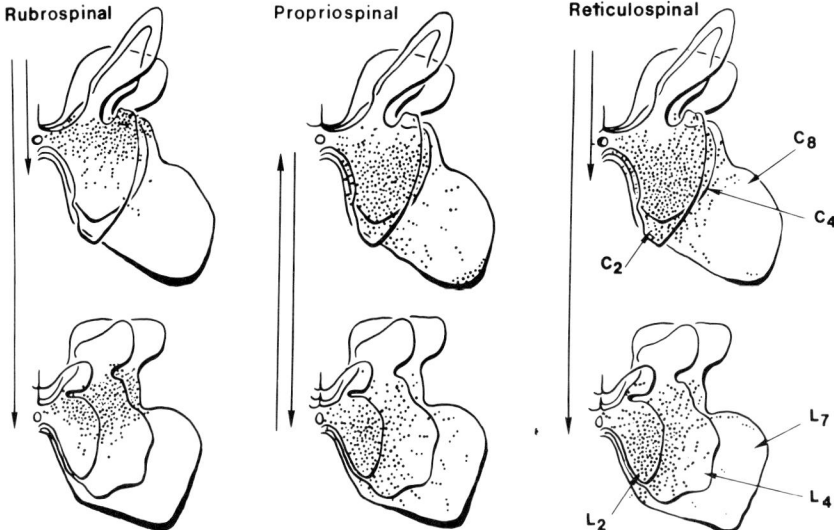

FIG. 5. Distribution of rubrospinal, long propriospinal, and bulbar reticulospinal fibers in gray matter of cat cervical and lumbosacral cord. Note that termination of long propriospinal and reticulospinal fibers in the enlargements occupy mainly the ventromedial part of intermediate zone, but in upper cervical and upper lumbar region occupy almost the entire width of ventral horn. Distributions of rubrospinal and reticulospinal fibers are represented according to Petras (553). [From Giovanelli-Barilari and Kuypers (216).]

[For a detailed review see Hultborn (307) as well as Burke and Rudomin (89); for a detailed review of propriospinal bundles in human beings see ref. 508.]

Brain Stem

LOWER BRAIN STEM. The lower brain stem represents the rostral continuation of the spinal cord. The arrangements of the fiber bundles and the neuronal populations are similar in these two portions of the neuraxis. Thus the fiber bundles of the spinal ventral funiculus can be traced rostrally as the paramedian fiber bundles, including the medial longitudinal fasciculus (MLF), into the mesencephalon. The bundles of the spinal lateral funiculus can be traced rostrally as a fiber band along the ventral aspect of the medulla oblongata into the deep pontine tegmentum dorsal to the pontine gray. In this band, in the brain stem, the relationship between the different fiber bundles as it exists in the spinal cord is largely maintained such that the bundles of the spinal dorsolateral funiculus (e.g., rubrospinal tract) are located laterally in the lower brain stem—i.e., close to the spinal V complex—whereas the bundles in the spinal ventrolateral funiculus (e.g., spinothalamic tract) are located more medially. In the brain stem the medial lemniscus and, more rostrally, the lateral lemniscus are added to this band of fiber bundles, which continues rostrally as a crescent through the ventral and lateral parts of the mesencephalon and extends in part into the diencephalon.

The gray matter in the lower brain stem also maintains the spinal arrangements. Thus the spinal dorsal horn continues rostrally as the laterally located spinal V complex and the trigeminal principle sensory nucleus. These cell groups together with the dorsal column nuclei also give rise to long ascending pathways to the thalamus (203, 287, 331, 636).

The spinal intermediate zone continues rostrally as the bulbar reticular formation, the medial parts of which in turn are continuous with the mesencephalic reticular formation. The spinal motoneuronal cell groups also have their counterpart in the lower brain stem. Thus the medial spinal motoneuronal aggregate continues rostrally as a supraspinal nucleus (532). This nucleus is contiguous with the hypoglossal nucleus, which may be regarded as the most rostral spinal motoneuronal cell group. The hypoglossal nucleus in turn is aligned with the more rostrally located eye muscle nuclei, i.e., the abducens, the trochlear, and the oculomotor nuclei. This entire group of motor nuclei is located immediately under the floor of the ventricle, in contrast to the arrangement in the spinal cord. Some cervical motoneurons innervating the neck muscles, however, are also located immediately under the central canal (592)—i.e., in the same position as the hypoglossal, abducens, trochlear, and oculomotor neurons in the brain stem. The lateral motoneuronal aggregate in the enlargements, which innervates extremity muscles, may have as a brain stem counterpart the facial nucleus. The medial facial subnuclei that innervate ear muscles (see later in this section) might then represent the bulbar homologues of the motoneurons in the ventral part of the lateral motoneuronal cell group, which innervate proximal extremity and girdle muscles, while the lateral facial subnuclei, which innervate perioral and periorbital muscles (see later) might then represent the bulbar counterpart of the dorsolateral spinal motoneuronal cell groups innervating muscles intrinsic to the limbs.

The band of autonomic preganglionic motoneurons in the thoracic lumbar and sacral cord (163, 556, 557), which extends laterally from the central canal, is converted in the brain stem into a radially oriented group comprising the medially located dorsal motor nucleus of glossopharyngeus and vagus (618, 696, 780) and the ventrolaterally located salvatory nuclei (616, 617) and nucleus ambiguus, some of the neurons of which also represent autonomic preganglionic motoneurons (468, 516, 666).

The reticular formation of the lower brain stem resembles in its cytoarchitecture the spinal intermediate zone with which it continues. In both, the neuronal dendritic trees tend to be oriented transversely (619), and the neurons with long axons are concentrated medially in both. In the spinal cord these neurons are located in lamina VIII and in the dorsally adjoining part of lamina VII next to the fiber bundles of the ventral funiculus; in the lower brain stem they are located in the bulbar medial tegmental field (45) next to the paramedian fiber bundles. The neurons in the bulbar lateral tegmental field are smaller (472, 680, 716) than in the medial field and may be regarded as the bulbar counterpart of the lateral portion of the spinal intermediate zone, comprising the lateral parts of laminae V and VI as well as the lateral and central parts of lamina VII.

In the caudal medulla oblongata the lateral tegmental field is relatively large and comprises the bulk of the reticular formation (dorsal and ventral reticular nuclei of the caudal medulla oblongata, refs. 472 and 532), while the medial tegmental field is represented only by the paramedian reticular nuclei and the interfascicular nuclei around the hypoglossal fiber bundles (680). Rostral to the obex the medial tegmental field enlarges and comprises in the medulla oblongata the gigantocellular and the dorsal and ventral paragigantocellular reticular nuclei (680) and in the pons the central pontine reticular nucleus (pars caudalis and pars oralis). The lateral tegmental field at pontine levels corresponds to area h (472, 532), which surrounds motor nucleus V. In the rostral pons the medial tegmental field is adjoined laterally by the nucleus subcoeruleus, whereas the lateral tegmental field seems to be replaced by the laterally located medial and lateral parabrachial areas surrounding the superior cerebellar peduncle (brachium conjunctivum).

The neurons in the medial tegmental field give rise to long ascending and descending fibers. Those in the lateral tegmental field give rise to relatively short (propriobulbar) fibers (Fig. 6), the descending members of which continue into the upper cervical segments, where they become intermixed with the propriospinal fibers in the deep parts of the dorsolateral and ventrolateral funiculi (92, 93, 292, 379, 451). Anterograde amino acid transport findings (295) indicate that the neurons in the medial parts of the lateral tegmental field distribute their fibers bilaterally (cf. neurons in the medial and central parts of lamina VII), while those in the lateral parts of the lateral tegmental field distribute their fibers mainly ipsilaterally (cf. neurons in the lateral parts of the spinal laminae V to VII). Propriobulbar neurons in both the medial and the lateral part of the lateral tegmental field also distribute fibers to motoneurons, i.e., to the trigeminal, facial, and hypoglossal motor nuclei (Fig. 5).

The bulbar motor nuclei are all somatotopically organized (29, 132, 160, 356, 406, 457, 458, 486, 543, 782). The facial nucleus is of special interest in this respect (132, 167, 361, 543, 572); this nucleus innervates the facial muscles, the external ear muscles, and the platysma. The motoneurons innervating the internal ear muscles, however, are located outside the nucleus (426, 427). In cat the facial nucleus is so organized that when viewed in cross sections the dorsomedial and ventromedial facial subnuclei innervate the auricular and platysma muscles, respectively, while the dorsolateral (intermediate) and the ventrolateral (lateral) subnuclei innervate the frontal and orbicularis oculi muscles and the muscles around the mouth, respectively. The facial nucleus in chimpanzee and the human being differs from that in cat and represents a vertically oriented cell group, the dorsal subnucleus of which apparently innervates the frontal and orbicularis oculi muscles, while the ventral subgroup innervates the muscles around the mouth (369). As in the spinal cord, the transversely oriented motoneuronal dendrites in the brain stem also tend to extend from the motor nuclei into the surrounding area. This is particularly pronounced with respect to the transverse hypoglossal dendrites, which radiate deeply into the bulbar lateral tegmental field (97).

Anterograde degeneration and amino acid transport findings (292, 295) indicate that the projections from the bulbar lateral tegmental field to the motor nuclei (Fig. 6) in cat are organized such that the propriobulbar neurons in the lateral parts of the lateral tegmental field in the caudal pons project especially to the motor nucleus V bilaterally; in the medulla oblongata at progressively more caudal levels they project preferentially to the lateral facial subnucleus (perioral muscles; cf. also ref. 167 for opossum and ref. 379 for monkey), the intermediate facial subnucleus (orbicularis oculi muscles), and the hypoglossal nucleus, respectively, the projections being distributed primarily ipsilaterally. This group of propriobulbar neurons is replaced caudally by neurons in the lateral part of lamina V of C_1 (295, 682), which project ipsilaterally to the dorsomedial facial subnucleus innervating the auricular muscles (132, 361). The neurons in the medial part of the bulbar lateral tegmental field project to the various bulbar motoneuronal cell groups bilaterally. These projections show relatively less spatial differentiations such that the neurons between the hypoglossal and the facial nuclei distribute fibers bilaterally to all three motor nuclei (295).

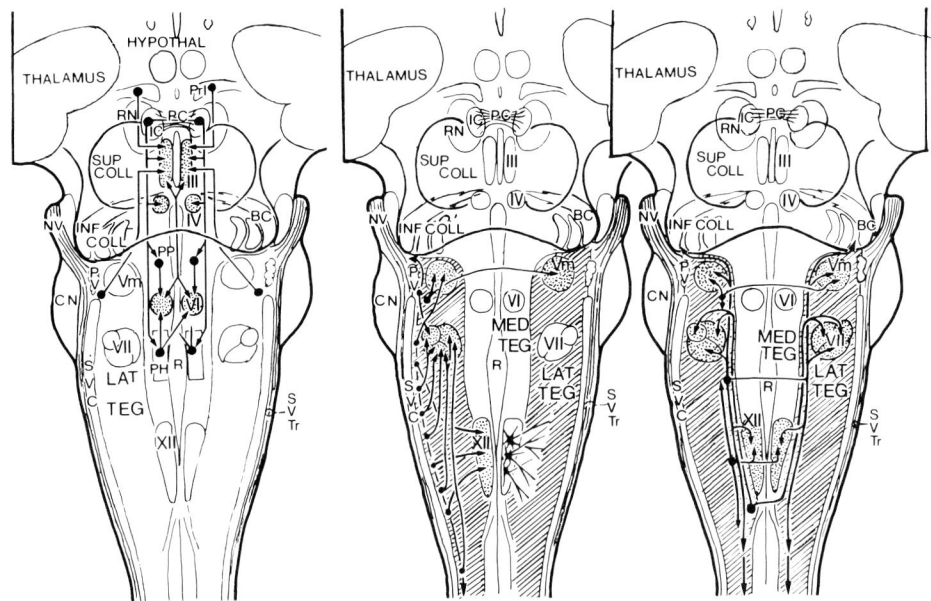

FIG. 6. *Left*: brain stem connections to eye muscle nuclei. *Middle* and *right*: distribution of propriobulbar fibers from medial and lateral parts of bulbar lateral tegmental field to bulbar motor nuclei V, VII, and XII. Prl, preinterstitial area; RN, red nucleus; PC, posterior commissure; BC, brachium conjunctivum; PP, pontine paramedian reticular formation; PH, prepositus hypoglossi nucleus; R, raphe nucleus; PV, principal sensory trigeminal nucleus; SVC, spinal V complex; CN, cochlear nuclei; NV, trigeminal nerve; MED TEG, bulbar medial tegmental field; LAT TEG, bulbar lateral tegmental field.

The eye muscle nuclei, which are also somatotopically organized (3, 55, 207, 504, 685, 750), do not receive fibers from the bulbar lateral tegmental field. They are under control of a different system of brain stem neurons, which are mainly incorporated in the medial tegmental field (see MESENCEPHALON, this page). The same applies to some degree to the motoneurons of the dorsomedial facial subnucleus, which innervates auricular muscles. These neurons receive projections from the bulbar medial tegmental field; the mesencephalic tegmentum (133, 175, 292, 431), including the caudal paralemniscal area (278); the superior colliculus (442); and the central gray (541). The intermediate facial subnucleus (orbicularis oculi muscles) also receives descending mesencephalic projections but mainly from the area of the contralateral red nucleus and from the pretectum (see discussions of pretectum in *Pathways distributing to long propriospinal neurons...*, p. 613).

MESENCEPHALON. Rostral to the decussation of the superior cerebellar peduncle, the mesencephalic tegmentum begins. At this level the colliculi develop and ventricle IV becomes transformed into the aqueduct surrounded by the central gray. The flat sheet of longitudinal fiber bundles along the ventral aspect of the medullary and pontine tegmentum containing ascending sensory pathways migrates laterally in the mesencephalon to form a crescent along both the ventral and the lateral aspects of the tegmentum. These fiber bundles separate the tegmentum from the substantia nigra, the cerebral peduncle, the medial geniculate body, and the posterior thalamus. On the other hand, the paramedian fiber bundles, including the MLF, maintain their bulbar position by continuing rostrally along the midline.

The mesencephalic tegmentum, which is thus enclosed between the paramedian fiber bundles and the laterally located crescent of fiber bundles, contains in its dorsal part the nuclei cuneiformis and subcuneiformis (532). These nuclei lay lateral and ventrolateral to the central gray and are transversed by many ascending and descending fiber bundles (central tegmental tract; cf. ref. 86). The descending bundles, after filtering through the superior cerebellar peduncle, converge into the medial tegmental field of the lower brain stem, and in the medulla oblongata they are located dorsal and dorsolateral to the inferior olive. The ventral part of the mesencephalic tegmentum contains caudally the ventral paralemniscal area and the nucleus tegmenti pedunculopontinus (532). This latter nucleus is replaced rostrally by the red nucleus, which extends rostrally into the mesodiencephalic junction. The rostral part of the red nucleus, which contains smaller neurons than the caudal part (see *Pathways distributing to short... neurons*, p. 619), is adjoined dorsomedially by the interstitial nucleus of Cajal, which is embedded in the MLF, and the adjoining bundles in the medial mesencephalic tegmentum. This tegmental area, dorsomedial to the red nucleus, continues rostrally into the subthalamic region, i.e., into the field of Forel and the zona incerta. The ventral tegmental area of Tsai (680) occupies the area ventral to the rostral half of the red nucleus. At these levels the mesencephalic tegmental decussations of the tectobulbar, reticulobulbar, and rubrospinal tracts have largely disappeared. As a consequence the central gray opens ventrally and becomes continuous with the ventral tegmental area. They extend together rostrally into the medial and the lateral hypothalamus, respectively.

The mesencephalon is capped dorsally by the inferior and superior colliculi, which border ventrally on the nucleus cuneiformis. The inferior colliculus is an oval cell group, while the superior colliculus is a laminated plate, the most ventral portion of which fades into the nucleus cuneiformis.

The superior colliculus contains a number of alternating white and gray layers: i.e., *1)* the superficial gray, including the stratum zonale; *2)* the fiber layer of the stratum opticum, which contains fibers of the optic tract; *3)* the intermediate gray, which contains several relatively large neurons; *4)* the fiber layer of the stratum lemnisci, which seems continuous with the crescent of fiber bundles along the ventral and lateral aspect of the mesencephalon containing the medial lemniscus; *5)* the deep gray, which also contains several large neurons; and *6)* the fiber layer of the stratum album profundum (532, 672), which separates the deep gray from the central gray.

The superior colliculus borders rostrally on the pretectal area (101). At this level the posterior commissure arches over the central gray. Some of the fibers of this commissure continue into the MLF; others fan out into the tegmentum. The nucleus of the posterior commissure is located dorsal and lateral to the central gray and adjoins dorsally the area of the interstitial nucleus of Cajal.

As pointed out already the eye muscle nuclei do not receive fibers from the propriobulbar lateral tegmental field, except for a small cell group close to the motor root of the trigeminal nerve. Instead they receive projections from the vestibular complex and the dorsolaterally adjoining nucleus y (see discussion of vestibular complex in *Pathway distributing to long propriospinal neurons ...*, p. 613) as well as from several of the medially located cell groups in brain stem already described (Fig. 6). Thus the oculomotor and trochlear nuclei receive fibers from the field of Forel rostral to the red nucleus (prerubral field), from the interstitial nucleus of Cajal, and from the nucleus of the posterior commissure (100, 238, 431). The prerubral field reportedly (330) functions mainly with respect to vertical gaze, while the area of the interstitial nucleus of Cajal steers mainly rotatory movements of the eyes (309, 673). The abducens nucleus receives fibers from the paramedian portion of the pontine medial tegmental field as well as from the dorsal part of the medullary medial tegmental field (94, 238, 433) and from the prepositus hypoglossi nucleus, which also projects to the oculomotor nuclei (239). The paramedian pontine reticular area, which has been implicated in steering of gaze (220), does not, however, project directly to the oculomotor nucleus but according to anterograde amino acid transport findings (94, 237, 238) distributes ascending fibers through the mesencephalic reticular formation to the interstitial nucleus of Cajal and the prerubral fields, which in turn project to the oculomotor (238) nuclei. In addition a third set of fibers exists linking the oculomotor with the abducens nuclei. These fibers are derived from neurons within the confines and the immediate vicinity of these nuclei, as demonstrated by anterograde and retrograde axonal transport findings (56, 94, 238, 239).

Throughout the brain stem a group of neurons is present in the midline raphe (189, 681), which in the medulla oblongata contains a vertically oriented bundle of dendrites (143). In the caudal medulla the group is small (nucleus raphe obscurus). More rostrally it progressively enlarges to form the nucleus raphe pallidus and the nucleus raphe magnus. The latter nucleus is located immediately above the pyramidal tract at the level of the facial nucleus. In the rostral pons the raphe contains the barrel-shaped nucleus centralis superior (532), which is bordered laterally by the paramedian fiber bundles and belongs to the caudal mesencephalic limbic area of Nauta (511). This nucleus continues rostrally to the level of the decussation of the superior cerebellar peduncles, where it extends dorsally into the central gray as the nucleus raphe dorsalis, which continues rostrally into the area between the trochlear nuclei. Rostral to the decussation the nucleus is called the nucleus linearis and at the level of the caudal red nucleus is replaced by two paramedian groups of neurons, the nucleus linearis rostralis. Retrograde HRP transport findings (381, 416) indicate that farther rostrally in the central gray another linear group of neurons exists, which in part occupies the nucleus of Edinger-Westphal. This group continues rostrally through the area around the floor of the third ventricle dorsal to mammillary bodies into the dorsal hypothalamus (381).

MONOAMINERGIC NEURONS. Histofluorescent studies have demonstrated two large monoaminergic cell populations in the brain stem, one being indolaminergic (serotonergic) and the other catecholaminergic (i.e., dopaminergic, noradrenergic, and adrenergic).

The serotonergic neurons (145, 190, 304, 515, 561, 563) in the pons and the medulla oblongata contribute to the descending pathways and are located mainly in the area of the raphe nuclei [groups B_1, B_2, and B_3; (145, 681)]. However, such neurons also occur around the pyramidal tract, along the ventral aspect of the medulla oblongata, and in the ventral part of the medullary medial tegmental field, the nucleus paragiganto cellularis lateralis (680). Serotonergic neurons are further present in the nucleus raphe pontis (group B_5), the nucleus raphe dorsalis (group B_7), the nucleus centralis superior (group B$_8$), the caudal mesencephalic ventral (paralemniscal) tegmental area, and in the caudal part of the interpeduncular nucleus (group B$_9$).

In the medulla oblongata and the pons the noradrenergic neurons, which also contribute to the descending pathways, are generally located laterally in the tegmentum (61, 116, 140, 145, 154, 190, 211, 302, 303, 313, 327, 404, 434, 515, 530, 561, 563, 615, 671). In the rostral pons a large accumulation of such neurons extends from the area of the nucleus coeruleus through the nucleus subcoeruleus [group A$_6$; (145)], i.e., between the parabrachial area and the nucleus centralis pontis (472, 532), into the area of the nucleus of Kölliker-Fuse [A$_7$; (145)] ventrolateral to the superior cerebellar peduncle. This accumulation continues in diminishing density caudally through the bulbar lateral tegmental field, where the noradrenergic neurons also tend to be arranged into a radially oriented group. Thus in the rostral medulla they are situated along the descending intramedullary limb of the facial nerve (group A$_5$) and at the level of the obex along a radially oriented line stretching from the area of the nucleus intercalatus and the solitary nucleus through the lateral tegmental field to the area of the lateral reticular nucleus (group A$_1$). Rostral to the coeruleus complex an accumulation of noradrenergic neurons occurs in the mesencephalic tegmentum dorsomedial to the medial lemniscus (group A$_8$) along the midline, in the ventral part of the caudal mesencephalic central gray, in the area of the nucleus linearis, and in the ventral tegmental area (group A$_{10}$). Catecholaminergic neurons are also present in the hypothalamus (groups A$_{11}$–A$_{13}$).

Adrenergic neurons have been demonstrated immunohistochemically (289) around the rostral part of the lateral reticular nucleus (group A$_1$ of Dahlström and Fuxe in ref. 145) and dorsomedially in the medullary tegmentum.

DESCENDING PATHWAYS

According to the data obtained by means of the techniques described in the preceding section the descending pathways consist of two parallel sets that are derived from the cerebral cortex and the brain stem, respectively. The bulk of these pathways is distributed to the spinal and bulbar interneurons and motoneurons and must represent the main instrument by which the brain steers movements. Transections of the different groups of descending pathways have been found to produce defects in motor control of different types of movements (373, 399, 400). From these findings it has been concluded that the medially descending group A brain stem pathways, which are especially derived from centrally located brain stem structures, characteristically steer body and integrated limb and body movements as well as movement synergisms of the individual limbs involving their various parts. Group B brain stem pathways also exist; these descend laterally. Components of this group appear to add further resolution to brain stem control, and provide the capacity to execute relatively independent movements of the limbs, especially of their distal parts. The cortical pathways to the spinal cord and lower brain stem, which parallel the descending brain stem pathways, further amplify the brain stem control but, especially in primates, also provide the unique capacity to execute highly fractionated movements, exemplified by individual finger movements.

These different motor capacities of the various descending pathways must be an expression of the differences in their relationships to interneurons and motoneurons. This is supported by several observations that will be discussed in detail in TRAJECTORY AND TERMINAL DISTRIBUTION, p. 613. Thus the fibers of the group A brain stem pathways, which according to the above findings steer body and integrated limb and body movements, give off a considerable number of axon collaterals along their trajectory through the spinal cord and characteristically terminate on "long" propriospinal neurons. Many of these pathways also maintain some monosynaptic connections with motoneurons. According to electrophysiological findings, however, these pathways mainly establish connections with motoneurons of axial and proximal limb muscles. Some of the laterally descending group B brain stem pathways, which provide the capacity to execute independent movements of the extremities and especially their distal parts, give off relatively few axon collaterals along their trajectory through the spinal cord and characteristically terminate on "short" propriospinal neurons. Moreover, according to electrophysiological findings, in monkey they also establish some monosynaptic connections with motoneurons and mainly with motoneurons of distal extremity muscles. The cortical pathways, which especially in primates characteristically provide the capacity to execute highly fractionated movements, terminate on both long and short propriospinal neurons and in addition distribute many fibers, with relatively few collaterals, in a highly organized fashion from different parts of the motor cortex directly to different motoneuronal cell groups. This suggests a parallelism between the anatomical connections of the descending pathways to interneurons and motoneurons in the lower brain stem and the spinal cord and the motor capacities of these pathways. For this reason in the present description the descending pathways are grouped according to their bulbar and spinal terminal distribution. Furthermore, after discussion of the descending pathways from this vantage point, an attempt is made in the last section of this chapter to synthesize the anatomical and functional data. In that framework a more detailed description of the motor defects resulting from the transection of the various groups of descending pathways is also presented.

Descending Brain Stem Pathways

CELLS OF ORIGIN. The following inventory of the cells of the descending brain stem pathways is based on retrograde HRP transport findings after HRP injections in the spinal white and gray matter at different spinal levels (34, 105, 141, 349, 381, 697, 698). Since HRP is taken up both by terminals and by broken axons (see ANATOMICAL TECHNIQUES, p. 597), fibers from the labeled neurons must be regarded as descending through the injected segment or as terminating there.

Unilateral HRP injections in T_1 in cat contralateral to a chronic C_1-C_2 hemisection label neurons retrogradely in the following areas (see Fig. 7): in the caudal medulla oblongata labeled neurons are located in the ipsilateral dorsal column nuclei (cf. refs. 91, 490), especially around the obex; in the contralateral retroambiguus nucleus from the pyramidal decussation to the obex; in the contralateral solitary nucleus; and dispersed in the lateral tegmental field between the solitary and the ambiguus nuclei (cf. ref. 615). In addition, in the upper part of C_1 a group of labeled neurons is present mainly ipsilaterally along the ventrolateral border of the spinal gray; this group continues rostrally into the area dorsomedial to the lateral reticular nucleus and around the hypoglossal root fibers. Around the level of the obex these neurons become accompanied medially by a large group of labeled neurons, which are located mainly in the ventral part of the medial tegmental field, i.e., in the nucleus reticularis gigantocellularis and paragigantocellularis (680) and in the raphe nuclei obscurus, pallidus, and magnus (681). Many labeled neurons are also present in the vestibular complex (see discussion of this in *Pathways distributing to long propriospinal neurons...*, p. 613), mainly ipsilaterally in the lateral vestibular nucleus and bilaterally in the medial and descending vestibular nuclei, including nucleus f (cf. ref. 548). In the pons labeled neurons are present ipsilaterally in the nucleus centralis pontis, partes caudalis and oralis (cf. ref. 532), but only few are present in the nucleus raphe pontis (cf. ref. 681). Furthermore, many labeled neurons occur mainly ipsilaterally in the monoaminergic nuclei coeruleus and subcoeruleus and in the area of the nucleus of Kölliker-Fuse (615) and mainly contralaterally in the ventrolateral portion of the pontine tegmentum, i.e., in the area close to the rubrospinal tract (Fig. 7). At the level of the decussation of the superior cerebellar peduncle only a few labeled neurons are present in the tegmentum, but more rostrally some are present in the area of the nucleus

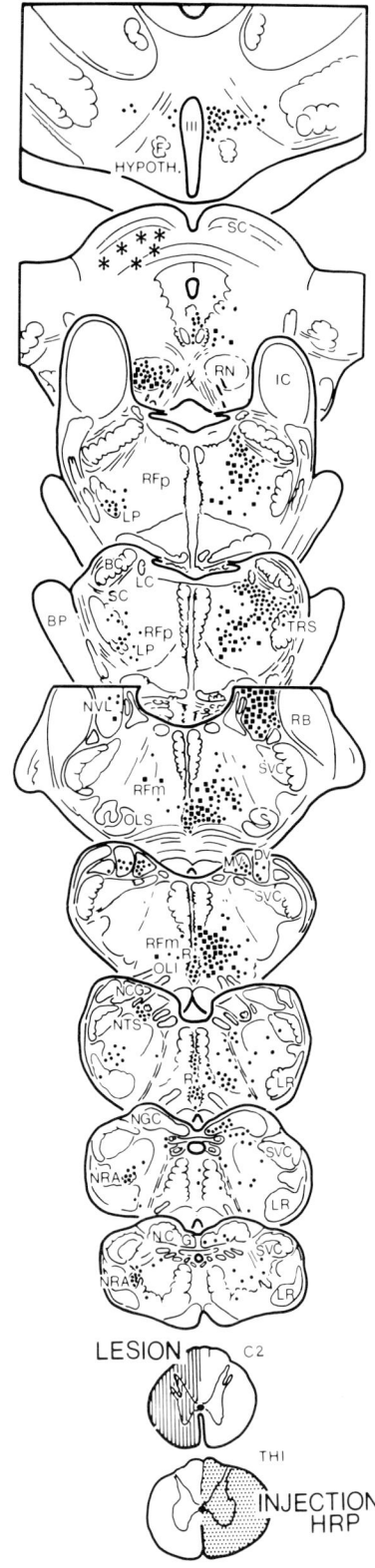

FIG. 7. Distribution of retrograde HRP-labeled neurons in a C_2 spinal hemisected cat after HRP injections on the other side at T_1. Asterisks in superior colliculus indicate locations of retrogradely labeled neurons after HRP injections at C_2. F, fornix; SC, superior colliculus; RN, red nucleus; IC, inferior colliculus; RFp, pontine reticular formation; LP, ventrolateral pontine tegmentum; BC, brachium conjunctivum; SC, nucleus subcoeruleus; TRS, rubrospinal tract; NVL, lateral vestibular nucleus; RB, restiform body; MV, medial vestibular nucleus; DV, descending vestibular nucleus; OLS, superior olive; OLI, inferior olive; R, raphe; SVC, spinal trigeminal complex; NTS, solitary nucleus; NCG, dorsal column nuclei cuneatus and gracilis; LR, lateral reticular nucleus; NRA, retroambiguus nucleus. [From Kuypers and Maisky (381).]

cuneiformis and in the adjoining lateral part of the central gray throughout the mesencephalon (106). Furthermore, many labeled neurons are present in the contralateral red nucleus. In addition at this level labeled neurons occur mainly ipsilaterally in the area of the interstitial nucleus of Cajal and the adjoining part of the nucleus of the posterior commissure (see *Brain Stem*, p. 607). In the rostral half of the mesencephalon some labeled neurons are also present in the midline, especially in the central gray, including the area of the nucleus of Edinger-Westphal (416, 665). This group of neurons in the central gray continues rostrally into the area along the ventral aspect of ventricle III, i.e., dorsal to the mammillary bodies and farther rostrally into the dorsal and lateral hypothalamus (611), including the area of the paraventricular nucleus. Retrograde axonal transport of fluorescent tracers has also demonstrated the existence of hypothalamospinal neurons in the ventral part of the hypothalamus, around the ventromedial nucleus, and in the retrochiasmatic area (L. W. Swanson and H. G. J. M. Kuypers, unpublished observations). Findings similar to those in cat have been obtained in monkeys [(349, 611); H. G. J. M. Kuypers and V. A. Maisky, unpublished observations] and opossum (141) as well as in lower vertebrates (687–689).

The findings in cat after HRP injections at C_1 and other spinal levels caudal to T_1 (381) indicate that long descending brain stem fibers, which travel throughout the length of the spinal cord, are derived from neurons in the dorsal column nuclei (490), the retroambiguus nucleus (91), the medullary and pontine medial tegmental field, the medullary raphe nuclei, the area around the lateral reticular nucleus, the lateral vestibular nucleus, and also in the medial and descending vestibular nuclei (548), the nucleus subcoeruleus, the ventrolateral pontine tegmentum, the red nucleus, and the hypothalamus. The findings further suggest that neurons in the solitary nucleus and in the mesencephalic tegmentum and central gray as well as in the interstitial nucleus of Cajal distribute their fibers mainly through the cervical, thoracic, and upper lumbar cord. The findings after C_1–C_2 HRP injections indicate that some fastigial and interpositus cerebellar neurons (201) and neurons in the intermediate and deep gray of the superior colliculus give rise to fibers that descend mainly into the cervical cord.

TRAJECTORY AND TERMINAL DISTRIBUTION. The brain stem pathways that are derived from the cell groups described are subdivided into five categories, according to their termination in the spinal cord: *1)* pathways characteristically distributing to long propriospinal neurons (laminae VII and VIII); *2)* pathways characteristically distributing to short propriospinal neurons (laminae V–VII); *3)* pathways to respiratory motoneurons; *4)* monoaminergic pathways and pathways to autonomic preganglionic neurons; *5)* pathways from the dorsal column nuclei to the spinal dorsal horn.

(For an earlier review of the descending pathways in human beings and in animals see ref. 507.)

Pathways distributing to long propriospinal neurons (laminae VII and VIII). Bulbar medial tegmental fields. According to retrograde HRP transport findings, long descending reticulospinal fibers in rat (785), cat (381), monkey (105), and opossum (141) are derived from the area of the bulbar medial tegmental field, i.e., the paramedian and interfascicular reticular nuclei at the level of the obex, the gigantocellular and paragigantocellular reticular nuclei at the level of the facial nucleus, and the nucleus centralis pontis, partes caudalis and oralis. According to retrograde HRP transport findings (209, 490) the descending fibers from the bulbar lateral tegmental field in cat and monkey are mainly distributed to the cervical cord (cf. refs. 295 and 379; and *Brain Stem*, p. 607).

The long reticulospinal fibers from the pontine and medullary medial tegmental field are present in a variety of animals (632, 687, 688). The existence of reticulospinal fibers in mammals was demonstrated in retrograde degeneration studies (42, 65, 679, 701) and in anterograde degeneration studies by using the Häggqvist technique (52, 92, 93). Their descent throughout the spinal cord was already suggested by anterograde degeneration findings in Marchi material (585–587) and has been confirmed in anterograde degeneration studies by using silver impregnation techniques (379, 447, 519, 553) and in antidromic electrical stimulation studies (172, 436, 547, 774). Häggqvist studies (92, 93) have shown that these reticulospinal fibers in cat are rather coarse. This is in keeping with their relatively high conduction velocity (315, 435), which, however, seems to be relatively lower in rat (198, 633).

Anterograde degeneration findings (447, 519) and anterograde amino acid transport findings (295, 451) indicate that the reticular fibers (Fig. 8) from the pontine medial tegmental field descend bilaterally through the medullary medial tegmental field but continue mainly ipsilaterally into the cervical ventral funiculus. The reticular fibers from the medullary medial tegmental field, however, descend bilaterally into the spinal cord, the ipsilateral distribution dominating. In the brain stem the ipsilaterally descending medullary reticulospinal fibers form a vertically oriented band that passes through the lateral part of the MLF and through the medial tegmental field. In the caudal medulla oblongata the ventral portion of this band is located dorsal and dorsolateral to the inferior olive. The fibers of this ventral portion descend into the cervical ventrolateral funiculus, whereas those of the dorsal portion continue into the cervical ventral funiculus (553). The contralaterally descending medullary reticulospinal fibers descend mainly through the dorsal portion of the contralateral MLF into the contralateral cervical ventral funiculus, while only very few descend into the contralateral ventrolateral funiculus (295, 447, 519, 553). Anterograde amino acid

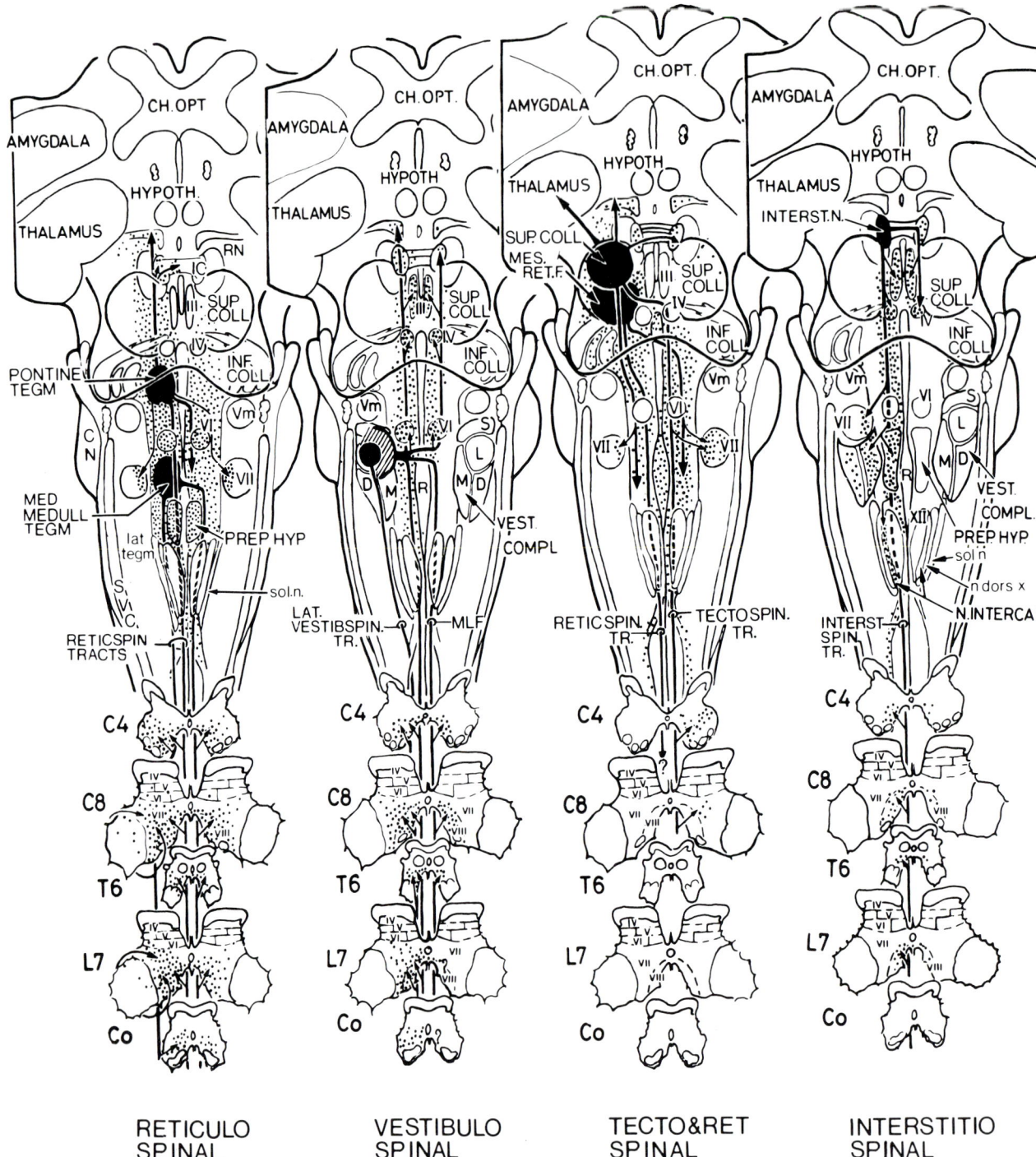

FIG. 8. Distribution of medially descending brain stem pathways, which terminate characteristically in area of long propriospinal neurons in intermediate one and in addition terminate also in bulbar medial reticular formation. Note that some of these pathways also project to medial part of facial nucleus, innervating external ear muscles and platysma. Note further that tectospinal fibers and medullary reticulospinal fibers also distribute to lateral parts of intermediate zone. CH OPT, optic chiasm; IC, interstitial nucleus of Cajal; RN, red nucleus; BC, brachium conjunctivum; Vm, trigeminal motor nucleus; VEST COMPL, vestibular complex; S, superior vestibular nucleus; L, lateral vestibular nucleus; M, medial vestibular nucleus; D, descending (spinal) vestibular nucleus; PREP HYP, nucleus prepositus hypoglossi; sol n, solitary nucleus; n dors x, dorsal motor nucleus of the vagus; N. INTERCAL., nucleus intercalatus.

transport findings (33) suggest that the ipsilaterally descending medullary fibers in the ventral funiculus are fewer in number than the contralaterally descending ones. These cervical funicular trajectories of the reticulospinal fibers also apply in the human being (215, 507). At caudal spinal levels, however, the reticulospinal fibers in the ventral and ventrolateral funiculi tend to migrate toward the dorsolateral funiculus (553).

With respect to the origin of the reticulospinal fibers, antidromic stimulation findings (549) and retrograde HRP transport findings (382, 697, 785) show that the reticulospinal fibers in the cervical ventral funiculus, contrary to earlier assumptions (519, 520), are derived from neurons in both the pontine and the medullary medial tegmental field, whereas the fibers in the ventrolateral funiculus are mainly derived from neurons in the medullary medial tegmental field. These studies also suggest that the fibers in the ventrolateral funiculus are mainly derived from neurons in the ventral part of the medullary medial tegmental field, while those in the ventral funiculus are mainly derived from neurons in its dorsal part. These respective groups of fibers roughly constitute the medial and the ventral reticulospinal tracts of Papez (542) and together form the medial reticulospinal tract of Busch (92, 93). Electrophysiological studies tend, however, to address the fibers in the ventral funiculus as the medial reticulospinal tract and those in the ventrolateral funiculus as the lateral one. The lateral reticulospinal tract thus defined therefore differs from the lateral reticulospinal tract of Papez (542), which is identical with the crossed pontospinal tract of Busch (92, 93) and descends in the dorsolateral funiculus together with the rubrospinal tract (see discussion of other laterally descending fiber systems in *Pathways distributing to short... neurons*, p. 619).

The reticulospinal projections display little somatotopic organization (701), and antidromic electrical stimulation studies (549) have shown that two-thirds of the reticulospinal neurons that distribute fibers to the cervical ventral gray also project to the lumbosacral cord. On the basis of retrograde HRP transport findings and antidromic stimulation findings (549, 551), however, it has been suggested that neurons in the rostrodorsal portion of the medullary medial tegmental field distribute fibers by way of the ventrolateral funiculus mainly to the upper cervical cord and may function in relation to the steering of neck movements.

The terminal distribution of the reticulospinal fibers (Fig. 8) is especially dense in the enlargements and, according to the anterograde degeneration and amino acid transport findings, involves mainly the ventral gray (33, 379, 447, 451, 519, 553, 581), i.e., lamina VIII and the medial and central parts of lamina VII in accordance with electrophysiological findings (725). Nevertheless, according to anterograde degeneration findings the medullary reticulospinal fibers have a wider distribution in the intermediate zone than the pontine reticulospinal fibers (519) and to some extent terminate also in the lateral parts of laminae VI and VII (553). The reticulospinal fibers are distributed bilaterally in the spinal gray. This bilateral distribution in part is because some of the ipsilaterally descending fibers in the spinal cord pass contralaterally by way of the spinal ventral commissure (519, 549, 553).

Recent anterograde transport findings in cat and opossum (294, 451) indicate that reticulospinal fibers from the medullary medial tegmental field at the levels between the facial nucleus and the obex, together with fibers from the medullary raphe (see discussion of serotonergic raphe neurons in *Monoaminergic and other pathways...*, p. 623), are distributed also to the medial and lateral motoneuronal cell groups in the spinal ventral horn. Only few pontine reticulospinal fibers are, however, distributed to these cell groups.

The medullary reticulospinal fibers to the motoneuronal cell groups probably establish the direct reticulomotoneuronal connections demonstrated electrophysiologically (550, 551, 766–768). According to the electrophysiological findings, however, such direct motoneuronal connections are established primarily with motoneurons of neck and back muscles and to a more limited degree also with motoneurons of limb muscles (550, 551, 766–768). According to electrophysiological findings in cat, the connections with motoneurons of limb muscles are established with both flexor and extensor motoneurons, proximal as well as distal (243, 245, 766, 767), while in monkey they are established mainly with motoneurons of proximal limb muscles (631). The direct reticulospinal connections to motoneurons of neck and back muscles are derived from the entire caudorostral extent of the medullary and caudal pontine medial tegmental field (550), although it has been observed that the connections from the dorsal part of this region are established primarily with motoneurons of neck muscles (550, 551). Furthermore, according to electrophysiological findings (550) the direct connections to motoneurons of limb muscles are derived mainly from a paramedian area in the medullary reticular formation: these connections may in part represent raphe spinal connections (see discussion of serotonergic raphe neurons in *Monoaminergic and other pathways...*, p. 623).

Vestibular complex. The vestibular complex distributes many fibers to the spinal cord. This complex comprises (73) the medial, descending (spinal), lateral (Deiters'), and superior vestibular nuclei, as well as several small cell groups: the interstitial nucleus of the vestibular nerve, nucleus y dorsal to the inferior cerebellar peduncle, and magnocellular group f in the caudolateral part of the descending nucleus. The medial vestibular nucleus is adjoined medially by the nucleus prepositus hypoglossi.

The vestibular complex receives primary sensory fibers from the vestibular nerve (418, 654, 741) in addition to other inputs from cell groups in different part of the neuraxis. It gives rise (Fig. 8) to ascending fibers to the mesencephalon and diencephalon as well as descending fibers to the spinal cord; it also distributes fibers to the lower brain stem, especially the bulbar medial tegmental field (386). The descending vestibular fibers to the spinal cord, according to retrograde HRP transport findings (141, 381, 548), are derived from the lateral vestibular (Deiters') as well as from the medial vestibular and descending (spinal) vestibular nuclei, including the magnocellular nucleus f; they travel through the ventral and ventrolateral funiculi (382).

Deiterospinal fibers from the lateral vestibular nucleus (Fig. 8) are derived from large and small cells (567) and are of varying diameter and conduction velocity (314). These fibers, which descend exclusively ipsilaterally, first traverse the upper part of the intramedullary descending limb of the facial nerve and then descend at the border between the medial and the lateral tegmental field. Farther caudally in the brain stem they migrate ventrally into the area dorsolateral to the inferior olive, whence they pass into the upper cervical ventrolateral funiculus. Along their trajectory through the spinal cord they migrate farther into the ventral part of the ventral funiculus at low cervical levels and into the medial part of the ventral funiculus, which adjoins the spinal ventral fissure at lumbar levels (52, 92, 93, 525, 553). These findings are in keeping with earlier anterograde degeneration findings in both animals and human beings (507).

Retrograde degeneration findings in cat (567) indicate that the population of Deiterospinal neurons is somatotopically organized such that the fibers to the cervical cord are derived mainly from neurons in the rostroventral part of the nucleus, while those to the lumbosacral cord are mainly derived from neurons in its dorsocaudal part. Retrograde degeneration findings (417) indicate that a similar but slightly modified arrangement exists in the human being. The retrograde degeneration findings in cat (567) are supported by anterograde degeneration findings (525) and are in keeping with antidromic electrical stimulation findings (314, 569, 763). The latter, however, show that the somatotopic organization in Deiters' nucleus is somewhat blurred by a considerable overlap between the populations of neurons projecting to the cervical and the lumbosacral segments, respectively. Moreover, according to antidromic electrical stimulation findings (1), 50% of the Deiterospinal fibers to the cervical enlargement represent collaterals of the fibers to the lumbosacral segments (cf. reticulospinal fibers in ref. 549).

Deiterospinal fibers in both cat and monkey terminate mainly ipsilaterally in the ventromedial part of the intermediate zone, i.e., lamina VIII and the medial parts of lamina VII (180, 379, 525, 553, 623, 646), while only a few fibers are distributed to this area contralaterally (180). Orthodromic stimulation findings indicate that Deiterospinal fibers establish polysynaptic excitatory connections with motoneurons of extensor muscles (243, 244, 421, 629, 766, 767). They also maintain with motoneurons of knee and ankle flexors polysynaptic inhibitory connections that are established by way of monosynaptic connections with Ia inhibitory interneurons (242, 422), which are located in the ventral part of the intermediate zone (307), where Deiterospinal fibers terminate. Anterograde degeneration studies have revealed few Deiterospinal fibers in the lateral motoneuronal cell group, although in opossum some are distributed to the ventromedial part of this cell group (443). In cat as in other animals many Deiterospinal fibers pass through the area of the medial motoneuronal cell groups (180, 525, 623). This may explain the orthodromic stimulation findings that indicate the existence of monosynaptic Deiterospinal connections to only some motoneurons of hindlimb extensor muscles (421, 766, 767) but to many motoneurons of neck and back muscles (766, 768).

Medial vestibulospinal fibers in the cat are of medium size (92, 93). According to anterograde degeneration findings they pass via the ipsilateral and contralateral MLF into the mediodorsal part of the spinal ventral funiculus along the spinal ventral fissure (92, 93, 471, 518, 553). According to these findings the medial vestibulospinal fibers are derived mainly from the medial vestibular nucleus. This has been confirmed by antidromic electrical stimulation findings (765) which, however, show that some of these fibers also come from the descending vestibular nucleus (764). The existence of descending fibers from the medial and descending vestibular nuclei (including group f) to the spinal cord has also been demonstrated by retrograde HRP transport findings (381, 548). According to the HRP findings some of these fibers reach the lumbosacral enlargement; this is in keeping with antidromic electrical stimulation findings (569). Anterograde degeneration data show that the medial vestibulospinal fibers in cat (518) and monkey (471) descend bilaterally into the spinal cord with an ipsilateral dominance. They also demonstrate that the ipsilaterally descending fibers at C_1 are located close to the gray matter, while the contralaterally descending fibers are located close to the medial surface of the ventral funiculus (92, 93). According to anterograde degeneration data (518) supported by orthodromic stimulation findings (646), the termination area of these fibers as observed in the cervical and the thoracic cord is more restricted than that of the Deiterospinal fibers and comprises mainly lamina VIII and the dorsally adjoining part of lamina VII (Fig. 8). Electrophysiological data in cat (766–768) show further that these medial vestibulospinal fibers also establish monosynaptic connections with many motoneurons of neck and back muscles; in contrast to the Deiterospinal connections these are inhibitory in nature (768).

Anterograde degeneration findings (386) and retrograde HRP transport findings (475) indicate that the vestibular complex also projects to the perihypoglossal nuclei and the bulbar medial tegmental field, especially to its medial part in the pons and to its dorsal part in the medulla oblongata. In addition it projects to a restricted portion of the medial part of the medullary lateral tegmental field (717). Anterograde degeneration and amino acid transport data (471, 584, 673, 683, 684) show further that fibers from the various vestibular nuclei (74) are distributed bilaterally to the eye muscle nuclei, the mesencephalic reticular formation, the nucleus of the posterior commissure, the interstitial nucleus of Cajal, and to the nucleus of Darkschewitsch in the rostral mesencephalic central gray (Fig. 8). Retrograde HRP transport data further show that cell group y, dorsally adjoining the vestibular complex, also projects to the oculomotor nucleus (239, 283) probably by way of the brachium conjunctivum (cf. ref. 102, 114). According to anterograde amino acid transport data (389, 584) some vestibular fibers ascend as far rostrally as the field of Forel and the ventromedial and lateral thalamus. Thus, the vestibular complex projects not only to the eye muscle nuclei but also to brain stem structures, which in turn project to these nuclei and have been implicated in the steering of gaze (see *Brain Stem*, p. 607). For a review of vestibular connections see ref. 70.

Mesencephalic reticular formation. The mesencephalic reticular formation comprises the nuclei cuneiformis and subcuneiformis. Retrograde HRP transport findings indicate that in cat (381), monkey (106), and opossum (141, 451) some neurons in the mesencephalic reticular formation lateral to the central gray, as well as in the lateral parts of the central gray itself, distribute fibers to the cervical cord and a few to the thoracic and lumbar cord (Fig. 8). The existence of such connections in the cat has been denied on the basis of retrograde degeneration (701) and anterograde degeneration findings (519). Their existence has been demonstrated, however, in sheep (679) and in monkey (65) by means of the former technique and in rat (745) and human beings (626) by means of the latter. According to the anterograde degeneration findings in the rat (745) and anterograde transport findings in opossum (451) these mesencephalic reticulospinal fibers descend through the medial part of the ventral funiculus and are distributed preferentially to laminae VII and VIII of the spinal gray.

The bulk of the descending fibers from the mesencephalic reticular formation is distributed to the lower brain stem bilaterally as demonstrated by retrograde HRP transport findings (C. E. Berrevoets and H. G. J. M. Kuypers, unpublished observations). According to anterograde amino acid transport findings (175) these descending fibers from the nucleus cuneiformis in the mesencephalic reticular formation are grouped into two main bundles. One bundle crosses the midline in the mesencephalon and descends through the paramedian fiber bundles ventral to the predorsal bundle, which contains fibers descending from the tectum to the lower brain stem and spinal cord (see discussion of superior colliculus, this subsection). This bundle of mesencephalic reticular fibers ventral to the predorsal bundles projects to the ventral part of the medial tegmental field in the pons and especially in the medulla oblongata. It also distributes fibers to the nucleus raphe magnus, to the motoneurons of the ear muscles (132, 361) in the dorsomedial subnucleus of the contralateral facial nucleus, and to the medial accessory olive. The other fiber bundle from the nucleus cuneiformis descends ipsilaterally and courses ventrolaterally through the mesencephalic tegmentum and the pontine medial tegmental field into the ventral parts of the medullary medial tegmental field and from there into the spinal cord (745). Along its bulbar trajectory this bundle distributes many fibers to the ventral portion of the bulbar medial tegmental field, the nucleus raphe magnus, and the spinal ventral gray at the level of the pyramidal decussation.

The distribution of the descending fibers from the nucleus subcuneiformis has not been described in detail. Earlier anterograde degeneration findings obtained by means of the Marchi technique (88) make it likely that these fibers descend mainly ipsilaterally through the ventral part of the bulbar medial tegmental field to the area of the inferior olive. This observation is further supported by some of the anterograde amino acid transport findings after midline mesencephalic injections (414). Further anterograde and retrograde transport studies are necessary, however, to clarify the course of these descending projections.

Interstitial nucleus of Cajal. Retrograde HRP transport findings (105, 141, 381, 382) show that fibers from the interstitial nucleus of Cajal descend mainly ipsilaterally into the spinal cord as far caudally as the lumbar segments. Anterograde degeneration supported by anterograde amino acid transport findings [Fig. 8; (414)] demonstrate that fibers from the area of this nucleus are distributed both through the ipsilateral MLF and by way of the posterior commissure through the contralateral MLF (cf. refs. 100, 431). By way of these two routes fibers are distributed bilaterally to the oculomotor and trochlear nuclei (cf. ref. 414). Other fibers are distributed ipsilaterally to the intermediate and deep gray of the superior colliculus. Caudal to the trochlear nucleus the descending fibers from the area of the interstitial nucleus of Cajal are present only ipsilaterally and are located in the most dorsomedial part of the MLF and in the adjoining tegmental bundles (92, 100). These fibers, which seem to be accompanied by some descending fibers from the medial part of the nucleus of the posterior commissure (46), pass through the lower brain stem into the spinal cord. In the lower brain stem none of the fibers from the area of the interstitial nucleus of Cajal are distributed to the abducens nuclei, but some are distributed to the bulbar medial tegmental field, the medial vestibular nucleus (431, 568), the descending vestibular nucleus, the nucleus prepositus hypoglossi, and the nucleus intercalatus (100, 431). In addition, according to the anterograde degeneration and amino acid transport findings a small number of fibers are distributed from the area of the interstitial nucleus and the adjoining central gray mainly to the dorsomedial facial subnuclei containing the ear muscle motoneurons as well as to the hypoglossal nucleus and the principal and medial accessory olivary nuclei (100, 431, 540, 541). According to anterograde degeneration findings the interstitiospinal fibers in the MLF continue into the most dorsal part of the spinal ventral funiculus (100, 521); this is in keeping with retrograde HRP transport findings (382). The fibers are distributed mainly ipsilaterally to the dorsal part of lamina VIII and the dorsally adjoining part of lamina VII throughout the spinal cord (521). Orthodromic electrical stimulation findings (200, 202) further indicate that the interstitiospinal fibers also establish some monosynaptic connections with neck muscle motoneurons, but connections with limb muscles motoneurons are mainly disynaptic (634).

Anterograde degeneration findings (431) show that the field of Forel, which is located rostral to the interstitial nucleus of Cajal, also projects to the oculomotor and trochlear nuclei as well as to the nucleus prepositus hypoglossi. However, the field of Forel does not project to the spinal cord as shown by retrograde HRP transport findings (see *Brain Stem*, p. 607).

Superior colliculus. According to retrograde HRP transport findings (105, 141, 381) the tectospinal fibers from the superior colliculus in cat, monkey, and opossum are only distributed to the cervical cord. This conclusion is in keeping with anterograde degeneration and anterograde amino acid transport findings (9, 262, 442, 517, 553, 745). The tectospinal neurons, which are labeled retrogradely after unilateral C_1 HRP injections in cat, are rather large and are located below the stratum opticum in the intermediate and deep gray of the contralateral superior colliculus (755), a finding in keeping with electrophysiological results (13). Similar retrograde HRP findings have been obtained in monkey, in which, however, the labeled neurons are less numerous than in cat (H. G. J. M. Kuypers and V. A. Maisky, unpublished observations). This is in accordance with anterograde amino acid transport findings (199, 262) that show relatively few tectal fibers descending into the spinal cord in monkey.

The intermediate and deep gray layers of the superior colliculus, which contain the tectospinal neurons, also distribute fibers to the diencephalon, mesencephalon, and lower brain stem (333). Thus according to anterograde degeneration and anterograde amino acid transport findings (39, 87, 231, 263) the deep layers of the colliculus project to the suprageniculate nucleus and the magnocellular portion of the medial geniculate body at the mesodiencephalic junction as well as to the intralaminar nuclei, the center median-parafascicular complex, and parts of the lateral thalamus in the diencephalon. Some fibers from the deep layers of the superior colliculus also pass to the zona incerta and the field of Forel and probably to the prerubral area, which projects to the eye muscle nuclei [(94, 238, 431); see *Brain Stem*, p. 607]. The fibers from the intermediate and deep collicular gray to the mesencephalon are distributed ipsilaterally to the pretectum, bilaterally to the nucleus of the posterior commissure (231) and interstitial nucleus of Cajal (9), and mainly ipsilaterally to the mesencephalic reticular formation, which comprises nuclei cuneiformis and subcuneiformis (332). In addition the intermediate gray and the deep gray of the superior colliculus (Fig. 8) give rise to two descending fiber bundles to the lower brain stem, one being located medially, the other laterally (9, 231, 262, 263, 332, 442, 575). These bundles follow much the same trajectory as the descending bundles from the mesencephalic reticular formation (175).

The medially descending tectal bundle (crossed tectobulbar and tectospinal tract) curves medially through the mesencephalic tegmentum. At this level many fibers are distributed to the ipsilateral mesencephalic reticular formation (332). It then passes through the dorsal mesencephalic tegmental decussation, at which level it distributes fibers to a group of neurons in the central gray dorsal to the oculomotor nuclei (176). Subsequently this bundle forms the contralaterally descending predorsal bundle, which is located in the paramedian fiber bundles immediately ventral to the MLF. This bundle descends through the brain stem into the cervical cord. Along its contralateral trajectory through the brain stem this bundle distributes some tectal fibers to an area close to the trochlear nucleus (176) and distributes many tectal fibers to the medial part of the pontine and medullary medial tegmental field, especially the dorsal part of the latter, including the para-abducens area. This portion of the bulbar medial tegmental field also receives many vestibular fibers (see discussion of vestibular complex, this subsection) and presumably contains neurons projecting to the eye muscle nuclei (see *Brain Stem*, p. 607). In this respect it is of interest to recall that the crossed mesencephalic reticulobulbar fibers that descend through the area ventral to the predorsal bundle are distributed differently in the lower brain stem and terminate mainly in the ventral parts of the medullary medial tegmental field, an area that does not seem to contribute substantially to projections to the eye muscle nuclei. The contralaterally descending tectal bundle also distributes a few fibers to the ear muscle motoneurons of the dorsomedial facial subnucleus, and in cat it distributes also to motoneurons of the periorbital and perioral muscles of the lateral facial subnuclei (176). Farther caudally in the medulla oblongata the contralaterally descending tectal bundle distributes fibers to the paramedian reticular nuclei, the interfascicular nucleus, and the medial accessory olive (199). The remaining crossed tectal fibers descend into the ventral part of the spinal ventral funiculus (93). These tectospinal fibers generally are reported to distribute to the medial parts of the ventral horn contralateral to their tectal origin (9, 262, 442, 745). Several anterograde degeneration studies (442, 517, 553) demonstrate, however, that some of these fibers also terminate in the lateral parts of laminae VI and VII in the upper cervical segments and in the medial and central parts of lamina VII at intermediate cervical levels (Fig. 8). Thus their distribution differs from that of vestibulospinal and interstitiospinal fibers, which terminate preferentially in lamina VIII and the adjoining parts of lamina VII. Moreover, according to orthodromic electrical stimulation findings (14) the tectospinal fibers, in contrast to the vestibulospinal and interstitiospinal fibers, do not establish monosynaptic connections with neck muscle motoneurons but only disynaptic or polysynaptic ones. These connections, which tend to be excitatory to contralateral neck muscle motoneurons and inhibitory to ipsilateral ones (14), are in part established by way of neurons in the caudal medulla oblongata.

The laterally descending tectal bundle (ipsilateral tectobulbar tract) passes through the outskirts of the mesencephalic tegmentum, i.e., medial to the brachium of the inferior colliculus and medial to the nuclei of the lateral lemniscus (Fig. 8). In the caudal mesencephalon this bundle distributes many fibers to the paralemniscal area (176, 279), which projects to the contralateral ear muscle motoneurons in the dorsomedial facial subnucleus (279). In the pons this bundle distributes fibers to the pontine cerebellar relay nuclei, including the nucleus reticularis tegmenti pontis, and to the ventrolateral part of the pontine tegmentum. According to some anterograde degeneration studies (263, 442) this bundle continues into the upper medulla oblongata and distributes fibers to the reticular formation as well as to ipsilateral ear muscle and platysma motoneurons of the medial facial subnuclei (132, 361, 541).

Horseradish peroxidase injections in the spinal cord and lower brain stem fail to label tectal neurons in the strata zonale and griseum superficiale [(268, 333); C. E. Berrevoets and H. G. J. M. Kuypers, unpublished observations]; parts of these layers receive retinotectal fibers (234, 305). Neurons in these superficial strata are, however, labeled retrogradely after HRP injections in the thalamus (5, 334, 574), indicating that they project rostrally. This difference in the projections from the superficial versus the intermediate and deep gray layers of the superior colliculus, which parallels functional differences (104), has also been demonstrated by means of anterograde degeneration and amino acid transport techniques in several animals (39, 231, 263).

The pretectum does not give rise to long descending fibers to the spinal cord (46). It does, however, project to the nucleus of the posterior commissure and the Edinger-Westphal nucleus and also gives rise to a group of laterally descending fibers, i.e., the pretectotegmental fasciculus of Bucher and Bürgi (83). According to anterograde amino acid transport findings (46, 235) these fibers are distributed to the nucleus reticularis tegmenti pontis and to an area laterally adjoining the red nucleus, which may also include the lateral part of the nucleus itself. Neurons in this area of the red nucleus probably project contralaterally to the bulbar lateral tegmental field, the trigeminal sensory nuclei, and to the motoneurons of periorbital and perioral muscles (361) of the intermediate and lateral facial subnuclei (174, 292, 562). According to anterograde amino acid transport findings, however, the pretectal area also distributes fibers directly to some of these facial motoneurons (A. M. Graybiel, personal communication).

Cerebellar fastigial nucleus. Many of the cell groups that give rise to descending brain stem pathways to long propriospinal neurons (laminae VII and VIII) receive fastigial cerebellar projections. Thus according to anterograde amino acid transport findings, neurons in the caudal part of the fastigial nucleus project mainly rostrally to the mesencephalic reticular formation, the deep layers of the superior colliculus, the nucleus of the posterior commissure, and probably also to the intersitital nucleus of Cajal (121, 692, 737). Neurons in the rostral part of the fastigial nucleus project mainly caudally, i.e., to the vestibular complex, the parasolitary nucleus, the prepositus hypoglossi nucleus, and the pontine and medullary medial tegmental field (35, 495, 692, 737, 743, 744). Some neurons in the rostral and intermediate parts of the fastigial nucleus and the adjoining portion of the interpositus nucleus also distribute fibers to the spinal cord, which fibers descend contralaterally (35, 201). According to the anterograde amino acid transport findings in monkey (35) these fibers descend through the uncinate fasciculus and after passing through the vestibular nuclei turn caudally and intermingle with the Deiterospinal fibers dorsolateral to the inferior olive. These fastigiospinal fibers mainly descend to the upper cervical segments (201), although in rat and tree shrew some fibers have been reported to reach the lumbar cord (2, 748). According to anterograde degeneration as well as amino acid transport findings (35, 692, 748) they are distributed to the intermediate zone and the ventral horn and possibly motoneuronal cell groups. Moreover, retrograde double-labeling findings indicate that some of these fibers in rat and cat are collaterals of fastigial fibers ascending to mesencephalon and thalamus (M. Bentivoglio, T. B. Bharos, and H. G. J. M. Kuypers, unpublished observations).

Pathways distributing to short propriospinal (laminae VII and VIII) and propriobulbar neurons. Red nucleus. The red nucleus is present in all mammals and in a variety of lower vertebrates (687, 688), but it is absent in snake (for general review see ref. 456). In higher primates such as monkeys, apes, and human

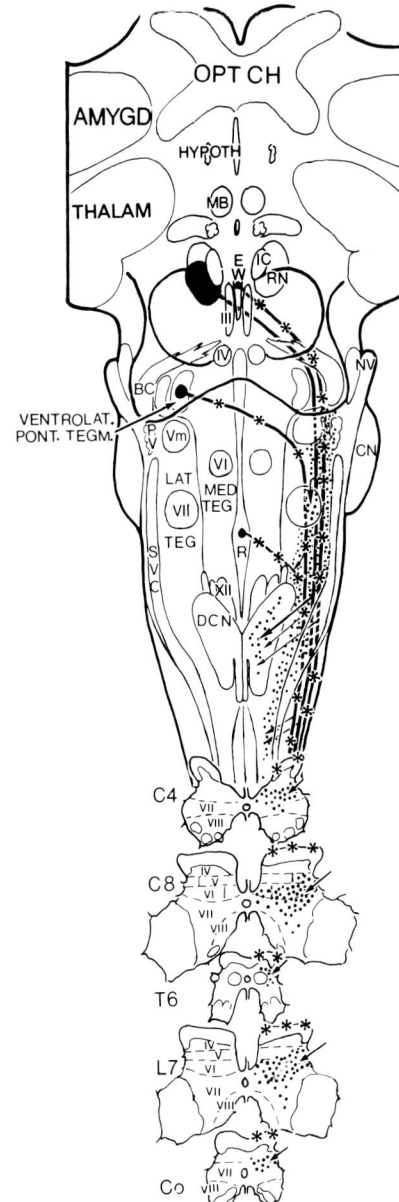

FIG. 9. Trajectory and terminal distribution of laterally descending brain stem pathway, which are derived from contralateral magnocellular red nucleus, Edinger-Westphal nucleus, ventrolateral pontine tegmentum, and raphe nuclei. Many of these pathways characteristically distribute fibers to bulbar lateral tegmental field, area of dorsal column nuclei, and dorsal and lateral part of the spinal intermediate zone, which contains short propriospinal neurons. Some of these pathways also distribute fibers to lamina I of spinal dorsal horn (asterisks). OPT CH, optic chiasm; HYPOTH, hypothalamus; THALAM, thalamus; EW, Edinger-Westphal nucleus; IC, interstitial nucleus of Cajal; RN, red nucleus; BC, brachium conjunctivum; PV, principal sensory trigeminal nucleus; R, raphe nuclei; DCN, dorsal column nuclei cuneatus and gracilis; LAT TEG, bulbar lateral tegmental field; CN, cochlear nuclei; MED TEG, medial tegmental field; SVC, spinal V complex.

beings it comprises a caudal magnocellular and a rostral parvocellular part (272); these parts receive many afferents from the contralateral interpositus and lateral cerebellar nuclei, respectively (16, 134, 197, 342). The parvocellular part in monkey consists of a dorsomedial and a ventrolateral portion (197, 204, 380, 532, 544), the former of which extends toward the central gray. In lower mammals such as rat and cat the magnocellular and parvocellular parts are less distinctly different than in the primates named (566).

Golgi and EM studies in monkey (345), cat (705), and opossum (341) have demonstrated the existence of three types of red nucleus neurons: 1) giganto- and magnocellular elements that are most numerous caudally in the nucleus and may show a pronounced cholinesterase reaction (249, 448); 2) large- to medium-size elements that possess relatively less Nissl substance and are most numerous rostrally in the nucleus (these latter neurons in the rostral part of the nucleus in cat and opossum differ from the truly parvocellular elements in the rostral part of the nucleus in monkey, which are characterized by a diffuse peripherally located Nissl substance and an eccentric nucleus); 3) very small neurons that have virtually no Nissl substance (343).

Two main fiber bundles descend from the red nucleus. One of these bundles decussates in the mesencephalon, descends contralaterally through the ventrolateral pontine tegmentum (Fig. 9), and continues along the ventral aspect of the bulbar lateral tegmental field, next to the spinal V complex, and then into the spinal dorsolateral funiculus. The other bundle proceeds ipsilaterally through the medial tegmental field toward the inferior olive. An ascending rubral fiber bundle leading to the ventral thalamic nuclei was assumed to exist in the past. However, anterograde degeneration and anterograde amino acid transport findings (174, 299), as well as antidromic electrical stimulation findings (12) in cat and rhesus monkey, make it likely that such ascending connections do not occur.

The crossed descending rubrobulbar and rubrospinal tract has been studied, for example, in rat (81), rabbit (487), opossum and other marsupials (445, 446, 541, 749), cat (27, 133, 174, 284, 292, 524, 553, 678, 739), galago (500), tree shrew (498, 501), monkey (373, 379, 481), and human being (215) by means of anterograde degeneration and anterograde amino acid transport techniques. In all these species this fiber bundle, after leaving the red nucleus from the ventral and medial aspect, passes through the ventral mesencephalic tegmental decussation. Subsequently in its descent through the mesencephalon the bundle gradually shifts laterally to occupy a position in the ventrolateral part of the rostral pontine tegmentum, i.e., next to the lower margin of the superior cerebellar peduncle. From this area the bundle descends medial to the trigeminal motor root into the medulla oblongata, where it is located ventromedial to the spinal V complex and ventrolateral to the facial nucleus. From the medulla oblongata the bundle continues into the spinal dorsolateral funiculus, medial to the dorsal spinocerebellar tract, a position it occupies throughout the length of the spinal cord.

In the upper pons this crossed bundle distributes

fibers via the brachium conjunctivum to the cerebellar anterior interpositus nucleus (135). In the lower pons and the medulla oblongata (Fig. 9) the fiber bundle distributes fibers to the lateral part of the pontine and medullary lateral tegmental field, including area h between the principal sensory and the motor nuclei V. Some fibers are also distributed to the principal sensory nucleus V itself as well as to some portions of the spinal V complex (27). In addition, fibers are distributed to the facial nucleus, especially to the periocular and periorbital motoneurons in the intermediate and in the lateral part of the lateral facial subnucleus. In the caudal medulla oblongata this bundle also distributes fibers to the subtrigeminal portion of the lateral reticular nucleus; the descending vestibular nucleus and especially nucleus f (174), which projects to the spinal cord (548); to nuclei x and z; and through the lateral tegmental field to the hilus of the dorsal column nuclei cuneatus and gracilis. This latter fiber trajectory apparently represents a standard route of access to the area of the dorsal column nuclei (378), since fibers from the mesencephalic central gray (416) to the dorsal column nuclei as well as those from the contralateral ventrolateral pontine tegmentum (see discussion of ventrolateral pontine tegmentum in this subsection) follow the same trajectory.

In the spinal cord the bulbar distribution pattern of the crossed rubral fibers is maintained such that the rubrospinal fibers are distributed from the dorsolateral funiculus to the lateral part of lamina V, lamina VI, and the dorsal parts of lamina VII, as demonstrated also by EM anterograde degeneration findings (354, 630). These findings are in keeping with orthodromic electrical stimulation findings in cat (297, 353, 630) that show in addition that rubrospinal fibers tend to excite flexor motoneurons (296, 565, 612, 693) and to inhibit extensor motoneurons [except for motoneurons of plantar muscles, which are also excited (296)]. Electrical stimulation findings further indicate that rubrospinal fibers in cat seldom establish direct synaptic contacts with motoneurons (296), whereas in rhesus monkey they establish some direct connections with motoneurons of distal extremity muscles (635).

Antidromic electrical stimulation findings in cat (638) demonstrate that individual rubrospinal fibers distribute collaterals to a group of adjoining spinal segments. In contrast to the collaterals of the individual vestibulospinal (1) and reticulospinal fibers (549), which are distributed throughout the cord, the collaterals of the rubrospinal fibers are largely restricted to specific levels, such that few rubrolumbar fibers distribute collaterals to the cervical segments (638).

The ipsilaterally descending rubral fiber bundle, according to anterograde degeneration studies in cat (284) and monkey (136, 481, 664), passes through the central tegmental tract into the pontine and upper medullary medial tegmental field. From the level of the superior olive this bundle gradually shifts ventrolaterally and terminates in the ipsilateral inferior olive:
in monkey in most of the principal olive, the dorsomedial cell column, and the middle portion of the medial accessory olive (136, 481); in cat mainly in the dorsal lamella of the principal olive (174, 284, 739). Along its course this bundle also distributes fibers to the medial tegmental field (481), probably including its paramedian reticular area (12).

The origin of descending rubral fibers may be concluded from antidromic electrical stimulation findings in cat (12) as well as from retrograde degeneration and transport findings in rat (249, 499), cat (381, 566), opossum (448), monkey (65, 106, 337, 349, 380, 562, 648), and human being (658). These findings indicate that the crossed rubrospinal fibers are mainly derived from neurons in the caudal part of the red nucleus. In rat, cat, and opossum, however, some are also derived from neurons in the rostral part, especially its ventral portion, as observed also in cat by means of retrograde HRP transport (H. G. J. M. Kuypers and V. A. Maisky, unpublished observations). In monkey (65, 106, 349, 380, 562, 648) and in human being (658), however, rubrospinal fibers appear to be derived only from the caudal magnocellular part of the nucleus. Antidromic electrical stimulation findings (12) show further that in cat some of the rubrocerebellar fibers are collaterals of rubrospinal fibers (cf. ref. 72) that originate from neurons in the caudal part of the red nucleus. Retrograde degeneration findings, as well as anterograde degeneration and anterograde amino acid transport findings in cat (174, 292) and opossum (448), suggest further that the crossed rubrobulbar fibers to the sensory trigeminal nuclei, the facial nucleus, and the bulbar lateral tegmental field are mainly derived from neurons in the rostral two-thirds of the red nucleus and the lateral extreme of its caudal one-third, possibly including the adjoining tegmental area (414, 562). Anterograde degeneration findings in opossum (448) also show that the fibers to the subtrigeminal portion of the lateral reticular nucleus and to the dorsal column nuclei are mainly derived from neurons in the caudal part of the nucleus.

Anterograde and retrograde degeneration findings in cat (524, 566), rat (249), and opossum (448) demonstrate that the population of rubrospinal neurons is somatopically organized. Thus the rubrospinal fibers to the cervical cord appear to be derived mainly from neurons in the medial and dorsal parts of the nucleus, while those to the lumbosacral cord appear to be derived mainly from neurons in its ventral and ventrolateral parts. This is supported by orthodromic and antidromic electrical stimulation findings (173, 213, 536, 712). Roughly the same arrangement exists in the rhesus monkey (106, 349, 648) and probably also in the chimpanzee, since corticorubral fibers from the precentral hand and foot representation areas to the magnocellular red nucleus in this species are distributed to the ventrolateral and the dorsomedial portions of the magnocellular part, respectively, as occurs also in monkey (267, 380, 383).

The ipsilaterally descending rubromedullary fibers, according to antidromic electrical stimulation findings (12) in cat, are mainly derived from neurons in the rostral part of the red nucleus, though some also come from neurons in its caudal part. This is in keeping with anterograde amino acid transport (174) and with anterograde degeneration findings (739). Retrograde and anterograde degeneration findings in monkey and opossum (337, 448, 481, 562) indicate that the same holds true in these animals, except that in monkey the ipsilateral rubromedullary fibers are almost exclusively derived from the parvocellular part of the nucleus. Antidromic electrical stimulation data (12) in cat indicate further that some of the ipsilateral rubromedullary fibers are collaterals of rubrospinal fibers.

The fiber diameter of the rubrospinal fibers is in general larger than that of the rubromedullary ones, as indicated by anterograde degeneration (215, 481) supported by antidromic electrical stimulation findings (12). With respect to the rubrospinal fibers, however, apparently some interspecies differences exist, because in rat (81) the majority of these fibers has a diameter of 1.5-2.0 µm, while in opossum (226), brush-tailed possum (749), and in tree shrew (501) the majority have a diameter from 2 to 6 µm. In higher primates such as gibbon (727) and human being (215) the rubrospinal fibers are few in number and are all rather thick, ranging in human being from 7 µm to 10 µm in diameter. These interspecies differences in diameter parallel differences in conduction velocity; they range in rat from 40 to 55 m/s [(248), quoted in ref. 632]; in cat from 40 to 150 m/s, the majority conducting from 40 to 90 m/s [(184), quoted in refs. 563, 632, 712]; and in rhesus monkey from 70 to 110 m/s (635). The shift toward thicker and faster conducting rubrospinal fibers in higher primates, combined with a diminution in their number, is probably related to their exclusive origin in the magnocellular red nucleus, which is rather small in these species, especially in gibbon (727), chimpanzee (731), and human being (658).

Ventrolateral pontine tegmentum. Retrograde degeneration findings in sheep (679) and retrograde HRP transport findings in cat (381, 697), monkey (258), and opossum (141) indicate that neurons in the ventrolateral part of the pontine tegmentum, close to the rubrospinal tract, give rise to long descending fibers that cross in the brain stem and distribute throughout the spinal cord (Fig. 7). Retrograde HRP findings (698), combined with large spinal lesions (382) and anterograde amino acid transport findings (293, 295, 451), indicate that these fibers descend mainly through the dorsolateral funiculus together with the rubrospinal and corticospinal tracts. This crossed pontine reticulospinal tract is probably identical with the lateral reticulospinal tract of Papez (542) and the crossed pontospinal tract of Busch (92, 93), which has been referred to earlier as the pontine component of the (rubrospinal) tract of Von Monakow (405). In recent anterograde amino acid transport studies in opossum and cat (293-295, 451) this tract has been traced from the pontine tegmentum through the contralateral bulbar lateral tegmental field into the spinal dorsolateral funiculus throughout the spinal cord and was found to terminate in some respects as the rubrobulbar and rubrospinal tract. Thus in the lower brain stem this tract seems to distribute fibers contralaterally to the bulbar lateral tegmental field and through this area to the area of the dorsal column nuclei. In the spinal cord in both cat (293-295) and opossum (451) this tract distributes fibers mainly to laminae V and VI of the spinal gray but distributes also some fibers to the area of the lateral cervical nucleus and to lamina I of the dorsal horn (Fig. 9).

Deep cerebellar nuclei. Cajal (97) observed the existence of a set of cerebellar fibers that descend ipsilaterally from the superior cerebellar peduncle into the lower brain stem. In Golgi material of newborn mouse the fibers were found to represent collaterals of fibers of the superior cerebellar peduncle (97). Anterograde degeneration (2, 186, 473, 474) and amino acid transport findings (114) show that such fibers also exist in guinea pig, rat, and monkey and terminate in the lateral parts of the pontine and medullary lateral tegmental field. According to the anterograde amino acid transport findings (114) those fibers are at least in part derived from the ipsilateral dentate nucleus and are also distributed to the area of the principal sensory nucleus V. Some of these ipsilaterally descending cerebellar fibers terminate densely in cell groups in the bulbar lateral tegmental field, which presumably project to the cerebellum and the oculomotor nuclei (cf. ref. 186).

Other laterally descending fiber systems. The trajectory of the rubrobulbar and rubrospinal tracts and of the crossed pontospinal tract is shared by several other descending suprabulbar fiber systems, which are also distributed to the area of the bulbar lateral tegmental field, the dorsal column nuclei, and by way of the spinal dorsolateral funiculus to the dorsal half of the spinal gray. Thus according to anterograde amino acid transport findings this trajectory is followed by fibers from the mesencephalic central gray (Fig. 9), especially the Edinger-Westphal nucleus (414); by fibers from the tegmental area close to the interstitial nucleus of Cajal (fibers that descend only to the bulbar lateral tegmental field; see ref. 414); by fibers from the pretectum to the intermediate facial subnucleus (A. M. Graybiel, personal communications); and by fibers from the amygdala (298) and the hypothalamus to the bulbar lateral tegmental field, the dorsal motor nucleus of the vagus, and the solitary nucleus (fibers that also descend mainly into the dorsolateral funiculus; see *Monoaminergic and other pathways...*, p. 623). Thus already in the upper pons the descending fibers tend to be segregated according to their terminal destination in the lower brain stem and the spinal cord, with the result that those to the bulbar medial tegmental field, the vestibular complex, and the long propriospinal neurons in the ventromedial part of the intermediate zone tend to be grouped medially, while those to the bulbar lateral tegmental field, the dorsal column nuclei, and the dorsal half of the spinal gray, including short propriospinal neurons, tend to be grouped laterally. Bagley's bundle (26, 253) of cortical fibers in ungulates (see CORTICOSPINAL AND CORTICO-BULBAR PATHWAYS, p. 627), which is destined mainly for the bulbar lateral tegmental field, conforms to this pattern and in the pontine tegmentum is also located relatively laterally, immediately dorsal to the rubrospinal tract. The raphespinal fibers and the subcoeruleospinal fibers (see *Monoaminergic and other pathways...*, this page) follow the same pattern such that the raphe spinal fibers to the dorsal horn occupy a lateral position and descend through the dorsolateral funiculus, while some of the other raphe spinal fibers and especially the subcoeruleospinal fibers that distribute to the spinal ventral horn are both located in the ventrolateral and ventral funiculi.

Pathways subserving respiratory activity; solitary and retroambiguus nuclei. According to retrograde HRP transport findings (381, 697) fibers from solitary and retroambiguus nuclei descend mainly contralaterally in the spinal cord. The HRP findings, as well as anterograde degeneration findings obtained in Marchi material (286) and retrograde degeneration findings (700), indicate that the fibers cross in the lower medulla oblongata. According to HRP transport findings in cat (381, 697), rat (615), and opossum (141) solitariospinal fibers are derived from neurons in the ventrolateral solitary subnucleus (cf. ref. 700) and also from a limited number of smaller monoaminergic neurons in the commissural nucleus interconnecting the caudal part of the solitary nuclei at the level of the pyramidal decussation.

Retrograde HRP transport findings combined with large spinal lesions (382) show that fibers from the ventrolateral solitary subnucleus and the retroambiguus nucleus are located at C_6–C_7 in the contralateral ventrolateral (cf. ref. 700), and ventral funiculi (cf. ref. 286). Correspondingly many neurons in both nuclei can be invaded antidromically from the contralateral cervical ventrolateral funiculus (53, 181, 476, 505). Unit recordings indicate that the activity of the neurons in the ventrolateral solitary subnucleus and the rostral part of the retroambiguus nucleus is mainly related to inspiration, while that of neurons in the caudal part of the latter nucleus is mainly related to expiration (53, 181, 476, 505). Anterograde amino acid transport findings in cat (412) show that the solitary neurons project to the retroambiguus nucleus, to phrenic motoneurons (cf. ref. 657) innervating the diaphragm, and to thoracic motoneuronal cell groups, which in part also innervate respiratory muscles. Physiological observations (53, 347) suggest that the retroambiguus nucleus projects to thoracic motoneurons. Bilateral transection of the upper cervical ventrolateral funiculus in cat and human beings (122, 506, 513) and low medullary midline transection ventral to the central canal in cat (609, 628) abolish rhythmic respiration. These data suggest that the solitary and retroambiguus connections to the contralateral spinal cord subserve automatic brain stem respiratory control. The contralaterality to these connections seems somewhat surprising, however, since it suggests that ipsilateral pulmonary afferents to the solitary nucleus would control mainly the activity of the contralateral diaphragm (for a general review see refs. 43, 485).

Monoaminergic and other pathways distributing to somatic motoneurons and autonomic preganglionic motoneurons. Hypothalamus. Retrograde degeneration findings (679) demonstrated that fibers from the hypothalamic paraventricular nucleus descend mainly ipsilaterally into the spinal cord. This is supported by retrograde transport findings in rat, cat, and monkey (58, 257, 349, 381, 611) that also indicate that these fibers are distributed throughout the spinal cord and are derived from neurons in the parvocellular part of the paraventricular nucleus (301) as well as from neurons in the dorsal and in the lateral hypothalamus (Fig. 7). Some of these neurons in the dorsal hypothalamus have been shown to be dopaminergic in nature (58, 60).

According to anterograde degeneration findings (cf. ref. 511) hypothalamic fibers descend caudally by way of the periventricular fiber systems to the mesencephalic central gray and by way of the ventral tegmental area of Tsai into the mesencephalic tegmentum. A portion of the latter fibers migrates medially to the raphe nuclei in the caudal mesencephalon and upper pons, while the remainder continues into the ventrolateral part of the mesencephalic tegmentum dorsally adjoining the medial lemniscus. This bundle (in the ventrolateral part of the mesencephalic tegmentum) distributes fibers to the caudal medial mesencephalic tegmentum and central gray. Anterograde degeneration findings in cat (119) as well as anterograde amino acid transport findings in rat (126) demonstrate that this bundle of hypothalamic fibers continues caudally into the pontine tegmental area adjoining the lateral lemniscus, whence they descend through the area of the lateral reticular nucleus of the medulla oblongata into the spinal lateral funiculus (611). Fibers are distributed along this trajectory (Fig. 10) in rat, cat, and monkey to the parabrachial area, the area of the locus coeruleus, and possibly the nucleus subcoeruleus. Farther caudally fibers are distributed to the bulbar lateral tegmental field, the solitary nucleus, the dorsal motor nucleus of the vagus, the nucleus ambiguus, and the medullary raphe nuclei (126, 611). It is of interest to note that this terminal distribution in the brain stem resembles that of the descending fibers from the central nucleus of the amygdala (Fig. 10), which follow roughly the same trajectory (298).

According to anterograde amino acid transport findings (611) the hypothalamospinal fibers are located

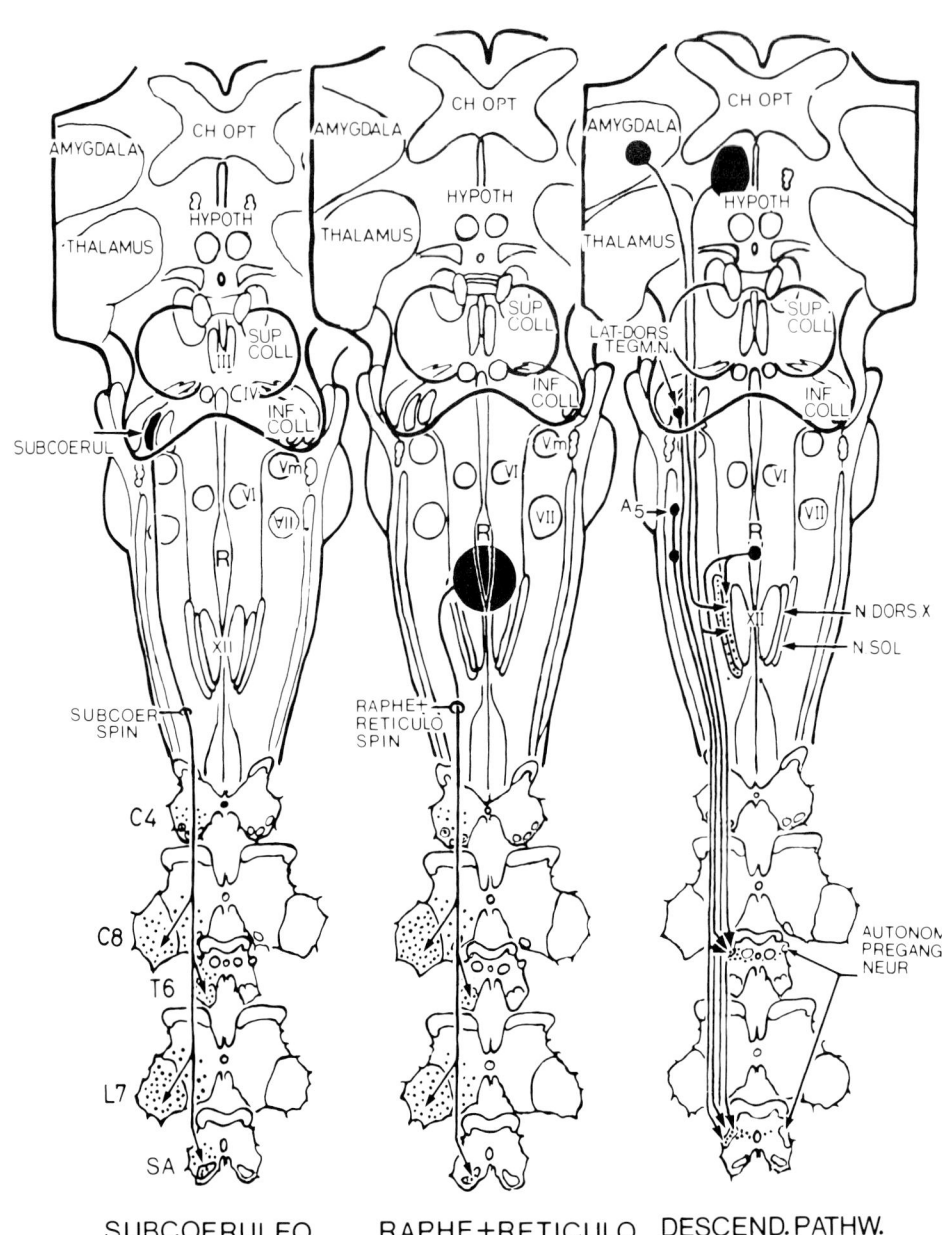

FIG. 10. Trajectory and terminal distribution of descending fibers from nucleus subcoeruleus (*left*) and from raphe nuclei and caudal medullary medial reticular formation (*middle*) to somatic motoneuronal cell groups in spinal cord. *Right*: descending brain stem fibers from amygdala, hypothalamus, nucleus laterodorsalis tegmenti, cell group A5, and raphe nuclei to autonomic motoneuronal cell groups of solitary-dorsal vagal complex and intermediolateral nuclei of thoracic and sacral cord. CH OPT, optic chiasm; HYPOTH, hypothalmus; SUP COLL, superior colliculus; INF COLL, inferior colliculus; SUBCOERUL, nucleus subcoeruleus; R, raphe nuclei; LAT-DORS TEGM. N, nucleus laterodorsalis tegmenti; N DORS X, dorsal motor nucleus of vagus; N SOL, solitary nucleus.

mainly in the spinal lateral funiculus. Retrograde HRP transport findings indicate, however, that at C_6–C_7 some hypothalamospinal fibers are also located in the ventral funiculus (382). According to anterograde amino acid transport findings in cat (611) the hypothalamospinal fibers terminate in the thoracic intermediolateral cell column. Anterograde degeneration findings (119) have suggested, however, that they are mainly distributed to the medial parts of the thoracic intermediate area, i.e., close to the central canal.

Immunohistochemical studies in rat (670) have shown that at least part of the hypothalamospinal neurons and their fibers contain neurophysine, which is synthesized by the paraventricular neurons and is also transported by their fibers to the posterior pituitary gland (28, 722, 723). The descending hypothalamospinal fibers containing neurophysine must at least in part be identical with the hypothalamic fibers to the spinal cord observed in anterograde amino acid transport studies (611), because they are distributed to the same brain stem areas. Moreover they are also located in the spinal lateral funiculus and are distributed to both the medial and lateral part of the thoracic autonomic intermediate region. Furthermore, fibers carrying neurophysine, oxytocin, and vasopressin are also distributed to lamina I of the dorsal horn (96, 670).

Catecholaminergic brain stem neurons. Histofluorescence and other studies have demonstrated the existence of several catecholaminergic neurons and fiber bundles in the caudal mesencephalon and the lower brain stem of rat, cat, monkey, and opossum (116, 140, 145, 190, 211, 289, 303, 313, 327, 434, 515, 530, 561). Yet in the spinal cord only catecholaminergic fibers but no catecholaminergic neurons are present. Since the catecholaminergic fibers in the spinal cord lose their fluorescence caudal to a spinal transection (99, 146), they are regarded as being derived from the catecholaminergic brain stem cell groups [e.g. A_7 to A_1 (145)]. This conclusion is supported by combined monoamine oxidase and HRP findings (615).

Catecholaminergic fibers are present in the lower brain stem, especially in the lateral tegmental field (434, 539, 671, 714). They continue rostrally through the area of the locus coeruleus and the nucleus subcoeruleus into the mesencephalon and forebrain. They continue caudally into the spinal dorsolateral funiculus as well as into the ventral funiculus and adjoining part of the ventrolateral funiculus (146).

In the lower brain stem catecholaminergic terminals are distributed to the motor nuclei of cranial nerves V, VII, and XII and especially to the solitary nucleus, the commissural nucleus, the dorsal motor nucleus of the vagus, and the raphe nuclei. Only relatively few such terminals are present in the trigeminal sensory nuclei (206, 539, 671). In the spinal cord catecholaminergic terminals are distributed according to the same pattern. Thus they are most numerous in the autonomic intermediolateral nucleus of the thoracic and sacral segments (99, 128, 146, 351), but they are present also in the dorsal horn, the intermediate zone, and the motoneuronal cell groups of the ventral horn (146).

Retrograde degeneration findings (42) as well as retrograde HRP transport findings (141, 258, 378, 381, 615) demonstrate that neurons in the nuclei coeruleus and subcoeruleus, as well as in the area of the lateral reticular nucleus, distribute fibers mainly ipsilaterally throughout the spinal cord (Fig. 7), and that many of these neurons are monoaminergic (615). According to retrograde HRP transport findings (698) combined with large spinal lesions (382) and in accordance with anterograde amino acid transport findings (56? the descending fibers from nuclei coeruleus and subcoeruleus are concentrated at C_6–C_7 in the ventrolateral funiculus, although some are also present in the dorsolateral and the ventral funiculi (294, 451). Correspondingly, lesions in the area of the nucleus coeruleus and subcoeruleus result in a loss of catecholaminergic fluorescent fibers from the ventral and ventrolateral funiculi and also result in a loss of fluorescent catecholaminergic fibers and terminals from the intermediate zone and the motoneuronal cell groups of the ventral horn (lamina V to lamina XI) (125, 527). After such lesions, however, there remain catecholaminergic fibers in the dorsolateral funiculus and catecholaminergic terminals in the autonomic intermediolateral and -medial cell groups as well as in the dorsal horn. This condition suggests that fibers from the nuclei coeruleus and subcoeruleus are distributed mainly to the spinal intermediate zone and motoneuronal cell groups (Fig. 10), as has been confirmed recently by anterograde transport findings (294, 451). Such findings also suggest that the catecholaminergic neurons in the area of the lateral reticular nucleus (group A_1 in ref. 145) and their descending fibers to the spinal cord (146) probably represent the main source of catecholaminergic fibers, which are distributed from the brain stem through the dorsolateral funiculus to the dorsal horn and especially to the autonomic intermediolateral nucleus [Fig. 10; (527)]. This conclusion has been confirmed recently by anterograde amino acid transport findings (413). Such findings (415) also showed that the nucleus tegmentalis laterodorsalis, which is located next to the locus coeruleus in the pontine central gray, distributes descending fibers (614) through the spinal lateral funiculus to the intermediolateral nucleus in the sacral cord (Fig. 10). These various descending connections to the preganglionic intermediolateral nucleus have only recently been clarified, because they could not be demonstrated convincingly by means of the classic anterograde degeneration technique (522). This is in keeping with the impression that many of the monoaminergic fibers escape detection when silver degeneration techniques are used.

Serotonergic raphe neurons. Cajal (97) observed in Golgi material that fibers from the raphe nuclei in the lower brain stem proceed to the ventral aspect of the medulla oblongata. Retrograde degeneration findings (76) have indicated that these fibers descend into the spinal cord (Fig. 7), and more recent retrograde HRP transport findings (381) show that they are distributed as far caudally as the lumbar and sacral segments. Retrograde HRP findings combined with large spinal lesions (382) as well as anterograde amino acid transport findings (451) and antidromic electrical stimulation findings (759) show that raphe spinal fibers descend through both the lateral and ventral funiculi.

According to anterograde amino acid transport findings (33) fibers from the rostrally located nucleus raphe magnus are distributed in the brain stem to the solitary nucleus and the dorsal motor nucleus of the vagus as well as to the marginal and gelatinous parts of the subnucleus caudalis of the spinal V complex. In the spinal cord many of the fibers from the nucleus raphe magnus descend through the dorsolateral funiculus, as shown also by retrograde HRP transport findings (34, 401, 455, 698), and are distributed to laminae I, II, and V, to the medial parts of lamina VI, and to parts of lamina VII (Fig. 9). This distribution pattern resembles that of the fibers from the ventral mesencephalic central gray, including midline neurons in the area of the Edinger-Westphal nucleus (414), which also distribute fibers through the dorsolateral funiculus.

In this respect it is important to note that electrical stimulation of the area of the nucleus raphe magnus and the rostrally adjoining raphe region produces an analgesic effect (529) that might be transmitted by upper medullary raphe spinal fibers. This analgesic effect may reflect the inhibition of dorsal horn neurons responsive to noxious stimuli; the inhibition is produced by electrical stimulation of the nucleus raphe magnus and the rostrally adjoining raphe region (37, 192, 247, 761). This relationship is also suggested because the inhibition of dorsal horn neurons and the analgesic effect produced by the raphe stimulation are both abolished by dorsolateral funicular transection (32). In this connection it is important to recall that earlier electrical stimulation findings (291) demonstrated a reticulospinal pathway in the dorsolateral funiculus, which exerts an inhibitory control over interneurons in the spinal flexion reflex arc and originates from neurons in the ventral portion of the rostral medullary medial tegmental field. This pathway, which possesses a conduction velocity of at least 20 m/s (179), probably originates in the serotonergic raphe nuclei, the fibers of which possess a conduction velocity that ranges from 6 m/s to 67 m/s (759). Nevertheless, the serotonergic raphe neurons apparently cannot be solely responsible for this control (179).

The raphe nuclei not only project to the spinal dorsal horn but also distribute many fibers to the autonomic lateral horn and the somatic motoneuronal cell groups of the ventral horn (Fig. 10). This conclusion is based on the following observations: *1*) Histofluorescence findings have showed (145, 190, 304, 561) that serotonergic neurons in the lower brain stem are concentrated in the raphe nuclei and their immediate vicinity, i.e., around and lateral to the pyramidal tract, and that serotonergic fibers from these neurons descend lateral to the inferior olive as well as through the paramedian fiber bundles into the spinal dorsolateral, ventrolateral, and ventral funiculi (99, 146, 206, 351). *2*) Retrograde HRP transport findings (34, 382, 455, 698) have further demonstrated that fibers from the nucleus raphe magnus descend mainly through the dorsolateral funiculus, while those from the raphe nuclei pallidus and obscurus descend mainly through the ventral and ventrolateral funiculus. *3*) The serotonergic raphespinal fibers distribute terminals not only to the substantia gelatinosa of the dorsal horn but also to the intermediomedial area around the central canal, and especially to the motoneuronal cell groups of the ventral horn (528) and the autonomic intermediolateral nucleus (Fig. 10) of the thoracic and lumbosacral cord (99, 206). This distribution to autonomic and somatic motoneuronal cell groups of the raphespinal fibers has recently been confirmed by anterograde amino acid transport findings (450, 451), which also showed (33) that raphe neurons also project to the motor nucleus of the vagus.

These novel anatomical findings indicate that the raphe nuclei, apparently together with neurons in the caudal part of the medullary medial tegmental field (294) and with neurons in the area of the nucleus subcoeruleus (294, 451, 527), distribute many brain stem fibers to the somatic motoneuronal cell groups throughout the spinal cord (Fig. 10), connections that escaped detection under use of the classic anterograde silver degeneration technique.

Pathways from dorsal column nuclei to spinal dorsal horn. Retrograde HRP and anterograde amino acid transport findings (91, 141, 381, 490) as well as antidromic electrical stimulation findings (149) indicate the existence of descending fibers from the dorsal column nuclei to the ipsilateral spinal dorsal horn. These fibers appear to be derived mainly from neurons in the rostral part of the nuclei as well as from neurons in the base and the hilus of the caudal two-thirds of the dorsal column nuclei, i.e., at the level of the dorsally located clusters of relay cells (228, 384). This may explain the paucity of retrogradely affected neurons in these areas after lemniscal transection (384). The fibers from these neurons in the dorsal column nuclei descend mainly through the dorsal funiculus and only to a limited extent through the dorsolateral funiculus (91, 149). In cervical segments these fibers, according to anterograde amino acid transport findings (91), terminate in the lateral cervical nucleus and in the spinal dorsal horn, especially in lamina IV and the medial and the lateral reticulated parts of lamina V. These areas in cat and monkey, according to retrograde HRP transport findings (706, 707), contain spinothalamic neurons. Furthermore, according to retrograde HRP transport findings (91, 490) the fibers to the cervical and lumbosacral segments tend to be derived mainly from the nuclei cuneatus and gracilis, respectively.

Neurons in the above-mentioned areas of the dorsal column nuclei receive many cortical fibers (384, 758) and many ascending spinal fibers (603, 607), the latter of which according to retrograde HRP transport findings (490, 604, 605) are derived mainly from neurons in lamina IV and the medial parts of laminae V and VI of the spinal dorsal horn. Thus descending fibers from the dorsal column nuclei contribute to the interconnections between the dorsal column nuclei and the spinal dorsal horn. Such interconnections probably also exist between the spinal V complex and the principal sensory nucleus V, the ascending components of which have been repeatedly observed in anterograde degeneration and anterograde amino acid transport studies (295, 379, 660).

Descending Cortical Pathways

The descending cortical pathways include the corticospinal and corticobulbar pathways, which pass directly to the lower brain stem and spinal cord, and cortical projections to the cell groups of the descending brain stem pathways, which thus establish indirect cortical connections to the lower brain stem and the spinal cord.

CORTICOSPINAL AND CORTICOBULBAR PATHWAYS. In contrast to the descending brain stem pathways the descending cortical pathways to lower brain stem and spinal cord vary in different animals with respect to both their trajectories and their terminal distribution.

Trajectory of the corticospinal and corticobulbar fibers. In mammals the cortical fibers to the spinal cord are distributed primarily contralaterally. They descend together with other cortical fibers via the internal capsule into the ipsilateral cerebral peduncle. According to anterograde degeneration findings (78, 742), however, some cortical fibers pass via the corpus callosum into the contralateral cerebral peduncle.

Many cortical fibers are distributed from the internal capsule and cerebral peduncle to the diencephalon and mesencephalon and thus establish contacts with cell groups of the descending brain stem pathways in these areas. These projections are discussed in the next subsection. Findings in normal Häggvist material as well as in anterograde degeneration studies further demonstrate that in several ungulates, e.g., goat, horse, cow, pig, and sheep (26, 253, 735) as well as in procavia, elephant, and hedgehog (78), a special bundle of cortical fibers detaches itself from the cerebral peduncle in the mesencephalon (see *Terminal distribution of corticobulbar fibers,* p. 631, and accompanying figure). This bundle, known as Bagley's bundle, has roughly the same fiber composition as the pyramidal tract (734) and descends ipsilaterally through the mesencephalic tegmentum lateral to the red nucleus into the lateral tegmental field of the lower brain stem. In the rostral pons Bagley's bundle is located in the lateral part of pontine tegmentum between the rubrospinal tract and the superior cerebellar peduncle and thus is situated in the same general area as other bundles destined for the bulbar lateral tegmental field, such as fiber bundles from the amygdala, red nucleus, and Edinger-Westphal nucleus. According to anterograde degeneration findings some dispersed cortical fiber bundles in rat (786) and opossum (444) follow the same course as Bagley's bundle.

In the human being and rhesus monkey another set of fiber bundles leaves the medial and intermediate parts of the cerebral peduncle (390) in the mesencephalon and descends through the medial lemniscus, or Pes lemnisci (732), into the lower brain stem, where some fibers rejoin the pyramidal tract (369). These bundles were originally thought to constitute the cortical fibers to the bulbar motor nuclei (151). In monkey, however, they appear to contain mainly cortical fibers from the area rostral to the precentral gyrus to the pontine and medullary medial tegmental field (371).

The bulk of the fibers of the cerebral peduncle continue caudally and terminate in the pontine gray. Many of the fibers in the intermediate portion of the cerebral peduncle, however, emerge at the caudal border of the pons (390) and are distributed to the lower brain stem and the spinal cord. These fibers constitute the pyramidal tract, which in general descends along the ventral surface of the medulla oblongata toward the pyramidal decussation at the caudal end of the brain stem. The corticobulbar and corticospinal fibers, however, do not always follow this standard pyramidal trajectory. Thus in some monotremes, e.g., *Tachyglossus* (echidna), the pyramidal tracts decussate in the pons and descend, fused with the spinal V tract, into the contralateral spinal dorsolateral funiculus (221, 731). In some chiroptera, e.g., bat and flying fox, they decussate immediately caudal to the pons and descend through the area lateral to the inferior olive into the spinal dorsolateral funiculus (78, 731). In other mammals, e.g., hedgehog (78) and procavia (klipdassie) (78, 730), the pyramidal tracts do not decussate but continue uncrossed into the ipsilateral spinal ventral funiculi. This arrangement also occurs in elephant (728), in which, however, some pyramidal fibers do cross at the spinomedullary junction and descend as the intracommissural bundle through the dorsal part of the spinal ventral funiculus. In several ungulates (e.g., horse, tapir, camel, and deer) the pyramidal fibers, after decussating, also descend mainly in the ventral funiculus (731). On the other hand, in marsupials—e.g., kangaroo, quokka, wallaby (752, 753), opossum (36), brush-tailed possum (453)—and in several rodents—e.g., rat (79, 168, 227), coypu rat (222), and capybara (78) as well as in tree shrew (*Tupaia*), an insectivore (319, 640, 729)—the bulk of the pyramidal fibers continue into the ventral part of the dorsal funiculus after a low medullary decussation. In certain other animals—e.g., sloth, an edentate (663); bat, a chiropter (78); rabbit (252)—and in several carnivores—e.g., cat (113, 523), dog, and raccoon (95)—as well as in primates, such as slow loris (319), galago (225), saimiri (265), rhesus monkey (371, 409), chimpanzee, and human being (205, 371, 731, 732), the pyramidal fibers after decussating descend mainly in the contralateral dorsolateral funiculus. In several of the species, however, some fibers also descend both crossed and uncrossed in the ipsilateral and contralateral ventral funiculus, and some uncrossed fibers descend in the ipsilateral dorsolateral funiculus (18, 218, 439). In armadillo, another edentate, however, the contralaterally descending fibers behave in the same way as in the elephant (728) and are mainly grouped into an intracommissural bundle (194, 663) in the most dorsal part of the ventral funiculus (Fig. 11).

In individual species some variations also occur, which are best known in human beings (507, 526). Thus, in human beings the pyramidal decussation may be absent (419, 733), or a ventrolateral pyramidal tract may exist (30) that leaves the corticobulbar and corticospinal tract in the pons and, as in bats, descends lateral to the inferior olive into the ipsilateral spinal ventrolateral funiculus. Frequently a Pick's bundle occurs. This bundle has also been reported in monkey, cat, and mouse (cf. ref. 719) and consists of recurrent pyramidal fibers, which after decussating in the lower medulla oblongata ascend in the bulbar lateral tegmental field. Furthermore, a circumolivary pyramidal bundle may occur (667, 668), a portion of which may descend as a ventrolateral pyramidal tract, while the remainder may terminate in the pontobulbar body. In some cases a bundle of pyramidal fibers may pass from the decussation into the dorsal funiculus (84), a trajectory similar to that found in marsupials and some rodents.

Terminal distribution of corticospinal fibers. Corticospinal fibers in different species differ in the rostrocaudal extent of their spinal terminal distribution (Fig. 11). For example, in the armadillo (194, 663), goat (252), rabbit (252), opossum (449), Tasmanian potoroo (452), brush-tailed possum (453), and tree shrew (319, 640, 729) the corticospinal fibers, according to anterograde degeneration findings, distribute either only to the cervical or to the cervical and thoracic cord (Fig. 11). In another group of mammals, such as primates, carnivores, and some rodents (e.g., rat) the corticospinal fibers, according to anterograde degeneration and anterograde transport findings (113, 168, 281, 371, 409, 523), are distributed throughout the length of the spinal cord. Interestingly enough these two groups of animals also differ with respect to the ratio between body weight and the number of pyramidal fibers (702).

The terminal distribution of the cortical fibers in the spinal gray of the individual segments also differs in various species (Figs. 11, 12). At first glance this difference seems to be related to the funicular trajectory of the cortical fibers, because in many of the animals (e.g., the marsupials, in which they descend in the dorsal funiculus) their densest termination occurs in the spinal dorsal gray. Yet the reverse does not hold, because in procavia or klipdassie (730) the cortical fibers descend without decussating into the ipsilateral ventral funiculus but terminate primarily in the dorsal half of the contralateral spinal gray. The extent of the terminal distribution area of the cortical fibers in the spinal gray of the individual segments seems to be correlated to some degree with the rostrocaudal extent of the distribution of the corticospinal fibers in the spinal cord; in the mammals in which the cortical fibers have a very widespread distribution within the spinal gray of the individual segments, including part of the motoneuronal cell groups, these fibers invariably are distributed throughout the length of the spinal cord, while in those mammals in which the cortical fibers terminate almost exclusively in the dorsal horn and the most dorsal part of the intermediate zone these fibers tend to be distributed only to the cervical and the thoracic segments (Fig. 11).

The various mammals that have been studied tend to fall into four groups that show an increasingly wider terminal distribution area of cortical fibers in the spinal gray matter of the individual segments (Fig. 12).

1. In the first group of mammals, commonly regarded as being primitive, the cortical fibers reach only the cervical and thoracic cord. According to anterograde degeneration findings they terminate mainly in the dorsal part of the contralateral spinal gray, i.e., the dorsal horn (lamina IV and the medial parts of laminae V and VI), and the dorsal part of the intermediate zone, i.e., lateral parts of laminae V and VI, while only very few fibers are distributed to lamina VII (Fig. 12). This group of animals comprises the following: sloth (663), elephant (728), goat (252, 253), rabbit (252), armadillo (194, 663), opossum (449), brush-tailed possum (453, 589), kangaroo (753), and tree shrew [(319, 640); Fig. 11]. Thus in these animals the bulk of the cortical fibers is distributed to the area of the dorsal horn, which contains neurons projecting to supraspinal levels, and to the area in the intermediate zone, which contains mainly short propriospinal neurons projecting mainly ipsilaterally.

2. In the second group of mammals the cortical fibers are distributed throughout the length of the spinal cord (Fig. 11) and according to anterograde degeneration and anterograde amino acid transport findings terminate mainly contralaterally in the dorsal horn as well as in laminae V, VI, and VII of the intermediate zone. Moreover, according to anterograde amino acid transport findings, in the cat (which belongs to this group) the fibers to the medial part of lamina VII (Fig. 12) are distributed bilaterally (195). This group of animals comprises, for example, rat (79, 168), slow loris (98, 319), procavia or klipdassie (730), cat (113, 195, 256, 523), and dog (95).

Anterograde degeneration and amino acid transport findings indicate that in these animals only very few cortical fibers are distributed to either the long propriospinal neurons in lamina VIII or to the motoneuronal cell groups of the ventral horn. This lack of cortical projections to spinal motoneuronal cell groups is supported in cat by orthodromic electrical stimulation findings (47, 410, 423), although similar studies in rat (177) suggest that in this animal corticomotoneuronal connections to forelimb motoneurons exist.

3. In the third group of mammals the terminal distribution of cortical fibers is dense throughout the intermediate zone (Fig. 12), including the area of the long propriospinal neurons in lamina VIII, and frequently on both sides. In some members of this group such as raccoon, however, the projection to lamina VIII occurs mainly at cervical levels (Fig. 11). This group of animals comprises some primates such as saimiri (265, 694), galago (225), rhesus macaque, and

CHAPTER 13: ANATOMY OF DESCENDING PATHWAYS 629

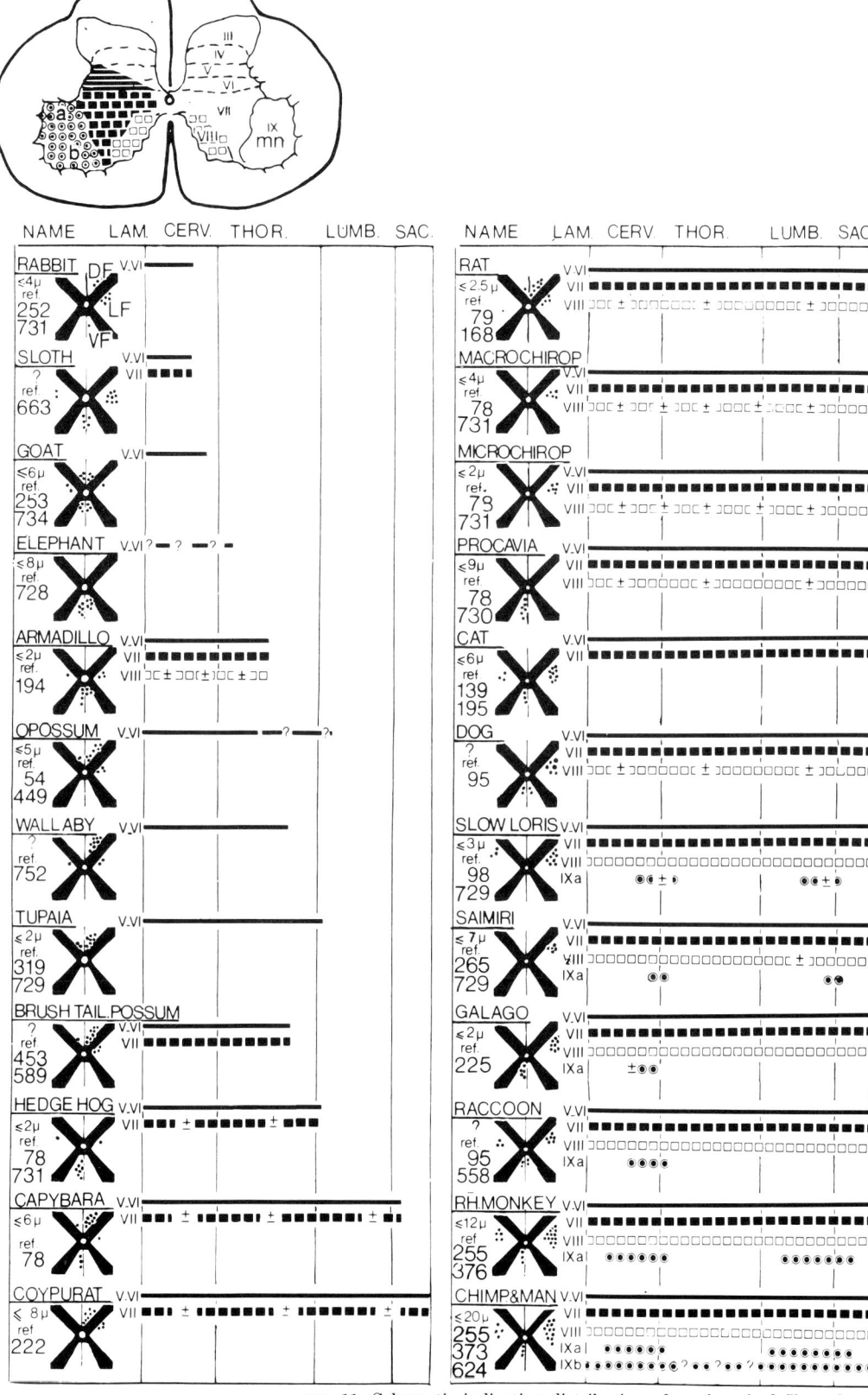

FIG. 11. Schematic indicating distribution of corticospinal fibers from left hemisphere over the various funiculi (DF, dorsal funiculus; LF, lateral funiculus; VF, ventral funiculus) in different mammalian species and distribution of these fibers to laminae V to VIII of intermediate zone and to motoneuronal cell groups in different parts of spinal cord. Notations at *left* for each animal: maximum diameter of pyramidal fibers, then reference number of work on which data are based.

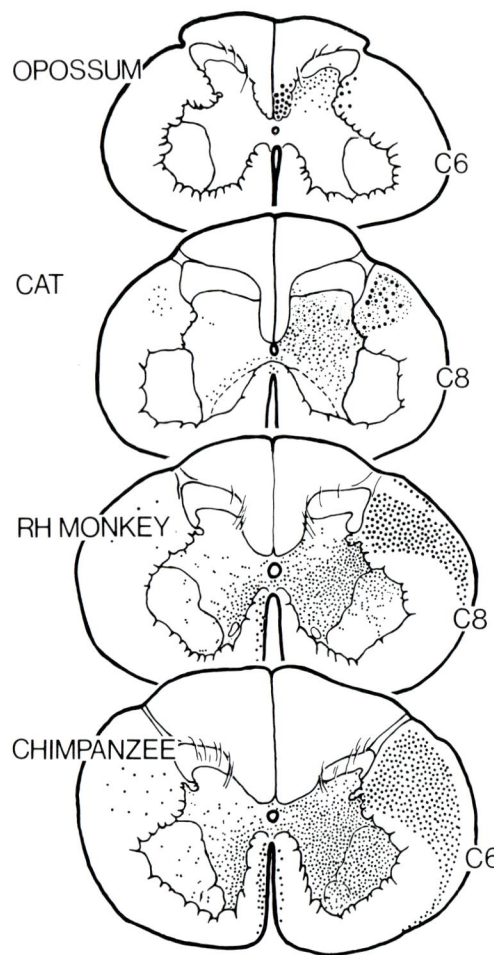

FIG. 12. Distribution of corticospinal fibers from left hemisphere to low cervical spinal gray matter in opossum, cat, rhesus monkey, and chimpanzee. [Drawing based on data of Flindt-Egebak (195), Kuypers and Brinkman (373, 376), and Martin and Fisher (449).]

other monkeys (371, 376, 409), as well as raccoon (95, 558, 769) and kinkajou (555). With respect to the distribution of corticospinal fibers to the intermediate zone in monkey, electrophysiological studies (324) show that corticospinal fibers in this animal establish direct connections with Ia inhibitory interneurons (cf. ref. 307); such connections in cat (310) tend to be disynaptic. This largely fits the difference in the distribution of corticospinal fibers to the intermediate zone in these two species, as observed in anterograde degeneration studies, because after sensory motor cortex lesions in cat relatively few degenerating cortical fibers are distributed to the ventral parts of lamina VII adjoining the motoneuronal cell groups (523) where the Ia inhibitory interneurons are located, while many such fibers are distributed to this area in rhesus monkey (376, 409).

In the animals of this third group, including the raccoon (95, 558, 769) and kinkajou (555), cortical fibers are also distributed contralaterally to motoneurons of distal extremity muscles (Fig. 11). This distribution is very limited in galago (225) and saimiri (265, 694) but is quite pronounced in several other monkeys, including rhesus monkeys [Fig. 12; (371, 376, 409, 555)], in which it has also been demonstrated by means of orthodromic electrical stimulation (23, 47, 191, 559, 571). In spider and woolly monkeys (554) cortical fibers are distributed in addition to motoneurons of tail muscles. According to orthodromic electrical stimulation (47) and anterograde degeneration findings (409) in rhesus monkey a few cortical fibers may also be distributed ipsilaterally to motoneurons of proximal limb muscles.

4. In the fourth group of mammals, which comprises the highest primates such as chimpanzee (373, 554) and human being (624, 625), the distribution of cortical fibers in the intermediate zone follows the same pattern as in the rhesus monkey (Fig. 11). Thus these fibers are distributed mainly contralaterally to the lateral parts of laminae V to VII and to the medial parts of lamina VII and bilaterally to lamina VIII. In chimpanzee (373, 554) and human being (625), however, the cortical fibers to the motoneuronal cell groups are much more abundant than in the rhesus monkey and are distributed in considerable numbers not only to motoneurons of distal extremity muscles but also to motoneurons of girdle and proximal extremity muscles (Figs. 11, 12). It is also of interest to note that in the human being (624), and probably also in chimpanzee (373), relatively few cortical fibers are distributed to the dorsal horn, which suggests that quantitatively the terminal distribution pattern of the cortical fibers in these species may be the reverse of that found in the first group of most primitive animals.

Corticospinal fibers give off collaterals at different spinal levels in the same way as fibers of the descending brain stem pathways. Thus, antidromic electrical stimulation findings (637) show that in cat 15% of cortical fibers to the cervical cord represent collaterals of fibers to levels between T_3 and L_1, and another 15% represent collaterals of fibers to levels below L_1. Corticospinal collateralization in cat therefore seems to be of a magnitude intermediate between that of the rubrospinal fibers (638), which project mainly to short propriospinal neurons, and that of the reticulospinal fibers (549), which project characteristically to long propriospinal neurons. In view of this relationship the corticospinal collaterals might be derived mainly from fibers projecting to relatively long propriospinal neurons, e.g., in the medial parts of lamina VII, rather than from fibers to short propriospinal neurons in the dorsal part of the intermediate zone. With respect to the branching of corticospinal fibers, electrophysiological data indicate that cortical fibers to the motoneuronal cell groups in monkey frequently give rise to branches to the dorsally and medially adjoining part of the intermediate zone (23), in keeping with anterograde degeneration findings after small precentral lesions [Fig. 17; (376)]. Electrophysiological studies also indicate that the cortical fibers to motoneuronal cell groups branch less to other segments than do other corticospinal fibers (639). Furthermore, recent electrophysiological findings suggest that corticomotoneuronal fibers, which are mainly distributed to α-motoneurons (120), may establish synaptic contacts with motoneurons (Fig. 13) of more than one anatomical muscle (23). In this respect it has to be kept in mind that an anatomical muscle may not represent a functional unit with respect to movements.

The influence exerted by the corticospinal fibers on motoneurons of cat hindlimb muscles results in inhibition of extensor and facilitation of flexor motoneurons (423). Roughly the same pattern occurs in cat forelimb muscles (570), except that among motoneurons of more distal forelimb muscles (cf. ref. 129) the contrast between facilitation of flexor and inhibition of extensor motoneurons is less pronounced than in the hindlimb, and that motoneurons of all muscles intrinsic to the hand are facilitated. In higher primates (e.g., baboon) the inhibition of extensor and facilitation of flexor motoneurons is even less pronounced and tends to be largely restricted to proximal muscles. More distally in the higher primate forelimb this difference may not occur, since motoneurons of elbow flexors are actually inhibited instead of facilitated, and motoneurons of all muscles around the wrist are facilitated (570).

Fiber diameter of the pyramidal tract. The pyramidal tract in the caudal medulla oblongata consists mainly of corticospinal fibers. At this level it contains in all mammals primarily fibers of small diameter (axon plus myelin sheath). Even in human being approximately 80% of the 0.5–1.0 million fibers (cf. refs. 392, 394) measure less than 2 μm in diameter, and approximately 90% range from 1 to 4 μm (732). Generally in the species in which the corticospinal fibers are distributed throughout the length of the spinal cord, e.g., primates and carnivores, the maximal fiber diameter tends to be larger than in species in which the corticospinal fibers descend only into the cervical and thoracic segments (Fig. 11), e.g., armadillo and tupaia (tree shrew). Yet the size of the animal presumably also must be considered, since in elephant, in which corticospinal fibers only reach upper thoracic segments, the maximum fiber diameter is apparently 8 μm (728), whereas in rat (79, 170) and loris (729), in which the cortical fibers descend throughout the length of the spinal cord (98), the fiber diameter ranges up to 3 μm. In higher primates such as rhesus monkey the maximum fiber diameter is approximately 12 μm (255), while in chimpanzee and human being according to the same study it may range up to approximately 20 μm (255, 732). Thick fibers therefore seem to occur especially in species that possess many direct corticomotoneuronal connections. Correspondingly, according to orthodromic electrical stimulation findings (47, 48), direct corticomotoneuronal connections in monkey are established by the fastest conducting corticospinal fibers, or 70 m/s. (For further data see refs. 396, 732.)

Postnatal development of corticospinal connections. Anterograde degeneration findings in rhesus monkey (372), dog (95), and rat (168) indicate that the full complement of corticospinal connections has not been established at birth. In newborn animals of these species only a limited number of cortical fibers is distributed from the funiculi into the gray matter, and these fibers are mainly distributed to the dorsal half of the intermediate zone (95, 168). Moreover, in newborn rhesus monkey (372) virtually no cortical fibers are distributed to the motoneuronal cell groups (Fig. 14), a finding in keeping with orthodromic electrical stimulation studies (188). According to anterograde degeneration studies (95, 168, 372) the full complement of corticospinal connections in rhesus monkey appears to be established at the age of approximately 8 months, in dog at an age of more than 3 months, and in rat at the age of 14–21 days. The increasingly wider distribution of cortical fibers in the spinal gray matter with increasing age probably represents a true outgrowth of cortical fibers and does not merely reflect an increased argentophilia of the degenerating fibers with increasing age (372). This conclusion may be reached because in rat virtually the same developmental findings have been obtained by means of the anterograde degeneration as by means of the anterograde amino acid transport technique (168).

During postnatal development of corticospinal connections in dog a gradual increase in the maximum conduction velocity of cortical fibers occurs (346). This probably reflects a postnatal increase in diameter of cortical fibers, as has been observed in the human being (393, 726) and in rat (50). In this respect it is of interest to note that direct corticomotoneuronal connections in monkey, which are established by the fastest pyramidal fibers (47), appear rather late in postnatal development and that the same is true for the very thick fibers in the pyramidal tract (393, 726).

Terminal distribution of corticobulbar fibers. The trigeminal sensory nuclei and the lateral tegmental field of the lower brain stem represent the bulbar homologues of the spinal dorsal horn and the lateral parts of the spinal intermediate zone (lateral parts of laminae V and VI and lamina VII). The neurons in the lateral parts of the lateral tegmental field distribute their fibers mainly ipsilaterally, except for some in the caudal pons, which distribute their fibers bilaterally (see ANATOMY OF ... BRAIN STEM, p. 601). In light of this homology it is important to emphasize that according to anterograde degeneration findings in tree shrew (640), rat (699), opossum and brush-tailed possum (443, 454), rabbit (252), goat (252, 253), cat (75, 368, 677), monkey (370), and human being (369, 625), corticobulbar fibers (Fig. 15) in virtually all these

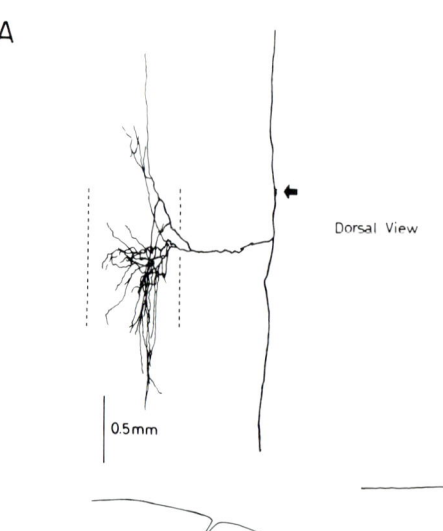

FIG. 13. *A*: Reconstruction of an axon collateral of corticospinal neuron at C_3 and C_4 in cat. Wide rostrocaudal extension of a single axon collateral is characteristic of corticospinal branches. *Broken lines* and *dashed* and *dotted line* show borders of gray matter at level of entry of the collateral into it and level of the central canal, respectively. *Arrow* indicates injection site of HRP. [Adapted from Futami et al. (205a).] *B*: Transverse reconstruction of a corticospinal axon originating from monkey motor cortex. Ulnar nerve motoneurons (*upper two* motor nuclei) and radial nerve motoneurons (*lower two* motor nuclei) labeled by method of retrograde transport of HRP. This axon branch projects to different motoneuron groups, and close contacts of terminal boutons with proximal dendrites of some of HRP-labeled motoneurons (presumably functional synapses) could be identified in these motor nuclei with light microscope. [From Shinoda et al. (639a).]

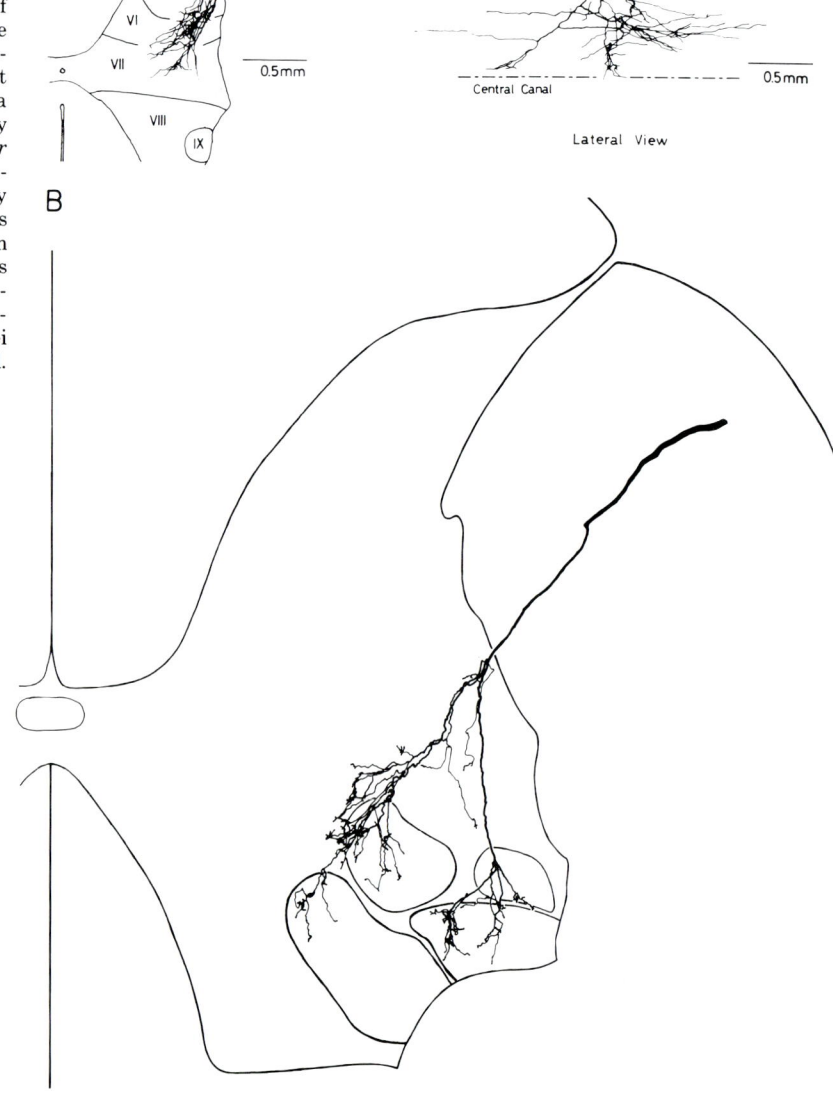

CHAPTER 13: ANATOMY OF DESCENDING PATHWAYS 633

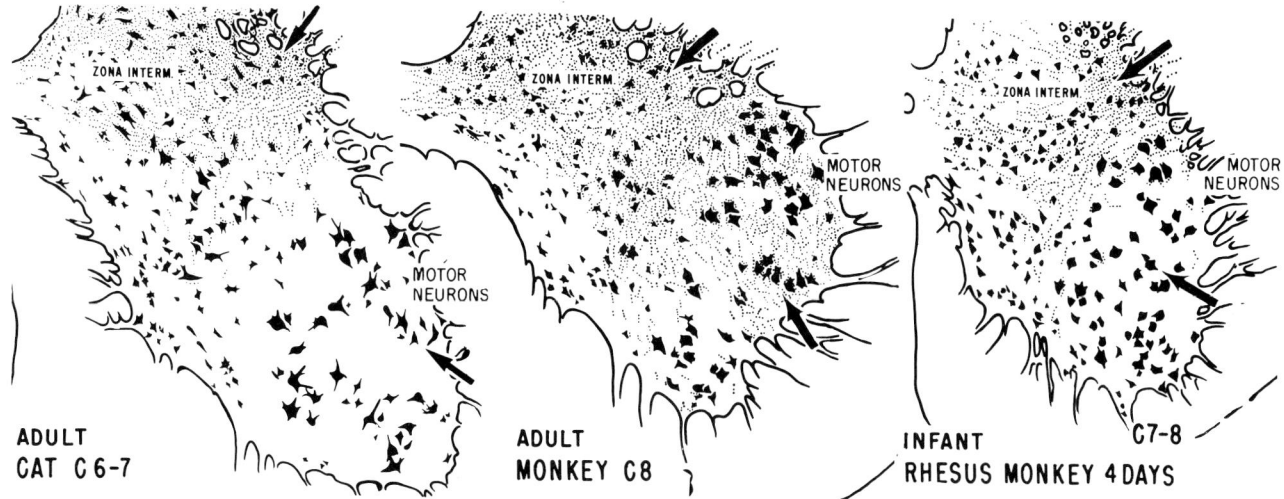

FIG. 14. Distribution of corticospinal fibers in low cervical intermediate zone and motoneuronal cell groups in cat, adult monkey, and 4-day-old monkey as observed in silver-impregnated anterograde fiber degeneration studies. [Adapted from Kuypers (372), copyright 1962 by the American Association for the Advancement of Science.]

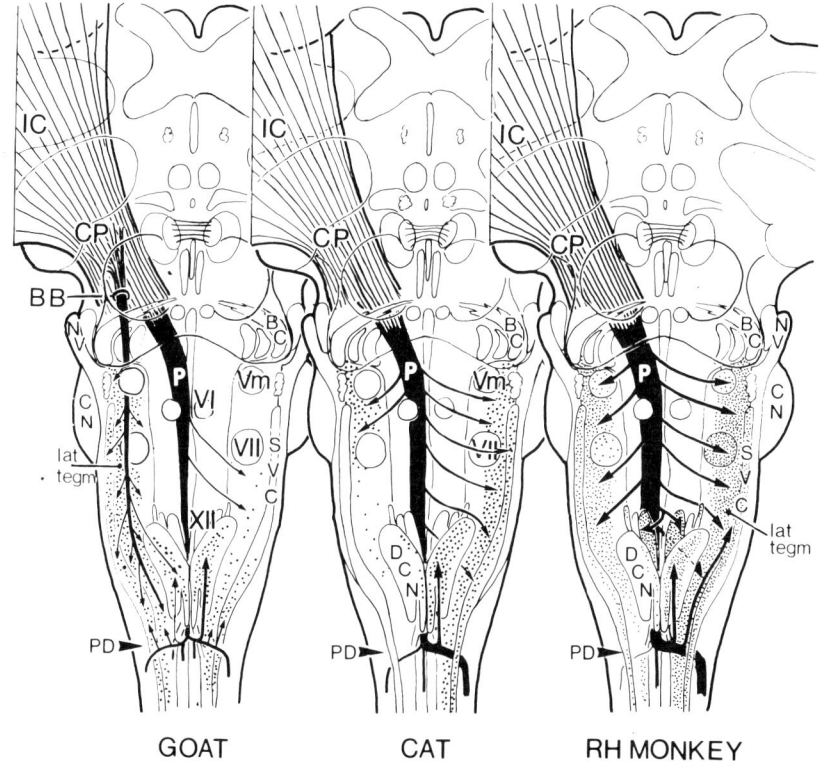

FIG. 15. Trajectory and terminal distribution of cortical fibers from left hemisphere to the various bulbar cell groups in goat, cat, and rhesus monkey. Note presence in goat of Bagley's bundle (BB), which distributes fibers mainly to ipsilateral lateral tegmental field. Note also absence of corticobulbar projections to bulbar Vm, motor nucleus VII, and motor nucleus XII in goat and cat, and presence of such connections in rhesus monkey. IC, internal capsule; CP, cerebral peduncle; BB, Bagley's bundle; P, pyramidal tract; BC, brachium conjunctivum; CN, cochlear nuclei; DCN, dorsal column nuclei; lat tegm, bulbar lateral tegmental field; SVC, spinal trigeminal complex; PD, pyramidal decussation.

species are distributed to the bulbar somatosensory nuclei (i.e., the spinal trigeminal complex, the area of the trigeminal main sensory nucleus, and the rostral part of the solitary nucleus) mainly contralaterally and to the lateral tegmental field to some extent bilaterally. In many of these species, except rhesus monkey, chimpanzee, and human being, the corticobulbar fibers to the bulbar lateral tegmental field seem to be distributed mainly to its lateral part. Moreover, except in the goat (252, 253), they are distributed bilaterally to the lateral part of the lateral tegmental field in the caudal pons and rostral medulla oblongata, but mainly contralaterally in the caudal medulla oblongata. This seems to fit the projections of the neurons in these areas (Fig. 6), since those in the lateral part of the lateral tegmental field in caudal pons and rostral medulla oblongata project to motor nucleus V bilaterally, while those in the lateral part of the lateral tegmental field in the caudal medulla project to the facial nucleus mainly ipsilaterally (see ANATOMY OF . . . BRAIN STEM, p. 601).

A major portion of cortical fibers to the lateral tegmental field descend through the pyramidal tract and reach their termination area by passing through the lower brain stem tegmentum, though some fibers may reach it by way of a recurrent trajectory (368). In the ungulate (e.g., goat), in which a large Bagley's bundle exists, however, corticobulbar fibers to the trigeminal sensory nuclei and lateral tegmental field arise mainly from this bundle (Fig. 15) and strikingly enough terminate mainly ipsilaterally in the lower brain stem (252).

In higher primates, e.g., rhesus monkey, chimpanzee, and human being, the corticobulbar fibers show a different distribution pattern from that in the above animals. Thus, according to anterograde degeneration findings (369, 370, 625), corticobulbar fibers from each hemisphere in monkey, chimpanzee, and human being are distributed bilaterally to the lateral tegmental field in both pons and medulla oblongata. Moreover in rhesus monkey the impression is gained that the cortical fibers are distributed to both the lateral and medial parts of the lateral tegmental field (H. G. J. M. Kuypers, unpublished observations). Furthermore, in these species, and especially in chimpanzee and human being, many corticobulbar fibers, like the corticospinal ones, are also distributed to the bulbar motor nuclei—predominantly contralaterally to the facial nucleus, but bilaterally to the trigeminal and hypoglossal nuclei (Fig. 15).

In this respect it is important to emphasize that according to anterograde degeneration findings (380, 625) in rhesus monkey and human being no direct cortical fibers are distributed to eye muscle nuclei.[1] Cortical influences on eye muscle motoneurons therefore appear to be exerted only by way of interneurons. This may be related to the fact that eye movements, in contrast to individual movements of the distal phalanges of the digits, for example, always involve conjugated movements of the two eyes.

One final comment should be made with respect to the anatomy of direct corticomotoneuronal connections. The transversely oriented dendrites of motoneurons in the brain stem as well as in the spinal cord extend from the motor nuclei into the surrounding structures. Thus the radially oriented dendrites of the hypoglossal motoneurons (Fig. 15) penetrate deeply into the lateral tegmental field (97), where many cortical fibers terminate. The same arrangement exists in the spinal cord (652)—for example, with respect to motoneurons of the small foot muscles, which distribute a group of dendrites dorsomedially into the lateral part of laminae V to VII (H. G. J. M. Kuypers, unpublished observations). Many cortical fibers terminate in this area also. As a consequence, even when cortical fibers are not distributed into motoneuronal cell groups they may still establish synaptic contacts with distal motoneuronal dendrites. In species in which such contacts would occur the corticomotoneuronal relationship would anatomically be only quantitatively different from that in monkey, chimpanzee, and human being in the sense that in these primates the synaptic contacts of the cortical fibers are not restricted to distal motoneuronal dendrites but also comprise increasing numbers of synaptic contacts with motoneuronal somata and proximal dendrites. However, such quantitative differences may in actuality still represent qualitative ones, since presumably the power of control exerted over the motoneurons by distal dendrite terminals is considerably less than that exerted by somatic terminals.

Areal origin of corticospinal and corticobulbar fibers. Retrograde degeneration findings after high cervical hemisections (290) in cat, dog, macaque, chimpanzee, and human being suggested that corticospinal fibers are derived exclusively from the large Betz cells of precentral area 4. It was shown subsequently, however, that the number of pyramidal tract fibers is approximately 30 times as large as that of the Betz cells (394). Even though the pyramidal tract at various levels in the medulla oblongata contains corticobulbar as well as corticospinal fibers, it seems most unlikely that the additional corticobulbar fibers could account for the enormous discrepancy between the number of Betz cells and the number of fibers in the pyramidal tract. It was therefore concluded (394-396) that a large portion of the corticospinal fibers is derived from neurons other than Betz cells. This is supported by antidromic electrical stimulation findings in rabbit, cat, and rhesus monkey (387, 777), which indicate that the pyramidal tract fibers (Fig. 16) are derived from a large cortical territory comprising not only area 4 but also area 6, especially its caudal part as well as the postcentral and parietal areas, including the secondary sensory cortex in the parietal operculum. This is in keeping with the changes in the fiber content of the pyramidal tract, which occur after ablation of different cortical areas in cat (139) and rhesus monkey (602). These findings indicate that in these species 60% of the pyramidal fibers including the largest ones (138, 395) are derived from area 4 and the rostrally adjoining area 6, while roughly 40% are derived from the postcentral and parietal areas, which contribute mainly thin fibers. In the human being, however, areas 4 and 6 seem to contribute 80% of the pyramidal tract fibers

---

[1] Recent anterograde horseradish peroxidase transport findings suggest that direct cortical connections to the oculomotor nuclei do exist (G. R. Leichnitz, *Brain Res.* 198: 440-445, 1980.)

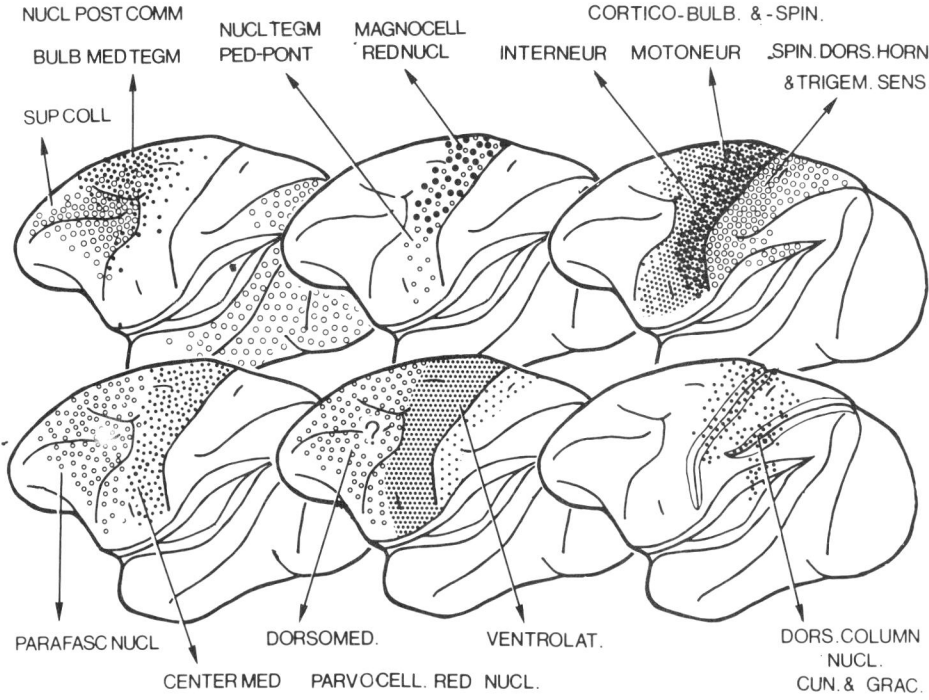

FIG. 16. Origin of cortical projections to different cell groups in brain stem and spinal cord in monkey. Note that cortical projections to superior colliculus, nucleus of posterior commissure, bulbar medial tegmental field, parafascicular nucleus, and dorsomedial part of parvocellular red nucleus (*left* and *middle* diagrams, *both rows*) are derived mainly from frontal areas rostral to precentral gyrus. Note that projections to magnocellular red nucleus, nucleus tegmenti pedunculopontinus, center median, and ventrolateral part of parvocellular red nucleus (*middle* diagram, *upper row*; *left* and *middle* diagrams, *lower row*) are primarily derived from precentral gyrus. Note also that cortical projections to bulbar lateral tegmental field and spinal intermediate zone (*upper row, right*) are derived from precentral gyrus and rostrally adjoining areas, whereas those of bulbar and spinal motoneuronal cell groups are mainly derived from caudal part of precentral gyrus. Note further that cortical projections to spinal V complex, spinal dorsal horn, and dorsal column nuclei (*left, both rows*) are derived mainly from postcentral and parietal areas and secondary sensory cortex but that projections to dorsal column nuclei are also derived from caudal part of precentral gyrus.

(320). This may be related to the relatively sparse distribution of corticospinal fibers, from the postcentral gyrus to the spinal dorsal horn in the human being (624).

The above-mentioned stimulation and anterograde degeneration findings are supported by recent retrograde HRP transport findings (107, 130) that show that corticospinal fibers in monkey are derived from the upper two-thirds of the pericentral cortex on the lateral convexity of the hemisphere, i.e., precentrally from area 4 and the caudal part of area 6 and postcentrally from areas 3a, 3b, 2, 1, and the rostral part of area 5, as well as from these same areas on the medial surface of the hemisphere, including the upper bank of the cingulate sulcus (Fig. 16). In rhesus monkey, therefore, the precentral corticospinal area largely coincides with the motor cortex as defined by electrical stimulation (779). The retrograde HRP transport findings further show that a limited number of corticospinal fibers are also derived from the supplementary motor cortex (779) from the area of the secondary somatic sensory cortex in the parietal operculum (497) and from the supplementary sensory area (306) on the medial surface of the hemisphere around the caudal end of the cingulate sulcus. Retrograde HRP transport findings (D. A. Hopkins, C. E. Catsman-Berrevoets, and H. G. J. M. Kuypers, unpublished observations) after injections in the bulbar lateral tegmental field support anterograde degeneration findings (371) and indicate that corticobulbar fibers to the trigeminal nuclei and the bulbar lateral tegmental field in rhesus monkey are mainly derived from the pericentral areas along the lower one-third of the central sulcus. An areal distribution of retrograde HRP-labeled corticospinal neurons, comparable to that observed in rhesus monkey (107), has been reported in cat (17, 51, 246) and rat (282). According to retrograde HRP transport findings, in cat (17, 51, 246) virtually no corticospinal neurons are present in area 6 (271), whereas in both monkey (107) and human being (484) this area contributes some fibers to the corticospinal pathway.[2]

Differences in spinal and bulbar distribution of precentral and postcentral cortical fibers. Anterograde degeneration findings (371, 409) indicate that in

---

[2] Recent findings obtained by means of fluorescent retrograde tracer (C. E. Catsman-Berrevoets and H. G. J. M. Kuypers, unpublished observations) indicate that in cat also corticospinal fibers are derived from area 6.

rhesus monkey the relatively thin fibers from the upper and middle one-third of the postcentral gyrus and the adjoining rostral part of the superior parietal lobule (395), are distributed mainly to the spinal dorsal horn (lamina IV and the medial parts of laminae V and VI) of the lumbosacral and the brachial cord, respectively (Fig. 16). The fibers from the lower one-third of the postcentral gyrus and the rostral parts of the inferior parietal lobule are distributed to the spinal V complex and the area of the main sensory trigeminal nucleus (371). Anterograde degeneration findings in cat (113) suggest that fibers from the secondary sensory cortex in the parietal operculum terminate also in the spinal dorsal horn.

Anterograde degeneration findings (371, 376, 409) further indicate that in rhesus monkey fibers from the precentral corticospinal area are distributed in a topographically organized fashion to the spinal intermediate zone and the bulbar lateral tegmental field and to motoneuronal cell groups. Thus the upper and middle third of the precentral gyrus project to intermediate zone and motoneuronal cell groups in the lumbosacral and the brachial cord, respectively, while the lower one-third of the precentral gyrus projects to the bulbar lateral tegmental field and motor nuclei (370, 371, 376, 380). These findings are supported by anterograde amino acid transport findings (131), which show that the postcentral corticospinal projections to the spinal dorsal horn in the monkey are derived from areas 3b, 1, 2, and 5 (Fig. 16) and that the projections from the caudal part of the precentral gyrus to the intermediate zone are derived from area 4 as well as from area 3a. According to these findings, however, projections to the motoneuronal cell groups, are derived mainly from area 3a. This is at variance with anterograde degeneration findings (371, 376) and antidromic as well as orthodromic electrical stimulation findings (23, 324), which indicate that the fibers to the motoneurons mainly come from area 4 (Fig. 16).

This differential distribution of precentral and postcentral cortical fibers in the spinal cord and the lower brain stem, observed first in the rhesus monkey (370, 371), seems to represent a general organizational principle, since it has also been found in several other species, e.g., cat (523), saimiri (265), galago (225), armadillo (194), and brush-tailed possum (443).

Anterograde degeneration studies (371, 376) indicate that the precentral corticobulbar and corticospinal projections to the motoneuronal cell groups, as well as those to the interneuronal areas of the intermediate zone in monkey and chimpanzee, also display a spatial organization. Thus cortical fibers to the bulbar, brachial, and lumbosacral motoneuronal cell groups are derived exclusively from the caudal parts of the lower, middle, and upper thirds of the precentral gyrus, respectively, the latter including the corresponding cortex on the medial surface of the hemisphere (Fig. 16). This is in keeping with several orthodromic electrical stimulation studies (47, 48, 324, 388, 559). Anterograde degeneration findings in monkey and chimpanzee (370) also indicate the existence of a further differentiation such that in the lower one-third of the precentral gyrus the cortical fibers to, for example, the hypoglossal and the facial nuclei, respectively, are largely derived from different areas.

The projections to the intermediate zone of the lumbosacral and brachial cord and to the bulbar lateral tegmental field in the rhesus monkey are derived from a wider cortical area than those to the motor nuclei (Fig. 16). This area comprises both the caudal and rostral parts of the precentral gyrus as well as the caudal part of area 6 above and below the arcuate sulcus (cf. anterograde amino acid transport findings in ref. 364). Anterograde degeneration findings (370) further indicate that in the lower one-third of the precentral gyrus of the chimpanzee the cortex along the central sulcus distributes fibers only to motoneuronal cell groups and virtually none to the interneuronal lateral tegmental field.

Anterograde degeneration findings (376) show that the precentral projections to the spinal intermediate zone in rhesus monkey are also spatially organized. Thus small lesions in the hand and foot representation areas (779), respectively, result in the distribution of degenerating fibers to the contralateral brachial and lumbosacral motoneuronal cell groups and to the adjoining dorsal and lateral parts of the intermediate zone (Fig. 17)—i.e., to those areas that contain mainly short and intermediate propriospinal neurons (490). A different distribution occurs, however, after lesions of the rostral bank of the central sulcus at the level of the superior precentral dimple, i.e., between the hand and the foot representation areas (Fig. 17). After lesions in this area, which carries representation of proximal limb and trunk movements (779), degenerating fibers are distributed not only to the lateral but also to the ventromedial parts of the intermediate zone containing long propriospinal neurons (lamina VIII), while relatively few fibers are distributed to motoneuronal cell groups (Fig. 17). A similar distribution pattern occurs after lesions that involve the rostral part of area 4 and the caudal part of area 6. As a consequence in rhesus monkey the cortical areas carrying primarily representations of axial and proximal limb movements (779) give rise to relatively few fibers to motoneuronal cell groups and characteristically project to those parts of the intermediate zone that contain long propriospinal neurons. In contrast, areas that carry primarily representation of distal extremity movements project to motoneuronal cell groups of distal extremity muscles and to those portions of the intermediate zone that mainly contain short and intermediate propriospinal neurons.

Corticospinal fibers in cat (637) and monkey (639) show some branching. Since the brain stem pathways to long propriospinal neurons show a higher degree of branching than those to short propriospinal neurons (see *Descending Brain Stem Pathways*, p. 612) it may

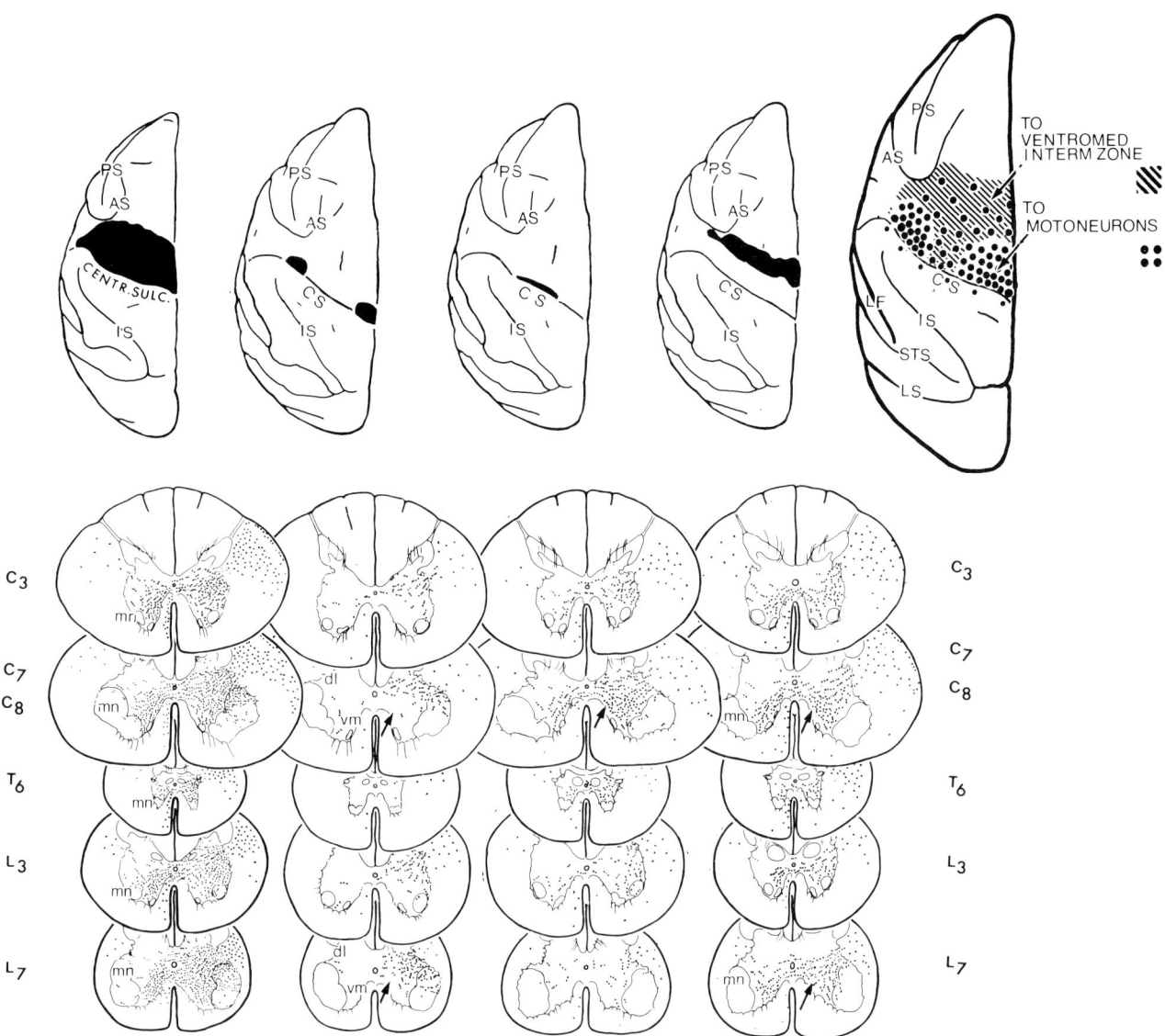

FIG. 17. Distribution of degenerating precentral corticospinal fibers to the different parts of spinal intermediate zone and motoneuronal cell groups in monkey after lesions in different parts of precentral corticospinal area. Note that after lesions of hand and foot representation areas the degenerating fibers are mainly distributed to dorsal and lateral parts, dl, of contralateral intermediate zone and to motoneuronal cell groups, mn, of distal extremity muscles. Note also that degenerating fibers, which are distributed bilaterally to ventromedial part, vm, of intermediate zone are most numerous after lesions along central sulcus between hand and foot representation areas and after lesions of anterior part of corticospinal area, in which cases only a few degenerating fibers are distributed to motoneuronal cell groups. *Upper right*: differential origin of projections to ventromedial part of intermediate zone and motoneuronal cell groups. [Adapted from Kuypers and Brinkman (376).]

be expected that precentral areas that characteristically project to long propriospinal neurons will also provide the bulk of the cortical fibers that distribute collateral branches to both the cervical and the lumbosacral segments. In view of the greater number of corticospinal fibers to long propriospinal neurons in monkey than in cat, the corticospinal tract in monkey therefore may turn out to contain a greater percentage of such branching fibers than in cat.

The organization of corticospinal and corticobulbar projections in cat (113, 195, 368, 523) differs in some respects from that in rhesus monkey, because in cat no fibers are distributed to bulbar and spinal motoneuronal cell groups. Moreover, according to antidromic stimulation (19) and retrograde HRP transport findings in cat (17, 51, 246), area 6 in the gyrus proreus, which as in monkey carries part of the representation of axial movements (514), does not project to the spinal cord.[3] This latter arrangement is not unusual, because the hindlimb representation in rabbit (776) and brush-tailed possum (300), according to anterograde degeneration findings, however, also does not project to the lumbosacral cord (252, 453, 589). In other respects, however, the corticospinal organization in cat resembles that in the rhesus monkey. This is especially suggested by retrograde HRP transport findings obtained after large spinal lesions (18). These findings show that the anterior as well as the middle portion of the feline motor cortex between the hand and foot representation areas characteristically distribute fibers bilaterally through the ventral funiculus; these portions carry representations of proximal arm movements and trunk movements just as in monkey (514). In view of their funicular position these fibers might terminate preferentially in the ventromedial parts of lamina VII (cf. ref. 195); this would render the arrangement in cat similar to that in monkey (Fig. 17).

CORTICAL PROJECTIONS TO CELL GROUPS OF DESCENDING BRAIN STEM PATHWAYS. *General organization.* Results of anterograde degeneration (380) and amino acid transport studies (267) indicate that the cerebral cortex in rhesus monkey also distributes many fibers to the brain stem by way of the cerebral peduncle and the pyramidal tract. When these projections are viewed in a temporal-occipital-parietal-frontal sequence, their target areas in the brain stem tend to shift from dorsal to ventral and medial. Thus the temporal and in particular the occipital areas project to superficial layers of the superior colliculus and to auditory cell groups, e.g., inferior colliculus, or medial geniculate body. The parietal and postcentral areas, in combination with the precentral gyrus, project to the area of the dorsolateral mesencephalic tegmentum immediately ventral to the superior colliculus, an area that includes the anterior pretectal nucleus (Fig. 18). This area also receives many cerebellar (187) and somatosensory afferents (44, 380, 384). The parietal and postcentral areas in combination with the precentral gyrus also project to trigeminal sensory nuclei and to the dorsal column nuclei (Fig. 16). The precentral gyrus, together with the frontal cortex above and below the arcuate sulcus and within its concavity, provides the bulk of the cortical projections to the mesencephalic and lower brain stem tegmentum and the red nucleus (Fig. 16). In addition, areas rostral to the precentral gyrus also project to the superior colliculus, especially to its deep layers (Fig. 16).

The cerebral cortex therefore distributes fibers to several of the cell groups that give rise to descending brain stem pathways, including cell groups that characteristically project to long propriospinal neurons (e.g., the intermediate and deep gray of the superior colliculus and lower brain stem medial tegmental field) as well as to cell groups that characteristically project contralaterally to short propriospinal and propriobulbar neurons (i.e., the magnocellular red nucleus). The bulk of these corticosubcortical projections in rhesus monkey are derived from the frontal cortex.

Frontal projections to superior colliculus. Frontocollicular projections are derived from an area (Fig. 16) that corresponds approximately to the area from which eye movements may be elicited by means of electrical stimulation (738). Thus according to anterograde degeneration findings (24, 380) such projections in rhesus monkey are derived from the area within the concavity of the arcuate sulcus and around the principal sulcus as well as from the area immediately above the upper limb of the arcuate sulcus (Fig. 16). According to anterograde degeneration (380) and amino acid transport findings (267), as well as retrograde HRP transport findings (111), however, only very few frontocollicular fibers are derived from the precentral gyrus.

Anterograde degeneration findings (24, 380) have demonstrated that in rhesus monkey the projections from the arcuate gyrus to the superior colliculus are directed mainly to the deep and intermediate collicular gray layers, through a few fibers spill over into the stratum opticum and a very few into the stratum griseum superficiale (Fig. 18). This termination pattern is followed also by the fibers from the upper bank of the middle one-third of the principal sulcus as demonstrated by anterograde amino acid transport findings (223). This pattern contrasts with that of the occipital fibers; according to anterograde degeneration findings (380, 762) these are distributed mainly to the superficial collicular layers. According to anterograde amino acid transport findings (365, 366), however, this contrast is less pronounced, since according to these findings the fibers from the rostral bank of the arcuate sulcus are distributed not only to the stratum griseum intermedium and stratum griseum opticum, but also to the stratum griseum superficiale, including the most superficially located stratum zonale.

Anterograde degeneration studies have also demonstrated the existence of frontocollicular projections in cat (210), rat (402), rabbit (252), goat (252), opossum (443), and several other animals (78). In rat, cat, and opossum these projections are derived in part from an area rostral to the corticospinal territory. In common with the frontocollicular projection area in rhesus monkey (340) this area also receives specific thalamic afferents mainly from the mediodorsal thalamic nucleus (402, 695). The frontal cortex in cat also projects to the superior colliculus as indicated by retrograde HRP transport findings [C. E. Catsman-Berrevoets and H. G. J. M. Kuypers, unpublished observations; (335)]. Anterograde degeneration findings (210), however, suggested that in cat corticocollicular fibers are also derived from sensory motor cortex. The existence of precentral projections to the area of the dorsolateral mesencephalic tegmentum and the anterior pretectal nucleus immediately ventral to the superior colliculus may be responsible for this discrepancy.

[3] See footnote[2], p. 635.

Projections to nucleus of posterior commissure and mesencephalic medial reticular formation. Anterograde silver degeneration findings in rhesus monkey (380) have confirmed earlier anterograde Marchi degeneration findings (357, 403, 479) and indicate that the frontal cortex projects mainly ipsilaterally to the area of the nucleus of the posterior commissure, the reticular formation of the medial mesencephalic tegmentum, and the adjoining lateral parts of the central gray (Fig. 18). These mesencephalic areas all contain neurons that project to the spinal cord (see *Descending Brain Stem Pathways*, p. 612). According to the anterograde degeneration findings (380) and anterograde amino acid transport findings (267, 364) only few cortical fibers are distributed to the interstitial nucleus of Cajal. The above-mentioned cortical projections to the mesencephalon have also been demonstrated by anterograde degeneration findings in cat (546, 677), rat (402, 718), goat (252), rabbit (252), and opossum (444), and also by means of orthodromic electrical stimulation in cat (436).

Cortical projections to the above-mentioned mesencephalic structures in rhesus monkey are derived mainly from the areas rostral to the precentral gyrus (Figs. 16 and 18), i.e., from area 6 and to a limited extent from the cortex of the rostral bank of the arcuate sulcus (area 8) and around the caudal half of the principal sulcus [Fig. 18; (380)]. Detailed anterograde degeneration studies in opossum indicate that these corticomesencephalic projections in this animal are derived from the area giving rise to corticospinal connections but especially from the rostrally adjoining area, which receives mediodorsal thalamic projections (573, 695). This latter area is therefore regarded as comparable to the area rostral to the precentral gyrus in monkey (340). In this respect it is of interest to note that retrograde double-labeling findings (110) indicate that some of the corticomesencephalic fibers that are derived from the intermediate and rostral part of the corticospinal area in actuality represent collaterals of corticospinal neurons. Projections to the reticular formation of the medial mesencephalic tegmentum in monkey, however, are also to some extent derived from the precentral gyrus. Yet, anterograde amino acid transport findings (267) indicate that these projections are especially directed to an area immediately dorsal to the red nucleus, a conclusion that seems to be compatible with the anterograde degeneration findings (380).

Projections to lower brain stem medial tegmental field. Anterograde degeneration findings (370, 371, 380) indicate that the frontal cortex in rhesus monkey projects by way of the pyramidal tract and pes lemnisci to the pontine and medullary medial tegmental field; according to these findings, however, these projections largely avoid the laterally located catecholaminergic nucleus subcoeruleus (Fig. 18). The cortical projections to the pontine and medullary medial tegmental field have also been demonstrated by means of anterograde degeneration in human beings (369, 625), cat (368, 600), opossum (444), goat (252), rabbit (252), rat (718, 786), brush-tailed possum (454), armadillo (264), tree shrew (640), and other animals (78).

The cortical projections to the pontine and medullary medial tegmental field in rhesus monkey and cat, according to anterograde degeneration findings (368, 380) and retrograde HRP transport findings (51, 642), are derived especially from the area rostral to the precentral gyrus, i.e., in monkey from the area above the arcuate sulcus, comprising area 6 and the rostral part of area 4 (Fig. 16). According to anterograde degeneration findings (380) and retrograde HRP transport findings (51, 642), however, some fibers to the medullary medial tegmental field in monkey are also derived from the precentral gyrus. Other anterograde degeneration findings suggest that in cat (600) these corticoreticular fibers are derived from an area that extends far beyond the sensory motor cortex. With respect to the laterality of the corticoreticular projections, anterograde degeneration findings (368) suggest that projections to the pontine medial tegmental field in cat are distributed mainly ipsilaterally, as shown also by electrical stimulation (547), while the projections to the medullary medial tegmental field are distributed bilaterally.

Anterograde degeneration studies (165, 380, 444) further indicate that cortical fibers are distributed not only to the medullary and pontine medial tegmental field but also to the raphe nuclei. The limited cortical projections from the convexity of the hemisphere to the rostral raphe nuclei (nucleus linearis and nucleus centralis superior) originate in monkey mainly from the most rostral part of the frontal lobe (165, 380, 444), whereas according to findings in cat (77) projections to the lower brain stem raphe nuclei are mainly derived from the area of the sensory motor cortex (77).

Corticorubral projections. Anterograde degeneration findings (380, 428) as well as orthodromic and antidromic electrical stimulation findings (308) show that the frontal cortex in the rhesus monkey distributes many fibers to the rostral parvocellular part of the red nucleus, to some degree bilaterally (Fig. 18). Anterograde degeneration (380, 428) and amino acid transport findings (267) further indicate that a relatively limited number of precentral corticorubral fibers are distributed (exclusively ipsilaterally) to the caudal magnocellular part (Fig. 18), which projects contralaterally to the spinal cord and lower brain stem (349, 380, 648). Anterograde degeneration findings have demonstrated similar projections in chimpanzee (383, 555) and human beings (625). In chimpanzee (383) and rhesus monkey (380, 555) the relatively small number of cortical fibers to the magnocellular red nucleus are mainly derived from the upper two-thirds of the precentral gyrus, especially its caudal half, and are topographically distributed. Thus, the upper one-third (the leg representation area) distributes fibers mainly to the ventrolateral part of the magnocellular red nu-

640 HANDBOOK OF PHYSIOLOGY ~ THE NERVOUS SYSTEM II

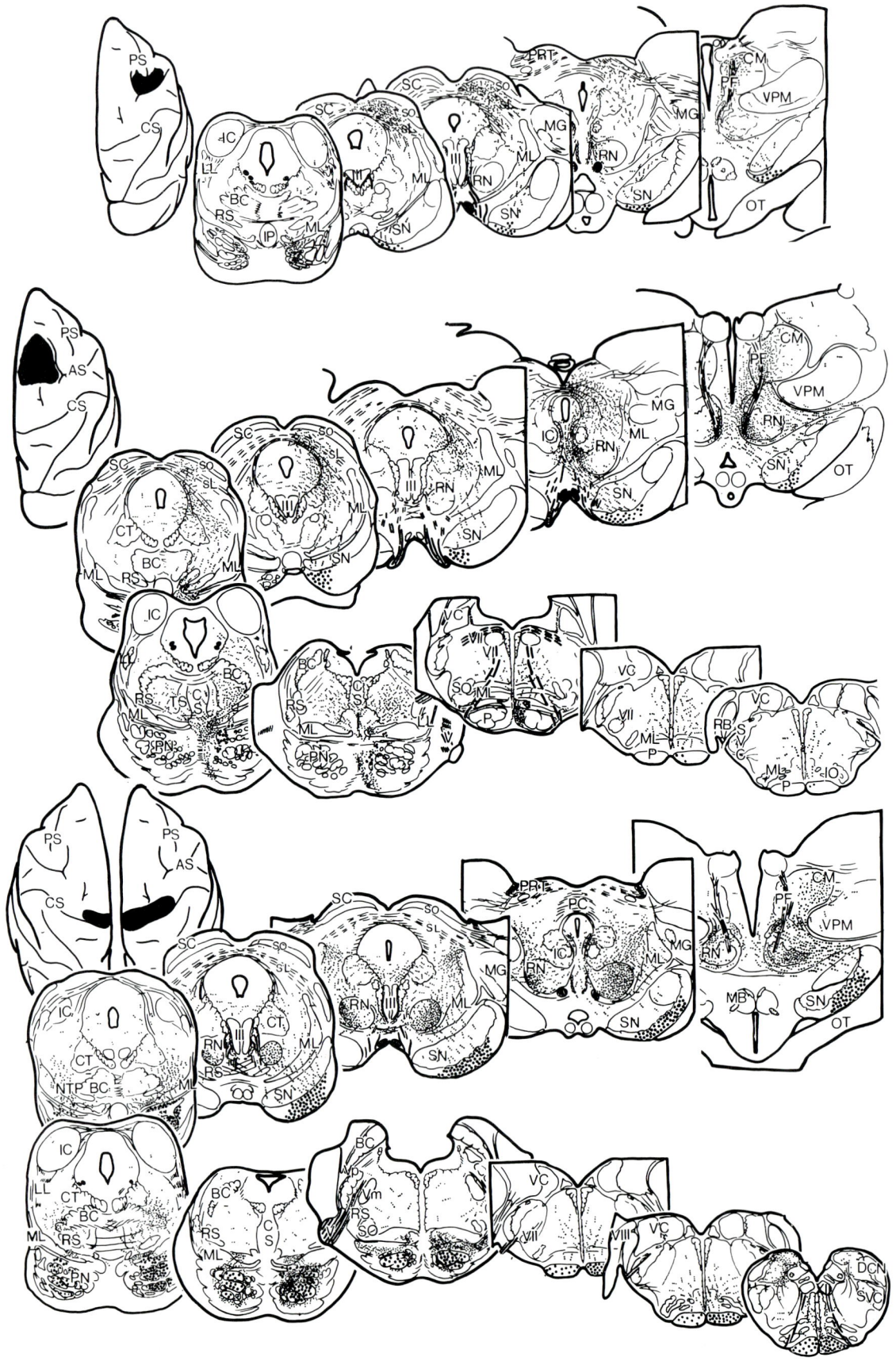

cleus, which in cat and monkey projects primarily to the lumbosacral segments (349, 566, 648), while fibers from the middle one-third (the arm representation area) are distributed primarily to more dorsal and medial parts of the nucleus, which project primarily to the cervical segments (349, 566, 648). These anterograde degeneration findings are supported by recent anterograde amino acid transport studies (267). Anterograde degeneration (430, 593, 608) and orthodromic as well as antidromic electrical stimulation findings (12, 537) indicate that a projection from area 4 to the magnocellular red nucleus also exists in cat and that this projection is also somatotopically organized. According to some anterograde degeneration findings (430), however, the somatic sensory cortex in cat also contributes to this corticorubral projection.

The cortical fibers to the parvocellular red nucleus are more numerous than to the magnocellular part and are derived from a wider frontal area, as indicated by anterograde degeneration findings in rhesus monkey (380, 555) and chimpanzee (383) and supported by anterograde amino acid transport findings (267, 364). These fibers originate (Fig. 16) in the precentral gyrus, the rostrally adjoining area 6, and according to the anterograde degeneration findings also in area 8 and in the cortex around the caudal part of the principal sulcus (380). These corticoparvocellular projections also display a topographical organization such that the areas rostral to the precentral gyrus project bilaterally to the dorsomedial part of the parvocellular red nucleus, while the precentral gyrus itself projects to the remainder of the parvocellular red nucleus (Fig. 18). The precentral projection itself is further topographically organized so that the fibers from the upper, middle, and lower one-third of the gyrus are distributed to the medial, intermediate, and lateral parts of the parvocellular red nucleus, respectively (380). Somewhat similar anterograde degeneration findings have been obtained in chimpanzee (383) and cat (373, 608). Anterograde amino acid transport findings (267) show in addition that the precentral projections to the parvocellular red nucleus in monkey are also distributed bilaterally, but mainly ipsilaterally.

Antidromic and orthodromic electrical stimulation studies (710) indicate that in cat two types of cortical connections to the rubrospinal neurons exist. One type is established by collaterals of fast-conducting cortical fibers, which continue into the pyramidal tract. These collaterals exert an inhibitory influence on rubrospinal neurons, probably by way of interneurons (97, 341, 343, 345, 709). They may be responsible for the retrograde HRP labeling of a few Betz cells in both cat and monkey after HRP injections in the area of the red nucleus [(111); C. E. Catsman-Berrevoets and H. G. J. M. Kuypers, unpublished observations]. The other type of cortical connections is excitatory in nature and is established by slowly conducting fibers that do not contribute to the pyramidal tract. According to electrical stimulation findings (710) these fibers establish direct synaptic contacts with distal dendrites of rubrospinal neurons. Thus excitatory collaterals from the corticospinal neurons to the red nucleus could not be demonstrated in cat (297). Electrophysiological findings (308), however, suggest that in monkey such excitatory collaterals exist. Other electrophysiological studies (711) have shown that in cat direct corticorubral fibers to distal dendrites of rubrospinal neurons may establish connections with proximal parts of the dendritic tree after destruction of the cerebellar interpositus nucleus, the fibers of which provide many terminals on the somata and proximal dendrites of these red nucleus neurons.

Anterograde degeneration findings suggest that in lower animals such as rat (80, 250) cortical fibers are distributed only to the rostral part of the red nucleus, which contains relatively small neurons, but not to the caudal rubrospinal (249) magnocellular part. A somewhat similar distribution pattern has been observed in the opossum (344), in which, however, some cortical fibers are distributed to the medium to large neurons in the lateral part of the caudal portion of the red nucleus; these neurons project in part to the spinal cord but especially to the bulbar lateral tegmental field and the facial nucleus (448).

Little is known about cortical projections to the recently identified cells of origin of the crossed pontospinal tract (93, 381), which also characteristically projects to relatively short propriospinal neurons (292–295, 451) and which has been referred to as the pontine component of the (rubrospinal) tract of von Monakow (405).

Cortical projections to dorsal column nuclei. Anterograde degeneration findings in cat and monkey have shown that the cortex also distributes fibers by way of the pyramidal tract to the dorsal column nuclei (113, 368, 370, 371, 740). These fibers first pass through the pyramidal decussation and then follow a recurrent trajectory. These projections are present in all mammals studied, from opossum (444) to human beings (369), and therefore seem to constitute a fundamental component of the corticobulbar and corticospinal pathways. In this respect it is of interest to note that cortical fibers are distributed not only to the nucleus cuneatus but also to the nucleus gracilis, even in those animals in which the corticospinal fibers themselves do not reach the lumbosacral cord (252, 444).

Anterograde degeneration (371, 409) and retrograde HRP transport (107, 757) findings indicate that corti-

FIG. 18. Distribution of degenerating cortical fibers from different parts of frontal lobe to brain stem in monkey. Note differences in distributions of cortical fibers to superior colliculus, red nucleus, and pontine and medullary reticular formation after lesions in different frontal areas. [From Kuypers and Lawrence (380).]

cal fibers to the dorsal column nuclei in rhesus monkey are derived from the caudal part of the precentral gyrus (areas 4 and 3a); from the postcentral gyrus (areas 3b, 1 and 2); from the adjoining superior parietal lobule (area 5), including the upper bank of the intraparietal sulcus; and from the area of the secondary sensory cortex in the parietal operculum (Fig. 16). Similar findings regarding the origin of the cortical fibers to the dorsal column nuclei have been obtained in other animals, e.g., in cat (51, 67, 113, 368, 756, 758), raccoon (555), and opossum (444). These various studies further indicate that fibers from the foot representation area are distributed mainly to nucleus gracilis and those from the hand representation area mainly to nucleus cuneatus.

The cortical fibers to the dorsal column nuclei terminate mainly in those parts of the nuclei populated by neurons with long radiating dendrites (384), and they largely avoid the cell clusters that contain relay neurons. Thus in cat (384, 758) cortical fibers are distributed to areas at the base of the caudal parts of the nuclei and to the rostral parts of the nuclei, areas that apparently do not contribute substantially to the medial lemniscus (115, 384). These areas may contain interneurons that distribute their fibers to the cell clusters (10). They also contain neurons that project to the cerebellum (115), however, and neurons that project to and receive ascending fibers from the spinal dorsal horn (see *Pathways from dorsal column nuclei to spinal dorsal horn*, p. 626). Thus the cortical fibers to the dorsal column nuclei as well as those to the spinal dorsal horn (see *Terminal distribution of corticospinal fibers*, p. 628) may in part be distributed to neurons interconnecting somatic sensory relay nuclei. In this light it is of interest to note that the cortical fibers to the area of the main sensory nucleus V, which also contains cell clusters, are distributed in the same way as in the area of the cuneatus and gracilis nuclei such that they also largely avoid the area of the cell clusters (384). Little information is available, however, regarding connections of the noncluster neurons in this trigeminal area.

Other corticosubcortical projections. The frontal cortex projects also to caudate putamen (224, 328), thalamus [i.e., specific thalamic nuclei (362, 364)], intralaminar nuclei and center median-parafascicular complex (164, 362, 380, 383), nucleus tegmenti pedunculopontinus (267, 380), and cerebellar relay nuclei such as pontine grey, nucleus reticularis tegmenti pontis, lateral reticular nucleus in the medulla oblongata, and inferior olive (Fig. 18). It is of interest to note that the frontal areas rostral to the precentral gyrus (Fig. 16), which project preferentially to brain stem cell groups that give rise to descending pathways to long propriospinal neurons, also project to the parafascicular nucleus (164, 267, 364, 380, 552), while the precentral gyrus, the upper two-thirds of which distributes fibers to the magnocellular red nucleus (267, 380), projects in a topographically organized fashion to the center median [Figs. 16, 18; (267, 380, 552)]. In addition the precentral gyrus projects to the subthalamic nucleus and represents the source of the frontal fibers to the nucleus tegmenti pedunculopontinus (267, 380), which also receives many fibers from the globus pallidus (512), the substantia nigra pars reticulata (38), and the subthalamic nucleus (509).

LAMINAR DISTRIBUTION OF CORTICAL NEURONS PROJECTING TO SUBCORTICAL AND SPINAL STRUCTURES. Retrograde HRP transport studies in rat (317, 770, 772), mouse (783), hamster (583), cat (214, 432, 480), and monkey (329, 420, 775) indicate that the supragranular cortical layers II and III mainly give rise to intrahemispheric and interhemispheric corticocortical connections, while the infragranular layers V and VI represent the main source of the descending cortical projections, e.g., to corpus striatum, thalamus, superior colliculus, brain stem tegmentum, dorsal column nuclei, and spinal and bulbar sensory relay nuclei (i.e., trigeminal complex and spinal dorsal horn), as well as spinal and bulbar interneurons and motoneurons. The infragranular layers, however, and especially layer V, also contribute to corticocortical connections (161, 329, 480) especially in rodents (317, 770, 771, 783).

Retrograde HRP transport findings further indicate that in rhesus monkey neurons projecting to various subcortical and spinal cell groups occupy a different position in the infragranular layers, suggesting that these respective projections are in part derived from different sets of cortical neurons; this is to some extent supported by antidromic stimulation findings (63, 67). Other such findings (62, 178, 710), however, indicate that cortical fibers to several subcortical structures in part represent collaterals of pyramidal fibers descending to the lower medulla oblongata and beyond. Some such collaterals have also been demonstrated anatomically by means of the retrograde double-labeling technique (110).

Some of the cortical neurons projecting from the motor and sensory areas to the *striatum* in monkey, according to retrograde HRP transport findings (329), are located superficially in the subgranular cortex (i.e., in the upper part of layer V), which is in keeping with antidromic stimulation findings in cat (480). Some of the neurons in question are also located in the deeper parts of layer V, below the Betz cells, and even in layer VI (329). This is compatible with antidromic stimulation findings (178, 480), which suggest that some corticostriate fibers represent collaterals of peduncular and pyramidal tract fibers that come from neurons in the deep part of layer V (see later in this subsection).

According to retrograde HRP transport findings (329) the cortical neurons projecting to the *red nucleus* in monkey are located in the precentral gyrus, including area 3a, in the bottom of the central sulcus, and in the areas immediately rostral to the precentral gyrus (Fig. 16), whereas a few seem to be derived also from postcentral areas (C. E. Catsman-Berrevoetts and H. G. J. M. Kuypers, unpublished observations); this is in accordance with anterograde degeneration (380) and amino acid transport findings (267, 364). In area 4 the corticorubral neurons are concentrated immediately above the Betz cells (329); this is in keeping with antidromic stimulation studies (63), which show that the corticorubral neurons are distinct from the corticothalamic neurons projecting to the ventrolateral nucleus, which are located deeper in the cortex (see later in this subsection). In cat and monkey a small number of Betz cells seems to contribute to this corticorubral projection, since a few of them are labeled after HRP injections in the area of the red nucleus (111) and since in cat and monkey some corticospinal neurons can be antidromically invaded by stimulation of the red nucleus (308, 710).

Cortical neurons projecting to the *dorsal column nuclei* in monkey are located (Fig. 16) in areas 4, 3a, 3b, 2, 1, and 5 as well as in the area of the secondary sensory cortex (107, 329, 371, 757). In the postcentral gyrus they are situated among the large neurons in the upper part of layer V; in the precentral gyrus they are located immediately above the Betz cells (107, 329, 757).

Neurons that project from the precentral gyrus to the *center median* in monkey (Fig. 16), according to retrograde HRP transport findings (108), are also located immediately above the Betz cells (i.e., together with those projecting to red nucleus and dorsal column nuclei). Antidromic stimulation findings in cat and monkey (62, 178) suggest, however, that some of the cortical fibers to these brain cell groups represent collaterals of pyramidal tract fibers. Neurons projecting to the *parafascicular nucleus* in monkey (Fig. 16) are located in areas rostral to the precentral gyrus (164, 267, 364, 380, 552) and according to retrograde HRP findings are also situated rather superficially in layer V (C. E. Catsman-Berrevoets and H. G. J. M. Kuypers, unpublished observations).

The neurons projecting to dorsal column nuclei and center median in cat display a slightly different laminar distribution than in monkey and are located among the Betz cells instead of above them (51, 109, 756). According to the HRP findings, however, the Betz cells do not contribute to these projections. This is in accordance with antidromic stimulation findings (67), indicating that corticonuclear neurons do not project to the spinal cord but may be at variance with other electrophysiological findings (62, 178).

The cortical neurons projecting to the *spinal cord*, according to retrograde HRP transport findings in monkey (107, 130, 329) and cat (17, 51, 246), are located in areas 4, 3a, 3b, 2, 1, and 5 and, in monkey, also in the caudal part of area 6 (Fig. 16). The bulk of these neurons in monkey, however, are located below those projecting to striatum, red nucleus, dorsal column nuclei, and center median, i.e., in the deeper parts of layer V; in area 4 they include the Betz cells. Neurons projecting to the *superior colliculus* and lower brain stem *medial tegmental field*, which in monkey and cat are mainly located in areas rostral to the precentral gyrus (Fig. 16) and in the rostral part of area 4 (51, 109, 642), are situated at roughly the same depth as the corticospinal neurons. Here it is of interest to note that according to double-labeling findings (110) some of the cortical fibers to the mesencephalon represent collaterals of corticospinal fibers.

Neurons projecting to *specific thalamic nuclei*, including the medial and lateral geniculate bodies, according to retrograde HRP transport findings are located in the infragranular cortex, i.e., in layer VI and the deep parts of layer V in rat (318, 770, 772), hamster (583), cat (214, 595), and monkey (108, 329, 420, 594). Antidromic stimulation findings in cat (178) suggest that some corticothalamic fibers represent collaterals of pyramidal fibers. This, however, is at variance with the findings of another electrophysiological study (63) as well as with recent retrograde double-labeling experiments (110).

In short, the cortical neurons projecting to spinal cord and to cell groups of descending brain stem pathways in monkey are situated between two groups of neurons: *1)* the more superficially located neurons projecting to the center median, red nucleus, and dorsal column nuclei and *2)* the more deeply located neurons projecting to the specific thalamic nuclei. It seems inconsistent, however, that neurons projecting to the red nucleus, which also gives rise to a descending pathway to spinal cord, are located superficial to the Betz cells. This inconsistency may be resolved by retrograde HRP transport findings (111) that indicate that the limited precentral projection to magnocellular red nucleus in monkey is derived from a very few Betz cells and from some smaller neurons situated either between or below them, i.e., at the same level as the corticospinal neurons (cf. antidromic stimulation findings in refs. 308 and 710). The many corticorubral neurons that are located superficial to the Betz cells (109, 329) may therefore mainly represent neurons projecting to parvocellular red nucleus.

SYNTHESIS

Grouping of Descending Pathways on the Basis of Their Terminal Distribution

DESCENDING BRAIN STEM PATHWAYS. The descending brain stem pathways surveyed in this chapter are distributed in roughly the same way in all mammals and terminate in the superficial parts of the dorsal horn, the interneuronal area of the intermediate zone, and the somatic and autonomic motoneuronal cell groups in the ventral and lateral horn. The brain stem pathways terminating in the intermediate zone as well as the motoneuronal cell groups probably subserve mainly motor functions. These pathways may be subdivided into two large groups on the basis of their terminal distribution.

Group A comprises those pathways that are characterized by their termination, which is frequently bilateral, in the ventromedial part of the intermediate zone (Fig. 8), an area that contains long and intermediate propriospinal neurons, the fibers of which are to some degree distributed bilaterally (Fig. 2). These brain stem pathways all descend through the medial and ventromedial parts of the medullary cross section and continue into the ventral and ventrolateral funiculi of the cervical cord. Group B comprises contralaterally descending pathways, which are characterized by their termination in the lateral parts of the bulbar lateral tegmental field and in the dorsal and lateral parts of the spinal intermediate zone (Fig. 9); these areas contain short propriobulbar and propriospinal neurons (Fig. 2), the fibers of which are distributed mainly ipsilaterally. These pathways descend through the ventrolateral part of the medullary cross section, i.e., close to the spinal V complex, and continue into the spinal dorsolateral funiculus.

Group A comprises the interstitiospinal tract, tectospinal tract, lateral and medial vestibulospinal tracts, the reticulospinal tracts from the pontine and medullary medial tegmental field and the medial mesencephalic tegmentum, as well as fibers from the area of the nucleus of the posterior commissure, which also descend in the ventral and ventrolateral funiculi (Fig. 8).

Group B comprises the contralaterally descending rubrospinal and rubrobulbar tracts as well as the contralaterally descending pontospinal tract from the ventrolateral pontine tegmentum (Fig. 9). The tectospinal and the medullary reticulospinal fibers, which are regarded as belonging to the group A pathways, however, share some characteristics with group B pathways in that some of their fibers also terminate in the more lateral parts of the intermediate zone that contain short propriospinal neurons.

Recent studies have demonstrated that in addition to the group A and group B brain stem pathways another group of pathways exist that are mainly derived from the area of the nucleus subcoeruleus and its immediate vicinity and from raphe nuclei. The descending pathways from these nuclei distributed many fibers to the intermediate zone and to the somatic motoneuronal cell groups of the spinal ventral horn throughout the spinal cord (Fig. 10). The functional contribution to the steering of movements of these descending brain stem pathways still remains largely obscure.

The members of the two respective groups of brain stem pathways (A and B) have several other characteristics in common. Thus all cell groups of group A pathways project to the reticular formation of the pontine and medullary medial tegmental field (Fig. 8), which in turn gives rise to long reticulospinal pathways belonging to this same group. Group B pathways apparently represent a different organization, because they characteristically avoid the pontine and medullary medial tegmental field (Fig. 9) and establish connections with the dorsal column nuclei, which have seldom been demonstrated for group A pathways. Moreover several of the group A pathways show a very high degree of collateralization, whereas the rubrospinal fibers of group B pathways do not.

The fiber components of group A pathways, because of their high degree of collateralization and their characteristic termination in areas containing long propriospinal neurons, seem to be especially well suited for synergistic activation of large numbers of muscular elements and can be expected to be characterized by a limited capacity for movement fractionation. The rubrospinal components of the group B pathways for the same reasons can be expected to be characterized by a relatively greater capacity for movement fractionation.

Both group A and group B pathways, in addition to terminating in the intermediate zone, establish some monosynaptic connections with motoneurons that have been demonstrated by means of electrophysiological and anatomical techniques. According to the anatomical findings these connections are mainly derived from the medial reticular formation of the lower medulla oblongata (group A pathways) and are distributed to the medial and lateral motoneuronal cell groups throughout the spinal cord. According to electrophysiological findings, however, the motoneuronal connections of the two groups of brain stem pathways tend to be established with different populations of motoneurons. Thus in cat several group A pathways establish monosynaptic connections with many motoneurons of neck and back muscles. In addition, some of these pathways establish some monosynaptic connections with limb extensor and flexor motoneurons; these connections in rhesus monkey, however, are largely restricted to motoneurons of proximal limb muscles. The rubrospinal components of the group B brain stem pathways in cat do not establish monosynaptic connections with motoneurons. Yet according to electrophysiological findings they do establish some direct connections with motoneurons of distal extremity muscles in rhesus monkey. Comparable differences exist in connections of these various brain stem pathways to the motoneuronal cell groups in the brain stem, because many group A pathways project in the brain stem to facial motoneurons of the ear muscles and to motoneurons of the external eye muscles, whereas the rubrobulbar components of group B pathways project mainly to facial motoneurons of perioral and periorbital muscles.

The cell populations, which give rise to the two groups of brain stem pathways, receive cortical projections that are preferentially derived from different frontal areas (Fig. 18). Thus the cell groups of group A brain stem pathways receive fibers mainly from areas rostral to the precentral gyrus (Fig. 16), while the rubrospinal components of group B brain stem pathways receive fibers mainly from this gyrus (Fig. 16). Thus in rhesus monkey, areas rostral to the precentral gyrus, by way of their connections to group A brain stem pathways, appear to be characteristically related to long propriospinal neurons and to motoneurons of eye and ear muscles, neck and back muscles, and proximal extremity muscles, while the precentral gyrus (at least by way of its connections with the rubrospinal components of group B pathways) is characteristically related to short propriospinal neurons and to motoneurons of periorbital and perioral facial muscles and of distal extremity muscles. These inferences are in keeping with the findings obtained by means of electrical stimulation of the frontal lobe (779).

CORTICOBULBAR AND CORTICOSPINAL PATHWAYS. The corticobulbar and corticospinal pathways parallel the brain stem pathways but possess different terminal distribution in different mammals. On this basis two groups of mammals may be distinguished: *1)* those in which the corticobulbar and corticospinal fibers are distributed to the lower brain stem and cervicothoracic segments, e.g., the edentates, elephants, marsupials, and lagomorphs; and *2)* those in which they are also distributed to the lumbar and sacral segments, e.g., the bats, certain rodents, carnivores, and primates.

The terminal distribution of the corticobulbar and corticospinal fibers in its most restricted form suggests that these pathways provide primarily a sensory rather than a motor control system. Thus in the first group of mammals and even in birds (784) the bulk of the cortical (forebrain) fibers are distributed to sensory nuclei, i.e., trigeminal complex, spinal dorsal horn, and dorsal column nuclei. These projections are accompanied in this group of mammals by a light projection to relatively short propriobulbar and propriospinal neurons in the most lateral part of the bulbar lateral tegmental field and the most dorsal and lateral parts of the spinal intermediate zone (Fig. 12). As a consequence the terminal distribution area of the cortical fibers to the intermediate zone in these species overlaps only that of group B brain stem pathways.

In the second group of mammals, in which cortical fibers are distributed throughout the length of the spinal cord, their distribution area in the spinal intermediate zone is wider than in the first group and, especially in higher primates, includes the area of the long propriospinal neurons (Fig. 12). As a consequence in these species the distribution area overlaps not only that of the group B but also that of the group A brain stem pathways.

In several primates and in two carnivore species cortical fibers are also distributed to spinal and bulbar motoneuronal cell groups. In the carnivores, prosimians, and monkey they are distributed mainly to motoneurons of distal extremity muscles, whereas in chimpanzee and the human being they are also distributed abundantly to motoneurons of proximal muscles.

The connections from the cortex to the motoneuronal cell groups show a high degree of topographical organization because the corticomotoneuronal fibers show little branching and the bulk of the cortical fibers to motoneurons of the various muscles are generally derived from distinctly different precentral areas (Fig. 17). This seems contrary to the motoneuronal connections established by the fibers from the brain stem, which according to the anatomical findings are distributed from relatively restricted brain stem cell groups to somatic motoneuronal cell groups at virtually all spinal levels (Fig. 10). The motoneuronal connections from the cerebral cortex therefore appear to represent a highly differentiated system as compared with those from the brain stem and probably provide to the descending cortical connections a critical increase in movement fractionation capacity as compared with the descending brain stem pathways.

Functional Epilogue

The cortical and brain stem pathways must represent the instruments by which the brain governs the activity of the spinal and bulbar motor mechanisms and thus steers movements. These pathways, which differ in their spinal termination, appear to be involved in the steering of different classes of movements, since their interruption produces different types of motor defects (399, 400).

Bilateral *pyramidotomy*, which interrupts the corticospinal fibers and some corticobulbar fibers, mainly interferes with steering of extremity movements in rhesus monkey. Immediately postoperatively the animals can sit with their heads up and can walk, run, and climb, but they cannot pick up pieces of food with their hands, which they only limply place on the food without grasping it. Yet they can use their hands and feet in clinging to the cage bars.

After some recovery the animals regain the capacity to pick up food morsels with their hands. Initially the reaching movements consist of a hooking circumduction of the whole arm, and the closure of the hand in grasping the food forms a part of this whole-arm movement. During further recovery, however, the closure of the hand, which consists of flexion of all fingers together, becomes progressively independent of the arm movements so that ultimately the animals can reach out and open and close the hand with a stable outstretched arm (Fig. 19). Yet closing of the hand always involves flexion of all fingers together, and even three to four years postoperatively, individual finger movements such as the thumb and index finger precision grip do not return (Fig. 20). After unilateral pyramidotomy roughly the same sequence of events occurs in the contralateral limb. When only the pyramidal tracts are interrupted no forward slumping of head and body occurs, as described by Tower (704) to

BILATERAL PYRAMIDOTOMY

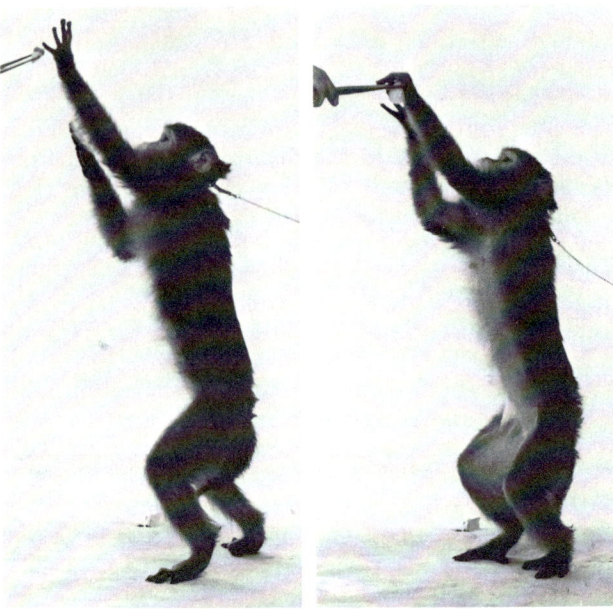

FIG. 19. Rhesus monkey, 5 mo after bilateral pyramidotomy, reaching for morsel of food held in forceps (*left*) and grasping it (*right*). Note opening and closing of hand relatively independent of arm movements. [From Lawrence and Kuypers (399).]

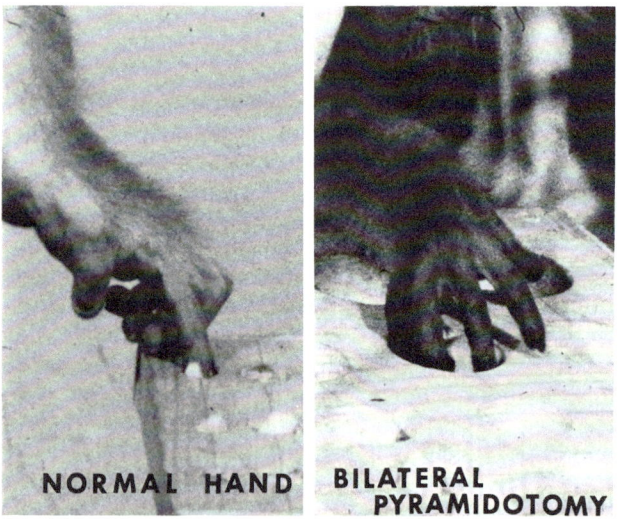

FIG. 20. *Left*: rhesus monkey with intact pyramidal tracts taking morsels of food from 8-mm diam food well using index finger alone. *Right*: rhesus monkey 2 mo after bilateral pyramidotomy taking morsel of food from large food well by flexing all fingers in concert. [From Lawrence and Kuypers (398a), copyright 1965 by the American Association for the Advancement of Science.]

indicate axial impairment. This only results from pyramidal lesions that extend into the medullary medial tegmental field, thus additionally involving group A brain stem pathways.

The capacity to execute relatively independent finger movements, which in view of the above findings is characteristically provided by the corticospinal pathway, probably reflects its high movement fractionation capacity inferred from its highly differentiated system of direct connections to the motoneurons of distal extremity muscles. This assumption is based on the following considerations: Cortical fibers are distributed to motoneuronal cell groups in those animals executing individual finger movements and displaying an unusual manipulatory agility (274). Thus such fibers are present in increasing numbers in slow loris, raccoon, rhesus monkey, chimpanzee, and human beings (Fig. 10) but are largely lacking in sloth, opossum, tree shrew, goat, cat, dog, and others (Fig. 10). Second, in newborn rhesus monkeys, which do not possess the capacity to execute relatively independent finger movements, no cortical fibers are distributed to the motoneuronal cell groups (Fig. 14). This distribution of cortical fibers to motoneuronal cell groups, however, gradually develops in the first six months of postnatal life, largely in parallel with development of the capacity to execute relatively independent finger movements (398); moreover, the development of this capacity in monkey depends exclusively on the presence of the pyramidal tract, because after its transection soon after birth this capacity does not develop and therefore is not provided vicariously by the descending brain stem pathways (398). Finally, the capacity to execute relatively independent finger movements is completely abolished in the rhesus monkey by a resection of the precentral arm area, which represents the major source of cortical projections to motoneurons of distal arm and hand muscles (374, 545).

In this context it is important to note that ablation of the precentral motor cortex is followed initially by a somewhat flaccid paresis. The severity and the duration of this flaccid paresis in various animals seem to parallel the quantitative development of the corticospinal tract but especially that of the corticomotoneuronal connections. Thus the flaccid paresis is rather limited in cat, is more pronounced in the rhesus monkey (especially in the distal extremity muscles), and is rather severe in chimpanzee and human beings (746). Moreover the flaccid paresis is largely lacking in the newborn rhesus monkey (338), in which the direct corticomotoneuronal connections have not yet developed. The flaccid paralysis gradually diminishes, however. This diminution progressively unmasks a remaining motor control, which is of considerable dimensions (156) and must be exerted by the various descending brain stem pathways.

The *brain stem motor control*, which returns after transection of the corticospinal pathways (399), has two different aspects that can be demonstrated in the bilaterally pyramidotomized monkey by additional transection of group A or group B descending brain stem pathways, respectively. These transections result in two contrasting motor defects (400).

Interruption of *group A descending brain stem pathways* in a bilaterally pyramidotomized monkey, by means of a bilateral transection of the brain stem pathways in the upper medullary medial tegmental field (cf. Fig. 8) typically produces postural changes of trunk and limbs, a prolonged inability to right itself, and a severe deficit in the steering of axial and proximal limb movements. At the same time distal extremity movements, as in picking up pieces of food with the hand, are considerably less impaired. Thus from the early stages of recovery on, there occurs a pronounced flexion of trunk and limbs that persists throughout the recovery period. In addition, the shoulders are elevated and the arms are held adducted to the body, especially when the animal is sitting or is held supine. Righting to a sitting position does not occur until one to several weeks later, and when the animals sit they tend to slump forward and are unsteady. Some time later they are able to walk, but they frequently veer from course and have grave difficulties in avoiding obstacles. In contrast to the severe impairment in righting and the immobility of the body axis and proximal parts of the extremities, the hands and the distal parts of the limbs are very active. Thus very soon after the operation the animals can hold pieces of food in their hands. Within a short time this manipulatory capacity returns to a level comparable to that after recovery from bilateral pyramidotomy such that they can pick up pieces of food from a board with their hands and can bring them to the mouth. In reaching for the food while sitting in the examining chair, however, the animals behave very differently from bilaterally pyramidotomized animals with intact brain stem pathways. When the latter are approached with food, they immediately turn toward it and eagerly reach for it with an outstretched arm and an open hand. In contrast the animals with an additional transection of the group A brain stem pathways follow the approaching food only with the eyes while the body and arms remain relatively stationary. They bring arm and hand to the food only when it is close to the hand and do so mainly by flexion in the elbow.

The behavior of pyramidotomized animals after transection of *group B brain stem pathways* strikingly contrasts with that after transection of group A brain stem pathways. Thus after transection of group B pathways at different brain stem levels and in the upper cervical dorsolateral funiculi, the animals are able to right immediately. They sit up in their cages, walk, and climb and do not have the axial and proximal limb flexion posture that occurs after transection of group A pathways. They show striking changes, however, in the use of the ipsilateral limb, especially the forelimb. When the animal is sitting in the examining chair the affected arm hangs loosely from the shoulder with the elbow slightly flexed and the fingers extended. Soon after the operation the fingers and wrists are noticeably limp. In reaching for food the elbow is held semiflexed and the hand is brought to the food by circumduction of the arm in the shoulder. The food is prehended by flexion of the fingers, but this in general occurs as part of the total arm movement. The affected limbs showed much less defect when used in walking and climbing. A defect similar to that occurring in the pyramidotomized animals after transection of the group B brain stem pathways has been observed after combining a unilateral lesion of the precentral hand area with a transection of the mesencephalic tegmental decussation, including that of the rubrospinal tract, the main component of the group B brain stem pathways (H. W. Hamersvelt and H. G. J. M. Kuypers, unpublished observations).

CONCLUSION. Group A brain stem pathways (Fig. 8) characteristically terminate on long propriospinal neurons, display a relatively high degree of collateralization, and according to physiological observations maintain some direct connections with motoneurons of many neck and back muscles and with some motoneurons of limb muscles; in the rhesus monkey connections are primarily with motoneurons of proximal extremity muscles. In view of the findings obtained in the freely moving monkey these brain stem pathways can be considered to represent the basic system by which the brain controls movements. This control is especially concerned with the maintenance of erect posture, with integration of movements of body and limbs and synergistic whole-limb movements, with orientation movements of body and head, and with direction of the course of progression. Group B brain stem pathways (Fig. 9) characteristically terminate in the area of relatively short propriospinal neurons. In monkey this group of brain stem pathways, by way of its rubrospinal components, maintains some direct connections with motoneurons of distal extremity muscles. In view of the above-mentioned findings in the freely moving animal, this group of brain stem pathways supplements the control exerted by the group A pathways and provides the capacity for independent, flexion-biased, movements of the extremities and of the shoulder but, in particular, of the elbow and hand. The findings obtained in the freely moving monkey further indicate that the corticospinal pathway, the termination area of which largely overlaps with those of the two groups of brain stem pathways, further amplifies the brain stem controls but in addition provides the capacity for a high degree of fractionation of movements as exemplified by individual finger movements. This capacity is probably provided by the direct corticomotoneuronal connections, which represents a highly differentiated system as compared with those of the brain stem pathways.

Previous observations support these conclusions. For example, stimulation of the superior colliculus (280, 601) and the interstitial nucleus of Cajal (270, 330), which contribute to the group A brain stem pathways (Fig. 8), produce turning movements and rotatory movements of head and trunk. Lesions in these areas or interruption of their descending pathways result in forced circling (155, 330, 429, 653). Stimulation as well as unilateral lesions of the mesencephalic and bulbar reticular formation, which also contribute to the group A brain stem pathways (Fig.

8), result in turning movements of the trunk accompanied by supporting flexion and extension of the extremities (185, 285, 311, 312, 493, 494, 502, 647, 651, 736, 760), and medullary reticular formation lesions interfere with the lordosis reflex in female rats (488). Moreover, unitary activity in the pontine and medullary reticular formation occurs in relation to movements of head and body (641, 643, 644). Further stimulation of the frontal cortical areas rostral to the precentral gyrus, areas that characteristically project to cells of origin of the group A brain stem pathways (Fig. 16), result in turning of eyes, body, and head (269, 738), while lesions in these areas give the opposite result (339). Furthermore, stimulation of the red nucleus (213, 565), which contributes to the group B brain stem pathways (Fig. 9), elicits movements of very restricted parts of the contralateral extremities, especially flexion. Lesions of the red nucleus in cat transiently impair the manipulatory capacity of the contralateral limb (229), and lesions of the laterally descending Group B pathways in monkey may produce hypokinesia of the ipsilateral extremities (535). Further stimulation of the precentral gyrus after pyramidotomy, leaving intact the corticosubcortical connections (e.g., to the magnocellular red nucleus; see Fig. 16) results mainly in movements of the limbs (407, 778). When the pyramidal tract is intact, however, electrical stimulation of the precentral gyrus, when applied to the areas that give rise to the corticospinal fibers to the dorsal and lateral parts of the intermediate zone and to motoneuronal cell groups [Fig. 17; (376)], elicits highly fractionated distal extremity movements, whereas stimulation of the precentral areas that give rise to corticospinal projections to long propriospinal neurons (376) elicits movements of trunk and the proximal parts of the extremities (779). Thus these various findings support the present concept with regard to the functional contributions of the various descending pathways to the steering of movements, a concept that has much in common with those brought forward earlier in clinical neurology (787). Yet these findings do not clarify the functional contribution to the steering of movements of the recently discovered direct brain stem projections from the raphe and the nucleus subcoeruleus to the somatic motoneuronal cell groups throughout the spinal cord (Fig. 10). Further research will have to elucidate these aspects.

REFERENCES

1. ABZUG, C., M. MAEDA, B. W. PETERSON, AND V. J. WILSON. Cervical branching of lumbar vestibulospinal axons. *J. Physiol. London* 243: 499-522, 1974.
2. ACHENBACH, K. E., AND D. C. GOODMAN. Cerebellar projections to pons, medulla and spinal cord in the albino rat. *Brain Behav. Evol.* 1: 43-57, 1968.
3. AKAGI, Y. The localization of the motor neurons innervating the extraocular muscles in the oculomotor nuclei of the cat and rabbit, using horseradish peroxidase. *J. Comp. Neurol.* 181: 745-762, 1978.
4. AKERT, K., AND C. SANDRI. Significance of the Maillet method for cytochemical studies of synapses. In: *Golgi Centennial Symposium: Perspectives in Neurobiology*, edited by M. Santini. New York: Raven Press, 1975, p. 387-399. (Golgi Centennial Symp., 1973.)
5. ALBANO, J. E., T. T. NORTON, AND W. C. HALL. Laminar origin of projections from the superficial layers of the superior colliculus in the tree shrew, *Tupaia glis. Brain Res.* 173: 1-11, 1979.
6. ALBE-FESSARD, D., J. BOIVIE, G. GRANT, AND A. LEVANTE. Labelling of the cells in the medulla oblongata and the spinal cord of the monkey after injections of horseradish peroxidase in the thalamus. *Neurosci. Lett.* 1: 75-80, 1975.
7. ALBE-FESSARD, D., A. LEVANTE, AND Y. LAMOUR. Origin of spinothalamic and spinoreticular pathways in cat and monkeys. *Adv. Neurol.* 4: 157-166, 1974.
8. ALSTERMARK, B., A. LUNDBERG, U. NORRSELL, AND E. SYBIRSKA. Role of C3-C4 propriospinal neurones in forelimb movements in the cat. *Acta Physiol. Scand.* 105: A24-A25, 1979.
9. ALTMAN, J., AND M. B. CARPENTER. Fiber projections of the superior colliculus in the cat. *J. Comp. Neurol.* 116: 157-177, 1961.
10. ANDERSEN, P., J. C. ECCLES, R. F. SCHMIDT, AND T. YOKOTA. Identification of relay cells and interneurons in the cuneate nucleus. *J. Neurophysiol.* 27: 1080-1095, 1964.
11. ANDERSON, F. D. The structure of a chronically isolated segment of the cat spinal cord. *J. Comp. Neurol.* 120: 297-315, 1963.
12. ANDERSON, M. E. Cerebellar and cerebral inputs to physiologically identified efferent cell groups in the red nucleus of cat. *Brain Res.* 30: 49-66, 1971.
13. ANDERSON, M. E., M. YOSHIDA, AND V. J. WILSON. Influence of superior colliculus on cat neck motoneurons. *J. Neurophysiol.* 34: 898-907, 1971.
14. ANDERSON, M. E., M. YOSHIDA, AND V. J. WILSON. Tectal and tegmental influences on cat forelimb and hindlimb motoneurons. *J. Neurophysiol.* 35: 462-470, 1972.
15. ANDERSON, W. J., M. W. STROMBERG, AND E. J. HINSMAN. Morphological characteristics of dendrite bundles in the lumbar spinal cord of the rat. *Brain Res.* 110: 215-227, 1976.
16. ANGAUT, P., AND D. BOWSHER. Cerebello-rubral connexions in the cat. *Nature London* 208: 1002-1003, 1965.
17. ARMAND, J., AND R. AURENTY. Dual organization of motor corticospinal tract in the cat. *Neurosci. Lett.* 6: 1-7, 1977.
18. ARMAND, J., AND H. G. J. M. KUYPERS. Organisation des projections contralatérales et bilatérales des faisceaux corticospinaux chez le chat. *C. R. Acad. Sci. Ser. D* 285: 1455-1458, 1977.
19. ARMAND, J., Y. PADEL, AND A. M. SMITH. Somatotopic organization of the corticospinal tract in cat motor cortex. *Brain Res.* 74: 209-227, 1974.
20. ARMSTRONG, D. M., AND R. F. SCHILD. Spino-olivary neurones in the lumbo-sacral cord of the cat demonstrated by retrograde transport of horseradish peroxidase. *Brain Res.* 168: 176-179, 1979.
21. ARMSTRONG, J., AND P. R. STEPHENS. A modified chrome-silver paraffin wax technique for staining neural end-feet. *Stain. Technol.* 35: 71-75, 1960.
22. ASANUMA, H., S. D. STONEY, JR., AND W. D. THOMPSON. Characteristics of cervical interneurons which mediate cortical motor outflow to distal forelimb muscles of cats. *Brain Res.* 27: 79-95, 1971.
23. ASANUMA, H., P. ZARZECKI, E. JANKOWSKA, T. HONGO, AND S. MARCUS. Projections of individual pyramidal tract neurons to lumbar motor nuclei of the monekey. *Exp. Brain Res.* 34: 73-89, 1979.
24. ASTRUC, J. Corticofugal connections of area 8 (frontal eye field)

in *Macaca mulatta. Brain Res.* 33: 241–256, 1971.
25. AXELSSON, S., A. BJORKLUND, B. FALCK, O. LINDVALL, AND L. A. SVENSSON. Glyoxylic acid condensation: a new fluorescence method for the histochemical demonstration of biogenic monoamines. *Acta Physiol. Scand.* 87: 57–62, 1973.
26. BAGLEY, C. Cortical motor mechanism of the sheep brain. *Arch. Neurol. Psychiatry* 7: 417–453, 1922.
27. BANDLER, R. Evidence for a bilateral "glomerular" projection from the red nucleus to the spinal nucleus of the trigeminal nerve in the cat. *Neurosci. Lett.* 8: 211–217, 1978.
28. BARGMANN, W. Neurosecretion. *Int. Rev. Cytol.* 19: 183–201, 1966.
29. BARNARD, J. W. The hypoglossal complex of vertebrates. *J. Comp. Neurol.* 72: 489–524, 1940.
30. BARNES, S. Degeneration in hemiplegia: with special reference to a ventrolateral pyramidal tract, the accessory fillet and Pick's bundle. *Brain* 24: 463–501, 1901.
31. BARONDES, S. M. On the site of synthesis of the mitochondrial protein of nerve endings. *J. Neurochem.* 13: 721–727, 1966.
32. BASBAUM, A. I., C. H. CLANTON, AND H. L. FIELDS. Opiate and stimulus-produced analgesia: functional anatomy of a medullospinal pathway. *Proc. Natl. Acad. Sci. USA* 73: 4685–4688, 1976.
33. BASBAUM, A. I., C. H. CLANTON, AND H. L. FIELDS. Three bulbospinal pathways from the rostral medulla of the cat: an autoradiographic study of pain modulating systems. *J. Comp. Neurol.* 178: 209–224, 1978.
34. BASBAUM, A. I., AND H. L. FIELDS. The origin of descending pathways in the dorsolateral funiculus of the spinal cord of the cat and rat: further studies on the anatomy of pain modulation. *J. Comp. Neurol.* 187: 513–532, 1979.
35. BATON, R. R., A. JAYARAMAN, D. RUGGIERO, AND M. B. CARPENTER. Fastigial efferent projections in the monkey: An autoradiographic study. *J. Comp. Neurol.* 174: 281–305, 1977.
36. BAUTISTA, N. S., AND H. A. MATZKE. A degeneration study of the course and extent of the pyramidal tract of the opossum. *J. Comp. Neurol.* 124: 367–376, 1965.
37. BEALL, J. E., R. F. MARTIN, A. E. APPLEBAUM, AND W. D. WILLIS. Inhibition of primate spinothalamic tract neurons by stimulation in the region of the nucleus raphe magnus. *Brain Res.* 114: 328–333, 1976.
38. BECKSTEAD, R. M., V. B. DOMESICK, AND W. J. H. NAUTA. Efferent connections of the substantia nigra and ventral tegmental area in rat. *Brain Res.* 175: 191–217, 1979.
39. BENEVENTO, L. A., AND J. H. FALLON. The ascending projections of the superior colliculus in the rhesus monkey (*Macaca mulatta*). *J. Comp. Neurol.* 160: 339–361, 1975.
40. BENTIVOGLIO, M., H. G. J. M. KUYPERS, C. E. CATSMAN-BERREVOETS, AND O. DANN. Fluorescent retrograde neuronal labeling in rat by means of substances binding specifically to adenine-thymine rich DNA. *Neurosci. Lett.* 12: 235–240, 1979.
41. BENTIVOGLIO, M., D. VAN DER KOOY, AND H. G. J. M. KUYPERS. The organization of the efferent projections of the substantia nigra in the rat: a retrograde fluorescent double labeling study. *Brain Res.* 174: 1–17, 1979.
42. BERAN, R. L., AND G. F. MARTIN. Reticulospinal fibers of the opossum, *Didelphis virginiana*. I. Origin. *J. Comp. Neurol.* 141: 453–466, 1971.
43. BERGER, A. J. Dorsal respiratory group neurons in the medulla of cat: spinal projections, responses to lung inflation and superior laryngeal nerve stimulation. *Brain Res.* 135: 231–254, 1977.
44. BERKLEY, K. J., AND D. C. MASH. Somatic sensory projections to the pretectum in the cat. *Brain Res.* 158: 445–449, 1978.
45. BERMAN, A. L. *The Brain Stem of the Cat. A Cytoarchitectonic Atlas with Stereotaxic Coordinates.* Madison: Univ. of Wisconsin Press, 1968.
46. BERMAN, N. Connections of the pretectum in the cat. *J. Comp. Neurol.* 174: 227–254, 1977.
47. BERNHARD, C. G., AND E. BOHM. Cortical representation and functional significance of the cortico-motoneuronal system. *Arch. Neurol. Psychiatry* 72: 473–502, 1954.
48. BERNHARD, C. G., E. BOHM, AND I. PETERSEN. Investigations on the organization of the corticospinal system in monkeys (*Macaca mulatta*). *Acta Physiol. Scand.* 29 Suppl. 106: 79–105, 1953.
49. BERNHARD, C. G., AND B. REXED. The localization of the premotor interneurons discharging through the peroneal nerve. *J. Neurophysiol.* 8: 387–392, 1945.
50. BERNSTEIN, J. J. Relationship of cortico-spinal tract growth to age and body weight in the rat. *J. Comp. Neurol.* 127: 207–218, 1966.
51. BERREVOETS, C. E., AND H. G. J. M. KUYPERS. Pericruciate cortical neurons projecting to brain stem reticular formation, dorsal column nuclei and spinal cord in the cat. *Neurosci. Lett.* 1: 257–262, 1975.
52. BEUSEKOM, G. T. *Fibre Analysis of the Anterior and Lateral Funiculi of the Cord in the Cat.* Leiden: Eduardo Ydo, 1955.
53. BIANCHI, A. L. Localisation et étude des neurones respiratoires bulbaires. Mise en jeu antidromique par stimulation spinale ou vagale. *J. Physiol. Paris* 63: 5–40, 1971.
54. BIEDENBACH, M. A., AND A. L. TOWE. Fiber spectrum and functional properties of pyramidal tract neurons in the American opossum. *J. Comp. Neurol.* 140: 421–430, 1970.
55. BIENFANG, D. C. Location of the cell bodies of the superior rectus and inferior oblique motoneurons in the cat. *Exp. Neurol.* 21: 455–466, 1968.
56. BIENFANG, D. C. The course of direct projections from the abducens nucleus to the contralateral medial rectus subdivision of the oculomotor nucleus in the cat. *Brain Res.* 145: 277–289, 1978.
57. BJORKLUND, A., O. LINDVALL, AND L. A. SVENSSON. Mechanisms of fluorophore formation in the histochemical glyoxylic acid method for monoamines. *Histochemie* 32: 113–131, 1972.
58. BJORKLUND, A., AND G. SKAGERBERG. Evidence for a major spinal cord projection from the diencephalic A11 dopamine cell group in the rat using transmitter-specific fluorescent retrograde tracing. *Brain Res.* 177: 170–176, 1979.
59. BJORKLUND, A., AND G. SKAGERBERG. Simultaneous use of retrograde fluorescent tracers and fluorescence histochemistry for convenient and precise mapping of monoaminergic projections and collateral arrangements in the CNS. *J. Neurosci. Methods* 1: 261–277, 1979.
60. BLESSING, W. W., AND J. P. CHALMERS. Direct projection of catecholamine (presumably dopamine)-containing neurons from hypothalamus to spinal cord. *Neurosci. Lett.* 11: 35–40, 1979.
61. BLESSING, W. W., J. P. CHALMERS, AND P. R. C. HOWE. Distribution of catecholamine-containing cell bodies in the rabbit central nervous system. *J. Comp. Neurol.* 179: 407–424, 1978.
62. BLUM, B. Microphysiological characterization of output channels and of impulse propagation from the sensorimotor cortex. Including through pyramidal tract collaterals to the center median nucleus of the cat and of the monkey. *Int. J. Neurol.* 8: 178–189, 1971.
63. BLUM, B., L. M. HALPERN, AND A. A. WARD. Microelectrode studies of the afferent connections and efferent projections of neurons in the sensorimotor cortex of the cat. *Exp. Neurol.* 20: 156–173, 1968.
64. BODIAN, D. A new method for staining nerve fibers and nerve endings in mounted paraffin sections. *Anat. Rec.* 65: 89–97, 1936.
65. BODIAN, D. Spinal projections of brain stem in rhesus monkey, deduced from retrograde chromatolysis. *Anat. Rec.* 94: 512–513, 1946.
66. BOK, S. T. Das Rückenmark. In: *Handbuch der mikroskopischen Anatomie des Menschen*, edited by W. von Mollendorf. Berlin: Springer-Verlag, 1928, p. 478–578.
67. BRECH, A. J., G. GORDON, AND T. P. S. POWELL. Corticofugal cells responding antidromically to stimulation of the cuneate or gracile nuclei of the cat. *Brain Res.* 128: 39–52, 1977.

68. BRINK, E. E., J. I. MORRELL, AND D. W. PFAFF. Localization of lumbar epaxial motoneurons in the rat. *Brain Res.* 170: 23-41, 1979.
69. BRODAL, A. Modification of Gudden method for study of cerebral localization. *Arch. Neurol. Psychiatry* 43: 46-58, 1940.
70. BRODAL, A. Anatomy of the vestibular nuclei and their connections. In: *Handbook of Sensory Physiology, Vestibular System, Basic Mechanisms*, edited by H. H. Kornhuber. Berlin: Springer-Verlag, 1974, vol. 6, pt. 1, p. 239-352.
71. BRODAL, A. *The Reticular Formation of the Brain Stem. Anatomical Aspects and Functional Correlations*. London: Oliver & Boyd, 1957.
72. BRODAL, A., AND A. GOGSTAD. Rubro-cerebellar connexions. An experimental study in the cat. *Anat. Rec.* 118: 455-485, 1954.
73. BRODAL, A., AND O. POMPEIANO. The vestibular nuclei in the cat. *J. Anat.* 91: 438-454, 1957.
74. BRODAL, A., AND O. POMPEIANO. The origin of ascending fibers of the medial longitudinal fasciculus from the vestibular nuclei. An experimental study in the cat. *Acta Morphol. Neerl. Scand.* 1: 306-328, 1958.
75. BRODAL, A., T. SZABO, AND A. TORVIK. Corticofugal fibers to sensory trigeminal nuclei and nucleus of solitary tract. An experimental study in the cat. *J. Comp. Neurol.* 106: 527-552, 1956.
76. BRODAL, A., E. TABER, AND F. WALBERG. The raphe nuclei of the brain stem in the cat. II. Efferent connections. *J. Comp. Neurol.* 114: 239-259, 1960.
77. BRODAL, A., F. WALBERG, AND E. TABER. The raphe nuclei of the brain stem in the cat. III. Afferent connections. *J. Comp. Neurol.* 114: 261-279, 1960.
78. BROERE, G. *Corticofugal Fibers in Some Mammals. An Experimental Study with Special Emphasis on the Cortico-Spinal System*. Oegstgeest, The Netherlands: De Kempenaer, 1971.
79. BROWN, L. T. Projections and termination of the corticospinal tract in rodents. *Exp. Brain Res.* 13: 432-450, 1971.
80. BROWN, L. T. Corticorubral projections in the rat. *J. Comp. Neurol.* 154: 149-168, 1974.
81. BROWN, L. T. Rubrospinal projections in the rat. *J. Comp. Neurol.* 154: 169-188, 1974.
82. BRYAN, R. N., D. L. TREVINO, AND W. D. WILLIS. Evidence for a common location of alpha and gamma motoneurons. *Brain Res.* 38: 193-196, 1972.
83. BUCHER, V. M., AND S. M. BÜRGI. Some observations on the fiber connections of the di- and mesencephalon in the cat. II. Fiber connections of the pretectal region and the posterior commissure. *J. Comp. Neurol.* 96: 139-177, 1952.
84. BUMKE, O. C. E. Ueber Variationen im Verlauf der Pyramidenbahn. *Arch. Psychiatr. Nervenkr.* 42: 1-18, 1907.
85. BUNT, A. H., R. D. LUND, AND J. S. LUND. Retrograde axonal transport of horseradish peroxidase by ganglion cells of albino rat retina. *Brain Res.* 73: 215-228, 1974.
86. BÜRGI, S. Ueber die zentralen Haubenbahnen. Studien an der Sammlung von W. R. Hess. *Schweiz. Med. Wochenschr.* 2: 57-67, 1954.
87. BÜRGI, S. Das Tectum Opticum. Seine Verbindungen bei der Katze und seine Bedeutung beim Menschen. *Dtsch. Z. Nervenheilk.* 176: 701-729, 1957.
88. BÜRGI, S., AND V. M. BUCHER. Some fiber systems passing through the mesencephalic tegmentum in the cat. In: *Progress in Neurobiology*, edited by J. A. Kapper. Amsterdam: Elsevier 1956, p. 256-263.
89. BURKE, R. E., AND P. RUDOMIN. Spinal neurons and synapses. In: *Handbook of Physiology. The Nervous System*, edited by J. M. Brookhart and V. B. Mountcastle. Bethesda, MD: Am. Physiol. Soc., 1977, sect. 1, vol. I, pt. 2, chapt. 24, p. 877-944.
90. BURKE, R. E., P. L. STRICK, K. KANDA, C. C. KIM, AND B. WALMSLEY. Anatomy of medial gastrocnemius and soleus motor nuclei in cat spinal cord. *J. Neurophysiol.* 40: 667-680, 1977.
91. BURTON, H., AND A. D. LOEWY. Projections to the spinal cord from medullary somatosensory relay nuclei. *J. Comp. Neurol.* 173: 773-792, 1977.
92. BUSCH, H. F. M. *An Anatomical Analysis of the White Matter in the Brain Stem of the Cat*. Assen, The Netherlands: Van Gorcum, 1961.
93. BUSCH, H. F. M. Anatomical aspects of the anterior and lateral funiculi at the spinobulbar junction. In: *Progress in Brain Research. Organization of the Spinal Cord*, edited by J. C. Eccles and J. P. Schadé. Amsterdam: Elsevier, 1964, vol. 11, p. 223-235.
94. BÜTTNER-ENNEVER, J. A. Pathways from the pontine reticular formation to structures controlling horizontal and vertical eye movements in the monkey. In: *Control of Gaze by Brain Stem Neurons. Development in Neurosciences*, edited by R. Baker and A. Berthoz. Amsterdam: Elsevier/North-Holland, 1977, vol. 1, p. 89-98.
95. BUXTON, D. F., AND D. C. GOODMAN. Motor function and the corticospinal tracts in the dog and raccoon. *J. Comp. Neurol.* 129: 341-360, 1967.
96. BUYS, R. M. Intra- and extrahypothalamic vasopressin and oxytocin pathways in the rat. Pathways to the limbic system, medulla oblongata and spinal cord. *Cell Tissue Res.* 192: 423-435, 1978.
97. CAJAL, S. R. *Histologie du Système Nerveux de l'Homme et des Vertébrés*. Madrid: Instituto Ramón y Cajal, 1952.
98. CAMPBELL, C. B. G., D. YASHON, AND J. A. JANE. The origin, course and termination of corticospinal fibers in the slow loris, *Nycticelus coucang* (Boddaert). *J. Comp. Neurol.* 127: 101-112, 1966.
99. CARLSSON, A., B. FALCK, K. FUXE, AND N. A. HILLARP. Cellular localization of monoamines in the spinal cord. *Acta Physiol. Scand.* 60: 112-119, 1964.
100. CARPENTER, M. B., J. W. HARBISON, AND P. PETER. Accessory oculomotor nuclei in the monkey: projections and effects of discrete lesions. *J. Comp. Neurol.* 140: 131-154, 1970.
101. CARPENTER, M. B., AND P. PETER. Accessory oculomotor nuclei in the monkey. *J. Hirnforsch.* 12: 405-418, 1970/1971.
102. CARPENTER, M. B., AND N. L. STROMINGER. Cerebello-oculomotor fibers in the rhesus monkey. *J. Comp. Neurol.* 123: 211-230, 1964.
103. CARSTENS, E., AND D. L. TREVINO. Laminar origins of spinothalamic projections in the cat as determined by the retrograde transport of horseradish peroxidase. *J. Comp. Neurol.* 182: 151-166, 1978.
104. CASAGRANDE, V. A., J. K. HARTING, W. C. HALL, I. T. DIAMOND, AND G. F. MARTIN. Superior colliculus of the tree shrew: a structural and functional subdivision into superficial and deep layers. *Science* 177: 444-447, 1972.
105. CASTIGLIONI, A. J., M. C. GALLAWAY, AND J. D. COULTER. Origins of descending spinal connections from brain stem in money. *Soc. Neurosci. Abstr.* 3: 268, 1977.
106. CASTIGLIONI, A. J., M. C. GALLAWAY, AND J. D. COULTER. Spinal projections from the midbrain in monkey. *J. Comp. Neurol.* 178: 329-346, 1978.
107. CATSMAN-BERREVOETS, C. E., AND H. G. J. M. KUYPERS. Cells of origin of cortical projections to dorsal column nuclei, spinal cord and bulbar medial reticular formation in the rhesus monkey. *Neurosci. Lett.* 3: 245-252, 1976.
108. CATSMAN-BERREVOETS, C. E., AND H. G. J. M. KUYPERS,. Differential laminar distribution of corticothalamic neurons projecting to the VL and the center median. An HRP study in the cynomolgus monkey. *Brain Res.* 154: 359-365, 1978.
109. CATSMAN-BERREVOETS, C. E., AND H. G. J. M. KUYPERS. The location of the precentral area 4 cortical neurons projecting to thalamic VL nucleus, centre median, red nucleus, brain reticular formation, dorsal column nuclei and spinal cord in cat and monkey. *Neurosci. Lett. Suppl.* 1: 157, 1978.
110. CATSMAN-BERREVOETS, C. E., AND H. G. J. M. KUYPERS. Differences in distribution of cortico-spinal axon collaterals to thalamus and midbrain tegmentum in cat, demonstrated by means of double retrograde fluorescent labeling of cortical

neurons. *Neurosci. Lett. Suppl.* 3: 133, 1979.
111. CATSMAN-BERREVOETS, C. E., H. G. J. M. KUYPERS, AND R. N. LEMON. Cells of origin of the frontal projections to magnocellular and parvocellular red nucleus and superior colliculus in cynomolgus monkey. An HRP study. *Neurosci. Lett.* 12: 41–46, 1979.
112. CESARO, P., J. NGUYEN-LEGROS, B. BERGER, C. ALVAREZ, AND D. ALBE-FESSARD. Double labelling of branched neurons in the central nervous system of the rat by retrograde axonal transport of horseradish peroxidase and iron dextran complex. *Neurosci. Lett.* 15: 1–7, 1979.
113. CHAMBERS, W. W., AND C. N. LIU. Cortico-spinal tract of the cat. An attempt to correlate the pattern of degeneration with deficits in reflex activity following neocortical lesions. *J. Comp. Neurol.* 108: 23–55, 1957.
114. CHAN-PALAY, V. *Cerebellar Dentate Nucleus: Organization, Cytology and Transmitters.* Berlin: Springer-Verlag, 1977.
115. CHEEK, M. D., A. RUSTIONI, AND D. L. TREVINO. Dorsal column nuclei projections to the cerebellar cortex in cats as revealed by the use of the retrograde transport of horseradish peroxidase. *J. Comp. Neurol.* 164: 31–46, 1975.
116. CHU, N. S., AND F. E. BLOOM. The catecholamine-containing neurons in the cat dorsolateral pontine tegmentum: distribution of the cell bodies and some axonal projections. *Brain Res.* 66: 1–21, 1974.
117. CHUNG, J. M., K. CHUNG, AND R. D. WURSTER. Sympathetic preganglionic neurons of the cat spinal cord: horseradish peroxidase study. *Brain Res.* 91: 126–131, 1975.
118. CHUNG, K., J. M. CHUNG, F. W. LAVELLE, AND R. D. WURSTER. Sympathetic neurons in the cat spinal cord projecting to the stellate ganglion. *J. Comp. Neurol.* 185: 23–30, 1979.
119. CIRELLO, J., AND F. R. CALARESU. Descending hypothalamic pathways with cardiovascular function in the cat: a silver impregnation study. *Exp. Neurol.* 57: 561–580, 1977.
120. CLOUGH, J. F. M., C. G. PHILLIPS, AND J. D. SHERIDAN. The short-latency projection from the baboon's motor cortex to fusimotor neurones of the forearm and hand. *J. Physiol. London* 216: 257–279, 1971.
121. COHEN, D., W. W. CHAMBERS, AND J. M. SPRAGUE. Experimental study of the efferent projections from the cerebellar nuclei to the brain stem of the cat. *J. Comp. Neurol.* 109: 233–259, 1958.
122. COHEN, F. L. Effects of various lesions on crossed and uncrossed descending inspiratory pathways in the cervical spinal cord of the cat. *J. Neurosurg.* 39: 589–595, 1973.
123. COLONNIER, M. Experimental degeneration in the cerebral cortex. *J. Anat.* 98: 47–53, 1964.
124. COLONNIER, M., AND E. G. GRAY. Degeneration in the cerebral cortex. In: *Electronmicroscopy*, edited by S. S. Breese, Jr. New York: Academic, 1962, vol. 2 p. 113–114. (Int. Congr. Electronmicroscopy, 5th, 1962.)
125. COMMISSIONG, J. W., S. O. HELLSTRÖM, AND N. H. NEFF. A new projection from locus coeruleus to the spinal ventral columns: histochemical and biochemical evidence. *Brain Res.* 148: 207–213, 1978.
126. CONRAD, L. C. A., AND D. W. PFAFF. Efferents from medial basal forebrain and hypothalamus in the rat. II. An autoradiographic study of the anterior hypothalamus. *J. Comp. Neurol.* 169: 221–261, 1976.
127. CONRADI, S., J. O. KELLERTH, AND C. H. BERTHOLD. Electron microscopic studies of serially sectioned cat spinal α-motoneurons. II. A method for the description of architecture and synaptology of the cell body and proximal dendritic segments. *J. Comp. Neurol.* 184: 741–754, 1979.
128. COOTE, J. H., AND V. H. MACLEOD. The influence of bulbospinal monoaminergic pathways on sympathetic nerve activity. *J. Phyisol. London* 241: 453–475, 1974.
129. CORAZZA, R., E. FADIGA, AND P. L. PERMEGGIANI. Patterns of pyramidal activation of cat's motoneurons. *Arch. Ital. Biol.* 101: 337–364, 1963.
130. COULTER, J. D., L. EWING, AND C. CARTER. Origin of primary sensorimotor cortical projections to lumbar spinal cord of cat and monkey. *Brain Res.* 103: 366–372, 1976.
131. COULTER, J. D., AND E. G. JONES. Differential distribution of corticospinal projections from individual cytoarchitectonic fields in the monkey. *Brain Res.* 129: 335–340, 1977.
132. COURVILLE, J. The nucleus of the facial nerve. The relation between cellular groups and peripheral branches of the nerve. *Brain Res.* 1: 338–354, 1966.
133. COURVILLE, J. Rubrobulbar fibres to the facial nucleus and the lateral reticular nucleus (nucleus of the lateral funiculus). An experimental study in the cat with silver impregnation methods. *Brain Res.* 1: 317–337, 1966.
134. COURVILLE, J. Somatotopical organization of the projection from the nucleus interpositus anterior of the cerebellum to the red nucleus. An experimental study in the cat with silver impregnation methods. *Exp. Brain Res.* 2: 191–215, 1966.
135. COURVILLE, J., AND A. BRODAL. Rubro-cerebellar connections in the cat: an experimental study with silver impregnation methods. *J. Comp. Neurol.* 126: 471–486, 1966.
136. COURVILLE, J., AND S. OTABE. The rubro-olivary projection in the macaque: an experimental study with silver impregnation methods. *J. Comp. Neurol.* 158: 479–495, 1974.
137. COWAN, W. M., D. I. GOTTLIEB, A. E. HENDRICKSON, J. L. PRICE, AND T. A. WOOLSEY. The autoradiographic demonstration of axonal connections in the central nervous system. *Brain Res.* 37: 21–51, 1972.
138. CREVEL, H., AND W. J. C. VERHAART. The "exact" origin of the pyramidal tract. A quantitative study in the cat. *J. Anat.* 97: 495–515, 1963.
139. CREVEL, H., AND W. J. C. VERHAART. The rate of secondary degeneration in the central nervous system. 1. Pyramidal tract of the cat. *J. Anat.* 97: 429–464, 1963.
140. CRUTCHER, K. A., AND A. O. HUMBERTSON. The organization of monoamine neurons within the brain stem of the North American opossum (*Didelphis virginiana*). *J. Comp. Neurol.* 179: 195–222, 1978.
141. CRUTCHER, K. A., A. O. HUMBERTSON, AND G. F. MARTIN. The origin of brain stem spinal pathways in the North American opossum (*Didelphis virginiana*). Studies using horseradish peroxidase method. *J. Comp. Neurol.* 179: 169–194, 1978.
142. CULLHEIM, S., AND J.-O. KELLERTH. Combined light and electron microscopic tracing of neurons, including axons and synaptic terminals, after intracellular injection of horseradish peroxidase. *Neurosci. Lett.* 2: 307–313, 1976.
143. CUMMINGS, J. P., AND D. L. FELTEN. A raphe dendrite bundle in the rabbit medulla. *J. Comp. Neurol.* 183: 1–24, 1979.
144. CZARKOWSKA, J., E. JANKOWSKA, AND E. SYBIRSKA. Axonal projections of spinal interneurones excited by group I afferents in the cat, revealed by intracellular staining with horseradish peroxidase. *Brain Res.* 118: 115–118, 1976.
145. DAHLSTRÖM, A., AND K. FUXE. Evidence for the existence of monoamine-containing neurons in the central nervous system. I. Demonstration of monoamines in the cell bodies of brain stem neurons. *Acta Physiol. Scand.* 62 Suppl. 232: 5–55, 1964.
146. DAHLSTRÖM, A., AND K. FUXE. Evidence for the existence of monoamine neurons in the central nervous system. II. Experimentally induced changes in the intraneuronal amine levels of bulbospinal neuron systems. *Acta Physiol. Scand.* 64 Suppl. 247: 6–36, 1965.
147. DALSGAARD, C. J., AND L. G. ELFVIN. Spinal origin of preganglionic fibers projecting onto the superior cervical ganglion and inferior mesenteric ganglion of the guinea pig, as demonstrated by the horseradish peroxidase technique. *Brain Res.* 172: 139–144, 1979.
148. DARIAN-SMITH, I., G. PHILLIPS, AND R. D. RYAN. Functional organization in trigeminal main sensory and rostral spinal nuclei of the cat. *J. Physiol. London* 168: 129–146, 1963.
149. DART, A. M. Cells of the dorsal column nuclei projecting down into the spinal cord. *J. Physiol. London* 219: 29P–31P, 1971.
150. DE GROAT, W. C., I. NADELHAFT, C. MORGAN, AND T. SCHAUBLE. Horseradish peroxidase tracing of visceral efferent and

primary afferent pathways in the cat's sacral spinal cord using benzidine processing. *Neurosci. Lett.* 10: 103-108, 1978.
151. DEJERINE, J. *Anatomie des Centres Nerveux.* Paris: Rueff, 1901.
152. DEKKER, J. J., AND H. G. J. M. KUYPERS. Quantitative EM study of projection terminals in the rat's AV thalamic nucleus. Autoradiographic and degeneration techniques compared. *Brain Res.* 117: 399-422, 1976.
153. DEKKER, J. J., D. G. LAWRENCE, AND H. G. J. M. KUYPERS. The location of longitudinally running dendrites in the ventral horn of the cat spinal cord. *Brain Res.* 51: 319-325, 1973.
154. DEMIRJIAN, C., R. GROSSMAN, R. MEYER, AND R. KATZMAN. The catecholamine pontine cellular groups locus coeruleus, A4, subcoeruleus in the primate *Cebus apella. Brain Res.* 115: 395-411, 1976.
155. DENNY-BROWN, D. *The Cerebral Control of Movement.* Springfield, IL: Thomas, 1966.
156. DENNY-BROWN, D., AND E. H. BOTTERELL. The motor functions of the agranular frontal cortex. *Res. Publ. Assoc. Nerv. Ment. Dis.* 27: 235-345, 1948.
157. DE OLMOS, J. A cupric-silver method for impregnation of terminal axon degeneration and its further use in staining granular argyrophilic structures. *Brain Behav. Evol.* 2: 213-237, 1969.
158. DE OLMOS, J., AND L. HEIMER. Mapping of collateral projections with the HRP method. *Neurosci. Lett.* 6: 107-114, 1977.
159. DE ROBERTIS, E. Submicroscopic changes of the synapse after nerve section in the acoustic ganglion of the guinea pig. An electron microscope study. *J. Biophys. Biochem Cytol.* 2: 503-512, 1956.
160. DESANTIS, M., V. LIMWONGSE, AND D. RIGAMONTI. Somatotopy in the trigeminal motor nucleus of the rat: field potentials recorded in the neuron pool after retrograde transport of horseradish peroxidase. *Neurosci. Lett.* 10: 95-98, 1978.
161. DESCHENES, M. Dual origin of fibers projecting from motor cortex to S1 in cat. *Brain Res.* 132: 159-162, 1977.
162. DESTOMBES, J., AND J. P. RIPERT. Ultrastructural observations of the abducens nucleus of the cat after injection of horseradish peroxidase into the lateral rectus muscle. *Exp. Brain Res.* 28: 63-71, 1977.
163. DEUSCHL, G., AND M. ILLERT. Location of lumbar preganglionic sympathetic neurones in the cat. *Neurosci. Lett.* 10: 49-54, 1978.
164. DE VITO, J. L. Projections from the cerebral cortex to the intralaminar nuclei in the monkey. *J. Comp. Neurol.* 136: 193-201, 1969.
165. DE VITO, J. L., AND O. A. SMITH. Subcortical projections of the prefrontal lobe of the monkey. *J. Comp. Neurol.* 123: 413-424, 1964.
166. DILLY, P. N., P. D. WALL, AND K. E. WEBSTER. Cells of origin of the spinothalamic tract in the cat and rat. *Exp. Neurol.* 21: 550-562, 1968.
167. DOM, R., W. FALLS, AND G. F. MARTIN. The motor nucleus of the facial nerve in the opossum (*Didelphis marsupialis virginiana*) its organization and connections. *J. Comp. Neurol.* 152: 373-402, 1973.
168. DONATELLE, J. M. Growth of the corticospinal tract and the development of placing reactions in the postnatal rat. *J. Comp. Neurol.* 175: 207-232, 1977.
169. DROZ, B., AND C. P. LEBLOND. Axonal migration of proteins in the central nervous system and peripheral nerves as shown by autoradiography. *J. Comp. Neurol.* 121: 325-346, 1963.
170. DUNKERLEY, G. B., AND D. DUNCAN. A light and electron microscopic study of the normal and the degenerating corticospinal tract in the rat. *J. Comp. Neurol.* 137: 155-184, 1969.
171. DURON, B., N. MARLOT, N. LARNICOL, M. C. JUNG-CAILLOL, AND J. M. MACRON. Somatotopy in the phrenic motor nucleus of the cat as revealed by retrograde transport of horseradish peroxidase. *Neurosci. Lett.* 14: 159-163, 1979.
172. ECCLES, J. C., R. A. NICOLL, T. RANTUCCI, H. TÁBOŘÍKOVÁ, AND T. J. WILLEY. Topographic studies on medial reticular nucleus. *J. Neurophysiol.* 39: 109-118, 1976.
173. ECCLES, J. C., T. RANTUCCI, P. SCHEID, AND H. TÁBOŘÍKOVÁ. Somatotopic studies on red nucleus: spinal projection level and respective receptive fields. *J. Neurophysiol.* 38: 965-980, 1975.
174. EDWARDS, S. B. The ascending and descending projections of the red nucleus in the cat: an experimental study using an autoradiographic tracing method. *Brain Res.* 48: 45-63, 1972.
175. EDWARDS, S. B. Autoradiographic studies of the projections of the midbrain reticular formation: descending projections of nucleus cuneiformis. *J. Comp. Neurol.* 161: 341-358, 1975.
176. EDWARDS, S. B., AND C. K. HENKEL. Superior colliculus connections with the extraocular motor nuclei in the cat. *J. Comp. Neurol.* 179: 451-467, 1978.
177. ELGER, C. E., E. J. SPECKMAN, H. CASPERS, AND R. W. C. JANZEN. Corticospinal connections in the rat. I. Monosynaptic and polysynaptic responses of cervical motoneurons to epicortical stimulation. *Exp. Brain Res.* 28: 385-404, 1977.
178. ENDO, K., T. ARAKI, AND N. YAGI. The distribution and pattern of axon branching of pyramidal tract cells. *Brain Res.* 57: 484-491, 1973.
179. ENGBERG, I., A. LUNDBERG, AND R. W. RYALL. Reticulospinal inhibition of transmission in reflex pathways. *J. Physiol. London* 194: 201-223, 1968.
180. ERULKAR, S. D., J. M. SPRAGUE, B. L. WHITSEL, S. DOGAN, AND P. J. JANNETTA. Organization of the vestibular projection to the spinal cord of the cat. *J. Neurophysiol.* 29: 626-664, 1966.
181. EULER, C., J. N. HAYWARD, I. MARTILLA, AND R. J. WYMAN. The spinal connections of the inspiratory neurones of the ventrolateral nucleus of the cat's solitarius. *Brain Res.* 61: 23-33, 1973.
182. FADEN, A. I., AND J. M. PETRAS. An intraspinal sympathetic preganglionic pathway: anatomical evidence in the dog. *Brain Res.* 144: 358-362, 1978.
183. FALCK, B., N. A. HILLARP, G. THIEME, AND A. TORP. Fluorescence of catecholamines and related compounds condensed with formaldehyde. *J. Histochem. Cytochem.* 10: 348-354, 1962.
184. FANARDJAN, V. V., AND D. S. SARKISJAN. Intracellular investigation of antidromic and synaptic activation of red nucleus neurons in the cat. *Sechenov Physiol. J. USSR* 55: 121-131, 1969.
185. FAULKNER, R. F., AND J. E. HYDE. Coordinated eye and body movements evoked by brainstem stimulation in decerebrated cats. *J. Neurophysiol.* 21: 171-182, 1958.
186. FAULL, R. L. M. The cerebellofugal projections in the brachium conjunctivum of the rat. II. The ipsilateral and contralateral descending pathways. *J. Comp. Neurol.* 178: 519-536, 1978.
187. FAULL, R. L. M., AND J. B. CARMAN. The cerebellofugal projections in the brachium conjunctivum of the rat. I. The contralateral ascending pathway. *J. Comp. Neurol.* 178: 495-518, 1978.
188. FELIX, D., AND M. WIESENDANGER. Pyramidal and non-pyramidal motor cortical effects on distal forelimb muscles of monkeys. *Exp. Brain Res.* 12: 81-91, 1971.
189. FELTEN, D. L., AND J. P. CUMMINGS. The raphe nuclei of the rabbit brain stem. *J. Comp. Neurol.* 187: 199-244, 1979.
190. FELTEN, D. L., A. M. LATIES, AND M. B. CARPENTER. Monoamine-containing cell bodies in the squirrel monkey brain. *Am. J. Anat.* 139: 153-166, 1974.
191. FETZ, E. E., P. D. CHENEY, AND D. C. GERMAN. Corticomotoneuronal connections of precentral cells detected by postspike averages of EMG activity in behaving monkeys. *Brain Res.* 114: 505-510, 1976.
192. FIELDS, H. L., A. I. BASBAUM, C. H. CLANTON, AND S. D. ANDERSON. Nucleus raphe magnus inhibition of spinal cord dorsal horn neurons. *Brain Res.* 126: 441-453, 1977.
193. FINK, R. P., AND L. HEIMER. Two methods for selective silver impregnation of degenerating axons and their synaptic endings in the central nervous system. *Brain Res.* 4: 369-374, 1967.
194. FISHER, A. M., J. K. HARTING, G. F. MARTIN, AND M. I. STUBER. The origin, course and termination of corticospinal fibers in the armadillo (*Dasypus novemcinctus mexicanus*). *J. Neurol. Sci.* 8: 347-361, 1969.

195. FLINDT-EGEBAK, P. Autoradiographical demonstration of the projections from the limb areas of the feline sensorimotor cortex to the spinal cord. *Brain Res.* 136: 153-156, 1977.
196. FLUMERFELT, B. A., AND P. R. LEWIS. Cholinesterase activity in the hypoglossal nucleus of the rat and changes produced by axotomy: a light and electron microscopic study. *J. Anat.* 119: 309-331, 1975.
197. FLUMERFELT, B. A., S. OTABE, AND J. COURVILLE. Distinct projections to the red nucleus from the dentate and interposed nuclei in the monkey. *Brain Res.* 50: 408-414, 1973.
198. FOX, J. E. Reticulospinal neurones in the rat. *Brain Res.* 23: 35-40, 1970.
199. FRANKFURTER, A., J. T. WEBER, G. J. ROYCE, N. L. STROMINGER, AND J. K. HARTING. An autoradiographic analysis of the tecto-olivary projection in primates. *Brain Res.* 118: 245-257, 1976.
200. FUKUSHIMA, K., N. HIRAI, AND S. RAPOPORT. Direct excitation of neck flexor motoneurones by the interstitiospinal tract. *Brain Res.* 160: 358-362, 1979.
201. FUKUSHIMA, K., B. W. PETERSON, Y. UCHINO, J. D. COULTER, AND V. J. WILSON. Direct fastigiospinal fibers in the cat. *Brain Res.* 126: 538-542, 1977.
202. FUKUSHIMA, K., N. G. PITTS, AND B. W. PETERSON. Responses of neck motoneurons to stimulation of the interstitial nucleus of Cajal. *Soc. Neurosci. Abstr.* 3: 154, 1977.
203. FUKUSHIMA, T., AND F. W. L. KERR. Organization of trigeminothalamic tracts and other thalamic afferent systems of brainstem in the rat: presence of gelatinosa neurons with thalamic connections. *J. Comp. Neurol.* 183: 169-184, 1979.
204. FUKUYAMA, U. Ueber eine substantielle Verschmelzung des roten Kerns mit den Nebenokulomotoriuskernen (Bechterew und Darkschewitsch) bei Affen. *Arb. Anat. Inst. Kais. Jpn. Univ. Sendai* 23: 1-122, 1940.
205. FULTON, J. F., AND D. SHEEHAN. Uncrossed lateral pyramidal tract in higher primates. *J. Anat.* 69: 181-187, 1935.
205a. FUTAMI, T., Y. SHINODA, AND J. YOKOTA. Spinal axon collaterals of corticospinal neurons identified by intracellular injection of horseradish peroxidase. *Brain Res.* 164: 279-284, 1979.
206. FUXE, K. Evidence for the existence of monoamine-containing neurons in the central nervous system. IV. The distribution of monoamine terminals in the central nervous system. *Acta. Physiol. Scand.* 64 Suppl. 247: 37-85, 1965.
207. GACEK, R. R. Localization of neurons supplying the extraocular muscles in the kitten using horseradish peroxidase. *Exp. Neurol.* 44: 381-403, 1974.
208. GALL, F. J., AND C. SPURZHEIM. *Anatomie et Physiologie du Système Nerveux en Général et du Cerveaux en Particulier.* Paris: Schoell, 1810-1819, vols I, II.
209. GALLAWAY, M. C., A. J. CASTIGLIONI, R. D. FOREMAN, AND J. D. COULTER. Origins of spinal projections from the caudal medulla in monkey. *Soc. Neurosci. Abstr.* 3: 271, 1977.
210. GAREY, L. J., E. G. JONES, AND T. P. S. POWELL. Interrelationships of striate and extrastriate cortex with the primary relay sites of the visual pathway. *J. Neurol. Neurosurg. Psychiatry* 31: 135-157, 1968.
211. GARVER, D. L., AND J. R. SLADEK. Monoamine distribution in primate brain. I. Catecholamine-containing perikarya in the brain stem of *Macaca speciosa*. *J. Comp. Neurol.* 159: 289-304, 1975.
212. GEFFEN, L. Biochemical and histochemical methods of tracing transmitter-specific neuronal molecules. In: *The Use of Axonal Transport for Studies of Neuronal Connectivity*, edited by M. Cowan and M. Cuénod. Amsterdam: Elsevier, 1975, p. 307-346.
213. GHEZ, C. Input-output relations of the red nucleus in the cat. *Brain Res.* 98: 93-108, 1975.
214. GILBERT, C. D., AND J. P. KELLY. The projections of cells in different layers of the cat's visual cortex. *J. Comp. Neurol.* 163: 81-105, 1975.
215. GIOK, S. P. *Localization of Fibre Systems Within the White Matter of the Medulla Oblongata and the Cervical Cord in Man*. Leiden: Eduardo Ydo, 1956.
216. GIOVANELLI-BARILARI, M., AND H. G. J. M. KUYPERS. Propriospinal fibers interconnecting the spinal enlargements in the cat. *Brain Res.* 14: 321-330, 1969.
217. GLEES, P. Terminal degeneration within the central nervous system as studied by a new silver method. *J. Neuropathol. Exp. Neurol.* 5: 54-59, 1946.
218. GLEES, P. *Experimental Neurology*. Oxford: Clarendon Press, 1961.
219. GOBEL, S., AND W. M. FALLS. Anatomical observations of horseradish peroxidase-filled terminal primary axonal arborizations in layer II of the substantia gelatinosa of Rolando. *Brain Res.* 175: 335-340, 1979.
220. GOEBEL, H. H., A. KOMATZUZAKI, M. B. BENDER, AND B. COHEN. Lesions of the pontine tegmentum and conjugate gaze paralysis. *Arch. Neurol. Chicago* 24: 431-440, 1971.
221. GOLDBY, F. An experimental investigation of the motor cortex and pyramidal tract of *Echidna aculeata*. *J. Anat.* 73: 509-524, 1939.
222. GOLDBY, F., AND G. N. KACKER. A survey of the pyramidal system in the coypu rat, *Myocastor coypus*. *J. Anat.* 97: 517-531, 1963.
223. GOLDMAN, P. S., AND W. J. H. NAUTA. Autoradiographic demonstration of a projection from the prefrontal association cortex to the superior colliculus in the rhesus monkey. *Brain Res.* 116: 145-149, 1976.
224. GOLDMAN, P. S., AND W. J. H. NAUTA. An intricately patterned prefrontocaudate projection in the rhesus monkey. *J. Comp. Neurol.* 171: 369-385, 1977.
225. GOODE, G. E., AND D. E. HAINES. Origin, course and termination of corticospinal fibers in a prosimian primate (*Galago*). *Brain Behav. Evol.* 12: 334-361, 1975.
226. GOODE, G. E., AND M. STREESAI. An electron microscopic study of rubrospinal projections to the lumbar spinal cord of the opossum. *Brain Res.* 143: 61-70, 1978.
227. GOODMAN, D. C., L. E. JARRARD, AND J. F. NELSON. Corticospinal pathways and their sites of termination in the albino rat. *Anat. Rec.* 154: 462-463, 1966.
228. GORDON, G., AND C. H. PAINE. Functional organization in nucleus gracilis of the cat. *J. Physiol. London* 153: 331-349, 1961.
229. GORSKA, T., AND E. SYBIRSKA. Effects of red nucleus and pyramidal lesions on forelimb movements in cats. *Neurosci. Lett. Suppl.* 1: 127, 1978.
230. GRAFSTEIN, B. Axonal transport: the intracellular traffic of the neuron. In: *Handbook of Physiology. The Nervous System*, edited by J. M. Brookhart and V. B. Mountcastle. Bethesda, MD: Am. Physiol. Soc., 1977, sect. 1, vol. I, pt. 1, chapt. 19, p. 691-717.
231. GRAHAM, J. An autoradiographic study of the efferent connections of the superior colliculus in the cat. *J. Comp. Neurol.* 173: 629-654, 1977.
232. GRAHAM, R. C., AND M. J. KARNOVSKY. The early stages of absorption of injected horseradish peroxidase in the proximal tubules of mouse kidney: ultra-structural cytochemistry by a new technique. *J. Histochem. Cytochem.* 14: 291-302, 1966.
233. GRAY, E. G., AND L. H. HAMLYN. Electron microscopy of experimental degeneration in the avian optic tectum. *J. Anat. London* 96: 309-316, 1962.
234. GRAYBIEL, A. M. Anatomical organization of retinotectal afferents in the cat: an autoradiographic study. *Brain Res.* 96: 1-23, 1975.
235. GRAYBIEL, A. M. Some efferents of pretectal region in cat. *Anat. Rec.* 178: 365, 1974.
236. GRAYBIEL, A. M. Wallerian degeneration and anterograde tracer methods. In: *The Use of Axonal Transport for Studies of Neuronal Connectivity*, edited by M. Cowan and M. Cuénod. Amsterdam: Elsevier, 1975, p. 173-216.
237. GRAYBIEL, A. M. Direct and indirect preoculomotor pathways of the brainstem: an autoradiographic study of the pontine reticular formation in the cat. *J. Comp. Neurol.* 175: 37-78, 1977.
238. GRAYBIEL, A. M. Organization of oculomotor pathways in the cat and rhesus monkey. In: *Control of Gaze by Brain Stem*

Neurons. Development in Neurosciences, edited by R. Baker and A. Berthoz. Amsterdam: Elsevier/North-Holland, 1977, vol. 1, p. 79–88.
239. GRAYBIEL, A. M., AND E. A. HARTWIEG. Some afferent connections of the oculomotor complex in the cat: an experimental study with tracer techniques. Brain Res. 81: 543–551, 1974.
240. GRAYBIEL, A. M., H. J. W. NAUTA, R. J. LASEK, AND W. J. H. NAUTA. A cerebello-olivary pathway in the cat: an experimental study using autoradiographic tracing techniques. Brain Res. 58: 205–211, 1973.
241. GRIFFIN, G., L. R. WATKINS, AND D. J. MAYER. HRP pellets and slow-release gels: two new techniques for greater localization and sensitivity. Brain Res. 168: 595–601, 1979.
242. GRILLNER, S., T. HONGO, AND S. LUND. Interaction between inhibitory pathways from the Deiter's nucleus and 1a afferents to flexor motoneurons. Acta Physiol. Scand. 68 Suppl. 277: 61, 1966.
243. GRILLNER, S., T. HONGO, AND S. LUND. Reciprocal effects between two descending bulbospinal systems with monosynaptic connections to spinal motoneurons. Brain Res. 10: 477–480, 1968.
244. GRILLNER, S., T. HONGO, AND S. LUND. The vestibulospinal tract. Effects on alpha-motoneurons in the lumbosacral cord in cat. Exp. Brain Res. 10: 94–120, 1970.
245. GRILLNER, S., AND S. LUND. The origin of a descending pathway with monosynaptic action on flexor motoneurons. Acta Physiol. Scand. 74: 274–284, 1968.
246. GROOS, W. P., L. K. EWING, C. M. CARTER, AND J. D. COULTER. Organization of corticospinal neurons in the cat. Brain Res. 143: 393–419, 1978.
247. GUILBAUD, G., J. L. OLIVERAS, G. GIESLER, JR., AND J. M. BESSON. Effects induced by stimulation of the centralis inferior nucleus of the raphe on dorsal horn interneurons in cat's spinal cord. Brain Res. 126: 335–360, 1977.
248. GUREVITCH, N. R., AND T. V. BELOZEROVA. Rubrospinal synaptic influences on lumbar motoneurons in the rat. Neurophysiology USSR 3: 274–284, 1971.
249. GWYN, D. G. Acetylcholinesterase activity in the red nucleus of the rat. Effects of rubrospinal tractotomy. Brain Res. 35: 447–461, 1971.
250. GWYN, D. G., AND B. A. FLUMERFELT. A comparison of the distribution of cortical and cerebellar afferents in red nucleus of the rat. Brain Res. 69: 130–135, 1974.
251. GWYN, D. G., AND J. H. WOLSTENCROFT. Ascending and descending cholinergic fibers in cat spinal cord: histochemical evidence. Science 153: 1543–1544, 1966.
252. HAARTSEN, A. B. Cortical Projections to Mesencephalon, Pons, Medulla Oblongata and Spinal Cord. An Experimental Study in the Goat and the Rabbit. Leiden: Eduardo Ydo, 1962.
253. HAARTSEN, A. B., AND W. J. C. VERHAART. Cortical projections to brain stem and spinal cord in the goat by way of the pyramidal tract and the bundle of Bagley. J. Comp. Neurol. 129: 189–202, 1967.
254. HAGGQVIST, G. Analyse der Faserverteilung in einem Rückenmarksquerschnitt (Th3). Z. Mikrosk. Anat. Forsch. 39: 1–34, 1936.
255. HAGGQVIST, G. Faseranalytischen Studien über die Pyramidenbahn. Acta Psychiatr. Neurol. 12: 457–466, 1937.
256. HANAWAY, J., AND J. M. SMITH. Synaptic fine structure and the termination of corticospinal fibers in the lateral basal region of the cat spinal cord. J. Comp. Neurol. 183: 471–486, 1979.
257. HANCOCK, M. B. Cells of origin of hypothalamo-spinal projections in the rat. Neurosci. Lett. 3: 179–184, 1976.
258. HANCOCK, M. B., AND C. L. FOUGEROUSSE. Spinal projections from the nucleus locus coeruleus and nucleus subcoeruleus in the cat and monkey as demonstrated by the retrograde transport of horseradish peroxidase. Brain Res. Bull. 1: 229–234, 1976.
259. HANCOCK, M. B., AND C. A. PEVETO. Preganglionic neurons in the sacral spinal cord of the rat: an HRP study. Neurosci. Lett. 11: 1–5, 1979.
260. HANKER, J. S., P. E. YATES, C. B. METZ, AND A RUSTIONI. A new specific sensitive and noncarcinogenic reagent for the demonstration of horseradish peroxidase (HRP). Histochem. J. 9: 789–792, 1977.
261. HARDY, H., AND L. HEIMER. A safer and more sensitive substitute for diaminobenzidine in the light microscopic demonstration of retrograde and anterograde axonal transport of HRP. Neurosci. Lett. 5: 235–240, 1977.
262. HARTING, J. K. Descending pathways from the superior colliculus: an autoradiographic analysis in the rhesus monkey (Macaca mulatta). J. Comp. Neurol. 173: 583–612, 1977.
263. HARTING, J. K., W. C. HALL, I. T. DIAMOND, AND G. F. MARTIN. Anterograde degeneration study of the superior colliculus in Tupaia glis: evidence for a subdivision between superficial and deep layers. J. Comp. Neurol. 148: 361–386, 1973.
264. HARTING, J. K., AND G. F. MARTIN. Neocortical projections to the pons and medulla oblongata of the nine-banded armadillo (Dasypus novemcinctus). J. Comp. Neurol. 138: 483–500, 1970.
265. HARTING, J. K., AND C. R. NOBACK. Corticospinal projections from the pre- and postcentral gyri in the squirrel monkey (Saimiri sciureus). Brain Res. 24: 322–328, 1970.
266. HARTMAN, B. K. Immunofluorescence of dopamine beta-hydroxylase: application of improved methodology to the localization of the peripheral and central noradrenergic nervous system. J. Histochem. Cyctochem. 21: 312–332, 1973.
267. HARTMAN-VON MONAKOW, K., K. AKERT, AND H. KÜNZLE. Projections of precentral and premotor cortex to the red nucleus and other midbrain areas in Macaca fascicularis. Exp. Brain Res. 34: 91–106, 1979.
268. HASHIKAWA, T., AND K. KAWAMURA. Identification of cells of origin of tectopontine fibers in the cat superior colliculus: an experimental study with the horseradish peroxidase method. Brain Res. 130: 65–79, 1977.
269. HASSLER, R. Thalamo-corticale Systeme der Körperhaltung und der Augenbewegungen. In: Structure and Function of the Cerebral Cortex, edited by D. B. Tower and J. P. Schadé. Amsterdam: Elsevier, 1960. p. 124–130. (Proc. Int. Mtng. Neurobiol., 2nd, Amsterdam, 1959.)
270. HASSLER, R., AND W. R. HESS. Experimentelle und anatomische Befunde über die Drehbewegungen und ihre nervösen Apparate. Arch. Psychiatr. Nervenkr. 192: 488–526, 1954.
271. HASSLER, R., AND K. MUHS-CLEMENT. Architektonischer Aufbau des sensomotorischen und parietalen Cortex der Katze. J. Hirnforsch. 6: 377–420, 1964.
272. HATSCHEK, R. Zur vergleichenden Anatomie des Nucleus ruber tegmenti. Arb. Neurol. Inst. Univ. Wien. 15: 89–136, 1907.
273. HAYES, N. L., AND A. RUSTIONI. Dual projections of single neurons are visualized simultaneously: use of enzymatically inactive (^{3}H) HRP. Brain Res. 165: 321–326, 1979.
274. HEFFNER, R., AND B. MASTERTON. Variation in form of the pyramidal tract and its relationship to digital dexterity. Brain Behav. Evol. 12: 161–200, 1975.
275. HENDRICKSON, A. Electronmicroscopic autoradiography: identification of origin of synaptic terminals in normal nervous tissue. Science 165: 194–196, 1969.
276. HENDRICKSON, A. E. Electronmicroscopic distribution of axoplasmic transport. J. Neurol. 144: 381–398, 1972.
277. HENDRY, I. A. Localization of horseradish peroxidase by in situ perfusion with substrate mixture. Brain Res. 156: 97–101, 1978.
278. HENKEL, C. K., AND S. B. EDWARDS. The paralemniscal reticular formation: secondary projections of the uncrossed connections of the superior colliculus. Anat. Rec. 187: 603, 1977.
279. HENKEL, C. K., AND S. B. EDWARDS. The superior colliculus control of pinna movements in the cat: possible anatomical connections. J. Comp. Neurol. 182: 763–776, 1978.
280. HESS, W. R., S. BÜRGI, AND V. BUCHER. Motorische Funktion des Tektal- und Tegmentalgebietes. Monatsschr. Psychiat. Neurol. 112: 1–52, 1946.

281. HICKS, S. P., AND C. J. D'AMATO. Motor-sensory and visual behavior after hemispherectomy in newborn and mature rats. *Exp. Neurol.* 29: 416-438, 1970.
282. HICKS, S. P., AND C. J. D'AMATO. Locating corticospinal neurons by retrograde axonal transport of horseradish peroxidase. *Exp. Neurol.* 56: 410-420, 1977.
283. HIGHSTEIN, S. M., M. YAMAMOTO, I. SHIMOYAMA, R. J. MACIEWICZ, AND A. STEINACKER. Cells relaying labyrinthine signals to the IIIrd nucleus through the brachium conjunctivum in the rabbit. *Soc. Neurosci. Abstr.* 3: 155, 1977.
284. HINMAN, A., AND M. CARPENTER. Efferent fiber projections of the red nucleus in the cat. *J. Comp. Neurol.* 113: 61-82, 1959.
285. HINSLEY, J. C., S. W. RANSON, AND H. H. DIXON. Responses elicited by stimulation of the mesencephalic tegmentum in the cat. *Arch. Neurol. Psychiatry* 24: 966-977, 1930.
286. HIROSE, K. Ueber eine bulbospinale Bahn. *Folia Neuro-Biol. Leipzig* 10: 371-382, 1916.
287. HOCKFIELD, S., AND S. GOBEL. Neurons in and near nucleus caudalis with long ascending projection axons demonstrated by retrograde labeling with horseradish peroxidase. *Brain Res.* 139: 333-339, 1978.
288. HOFF, E. C. Central nerve terminals in the mammalian spinal cord and their examination by experimental degeneration. *Proc. Roy Soc. London* 111: 175-188, 1932.
289. HÖKFELT, T., K. FUXE, M. GOLDSTEIN, AND O. JOHANSSON. Immunohistochemical evidence for the existence of adrenaline neurons in the rat brain. *Brain Res.* 66: 235-251, 1974.
290. HOLMES, G., AND W. P. MAY. On the exact origin of the pyramidal tracts in man and other mammals. *Brain* 132: 1-43, 1909.
291. HOLMQUIST, B., AND A. LUNDBERG. On the organization of the supraspinal inhibitory control of interneurons in various spinal reflex arcs. *Arch. Ital. Biol.* 97: 340-356, 1959.
292. HOLSTEGE, G., AND H. G. J. M. KUYPERS. Propriobulbar fibre connections to the trigeminal, facial and hypoglossal motor nuclei. I. An anterograde degeneration study in the cat. *Brain* 100: 239-264, 1977.
293. HOLSTEGE, G., AND H. G. J. M. KUYPERS. Descending brain stem pathways from the nucleus subcoeruleus and the pontine tegmentum to the spinal cord in the cat, a labeled leucine tracing study. *Neurosci. Lett. Suppl.* 1: 128, 1978.
294. HOLSTEGE, G., H. G. J. M. KUYPERS, AND R. C. BOER. Anatomical evidence for direct brain stem projections to the somatic motoneuronal cell groups and autonomic preganglionic cell groups in cat spinal cord. *Brain Res.* 171: 329-333, 1979.
295. HOLSTEGE, G., H. G. J. M. KUYPERS, AND J. J. DEKKER. The organization of the bulbar fibre connections to the trigeminal, facial and hypoglossal motor nuclei. II. An autoradiographic study in cat. *Brain* 100: 265-286, 1977.
296. HONGO, T., E. JANKOWSKA, AND A. LUNDBERG. The rubrospinal tract. I. Effects on alpha-motoneurons innervating hindlimb muscles in cats. *Exp. Brain Res.* 7: 344-364, 1969.
297. HONGO, T., E. JANKOWSKA, AND A. LUNDBERG. The rubrospinal tract. IV. Effects on interneurons. *Exp. Brain Res.* 15: 54-78, 1972.
298. HOPKINS, D. A., AND G. HOLSTEGE. Amygdaloid projections to the mesencephalon, pons and medulla oblongata in the cat. *Exp. Brain Res.* 32: 529-547, 1978.
299. HOPKINS, D. A., AND D. G. LAWRENCE. On the absence of a rubrothalamic projection in the monkey with observations on some ascending mesencephalic projections. *J. Comp. Neurol.* 161: 269-293, 1975.
300. HORE, J., AND R. PORTER. The role of the pyramidal tract in the production of cortically evoked movements in the brushtailed possum (*Trichosurus vulpecula*). *Brain Res.* 30: 232-234, 1971.
301. HOSOYA, Y., AND M. MATSUSHITA. Identification and distribution of the spinal and hypophyseal projection neurons in the paraventricular nucleus of the rat. A light and electron microscopic study with the horseradish peroxidase method. *Exp. Brain Res.* 35: 315-331, 1979.
302. HUBBARD, J. E., AND V. DI CARLO. Fluorescence histochemistry of monoamine-containing cell bodies in the brain stem of the squirrel monkey (*Saimiri sciureus*). I. The locus coeruleus. *J. Comp. Neurol.* 147: 553-566, 1973.
303. HUBBARD, J. E., AND V. DI CARLO. Fluorescence histochemistry of monoamine-containing cell bodies in the brain stem of the squirrel monkey (*Saimiri sciureus*). II. Catecholamine-containing groups. *J. Comp. Neurol.* 153: 369-384, 1974.
304. HUBBARD, J. E., AND V. DI CARLO. Fluorescence histochemistry of monoamine-containing cell bodies in the brain stem of the squirrel monkey (*Saimiri sciureus*). III. Serotonin-containing groups. *J. Comp. Neurol.* 153: 385-398, 1974.
305. HUBEL, D. H., S. LEVAY, AND T. N. WIESEL. Mode of termination of retinotectal fibers in macaque monkey: an autoradiographic study. *Brain Res.* 96: 25-40, 1975.
306. HUGHES, J. R., AND J. A. MAZUROWSKI. Studies on the supracallosal mesial cortex of unanesthetized, conscious mammals II. Monkey. A. Movements elicited by electrical stimulation. *Electroencephalogr. Clin. Neurophysiol.* 14: 477-485, 1962.
307. HULTBORN, H. Transmission in the pathway of reciprocal Ia inhibition to motoneurones and its control during the tonic stretch reflex. In: *Progress in Brain Research. Understanding the Stretch Reflex,* edited by S. Homma. Amsterdam: Elsevier, 1976, vol. 44, p. 235-255.
308. HUMPHREY, D. R., AND R. R. RIETZ. Cells of origin of corticorubral projections from the arm area of primate motor cortex and their synaptic actions in the red nucleus. *Brain Res.* 110: 162-169, 1976.
309. HYDE, J. E., AND S. TOCZEK. Functional relation of interstitial nucleus to rotatory movements evoked from zona incerta stimulation. *J. Neurophysiol.* 25: 455-466, 1962.
310. ILLERT, M., AND R. TANAKA. Integration in descending motor pathways controlling the forelimb in the cat. 4. Corticospinal inhibition of forelimb motoneurones mediated by short propriospinal neurones. *Exp. Brain Res.* 31: 131-141, 1978.
311. INGRAM, W. R., S. W. RANSOM, AND F. I. HANNETT. The direct stimulation of the red nucleus in cats. *J. Neurol. Psychopathol.* 12: 219-230, 1932.
312. INGRAM, W. R., S. W. RANSON, F. I. HANNETT, F. R. ZEISS, AND E. T. TERWILLIGER. Results of stimulation of the tegmentum with the Horseley-Clarke stereotaxic apparatus. *Arch. Neurol. Psychiatry* 28: 513-541, 1932.
313. ISHIKAWA, M., S. SHIMADA, AND C. TANAKA. Histochemical mapping of catecholamine neurons and fiber pathways in the pontine tegmentum of the dog. *Brain. Res.* 86: 1-16, 1975.
314. ITO, M., T. HONGO, M. YOSHIDA, Y. OKADA, AND K. OBATA. Antidromic and trans-synaptic activation of Deiters' neurones induced from the spinal cord. *Jpn. J. Physiol.* 14: 638-658, 1964.
315. ITO, M., M. UDO, AND N. MANO. Long inhibitory and excitatory pathways converging onto cat reticular and Deiters' neurons and their relevance to reticulofugal axons. *J. Neurophysiol.* 33: 210-226, 1970.
316. ITOH, K., A. KONISHI, S. NOMURA, N. MIZUNO, Y. NAKAMURA, AND T. SUGIMOTO. Application of coupled oxidation reaction to electron microscopic demonstration of horseradish peroxidase: cobalt-glucose oxidase method. *Brain Res.* 175: 341-346, 1979.
317. JACOBSON, S., AND J. Q. TROJANOWSKI. The cells of origin of the corpus callosum in rat, cat and rhesus monkey. *Brain Res.* 74: 149-155, 1974.
318. JACOBSON, S., AND J. Q. TROJANOWSKI. Cortico-thalamic neurons and thalamocortical terminal fields: an investigation in rat using horseradish peroxidase and autoradiography. *Brain Res.* 85: 385-401, 1975.
319. JANE, J. A., C. B. G. CAMPBELL, AND D. YASHON. Pyramidal tract: a comparison of two prosimian primates. *Science* 147: 153-155, 1965.
320. JANE, J. A., D. YASHON, W. DE MEYER, AND P. C. BUCY. The contribution of the precentral gyrus to the pyramidal tract of man. *J. Neurosurg.* 26: 244-248, 1967.

321. JANKOWSKA, E., AND S. LINDSTRÖM. Morphological identification of Renshaw cells. *Acta Physiol. Scand.* 81: 428–430, 1971.
322. JANKOWSKA, E., AND S. LINDSTRÖM. Morphology of interneurones mediating 1a reciprocal inhibition of montoneurones in the spinal cord of the cat. *J. Physiol. London* 226: 805–823, 1972.
323. JANKOWSKA, E., A. LUNDBERG, W. J. ROBERTS, AND D. STUART. A long propriospinal system with direct effect on motoneurones and on interneurones in the cat lumbosacral cord. *Exp. Brain Res.* 21: 169–194, 1974.
324. JANKOWSKA, E., Y. PADEL, AND R. TANAKA. Disynaptic inhibition of spinal motoneurones from the motor cortex in the monkey. *J. Physiol. London* 258: 467–487, 1976.
325. JANKOWSKA, E., J. RASTAD, AND J. WESTMAN. Intracellular application of horseradish peroxidase and its light and electron microscopical appearance in spinocervical tract cells. *Brain Res.* 105: 557–562, 1976.
326. JANKOWSKA, E., AND D. O. SMITH. Antidromic activation of Renshaw cells and their axonal projections. *Acta Physiol. Scand.* 88: 198–214, 1973.
327. JONES, B. E., AND R. Y. MOORE. Catecholamine-containing neurons of the nucleus locus coeruleus in the cat. *J. Comp. Neurol.* 157: 43–52, 1974.
328. JONES, E. G., J. D. COULTER, H. BURTON, AND R. PORTER. Cells of origin and terminal distribution of corticostriatal fibers arising in the sensory-motor cortex of monkeys. *J. Comp. Neurol.* 173: 53–80, 1977.
329. JONES, E. G., AND S. P. WISE. Size, laminar and columnar distribution of efferent cells in the sensory-motor cortex of monkeys. *J. Comp. Neurol.* 175: 391–438, 1977.
330. JUNG, R., AND R. HASSLER. The extrapyramidal motor system. In: *Handbook of Physiology. Neurophysiology,* edited by H. W. Magoun. Washington, DC: Am. Physiol. Soc., 1960, sect. 1., vol. II, chapt. 35, p. 863–927.
331. KARAMANLIDIS, A. N., H. MICHALOUDI, O. MANGANA, AND R. P. SAIGAL. Trigeminal ascending projections in the rabbit, studied with horseradish peroxidase. *Brain Res.* 156: 110–116, 1978.
332. KAWAMURA, K., A. BRODAL, AND G. HODDEVIK. The projection of the superior colliculus onto the reticular formation of the brain stem. An experimental anatomical study in the cat. *Exp. Brain Res.* 19: 1–19, 1974.
333. KAWAMURA, K., AND T. HASHIKAWA. Cell bodies of origin of reticular projections from the superior colliculus in the cat: an experimental study with the use of horseradish peroxidase as a tracer. *J. Comp. Neurol.* 182: 1–16, 1978.
334. KAWAMURA, S., AND E. KOBAYASHI. Identification of laminar origin of some tecto-thalamic fibers in the cat. *Brain Res.* 91: 281–285, 1975.
335. KAWAMURA, K., T. KONNO, AND M. CHIBA. Cells of origin of corticopontine and corticotectal fibers in the medial and lateral banks of the middle suprasylvian sulcus in the cat. An experimental study with the horseradish peroxidase method. *Neurosci. Lett.* 9: 129–135, 1978.
336. KAWANA, E., K. AKERT, AND H. BRUPPACHER. Enlargement of synaptic vesicles as an early sign of terminal degeneration in the rat caudate nucleus. *J. Comp. Neurol.* 142: 297–308, 1971.
337. KELLER, A. D., AND W. K. HARE. The rubrospinal tracts in the monkey. Effects of experimental section. *Arch. Neurol. Psychiatry* 32: 1253–1272, 1934.
338. KENNARD, M. A. Reorganization of motor function in the cerebral cortex of monkeys deprived of motor and premotor areas in infancy. *J. Neurophysiol.* 1: 477–496, 1938.
339. KENNARD, M. A., AND L. ECTORS. Forced circling in monkeys following lesions of the frontal lobes. *J. Neurophysiol.* 1: 45–54, 1938.
340. KIEVIT, J., AND H. G. J. M. KUYPERS. Organization of the thalamo-cortical connexions to the frontal lobe in the rhesus monkey. *Exp. Brain Res.* 29: 299–322, 1977.
341. KING, J. S., M. H. BOWMAN, AND G. F. MARTIN. The red nucleus of the opossum (*Didelphis marsupialis virginiana*): a light and electron microscopic study. *J. Comp. Neurol.* 143: 157–184, 1971.
342. KING, J. S., R. M. DOM, J. B. CONNER, AND G. F. MARTIN. An experimental light and electron microscopic study of cerebellorubral projections in the opossum. *Didelphis marsupialis virginiana.* *Brain Res.* 52: 61–78, 1973.
343. KING, J. S., R. M. DOM, AND G. F. MARTIN. Anatomical evidence for an intrinsic neuron in the red nucleus. *Brain Res.* 67: 317–323, 1974.
344. KING, J. S., G. F. MARTIN, AND J. B. CONNER. A light and electron microscopic study of corticorubral projections in the opossum (*Didelphis marsupialis virginiana*). *Brain Res.* 38: 251–265, 1972.
345. KING, J. S., R. C. SCHWYN, AND C. A. FOX. The red nucleus in the monkey (*Macaca mulatta*): a Golgi and an electron microscopic study. *J. Comp. Neurol.* 142: 75–108, 1971.
346. KIRK, G. R., AND J. E. BREAZILE. Maturation of the corticospinal tract in the dog. *Exp. Neurol.* 35: 394–397, 1972.
347. KIRKWOOD, P. A., AND T. A. SEARS. Monosynaptic excitation of thoracic expiratory motoneurones from lateral respiratory neurones in the medulla of the cat. *J. Physiol. London.* 234: 87–89, 1973.
348. KLÜVER, H., AND E. BARRERA. A method for the combined staining of cells and fibers in the nervous system. *J. Neuropathol. Exp. Neurol.* 12: 400–403, 1953.
349. KNEISLEY, L. W., M. P. BIBER, AND J. H. LAVAIL. A study of the origin of brain stem projections to monkey spinal cord using the retrograde transport method. *Exp. Neurol.* 60: 116–139, 1978.
350. KONISHI, A., M. SATO, N. MIZUNO, K. ITHOH, S. NOMURA, AND T. SUGIMOTO. An electron microscope study of the Onuf's nucleus in the cat. *Brain Res.* 156: 333–338, 1978.
351. KONISHI, M. Fluorescence microscopy of the spinal cord of the dog, with special reference to the autonomic lateral horn cells. *Arch. Histol. Jpn. Niigata Jpn.* 30: 33–44, 1968.
352. KOSTYUK, P. G., AND V. A. MAISKY. Propriospinal projections in the lumbar spinal cord of the cat. *Brain Res.* 39: 530–535, 1972.
353. KOSTYUK, P. G., AND A. I. PILYAVSKY. A possible direct interneuronal pathway from rubrospinal tract to motoneurones. *Brain Res.* 14: 526–529, 1969.
354. KOSTYUK, P. G., AND G. G. SKIBO. An electron microscopic analysis of rubrospinal tract termination in the spinal cord of the cat. *Brain Res.* 85: 511–516, 1975.
355. KOSTYUK, P. G., D. A. VASILENKO, AND E. LANG. Propriospinal pathways in the dorsolateral funiculus and their effects on lumbosacral motoneuronal pools. *Brain Res.* 28: 233–249, 1971.
356. KRAMMER, E. B., T. RATH, AND M. F. LISCHKA. Somatotopic organization of the hypoglossal nucleus: a HRP study in the rat. *Brain Res.* 170: 533–537, 1979.
357. KRIEG, W. J. S. *Connections of the Frontal Cortex of the Monkey.* Springfield, IL: Thomas, 1954.
358. KRISTENSSON, K., AND Y. OLSSON. Retrograde axonal transport of protein. *Brain Res.* 29: 363–365, 1971.
359. KRISTENSSON, K., AND Y. OLSSON. Uptake and retrograde transport of horseradish peroxidase in hypoglossal neurons. Electron microscopic localization in the neuronal perikaryon. *Acta Neuropathol.* 19: 1–9, 1971.
360. KRISTENSSON, K., AND Y. OLSSON. Retrograde transport of horseradish peroxidase in transected axons. I. Time relationships between transport and induction of chromatolysis. *Brain Res.* 79: 101–109, 1974.
361. KUME, M., M. UEMURA, K. MATSUDA, R. MATSUSHIMA, AND N. MIZUNO. Topographical representation of peripheral branches of the facial nerve within the facial nucleus. A HRP study in the cat. *Neurosci. Lett.* 8: 5–8, 1978.
362. KÜNZLE, H. Thalamic projections from the precentral motor cortex in *Macaca fascicularis*. *Brain Res.* 105: 253–267, 1976.
363. KÜNZLE, H. Evidence for selective axon-terminal uptake and retrograde transport of label in cortico- and rubropsinal systems after injections of 3H-Proline. *Exp. Brain Res.* 28: 125–132, 1977.

364. KÜNZLE, H. An autoradiographic analysis of the efferent conections from premotor and adjacent prefrontal regions (areas 6 and 9) in *Macaca fascicularis*. *Brain Behav. Evol.* 15: 185-234, 1978.

365. KÜNZLE, H., AND K. AKERT. Efferent connections of cortical area 8 (frontal eye field) in *Macaca fascicularis*. A reinvestigation using the autoradiographic technique. *J. Comp. Neurol.* 173: 147-164, 1977.

366. KÜNZLE, H., K. AKERT, AND R. H. WURTZ. Projection of area 8 (frontal eye field) to superior colliculus in the monkey. An autoradiographic study. *Brain Res.* 117: 487-492, 1976.

367. KÜNZLE, H., AND M. CUENOD. Differential uptake of (^{3}H) proline and (^{3}H) leucine by neurons: its importance for the autoradiographic tracing of pathways. *Brain Res.* 62: 213-217, 1973.

368. KUYPERS, H. G. J. M. An anatomical analysis of cortico-bulbar connexions to the pons and lower brain stem in the cat. *J. Anat.* 92: 189-218, 1958.

369. KUYPERS, H. G. J. M. Corticobulbar connexions to the pons and lower brain stem in man. An anatomical study. *Brain* 81: 364-388, 1958.

370. KUYPERS, H. G. J. M. Some projections from the peri-central cortex to the pons and lower brain stem in monkey and chimpanzee. *J. Comp. Neurol.* 110: 221-255, 1958.

371. KUYPERS, H. G. J. M. Central cortical projections to motor and somato-sensory cell groups. An experimental study in the rhesus monkey. *Brain* 83: 161-184, 1960.

372. KUYPERS, H. G. J. M. Corticospinal connections: postnatal development in the rhesus monkey. *Science* 138: 678-680, 1962.

373. KUYPERS, H. G. J. M. The descending pathways to the spinal cord, their anatomy and function. In: *Progress in Brain Research. Organization of the Spinal Cord*, edited by J. C. Eccles and J. P. Schadé. Amsterdam: Elsevier, 1964, vol. 11, p. 178-200.

373a. KUYPERS, H. G. J. M. The anatomical organization of the descending pathways and their contributions to motor control especially in primates. In: *Human Reflexes, Pathophysiology of Motor Systems, Methodology of Human Reflexes. New Developments in Electromyography and Clinical Neurophysiology*, edited by J. E. Desmedt. Basel: Karger, 1973, vol. 3, p. 38-68.

374. KUYPERS, H. G. J. M. From motor control to conscious experience. In: *Cerebral Correlates of Conscious Experience*, edited by P. A. Buser and A. Rougeul-Buser. Amsterdam: Elsevier/North-Holland, 1978, p. 95-110. (INSERM Symp. 6th.)

375. KUYPERS, H. G. J. M., M. BENTIVOGLIO, D. VAN DER KOOY, AND C. E. CATSMAN-BERREVOETS. Retrograde transport of bisbenzimide and propidium iodide through axons to their parent cell bodies. *Neurosci. Lett.* 12: 1-7, 1979.

376. KUYPERS, H. G. J. M., AND J. BRINKMAN. Precentral projections to different parts of the spinal intermediate zone in the rhesus monkey. *Brain Res.* 24: 29-48, 1970.

377. KUYPERS, H. G. J. M., C. E. CATSMAN-BERREVOETS, AND R. E. PADT. Retrograde axonal transport of fluorescent substances in the rat's forebrain. *Neurosci. Lett.* 6: 127-135, 1977.

378. KUYPERS, H. G. J. M., W. R. FLEMING, AND J. W. FARINHOLT. Descending projections to spinal motor and sensory cell groups in the monkey: cortex versus subcortex. *Science* 132: 38-40, 1960.

379. KUYPERS, H. G. J. M., W. R. FLEMING, AND J. W. FARINHOLT. Subcorticospinal projections in the rhesus monkey. *J. Comp. Neurol.* 118: 107-137, 1962.

380. KUYPERS, H. G. J. M., AND D. G. LAWRENCE. Cortical projections to the red nucleus and the brain stem in the rhesus monkey. *Brain Res.* 4: 151-188, 1967.

381. KUYPERS, H. G. J. M., AND V. A. MAISKY. Retrograde axonal transport of horseradish peroxidase from spinal cord to brain stem cell groups in the cat. *Neurosci. Lett.* 1: 9-14, 1975.

382. KUYPERS, H. G. J. M., AND V. A. MAISKY. Funicular trajectories of descending brain stem pathways in cat. *Brain Res.* 136: 159-165, 1977.

383. KUYPERS, H. G. J. M., AND D. PANDYA. Comments on the cortical projections to the center median in the chimpanzee. In: *The Thalamus*, edited by D. P. Purpura and M. D. Yahr. New York: Columbia Univ. Press, 1966, p. 122-127.

384. KUYPERS, H. G. J. M., AND J. D. TUERK. The distribution of the cortical fibres within the nuclei cuneatus and gracilis in the cat. *J. Anat.* 98: 143-162, 1964.

385. KUZUHARA, S., I. KANAZAWA, AND T. NAKANISHI. Topographical localization of the Onuf's nuclear neurons innervating the rectal and vesical striated muscles: a retrograde fluorescent double labeling in cat and dog. *Neurosci. Lett.* 6: 125-130, 1980.

386. LADPLI, R., AND A. BRODAL. Experimental studies of commissural and reticular formation projections from the vestibular nuclei in the cat. *Brain Res.* 8: 65-96, 1968.

387. LANCE, J. W., AND R. L. MANNING. Origin of the pyramidal tract in cat. *J. Physiol. London* 124: 385-399, 1954.

388. LANDGREN, S., C. G. PHILLIPS, AND R. PORTER. Cortical fields of origin of the monosynaptic pyramidal pathways to some alpha motoneurones of the baboon's hand and forearm. *J. Physiol. London* 161: 112-125, 1962.

389. LANG, W., J. A. BÜTTNER-ENNEVER, AND U. BÜTTNER. Vestibular projections to the monkey thalamus: an autoradiographic study. *Brain Res.* 177: 3-18, 1979.

390. LANKAMP, D. J. *Fiber Composition of the Pedunculus Cerebri (Crus cerebri) in Man*. Leiden: Luctor et Emergo, 1967.

391. LASEK, R., B. S. JOSEPH, AND D. G. WHITLOCK. Evaluation of a radioautographic neuroanatomical tracing method. *Brain Res.* 8: 319-336, 1968.

392. LASSEK, A. M. The human pyramidal tract. IV. A study of the mature, myelinated fibers of the pyramid. *J. Comp. Neurol.* 76: 217-225, 1942.

393. LASSEK, A. M. The human pyramidal tract. V. Postnatal changes in the axons of the pyramids. *Arch. Neurol. Psychiatry* 47: 422-427, 1942.

394. LASSEK, A. M. The pyramidal tract: basic considerations of corticospinal neurons. *Res. Publ. Assoc. Res. Nerv. Ment. Dis.* 27: 106-128, 1948.

395. LASSEK, A. M. A study of the effect of complete frontal lobe extirpations on the fiber components of the pyramidal tract. *J. Comp. Neurol.* 96: 121-125, 1952.

396. LASSEK, A. M. *The Pyramidal Tract. Its Status in Medicine*. Springfield IL: Thomas, 1955.

397. LA VAIL, J. H., AND M. M. LA VAIL. Retrograde axonal transport in the central nervous system. *Science* 176: 1416-1417, 1972.

398. LAWRENCE, D. G., AND D. A. HOPKINS. The development of motor control in the rhesus monkey: evidence concerning the role of corticomotoneuronal connections. *Brain* 99: 235-254, 1976.

398a. LAWRENCE, D. G., AND H. G. J. M. KUYPERS. Pyramidal and non-pyramidal pathways in monkeys: anatomical and functional correlation. *Science* 148: 973-975, 1965.

399. LAWRENCE, D. G., AND H. G. J. M. KUYPERS. The functional organization of the motor system in the monkey. I. The effects of bilateral pyramidal lesions. *Brain* 91: 1-14, 1968.

400. LAWRENCE, D. G., AND H. G. J. M. KUYPERS. The functional organization of the motor system in the monkey. II. The effects of lesions of the descending brain-stem pathways. *Brain* 91: 15-36, 1968.

401. LEICHNETZ, G. R., L. WATKINS, G. GRIFFIN, R. MURFIN, AND D. J. MAYER. The projection from nucleus raphe magnus and other brainstem nuclei to the spinal cord in the rat: a study using the HRP blue-reaction. *Neurosci. Lett.* 8: 119-124, 1978.

402. LEONARD, C. M. The prefrontal cortex of the rat. I. Cortical projection of the mediodorsal nucleus. II. Efferent connections. *Brain Res.* 12: 321-343, 1969.

403. LEVIN, P. M. The efferent fibers of the frontal lobe of the monkey *Macaca mulatta*. *J. Comp. Neurol.* 63: 369-419, 1936.

404. LEVITT, P., AND R. Y. MOORE. Origin and organization of brainstem catecholamine innervation in the rat. *J. Comp. Neurol.* 186: 505-528, 1979.

405. LEWANDOWSKY, M. Untersuchungen über die Leitungsbahnen des Truncus cerebri und ihren Zusammenhang mit denen der Medulla spinalis und des Cortex cerebri. In: *Weitere Beitrage zur Hirnanatomie. Neurol*, edited by O. v. Vogt. Jena: Fischer, 1904. Arb. II., p. 60-150.

406. LEWIS, P. R., B. A. FLUMERFELT, AND C. C. D. SHUTE. The use of cholinesterase techniques to study topographical localization in the hypoglossal nucleus of the rat. *J. Anat.* 110: 203-213, 1971.

407. LEWIS, R., AND G. S. BRINDLEY. The extrapyramidal cortical motor map. *Brain* 88: 397-406, 1965.

408. LIGHT, A. R., AND C. B. METZ. The morphology of the spinal cord efferent and afferent neurons contributing to the ventral roots of the cat. *J. Comp. Neurol.* 179: 501-516, 1978.

409. LIU, C. N., AND W. W. CHAMBERS. An experimental study of the corticospinal system in the monkey (*Macaca mulatta*). *J. Comp. Neurol.* 123: 257-284, 1965.

410. LLOYD, D. P. C. The spinal mechanism of the pyramidal system in cats. *J. Neurophysiol.* 4: 525-546, 1941.

411. LLOYD, D. P. C. Mediation of descending long spinal reflex activity. *J. Neurophysiol.* 5: 435-458, 1942.

412. LOEWY, A. D., AND H. BURTON. Efferent projections from nuclei of the solitary tract in the cat. *Soc. Neurosci. Abstr.* 3: 23, 1977.

413. LOEWY, A. D., S. MCKELLAR, AND C. B. SAPER. Direct projections from the A5 catecholamine cell group to the intermediolateral cell column. *Brain Res.* 174: 309-314, 1979.

414. LOEWY, A. D., AND C. B. SAPER. Edinger-Westphal nucleus: projections to the brain stem and spinal cord in the cat. *Brain Res.* 150: 1-27, 1978.

415. LOEWY, A. D., C. B. SAPER, AND R. P. BAKER. Descending projections from the pontine micturition center. *Brain Res.* 172: 533-539, 1979.

416. LOEWY, A. D., C. B. SAPER, AND N. D. YAMODIS. Re-evaluation of the efferent projections of the Edinger-Westphal nucleus in the cat. *Brain Res.* 141: 153-159, 1978.

417. LØKEN, A. C., AND A. BRODAL. A somatotopic pattern in the human lateral vestibular nucleus. *Arch. Neurol. Chicago* 23: 350-357, 1970.

418. LORENTE DE NO, R. Anatomy of the eighth nerve. The central projections of the nerve endings of the internal ear. *Laryngoscope* 43: 1-38, 1933.

419. LUHAN, J. A. Long survival after unilateral stab wound of medulla with unusual pyramidal tract distribution. *Arch. Neurol. Chicago* 1: 427-434, 1959.

420. LUND, J. S., R. D. LUND, A. E. HENDRICKSON, A. H. BUNT, AND A. F. FUCHS. The origin of efferent pathways from the primary visual cortex. Area 17 of the Macaque monkey as shown by retrograde transport of horseradish peroxidase. *J. Comp. Neurol.* 164: 287-303, 1975.

421. LUND, S., AND P. POMPEIANO. Descending pathways with monosynaptic action on motoneurones. *Experientia* 21: 602-603, 1965.

422. LUNDBERG, A. The excitatory control of the 1a inhibitory pathway. In: *Excitatory Synaptic Mechanisms*, edited by P. Andersen and J. K. S. Jansen. Oslo: Universiteitsforlaget, 1970, p. 330-340.

423. LUNDBERG, A., AND P. VOORHOEVE. Effects from the pyramidal tract on spinal reflex arcs. *Acta Physiol. Scand.* 56: 201-219, 1962.

424. LYNCH, G., C. GALL, P. MENSAH, AND C. W. COTMAN. Horseradish peroxidase histochemistry: a new method for tracing efferent projections in the central nervous system. *Brain Res.* 65: 373-380, 1974.

425. LYNCH, G., R. L. SMITH, P. MENSAH, AND C. W. COTMAN. Tracing the dentate gyrus mossy fiber system with horseradish peroxidase histochemistry. *Exp. Neurol.* 40: 516-524, 1973.

426. LYON, M. J. Localization of the efferent neurons of the tensor tympani muscle of the newborn using horseradish peroxidase. *Exp. Neurol.* 49: 439-455, 1975.

427. LYON, M. J. The central location of the motor neurons to the stapedius muscle in the cat. *Brain Res.* 143: 437-444, 1978.

428. MABUCHI, M. Corticofugal projections to the subthalamic nucleus, the red nucleus and the adjacent areas in the monkey. *Proc. Jpn. Acad.* 43: 818, 1967.

429. MABUCHI, M. Rotatory head response evoked by stimulating and destroying the interstitial nucleus and surrounding region. *Exp. Neurol.* 27: 175-193, 1970.

430. MABUCHI, M., AND T. KUSAMA. The cortico-rubral projection in the cat. *Brain Res.* 2: 254-273, 1966.

431. MABUCHI, M., AND T. KUSAMA. Mesodiencephalic projections to the inferior olive and the vestibular and perihypoglossal nuclei. *Brain Res.* 17: 133-136, 1970.

432. MACIEWICZ, R. J. Afferents to the lateral suprasylvian gyrus of the cat traced with horseradish peroxidase. *Brain Res.* 78: 139-143, 1974.

433. MACIEWICZ, R. J., K. EAGER, C. R. S. KANEKO, AND S. M. HIGHSTEIN. Vestibular and medullary brain stem afferents to the abducens nucleus in the cat. *Brain Res.* 123: 229-240, 1977.

434. MAEDA, T., C. PIN, D. SALVERT, M. LIGIER, AND M. JOUVET. Les neurones contenant des catécholamines du tegmentum pontique et leurs voies de projection chez le chat. *Brain Res.* 57: 119-152, 1973.

435. MAGNI, F., AND W. D. WILLIS. Antidromic activation of neurones of the reticular formation of the brain stem. *Nature* 198: 592-594, 1963.

436. MAGNI, F., AND W. D. WILLIS. Identification of reticular formation neurons by intercellular recording. *Arch. Ital. Biol.* 101: 681-702, 1963.

437. MALMGREN, L., AND Y. OLSSON. A sensitive method for histochemical demonstration of horseradish peroxidase in neurons following retrograde axonal transport. *Brain Res.* 148: 279-294, 1978.

438. MALMGREN, L., Y. OLSSON, T. OLSSON, AND K. KRISTENSSON. Uptake and retrograde axonal transport of various exogenous macromolecules in normal and crushed hypoglossal neurones. *Brain Res.* 153: 477-494, 1978.

439. MANGHI, E. Il fascio piramidale laterale diretto nel gatto. *Boll. Soc. Ital. Biol. Sper.* 32: 1491-1493, 1956.

440. MANNEN, H. Morphological analysis of an individual neuron with Golgi's method. In: *Golgi Centennial Symposium: Perspectives in Neurobiology*, edited by M. Santini. New York: Raven Press, 1975, p. 61-70. (Golgi Centennial Symp., 1973.)

441. MARINESCO, G. Recherches sur les localisations motrices spinales. *Semaine Méd. Paris* 29: 225-231, 1904.

442. MARTIN, G. F. Efferent tectal pathways of the opossum (*Didelphis virginiana*). *J. Comp. Neurol.* 135: 209-224, 1969.

443. MARTIN, G. F., M. S. BEATTIE, J. C. BRESNAHAN, C. K. HENKEL, AND H. C. HUGHES. Cortical and brain stem projections to the spinal cord of the american opossum (*Didelphis marsupialis virginiana*). *Brain Behav. Evol.* 12: 270-310, 1975.

444. MARTIN, G. F., J. C. BRESNAHAN, C. K. HENKEL, AND D. MEGIRIAN. Corticobulbar fibres in the North American opossum (*Didelphis marsupialis virginiana*) with notes on the Tasmanian brush-tailed possum (*Trichosurus vulpecula*) and other marsupials. *J. Anat.* 120: 439-484, 1975.

445. MARTIN, G. F., AND R. DOM. Rubrobulbar projections of the opossum (*Didelphis virginiana*). *J. Comp. Neurol.* 139: 199-214, 1970.

446. MARTIN, G. F., AND R. DOM. The rubro-spinal tract of the opossum (*Didelphis virginiana*). *J. Comp. Neurol.* 138: 19-30, 1970.

447. MARTIN, G. F., AND R. DOM. Reticulospinal fibers of the opossum (*Didelphis virginiana*). II. Course, caudal extent and distribution. *J. Comp. Neurol.* 141: 467-484, 1971.

448. MARTIN, G. F., R. DOM, S. KATZ, AND J. S. KING. The organization of projection neurons in the opossum red nucleus. *Brain Res.* 78: 17-34, 1974.

449. MARTIN, G. F., AND A. M. FISHER. A further evaluation of the origin, the course and the termination of the opossum corticospinal tract. *J. Neurol. Sci.* 7: 177-187, 1968.

450. MARTIN, G. F., A. O. HUMBERTSON, C. LAXSON, AND W. M. PANNETON. Evidence for direct bulbospinal projections to lam-

inae IX, X and the intermediolateral cell column. Studies using axonal transport techniques in the North American opossum. *Brain Res.* 170: 165-171, 1979.
451. MARTIN, G. F., A. O. HUMBERTSON, L. C. LAXSON, W. M. PANNETON, AND I. TSCHISMADIA. Spinal projections from mesencephalic and pontine reticular formation in North American opossum: a study using axonal transport techniques. *J. Comp. Neurol.* 187: 373-400, 1979.
452. MARTIN, G. F., D. MEGIRIAN, AND J. B. CONNER. The origin course and termination of the corticospinal tract of the Tasmanian potoroo (*Potorous apicalis*). *J. Anat.* 111: 263-281, 1972.
453. MARTIN, G. F., D. MEGIRIAN, AND A. ROEBUCK. The corticospinal tract of the marsupial phalanger (*Trichosurus vulpecula*). *J. Comp. Neurol.* 139: 245-258, 1970.
454. MARTIN, G. F., D. MEGIRIAN, AND A. ROEBUCK. Corticobulbar projections of the marsupial phalanger (*Trichosurus vulpecula*). I. Projections to the pons and medulla oblongata. *J. Comp. Neurol.* 142: 275-296, 1971.
455. MARTIN, R. F., L. M. JORDAN, AND W. D. WILLIS. Differential projections of cat medullary raphe neurons demonstrated by retrograde labelling following spinal cord lesions. *J. Comp. Neurol.* 182: 77-88, 1979.
456. MASSION, J. The mammalian red nucleus. *Physiol. Rev.* 47: 383-436, 1967.
457. MATSUDA, K., M. UEMURA, M. KUME, R. MATSUSHIMA, AND N. MIZUNO. Topographical representation of mosticatory muscles in the motor trigeminal nucleus in the rabbit: a HRP study. *Neurosci. Lett.* 8: 1-14, 1978.
458. MATSUDA, K., M. UEMURA, Y. TAKEUCHI, M. KUME, R. MATSUSHIMA, AND N. MIZUNO. Localization of motoneurons innervating the posterior belly of the digastric muscle: a comparative anatomical study by the HRP method. *Neurosci. Lett.* 12: 47-52, 1979.
459. MATSUSHITA, M. Some aspects of the interneuronal connections in cat's spinal gray matter. *J. Comp. Neurol.* 136: 57-80, 1969.
460. MATSUSHITA, M. The axonal pathways of spinal neurons in the cat. *J. Comp. Neurol.* 138: 391-418, 1970.
461. MATSUSHITA, M., AND Y. HOSOYA. Cells of origin of the spinocerebellar tract in the rat, studied with the method of retrograde transport of horseradish peroxidase. *Brain Res.* 173: 185-200, 1979.
462. MATSUSHITA, M., Y. HOSOYA, AND M. IKEDA. Anatomical organization of the spinocerebellar system in the cat, as studied by retrograde transport of horseradish peroxidase. *J. Comp. Neurol.* 184: 81-106, 1979.
463. MATSUSHITA, M., AND M. IKEDA. Propriospinal fiber connections of the cervical motor nuclei in the cat: a light and electron microscope study. *J. Comp. Neurol.* 150: 1-32, 1973.
464. MATSUSHITA, M., M. IKEDA, AND Y. HOSOYA. The location of spinal neurons with long descending axons (long descending propriospinal tract neurons) in the cat: a study with the horseradish peroxidase technique. *J. Comp. Neurol.* 184: 63-80, 1979.
465. MATSUSHITA, M., AND T. UEYAMA. Ventral motor nucleus of the cervical enlargement in some mammals; its specific afferents from the lower cord levels and cytoarchitecture. *J. Comp. Neurol.* 150: 33-52, 1973.
466. MATTHEWS, M. A., W. D. WILLIS, AND V. WILLIAMS. Dendrite bundles in lamina IX of cat spinal cord: a possible source for electrical interaction between motoneurons? *Anat. Rec.* 171: 313-328, 1971.
467. MAUNZ, R. A., N. G. PITTS, AND B. W. PETERSON. Cat spinoreticular neurons: locations, responses and changes in responses during repetitive stimulation. *Brain Res.* 148: 365-379, 1978.
468. MCALLEN, R. M., AND K. M. SPYER. The location of cardiac vagal preganglionic motoneurones in the medulla of the cat. *J. Physiol. London* 258: 187-204, 1976.
469. MCLAUGHLIN, B. J. Propriospinal and supraspinal projections to the motor nuclei in the cat spinal cord. *J. Comp. Neurol.* 144: 475-500, 1972.

470. MCLAUGHLIN, B. J., R. BARBER, K. SAITO, E. ROBERTS, AND J. Y. WU. Immunocytochemical localization of glutamate decarboxylase in rat spinal cord. *J. Comp. Neurol.* 164: 305-321, 1975.
471. MCMASTERS, R. E., A. H. WEISS, AND M. B. CARPENTER. Vestibular projections to the nuclei of the extraocular muscles. Degeneration resulting from discrete partial lesions of the vestibular nuclei in the monkey. *Am. J. Anat.* 118: 163-194, 1966.
472. MEESSEN, H., AND J. OLZEWSKI. *A Cytoarchitectonic Atlas of the Rhombencephalon of the Rabbit.* Basel: Karger, 1949.
473. MEHLER, W. R. Double descending pathways originating from the superior cerebellar peduncle. An example of neural species differences. *Anat. Rec.* 157: 374, 1967.
474. MEHLER, W. R. Some neurological species differences—a posteriori. *Ann. NY Acad. Sci.* 167: 424-468, 1969.
475. MERGNER, T., O. POMPEIANO, AND N. CORVAJA. Vestibular projections to the nucleus intercalatus of Staderini mapped by retrograde transport of horseradish peroxidase. *Neurosci. Lett.* 5: 309-314, 1977.
476. MERRILL, E. G. The lateral respiratory neurones of the medulla: their associations with nucleus ambiguus, nucleus retroambigualis, the spinal accessory nucleus and the spinal cord. *Brain Res.* 24: 11-28, 1970.
477. MESULAM, M. M. The blue reaction product in horseradish peroxidase neurohistochemistry: incubation parameters and visibility. *J. Histochem. Cytochem.* 24: 1273-1280, 1976.
478. MESULAM, M. M. A horseradish peroxidase method for the identification of the efferents of acetyl cholinesterase-containing neurons. *J. Histochem. Cytochem.* 24: 1281-1286, 1976.
479. METTLER, F. A. Extracortical connections of the primate frontal cerebral cortex. II. Corticofugal connections. *J. Comp. Neurol.* 86: 119-166, 1947.
480. MILLER, R. Distribution and properties of commissural and other neurons in cat sensory motor cortex. *J. Comp. Neurol.* 164: 361-373, 1975.
481. MILLER, R. A., AND N. L. STROMINGER. Efferent connections of the red nucleus in the brainstem and spinal cord of the Rhesus monkey. *J. Comp. Neurol.* 152: 327-345, 1973.
482. MILLER, S. Excitatory and inhibitory propriospinal pathways from lumbosacral to cervical segments in the cat. *Acta Physiol. Scand.* 80: 25A-26A, 1970.
483. MILLER, S., D. J. REITSMA, AND F. G. A. VANDER MECHÉ. Excitatory ascending propriospinal actions between lumbosacral and cervical segments in the cat. *J. Physiol. London* 218: 76P-77P, 1971.
484. MINCKLER, J., R. M. KLEMME, AND D. MINCKLER. The course of efferent fibers from the human premotor cortex. *J. Comp. Neurol.* 81: 259-277, 1944.
485. MITCHELL, R. A., AND A. J. BERGER. Neural regulation of respiration. *Am. Rev. Respir. Dis.* 3: 206-224, 1975.
486. MIZUNO, N., A. KONISHI, AND M. SATO. Localization of masticatory motoneurons in the cat and rat by means of retrograde axonal transport of horseradish peroxidase. *J. Comp. Neurol.* 164: 105-115, 1975.
487. MIZUNO, N., AND Y. NAKAMURA. Rubral fibers to the facial nucleus in the rabbit. *Brain Res.* 28: 545-549, 1971.
488. MODIANOS, D., AND D. PFAFF. Medullary reticular formation lesions and lordosis reflex in female rats. *Brain Res.* 171: 334-338, 1979.
489. MOLENAAR, I. The distribution of propriospinal neurons projecting to different motoneuronal cell groups in the cat's brachial cord. *Brain Res.* 158: 203-206, 1978.
490. MOLENAAR, I., AND H. G. J. M. KUYPERS. Cells of origin of propriospinal fibers and of fibers ascending to supraspinal levels. A HRP study in cat and rhesus monkey. *Brain Res.* 152: 429-450, 1978.
491. MOLENAAR, I., A. RUSTIONI, AND H. G. J. M. KUYPERS. The location of cells of origin of the fibers in the ventral and the lateral funiculus of the cat's lumbo-sacral cord. *Brain Res.* 78: 239-254, 1974.
492. MOLL, L., AND H. G. J. M. KUYPERS. Premotor cortical abla-

tions in monkeys: contralateral changes in visually guided reaching behavior. *Science* 198: 317-319, 1977.
493. MONNIER, M. Syndromes déviationnels provoqués par l'excitation et la destruction du système réticulaire bulbo-protubérantiel chez le chat. *Monatsschr. Psychiatr. Neurol.* 107: 84-102, 1943.
494. MONNIER, M. L'organisation des fonctions motrices chez les primates. *Schweiz. Arch. Neurol. Psychiatr.* 57: 325-349, 1946.
495. MOOLENAAR, G. M., AND H. K. RUCKER. Autoradiographic study of brain stem projections from fastigial pressor areas. *Brain Res.* 114: 492-496, 1976.
496. MORGAN, C., I. NADELHAFT, AND W. C. DE GROAT. Location of bladder preganglionic neurons within the sacral parasympathetic nucleus of the cat. *Neurosci. Lett.* 14: 189-194, 1979.
497. MURRAY, E. A., AND J. D. COULTER. Corticospinal projections from the medial cerebral hemisphere in monkey. *Soc. Neurosci. Abstr.* 3: 275, 1977.
498. MURRAY, H. M. Rubrobulbar projections in the tree shrew (*Tupaia*). *Soc. Neurosci. Abstr.* 3: 59, 1977.
499. MURRAY, H. M., AND M. E. GURULE. Origin of the rubrospinal tract of the rat. *Neurosci. Lett.* 14: 19-24, 1979.
500. MURRAY, H. M., AND D. E. HAINES. The rubrospinal tract in a Prosimian primate (*Galago senegalensis*). *Brain Behav. Evol.* 12: 311-333, 1975.
501. MURRAY, H. M., D. E. HAINES, AND I. COTE. The rubrospinal tract of the tree shrew (*Tupaia glis*). *Brain Res.* 116: 317-322, 1976.
502. MUSSEN, A. T. Cerebellum and red nucleus. *Arch. Neurol. Psychiatry* 31: 110-126, 1934.
503. NADELHAFT, I., C. MORGAN, I. SCHAUBLE, AND W. C. DE GROAT. Localization of the sacral autonomic (parasympathetic) nucleus in the spinal cord of cat and monkey by the horseradish peroxidase technique. *Soc. Neurosci. Abstr.* 3: 24, 1977.
504. NAITO, H., K. TANIMURA, N. TAGA, AND Y. HOSOYA. Microelectrode study on the subnuclei of the oculomotor nucleus in the cat. *Brain Res.* 81: 215-231, 1974.
505. NAKAYMA, S., AND R. VON BAUMGARTEN. Lokalisierung absteigender Atmungsbahnen im Rückenmark der Katze mittels antidromer Reizung. *Pfluegers Arch. Gesamte Physiol. Menschen Tiere* 281: 231-244, 1964.
506. NATHAN, P. W. The descending respiratory pathway in man. *J. Neurol. Neurosurg. Psychiatry* 26: 487-499, 1963.
507. NATHAN, P. W., AND M. C. SMITH. Long descending tracts in man I. Review of present knowledge. *Brain* 78: 248-303, 1955.
508. NATHAN, P. W., AND M. C. SMITH. Fasciculi proprii of the spinal cord in man. *Brain* 82: 610-668, 1959.
509. NAUTA, H. J. W., AND M. COLE. Efferent projections of the subthalamic nucleus: an autoradiographic study in monkey and cat. *J. Comp. Neurol.* 180: 1-16, 1978.
510. NAUTA, W. J. H., AND P. A. GYGAX. Silver impregnation of degenerating axons in the central nervous system: a modified technique. *Stain Technol.* 29: 91-94, 1954.
511. NAUTA, W. J. H., AND W. HAYMAKER. Hypothalamic nuclei and fiber connections. In: *The Hypothalamus*, edited by W. Haymaker, E. Anderson, and W. J. H. Nauta. Springfield, IL: Thomas, 1969. p. 136-209.
512. NAUTA, W. J. H., AND W. R. MEHLER. Projections of the lentiform nucleus in the monkey. *Brain Res.* 1: 3-42, 1966.
513. NEWSON DAVIS, J., AND F. PLUM. Separation of descending spinal pathways to respiratory motoneurons. *Exp. Neurol.* 34: 78-94, 1972.
514. NIEOULLON, A., AND L. RISPAL-PADEL. Somatotopic localization in cat motor cortex. *Brain Res.* 105: 405-422, 1976.
515. NOBIN, A., AND A. BJÖRKLUND. Topography of the monoamine neuron systems in the human brain as revealed in fetuses. *Acta Physiol. Scand. Suppl.* 388: 1-40, 1973.
516. NOSAKA, S., T. YAMAMOTO, AND K. YASANUGA. Localization of vagal cardioinhibitory preganglionic neurons within rat brain stem. *J. Comp. Neurol.* 186: 79-92, 1979.
517. NYBERG-HANSEN, R. The location and termination of tectospinal fibers in the cat. *Exp. Neurol.* 9: 212-227, 1964.
518. NYBERG-HANSEN, R. Origin and termination of fibers from the vestibular nuclei descending in the medial longitudinal fasciculus. An experimental study with silver impregnation methods in the cat. *J. Comp. Neurol.* 122: 355-367, 1964.
519. NYBERG-HANSEN, R. Sites and mode of termination of reticulo-spinal fibers in the cat. An experimental study with silver impregnation methods. *J. Comp. Neurol.* 124: 71-100, 1965.
520. NYBERG-HANSEN, R. Functional organization of descending supraspinal fibre systems to the spinal cord. Anatomical observations and physiological correlations. *Ergeb. Anat. Entwicklungsesch.* 39: 6-47, 1966.
521. NYBERG-HANSEN, R. Sites of termination of interstitiospinal fibers in the cat. An experimental study with silver impregnation methods. *Arch. Ital. Biol.* 104: 98-111, 1966.
522. NYBERG-HANSEN, R. Do cat spinal motoneurones receive direct supraspinal fibre connections? A supplementary silver study. *Arch. Ital. Biol.* 107: 67-78, 1969.
523. NYBERG-HANSEN, R., AND A. BRODAL. Sites of termination of corticospinal fibers in the cat. An experimental study with silver impregnation methods. *J. Comp. Neurol.* 120: 369-391, 1963.
524. NYBERG-HANSEN, R., AND A. BRODAL. Sites and mode of termination of rubrospinal fibres in the cat. An experimental study with silver impregnation methods. *J. Anat.* 98: 235-253, 1964.
525. NYBERG-HANSEN, R., AND T. A. MASCITTI. Sites and mode of termination of fibers of the vestibulospinal tract in the cat. An experimental study with silver impregnation methods. *J. Comp. Neurol.* 122: 369-383, 1964.
526. NYBERG-HANSEN, R., AND E. RINVIK. Some comments on the pyramidal tract, with special reference to its individual variations in man. *Acta Neurol. Scand.* 39: 1-30, 1963.
527. NYGREN, L. G., AND L. OLSON. A new major projection from locus coeruleus: the main source of noradrenergic nerve terminals in the ventral and dorsal columns of the spinal cord. *Brain Res.* 132: 85-93, 1977.
528. OLIVERAS, J. L., S. BOURGOIN, F. HERY, J. M. BESSON, AND M. HAMON. The topographical distribution of serotoninergic terminals in the spinal cord of the cat: biochemical mapping by the combined use of microdissection and microassay procedures. *Brain Res.* 138: 393-406, 1977.
529. OLIVERAS, J. L., F. REDJEMI, G. GUILBAUD, AND J. M. BESSON. Analgesia induced by electrical stimulation of the inferior centralis nucleus of the raphe in the cat. *Pain* 1: 139-145, 1975.
530. OLSON, L., AND K. FUXE. On the projections from the locus coeruleus noradrenaline neurons: the cerebellar innervation. *Brain Res.* 28: 165-171, 1971.
531. OLSSON, T., AND K. KRISTENSSON. A simple histochemical method for double labelling of neurons by retrograde axonal transport. *Neurosci. Lett.* 8: 265-268, 1978.
532. OLZEWSKI, J., AND D. BAXTER. *Cytoarchitecture of the Human Brain Stem.* Basel: Karger, 1954.
533. ONUF, B. Notes on the arrangement and function of the cell groups in the sacral region of the spinal cord. *J. Nerv. Ment. Dis.* 26: 498-504, 1899.
534. ONUF, B. On the arrangement and function of the cell groups of the sacral region of the spinal cord in man. *Arch. Neurol. Psychopathol.* 3: 387-411, 1900.
535. ORIOLI, F. L., AND F. A. METTLER. The rubro-spinal tract in *Macaca mulatta*. *J. Comp. Neurol.* 106: 299-318, 1956.
536. PADEL, Y., J. ARMAND, AND A. M. SMITH. Topography of rubrospinal units in the cat. *Exp. Brain Res.* 14: 363-371, 1972.
537. PADEL, Y., A. M. SMITH, AND J. ARMAND. Topography of projections from the motor cortex to rubrospinal units in the cat. *Exp. Brain Res.* 17: 315-332, 1973.
538. PALAY, S. L., AND V. CHAN-PALAY. General morphology of neurons and neuroglia. In: *Handbook of Physiology. The Nervous System*, edited by J. M. Brookhart and V. B. Mountcastle. Bethesda, Maryland: Am. Physiol. Soc., 1977, sect. 1, vol. I., pt. 1, chapt. 2, p. 5-38.
539. PALKOVITS, M., AND D. M. JACOBOWITZ. Topographic atlas of

catecholamine and acetylcholinesterase-containing neurons in the rat brain. II. Hindbrain (mesencephalon, rhombencephalon). *J. Comp. Neurol.* 157: 29-42, 1974.
540. PANNETON, W. M., AND G. F. MARTIN. The organization of midbrain-facial systems. *Soc. Neurosci. Abstr.* 3: 276, 1977.
541. PANNETON, W. M., AND G. F. MARTIN. Midbrain projections to the trigeminal, facial and hypoglossal nuclei in the opossum. A study using axonal transport techniques. *Brain Res.* 168: 493-511, 1979.
542. PAPEZ, J. W. Reticulo-spinal tracts in the cat. Marchi method. *J. Comp. Neurol.* 41: 365-399, 1926.
543. PAPEZ, J. W. Subdivisions of the facial nucleus. *J. Comp. Neurol.* 43: 159-191, 1927.
544. PAPEZ, J. W., AND W. A. STOTLER. Connections of the red nucleus. *Arch. Neurol. Psychiatry* 44: 776-791, 1940.
545. PASSINGHAM, R., H. PERRY, AND F. WILKINSON. Failure to develop a precision grip in monkeys with unilateral neocortical lesions made in infancy. *Brain Res.* 145: 410-414, 1978.
546. PEARCE, G. W. Some cortical projections to the midbrain reticular formation. In: *Structure and Function of the Cerebral Cortex*, edited by D. B. Tower and J. P. Schadé. Amsterdam: Elsevier, 1960, p. 131-138. (Proc. Int. Mtng. Neurobiol., 2nd, Amsterdam, 1959.)
547. PETERSON, B. W., M. E. ANDERSON, AND M. FILION. Responses of ponto-medullary reticular neurons to cortical, tectal and cutaneous stimuli. *Exp. Brain Res.* 21: 19-44, 1974.
548. PETERSON, B. W., AND J. D. COULTER. A new long projection from the vestibular nuclei in the cat. *Brain Res.* 122: 351-356, 1977.
549. PETERSON, B. W., R. A. MAUNZ, N. G. PITTS, AND R. G. MACKEL. Patterns of projection and branching of reticulospinal neurons. *Exp. Brain Res.* 23: 333-351, 1975.
550. PETERSON, B. W., N. G. PITTS, AND K. FUKUSHIMA. Reticulospinal connections with limb and axial motoneurons. *Exp. Brain Res.* 36: 1-20, 1979.
551. PETERSON, B. W., N. G. PITTS, K. FUKUSHIMA, AND R. MACKEL. Reticulospinal excitation and inhibition of neck motoneurons *Exp. Brain Res.* 32: 471-489, 1978.
552. PETRAS, J. M. Some fiber connections of the precentral and postcentral cortex with the basal ganglia, thalamus and subthalamus. *Trans. Am. Neurol. Assoc.* 90: 274-275, 1965.
553. PETRAS, J. M. Cortical, tectal and tegmental fiber connections in the spinal cord of the cat. *Brain Res.* 6: 275-324, 1967.
554. PETRAS, J. M. Corticospinal fibers in New World and Old World simians. *Brain Res.* 8: 206-208, 1968.
555. PETRAS, J. M. Some efferent connections of the motor and somatosensory cortex of simian primates and felid, canid and procyonid carnivores. *Ann. NY Acad. Sci.* 167: 469-505, 1969.
556. PETRAS, J. M., AND J. F. CUMMINGS. Autonomic neurons in the spinal cord of the Rhesus monkey: a correlation of the findings of cytoarchitectonics and sympathectomy with fiber degeneration following dorsal rhizotomy. *J. Comp. Neurol.* 146: 189-218, 1972.
557. PETRAS, J. M., AND A. I. FADEN. The origin of sympathetic preganglionic neurons in the dog. *Brain Res.* 144: 353-357, 1978.
558. PETRAS, J. M., AND R. A. W. LEHMAN. Corticospinal fibers in the raccoon. *Brain Res.* 3: 195-197, 1966.
559. PHILIPS, C. G., AND R. PORTER. The pyramidal projection to motoneurones of some muscle groups of the baboon's forelimb. In: *Progress in Brain Research. Physiology of Spinal Neurons*, edited by J. C. Eccles and J. P. Schadé. Amsterdam: Elsevier, 1964, vol. 12, p. 222-242.
560. PICKEL, V. M., M. SEGAL, AND F. E. BLOOM. A radioautographic study of the efferent pathways of the nucleus locus coeruleus. *J. Comp. Neurol.* 155: 15-42, 1974.
561. PIN, C., B. JONES, AND M. JOUVET. Topographie des neurones monoaminergiques du tronc cérébral du chat: étude par histofluorescence. *C. R. Soc. Biol.* 162: 2136-2141, 1968.
562. POIRIER, L. J., AND G. BOUVIER. The red nucleus and its efferent nervous pathways in the monkey. *J. Comp. Neurol.* 128: 223-243, 1966.

563. POITRAS, D., AND A. PARENT. Atlas of the distribution of monoamine-containing nerve cell bodies in the brain stem of the cat. *J. Comp. Neurol.* 179: 699-718, 1978.
564. POLJAK, S. Die Struktureigentümlichkeiten des Rückenmarkes bei den Chiropteren. *Z. Anat. Entwicklungsgesch.* 74: 507-576, 1924.
565. POMPEIANO, O. Analisi degli effetti della stimolazione elettrica del nucleo rosso nel gatto decerebrato. *Atti Accad. Naz. Lincei Cl. Sci. Fis. Mat. Nat. Rend.* 22: 100-103, 1957.
566. POMPEIANO, O., AND A. BRODAL. Experimental demonstration of a somatotopical origin of rubrospinal fibers in the cat. *J. Comp. Neurol.* 108: 225-252, 1957.
567. POMPEIANO, O., AND A. BRODAL. The origin of the vestibulospinal fibers in the cat. An experimental-anatomical study, with comments on the descending medial longitudinal fasciculus. *Arch. Ital. Biol.* 95: 166-195, 1957.
568. POMPEIANO, O., AND F. WALBERG. Descending connections to the vestibular nuclei. An experimental study in the cat. *J. Comp. Neurol.* 108: 465-504, 1957.
569. PRECHT, W., J. GRIPPO, AND A. WAGNER. Contribution of different types of central vestibular neurons to the vestibulospinal system. *Brain Res.* 4: 119-123, 1967.
570. PRESTON, J. B., M. C. SHENDE, AND K. UEMURA. The motor cortex-pyramidal system: patterns of facilitation and inhibition on motoneurons innervating limb musculature of cat and baboon and their possible adaptive significance. In: *Neurophysiological Basis of Normal and Abnormal Motor Activities*, edited by M. D. Yahr and D. P. Purpura. New York: Raven, 1967, p. 61-72. (Symp. Parkinsons's Dis. Info. Res. Ctr., 3rd, New York, 1966.)
571. PRESTON, J. B., AND D. G. WHITLOCK. Intracellular potentials recorded from motoneurons following precentral gyrus stimulation in primate. *J. Neurophysiol.* 24: 91-100, 1961.
572. PROVIS, J. The organization of the facial nucleus of the brushtailed possum (*Trichosurus vulpecula*). *J. Comp. Neurol.* 172: 177-188, 1977.
573. PUBOLS, B. H. Retrograde degeneration study of somatic sensory thalamocortical connections in brain of Virginia opossum. *Brain Res.* 7: 232-251, 1968.
574. RACZKOWSKI, D., AND I. T. DIAMOND. Cells of origin of several efferent pathways from the superior colliculus in *Galago senegalensis*. *Brain Res.* 146: 351-357, 1978.
575. RAFOLS, J. A., AND H. A. MATZKE. Efferent projections of the superior colliculus in the opossum. *J. Comp. Neurol.* 138: 147-160, 1970.
576. RAISMAN, G., AND M. R. MATTHEWS. Degeneration and regeneration of synapses. In: *Structure and Function of Nervous Tissue*, edited by G. H. Bourne. New York: Academic, 1972, vol. V, p. 61-104.
577. RALL, W. Core conduction theory and cable properties of neurons. In: *Handbook of Physiology. The Nervous System*, edited by J. M. Brookhart and V. B. Mountcastle, Bethesda, MD: Am. Physiol. Soc., 1977, sect. 1, vol. I, pt. 1, chapt. 3, p. 36-97.
578. RAMON-MOLINER, E. The Golgi-Cox technique. In: *Contemporary Research Methods in Neuroanatomy*, edited by W. J. H. Nauta and O. E. Ebbeson, Berlin: Springer-Verlag, 1970, p. 32-55. (Proc. Int. Conf. Inst. Perinatal Physiol., San Juan, 1969.)
579. RAPOPORT, S. Location of sternocleidomastoid and trapezius motoneurons in the cat. *Brain Res.* 156: 339-344, 1978.
580. RASDOLSKY, I. Beiträge zur Architektur der grauen Substanz des Rückenmarks (Unter Benutzung einer neuen Methode der Färbung der Nervenfasernkollateralen). *Virchows Arch. Pathol. Anat. Physiol.* 257: 356-363, 1925.
581. RASDOLSKY, J. Über die Endigung der extraspinalen Bewegungssysteme im Rückenmark. *Z. Gesamte. Neurol. Psychiatr.* 86: 360-374, 1923.
582. RASMUSSEN, G. L. Selective silver impregnation of synaptic endings. In: *New Research Techniques of Neuroanatomy*, edited by W. F. Windle. Springfield, IL: Thomas, 1957, p. 27-39.

583. RAVIZZA, R. J., R. B. STRAW, AND P. D. LONG. Laminar origin of efferent projections from auditory cortex in the golden Syrian hamster. *Brain Res.* 114: 497-500, 1976.
584. RAYMOND, J., D. DEMEMES, AND R. MARTY. Voies et projections vestibulaires ascendantes emanant des noyaux primaires: étude radioautographique. *Brain Res.* 111: 1-12, 1976.
585. REDLICH, E. Beiträge zur Anatomie und Physiologie der motorischen Bahnen bei der Katze. *Monatsschr. Psychiatr. Neurol.* 5: 41-51, 1899.
586. REDLICH, E. Beiträge zur Anatomie und Physiologie der motorischen Bahnen bei der Katze. *Monatsschr. Psychiatr. Neurol.* 5: 112-128, 1899.
587. REDLICH, E. Beiträge zur Anatomie und Physiologie der motorischen Bahnen bei der Katze. *Monatsschr. Psychiatr. Neurol.* 5: 192-206, 1899.
588. REED, A. F. The nuclear masses in the cervical spinal cord of Macaca mulatta. *J. Comp. Neurol.* 72: 187-206, 1940.
589. REES, S., AND J. HORE. The motor cortex of the brush-tailed possum (*Trichosurus vulpecula*): motor representation, motor function and the pyramidal tract. *Brain Res.* 20: 439-451, 1970.
590. REXED, B. The cytoarchitectonic organization of the spinal cord in the cat. *J. Comp. Neurol.* 96: 415-493, 1952.
591. REXED, B. A cytoarchitectonic atlas of the spinal cord in the cat. *J. Comp. Neurol.* 100: 297-379, 1954.
592. RICHMOND, F. J. R., D. A. SCOTT, AND V. C. ABRAHAMS. Distribution of motoneurones to the neck muscles, biventer cervicis, splenius and complexus in the cat. *J. Comp. Neurol.* 181: 451-464, 1978.
593. RINVIK, E., AND F. WALBERG. Demonstration of a somatotopically arranged cortico-rubral projection in the cat. An experimental study with silver methods. *J. Comp. Neurol.* 120: 393-407, 1963.
594. ROBSON, J. A., AND W. C. HALL. Connections of layer VI in striate cortex of grey squirrel. (*Scirus carolinensis*). *Brain Res.* 93: 133-139, 1975.
595. ROMAGNANO, M. A., AND R. J. MACIEWICZ. Peroxidase labeling of motor cortex neurons projecting to the ventrolateral nucleus in the cat. *Brain Res.* 83: 469-473, 1975.
596. ROMANES, G. J. The motor cell columns of the lumbo-sacral spinal cord of the cat. *J. Comp. Neurol.* 94: 313-363, 1951.
597. ROMEIS, B. *Mikroscopische Technik.* Munich: R. Oldenbourg, 1948.
598. ROSE, P. K. Morphology of motoneurones in the upper cervical spinal cord of the adult cat. *J. Physiol. London* 272: 37P-38P, 1977.
599. ROSE, P. K., AND F. J. R. RICHMOND. A morphological description of motoneurons in the upper cervical spinal cord of the adult cat. *Soc. Neurosci. Abstr.* 3: 277, 1977.
600. ROSSI, G. F., AND A. BRODAL. Corticofugal fibers to the brain stem reticular formation. An experimental study in the cat. *J. Anat.* 90: 42-62, 1956.
601. ROUCOUX, A., AND M. CROMMELINCK. Eye movements evoked by superior colliculus stimulation in the alert cat. *Brain Res.* 106: 349-363, 1976.
602. RUSSELL, J. R., AND W. DEMEYER. The quantitive cortical origin of pyramidal axons of Macaca rhesus, with some remarks on slow rate of axolysis. *Neurology* 11: 96-108, 1961.
603. RUSTIONI, A. Non-primary afferents to the nucleus gracilis from the lumbar cord of the cat. *Brain Res.* 51: 81-95, 1973.
604. RUSTIONI, A. Spinal neurons project to the dorsal column nuclei of rhesus monkeys. *Science* 196: 656-658, 1977.
605. RUSTIONI, A., AND A. B. KAUFMAN. Identification of cells of origin of non-primary afferents to the dorsal column nuclei of the cat. *Exp. Brain Res.* 27: 1-14, 1977.
606. RUSTIONI, A., H. G. J. M. KUYPERS, AND G. HOLSTEGE. Propriospinal projections from the ventral and lateral funiculi to the motoneurons of the lumbosacral cord of the cat. *Brain Res.* 34: 255-275, 1971.
607. RUSTIONI, A., AND I. MOLENAAR. Dorsal column nuclei afferents in the lateral funiculus of the cat: distribution pattern and absence of sprouting after chronic deafferentation. *Exp. Brain Res.* 23: 1-12, 1975.
608. SADUN, A. Differential distribution of cortical terminations in the cat red nucleus. *Brain Res.* 99: 145-151, 1975.
609. SALMOIRAGHI, G. C., AND B. D. BURNS. Notes on mechanism of rhythmic respiration. *J. Neurophysiol.* 23: 14-26, 1960.
610. SANDRI, C., H. RIS, AND K. AKERT. Comparison of active zones in spinal cord of anesthetized and unanesthetized rats: a high voltage electron microscope study. *Brain Res.* 159: 247-253, 1978.
611. SAPER, C. B., A. D. LOEWY, L. W. SWANSON, AND W. M. COWAN. Direct hypothalamo-autonomic connections. *Brain Res.* 117: 305-312, 1976.
612. SASAKI, K., A. NAMIKAWA, AND S. HASHIRAMOTO. The effect of midbrain stimulation upon alpha motoneurones in lumbar spinal cord of the cat. *Jpn. J. Physiol.* 10: 303-316, 1960.
613. SATO, M., N. MIZUNO, AND A. KONISHI. Localization of motoneurons innervating perineal muscles: a HRP study in cat. *Brain Res.* 140: 149-154, 1978.
614. SATOH, K., M. TOHYAMA, K. SAKUMOTO, K. YAMAMOTO, AND N. SHIMIZU. Descending projection of the nucleus tegmentalis latero-dorsalis to the spinal cord: studied by the horseradish peroxidase method following 6-hydroxy-dopa administration. *Neurosci. Lett.* 8: 9-15, 1979.
615. SATOH, K., M. TOHYAMA, K. YAMAMOTO, T. SAKUMOTO, AND N. SHIMIZU. Noradrenaline innervation of the spinal cord studied by the horseradish peroxidase method combined with monoamine oxidase staining. *Exp. Brain Res.* 30: 175-186, 1977.
616. SATOMI, H., K. TAKAHASHI, H. ISE, AND T. YAMAMOTO. Identification of the superior salivatory nucleus in the cat as studied by the HRP method. *Neurosci. Lett.* 14: 135-139, 1979.
617. SATOMI, H., T. YAMAMOTO, H. ISE, AND K. TAKAHASHI. Identification of the inferior salivatory nucleus in the cat as studied by HRP bathings of the transected glossopharyngeal nerve root. *Neurosci. Lett.* 11: 259-263, 1979.
618. SATOMI, H., T. YAMAMOTO, H. ISE, AND H. TAKATAMA. Origins of the parasympathetic preganglionic fibers to the cat intestine as demonstrated by the horseradish peroxidase method. *Brain Res.* 151: 571-578, 1978.
619. SCHEIBEL, M. E., AND A. B. SCHEIBEL. Structural substrates for integrative patterns in the brain stem reticular core. In: *Reticular Formation of the Brain*, edited by H. H. Jasper, L. D. Proctor, A. S. Knighton, W. C. Noshap, and R. T. Costello, Boston: Little Brown, 1958, p. 31-55.
620. SCHEIBEL, M. E., AND A. B. SCHEIBEL. Spinal motoneurons, interneurons and Renshaw cells. A Golgi study. *Arch. Ital. Biol.* 104: 328-353, 1966.
621. SCHEIBEL, M. E., AND A. B. SCHEIBEL. Organization of spinal motoneuron dendrites in bundles. *Exp. Neurol.*, 28: 106-112, 1970.
622. SCHEIBEL, M. E., AND A. B. SCHEIBEL. Inhibition and the Renshaw cell a structural critique. *Brain Behav. Evol.* 4: 53-93, 1971.
623. SCHIMERT, J. S. Die Endigungsweise des Tractus vestibulospinalis. *Z. Anat. Entwicklungsgesch.* 108: 761-767, 1938.
624. SCHOEN, J. H. R. Comparative aspects of the descending fiber systems in the spinal cord. In: *Progress in Brain Research. Organization of the Spinal Cord*, edited by J. C. Eccles and J. P. Schadé. Amsterdam: Elsevier, 1964, vol. 11, p. 203-222.
625. SCHOEN, J. H. R. The corticofugal projection in the brain stem and spinal cord in man. *Psychiatr. Neurol. Neurochir.* 72: 121-128, 1969.
626. SCHOEN, J. H. R. Some supplementary data concerning the central tegmental tract in man. *Acta Morphol. Neerl. Scand.* 10: 380-381, 1972.
627. SCHONBACH, J., C. SCHONBACH, AND M. CUENOD. Rapid phase of exoplasmic flow and synaptic proteins: an electron microscopical autoradiographic study. *J. Comp. Neurol.* 141: 485-498, 1971.
628. SEARS, T. A. Pathways of supra-spinal origin regulating the activity of respiratory motoneurones. In: *Muscular Afferents and Motor Control*, edited by R. Granit. Stockholm: Almqvist

and Wiksell, 1966, p. 187-196. (Proc. Nobel Symp. I. Stockholm, 1965.)
629. SHAPOVALOV, A. I. Posttetanic potentiation of monosynaptic and disynaptic actions from supraspinal structures on lumbar motoneurons. *J. Neurophysiol.* 32: 948-959, 1969.
630. SHAPOVALOV, A. I. Extrapyramidal monosynaptic and disynaptic control of mammalian alpha-motoneurons. *Brain Res.* 40: 105-115, 1972.
631. SHAPOVALOV, A. I. Extrapyramidal control of primate motoneurons. In: *New Developments in Electromyography and Clinical Neurophysiology,* edited by J. E. Desmedt. Basel: Karger, 1973, vol. 3, p. 145-158.
632. SHAPOVALOV, A. I. Neuronal organization and synaptic mechanisms of supraspinal motor control in vertebrates. *Rev. Physiol. Biochem. Pharmacol.* 72: 1-54, 1975.
633. SHAPOVALOV, A. I., AND N. R. GUREVITCH. Monosynaptic and disynaptic reticulospinal actions on lumbar motoneurons of the rat. *Brain Res.* 21: 249-263, 1970.
634. SHAPOVALOV, A. I., AND O. A. KARAMIAN. Short-latency interstitiospinal and rubrospinal synaptic influences on alpha-motoneurons. *Byull. Eksp. Biol. Med.* 66: 1297-1300, 1968.
635. SHAPOVALOV, A. I., O. A. KARAMJAN, G. G. KURCHAVYI, AND Z. A. REPINA. Synaptic actions evoked from the red nucleus on spinal alpha-motoneurons in the Rhesus monkey. *Brain Res.* 32: 325-348, 1971.
636. SHIGENAGA, Y., M. TAKABATAKE, T. SUGIMOTO, AND A. SAKAI. Neurons in marginal layer of trigeminal nucleus caudalis project to ventrobasal complex (VB) and posterior nuclear group (PO) demonstrated by retrograde labeling with horseradish peroxidase. *Brain Res.* 166: 391-396, 1979.
637. SHINODA, Y., A. P. ARNOLD, AND H. ASANUMA. Spinal branching of corticospinal axons in the cat. *Exp. Brain Res.* 26: 215-234, 1976.
638. SHINODA, Y., C. GHEZ, AND A. ARNOLD. Spinal branching of rubrospinal axons in the cat. *Exp. Brain Res.* 30: 203-218, 1977.
639. SHINODA, Y., P. ZARZECKI, AND H. ASANUMA. Spinal branching of pyramidal tract neurons in the monkey. *Exp. Brain Res.* 34: 59-72, 1979.
639a.SHINODA, Y., J. YOKOTA, AND T. FUTAMI. Divergent projection of individual corticospinal axons to motoneurons of multiple muscles in the monkey. *Neurosci. Lett.* In press.
640. SHRIVER, J. E., AND C. R. NOBACK. Cortical projections to the lower brain stem and spinal cord in the three shrew (*Tupaia glis*). *J. Comp. Neurol.* 130: 25-54, 1967.
641. SIEGEL, J. Behavioral relations of medullary reticular formation cells. *Exp. Neurol.* 65: 691-698, 1979.
642. SIEGEL, J., P. M. SAXTON, AND T. HAGEMAN. Descending projections to the region of the gigantocellular tegmental field of the medulla oblongata. *Soc. Neurosci. Abstr.* 3: 71, 1977.
643. SIEGEL, J. M., AND D. J. MCGINTY. Pontine reticular formation neurons: relationship of discharge to motor activity. *Science* 196: 678-680, 1977.
644. SIEGEL, J. M., AND D. J. MCGINTY. Pontine reticular formation and motor activity. *Science* 199: 207-208, 1978.
645. SKINNER, R. D., J. D. COULTER, AND A. B. CHATT. Origins of the long descending and ascending propriospinal pathways in cat and monkey. *Soc. Neurosci. Abstr.* 3: 508, 1977.
646. SKINNER, R. D., AND R. S. REMMEL. Monosynaptic inputs to lumbar interneurons from the lateral vestibulospinal tract and the medial longitudinal fasciculus. *Neurosci. Lett.* 10: 259-264, 1978.
647. SKULTETY, F. M. Circus movements in cats following midbrain stimulation through chronically implanted electrodes. *J. Neurophysiol.* 25: 152-164, 1962.
648. SMITH, A. M., AND J. COURVILLE. The origin of the rubrospinal tract in primates as shown by the retrograde transport of horseradish peroxidase. *Soc. Neurosci. Abstr.* 2: 551, 1976.
649. SNOW, P. J., P. K. ROSE, AND A. BROWN. Tracing axons and axon collaterals of spinal neurones using intracellular injection of horseradish peroxidase. *Science* 191: 312-313, 1976.
650. SPRAGUE, J. M. A study of motor cell localization in the spinal cord of the rhesus monkey. *Am. J. Anat.* 82: 1-26, 1948.
651. SPRAGUE, J. M., AND W. W. CHAMBERS. Control of posture by reticular formation and cerebellum in the intact, anesthetized and unanesthetized and in the decerebrated cat. *Am. J. Physiol.* 176: 52-64, 1954.
652. SPRAGUE, J. M., AND H. HA. The terminal fields of dorsal root fibers in the lumbosacral cord of the cat, and the dendritic organization of the motor nuclei. In: *Progress in Brain Research. Organization of the Spinal Cord,* edited by J. C. Eccles and J. P. Schadé. Amsterdam: Elsevier, 1964, vol. 11, p. 120-154.
653. SPRAGUE, J. M., AND T. H. MEIKLE. The role of the superior colliculus in visually guided behavior. *Exp. Neurol.* 11: 115-146, 1965.
654. STEIN, B. M., AND M. B. CARPENTER. Central projections of portions of the vestibular ganglion innervating specific parts of the labyrinth in the rhesus monkey. *Am. J. Anat.* 120: 281-318, 1967.
655. STERLING, P., AND H. G. J. M. KUYPERS. Anatomical organization of the brachial spinal cord of the cat. I. Distribution of dorsal root fibers. *Brain Res.* 4: 1-15, 1967.
656. STERLING, P., AND H. G. J. M. KUYPERS. Anatomical organization of the brachial spinal cord of the cat. II. The motoneuron plexus. *Brain Res.* 4: 16-32, 1967.
657. STERLING, P., AND H. G. J. M. KUYPERS. Anatomical organization of the brachial spinal cord of the cat. III. The propriospinal connections. *Brain Res.* 7: 419-443, 1968.
658. STERN, K. Note on nucleus ruber magnocellularis and its efferent pathway in man. *Brain* 61: 284-289, 1938.
659. STEWARD, O., S. A. SCOVILLE, AND S. L. VINSANT. Analysis of collateral projections with a double retrograde labeling technique. *Neurosci. Lett.* 5: 1-6, 1977.
660. STEWART, W. A., AND R. B. KING. Fiber projections from the nucleus caudalis of the spinal trigeminal nucleus. *J. Comp. Neurol.* 121: 271-286, 1963.
661. STREIT, P., AND J. C. REUBI. A new and sensitive staining method for axonally transported horseradish peroxidase in the pigeon visual system. *Brain Res.* 126: 530-537, 1977.
662. STRICK, P. L., R. E. BURKE, K. KANDA, C. C. KIM, AND B. WALMSLEY. Differences between alpha and gamma motoneurons labeled with horseradish peroxidase by retrograde transport. *Brain Res.* 113: 582-588, 1976.
663. STROMINGER, N. L. A comparison of the pyramidal tracts in two species of edentate. *Brain Res.* 15: 259-262, 1969.
664. STROMINGER, N. L., T. C. TRUSCOTT, R. A. MILLER, AND G. J. ROYCE. An autoradiographic study of the rubroolivary tract in the rhesus monkey. *J. Comp. Neurol.* 183: 33-46, 1979.
665. SUGIMOTO, T., K. ITOH, AND N. MIZUNO. Direct projections from the Edinger-Westphal nucleus of the cerebellum and spinal cord in the cat: an HRP study. *Neurosci. Lett.* 9: 17-22, 1978.
666. SUGIMOTO, T., K. ITOH, N. MIZUNO, S. NOMURA, AND A. KONISHI. The site of origin of the cardiac preganglionic fibers of the vagus nerve: an HRP study in the cat. *Neurosci. Lett.* 12: 53-58, 1979.
667. SWANK, R. L. Aberrant pyramidal fascicles in the cat. *J. Comp. Neurol.* 60: 355-359, 1934.
668. SWANK, R. L. The relationship between the circumolivary pyramidal fascicles and the pontobulbar body in man. *J. Comp. Neurol.* 60: 309-317, 1934.
669. SWANK, R. L., AND H. A. DAVENPORT. Marchis staining method: studies of some of the underlying mechanism involved. *Stain Technol.* 9: 11-19, 1934.
670. SWANSON, L. W. Immunohistochemical evidence for a neurophysin containing autonomic pathway arising in the paraventricular nucleus of the hypothalamus. *Brain Res.* 128: 346-353, 1977.
671. SWANSON, L. W., AND B. K. HARTMAN. The central adrenergic system. An immunofluorescence study of the location of cell bodies and their efferent connections in the rat utilizing dopamine-beta-hydroxylase as a marker. *J. Comp. Neurol.* 163: 467-505, 1975.

672. SZEKELY, G. Anatomy and synaptology of the optic tectum. In: *Handbook of Sensory Physiology. Central Processing of Vision Information*, edited by R. Jung. Berlin: Springer-Verlag, 1973, vol. 7, pt. 3, sect. B, p. 1-26.
673. SZENTAGOTHAI, J. Die zentrale Innervation der Augenbewegungen. *Arch. Psychiatr. Nervenkr.* 116: 721-760, 1943.
674. SZENTAGOTHAI, J. Short propriospinal neurons and intrinsic connections of the spinal gray matter. *Acta Morphol. Acad. Sci. Hung.* 1: 81-94, 1951.
675. SZENTAGOTHAI, J. Synaptic architecture of the spinal motoneuron pool. In: *Recent Advances in Clinical Neurophysiology*, edited by L. Widén. Amsterdam: Elsevier, 1967, p. 4-19.
676. SZENTAGOTHAI, J. Propriospinal pathways and their synapses. In: *Progress in Brain Research. Organization of the Spinal Cord*, edited by J. C. Eccles and J. P. Schadé. Amsterdam: Elsevier, 1969, vol. 11, p. 155-177.
677. SZENTAGOTHAI, J., AND K. RAJKOVITS. Der Hirnnervenanteil der Pyramidenbahn und der prämotorische Apparat motorischer Hirnnervenkerne. *Arch. Psychiatr. Nervenkr.* 197: 335-354, 1958.
678. SZENTAGOTHAI-SCHIMERT, J. Die Endigungsweise der absteigenden Rückenmarksbahnen. *Z. Anat. Entwicklungsgesch.* 11: 322-330, 1941.
679. SZTEYN, S., J. WELENTO, AND Z. MILART. Centres of efferent tracts of the brain stem in the sheep. *Anat. Anz.* 121: 29-37, 1967.
680. TABER, E. The cytoarchitecture of the brain stem of the cat. 1. Brain stem nuclei of cat. *J. Comp. Neurol.* 116: 27-69, 1961.
681. TABER, E., A. BRODAL, AND F. WALBERG. The raphe nuclei of the brain stem in the cat. 1. Normal topography and cytoarchitecture and general discussion. *J. Comp. Neurol.* 114: 161-187, 1960.
682. TANAKA, T., Y. TAKEUCHI, AND K. NAKANO. Cells of origin of the spina-facial pathway in the cat: a horseradish peroxidase study. *Brain Res.* 142: 580-585, 1978.
683. TARLOV, E. The rostral projections of the primate vestibular nuclei. An experimental study in the macaque baboon and chimpanzee. *J. Comp. Neurol.* 135: 27-56, 1969.
684. TARLOV, E. Organization of vestibulo-oculomotor projections in the cat. *Brain Res.* 20: 159-179, 1970.
685. TARLOV, E., AND S. R. TARLOV. The representation of extraocular muscles in the oculomotor nuclei: experimental studies in the cat. *Brain. Res.* 34: 37-52, 1971.
686. TAYLOR, A. C., AND P. WEISS. Demonstration of axonal flow by the movement of tritium-labeled protein in mature optic nerve fibers. *Proc. Natl. Acad. Sci. USA* 54: 1521-1527, 1965.
687. TEN DONKELAAR, H. J. Descending pathways from the brain stem to the spinal cord in some reptiles. I. Origin. *J. Comp. Neurol.* 167: 421-442, 1976.
688. TEN DONKELAAR, H. J. Descending pathways from the brain stem to spinal cord in some reptiles. II. Course and site of termination. *J. Comp. Neurol.* 167: 443-464, 1976.
689. TEN DONKELAAR, H. J., AND R. DE BOER-VAN HUIZEN. Cells of origin of pathways descending to the spinal cord in a lizard (*Lacerta gallotti*). *Neurosci. Lett.* 9: 123-128, 1978.
690. TEN DONKELAAR, H. J., AND R. DE BOER-VAN HUIZEN. Cells of origin of propiospinal and ascending supraspinal fibres in a lizard (*Lacerta gallotti*). *Neurosci. Lett.* 4: 285-290, 1978.
691. TESTA, C. Functional implications of the morphology of spinal ventral horn neurons of the cat. *J. Comp. Neurol.* 123: 425-444, 1964.
692. THOMAS, D. M., R. P. KAUFMANN, J. M. SPRAGUE, AND W. W. CHAMBERS. Experimental studies of the vermal cerebellar projections in the brain stem of the cat (fastigiobulbar tract). *J. Anat.* 90: 371-385, 1956.
693. THULIN, C. A. Effects of electrical stimulation of the red nucleus on the alpha motor system. *Exp. Neurol.* 7: 464-480, 1963.
694. TIGGES, J., S. NAKAGAWA, AND M. TIGGES. Effects of area 4 in a South American monkey (Saimiri). I. Terminations in the spinal cord. *Brain Res.* 171: 1-11, 1979.
695. TOBIAS, T. J., AND F. F. EBNER. Thalamocortical projections from the mediodorsal nucleus in the Virginia opossum. *Brain Res.* 52: 79-96, 1973.
696. TODO, K., T. YAMAMOTO, H. SATOMI, H. ISE, H. TAKATAMA, AND K. TAKAHASHI. Origins of vagal preganglionic fibers to the sino-atrial and atrio-ventricular node regions in the cat heart as studied by the horseradish peroxidase method. *Brain Res.* 130: 545-550, 1977.
697. TOHYAMA, M., K. SAKAI, D. SALVERT, M. TOURET, AND M. JOUVET. Spinal projections from the lower brain stem in the cat as demonstrated by the horseradish peroxidase technique. I. Origins of the reticulo-spinal tracts and their funicular trajectories. *Brain Res.* 173: 383-404, 1979.
698. TOHYAMA, M., K. SAKAI, M. TOURET, D. SALVERT, AND M. JOUVET. Spinal projections from the lower brain stem in the cat as demonstrated by the horseradish peroxidase technique. II. Projections from the dorsolateral pontine tegmentum and raphe nuclei. *Brain Res.* 176: 215-231, 1979.
699. TORVIK, A. Afferent connections to the sensory trigeminal nuclei, the nucleus of the solitary tract and adjacent structures. An experimental study in the rat. *J. Comp. Neurol.* 106: 51-132, 1956.
700. TORVIK, A. The spinal projection from the nucleus of the solitary tract. An experimental study in the cat. *J. Anat.* 91: 314-322, 1957.
701. TORVIK, A., AND A. BRODAL. The origin of reticulospinal fibers in the cat. An experimental study. *Anat. Rec.* 128: 113-137, 1957.
702. TOWE, A. L. Motor cortex and the pyramidal system. In: *Efferent Organization and the Integration of Behavior*, edited by J. D. Maser. New York: Academic, 1973, p. 67-97.
703. TOWER, S., D. BODIAN, AND H. HOWE. Isolation of intrinsic and motor mechanism of the monkey's spinal cord. *J. Neurophysiol.* 4: 388-397, 1941.
704. TOWER, S. S. Pyramidal lesion in the monkey. *Brain* 63: 36-90, 1940.
705. TREDICI, G., G. PIZZINI, AND A. MIANI. The ultrastructure of the red nucleus of the cat. *J. Submicrosc. Cytol.* 5: 29-48, 1973.
706. TREVINO, D. L., AND E. CARSTENS. Confirmation of the location of spinothalamic neurons in the cat and monkey by the retrograde of horseradish peroxidase. *Brain Res.* 98: 177-182, 1975.
707. TREVINO, D. L., J. D. COULTER, AND W. D. WILLIS. Location of cells of origin of spinothalamic tract in lumbar enlargement of the monkey. *J. Neurophysiol.* 36: 750-761, 1973.
708. TREVINO, D. L., R. MAUNZ, R. N. BRYAN, AND W. D. WILLIS. Location of cells of origin of the spinothalamic tract in the lumbar enlargement of cat. *Exp. Neurol.* 34: 64-77, 1972.
709. TSUKAHARA, N., AND D. R. G. FULLER. Conductance changes during pyramidally induced postsynaptic potentials in red nucleus neurons. *J. Neurophysiol.* 32: 35-42, 1969.
710. TSUKAHARA, N., D. R. G. FULLER, AND V. B. BROOKS. Collateral pyramidal influences on the corticorubrospinal system. *J. Neurophysiol.* 31: 467-484, 1968.
711. TSUKAHARA, N., H. HULTBORN, F. MURAKAMI, AND Y. FUJITO. Electrophysiological study of formation of new synapses and collateral sprouting in red nucleus neurons after partial denervation. *J. Neurophysiol.* 38: 1359-1372, 1975.
712. TSUKAHARA, N., K. TOYAMA, AND K. KOSAKA. Electrical activity of red nucleus neurones investigated with intracellular microelectrodes. *Exp. Brain Res.* 4: 18-33, 1967.
713. ULLAH, M. Localization of the phrenic nucleus in the spinal cord of the rabbit. *J. Anat.* 125: 377-386, 1978.
714. UNGERSTEDT, U. Stereotaxic mapping of the monoamine pathways in the rat brain. *Acta Physiol. Scand. Suppl.* 367: 1-48, 1971.
715. VACCA, L. L., S. L. ROSARIO, E. A. ZIMMERMAN, P. TOMASHEFSKY, N. G. PY, AND K. C. HSU. Application of immunoperoxidase techniques to localize horseradish peroxidase-tracer in the central nervous system. *J. Histochem. Cytochem.* 23: 208-215, 1975.

716. VALVERDE, F. A new type of cell in the lateral reticular formation of the brain stem. *J. Comp. Neurol.* 117: 189–195, 1961.
717. VALVERDE, F. Reticular formation of the pons and medulla oblongata. A Golgi study. *J. Comp. Neurol.* 116: 71–100, 1961.
718. VALVERDE, F. Reticular formation of the albino rat's brain stem cytoarchitecture and corticofugal connections. *J. Comp. Neurol.* 119: 25–49, 1962.
719. VALVERDE, F. The pyramidal tract in rodents. A study of its relations with the posterior column nuclei, dorsolateral reticular formation of the medulla oblongata, and cervical spinal cord. *Z. Zellforsch. Mikrosk. Anat.* 71: 297–363, 1966.
720. VAN DER KOOY, D., H. G. J. M. KUYPERS, AND C. E. CATSMAN-BERREVOETS. Single mammillary body cells with divergent axon collaterals. Demonstration by a simple fluorescent retrograde double labeling technique in the rat. *Brain Res.* 158: 189–196, 1978.
721. VANDESANDE, F. A critical review of immunocytochemical methods for light microscopy. *J. Neurosci. Methods* 1: 3–23, 1979.
722. VANDESANDE, F., J. DEMEY, AND K. DIERICKX. Identification of neurophysin producing cells. I. The origin of neurophysin-like substance containing nerve fibers of external region of median eminence of the rat. *Cell Tissue Res.* 151: 187–200, 1974.
723. VANDESANDE, F., K. DIERICKX, AND J. DEMEY. Identification of the vasopressin-neurophysin II and the oxytocin-neurophysin I producing neurons in the bovine hypothalamus. *Cell Tissue Res.* 156: 189–200, 1975.
724. VASILENKO, D. A. Propriospinal pathways in the ventral funicles of the cat spinal cord: their effects on lumbosacral motoneurones. *Brain Res.* 93: 502–506, 1975.
725. VASILENKO, D. A., AND A. I. KOSTYUKOV. Brain stem and primary afferent projections to the ventromedial group of propriospinal neurones in the cat. *Brain Res.* 117: 141–146, 1976.
726. VERHAART, W. J. C. Hypertrophy of pes penduculi and pyramid as result of degeneration of contralateral corticofugal fiber tracts. *J. Comp. Neurol.* 92: 1–15, 1950.
727. VERHAART, W. J. C. The rubrospinal tract in the cat, the monkey and the ape, its location and fibre content. *Monatsschr. Psychiatr. Neurol.* 129: 487–500, 1955.
728. VERHAART, W. J. C. Pyramidal tract in the cord of the elephant. *J. Comp. Neurol.* 121: 45–49, 1963.
729. VERHAART, W. J. C. The pyramidal tract of tupaia, compared to that in other primates. *J. Comp. Neurol.* 126: 43–50, 1966.
730. VERHAART, W. J. C. The non-crossing of the pyramidal tract in procavia capensis (Storr) and other instances of absence of the pyramidal crossing. *J. Comp. Neurol.* 131: 387–392, 1967.
731. VERHAART, W. J. C. *Comparative Anatomical Aspects of the Mammalian Brain Stem and the Cord.* Assen, The Netherlands: Van Gorcum, 1970, vol. 1.
732. VERHAART, W. J. C. The pyramidal tract in the primates. In: *Advances in Primatology. The Primate Brain,* edited by C. R. Noback and W. Montagna. New York: Appleton, 1970, vol. 1, p. 83–108.
733. VERHAART, W. J. C., AND W. KRAMER. The uncrossed pyramidal tract. *Acta Psychiatr. Neurol. Scand.* 27: 181–200, 1952.
734. VERHAART, W. J. C., AND N. J. A. NOORDUYN. The cerebral peduncle and the pyramid. *Acta Anat.* 45: 315–343, 1961.
735. VERHAART, W. J. C., AND M. R. SOPERS-JURGENS. Aspects of comparative anatomy of the mammalian brainstem. *Acta Morphol. Neerl. Scand.* 1: 246–255, 1957.
736. VIERCK, C. J., JR., R. H. BROOKS, AND D. C. GOODMAN. Forced movement resulting from midbrain stimulation in the rat. *Brain Behav. Evol.* 1: 519–528, 1968.
737. VOOGD, J. *The Cerebellum of the Cat.* Assen, The Netherlands: Van Gorcum, 1964.
738. WAGMAN, I. H. Eye movements induced by electrical stimulation of cerebrum in monkeys and their relationship to bodily movements. In: *The Oculomotor System,* edited by M. B. Bender. New York: Harper, 1964, p. 18–39.
739. WALBERG, F. Descending connections to the inferior olive. An experimental study in the cat. *J. Comp. Neurol.* 104: 77–174, 1956.
740. WALBERG, F. Corticofugal fibres to the nuclei of the dorsal columns. An experimental study in the cat. *Brain* 80: 273–287, 1957.
741. WALBERG, F., D. BOWSHER, AND A. BRODAL. The termination of primary vestibular fibers in the vestibular nuclei in cat. An experimental study with silver methods. *J. Comp. Neurol.* 110: 391–419, 1958.
742. WALBERG, F., AND A. BRODAL. Pyramidal tract fibres from temporal and occipital lobes. An experimental study in the cat. *Brain* 76: 491–508, 1953.
743. WALBERG, F., O. POMPEIANO, A. BRODAL, AND J. JANSEN. The fastigiovestibular projection in the cat. An experimental study with silver impregnation methods. *J. Comp. Neurol.* 118: 49–76, 1962.
744. WALBERG, F., O. POMPEIANO, L. E. WESTRUM, AND E. HAUGLIEH-HANSSEN. Fastigioreticular fibers in the cat. An experimental study with silver methods. *J. Comp. Neurol.* 119: 187–199, 1962.
745. WALDRON, H. A., AND D. G. GWYN. Descending nerve tracts in the spinal cord of the rat. I. Fibers from the midbrain. *J. Comp. Neurol.* 137: 143–154, 1969.
746. WALKER, E. A., AND J. F. FULTON. Hemidecortication in chimpanzee, baboon, macaque, cat and coati: a study in encephalization. *J. Nerv. Ment. Dis.* 87: 677–700, 1938.
747. WALLER, A. Experiments on the section of the glossopharyngeal and hypoglossal nerves of the frog and observations of the alterations produced thereby in the structure of their primitive fibers. *Philos. Trans. R. Soc. London Ser. B.* 140: 423–469, 1850.
748. WARE, C. B., AND E. J. MUFSON. Spinal cord projections from the medial cerebellar nucleus in tree shrew (*Tupaia glis*). *Brain Res.* 171: 383–400, 1979.
749. WARNER, G., AND C. R. R. WATSON. The rubrospinal tract in a diprotodont marsupial (*Trichosurus vulpecula*). *Brain Res.* 41: 180–183, 1972.
750. WARWICK, R. Representation of the extra-ocular muscles in the oculomotor nuclei of the monkey. *J. Comp. Neurol.* 98: 449–504, 1953.
751. WARWICK, R., AND G. A. G. MITCHELL. The phrenic nucleus of the rhesus monkey. *J. Anat.* 89: 562–563, 1955.
752. WATSON, C. R. R. The corticospinal tract of the quokka wallaby (*Setonix brachyurus*). *J. Anat.* 109: 127–133, 1971.
753. WATSON, C. R. R. An experimental study of the corticospinal tract of the kangaroo. *J. Anat.* 110: 501, 1971.
754. WEBBER, CH.L., JR., R. D. WURSTER, AND J. M. CHUNG. Cat phrenic nucleus architecture as revealed by horseradish peroxidase mapping. *Exp. Brain Res.* 35: 395–406, 1979.
755. WEBER, J. T., G. F. MARTIN, M. BEHAN, M. F. HUERTA, AND J. K. HARTING. The precise origin of the tectospinal pathway in three common laboratory animals: a study using the horseradish peroxidase method. *Neurosci. Lett.* 11: 121–127, 1979.
756. WEISBERG, J. A., AND A. RUSTIONI. Cortical cells projecting to the dorsal column nuclei of cats. An anatomical study with the horseradish peroxidase technique. *J. Comp. Neurol.* 168: 425–437, 1976.
757. WEISBERG, J. A., AND A. RUSTIONI. Cortical cells projecting to the dorsal column nuclei of rhesus monkeys. *Exp. Brain Res.* 28: 521–528, 1977.
758. WEISBERG, J. A., AND A. RUSTIONI. Differential projections of cortical sensorimotor areas upon the dorsal column nuclei of cats. *J. Comp. Neurol.* 184: 401–422, 1979.
759. WEST, D. C., AND J. H. WOLSTENCROFT. Location and conduction velocity of raphespinal neurones in nucleus raphe magnus and raphe pallidus in the cat. *Neurosci. Lett.* 5: 147–151, 1977.
760. WHITE, R. P., AND H. E. HIMWICH. Circus movements and excitation of striatal and mesodiencephalic centers in rabbits.

J. Neurophysiol. 20: 81–90, 1957.

761. WILLIS, W. D., L. H. HABER, AND R. F. MARTIN. Inhibition of spinothalamic tract cells and interneurons by brain stem stimulation in the monkey. *J. Neurophysiol.* 40: 968–981, 1977.
762. WILSON, M. E., AND M. J. TOYNE. Retino-tectal and corticotectal projections in *Macaca mulatta*. *Brain Res.* 24: 395–406, 1970.
763. WILSON, V. J., M. KATO, B. W. PETERSON, AND R. M. WYLIE. A single-unit analysis of the organization of Deiters' nucleus. *J. Neurophysiol.* 30: 603–619, 1967.
764. WILSON, V. J., R. M. WYLIE, AND L. A. MARCO. Projection to spinal cord from the medial and the descending vestibular nuclei of the cat. *Nature* 215: 429–430, 1967.
765. WILSON, V. J., R. M. WYLIE, AND L. A. MARCO. Organization of the medial vestibular nucleus. *J. Neurophysiol.* 31: 166–175, 1968.
766. WILSON, V. J., AND M. YOSHIDA. Comparison of effects of stimulation of Deiters' nucleus and medial longitudinal fasciculus on neck, forelimb, and hindlimb motoneurons. *J. Neurophysiol.* 32: 743–758, 1969.
767. WILSON, V. J., AND M. YOSHIDA. Monosynaptic inhibition of neck motoneurones by the medial vestibular nucleus. *Exp. Brain Res.* 9: 365–380, 1969.
768. WILSON, V. J., M. YOSHIDA, AND R. H. SCHOR. Supraspinal monosynaptic excitation and inhibition of thoracic back motoneurons. *Exp. Brain Res.* 11: 282–295, 1970.
769. WIRTH, F. P., J. L. O'LEARY, J. M. SMITH, AND A. B. JENNY. Monosynaptic corticospinal-motoneuron path in the raccoon. *Brain Res.* 77: 344–348, 1974.
770. WISE, S. P. The laminar organization of certain afferent and efferent fiber systems in the rat somatosensory cortex. *Brain Res.* 90: 139–142, 1975.
771. WISE, S. P., AND E. G. JONES. The organization and postnatal development of the commissural projection of the rat somatic sensory cortex. *J. Comp. Neurol.* 168: 313–344, 1976.
772. WISE, S. P., AND E. G. JONES. Somatotopic and columnar organization in the corticotectal projection of the rat somatic sensory cortex. *Brain Res.* 133: 223–235, 1977.
773. WITANEN, J. T. Selective silver impregnation of degenerating axons and axon terminals in the central nervous system of the monkey (*Macaca mulatta*). *Brain Res.* 14: 546–548, 1969.
774. WOLSTENCROFT, J. H. Reticulospinal neurones. *J. Physiol. London* 174: 91–108, 1964.
775. WONG-RILEY, M. T. T. Demonstration of geniculocortical and callosal projection neurons in the squirrel monkey by means of retrograde axonal transport of horseradish peroxidase. *Brain Res.* 79: 267–272, 1974.
776. WOOLSEY, C. N. Organization of somatic sensory and motor areas of the cerebral cortex. In: *Biological and Biochemical Bases of Behavior*, edited by H. F. Harlow and C. N. Woolsey. Madison: Univ. of Wisconsin Press, 1958, p. 63–81.
777. WOOLSEY, C. N., AND H. T. CHANG. Activation of the cerebral cortex by antidromic volleys in the pyramidal tract. *Res. Publ. Assoc. Res. Nerv. Ment. Dis.* 27: 146–162, 1948.
778. WOOLSEY, C. N., T. GORSKA, A. WETZEL, T. C. ERICKSON, F. EARLS, AND J. M. ALLMAN. Complete unilateral section of the pyramidal tract at the medullary level in *Macaca mulatta*. *Brain Res.* 40: 119–123, 1972.
779. WOOLSEY, C. N., P. H. SETTLAGE, D. R. MEYER, W. SPENCER, P. HAMUY, AND A. M. TRAVIS. Patterns of localization in the precentral and "supplementary" motor areas and their relation to the concept of a premotor area. *Res. Publ. Assoc. Res. Nerv. Ment. Dis.* 30: 238–264, 1950.
780. YAMAMOTO, T., H. SATOMI, H. ISE, AND K. TAKAHASHI. Evidence of the dual innervation of the cat stomach by the vagal dorsal motor and medial solitary nuclei as demonstrated by the horseradish peroxidase method. *Brain Res.* 122: 125–131, 1977.
781. YAMAMOTO, T., H. SATOMI, H. ISE, H. TAKATOMA, AND K. TAKAHASHI. Sacral spinal innervations of the rectal and vesical smooth muscles and the sphincteric striated muscles as demonstrated by the horseradish peroxidase method. *Neurosci. Lett.* 7: 41–47, 1978.
782. YASSIN, I. B. H. M., AND S. K. LEONG. Localization of neurons supplying the temporalis muscle in the rat and monkey. *Neurosci. Lett.* 11: 63–68, 1979.
783. YORKE, C. H., AND V. S. CAVINESS. Interhemispheric neocortical connections of the corpus callosum in the normal mouse: a study based on anterograde and retrograde methods. *J. Comp. Neurol.* 164: 233–246, 1975.
784. ZECHA, A. The "pyramidal tract" and other telencephalic efferents in birds. *Acta Morphol. Neerl. Scand.* 5: 194–195, 1962.
785. ZEMLAN, F. P., AND D. W. PFAFF. Topographical organization in medullary reticulospinal systems as demonstrated by the horseradish peroxidase technique. *Brain Res.* 174: 161–166, 1979.
786. ZIMMERMAN, E. A., W. W. CHAMBERS, AND C. N. LIU. An experimental study of the anatomical organization of the corticobulbar system in the albino rat. *J. Comp. Neurol.* 123: 301–324, 1964.
787. ZULCH, K. J. Pyramidal and parapyramidal motor systems in man. In: *Cerebral Localization: An Otrified Foerster Symposium*, edited by K. J. Zulch, O. Creutzfeldt, and G. C. Galbraith. Berlin: Springer-Verlag, 1975, p. 32–47.

CHAPTER 14

Vestibulospinal and reticulospinal systems

VICTOR J. WILSON
BARRY W. PETERSON

The Rockefeller University, New York, New York

CHAPTER CONTENTS

Vestibular and Neck Reflexes
  Vestibular reflexes
    Semicircular canal reflexes
    Otolith reflexes
  Neck reflexes
  Interaction of vestibular and neck reflexes
Central Pathways for Vestibular Reflexes
  Pathways linking vestibular nuclei to spinal cord
  Vestibulospinal tracts
    Origin and destination of tracts
    Inputs to vestibulospinal tract neurons
    Synapses of vestibulospinal tract fibers with spinal neurons
    Summary
  Reticulospinal tracts
    Origin and destinations of tracts
    Inputs to reticulospinal tract neurons
    Reticulospinal actions on spinal motoneurons
    Summary
  Connections between labyrinthine and spinal motoneurons
    Stimulation of whole vestibular nerve
    Stimulation of vestibular nerve branches
Central Pathways for Neck Reflexes
Functional Studies of Vestibulospinal Reflexes
  Semicircular canal reflexes
  Otolith reflexes
  Central pathways for vestibulospinal reflexes
    Canal reflexes
    Otolith reflexes
  Vestibulospinal reflexes and γ-loop
  Cerebellum and vestibulospinal reflexes
Conclusion

SIGNALS ARISING IN vestibular receptors activate an important motor system producing vestibulospinal and vestibuloocular reflexes that maintain body equilibrium, the position of the head in space, and the direction of gaze. This chapter deals with vestibulospinal reflexes acting on the body and limb musculature and also with the reflexes arising from neck receptors, with which vestibulospinal reflexes are closely linked. Our goal is to describe the reflexes and the central circuitry that underlies them. We focus on the descending tracts that must carry premotor signals from brain stem to spinal cord, on dynamic properties of vestibulospinal reflexes, and on the role that the tracts have in the execution of these reflexes. Vestibuloocular reflexes are considered in the chapter by Robinson in this *Handbook*. Descriptions of the vestibular periphery and the first stage in central processing of afferent impulses in the vestibular nuclei are presented in reference 71. Various aspects of the anatomy and physiology of the vestibular system are discussed in references 112 and 222.

VESTIBULAR AND NECK REFLEXES

Vestibular Reflexes

Vestibular (labyrinthine) reflexes, studied in detail by Magnus (131), are elicited by signals from the semicircular canal or otolith receptors of the vestibular labyrinth and are organized to counter or damp out movements of the head and consequent changes in the direction of gaze caused by external forces. In adult humans, where visual cues play a preeminent role in maintenance of posture, the action of these reflexes is often difficult to detect. Vestibular reflexes acting to maintain the position of the head in space are, however, readily observed in human infants and in animals.

Under carefully controlled conditions it is possible to activate a single type of labyrinthine receptor and to study the resulting pattern of muscle activity. Under most circumstances, however, compensatory vestibular reflex movements are produced by simultaneous activation of canal and otolith receptors. In addition, when there is movement of the head relative to the body, neck reflexes combine with and modify the pattern of vestibular reflexes as is discussed in subsection *Interaction of Vestibular and Neck Reflexes*, p. 670. As a result of these complexities, most experimenters have attempted to devise ways to isolate and study the reflexes evoked by a single type of receptor.

SEMICIRCULAR CANAL REFLEXES. The semicircular canals are inertial receptors activated by angular acceleration of the head, but as a result of the dynamics of fluid movement within the canal the signal carried by semicircular canal afferent fibers is related to head angular velocity during typical brief head movements (71). The reflex muscle activity produced by the semicircular canal afferent signal can be studied in the absence of otolith and neck reflexes by fixing the head relative to the body and applying an angular acceleration to both head and body in the horizontal plane. When this is done, vestibular reflexes cause the eyes to move in the direction opposite the applied motion and elicit contraction of neck muscles that would act to move the head in the same direction as the eyes (50, 133, 197).

To obtain quantitative measurements of vestibular reflex movements, a sinusoidal angular rotation is often applied to the experimental subject. When this is done, amplitude and timing of the reflex movement can be compared with the same parameters of the applied rotatory stimulus. Timing is usually measured as a fraction of the period of the applied sinusoidal stimulus and expressed as a phase angle where 360° represents a full cycle. In the discussion that follows, all phase angles are expressed relative to a perfect compensatory movement that is exactly opposite the applied rotation.

In an alert monkey, in darkness, the eye movement evoked by a sinusoidal angular acceleration has an amplitude approaching that of the applied movement, and over a broad frequency range (0.04–1.5 Hz) it is approximately in phase with the ideal compensatory movement (197). With the head fixed with respect to the body, only the timing of neck-muscle activation can be observed. In the decerebrate cat, activity in muscles that turn the head to the left peaks about 40° before the maximum rightward deviation of the turntable when a 0.05–0.15-Hz sinusoidal motion is applied (50). Both vestibuloocular and vestibular-neck (vestibulocollic) reflex pathways, therefore, produce a pattern of muscle action that tends to move the eyes and head in a direction opposite the applied movement.

Reflex responses to horizontal angular acceleration have also been studied in human subjects who were free to move their heads (151). Under these circumstances the vestibulocollic reflex operates in its closed-loop mode: vestibular reflex activity tends to counter the rotation of the head produced by the turntable, thus reducing the afferent signal from the horizontal semicircular canals. Rotation of the head on the neck also gives rise to neck reflexes acting on the body and limbs that may contribute to the overall response pattern. When the applied stimulus is a sudden angular acceleration, both eyes and head move in the direction opposite the applied rotation, with the head movement accounting for over half of the compensatory shift of gaze. If slower 0.01-Hz sinusoidal rotations are applied, both the eyes and head show slow movements, in a direction counter to the applied rotation, interrupted by rapid resetting movements in the opposite direction (eye and head nystagmus). When the resetting movements are subtracted, the remaining slow movement of the eyes leads the ideal compensatory motion by 60°, while the head, operating in its closed-loop mode, does somewhat better, leading by only 30°.

Horizontal angular acceleration also evokes responses in the limbs, but the pattern of these responses is not clear from the available data. Observations of forelimb muscle activity produced by hydraulic (204) or electrical (201) activation of a single horizontal canal suggest that increased extensor activity is evoked in the ipsilateral forelimb while the contralateral forelimb flexes. In experiments by Suzuki and Cohen (201), the head was free to move and neck reflexes could have contributed to those response patterns. Because horizontal canal stimulation causes contralateral head movement, however, the neck reflex should cause excitation of contralateral forelimb extensors (see subsection *Neck Reflexes*, p. 669) and the excitation of ipsilateral extensors is most likely due to vestibular reflexes. On the other hand, observations of activity in the triceps muscles during horizontal rotation of decerebrate cats indicate that stimuli that activate the horizontal semicircular canal on one side lead to enhanced activity in the contralateral triceps muscle and decreased activity in the ipsilateral triceps (16). The reasons for the discrepancy between the two sets of data are not clear at this time; a difference between experimental preparations is one possibility.

OTOLITH REFLEXES. The weighted otolith membranes of the utriculus and sacculus render these two receptor organs sensitive to linear accelerations in the horizontal and parasagittal planes, respectively (71). These receptor organs thus inform the central nervous system about linear head movements and in addition provide a means of sensing the linear acceleration of gravity and thereby determining the position of the head with respect to the gravitational vertical. Because some otolith afferents are sensitive to the rate of change of linear acceleration, the otolith organs also provide information about rate of change of linear acceleration or head position.

Essentially pure otolith reflexes can be observed during maintained tilting of the head about roll (longitudinal) or pitch (side-to-side) axes, provided care is taken to eliminate neck reflexes by immobilizing the spinal column or cutting the cervical dorsal roots. Static roll tilt causes extension of the limbs on the side tilted downward, flexion of the opposite limbs (upper half of Fig. 1; Fig. 3), and counterrolling of the eyes (117, 142, 183). Forward pitch evokes extension of the forelimbs, flexion of the hindlimbs (Fig. 2C, F), and upward eye movement, whereas backward pitch evokes the opposite pattern (Fig. 2D, G; see refs. 117, 183). In all cases the reflex actions are those that tend to restore the normal orientation of the head and eyes.

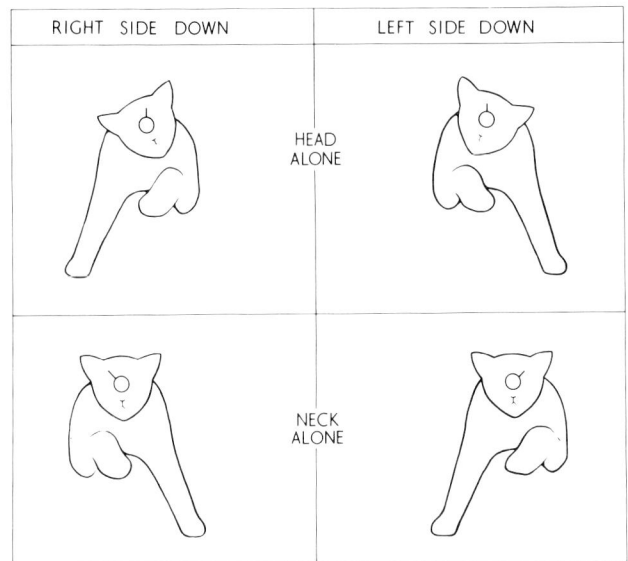

FIG. 1. Neck and vestibular reflexes in animal with C_1 and C_2 denervated. *Top*, rotation of head with axis clamped evokes vestibular reflexes. *Bottom*, rotation of axis (*line* shows tilt of spinal process) evokes neck reflexes. [From Roberts (182).]

The otolith organs also play a role in reflexes elicited by vertical linear acceleration. When a human or animal subject is dropped, the sudden change in such acceleration leads to a rapid activation of extensor muscles in the limbs that prepares the subject for landing (73, 74, 140, 211). In the cat this early reflex activation disappears after destruction of the labyrinths but survives procedures that render the semicircular canals inoperative, indicating that the response is mediated by the otolith organs (211). The receptor involved is presumably the sacculus, because its orientation renders it selectively sensitive to vertical accelerations.

Otolith reflexes have also been studied during experimentally produced linear accelerations in the horizontal plane (15). Such accelerations might be expected to evoke reflex activity similar to that evoked by static tilt, but in fact the pattern of muscle activity in the triceps muscles is opposite to that described above. The variation in reflex response is hard to explain but might be related to the inherent ambiguity of linear acceleration as a reflex cue. The reflex responses evoked by static roll tilt to the right have been described above and are illustrated in Figure 1. Similar responses seem appropriate for an animal swaying to its right, but in this case, because the head is above the center of gravity of the body, the downward acceleration of the body tends to accelerate the head at a rate exceeding that of gravity so that the net acceleration sensed by the otoliths is in the opposite direction to that sensed during static tilt (143). The ambiguity of these otolith signals can be resolved by signals from the semicircular canals or from otolith afferents sensitive to rate of change of linear acceleration. The latter might contribute to the reversed responses seen during horizontal linear accelerations.

Under ordinary circumstances, where the head is subjected to dynamic pitch and roll movements, vestibular reflexes are the result of combined canal and otolith input. In such combined responses the otolith signal might be expected to contribute to stabilization of the head during slow movements while signals from the canals provide a velocity feedback to damp out higher frequency movements. The otoliths might contribute to stabilization at the higher frequencies as well. Roberts (183) has pointed out that the velocity feedback of the canals would be expected to lead to a type of head stabilization analogous to viscous damping in a mechanical system. Such damping has the disadvantage of a phase lag between the command signal and the output. This lag can be reduced by a feedforward signal related to head velocity that might be derived from otolith afferents sensitive to rate of change of head tilt. Alternatively the lag at higher frequencies might be compensated for by canal afferents sensitive to the rate of change of angular velocity (71).

Neck Reflexes

Neck reflexes can be subdivided into several categories. The best known are the tonic neck reflexes acting on the limbs; they arise from receptors in the region of the upper cervical joints. In addition there are the neck righting reflexes and reflexes due to activity in proprioceptors in the large neck muscles.

Tonic neck reflexes were first described by Magnus and de Kleijn [(133); see also refs. 126, 183]. In order to study them in isolation it is necessary to destroy the labyrinths bilaterally or to fix the head in space when rotating the neck. Under such conditions movement of the body with respect to the head has two distinct effects (as observed in rabbits, cats, dogs, and humans with defective labyrinths). First, it evokes cervicoocular reflexes (131). These are not within the scope of this article and are not discussed further. Second, it has reflex effects on the limb muscles, some of which are illustrated in Figure 2. When the neck is dorsiflexed, there is extension of the forelimbs and flexion of the hindlimbs (Fig. 2*B*); the reverse occurs when the neck is ventriflexed (Fig. 2*H*). When the head is rotated, the two limbs on the side to which the chin points extend while the contralateral limbs flex. This effect of head rotation with respect to the body is illustrated in the lower half of Figure 1. Here the head is fixed in space and only the axis is rotated. Observe that rotation of the axis normally accompanying head rotation that brings the chin to the animal's left causes extension of the left forelimb (*lower left*, Fig. 1) and vice versa. The reflex responses to this lateral rotation are more powerful than those evoked by movement in the dorsoventral direction. In recent years this classic description of the pattern of

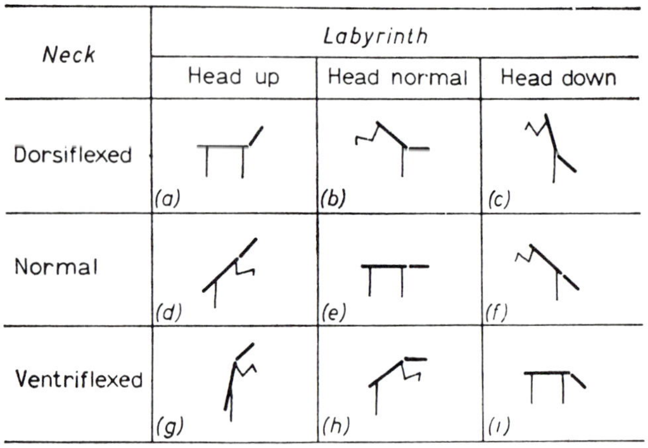

Neck	Labyrinth		
	Head up	Head normal	Head down
Dorsiflexed	(a)	(b)	(c)
Normal	(d)	(e)	(f)
Ventriflexed	(g)	(h)	(i)

FIG. 2. Scheme of combined effects upon limbs produced by tonic neck reflexes and vestibular otolith reflexes. With head normal (b, e, h) only neck reflexes are evoked. With neck normal (d, e, f) only vestibular reflexes are evoked. The 4 corners show combined effects of vestibular and neck reflexes. [From Roberts (183).]

tonic neck reflex actions has been confirmed in studies utilizing monosynaptic testing or electromyogram (EMG) recording in decerebrate cats (e.g., refs. 117, 212, 213). As indicated above, vestibular reflexes are clearly visible in human infants. Contrary to this, tonic neck reflexes become obvious only under pathological conditions, even in infants. From observations of athletes, however, it has been concluded that neck reflexes are present in the normal adult and that they make a contribution to posture that becomes clearly visible at times of strong exertion (59).

Tonic neck reflexes are present in the decerebrate cat and even in the high spinal cat (131). In the midbrain animal there is also a group of righting reflexes to which the neck righting reflexes (which orient the body with respect to the head) belong (132). For example, if the head of an animal lying on its side is restored to its usual position, the neck reflexes bring the thorax into symmetry with the head; the lower parts of the body follow (183). There is no evidence indicating whether activation of the same receptors evokes both tonic neck reflexes and neck righting reflexes.

Although the large neck muscles involved in head movement are very rich in spindles (72, 180), receptors in these muscles are neither necessary nor sufficient to produce tonic neck reflexes. This was demonstrated by McCouch et al. (126), who identified the location of receptors that give rise to the reflex. Sectioning muscle nerves or muscles connecting neck with occiput did not affect the typical responses to horizontal rotation of the head of labyrinthectomized cats. The reflexes were abolished by incisions around the upper cervical dorsal roots, particularly C_1 and C_2. Such cuts interrupt nerve fibers from receptors in the region of the upper neck joints before they reach the dorsal root ganglion. This led to the widespread belief that joint receptors are responsible for the tonic neck reflex (this was not specifically claimed by McCouch and his colleagues). Unfortunately for this notion no specific intravertebral receptors have so far been found near the upper cervical joints (181). There are, however, numerous spindles in the small perivertebral muscles in this region (179, 181). Afferents from these spindles could form the afferent limb of the tonic neck reflex; they most likely would have been transected by McCouch et al. (126).

Activation of proprioceptors in the large dorsal neck muscles also has reflex effects on limb muscles, but only in intact cats (2). In anesthetized preparations stimulation of the biventer cervicis nerve facilitates hindlimb monosynaptic reflexes and even causes motoneuron firing. This facilitation is abolished by small lesions of the anterior pole of the suprasylvian gyrus, a region receiving proprioceptive input from neck muscles (1). Although the reflex originates in the biventer cervicis muscle, there is no evidence suggesting a role for any particular receptor in the muscle.

The various experiments just described show that activation of receptors in the neck by movement of the head can profoundly affect limb muscles. It is therefore not surprising that interruption of upper cervical afferents has serious consequences. Section or anesthetic block of the C_1, C_2, and C_3 dorsal roots results in nystagmus, ataxia, and, in humans, a sensation of falling or tilting (39, 40). It is of particular interest that these symptoms resemble those of labyrinthectomy, suggesting convergence of neck and labyrinth activity on common neural elements. Even section of only the biventer cervicis nerve in C_2 and C_3 leads to ataxia of the hindlegs (2).

Interaction of Vestibular and Neck Reflexes

Rotation of the head on the body evokes both labyrinthine and neck reflexes, and these two sets of reflexes typically have opposite effects on the limbs. It follows that they interact; various demonstrations of this interaction do, in fact, exist. For example, ventriflexion of the head gradually depresses the activity evoked in the radial nerve by vestibular nerve stimulation (66). This depression can also be obtained by squeezing the dorsal neck muscles; therefore it is not necessarily due to the receptors responsible for tonic neck reflexes. Not only is activity of vestibular origin affected: neck ventriflexion decreases forelimb nerve discharge elicited by stimulation of either the motor cortex or the dorsal roots; the segmental discharge is inhibited even after spinalization, and at least some of the inhibition is therefore exerted at the spinal level (67).

The best studies on interaction between tonic labyrinthine and tonic neck reflexes are those of Lindsay et al. (117). In ingenious experiments C_1 and C_2 were denervated, leaving C_3 as the afferent channel for neck reflexes. (This removes an important afferent input,

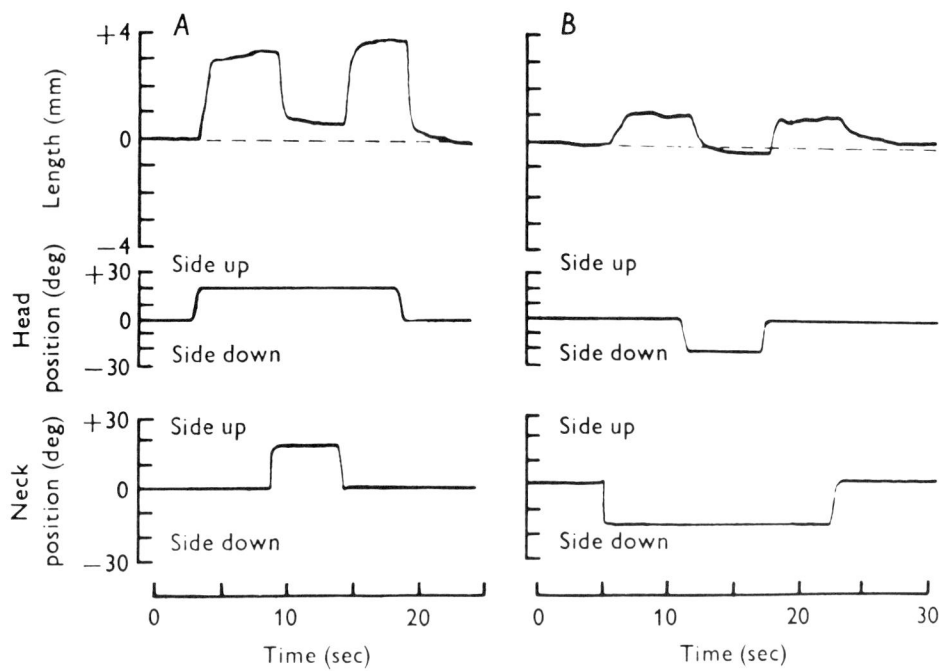

FIG. 3. Isotonic length changes in medial triceps elicited by combinations of head tilt and neck torsion (given in degrees) in same direction. Decerebrate cat: upper cervical dorsal roots (C_1 and C_2) cut. A: neck reflex superimposed on labyrinthine reflex. B: labyrinthine reflex superimposed on neck reflex. [From Lindsay et al. (117).]

but the remaining neck reflexes, while weaker, should not differ qualitatively from reflexes obtained with C_1 and C_2 intact.) With the axis clamped, the head can be rotated to produce tonic otolith reflexes as described earlier; on the other hand the axis can be rotated with the head fixed, producing the tonic neck reflex (lower half of Fig. 1). The two reflexes can also be produced in combination (Fig. 3). For example, when the head is rotated 20° (ear up) and fixed in place, the ipsilateral triceps lengthens (Fig. 3A). Subsequently rotating the axis 20° in the same direction causes an almost complete return of the muscle to resting length because of the tonic neck reflex. In other words the effects of head tilt and neck torsion in the same direction essentially cancel each other. Because of this interaction, Roberts (see ref. 117) points out that labyrinthine and neck reflexes must be considered as one system and suggests that "the function of the opposed action of the labyrinth and neck reflexes was to provide an effective stabilizing action of the limbs on the trunk, while permitting movements of the head with respect to the body."

CENTRAL PATHWAYS FOR VESTIBULAR REFLEXES

Vestibular afferent activity is transmitted to the vestibular nuclei in the medulla and pons. The anatomical organization of these nuclei has already been described in great detail (28, 71). It is sufficient to note that there are four principal vestibular nuclei (superior, lateral or Deiters', medial, and descending) and several small related cell groups (f, l, x, y, z). Of the main nuclei, all but the superior project to the spinal cord. The responses of neurons in all four nuclei to natural vestibular stimulation and to electrical stimulation of the vestibular nerve have been described by Goldberg and Fernandez (71) and are discussed in this chapter only as necessary.

Pathways Linking Vestibular Nuclei to Spinal Cord

Activity evoked in the lateral, medial, and descending nuclei by impulses in vestibular afferent fibers can be transmitted to the spinal cord by several descending fiber systems. The most direct pathways are the lateral and medial vestibulospinal tracts (LVST and MVST). Many LVST and MVST neurons can be activated at short latency, often monosynaptically, by electrical stimulation of the vestibular nerve or of its branches. The caudal vestibulospinal tract comes from cells located very caudally in the nuclei; little is known about it.

There is no direct (monosynaptic) connection between the vestibular nerve and the neurons giving rise to the medial and lateral reticulospinal tracts, but these tracts nevertheless may play an important role in the execution of vestibulospinal reflexes; that activity originating in the labyrinth can be transmitted to the spinal cord by reticulospinal tracts has long been recognized (65, 68, 123).

Vestibulospinal Tracts

ORIGIN AND DESTINATION OF TRACTS. The cells of origin of the mammalian vestibulospinal tracts have been identified in a number of ways. For instance, the tracts in the spinal cord have been transected, and then retrograde changes in brain stem neurons have been investigated. Localized lesions in the vestibular nuclei have been made and degenerating axons in the spinal cord examined. Injecting horseradish peroxidase in the region of vestibulospinal tract axon terminals and then searching for traces of the enzyme after retrograde transport is another means of identifying cells of origin, as is mapping the locations of neurons activated antidromically with electrodes placed at different spinal cord levels. Most of the work has been done in the cat, although some key experiments have been performed on rabbits. Additional detail regarding anatomical studies on the origin and course of the LVST and MVST can be found in references 28 and 222.

Lateral vestibulospinal tract. As partly illustrated in Figure 4A, C, and E, the LVST originates mainly in Deiters' nucleus (LV), with a small contribution from the descending nucleus (DV); see references 6, 29, 146, 166, 175. It is ipsilateral, extends the length of the cord, and contains for the most part rapidly conducting fibers. Conduction velocities range from 20–140 m/s, with a modal value of 90 m/s (8, 97, 219). In the cervical and lumbar enlargements, LVST terminals are found not near the motor nuclei in Rexed's lamina IX but mainly medially, in laminae VII and VIII (146, 166). Nevertheless in both hindlimb and neck segments, tract axons make synapses with motoneurons (see subsection SYNAPSES OF VST FIBERS WITH SPINAL NEURONS, p. 676).

The axons of some LVST neurons extend to the lumbosacral cord while others terminate more rostrally. These different neuron types are not distributed in random fashion, leading experimenters to believe that Deiters' nucleus is somatotopically organized. It was first suggested, on the basis of retrograde changes, that cells projecting to the lumbosacral cord were located in the dorsocaudal part of the nucleus, cells projecting to the thoracic cord were situated in the ventral region of the caudal one-third, cells projecting to the cervical cord were found in the rostral one-third and the ventral part of the middle one-third (168). Subsequent electrophysiological studies, in which neurons were identified by antidromic stimulation with electrodes at different spinal levels, modified this picture somewhat and placed more emphasis on a dorsoventral gradient, with cells with long axons found predominantly dorsally and cells with short axons found ventrally (52, 97, 153, 219).

The distinction between these populations is far from rigid: there is considerable overlap between neurons projecting to different levels (153, 175, 219). Furthermore another pattern of organization is superimposed on the somatotopic distribution of different LVST neurons. By activating the branch of an LVST neuron in the gray matter of the cervical enlargement

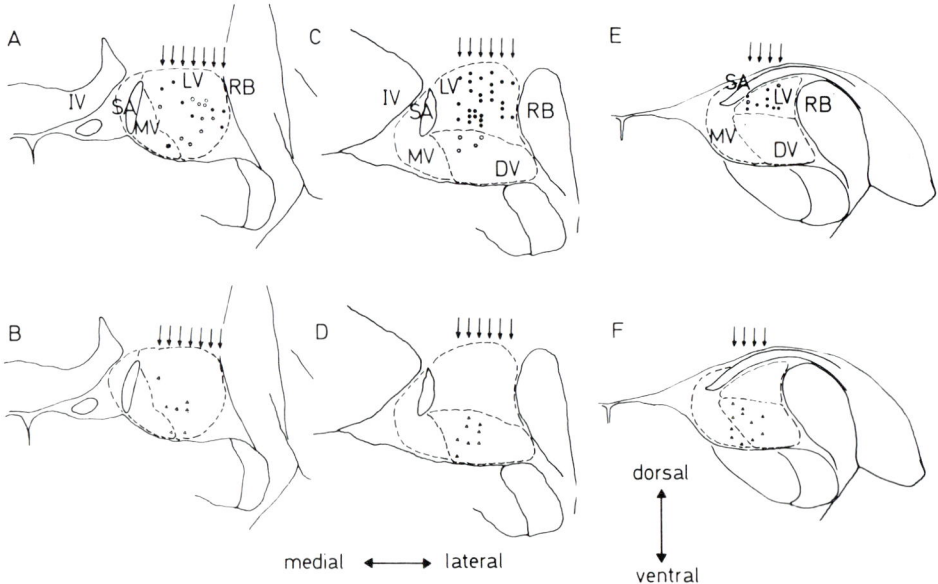

FIG. 4. Location of lateral vestibulospinal tract (LVST) and medial vestibulospinal tract (MVST) cells in cat. *A, C,* and *E* show spacing of LVST cells on 3 transverse sections of medulla obtained from 3 cats. IV, 4th ventricle; DV, descending vestibular nucleus; LV, Deiters' nucleus; MV, medial vestibular nucleus; RB, restiform body; SA, stria acoustica. *Arrows* indicate microelectrode tracks, each 0.25 mm apart. *Open circles,* second-order LVST cells. *Closed circles,* non-second-order LVST cells. *B, D,* and *F* show spacing of MVST cells on same sections as *A, C,* and *E. Open triangles,* second-order MVST cells. No non-second-order MVST cells were sampled in these preparations. In both rows most rostral sections are on *left.* [From Akaike (6).]

with microstimulation and testing for a more caudal projection of the same neuron (branching), Abzug, Maeda, Peterson, and Wilson (4) have demonstrated that at least 50% of the neurons with axons that give off branches to the cervical enlargement also project to the lumbosacral cord.

Branching neurons can potentially influence widely separated muscles. This is appropriate for neurons that may contribute to reflexes that involve many muscles. Neurons with terminals in the upper cervical (neck) segments also branch. At least 62% project to the cervical enlargement but not to the lumbar cord (175). The presence of two different populations of branching neurons, in addition to any neurons that do not branch, shows that the organization of the LVST is very complex. It might be expected that the different cell groups serve different functions, but to date there is no evidence for or against this.

After branching was demonstrated for LVST axons (4), it was found for reticulospinal (163), pyramidal (194), rubrospinal (195), and interstitiospinal (61) axons. It is obviously a shared property of descending systems with widely different functions and deserves further investigation.

Medial vestibulospinal tract. The MVST originates from neurons in the medial, descending, and Deiters' nuclei. The contribution of the medial nucleus was identified first, by anatomical methods (29, 144). Antidromic stimulation of tract axons in the spinal cord later confirmed that many neurons in the medial nucleus, particularly in its rostral part, project to the spinal cord (226). In addition this technique revealed the presence of tract neurons, first in the descending nucleus (109, 175, 225) and then in Deiters' nucleus (Fig. 4B, D, F). The surprising finding that Deiters' nucleus contributed to the MVST was first made in the rabbit, where a substantial number of MVST neurons are found intermingled with LVST cells (7). Neurons of the LVST and the MVST are more distinctly separated in the cat (6), where it has also been shown that the Deiters' contribution to the tract is bilateral (175).

Unlike the LVST, the MVST is bilateral and projects mainly to the more rostral segments of the spinal cord. In the cat, lesions of the medial nucleus are followed by heavy degeneration in laminae VII and VIII in the upper cervical segments; there is relatively little degeneration below this level (144, 166). In agreement with this finding, only 11% of MVST axons can be activated antidromically below the first thoracic segment in the cat, although many more project to caudal levels in the rabbit (6, 10). The MVST contains both rapidly and slowly conducting axons. At least one population of relatively slowly conducting fibers (average conduction velocity, 69 m/s) is inhibitory (231). On the whole the MVST appears more heterogeneous than the LVST and more closely related to the rostral cervical segments of the spinal cord, which control the neck and upper back musculature (177).

Caudal vestibulospinal tract. The CVST was found by injecting horseradish peroxidase into the spinal cord (158) and studied further by antidromic activation of tract neurons (162). Its cells of origin are in the caudal poles of the medial and descending nuclei and in cell group f. The axons, many of which extend to the lumbar segments, have relatively slow conduction velocities (median, 12 m/s).

INPUTS TO VESTIBULOSPINAL TRACT NEURONS. Vestibular neurons generally receive a variety of inputs other than those from the labyrinth; for example, there is input from the cerebellum, peripheral somatic nerves, and the visual or oculomotor systems (19, 71, 223). In some preparations the neurons are the site of complex interaction between these inputs. This is also true for vestibulospinal neurons. The vestibulospinal tracts, therefore, may participate in motor acts other than vestibulospinal reflexes. In a mesencephalic cat walking on a treadmill with head immobilized and labyrinthine reflexes absent, for instance, the activity of LVST neurons is modulated during the different phases of the step cycle (149). While the focus of this chapter is on the role of the vestibulospinal tracts in labyrinthine reflexes, information is also presented on the nature of somatic and cerebellar signals that reach the vestibulospinal tract neurons identified by antidromic stimulation.

Vestibular inputs. 1. Lateral vestibulospinal tract. Anatomical studies and field potentials, unit activity, and synaptic potentials evoked by vestibular nerve stimulation show that vestibular afferent fibers terminate mainly in the ventral portion of Deiters' nucleus, where they excite a substantial fraction of the neurons (28, 52, 96, 153, 219). It follows that ventrally located LVST neurons are more likely to receive monosynaptic vestibular input than dorsally located ones. An example of this can be seen in Figure 4, where Deiters' neurons receiving monosynaptic input (second-order cells) are present ventrally in the more rostral section (Fig. 4A) and are almost absent from the more dorsal, caudal regions (Fig. 4C, E); the separation of second-order and non-second-order neurons is usually not so complete. Because ventral LVST neurons tend to have shorter axons than dorsal LVST neurons, the proportion of second-order neurons is particularly high among LVST neurons projecting to the cervical cord. For example, in the cat, stimulating the whole vestibular nerve with single stimuli evoked monosynaptic (latency 1–1.3 ms) firing in 51% of neurons projecting to the cervical enlargement, but in only 21% of those projecting to the lumbar cord (219). These values are likely underestimates because they are based on firing, which does not reveal subthreshold inputs. They also vary from mammal to mammal and are somewhat different in the rabbit (10). A general conclusion is that a fraction of LVST neurons receives monosynaptic input from the labyrinth while the remainder does not, and in the cat, second-order neurons predominate among the neurons with shorter axons. It might therefore seem that the LVST relays vestibular activity mainly to the neck and forelimb segments. This is an oversimplification, however. Many neurons receive additional, less direct input that could become important when the stimulus consists of linear or angular acceleration instead of single electric shocks. Even Deiters' neurons that do not respond to single stimuli or to short trains of stimuli respond to sinusoidal polarization of ampullary nerves (161) and, no doubt, to natural stimulation (cf. ref. 193).

Although Deiters' nucleus has always been considered a target of utricular afferents, it also receives afferents from both the sacculus and the semicircular canals (71, 223). Activity originating in all of these receptors has been shown to influence LVST neurons, which can be facilitated or inhibited by lateral tilt [i.e., by activation of the utricle (150, 153, 193)] and by stimulation of the saccular nerve (218). That LVST neurons receive input from semicircular canals is shown by their response to horizontal rotation (171) and to stimulation of ampullary nerves (161), and by the disappearance of anterior canal nerve-evoked excitatory postsynaptic potentials (EPSPs) from neck motoneurons when the LVST is cut (221).

2. Medial vestibulospinal tract. Many neurons with axons in the MVST are excited monosynaptically or polysynaptically by vestibular afferents. In one series of experiments, stimulating the vestibular nerve with single stimuli caused monosynaptic firing of 32 of 40 MVST neurons in the medial nucleus and 7 of 11 MVST neurons in the descending nucleus (225, 227). Many Deiters' MVST neurons projecting to various spinal levels are similarly driven (6, 10). The population of neurons that is not second order is much smaller in the MVST than in the LVST. At least on the basis of monosynaptic input, the MVST as a whole transmits vestibular activity to the segments it innervates. If there are any indirect inputs to MVST neurons, they have not been investigated so far and their importance cannot be assessed.

The nuclei giving rise to the MVST receive canal and macular inputs (71, 223), but there is little direct information about connections between different vestibular receptors and MVST neurons. Some tract neurons are influenced by horizontal rotation, responding in type I or type III fashion (171, 193); that is, they are excited by ipsilateral and inhibited by contralateral angular acceleration or excited by acceleration in both directions respectively (71, 192). Indirect evidence shows that even though individual vestibular neurons are typically influenced monosynaptically from only one canal (107, 135, 215), MVST cells as a group are excited by afferents from all three ipsilateral semicircular canals. When any of the three ampullary nerves is stimulated selectively, disynaptic potentials are seen in neck motoneurons; these potentials disappear when the MVST is transected (221). The MVST neurons are also under the influence of the maculae. A few have been excited by stimulation of the saccular nerve (218). In addition all disynaptic potentials evoked in contralateral C_1 motoneurons by vestibular nerve stimulation disappear when the MVST is cut (9). This suggests that the tract also relays utricular information.

Somatosensory inputs. 1. Lateral vestibulospinal tract. In decerebellate cats stimulation of peripheral nerves in limbs and neck usually causes a long-lasting facilitation of LVST neurons (141, 219, 220). The latency of the facilitation is as long as 10–35 ms from the hindlimb and somewhat shorter from more rostral sites. The connections between some ascending fibers and LVST neurons are very direct (99, 101); this implies several synaptic delays at the spinal level. Because facilitation can be evoked by stimulating cutaneous nerves and muscle nerves of various sizes, it presumably can be produced by activation of a variety of receptors. Primary spindle afferents and tendon organs are not usually among these because muscle nerves [with the exception of the quadriceps nerve (11, 33, 233)] must receive stimulation of at least group II strength to produce facilitation (70, 219, 220).

There is no sign of any somatotopic organization when the distribution of the facilitation is studied in decerebellate cats. Both facilitation of cell firing and EPSPs are observed throughout Deiters' nucleus, and stimulation of either forelimb or hindlimb nerves acts on LVST neurons projecting to the cervical or to the lumbar cord (33, 219). When the cerebellum is intact, introduction of the circuitry described in the next section brings about marked changes in the effects of peripheral nerve stimulation. This produces both facilitation and inhibition in a meaningful pattern (11, 12, 32, 33). Most striking is the result of activation of anterior lobe Purkinje cells by climbing-fiber inputs to the cerebellum. There is a strong tendency for some LVST neurons to be inhibited only by stimulation of hindlimb nerves, and for others to be inhibited solely by stimulation of forelimb nerves. Generally the former project to the lumbar cord whereas the latter project only to the cervical cord.

2. Medial vestibulospinal tract. The somatic input to neurons contributing to this tract has not been studied extensively. Those in Deiters' nucleus are often excited by stimulation of the cervical spinal cord (8). Very few MVST neurons were fired by similar stimulation in a study of the cat (227), but extracellular recording was used and subthreshold inputs may have been overlooked.

Cerebellum and vestibulospinal tracts. There are extensive interconnections between the cerebellar cortex and nuclei and the vestibular nuclei (28, 71). Both the cerebellar cortex and the fastigial nucleus project to the vestibular nuclei. The anterior lobe of the cortex, and to a lesser extent the posterior lobe, provide a significant input to Deiters' nucleus (28). The flocculus and nodulus project to the vestibular nuclei in an organized fashion (28); of the three nuclei relevant to the vestibulospinal system, Deiters' is poorly supplied whereas the others receive dense terminations. The rostral parts of the medial and the descending nuclei get fibers from the flocculus and their caudal parts from the nodulus. From the anatomy, therefore, we see the possibility of anterior lobe control of the LVST and MVST and floccular control of the MVST. Because Purkinje cells are inhibitory neurons (104), direct control would be inhibitory although more complex influences, for example disinhibition, also exist (100, 214).

Fastigial nucleus efferents terminate in all four vestibular nuclei; the caudal part of the nucleus projects contralaterally, the rostral part ipsilaterally (29). Fastigial axons excite the neurons on which they terminate (103, 193).

1. Lateral vestibulospinal tract. Stimulation of the anterior and posterior lobes evokes monosynaptic inhibitory postsynaptic potentials (IPSPs) in antidromically identified LVST neurons, particularly in the dorsal part of Deiters' nucleus [(8, 98); see also ref. 193]. Many second-order (86%; see ref. 8) and non-second-order LVST neurons are inhibited. The inhibitory projection can be activated from several sources. There is convergence in the vermis of a variety of inputs, including those from the periphery (27), including the neck (25), and the labyrinth (5, 53, 172). Contrary to earlier belief, the labyrinth projection is relayed not only by very indirect pathways but also by first- and second-order vestibular fibers (113, 114, 172). As first shown by Ito et al. (101) and discussed in connection with somatic inputs, activity ascending in spinal tracts fires Purkinje cells inhibiting LVST neurons, and very likely the same is true for activity of vestibular origin.

Stimulation of the flocculus does not evoke IPSPs in LVST neurons (8). There has been no conclusive work on the effects of nodulus stimulation. There is evidence that nodulus Purkinje cells inhibit vestibular neurons projecting to the cerebellum (173), but satisfactory testing of their effects on neurons projecting to the spinal cord has not been possible (8).

Both somatic (44-46) and vestibular (63, 64, 69) inputs excite fastigial neurons, some of which can excite LVST neurons monosynaptically. The fastigial nucleus therefore provides an excitatory channel from periphery or labyrinth to LVST neurons. Somatic and vestibular activity reaching the fastigial nucleus also contributes to the maintenance of tonic excitatory fastigial bombardment of LVST neurons. Because Purkinje cells inhibit fastigial neurons (105), the tonic depolarization can be modulated by Purkinje cell impulses triggered by activity originating in the same sites that give rise to activation of fastigial neurons.

2. Medial vestibulospinal tract. Cerebellar control of MVST neurons has been studied primarily in Deiters' nucleus, where it is very similar to control of LVST neurons. Monosynaptic inhibitory postsynaptic potentials (IPSPs) can be evoked from the anterior and posterior lobes; the inhibition is somewhat less frequent in slowly conducting neurons (8). There is no inhibition from the flocculus, and no information regarding the nodulus (8). Monosynaptic excitation can often be evoked from the fastigial nucleus (193).

3. Functional aspects of cerebellar control of vestibulospinal tracts. Two things emerge from neuroanatomical and neurophysiological investigations of cerebellar action on vestibulospinal tract (VST) neurons. First, activity of VST cells is inhibited by the Purkinje cells of the anterior and posterior cerebellar vermis (8); this is reflected in inhibition of labyrinth-evoked vestibulospinal volleys recorded in the spinal cord. The inhibition is brought about by the various inputs that converge upon vermal Purkinje cells. As noted, these include somatic inputs whose effect on VST neurons is modified by transcerebellar pathways; it may include vestibular inputs as well. Second, there is no inhibition of the VSTs by the flocculus. Apparently the flocculus is selectively involved in control of vestibuloocular reflexes (19, 94, 95). Because eye and head movements are so closely related, it might be expected that there is also floccular control of vestibular pathways to the neck segments, but there is no evidence that this is so: Akaike et al. (8) failed to inhibit vestibular-evoked activity in the C_1 segment by stimulation of the flocculus.

Cerebellar cortical input is particularly prominent in the dorsal part of Deiters' nucleus, and this area contains a concentration of LVST neurons projecting to the lumbar cord. Under behavioral conditions transcerebellar circuits modify the activity of these neurons in various ways. We saw earlier that the firing of many lumbar LVST neurons is modulated with the phases of the step, peaking during stance (149). This modulation is abolished by decerebellation. In decerebrate cats many LVST neurons projecting to the hindlimb segments respond to lateral tilt only with a phasic response, although there is a static response in decerebellate animals (150). This modification of the dynamics of vestibular neuron response is presumably executed by anterior lobe Purkinje cells receiving otolith input (172).

It is not only vestibular actions on lumbar neurons that are under the control of the cerebellar cortex. Because LVST neurons projecting to various spinal levels intermingle, many neurons projecting only to the cervical enlargement are inhibited via the anterior lobe (11, 12); the actions previously described regarding step-related modulation and tilt responses of lumbar LVST neurons are probably present in cervical LVST neurons also. In addition to LVST neurons projecting to hindlimb and forelimb segments, dorsal Deiters' nucleus also contains neurons projecting to the neck segments. That such neurons, whatever their location, must be subject to cerebellar inhibition follows from the observation that decerebellation of a decerebrate cat causes strong extension of the head, apparently by release of tonic vestibular reflexes (167).

Ito (95) has postulated that the anterior lobe controls a feedforward circuit that includes both vestibulospinal neurons not receiving primary vestibular input and ascending tracts carrying the spinal afferent activity resulting from the head, trunk, and limb movements that are a consequence of vestibulospinal or other reflexes. "Positional change or movement in limbs and trunk will provide compensatory adjustment in certain combination of muscles through the spinovestibulospinal reflexes which will be optimized by the cerebellar action." Any compensatory head movement itself, of course, is sensed by vestibular receptors and is performed by a loop that includes VST neurons receiving primary vestibular input. This closed loop was postulated not to require cerebellar control. Originally a clear distinction was drawn between the flocculus, which receives primary vestibular input and inhibits open-loop vestibuloocular reflexes, and the anterior lobe, which inhibits the feedforward system previously described (95) but was not believed to receive primary vestibular input. The results of recent studies (113, 114, 172) revealing that vestibular afferents do reach the anterior lobe necessitate a change in this view.

SYNAPSES OF VESTIBULOSPINAL TRACT FIBERS WITH SPINAL NEURONS. The monosynaptic (or at any rate, fairly direct) pathways to motoneurons are the shortest available links between the vestibular nuclei and spinal motor centers. Impulses from these nuclei, however, can reach the spinal cord by other routes; for example, they may travel by projections to the reticular formation. Thus the functional significance of these various pathways still remains to be defined.

Vestibulospinal axons synapse with spinal neurons that are not directly related to motor output, such as ventral spinocerebellar and spinoreticular neurons (e.g., refs. 20, 76, 86). These connections are not relevant to the focus of this chapter and will not be considered further.

The actions that vestibulospinal axons exert on spinal neurons have been extensively studied by localized stimulation within the vestibular nuclei. This method has the serious drawback that the stimulus may activate not only the intended cell bodies or their axons, but also fibers of passage or nearby neurons belonging to other cell groups. Nevertheless there has been satisfactory agreement between results of various investigations, including stimulation experiments and experiments in which the vestibular nerve was stimulated and a specific tract interrupted (e.g., see refs. 78, 87, 128, 229).

Connections of LVST axons. The LVST, which extends ipsilaterally the length of the spinal cord, has long been known to excite ipsilateral extensor muscles (29). Studies with fairly localized stimulation of Deiters' nucleus were begun by Lund and Pompeiano (124), and the actions of the tract have since been studied at levels ranging from upper cervical to lumbosacral. In all cases the monosynaptic effects observed have been excitatory.

Stimulation of Deiters' nucleus may activate the MVST as well as the LVST. This should not distort results of studies involving limb motoneurons because in the cat the MVST has only a minor projection to limb segments. It is also unlikely to be a factor in the study of neck motoneurons because, as is discussed later, the known ipsilateral MVST actions on these neurons are inhibitory.

1. Limb segments. a. Alpha motoneurons. Stimulation of Deiters' nucleus causes EPSPs in many limb extensor motoneurons; in some hindlimb motoneurons the calculated segmental delay between EPSP onset and arrival of the fastest descending volleys is monosynaptic [(78); see also refs. 124 and 229]. Monosynaptic EPSPs, similar to those shown by the arrows in Figure 5A, are found mainly in gastrocnemius-soleus and quadriceps motoneurons in the hindlimb and are absent from forelimb motoneurons (78, 229). Their amplitude is small, generally less than a millivolt in response to single stimuli; there is summation with higher frequencies of stimulation (Fig. 5A). The limited distribution of monosynaptic EPSPs shows that this direct route is not the main pathway from Deiters' nucleus to limb extensors, although the input to gastrocnemius-soleus and quadriceps can be expected to have some specific function.

Whereas Deiters' stimulation evokes monosynaptic EPSPs only in certain cases, polysynaptic EPSPs (disynaptic or later) are widespread among limb extensor motoneurons and are also found in some flexor motoneurons such as those of the deep peroneal muscle in the hindlimb and forearm flexors in the forelimb (78, 229). As illustrated in Figure 5B–D, these potentials grow markedly with lengthening trains of shocks and with increases in frequency within the train and can cause significant levels of depolarization. This, plus their broad distribution, indicates that whatever the function of short-latency pathways in limb vestibulospinal reflexes, it is mainly carried out by the polysynaptic route.

Vestibulospinal excitation of extensor motoneurons is often accompanied by reciprocal inhibition of flexors (78, 229); IPSPs are observed in various types of flexor motoneurons but are only rarely seen in extensors, with the exception of some hip extensor cells. The IPSPs are evoked disynaptically by rapidly conducting fibers (78). Inhibition of knee flexors and hip extensors, but not of pretibial flexors, is via the segmental Ia-interneuron (31, 89, 90).

The point has already been made that LVST axons exert their effects on motoneurons directly or via interneurons. The interneuronal pathways often cause measurable changes in motoneuron excitability, but this is not always the case. Stimulation of Deiters' nucleus can facilitate a variety of segmental reflex actions without evoking obvious changes in motoneurons. In addition to synapsing with some Ia inhibitory interneurons, LVST fibers converge on interneurons that receive input from contralateral high-threshold muscle afferents and cutaneous afferents (31).

b. Gamma motoneurons. It was first deduced on the basis of indirect evidence that the LVST excites not only α- but also γ-motoneurons (34). Stimulation of Deiters' nucleus was later shown to cause facilitation of extensor γ-motoneurons and inhibition of flexor γ-motoneurons (108); in some cases the facilitation is due to a monosynaptic pathway (77). The general pattern of excitation and inhibition of α- and γ-motoneurons is similar, allowing α-γ-coactivation in vestibulospinal reflexes (see subsection *Vestibulospinal Reflexes and γ-Loop*, p. 695).

c. Contralateral actions. Although the LVST is entirely ipsilateral, stimulation of Deiters' nucleus affects contralateral motoneurons by commissural interneurons, the axons of which cross the cord at or near the level of the motoneurons (87, 128). Potentials in contralateral motoneurons are smaller and of longer latency than those recorded in ipsilateral motoneurons, but the pattern of activity is very similar on the two sides (87). There is usually bilateral excitation in extensor motoneurons and sometimes bilateral inhibition in flexors. Effects in flexor motoneurons, however, are often mixed and sometimes reciprocal on the two sides. The bilaterally similar effects are produced by convergence on common interneurons (18).

2. Axial motoneurons. The LVST makes monosynaptic excitatory connections with many motoneurons innervating the biventer cervicis, the complexus, and the splenius muscles, which extend the head. Stimulation of Deiters' nucleus evokes small (0.8 mV) EPSPs with a latency of 1.0–1.5 ms in many motoneurons in the upper cervical segments (229). Polysynaptic EPSPs are present but are less conspicuous than in limb motoneurons. Monosynaptic EPSPs are also seen in back motoneurons (231).

Connections of MVST axons. The MVST fibers have been activated by stimuli localized to the medial vestibular nucleus. This stimulation has no effect on limb motoneurons but does evoke IPSPs in many neck motoneurons (230). Intrasegmental delays measured from the arrival of the fastest descending volleys range from 0.5–1.0 ms, peaking at 0.7 ms. This demonstrates that the IPSPs are monosynaptic, due to inhibitory fibers in the MVST; the result has been confirmed in two ways. First, stimulation of the vestibular nerve in rabbits causes disynaptic IPSPs in C_1 motoneurons that are abolished by transection of the MVST (9). Second, the action of medial nucleus neurons on neck motoneurons has been studied by spike-triggered signal averaging (176). For example, Figure 6C and D shows the IPSPs produced in two neck motoneurons by the activity of a medial nucleus neuron (firing frequency was enhanced by leakage of glutamate from one barrel of the recording electrode). The neuron, which received monosynaptic vestibular input (Fig. 6A2), was identified by its antidromic firing to microstimulation in the C_3 gray matter (Fig. 6A1). With this technique inhibitory neurons were identified not only in the medial nucleus, but also in the descending nucleus and even in Deiters'.

Monosynaptic IPSPs are evoked in back motoneurons by stimulation of the medial longitudinal fasciculus (MLF), and indirect evidence suggests that they are due to the MVST (231). In agreement with this, the disynaptic IPSPs that are observed in thoracic motoneurons when the vestibular nerve is stimulated disappear when the MLF is cut (9).

Inhibitory MVST fibers are of medium conduction velocity, about 60–79 m/s (9, 231). The rapidly conducting ($\approx$ 100 m/s) fibers in the tract are excitatory, as demonstrated by a combination of vestibular nerve stimulation and MVST transection. There is monosynaptic excitation of contralateral neck motoneurons (9, 221) and bilateral excitation of lower cervical motoneurons (9).

SUMMARY. The vestibular nuclei are linked to the spinal cord by the lateral, medial, and caudal vestibulospinal tracts. The first two have been studied extensively but very little is known about the third. The LVST originates mainly in Deiters' nucleus and extends to the ipsilateral sacral segments. Cells of origin of the tract receive inputs from many sources, including the somatic periphery; the labyrinth provides a dominant input for many of these cells. Monosynaptic connections from otolith or canal receptors are for the most part located ventrally in Deiters' nucleus; dorsal cells are activated by less direct pathways. The LVST as a whole can transmit activity originating in various receptors in the labyrinth, as well as activity from other sources, to all rostrocaudal levels of the spinal cord.

The MVST originates in the medial, descending, and Deiters' nuclei and is bilateral, terminating mostly in the upper cervical cord. The most prominent input to neurons of this tract is from the labyrinth, including canal and otolith receptors. This tract transmits labyrinth activity mainly to the more rostral spinal segments.

The two vestibulospinal tracts make synapses with a variety of spinal neurons. The LVST consists of excitatory fibers, some of which excite neck and hindlimb α-extensor motoneurons monosynaptically. There are also some terminations on γ-motoneurons, allowing α-γ-coactivation in vestibulospinal reflexes. Despite the presence of monosynaptic connections on some motoneurons, it seems likely that the ipsilateral actions of the LVST, which are generally excitatory to neck and limb extensors and inhibitory to limb flexors, are exerted mainly via interneurons. Pathways that include commissural interneurons cause similar effects in contralateral limb motoneurons. The MVST consists of excitatory and inhibitory fibers that synapse with neck and back motoneurons.

Both vestibulospinal tracts are under the inhibitory

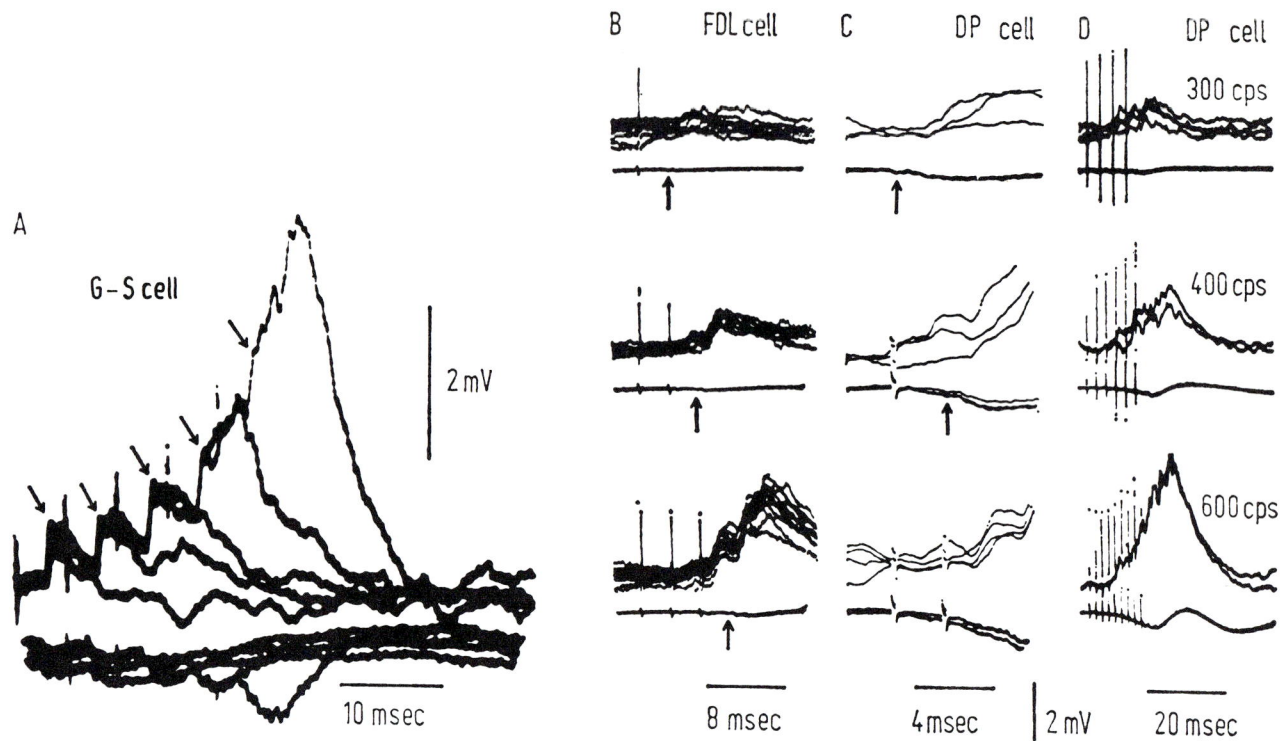

FIG. 5. Monosynaptic and polysynaptic excitatory postsynaptic potentials (EPSPs) evoked from Deiters' nucleus. *Upper traces* are intracellular potentials, *lower traces* are cord dorsum potentials. DP, deep peroneal; FDL, flexor digitorum longus; G-S, gastrocnemius. *A*: G-S cell. Photographic superimposition of vestibulospinal EPSPs evoked by 1–5 stimuli applied to Deiters' nucleus. Monosynaptic EPSPs indicated by *arrows*. *B*: FDL cell; EPSPs evoked by single, double, and triple shocks to Deiters' nucleus. *C*: DP cell; same as *B*. First stimulus was given just before onset of sweep. *Arrows* in *B* and *C* indicate arrival of descending volley (peak of initial positivity in cord dorsum potential). *D*: another DP cell; polysynaptic EPSPs produced by repetitive stimulation of Deiters' nucleus at different frequencies. [From Grillner et al. (78).]

control of Purkinje cells of the anterior and posterior vermis. To date no inhibitory effects have been obtained by stimulating the flocculus, the only part of the vestibulocerebellum tested.

Reticulospinal Tracts

ORIGIN AND DESTINATIONS OF TRACTS. The same anatomical and electrophysiological methods used to identify VST neurons have been used in experiments on reticulospinal tract (RST) neurons. These studies, performed primarily in the cat, indicate that four reticular nuclei in the medial pontomedullary brain stem—nucleus reticularis (n.r.) pontis oralis, n.r. pontis caudalis, n.r. gigantocellularis, and n.r. ventralis—contain large- and medium-sized neurons that send axons to the spinal cord via the medial reticulospinal tract (MRST) in the ventromedial funiculus and the lateral reticulospinal tract (LRST) in the ventrolateral funiculi. The brain stem tegmentum also contains a number of other regions containing smaller neurons projecting to the spinal cord.

Medial reticulospinal tract. Figure 7B shows that the MRST originates primarily in the rostral part of the region that gives rise to reticulospinal projections, which includes n.r. pontis oralis, n.r. pontis caudalis, and the dorsorostral part of n.r. gigantocellularis (102, 145, 163, 166). It is primarily ipsilateral, extends the length of the cord, and contains mainly rapidly conducting fibers [conduction-velocity range, 14–150 m/s; median, 101 m/s; (163)]. Most MRST neurons project to lumbar levels or beyond, but some extend only to cervical or thoracic levels (Fig. 7B). In contrast to results on the LVST and the LRST (see next subsection, *Lateral reticulospinal tract*), there is no evidence of a somatotopic organization of MRST neurons projecting different distances down the spinal cord. Many MRST neurons have axon branches that terminate at more than one spinal level (163). The diagram in Figure 8B illustrates the course of an axon collateral of one MRST neuron that leaves the ventromedial funiculus and courses through the ventral horn of the cervical enlargement toward the lateral motoneuron pools. The parent axon of this neuron continues to lumbar levels. The MRST terminals are found throughout the ventral horn but are particularly concentrated in its medial portion (145, 166).

Lateral reticulospinal tract. The LRST (Fig. 7A, C) originates in the medial medullary reticular formation: n.r. gigantocellularis and n.r. ventralis (102,

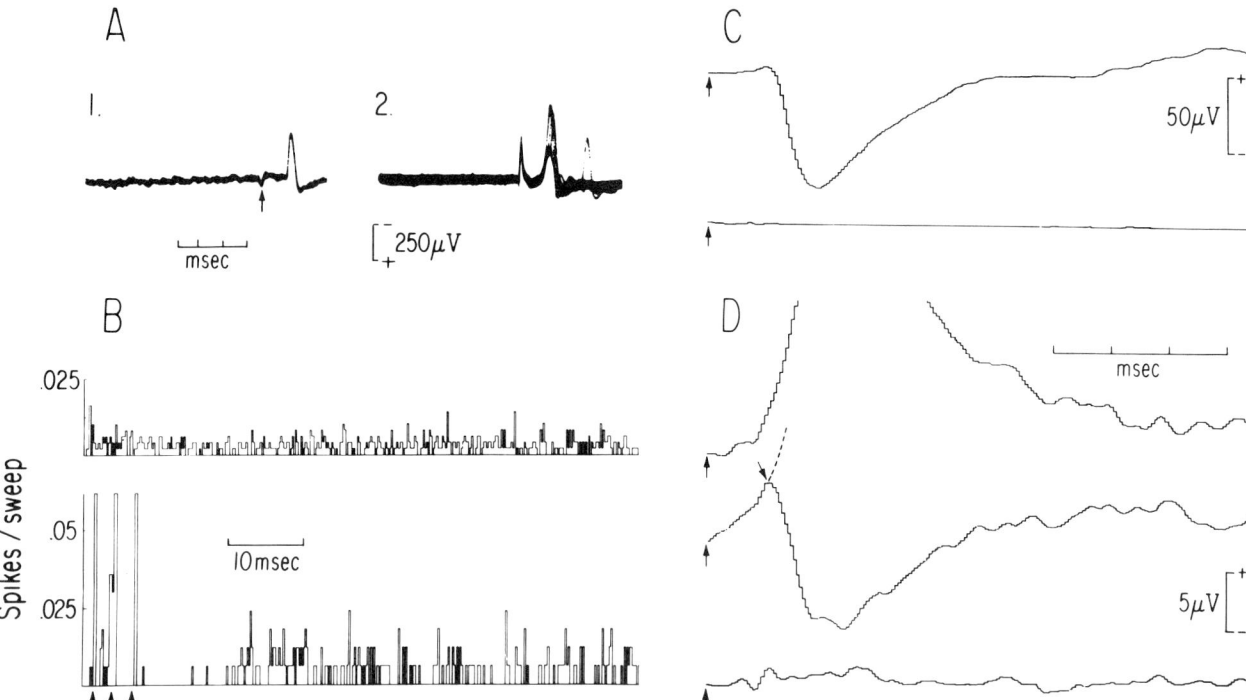

FIG. 6. Properties of inhibitory neuron in vestibular nuclei, and unitary inhibitory postsynaptic potentials (IPSPs) evoked by activity of this neuron in 2 neck motoneurons. *A1*: antidromic spike of neuron evoked by 8-μA stimulus (*arrow*) to electrode in C$_3$ dorsal ramus motoneuron pool. *A2*: monosynaptic response of neuron to stimulation of ipsilateral vestibular nerve at 1.4 times N$_1$ threshold. *B*: *upper trace* shows spontaneous activity of neuron as poststimulus time histogram (440 sweeps). *Lower trace* shows effect of 150-μA triple shock to contralateral vestibular nerve (150 sweeps). *C*: unitary IPSP evoked in 1 motoneuron by activity of inhibitory neuron; *lower trace*, extracellular record. *D*: unitary IPSP (*middle trace*) evoked in another motoneuron. IPSP was reversed by injection of 10-μA hyperpolarizing current; part of this reversed IPSP is shown in *upper trace*. Downward arrow in *middle trace* shows divergence between IPSPs recorded with and without current injection. *Lower trace*, extracellular record. All records in *C* and *D* are averages of 600–1,000 sweeps; *upward arrows* indicate time of discriminator output pulses. [From Rapoport, Wilson, et al. (176).]

145, 163, 166). Its fibers descend in the ipsilateral ventrolateral funiculus and to a lesser extent in the contralateral ventrolateral funiculus to all levels of the spinal cord and, like MRST fibers, have a wide range of conduction velocities (11–150 m/s). The median conduction velocity (69 m/s) is smaller than that of the MRST (163). There is some indication of a topographic organization of the LRST neurons projecting to different spinal levels (Fig. 7C): cells of origin of LRST axons extending beyond the neck are primarily restricted to the ventrocaudal part of n.r. gigantocellularis whereas cells of origin of LRST fibers projecting only to the neck are found throughout n.r. gigantocellularis and in the anterior part of n.r. ventralis (154, 163). The region of termination of LRST fibers is very extensive and includes the entire ventral horn and the base of the dorsal horn (145, 166). Because of axon branching, the terminal field of an individual LRST neuron may also be quite extensive: for instance, Figure 8C illustrates an LRST neuron that projects to the lumbar spinal cord and also sends terminal branches to the ipsilateral and contralateral cervical enlargement.

INPUTS TO RETICULOSPINAL TRACT NEURONS. Reticular neurons receive input from many sources; vestibular, peripheral somatic, and cerebellar inputs are likely to be important in the control of posture and equilibrium. Input from other sources such as the cerebral cortex (115, 129, 157) and spinal cord (129, 138) are not considered.

Vestibular inputs. Experiments with natural vestibular stimulation show that neurons in the reticular formation respond to activation of both semicircular canal and otolith receptors (42, 150, 200). Electrical stimulation of the whole vestibular nerve does not excite reticular neurons monosynaptically but elicits di- and polysynaptic excitation and inhibition of neurons within the reticulospinal projection area (156, 159).

The actions of the labyrinth on the reticular formation are bilateral and tend to excite reticulospinal neurons, which receive di- and polysynaptic excitation but only polysynaptic inhibition. In one study, 34 of 51 reticulospinal neurons exhibited EPSPs following stimulation of the whole ipsilateral vestibular nerve while only 5 of 51 exhibited IPSPs (159). With contra-

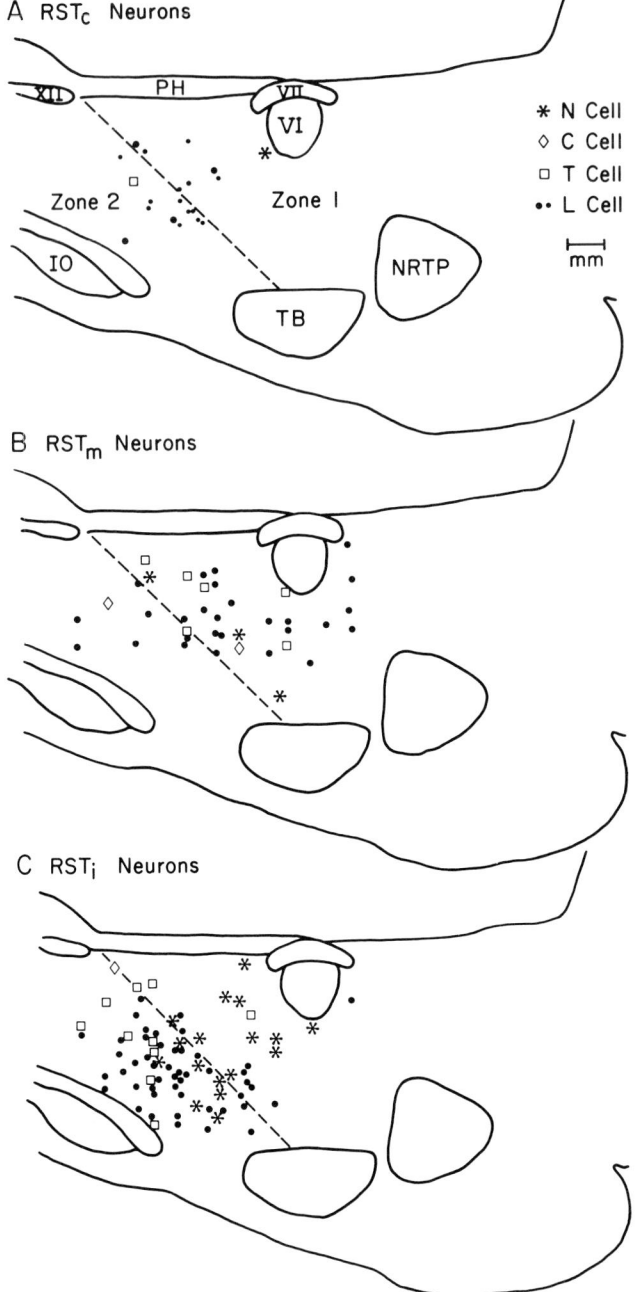

FIG. 7. Locations of reticulospinal neurons in cat. Histologically determined locations of neurons projecting in medial reticulospinal tract (RST$_m$) and in the ipsilateral (RST$_i$) and contralateral (RST$_c$) lateral reticulospinal tracts are shown on drawings of a parasagittal section through pons and medulla. Symbols indicate neurons projecting to different spinal levels (N, neck; C, cervical; T, thoracic; and L, lumbar cord). The L cells found in experiments in which spinal cord was stimulated at 4 levels are shown by *large, closed circles* in *A*, *B*, and *C*. An additional group of L cells, found in experiments where stimuli were applied at fewer spinal levels, are shown by *small, filled circles*. These L cells were included only in *A*. *Dashed lines* indicate border between 2 reticular regions labeled zone 1 and zone 2 in *A*. Zone 1 contains primarily medial, and zone 2 primarily lateral, reticulospinal neurons. IO, inferior olivary nucleus; NRTP, nucleus reticularis tegmenti pontis; PH, nucleus prepositus hypoglossi; TB, trapezoid body; VI, abducens nucleus; VII, genu of facial nerve; XII, hypoglossal nucleus. [From Peterson et al. (163).]

lateral stimulation 29 of 50 exhibited EPSPs and 7 of 50 IPSPs. Figure 9 shows that the shortest latency disynaptic responses were considerably more prevalent in the medullary reticular formation than in the pontine reticular formation, suggesting that LRST neurons are more closely linked to labyrinthine afferents than are MRST neurons. Responses obtained with stimulation of the whole nerve are difficult to interpret, however, since they reflect the superimposed action of fibers from a variety of labyrinthine receptors. Responses evoked by stimulation of a single canal nerve are quite different from those evoked by whole nerve stimulation. Activation of the horizontal canal nerve with multiple stimuli elicits firing primarily of reticulospinal neurons located in the vicinity of the contralateral abducens nucleus near the pontomedullary border (155). As expected from their locations, most of these responding neurons are MRST neurons. Thus while the LRST is more responsive to activation of the whole nerve, the MRST plays an important role in transmitting semicircular canal signals to the spinal cord.

One pathway from the labyrinth to the reticular formation is via the vestibular nuclei. This route has been investigated by studying the properties of vestibular neurons that could be activated antidromically by electrical stimulation of the medial reticular formation (156). Apparently these neurons do not function only as direct relays of labyrinthine activity, since just a small fraction (4/45) receives monosynaptic input from vestibular afferent fibers. Thus the majority of vestibuloreticular neurons transmit only higher order labyrinthine activity, possibly combined with other inputs reaching the vestibular nuclei, to the reticular formation. Whatever the signals it carries, the vestibuloreticular projection is quite extensive; all four main vestibular nuclei project to the reticular formation (116, 156) and most reticulospinal neurons are monosynaptically excited or inhibited following stimulation of one or more of the vestibular nuclei (156).

Another path from the labyrinth to the reticular formation involves the fastigial nucleus, which is known to receive vestibular input. This path is described in the subsection *Cerebellar inputs*, p. 681.

Somatosensory inputs. When electrical stimuli are applied to the body surface, reticular neurons are excited or inhibited at latencies ranging from 5 to over 30 ms (43, 130, 157, 190, 232). The earliest responses are probably disynaptic, but the great majority appear to involve more complex pathways. Figure 10*G* and *H* illustrate the responses of a reticulospinal neuron to stimulation of forelimb (iSR, cSR) and hindlimb (iPER, cPER) nerves. The responses consist of a weak initial inhibition followed by strong excitation. In some cases there is a later phase of inhibition as well. The predominant response of the neuron, however, is excitation originating from nerves in all four limbs. Similar excitation has been elicited by taps or airjets applied to the four limbs or body surface (Fig. 10*I*, *J*). The neuron in Figure 10 is a typical reticulospinal

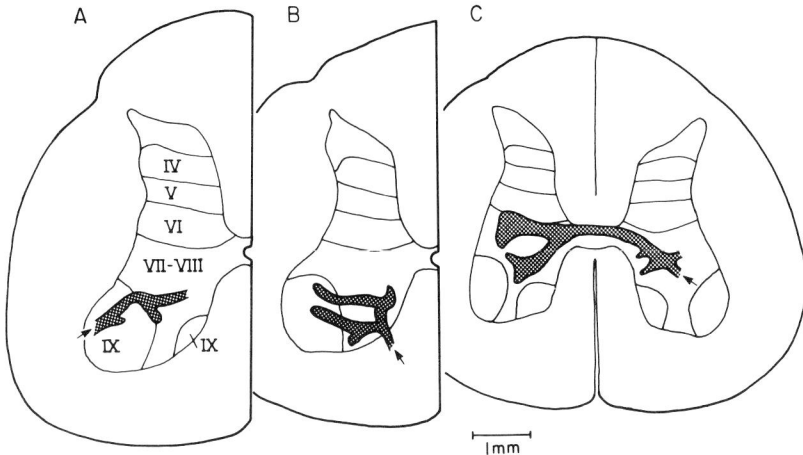

FIG. 8. Localization of reticulospinal axon branches within cervical enlargement. Shaded areas in A, B, and C indicate regions within which stimuli of 20 μA or less produced antidromic activation of 3 reticulospinal neurons found in left nucleus reticularis gigantocellularis. Open ends of shaded profiles indicate points where axon branch extended to edge of region explored and possibly beyond. *Arrows* indicate part of branch that was closest to parent axon as shown by latency measurements. Neuron in A projected into ipsilateral reticulospinal tract (RST), neuron in B into medial RST, and neuron in C into contralateral RST. Numbers in A indicate spinal laminae. [From Peterson et al. (163).]

neuron, receiving excitation from a wide area often covering most of the body surface. A smaller number of reticulospinal neurons exhibits predominantly inhibitory or mixed excitatory-inhibitory responses or excitatory responses originating from more restricted receptive fields (157, 232).

Studies involving natural stimulation or stimulation of peripheral nerves indicate that reticular neurons receive input from a wide variety of cutaneous and deep receptors and from high-threshold muscle afferents. They receive no input, however, from muscle spindle primary receptors or Golgi tendon organs (169, 170, 190). Responses to natural stimulation are typically graded over a wide range of stimulus intensities indicating that activity from receptors with very different thresholds converges upon individual reticular neurons. Another prominent feature of reticular responses to somatic stimulation is the strong decrement in response amplitude that occurs during repetitive stimulation (160, 188, 190). This decrement, illustrated in Figure 11, has many of the properties of behavioral and neural habituation defined by Thompson and Spencer (208). It appears to be a property of inputs to the reticular formation from various peripheral receptors because it also is observed during repetitive activation of the whole vestibular nerve (160). On the other hand, repetitive stimulation of corticoreticular or spinoreticular pathways that synapse directly with reticular neurons typically produces a response increment rather than a decrement (160). These findings lead to the hypothesis that the response decrement occurs within afferent pathways leading to the reticular formation rather than within the reticular formation itself. This has recently been verified in the case of somatoreticular pathways by recording from identified spinoreticular neurons in the lumbar enlargement. When repetitive electrical stimuli were applied to the skin of the hindlimb or to hindlimb nerves, the responses of these neurons decremented in much the same way as did responses of neurons in the medial reticular formation (137). The somatoreticular pathway thus provides the reticular formation with information about novel stimuli occurring over wide receptive fields, with the most vigorous responses being elicited by strong stimuli. This appears appropriate for triggering motor responses such as the startle or orientation reflexes.

Cerebellar inputs. The medial pontomedullary reticular formation receives cerebellar input via projections from the fastigial and dentate, deep cerebellar nuclei. Dentatoreticular fibers originate in the ventral part of the dentate nucleus and project via the superior cerebellar peduncle to the ventral part of the ipsilateral pontine reticular formation (22, 38). Stimulation of the dentate nucleus elicits monosynaptic excitation of neurons in the medial pontine reticular formation, including reticulospinal neurons that, from their location, are likely to project into the MRST (22). It is hard to rule out the possibility that axon reflex activation of cerebellar afferents with collaterals to the reticular formation might have contributed to the excitation evoked by dentate stimulation. However, the results suggest that a dentatoreticulospinal pathway contributes to modulation of spinal motor activity by the lateral cerebellum (21).

Although lesions within the fastigial nucleus give rise to degenerating fibers in the medial pontomedullary reticular formation on both sides of the brain stem, careful analysis indicates that the primary fastigioreticular projection is a crossed pathway via the hook bundle, which includes fibers terminating throughout the contralateral medial pontomedullary reticular formation (207, 210). Although a sparse ipsilateral projection cannot be ruled out, ipsilateral de-

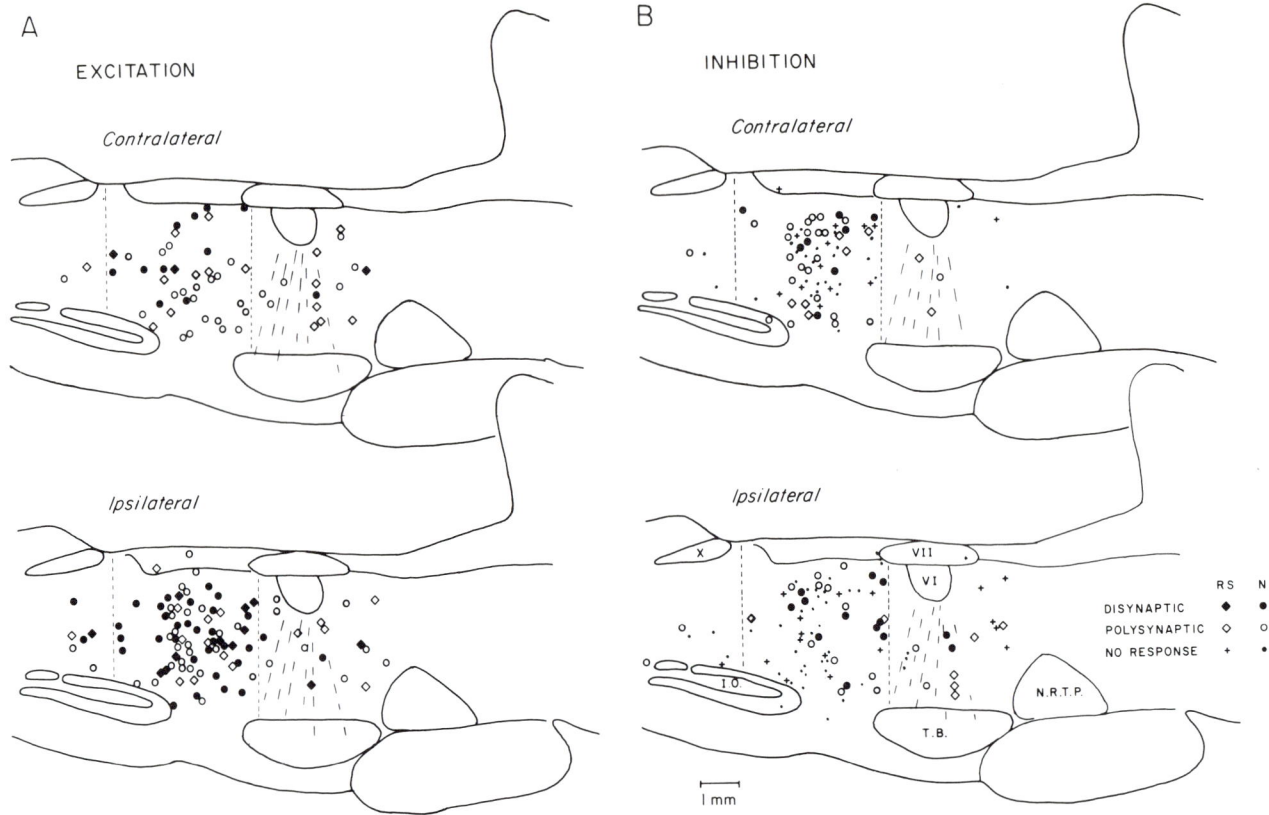

FIG. 9. Locations within medial reticular formation of neurons responding to vestibular nerve stimulation. Histologically determined locations of neurons whose responses were studied with intracellular recording are superimposed on 4 identical schematic parasagittal sections through pons and medulla. *Dashed lines* indicate rostral and caudal borders of nucleus reticularis gigantocellularis. Symbols indicate whether each neuron was reticulospinal (RS) or nonreticulospinal (N) neuron and whether it exhibited a di- or polysynaptic postsynaptic potential (PSP) or had no response to vestibular nerve stimulation. *A*: locations of neurons that responded with excitatory PSPs to stimulation of ipsilateral vestibular nerve (*lower section*) and contralateral vestibular nerve (*upper section*). *B*: locations of neurons that exhibited inhibitory PSPs or no response following stimulation of ipsilateral vestibular nerve (*lower section*) or contralateral vestibular nerve (*upper section*). I.O., inferior olivary nucleus; N.R.T.P, nucleus reticularis tegmenti pontis; T.B., trapezoid body; VI, abducens nucleus; VII, genu of facial nerve; X, dorsal nucleus of vagus. [From Peterson et al. (159).]

generation is likely due to interruption of hook-bundle fibers from the contralateral fastigial nucleus as they pass through the fastigial nucleus on the ipsilateral side.

As illustrated in Figure 10*F*, activation of the crossed fastigioreticular pathway by stimulation of the fastigial nucleus gives rise to monosynaptic excitation and causes firing of many neurons in the contralateral medial reticular formation, including reticulospinal neurons (43, 103). Responding reticulospinal neurons are located in both the pontine and medullary reticular formation, which suggests that fastigial excitation reaches both MRST and LRST neurons. Reticular neurons also respond to stimulation of the ipsilateral fastigial nucleus (Fig. 10*E*), but this cannot be taken as conclusive evidence for an ipsilateral fastigioreticular projection because the responses may have been produced by axon reflex activation of cerebellar afferent fibers (43, 103).

Little is known about the functional role of cerebellar projections to the medial reticular formation. The pattern of afferent input to cerebellar nuclei suggests that the fastigioreticular pathway relays information reaching the fastigial nucleus from somatic (44–46) or vestibular (63, 64, 69) receptors, while the dentatoreticular pathway carries information related to cortical motor systems (205). In each case the relayed information is modulated by Purkinje cell inhibition playing upon the deep nuclear neurons. Comparison of responses to somatic activation of reticulospinal neurons with and without fastigial input suggests that the fastigioreticular system contributes an early phase of depression and a later phase of excitation to the response of neurons receiving fastigial excitation (43). The timing of the depression and excitation suggests that the former is produced by Purkinje inhibition of fastigial neurons (resulting in disfacilitation) and the latter by somatic excitation of those neurons.

Comparison of the behavior of reticulospinal neurons in intact and cerebellectomized animals shows that the cerebellum plays an important role in controlling the activity of reticulospinal neurons during locomotion and static tilt. In decerebrate animals with an intact cerebellum, 31 of 89 reticulospinal neurons were activated in phase with stepping (while the animal was walking on a treadmill), whereas only 8% of the reticulospinal neurons studied in decerebrate, cerebellectomized animals showed such modulation (147, 148). Cerebellectomy correspondingly caused a significant decrease in the number of reticulospinal neurons that responded to roll tilt and converted many of the remaining responses from phasic to static (150). These changes are similar to those observed in the behavior of vestibulospinal neurons during locomotion and roll tilt following cerebellectomy (see subsection INPUTS TO VESTIBULOSPINAL TRACT NEURONS, p. 673).

RETICULOSPINAL ACTIONS ON SPINAL MOTONEURONS. Stimulation of the medial pontomedullary reticular formation produces a variety of effects at spinal levels including modulation of sensory pathways (30, 81, 127), depolarization of primary afferent fibers (35, 125),

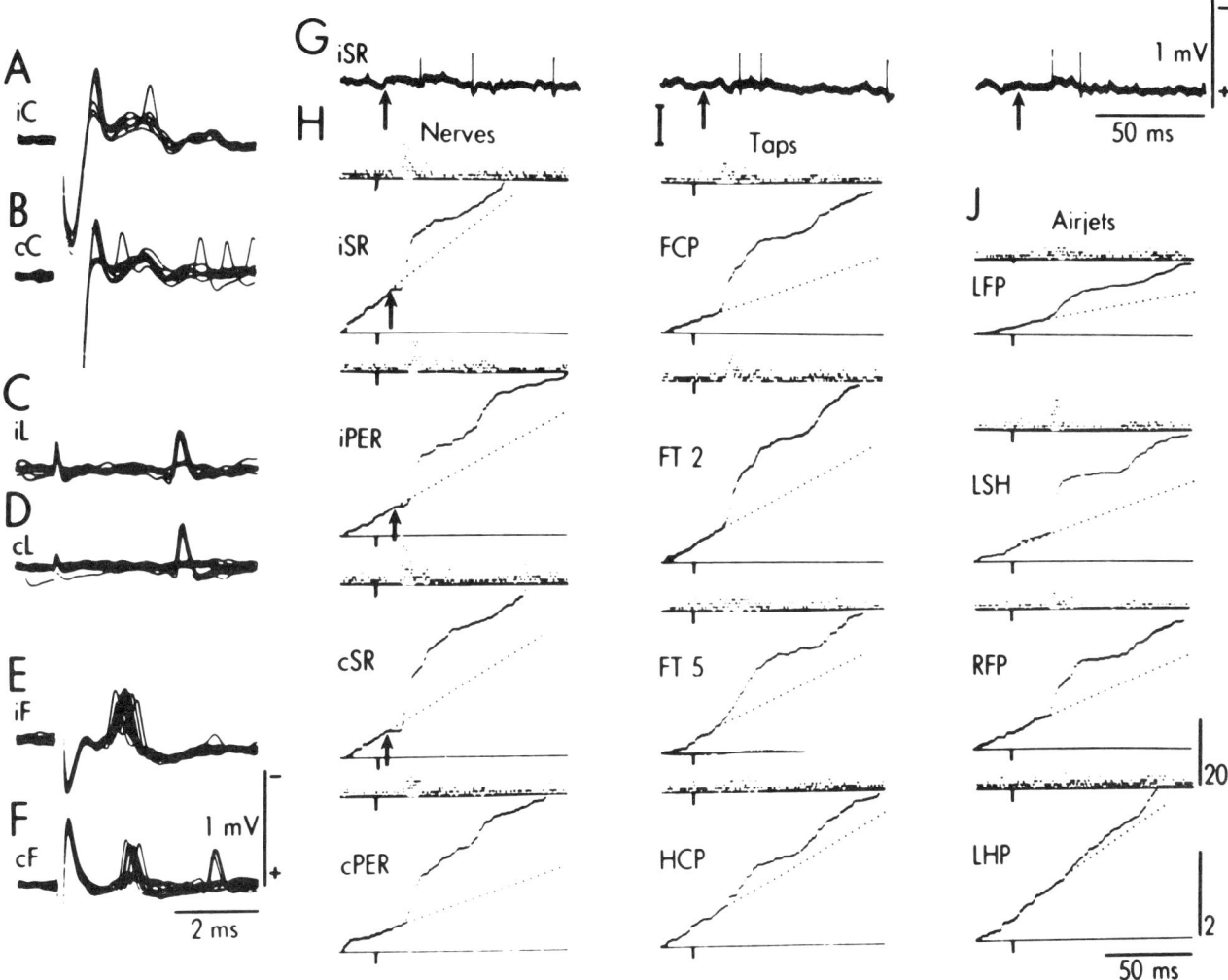

FIG. 10. Responses of reticulospinal neuron evoked antidromically and orthodromically with nerve and adequate stimulation. A-D are antidromic responses to juxtathreshold stimulation of ipsi- and contralateral cervical (A and B) and lumbar (C and D) spinal cord (i indicates ipsilateral, c denotes contralateral). E and F are monosynaptic responses to fastigial stimulation. G and H illustrate responses evoked by stimulation of superficial radial (SR) and peroneal (PER) nerves. Specimen records to iSR are shown in G; H displays poststimulus time histograms (PSTHs) and cumulative frequency distributions (CFDs) for responses to iSR and 3 other limb nerves as indicated. In I are PSTHs and CFDs for responses to brief taps (16 ms and 1.6 mm) to indicated foot pads on ipsilateral side: FCP, forelimb central pad; FT2 and FT5, forelimb toes 2 and 5; HCP, hindlimb central pad. In J are PSTHs and CFDs to airjet stimulation applied to hairy skin at indicated sites as defined in text. Same time and voltage scales for A-F. Same time scale for all PSTHs and CFDs. In H, arrows mark onsets of initial inhibition. [From Eccles et al. (43).]

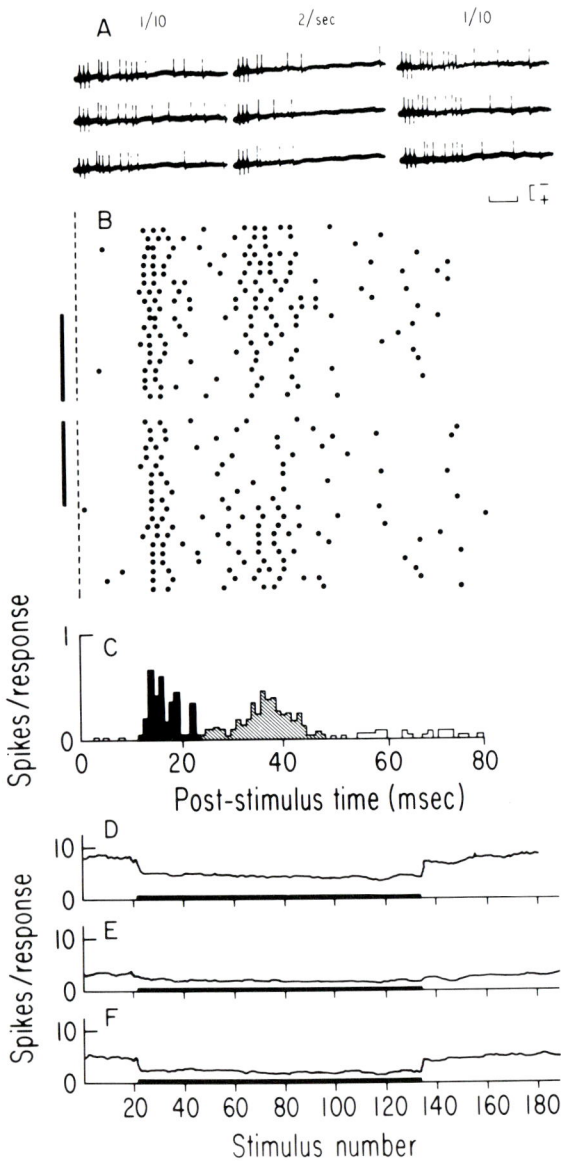

FIG. 11. Response of neuron in nucleus reticularis gigantocellularis during stimulation of ipsilateral hindpaw at rates of 0.1/s (control rate) and 2/s. *A*: oscilloscope traces showing firing of neuron during initial control period, during 2/s stimulation, and at end of final control period. Horizontal scale, 10 ms; vertical scale, 0.5 mV. *B*: raster display showing changes in neuronal firing during transition from 0.1/s to 2/s stimulation and from 2/s back to 0.1/s. Each *dot* represents an action potential and each *row of dots* shows neuronal firing in the first 80 ms after stimulus, which was given at point marked by *vertical dash*. Time scale is given below *C*. *Heavy vertical bars* indicate period of 2/s stimulation. First and second groups of responses were separated by 95 responses at 2/s. *C*: poststimulus time histogram of firing during initial control period. Abscissa is divided into 80 1-ms bins. Ordinate indicates average number of action potentials per bin per response. *Filled* and *shaded areas* show how response was divided into early and late components for further analysis. *D*: plot of number of action potentials occurring between 10 and 50 ms after each stimulus. *Filled bar* on base line indicates period of 2/s stimulation. *E*: plot similar to D of action potentials occurring within early response component (*solid area*) shown in *C*. *F*: plot of action potentials occurring within late response component (*shaded area* in *C*). [From Peterson et al. (160).]

control of autonomic functions (82–84), and excitation or inhibition of spinal motoneurons or interneurons (47, 123, 134, 178, 199). We will consider only those effects related to motor control.

Early investigations of reticular action on the motor apparatus suggested that the medial reticular formation could be divided into anterior and posterior regions. Stimulation of the former produced facilitation of reflexes in all four limbs while stimulation of the latter produced inhibition of those reflexes (134, 178). It has been shown, however, that carefully controlled stimulation of the medial reticular formation can elicit more localized changes in motor activity (199). At the lowest stimulus intensities, changes in position of one limb or body part can sometimes be observed, and with slightly stronger stimuli flexion of ipsilateral limbs, extension of contralateral limbs, and turning of the head toward the stimulated side are often seen. Only when stimulus intensities are increased still further is there global facilitation or inhibition of muscles in all four limbs. Stimulation of the reticular formation can therefore elicit fractionated body movements that might form components of a variety of motor behaviors.

Experiments involving monosynaptic reflex testing and recording from interneurons have emphasized that indirect pathways involving spinal interneurons play an important and often preeminent role in reticulospinal action on hindlimb motoneurons (47, 48, 123). More recent experiments with intracellular recording have shown that reticulospinal neurons also establish direct, monosynaptic connections with both α- and γ-motoneurons (77, 79, 80, 164, 165, 191, 229, 231). Monosynaptic reticulospinal excitation has been observed in a wide variety of motoneurons supplying muscles of the neck, back, and limbs. This phenomenon is common in limb motoneurons innervating flexors and the most proximal or distal extensor muscles. It is somewhat less common in motoneurons innervating extensor muscles acting about intermediate joints such as the elbow, knee, and ankle (Fig. 12). Hindlimb motoneurons in this latter group, such as gastrocnemius-soleus and quadriceps motoneurons, receive monosynaptic excitation from the LVST. Motoneurons receiving this excitation are generally not directly excited by reticulospinal fibers (79, 229). The limited data available on γ-motoneurons supplying spindles in hindlimb muscles indicates that direct reticulospinal excitation of these motoneurons has a pattern similar to that observed in hindlimb α-motoneurons (77). Reticulospinal action therefore tends to produce coactivation of α- and γ-motoneurons. In addition to monosynaptic excitation, activation of reticulospinal pathways also produces polysynaptic excitation of motoneurons with a generally similar distribution (79). As originally emphasized by Lloyd (123), this polysynaptic excitation is often more potent than direct excitation, particularly when reticulospinal neurons are activated repetitively.

Reticulospinal inhibition of motoneurons is also produced in part by direct, monosynaptic connections, but such connections appear to be restricted to neck motoneurons, which are monosynaptically inhibited by neurons in n.r. ventralis and dorsal n.r. gigantocellularis (165). Motoneurons at lower spinal levels receive polysynaptic IPSPs following stimulation of the medullary reticular formation (79, 106, 119, 120, 164). In the hindlimb these IPSPs are especially prevalent in motoneurons innervating extensors of the knee and ankle, a population receiving little reticulospinal excitation. Inhibition is also found in hamstring motoneurons; this population is therefore both excited and inhibited (Fig. 12).

Which of the reticulospinal tracts is responsible for direct excitation and inhibition of motoneurons? This question can be answered in part by analyzing the location of reticular regions from which excitation or inhibition of different motoneuron populations can be evoked, as shown in Figure 13. Stimulation of n.r. pontis caudalis and dorsal n.r. gigantocellularis (the region lying to the right of the dashed line in Fig. 13D) produces excitation of neck, back, and limb motoneurons. Because these reticular regions contain primarily MRST neurons, it appears that the MRST has a direct excitatory action on motoneurons supplying muscles throughout the body. Further evidence supporting this comes from observations that stimulation of the MLF, through which many MRST fibers run, elicits a similar widespread pattern of excitation (155, 164, 229, 231). By contrast, stimulation of n.r. ventralis and ventrocaudal n.r. gigantocellularis (the region lying to the left of the dashed line in Fig. 13D), which project to the spinal cord via the LRST, elicits direct excitation of neck and back motoneurons (Fig. 13A, C) and direct inhibition of neck motoneurons but has no direct action on limb motoneurons (Fig. 13B, D). It thus appears that the direct motor action of the LRST is restricted to axial motoneurons. There is also evidence that this pathway contains neurons that act selectively on neck motoneurons. These neurons include the inhibitory reticulospinal neurons previously described and excitatory neurons situated in dorsal n.r. gigantocellularis, which is within the effective zone for excitation of neck motoneurons (Fig. 13A) but outside the effective zones for excitation of other motoneuron groups (Fig. 13B–D). Thus with regard to their direct motor actions, the MRST and LRST are quite different. The former has a widespread excitatory action with no sign of intrinsic topographic organization whereas the latter has topographically segregated groups of excitatory and inhibitory neurons that act only on neck and back motoneurons.

SUMMARY. Two rapidly conducting fiber systems link the medial pontomedullary reticular formation to the spinal cord: the medial and lateral reticulospinal tracts. The MRST originates primarily from anterior and dorsal regions, including the medial pontine reticular formation and the anterior n.r. gigantocellularis, and descends in the ventromedial funiculus. The LRST fibers originate in the more posterior medullary reticular formation and descend in the ipsilateral and contralateral ventrolateral funiculi. Both pathways extend the entire length of the spinal cord and the majority of neurons in each reach lumbar levels, often after giving off terminal branches at higher spinal levels.

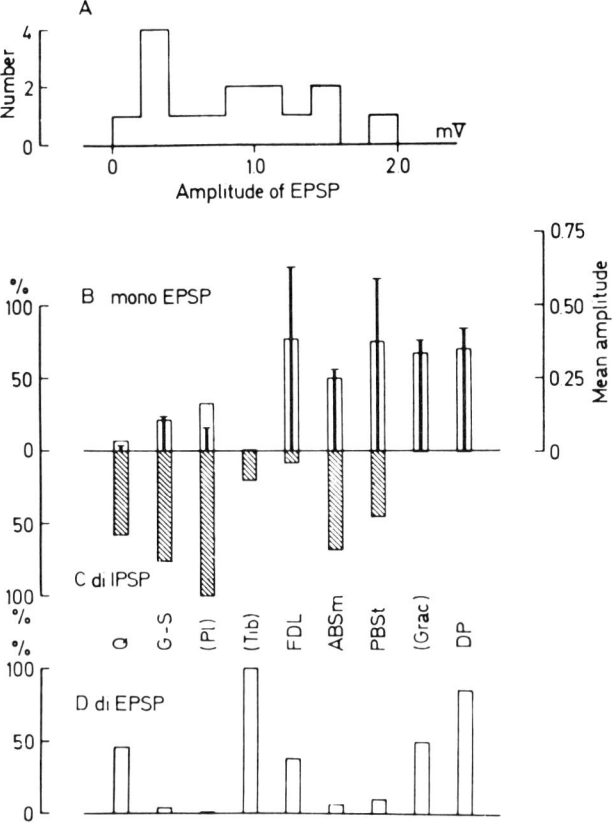

FIG. 12. Amplitude distribution of monosynaptic excitatory postsynaptic potentials (EPSPs) in α-motoneurons (A) and distribution of monosynaptic EPSPs (B), disynaptic inhibitory PSPs (C) and disynaptic EPSPs (D) evoked by stimulation of medial longitudinal fasciculus (MLF) in different species of α-motoneurons. A: frequency histogram of amplitude of maximal monosynaptic EPSP evoked by MLF stimulation, from 15 cells sampled in same cat. B–D: percentages of occurrence, indicated by height of columns (left ordinates). Bars in B show mean amplitude of monosynaptic EPSPs (right ordinate). Q, quadriceps; G-S, gastrocnemius-soleus; Pl, plantaris; Tib, tibial; FDL, flexor digitorum and hallucis longus; ABSm, anterior biceps-semimembranosus; PBSt, posterior biceps-semitendinosus; Grac, gracilis; DP, deep peroneal. (Parentheses indicate that data are based on less than 10 cells.) Motoneurons with spike and resting potentials below 40 mV were discarded. [From Grillner et al. (79).]

The two tracts establish synaptic connections with a wide variety of spinal neurons including motoneurons. Fibers of the MRST directly excite motoneurons supplying both axial muscles and limb flexor and extensor muscles. The more circumscribed direct connections of LRST fibers include excitatory and inhib-

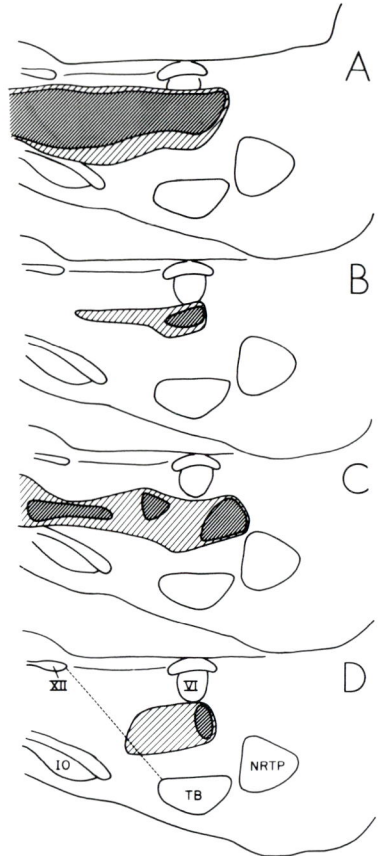

FIG. 13. Reticular regions from which monosynaptic excitation of spinal motoneurons could be evoked. Effectiveness of 100-μA stimuli (applied at points located 0.5 mm from midline) in evoking monosynaptic excitation of ipsilateral neck (A), forelimb (B), back (C), and hindlimb (D) motoneurons is indicated by *shaded areas* in each schematic parasagittal section. *Light shading* indicates regions that contained a few effective points (i.e., points at which 100-μA stimulus produced monosynaptic excitation in more than 10% of motoneurons tested). *Dark shading* indicates areas within which more than half of points were effective. *Dotted line* in D separates zone 1 (which contains primarily medial reticulospinal neurons) and zone 2 (comprised of mainly lateral reticulospinal neurons). IO, inferior olive; NRTP, nucleus reticularis tegmenti pontis; TB, trapezoid body; VI, abducens nucleus; XII, hypoglossal nucleus. [From Peterson (155).]

itory connections with neck motoneurons and excitatory connections with back motoneurons. These fibers have no direct action upon limb motoneurons, although both LRST and MRST neurons have substantial indirect, polysynaptic actions on all types of somatic motoneurons.

Inputs to reticulospinal neurons arise from many sources, including the vestibular system, somatosensory system, and cerebellum. Vestibular signals, which may originate in either semicircular canal or otolith receptors, reach reticulospinal neurons indirectly via relays in the vestibular or cerebellar nuclei. Somatosensory inputs, which originate in cutaneous and high-threshold muscle receptors, are also indirect, involving relays in spinal cord or brain stem. Interneurons in these pathways likely cause a decrement in response of reticulospinal neurons to stimuli that are applied repetitively. Reticulospinal neurons also receive direct, excitatory input from two deep cerebellar nuclei: the ipsilateral dentate nucleus and contralateral fastigial nucleus. Input from these nuclei, which are under the inhibitory control of the cerebellar cortex, contributes to modulation of the activity of reticulospinal neurons by vestibular, somatic, and proprioceptive inputs.

Connections Between Labyrinthine and Spinal Motoneurons

When the vestibular nerve or its branches are stimulated by single stimuli or by trains of stimuli, this evokes synaptic potentials in motoneurons and head, body, and limb movements in unrestrained animals. All of these motor phenomena begin with activation of the vestibular nuclei. It is the role of the vestibulospinal and reticulospinal tracts in the production of such synaptic potentials and movements that is now discussed.

STIMULATION OF WHOLE VESTIBULAR NERVE. Vestibular nerve stimulation evokes EPSPs and IPSPs with latencies shorter than 2.5 ms in ipsilateral and contralateral neck motoneurons (228–230). Transection of the MVST confirms that, as may be expected, ipsilateral EPSPs are mediated by the LVST, and contralateral EPSPs and bilateral IPSPs are mediated by the MVST (9). There are also disynaptic connections between labyrinthine and back motoneurons (9, 231). On the other hand, there are no disynaptic connections between labyrinthine and limb motoneurons (228). This shows that the LVST neurons that make monosynaptic contact with gastrocnemius and quadriceps motoneurons do not receive monosynaptic vestibular input. In decerebrate cats, but not in barbiturate-anesthetized cats, stimulation with short trains of stimuli, and sometimes with single stimuli, evokes potentials that are at least trisynaptic in forelimb motoneurons (128). These potentials, which may have smooth rising phases or steplike components, are illustrated in Figure 14. The pattern of effects consists predominantly of bilateral excitation of the tested shoulder and elbow extensors and bilateral inhibition of elbow flexors (128). The potentials survive transection of the medial longitudinal fasciculus (MLF) (Fig. 14A) but not of the LVST (Fig. 14B) and are therefore due to activity in the latter tract. There have not been comparable experiments on hindlimb motoneurons, but the pattern of the synaptic actions and the appearance of the potentials evoked in these motoneurons by stimulation of Deiters' nucleus (87) suggest that they may receive labyrinthine inputs similar to those received by forelimb motoneurons.

STIMULATION OF VESTIBULAR NERVE BRANCHES. A big step forward in the study of central vestibular connec-

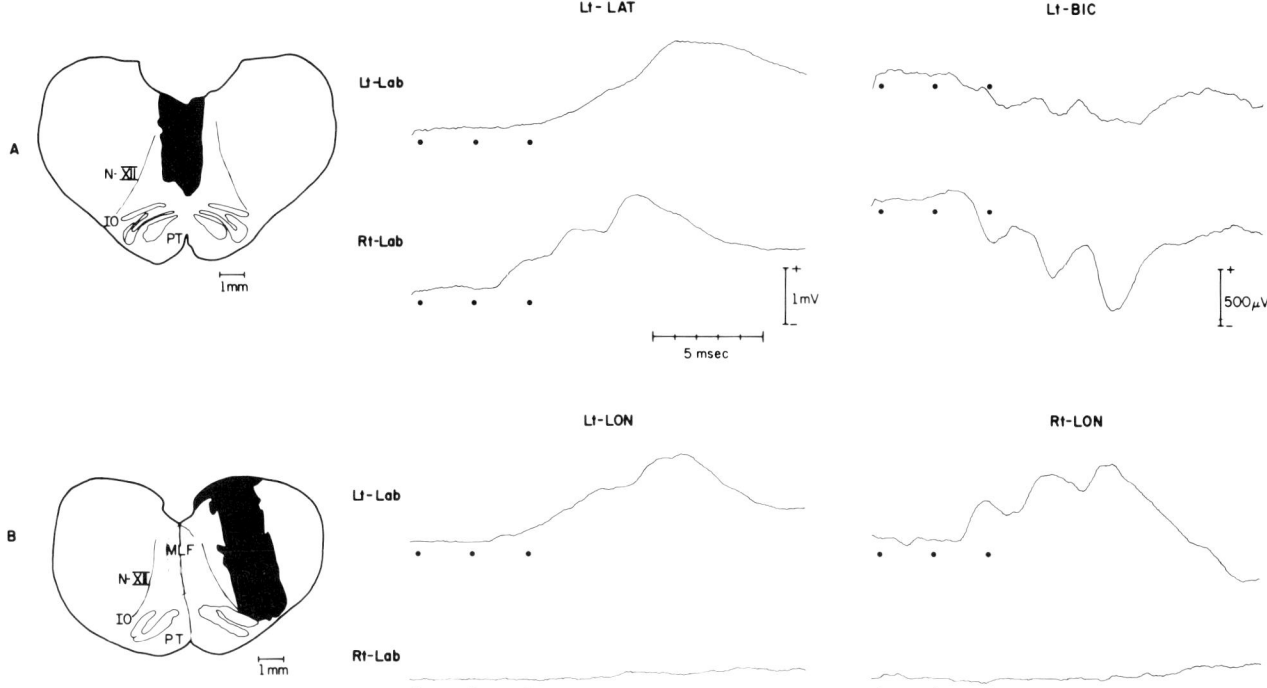

FIG. 14. Synaptic potentials evoked in forelimb motoneurons. *A*: after transection of medial longitudinal fasciculus (MLF), as illustrated in drawing, typical potentials are still evoked in motoneurons of left lateral head of triceps (LAT) or biceps (BIC) by stimulation of either vestibular nerve. After large lateral lesion of brain stem that interrupts right lateral vestibulospinal tract, stimulation of right vestibular nerve is no longer effective, although stimulation of left vestibular nerve still evokes excitatory postsynaptic potentials bilaterally in motoneurons of long head of triceps (LON). IO, inferior olive; NXII, hypoglossal nerve; PT, pyramidal tract. [From Maeda, Maunz, and Wilson (128).]

tions was the development of the Suzuki technique for selective stimulation of individual ampullary nerves (202). Although it is also possible to stimulate the utricular nerve and the saccular macula selectively (55, 56, 203), the danger of stimulus spread appears greater than with ampullary nerve stimulation. While selective stimulation of the saccular macula has been used for the study of vestibuloocular connections (91), there have been no attempts at selective stimulation of the otoliths or otolith nerves (in a normal labyrinth) for study of vestibulospinal connections. Instead the utricular or saccular nerve has been stimulated in cats in which the other nerve branches have been chronically severed (217).

Neck motoneurons. Stimulation of individual semicircular canal nerves with trains of stimuli causes stereotyped movements of the head [Fig. 15; (201)]. Whichever canal is stimulated, the movements observed are the same as the compensatory movements that would be evoked by natural activation of that particular canal. For example, ipsilateral horizontal rotation or horizontal canal nerve stimulation produces contralateral movement of the head relative to the body in the horizontal plane (Fig. 15C). When the same nerves are stimulated in anesthetized cats, a regular pattern of synaptic potentials is observed in motoneurons innervating neck muscles. Horizontal canal nerve stimulation evokes IPSPs ipsilaterally and EPSPs contralaterally. In this instance, and with stimulation of other nerves, the pattern of potentials is fully consistent with the head movements observed in alert cats [Fig. 16; (221)]. Both EPSPs and IPSPs have latencies of 2.5 ms or less, and are disynaptic. Section of the MVST in the MLF, or a lesion of the area of the LVST in the lower medulla, reveals the role of the two tracts in the production of the potentials. The contributions of the two tracts, as well as the pattern of potentials, are summarized in Figure 16: excitatory LVST fibers transmit ipsilateral excitation from the anterior canal, inhibitory MVST fibers transmit ipsilateral inhibition from the horizontal canal and bilateral inhibition from the posterior canal, and excitatory MVST fibers transmit contralateral excitation from the anterior canal (221). Complementary results have been recently obtained for neck flexor motoneurons by Fukushima, Hirai, and Rapoport (see ref. 60). These motoneurons receive all their short-latency connections via the MVST. The electrophysiological approach therefore shows that canal nerve-evoked synaptic potentials of disynaptic latency are transmitted by the two vestibulospinal tracts, and that the pattern of the potentials is the same as the pattern of head movement produced by electrical stimulation of the same canal nerves. Whether the short latency poten-

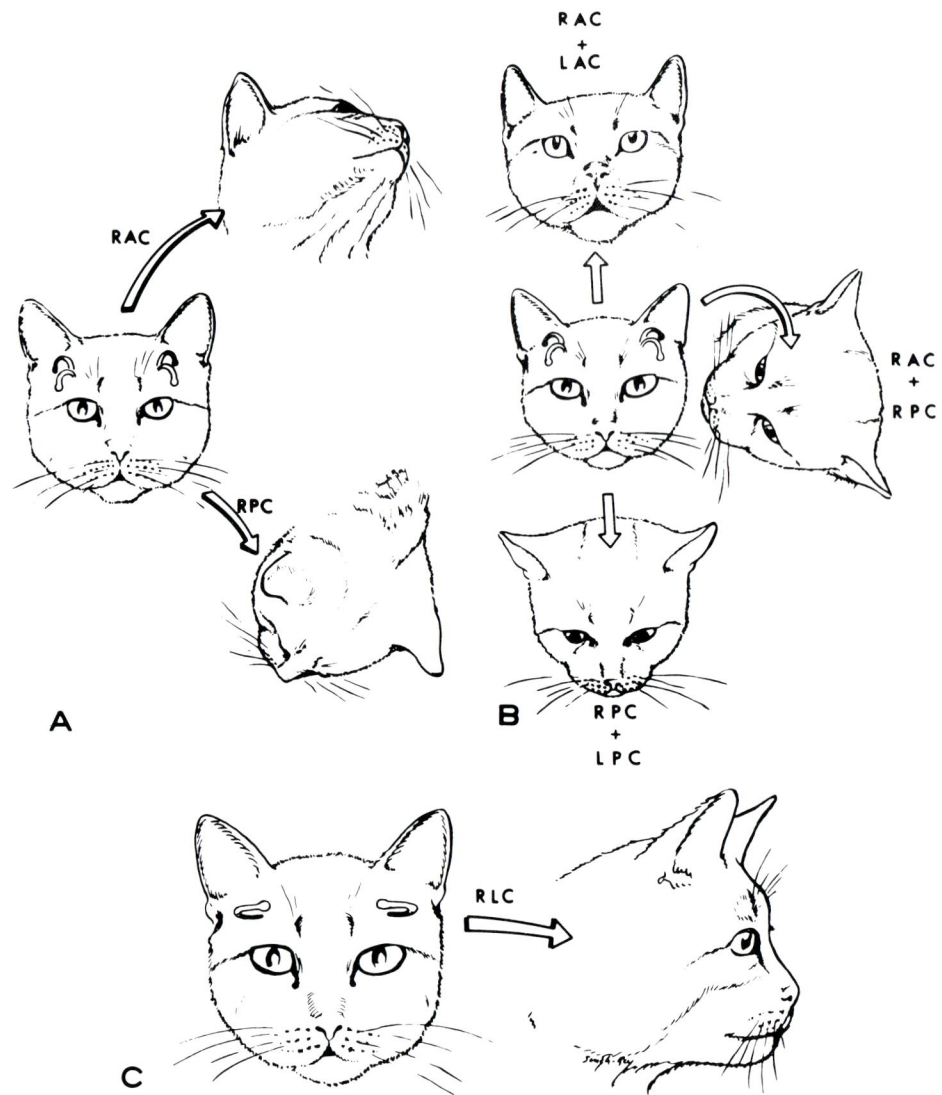

FIG. 15. Schematic drawings of semicircular canals and head movements induced in cat by stimulation of ampullary nerves. *Arrows* show direction of induced head movements. RAC and LAC, right and left anterior canals, respectively; RPC and LPC, right and left posterior canals, respectively; RLC, right lateral (horizontal) canal. [From Suzuki and Cohen (201).]

tials are necessary or sufficient to produce the movements is another question. It seems likely that they at least contribute to production of the movement because with trains of stimuli the level of depolarization due to the summed monosynaptic potentials may be large enough to cause firing (221). Even with single stimuli, however, somewhat later small potentials of the same polarity as the disynaptic potentials can still be evoked in neck motoneurons after MVST section (221). The pathways that produce these potentials, perhaps the reticulospinal tracts, may be very important in unanesthetized, intact animals.

Compared to the wealth of electrophysiological information available about pathways from semicircular canals to neck motoneurons, little is known about pathways from otolith organs. Micromanipulation of the utricular macula causes contraction of neck muscles (204). Stimulation of both the saccular and utricular nerves evokes disynaptic and trisynaptic (as well as later) potentials in neck motoneurons (218), showing the existence of quite direct otolith-spinal pathways. The patterns of short-latency effects produced by stimulation of the utricular and saccular nerves differ: saccular stimulation evokes mainly ipsilateral EPSPs and contralateral IPSPs, while the reverse is true for stimulation of the utricular nerve (218).

Limb motoneurons. When any one of the semicircular canal nerves is stimulated, there is usually ipsilateral forelimb extension and contralateral flexion (201, 204). In decerebrate cats, stimulation of canal nerves evokes synaptic potentials in forelimb moto-

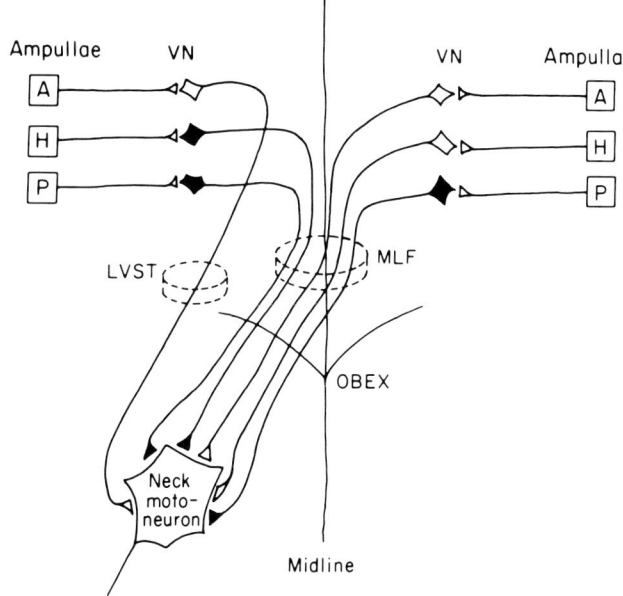

FIG. 16. Schematic drawing of connections between ipsilateral and contralateral ampullae and neck motoneurons. A, H, and P are anterior, horizontal, and posterior ampullae, respectively; VN, vestibular nuclei; LVST, lateral vestibulospinal tract; MLF, medial longitudinal fasciculus. Inhibitory neurons and their terminals shown in black, excitatory in white. [From Wilson and Maeda (221).]

neurons; there are EPSPs bilaterally in extensors, IPSPs in flexors (128). The pattern of these potentials does not fit with the movements observed by others (201, 204). This suggests that long lasting stimulation or natural activation of canal afferents activates more complex pathways that are responsible for the movements described.

CENTRAL PATHWAYS
FOR NECK REFLEXES

Tonic neck reflexes survive transection at the rostral edge of C_1 [(131), but see ref. 212]; accordingly, intraspinal pathways should be sufficient to produce them. This is supported by recent experiments in which neck muscle and cutaneous afferents, and the C_2 dorsal root ganglion, were stimulated (111). Stimulation of cutaneous and muscle nerves evoked EPSPs with a latency of 14–25 ms in various types of hindlimb motoneurons (Fig. 17D–F). Stimulation of the dorsal root ganglion, which should excite afferents from the region of the neck joints as well as muscle and cutaneous afferents, evoked similar potentials plus an early EPSP with a latency as short as 6 ms (Fig. 17A–C). Spinalization at C_1 abolished the EPSPs evoked from muscle and cutaneous nerves; these postsynaptic potentials may be related to the long loop reflexes that require the cerebral cortex (1, 2). The EPSPs evoked from the dorsal root ganglia survived the transection and may be related to tonic neck reflexes. It is reasonable to assume that similar results would be obtained for forelimb motoneurons. Experiments such as these (111, 131) obviously do not rule out a contribution to tonic neck reflexes by supraspinal pathways.

Little else is known about the pathways leading from neck receptors to motoneurons. The shortest latency of 6 ms for C_2 dorsal root ganglion-evoked EPSPs in hindlimb motoneurons suggests a polysynaptic connection to these motoneurons. There is probably such a connection to forelimb motoneurons as well. The interneurons that may be involved have not been identified. There is a population of propriospinal neurons in the C_3-C_4 segments that excite forelimb motoneurons monosynaptically and receive converging excitation from many sources including motor cortex, red nucleus, and superior colliculus (93). Stimulation of the cervical dorsal columns, which may excite not only ascending but also descending fibers, evokes monosynaptic EPSPs in these propriospinal neurons (Fig. 18E–H). Stimulation of C_2-C_3 muscular and cutaneous nerves often evokes late synaptic potentials while stimulation near the dorsal root ganglion may evoke monosynaptic EPSPs (Fig. 18J–M). This propriospinal pathway may be part of the neural substrate of tonic, or other, neck reflexes.

Until more elements of the pathway(s) from neck receptors to limb motoneurons are identified, one can only speculate on the loci for interaction of neck and vestibular reflexes. The interaction may take place at several levels. First, there is convergence of neck and vestibular input on cells in the vestibular nuclei. Activation of neck joint afferents and stimulation of the labyrinth can excite the same vestibular neurons, including those with unknown projections (57, 85, 206), those that project to the abducens nucleus (85), and those that project to the spinal cord (27). Second, there may be convergence on spinal interneurons. Propriospinal neurons are not good candidates for convergence, since present evidence suggests lack of vestibulospinal input (93). Finally, there may be direct convergence on motoneurons.

FUNCTIONAL STUDIES OF
VESTIBULOSPINAL REFLEXES

The section CENTRAL PATHWAYS FOR VESTIBULAR REFLEXES, p. 671, reviewed the extensive information regarding the vestibulospinal system that has been accumulated by reductionist techniques, that is, the physiological and anatomical methods that concentrate on direct connections. In summary this work has shown that different receptors in the labyrinth are connected to the spinal cord via the vestibular nuclei by two tracts, the LVST and MVST. When different nerves in the labyrinth are stimulated, disynaptic potentials and others of somewhat longer latency are evoked in motoneurons. Disynaptic and many trisynaptic potentials, and potentials of even longer la-

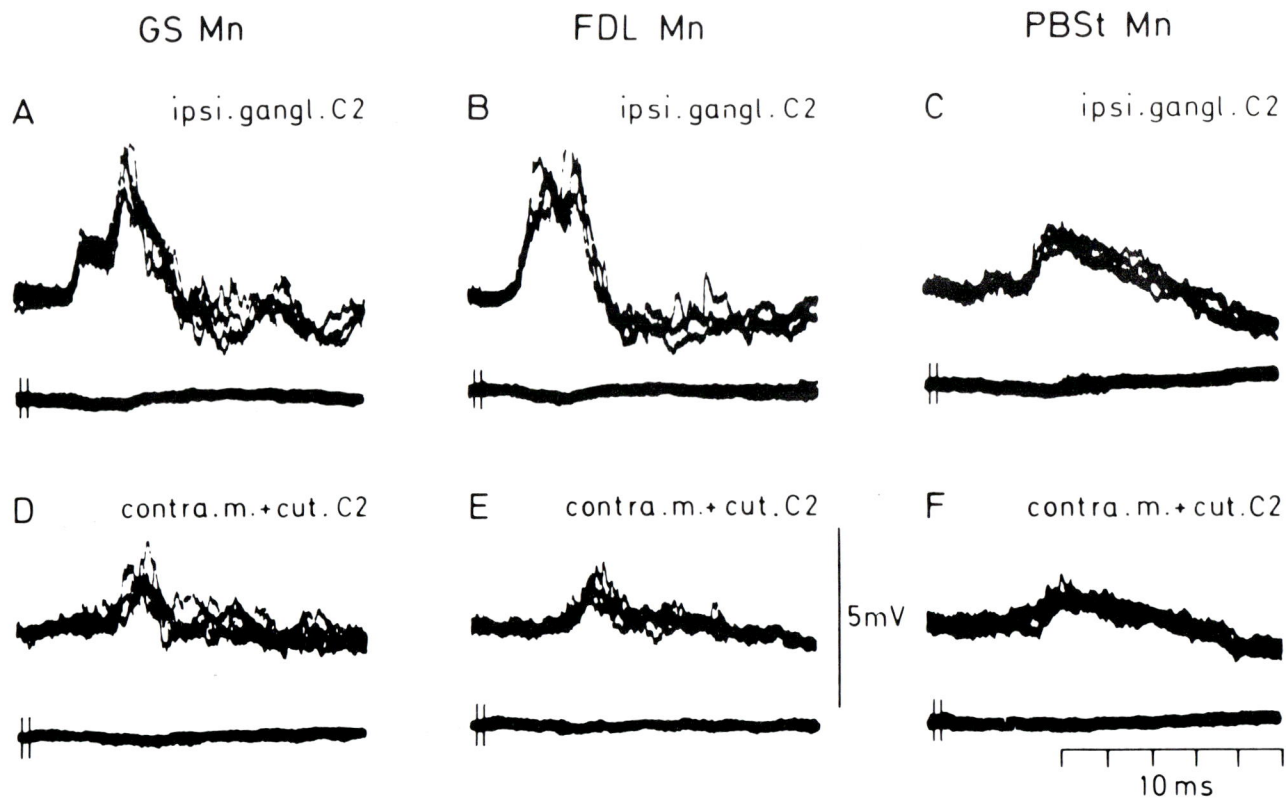

FIG. 17. Early and late excitation evoked from cervical dorsal root ganglion stimulation but only late excitation from combined muscle-skin stimulation in cat with intact CNS. Intracellular records from gastrocnemius (*A* and *D*), flexor digitorum longus (*B* and *E*), and posterior biceps-semitendinosus (*C* and *F*) motoneuron (*upper beam*). Records of extracellular potential on *lower beam*. Stimulation of ipsilateral C₂ dorsal root ganglion (*A–C*), and contralateral muscle and skin nerves (*D–F*) with double stimuli; stimuli marked on *lower beam*. [From Kenins et al. (111).]

tency, are evoked via the vestibulospinal tracts. Some potentials that are trisynaptic or later may be evoked via the reticulospinal tracts. When canal nerves are stimulated with trains of stimuli, the pattern of head movements produced is the same as the pattern of disynaptic potentials in neck motoneurons (Figs. 15 and 16). On the other hand, there is no such agreement between movement and the potential pattern in the forelimb. This raises a question as to the extent to which the reflex movements evoked by natural stimulation are due to short-latency potentials.

A very different approach to the study of vestibulospinal reflexes concentrates on the dynamics of reflexes evoked by natural stimulation. From the behavior of the reflexes, it is possible to see what processing the afferent input must be subjected to in order to produce the appropriate responses, and to deduce some of the properties of the central circuitry involved. Sinusoidal analysis, which was described briefly in the section VESTIBULAR AND NECK REFLEXES; subsection SEMICIRCULAR CANAL REFLEXES, p. 667, has been used extensively to study the behavior of vestibular afferents and second-order neurons (71) and of vestibuloocular reflexes. It has been recently used for investigations of vestibulospinal reflexes. The earliest experiments were not with natural but with electrical modulation. Partridge and Kim (152) delivered frequency-modulated pulses to the whole vestibular nerve and recorded the resulting tension changes in the gastrocnemius muscle. Subsequent work has employed natural sinusoidal stimulation to investigate vestibulocollic and vestibular-forelimb reflexes. As already pointed out, the vestibulocollic reflex is a closed-loop system: movement of the head is detected by the relevant labyrinth receptor and the appropriate compensatory movement is evoked. To date, however, all animal experiments involving this reflex have been done in the open-loop mode, with the head restrained. The reflex dynamics observed under these conditions are not necessarily the same as those in an animal whose head is free to move. This experimental arrangement is less artificial for vestibular-limb reflexes because the relation of limb movement to head position is less direct.

Semicircular Canal Reflexes

As was described earlier, when a cat is rotated to the right around its vertical axis, the left neck muscles contract. The dynamics of this vestibulocollic reflex have been analyzed by oscillating decerebrate cats in the plane of the horizontal canal and recording the responses of neck muscle motor units or of the compound EMG (24, 50). The effects of oscillation at frequencies up to 0.4 Hz are illustrated in Figure 19. The Bode plot of Figure 19C shows that there is a considerable phase lag (measured as in Fig. 19B) between the input acceleration and the response of the motor units. The phase lag is as large as 150° at 0.2 Hz. Over the range of frequencies studied, gain decreases with a slope of 40 dB/decade (50). These results are generally similar to those of Berthoz and Anderson (24), who worked over a wider frequency range but observed smaller phase lags.

It is instructive to compare the behavior of the muscle with that of second-order type I neurons in the horizontal canal system. These neurons have the same response pattern as contralateral neck muscles and are the first brain stem neurons in the pathway to those muscles. In decerebrate cats second-order neurons fire approximately in phase with the velocity of the stimulus, that is, with a phase lag re acceleration approaching 90° for frequencies between 0.05 and 0.5 Hz; at lower frequencies the phase lag is even smaller (71, 196). Hence there is a considerable central phase lag between the responses of second-order neurons and muscle, as illustrated in Figure 20. The lag increases to approximately 70°–80° at 0.05 Hz and then decreases as the frequency increases.

Comparable results have been obtained by using sinusoidal polarizing current (applied to branches of the vestibular nerve) as a stimulus instead of natural stimulation (216, 224). With this method it is easy to deliver high-frequency stimuli, and the experiments, performed by stimulating vertical and horizontal canal nerves, show that central phase lags are much smaller (about 20° at 3-6 Hz). This higher part of the frequency range is of particular interest: for passive movements of a human walking, running, or jumping, and for voluntary movements, the principal sine wave frequency components of vertical head movement lie between 1 and 4 Hz (75).

A central phase lag approaching 90° at some frequencies indicates the presence of a circuit that performs the equivalent of a step of mathematical integration on the signal between second-order neurons and muscle, that is, a neural integrator (197). Because the vestibulocollic reflex compensates for head position, it may be appropriate that a neural network transforms the signal that will eventually result in muscular contraction from one in phase with velocity to one in phase with position. We do not know, however, how the system functions in the closed-loop mode and to what extent the transformation of the

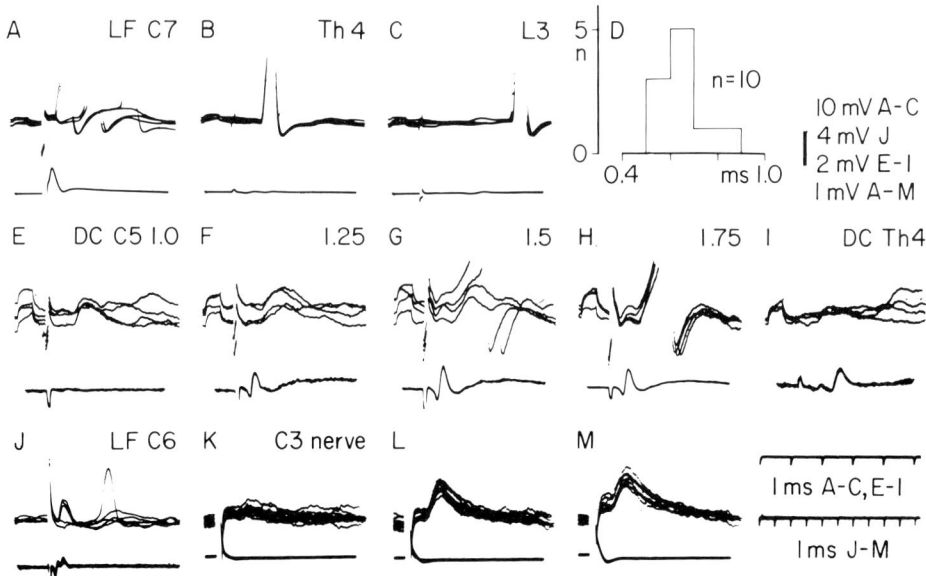

FIG. 18. Monosynaptic excitatory postsynaptic potentials (EPSPs) evoked from cervical primary afferents in propriospinal neurons in 3rd cervical segment (C_3). Cell 1 (*A–I*) projected beyond 3rd lumbar segment (L_3 in *C*). Cell 2 (*J–M*) was only tested for antidromic invasion from C_6 (*J*). The EPSPs in *upper traces* of *E–H* were evoked by bipolar stimulation of dorsal column (DC) in C_5. *Lower traces* recorded from surface of lateral funiculus (LF). Stimulus strengths are given in multiples of threshold. Observe that DC stimulation in 4th thoracic segment (Th_4) does not evoke monosynaptic EPSP (*I*) at a strength giving slight coactivation of LF, from which can be seen a small discharge preceding main volley. Amplification of surface record in *H* is one-half of that in *E–G*. Histogram in *D* gives distribution of segmental latencies of EPSPs evoked from DC. Monosynaptic EPSP in cell 2 was evoked by stimulation of C_3 dorsal rami close to spinal ganglion; graded stimulation in *K–M*. [From Illert et al. (92).]

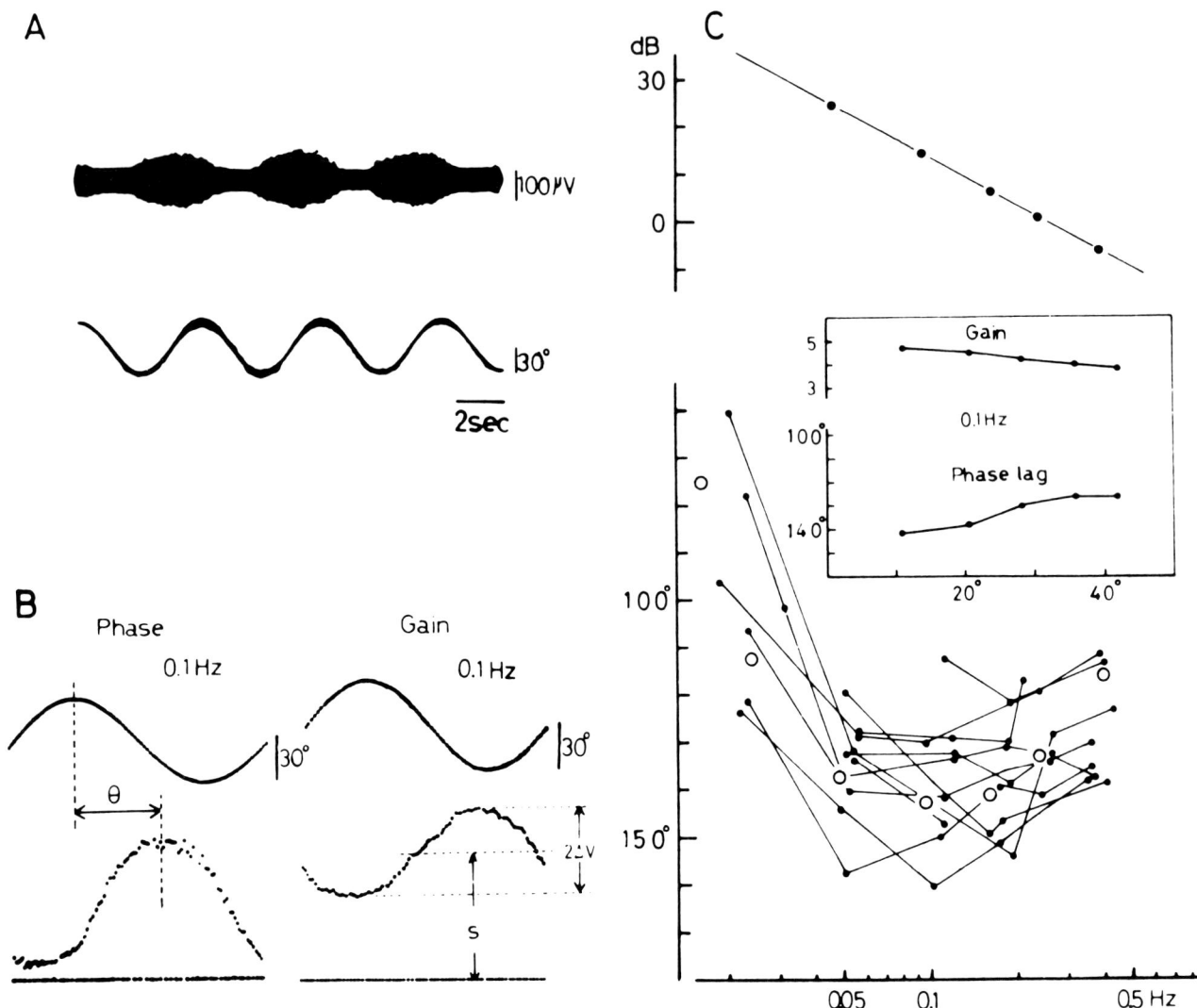

FIG. 19. Response of compound electromyograms (EMGs) to sinusoidal oscillation. *A*: *top*, compound EMG activity of right extensor muscles; *bottom*, position of turntable, downward displacement indicating rightward movement. *B*: methods of measurement of phase lag and gain. *Top*, position of turntable, upward displacement indicating rightward rotation. For measurement of phase lag, rectified EMGs were averaged (*left*); for measurement of gain, rectified EMGs were integrated through low-pass filter and then averaged (*right*). S, level of spontaneous activity. *C*: Bode diagram. Phase lags were plotted from 11 cats; *open circles*, averaged phase lag of motor units. Gain was obtained from cat whose spontaneous activity was maintained constant during whole period of recording (normalized at 0.25 Hz). *Inset*: linearity of compound EMG responses, abscissa showing amplitude of oscillation (turntable position). [From Ezure and Sasaki (50).]

signal is performed by the mechanics of the head movement system in intact animals.

Vestibular-forelimb reflexes have also been studied with sinusoidal angular acceleration (16, 23, 198). In contrast with movements evoked by trains of pulses, activation of the horizontal canal, even with pulses of angular acceleration, causes excitation of contralateral forelimb extensors (see section VESTIBULAR AND NECK REFLEXES; subsection SEMICIRCULAR CANAL REFLEXES, p. 667). As with vestibulocollic reflexes, there is a considerable phase lag between input (contralateral) acceleration and muscle response (Fig. 21). The estimated phase lag vs. the responses of peripheral afferents, and therefore second-order neurons, is shown by the stippled area in Figure 21. When vertical angular acceleration is used and the contribution of macular afferents subtracted, similar results are obtained for vertical canal reflexes (198). While the central lag in the vestibulocollic reflex decreases at higher frequencies, the lag in the vestibular-forelimb horizontal reflex is still increasing at 1 Hz. Similar results are obtained when the responses of neck and forelimb muscles to sinusoidal polarization of the horizontal canal nerve at frequencies up to 3 Hz are compared in

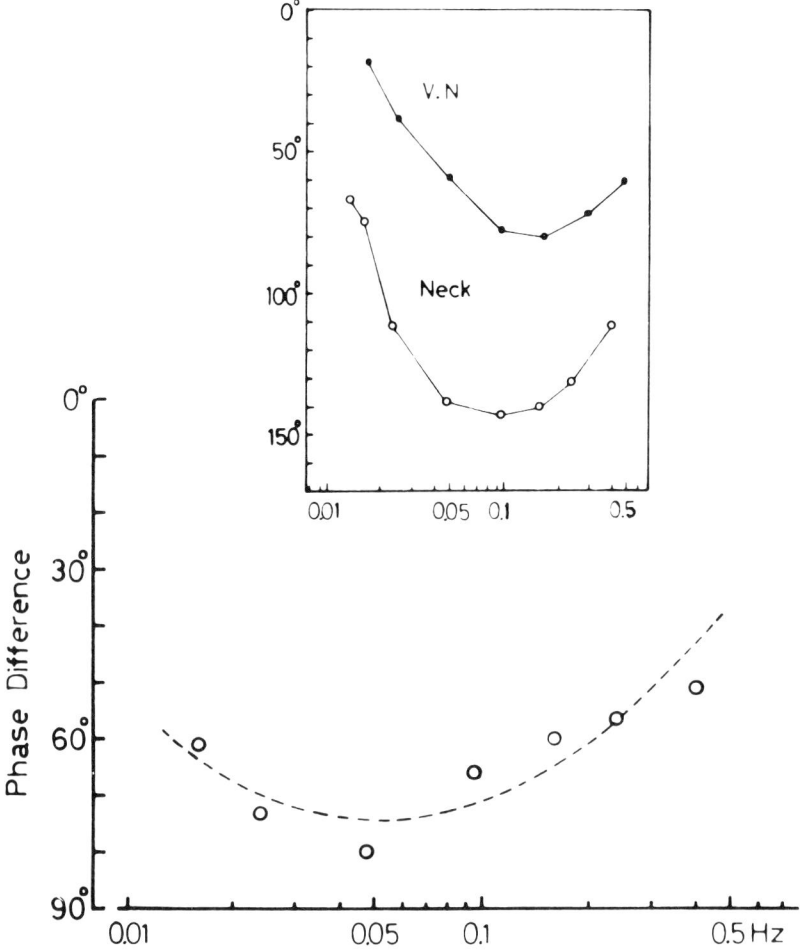

FIG. 20. Averaged phase differences (as function of frequency) between vestibular nucleus neurons and neck motor units. Best-fit curve is drawn with least-square methods (*broken lines*). *Inset*: upper curve, from data of Shinoda and Yoshida (196) on neurons in vestibular nuclei (VN); lower curve, neck motor unit responses. [From Ezure and Sasaki (50).]

the same preparation (85a). There is apparently a difference in the central processing of vestibular (canal) reflexes of neck and forelimb.

Otolith Reflexes

The effects of static tilt (position change) on the musculature are well known and have already been described. The dynamics of otolith vestibulospinal reflexes, however, have not been studied extensively. Recent work shows that activity in the triceps muscles of decerebrate cats is modulated by sinusoidal linear acceleration applied along the horizontal or vertical axes, that is, in the plane of the utricular or saccular maculae (15). For both directions of acceleration the motor output is in phase with input acceleration below 0.2 Hz. A lag then develops that reaches 40°–60° at 1 Hz. Over the same range of frequencies otolith afferents in monkey and cat either lead acceleration somewhat or fire in phase with it (14, 71). Little is known about the dynamics of second-order otolith neurons, although otherwise unidentified neurons in the vestibular nuclei may have considerable phase lags with respect to input linear acceleration (139). The firing rate of LVST neurons is sensitive to the frequency of tilt in cats in which the canals are not functional (189). Phase was not studied in these latter experiments but gain increased with frequency, whereas the gain of the reflex response to linear acceleration drops as the frequency is increased (15). The results of studies of afferents and these fragmentary data on central neurons indicate extensive central processing in otolith-spinal reflexes.

Central Pathways for Vestibulospinal Reflexes

CANAL REFLEXES. The dynamic properties of the canal vestibulocollic reflex in the decerebrate cat may be summarized as follows: there is a considerable central phase lag at low frequencies with the response dominated by the output of the neural integrator. The

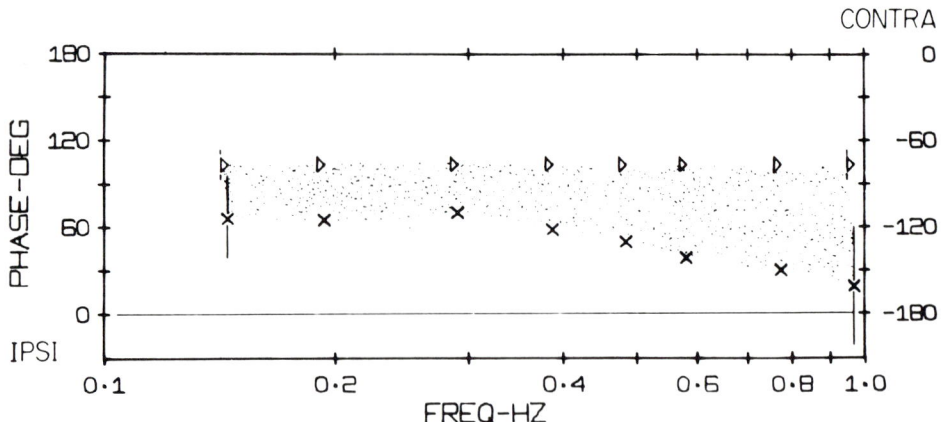

FIG. 21. Phase relation between excitatory acceleration for horizontal semicircular canals and motor output to forelimb extensor. Comparison between canal afferent activity (▷) and motor output (×). Phase reference on left ordinate is ipsilateral angular acceleration. Phase reference on right ordinate is contralateral angular acceleration, that is, positive acceleration for horizontal canal afferents of labyrinth opposite each forelimb. Output of this canal was shown to be adequate input that excites triceps muscle of opposite forelimb. Data points for afferent activity were obtained from transfer function for canal afferents given by Fernandez and Goldberg (54). *Stippled area* is difference in phase introduced by central processing. [From Anderson et al. (16).]

central phase lag decreases sharply at higher frequencies. In the vestibular-forelimb reflex the situation is similar at low frequencies but different at the higher frequencies where the phase lag is maintained.

As already stated, present evidence shows that in decerebrates second-order neurons fire essentially in phase with velocity during sinusoidal rotation at frequencies on the order of 0.2 Hz; in other words, they fire with the afferent signal. Just as the properties of the reflex may be different in intact cats, so may the behavior of second-order neurons. In alert preparations many vestibular nucleus neurons are influenced by the visuomotor system and do not simply reflect vestibular input (58, 209, 222). However, identified second-order neurons in alert animals do fire more or less in phase with stimulus velocity, although firing of higher order neurons may lag behind velocity considerably (110). A priori, therefore, disynaptic pathways between canals and motoneurons would not be expected to play an important role in relaying a phase-lagging signal to the spinal cord in decerebrates or in other preparations. This hypothesis has been tested for the vestibulocollic reflex. The disynaptic pathways from canal to contralateral neck motoneurons are all in the MVST, which can be interrupted by a lesion of the MLF near the obex (Fig. 16). Figure 22 shows that such a lesion, which interrupts more than the axons of second-order vestibular neurons, has no effect on phase (Fig. 22C) or gain (Fig. 22B) of neck motor units or compound EMGs at low frequencies, even though the short-latency EMG evoked by brief trains of shocks to the canal nerve is abolished (51, 216, 224). The MVST may contribute to the reflex, but another pathway(s) must be mainly responsible for transmitting the phase-lagging reflex signal to the spinal cord. Judging from electrophysiological experiments, the MVST does not make a significant contribution to vestibular-limb reflexes, but the role of this tract, or of the LVST, on responses of limb muscles to angular acceleration has not been tested.

There are two questions to be answered. What circuits produce the shift in phase between second-order neurons and muscle activity? Also, what are the output pathways to motoneurons (or where are the premotor neurons)? There has been speculation that the pontomedullary reticular formation may function as the neural integrator for vestibuloocular or vestibulospinal reflex signals (e.g., ref. 50), but different classes of neurons are probably involved and identification of a specific integrator may be difficult or impossible. Reticular neurons that fire with phase lags in response to horizontal rotation have been observed (62) as have identified reticulospinal and higher order vestibulospinal neurons that fire with phase lags in response to sinusoidal polarization (161). Phase-lagging premotor neurons for canal-neck and canal-limb reflexes may be located in the vestibular nuclei and reticular formation, and they may act on neck and limb motoneurons via vestibulospinal and reticulospinal tracts.

While the most direct pathways are not required for transmission of the phase-lagging signal, it may be suggested on theoretical grounds that in the vestibulocollic reflex these pathways become more important at higher frequencies where the phase of the output to muscle approaches that of the afferent signal [(51); see also ref. 197]. However, MLF cuts have no consistent, specific effects on the phase and gain of the response to high-frequency sinusoidal stimulation (216, 224). While the MVST may make a contribution, possibly an important one, to the response observed at high frequencies of stimulation, one or more parallel path-

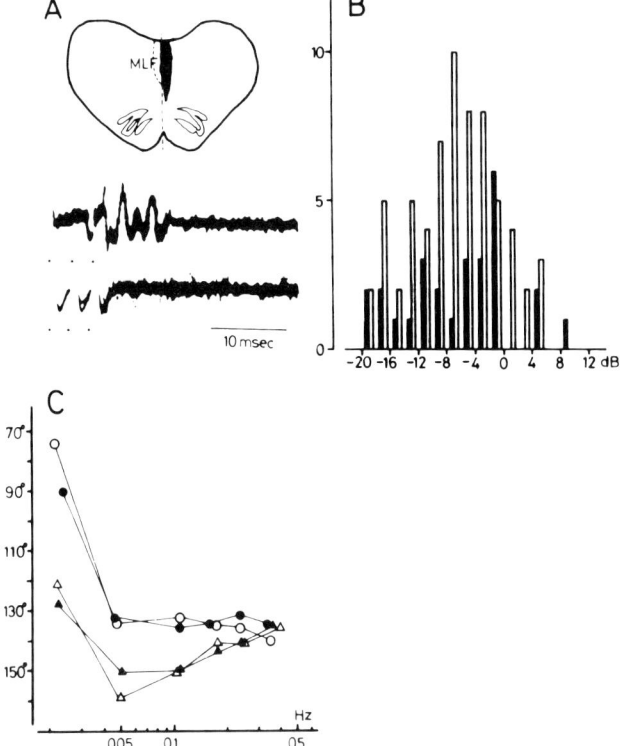

FIG. 22. Effect of sectioning medial longitudinal fasciculus (MLF) on dynamic characteristics of neck electromyogram (EMG) response. A: typical lesion. Bottom, 2 recordings are compound EMG potentials (from right neck extensor muscles) evoked by stimulation of contralateral horizontal canal nerve (trains of 3 pulses are indicated by dots). Recording taken after MLF cut (below) does not show EMG activity that is seen in control record (above). B: distribution of gain of motor-unit response at 0.17 Hz. White columns, before cut (means ± SD: −6.75 ± 6.14 dB; n = 65). Filled columns, after cut (means ± SD: −6.26 ± 7.47 dB; n = 27). C: phase characteristics of compound EMG response from 2 cats. Phase lags (ordinate, in degrees) are plotted (open symbols, before cut; filled symbols, after cut) against angular frequency (abscissa). [Modified from Ezure, Wilson, et al. (51).]

ways are obviously able to transmit the high-frequency signal effectively in the absence of the MVST. The pathways may be the LVST and/or the RSTs.

OTOLITH REFLEXES. On anatomical and electrophysiological grounds, the LVST would be expected to participate in otolith reflexes of the limbs. Indeed the variety of responses of LVST neurons to lateral and fore-aft tilt (153) makes it likely that they contribute to the responses to position change observed in experimental animals (e.g. refs. 49, 117, 142). However, work on canal reflexes shows that it is dangerous to infer the role of tracts on the basis of the pattern of effects obtained when they are stimulated electrically. The scant neuron data described in the section FUNCTIONAL STUDIES OF VESTIBULOSPINAL REFLEXES; subsection *Otolith Reflexes*, p. 693, indicate that tracts other than the vestibulospinal, perhaps the reticulospinal, generate the motor output of otolith reflexes (15). The difference between the pattern of forelimb reflexes elicited in response to horizontal linear acceleration (excitation and inhibition of ipsilateral and contralateral extensors, respectively) and the pattern of synaptic potentials seen when the LVST is activated by stimulation of the whole vestibular nerve (bilateral EPSPs in extensors; see ref. 128) supports this view. However, the same hazards that make it difficult to conclude on the basis of electrophysiological experiments that a tract is instrumental in producing a response apply when making the opposite conclusion. The role of the VSTs in otolith reflexes remains to be studied in more definitive experiments.

Vestibulospinal Reflexes and γ-Loop

While it is no longer believed that impulses in descending pathways evoke movement by first activating γ-motoneurons (fusimotor neurons) and causing firing of α-motoneurons indirectly via the γ-loop, it is established that α- and γ-motoneurons are often coactivated [α-γ-linkage; (72, 136)]. Excitation of γ-motoneurons and the resulting intrafusal fiber contraction can keep muscle spindles active during contraction of the muscle, thereby contributing to increased α-motoneuron discharge (72, 136). How important is α-γ-coactivation, and peripheral afferent input in general, in vestibulospinal reflexes?

In the spinal segments that control the limbs, vestibulospinal and reticulospinal fibers make synapses with both α- and γ-motoneurons (see subsections *Vestibulospinal Tracts*, p. 672, and *Reticulospinal Tracts*, p. 678) and local circuitry required to make α-γ-coactivation significant exists and has been well studied (72, 136). Much of the needed information has only recently become available for the segments controlling the neck. Neck muscles have a high density and content of spindles (72, 180), and there are monosynaptic connections between low-threshold muscle afferents and motoneurons of neck extensor and flexor muscles (17, 51, 174, 221). On the other hand, monosynaptic potentials are small and monosynaptic firing is apparently present only in very excitable preparations (3, 51). In agreement with these data, responses to unexpected loads applied during head movement suggest that the stretch reflex in neck muscles is present but weak (26). While there is no electrophysiological evidence for or against connections between LVST, MVST, or RST fibers and neck γ-motoneurons, Ia spindle afferents are modulated by horizontal angular oscillation, some in phase with the compound neck muscle EMG (51). All of these results show that the neural basis for functionally meaningful α-γ-coactivation in vestibulospinal control of neck and limb muscles exists, although the gain of the loop appears weak in the neck.

When the γ-loop is opened by cutting the dorsal roots, a procedure that of course interrupts all other peripheral input, both vestibulocollic and vestibular

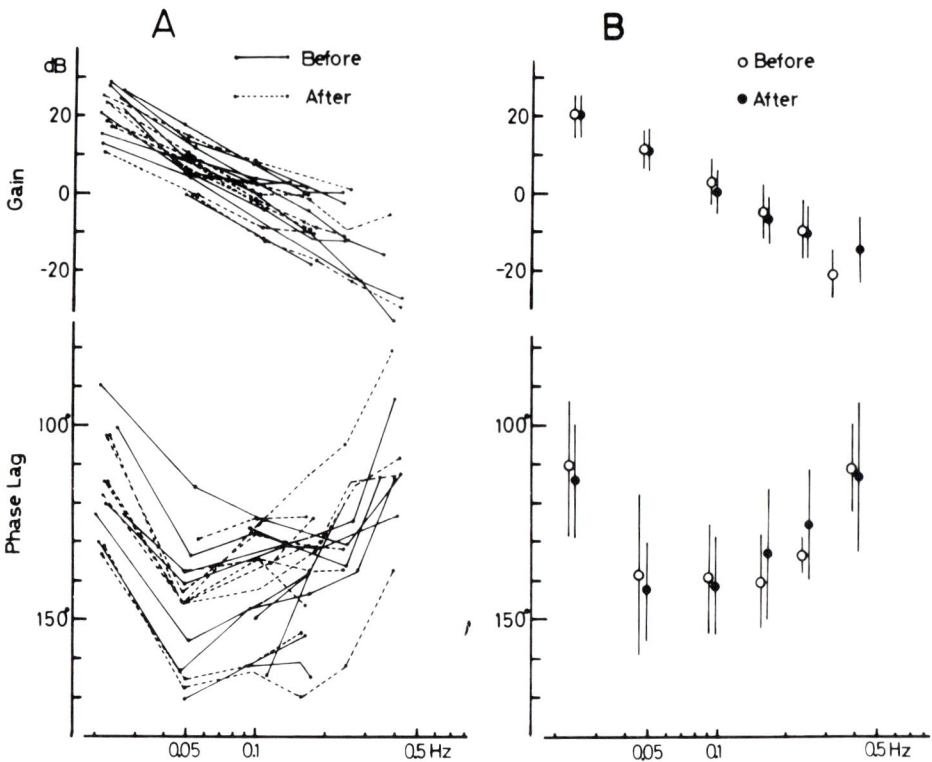

FIG. 23. Effect of dorsal root section on neck extensor motor-unit response. *A*: motor units that were examined at more than 3 different frequencies are plotted on Bode diagram. *Solid lines*, before deafferentation (*n* = 11). *Dotted lines*, after deafferentation (*n* = 10). *B*: mean and standard deviation at each frequency. [From Ezure, Wilson, et al. (51).]

forelimb reflexes are relatively unaffected (13, 51). When the C_1 through C_4 dorsal roots are cut on the recording side, and modulation of neck muscle motor units is sampled before and after the cut, no obvious change in gain or phase is observed in response to horizontal angular acceleration over the range of frequencies studied, up to 0.4 Hz (Fig. 23). Deafferentation, however, causes a drop in the spontaneous activity level. This in turn can lead to a drop in the gain of the compound EMG response because fewer motor units participate in the reflex. The phase of forelimb extensor responses to horizontal or vertical linear acceleration and to horizontal angular acceleration at frequencies up to 1 Hz also remains unchanged after dorsal rhizotomy (13). There may be changes in gain; if so, they are probably due to changes in excitability resulting from deafferentation.

Results from experiments on neck and forelimb responses therefore show that, at least at frequencies up to 1.0 Hz, vestibular modulation of muscle activity takes place in the absence of the γ-loop. Opening this loop, indeed completely interrupting afferent input to the spinal segments involved, has no clear-cut effect on the dynamics of the reflex response although it may affect its amplitude. However, α-γ-coactivation is present and may be of more importance in behaving animals.

Cerebellum and Vestibulospinal Reflexes

It was shown earlier that there is close linkage between neocerebellum, vestibulocerebellum (flocculus, nodulus, uvula), fastigial nucleus, and vestibular nuclei. The functional importance of these links is reflected in the effects of cerebellar lesions. In primates, for example, removal of the nodulus and uvula, or the flocculus, leads to disequilibrium, head oscillation, and postural disturbance (37, 41). Total nodulus and uvula removal has no effect if performed after bilateral labyrinthectomy, suggesting that the symptoms of this cerebellar lesion are largely due to an effect on vestibular reflexes (41). There are more specific instances of cerebellar influence on several aspects of vestibulospinal reflexes such as dynamics, pattern, and compensation following unilateral labyrinthectomy. Some examples are given below.

Although the role of neural integrator is presumably played by the pontomedullary reticular formation, the question arises whether cerebellar circuits are required for its optimal performance, as they may be in the vestibuloocular reflex (36, 184). Integration in the vestibulocollic reflex is present with much of the cerebellum removed (161, 216, 224), but quantitative studies are required to determine whether the performance of the integrator is as effective as in animals with the cerebellum intact.

As already described horizontal linear acceleration or lateral tilt causes reciprocal effects on forelimb muscles. The extensors on the side to which acceleration is directed are facilitated while the contralateral extensors are inhibited. This pattern persists after unilateral labyrinthectomy (15). If the cerebellar nuclei and surrounding white matter are then destroyed chronically, however, there is bilateral extensor facilitation (15). With only one labyrinth functioning, the inhibitory cerebellar output, presumably from anterior lobe Purkinje cells whose axons are interrupted by the lesion, is required to produce reciprocal facilitation and inhibition. The cerebellum is also required for production of the normal response to lateral tilt, even with both labyrinths intact. Side-down tilt excites ipsilateral and inhibits contralateral extensor muscles. Following acute cerebellectomy, there is simultaneous bilateral shortening of the triceps muscles (118). In this case the required circuitry probably also involves anterior lobe Purkinje cells.

Unilateral labyrinthectomy leads to severe postural disturbance, including the turning of the head and body to the operated side, which is largely compensated for within a short period of time (187). Vestibular compensation, that is, motor learning, is outside the scope of this chapter except insofar as it has been suggested that olivocerebellar circuits, specifically those through the cerebellar nuclei, are required for compensation to take place and be maintained in the rat. Chemical destruction of the inferior olive prevents compensation, and its destruction in compensated animals results in the return of the symptoms (122). During the compensation period, activity in the cerebellar nuclei is greater than normal (121). Studies of the cat, however, show that compensation can take place even though the cerebellar nuclei and surrounding white matter are destroyed chronically, and that the vestibular syndrome does not return when the cerebellar nuclei are destroyed in a compensated animal (186). Future work may resolve these conflicting results and the role of the cerebellum in the central readjustments that produce vestibular compensation.

CONCLUSION

In this chapter we have described both vestibular reflexes acting on axial and limb muscles and tonic neck reflexes acting on the limbs. These two groups of reflexes are very closely related but the former have been studied much more extensively with modern neurophysiological techniques. What we know about the neural machinery underlying the reflexes has been obtained by two different approaches. The first is the traditional method of circuit tracing, which employs mainly single-unit analysis. It has revealed the properties of the fairly direct connections between different receptors in the labyrinth and motoneurons via the lateral and medial vestibulospinal and reticulospinal tracts. The second is linear systems analysis; sinusoidal natural stimulation and sinusoidal electrical stimulation of vestibular nerve branches have revealed the dynamic properties of vestibular reflexes and given some insight into the central processing that takes place between second-order vestibular neurons and motoneurons. At this time it is necessary to reconcile the results obtained by the two methods. For example, the vestibulospinal tracts cannot by themselves account for the dynamic properties of the vestibulocollic reflex in decerebrate cats with the head immobilized, and the reticulospinal tracts may play an important role in producing the reflex response. Further experiments combining single-unit recording and systems analysis are required to identify the neurons and tracts responsible for different aspects of vestibulospinal reflexes.

REFERENCES

1. ABRAHAMS, V. Cervico-lumbar reflex interactions involving a proprioceptive receiving area of the cerebral cortex. *J. Physiol London* 209: 45–56, 1970.
2. ABRAHAMS, V., AND S. FALCHETTO. Hind leg ataxia of cervical origin and cervico-lumbar spinal interactions with a supratentorial pathway. *J. Physiol. London* 203: 435–447, 1969.
3. ABRAHAMS, V. C., F. RICHMOND, AND P. K. ROSE. Absence of monosynaptic reflex in dorsal neck muscles of the cat. *Brain Res.* 92: 130–131, 1975.
4. ABZUG, C., M. MAEDA, B. W. PETERSON, AND V. J. WILSON. Cervical branching of lumbar vestibulospinal axons. *J. Physiol. London* 243: 499–522, 1974.
5. AJALA, G. F., AND R. E. POPPELE. Some problems on the central actions of vestibular inputs. In: *Neurophysiological Basis of Normal and Abnormal Motor Activities*, edited by M. D. Yahr and D. P. Purpura. Hewlett, NY: Raven, 1967, p. 141–154.
6. AKAIKE, T. Comparison of neuronal composition of the vestibulospinal system between cat and rabbit. *Exp. Brain Res.* 18: 429–432, 1973.
7. AKAIKE, T., V. V. FANARDJIAN, M. ITO, M. KUMADA, AND H. NAKAJIMA. Electrophysiological analysis of the vestibulospinal reflex pathway of rabbit. I. Classification of tract cells. *Exp. Brain Res.* 17: 477–496, 1973.
8. AKAIKE, T., V. V. FANARDJIAN, M. ITO, AND H. NAKAJIMA. Cerebellar control of vestibulospinal tract cells in rabbit. *Exp. Brain Res.* 18: 446–463, 1973.
9. AKAIKE, T., V. V. FANARDJIAN, M. ITO, AND T. OHNO. Electrophysiological analysis of the vestibulospinal reflex pathway of rabbit. II. Synaptic actions upon spinal neurones. *Exp. Brain Res.* 17: 497–515, 1973.
10. AKAIKE, T., AND R. A. WESTERMAN. Spinal segmental levels innervated by different types of vestibulospinal tract neurons in rabbit. *Exp. Brain Res.* 17: 443–446, 1973.
11. ALLEN, G. I., N. H. SABAH, AND K. TOYAMA. Synaptic actions of peripheral nerve impulses upon Deiters' neurones via the climbing fiber afferents. *J. Physiol. London* 226: 311–333, 1972.
12. ALLEN, G. I., N. H. SABAH, AND K. TOYAMA. Synaptic actions of peripheral nerve impulses upon Deiters' neurones via the mossy fiber afferents. *J. Physiol. London* 226: 335–351, 1972.

13. ANDERSON, J. H., A. BERTHOZ, J. F. SOECHTING, AND C. A. TERZUOLO. Motor output to deafferented forelimb extensors in the decrebrate cat during natural vestibular stimulation. *Brain Res.* 122: 150–153, 1977.
14. ANDERSON, J. H., R. H. BLANKS, AND W. PRECHT. Response characteristics of primary vestibular fibers. *Exp. Brain Res.* 32: 491–507, 1978.
15. ANDERSON, J. H., J. F. SOECHTING, AND C. A. TERZUOLO. Dynamic relations between natural vestibular inputs and activity of forelimb extensor muscles in the decrebrate cat. I. Motor output during sinusoidal linear accelerations. *Brain Res.* 120: 1–16, 1977.
16. ANDERSON, J. H., J. F. SOECHTING, AND C. A. TERZUOLO. Dynamic relations between natural vestibular inputs and activity of forelimb extensor muscles in the decrebrate cat. II. Motor output during rotations in the horizontal plane. *Brain Res.* 120: 17–34, 1977.
17. ANDERSON, M. E. Segmental reflex inputs to motoneurons innervating dorsal neck musculature in the cat. *Exp. Brain Res.* 28: 175–187, 1977.
18. AOYAMA, M., T. HONGO, N. KUDO, AND R. TANAKA. Convergent effects from bilateral vestibulospinal tracts on spinal interneurons. *Brain Res.* 35: 250–253, 1971.
19. BAKER, R., AND A. BERTHOZ (editors). *Control of Gaze by Brainstem Neurons.* New York: Elsevier, 1977.
20. BALDISSERA, F., AND W. J. ROBERTS. Effects on the ventral spinocerebellar tract neurones from Deiters' nucleus and the medial longitudinal fascicle in the cat. *Acta Physiol. Scand.* 93: 228–249, 1975.
21. BANTLI, H., AND J. R. BLOEDEL. The action of the dentate nucleus on the excitability of spinal motoneurons via pathways which do not involve the primary sensorimotor cortex. *Brain Res.* 88: 86–90, 1975.
22. BANTLI, H., AND J. R. BLOEDEL. Monosynaptic activation of a direct reticulospinal pathway by the dentate nucleus. *Pfluegers Arch.* 357: 237–242, 1975.
23. BERTHOZ, A., AND J. H. ANDERSON. Frequency analysis of vestibular influence on extensor motoneurons. I. Response to tilt in forelimb extensors. *Brain Res.* 34: 370–375, 1971.
24. BERTHOZ, A., AND J. H. ANDERSON. Frequency analysis of vestibular influence on extensor motoneurons. II. Relationship between neck and forelimb extensors. *Brain Res.* 34: 376–380, 1971.
25. BERTHOZ, A., AND R. LLINÁS. Afferent neck projection to the cat cerebellar cortex. *Exp. Brain Res.* 20: 385–402, 1974.
26. BIZZI, E., P. DEV, P. MORASSO, AND A. POLIT. Effects of load disturbances during centrally initiated movements. *J. Neurophysiol.* 41: 542–556, 1978.
27. BRINK, E. E., N. HIRAI, AND V. J. WILSON. Influence of neck afferents on vestibulospinal neurons. *Exp. Brain Res.* In press.
28. BRODAL, A. Anatomy of the vestibular nuclei and their connections. In: *Handbook of Sensory Physiology. Vestibular System,* edited by H. H. Kornhuber. Berlin: Springer-Verlag, 1974, vol. 6, pt. 1, p. 239–352.
29. BRODAL, A., O. POMPEIANO, AND F. WALBERG. *The Vestibular Nuclei and Their Connections.* London: Oliver & Boyd, 1962.
30. BROWN, A. G. Descending control of the spinocervical tract in decerebrate cats. *Brain Res.* 17: 152–155, 1970.
31. BRUGGENCATE, G. TEN, AND A. LUNDBERG. Facilitatory interaction in transmission to motoneurons from vestibulospinal fibres and contralateral primary afferents. *Exp. Brain Res.* 19: 248–270, 1974.
32. BRUGGENCATE, G. TEN, J. SCHERER, AND R. TEICHMANN. Neuronal activity in the lateral vestibular nucleus of the cat. V. Topographical distribution of inhibitory effects mediated by the spino-olivocerebellar pathway. *Pfluegers Arch.* 360: 321–336, 1975.
33. BRUGGENCATE, G. TEN, R. TEICHMANN, AND E. WELLER. Neuronal activity in the lateral vestibular nucleus of the cat. IV. Postsynaptic potentials evoked by stimulation of peripheral somatic nerves. *Pfluegers Arch.* 360: 301–320, 1975.
34. CARLI, G., K. DIETE-SPIFF, AND O. POMPEIANO. Responses of the muscle spindles and the extrafusal fibres in an extensor muscle to stimulation of the lateral vestibular nucleus in the cat. *Arch. Ital. Biol.* 105: 209–242, 1967.
35. CARPENTER, D., I. ENGBERG, AND A. LUNDBERG. Primary afferent depolarization evoked from the brain stem and the cerebellum. *Arch. Ital. Biol.* 104: 73–85, 1966.
36. CARPENTER, R. H. S. Cerebellectomy and the transfer function of the vestibulo-ocular reflex in the decerebrate cat. *Proc. R. Soc. London Ser. B* 181: 353–374, 1972.
37. CARREA, R. M. E., AND F. A. METTLER. Physiologic consequences following extensive removals of the cerebellar cortex and deep cerebellar nuclei and effect of secondary cerebral ablations in the primate. *J. Comp. Neurol.* 87: 169–288, 1947.
38. COHEN, F., W. W. CHAMBERS, AND J. M. SPRAGUE. Experimental study of efferent projections from the cerebellar nuclei to the brainstem of the cat. *J. Comp. Neurol.* 109: 233–259, 1958.
39. COHEN, L. A. Role of eye and neck proprioceptive mechanisms in body orientation and motor coordination. *J. Neurophysiol.* 24: 1–11, 1961.
40. DE JONG, P. T. V. M., J. M. B. V. DE JONG, B. COHEN, AND L. B. W. JONGKEES. Ataxia and nystagmus induced by injection of local anesthetics in the neck. *Ann. Neurol.* 1: 240–246, 1977.
41. DOW, R. S. Effects of lesions in the vestibular part of the cerebellum in primates. *Arch. Neurol. Psychiatry* 40: 500–520, 1938.
42. DUENSING, F., AND K. P. SCHAEFFER. Die Aktivität einzelner Neurone der Formatio reticularis des nicht gefesselten Kaninchens bei Kopfwendungen und vestibulären Reizen. *Arch. Psychiatr. Nervenkr.* 201: 97–122, 1960.
43. ECCLES, J. C., R. A. NICOLL, W. F. SCHWARZ, H. TÁBOŘÍKOVÁ, AND T. J. WILLEY. Reticulospinal neurons with and without monosynaptic inputs from cerebellar nuclei. *J. Neurophysiol.* 38: 513–530, 1975.
44. ECCLES, J. C., T. RANTUCCI, N. H. SABAH, AND H. TÁBOŘÍKOVÁ. Somatotopic studies on cerebellar fastigial cells. *Exp. Brain Res.* 19: 100–118, 1974.
45. ECCLES, J. C., N. H. SABAH, AND H. TÁBOŘÍKOVÁ. Excitatory and inhibitory responses of neurones of the cerebellar fastigial nucleus. *Exp. Brain Res.* 19: 61–74, 1974.
46. ECCLES, J. C., N. H. SABAH, AND H. TÁBOŘÍKOVÁ. The pathways responsible for excitation and inhibition of fastigial neurones. *Exp. Brain Res.* 19: 78–99, 1974.
47. ENGBERG, I., A. LUNDBERG, AND R. W. RYALL. Reticulospinal inhibition of transmission in reflex pathways. *J. Physiol. London* 194: 201–223, 1968.
48. ENGBERG, I., A. LUNDBERG, AND R. W. RYALL. Reticulospinal inhibition of interneurones. *J. Physiol. London* 194: 225–236, 1968.
49. ERHARDT, K. J., AND A. WAGNER. Labyrinthine and neck reflexes recorded from spinal single motoneurons in the cat. *Brain Res.* 19: 87–104, 1970.
50. EZURE, K., AND S. SASAKI. Frequency-response analysis of vestibular-induced neck reflex in cat. I. Characteristics of neural transmission from horizontal semicircular canal to neck motoneurons. *J. Neurophysiol.* 41: 445–458, 1978.
51. EZURE, K., S. SASAKI, Y. UCHINO, AND V. J. WILSON. Frequency-response analysis of vestibular-induced neck reflex in cat. II. Functional significance of cervical afferents and polysynaptic descending pathways. *J. Neurophysiol.* 41: 459–471, 1978.
52. FANARDJIAN, V. V., J. S. SARKISSIAN, V. A. SARGSIAN, AND K. Z. PAKHLEVANIAN. Electrophysiological investigation into topographical organization of the Deiters' lateral vestibular nucleus. *Sechenov Physiol. J. USSR* 58: 1827–1833, 1972.
53. FERIN, M., R. A. GRIGORIAN, AND P. STRATA. Mossy and climbing fibre activation in the cat cerebellum by stimulation of the labyrinth. *Exp. Brain Res.* 12: 1–17, 1971.
54. FERNANDEZ, C., AND J. M. GOLDBERG. Physiology of peripheral neurons innervating semicircular canals of the squirrel

monkey. II. Response to sinusoidal stimulation and dynamics of peripheral vestibular system. *J. Neurophysiol.* 34: 661–675, 1971.
55. FLUUR, E., AND A. MELLSTRÖM. Utricular stimulation and oculomotor reactions. *Laryngoscope* 80: 1701–1712, 1970.
56. FLUUR, E., AND A. MELLSTRÖM. Saccular stimulation and oculomotor reactions. *Laryngoscope* 80: 1713–1721, 1970.
57. FREDERICKSON, J. M., D. SCHWARZ, AND H. H. KORNHUBER. Convergence and interaction of vestibular and deep somatic afferents upon neurons in the vestibular nuclei of the cat. *Acta Oto Laryngol.* 61: 168–188, 1966.
58. FUCHS, A., AND J. KIMM. Unit activity in vestibular nucleus of the alert monkey during horizontal angular acceleration and eye movement. *J. Neurophysiol.* 38: 1140–1161, 1975.
59. FUKUDA, T. Studies on human dynamic postures from the viewpoint of postural reflexes. *Acta Oto Laryngol. Suppl.* 161: 1–52, 1961.
60. FUKUSHIMA, K., B. W. PETERSON, AND V. J. WILSON. Vestibulospinal, reticulospinal and interstitiospinal pathways in the cat. In: *Progress in Brain Research. Reflex Control of Posture and Movements*, edited by R. Granit and O. Pompeiano. Amsterdam: Elsevier, 1979, vol. 50, p. 121–136.
61. FUKUSHIMA, K., N. G. PITTS, AND B. W. PETERSON. Direct excitation of neck motoneurons by interstitiospinal fibers. *Exp. Brain Res.* 33: 565–581, 1979.
62. FUKUSHIMA, Y., Y. IGUSA, AND K. YOSHIDA. Characteristics of responses of medial brain stem neurons to horizontal head angular acceleration and electrical stimulation of the labyrinth in the cat. *Brain Res.* 120: 564–570, 1977.
63. FURUYA, N., K. KAWANO, AND H. SHIMAZU. Functional organization of vestibulo-fastigial projection in the horizontal semicircular canal system in the cat. *Exp. Brain Res.* 24: 75–87, 1975.
64. GARDNER, E. P., AND A. F. FUCHS. Single-unit responses to natural vestibular stimuli and eye movements in deep cerebellar nuclei of the alert rhesus monkey. *J. Neurophysiol.* 38: 627–649, 1975.
65. GERNANDT, B. E. Vestibulo-spinal mechanisms. In: *Handbook of Sensory Physiology. Vestibular System*, edited by H. H. Kornhuber. Berlin: Springer-Verlag, 1974, vol. 6, pt. 1, p. 541–564.
66. GERNANDT, B. E., AND S. GILMAN. Descending vestibular activity and its modulation by proprioceptive, cerebellar and reticular influences. *Exp. Neurol.* 1: 274–304, 1959.
67. GERNANDT, B. E., AND S. GILMAN. Differential supraspinal controls of spinal centers. *Exp. Neurol.* 3: 307–324, 1961.
68. GERNANDT, B. E., M. IRANYI, AND R. B. LIVINGSTON. Vestibular influence on spinal mechanisms. *Exp. Neurol.* 1: 248–273, 1959.
69. GHELARDUCCI, B. Responses of cerebellar fastigial neurons to tilt. *Pfluegers Arch.* 344: 195–206, 1973.
70. GIAQUINTO, S., O. POMPEIANO, AND M. SANTINI. Riposta de unita Deitersiana a stimolazione graduata di-nervi cutanei e muscolari in animali decerebrati a cervelleto integro. *Boll. Soc. Ital. Biol. Sper.* 39: 524–527, 1963.
71. GOLDBERG, J. M., AND C. FERNANDEZ. Vestibular system. In: *Handbook of Physiology. Sensory Processes*, edited by I. Darian-Smith. Bethesda, MD: Am. Physiol. Soc. In press.
72. GRANIT, R. *The Basis of Motor Control.* New York: Academic, 1970.
73. GREENWOOD, R., AND A. HOPKINS. Landing from an unexpected fall and a voluntary step. *Brain* 99: 375–386, 1976.
74. GREENWOOD, R., AND A. HOPKINS. Muscle responses during sudden falls in man. *J. Physiol. London* 254: 507–518, 1976.
75. GRESTY, M. A., K. HESS, AND J. LEECH. Disorders of the vestibulo-ocular reflex producing oscillopsia and mechanisms compensating for loss of labyrinthine function. *Brain* 100: 693–716, 1977.
76. GRILLNER, S., T. HONGO, AND S. LUND. The origin of descending fibers monosynaptically activating spinoreticular neurones. *Brain Res.* 10: 259–262, 1968.
77. GRILLNER, S., T. HONGO, AND S. LUND. Descending monosynaptic and reflex control of gamma motoneurons. *Acta Physiol. Scand.* 75: 592–613, 1969.
78. GRILLNER, S., T. HONGO, AND S. LUND. The vestibulospinal tract. Effects on alpha motoneurones in the lumbosacral spinal cord in the cat. *Exp. Brain Res.* 10: 94–120, 1970.
79. GRILLNER, S., T. HONGO, AND S. LUND. Convergent effects on alpha motoneurones from the vestibulospinal tract and a pathway descending in the medial longitudinal fasciculus. *Exp. Brain Res.* 12: 457–479, 1971.
80. GRILLNER, S., AND S. LUND. The origin of a descending pathway with monosynaptic action on flexor motoneurons. *Acta Physiol. Scand.* 74: 274–284, 1968.
81. HABER, L. H., R. F. MARTIN, A. B. CHATT, AND W. D. WILLIS. Effects of stimulation in nucleus reticularis gigantocellularis on the activity of spinothalamic tract neurons in the monkey. *Brain Res.* 153: 163–168, 1978.
82. HENRY, J. L., AND F. R. CALARESU. Excitatory and inhibitory inputs from medullary nuclei projecting to spinal cardioacceleratory neurons in the cat. *Exp. Brain Res.* 20: 495–504, 1974.
83. HENRY, J. L., AND F. R. CALARESU. Pathways from medullary nuclei to spinal cardioacceleratory neurons in the cat. *Exp. Brain Res.* 20: 505–514, 1974.
84. HENRY, J. L., AND F. R. CALARESU. Origin and course of crossed medullary pathways to spinal sympathetic neurons in the cat. *Exp. Brain Res.* 20: 515–526, 1974.
85. HIKOSAKA, O., AND M. MAEDA. Cervical effects on abducens motoneurons and their interaction with vestibulo-ocular reflex. *Exp. Brain Res.* 18: 512–530, 1973.
85a. HIRAI, N., J. C. HWANG, AND V. J. WILSON. Comparison of dynamic properties of canal-evoked vestibulospinal reflexes of the neck and forelimb in the decerebrate cat. *Exp. Brain Res.* 36: 393–397, 1979.
86. HOLMQUIST, B., A. LUNDBERG, AND O. OSCARSSON. A supraspinal control system monosynaptically connected with an ascending spinal pathway. *Arch. Ital. Biol.* 98: 402–422, 1960.
87. HONGO, T., M. KUDO, AND R. TANAKA. The vestibulospinal tract: crossed and uncrossed effects on hindlimb motoneurones in the cat. *Exp. Brain Res.* 24: 37–55, 1975.
89. HULTBORN, H., M. ILLERT, AND M. SANTINI. Convergence on interneurones mediating the reciprocal Ia inhibition of motoneurones. III. Effects from supraspinal pathways. *Acta Physiol. Scand.* 96: 368–391, 1976.
90. HULTBORN, H., AND M. UDO. Recurrent depression from motor axon collaterals of supraspinal inhibition in motoneurones. *Acta Physiol. Scand.* 85: 44–57, 1972.
91. HWANG, J. C., AND W. F. POON. An electrophysiological study of the sacculo-ocular pathways in cat. *Jpn. J. Physiol.* 25: 241–251, 1975.
92. ILLERT, M., A. LUNDBERG, Y. PADEL, AND R. TANAKA. Integration in descending motor pathways controlling the forelimb in the cat. V. Properties of and monosynaptic excitatory convergence on C3-C4 propriospinal neurones. *Exp. Brain Res.* 33: 101–130, 1978.
93. ILLERT, M., A. LUNDBERG, AND R. TANAKA. Integration in descending motor pathways controlling the forelimb in the cat. III. Convergence on propriospinal neurones transmitting disynaptic excitation from the corticospinal tract and other descending tracts. *Exp. Brain Res.* 29: 323–346, 1977.
94. ITO, M. Neural design of the cerebellar motor control system. *Brain Res.* 40: 81–85, 1971.
95. ITO, M. Cerebellar control of the vestibular neurones: physiology and pharmacology. In: *Progress in Brain Research. Basic Aspects of Central Vestibular Mechanisms*, edited by A. Brodal and O. Pompeiano. Amsterdam: Elsevier, 1972, vol. 37, p. 377–390.
96. ITO, M., T. HONGO, AND Y. OKADA. Vestibular-evoked postsynaptic potentials in Deiters' neurones. *Exp. Brain Res.* 7: 214–230, 1969.
97. ITO, M., T. HONGO, M. YOSHIDA, Y. OKADA, AND K. OBATA.

Antidromic and trans-synaptic activation of Deiters' neurones induced from the spinal cord. *Jpn. J. Physiol.* 14: 638-658, 1964.
98. ITO, M., N. KAWAI, AND M. UDO. The origin of cerebellar-induced inhibition of Deiters' neurones. III. Localization of the inhibitory zone. *Exp. Brain Res.* 4: 310-320, 1968.
99. ITO, M., N. KAWAI, M. UDO, AND N. MANO. Axon reflex activation of Deiters' neurones from the cerebellar cortex through collaterals of the cerebellar afferents. *Exp. Brain Res.* 8: 249-268, 1969.
100. ITO, M., N. KAWAI, M. UDO, AND N. SATO. Cerebellar-evoked disinhibition in dorsal Deiters' neurones. *Exp. Brain Res.* 6: 247-264, 1968.
101. ITO, M., K. OBATA, AND R. OCHI. The origin of cerebellar-induced inhibition of Deiters' neurones. II. Temporal correlation between the trans-synaptic activation of Purkinje cells and the inhibition of Deiters' neurones. *Exp. Brain Res.* 2: 350-364, 1966.
102. ITO, M., M. UDO, AND N. MANO. Long inhibitory and excitatory pathways converging onto cat reticular and Deiters' neurons and their relevance to reticulofugal axons. *J. Neurophysiol.* 33: 210-226, 1970.
103. ITO, M., M. UDO, N. MANO, AND N. KAWAI. Synaptic action of the fastigiobulbar impulses upon neurones in the medullary reticular formation and vestibular nuclei. *Exp. Brain Res.* 11: 29-47, 1970.
104. ITO, M., AND M. YOSHIDA. The origin of cerebellar-induced inhibition of Deiters' neurones. I. Monosynaptic initiation of the synaptic potentials. *Exp. Brain Res.* 2: 330-349, 1966.
105. ITO, M., M. YOSHIDA, K. OBATA, N. KAWAI, AND M. UDO. Inhibitory control of intracerebellar nuclei by the Purkinje cell axons. *Exp. Brain Res.* 10: 64-80, 1970.
106. JANKOWSKA, E., S. LUND, A. LUNDBERG, AND O. POMPEIANO. Inhibitory effects evoked through ventral reticulospinal pathways. *Arch. Ital. Biol.* 106: 124-140, 1968.
107. KASAHARA, M., AND Y. UCHINO. Bilateral semicircular canal inputs to neurons in cat vestibular nuclei. *Exp. Brain Res.* 20: 285-296, 1974.
108. KATO, M., AND J. TANJI. The effects of electrical stimulation of Deiters' nucleus upon hindlimb γ motoneurons in the cat. *Brain Res.* 30: 385-395, 1971.
109. KAWAI, N., M. ITO, AND M. NOZUE. Postsynaptic influences on the vestibular non-Deiters' nuclei from primary vestibular nerve. *Exp. Brain Res.* 8: 190-200, 1969.
110. KELLER, E. L., AND B. Y. KAMATH. Characteristics of head rotation and eye movement-related neurons in alert monkey vestibular nucleus. *Brain Res.* 100: 182-187, 1975.
111. KENINS, K., H. KIKILLUS, AND E. D. SCHOMBURG. Short and long-latency reflex pathways from neck afferents to hindlimb motoneurones in the cat. *Brain Res.* 149: 235-238, 1978.
112. KORNHUBER, H. H. (editor). *Handbook of Sensory Physiology. Vestibular System.* Berlin: Springer-Verlag, 1974, vol. 6, pts. 1 and 2.
113. KOTCHABHAKDI, N., AND F. WALBERG. Cerebellar afferent projections from the vestibular nuclei in the cat: an experimental study with the method of retrograde axonal transport of horseradish peroxidase. *Exp. Brain Res.* 31: 591-604, 1978.
114. KOTCHABHAKDI, N., AND F. WALBERG. Primary vestibular afferent projections to the cerebellum as demonstrated by retrograde axonal transport of horseradish peroxidase. *Brain Res.* 142: 142-146, 1978.
115. KUYPERS, H. G. J. M. An anatomical analysis of cortico-bulbar connexions of the pons and lower brain stem in the cat. *J. Anat.* 92: 198-218, 1958.
116. LADPLI, R., AND A. BRODAL. Experimental studies of commissural and reticular formation projections from the vestibular nuclei in the cat. *Brain Res.* 8: 65-96, 1968.
117. LINDSAY, K. W., T. D. M. ROBERTS, AND J. R. ROSENBERG. Asymmetrical tonic labyrinth reflexes and their interaction with neck reflexes in the decerebrate cat. *J. Physiol. London* 261: 583-601, 1976.
118. LINDSAY, K. W., AND J. R. ROSENBERG. The effects of cerebellectomy on tonic labyrinth reflexes in the forelimb of the decerebrate cat. *J. Physiol. London* 273: 76P-77P, 1977.
119. LLINÁS, R., AND C. A. TERZUOLO. Mechanisms of supraspinal actions upon spinal cord activities. Reticular inhibitory mechanisms on alpha extensor motoneurons. *J. Neurophysiol.* 27: 579-591, 1964.
120. LLINÁS, R., AND C. A. TERZUOLO. Mechanisms of supraspinal actions upon spinal cord activities. Reticular inhibitory mechanisms upon flexor motoneurons. *J. Neurophysiol.* 28: 413-422, 1965.
121. LLINÁS, R., AND K. WALTON. Vestibular compensation: a distributive property of the central nervous system. In: *Integration in the Nervous System*, edited by H. Asanuma and V. J. Wilson. Tokyo: Igaku Shoin, 1979, p. 145-166.
122. LLINÁS, R., K. WALTON, D. E. HILLMAN, AND C. SOTELO. Inferior olive: its role in motor learning. *Science* 190: 1230-1231, 1975.
123. LLOYD, D. P. C. Activity in neurons of the bulbospinal correlation system. *J. Neurophysiol.* 4: 115-134, 1941.
124. LUND, S., AND O. POMPEIANO. Monosynaptic excitation of alpha motoneurones from supraspinal structures in the cat. *Acta Physiol. Scand.* 73: 1-21, 1968.
125. LUNDBERG, A., AND L. VYKLICKY. Inhibition of transmission to primary afferents by electrical stimulation of the brain stem. *Arch. Ital. Biol.* 104: 86-96, 1966.
126. MCCOUCH, G. P., I. D. DEERING, AND T. H. LING. Location of receptors for tonic neck reflexes. *J. Neurophysiol.* 14: 191-195, 1951.
127. MCCREERY, D., AND J. R. BLOEDEL. Reduction of the response of cat spinothalamic neurons to graded mechanical stimuli by electrical stimulation of the lower brain stem. *Brain Res.* 97: 151-156, 1975.
128. MAEDA, M., R. A. MAUNZ, AND V. J. WILSON. Labyrinthine influence on cat forelimb motoneurons. *Exp. Brain Res.* 22: 69-86, 1975.
129. MAGNI, F., AND W. D. WILLIS. Cortical control of brain stem reticular neurons. *Arch. Ital. Biol.* 102: 418-433, 1964.
130. MAGNI, F., AND W. D. WILLIS. Subcortical and peripheral control of brain stem reticular neurons. *Arch. Ital. Biol.* 102: 434-448, 1964.
131. MAGNUS, R. *Körperstellung.* Berlin: Julius Springer, 1924.
132. MAGNUS, R. Some results of studies in the physiology of posture. II. General static reactions of the mid-brain animal. *Lancet* 211: 585-588, 1926.
133. MAGNUS, R., AND A. DE KLEIJN. Die Abhängigkeit des Tonus der Extremitätenmuskeln von der Kopfstellung. *Pfluegers Arch.* 145: 455-548, 1912.
134. MAGOUN, H. W., AND R. RHINES. An inhibitory mechanism in the bulbar reticular formation. *J. Neurophysiol.* 9: 165-171, 1946.
135. MARKHAM, C. H., AND I. S. CURTHOYS. Convergence of labyrinthine influences on units in the vestibular nuclei of the cat. II. Electrical stimulation. *Brain Res.* 43: 383-397, 1972.
136. MATTHEWS, P. B. C. *Mammalian Muscle Receptors and Their Central Actions.* London: Arnold, 1972.
137. MAUNZ, R. A., N. G. PITTS, AND B. W. PETERSON. Cat spinoreticular neurons: locations, responses and changes in responses during repetitive stimulation. *Brain Res.* 148: 365-379, 1978.
138. MEHLER, W. R., M. E. FEFERMAN, AND W. J. H. NAUTA. Ascending axon degeneration following anterolateral cordotomy: an experimental study in the monkey. *Brain* 83: 719-750, 1960.
139. MELVILL-JONES, G., AND J. H. MILSUM. Neural response of the vestibular system to translational acceleration. In: *Systems Analysis Approach to Neurophysiological Problems.* Brainerd, MN: Lab. Neurophysiol., 1969, p. 105-107.
140. MELVILL-JONES, G., AND D. G. D. WATT. Muscular control of landing from unexpected falls in man. *J. Physiol. London* 219: 729-737, 1971.

141. MORI, S., AND S. MIKAMI. Excitation of Deiters' neurones by stimulation of the nerves to neck extensor muscles. *Brain Res.* 56: 331-334, 1973.
142. NAGAKI, J. Effects of natural vestibular stimulation on alpha extensor motoneurons of the cat. *Kumamoto Med. J.* 20: 102-111, 1967.
143. NASHNER, L. M. *Sensory Feedback in Human Posture Control.* Cambridge: MIT Press, MVT-70-3, 1970.
144. NYBERG-HANSEN, R. Origin and termination of fibers from the vestibular nuclei descending in the medial longitudinal fasciculus. An experimental study with silver impregnation methods in the cat. *J. Comp. Neurol.* 122: 355-367, 1964.
145. NYBERG-HANSEN, R. Sites and mode of termination of reticulo-spinal fibers in the cat. An experimental study with silver impregnation methods. *J. Comp. Neurol.* 124: 71-99, 1965.
146. NYBERG-HANSEN, R., AND T. A. MASCITTI. Sites and mode of termination of fibers of the vestibulospinal tract in the cat. An experimental study with silver impregnation methods. *J. Comp. Neurol.* 122: 369-388, 1964.
147. ORLOVSKY, G. N. Work of the reticulospinal neurons during locomotion. *Biofizika* 15: 728-737, 1970.
148. ORLOVSKY, G. N. Influence of the cerebellum on the reticulospinal neurones during locomotion. *Biofizika* 15: 894-904, 1970.
149. ORLOVSKY, G. N. Activity of vestibulospinal neurons during locomotion. *Brain Res.* 46: 85-98, 1972.
150. ORLOVSKY, G. N., AND G. A. PAVLOVA. Vestibular responses of neurons of different descending pathways in cats with intact cerebellum and in decerebellated ones [in Russian]. *Neirofiziologiya* 4: 303-310, 1972.
151. OUTERBRIDGE, J. S., AND G. MELVILL JONES. Reflex vestibular control of head movements in man. *Aerosp. Med.* 42: 935-940, 1971.
152. PARTRIDGE, L. D., AND J. H. KIM. Dynamic characteristics of response in a vestibulomotor reflex. *J. Neurophysiol.* 32: 485-495, 1969.
153. PETERSON, B. W. Distribution of neural responses to tilting within vestibular nuclei of the cat. *J. Neurophysiol.* 33: 750-767, 1970.
154. PETERSON, B. W. Identification of reticulospinal projections that may participate in gaze control. In: *Control of Gaze by Brainstem Neurons*, edited by R. Baker and A. Berthoz. New York: Elsevier, 1977, p. 143-152.
155. PETERSON, B. W. Reticulo-motor pathways: their connections and possible roles in motor behavior. In: *Integration in the Nervous System*, edited by H. Asanuma and V. J. Wilson. Tokyo: Igaku Shoin, 1979, p. 185-200.
156. PETERSON, B. W., AND C. ABZUG. Properties of projections from vestibular nuclei to medial reticular formation in the cat. *J. Neurophysiol.* 38: 1421-1435, 1975.
157. PETERSON, B. W., M. E. ANDERSON, AND M. FILION. Responses of pontomedullary reticular neurons to cortical, tectal, and cutaneous stimuli. *Exp. Brain Res.* 21: 19-44, 1974.
158. PETERSON, B. W., AND J. D. COULTER. A new long spinal projection from the vestibular nuclei in the cat. *Brain Res.* 122: 351-356, 1977.
159. PETERSON, B. W., M. FILION, L. P. FELPEL, AND C. ABZUG. Responses of medial reticular neurons to stimulation of the vestibular nerve. *Exp. Brain Res.* 22: 335-350, 1975.
160. PETERSON, B. W., J. I. FRANCK, N. G. PITTS, AND N. G. DAUNTON. Changes in responses of medial pontomedullary reticular neurons during repetitive cutaneous, vestibular, cortical, and tectal stimulation. *J. Neurophysiol.* 39: 564-581, 1976.
161. PETERSON, B. W., K. FUKUSHIMA, N. HIRAI, R. H. SCHOR, AND V. J. WILSON. Activation of vestibular and reticular neurons by sinusoidal polarization of semicircular canal afferents. *Soc. Neurosci. Abstr.* 4: 613, 1978.
162. PETERSON, B. W., R. A. MAUNZ, AND K. FUKUSHIMA. Properties of a new vestibulospinal projection, the caudal vestibulospinal tract. *Exp. Brain Res.* 32: 287-292, 1978.
163. PETERSON, B. W., R. A. MAUNZ, N. G. PITTS, AND R. MACKEL. Patterns of projection and branching of reticulospinal neurons. *Exp. Brain Res.* 23: 333-351, 1975.
164. PETERSON, B. W., N. G. PITTS, AND K. FUKUSHIMA. Reticulospinal connections with limb and axial motoneurons. *Exp. Brain Res.* 36: 1-20, 1979.
165. PETERSON, B. W., N. G. PITTS, K. FUKUSHIMA, AND R. MACKEL. Reticulospinal excitation and inhibition of neck motoneurons. *Exp. Brain Res.* 32: 471-489, 1978.
166. PETRAS, J. M. Cortical, tectal and tegmental fiber connections in the spinal cord of the cat. *Brain Res.* 6: 275-324, 1967.
167. POLLOCK, L. J., AND L. DAVIS. The influence of the cerebellum upon the reflex activities of the decerebrate animal. *Brain* 50: 277-312, 1927.
168. POMPEIANO, O., AND A. BRODAL. The origin of vestibulospinal fibres in the cat. An experimental-anatomical study, with comments on the descending medial longitudinal fasciculus. *Arch. Ital. Biol.* 95: 166-195, 1957.
169. POMPEIANO, O., AND J. E. SWETT. Actions of graded cutaneous and muscle afferent volleys on brain stem units in the decerebrate, cerebellectomized cat. *Arch. Ital. Biol.* 101: 552-583, 1963.
170. POMPEIANO, O., AND J. E. SWETT. Cerebellar potentials and responses of reticular units evoked by muscle afferent volleys in the decerebrate cat. *Arch. Ital. Biol.* 101: 584-613, 1963.
171. PRECHT, W., J. GRIPPO, AND A. WAGNER. Contribution of different types of central vestibular neurons to the vestibulospinal system. *Brain Res.* 4: 119-123, 1967.
172. PRECHT, W., R. VOLKIND, AND R. H. I. BLANKS. Functional organization of the vestibular input to the anterior and posterior cerebellar vermis of cat. *Exp. Brain Res.* 27: 143-160, 1977.
173. PRECHT, W., R. VOLKIND, M. MAEDA, AND M. L. GIRETTI. The effects of stimulating the cerebellar nodulus in the cat on the response of vestibular neurons. *Neuroscience* 1: 301-312, 1976.
174. RAPOPORT, S. Reflex connections of motoneurons of muscles involved in head movement in the cat. *J. Physiol. London* 289: 311-327, 1979.
175. RAPOPORT, S., A. SUSSWEIN, Y. UCHINO, AND V. J. WILSON. Properties of vestibular neurones projecting to neck segments of the cat spinal cord. *J. Physiol. London* 268: 493-510, 1977.
176. RAPOPORT, S., A. SUSSWEIN, Y. UCHINO, AND V. J. WILSON. Synaptic actions of individual vestibular neurones on cat neck motoneurones. *J. Physiol. London* 272: 367-382, 1977.
177. REIGHARD, J., AND H. S. JENNINGS. *Anatomy of the Cat* (3rd ed.). New York: Holt, 1935.
178. RHINES, R., AND H. W. MAGOUN. Brain stem facilitation of cortical motor response. *J. Neurophysiol.* 9: 219-229, 1946.
179. RICHMOND, F. J. R. Physiological characteristics of neck muscle receptors in the cat. *J. Physiol. London* 272: 67P-68P, 1977.
180. RICHMOND, F. J. R., AND V. C. ABRAHAMS. Morphology and distribution of muscle spindles in dorsal muscles of the cat neck. *J. Neurophysiol.* 38: 1322-1339, 1975.
181. RICHMOND, F. J. R., D. A. LAKANEN, AND V. C. ABRAHAMS. Receptors around vertebrae in the cat neck. *Soc. Neurosci. Abstr.* 4: 516, 1978.
182. ROBERTS, T. D. M. The behavioural vertical. *Fortschr. Zool.* 23: 192-198, 1975.
183. ROBERTS, T. D. M. *Neurophysiology of Postural Mechanisms* (2nd ed.). London: Butterworths, 1978.
184. ROBINSON, D. A. The effect of cerebellectomy on the cat's vestibulo-ocular integration. *Brain Res.* 71: 195-207, 1974.
186. SANCHEZ ROBLES, S., AND J. H. ANDERSON. Compensation of vestibular deficits in the cat. *Brain Res.* 147: 183-187, 1978.
187. SCHAEFER, K. P., AND D. L. MEYER. Compensation of vestibular lesions. In: *Handbook of Sensory Physiology. Vestibular System*, edited by H. H. Kornhuber. Berlin: Springer-Verlag, 1974, vol. 6, pt. 2, p. 463-490.
188. SCHEIBEL, M. E., AND A. B. SCHEIBEL. The response of reticular units to repetitive stimuli. *Arch. Ital. Biol.* 103: 279-299, 1965.
189. SCHOR, R. H. Responses of cat vestibular neurons to sinusoidal roll tilt. *Exp. Brain Res.* 20: 347-362, 1974.

190. SEGUNDO, J. P., T. TAKENAKA, AND H. ENCABO. Somatic sensory properties of bulbar reticular neurons. *J. Neurophysiol.* 30: 1221–1238, 1967.
191. SHAPOVALOV, A. I., AND N. R. GUREVITCH. Monosynaptic and disynaptic reticulospinal actions on lumbar motoneurons of the rat. *Brain Res.* 21: 249–263, 1970.
192. SHIMAZU, H., AND W. PRECHT. Tonic and kinetic responses of cat's vestibular neurons to horizontal angular acceleration. *J. Neurophysiol.* 28: 989–1013, 1965.
193. SHIMAZU, H., AND C. M. SMITH. Cerebellar and labyrinthine influences on single vestibular neurons identified by natural stimuli. *J. Neurophysiol.* 34: 493–508, 1971.
194. SHINODA, Y., A. P. ARNOLD, AND H. ASANUMA. Spinal branching of corticospinal axons in the cat. *Exp. Brain Res.* 26: 215–234, 1976.
195. SHINODA, Y., C. GHEZ, AND A. ARNOLD. Spinal branching of rubrospinal axons in the cat. *Exp. Brain Res.* 30: 203–218, 1977.
196. SHINODA, Y., AND K. YOSHIDA. Dynamic characteristics of responses to horizontal head angular acceleration in vestibuloocular pathway in the cat. *J. Neurophysiol.* 37: 653–673, 1974.
197. SKAVENSKI, A. A., AND D. A. ROBINSON. Role of abducens neurons in vestibuloocular reflex. *J. Neurophysiol.* 36: 724–738, 1973.
198. SOECHTING, J. F., J. H. ANDERSON, AND A. BERTHOZ. Dynamic relations between natural vestibular inputs and activity of forelimb extensor muscles in the decerebrate cat. III. Motor output during rotations in the vertical plane. *Brain Res.* 120: 35–47, 1977.
199. SPRAGUE, J. M., AND W. W. CHAMBERS. Control of posture by reticular formation and cerebellum in the intact, anesthetized and unanesthetized and in the decerebrated cat. *Am. J. Physiol.* 176: 52–64, 1954.
200. SPYER, K. M., B. GHELARDUCCI, AND O. POMPEIANO. Gravity responses of neurons in main reticular formation. *J. Neurophysiol.* 37: 705–721, 1974.
201. SUZUKI, J. I., AND B. COHEN. Head, eye, body and limb movements from semicircular canal nerves. *Exp. Neurol.* 10: 393–405, 1964.
202. SUZUKI, J. I., K. GOTO, K. TOKUMASU, AND B. COHEN. Implantations of electrodes near individual nerve branches in mammals. *Ann. Otol. Rhinol. Laryngol.* 78: 815–826, 1969.
203. SUZUKI, J. I., K. TOKUMASU, AND K. GOTO. Eye movements from single utricular nerve stimulation in the cat. *Acta Oto Laryngol.* 68: 350–362, 1969.
204. SZENTÁGOTHAI, J. *Die Rolle der Einzelnen Labyrinthrezeptoren bei der Orientation von Augen und Kopf im Raume.* Budapest: Akademiai Kiado, 1952.
205. THACH, W. T. Timing of activity in cerebellar dentate nucleus and cerebral motor cortex during prompt volitional movement. *Brain Res.* 88: 233–241, 1975.
206. THODEN, U., R. GOLSONG, AND J. WIRBITZKY. Cervical influence on single units of vestibular and reticular nuclei in cats. *Pfluegers Arch.* 355: R101, 1975.
207. THOMAS, D. M., R. P. KAUFMAN, J. M. SPRAGUE, AND W. W. CHAMBERS. Experimental studies of the vermal cerebellar projections in the brain stem of the cat (fastigiobulbar tract). *J. Anat.* 90: 371–385, 1956.
208. THOMPSON, R. F., AND W. A. SPENCER. Habituation: a model phenomenon for the study of neuronal substrates of behavior. *Psychol. Rev.* 173: 16–43, 1966.
209. WAESPE, W., AND V. HENN. Neuronal activity in the vestibular nuclei of the alert monkey during vestibular and optokinetic stimulation. *Exp. Brain Res.* 27: 523–538, 1977.
210. WALBERG, F., O. POMPEIANO, L. E. WESTRUM, AND E. HAUGLIE-HANSSEN. Fastigioreticular fibers in the cat. An experimental study with silver methods. *J. Comp. Neurol.* 119: 187–199, 1962.
211. WATT, D. G. D. Response of cats to sudden falls: an otolith-originating reflex assisting landing. *J. Neurophysiol.* 39: 257–265, 1976.
212. WENZEL, D., AND U. THODEN. Modulation of hindlimb reflexes by tonic neck positions in cats. *Pfluegers Arch.* 370: 277–282, 1977.
213. WENZEL, D., U. THODEN, AND A. FRANK. Forelimb reflexes modulated by tonic neck positions in cats. *Pfluegers Arch.* 374: 107–113, 1978.
214. WILSON, V. J., AND P. R. BURGESS. Disinhibition in the cat spinal cord. *J. Neurophysiol.* 25: 392–404, 1962.
215. WILSON, V. J., AND L. P. FELPEL. Specificity of semicircular canal input to neurons in the pigeon vestibular nuclei. *J. Neurophysiol.* 35: 253–264, 1972.
216. WILSON, V. J., K. FUKUSHIMA, N. HIRAI, B. W. PETERSON, AND Y. UCHINO. Analysis of central vestibulocollic pathways by means of modulated polarization of vestibular afferents. *Soc. Neurosci. Abst.* 4: 616, 1978.
217. WILSON, V. J., R. R. GACEK, M. MAEDA, AND Y. UCHINO. Saccular and utricular input to cat neck motoneurons. *J. Neurophysiol.* 40: 63–73, 1977.
218. WILSON, V. J., R. R. GACEK, Y. UCHINO, AND A. M. SUSSWEIN. Properties of central vestibular neurons fired by stimulation of the saccular nerve. *Brain Res.* 143: 251–261, 1978.
219. WILSON, V. J., M. KATO, B. W. PETERSON, AND R. M. WYLIE. A single-unit analysis of the organization of Deiters' nucleus. *J. Neurophysiol.* 30: 603–619, 1967.
220. WILSON, V. J., M. KATO, R. C. THOMAS, AND B. W. PETERSON. Excitation of lateral vestibular neurons by peripheral afferent fibers. *J. Neurophysiol.* 29: 508–529, 1966.
221. WILSON, V. J., AND M. MAEDA. Connections between semicircular canals and neck motoneurons in the cat. *J. Neurophysiol.* 37: 346–357, 1974.
222. WILSON, V. J., AND G. MELVILL-JONES. *Mammalian Vestibular Physiology.* New York: Plenum, 1979.
223. WILSON, V. J., AND B. W. PETERSON. Peripheral and central substrates of vestibulospinal reflexes. *Physiol. Rev.* 58: 80–105, 1978.
224. WILSON, V. J., B. W. PETERSON, K. FUKUSHIMA, N. HIRAI, AND Y. UCHINO. Analysis of vestibulocollic reflexes by sinusoidal polarization of vestibular afferent fibers. *J. Neurophysiol.* 42: 331–346, 1979.
225. WILSON, V. J., R. M. WYLIE, AND L. A. MARCO. Projection to the spinal cord from the medial and descending vestibular nuclei of the cat. *Nature London* 215: 429–430, 1967.
226. WILSON, V. J., R. M. WYLIE, AND L. A. MARCO. Organization of the medial vestibular nucleus. *J. Neurophysiol.* 31: 166–175, 1968.
227. WILSON, V. J., R. M. WYLIE, AND L. A. MARCO. Synaptic inputs to cells in the medial vestibular nucleus. *J. Neurophysiol.* 31: 176–185, 1968.
228. WILSON, V. J., AND M. YOSHIDA. Bilateral connections between labyrinths and neck motoneurons. *Brain Res.* 13: 603–607, 1969.
229. WILSON, V. J., AND M. YOSHIDA. Comparison of effects of stimulation of Deiters' nucleus and medial longitudinal fasciculus on neck, forelimb, and hindlimb motoneurons. *J. Neurophysiol.* 32: 743–758, 1969.
230. WILSON, V. J., AND M. YOSHIDA. Monosynaptic inhibition of neck motoneurons by the medial vestibular nucleus. *Exp. Brain Res.* 9: 365–380, 1969.
231. WILSON, V. J., M. YOSHIDA, AND R. H. SCHOR. Supraspinal monosynaptic excitation and inhibition of thoracic back motoneurons. *Exp. Brain Res.* 11: 282–295, 1970.
232. WOLSTENCROFT, J. H. Reticulospinal neurones. *J. Physiol. London* 174: 91–108, 1964.
233. WYLIE, R. M., AND L. P. FELPEL. The influence of the cerebellum and peripheral somatic nerves on the activity of Deiters' cells in the cat. *Exp. Brain Res.* 12: 528–546, 1971.

CHAPTER 15

The pyramidal tract

HIROSHI ASANUMA | *The Rockefeller University, New York, New York*

CHAPTER CONTENTS

Organization of Projection From Cerebral Cortex to Spinal Cord
   Studies by cortical surface stimulation
   Studies by cortical depth stimulation
   Microstructure of corticospinal projection
   Projection to γ-motoneurons
   Projections to spinal interneurons
   Pyramidal collaterals and branches within brain
Afferent Inputs to Motor Cortex and Pyramidal Tract Neurons
   General problems
   Inputs from nucleus ventralis lateralis of thalamus
   Peripheral inputs to motor cortex and pyramidal tract cells
      Pathways from periphery to motor cortex
      Functional significance of peripheral inputs to motor cortex
   Inputs through association fibers
      Inputs from sensory cortex
      Inputs from association cortex
   Inputs through commisural fibers
Function of Pyramidal Tract
Summary

THE PYRAMIDAL TRACT is by definition made up of all those fibers that course longitudinally in the pyramids of the medulla oblongata, regardless of their site of origin or termination. These fibers are thought to originate from cell bodies in the cerebral cortex, and most of them continue into the spinal cord to constitute the corticospinal tract. Some pyramidal tract fibers leave the tract in the medulla and terminate at cranial nerve nuclei in the brain stem. The existence of the pyramidal fiber bundle had been known for a long time, but the importance of this tract was gradually recognized after the discovery of localization of motor function within the cerebral cortex by Fritsch and Hitzig in 1870 (53). After the introduction of the Marchi method around 1880 (25), the origin and the course of the pyramidal tract fibers were studied extensively. As early as 1889 Sherrington observed that after lesion of the leg or arm area of the "motor" cortex in monkeys and dogs, the number of degenerating fibers markedly diminished at the lower portions of the lumbar or cervical enlargment, respectively (135, 136). After repeated experiments by a number of investigators using this method, it became clear that although the majority of the fibers originate from the classic motor cortex (or area 4 of Brodmann), a considerable fraction of them arise from the primary "sensory" cortex (areas 1, 2, and 3) as well as from regions located anterior to the motor cortex (e.g., area 6). Details of the distribution of cells of origin of the corticospinal tract are described in the chapter by Kuypers in this *Handbook*.

Studies carried out by the Marchi method left many unanswered questions, because this method necessitates relatively large lesions in the cortex and stains only degenerating myelinated fibers. The pyramidal tract, however, contains a large number of nonmyelinated or thinly myelinated fibers, and myelinated fibers lose their myelin sheath at their terminal branches. The use of the Nauta method (118) to trace unmyelinated as well as the terminal branches of degenerating fibers revealed finer details of pyramidal tract organization. At about the same time, advances in electrical recording techniques made it possible to trace single as well as groups of pyramidal tract fibers electroanatomically. Furthermore the recent development of the horseradish peroxidase technique has made it possible to determine the origin of neurons projecting to limited areas in the spinal cord. As a result of the application of these techniques, our knowledge of the structure and function of the pyramidal tract system is growing rapidly. The interpretation of the results, however, needs to be done carefully because the structure and possibly the function of the pyramidal tract vary with the species studied. For example, in carnivores all or nearly all of the pyramidal tract fibers terminate on spinal interneurons (98), whereas in primates (22) and rodents (39) some terminate directly on motoneurons. Because most of the relevant experiments have been performed using cats and monkeys, results with these animals are emphasized. The description of the experiments is limited in this chapter; therefore readers interested in the details should refer to the original reports. Some of the excellent reviews published recently are listed in GENERAL REFERENCES.

ORGANIZATION OF PROJECTION FROM
CEREBRAL CORTEX TO SPINAL CORD

Studies by Cortical Surface Stimulation

   After the discovery in 1870 of a motor representation

in the cerebral cortex by Fritsch and Hitzig (53), attempts were made to define the location of the motor cortex using electrical current. As early as 1875 Ferrier (45) was able to draw a remarkably detailed "motor map" (using faradic current instead of galvanic current, as used earlier by Fritsch and Hitzig), although this map included precentral, parietal, and also temporal lobes (Fig. 1A). As time went on the methods of stimulation and anesthesia were progressively improved, so that by the turn of the century the area representing motor function had shrunk to roughly that seen in current textbooks (Fig. 1B). During this early stage of investigation, it was frequently asked whether the structural organization of the motor cortex is in accord with Hughlings Jackson's idea of "minute representation." Strongly influenced by his contemporary evolutionists, Jackson proposed that the central nervous system is organized in a hierarchical fashion, i.e., the cerebral cortex controls the least automatic movements, whereas automatic movements are controlled by lower levels. According to this theory there is widespread overlap in the representation of muscles within the motor cortex. Each muscle would be represented repeatedly in various parts of the motor cortex, and a group of corticofugal neurons located in a small area of the cortex would project to various motor nuclei at several levels of the spinal cord. Hence stimulation of a small area of the cortex would produce contraction of a group of muscles (158). During the course of his study with the chimpanzee and gorilla, Sherrington (137) noted that the effect produced by cortical stimulation was always coordinated contraction of muscles. He also stated that "by cortical stimulation, the true antagonists were never thrown into simultaneous activity." Similar observations were reported by other investigators, and it was agreed that to produce solitary contraction of a muscle by cortical (surface) stimulation was very difficult. It should be noted, however, that there were many limitations in pursuing these experiments. The stimulation used at that time was faradic current produced by induction coils. With this instrument, frequency and duration of the pulses were determined by the rate of vibration of the contact breaker, whereas the intensity was varied by changing the distance between two coils. Because of the sparking at the make and break of the circuit, however, accurate control of stimulus parameters was impossible. To make the situation worse, the only anesthetics available were chloroform and ether, with which control of the depth of anesthesia was very difficult. Altogether the results supported Jackson's notion that movements rather than muscles are represented in the motor cortex, i.e., "the nervous system knows nothing of muscles and thinks in terms of movement" (158).

In 1947 Chang et al., aided by the rapid progress of

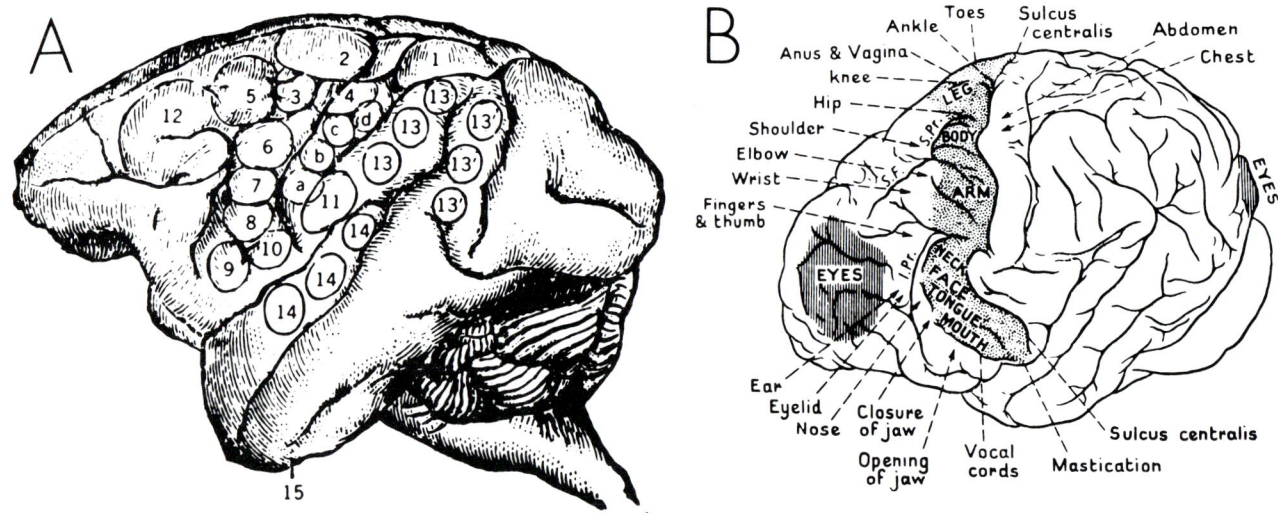

FIG. 1. A: Ferrier's historic map of motor representation of monkey brain (46). 1, Opposite hindlimb is advanced as in walking. 2, Flexion with outward rotation of thigh, rotation inward of leg, with flexion of toes. 3, Tail. 4, Opposite arm is adducted, extended, and retracted; hand pronated. 5, Extension forward of opposite arm; a, b, c, d, movements of fingers and wrists. 6, Flexion and spination of forearm. 7, Retraction and elevation of angle of mouth. 8, Elevation of ala of nose and upper lip. 9 and 10, Opening of mouth with protrusion, 9, and retraction, 10, of tongue. 11, Retraction of angle of mouth. 12, Eyes open widely, pupils dilate, and head and eyes turn to opposite side. 13 and 13′, Eyes move to opposite side. 14, Pricking of opposite ear, head and eyes turn to opposite side, pupils dilate widely. B: motor representation in brain of chimpanzee. Left hemisphere viewed from side and above to obtain best configuration of sulcus centralis area. Motor area indicated by *stippling*. Shaded *regions*, marked EYES, indicate portions of cortex that yield conjugate movements of eyeballs under faradization. S.F., superior frontal sulcus; S.Pr., superior precentral sulcus; I.Pr., inferior precentral sulcus. [A from Ferrier (46); B from Sherrington (137).]

electrical techniques, made an important observation (33). They were able to control the stimulus parameters, i.e., frequency, intensity, and pulse duration, independently and were able to elicit an isolated response of a single muscle without the simultaneous contraction of any of the other muscles under observation (Fig. 2). The results clearly demonstrated topographical representation of muscles within the motor cortex, although the mode of representation was difficult to assess. They concluded that the Betz cells (by which they meant pyramidal tract cells) for a particular muscle were distributed over an area of the cortex with the highest cell concentration located at a particular focus within this area.

Another complication relating to the use of cortical surface stimulation is the difficulty of determining which neuronal element is activated when electrical current is passed from the surface. Patton and Amassian (123), using monkeys, studied this problem by recording corticofugal volleys elicited by bipolar cortical stimulation. They recorded a stable, short-latency, short-duration, positive deflection (D-wave), which was followed by a series of irregular rhythmic waves (I-waves) lasting for several milliseconds (Fig.

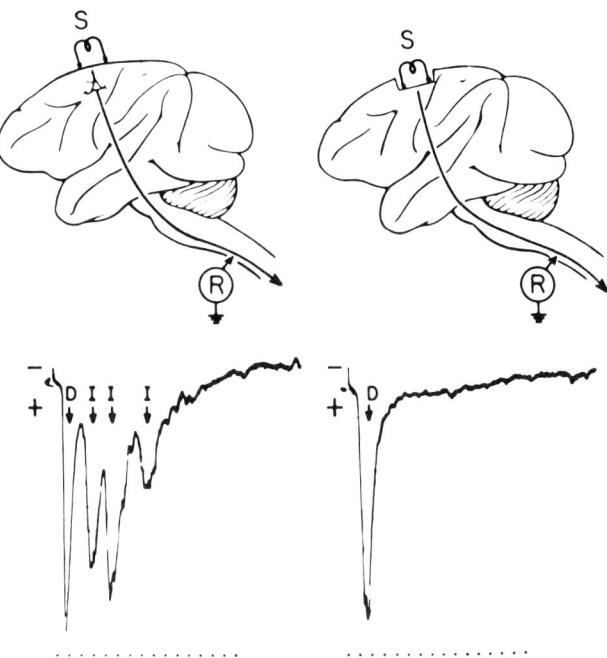

FIG. 3. Pyramidal tract responses (R) to stimulation (S) of motor cortex and white matter in monkey. Recording electrode in lateral column of spinal cord at first cervical segment. Downward deflection indicates positivity at electrode in pyramidal tract. Time: 1 ms. Direct (D) and indirect (I) waves present at *left*, whereas only D-wave at *right*. [From Patton and Amassian (123).]

3). They presented convincing evidence that the first wave was elicited by direct activation of pyramidal tract neurons and the later waves were caused by their indirect excitation. The results clearly indicated that "bipolar" cortical surface stimulation excites pyramidal tract neurons directly and also synaptically through cortical interneurons.

This combined direct and synaptic activation of pyramidal tract neurons would complicate the interpretation of experiments using cortical surface stimulation. These interpretative difficulties were reduced by the efforts of Phillips and his collaborators (67, 87). Instead of using bipolar stimulation, Hern et al. (67) used monopolar anodal stimulation and were able to activate pyramidal tract neurons only directly. Using this technique of monopolar stimulation, Landgren et al. (87) recorded monosynaptic excitatory postsynaptic potentials (EPSPs) from cervical motoneurons in the monkey. Instead of simply mapping the low-threshold areas on the cortex, they measured the size of EPSPs elicited in a given motoneuron by an electrode moved over the cortical surface to determine the extent of current spread within the cortex. Then they calculated the focal areas. They concluded that in about one-half of the instances studied, colonies of pyramidal tract neurons that projected monosynaptically to single spinal motoneurons were confined within narrow foci having a cross-sectional diameter of the order of 1.0 mm (Fig. 4). In the remainder of

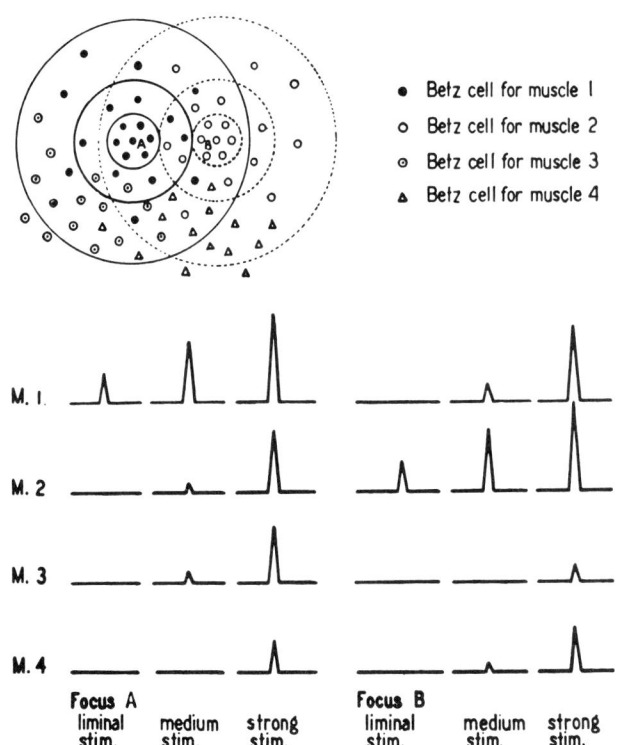

FIG. 2. Diagrammatic representation of hypothetical distribution of pyramidal tract cells for individual muscles. Cell group for each muscle has focal distribution and overlapping fringe. Each symbol represents a pyramidal tract cell. *Large concentric circles* are spheres of excitation. Expected contraction of muscles to cortical stimulation at different strength shown by myograms in *lower portion*, in which magnitude of contraction is determined by number of pyramidal tract cells involved in sphere of excitation. [From Chang et al. (33).]

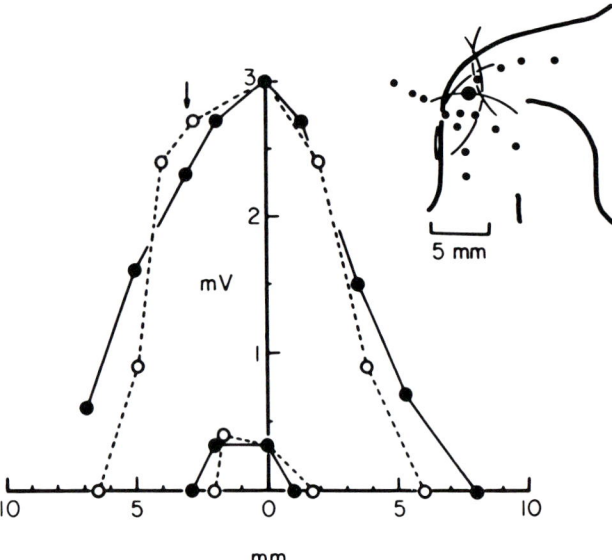

FIG. 4. Amplitude change of monosynaptic excitatory postsynaptic potentials (EPSPs) recorded in radial motoneuron of baboon. Amplitude plotted against distance from best point. *Large curves*, stimulus 1.3 mA; *small curves*, stimulus 0.75 mA; membrane potential −66 mV. *Dotted line*, points along line at right angles to Rolandic fissure; *unbroken line*, points parallel to Rolandic fissure. *Upper right*: points of stimulation around Rolandic fissure. *Large circle*, best point. *Arcs* show farthest limits of cell populations excited by stimuli applied at points of zero synaptic action on test motoneuron. [From Landgren et al. (87).]

the cases, however, these colonies were widespread in the motor cortex. Jankowska et al. (75) restudied the same problem in lumbar motoneurons of the monkey using computer averaging technique. They stimulated the surface of the cortex with single anodal pulses of near-threshold strength for pyramidal tract cells (0.4–0.5 mA), assuming that the spread of current was limited to within a distance of 1.0 mm from the electrode. The area of origin of pyramidal tract cells projecting to a given motoneuron was defined as that area from which were evoked EPSPs of at least 30% the amplitude of the largest monosynaptic EPSPs. They reported that cortical areas projecting to a motoneuron were remarkably large, most often between 3 mm^2 and 7 mm^2 (Fig. 5). They also reported that areas of location of pyramidal tract cells projecting to various motoneurons innervating one muscle were usually not identical. These areas often overlapped only partially or did not overlap at all. A problem in the interpretation of their results (75) is that if each area actually occupies 3–7 mm^2 (average of 5 mm^2) and there is no overlap, then the total area necessary for innervating even one motoneuron pool [260 α-motoneurons in medial gastrocnemius nucleus (31)] becomes so large that it cannot be fitted into the motor cortex. Therefore some assumptions are necessary, such as the possibility that only a small fraction of motoneurons receives cortical innervation. Another difficulty is that the results apparently differ from those of Landgren et al. (87), who reported that about one-half of cervical motoneurons studied received monosynaptic inputs from a restricted cortical area. The results also are not concordant with those of Chang et al. (33), who reported that isolated contraction of single muscles could be elicited by stimulation of circumscribed cortical areas. These apparently contradictory results have been to some extent resolved by Asanuma et al. (13), who demonstrated that the surface threshold currents (0.3 mA) for activating a given pyramidal tract cell did not change within an area of 2.0 mm in diameter. With 0.4 mA, individual pyramidal tract cells could be activated from areas as wide as 4 mm in diameter. This was partly due to the activation of pyramidal axon collaterals that were found to spread nearly 1.0 mm from the cell body and to have an excitability as high as the cell or initial segment of the axon. These experiments were carried out using cats. Because it is known that minimum thresholds for activating pyramidal tract cells from the surface of the cortex are approximately equal in cats (67) and monkeys (66), the projection areas reported by Jankowska et al. (75) could have been smaller than they estimated. Asanuma et al. (13) concluded that surface stimulation could not resolve the question as to whether a single muscle is represented in the motor cortex.

Apart from this question of single muscle representation, investigators have generally agreed that motor function is represented topographically within the cortex. This organization has been studied most extensively by Woolsey and his collaborators (163), who performed comparative studies on the localization of cortical sensory and motor functions. A typical example of their results is shown in Figure 6. They also studied the origin of the pyramidal tract. As already stated, the Marchi method reveals only the degenerating myelinated fibers. In addition, because only about 10% of the pyramidal fibers are large enough (> 5 µm) to show up with this technique (89), accurate location of the origin of the smaller fibers was uncertain. Woolsey and Chang (162) developed an elegant method of stimulating the medullary pyramid and then examined the distribution of antidromically evoked potentials on the surface of the cortex. As shown in Figure 7, these potentials are not restricted to the precentral (primate) or pericruciate (carnivore) gyrus, the sites of the classic motor cortex, but spread over the sensory as well as premotor areas. From these findings, as well as from the known evidence that stimulation of the sensory cortex with stronger currents can produce movements and that peripheral nerve stimulation evoked potential changes in the motor cortex, Woolsey (161) proposed the terminology *sensory-motor* and *motor-sensory* to describe the classic *sensory* and *motor* cortices, respectively. These terms are still used by many investigators and need to be distinguished from the also-common term *sensorimotor*, which refers to the sensory plus motor cortices.

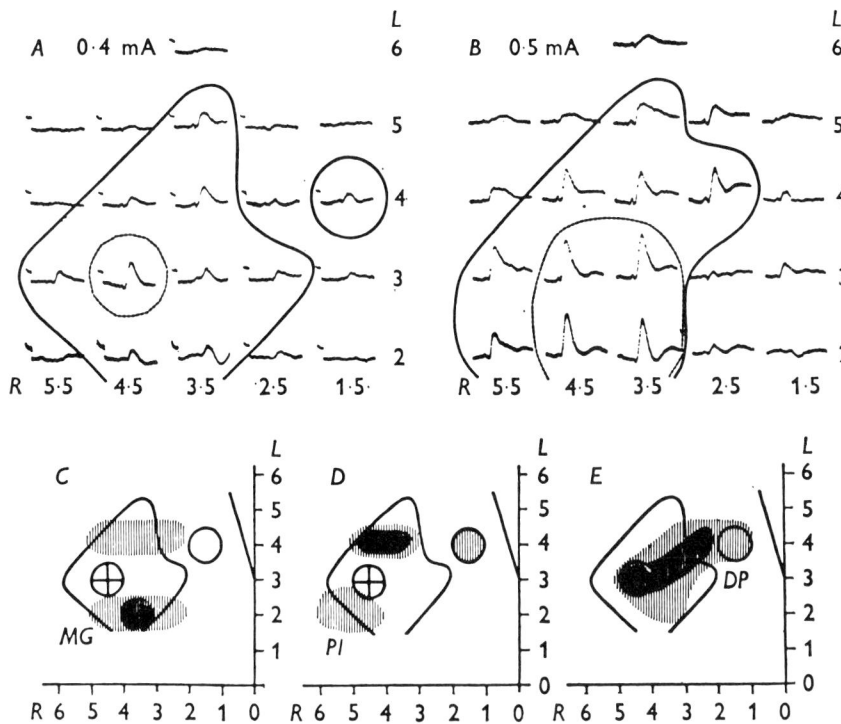

FIG. 5. Area of origin of pyramidal tract cells projecting to a lateral gastrocnemius motoneuron in monkey. *A, B*: averaged records of postsynaptic potentials evoked from indicated electrode positions by 0.4 and 0.5 mA, respectively. *C, D, E*: comparison of total projection areas and areas from which largest excitatory postsynaptic potentials (EPSPs) were evoked at 0.4-mA strength for illustrated lateral gastrocnemius motoneuron and for motoneurons to synergistic muscles (MG, medial gastrocnemius; Pl, plantaris) and to antagonistic muscle (DP, deep peroneal). [From Jankowska et al. (75).]

Studies by Cortical Depth Stimulation

Although Betz cells are known as the origin of fibers in the pyramidal tract, these cells contribute only 3% or 4% of the total pyramidal fibers (89). They have been identified as a part of the origin of the tract by the occurrence of retrograde cellular changes after pyramidal section. The difficulty intrinsic to this method is that not all affected cells present changes that are definite enough to permit recognition. This is particularly true with small pyramidal tract cells. Because of these limitations, the analysis of the laminar distribution of pyramidal tract cells had been limited to physiological experiments in which the depth distribution of antidromic unitary activities was examined. In the early stages of microelectrode experiments, there were reports that pyramidal tract cells were located in both layer III and layer V. The latest and most extensive analysis made using microelectrode techniques (71), however, suggests that at least the majority of pyramidal tract cells, both large and small, are located in layer V in the monkey. Using retrograde transport of horseradish peroxidase after injections into the spinal cord, Coulter et al. (36) were able to stain large- and medium-sized pyramidal tract cells in cats and monkeys and reported that they were all located in layer V. This study strongly supported the conclusion that all corticospinal tract fibers originate from pyramidal-shaped cells in layer V. They are located at a depth of 1.2–2.0 mm from the surface in the monkey and slightly shallower in the cat because of its thinner motor cortex.

These findings may explain some of the difficulties of interpretation of the results of surface stimulation experiments mentioned earlier. To activate pyramidal tract neurons, the current has to travel at least 1.2 mm from the surface and when the neuron is located deep in the sulcus, the distance is even greater. This large distance created ambiguity in the attempts to localize motor function because of uncertainties about the effective current spread. The difficulty has been overcome by directly stimulating the depth of the cortex through metal microelectrodes. Stoney et al. (141) could excite pyramidal tract cells directly and/or synaptically through a microelectrode with currents of only microamperes, less than one-hundredth of the current necessary to activate the same cells from the surface. Because the current necessary for activating pyramidal tract cells was so weak, it could be delivered through fine microelectrodes that were also able to record unit spikes. By using a pair of microelectrodes, one for microstimulation of and the other for extracellular recording from a given pyramidal tract cell, Stoney et al. were able to examine the spread of stimulating current within the cortex. Negative current was found to be more effective for depth stimulation. When the stimulating current was restricted to 10 μA or less (0.2-ms duration), direct excitation was limited to those cells located within a distance of less than 0.1 mm, and synaptic activation was limited to within a radius of less than 0.5 mm.

Utilizing the intracortical microstimulation technique, Asanuma and his collaborators examined the localization of motor function in the cat (12) and the monkey (10). Figure 8 shows an example of the results obtained using anesthetized cats, where the effects of

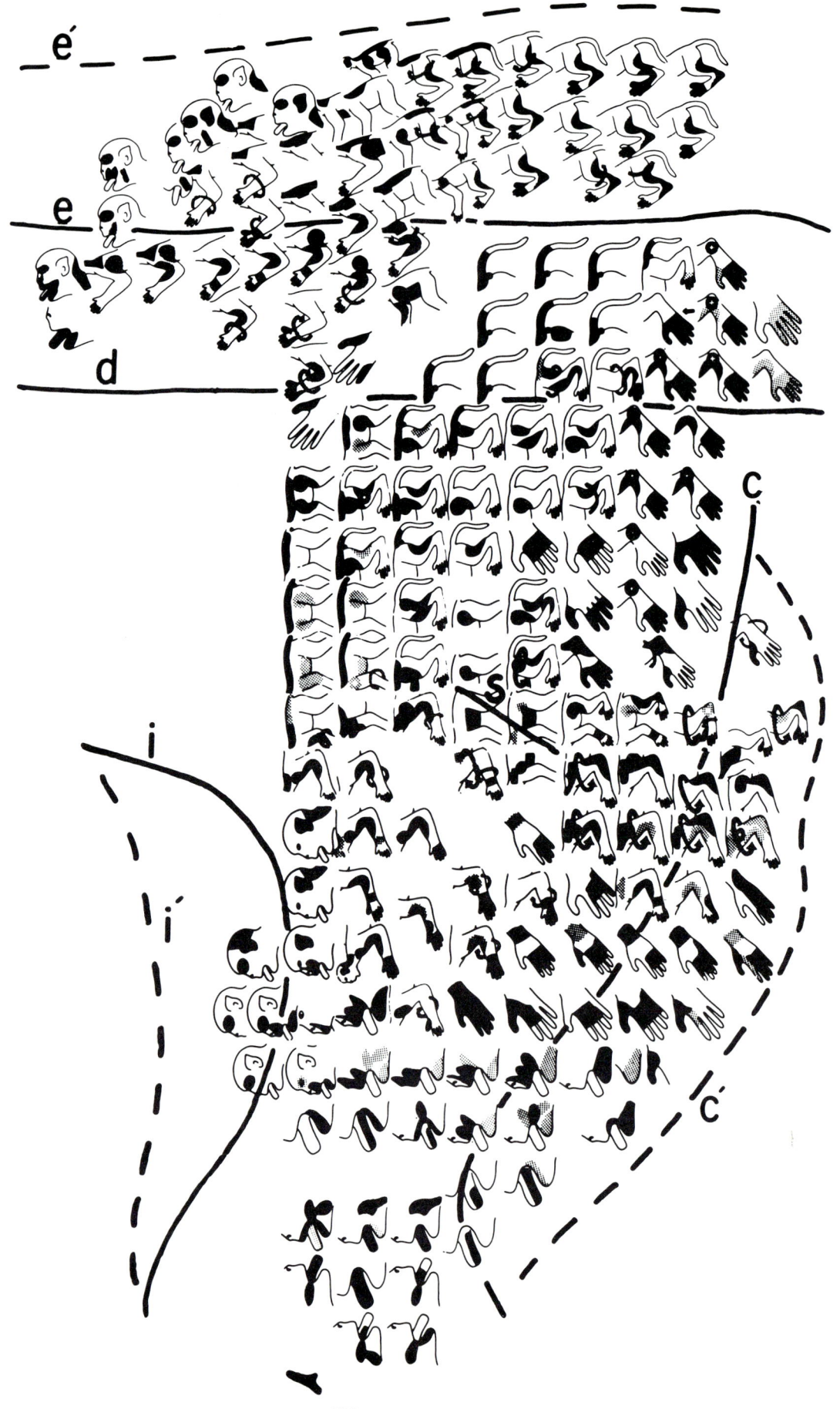

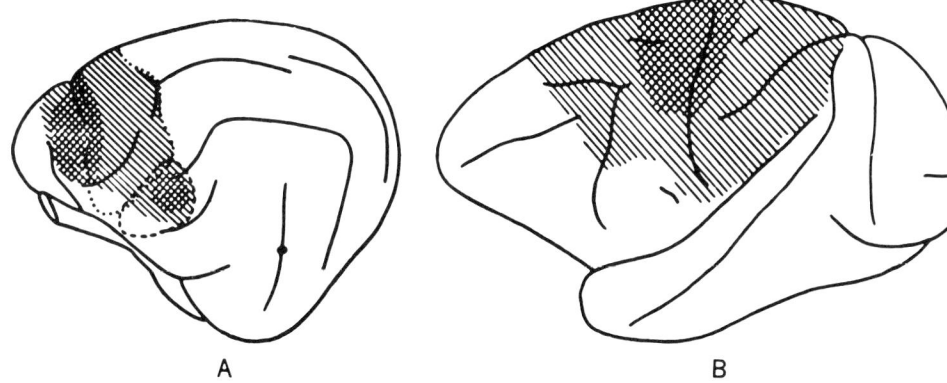

FIG. 7. Distribution of potentials produced by antidromic activation of pyramidal tract neurons by stimulation of medullary pyramid in cat, A, and monkey, B. Potentials are not restricted to motor cortex. [From Woolsey and Chang (162).]

microstimulation were monitored by its facilitation or inhibition of spinal monosynaptic reflexes. At the depths from 0.5 mm to 1.1 mm, 20-μA stimulation facilitated extensor digitorum longus (wrist dorsiflexor) reflexes with the lowest threshold at 1.0 mm. At this depth, stimulation with 20 μA also facilitated extensor carpi ulnaris and extensor carpi radialis reflexes. Weak stimulation (less than 10 μA), however, produced the effect only on extensor digitorum longus reflexes. This is the major difference between the effects of microstimulation and surface stimulation. Usually threshold microstimulation produces the effect only in one motoneuron pool, whereas surface stimulation, even with threshold intensity, produces effects in more than one motoneuron pool. It was also shown that the effect of microstimulation was abolished by pyramidal section (12). Altogether, the results suggested that there are aggregates of pyramidal tract cells in small areas of the cortex which send their axons to particular motoneuron pools, and also suggested that these cells are intermixed with others projecting to different motoneuron pools. In the example shown in Figure 8, the area for the extensor digitorum longus was limited to a small focus, but the area for the extensor carpi ulnaris was wider and had two foci.

Asanuma and Sakata (12) were also able to delineate the extent of low-threshold cortical areas that facilitated a particular monosynaptic reflex in the cat. The lowest threshold sites were confined within a sector that extended along the direction of the radial fibers in the gray substance. The diameter of the sectors ranged from 0.5 mm to a few millimeters, the average being about 1.0 mm, and the fringes overlapped with those of neighboring sectors. Figure 9 shows an example of such a sector, which was termed a "cortical efferent zone." The lowest threshold points in adjacent penetrations were located along a line parallel to the radial fibers, and the threshold increased rapidly as the electrode was moved. At the fringes thresholds suddenly rose to greater than 20 μA. A similar arrangement was found in the monkey cortex. In these experiments (10) the effect of cortical stimulation was monitored by electromyographic recordings as well as by observing movement of fingers. In adjacent penetrations the effective sites for eliciting extension and adduction of the thumb were located in an area parallel to the radial fibers in the gray matter (Fig. 10A). When the stimulus intensity was doubled (Fig. 10B), the distribution of the effective sites was more complicated. The area for thumb flexion expanded into an irregular shape, and two areas for thumb abduction were found. The authors suggested that the abduction of the thumb produced by stimulation of the second area was possibly due to the sum of the contractions caused by simultaneous activation of neighboring extension and flexion zones.

In their experiments Asanuma and collaborators (10, 12) used only weak intracortical microstimulation of 10 μA or less and identified only the lowest threshold efferent zones. On the other hand, Andersen et al. (7), using stronger intracortical stimuli (80 μA or less) in the lightly anesthetized monkey, were able to activate the same muscle units from different cortical foci,

FIG. 6. Composite figurine charts of precentral and supplementary motor areas of monkey brain derived from several experiments in which left cortex was mapped by systemic punctuate electrical stimulation. C, central sulcus; area between C and C' folds down to depth of sulcus. d, Medial edge of hemisphere; area between e and e' is supplementary motor area located on medial surface of hemisphere. Except for responses from points in ipsilateral motor face area (at *extreme left*), muscle responses are on right side of body. Strongest and earliest movements indicated in *solid*, intermediate in *cross-hatching*, and weakest in *stippling*. Symbols with crosses on ankles indicate eversion of foot; *symbols with open centers* on hip and ankle signify adduction and inversion; *curved lines with arrows* designate rotation. e, Sulcus cinguli; i, inferior precentral sulcus. [From Woolsey et al. (163).]

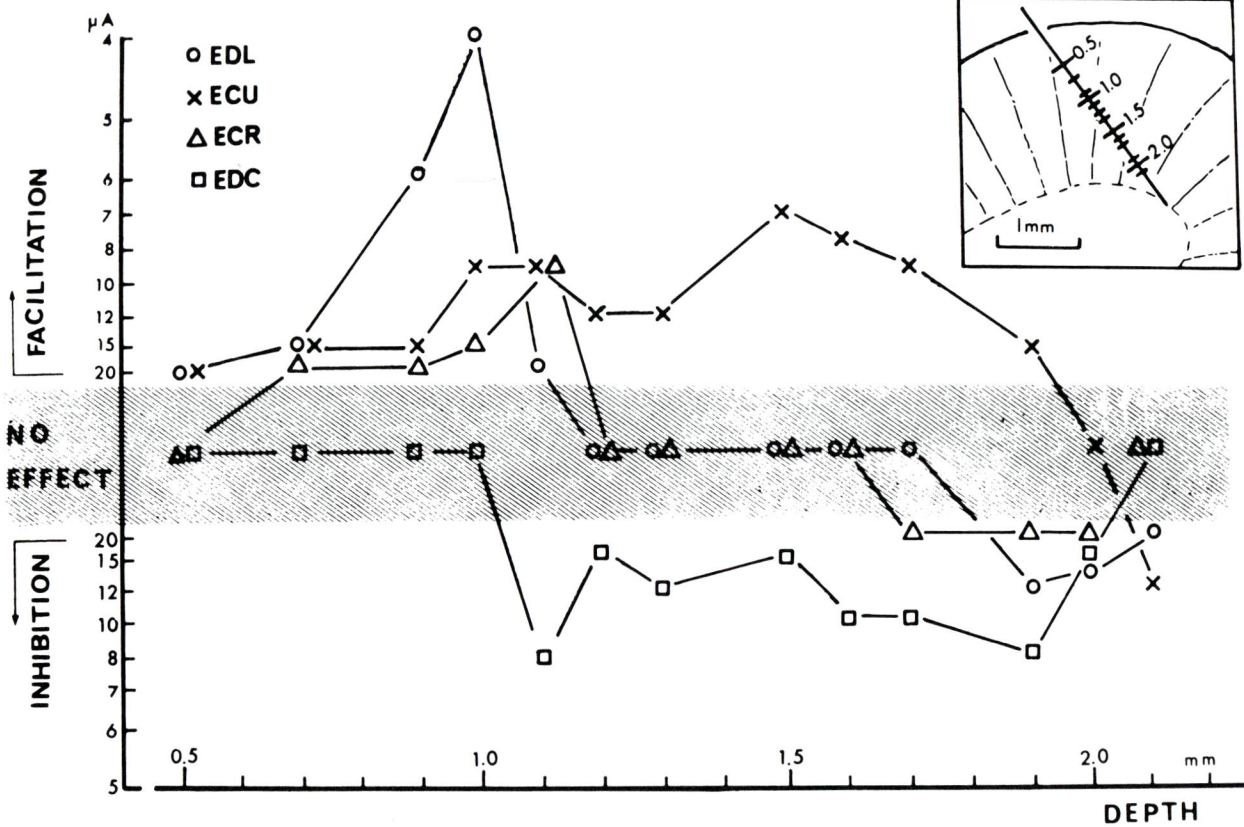

FIG. 8. Threshold changes for facilitation or inhibition of 4 spinal monosynaptic reflexes during insertion of stimulating microelectrode into cortex in cat (*top right inset*). Ordinates, threshold currents (μa) for just-observable facilitation (*upper graph*) and inhibition (*lower graph*). Note that graphs symmetrically reach maximum current of 20 μa bordering *hatched area*, which indicates no effects with stimulation of 20 μa. EDL, extensor digitorum longus; ECU, extensor carpi ulnaris; ECR, extensor carpi radialis; EDC, extensor digitorum communis. [From Asanuma and Sakata (12).]

although with different thresholds. Using squirrel monkeys, Strick and Preston (147) examined the distribution of efferent zones with weaker current of 10 μA or less. They reported that finger areas and wrist areas were mutually intercalated with small bands of 0.25-mm width. The same movement was represented twice in the small area of the motor cortex. The difference in thresholds reported by Andersen et al. (7) may indicate that the density of neurons projecting to a particular motoneuron pool varies among the different foci. Kwan et al. (86), using unanesthetized awake monkeys, mapped motor representation with the microstimulation technique. They reported that finger zones were tightly clustered in a central area surrounded by loci evoking movement about the wrist. They concluded that there is a nested-ring organization of the forelimb zones in the motor cortex such that a cortical zone controlling movement of a distal joint is partly encircled by the zone controlling a more proximal joint. The microstimulation method has thus enabled the delineation of progressively finer details of organization of efferent zones in the motor cortex.

To evoke motor effects from the cortex necessitates repetitive stimulation. Therefore consideration must be given to the extent of effective spread of such repetitive stimulation and to the means by which it activates corticofugal neurons. From the time of some of the earliest studies utilizing intracortical microstimulation, it has been known that even weak stimuli may excite pyramidal tract neurons not only directly but also synaptically (141). For the purpose of examining the relative contributions of these modes of activation, Jankowska et al. (74) recorded descending volleys from the lateral funiculus of the spinal cord following cortical stimulation. As shown in Figure 11, the direct response did not change much during repetitive stimulation, but the indirect (synaptic) responses to the second and third stimulus presentations were much larger. Similar results were reported by Asanuma et al. (13), whose studies showed that microstimulation delivered to the pyramidal tract cell layer produced both direct and indirect descending volleys, but only indirect waves when delivered to the superficial layers. During repetitive stimulation, the synaptic responses were grouped in one volley after each stimulus. Judging from the latencies, Jankowska et al. (74) concluded that "practically all of the earliest indirect and a great part of the later responses" were

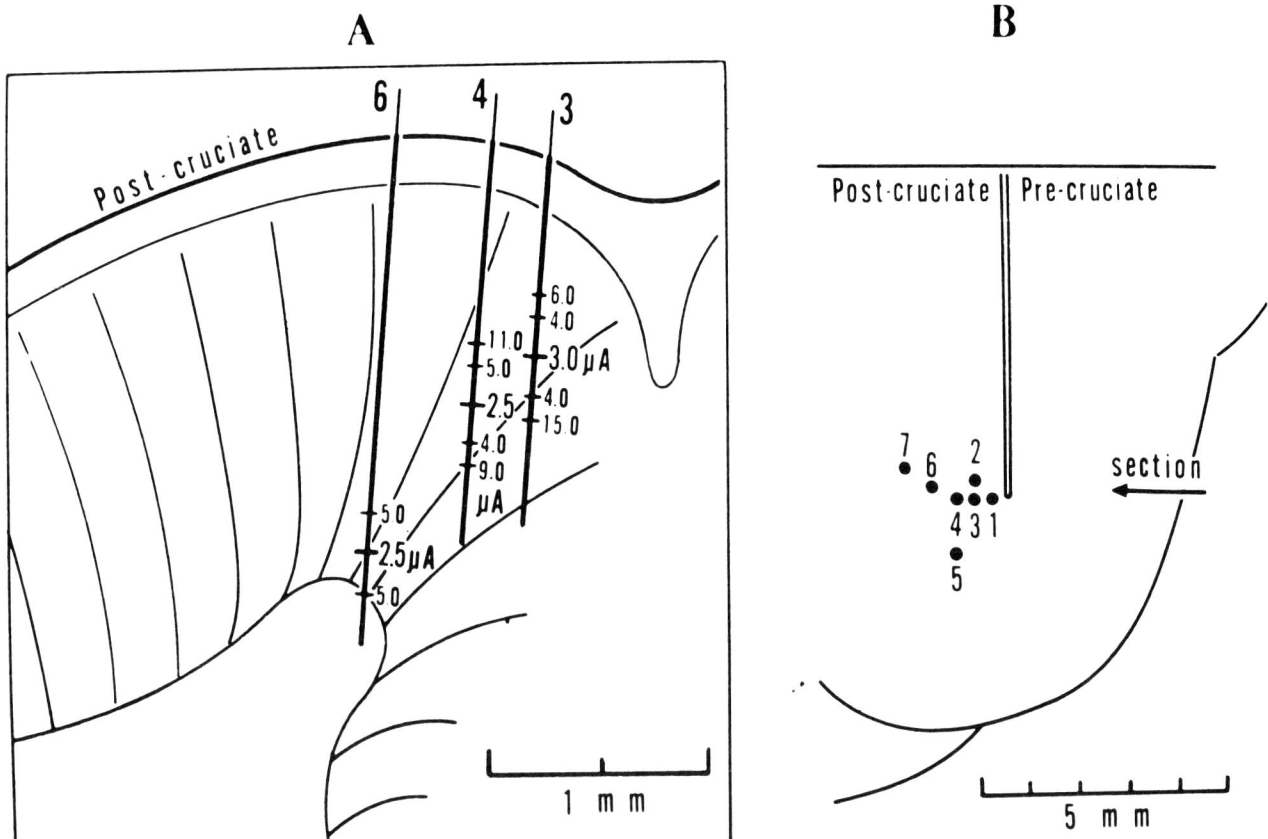

FIG. 9. Distribution of low-threshold points for facilitation of monosynaptic reflexes in medianus pronator nerve (pronator of wrist). *A*: tracks that passed low-threshold points of less than 20 μa. Each track number corresponds to surface position shown in *B*. Numbers along penetrations show threshold currents. [From Asanuma and Sakata (12).]

induced monosynaptically. If an indirect (and mainly monosynaptic) activation of pyramidal tract cells is the predominant effect of intracortical microstimulation, it becomes important to consider the extent of the monosynaptic spread from the site of stimulation. It is known that neurons in the cerebral cortex are connected predominantly in the radial direction (99), with the spread of fibers in the horizontal direction being limited to a short distance (35, 99, 149) except for layer I. Figure 12 shows cells and their interconnections in the neocortex as drawn by Szentágothai (149). The connections are mostly in the radial direction, and the only horizontal spread is in the deep layer by basket cells, which probably act as inhibitory neurons. As the motor effects of microstimulation appear from layer II or deeper, the horizontal spread of impulses in these layers is of interest. This has been studied by Asanuma and Rosén (11) by stimulating the cat cortex with a microelectrode at various depths and recording postsynaptic potentials from nearby neurons through another electrode. They found that monosynaptic spread from the superficial layers (II, III) was limited to neurons located within a horizontal distance of 0.5 mm from the stimulation site. Stimulation of the deep layers (V and VI) produced monosynaptic postsynaptic potentials (PSPs) in neurons of the same layer as well as in the superficial layers, and the horizontal spread was wider. This wider spread was mostly inhibitory, however. Microstimulation also produced polysynaptic PSPs in neurons of wider areas, but the effects beyond the monosynaptic range were predominantly inhibitory. Hess et al. (68) microiontophoretically ejected small amounts of glutamate into the visual cortex in the cat to excite a small group of neurons and reported that the effects upon neighboring cells were predominantly inhibitory. The possibility that association fibers produce corollary activation of neurons in distant regions of the motor cortex seems small, because a microlesion of the motor cortex produces degenerating fibers only in the vicinity of the lesion (55). Taken together, the results suggest that a train of microstimulation pulses activates corticofugal neurons mostly transsynaptically, but also suggest that these activated neurons are located within a horizontal radius of about 0.5 mm from the stimulating electrode.

Recent development in anatomic techniques has made it possible to examine the structural basis for the localization of motor function. Using the Nauta method, Kuypers and Brinkman (85) showed that a

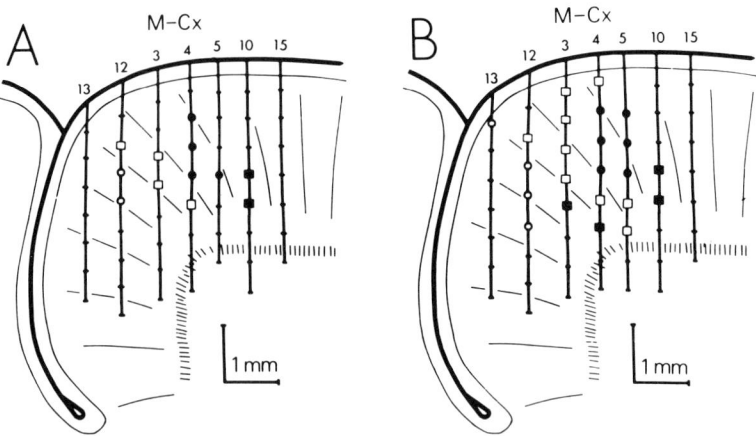

FIG. 10. Distribution of effective spots for producing thumb movements within depth of motor cortex. Effects examined at 100-μm steps in each penetration. *A*: Examined with stimulating current of 5 μa. *B*: examined with 10 μa; ○, thumb flexion; □, thumb extention; ●, thumb adduction; ■, thumb abduction; -, spots of no effect. [From Asanuma and Rosén (10).]

lesion in either the forelimb or hindlimb area of the precentral cortex produced degeneration of fibers at all levels of the spinal cord but that the common regions of distribution were restricted to parts of the spinal gray matter outside the motor nuclei. Those fibers terminating within the cervical or lumbar motor nuclei originated only from the respective forelimb or hindlimb area of the precentral cortex. More recently, Groos et al. (60) injected horseradish peroxidase into different spinal segments in the cat and observed that 5-10 labeled neurons formed clusters having diameters of 0.3-0.5 mm, which they interpreted as a sign of functional subdivision within the motor cortex. Neurons projecting to the spinal enlargements were most abundant in area 4, the primary motor cortex; but substantial populations of neurons were located also in areas 1, 2, 3, and 6, and labeled neurons included large and small pyramidal cells of layer V.

Microstructure of Corticospinal Projection

Data presented in the preceding section lead to the conclusion that there is a fine localization of cortical motor function at the level of individual muscles, especially for the distal limb muscles. It cannot be concluded, however, that all projection neurons within a given cortical efferent zone terminate only in a particular motoneuron pool. On the contrary, the observation that stronger microstimulation even at the center of a cortical efferent zone produces contraction of more than one muscle suggests that neurons projecting to different motoneuron pools are intermixed in a given efferent zone.

In addition to this issue of the projections of neighboring corticospinal neurons, there is the remaining fundamental question of whether or not individual corticospinal neurons synapse only with motoneurons innervating one muscle (41). Several attempts have been made to answer this question. Scheibel and Scheibel (134) stained terminal branches of presumed corticospinal fibers of the cat using the Golgi-Cox method. They observed that both collateral and terminal branches of individual fibers left the body of the corticospinal tract and entered the spinal gray matter at right angles over a distance of one to three segments and terminated on interneurons within the intermediate zone (Fig. 13). These interneurons, in turn, projected from one to four segments rostral and caudal, and frequently in both directions. Futami et al. (54) observed similar patterns of branching following injections of horseradish peroxidase into single pyramidal tract fibers in the spinal cord in the cat. These findings could be interpreted to indicate that some pyramidal tract neurons exert influences on spinal motoneurons located in a small area within one segment, whereas others can exert the effects over as many as 6-8 segments through interneurons. As a given motor nucleus that innervates a muscle extends from one to three segments along the spinal cord (31, 132), the results suggest that some pyramidal tract neurons can influence more than one motor nucleus. However, these studies were made with the cat, in which the pyramidal tract is known not to make direct synaptic connections with motoneurons (98), and there is a possibility that some interneurons on which the pyramidal tract axons terminate do not have connections with motoneurons. Subsequently Shinoda et al. (139) performed electroanatomic experiments in monkeys in which pyramidal tract cells were activated antidromically from branches located within spinal motor nuclei. They found that about one-third of the pyramidal tract neurons sending axons to cervical motor nuclei also sent other axon branches to the lower levels of the spinal cord. Those pyramidal tract neurons terminating only within the cervical cord branched extensively, and nearly one-half of the neurons distributed axons to more than one segment. Some sent branches as widely as three segments of the cervical ventral horn. It was also found, however, that pyramidal tract neurons activated from the various motor nuclei were not alike, i.e., those activated from within motor nuclei innervating distal forelimb muscles branched significantly less than those activated from nuclei innervating proximal muscles.

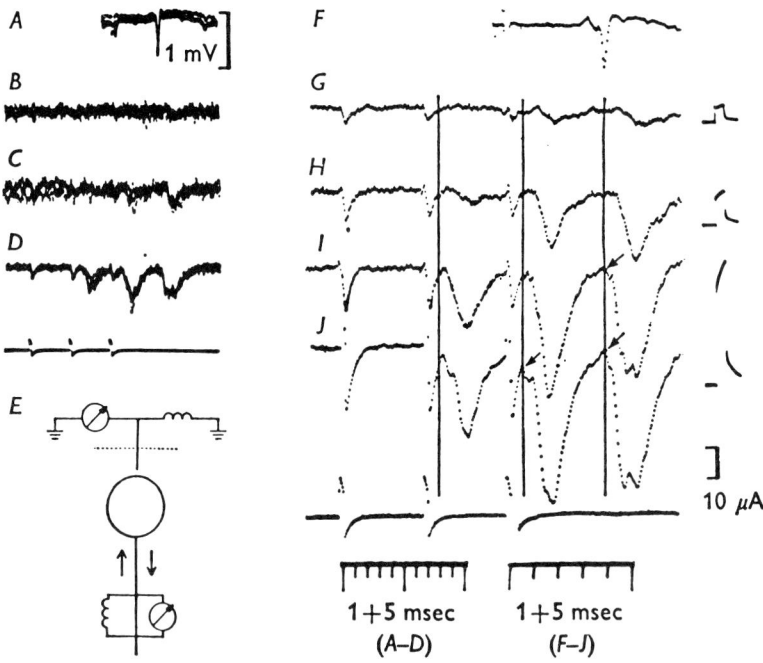

FIG. 11. Descending volleys evoked by repetitive intracortical stimulation in monkey. *A, F*: antidromic potential from pyramidal tract cell. *B–D, G–J*: descending volleys evoked by increasing strength of stimulation at same electrode position as in *A* and *F*, recorded from lateral funiculus at L_1–L_2. *J*: intracortical stimulation with same strength as for *D* and *I*, but 300 μm deeper. Superimposed traces at *left* and corresponding averaged records at *right*. Amplitude of stimuli shown at right, and their timing on *lower traces* in *D* and *J*. Arrows indicate direct responses to cortical stimulation, negativity downward. [From Jankowska et al. (74).]

Fetz et al. (48, 49) studied this problem using a different approach. Their rationale was that because pyramidal tract neurons have direct connections with motoneurons in primates, the activity of a given pyramidal tract neuron would change the excitability of the motoneurons upon which it terminated, so that following the pyramidal tract neuron discharge, the firing probability of these motoneurons would be increased. This change of motoneuronal firing frequency would be detectable by averaging unitary electromyograms. With this assumption, they implanted electrodes into various muscles of awake monkeys and could observe transient increases of electromyographic activity in more than one muscle following discharges of individual pyramidal tract cells in the motor cortex. The results suggested that at least some pyramidal tract neurons send terminal branches to more than one group of motoneurons innervating different muscles. The results have to be interpreted with some caution, however. It is known that a group of cortical neurons located within a limited area receive similar inputs in the sensory (70, 113) as well as in the motor (27, 28, 133) cortices in both cats and monkeys. It is possible that some pyramidal tract cells receive the same inputs from the same source and produce synchronous discharges, even if only occasionally. Because the averaging of the electromyograms was made for several thousands of pyramidal tract cell discharges, a possibility exists that the transient facilitation in different muscles was produced by different pyramidal tract neurons. Although the authors (49) were aware of the problem, it is difficult to exclude this possibility completely. Thus, all the results until now are inconclusive as to whether a single pyramidal tract neuron terminates upon different groups of motoneurons innervating different muscles, but they suggest that at least some pyramidal tract neurons do so.

A natural question then arises regarding how these pyramidal tract neurons innervating various groups of motoneurons are organized within the motor cortex to produce movements. To investigate this question, Asanuma et al. (20), using anesthetized monkeys, recorded antidromic spikes simultaneously from a group of pyramidal tract cells through an electrode placed in a fixed position in the motor cortex and traced the branches of these pyramidal tract neurons in the spinal cord. They made a grid of microelectrode insertions into the spinal cord and delivered weak stimulating currents to activate these pyramidal tract cells antidromically. By adjusting the dimensions of the grid and the intensity of stimuli, they could activate all branches within given areas. Because the stimulating electrode could also be used to record antidromic field potentials from spinal motor nuclei, they could relate the locations of pyramidal tract branches and of motor nuclei. An example of the results is shown in Figure 14. Four pyramidal tract cells were simultaneously recorded through the same electrode, indicating that these cells were located close together. Three of them sent branches to the spinal motor nuclei as well as outside the nuclei, and one, marked by the parallelogram, sent branches outside the nuclei only. As shown in Figure 14*A* and summarized in Figure 14*B*, all three neurons sent terminal branches to nucleus extensor digitorum brevis and all three passed through nucleus flexor digitorum longus. If the sites of synaptic contacts between pyramidal tract axons and motoneurons is limited only to soma or proximal dendrites, the results could indicate that a given pyramidal tract neuron synapses with motoneurons innervating differ-

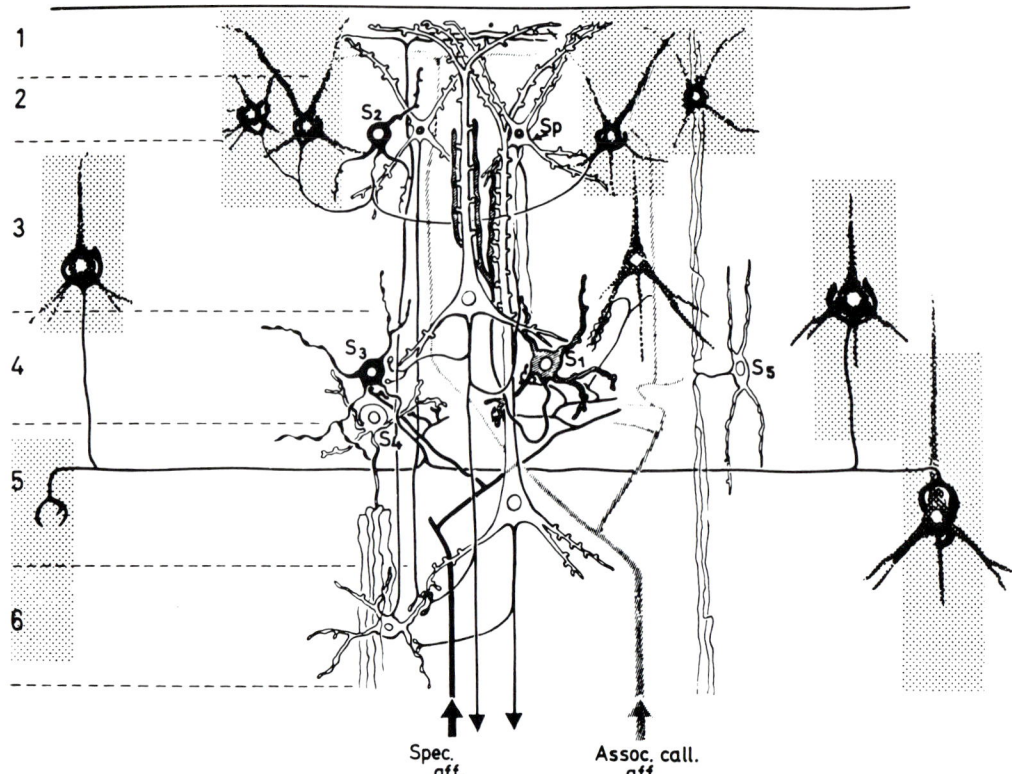

FIG. 12. Interconnections of some cell types in cerebral cortex. Two pyramidal cells shown in laminae 3 and 5. Specific afferent fiber (spec. aff.) shown to excite stellate cell (S_1), the axon of which establishes cartridge-type synapses on apical dendrites. Specific afferent fiber also excites stellate interneurons (S_3) that give inhibition to pyramidal cells in adjacent cortical columns, indicated by *shadings*. Sp, stellate pyramidal cells; S_2, short axon inhibitory cells in lamina 2; S_5, S_6, interneurons with ascending and descending axons. [From Szentágothai (149).]

ent muscles. The exact site of synaptic contact, however, is unknown, and if some pyramidal tract fibers synapse on distal dendrites, the location of apparent terminal branches does not reflect a connection between the pyramidal tract fibers and identified motor nuclei. This caution is necessary because motoneurons, especially those with large cell bodies, send dendritic branches several millimeters from the soma, spreading even into the intermediate zone of the spinal cord (134). With these limitations in mind, Asanuma et al. (20) examined the distribution of spinal branches of four groups of pyramidal neurons and found that in all cases there was at least one motor nucleus in which the majority of the neurons sent branches that either terminated there or passed through. Because of technical limitations they could not determine if those fibers that passed through a common nucleus made synaptic contacts with nearby neurons by short branches, but the possibility does exist. A similar organization has been reported in the pyramidal tract system of the cat in which a group of pyramidal tract neurons located close together tended to be activated antidromically by stimulation through the same electrode in the spinal cord (138). The results altogether suggest that although pyramidal tract axons from a

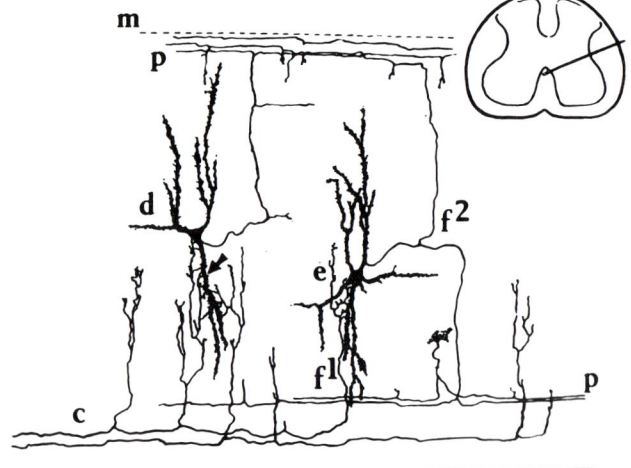

FIG. 13. Terminal branches of pyramidal tract axons in lumbar cord of cat. Horizontal section cut slightly obliquely (*inset diagram*) showing relations of lateral corticospinal terminals (f^1) to proprioneurons. Terminating corticospinal elements, c, project synaptically upon lateral dendrites and somata of propriospinal neurons d and e. At *arrow*, terminals from two different corticospinal fibers converge on same dendrite. Propriospinal neurons d and e project axons toward midline, m, and/or lateral propriospinal bundles, p, to form secondary terminals, f^2. [From Scheibel and Scheibel (134).]

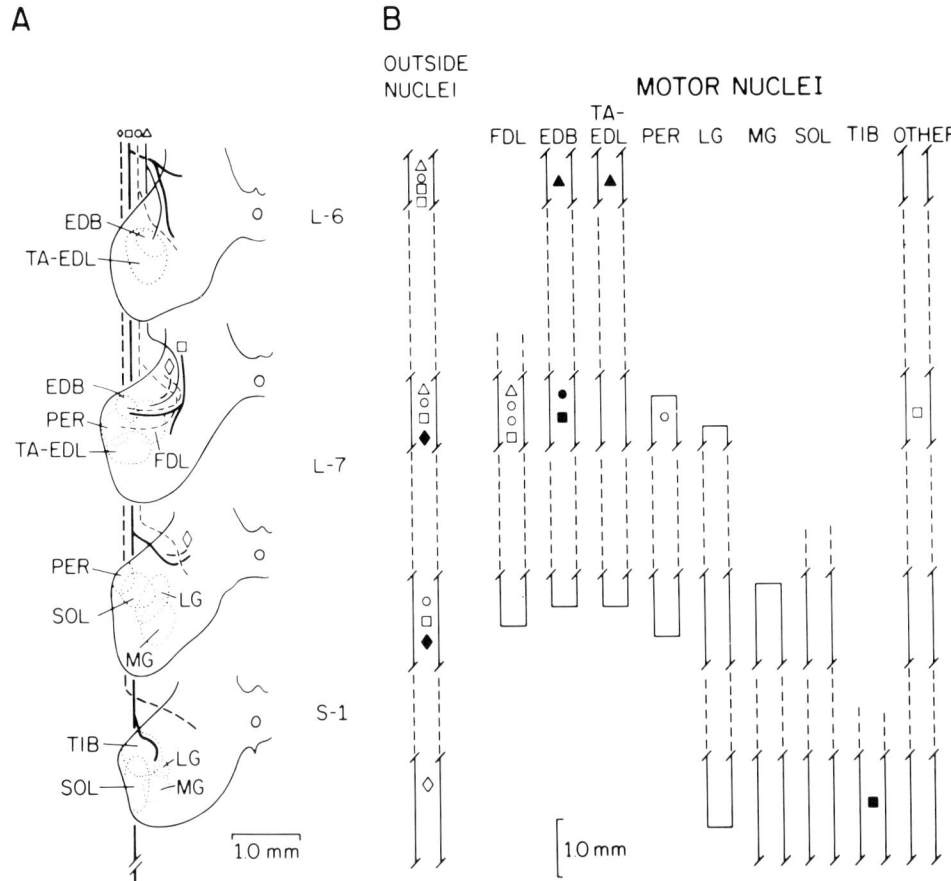

FIG. 14. Distribution of terminal branches of 4 pyramidal tract neurons in spinal cord. These 4 neurons recorded simultaneously through same cortical electrode. A: likely course of axonal branches summarized in 4 representative transverse planes. Each neuron represented by different line and symbol. B: areas of passage (*open symbols*) and termination (*filled symbols*) of axon collaterals in ventral horn in relation to motor nuclei identified by antidromically evoked potentials. *Continuous bars*, explored parts of spinal cord; *dashed bars*, unexplored areas; OTHER, those sites that histological examination indicated as ventral horn, but antidromic stimulation of isolated motor nerves did not identify nuclei. FDL, flexor digitorum longus; EDB, extensor digitorum brevis; EDL, extensor digitorum longus; PER, peroneus; LG, lateral gastrocnemius; MG, medial gastrocnemius; SOL, soleus; TIB, tibialis; L_6, sixth lumbar segment; L_7, seventh lumbar segment; S_1, first sacral segment. [From Asanuma et al. (20).]

small area in the motor cortex project to a wide area in the spinal cord, there is a focal area to which they project most heavily. Figure 15 illustrates the above conclusion in a simplified form.

Projection to γ-Motoneurons

The cortical representation of γ-motoneurons was first studied by Mortimer and Akert (111) in anesthetized cats and monkeys. They recorded unitary activities from lumbosacral ventral root filaments and differentiated α- and γ-motoneurons by their physiological properties. They reported that the cortical area, which activated γ-motoneurons, was comparable to the one for α-motoneurons in both species. Because they did not section the pyramidal tract, however, it still remained in question whether the effect was mediated by this tract. Fidone and Preston (50), using pyramidal cats, and Grigg and Preston (59), using pyramidal monkeys, examined cortical effects on γ-motoneurons. They dissected hindlimb nerves and recorded unitary activities of both α- and γ-fibers that innervated the same muscle. They reported parallel predominances of facilitation or inhibition on α- and γ-motoneurons of the same muscle. They also showed (59) that there were monosynaptic connections made by fibers of the pyramidal tract upon γ-motoneurons in primates. Clough et al. (34) stimulated the motor cortex in the baboon and recorded intracellularly from γ-motoneurons that innervated distal forelimb muscles. Of 19 γ-motoneurons that they recorded, 6 showed EPSPs at monosynaptic latencies and 4 showed short-latency inhibitory postsynaptic poten-

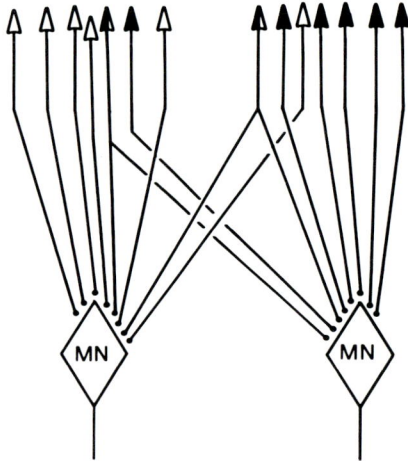

FIG. 15. Simplified diagram showing mode of pyramidal projection from motor cortex to spinal motor nuclei (MN). Group of pyramidal tract neurons located in small area of cortex project primarily to given motor nucleus, but some send axons to another motor nucleus and some send branches to more than one motor nucleus.

tials (IPSPs), probably elicited by disynaptic connections. Although they did not use pyramidal baboons, the monosynaptic EPSPs indicated that the transmission was via the pyramidal tract. Thus the results demonstrate the existence of γ-representation in the motor cortex and show that at least some corticofusimotor connections are made through the pyramidal tract. The overlap of alpha and gamma representations suggests that there is an α-γ-linkage at the cortical level.

The activity of γ-motoneurons may be inferred by monitoring discharges of spindle afferents. Koeze et al. (83) examined cortical effects on spindle afferents using prolonged repetitive stimulation in the baboon. They found both excitatory and inhibitory effects, but because they did not use pyramidal animals, other pathways may have been responsible for the effects.

Projections to Spinal Interneurons

Although there are direct connections between pyramidal tract fibers and motoneurons in primates (22), the majority of the fibers terminate on spinal interneurons (25). Those terminating on motoneurons arise primarily from pyramidal tract cells in the limb area and terminate on motoneurons innervating limb muscles (84, 96). Recent evidence indicates that even those innervating motoneurons send other branches outside the motor nuclei (Fig. 14). In cats the direct connection to motoneurons has not been demonstrated (98, 119). In his pioneering study, Lloyd (98) elegantly demonstrated, using the pyramidal cat, that pyramidal volleys reached motoneurons through interneurons located in the intermediate region of the spinal cord. The distributions of pyramidal tract axons arising from the motor and the sensory cortices are different in both the cat and the monkey, suggesting a difference of function between the two groups: those arising from the sensory cortex end dorsomedially in the cord, in laminae IV, V, and VI of Rexed (131). Neurons in these laminae transfer afferent impulses from the periphery to local spinal segments and to higher levels of the central nervous system. The fibers from the motor cortex end in laminae V, VI, and VII in the cat (119) and end further ventrally to lamina IX in the monkey (84), where motoneurons are located. These branching patterns suggest that the pyramidal tract functions not only in transferring corticofugal impulses directly to motoneurons, but also functions in modulating reflex activities of the spinal cord. Furthermore, those pyramidal tract fibers arising from the sensory cortex may influence the transmission of afferent impulses to higher centers, including the motor cortex.

This problem was studied most intensively by Lundberg and collaborators (102, 103). They produced convincing evidence that the pyramidal tract and group Ia muscle afferents converge on the group Ia inhibitory pathway in cats (103). They used the conventional method of conditioning monosynaptic reflexes by various stimuli. As shown in Figure 16, the inhibitory effect produced by deep peroneal nerve stimulation is greatly enhanced by cortical stimulation. Because the cortical effect disappeared after pyramidal section, they attributed the effect to the pyramidal tract. In the succeeding study (102), in which recordings were made intracellularly from spinal interneurons, they were able to demonstrate the convergence of inputs from the motor cortex with those from skin and muscle afferents. Although they did not use pyramidal cats in this experiment, they concluded that the effect was mediated by the pyramidal tract based on the short latencies of the PSPs, which did not allow time for a disynaptic connection from the cortex to the target interneurons. The control of the spinal cord from the higher centers, including the pyramidal tract, has been reviewed by Lundberg (100, 101).

The effects of cortical stimulation on spinal reflexes in pyramidal cats and baboons were studied extensively by Preston and collaborators (130). Using the conditioning-testing method, they reported that the amount of facilitation or inhibition produced by cortical stimulation was different in different motoneuron populations. The pyramidal effect was predominantly inhibitory for extensor motoneurons and predominantly facilitatory for flexor motoneurons in both cats and monkeys. This pattern, however, was reversed in motoneurons of the baboon. Preston et al. argued that, although both the cat and the baboon are considered to be quadrupeds, the baboon uses the forelimb in a manner similar to that of the erect primates. Because of these considerations, they suggested that the motor cortex inhibits the tonic activities of postural mechanisms to permit volitional movements to occur.

Thus results from various laboratories demonstrated that the pyramidal tract not only excites particular motor nuclei, but also exerts influences on postural mechanisms of the spinal cord through interneurons. The manner in which these specific and

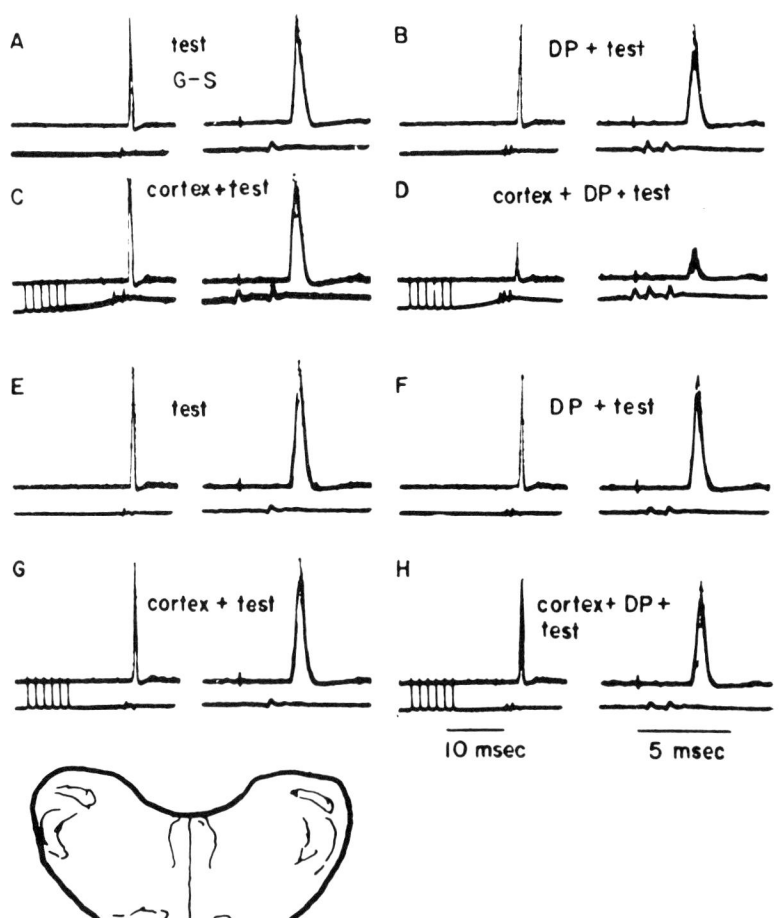

FIG. 16. Pyramidal effects on gastrocnemius-soleus, G-S, and deep peroneal, DP, monosynaptic reflexes. Reflexes were recorded simultaneously at two different sweep speeds. *Upper traces,* reflex discharges in ventral root; *lower traces,* potentials at dorsal root entry zone. *A*: unconditioned test reflex. *B*: effect of conditioning G-S reflex with maximal group Ia volley in DP. *C, D*: effect of train of 6 stimuli to motor cortex on *A* and *B*. *E–H*: repetition of same series after transection of pyramidal tract shown in *inset*. [From Lundberg and Voorhoeve (103).]

general effects interact during natural movements is, at present, rather difficult to assess. One of the seeming paradoxes is that, although the electrophysiological method has demonstrated connections between the pyramidal tract and various spinal neurons, a lesion of the pyramidal tract leaves very little functional deficiency. As is discussed in more detail in section FUNCTION OF PYRAMIDAL TRACT, p. 727, within the first 24 h after a properly placed lesion, monkeys can stand, grip the cage, and take a few climbing steps (92). The only permanent deficiency is the loss of discrete usage of individual digits. These findings serve to remind us that the pyramidal tract is not the only pathway from the higher central nervous system controlling the movements or modulating the postural mechanisms of the spinal cord. To what extent the pyramidal tract participates in the postural control in normal animals during willed movement is still in question.

Pyramidal Collaterals and Branches Within Brain

The pyramidal cells in layer V, including Betz cells, are known to send axon collaterals as far as layer II. The horizontal spread of these axon collaterals, however, is limited to a narrow range of less than 1.0 mm (99). Physiological experiments (13) have also demonstrated that some pyramidal tract cells can be activated antidromically only from a horizontal distance of less than 1.0 mm. The excitability of these axon collaterals is as high as the neuron somata or axon hillocks, and any cortical stimulation excites cell bodies and axon collaterals indiscriminately (13). A question then arises as to the manner in which these axon collaterals influence neighboring corticofugal neurons. Do they excite the neighboring pyramidal tract cells or do they inhibit them in a way similar to that in which spinal motoneurons inhibit the neighboring motoneurons? Phillips (125) studied the problem by stimulating the pyramidal tract with a strength subthreshold for an intracellularly recorded pyramidal tract cell. Unlike ventral root stimulation, pyramidal stimulation produced early depolarization followed by hyperpolarization in the target cell. Later, Takahashi et al. (150) demonstrated that this early EPSP is produced by axon collaterals of slow pyramidal tract cells, which synapse directly on the fast pyramidal tract cells. Using lightly anesthetized cats or nonanesthetized cats immobilized by coagulation of the brain stem, Stefanis and Jasper (140) examined the effect of repetitive stimulation of the pedunculus upon pyramidal tract neurons. They found that repetitive antidromic stimulation greatly enhanced the recurrent inhibitory effect, which lasted several tens of milliseconds after stimulation. These inhibitory effects were frequently interrupted by facilitatory effects. They suggested that the recurrent inhibition by pyramidal tract axon collaterals functions to increase the contrast between a central group of most active cells and the surrounding neurons. Using unanesthetized cats, Brooks and Asanuma (26) examined the effect of pyramidal stimulation on the receptive fields of cortical neurons. They demonstrated that the size of receptive fields of pyramidal tract neurons were reduced to the center of the fields during and after repetitive stimulation of the medullary pyramid.

Besides the recurrent axon collaterals, pyramidal tract axons send branches to various subcortical nuclei. Until recently it was difficult to determine whether the projection fibers to subcortical nuclei were branches of pyramidal tract neurons or independent fibers. Advances in electrophysiological techniques have made it possible to determine whether some of these projections are made by branches of pyramidal tract axons. Tsukahara et al. (155) stimulated the red nucleus in cats and were able to antidromically activate pyramidal tract cells identified by prior pyramidal stimulation. They also demonstrated that pyramidal stimulation could produce EPSPs and IPSPs in red nucleus neurons. Humphrey and Corrie made an extensive study on the branching of pyramidal tract axons by activating pyramidal tract cells from the red nucleus in the monkey (71). They found that the pattern of branching was different between fast and slow pyramidal tract cells. About 20% of fast pyramidal tract cells that they examined sent branches to the red nucleus, whereas only 8% of slow pyramidal tract cells sent branches. Because slow pyramidal tract cells are more numerous than fast pyramidal tract cells, they estimated that only about 10% of total pyramidal tract cells send branches to the red nucleus. In another study (72) they stimulated the pyramidal tract and subcortical white matter after ablation of the motor cortex in the monkey and reported that subcortical stimulation exerted much bigger facilitatory effects upon red nucleus neurons. As subcortical stimulation activated pyramidal as well as nonpyramidal inputs to the red nucleus, they concluded that the pyramidal collateral route is of only minor significance in activating red nucleus neurons. Endo et al. (40) reported that some identified pyramidal tract cells could also be antidromically activated from the corpus striatum, ventrolateral or ventral posterolateral nucleus of the thalamus, the red nucleus, the reticular formation, or the pontine nucleus. Some pyramidal tract cells could be activated from more than one of these nuclei. In addition to the subcortical motor nuclei, pyramidal tract branches reach sensory relay nuclei. Jabbur and Towe (73) stimulated the sensorimotor cortex in pyramidal cats and could excite or inhibit neurons in the dorsal column nuclei, clearly demonstrating that the pyramidal tract can modulate activities of the sensory relay nuclei. Andersen et al. (6) showed that cortical stimulation could evoke depolarization of primary afferent fibers in the cat, and Fetz (47), using the same species, demonstrated that at least a part of the depolarization was mediated by the pyramidal tract. The latter investigator also demonstrated that pyramidal tract stimulation could excite or inhibit neurons in the dorsal horn. From these experiments it has become clear that some pyramidal tract neurons can influence the activities of various subcortical motor nuclei or sensory relay nuclei. Furthermore, Zarzecki et al. (165) have shown that some pyramidal tract cells in area 3a (63) send long axon collaterals to the motor cortex. Yet there are demonstrations that some corticofugal neurons projecting to the ventrolateral nucleus (23) and the dorsal column nuclei (57) do not project to the spinal cord. Anatomic studies with horseradish peroxidase have revealed that cortical cells projecting to the corpus striatum are located in the superficial part of layer VI and also in the deeper part of layer V in the monkey (76), whereas the majority of corticocaudate projection cells are located in layer III in the cat (81). Thus the results are still controversial, but it seems that at least some pyramidal tract fibers give off collaterals before reaching the medullary pyramid and send branches to various subcortical nuclei. The functional significance of these collateral branches are still unknown, but it may be said that activities of the pyramidal system are accompanied by corollary activities of the sensory and other motor systems to produce purposeful movements.

AFFERENT INPUTS TO MOTOR CORTEX
AND PYRAMIDAL TRACT NEURONS

General Problems

Inputs to the motor cortex have been studied less extensively than the outputs from the motor cortex, and they have been studied more anatomically than physiologically. Various methods, each with its own limitations, have been used to determine the connections. It is generally agreed that the motor cortex receives its main inputs from the thalamus. It also receives projections from the ipsilateral hemisphere through association fibers and from the contralateral hemisphere through commissural fibers. Recent developments in autoradiography and horseradish peroxidase techniques have made it possible to study further details of projections from various areas, and our knowledge is increasing rapidly.

Inputs From Nucleus Ventralis Lateralis of Thalamus

The motor cortex receives its major inputs from the nucleus ventralis lateralis of the thalamus. Olszewski

(120) subdivided this nucleus into three main parts: pars oralis, pars medialis, and pars caudalis in the monkey. The largest subdivision is the pars oralis, and it receives fiber connections from the cerebellar nuclei and the globus pallidus. The pars medialis receives fibers from the globus pallidus and the substantia nigra. Corticofugal fibers from the precentral cortex project to the pars oralis and the pars caudalis, constituting reciprocal connections between the nucleus ventralis lateralis and the cortex. It has been suggested that there is a crude topographic organization within the nucleus ventralis lateralis (157). Medial parts of the nucleus send fibers to the face area, intermediate parts to the arm and trunk area, and lateral parts to the leg area of the cortex. Using the Fink-Heimer method, Strick (142) studied the distribution of degenerating fibers from small regions of the nucleus ventralis lateralis in the cat. He confirmed the existence of crude topographic projection to the motor cortex, and reported that the projection from a small area of the nucleus ventralis lateralis was not restricted to a small area of the motor cortex. A small lesion in the nucleus ventralis lateralis produced sparse degeneration spread over a relatively wide area of the motor cortex. Larger lesions increased the density of degeneration within the same cortical area, indicating an extensive arborization of individual ventrolateral fibers in the motor cortex. Massion and Rispal-Padel (108) examined the projection from nucleus ventralis lateralis in cats using physiological methods. They implanted several (12–16) stimulating electrodes into the depths of the motor cortex and examined the distribution of neurons in the nucleus ventralis lateralis activated antidromically from the individual electrodes. They also confirmed the existence of topographical relationships between the motor cortex and the nucleus ventralis lateralis and in addition found that some ventrolateral neurons (8 of 29) could be activated from more than one cortical stimulating site, clearly indicating that some neurons send branches to different parts of the motor cortex. Because the number of the cortical electrodes was limited, it is likely that the actual ratio of the neurons with bifurcating axons is higher than they had observed. Subsequently Asanuma and Fernandez, in collaboration with Scheibel and Scheibel (19), studied the characteristics of these projections in cats using physiological and anatomic methods. They found that each terminal bush of these multiple branching neurons covers a much wider area than that covered by the specific projection fibers originating from the thalamic sensory relay nuclei and project to their respective sensory cortices (99). Scheibel and Scheibel (19) were able to stain these terminal bushes of young cats using the Golgi method (Fig. 17). The width of these terminal bushes measured in the horizontal direction was 1.16 ± 0.27 mm in diameter, and the terminal fibers reached to the upper part of the second cortical layer. The predominantly oblique direction of the components of the

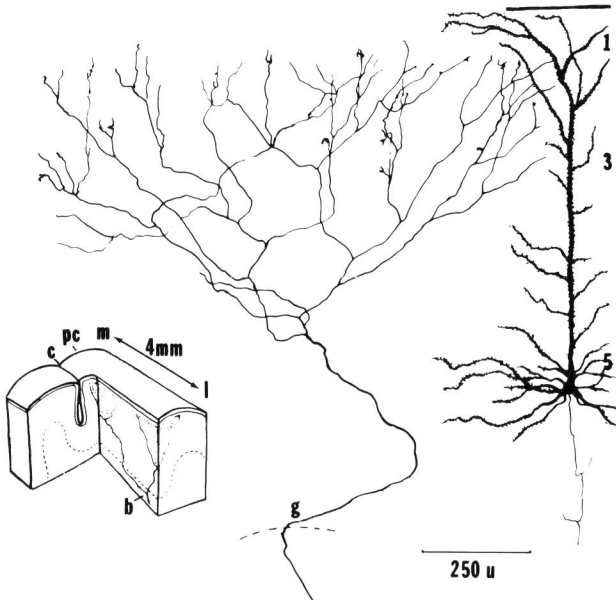

FIG. 17. Terminal intracortical domain generated by axon of single thalamic ventrolateral neuron shown in relation to large fifth-layer pyramidal neuron. g, Gray matter–white matter junction. Reconstruction at *lower left* shows single ventrolateral fiber system projecting onto pericruciate gyrus, pc. Two of these tridimensional plexuses are shown developing from same fiber via branch point, b; young kitten cortex. c, Cruciate sulcus; m, medial; l, lateral. [From Scheibel and Scheibel, in Asanuma et al. (19).]

axonal plexus in the lower two-thirds of the terminal arbor suggested that contacts were most likely made with some of the basal dendrites of pyramidal cells and with some of the oblique branches of the apical shafts. The majority of terminal branches were located in the superficial layers, which suggested that they might have synaptic contacts with or climb along the apical dendrites of large- and medium-sized pyramids. Strick and Sterling (148) examined synaptic terminations of afferent fibers from the ventrolateral nucleus in cats using light microscopy and electron microscopy. They reported that following the ventrolateral lesion, degenerating synapses were mainly found in three layers: the upper one-third of layer I (18%), layer III (66%), and layer VI (13%). Some of the synapses were found on the dendritic shafts or cell bodies of stellate cells, but most (91%) were found on the dendritic spines. Because it is known that ventrolateral stimulation produces mono- and polysynaptic activation of pyramidal tract cells (5), it is likely that some of these degenerating fibers made synapses on the dendritic spines of pyramidal tract cells.

The nature of the afferent inputs to ventrolateral neurons has been studied repeatedly (19, 106, 107), and all the investigators agree that these neurons do not receive specific peripheral inputs. This excludes the possibility that receptive fields of neurons in the motor cortex are transferred through ventrolateral neurons. Activities of neurons in the nucleus ventralis lateralis during natural movements were studied by

Evarts (43) and Strick (144) in the monkey. They found that some ventrolateral neurons discharged prior to movements, suggesting that they were related to the initiation of movements. Unlike many motor cortex neurons that receive peripheral inputs, however, most of them were not influenced by natural stimulation in the periphery.

Peripheral Inputs to Motor Cortex and Pyramidal Tract Cells

During the several decades following the discovery of the motor representation within the cortex (53), the major interest among neurologists and neurophysiologists was the localization of motor function; little attention was paid to the sensory inputs to the precentral cortex (124). With the advancement of electrical techniques, Adrian and Moruzzi (1) were able to record discharges in the pyramidal tract in response to peripheral stimulation, which clearly demonstrated that pyramidal tract cells received peripheral inputs. As already stated, Woolsey and his collaborators (163) studied the distribution of evoked potentials in both the sensory and motor cortices in combination with stimulation of the cortex, and they reported that there were rough topographical relationships between afferent input and efferent outflow. They observed that the area of the motor cortex where the largest evoked potential was recorded by stimulation of a particular part of the body had the lowest threshold for the movement of the same part of the body. Following the development of the microelectrode technique, the nature of the inputs was studied extensively. In the early stage of these experiments, however, the results were confusing. The experiments were frequently carried out under chloralose anesthesia using electrical stimulation instead of with unanesthetized animals and natural stimulation. Under the former conditions, motor and sensory cortical cells received widespread convergence of inputs without recognizable patterns of spatial localization or sensory modality. Most cells responded to electrical stimulation applied to any part of the body (153). It was noticed later that chloralose enhances the activity of the nonspecific system (2). These widespread responses could therefore have been produced by abnormal activities of the system.

The receptive fields of neurons in the motor cortex were studied extensively with cats by Brooks et al. (27, 28) and by Buser and Imbert (32). The experiments were carried out under local anesthesia with natural stimulation. These authors found that the pattern of sensory activation was similar in pyramidal tract and nonpyramidal tract cells. About 65% of cells responded to cutaneous stimulation, 20% to passive joint movement, and the remainders were not driven. More than one-half of driven cells received modality-specific inputs from a fixed small area of the body. The rest received inputs from wide areas of the body, and some of these had labile receptive fields. In a subsequent study by Welt et al. with cats (159), it was found that cells with similar receptive fields were grouped together in a small area of the cortex. These cells were intermixed with other groups of cells that received inputs of different modalities but that had receptive fields located in the same area of the body. These groups of cells were located in a small area extended along the direction of radial fibers in the cortex, and their diameters ranged from 0.1 mm to 0.4 mm. An example of these aggregates of cells is shown in Figure 18.

A natural question following these observations is whether a group of afferent inputs converging from a particular part of the body to a small area of the cortex is related to the motor function of the cortex. The problem has been studied by Asanuma and his collaborators in cats (18) and monkeys (133) using a closed-chamber system that allowed recordings from single cortical neurons while animals were awake and able to move. The receptive fields of neurons were examined first, then the same electrode was used to stimulate these neurons and their neighbors to produce contraction of individual limb muscles. It was then possible to relate the afferent inputs to a small area of the cortex with the motor effects elicited from the same area. They found that a given efferent zone received polymodal inputs from skin as well as from deep structures. Figure 19 shows an example of the results in the cat. The cutaneous receptive fields of neurons in a given efferent zone were spread over a relatively wide area surrounding the target muscle, but most of them were located on a skin region that lay in the path of the limb movement produced by contraction of the target muscle. The inputs from the deep structures arose mostly from the joint where the target muscle was inserted (18). This input-output relationship is more elaborate in the monkey motor cortex (133). As illustrated in Figure 10, cortical efferent zones that produced contraction of individual muscles were located along the direction of radial fibers within the depth of the motor cortex. While delineating these efferent zones, Rosén and Asanuma (133) examined the peripheral inputs to neurons in each efferent zone. As in the cat, a single zone received various inputs arising from deep as well as superficial receptors. Figure 20 illustrates the input-output relations of cortical efferent zones in a sagittal row of penetrations through the thumb area of the cortex. In addition to passive movements of thumb, two cells in the thumb flexion zone responded to touch of the skin, and the receptive fields of both cells were on the ventral aspect of the thumb. The cells in the zones producing extension, adduction, and abduction of the thumb were activated by touch of the distal tip, medial surface, and lateral surface of the thumb, respectively. The characteristics of this input-output relationship suggested that each zone received afferent inputs related to movement produced by the activity of the same zone, because the receptors were located in the

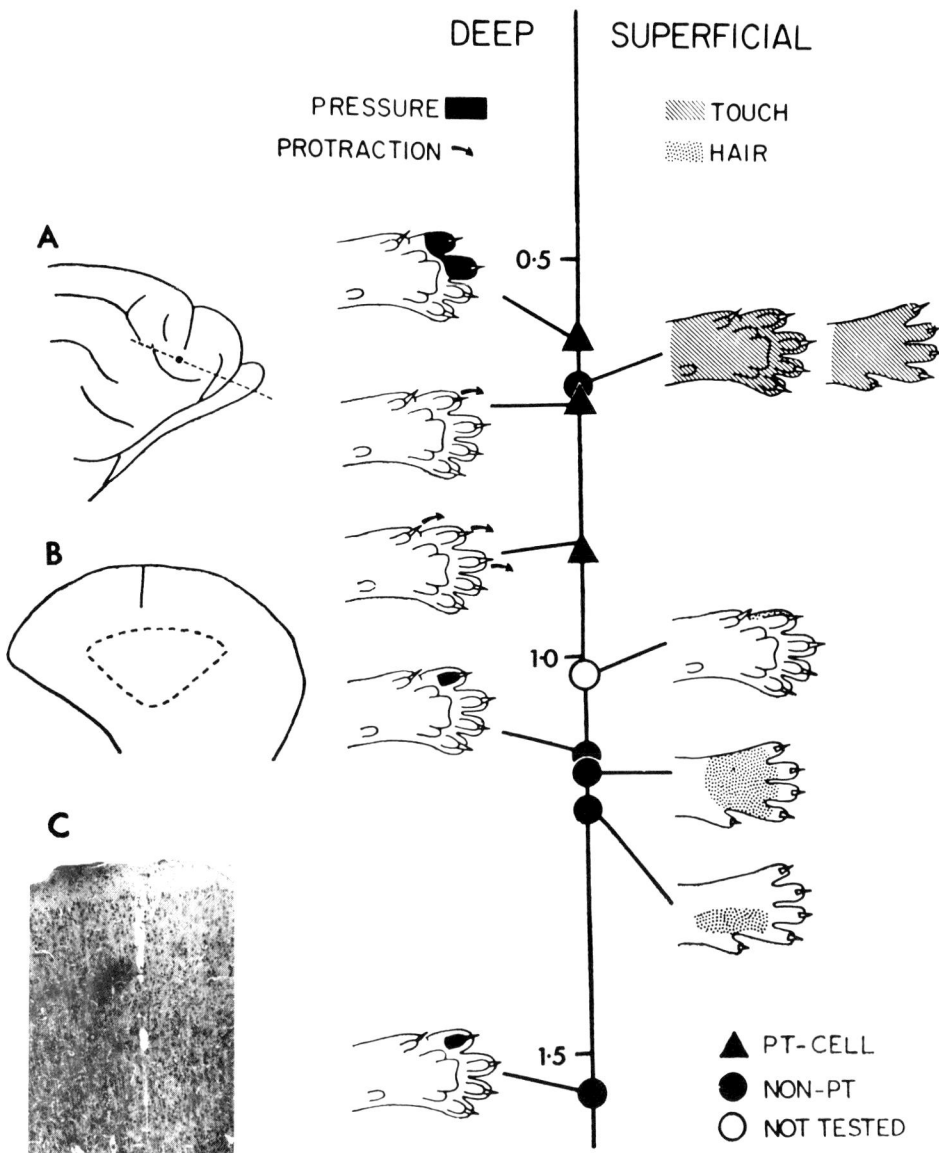

FIG. 18. Example of multimodal sensory inputs from small area in periphery to cortical column in cat. *A*: location of penetration on pericruciate cortex. *Dotted line* indicates sagittal plane of section. *B*: diagram of sagittal section and of radial penetration in gray matter. *C*: photomicrograph of part of section containing penetration. Figurines show peripheral receptive fields. Adequate stimuli to deep structures shown at *left* and those to the superficial structure shown at *right*. [From Welt et al. (159).]

region that tended to be stimulated by contraction of the target muscle. From these experiments in cats and monkeys, it was concluded that a cortical efferent zone receives feedback information related to the contraction of the target muscle.

Lemon et al. (93, 95) studied the input-output relationship with a different approach, using awake monkeys. They recorded activities of precentral neurons while the monkey performed a wide variety of movements in order to collect a food reward placed in a number of different positions. They selected those neurons that showed definite modulation of their discharge frequency related to specific movements about one joint and then examined receptive fields of these neurons by natural stimulation. They reported that the majority of neurons examined received afferent inputs from areas that were anatomically closely related to the joint involved in the movement with which the discharges of the neuron were modulated. These results are in agreement with those obtained using microstimulation methods (133), but Lemon et al. (93, 95) also reported that not all the members of a restricted local population shared the same peripheral territory. These latter results may contradict the previous study (133) in which neurons in a given efferent zone received inputs related to the movements produced by microstimulation of the same zone. This problem was restudied by Murphy and his collabora-

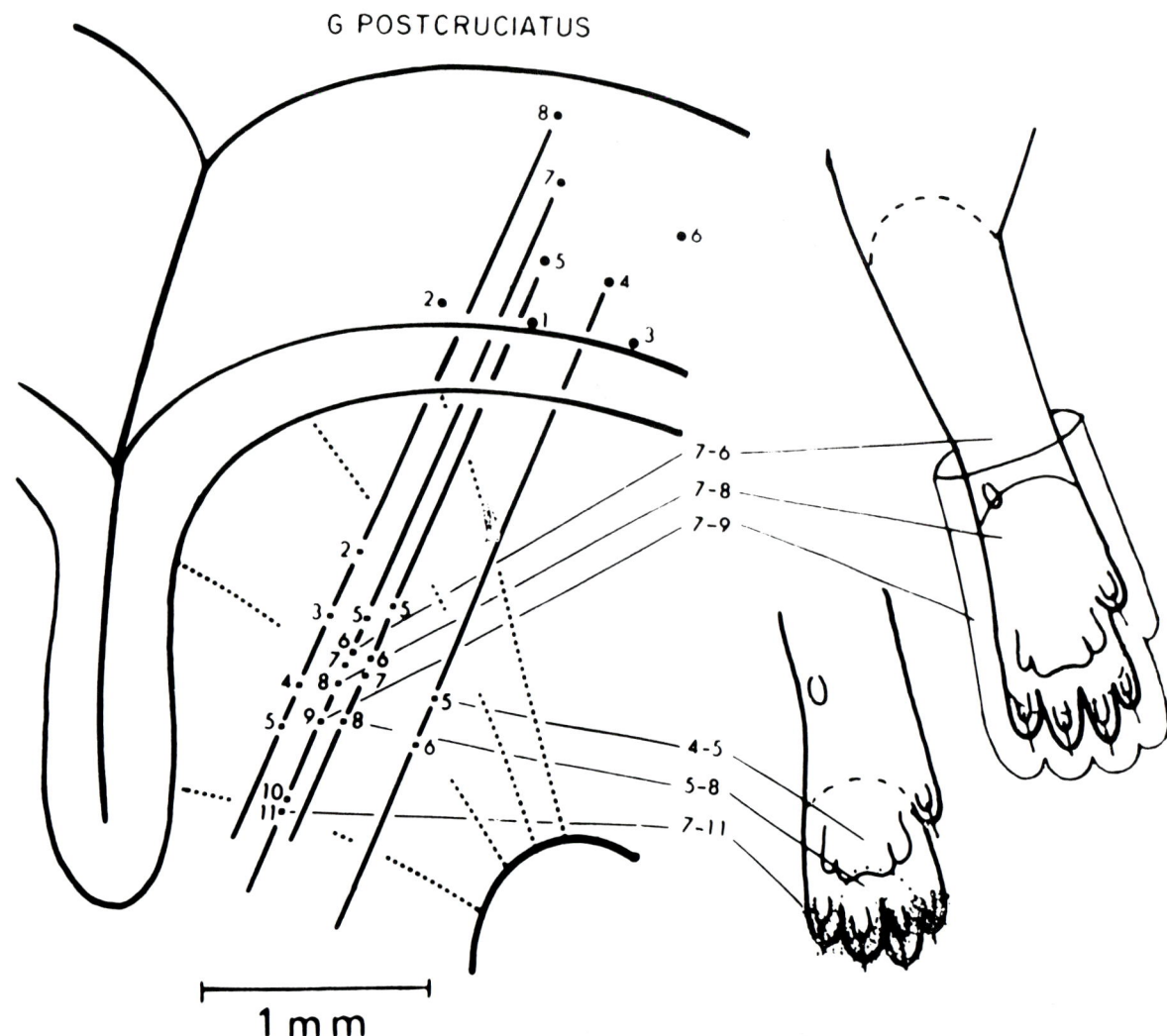

FIG. 19. Afferent inputs converging into cortical efferent zone for palmar muscle. Of 8 penetrations, 4 passed through palmar zone, and 17 cells could be isolated within the zone. Six of 17 cells responded to natural stimulation of skin; receptive fields shown by figurines connected to cell locations by respective lines interrupted by penetration and cell number. These 6 neurons shared common receptive field on ventral surface of paw. [From Asanuma et al. (18).]

tors (115) using awake monkeys and the microstimulation technique. They studied the same monkey over a period of 18 mo and made a detailed map of cortical efferent zones in relation to their afferent inputs. They confirmed the results of Rosén and Asanuma (133) and concluded that the results of Lemon et al. (93) could occur if penetrations were made in the boundary areas of adjacent zones or if they were made in a direction parallel to the cortical surface in the sulcus, which would sequentially traverse several vertical aggregates representing different limb joints. Murphy et al. (115), however, also reported that when neurons received cutaneous inputs the movements induced by microstimulation of the same sites were, in about one-half of the cases, in the direction which withdrew the limb away from the loci of adequate peripheral stimuli. These results were somewhat contradictory to the previous results, because Rosén and Asanuma (133) reported that cells activated by tactile stimuli had receptive fields almost exclusively on the glabrous volar surface of the hand and lay within cortical efferent zones projecting to finger flexor muscles. The controversy might have stemmed from the following differences. In their study, Rosén and Asanuma (133) restricted the stimulating current to 10 μA or less because current beyond this range frequently produced complicated finger movements, making analysis of the results difficult. Because the thresholds for contraction of proximal limb muscles were higher, their study was restricted to areas that induced movement of the hand and fingers. Murphy et al. (115) used stronger current of up to 30 μA and examined input-output relationships not only in the distal, but also in the proximal limb area. These zones from which move-

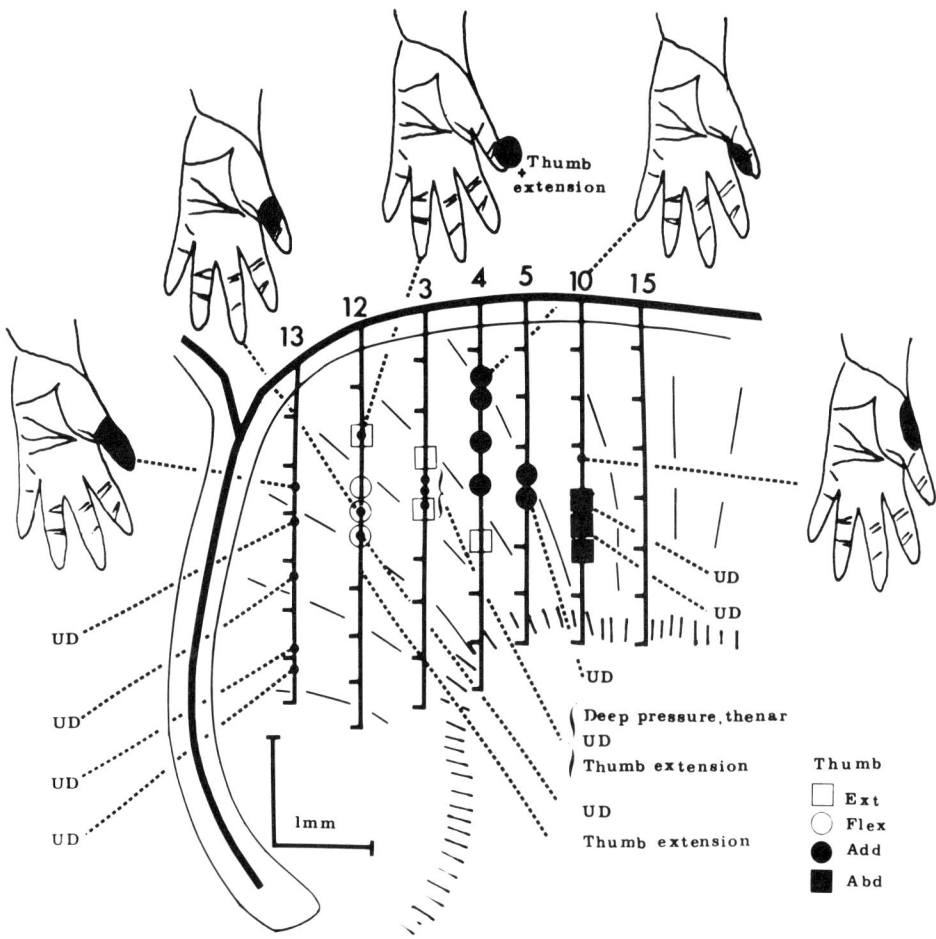

FIG. 20. Afferent inputs converging to thumb area of monkey motor cortex. Several penetrations passed through areas, which when stimulated produced extension, flexion, adduction, or abduction of thumb. Each area marked by symbols explained at *lower right*. Cortical sites from which movement could not be produced are shown by *small bars* on electrode tracks. Locations of isolated cells are indicated by *dots*, and are connected to descriptions of receptive fields and adequate stimuli by *dotted lines*. *Filled areas* on figurines are superficial receptive fields. UD, undriven cells. [From Rosén and Asanuma (133).]

ments were induced away from the peripheral receptive fields were located in the rostral part of the motor cortex and represented proximal limb muscles where cutaneous inputs have not been reported by previous investigations (133, 93). In the results of Murphy et al. obtained from the area near the central sulcus, however, the relationship was the same as that reported by the previous investigators (133). This seems to suggest that the input-output relationship in the proximal limb area is more variable than that in the distal limb area.

In their study, Rosén and Asanuma (133) recorded from a total of 192 cells, and about one-half (45%) responded to peripheral stimulation. The distribution of these responsive cells was not uniform within the motor cortex, however. As already described, not all areas of the motor cortex, even in the distal limb area, produced contraction of muscles with intracortical microstimulation of limited intensity. The low-threshold efferent zones (10 μA or less) were clustered in some parts of the motor cortex constituting an overlapping mosaic, and in other parts the zones were scattered with intercalating silent areas. Peripheral afferent inputs projected more heavily into the low-threshold zones. In the efferent zones 52% of all isolated cells responded to peripheral stimulation, whereas in the silent areas (threshold > 10 μA) only 32% responded. Although an increase in the stimulus intensity delivered within a silent area could produce muscle contractions, the effect then tended to appear in more than one muscle and the input-output relationship became less clear, even in the distal limb area (133).

Asanuma et al. (19, 133) did not identify the receptors located in the muscle. The identity of these receptors has been studied by Murphy et al. (116, 117) using locally anesthetized cats. They denervated the forelimb except for those nerves innervating the extensor digitorum communis muscle and the flexor palmaris longus muscle. After fixation of the elbow joint, the distal tendons of these muscles were severed, and the muscles were stretched by pulling the tendons. Murphy et al. observed that neurons in the motor cortex responded to both low-velocity stretches, which activate primary endings of muscle spindles, and high-velocity stretches, which principally activate secondary spindle endings and Golgi tendon organs. Because they combined intracortical microstimulation with these recordings, they were able to relate the location of these neurons to the cortical efferent zones. They found that neurons showing threshold responses to low-velocity stretches were located exclusively within the cortical efferent zones that projected to the same muscle. Neurons responding to high-velocity stretches were found not only in the same zone, but also—although sparsely—outside of the zone. The results revealed that the cortical efferent zones receive peripheral inputs not only from receptors in the skin, joint, and connective tissues, but also from those located in the muscle itself.

PATHWAYS FROM PERIPHERY TO MOTOR CORTEX. Until recently it has been controversial as to whether the motor cortex receives peripheral inputs directly from the thalamus or only via the sensory cortex (160). There were observations that indicated that some of the inputs from the periphery arrive at the motor cortex directly from the thalamus. Using evoked potential methods, Malis et al. (104) were able to record peripherally evoked potentials in the monkey motor cortex after removal of the sensory cortex. In the cat, Thompson et al. (152) reported that receptive fields of neurons in the motor cortex did not change before and during the cooling of the sensory cortex. The nucleus ventralis posterolateralis of the thalamus, which relays peripheral inputs to the sensory cortex, does not project to the motor cortex, and the nucleus ventralis lateralis, which sends the major inputs to the motor cortex, does not receive peripheral inputs in either cats (19, 106, 107) or monkeys (144). Hence the pathway for direct inputs to the motor cortex was uncertain. Recent development of horseradish peroxidase technique made it possible to reveal finer features of projection than were revealed by the degeneration methods. It has been shown in both cats (88) and monkeys (143) that a small area between the ventralis lateralis and ventralis posterolateralis [(pars oralis of ventralis posterolateralis of Olszewski; (77)] sends fibers directly to the motor cortex. Subsequently the physiological properties of neurons in this border area have been studied in both cats (14) and monkeys (15, 94). In these experiments the thalamic projection neurons were antidromically activated from the motor cortex and then the receptive fields of these identified neurons were examined. In both species, neurons in the border area between the ventralis lateralis and ventralis posterolateralis received somesthetic inputs similar to those received by neurons in the motor cortex. In the example shown in Figure 21, 56 neurons were isolated, and 3 of them were activated antidrom-

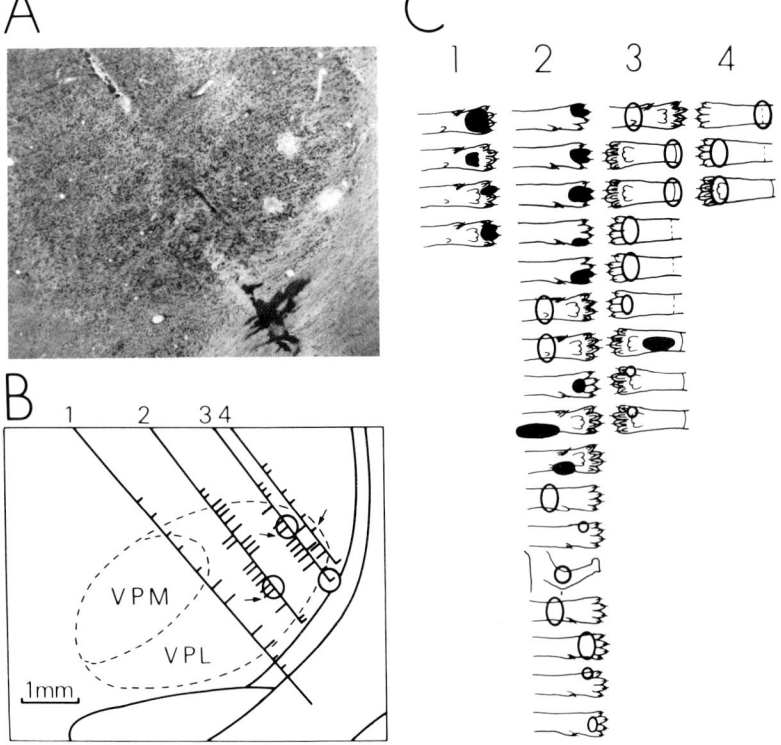

FIG. 21. Thalamic neurons that transfer peripheral somesthetic inputs directly to motor cortex in cat. *A*: sagittal section of ventral thalamus showing electrode tracks and lesions. *B*: reconstruction of tracks from histological preparations. *Short bars* on tracks show locations of neurons with no receptive fields. *Long bars* at *right* are locations of neurons activated from skin receptors. *Long bars* at *left* are those activated from deep receptors. *Circles* indicate lesions made during experiment. *Arrows* indicate neurons activated antidromically from motor cortex. *C*: receptive fields of neurons shown in *B*. *Solid areas* indicate receptive fields for hair bending or light touch. *Circles* indicate deep receptive fields such as pressure or passive joint movement. Numbers on column correspond to track numbers, and each figurine corresponds to respective *long bar* on the track. [From Asanuma et al. (14).]

ically from the motor cortex. Of these 3, 2 were activated by passive movement of joints. Of 40 cells projecting to the motor cortex from the border area, 12 received inputs from the skin, 20 from deep structures, and 8 were undriven from the periphery. Furthermore it has also been shown that ablation of the sensory cortex does not significantly change the characteristics of the receptive field of neurons in the motor cortex in either cats (14) or monkeys (15). It was concluded that at least some of the peripheral somesthetic inputs arrived in the motor cortex directly from the thalamus without passing through the sensory cortex in both cats and monkeys (15).

Pathways conveying the inputs to the motor cortex were studied by making lesions in the spinal cord. Asanuma et al. (17) reported that in the cat the amplitudes of potentials evoked in the motor cortex by stimulation of either skin or muscle afferents were reduced by section of the spinocervical tract or dorsal column. In the monkey (16), section of the dorsal column abolished the evoked potentials in the motor cortex, but spinothalamic tract section reduced the amplitude of the potentials only in the sensory cortex. Brinkman et al. (24) observed that the receptive fields of neurons in the monkey motor cortex disappeared almost completely after dorsal column lesions. From the above experiments it became clear that the dorsal column plays the major role in transferring peripheral inputs to the motor cortex in the monkey, whereas both spinocervical tract and dorsal column are involved in the cat.

The simplest connections between the motor cortex and the periphery are shown diagrammatically in Figure 22. This diagram is meant to illustrate only a part of the connections between the cortex and the periphery. Pathways are shown by which cortically induced movements send peripheral information directly back to the original cortical areas continuously during movements.

FUNCTIONAL SIGNIFICANCE OF PERIPHERAL INPUTS TO MOTOR CORTEX. It has been shown that voluntary movement is severely disturbed by interrupting inputs from the periphery. Mott and Sherrington (112) reported that deafferentation of the upper limb resulted in a loss of the use of the hand, closely resembling the symptoms that follow ablation of the motor cortex, although the responses to electrical stimulation of the cortex were not impaired. This experiment was repeated by many investigators, and it was found that the loss of the movement is not permanent. It became clear that in certain circumstances the monkey can eventually ambulate with the deafferented arm and can also learn to reach for food using visual guidance, although the movement is not as smooth as in the normal animal (82). These observations demonstrate the importance of afferent inputs for voluntary movements, but the role of afferent inputs arriving directly at the motor cortex is still in question. In normal

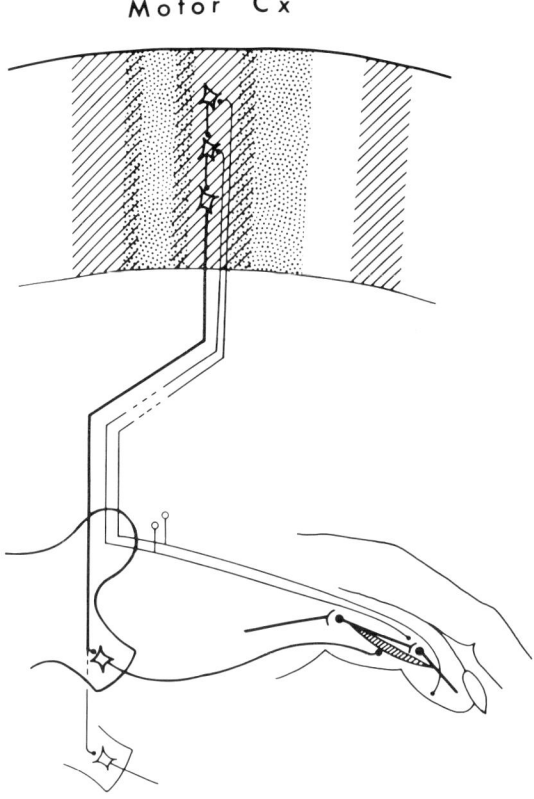

FIG. 22. Simplified diagram of connections between motor cortex (motor Cx) and periphery. Neurons in motor cortex are connected predominantly in radial direction and are subdivided into cortical efferent zones marked by *hatched* and *dotted* areas. Fringes of these efferent zones overlap with fringes of others, constituting overlapping mosaic within cortex. These efferent zones are intercalated with silent areas where threshold for motor effect is high. Corticospinal fibers from given efferent zone project most heavily to given motor nuclei to produce contraction of a muscle, but they also project to other motor nuclei to produce subliminal fringes of excitation. Afferent inputs originated by contraction of target muscle ascend spinal cord and project to original efferent zone directly through nucleus ventralis pars oralis, constituting a closed loop between cortex and periphery. This corticoperipheral loop circuit is well developed for distal limb muscles but is less clear for proximal muscles.

animals the reflexes in which the motor cortex is known to participate are the placing (21) and grasping (37) reactions. Both reactions can be elicited by tactile stimulation of a part of a limb. Although it is possible that the peripheral inputs arriving directly at the motor cortex play some role in these reflexes, it is unlikely that they play a major role. Both reflexes persist as long as sensory and motor cortices are intact, but disappear after either the sensory or the motor cortex is removed, whereas the peripheral inputs to the motor cortex persist after ablation of the sensory cortex. Furthermore it has been shown recently in the kitten (52) that the tactile placing reaction persisted in the hindlimb after transection to the spinal cord at the level of the first lumbar segment. Amassian (3) reported that in the kitten tactile placing was subserved by a subcortical circuit, and the subsequent involvement of the cerebral cortex started to occur through tonic rather than dynamic activity. The results suggest that tactile placing is a subcortical or even a spinal reflex. As the tactile placing reaction disappears with pyramidal section in adult monkeys (154), the role of the pyramidal tract in the adult monkey may be to modulate the activity of subcortical circuits. These circuits may be activated not by the direct inputs to the motor cortex, but by the inputs to the sensory cortex, which are then relayed to the motor cortex via corticocortical and/or subcortical pathways.

It was proposed that the direct sensory inputs to the motor cortex function as positive feedback information related to movements (15). As the type of inputs to the cortex and the nature of efferent projection to the muscle indicate the existence of loop circuits between the motor cortex and the periphery, it is possible that impulses circulate within a set of circuits during a particular movement. This circulation of the impulses could result in an increase of the excitability of efferent and afferent relay nuclei involved in these circuits and subsequently further increase the excitability of related cortical efferent zones. Such an increased excitability of these loop circuits including the cortical efferent zones could alter the efficacy of excitatory and inhibitory inputs from other pathways. Because the motor cortex is known to be involved in multiple-loop circuits with various sites in the central nervous system, such as other areas of the cerebral cortex, subcortical nuclei, and cerebellum, there is the possibility for an interaction of these circuits, including the one between the cortex and the periphery, in the production of various combinations of muscle contractions during normal movements.

Inputs Through Association Fibers

The existence of interconnections between various parts of the cortex has been known for a long time, but detailed studies were made after the introduction of the Nauta method (118). The development of autoradiography and horseradish peroxidase methods have made it possible to reveal yet a finer structure of the connections between various areas, and these studies are progressing rapidly. Stimulated by these findings, physiological experiments are also vigorously being carried out. The following section describes the recent information concerning the fine connections between the motor cortex and other areas of the cortex.

INPUTS FROM SENSORY CORTEX. The connections between the motor and the sensory cortices have been studied extensively. Using the Nauta method, Jones and Powell (78, 80) studied these connections in the cat and the monkey. They found that in both species the first and second somatic sensory area and the motor cortex are all reciprocally interconnected by association fibers. Physiological studies in the monkey have revealed that different areas of the primary sensory cortex receive different inputs from the periphery. Areas 1 and 2 receive inputs primarily from receptors located in deep structures such as those excited by rotation of or pressure on joints, whereas area 3b receives inputs from receptors in the skin (129). In both cats and monkeys, neurons in area 3a receive inputs primarily from group I muscle afferent fibers (4, 121, 128). Projections from these subdivisions of the sensory cortex to the motor cortex have been studied subsequently. Grant et al. (58), using cats, made a needle-stitch lesion in area 3a where the maximal group I–evoked potential was recorded. They found that degenerating U-fibers originating from the lesion traveled in the white matter to the cortex of areas 4γ, 3b, and 2. These fibers branched in layer III, and some of them reached layer I. The degenerated fibers were distributed as distinct columns with a diameter of about 1 mm, the same diameter as the cortical efferent zones in the motor cortex. Zarzecki et al. (164), using anesthetized cats, studied the physiological properties of projection neurons in area 3a, which were identified by their antidromic activation from the motor cortex (area 4γ). They showed that most of the projection neurons were located in layer III, with some in layer V. By recording intracellularly from those neurons, they were able to demonstrate strong excitatory synaptic inputs from group I afferents. The information transferred by these corticocortical fibers may contribute to the formation of receptive fields of neurons in the motor cortex, but it probably does not play a major role because cooling area 3a does not abolish inputs from a specific muscle to neurons in a given efferent zone (116).

Theories concerning the functional significance of this projection are still controversial. One of the suggested functions has been a participation in cortical regulation of muscle contraction. It has been shown that the sudden extension of the forearm of a human subject could evoke two separate bursts of electromyographic activity in the biceps muscle (62). The first was identified as the tendon jerk by its short latency. The second burst had a latency of about 50 ms, and the magnitude of this component increased when the subject resisted the tension and decreased when he was told to "let go" (61). This second burst was termed "function stretch reflex" (109), and Marsden et al. (105) suggested that this reflex might serve to counteract unexpected loads encountered in the course of a willed movement. They proposed that this reflex was mediated by a relatively simple transcortical loop. Several studies have been carried out to clarify the role of sensory and motor cortices in this reflex using chronically trained monkeys (42, 44, 151). It was shown later (56), however, that the two separate bursts of electromyographic activity persisted in decerebrate and spinal cats. These results indicate that the second burst does not necessitate the transcortical loop that carries group I muscle afferents. One possibility is that the cortex influences the functional stretch reflex by tonically changing the excitability of the lower centers. Another suggestion has been made by Phillips (127) based on the following evidence. Foerster (51) reported that rhizotomy performed on patients with intractable pain impaired most severely the manipulation of individual fingers, although the patients could move their arms and hands. On the other hand, Merton (110) reported that deprivation of all inputs other than the spindle feedback did not impair the movement of the thumb in a normal subject. In this experiment a sphygmomanometer cuff was kept inflated at the wrist until all sensation was lost from the hand. Skin and joints and intrinsic hand muscles were thus reversibly denervated, but the spindle feedback from the long flexors and extensors of the fingers remained intact. In this condition the subject was still able to move his thumb voluntarily and even to move a pointer attached to it through a prescribed angle. Eklund and Hagbarth (38) reported the following experiments. A normal subject was instructed to try to maintain a steady isometric force, flexing the elbow against a restraining strain-gauge dynamometer at the wrist. When the biceps tendon was vibrated, there was a large increase in force of which the subject was quite unaware. As longitudinal vibration is a highly selective stimulus to the primary endings of the muscle spindles (29), it is likely that the artificially disturbed spindle feedback provided the wrong information. Based on these evidences and on the results of his group (87) that colonies of corticomotoneuronal neurons have a direct and powerful connection with the motoneurons innervating the hand muscles in the baboon, Phillips (127) proposed that inputs from muscle spindles to the cortex may function as part of a transcortical servo loop that signals the discrepancy between intended and actual movements.

Jones et al. (77), using anterograde and retrograde transport methods, and Vogt and Pandya (156), using a degeneration method, have more detailed studies of projections from the somatic sensory areas in the monkey. Both groups reported that area 3b, which is known to receive inputs primarily from skin receptors, did not project to the motor cortex but projected to areas 1 and 2. Area 1 was reciprocally connected to area 3 but sent the strongest projection to area 2, and area 2 was reciprocally connected to the motor cortex. Neurons in area 2 receive inputs predominantly from receptors in deep structures (129) in the monkey, and it is possible that area 2 transfers these inputs to the motor cortex. It is also known, however, that in the monkey, receptive fields of neurons in the motor cortex do not change significantly after removal of the sensory cortex, including area 2 (15). In addition the virtual absence of projection from areas 3b and 1 to the motor cortex makes it unlikely that corticocortical projections play an important role in forming cutaneous receptive fields of neurons in the motor cortex.

INPUTS FROM ASSOCIATION CORTEX. Strick and Kim (146), using the horseradish peroxidase method, and Zarzecki et al. (165), using physiological methods, demonstrated that there was a rather heavy projection from area 5 to area 4 in the monkey, and that the projection was topographically arranged. It has been reported by Mountcastle et al. (114) that some neurons in areas 5 and 7 of the monkey cortex were not activated by sensory stimuli but were discharged at high rates when the animal moved its arm to obtain an object. They proposed that these neurons function in a command fashion, directing visual attention to and the exploration of the immediately surrounding extrapersonal space. The strong connection between area 5 and the motor cortex suggests a functional coupling between the two areas, but whether or not this connection plays an important role in the command of movement, which is a complex function, is still in question.

Inputs Through Commissural Fibers

Much is known about the commissural connections for the visual and association cortices, but few studies have been carried out concerning the connections between the motor cortices. Using cats, Asanuma and Okuda (19) reported that orthodromic excitation of pyramidal tract cells could be evoked from a circumscribed area of the contralateral cortex. The excitatory point was surrounded by an area, the stimulation of which inhibited the discharges that were evoked from the center. The results suggested the existence of topographic projections between cortices with a general feature of an on-center, off-periphery arrangement. This, however, does not seem to be the general scheme of connection between the motor cortices, because it was later found in the monkey (122) that although axial and limb girdle areas of the precentral areas are mutually interconnected, the neurons in the hand and foot areas do not project to the contralateral cortex. There is a somewhat similar arrangement in the somatosensory area in the cat in which the callosal connections are limited to areas representing the face, trunk, and limb girdles (79). These results are interesting because they suggest that distal limb areas controlling the fine movements of limbs are mutually independent, which may be important for the production of a variety of combinations of independent limb movements.

FUNCTION OF PYRAMIDAL TRACT

The traditional methods of studying the functions of the central nervous system are to stimulate or ablate a part of the system and to observe the effects. Stimulation experiments were dealt with in the preceding sections, and only ablation experiments are described in this section. A new method introduced recently in which activities of individual neurons are studied in relation to trained movements of the animal (41) are not discussed here. The results from this latter type of experiment are described fully in the chapter by Evarts in this *Handbook*.

To study the genesis of the symptoms of hemiplegia has been one of the most intriguing challenges to the neurologist and neurophysiologist. Hemiplegia, caused by damage to the internal capsule, is typified by paralysis with spasticity. It is accompanied by exaggerated deep tendon reflexes, the Babinski sign, and absence of abdominal and cremasteric reflexes. All of these symptoms were once thought to be caused by a lesion of the pyramidal tract. Accumulation of careful clinical observations had cast some doubt on this interpretation, although the controversy continued as to whether the lesion of the pyramidal tract contributed to the spasticity of the muscles. It was Tower (154) who clearly demonstrated that a pyramidal lesion did not produce spastic paralysis. The main deficits after pyramidal section were diminished muscle tone, diminished cutaneous reflexes, slow tendon reflexes restricted to the stimulated muscle, and defective initiation and execution of all performance by skeletal musculature, particularly the loss of all discrete usage of digits. The tactile placing reaction was lost permanently, but a Babinski sign did not develop although it was later shown that the Babinski sign could develop in the chimpanzee after pyramidal section (69). Tower summarized pyramidal functions in space and time as follows: "The spatial function is the ability to bring into action any portion of the skeletal musculature, and in all combinations. This detailed control of the skeletal musculature enables the discrete usage of musculature, especially of the digits, and the modulation of extrapyramidal activity, which are outstanding pyramidal functions. In time, the pyramidal tract operates in two phases. One is a continuous, or tonic, action in effect at all times in the waking state. The other is a specifically timed increase of discharge, or phasic action, which is evoked in relation to particular situations." She concluded that "together, the tonic function provides for smooth, continuous, efficient action while the phasic function contributes, outstandingly, precision and lability to total performance."

The pioneering work of Tower has been repeated, and the results have been confirmed by many investigators, but there were some controversies. One of the problems was whether or not the loss of control of fine movements was permanent. Bucy et al. (30) cut the cerebral peduncles bilaterally, although not always completely. They observed that some of the fully recovered animals were able to use the thumb and index finger along to pick up food, although others could not. The difficulty in these experiments was determining the extent of the pyramidal section. Lawrence and Kuypers (92) argued that the recovery was caused by incomplete section of the pyramidal tract. They interrupted the pyramidal tract bilaterally in 39 monkeys, and in 8 of them the lesion was virtually limited to the pyramidal tracts. These animals could sit with head up and could stand, walk, run, and climb immediately following the operation. They soon regained the capacity for independent use of their extremities, and within 3 wk they could reach accurately with either hand to pick up morsels of food by closure of all fingers in concert. Individual finger movements never returned, however, even after recovery periods of up to 11 mo. In addition all movements were slower, and the monkeys fatigued more rapidly than normal animals. These results virtually confirmed the observations reported by Tower, except for their emphasis that pyramidal deficits were more restricted to the manipulation of distal extremities. Using the monkey, Hepp-Reymond and Wiesendanger (64) and Hepp-Reymond et al. (65) examined the effect of pyramidal section on the reaction time and force exerted during precision tasks. The monkeys were trained to squeeze a transducer between the thumb and index finger and were tested before and after unilateral or bilateral pyramidotomy. After partial pyramidotomy there was a long-lasting slowing in the performance of the finger grip. This delay was due not only to weakness of the muscle contraction, but also to delay in the initiation of the movement. These results partially conflict with the results reported by Laursen and Wiesendanger (91) on cats and Laursen (90) on monkeys. In both of these experiments, the animal was trained to react to the test stimulus in different fashions, depending on the conditioning stimulus. After partial pyramidotomy it was found that the reaction time was increased when a choice was involved but not when discrimination was unnecessary. It should be noted that in these discrimination experiments (90, 91), arm and wrist movements were studied, whereas for the precision tasks described above (64, 65), finger movements were necessary. The involvement of different muscle groups in the two experimental situations may account for the difference in conclusions. The experiments of Laursen and Wiesendanger (91) and Laursen (90) are important because they suggest that the pyramidal tract participates in movements that involve learning and selection.

In this section only representative studies that examined the permanent deficits produced by pyramidal section were discussed. It should be noted, however, that a well-known feature of the central nervous system is "redundancy of function," and loss of function produced by ablation of one system is rapidly compensated for by other systems. Thus it is obvious that the permanent functional deficits produced by pyramidal section reveal only a part of pyramidal functions, all of which cannot be explored by simply destroying the pyramidal tract. However, whether the initial deficits that recover as time passes are also due to the loss of pyramidal function or to other factors such as pressure temporarily produced by acute hemorrhage is difficult to determine (37). This is one of the reasons why there is still controversy between the interpretation of the results of stimulation experiments and ablation experiments.

SUMMARY

Twenty years have passed since the publication of the chapter on the pyramidal tract by Patton and Amassian in the *Handbook of Physiology's* first edition of the nervous system (123a). During this time a remarkable progress has been made in our understandings of the structure and function of this tract. Detailed distribution of the origin and the termination of the pyramidal tract neurons has been worked out. Progress in recording techniques have enabled us to study the nature of afferent inputs to individual pyramidal tract neurons. Microstimulation technique revealed columnar organization of cortical efferent zones. Introduction of the horseradish peroxidase method is still exploring various connections to the motor cortex. Thus the wealth of knowledge we have accumulated becomes incomparable to that which we possessed 20 years ago, as is evidenced by the richness of description in this chapter. We hope that the progress in the coming 20 years will be as fruitful as in the past and will explore further the details of the pyramidal functions.

GENERAL REFERENCES*

ASANUMA, H. Recent developments in the study of the columnar arrangement of neurons within the motor cortex. *Physiol. Rev.* 55: 143-156, 1975.

BROOKS, V. B., AND S. D. STONEY, JR. Motor mechanisms: the role of the pyramidal system in motor control. *Annu. Rev. Physiol.* 33: 337-392, 1971.

HENNEMAN, E. Motor functions of the cerebral cortex. In: *Medical Physiology* (14th ed.), edited by V. B. Mountcastle. St. Louis: Mosby, 1980, vol. 1, pt. VII, p. 859-889.

PATTON, H. D., AND V. E. AMASSIAN. The pyramidal tract: its excitation and functions. In: *Handbook of Physiology. Neurophysiology*, edited by J. Field. Washington, DC: Am. Physiol. Soc., 1960, sect. I, vol. 2, p. 837-861.

PHILLIPS, C. G., AND R. PORTER. *Corticospinal Neurons: Their Role in Movement.* London: Academic, 1977.

WIESENDANGER, M. The pyramidal tract: recent investigations on its morphology and function. *Ergeb. Physiol.* 61: 73-135, 1969.

REFERENCES

1. ADRIAN, E. D., AND G. MORUZZI. Impulses in the pyramidal tract. *J. Physiol. London* 97: 153-199, 1939.
2. ALBE-FESSARD, D., J. M. BESSON, AND M. ABDELMOUNENE. Action of anesthetics on somatic evoked activities. In: *Anesthesia and Neurophysiology*, edited by H. Yamamura. Boston: Little, Brown, 1970, p. 129-158.
3. AMASSIAN, V. E. The use of contact placing in analytical and synthetic studies of the higher sensorimotor control system. In: *Integration in the Nervous System*, edited by H. Asanuma and V. J. Wilson. Tokyo: Igaku Shoin, 1979, p. 279-304.
4. AMASSIAN, V. E., AND L. BERLIN. Early cortical projection or group 1 afferents in the forelimb muscle nerves of cat. *J. Physiol. London* 143: 61, 1958.
5. AMASSIAN, V. E., AND H. WEINER. Monosynaptic and polysynaptic activation of pyramidal tract neurons by thalamic stimulation. In: *The Thalamus*, edited by D. P. Purpura and M. D. Yahr. New York: Columbia Univ. Press, 1966, p. 255-282.
6. ANDERSEN, P., J. C. ECCLES, AND T. A. SEARS. Cortically evoked depolarization of primary afferent fibers in the spinal cord. *J. Neurophysiol.* 27: 62-77, 1964.
7. ANDERSEN, P., P. J. HAGAN, C. G. PHILLIPS, AND T. P. S. POWELL. Mapping by microstimulation of overlapping projections from area 4 to motor units of the baboon's hand. *Proc. R. Soc. London Ser. B* 188: 31-60, 1975.
8. ASANUMA, H., AND A. P. ARNOLD. Noxious effects of excessive currents used for intracortical microstimulation. *Brain Res.* 96: 103-107, 1975.
9. ASANUMA, H., AND O. OKUDA. Effects of transcallosal volleys on pyramidal tract cell activity of cat. *J. Neurophysiol.* 25: 198-208, 1962.
10. ASANUMA, H., AND I. ROSÉN. Topographical organization of cortical efferent zones projecting to distal forelimb muscles in the monkey. *Exp. Brain Res.* 14: 243-256, 1972.

11. ASANUMA, H., AND I. ROSÉN. Spread of mono- and polysynaptic connections within cat's motor cortex. *Exp. Brain Res.* 16: 507-520, 1973.
12. ASANUMA, H., AND H. SAKATA. Functional organization of a cortical efferent system examined with focal depth stimulation in cats. *J. Neurophysiol.* 30: 35-54, 1967.
13. ASANUMA, H., A. ARNOLD, AND P. ZARZECKI. Further study on the excitation of pyramidal tract cells by intracortical microstimulation. *Exp. Brain Res.* 26: 443-461, 1976.
14. ASANUMA, H., K. D. LARSEN, AND H. YUMIYA. Somatosensory inputs from the thalamus to the motor cortex in the cat. *Brain Res.* 172: 217-228, 1979.
15. ASANUMA, H., K. D. LARSEN, AND H. YUMIYA. Direct sensory pathways to the motor cortex in the monkey: a basis of cortical reflexes. In: *Integration in the Nervous System*, edited by H. Asanuma and V. J. Wilson. Tokyo: Igaku Shoin, 1979, p. 223-238.
16. ASANUMA, H., K. D. LARSEN, AND H. YUMIYA. Peripheral input pathways to the monkey motor cortex. *Exp. Brain Res.* 38: 349-355, 1980.
17. ASANUMA, H., K. D. LARSEN, AND P. ZARZECKI. Peripheral input pathways projecting to the motor cortex in the cat. *Brain Res.* 172: 197-208, 1979.
18. ASANUMA, H., S. D. STONEY, JR., AND C. ABZUG. Relationship between afferent input and motor outflow in cat motorsensory cortex. *J. Neurophysiol.* 31: 670-681, 1968.
19. ASANUMA, H., J. FERNANDES, M. E. SCHEIBEL, AND A. B. SCHEIBEL. Characteristics of projections from the nucleus ventralis lateralis to the motor cortex in the cats: an anatomical and physiological study. *Exp. Brain Res.* 20: 315-330, 1974.
20. ASANUMA, H., P. ZARZECKI, E. JANKOWSKA, T. HONGO, AND S. MARCUS. Projection of individual pyramidal tract neurons to lumbar motoneuron pools of the monkey. *Exp. Brain Res.* 34: 73-89, 1979.
21. BARD, P. Studies on the cortical representation of somatic sensibility. *Bull. NY Acad. Med.* 14: 585-607, 1938.

* These general references provide an excellent overview of the field; specific references cited in the text follow.

22. BERNARD, C. G., AND E. BOHM. Cortical representation and functional significance of the corticomotoneuronal system. *Arch. Neurol. Psychiatry* 72: 473-502, 1954.
23. BLUM, B., L. M. HALPERN, AND A. A. WARD, JR. Microelectrode studies of the afferent connections and efferent projections of neurons in the sensorimotor cortex of the cat. *Exp. Neurol.* 20: 156-173, 1968.
24. BRINKMAN, J., B. M. BUSH, AND R. PORTER. Deficient influences of peripheral stimuli on precentral neurons in monkeys with dorsal column lesions. *J. Physiol. London* 276: 27-48, 1978.
25. BRODAL, A. *Neurological Anatomy* (2nd ed.). London: Oxford Univ. Press, 1969.
26. BROOKS, V. B., AND H. ASANUMA. Recurrent effects following stimulation of medullary pyramid. *Arch. Ital. Biol.* 103: 247-278, 1965.
27. BROOKS, V. B., P. RUDOMIN, AND C. L. SLAYMAN. Sensory activation of neurons in the cat's cerebral cortex. *J. Neurophysiol.* 24: 286-301, 1961.
28. BROOKS, V. B., P. RUDOMIN, AND C. L. SLAYMAN. Peripheral receptive fields of neurons in the cat's cerebral cortex. *J. Neurophysiol.* 24: 302-325, 1961.
29. BROWN, M. C., I. ENGBERG, AND P. B. C. MATHEWS. The relative sensitivity to vibration of muscle receptors in the cat. *J. Physiol. London* 192: 773-800, 1967.
30. BUCY, P. C., R. LADPLI, AND A. EHRLICH. Destruction of the pyramidal tract in the monkey. The effects of bilateral section of the cerebral peduncles. *J. Neurosurg.* 25: 1-23, 1966.
31. BURKE, R. E., P. L. STRICK, K. KANDA, C. C. KIN, AND B. WALMSLEY. Anatomy of medial gastrocnemius and soleus motor nuclei in cat spinal cord. *J. Neurophysiol.* 40: 667-680, 1977.
32. BUSER, P., AND M. IMBERT. Sensory projections to the motor cortex in cats. In: *Sensory Communication*, edited by W. A. Rosenblith. New York: Wiley, 1961, p. 607-626.
33. CHANG, H-T., T. C. RUCH, AND A. A. WARD, JR. Topographical representation of muscles in motor cortex of monkeys. *J. Neurophysiol.* 10: 39-56, 1947.
34. CLOUGH, J. F. M., C. G. PHILLIPS, AND J. D. SHERIDAN. The short latency projection from the baboon's motor cortex to fusimotor neurons of the forearm and hand. *J. Physiol. London* 216: 257-279, 1971.
35. COLONNIER, M. L. The structural design of the neocortex. In: *Brain and Conscious Experience*, edited by J. C. Eccles. New York: Springer-Verlag, 1966, p. 1-23.
36. COULTER, J. D., L. EWING, AND C. CARTER. Origin of primary sensorimotor cortical projection to lumbar spinal cord of cat and monkey. *Brain Res.* 103: 366-372, 1976.
37. DENNY-BROWN, D. *The Cerebral Control of Movement*. Springfield, IL: Thomas, 1966.
38. EKLUND, G., AND K-E. HAGBARTH. Normal variability of tonic vibration reflexes in man. *Exp. Neurol.* 16: 80-92, 1966.
39. ELGER, C. E., E.-J. SPECKMAN, H. CASPERS, AND R. W. C. JANZEN. Cortico-spinal connections in the rat. I. Monosynaptic and polysynaptic responses of cervical motoneurons to epicortical stimulation. *Exp. Brain Res.* 28: 385-404, 1977.
40. ENDO, K., T. ARAKI, AND N. YAGI. The distribution and pattern of axon branching of pyramidal tract cells. *Brain Res.* 57: 484-491, 1973.
41. EVARTS, E. V. Representation of movements and muscles by pyramidal tract neurons of the precentral motor cortex. In: *Neurophysical Basis of Normal and Abnormal Motor Activities*, edited by D. P. Purpura and M. D. Yahr. Hewlett, NY: Raven, 1967, p. 215-251.
42. EVARTS, E. V. Motor cortex reflexes associated with learned movements. *Science* 179: 501-503, 1973.
43. EVARTS, E. V. Activity of thalamic and cortical neurons in relation to learned movement in the monkey. *Int. J. Neurol.* 8: 321-326, 1971.
44. EVARTS, E. V., AND J. TANJI. Gating of motor cortex reflexes by prior instruction. *Brain Res.* 71: 479-494, 1974.
45. FERRIER, D. Experiments on the brain of monkeys. *Proc. R. Soc. London* 23: 409-430, 1875.
46. FERRIER, D. *The Functions of the Brain*. London: Smith, Elder, 1876.
47. FETZ, E. E. Pyramidal tract effects on interneurons in the cat lumbar dorsal horn. *J. Neurophysiol.* 31: 69-80, 1968.
48. FETZ, E. E., AND P. D. CHENEY. Muscle fields of primate corticomotoneuronal cells. *J. Physiol. Paris* 74: 239-245, 1978.
49. FETZ, E. E., P. D. CHENEY, AND D. C. GERMAN. Corticomotoneuronal connections of precentral cells detected by postspike averaging of EMG activity in behaving monkeys. *Brain Res.* 114: 505-510, 1976.
50. FIDONE, S. J., AND J. B. PRESTON. Patterns of motor cortex control of flexor extensor cat fusimotor neurons. *J. Neurophysiol.* 32: 103-115, 1969.
51. FOERSTER, O. Schlaffe und spastische Lämung. In: *Handbuch der Normalen und Pathologishen Physiologie*, edited by A. Bethe, G. V. Bergman, G. Embden, and A. Ellinger. Berlin: Springer-Verlag, 1927, p. 900-901.
52. FORSSBERG, H., S. GRILLNER, AND A. SJÖSTRÖM. Tactile placing reactions in chronic spinal kittens. *Acta Physiol. Scand.* 92: 114-120, 1974.
53. FRITSCH, G., AND E. HITZIG. Ueber die elektrische Erregbarkeit des Grosshirns. *Arch. Anat. Physiol. Wiss. Med.* 37: 300-332, 1870.
54. FUTAMI, T., Y. SHINODA, AND J. YOKOTA. Spinal axon collaterals of corticospinal neurons identified by intracellular injection of horseradish peroxidase. *Brain Res.* 164: 279-284, 1979.
55. GATTER, K. C., AND T. P. S. POWELL. The intrinsic connections of the cortex of area 4 of the monkey. *Brain* 101: 513-541, 1978.
56. GHEZ, C., AND Y. SHINODA. Spinal mechanisms of the functional stretch reflex. *Exp. Brain Res.* 32: 55-68, 1978.
57. GORDON, G., AND R. MILLER. Identification of cortical cells projecting to the dorsal column nuclei of the cat. *Q. J. Exp. Physiol.* 54: 85-98, 1969.
58. GRANT, G., S. LANDGREN, AND H. SILFVENIUS. Columnar distribution of U-fibers from the postcruciate cerebral projection area of the cat's group I muscle afferents. *Exp. Brain Res.* 24: 57-74, 1975.
59. GRIGG, P., AND J. B. PRESTON. Baboon flexor and extensor fusimotor neurons and their modulation by motor cortex. *J. Neurophysiol.* 34: 428-436, 1971.
60. GROOS, W. P., L. K. EWING, C. M. CARTER, AND J. D. COULTER. Organization of corticospinal neurons in the cat. *Brain Res.* 143: 393-419, 1978.
61. HAMMOND, P. H. The influence of prior instruction to the subject on an apparently involuntary neuromuscular response. *J. Physiol. London* 132: 17, 1956.
62. HAMMOND, P. H. Experimental study of servo action in human muscular control. *Proc. III Int. Congr. Med. Elect. London, 1960*, p. 190-191. (Inst. Electr. Eng.)
63. HASSLER, R., AND K. MUHS-CLEMENT. Architektonisher Aufbau der sensomotorischen und parietalen Cortex der Katze. *J. Hirnforsch.* 6: 377-420, 1964.
64. HEPP-REYMOND, M.-C., AND M. WIESENDANGER. Unilateral pyramidotomy in monkeys; effect on force and speed of a conditioned precision grip. *Brain Res.* 36: 117-131, 1972.
65. HEPP-REYMOND, M.-C., E. TROUCHE, AND M. WIESENDANGER. Effects of unilateral and bilateral pyramidotomy on a conditioned rapid precision grip in monkeys (*Macaca fascicularis*). *Exp. Brain Res.* 21: 519-527, 1974.
66. HERN, J. E. C., S. LANDGREN, C. G. PHILLIPS, AND R. PORTER. Selective excitation of corticofugal neurones by surface-anodal stimulation of the baboon's motor cortex. *J. Physiol. London* 161: 73-90, 1962.
67. HERN, J. E. C., C. G. PHILLIPS, AND R. PORTER. Electrical thresholds of unimpaled corticospinal cells in the cat. *Q. J. Exp. Physiol.* 47: 134-140, 1962.
68. HESS, R., K. NEGISHI, AND O. CREUTZFELDT. The horizontal spread of intracortical inhibition in the visual cortex. *Exp. Brain Res.* 22: 415-419, 1975.
69. HINES, M. Significance of the precentral motor cortex. In: *The Precentral Motor Cortex*, edited by P. C. Bucy. Urbana: Univ. of Illinois Press, 1944, p. 461-494.

70. HUBEL, D. H., AND T. N. WIESEL. Shape and arrangement of columns in cat's striate cortex. *J. Physiol. London* 165: 559-568, 1963.
71. HUMPHREY, D. R., AND W. S. CORRIE. Properties of pyramidal tract neuron system within a functionally defined subregion of primate motor cortex. *J. Neurophysiol.* 41: 216-243, 1978.
72. HUMPHREY, D. R., AND R. R. RIETZ. Cells of origin of corticorubral projections from the arm area of the primate motor cortex and their synaptic actions in the red nucleus. *Brain Res.* 110: 162-169, 1976.
73. JABBUR, S. J., AND A. L. TOWE. Cortical excitation of neurons in dorsal column nuclei of cat, including an analysis of pathways. *J. Neurophysiol.* 24: 499-509, 1961.
74. JANKOWSKA, E., Y. PADEL, AND Y. TANAKA. The mode of activation of pyramidal cells by intracortical stimuli. *J. Physiol. London* 249: 617-636, 1975.
75. JANKOWSKA, E., Y. PADEL, AND R. TANAKA. Projections of pyramidal tract cells to α-motoneurons innervating hindlimb muscles in the monkey. *J. Physiol. London* 249: 637-669, 1975.
76. JONES, E. G., J. D. COULTER, AND H. BURTON. Cells of origin and terminal distribution of corticostriatal fibers arising in the sensory-motor cortex of monkeys. *J. Comp. Neurol.* 173: 53-80, 1977.
77. JONES, E. G., J. D. COULTER, AND S. H. C. HENDRY. Intracortical connectivity of architechtonic fields in the somatic sensory, motor, and parietal cortex of monkeys. *J. Comp. Neurol.* 181: 291-348, 1978.
78. JONES, E. G., AND T. P. S. POWELL. The ipsilateral cortical connections of the somatic sensory area in the cat. *Brain Res.* 9: 71-94, 1968.
79. JONES, E. G., AND T. P. S. POWELL. The commisural connections of the somatic sensory cortex in the cat. *J. Anat.* 103: 433-455, 1968.
80. JONES, E. G., AND T. P. S. POWELL. Connections of the somatic sensory cortex of the rhesus monkey. I. Ipsilateral cortical connections. *Brain* 92: 477-502, 1969.
81. KITAI, S. T., J. D. KOCSIS, AND J. WOOD. Origin and characteristics of the cortico-caudate afferents: an anatomical and electrophysiological study. *Brain Res.* 118: 137-141, 1976.
82. KNAPP H. E., E. TAUB, AND A. J. BERMAN. Movements in monkeys with deafferented forelimbs. *Exp. Neurol.* 7: 305-315, 1963.
83. KOEZE, T. H., C. G. PHILLIPS, AND J. D. SHERIDAN. Thresholds of cortical activation of muscle spindles and motoneurons of the baboon's hand. *J. Physiol. London* 195: 419-449, 1968.
84. KUYPERS, H. G. J. M. Central cortical projections to motor and somatosensory cell groups. *Brain* 83: 161-184, 1960.
85. KUYPERS, H., AND J. BRINKMAN. Precentral projections to different parts of the spinal intermediate zone in the rhesus monkey. *Brain Res.* 24: 29-48, 1970.
86. KWAN, H. C., W. A. MACKAY, J. T. MURPHY, AND Y. C. WONG. Spatial organization of precentral cortex in awake primates. II. Motor outputs. *J. Neurophysiol.* 41: 1120-1131, 1978.
87. LANDGREN, S., C. G. PHILLIPS, AND R. PORTER. Cortical fields of origin of the monosynaptic pyramidal pathways to some alpha motoneurons of the baboon's hand and forearm. *J. Physiol. London* 161: 112-125, 1962.
88. LARSEN, K. D., AND H. ASANUMA. Thalamic projections to the feline motor cortex studied with horseradish peroxidase. *Brain Res.* 172: 209-215, 1979.
89. LASSEK, A. M. The pyramidal tract: basic considerations of corticospinal neurons. *Res. Publ. Assoc. Res. Nerv. Ment. Dis.* 27: 106-128, 1948.
90. LAURSEN, A. M. Selective increase in choice latency after transsection of a pyramidal tract in monkeys. *Brain Res.* 24: 544-545, 1970.
91. LAURSEN, A. M., AND M. WIESENDANGER. Motor deficit after transection of a bulbar pyramid in the cat. *Acta Physiol. Scand.* 68: 118-126, 1966.
92. LAWRENCE, D. G., AND H. G. J. M. KUYPERS. The functional organization of the motor system in the monkey. I. The effects of bilateral pyramidal lesions. *Brain* 91: 1-14, 1968.

93. LEMON, R. N., AND R. PORTER. Afferent input to movement-related precentral neurons in conscious monkeys. *Proc. R. Soc. London Ser. B* 194: 313-339, 1976.
94. LEMON, R. N., AND J. VAN DER BURG. Short-latency peripheral inputs to thalamic neurons projecting to the motor cortex in the monkey. *Exp. Brain Res.* 36: 445-462, 1979.
95. LEMON, R. N., J. A. HANBY, AND R. PORTER. Relationship between the activity of precentral neurons during active and passive movements in conscious monkeys. *Proc. R. Soc. London. Ser. B* 194: 341-373, 1976.
96. LIDDELL, E. G. T., AND C. G. PHILLIPS. Pyramidal section in the cat. *Brain* 67: 1-100, 1944.
97. LIU, C. N., AND W. W. CHAMBERS. An experimental study of the corticospinal system in the monkey (*Macaca mulatta*): the spinal pathways and preterminal distribution of degenerating fibers following discrete lesions of the pre- and postcentral gyri and bulbar pyramid. *J. Comp. Neurol.* 123: 257-284, 1964.
98. LLOYD, D. P. C. The spinal mechanism of the pyramidal system in cats. *J. Neurophysiol.* 4: 525-546, 1941.
99. LORENTE DE NÓ, R. Cerebral cortex: architecture, intercortical connections, motor projection. In: *Physiology of the Nervous System* (3rd ed.), edited by J. F. Fulton. New York: Oxford Univ. Press, 1949, p. 274-298.
100. LUNDBERG, A. Integration in a propriospinal motor center controlling the forelimb in the cat. In: *Integration in the Nervous System*, edited by H. Asanuma and V. J. Wilson. Tokyo: Igaku Shoin, 1979, p. 47-64.
101. LUNDBERG, A. Control of spinal mechanisms from the brain. In: *The Nervous System*, edited by D. B. Tower. New York: Raven, 1975, vol. 1, p. 253-265.
102. LUNGBERG, A., U. NORRSELL, AND P. VOORHOEVE. Pyramidal effects on lumbo-sacral interneurons activated by somatic afferents. *Acta Physiol. Scand.* 56: 220-229, 1962.
103. LUNDBERG, A., AND P. VOORHOEVE. Effects from the pyramidal tract on spinal reflex arcs. *Acta Physiol. Scand.* 56: 201-219, 1962.
104. MALIS, L. I., K. H. PRIBRAM, AND L. KRUGER. Action potentials in "motor" cortex evoked by peripheral nerve stimulation. *J. Neurophysiol.* 16: 161-167, 1953.
105. MARSDEN, C. D., P. A. MERTON, AND H. B. MORTON. Servo action in human voluntary movement. *Nature London* 238: 140-143, 1972.
106. MASSION, J., AND P. A. ALBE-FESSARD. Activités évoquées chez le chat dans la région du nucleus ventralis lateralis par diverses stimulations sensorielles. I. Etude macrophysiologique. *Electroencephalogr. Clin. Neurophysiol.* 19: 433-451, 1965.
107. MASSION, J., AND P. A. ALBE-FESSARD. Activités évoquées chez le chat dans la région du nucleus ventralis lateralis par diverses stimulations sensorielles. II. Etude microphysiologique. *Electroencephalogr. Clin. Neurophysiol.* 19: 452-469, 1965.
108. MASSION, J., AND L. RISPAL-PADEL. Differential control of motor cortex and sensory areas on ventrolateral nucleus of the thalamus. In: *Corticothalamic Projections and Sensory-Motor Activities*, edited by T. L. Frigyesi, E. Rinvic, and M. D. Yahr. New York: Raven, 1973, p. 357-374.
109. MELVIL-JONES, G., AND D. G. D. WATT. Observations on the control of stepping and hopping movements in man. *J. Physiol. London* 219: 709-727, 1971.
110. MERTON, P. A. Human position sense and sense of effort. *Symp. Soc. Exp. Biol.* 18: 387-400, 1964.
111. MORTIMER, E. M., AND K. AKERT. Cortical control and representation of fusimotor neurons. *Am. J. Phys. Med.* 40: 228-248, 1961.
112. MOTT, F. W., AND C. S. SHERRINGTON. Experiments upon the influence of sensory nerves upon movement and nutrition of the limb. *Proc. R. Soc. London* 57: 481-488, 1895.
113. MOUNTCASTLE, V. B., P. W. DAVIES, AND A. L. BERMAN. Response properties of neurons of cat's somatic sensory cortex to peripheral stimuli. *J. Neurophysiol.* 20: 374-407, 1957.
114. MOUNTCASTLE, V. B., J. C. LYNCH, A. GEORGOPOULOS, H.

SAKATA, AND C. ACUNA. Posterior parietal association cortex of the monkey: command functions for operations within extrapersonal space. *J. Neurophysiol.* 38: 871–908, 1975.
115. MURPHY, J. T., H. C. KWAN, W. A. MACKAY, AND Y. C. WONG. Spatial organization of precentral cortex in awake primates. III. Input-output coupling. *J. Neurophysiol.* 41: 1132–1139, 1978.
116. MURPHY, J. T., Y. C. WONG, AND H. C. KWAN. Distributed feedback systems for muscle control. *Brain Res.* 71: 495–505, 1974.
117. MURPHY, J. T., Y. C. WONG, AND H. C. KWAN. Afferent-efferent linkages in motor cortex for single forelimb muscles. *J. Neurophysiol.* 38: 990–1014, 1975.
118. NAUTA, W. H. J., AND P. A. GYGAX. Silver impregnation of degenerating axons in the central nervous system: a modified technique. *Stain Tech.* 29: 91–93, 1954.
119. NYBERG-HANSEN, R., AND A. BRODAL. Sites of termination of corticospinal fibers in the cat. *J. Comp. Neurol.* 120: 369–391, 1963.
120. OLSZEWSKI, J. The thalamus of the *Macaca mulatta*. Basel: Karger, 1952.
121. OSCARSSON, O., AND I. ROSÉN. Projection to cerebral cortex of large muscle-spindle afferents in forelimb nerves of the cat. *J. Physiol. London* 169: 924–945, 1963.
122. PANDIA, D. N., D. GOLD, AND T. BERGER. Interhemispheric connections of the precentral motor cortex in the rhesus monkey. *Brain Res.* 15: 594–596, 1969.
123. PATTON, H. D., AND V. E. AMASSIAN. Single- and multiple-unit analysis of cortical stage of pyramidal tract activation. *J. Neurophysiol.* 17: 345–363, 1954.
123a. PATTON, H. D., AND V. E. AMASSIAN. The pyramidal tract: its excitation and functions. In: *Handbook of Physiology. Neurophysiology*, edited by H. W. Magoun. Washington, DC: Am. Physiol. Soc., 1960, sect. 1, vol. II, chapt. 34, p. 837–861.
124. PENFIELD, W. The excitable cortex in conscious man. Liverpool: Liverpool Univ. Press, 1958.
125. PHILLIPS, C. G. Actions of antidromic pyramidal volleys on single Betz cells in the cat. *Q. J. Exp. Physiol.* 44: 1–25, 1959.
126. PHILLIPS, C. G. Cortical motor threshold and the thresholds and distribution of excited Betz cells in the cat. *Q. J. Exp. Physiol.* 41: 70–84, 1956.
127. PHILLIPS, C. G. Motor apparatus of the baboon's hand. *Proc. R. Soc. London Ser. B* 173: 141–174, 1969.
128. PHILLIPS, C. G., T. P. S. POWELL, AND M. WIESENDANGER. Projection from low-threshold muscle afferents of hand and forearm to area 3a of baboon's cortex. *J. Physiol London* 217: 419–446, 1971.
129. POWELL, T. P. S., AND V. B. MOUNTCASTLE. Some aspects of the functional organization of the cortex of the postcentral gyrus of the monkey: a correlation of findings obtained in a single-unit analysis with cytoarchitecture. *Johns Hopkins Hosp. Bull.* 105: 133–162, 1959.
130. PRESTON, J. B., M. C. SHENDE, AND K. UEMURA. The motor cortex-pyramidal system: patterns of facilitation and inhibition on motoneurons innervation limb musculature of cat and baboon and their adaptive significance. In: *Neurophysiological Basis of Normal and Abnormal Motor Activities*, edited by D. H. Purpura and M. D. Yahr. Hewlett, NY: Raven, 1967, p. 61–72.
131. REXED, B. A cytoarchitectonic atlas of the spinal cord in the cat. *J. Comp. Neurol.* 100: 297–380, 1954.
132. ROMANES, G. J. The motor cell columns of the lumbo-sacral spinal cord of the cat. *J. Comp. Neurol.* 94: 313–364, 1951.
133. ROSÉN, I., AND H. ASANUMA. Peripheral afferent inputs to the forelimb area of the monkey motor cortex: input-output relations. *Exp. Brain Res.* 14: 257–273, 1972.
134. SCHEIBEL, M. E., AND A. B. SCHEIBEL. Terminal axonal patterns in cat spinal cord. I. The lateral corticospinal tract. *Brain Res.* 2: 333–350, 1966.
135. SHERRINGTON, C. S. On secondary and tertiary degenerations in the spinal cord of the dog. *J. Physiol. London* 6: 177–191, 1885.
136. SHERRINGTON, C. S. On nerve-tracts degenerating secondarily to lesions of the cortex cerebri. *J. Physiol. London* 10: 429–432, 1889.
137. SHERRINGTON, C. S. *The Integrative Action of the Nervous System.* New Haven, CT: Yale Univ. Press, 1906. Reprinted in 1947.
138. SHINODA, Y., A. P. ARNOLD, AND H. ASANUMA. Spinal branching of corticospinal axons in the cat. *Exp. Brain Res.* 26: 215–234, 1976.
139. SHINODA, Y., P. ZARZECKI, AND H. ASANUMA. Spinal branching of pyramidal tract neurons in the monkey. *Exp. Brain Res.* 34: 59–72, 1979.
140. STEPHANIS, C., AND H. JASPER. Recurrent collateral inhibition in pyramidal tract neurons. *J. Neurophysiol.* 27: 855–877, 1964.
141. STONEY, S. D., JR., W. D. THOMPSON, AND H. ASANUMA. Excitation of pyramidal tract cells by intracortical microstimulation: effective extent of stimulating current. *J. Neurophysiol.* 31: 659–669, 1968.
142. STRICK, P. L. Light microscopic analysis of the cortical projection of the thalmic ventrolateral nucleus in the cat. *Brain Res.* 55: 1–24, 1973.
143. STRICK, P. L. Anatomical analysis of ventrolateral thalamic input to primate motor cortex. *J. Neurophysiol.* 39: 1020–1031, 1976.
144. STRICK, P. L. Activity of ventrolateral thalamic neurons during arm movement. *J. Neurophysiol.* 39: 1032–1044, 1976.
145. STRICK, P. L., R. E. BURKE, K. KANDA, C. C. KIM, AND B. WALMSLEY. Differences between alpha and gamma motoneurons labeled with horseradish peroxidase by retrograde transport. *Brain Res.* 113: 582–588, 1976.
146. STRICK, P. L., AND C. C. KIM. Input to primate motor cortex from posterior parietal cortex (area 5). I. Demonstration by retrograde transport. *Brain Res.* 157: 325–330, 1978.
147. STRICK, P. L., AND J. B. PRESTON. Multiple representation in the primate motor cortex. *Brain Res.* 154: 366–370, 1978.
148. STRICK, P. L., AND P. STERLING. Synaptic termination of the ventrolateral nucleus of the thalamus in the cat motor cortex. A light and electron microscope study. *J. Comp. Neurol.* 153: 77–106, 1974.
149. SZENTÁGOTHAI, J. Architecture of the cerebral cortex. In: *Basic Mechanisms of the Epilepsies*, edited by H. Jasper, A. Ward, and A. Pope. Boston: Little, Brown, 1969.
150. TAKAHASHI, K., K. KUBOTA, AND M. UNO. Recurrent facilitation in cat pyramidal cells. *J. Neurophysiol.* 30: 22–34, 1967.
151. TATTON, E. G., S. D. FORNER, G. L. GERSTEIN, W. W. CHAMBERS, AND C. M. LIU. The effect of postcentral cortical lesions on motor responses to sudden upper limb displacements in monkeys. *Brain Res.* 96: 108–113, 1975.
152. THOMPSON, E. D., S. D. STONEY, JR., AND H. ASANUMA. Characteristics of projections from primary sensory cortex to motor-sensory cortex in cats. *Brain Res.* 22: 15–27, 1970.
153. TOWE, A. L., H. D. PATTON, AND T. T. KENNEDY. Response properties of neurons in the pericruciate cortex of the cat following electrical stimulation of the appendages. *Exp. Neurol.* 10: 325–344, 1964.
154. TOWER, S. S. Pyramidal lesion in the monkey. *Brain* 63: 36–90, 1940.
155. TSUKAHARA, N., D. R. G. FULLER, AND V. B. BROOKS. Collateral pyramidal influences on the corticorubrospinal system. *J. Neurophysiol.* 31: 467–484, 1968.
156. VOGT, V. A., AND D. N. PANDYA. Cortico-cortical connections of somatic sensory cortex (areas 3, 1, and 2) in the rhesus monkey. *J. Comp. Neurol.* 177: 179–192, 1978.
157. WALKER, A. E. Internal structure and afferent-efferent relations of thalamus. In: *The Thalamus*, edited by D. P. Purpura and M. D. Yahr. New York: Columbia Univ. Press, 1966, p. 1–12.
158. WALSHE, F. M. R. The mode of representation of movements in the motor cortex, with special reference to "convulusions beginning unilaterally." *Brain* 66: 104–139, 1943.
159. WELT, C., J. ASCHOFF, K. KAMEDA, AND V. B. BROOKS. Intracortical organization of cat's sensory motor neurons. In: *Sym-*

posium on Neurophysiological Basis of Normal and Abnormal Motor Activities, edited by D. P. Purpura and M. D. Yahr. Hewlett, NY: Raven, 1967, p. 255–293.
160. WIESENDANGER, M. Input from muscle and cutaneous nerves of the hand and forearm to neurones of the precentral gyrus of baboons and monkeys. *J. Physiol. London* 228: 203–219, 1973.
161. WOOLSEY, C. N. Organization of somatic sensory and motor areas of the cerebral cortex. In: *Biological and Biochemical Bases of Behavior*, edited by H. R. Harlow and C. N. Woolsey. Madison: Univ. of Wisconsin Press, 1958, p. 63–82.
162. WOOLSEY, C. N., AND H-T. CHANG. Activation of the cerebral cortex by antidromic volleys in the pyramidal tract. *Res. Publ. Assoc. Res. Nerv. Ment. Dis.* 27: 146–161, 1948.
163. WOOLSEY, C. N., P. H. SETTLAGE, D. R. MEYER, W. SENCER, T. P. HAMUY, AND A. M. TRAVIS. Pattern of localization in precentral and 'supplementary' motor area and their relation to the concept of a premotor area. *Res. Publ. Assoc. Res. Nerv. Ment. Dis.* 30: 238–264, 1952.
164. ZARZECKI, P., Y. SHINODA, AND H. ASANUMA. Projection from area 3a to the motor cortex by neurons activated from group I muscle afferents. *Exp. Brain Res.* 33: 269–282, 1978.
165. ZARZECKI, P., P. L. STRICK, AND H. ASANUMA. Input to primate motor cortex from posterior parietal cortex (area 5). II. Identification by antidromic activation. *Brain Res.* 157: 331–335, 1978.

INDEX

Index

Acoustic nerve
  lesions of, recovery from, 1310
Action potentials
  extracellular potentials from mammalian Purkinje cells, 842
  of Purkinje cells, ionic basis of, 842-844
    action potentials at dendritic level, 843-844
    action potentials at somatic level, 842-843
Adenosine triphosphatase
  myofibrillary ATPase in animal motor units in relation to twitch-contraction times, 355-358
Afferent fibers
  jaw muscle spindle afferents, effects of their destruction on mastication, 1253-1254
  mesencephalic V afferents, activity patterns during mastication, 1254-1255
  muscle spindle afferent activity in limb response to sinusoidal movements, timing of, 239
  peripheral receptors transmitting to motor cortex, 1073-1077
    influence of peripheral afferent input to individual cortical elements, 1076
    input from peripheral receptors to pyramidal tract neurons, 1077
    projection from peripheral afferents to motor cortex, 1074-1075
    relation between afferent input zone and motor effect field, 1075-1076
  primary and secondary spindle afferent endings, functional properties of, 193-200
    amplitude nonlinearity, 196-197
    assessment, 199
    different responses to various stimuli, 193-196
    linear responses to sinusoidal stretching, 197-199
    mode of summation of signal components, 196
    possible intermediate endings, 199-200
  single fibers, amplitudes of EPSPs elicited by impulses in, 465-468
  single fibers, techniques for study of EPSPs elicited by impulses in, 464-465
  stretch afferents in oculomotor muscles, 1282-1283
  thalamic afferents, input to motor cortex, 1065-1068
    collaterals of pyramidal cells, 1068
    corticocortical afferents, 1067
    excitatory interneurons, 1067-1068
    inhibitory interneurons, 1067
Afferent pathways
  aminergic afferent projections to cerebellum, 783-786
    noradrenergic system, 783-785
    serotonergic afferent system, 785
  cerebellar afferent systems, 735-829
    question of somatotopy, 804-808
    responses of cerebellar neurons to exteroceptive and proprioceptive stimuli, 786-795
    responses of cerebellar neurons to visual, auditory, and vestibular stimuli, 795-804
  climbing fiber afferent systems, 764-783
    afferent projections to inferior olive, 765-771
    olivocerebellar projection, 771-779
    physiology of inferior olive, 779-783
    similarities and differences with mossy fiber system, 808-810
    structure and ultrastructure of inferior olive, 764-765
  for afferent projections to motor cortex, 1078
    thalamic relay for inputs to motor cortex, 1078
  mossy fiber afferent systems in cerebellar cortex, 736-764
    direct spinocerebellar systems, 736-748
    nucleocortical projection, 761-764
    pontocerebellar system, 750-754
    reticulocerebellar projections, 754-761
    similarities and differences with climbing fiber system, 808-810
    trigeminocerebellar projection, 749-750
    vestibulocerebellar projection, 748-749
  nigral afferent fibers, 971-972
    other nigral afferent fibers, 972
    pallidonigral projections, 967-968, 972
    strionigral fibers, 971-972
  of red nucleus, 983-985
    cerebellorubral projections, 984-985
    corticorubral fibers, 983-984
  pallidal afferent projections, 961-963
    striopallidal fibers, 961-962
    subthalamopallidal fibers, 962-963
  pallidofugal fiber systems, 963-969
    pallidohabenular fibers, 968-969
    pallidonigral projections, 967-968
    pallidosubthalamic projections, 137, 963
    pallidotegmental fibers, 969
    pallidothalamic projections, 963-967
  striatal afferent systems, 950-960, 997-1003
    convergence of extrinsic inputs to striatal neurons, 1002-1003
    corticostriatal afferents, 997-998
    corticostriatal fibers, 950-954
    nigrostriatal afferents, 999-1002, 1010
    nigrostriatal fibers, 957-958
    nigrostriatal pathway, transmitters in, 134-135
    other striatal afferents, 135, 1002
    striatal brain stem afferents, 958-960
    thalamostriatal afferents, 998-999
    thalamostriatal fibers, 954-957
  to motor cortex and pyramidal tract neurons, 718-727
    general problems, 718
    input through association fibers, 726-727
    input through commissural fibers, 727
    inputs from association cortex, 727
    inputs from nucleus ventralis lateralis of thalamus, 718-720
    inputs from sensory cortex, 726-727
    peripheral inputs to motor cortex and pyramidal tract cells, 720-726
ATPase: *see* Adenosine triphosphatase
Atrophy
  disuse atrophy, clinical application of functional electrical stimulation in, 180
Auditory nerve: *see* Acoustic nerve
Axons
  axon collaterals of α-motoneurons, 427-428

Axons (*continued*)
  diameter of and motoneuron size, relation of critical firing level to, 443–445
  α-motor axons, initial segment of, 427
  β-motor axons or skeletofusimotor axons to muscle spindles, 210–211
  γ-motor axons to muscle spindles, 200
  of descending pathways, tracing of them and identification of their terminals by techniques of anterograde labeling, 598–600
  of neurons of descending pathways, tracing by histofluorescence and immunohistochemistry, 600–601
  static and dynamic axons, intrafusal destination of, 203–208, 223
    assessment of position, 207–208
    glycogen depletion analysis, 205–206
    histological tracing of individual fusimotor fibers, 204–205
    initial ideas, 203–204
    studies on single living spindles, visual observation and intracellular recordings, 206–207
  static and dynamic fusimotor axons, delimitation of, 200–203, 223
    main differences, 200–202
    recent reexamination, 202–203
    speed of action, 202

Behavior
  behavioral analysis of movement, 1391–1414
  complex or cognitive behavior, effects of lesions of corpus striatum on, 1027–1028
  emotional behavior changes produced by prefrontal cortex lesions, 1158–1159
  interference control function of prefrontal cortex, 1167–1168
  studies suggesting that spinal centers generate locomotor movements, 1197–1199
  temporal synthesis of behavior affected by prefrontal cortex lesions, 1165–1168
Biomechanics
  dynamics of body, 33–35
  of skeleton and tendons, 17–42
    dynamics of skeleton, 30–33
    engineering design of bones, 36–41
    kinematics of joints, 19–26
    statics of skeleton, 28–30
    stresses and strains in bones, 36–41
    stresses and strains in tendons, 35–36
Bone and bones
  properties of, 27–28
  stresses and strains in, 36–41
    engineering design of bones, 36–41
Brain
  see also Brain stem; Cerebellum; Decerebrate state; Mesencephalon
  association fibers, input to motor cortex through, 726–727
  commissural fibers, input to motor cortex through, 727
  subcortical mastication pattern generator, 1256–1260
    local interneurons possibly involved in, 1258–1260
    rhythmic jaw movements evoked in reduced or anesthetized animals, 1256–1257
    rhythmic neural activity in absence of peripheral feedback, 1257–1258
  tissue reaction to surface electrodes used in functional electrical stimulation, 163
Brain stem
  see also Medulla oblongata; Pons; Reticular formation
  anatomy of, 607–611
    lower brain stem, 607–609
    mesencephalon, 609–610
    monoaminergic neurons, 610–611
  caudal brain stem projections to olive, 768
  cell types involved in vestibuloocular reflex, 1291–1292
    burst cells, 1291–1292
    burst-tonic cells, 1292
  certain neuronal activity during locomotion, 1203–1207
  circuitry for initiation of locomotion, 1194–1222
    background excitability, 1213
    corticobulbar control, 1209
    mesencephalic and pontine locomotor regions, 1210–1213
    specific control systems, 1213
    subthalamic locomotor region, 1209–1210
  descending pathways of, 612–627
    catecholaminergic brain stem neurons, 625
    cells of origin, 612–613
    cerebellar fastigial nucleus, 619
    cortical projections to cell groups of descending brain stem pathways, 638–642
    corticobulbar pathways, 627–638
    deep cerebellar nuclei, 622
    grouping of pathways on basis of their terminal distribution, 643–645
    interstitial nucleus of Cajal, 617–618
    monoaminergic and other pathways distributing to somatic motoneurons and autonomic preganglionic motoneurons, 623–625
    other laterally descending fiber systems, 622–623
    pathways distributing to short propriospinal and propriobulbar neurons, 619–622
    pathways from dorsal column nuclei to spinal dorsal horn, 626–627
    pathways subserving respiratory activity and solitary and retroambiguus nuclei, 623
    serotonergic raphe neurons, 625–626
    superior colliculus, 618–619
    trajectory and terminal distribution, 613–627
    ventrolateral pontine tegmentum, 622
    vestibular complex, 615–617
  integrating systems of, anatomy, 970–986
  integrating systems of, electrophysiology, 997–1015
  motor systems of, transmitters in, 127–130
    cranial motoneurons, 127
    red nucleus, 127–128
    reticulospinal cells, 128
    vestibulospinal cells, 128–130
  rubrobulbar efferent projections, 985–986
  striatal brain stem afferents, 958–960

Calcium
  high-threshold calcium spike in inferior olive, 862
  low-threshold calcium-dependent spikes in inferior olive, 862
Catecholamines
  catecholaminergic inhibitory system in cerebellar cortex, 855
Caudate nucleus
  anatomy of, 948–949
  cytology of, 949–950
Central nervous system
  see also Brain; Spinal cord
  central oscillations in generation of tremor, 338–340
    central feedback onto motoneurons, 339
    interneuronal networks, 339
    single pacemakers, 338–339
    supraspinal oscillators, 339–340
  descending pathways of, anatomy of, 597–666
    cortical projections to cell groups of descending brain stem pathways, 638–642
    corticospinal and corticobulbar pathways, 627–638
    descending brain stem pathways, 612–627
    descending cortical pathways, 627–643
    grouping of descending pathways on basis of their terminal distribution, 643–645
    identification of cells of origin of fiber systems by retrograde labeling, 600

Central nervous system (*continued*)
  identification of neurons and tracing of their axons, 600–601
  laminar distribution of cortical neurons projecting to subcortical and spinal structures, 642–643
  tracing of axons and identification of their terminals by techniques of anterograde labeling, 598–600
  visualization of neurons and their processes, 597–598
  how does it use motoneuron pool? 498–499
  in generation of basic locomotor synergy, 1194–1196
  parts of CNS of primary importance for neural control of basic locomotor synergy, 1196–1197
Central nervous system diseases
  causing disturbances in gait, 1193
Central pathways: *see* Neural pathways
Cerebellar cortex
  see also Purkinje cells
  climbing fiber afferent systems, 764–783, 839–840, 845–848
    activation by electrical stimulation of cerebellar white matter, 839–840
    activation of Purkinje cells, comparative aspects of, 847–848
    afferent projections to inferior olive, 765–771
    functional properties of, 846–847
    olivocerebellar projection, 771–779
    physiology of inferior olive, 779–783
    role in cerebellar control of movement, 918
    similarities and differences with mossy fiber system, 808–810
    structure and ultrastructure of inferior olive, 764–765
  field potentials of, 832–841
    evoked by surface stimulation, comparative aspects of, 835–838
    generated by white matter stimulation of cerebellar cortex, 838–841
    local stimulation of cerebellar cortex, 833–838
    parallel fiber field potentials, 833–835
  inhibitory systems in, 852–857
    basket cell inhibition, 853–854
    catecholaminergic inhibitory system, 855
    comparative aspects, 855–857
    inhibitory system of granular layer and Golgi cells, 855
    inhibitory systems of molecular layer, 853–855
    spatial distribution of basket cell inhibition, 854
    stellate cell inhibition, 854–855
  mossy fiber afferent systems, 736–764, 839–840, 848–852
    activation by electric stimulation of cerebellar white matter, 839–840
    direct spinocerebellar systems, 736–748
    nucleocortical projection, 761–764
    parallel fiber action on Purkinje cells, 852
    pontocerebellar system, 750–754
    radial organization of molecular-layer afferents, 851–852
    reticulocerebellar projections, 754–761
    role in cerebellar control of movement, 916–918
    similarities and differences with climbing fiber system, 808–810
    trigeminocerebellar projection, 749–750
    vestibulocerebellar projection, 748–749
  networks and circuits of, electrophysiology of, 831–876
    comparative aspects of, 831–832
    field potentials of, 832–841
    inhibitory systems in cortex, 852–857
    Purkinje cell target neurons, cerebellar nuclei, and Deiters' nucleus, 857–859
    unitary cell recording from cortex, 841–857
  neuron responses to exteroceptive and proprioceptive stimuli, 786–792
    neurons in vermis and paravermis, 786–788
  neuron responses to visual, auditory, and vestibular stimuli, 795–804
    responses to auditory stimuli, 797

  responses to vestibular stimuli, 797–804
  responses to visual stimuli, 795–797
Cerebellar nuclei
  activity of, relation to sequencing of movements and to postural holds, 920–925
  deep nuclei, neuronal responses to exteroceptive and proprioceptive stimuli, 792–795
  intracerebellar nuclei, neuronal responses to activation of descending pathways, 794–795
  intracerebellar nuclei, responses to peripheral stimuli, 793–794
  organization of nucleocortical afferent system, 761–764
  projection to olive, 768–769
  relation to Purkinje cell target neurons and Deiters' nucleus, 857–859
Cerebellum
  see also Cerebellar cortex
  cerebellar afferent systems, 735–829
    aminergic afferent projections to cerebellum, 783–786
    cerebellorubral projections, 984–985
    climbing fiber afferent systems, 764–783, 808–810
    mossy fiber afferent systems, 736–764, 808–810
    noradrenergic afferent projections, 783–785
    question of somatotopy, 804–808
    responses of cerebellar neurons to exteroceptive and proprioceptive stimuli, 786–795
    responses of cerebellar neurons to visual, auditory, and vestibular stimuli, 795–804
    serotonergic afferent projections, 785
  cerebellar connections in vestibuloocular reflex, 1292–1293
  certain neuronal activity during locomotion, 1203–1207
  control of posture and movement, 877–946
    analysis of α- and γ-motoneurons in, 910–912
    aspects of control, 882–912, 936–937
    ballistic movements, 883–887, 895–897
    classification of movements, 883–887
    comment on strategy and tactics, 901–904
    compound movements, 887, 892–895
    frame of reference in understanding control, 887–891
    motor programs and cerebellar circuit, 888–889
    movement initiation, 897–899
    muscle tone and force in, 909–912
    ongoing control of simple movements, 899–901
    self-terminated simple movements, 897
    servo control of movements examined by perturbations, 904–906
    simple movements, 883–887, 895–908
    speed and accuracy in, 887–888
    termination of simple movements, 906–908
  function of, cellular roles in, 912–936
    climbing fibers, 918
    discharge properties, 912–918
    firing frequencies, 914–915
    mossy fibers, 916–918
    α-motoneurons, γ-motoneurons, and interneurons as output targets, 928–931
    mystery of climbing fiber and theory of adaptive motor control, 931–934
    parameters of movement, 926–928
    rapid vs. slow movements and reciprocal contraction vs. cocontraction, 925–926
    relation of cerebellar nuclear activity to sequencing of movements and to postural holds, 920–925
    relation of discharge to behavioral events, 918–936
    role of individual cells within cerebellar circuit, 938
    role of Purkinje cell, 915–916
    topographic relation between body parts and cerebellum, 919–920
  function of, concepts of, 877–878
  functional anatomy of, 878–882
  localization of bodily functions in, 878–882

Cerebellum (*continued*)
   microanatomy and fundamental cerebellar circuitry, 912
   motor systems of, transmitters in, 130–134
      cerebellar inputs, 132–134
      excitatory interneurons, 132
      Purkinje cells, 130–131
   overall function of, 863–870
      Boylls' synergic parameterization theory, 869–870
      Braitenberg's timing model, 866
      Marr's learning model, 866–867
      Pellionisz-Llinás tensor model, 867–869
   role in locomotion, 1207–1208
   role in vestibulospinal reflexes, 696–697
   rubrocerebellar efferent fibers, 986
   trigeminal inputs and involvement in control of mandibular movements, 1265–1267
   white matter electrical stimulation generating field potentials in cerebellar cortex, 838–841
      activation of mossy fiber and climbing fiber afferents, 839–840
      interactions, 840–841
Cerebral cortex
   see also Motor cortex; Prefrontal cortex; Sensorimotor cortex; Somatosensory cortex
   association cortex, inputs to motor cortex from, 727
   cortical localization, classic concept in early research on motor control, 10–12
   corticobulbar control of locomotion, 1209
   corticoolivary afferent fibers, 770
   corticorubral afferent fibers, 983–984
   corticostriatal afferents, 997–998
   corticostriatal fibers, 950–954
   descending cortical pathways, 612–627
      cortical projections to cell groups of descending brain stem pathways, 638–642
      corticospinal and corticobulbar pathways, 627–638
      grouping of corticobulbar and corticospinal pathways on basis of their terminal distribution, 645
      laminar distribution of cortical neurons projecting to subcortical and spinal structures, 642–643
   premotor area, 1124–1129
      electrical activity recorded in premotor cortex of unconscious animals, 1128
      electrical stimulation of premotor cortex, 1127–1128
      lesions of premotor cortex, 1126–1127
      single-unit recordings in premotor cortex of conscious monkeys, 1128
      structure and general considerations, 1124–1126
   primary and secondary motor areas, cytoarchitectonic maps and terminology of, 1123–1124
   projection to spinal cord via pyramidal tract, organization of, 703–718
      microstructure of corticospinal projection, 712–715
      projection to γ-motoneurons, 715–716
      projections to spinal interneurons, 716–717
      pyramidal collaterals and branches within brain, 717–718
      studies by cortical depth stimulation, 707–712
      studies by cortical surface stimulation, 703–707
   secondary motor areas, organization of, 1121–1147
      methodological approach in historical perspective, 1122–1123
   subcortical motor centers, stereotactic experiments in early research on motor control, 8–9
   supplementary motor area, 1129–1137
      activation of, studies in humans, 1135–1137
      definition and historical note, 1129
      direct corticospinal connections, 1130–1131
      effects of electrical stimulation of SMA and epilepsy, 1131–1133
      electrophysiology of, 1134–1135
      indirect connections with motor apparatus, 1131
      inputs to, 1131
      lesions of, deficits after, 1133–1134
      movement-associated discharge of neurons in, 1134–1135
      possible implication of SMA neurons in transcortical reflexes, 1135
      responses to sensory input, 1134
      structural relationship, 1129–1131
   thalamocortical projections, 1019–1020
Climbing fibers: *see* Cerebellar cortex
Clonus: *see* Myoclonus
Colliculus, superior: *see* Superior colliculus
Corpus striatum
   see also Caudate nucleus; Globus pallidus; Putamen
   anatomy of, 947–969, 1018–1019
      cytology of, 949–950
      striatal connections, 950–960
   electrophysiology of, 997–1015
   lesions of, 1025–1028
      effects on "complex" behavior, 1027–1028
      effects on motor functions, 1025–1027
   striatal afferent systems, 950–960, 997–1003
      convergence of extrinsic inputs to striatal neurons, 1002–1003
      corticostriatal afferents, 997–998
      corticostriatal fibers, 950–954
      nigrostriatal afferents, 999–1002, 1010
      nigrostriatal fibers, 957–958
      nigrostriatal pathway, transmitters in, 134–135
      other striatal afferents, 135, 1002
      striatal brain stem afferents, 958–960
      thalamostriatal afferents, 998–999
      thalamostriatal fibers, 954–957
   striatal efferent systems, 1003–1009
      other striatal efferent pathways, 137
      striatal projection neurons, 1006–1009
      striatonigral fibers, 971–972
      striatonigral pathways, transmitters in, 135–137
      striatonigral system, 1004–1006
      striatopallidal fibers, 961–962
      striatopallidal system, 1004
   striatal interneurons, 137–138
Cybernetics
   impact on research on motor control, 6–7
   place of brain theory within cybernetics, 1450–1451

Decerebrate state
   animal models for study of neural control of muscle length and tension, 282–283
   tonic inhibitory control of segmental reflex transmission in, 564–567
Deiters' nucleus: *see* Pons
Dendrites
   basal dendrites of pyramidal cells of motor cortex, 1071
   dendritic level of Purkinje cells, ionic basis of action potentials at, 843–844

Efferent pathways
   see also Pyramidal tracts
   descending pathways, anatomy of, 597–666
      cortical projections to cell groups of descending brain cell pathways, 638–642
      corticospinal and corticobulbar pathways, 627–638
      descending brain stem pathways, 612–627
      descending cortical pathways, 627–643
      grouping of descending pathways on basis of their terminal distribution, 643–645
      identification of cells of origin of fiber systems by retrograde labeling, 600
      identification of neurons and tracing of their axons, 600–601
      laminar distribution of cortical neurons projecting to subcortical and spinal structures, 642–643

Efferent pathways (*continued*)
    tracings of axons and identification of their terminals by techniques of anterograde labeling, 598–600
    visualization of neurons and their processes, 597–598
  nigral efferent fibers, 972–975, 1010–1012
    nigrostriatal fibers, 957–958
    nigrostriatal pathway, transmitters in, 134–135
    nigrostriatal projection, 999–1002, 1010
    nigrostriatal system, 999–1002
    nigrotectal fibers, 973–975
    nigrotectal projection, 1011–1012
    nigrothalamic fibers, 972–973
    nigrothalamic projection, 1010–1011
  of red nucleus, 985–986
    rubrobulbar projections, 985–986
    rubrocerebellar fibers, 986
    rubrospinal fibers, 985
  pallidal efferent systems, 963–969, 1009–1010
    pallidohabenular fibers, 968–969
    pallidonigral projections, 967–968, 972
    pallidosubthalamic projections, 137, 963, 1009–1010
    pallidotegmental fibers, 969
    pallidothalamic projections, 963–967, 1009
  striatal efferent systems, 1003–1009
    other striatal efferent pathways, 137
    striatal projection neurons, 1006–1009
    striatonigral fibers, 971–972
    striatonigral pathways, transmitters in, 135–137
    striatonigral system, 1004–1006
    striatopallidal fibers, 961–962
    striatopallidal system, 1004
Electrical stimulation
  see also Functional electrical stimulation
  early use of microelectrodes in research on motor control, 4–5
  in tracing of inputs and outputs of prefrontal cortex, 1159–1160
  injected currents, differential responses of motoneurons to, 489
  intracellular electrodes applied to motoneurons in early research on motor control, 5–6
  local stimulation of cerebellar cortex generating field potentials, 833–838
    comparative aspects of field potentials evoked by surface stimulation, 835–838
    general description, 833
    parallel fiber field potentials, 833–835
  of basal ganglia, motor effects of, 1028–1033
    effects on cortically induced movements in anesthetized animals, 1031–1032
    effects on spinal motor mechanisms in anesthetized animals, 1032
    inhibitory influences, 1032–1033
    observations in alert humans, 1030–1031
    spontaneous motor behavior in alert animals, 1028–1030
  of cerebellar white matter generating field potentials in cerebellar cortex, 838–841
    activation of mossy fiber and climbing fiber afferents, 839–840
    interactions, 840–841
  of cortical depth in study of projection from cerebral cortex to spinal cord via pyramidal tract, 707–712
  of cortical surface in study of projection from cerebral cortex to spinal cord via pyramidal tract, 703–707
  of motor cortex in study of internal organization for input-output arrangements, 1071–1073
    contributions of different output elements to response produced, 1072–1073
    cortical distribution of output elements, 1071–1072
  of parietal association cortex eliciting movements, 1140–1141
  of prefrontal cortex, effects on frontal eye fields and oculomotor control, 1160–1161
  of premotor cortex, 1127–1128

  of supplementary motor area, effects and relation to epilepsy, 1131–1133
Electrochemistry
  electrochemical aspects of functional electrical stimulation to restore lost or impaired body function, 156–161
    biphasic stimulation, 159–161
    metal-tissue interface without applied field, 156–157
    monophasic stimulation, 159
    regulated voltage vs. regulated current, 158
    relationship between electrode potential and charge density, 157–158
    system for electrical excitation, 157
Electrodes
  coiled wire electrodes to muscles, tissue reaction during functional electrical stimulation, 163–166
  component materials, role in tissue damage during functional electrical stimulation, 162–163
  cuff electrodes to nerves, in electrical activation of normal muscle, 173–174
  cuff electrodes to nerves, tissue reaction during functional electrical stimulation, 163
  intramuscular electrode in electrical activation of normal muscle, 174
  surface electrode in electrical activation of normal muscle, 174
  surface electrodes to brain, tissue reaction during functional electrical stimulation, 163
Electromyography
  activity in limb muscles during locomotion, 1185–1186
Electronics
  early influence in research on motor control, 4–5
Embryology
  developmental considerations of muscle fiber types, 364–365
Emotions
  behavioral changes produced by prefrontal cortex lesions, 1158–1159
Epilepsy
  relation to effects of electrical stimulation of supplementary motor area, 1131–1133
EPSP: *see* Postsynaptic potentials
Excitatory postsynaptic potentials: *see* Postsynaptic potentials
Extremities
  see also Joints
  complex motor patterns, representation of, 1400–1413
    constraints on coordination, 1409–1413
    human evidence for a program concept, 1401–1409
  forelimb afferent systems to cerebellum, 745–747
  interlimb coordination during locomotion, 1187–1189, 1215–1216
    alternating gaits, 1188
    nonalternating gaits, 1188–1189
  limb positioning in each step during locomotion, 1224–1225
  limb response to sinusoidal movements, negative stiffness and spontaneous oscillations, 240–246
    comparison of stretch reflex with man-made control system, 244–245
    factors affecting stability of stretch reflexes, 242
    level of muscle activation, 242–243
    nature of external load, 242
    resistance to movements of different amplitudes, 243–244
    stability and gain in stretch reflex, 245–246
    stability of man-made system, 245
  limb response to sinusoidal movements, servo-control mechanisms in, 234–240
    effects of limb mass, 236
    muscles as low-pass filters, 238–239
    reflex delay, 239–240
    resistance of muscles to movement, 236–237
    timing of muscle spindle afferent activity, 239
    timing of reflex force, 239

Extremities (*continued*)
    two components of muscle force, 237–238
    manual control in humans, 1337–1389
        bias from transfer, 1343–1346
        comparison with tracking by eye, 1384–1385
        measures of error, 1346–1349
        nonvisual memory for single movements, 1350–1358
        prediction and preprogramming replace error correction in complex skills, 1380–1384
        preparation and time sharing, 1364–1379
        preprogramming and error correction, 1349–1350
        reaction time for correcting a limb movement, 1358–1364
        simple model for voluntary control, 1338–1343
    single limb, biomechanics during locomotion, 1180–1187
        active and passive factors controlling a limb, 1186–1187
        central organization of spinal pattern generation in, 1213–1215
        electromyographical activity in limb muscles, 1185–1186
        force factors, 1183–1185
        step cycle at different velocities, 1180–1183
    single-movement control of, 1392–1400
        Fitts' law, 1392–1393
        theoretical interpretations of, 1393–1399
Eye movements
    see also Nystagmus; Vestibuloocular reflex
    afoveate saccadic system, 1276–1277
    control of, 1275–1320
    corollary discharges and, 1433–1440
        corollary discharges and kinesthetic sensibility in eye, 1433–1435
        corollary discharges and visual perception, 1435–1440
    effect of electrical stimulation of prefrontal cortex on, 1160–1161
    eye-head coordination after appearance of unexpected and stationary target in space, 1321–1330
        compensatory eye movements, 1324–1325
        head movement, 1325–1329
        saccades during head movement, 1321–1323
        schematic outline of, 1329–1330
    eye-head coordination during smooth pursuit, 1330–1331
    eye-head coordination, other strategies of, 1331–1332
    eye-head coordination, plastic changes in central organization of, 1332–1334
        centrally generated slow phases, 1333–1334
        modification of saccades, 1334
    in visual stabilization, 1278, 1304–1305
    measurement of, 1311–1313
        contact methods, 1313
        corneal reflection, 1312
        differential limbus reflection, 1312
        double-image tracking devices, 1312–1313
        electrooculogram, 1311–1312
        magnetic search coil method, 1313
        noncontact methods, 1311–1313
        optical lever, 1313
        photography, 1311
    oculomotor plant, 1279–1284
        motoneuron behavior, 1279–1282
        movement and muscle fiber types, 1282
        muscle mechanics, 1283–1284
        plasticity and repair of oculomotor system, 1309–1311
        stretch afferents, 1282–1283
    optokinetic system, 1278, 1293–1297
        model of optokinetic-vestibular cooperation, 1295–1296
        neurophysiology of, 1296–1297
        properties of optokinetic nystagmus, 1293–1295
    purposes of, 1276–1279
    pursuit system, 1278–1279, 1304–1306
        models of pursuit, 1306
        neurophysiology of pursuit, 1305–1306
        properties of pursuit, 1305
        stabilization system, 1304–1305
    saccadic system, 1279, 1297–1304
        coordinate systems, 1300
        microsaccades, 1299
        neurophysiology of saccades, 1301–1304
        perception of visual direction, 1300
        properties of quick-phase system, 1299
        properties of rapid eye movements, 1297–1299
        saccadic plasticity, 1310–1311
        sampled-datalike behavior, 1299–1300
    tracking by eye, 1384–1385
    vergence system, 1279, 1306–1309
        neurophysiology of vergence, 1307–1309
        plasticity of vergence tone, 1311
        properties of vergence movements, 1306–1307

Feedback
    and learning of motor skills, 252–253
    central feedback onto motoneurons in generation of tremor, 339
    control and precomputed movements, 251–252
    forward-looking control systems, 253–254
    in motor control systems, 260–261
        simplified animal models for study of, 282–283
    man-made servo-control system, comparison of stretch reflex with, 244–245
    stability of man-made system, 245
    motor servo dynamic responses to mechanical disturbances in muscles, 297–308
        amplitude dependence and linearity, 299–301
        asymmetry of motor servo response, 301–302
        compensation for yielding, 302–304
        dependence of transient responses on initial force, 298–299
        dynamic features of force development, 297–298
        predictive compensation, feedforward vs. nonlinear feedback viewpoints, 304
        velocity dependence and damping, 306–307
        vibration and stretch reflex, 304–306
    motor servo function, hypotheses of, 264–270
        adaptive models, 269
        conditional feedback and servo assistance, 265–266
        follow-up servo hypothesis, 264–265
        salient features of available sensors, 264
        spindle receptors as model-reference error detectors, 265
        stiffness regulation, 266–268
        summary model, 268–269
        β-system and possibility for zero sensitivity, 266
    motor servo operations in muscles of intact subjects, 290–297
        effect of instructional set, 294–296
        equivalent stiffness and concept of composite motor servos, 293–294
        gain variation vs. gain control, 296–297
        skeletal mechanics and coordinate systems, 291
        steady-state responses to changes in load force, 291–292
        torque-angle relations, 292–293
    motor servos in implementation of movement commands, 308–316
        analytical approaches to actions of α-, β-, and γ-motoneurons, 310–311
        compliance, load compensation, and biological design, 315–316
        equilibrium point control, 311–313
        β-innervation of muscle spindles, 310
        perturbations during movement, 314–315
        positional stiffness deduced from spindle relations, 309–310
        α-γ-relations, 308–309
        stiffness regulations vs. stiffness control, 313–314
    negative feedback principle in motor control theory, 261–262
    problems in early research on motor control, 7–8
    recurrent inhibitory feedback from motoneurons, 429

PART 1: pages 1–733; PART 2: pages 735–1480

Feedback (*continued*)
  servo assistance of voluntary movements, 250-251
  servo-control mechanisms in limb response to sinusoidal movements, 234-240
    effects of limb mass, 236
    muscles as low-pass filters, 238-239
    reflex delay, 239-240
    resistance of muscles to movement, 236-237
    timing of muscle spindle afferent activity, 239
    timing of reflex force, 239
    two components of muscle force, 237-238
  servomechanisms, some properties of, 230-234
    combination of different vectors, 233
    frequency transfer function, 231
    loop gain, 231
    low-pass filters, 234
    nonlinear systems, 234
    properties of different loads, 231
    stability, 234
    vector representation of a delay, 232-233
    vector representation of frequency transfer function, 231-232
    velocity-sensitive transducer, 233-234
Feeding
  relation of single-cell activity in basal ganglia to, 1040
FES: *see* Functional electrical stimulation
Field potentials
  of cerebellar cortex, 832-841
    evoked by surface stimulation, comparative aspects of, 835-838
    generated by white matter stimulation of cerebellar cortex, 838-841
    local stimulation of cerebellar cortex, 833-838
    parallel fiber field potentials, 833-835
Fishes
  trunk movements during locomotion in, 1190-1191
Functional electrical stimulation
  clinical applications of, 179-184
    disuse atrophy, 180
    hemiplegia, 180-181
    paralyzed muscle, 179-182
    respiratory problems, 182
    scoliosis, 182-184
    spinal cord injury, 181-182
  electrical activation of normal muscle, 173-174
    intramuscular electrode, 174
    nerve cuff electrode, 173-174
    surface electrode, 174
  electrical activation of skeletal muscle, 172-179
  electrochemical aspects of, 156-161
    biphasic stimulation, 159-161
    metal-tissue interface without applied field, 156-157
    monophasic stimulation, 159
    regulated voltage vs. regulated current, 158
    relationship between electrode potential and charge density, 157-158
    system for electrical excitation, 157
  for restoration of lost or impaired body function, 155-187
  muscle alterations induced by, 174-179
    changes in contractile properties, 174-175
    fatigue resistance, 176-177
    force modulation, 177-179
    metabolic changes, 175-176
    reversibility of changes, 177
    time course of changes, 176
  nerve excitation in, 166-172
    effects of electrode configuration on threshold and excitation site, 170-171
    excitation of myelinated nerve, 168-169
    membrane response to applied electrical field, 166-168
    neural fatigue or loss of electrical excitability, 172
    threshold relationship between nerve and muscle, 169-170
  tissue damage from, factors in, 161-166
    brain reaction to surface electrodes, 163
    electrode materials, 162-163
    muscle reaction to coiled wire electrodes, 163-166
    nerve reaction to cuff electrodes, 163

Ganglia, basal
  see also Corpus striatum
  anatomical background, 1018-1020
  electrical stimulation of, motor effects, 1028-1033
    effects on cortically induced movements in anesthetized animals, 1031-1032
    effects on spinal motor mechanisms in anesthetized animals, 1032
    inhibitory influences, 1032-1033
    observations in alert humans, 1030-1031
    spontaneous motor behavior in alert animals, 1028-1030
  lesioning and recording in humans, 1041-1043
  lesions of, motor effects of, 1020-1028
    acute vs. chronic effects, 1020
    general considerations, 1020
    lesion specificity, 1020
    lesions of individual nuclei, 1020-1028
    methods of observation and examination, 1020
    species differences, 1020
  motor functions of, 1017-1061
    motor behavior studies in Parkinson's disease, 1043-1044
  motor systems of, transmitters in, 134-138
    nigrostriatal pathway, 134-135
    other striatal afferents, 135
    other striatal efferent pathways, 137
    pallidosubthalamic projection, 137
    striatal interneurons, 137-138
    striatonigral pathways, 135-137
    transmitters in various striatal pathways, 134
  output of, 1019
  pathophysiological mechanisms of disorders of, 1044-1048
    akinesia and hyperactivity, 1045-1046
    dyskinesias and stereotyped behavior, 1046-1047
    resting tremor, 1048
    rigidity, 1047-1048
  single-cell studies in ganglia during movement, 1033-1041
    relation to delayed response task, 1041
    relation to feeding behavior, 1040
    relations to parameters of movement, 1037-1038
    responses to peripheral stimuli, 1040
    somatotopic organization, 1035-1037
    spontaneous activity, 1033-1034
    temporal relation to movement, 1034-1035
    vestibular and postural mechanisms, 1038-1040
Globus pallidus
  anatomy of, 960-969
    cytology of, 961
    pallidal connections, 961-969
    pallidal-subthalamic relations, 1019
  lesions of, motor effects of, 1020-1022
    combined pallidal and nigral lesions, 1024
  pallidal afferent projections, 961-963
    striopallidal fibers, 961-962
    subthalamopallidal fibers, 962-963
  pallidal efferent systems, 963-969, 1009-1010
    pallidohabenular fibers, 968-969
    pallidonigral projections, 967-968, 972
    pallidosubthalamic projections, 137, 963, 1009-1010
    pallidotegmental fibers, 969
    pallidothalamic projections, 963-967, 1009

PART 1: pages 1-733; PART 2: pages 735-1480

Golgi cells
    representation in inhibitory system of granular layer of cerebellar cortex, 855
Golgi tendon organs: *see* Tendons

Habenula
    pallidohabenular fibers, 968–969
Hand: *see* Extremities
Head
    eye-head coordination after appearance of unexpected and stationary target in space, 1321–1330
        compensatory eye movements, 1324–1325
        head movement, 1325–1329
        saccades during head movement, 1321–1323
        schematic outline of, 1329–1330
    eye-head coordination during smooth pursuit, 1330–1331
    eye-head coordination, other strategies of, 1331–1332
    eye-head coordination, plastic changes in central organization of, 1332–1334
        centrally generated slow phases, 1333–1334
        modification of saccades, 1334
Hearing
    auditory stimuli and responses evoked in neurons of cerebellar cortex, 797
Hemiplegia
    clinical application of functional electrical stimulation in, 180–181
Histochemistry
    of muscle fiber types, 347–351
    of muscle motor units, 354–355
Hormones
    as chemical messengers in motor systems, 109–110

Inferior olive: *see* Olive, inferior
Interneurons
    see also Renshaw cells
    as output targets in cerebellar control of movement, 928–931
    central interneuronal networks in generation of tremor, 339
    cerebellar excitatory interneurons, 132
    cerebellar inhibitory interneurons, 131–132
    excitatory interneurons in input of thalamic afferents to motor cortex, 1067–1068
    Ia inhibitory interneurons, 480–481
    inhibitory interneurons in input of thalamic afferents to motor cortex, 1067
    local interneurons possibly involved in subcortical mastication pattern generator, 1258–1260
    of spinal cord, projection from cerebral cortex via pyramidal tract to, 716–717
    segmental activity, ascending pathways that monitor it, 569–576
        evidence that ascending flexor-reflex afferent pathways monitor activity in interneurons of reflex pathways, 569–570
        information via ascending collaterals of interneurons, 571–572
        ventral flexor-reflex tracts, 572–573
        ventral spinocerebellar tract, 573–576
    striatal interneurons, 137–138
Ions
    ionic basis of Purkinje cell action potentials, 842–844
        action potentials at dendritic level, 843–844
        action potentials at somatic level, 842–843
        noninactivating Na-dependent plateau potentials, 844
    ionic mechanisms in spike generation in inferior olive, 862

Jaws
    see also Mandible
    jaw reflexes, evidence concerning their contribution to mastication, 1253–1256
        activity patterns of mesencephalic V afferents during mastication, 1254–1255
        effects of destruction of jaw muscle spindle afferents, 1253–1254
        possible contribution of low-threshold mechanoreceptors to load regulation during chewing, 1255–1256
    reflexes possibly involved in chewing, 1247–1253
        jaw-opening reflex, 1248–1251
        jaw-stretch reflex, 1247–1248
    rhythmic jaw movements evoked in reduced or anesthetized animals, 1256–1257
    voluntary isometric jaw muscle contraction in control of mandibular movements, 1263–1265
    voluntary movements of, role of sensorimotor cortex in, 1260–1263
Joints
    hip position and movement, influence on reflex control of basic locomotor synergy, 1200–1202
    joint afferents, reflex pathways from groups II and III muscle afferents and from, 535–549
    kinematics of, 19–26

Labyrinth
    see also Vestibular apparatus
    motoneurons of, connections with spinal motoneurons, 686–689
    otolith reflexes, 668–669, 693, 1288
Learning
    of motor skills, feedback in, 252–253
Limbs: *see* Extremities
Locomotion
    basic locomotor synergy, adaptation to animal's needs, 1222–1226
        changing speed, 1222–1223
        goal-directed locomotion such as turning and walking along curvatures, 1223
        modifications of "locomotor posture," 1223–1224
        positioning of limb in each step, 1224–1225
        reflex adaptation of step, 1225–1226
    basic locomotor synergy, neural generation of, 1194–1222
        activity in certain spinal, cerebellar, and brain stem neurons and in certain reflex pathways during locomotion, 1203–1207
        brain stem circuitry for initiation of locomotion, 1209–1222
        central organization of spinal pattern generation, 1213–1216
        central vs. peripheral, 1194–1196
        cerebellum and locomotion, 1207–1208
        developmental aspects, 1220–1221
        parts of CNS of primary importance for neural control of basic locomotor synergy, 1196–1197
        possible rhythm-generating mechanisms and models, 1216–1220
        reflex control, 1199–1203
        spinal centers for locomotion, behavioral results, 1197–1199
    biomechanical and electromyographical aspects, 1180–1194
        active and passive factors controlling a limb, 1186–1187
        dorsoventral movements of spine in gallop and leaping, 1192–1193
        electromyographical activity in limb muscles during locomotion, 1185–1186
        force factors, 1183–1185
        gait disturbances due to CNS damage, 1193
        gait disturbances due to peripheral damage, 1193
        interlimb coordination, 1187–1189
        lateral trunk movements in alternating gaits, 1191–1192
        single limb during locomotion, 1180–1187
        step cycle at different velocities, 1180–1183
        torsion around longitudinal axis in walking humans, 1193
        treadmill vs. overground locomotion, 1189–1190
        trunk movements during locomotion, 1190–1193
    control in bipeds, tetrapods, and fish, 1179–1236
    initiation of, brain stem circuitry for, 1194–1222
        background excitability, 1213
        corticobulbar control, 1209

PART 1: pages 1–733; PART 2: pages 735–1480

Locomotion (*continued*)
  mesencephalic and pontine locomotor regions, 1210–1213
  specific control systems, 1213
  subthalamic locomotor region, 1209–1210
Mandible
  mandibular control, neural mechanisms for mastication and voluntary biting, 1237–1274
  masticatory system, neuroanatomy of, 1241–1243
  movements of, initiation and control of, 1260–1267
    peripheral systems and voluntary isometric jaw muscle contraction, 1263–1265
    role of sensorimotor cortex in mastication and voluntary jaw movements, 1260–1263
    trigeminal relationships in cerebellum, 1265–1267
  muscles of, 1238–1241
    anatomy, 1238–1240
    physiology and histochemistry, 1240–1241
Mastication
  characteristics of normal mastication, 1243–1247
  evidence concerning contribution of jaw reflexes to, 1253–1256
    activity patterns of mesencephalic V afferents during mastication, 1254–1255
    effects of destruction of jaw muscle spindle afferents, 1253–1254
    possible contribution of low-threshold mechanoreceptors to load regulation during chewing, 1255–1256
  mandibular movements, initiation and control of, 1260–1267
    peripheral systems and voluntary isometric jaw muscle contraction, 1263–1265
    role of sensorimotor cortex in mastication and voluntary jaw movements, 1260–1263
    trigeminal relationships in cerebellum, 1265–1267
  masticatory system, neuroanatomy of, 1241–1243
  reflexes possibly involved in, 1247–1253
    excitatory effects from oral mechanoreceptors, 1251
    jaw-opening reflex, 1248–1251
    jaw-stretch reflex, 1247–1248
    modulation of trigeminal reflexes by primary afferent depolarization, 1251–1253
  subcortical mastication pattern generator, 1256–1260
    local interneurons possibly involved in, 1258–1260
    rhythmic jaw movements evoked in reduced or anesthetized animals, 1256–1257
    rhythmic neural activity in absence of peripheral feedback, 1257–1258
Medulla oblongata
  gracilocerebellar tract, 745
Membrane potentials
  of intrafusal muscle fibers, 209–210
Memory
  provisional memory function of prefrontal cortex, 1166
Mesencephalon
  see also Red nucleus; Substantia nigra
  mesencephalic locomotor region, 1210–1213
  mesencephalolivary projection, 769–770
  pallidotegmental fibers, 969
Metals
  electrode materials, role in tissue damage during functional electrical stimulation, 162–163
Microscopy, electron
  of neurons and their processes in descending pathways, 598
Models
  of motor control systems, 258–259
  of motor servo function, 268–269
    adaptive models, 269
    summary model, 268–269
  simple model for voluntary motor control functions of brain, 1338–1343

coding of words in working memory, 1339–1341
computer of limited capacity, 1341–1342
long-term memory and automation of skill, 1342–1343
single-channel input selector, 1342
working memory and internal rehearsal, 1339
simplified animal models for study of neural control of muscle length and tension, 282–283
Mossy fibers: *see* Cerebellar cortex
Motoneuron pools
  firing patterns of individual motoneurons and motor units, 435–460
    critical firing levels of motoneurons, 440–443
    effects of inhibitory input on critical firing level and rank order during repetitive firing, 445–448
    evidence regarding alternative patterns of recruitment, 452–457
    evidence regarding voluntary selective control of motor units, 457–458
    functional significance of size of motoneurons, 435–439
    measurement of total output of pools, 439–440
    modulation of firing rate, 459–460
    recruitment of motor units in humans, 448–452
    relation of critical firing level to axon diameter and motoneuron size, 443–445
    size principle in other species, 458–459
  functional organization and their inputs, 423–507
  how size of motoneurons determines their susceptibility to discharge, 491–494
    properties of motoneurons that influence susceptibility to discharge, 491–493
    role of input in determining susceptibility to discharge, 493–494
  morphological considerations of, 424–435
    axon collaterals of α-motoneurons, 427–428
    columnar arrangement of motoneuron pool, 424–425
    dimensions of α-motoneurons and distribution of cell size, 425
    direct synaptic interconnections between spinal motoneurons, 429
    initial segment of α-motor axons, 427
    matching properties of motoneurons and muscle fibers they supply, 433–434
    morphology of neuromuscular junctions, 432–433
    recurrent inhibitory feedback from motoneurons, 429
    scaling of motoneurons, 425–426
    species of motoneurons, 429–430
    terminals of motoneurons in muscle, 430–432
  nonuniformity of motoneurons, 485–491
    differential responses of motoneurons to injected currents, 489
    early classification of tonic and phasic types of motoneurons, 486–487
    evidence from human disease, 490–491
    influence of muscle on developing and mature motoneurons, 489–490
    motoneuron properties independent of size, 487–489
    significance of nonuniformity of muscle fibers, 487
  organization of input to, 460–485
    amplitudes of EPSPs elicited by impulses in single fibers, 465–468
    anatomical studies, 461–464
    boutons of Ia-fibers on motoneurons, 468–472
    comparison of projections to homonymous and heteronymous motoneurons, 474–476
    distribution of Ia excitation to pools, 473–474
    group Ib input from Golgi tendon organs, 482–483
    group II input from secondary endings in muscle spindles, 479–480
    Ia-projections to motoneurons controlling other parts of body, 478–479
    correlations between morphology and function, 476–477

PART 1: pages 1–733; PART 2: pages 735–1480

Motoneuron pools (*continued*)
    inhibitory inputs to motoneurons, 480–482
    latency of EPSPs, 477–478
    monosynaptic input from descending pathways, 483
    other examples of divergence in inputs to motoneurons, 478
    physiology of Ia-terminals, 472–473
    techniques used to study EPSPs elicited by impulses in single afferent fibers, 464–465
    topographic factors governing development of connections of Ia-fibers to motoneurons, 483–484
  some principles underlying organization of, 494–499
    actual sensitivity in grading muscular tension, 497
    basis for relation between motoneuron size and force its motor unit develops, 496–497
    collective action of pool and role of input, 498
    how does CNS use pool? 498–499
    how sensitivity in gradation of tension is achieved, 494–496
    mathematical derivation of "principle of maximum grading sensitivity," 497–498
    recruitment order and minimum energy principle, 498
    size principle in Ia and group II sensory fibers, 498
Motoneurons
  α-, analysis in study of cerebellar control of movement, 910–912
  α-, as output targets in cerebellar control of movement, 928–931
  α-, axon collaterals of, 427–428
  α-, dimensions and distribution of cell size, 425
  α-, direct projections of descending spinal pathways to, 567–569
  α-, motoneuron actions, in implementation of movement commands, 310–311
  α-, physiology and synaptic inputs in relation to motor unit type, 378–385
    electrophysiological properties intrinsic to motoneurons, 379–381
    group Ia synaptic efficacy, 381–382
    interactive factors in control of motoneuron excitability, 383–385
    monosynaptic supraspinal inputs, 382
    organization of synaptic input, 381–383
    polysynaptic input systems, 382–383
  α-γ-relations in implementation of movement commands, 308–309
  β-motoneuron actions, in implementation of movement commands, 310–311
  γ-, analysis in study of cerebellar control of movement, 910–912
  γ-, as output targets in cerebellar control of movement, 928–931
  γ-, control of pathways from Ia-afferents of muscle spindles, 519–530
  γ-, cortical representation via pyramidal tract to, 715–716
  γ-motoneuron actions, in implementation of movement commands, 310–311
  anatomy in relation to motor unit type, 377–378
  anatomy of, 461
  application of microelectrodes in early research on motor control, 5–6
  autonomic preganglionic motoneuronal cell groups of spinal cord, anatomy of, 603
  boutons of Ia-fibers on, 468–472
  central feedback onto, in generation of tremor, 339
  cranial motoneurons in brain stem motor systems, 127
  homonymous and heteronymous inputs to, comparison of, 474–476
  Ia-branches to, anatomy of, 461–462
  Ia excitation to, distribution of, 473–474
  Ia-fiber connections to, topographic factors governing development of, 483–484
  Ia-synapses on, 462–464
  Ia-terminals, physiology of, 472–473
  innervation ratio for muscle fibers and motor unit "size," 369–372
  input role in determining susceptibility to discharge, 493–494
  morphology and function of, correlations between, 476–477
  motor nuclei, anatomy of, 372–377
    numbers of motoneurons and motor units, 376–377
  oculomotor motoneurons, behavior of, 1279–1282
  of labyrinth and spinal cord, connections between, 686–689
  properties independent of their size, 487–489
  properties that influence their susceptibility to discharge, 491–493
  rate and pattern of firing of, control of muscular action by modulation of, 394–402
    effects of firing rate and firing pattern on muscle unit output, 397–402
    motoneuron firing characteristics, 394–397
  size and force its motor unit develops, relation between, 496–497
  size of, correlation with susceptibility to discharge, 491–494
  size of, functional significance of, 435–439
  size of, relation of critical firing level to axon diameter and, 443–445
  size principle in Ia and group II sensory fibers, 498
  somatic motoneuronal cell groups of ventral horn, anatomy of, 601–603
  spinal motoneurons and their synaptic control, 115–127
    inhibitory inputs on motoneurons, 120–122
    monosynaptic reflex, 115–119
    other excitatory inputs on motoneurons, 119–120
    other relevant spinal mechanisms, 123–127
    presynaptic inhibition, 122–123
  spinal motoneurons, reticulospinal tract actions on, 683–685
  tonic and phasic types of, early classification of, 486–487
Motor activity
  chemical transmitters in motor systems, 108–115
    definition of, 108
    hormones, 109–110
    identification of transmitters, 111–115
    intercellular communication, 109–111
    intracellular mediators, 108–109
    neuromodulators, 110–111
    synaptic transmitters, 110
    varieties of transmitters, 108–111
  learning of motor skills, feedback in, 252–253
  lost or impaired body function, restoration by functional electrical stimulation, 155–187
  motor area features of parietal association cortex, 1140–1143
    command functions of parietal lobe, 1141–1143
    parietal lesions and electrical stimulation, 1140–1141
    structural relationships with motor areas, 1141
  motor behavior studies in Parkinson's disease, 1043–1044
    continuous pursuit movements, 1044
    other aspects of motor performance, 1044
    reaction time, 1043
    speed of movement, 1043–1044
  motor effects of electrical stimulation of basal ganglia, 1028–1033
    effects on cortically induced movements in anesthetized animals, 1031–1032
    effects on spinal motor mechanisms in anesthetized animals, 1032
    inhibitory influences, 1032–1033
    observations in alert humans, 1030–1031
    spontaneous motor behavior in alert animals, 1028–1030
  motor effects of lesions of basal ganglia, 1020–1028
    acute vs. chronic effects, 1020
    combined pallidal and nigral lesions, 1024
    corpus striatum lesions, 1025–1028
    general considerations, 1020
    globus palidus lesions, 1020–1022
    lesion specificity, 1020
    lesions of individual nuclei, 1020–1028
    methods of observation and examination, 1020

PART 1: pages 1–733; PART 2: pages 735–1480

INDEX xxiii

Motor activity (*continued*)
    species differences, 1020
    subthalamic nucleus lesions, 1024-1025
  motor features of somatosensory cortex areas I and II, critical review of evidence for, 1137-1139
  motor functions of basal ganglia, 1017-1061
    single-cell studies in ganglia during movement, 1033-1041
  muscle as producer of, 43-106
    motor functions of muscles, 87
    units for measure of motor function, 88-94
  representation of muscle properties in relation to, 44-55
    dimensions used, 44-45
    models, 45-49
    real motor systems, 49-55
  spinal motoneurons and their synaptic control, 115-127
    inhibitory inputs on motoneurons, 120-122
    monosynaptic reflex, 115-119
    other excitatory inputs on motoneurons, 119-120
    other relevant spinal mechanisms, 123-127
    presynaptic inhibition, 122-123
  transmitters in basal ganglia, 134-138
    nigrostriatal pathway, 134-135
    other striatal afferents, 135
    other striatal efferent pathways, 137
    pallidosubthalamic projection, 137
    striatal interneurons, 137-138
    striatonigral pathways, 135-137
    transmitters in various striatal pathways, 134
  transmitters in brain stem, 127-130
    cranial motoneurons, 127
    red nucleus, 127-128
    reticulospinal cells, 128
    vestibulospinal cells, 128-130
  transmitters in cerebellum, 130-134
    cerebellar inhibitory interneurons, 131-132
    cerebellar inputs, 132-134
    excitatory interneurons, 132
    Purkinje cells, 130-131
  transmitters in motor cortex, 138-142
    cortical inhibitory mechanisms, 141-142
    other transmitters in cortex, 142
    pyramidal tract neurons, 138-141
  transmitters in motor systems, 107-154
  transmitters in peripheral motor systems, 115
  transmitters in spinal motor mechanisms, 115-127
  transmitters in supraspinal motor systems, 127-142
Motor control
  central pathways in neural control of muscle length and tension, 276-282
    clasp-knife reflex, 279-280
    long-loop reflexes, 280-282
    primary ending projections, 276-277
    projections from groups III and IV free nerve endings, 279
    projections from secondary endings and group II free nerve endings, 278-279
    tendon organ projections, 277-278
  cerebellar control of posture and movement, 877-946
  complex motor patterns, representation of, 1400-1413
    constraints on coordination, 1409-1413
    human evidence for a program concept, 1401-1409
  control of eye movements, 1275-1320
  control theory concepts, 258-264
    control configurations, 262-264
    control systems, 259-260
    feedback, feedforward, and adaptive systems, 260-261
    principle of negative feedback, 261-262
    regulated variables and properties, 262
    systems and models, 258-259

  distributed motor control, perceptual structures and, 1449-1480
    concepts from computer science and control theory, 1452-1453
    coordinated control programs, 1465-1471
    motor schemas, 1463-1465
    optic flow and control of movement, 1461-1463
    perceptual schemas and the action-perception cycle, 1458-1461
    perspective of artificial intelligence, 1471-1477
    place of brain theory within cybernetics, 1450-1451
  evidence regarding voluntary selective control of motor units, 457-458
  eye head coordination, 1321-1336
  history of research on, 1-16
    back to muscular end organs, 6
    classic concept of cortical localization in, 10-12
    early attempts at quantifying control functions, 2-3
    early influence of electronics and microelectrodes, 4-5
    feedback problems, 7-8
    impact of cybernetics on motor physiology, 6-7
    intracellular approach, 5-6
    modern-day reorientation in concepts and interests, 12-13
    reflex origin in basic ideas, 3-4
    stereotactic experiments and study of subcortical motor centers, 8-9
    stretch reflex studies, 9-10
  mandibular control, neural mechanisms for mastication and voluntary biting, 1237-1274
    characteristics of normal mastication, 1243-1247
    evidence concerning contribution of jaw reflexes to mastication, 1253-1256
    peripheral systems and voluntary isometric jaw muscle contraction, 1263-1265
    reflexes possibly involved with chewing, 1247-1253
    role of sensorimotor cortex in mastication and voluntary jaw movements, 1260-1263
    subcortical mastication pattern generator, 1256-1260
    trigeminal relationships in cerebellum, 1265-1267
  manual control in humans, 1337-1389
    bias from transfer, 1343-1346
    comparison with tracking by eye, 1384-1385
    measures of error, 1346-1349
    nonvisual memory for single movements, 1350-1358
    prediction and preprogramming replace error correction in complex skills, 1380-1384
    preparation and time sharing, 1364-1379
    preprogramming and error correction, 1349-1350
    reaction time for correcting a limb movement, 1358-1364
    simple model for voluntary control, 1338-1343
  motor commands and their perceptual consequences, 1415-1447
    corollaries of motor commands to limb and trunk muscles, 1421-1433
    corollary discharges and eye movements, 1433-1440
    corollary discharges and somatosensory afferents, 1428
    electrophysiological correlates of motor commands, 1440-1441
    historical development, 1416-1420
    interactions between corollary discharges and kinesthetic afferent inputs, 1425-1428
    other instances of central irradiation by motor commands, 1441-1442
    sensations of movement, 1422-1425
    sensations of muscular force or heaviness, 1428-1433
    terminology, 1420-1421
  motor prostheses by means of functional electrical stimulation, 155-187
  motor servo function, hypotheses of, 264-270
    adaptive models, 269
    conditional feedback and servo assistance, 265-266
    follow-up servo hypothesis, 264-265
    salient features of available sensors, 264

PART 1: pages 1-733; PART 2: pages 735-1480

Motor control (*continued*)
    spindle receptors as model-reference error detectors, 265
    stiffness regulation, 266–268
    summary model, 268–269
    β-system and possibility for zero sensitivity, 266
  motor unit recruitment, 386–394
    evidence regarding alternative patterns of recruitment, 452–457
    in humans, 448–452
    possibility of major shifts in recruitment order, 391–394
    precision and stereotypy in recruitment process, 390–391
    recruitment patterns and motor unit types, 386–390
  neural control of muscle length and tension, 257–323
    decerebrate preparation for study of, 282–283
    simplified animal models for study of, 282–283
    spinal preparation for study of, 283
  prefrontal cortex in, 1149–1178
    electrical correlates of performance, 1161–1164
    frontal eye fields and oculomotor control, 1160–1161
    inhibition from orbital prefrontal cortex, 1160
    inputs and outputs electrically traced, 1159–1160
    lesion studies of, 1154–1159
  single-movement control of limbs, 1392–1400
    Fitts' law, 1392–1393
    theoretical interpretations of, 1393–1399
  spinal neuronal circuits used in common by segmental afferents and supraspinal motor centers, 512–560
    pathways from Ia-afferents and their control by γ-motoneurons, 519–530
    presynaptic inhibition of transmission from primary afferents, 554–560
    propriospinal neurons, 549–554
    recurrent inhibition, 513–519
    reflex pathways from cutaneous and joint afferents and from groups II and III muscle afferents, 535–549
    reflex pathways from group Ib tendon organ afferents, 530–535
  spinal neuronal systems, integration in, 509–595
    ascending pathways that monitor segmental interneuronal activity, 569–576
    direct projections of descending pathways to α-motoneurons, 567–569
    methodological considerations, 510–512
    reticulospinal inhibition of segmental reflex transmission, 560–567
  static regulatory characteristics in intact subjects, 290–297
    effect of instructional set, 294–296
    equivalent stiffness and concept of composite motor servos, 293–294
    gain variation vs. gain control, 296–297
    skeletal mechanics and coordinate systems, 291
    steady-state responses to changes in load force, 291–292
    torque-angle relations, 292–293
  visuomotor coordination in frog and toad, 1453–1458
    maps as control surfaces, 1453–1454
    model of frog snapping, 1454–1457
    the many visual systems, 1457

Motor cortex
  see also Sensorimotor cortex
  afferent inputs to, 718–727
    general problems, 718
    inputs from nucleus ventralis lateralis of thalamus, 718–720
    inputs from sensory cortex, 726–727
    inputs through association cortex, 727
    inputs through association fibers, 726–727
    inputs through commissural fibers, 727
    peripheral inputs, 720–726
  arrangement of cells in, 1064–1071
    basal dendrites of pyramidal cells, 1071
    complex local interactions affecting output cells, 1069–1071
    dynamic input-output relations for individual output elements, 1071
    input of thalamic afferents to cortex, 1065–1068
    output cells with separate axonal destinations, 1069
    stratification of output elements, 1068–1069
  cytoarchitectonic maps and terminology of, 1123–1124
  electrical stimulation eliciting movement in anesthetized animals, effects of electrical stimulation of basal ganglia on, 1031–1032
  input of thalamic afferents to, 1065–1068
    collaterals of pyramidal cells, 1068
    corticocortical afferents, 1067
    excitatory interneurons, 1067–1068
    inhibitory interneurons, 1067
  internal organization for input-output arrangements, 1063–1081
    arrangement of cells in motor cortex, 1064–1071
    contributions of different output elements to response produced by electrical stimulation, 1072–1073
    cortical distribution of output elements, 1071–1072
    electrical stimulation studies, 1071–1073
    influences of natural activation of peripheral receptors, 1073–1077
    modification of cortical responses to peripheral stimuli, 1078
    pathways for afferent projections, 1078
  motor systems of, transmitters in, 138–142
    cortical inhibitory mechanisms, 141–142
    other transmitters in cortex, 142
    pyramidal tract neurons, 138–141
  role in voluntary movements in primates, 1083–1120
    historical considerations, 1083–1084

Motor units
  anatomy of, 367–372
    innervation ratios and muscle unit "size," 369–372
    regionalization within a muscle, 368–369
  anatomy, physiology, and functional organization of, 345–422
  control of muscular action, 385–402
    evidence regarding alternative patterns of recruitment, 452–457
    evidence regarding voluntary selective control of motor units, 457–458
    motor unit recruitment, 386–394
    motor unit recruitment and minimum energy principle, 498
    motor unit recruitment in humans, 448–452
    output modulation by rate and pattern of motoneuron firing, 394–402
    recruitment or rate and pattern modulation? 402
  firing patterns of, 435–460
  force developed in relation to motoneuron size, 496–497
  motor nuclei, anatomy of, 372–377
    numbers of motoneurons and motor units, 376–377
  Sherrington's notion of, 345–346
  types of, 346–367
    alterations of demand within physiological range, 362–363
    developmental considerations, 364–365
    in human muscle, 359–361
    motoneuron anatomy in relation to, 377–378
    nonphysiological alterations, 363–364
    skeletofusimotor units, 365–366
    stability of, 361–364
  types, physiological profiles in experimental animals, 351–359
    fatigability and metabolic profiles, 358–359
    methodology, 352–353
    motor unit population of cat medial gastrocnemius muscle, 353–354
    physiological and histochemical profiles of units, 354–355
    twitch-contraction times and myofibrillary ATPase, 355–358
  types, physiology of α-motoneurons and their synaptic inputs in relation to, 378–385

Motor units (*continued*)
  electrophysiological properties intrinsic to motoneurons, 379–381
  group Ia synaptic efficacy, 381–382
  interactive factors in control of motoneuron excitability, 383–385
  monosynaptic supraspinal inputs, 382
  organization of synaptic input, 381–383
  polysynaptic input systems, 382–383
Movement
  see also Eye movements; Locomotion; Motor activity
  basic kinematics, 17–19
  behavioral analysis of, 1391–1414
  causing discharge of neurons in supplementary motor area in monkeys, 1134–1135
  cerebellar control of, 877–946
    analysis of α- and γ-motoneurons in, 910–912
    aspects of control, 882–912, 936–937
    ballistic movements, 883–887, 895–897
    cellular roles, 912–936
    classification of movements, 883–887
    comment on strategy and tactics, 901–904
    compound movements, 887, 892–895
    discharge properties, 912–918
    firing frequencies, 914–915
    frame of reference in understanding control, 887–891
    α-motoneurons, γ-motoneurons, and interneurons as output targets, 928–931
    motor programs and cerebellar circuit, 888–889
    movement initiation, 897–899
    muscle tone and force in, 909–912
    mystery of climbing fiber and theory of adaptive motor control, 931–934
    ongoing control of simple movements, 899–901
    parameters of movement, 926–928
    rapid vs. slow movements and reciprocal contraction vs. cocontraction, 925–926
    relation of cerebellar nuclear activity to sequencing of movements and to postural holds, 920–925
    relation of discharge to behavioral events, 918–936
    role of climbing fibers, 918
    role of individual cells within cerebellar circuit, 938
    role of mossy fibers, 916–918
    role of Purkinje cell, 915–916
    self-terminated simple movements, 897
    servo control of movement examined by perturbations, 904–906
    simple movements, 883–887, 895–908
    speed and accuracy in, 887–888
    termination of simple movements, 906–908
    topographic relation between body parts and cerebellum, 919–920
  complex motor patterns, representation of, 1400–1413
    constraints on coordination, 1409–1413
    human evidence for a program concept, 1401–1409
  continuous pursuit movements in Parkinson's disease, 1044
  control of, limitations of somatosensory feedback in, 229–256
  dynamics of skeleton, 30–33
  effect of bilateral pyramidotomy in monkeys on, 645–647
  elicited by cortical stimulation in anesthetized animals, effects of electrical stimulation of basal ganglia on, 1031–1032
  elicited by electrical stimulation of parietal association cortex, 1140–1141
  eye-head coordination, 1321–1336
  kinematics of joints, 19–26
    muscle attachments, 24–26
    number of muscles required to work joints, 23–24
  mandibular movements, initiation and control of, 1260–1267
    peripheral systems and voluntary isometric jaw muscle contraction, 1263–1265

role of sensorimotor cortex in mastication and voluntary jaw movements, 1260–1263
    trigeminal relationships in cerebellum, 1265–1267
  mechanics of skeleton and tendons, 17–42
  motor commands and their perceptual consequences, 1415–1447
    corollaries of motor commands to limb and trunk muscles, 1421–1433
    corollary discharges and eye movements, 1433–1440
    corollary discharges and somatosensory afferents, 1428
    electrophysiological correlates of motor commands, 1440–1441
    historical development, 1416–1420
    interactions between corollary discharges and kinesthetic afferent inputs, 1425–1428
    other instances of central irradiation by motor commands, 1441–1442
    sensations of movement, 1422–1425
    sensations of muscular force or heaviness, 1428–1433
    terminology, 1420–1421
  movement commands, implementation of, 308–316
    analytical approaches to actions of α-, β-, and γ-motoneurons, 310–311
    compliance, load compensation, and biological design, 315–316
    equilibrium point control, 311–313
    β-innervation of muscle spindles, 310
    perturbations during movement, 314–315
    positional stiffness deduced from spindle relations, 309–310
    α-γ-relations, 308–309
    stiffness regulation vs. stiffness control, 313–314
  precomputed movements, control and reflex mechanisms in, 251–252
  rhythmic jaw movements evoked in reduced or anesthetized animals, 1256–1257
  single-cell studies in basal ganglia during, 1033–1041
    relation to delayed response task, 1041
    relation to feeding behavior, 1040
    relations to parameters of movement, 1037–1038
    responses to peripheral stimuli, 1040
    somatotopic organization, 1035–1037
    spontaneous activity, 1033–1034
    temporal relation to movement, 1034–1035
    vestibular and postural mechanisms, 1038–1040
  single-movement control of limbs, 1392–1400
    Fitts' law, 1392–1393
    theoretical interpretations of, 1393–1399
  sinusoidal movements of limbs, negative stiffness and spontaneous oscillations, 240–246
    comparison of stretch reflex with man-made control system, 244–245
    factors affecting stability of stretch reflexes, 242
    level of muscle activation, 242–243
    nature of external load, 242
    resistance to movements of different amplitudes, 243–244
    stability and gain in stretch reflex, 245–246
    stability of man-made system, 245
  sinusoidal movements of limbs, reflex responses or precomputed motor activity, 246–250
    response to sudden disturbance, 246–247
    triggered responses to disturbance, 249–250
    tuning of neuromuscular system, 247–249
  sinusoidal movements, servo-control mechanisms in limb response to, 234–240
    effects of limb mass, 236
    muscles as low-pass filters, 238–239
    reflex delay, 239–240
    resistance of muscles to movement, 236–237
    timing of muscle spindle afferent activity, 239
    timing of reflex force, 239
    two components of muscle force, 237–238
  speed of movement in Parkinson's disease, 1043–1044
  stresses and strains in tendons, 35–36

PART 1: pages 1–733; PART 2: pages 735–1480

Movement (*continued*)
  trunk movements during locomotion, 1190–1193
    dorsoventral movements of spine in gallop and leaping, 1192–1193
    in fishes, 1190–1191
    lateral trunk movements in alternating gaits, 1191–1192
    torsion around longitudinal axis in walking humans, 1193
  voluntary movements in primates, role of motor cortex in, 1083–1120
    centrally programmed movement, 1103–1110
    coding of output of precentral motor cortex in relation to parameters of movement, 1086–1089
    contrasts between precentral motor cortex and sensorimotor cortex in relation to voluntary movement, 1110–1112
    corollary discharge and efference copy in sensorimotor cortex, 1112
    foci for afferent submodalities, 1097–1098
    functional analogies between segmental and suprasegmental reflexes in, 1101–1102
    historical considerations, 1083–1084
    parallels between servo responses in humans and subhuman primates, 1098–1101
    precision, fractionation, and dynamic range of motor control, 1112–1114
    reflexes of precentral motor cortex in course of volitional movements, 1095–1097
    responses of precentral motor cortex neurons to afferent input, 1089–1091
    topography of cortex and spatial distribution of its functional components in relation to generation of different movements, 1114–1116
    transcortical reflexes in, 1093–1103
  voluntary movements, servo assistance of, 250–251
Movement disorders
  akinesia and hyperactivity, role of basal ganglia in, 1045–1046
  dyskinesias and stereotyped behavior, role of basal ganglia in, 1046–1047
  produced by lesions of prefrontal cortex, 1154–1155
  rigidity, role of basal ganglia in, 1047–1048
Muscle contraction
  changes induced by electrically induced exercise, 174–175
  differences in contractility of intrafusal muscle fibers, 208–209
  gradation of tension, how this sensitivity is achieved, 494–496
  grading of tension, actual sensitivity in, 497
  multiple units of muscle, 79–83
    relationships in multiunit function, 81–83
    unit of muscle function, 79–81
  properties of contractile unit, 55–79
    functional variations, 72–79
    interaction between neural and other inputs, 62–72
    passive mechanical contributions, 55–56
    response to neural signals, 56–62
  some measures of muscle function, 83–87
  twitch-contraction times and myofibrillar ATPase in animal motor units, 355–358
  voluntary isometric jaw muscle contraction in control of mandibular movements, 1263–1265
Muscle spindles: *see* Neuromuscular spindles
Muscles
  see also Neuromuscular junction; Neuromuscular spindles; Oculomotor muscles; Tendons
  alterations induced by electrical activation, 174–179
    changes in contractile properties, 174–175
    fatigue resistance, 176–177
    force modulation, 177–179
    metabolic changes, 175–176
    reversibility of changes, 177
    time course of changes, 176
  as low-pass filters in servo-control mechanism of response to sinusoidal stretching, 238–239

  as producer of motor function, 43–106
    some measures of motor function, 83–87
    units for measure of, 88–94
  attachments to bones, 24–26
  dynamic responses of motor servo to mechanical disturbances, 297–308
    amplitude dependence and linearity, 299–301
    asymmetry of motor servo response, 301–302
    compensation for yielding, 302–304
    dependence of transient responses on initial force, 298–299
    dynamic features of force development, 297–298
    predictive compensation, feedforward vs. nonlinear feedback viewpoints, 304
    velocity dependence and damping, 306–307
    vibration and stretch reflex, 304–306
  fiber types, histochemical profiles and ultrastructural correlations, 347–351
    anatomy and ultrastructure, 350
    neuromuscular junction specializations, 350–351
  fibers and motor units, significance of nonuniformity of, 487
  fibers in relation to properties of motoneurons which supply them, 433–434
  fibrillary ATPase in animal motor units in relation to twitch-contraction times, 355–358
  functional electrical stimulation of, 172–179
    in treatment of scoliosis, 182–184
  functionally isolated muscles, tonic stretch reflex in, 283–290
    actions of control signals on motor servo, 286–287
    basic features of reflex, 283–284
    dependence of incremental stiffness on initial force, 287–288
    loop gain or force feedback, 288–289
    mechanically and neurally mediated components, 285–286
    normalized stiffness, 285
    static force-length relations, 284–285
  influence on developing and mature motoneurons that innervate them, 489–490
  intrafusal muscle fibers, properties of, 208–210
    creep, 209
    differences in contractility, 208–209
    membrane potentials, 209–210
  length and tension of, neural control of, 257–323
    central pathways for, 276–282
    dynamic responses to mechanical disturbances, 297–308
    hypotheses of motor servo function, 264–270
    implementation of movement commands, 308–316
    muscular mechanical stiffness, 270–276
    simplified animal models for study of, 282–283
    static regulatory characteristics in intact subjects, 290–297
    tonic stretch reflex in functionally isolated muscles, 283–290
  level of activation in limb response to sinusoidal movements, 242–243
  medial gastrocnemius of cat, motor unit population of, 353–354
  moment arms and pennation patterns, 26–27
  movement commands, implementation of, 308–316
    analytical approaches to actions of α-, β-, and γ-motoneurons, 310–311
    compliance, load compensation, and biological design, 315–316
    equilibrium point control, 311–313
    β-innervation of muscle spindles, 310
    perturbations during movement, 314–315
    positional stiffness deduced from spindle relations, 309–310
    α-γ-relations, 308–309
    stiffness regulation vs. stiffness control, 313–314
  multiple units of, 79–83
    relationships in multiunit function, 81–83
    unit of muscle function, 79–81
  normal muscles, electrical activation of, 173–174
    intramuscular electrode, 174
    nerve cuff electrode, 173–174
    surface electrode, 174

PART 1: pages 1–733; PART 2: pages 735–1480

Muscles (*continued*)
  number required to work joints, 23–24
  of mandible, 1238–1241
    anatomy, 1238–1240
    physiology and histochemistry, 1240–1241
  physiology of, brief review, 172–173
    motor-unit properties, 173
    muscle-fiber type, 172–173
  properties, representation of, 44–55
    dimensions used, 44–45
    models, 45–49
    real motor systems, 49–55
  regionalization of motor units within, 368–369
  resistance to sinusoidal movement, 236–237
  static regulatory characteristics in intact subjects, 290–297
    effect of instructional set, 294–296
    equivalent stiffness and concept of composite motor servos, 293–294
    gain variation vs. gain control, 296–297
    skeletal mechanics and coordinate systems, 291
    steady-state responses to changes in load force, 291–292
    torque-angle relations, 292–293
  stiffness of, 270–276
    instantaneous stiffness and short-range elasticity, 272–273
    instantaneous stiffness beyond short-range region, 274
    length dependence, 271
    natural combinations of recruitment and rate modulation, 276
    ramp responses, transient properties and nonlinearity, 274–276
    rate modulation of motor units, 272
    recruitment of motor units, 271–272
    regulation in hypothesis of motor servo function, 266–268
    stiffness definitions, 270–271
    stiffness regulation vs. stiffness control in implementation of movement commands, 313–314
  terminals of motoneurons in, 430–432
  tissue reaction to coiled wire electrodes used in functional electrical stimulation, 163–166
  tone and force, role in cerebellar control of movement, 909–912
  two components of muscle force in response to sinusoidal stretching, 237–238
Muscular diseases
  clinical evidence of nonuniformity of motoneurons in a pool, 490–491
Myoclonus
  review of, 331–332

Neck
  neck reflexes, 669–670
    central pathways for, 689
    interaction with vestibular reflexes, 670–671
Neostriatum: *see* Caudate nucleus; Putamen
Nerve endings
  see also Neural transmission; Receptors, neural
  groups III and IV free nerve endings, projections in neural control of muscle length and tension, 279
  primary ending projections in neural control of muscle length and tension, 276–277
  secondary endings and group II free nerve endings, projections in neural control of muscle length and tension, 278–279
Nerve fibers
  see also Axons
  excitation in functional electrical stimulation, 166–172
    effects of electrode configuration on threshold and excitation site, 170–171
    excitation of myelinated nerve, 168–169
    membrane response to applied electrical field, 166–168
    neural fatigue or loss of electrical excitability, 172
    threshold relationship between nerve and muscle, 169–170
Neural pathways
  see also Afferent pathways; Efferent pathways

central pathways for neck reflexes, 689
central pathways for vestibular reflexes, 671–689
  connections between labyrinthine and spinal motoneurons, 686–689
  pathways linking vestibular nuclei to spinal cord, 671
  reticulospinal tracts, 678–686
  vestibulospinal tracts, 672–678
central pathways for vestibuloocular reflex, 1287–1288
  neural integrator, 1288
  transforming cupula time constant, 1287–1288
central pathways for vestibulospinal reflexes, 693–695
  canal reflexes, 693–695
  otolith reflexes, 695
central pathways in neural control of muscle length and tension, 276–282
  clasp-knife reflex, 279–280
  long-loop reflexes, 280–282
  primary ending projections, 276–277
  projections from groups III and IV free nerve endngs, 279
  projections from secondary endings and group II free nerve endings, 278–279
  tendon organ projections, 277–278
descending pathways projecting monosynaptically to motoneurons, 483
Neural transmission
see also Neuroregulators
transmitters in motor systems, 107–154
Neuromuscular junction
  contractile unit response to neural signals, 56–62
    dynamic stimulus, 61–62
    repetitive stimulus, 59–61
    single stimulus, 57–59
  morphology of, 432–433
  specializations in relation to muscle fiber types, 350–351
Neuromuscular spindles
  fusimotor system, possible functional roles for, 211–222, 223–224
    assessment, 219–222
    central regulation of spindle sensitivity or parameter control, 212–217
    fusimotor biasing and suggested role as servo input, 217–219
    maintenance of sensitivity, 211–212
  groups II and III muscle afferents, reflex pathways from cutaneous and joint afferents and from, 535–549
  β-innervation of, in implementation of movement commands, 310
  jaw muscle spindle afferents, effects of their destruction on mastication, 1253–1254
  motor supply to, 200–211
    delimitation of static and dynamic fusimotor axons, 200–203, 223
    intrafusal destination of static and dynamic axons, 203–208, 223
    γ-motor axons, 200
    β- or skeletofusimotor axons, 210–211
    properties of intrafusal muscle fibers, 208–210
  primary and secondary spindle afferent endings, functional properties of, 193–200
    amplitude nonlinearity, 196–197
    assessment, 199
    different responses to various stimuli, 193–196
    linear responses to sinusoidal stretching, 197–199
    mode of summation of signal components, 196
    possible intermediate endings, 199–200
  primary endings of Ia-afferents and their control by γ-motoneurons, 519–530
  secondary endings in, group II input from, 479–480
  spindle afferent activity in limb response to sinusoidal movements, timing of, 239
  spindle receptors as model-reference error detectors in motor servo system, 265

PART 1: pages 1–733; PART 2: pages 735–1480

Neuromuscular spindles (*continued*)
   structure of, 191–193, 222
      classic view, 191
      recognition of motor duality, 191–192
      subdivision of nuclear-bag fibers, 192–193
   study in early research on motor control, 6
   their messages and their fusimotor supply, 189–228
Neurons
   see also Axons; Dendrites; Interneurons; Motoneurons; Nerve fibers; Purkinje cells; Synapses
   certain spinal, cerebellar, and brain stem neurons, activity during locomotion, 1203–1207
   monoaminergic neurons of brain stem, anatomy of, 610–611
   of cerebellum, responses to exteroceptive and proprioceptive stimuli, 786–795
      responses of neurons in cerebellar cortex, 786–792
      responses of neurons in deep cerebellar nuclei, 792–795
      responses of neurons in intracerebellar nuclei to activation of descending pathways, 794–795
      responses of neurons in intracerebellar nuclei to peripheral stimuli, 793–794
      responses of neurons in lateral cerebellum to spinal inputs, 788–790
      responses of neurons in vermis and paravermis to spinal inputs, 786–788
      responses to activation of descending pathways, 791–792
      responses to trigeminal inputs, 790–791
   of cerebellum, responses to visual, auditory, and vestibular stimuli, 795–804
      responses to auditory stimuli, 797
      responses to vestibular stimuli, 797–804
      responses to visual stimuli, 795–797
   of corpus striatum, convergence of extrinsic inputs to, 1002–1003
   of descending pathways, light and electron microscopy of, 597–598
      identification of cells of origin of fiber systems by retrograde labeling, 600
      identification of neurons and tracing of their axons, 600–601
      tracing of axons and identification of their terminals by techniques of anterograde labeling, 598–600
   of inferior olive, long-term changes in excitability of, 862–863
   of inferior olive, peripheral inputs to, 781
   of inferior olive, responses to depolarizing inputs, 779–781
   of precentral motor cortex, responses to afferent input, 1089–1091
   of prefrontal cortex, unit discharge during delayed-response and delayed-alternation tasks, 1162–1164
   of premotor cortex, single-unit recordings in conscious monkeys, 1128
   of pyramidal tract, afferent inputs to, 718–727
   of pyramidal tract, input from peripheral receptors to, 1077
   of pyramidal tract, transmitters in, 138–141
   of reticulospinal tract, inputs to, 679–683
      cerebellar inputs, 681–683
      somatosensory inputs, 680–681
      vestibular inputs, 679–680
   of supplementary motor area, movement-associated discharge of, 1134–1135
   Purkinje cell target neurons, cerebellar nuclei, and Deiters' nucleus, 857–859
   spinal neuronal circuits used in common by segmental afferents and supraspinal motor centers, 512–560
      pathways from Ia-afferents and their control by γ-motoneurons, 519–530
      presynaptic inhibition of transmission from primary afferents, 554–560
      propriospinal neurons, 549–554
      recurrent inhibition, 513–519
      reflex pathways from cutaneous and joint afferents and from groups II and III muscle afferents, 535–549
      reflex pathways from group Ib tendon organ afferents, 530–535
   spinal neuronal systems, integration in, 509–595
      ascending pathways that monitor segmental interneuronal activity, 569–576
      direct projections of descending pathways to α-motoneurons, 567–569
      methodological considerations, 510–512
      reticulospinal inhibition of segmental reflex transmission, 560–567
   striatal projection neurons, 1006–1009
Neuroregulators
   see also Neural transmission
   chemical transmitters in motor systems, 108–115
      definition of, 108
      hormones, 109–110
      identification of transmitters, 111–115
      intercellular communication, 109–111
      intracellular mediators, 108–109
      neuromodulators, 110–111
      synaptic transmitters, 110
      varieties of transmitters, 108–111
   spinal motoneurons and their synaptic control, 115–127
      inhibitory inputs on motoneurons, 120–122
      monosynaptic reflex, 115–119
      other excitatory inputs on motoneurons, 119–120
      other relevant spinal mechanisms, 123–127
      presynaptic inhibition, 122–123
   transmitters in basal ganglia, 134–138
      nigrostriatal pathway, 134–135
      other striatal afferents, 135
      other striatal efferent pathways, 137
      pallidosubthalamic projection, 137
      striatal interneurons, 137–138
      striatonigral pathways, 135–137
      transmitters in various striatal pathways, 134
   transmitters in brain stem, 127–130
      cranial motoneurons, 127
      red nucleus, 127–128
      reticulospinal cells, 128
      vestibulospinal cells, 128–130
   transmitters in cerebellum, 130–134
      cerebellar inhibitory interneurons, 131–132
      cerebellar inputs, 132–134
      excitatory interneurons, 132
      Purkinje cells, 130–131
   transmitters in motor cortex, 138–142
      cortical inhibitory mechanisms, 141–142
      other transmitters in cortex, 142
      pyramidal tract neurons, 138–141
   transmitters in motor systems, 107–154
   transmitters in peripheral motor systems, 115
   transmitters in spinal motor mechanisms, 115–127
   transmitters in supraspinal motor systems, 127–142
Neurotransmitters: *see* Neuroregulators
Norepinephrine
   noradrenergic afferent projections to cerebellum, 783–785
Nystagmus
   optokinetic, properties of, 1293–1295

Oculomotor muscles
   see also Eye movements
   mechanics of, 1283–1284
      dynamics, 1284
      statics, 1283–1284
   muscle fiber types in relation to eye movements, 1282
   stretch afferents in, 1282–1283
Olive, inferior
   afferent projections to, 765–771
      afferent fibers from spinal cord, 765–768

PART 1: pages 1–733; PART 2: pages 735–1480

Olive, inferior (*continued*)
    aminergic projections, 769
    cortico-olivary fibers, 770
    dorsal column nuclei projections, 768
    mesencephalo olivary projection, 769–770
    other caudal brain stem projections, 768
    other descending projections to olive, 770
    pretectal projections, 769
    projections from cerebellar nuclei to olive, 768–769
    projections from superior colliculus, 769
  electrophysiology of, 779–783, 859–863
    electrotonic coupling, 863
    inferior olivary cell as single-cell oscillator, 862
    intracellular recording from cells in vivo and in vitro, 861–862
    ionic mechanisms in spike generation, 862
    long-term changes in inferior olive neuronal excitability, 862–863
    peripheral inputs to olivary neurons, 781
    proposed function of, 781–783
    responses of olivary neurons, 779–781
  olivocerebellar projection, 771–779
    olivocerebellar topography, 772–778
    origin and course of olivocerebellar fibers, 771–772
    sagittal organization of cerebellum, 778–779
  structure and ultrastructure of, 764–765
Optic tectum
  nigrotectal efferent fibers, 973–975, 1011–1012
  pretectal projections to inferior olive, 769
Otoliths: *see* Labyrinth

Paleostriatum: *see* Globus pallidus
Paralysis
  see also Hemiplegia; Respiratory paralysis
  clinical application of functional electrical stimulation in, 179–182
Parietal lobe
  see also Somatosensory cortex
  parietal association cortex viewed as motor area, 1140–1143
    command functions of parietal lobe, 1141–1143
    parietal lesions and electrical stimulation, 1140–1141
    structural relationships with motor areas, 1141
Parkinson's disease
  continuous pursuit movements in, 1044
  other aspects of motor performance, in 1044
  reaction time in, 1043
  resting tremor in, pathophysiological basis of, 1048
  rigidity in, pathophysiological basis of, 1047–1048
  speed of movement in, 1043–1044
  tremor in, mechanism of, 331, 336–337, 339–340
Perception
  see also Visual perception
  perceptual influences of corollary discharges arising from motor commands, 1415–1447
    corollaries of motor commands to limb and trunk muscles, 1421–1433
    corollary discharges and eye movements, 1433–1440
    corollary discharges and somatosensory afferents, 1428
    electrophysiological correlates of motor commands, 1440–1441
    historical development, 1416–1420
    interactions between corollary discharges and kinesthetic afferent inputs, 1425–1428
    other instances of central irradiation by motor commands, 1441–1442
    sensations of movement, 1422–1425
    sensations of muscular force or heaviness, 1428–1433
    terminology, 1420–1421
  perceptual structures and distributed motor control, 1449–1480
    concepts from computer science and control theory, 1452–1453
    coordinated control programs, 1465–1471
    motor schemas, 1463–1465
    optic flow and control of movement, 1461–1463
    perceptual schemas and the action-perception cycle, 1458–1461
    perspective of artificial intelligence, 1471–1477
    place of brain theory within cybernetics, 1450–1451
Peripheral nerve diseases
  causing disturbances in gait, 1193
Peripheral nerves
  see also Nerve endings
  in generation of basic locomotor synergy, 1194–1196
  peripheral motor systems, transmitters in, 115
  tissue reaction to cuff electrodes used in functional electrical stimulation, 163
Phylogeny
  of cerebellar networks and circuits, 831–832
  of climbing fiber activation of Purkinje cells, 847–848
  of field potentials evoked by surface stimulation of cerebellar cortex, 835–838
  of inhibitory interneuronal systems in cerebellar cortex, 855–857
  of Purkinje cell spontaneous firing, 845
Pons
  Deiters' nucleus in relation to Purkinje cell target neurons and cerebellar nuclei, 857–859
  pontine locomotor region, 1210–1213
  pontocerebellar afferent system, 750–754
    inputs to pontine nuclei, 751–753
    organization of pontocerebellar projection, 750–751
Postsynaptic potentials
  EPSPs elicited by impulses in single afferent fibers, amplitudes of, 465–468
  EPSPs elicited by impulses in single afferent fibers, latency of, 477–478
  EPSPs elicited by impulses in single afferent fibers, techniques for study of, 464–465
Posture
  cerebellar control of, 877–946
    aspects of control, 882–912
    compound movements, 887, 892–908
    simple movements, 883–887, 895–908
  control of, limitations of somatosensory feedback in, 229–256
  postural and vestibular mechanisms, possible association of basal ganglia with, 1038–1040
  postural tremor, 328–329
Precentral motor cortex: *see* Sensorimotor cortex
Prefrontal cortex
  anatomy of, 1149–1154
    connections, 1151–1153
    developmental and comparative anatomy, 1149–1151
  electrophysiology of, 1159–1165
    electrical correlates of performance, 1161–1164
    frontal eye fields and oculomotor control, 1160–1161
    inhibition from orbital prefrontal cortex, 1160
    inputs and outputs electrically traced, 1159–1160
    slow potentials, 1161–1162
    unit activity during delayed-response and delayed-alternation task performance, 1162–1164
  function in organization of behavior, 1165–1168
  in motor control, 1149–1178
  lesion studies of, 1154–1159
    ablations producing difficulties in discrimination task performance, 1155
    ablations producing hyperactivity, 1154–1155
    emotional behavior changes, 1158–1159
    producing difficulties in performance of delay tasks, 1155–1158
    suggestion of anticipatory function of prefrontal cortex, 1166–1167
  provisional memory function of, 1166
Premotor area: *see* Cerebral cortex

Purkinje cells
  electrophysiology of, 841–845
    climbing fiber activation of Purkinje cells, comparative aspects, 847–848
    comparative aspects of Purkinje cell spontaneous firing, 845
    extracellular action potentials, 842
    integrative properties of Purkinje cells, 845
    intracellular studies, 842
    ionic basis of Purkinje cell action potentials, 842–844
    mossy fiber inputs and parallel fiber action on Purkinje cells, 852
    spontaneous activity, 842
  output in cerebellar motor systems, 130–131
  Purkinje cell target neurons, cerebellar nuclei, and Deiters' nucleus, 857–859
  role in cerebellar function, 915–916
Putamen
  anatomy of, 949
  cytology of, 949–950
Pyramidal cells
  basal dendrites of pyramidal cells of motor cortex, 1071
  collaterals of pyramidal cells of motor cortex, role in input-output arrangements, 1068
Pyramidal tracts
  bilateral pyramidotomy in monkeys, effect on movement, 645–647
  function of, 727–729
  neurons of, afferent inputs to, 718–727
  neurons of, input from peripheral receptors to, 1077
  neurons of, transmitters in, 138–141
  projection from cerebral cortex to spinal cord, organization of, 703–718
    microstructure of corticospinal projection, 712–715
    projection to γ-motoneurons, 715–716
    projections to spinal interneurons, 716–717
    pyramidal collaterals and branches within brain, 717–718
    studies by cortical depth stimulation, 707–712
    studies by cortical surface stimulation, 703–707

Reaction time
  for multiple choices in manual task performance, 1364–1366
  for voluntary corrections of errors in limb movement, 1358–1364
    additional artifacts in measuring reaction times to steps, 1363–1364
    advance correction of direction, 1361
    corrected anticipatory response, 1361–1362
    deliberate and automatic corrections, 1358–1359
    difficulties of interpretation, 1362–1363
    kinesthetic reaction time, 1359–1360
    reaction time for correction in tracking steps, 1360–1361
    visual correction of quick movements, 1360
  in Parkinson's disease, 1043
Receptors, neural
  group Ib tendon organ afferents, reflex pathways from, 530–535
  low-threshold mechanoreceptors, possible contribution to load regulation during chewing, 1255–1256
  oral mechanoreceptors, excitatory effects on jaw-closing muscles in chewing, 1251
  tendon organ projections in neural control of muscle length and tension, 277–278
  tendon organs, 190–191
Recruitment
  of motor units, 386–394
    evidence regarding alternative patterns of recruitment, 452–457
    in humans, 448–452
    possibility of major shifts in recruitment order, 391–394
    precision and stereotypy in recruitment process, 390–391
    recruitment order and minimum energy principle, 498
    recruitment patterns and motor unit types, 386–390
    vs. rate and pattern modulation in control of muscular action, 402
Red nucleus
  afferent fiber systems of, 983–985
    cerebellorubral projections, 984–985
    corticorubral fibers, 983–984
  anatomy of, 979–986
  cytology of, 980–983
  efferent projections of, 985–986
    rubrobulbar projections, 985–986
    rubrocerebellar fibers, 986
    rubrospinal fibers, 985
  transmitters in supraspinal motor systems, 127–128
Reflex
  see also Stretch reflex; Vestibuloocular reflex
  adaptation of step during locomotion, 1225–1226
  certain reflex pathways, activity during locomotion, 1203–1207
  clasp-knife reflex in central pathways of control of muscle length and tension, 279–280
  control and precomputed movements, 251–252
  in origin of basic ideas on motor control, 3–4
  jaw reflexes, evidence concerning their contribution to mastication, 1253–1256
    activity patterns of mesencephalic V afferents during mastication, 1254–1255
    effects of destruction of jaw muscle spindle afferents, 1253–1254
    possible contribution of low-threshold mechanoreceptors to load regulation during chewing, 1255–1256
  long-loop reflexes in central pathways of control of muscle length and tension, 280–282
  monosynaptic reflex mediated by spinal motoneurons, 115–119
  neck reflexes, 669–670
    central pathways for, 689
  otolith reflex, 668–669, 693, 1288
  reflex control of basic locomotor synergy, 1199–1203
    feedback on fish central pattern generator, 1202–1203
    influence of hip position and movement, 1200–1202
    load sensitivity, 1200
  reflex delay in limb response to sinusoidal movements, 239–240
  reflex force in limb response to sinusoidal movements, timing of, 239
  reflex oscillations in mechanism of tremor, 334–337
    gain, 334–335
    interaction of mechanisms, 335–336
    latency, 335
    resetting, 336–337
    stability, 335
  reflexes of precentral motor cortex in course of volitional movements, 1095–1097
  reflexes possibly involved in chewing, 1247–1253
    excitatory effects from oral mechanoreceptors, 1251
    jaw-opening reflex, 1248–1251
    jaw-stretch reflex, 1247–1248
    modulation of trigeminal reflexes by primary afferent depolarization, 1251–1253
  segmental and suprasegmental reflexes in motor cortex role in voluntary movements in primates, 1101–1102
  spinal neuronal circuits used in common by segmental afferents and supraspinal motor centers, 512–560
    pathways from Ia-afferents and their control by γ-motoneurons, 519–530
    presynaptic inhibition of transmission from primary afferents, 554–560
    propriospinal neurons, 549–554
    recurrent inhibition, 513–519
    reflex pathways from cutaneous and joint afferents and from groups II and III muscle afferents, 535–549

PART 1: pages 1–733; PART 2: pages 735–1480

Reflex (continued)
  reflex pathways from group Ib tendon organ afferents, 530–535
  spinal neuronal systems, integration in, 509–595
    ascending pathways that monitor segmental interneuronal activity, 569–576
    direct projections of descending pathways to α-motoneurons, 567–569
    methodological considerations, 510–512
    reticulospinal inhibition of segmental reflex transmission, 560–567
  transcortical reflexes and role of motor cortex in voluntary movements in primates, 1093–1103
  transcortical reflexes, possible implication of neurons of supplementary motor area in, 1135
  vestibular and neck reflexes, interaction of, 670–671
  vestibular reflexes, 667–669
    central pathways for, 671–689
    otolith reflexes, 668–669
    semicircular canal reflexes, 667–668
  vestibulospinal reflexes, functional studies of, 689–697
    central pathways for vestibulospinal reflexes, 693–695
    cerebellum and vestibulospinal reflexes, 696–697
    otolith reflexes, 693
    semicircular canal reflexes, 690–693
    vestibulospinal reflexes and γ-loop, 695–696
Renshaw cells
  in recurrent inhibition of spinal neuronal circuits, 513–519
  providing inhibitory input to α-motoneurons, 482
Respiratory paralysis
  clinical application of functional electrical stimulation in, 182
Reticular formation
  reticulocerebellar afferent projections, 754–761
    lateral reticular nucleus, 755–758
    nucleus reticularis tegmenti pontis, 758–760
    paramedian reticular nucleus, 754–755
    proposed functions of reticulocerebellar projections, 760–761
  reticulospinal inhibition of segmental reflex transmission, 560–567
    decerebrate preparation, 564–567
    dorsal reticulospinal system, 560–562
    monoaminergic reticulospinal pathways, 562–564
    ventral reticulospinal pathways, 562
  reticulospinal system, 667–702
  reticulospinal tracts, 678–686
    inputs to reticulospinal tract neurons, 679–683
    origin and destination of tracts, 678–679
    reticulospinal actions on spinal motoneurons, 683–685

Saccades: see Eye movements
Scoliosis
  clinical application of functional electrical stimulation in, 182–184
Semicircular canals
  in vestibuloocular reflex, 1285–1287
  semicircular canal reflexes, 667–668, 690–693
Sensorimotor cortex
  hierarchical organization within, 1091–1092
  precentral motor cortex in voluntary movements in primates, 1084–1116
    activity in relation to input and output, 1086–1093
    boundaries of, 1084–1085
    centrally programmed movement, 1103–1110
    coding of output in relation to parameters of movement, 1086–1089
    contrasts between precentral motor cortex and sensorimotor cortex in relation to voluntary movement, 1110–1112
    corollary discharge and efference copy in sensorimotor cortex, 1112

    foci for afferent submodalities, 1097–1098
    functional analogies between segmental and suprasegmental reflexes, 1101–1102
    parallels between servo responses in humans and subhuman primates, 1098–1101
    pathways transmitting central programs to precentral motor cortex, 1108–1110
    precision, fractionation, and dynamic range of motor control, 1112–1114
    responses of precentral motor cortex neurons to afferent input, 1089–1091
    reviews of, 1085–1086
    topography of cortex and spatial distribution of its functional components in relation to generation of different movements, 1114–1116
    transcortical reflexes, 1093–1103
  role in mastication and voluntary jaw movements, 1260–1263
Serotonin
  serotonergic afferent projections to cerebellum, 785
Servomechanisms: see Feedback
Skeleton
  see also Bone and bones
  dynamics of, 30–33
  mechanics and coordinate systems in motor servo functions of intact subjects, 291
  mechanics of, 17–42
  skeletal materials, properties of, 27–28
  statics of, 28–30
Skin
  cutaneous afferents, reflex pathways from groups II and III muscle afferents and from, 535–549
Sodium
  noninactivating Na-dependent plateau potentials in Purkinje cells, 844
Somatosensory cortex
  areas I and II, 1137–1140
    concept of corticofugal control of somatosensory transmission, 1139
    major features of, critical review of evidence for, 1137–1139
  inputs to motor cortex from, 726–727
Sound
  auditory stimuli and responses evoked in neurons of cerebellar cortex, 797
Spinal cord
  see also Pyramidal tracts
  afferent fibers projected to inferior olive, 765–768
  anatomy of, 601–607
    autonomic preganglionic motoneuronal cell groups, 603
    dorsal horn, 601
    intermediate zone, 603–607
    somatic motoneuronal cell groups, 601–603
  certain neuronal activity during locomotion, 1203–1207
  descending pathways projecting monosynaptically to motoneurons, 483
  direct corticospinal connections of supplementary motor area of cerebral cortex, 1130–1131
  direct spinocerebellar systems, 736–748
    dorsal spinocerebellar tract, 736–742
    forelimb afferent systems to cerebellum, 745–747
    other direct spinocerebellar projections, 747
    ventral spinocerebellar tract, 742–745
  dorsal column nuclei projections to olive, 768
  input to lateral cerebellum, neuronal responses to, 788–790
  inputs to vermis and paravermis, neuronal responses to, 786–788
  motoneuron pool, functional organization and its inputs, 423–507
    firing patterns of individual motoneurons and motor units, 435–460
    how size of motoneurons determines their susceptibility to discharge, 491–494

PART 1: pages 1–733; PART 2: pages 735–1480

Spinal cord (*continued*)
    morphological considerations, 424-435
    nonuniformity of motoneurons, 485-491
    organization of input to motoneuron pools, 460-485
    some principles underlying organization of motoneuron pools, 494-499
    motor mechanisms in anesthetized animals, effects of electrical stimulation of basal ganglia on, 1032
    neuronal circuits used in common by segmental afferents and supraspinal motor centers, 512-560
        pathways from Ia-afferents and their control by γ-motoneurons, 519-530
        presynaptic inhibition of transmission from primary afferents, 554-560
        propriospinal neurons, 549-554
        recurrent inhibition, 513-519
        reflex pathways from cutaneous and joint afferents and from groups II and III muscle afferents, 535-549
        reflex pathways from group Ib tendon organ afferents, 530-535
    projection from cerebral cortex via pyramidal tract, organization of, 703-718
        microstructure of corticospinal projection, 712-715
        projection to γ-motoneurons, 715-716
        projection to spinal interneurons, 716-717
        pyramidal collaterals and branches within brain, 717-718
        studies by cortical depth stimulation, 707-712
        studies by cortical surface stimulation, 703-707
    reticulospinal cells in supraspinal motor systems, 128
    reticulospinal tracts, 678-686
        inputs to reticulospinal tract neurons, 679-683
        origin and destination of tracts, 678-679
        reticulospinal actions on spinal motoneurons, 683-685
    rubrospinal efferent fibers, 985
    spinal centers in generation of locomotor movements, behavioral results, 1197-1199
    spinal motoneurons and their synaptic control, 115-127
        inhibitory inputs on motoneurons, 120-122
        monosynaptic reflex, 115-119
        other excitatory inputs on motoneurons, 119-120
        other relevant spinal mechanisms, 123-127
        presynaptic inhibition, 122-123
    spinal neuronal systems, integration in, 509-595
        ascending pathways that monitor segmental interneuronal activity, 569-576
        direct projections of descending pathways to α-motoneurons, 567-569
        methodological considerations, 510-512
        reticulospinal inhibition of segmental reflex transmission, 560-567
    spinal pattern generation in locomotion, central organization of, 1213-1216
        interlimb coordination, 1215-1216
        single-limb control, 1213-1215
    spinal preparation animals for study of neural control of muscle length and tension, 283
    vestibulospinal and reticulospinal systems, 667-702
    vestibulospinal cells in supraspinal motor systems, 128-130
    vestibulospinal reflexes, functional studies of, 689-697
        central pathways for vestibulospinal reflexes, 693-695
        cerebellum and vestibulospinal reflexes, 696-697
        otolith reflexes, 693
        semicircular canal reflexes, 690-693
        vestibulospinal reflexes and γ-loop, 695-696
    vestibulospinal tracts, 672-678
        inputs to vestibulospinal tract neurons, 673-676
        origin and destination of, 672-673
        pathways linking vestibular nuclei to spinal cord, 671
        synapses of vestibulospinal tract fibers with spinal neurons, 676-677

Spinal cord injuries
    clinical application of functional electrical stimulation in, 181-182

Spine
    dorsoventral movements during gallop and leaping in carnivores and ungulates, 1192-1193

Stereotaxic techniques
    advent in early research on motor control, 8-9

Stretch
    sinusoidal stretching of muscle, linear responses of primary and secondary spindle afferent endings to, 197-199
    stretch afferents in oculomotor muscles, 1282-1283

Stretch reflex
    comparison with man-made control system, 244-245
    dynamic responses of motor servo to, 304-306
    in functionally isolated muscles, 283-290
        actions of control signals on motor servo, 286-287
        basic features of reflex, 283-284
        dependence of incremental stiffness on initial force, 287-288
        loop gain or force feedback, 288-289
        mechanically and neurally mediated components, 285-286
        normalized stiffness, 285
        static force-length relations, 284-285
    reflex responses or precomputed motor activity, 246-250
        response to sudden disturbance, 246-247
        triggered responses to disturbance, 249-250
        tuning of neuromuscular system, 247-249
    stability and gain in, 245-246
    stability in limb response to sinusoidal movements, factors in, 242
    studies in early research on motor control, 9-10

Substantia nigra
    anatomy of, 970-975
    cytology of, 970-971
    lesions of, motor effects of, 1022-1024
        combined pallidal and nigral lesions, 1024
    nigral afferent fibers, 971-972
        other nigral afferent fibers, 972
        pallidonigral projections, 967-968, 972
        striatonigral pathways, transmitters in, 135-137
        strionigral fibers, 971-972
    nigral efferent fibers, 972-975, 1010-1012
        nigrostriatal fibers, 957-958
        nigrostriatal pathway, transmitters in, 134-135
        nigrostriatal projection, 999-1002, 1010
        nigrostriatal system, 999-1002
        nigrotectal fibers, 973-975
        nigrotectal projection, 1011-1012
        nigrothalamic fibers, 972-973
        nigrothalamic projection, 1010-1011

Subthalamic nucleus
    anatomy of, 975-979
    connections of, 976-979
    cytology of, 976
    lesions of, motor effects, of, 979, 1024-1025
    pallidal-subthalamic relations, 1019
    pallidosubthalamic projections, 137, 963, 1009-1010
    subthalamic locomotor region in initiation of locomotion, 1209-1210
    subthalamopallidal fibers, 962-963

Superior colliculus
    see also Optic tectum
    projections to inferior olive, 769

Supplementary motor area: *see* Cerebral cortex

Synapses
    see also Receptors, neural
    direct synaptic interconnections between spinal motoneurons, 429
    Ia-synapses on motoneurons, 462-464
    of vestibulospinal tract fibers with spinal neurons, 676-677

PART 1: pages 1-733; PART 2: pages 735-1480

Synapses (*continued*)
   synaptic control of spinal motoneurons, 115–127
      inhibitory inputs on motoneurons, 120–122
      monosynaptic reflex, 115–119
      other excitatory inputs on motoneurons, 119–120
      other relevant spinal mechanisms, 123–127
      presynaptic inhibition, 122–123
   synaptic inputs of α-motoneurons in relation to motor unit types, 378–385
      group Ia synaptic efficacy, 381–382
      monosynaptic supraspinal inputs, 382
      organization of synaptic input, 381–383
      polysynaptic input systems, 382–383
      synaptic efficacy in control of motoneuron excitability, 383–384
   synaptic transmitters in motor systems, 110

Task performance
   complex motor patterns, representation of, 1400–1413
      constraints on coordination, 1409–1413
      human evidence for a program concept, 1401–1409
   delay task performance, difficulties produced by prefrontal cortex lesions, 1155–1158
   delayed-response and delayed-alternation tasks, unit activity in prefrontal cortex during performance of, 1162–1164
   difficulties produced by ablations of prefrontal cortex, 1155
   manual control in humans, 1337–1389
      bias from transfer, 1343–1346
      comparison with tracking by eye, 1384–1385
      measures of error, 1346–1349
      nonvisual memory for single movements, 1350–1358
      prediction and preprogramming replace error correction in complex skills, 1380–1384
      preparation and time sharing, 1364–1379
      preprogramming and error correction, 1349–1350
      reaction time for correcting a limb movement, 1358–1364
   tracking by eye, 1384–1385
Tegmentum mesencephali: *see* Mesencephalon
Tendons
   Golgi tendon organs, group Ib input from, 482–483
   group Ib tendon organ afferents, reflex pathways from, 530–535
   mechanics of, 17–42
   properties of, 27–28
   stresses and strains in, 35–36
   tendon organ projections in neural control of muscle length and tension, 277–278
   tendon organs, 190–191
   vibration of, dynamic responses of motor servo to, 304–306
Thalamus
   see also Subthalamic nucleus
   nigrothalamic efferent fibers, 972–973, 1010–1011
   nucleus ventralis lateralis, inputs to motor cortex from, 718–720
   pallidothalamic projections, 963–967, 1009
   thalamic afferents, input to motor cortex, 1065–1068
      collaterals of pyramidal cells, 1068
      corticocortical afferents, 1067
      excitatory interneurons, 1067–1068
      inhibitory interneurons, 1067
   thalamic relay for input to motor cortex, 1078
   thalamocortical projections, 1019–1020
   thalamostriatal afferents, 998–999
   thalamostriatal fibers, 954–957
Time
   temporal relation between neuronal activity in basal ganglia and onset of movement, 1034–1035
   temporal synthesis of behavior affected by prefrontal cortex lesions, 1165–1168
   time course of changes in electrically activated muscles, 176
Tremor
   generation of, anatomic relationships in, 330–331
   mechanisms of, 332–340
      central oscillations, 338–340
      mechanical oscillations, 332–334
      reflex oscillations, 334–337
   resting tremor in Parkinson's disease, pathophysiological basis of, 1048
   review of, 325–343
   types of, 326–330
      intention tremor, 329–330
      pathological tremors, 327–330
      physiological tremor, 326–327
      postural tremor, 328–329
      resting tumor, 328
Trigeminal nucleus
   inputs to cerebellar cortex, neuronal responses to, 790–791
   trigeminocerebellar afferent projection, 749–750

Vestibular apparatus
   see also Semicircular canals
   optokinetic-vestibular cooperation, model of, 1295–1296
   stimulation and responses evoked in neurons of cerebellum, 797–804
      afferent projections from perihypoglossal nuclei, 802–803
   vestibular and postural mechanisms, possible association of basal ganglia with, 1038–1040
   vestibular inputs to neurons of reticulospinal tract, 679–680
   vestibular reflexes, 667–669
      central pathways for, 671–689
      interaction with neck reflexes, 670–671
      otolith reflexes, 668–669
      semicircular canal reflexes, 667–668
   vestibulocerebellar afferent projections, 748–749
      primary afferents, 748–749
      secondary fibers, 749
   vestibulospinal reflexes, functional studies of, 689–697
      central pathways for vestibulospinal reflexes, 693–695
      cerebellum and vestibulospinal reflexes, 696–697
      otolith reflexes, 693
      semicircular canal reflexes, 690–693
      vestibulospinal reflexes and γ-loop, 695–696
Vestibular nerve
   see also Vestibuloocular reflex
   vestibulospinal cells in supraspinal motor systems, 128–130
   vestibulospinal system, 667–702
   vestibulospinal tracts, 672–678
      inputs to vestibulospinal tract neurons, 673–676
      origin and destination of, 672–673
      synapses of vestibulospinal tract fibers with spinal neurons, 676–677
Vestibular nuclei
   pathways linking them to spinal cord, 671
Vestibuloocular reflex
   central pathways in, 1287–1288
      neural integrator, 1288
      transforming cupula time constant, 1287–1288
   description and function, 1276, 1284–1293
   neurophysiology of, 1288–1293
      cell types in brain stem, 1291–1292
      cerebellar connections, 1292–1293
      horizontal reflex signals, 1290–1291
      signal conversions, 1292
      spatial organization, 1288–1289
      vertical reflex signals, 1289–1290
   otolith reflex, 1288
   properties of, 1284–1285
      gain, 1285, 1309–1310
      high frequencies, 1284
      low frequencies, 1284–1285
   semicircular canals in, 1285–1287

Vibration
    tendon vibration, dynamic responses of motor servo to, 304–306
Vision
    visual stabilization as one purpose of eye movements, 1278
    visual stimuli and responses evoked in neurons of cerebellar cortex, 795–797
    visuomotor coordination in frog and toad, 1453–1458
        maps as control surfaces, 1453–1454
        model of frog snapping, 1454–1457
        the many visual systems, 1457
Visual perception
    corollary discharges in, 1435–1440